Prakash's

Notebook of Microbiology

Including Parasitology and Entomology

Third Edition

for Undergraduate Students and PG Aspirants

Prakash Modi
MD (Microbiology)

Professor and Head
Department of Microbiology
PDU Government Medical College
Rajkot 360001, Gujarat, India
E-mail: drprakash_md @yahoo.co.in

Ex-Assistant Professor and Ex-Associate Professor
Department of Microbiology
Shri M P Shah Government Medical College
Jamnagar 361001, Gujarat, India

Ex-Assistant Professor
Department of Microbiology
Government Medical College
Bhavnagar 364001, Gujarat, India

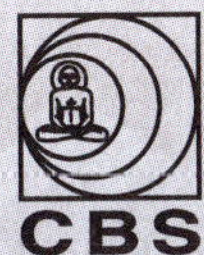

CBS Publishers & Distributors Pvt Ltd
New Delhi • Bengaluru • Chennai • Kochi • Kolkata • Mumbai
Bhopal • Bhubaneswar • Hyderabad • Jharkhand • Nagpur • Patna • Pune • Uttarakhand • Dhaka (Bangladesh) • Kathmandu (Nepal)

Disclaimer

Science and technology are constantly changing fields. New research and experience broaden the scope of information and knowledge. The author has tried his best in giving information available to them while preparing the material for this book. Although, all efforts have been made to ensure optimum accuracy of the material, yet it is quite possible some errors might have been left uncorrected. The publisher, the printer and the author will not be held responsible for any inadvertent errors, omissions or inaccuracies.

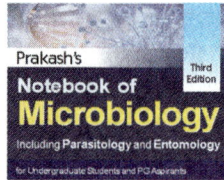

ISBN: 978-93-88725-60-6

Third Edition: 2020

First Edition: 2015
Second Edition: 2017

Published by Satish Kumar Jain and produced by Varun Jain for

CBS Publishers & Distributors Pvt Ltd
4819/XI Prahlad Street, 24 Ansari Road, Daryaganj, New Delhi 110 002
Ph: 011-23289259, 23266861, 23266867 Fax: 011-23243014 Website: www.cbspd.com
e-mail: delhi@cbspd.com; cbspubs@airtelmail.in

Corporate Office: 204 FIE, Industrial Area, Patparganj, Delhi 110 092
Ph: 011-49344934 Fax: 011-49344935 e-mail: publishing@cbspd.com; publicity@cbspd.com

Branches

- **Bengaluru:** Seema House 2975, 17th Cross, K.R. Road, Banasankari 2nd Stage, Bengaluru 560 070, Karnataka
  Ph: +91-80-26771678/79 Fax: +91-80-26771680 e-mail: bangalore@cbspd.com
- **Chennai:** 7, Subbaraya Street, Shenoy Nagar, Chennai 600 030, Tamil Nadu
  Ph: +91-44-26260666, 26208620 Fax: +91-44-42032115 e-mail: chennai@cbspd.com
- **Kochi:** 42/1325, 1326, Power House Road, Opp KSEB Power House, Eranakulam 682 018, Kochi, Kerala
  Ph: +91-484-4059061-65 Fax: +91-484-4059065 e-mail: kochi@cbspd.com
- **Kolkata:** No. 6/B, Ground Floor, Rameswar Shaw Road, Kolkata-700014 (West Bengal), India
  Ph: +91-33-2289-1126, 2289-1127, 2289-1128 e-mail: kolkata@cbspd.com
- **Mumbai:** 83-C, Dr E Moses Road, Worli, Mumbai-400018, Maharashtra
  Ph: +91-22-24902340/41 Fax: +91-22-24902342 e-mail: mumbai@cbspd.com

Representatives

- **Bhopal** 0-8319310552
- **Jharkhand** 0-9811541605
- **Pune** 0-9623451994
- **Kathmandu (Nepal)** 977-9818742655
- **Bhubaneswar** 0-9911037372
- **Nagpur** 0-9421945513
- **Uttarakhand** 0-9716462459
- **Hyderabad** 0-9885175004
- **Patna** 0-9334159340
- **Dhaka (Bangladesh)** 01912-003485

Printed At : Goyal Offset Works (P) Limited

to

---

my elder brothers, Mr Asvin and Mr Arvind and
to all those who believe in hardwork, self-confidence, dedication, adventure and courage and
who are having sharp weapons like passion and consistency

Preface to the Third Edition

Do not underestimate the power of microbes, absolutely true because human is trying to beat them since long time but they escape the human defence and continuously creating a problem to treat the infectious diseases. Clinical knowledge on infectious diseases served in this book shall help the clinicians to come out from these issues.

There are many books existing on the subjects but author is not satisfied with the way of presentation in all of them, that's why an attempt has been made to serve the entire material of microbiology including theory, practical, journal preparation, MCQs for pre-PG preparation, parasitology and entomology in one book like "ALL IN ONE" with presentation in point-wise, organised and in proper orderial manner like notes hence title prefix is "notebook". This book will sort out many questions of students such as how to make examination effective, how to score high, why multiple books for one subject, why different books for UG and PG entrance examination, which are the important questions for examination, etc. After reading this book, all the students will surely realise that medical science wouldn't be tough if all books of medical subjects could be available in same format as *Prakash's Notebook of Microbiology including Parasitology and Entomology*.

This book is written in simple language and in precise manner. Changes made in this edition are placement of **"Learning heading and subheadings"** at the beginning of each chapter and addition of six new chapters like **miscellaneous topics (world days, health care related symbols), medical entomology, oncogenic microbes, bioterrorism, microbiology of water, milk and air,** and **image based MCQs**. Attempts have been made to guide the microbiologist from the laboratory to the bed side by putting clinical pictures of infectious diseases in chapters and by putting clinical case study at the end of chapter. **Question bank** is available at the end of each chapter, so no need to search extra sources of question papers (sample papers) for important questions for preparation of examinations. Extra efforts have been made to strengthen the PG entrance preparation from the time of undergraduation by increasing the numbers of MCQs (with answers and explanations) in three forms like MCQs for chapter review (given at the end of each chapter), MCQs for system review (chapter no. 108) and image based MCQs (chapter no. 109).

After the publication of 1st and 2nd editions, I got tremendous response from everywhere, especially from medical students and my friends/seniors who are serving as medical teachers in different colleges, I am thankful to all of them for encouraging me to go for 3rd edition. This task could not be possible without an eternal support from my wife Shweta Modi and my daughter Aarya Modi. Last but not least, again thank you to all those who were always at there for me to make this journey successful.

Attempt has been made to serve the complete knowledge but I don't claim for perfection. Suggestions are welcome from all students and teachers for any shortcomings in contents, which will help me to improve my work and to serve more quality material to students in subsequent editions.

Prakash Modi
MD (Microbiology)

Preface to the First Edition

Microbiology is a link between clinical subjects and non-clinical subjects like anatomy, physiology, pharmacology, biochemistry. In a busy curriculum of medical students, it is very difficult to spare enough time for textbook type material, where point-wise presentation is lacking and also to spare time for reference books. In last 10 years of my journey as a medical teacher, I always felt that medical students are looking for such books which having not only knowledge but also have exam-oriented approach, covering of practical aspects and detailed knowledge about a particular point on single platform which minimise the use of reference books. I kept all this in my mind when I was writing the book. Present knowledge is prepared with use of multiple cross references and attempt was made to put complete knowledge about a particular point on single platform. Book is useful for medical students and also for clinician to diagnose, to prevent and to treat the infectious diseases.

Effort is made to cover entire subject, however nobody is perfect and complete one. This book is also lack at somewhere. Suggestions, instructions and advice are invited from students, seniors and all readers to make the effort perfect and complete. During the journey of organisation of this book, I required help and support from friends, colleagues and family. I am very grateful to all of them for sparing their valuable time for me.

Prakash Gelotar (Modi)
MD (Microbiology)

Contents

Section III: Systemic Bacteriology

Gram Positive Cocci (GPC)

Gram Negative Cocci (GNC)

Gram Positive Bacilli (GPB)

Gram Negative Bacilli (GNB)

Miscellaneous Bacteria

Section IV: Virology

General Virology

Systemic Virology: DNA viruses

Systemic Virology: RNA viruses

Systemic Virology: Miscellaneous viruses

Section V: Mycology

General Mycology

Systemic Mycology

Section VI: Parasitology

General Parasitology

Systemic Parasitology: Protozoa

Systemic Parasitology: Metazoa (Helminths/worms)

Cestodes

Trematodes

Tips to Start PG Entrance Preparation from the Time of Undergraduation

- **Theory:** Read theory first to clear the basics → Solve all questions (like case study, full questions, short notes and short questions) of "**question bank**" given at the end of each chapter → Check **"chapterwise MCQs"** given at the end of each chapter, by that way cover the all chapters of particular system and then → Solve the system-wise MCQs.
- **Group/pair study:** You will know which you don't know from the discussion with partner.
- **Mnemonic:** Should be limited.
- **Abbreviations:** Abbreviations are used in many MCQs, so remember the full forms.
- **Assessments:** Regular solving the NEET PG sample paper within the allotted time. This technique will help students in improving their speed and accuracy level. By this way, candidates can analyse their performance, expected score they can score and focus on weaker section.
- **Coaching:** Better to attend the coaching class than preparing at home.
- **MCQs pattern:** Few MCQs required knowledge of one chapter while few required knowledge of multiple chapters, so better to read all chapters (of particular system) before solving the MCQs.
- **Microbiology weightage in PG entrance:** Microbiology carrying approximately 20 marks in NEET PG, but questions based on infectious disease of other subjects such as community medicine, general medicine, surgery, skin, paediatrics etc., are also required basic knowledge of this subject, so eventually microbiology carrying around 40–50 marks burden.
- **Section ignored by students:** Epidemiology (covered in my second edition along with pathogenicity), resistance, virulence factors, prevention, treatment etc., sections are ignored by many students in microbiology but many MCQs are also the part of the section, so read it with university exam.

  Example:

  Q. Risk of pneumococcal meningitis is seen in - (AIIMS-1999)

  (a) Post splenectomy patient; (b) Patient undergoes neurological intervention; (c) Patient following cardiac surgery; (d) Patient with hypoplasia of lung.

  Ans. (a) is the answer: Splenectomy is the precipitating factor for capsulated bacterial infection, but students are rarely reading such topics.

  Must read: Remember food poisoning by heart because, almost in every year exam, there is a MCQ on food poisoning or microbes causing food poisoning.

Tips to Attend the Answers of MCQs

- **Time Management:** Don't waste the time to read the all MCQs at a time but read and attend the answer one by one.
- **Read all options:** Read all options at first, before encircling initial option, because some time after encircling first option you may realise that later option is more correct answer.
- **–ve marking:** Don't attend if you don't know the answer.
- **Most right answer:** Sometimes MCQ has more than one right options, but if it is required to tick only one option, then go for most right option.

  Example:

  Q. The most avidly complement fixing antibody is— (AIIMS, May 2002)

  (a) IgA (b) IgG (c) IgM (d) IgE

  Ans. Options a, b and c are the right answers because IgA fixes the alternative pathway while IgG (++) and IgM (+++) fix the classical pathway. But IgM (option 'c') is the most correct answer, if single option is required to encircle.
- **Wrong options:** Options given along with MCQs are sometimes partially or completely written wrong due to any reasons but it may confuse the students and in this situation believe only in yourself and put confidence on your knowledge.

  Example-1:

  Q. All the following statements about staphylococci are true, except— (AI 2010)

  (a) Most common source of infection is cross infection from infected people; (b) About 30% of general population is healthy nasal carrier; (c) Epidermolysin and TSS toxin are superantigen; (d) Methicillin resistance is chromosomally mediated

  Ans. Option 'a' is the right answer, but option 'c' is partially correct because epidermolysin is not superantigen, only TSS toxin is a superantigen.

  Example-2:

  Q: C-reactive protein stands for— (AI 2011)

  (a) Capsular polysaccharide in Pneumococcus; (b) Concanavalin-A; (c) Calretin; (d) Cellular

  Ans. All options are wrong

  In CRP, C stands for carbohydrate antigen of cell wall of Pneumococcus neither the capsular polysaccharide Ag nor other.
- **Confusing options:** Options given along with MCQs are sometimes look right but systematically not right.

  Example:

  Q. Hepatitis C virus is a— (AIIMS, May 2004)

  (a) Toga virus; (b) *Flavivirus;* (c) Filo virus; (d) Retro virus

  Ans. Option 'c' looks right but Flaviridae family has four genera like *Hepacivirus*, *Pegivirus*, *Pestivirus* and *Flavivirus* of which hepatitis C virus belong to genus *Hepacivirus* not *Flavivirus.* However, many authors considered common name as flavi virus to all virues belong to Flaviridae family, so option 'c' is right.
- **No time waste:** If you don't know the answer, then don't waste the time, move to the next question. Also don't waste the time for MCQs with confusing options and wrong options.

Section I
General Microbiology

Preview of General Microbiology

Prakash

❖ **Important scientists:** Like Louis Pasteur & Robert Koch are mentioned with following common headings

➢ **Birth:**

➢ **Contribution in Microbiology:**

❖ **Staining techniques:** Like gram stain, acid fats stains etc. are written with following main headings

➢ **History:**

➢ **Meaning:**

➢ **Principle:**

➢ **Modifications:** Each modified method (like KB method or ZN stain) is described by following subheadings

- **Full form/synonym:**
- **History:**
- **Principle:**
- **Steps:**
- **Precautions:**
- **Action of ingredients:**
- **Results:**

➢ **Control:**

➢ **Theories of stain:**

➢ **Uses:**

➢ **Summary**

❖ **Media:** All the media like simple/basal media, enriched media, enrichment media, transport (holding) media, selective media, sugar media, anaerobic media, differential media, composite media etc. are described in **table form** with following columns

- **No. (Number)**
- **Name of medium**
- **Important ingredients**
- **Action of important ingredients**
- **Uses**

❖ **Biochemical reactions (B/Rs):** Almost all the B/Rs are mentioned by using following common headings & subheadings

✪ **Principle:**

✪ **Medium:**

✪ **Reagent(s):**

✪ **Control:**

- **+Ve control:**
- **- Ve control:**

✪ **Methods / steps:**

✪ **Result: With appropriate figures**

- **+Ve test:**
- **-Ve test:**

✪ **Uses:**

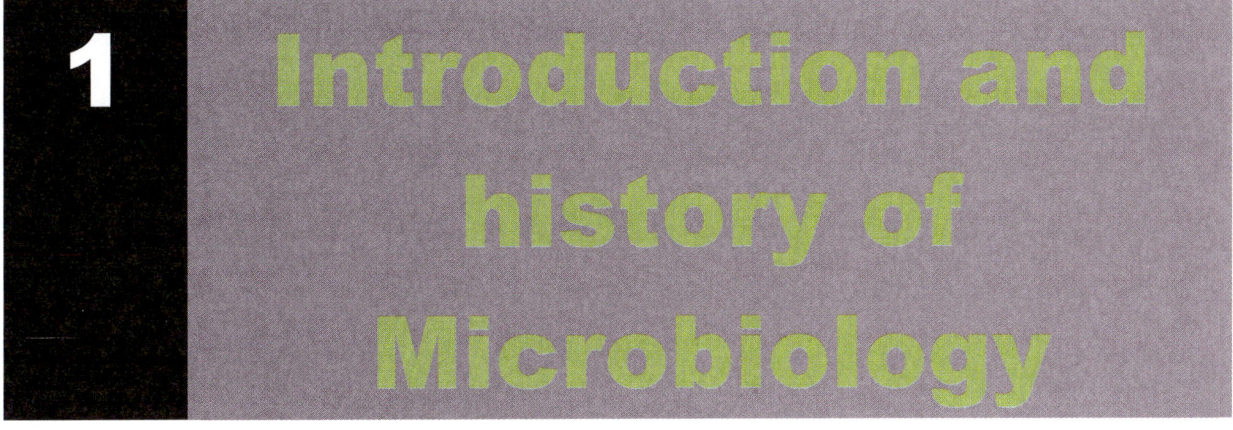

1 Introduction and history of Microbiology

Learning heading & subheadings

- Introduction
- Scientists & their role (History)

Introduction

❖ **Microbiology:** It is branch of medical science which related with study of microorganisms & disease produced by them. It includes diagnosis, prevention & treatment of disease & host response against microorganisms and or their products.

❖ **Branches of Microbiology:**

1. Medical Microbiology: Immunology, Bacteriology, Virology, Mycology, Parasitology & Molecular Microbiology
2. Food Microbiology
3. Industrial Microbiology
4. Soil Microbiology
5. Plant Microbiology

Scientists & their role (History)

❖ **Antony Philips Van Leeuwenhoek: [Delft, Holland, 1632-1723, Fig.1(a)]**

1. The Dutchman was draper, who 1st prepared the single lens microscope (by own) & observe the diverse materials through it. He observed the minute organisms & other materials in rain water through an instrument (single lens microscope) with 40-300 magnification power and designated them as **animalcules.** He communicated his observation to the Royal Society of London in 1676. However he did not realise the importance of these **animalcules.** As he worked on inventing different types of microscopes and improving the existing ones. Sure, his work helped to microbiology to achieve new heights because without a microscope, Microbiology cannot exist, so he can be **called as father of microscopy.**
2. In 1678, **Robert Koch** developed a compound microscope & confirmed Leeuwenhoek's observation.

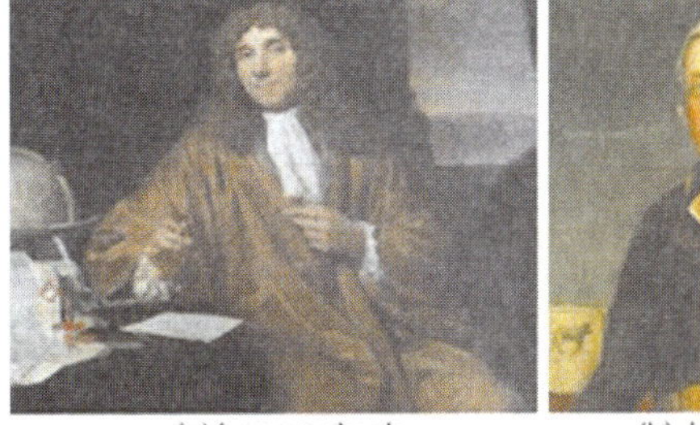

Figure-1: (a) Antony Van Leeuwenhoek & (b) Edward Jenner

3. Almost after a century & after research of many people it was accepted that **animalcules** are the causes of many contagious disease.
4. He observed the *Giardia lamblia* in his own stool in 1681.
5. He defined the shape of bacteria as cocci, bacilli & spirochetes.

❖ **Abiogenesis (Theory of spontaneous generation):** In an earliest time people had believed that living organisms could develop from non living thing like soil, elements etc. **called spontaneous generation or Abiogenesis.** In later part this theory was challenged by many scientists.

❖ **Edward Jenner: [England, 1749-1823, Fig.-1(b)]**

1. **Small pox vaccine:** He discovered the prophylactic preparation for small pox from cow lesion or cowpox. Such prophylactic preparation was labelled as **Vaccine (in Latin cow means Vacca)** by **Pasteur.**
2. **Father of Immunology:** He is awarded as **father of Immunology** for his contribution in the field of immunology

❖ **Louis Pasteur: [Dole, Jura, France 27th December 1822- 28th September, 1895, Fig.-2(a)]**

➢ **Birth:** He was born in the village Dole, France in 27th December 1822. His father was a tanner.

➢ **Contribution in Microbiology:**

1. **Profession:** He was trained as chemist, but his studies on fermentation led him to take interest in microorganisms.
2. **Father of microbiology:** His study on microorganisms leads the development of Microbiology & he is awarded as **father of Microbiology (medical Microbiology, modern Microbiology).**

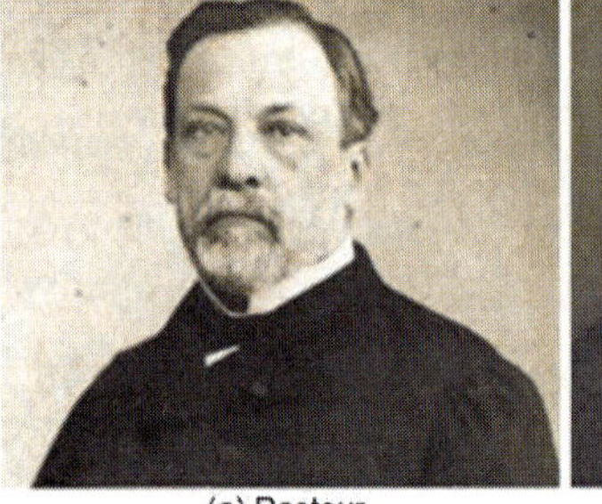
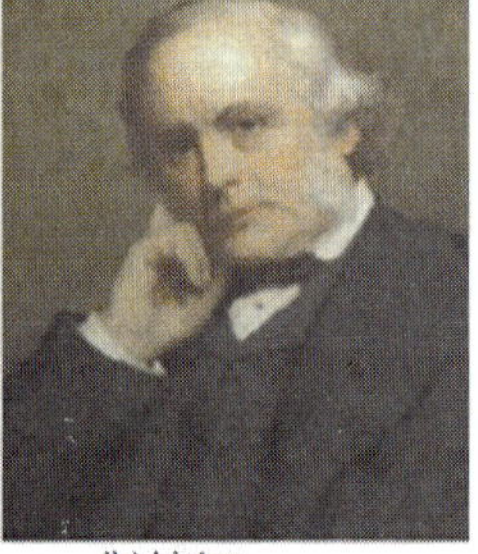

(a) Pasteur (b) Lister

Figure-2: (a) Louis Pasteur & (b) Joseph Lister

3. **Germ theory of disease (biogenesis) (1857):** He established that putrefaction & fermentation was the result of microorganisms & their activities (Biogenesis).
4. **Disapproved abiogenesis (1860-61):** With series of classical experiments, he proved that all forms of life, even microbes, arouse only from their like & not *de novo* & disapproved abiogenesis.
5. **Sterilisation technique:**
   - He developed the steam steriliser, hot air oven & autoclave.
   - He invented the pasteurisation (1863-65) useful for milk sterilisation.
6. **Cultivation technique:** He showed that growth medium, temperature, acidity, alkalinity & O_2 are required for successful cultivation.
7. **Studies on different diseases:**
   - **Pebrine or silk worm disease:** It was Pasteur who identify the Microspora (*Nosema bombycis*) as a causative agent of **pebrine (Silkworm disease)** in 1863 in France
   - **Anthrax:**
   - **Chicken cholera:**
   - **Hydrophobia (rabies):**
8. **Coined the term vaccine:** Edward Jenner developed the prophylactic preparation for smallpox from cow **(in Latin cow means Vacca)** lesion. Pasteur termed the **word vaccine** for such prophylactic preparation.
9. **Discovery of theory of attenuation & chicken cholera vaccine:** when chicken cholera culture left on the bench for several weeks it lost their pathogenicity but retains their ability to protect the bird against subsequent infection by them, led the discovery of theory of attenuation & lives chicken cholera vaccine.
10. **Discovered live attenuated anthrax vaccine:** He attenuated the *Anthrax bacilli* by incubating at 42-43^{0}C & proved that inoculation of such culture in animals induced specific protection against anthrax. The success of such immunisation was dramatically demonstrated by a experiment on a farm at Pouilly-Ie- Fort in 1881 during which vaccinated sheep, cows & goats were challenged with a virulent anthrax bacillus culture. All the vaccinated animals were survived while simultaneously unvaccinated animals died.
11. **Development of rabies vaccine:** He developed rabies vaccine (hydrophobia in human) in 1885
12. **Pasteur institute Paris:** It is built in honour of Louis Pasteur in Paris by public contribution. Similar institute were established in other regions for vaccine preparation & diagnosis of infectious diseases.
13. **Pneumococci** were 1st noticed by Pasteur & Stenberg

✓ **Notes: Who is the actual father of microbiology, A. Leeuwenhoek or Louis Pasteur? (link: https://www.quora.com/Who-is-the-actual-father-of-microbiology-A-Leeuwenhoek-or-Louis-Pasteur)**

- Antony van Leeuwenhoek can be considered more specifically as the "father of Microscopy" because of his contribution as mentioned earlier. But, having said that, the contributions of Louis Pasteur are far more than A. Leeuwenhoek's. He single handedly explored all the fields of Microbiology; right from proving that life arises from a pre-existing life to industrial Microbiology. His studies and sincere work is what makes Microbiology one of the most interesting subjects to study. So, Louis Pasteur can rightly be **called the "Father of Microbiology"**

❖ **Joseph Lister: [Scotland, 1827 –1912, Fig.-2(b)]**

1. Pasteur work was immediately followed by Joseph Lister in 1867 with introduction of antiseptic techniques in surgery resulting decreased morbidity & mortality due to surgical sepsis.
2. He 1st used the carbolic acid as antiseptic agents in surgery (1865).
3. He was awarded as **father of antiseptic surgery.**
4. **Lister institute London:** Was built in honour of Joseph Lister in London in 1891. It works for vaccine preparation & diagnosis of infectious diseases.

❖ Robert Koch: [Clausthal, Hanover, Germany, 11th December 1843 – 27th May 1910, Fig.-3(a)]

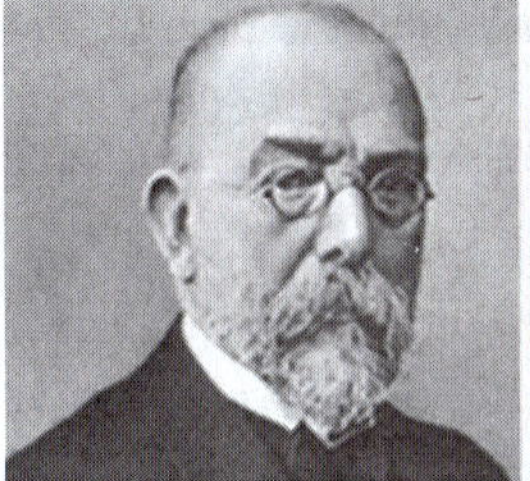
(a) Koch

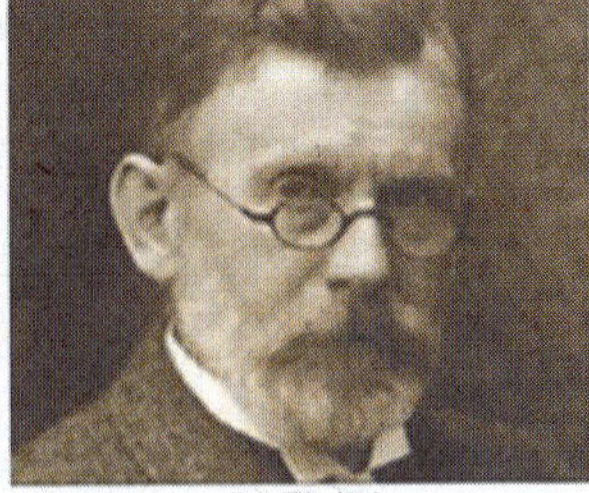
(b) Ehrlich

Figure-3: (a) Robert Koch, (b) Ehrlich

➢ **Birth:** He was born in Clausthal, Hanover, Germany, on 11th December 1843.

➢ **Contribution in Microbiology:**

a. **Father of bacteriology:**
- He was German physician & pioneering microbiologist.
- The founder of role of bacteria in production of diseases.
- Identify the causative agents of cholera (*Vibrio cholerae* in 1883), anthrax (*Bacillus anthracis* in 1876) and tuberculosis (*M tuberculosis* in 1882).
- Winner of **Nobel Prize** in 1905 & known as **father of Bacteriology.**

b. **Role in microscopy:** In 1678, **Robert Koch** developed a compound microscope & confirmed Leeuwenhoek's observation.

c. **Staining technique:** He described the staining method for identification of bacteria in dried fixed films stained with aniline dyes.

d. **Cultivation technique:**
- Robert Koch invented the culture method for pure isolation of bacteria over solid media. Earliest solid medium was **cooked cut potato** used by him, later he used gelatin for solidification of media, but gelatin is not satisfactory as it has tendency to get liquefy at 24^0C & by proteolytic bacteria.
- Use of agar in solidification of media was suggested by Frau Hesse, the wife of one investigator in Koch laboratory, who had seen her mother using agar to make jellies.

e. **Hanging drop technique:** He was the 1st to use hanging drop method to detect bacterial motility.

f. **Koch's postulates (1876):**
- **Principles:** Any organism will be accepted as causative agent of disease if it satisfied following four generalized principles **called Koch's postulates**.

1. The organism must be **present** in disease.
2. The organism must be **isolated** from the disease in pure culture.
3. Samples of the organism taken from pure culture must cause the same disease when inoculated into a healthy, susceptible **animal** in the laboratory.
4. The organism must be **re-isolated** from the inoculated animal

- **Additional principles in Koch's postulates:** Later one more principle is added, which is **detection of antibody (Ab)** from patient's serum.
- **Limitations (clinical applications) of Koch's postulates:** Some bacteria are not satisfying the Koch's postulates like
  - *M. leprae*: Not growing over artificial media.
  - *T. pallidum*: Pathogenic strains are not growing over artificial media, but non pathogenic can grow.
  - *N. gonorrhoea*: No animal model

> **Mnemonic:**
> - **Vaccines discovered by Louis Pasture:** CAR→ Cholera, Anthrax & Rabies
> - **Agents discovered by Robert Koch:** CAT→ Cholera, Anthrax & Tuberculosis

g. **Koch's phenomenon (1890):** Koch observed that a guinea pig already infected with tubercle bacillus gives exaggerated response when injected with tubercle bacilli or tuberculin protein. This hypersensitivity or allergic reaction **called Koch's phenomenon.**

❖ Paul Ehrlich: [Germany, 1854 –1915, Fig.-2(b)]

➢ **Profession:** German scientist

➢ **Contribution in Microbiology:**

1. **Stain** the cells & tissues to reveal their function.
2. He reported the **acid fastness of tubercle bacilli.**
3. He introduced the method for **standardisation of toxin & antitoxin** & coined the term **Minimum Lethal Dose (MLD).**
4. **Father of chemotherapy:** He used **salvarsanl** (an arsenical compound) sometimes called '**magic bullet** 'to kill spirochetes of syphilis with moderate toxic effect. He continued with his experiments till 1912 & discovered **neosalvarsan** & new branch in medicine **called chemotherapy**. Because of his extraordinary activities in medicine he is **called father of chemotherapy.**

❖ Other important scientists & their contribution in the field of Microbiology:

➢ **Hans Christian Gram:** A histologist developed the technique to identify the bacteria in tissue in 1884

➢ **Ziehl & Neelsen:** Initially Ehrlich developed the acid fast stain in 1882 & later modified by Ziehl & Neelsen in 1882

➢ **Ernst Ruska & co:** Invented the electron microscope in 1931 for which he won the Nobel Prize in Physics in 1986.

➢ **Alexander Fleming:** He discovered the penicillin from the fungus *Penicillium notatum* in 1928 & got Nobel Prize in 1945

- **Good Pasture:** He developed the viral culture method in chick embryo in 1931

Nobel Laureate	Year	Contribution
Emil A Behring	1901	Developed antitoxin to Diphtheria
Sir Ronald Ross	1902	Studied life cycle of *Plasmodium* in Mosquito
Robert Koch	1905	Discovered the *M. tuberculosis*
Charles LA Laveran	1907	Studied the *Plasmodium* under unstained preparation of blood
Paul Ehrlich & Elie Metchnikoff	1908	Discovered the selective theory of antibody formation
Charles Richet	1913	Discovered the anaphylaxis
Jules Bordet	1919	Role in Complement & CFT
Kleinberger	1941	Defined the L-Forms
Alexander Fleming	1945	Discovered the penicillin from the *P. notatum*
F Enders, FC Robbins, TH Weller	1954	Developed the tissue culture of Polio virus
JL Lederberg & EL Tatum	1958	Discovered conjugation theory in bacteria
Sir M Burnet & Sir PB Medawar	1960	Immunological tolerance
Watson & Crick	1960	Discovered the double helix DNA structure
Peyton Rous	1966	Discovered viral oncogenesis
Holley, Khurana & Nirenberg	1968	Discovered the genetic model
BS Blumberg	1976	Discovered the HBsAg
Barbara Mc Clintoch	1983	Discovered the transposon
George Kohler	1984	Discovered the hybridoma technique for mononclonal antibodies production
Karry B Mullis	1993	Discovered the PCR method
Stanley B Prusiner	1997	Discovered Prions
J Robin Warren & Barry J Marshal	2005	Discovered the *H. pylori* & its role in peptic ulcer
Harald Zur Hausen	2008	Discovery of HPV
Luc Montagnier & F Barre Sinoussi	2008	Discovery of HIV
Bruce A Beutler & Jules A Hoffmann	2011	Discovery of the theory of innate immunity
Ralph M Steinman	2011	Discovery of Dendritic cells & its role in adaptive immunity
Sir John B Gurdon & Shinya Yamanaka	2012	Mature cell can be reprogrammed to become pluripotent

Table-1: Noble Laureate

✓ **Note:** Year in **table -1** indicates the time of Nobel Prize given

Scientists	Common name	Scientific name
Victor Morax & Theodor Axenfeld	Morax - Axenfeld bacillus	*Moraxella lacunata*
Klebs & Loeffler	Klebs-Loeffler Bacill us (KLB)	*Corynebacterium diphtheriae*
Preisz & Nocard	Preisz-Nocard Bacillus	*Corynebacterium pseudotuberculosis*
Arthur Nicolaier	Nicolaier's bacillus	*Clostridium tetani*
Robert Koch	Koch's bacillus	*Mycobaterium tuberculosis*
Heinrich A. Johne	Johne's bacillus	*Mycobaterium paratuberculosis*
Gerard HA Hansen	Hansen's bacillus	*Mycobaterium leprae*
Heinrich A. Johne	Johne's bacillus	*Mycobaterium paratuberculosis*
George Hoyt Whipple	Whipple's bacillus	*Trophyrema whipplei*
Carl Friedlander	Friedlander's bacillus	*Klebsiella pneumoniae*
Abel Rudolf	Abel's bacillus	*Klebsiella pneumoniae* subsp. *ozaenae*
Anton Von Frisch	Frisch's bacillus	*Klebsiella pneumoniae* subsp. *rhinisclerοmatis*
Gaffky & Eberth	Gaffky-Eberth bacillus	*Salmonella typhi*
Alexander Yersin	Yersin bacillus (Plague bacillus)	*Yersinia pestis*
Whitmore	Whitmore's bacillus	*Burkholderia pseudomallei*
Pfeiffer	Pfeiffer's bacillus	*Haemophilus influenzae*
Koch & Weeks	Koch Weeks bacillus	*Haemophilus aegypticus*
Jules Bordet & Octave Gengou	Bordet – Gengou bacillus	*Bordetella pertusis*
Albert Doderlein	Doderlein's bacillus	*Lactobacillus acidophilus*
Eaton	Eaton agent	*Mycoplasma pneumoniae*

Table-2: Common name of the microorganisms from the name of scientists

- **Kleinberger:** He described the cell wall deficient form of bacteria in 1935 while studying the culture of *Streptobacillus moniliformis* in the Lister institute, London **called L-forms** after the Lister institute. He won Nobel Prize in 1941.
- **Von Behring Kitasato:** Described antibody

- **Karry B Mullis:** Invented the PCR technique in 1993

❖ **Nobel prizes:** Number of scientists have been awarded with Nobel Prizes for their significant contribution & research work in the field of Microbiology as shown in **Table-1**

❖ **Common name of the microorganisms from the name of scientists:** →**Table-2**

❖ **Scientific name of the microorganisms from the name of scientists:** →**Table-3**

❖ **Special honour to scientists:**

- **Father of microscopy:** Antony van Leeuwenhoek
- **Father of microbiology (medical microbiology, modern microbiology):** Louis Pasteur
- **Father of immunology:** Edward Jenner
- **Father of antiseptic surgery:** Joseph Lister
- **Father of bacteriology:** Robert Koch
- **Father of virology:** WM Stanely
- **Father of tumour virology:** Peyton Rous
- **Father of mycology**: Raymond Jacques Sabouraud
- **Father of chemotherapy:** Paul Ehrlich

Scientists	Scientific name
Bacteria	
Shiga & Flexner	*Shigella flexneri*
Shiga & Boyd	*Shigella boydii*
Shiga & Sonne	*Shigella sonnei*
Amedee Borrel & Bergdorfer	*Borrelia burgdorferi*
Cox & Burnet	*Coxiella burnetii*
Parasites	
Leishman & Donovan	*Leishmania donovani*
Wucherer & Bancroft	*Wucheria bancrofti*

Table-3: Scientific name of the microorganisms from the name of scientists

Question bank

Short notes

1) Robert Koch
2) Louis Pasteur

Short questions for theory/viva questions

1) What are Koch's postulates?
2) Name the bacteria which are not satisfying the criteria of Koch's postulates
3) Comment: *M. leprae* is excluded from the Koch's postulates
4) Write the common name for following bacterium
   - *C. diphtheriae* - *M. tuberculosis*
   - *S. typhi* *L. acidophilus*
5) Name the following
   - Father of Microbiology - Father of Immunology
   - Father of antiseptic surgery - Father of Bacteriology

MCQs for chapter review

Antony Philips Van Leeuwenhoek

1) **Antony Van Leeuwenhoek is associated with**
(a) Telescope (b) Microscope (c) Stains (d) Immunisation

Louis Pasteur

2) **Louis Pasteur is not associated with**
(a) Introduction of complex media (b) Discovery of rabies vaccine (c) Discovery of *M tuberculosis* (d) Disproved spontaneous generation theory
3) **Louis Pasteur is associated with**
(a) Discovery of the bacillus of tuberculosis (b) The cellular concept of immunity (c) Introduction of anthrax vaccine (d) Discovery of penicillin
4) **Vaccine of rabies was first discovered by**
(a) Louis Pasteur (b) Robert Koch (c) Edward Jener (d) Landsteiner
5) **Pasteur developed vaccine for**
(a) Anthrax (b) Rabies (c) Chicken cholera (d) All of the above

Robert Koch

6) **Microorganisms that does not obey Koch's postulates:** (AI-89)
(a) *M tuberculosis* (b) Polio virus (c) *M leprae* (d) *Streptococcus*
7) ***Vibrio cholerae* was discovered by**
(a) Koch (b) Meknitoff (c) John snow (d) Virchow

Other important scientists & their contribution in the field of Microbiology

8) **Electronic microscope was invented by**
(a) Ruska (b) Robert Koch (c) Antony van Leeuvenhock (d) Louis Pastuer

Common name of the microorganisms from the name of scientists

9) ***C. diphtheriae* is also called as-**
(a) Klebs-Loeffler Bacilli (KLB) (b) Roux bacilli
(c) Koch's bacilli (d) Yersin bacilli
10) **Which of the following is called Preisz-Nocard Bacillus**
(a) *C. diphtheriae* (b) *C. pseudotuberculosis* (c) *M tuberculosis* (d) *Mycoplasma*
11) **Eaton agent is**
(a) *Chlamydia* (b) *Mycoplasma pneumoniae* (c) *Klebsiella* (d) *H influenzae*

Answers of MCQs & explanation

1) **(b)**
- Follow section, **Antony Philips Van Leeuwenhoek** for explanation

2) **(c)**
- *M tuberculosis* was discovered by Robert Koch
- Follow section, **Louis Pasteur** for explanation of other options

3) **(c)**
4) **(a)** } Follow section, **Louis Pasteur** for explanation
5) **(d)**
6) **(c)**
- Follow section, **Robert Koch (limitation of Koch's postulates)** for explanation

7) **(a)**
- Follow section, **Robert Koch** for explanation

8) **(a)**
- Ernst Ruska & co: Invented the electron microscope in 1931 for which he won the Nobel Prize in Physics in 1986.

9) **(a)**
- *C. diphtheriae* was 1st identified by **Klebs** in 1883 but 1st cultivated by **Loeffler** in 1884 hence commonly **called Klebs-Loeffler Bacillus (KLB).**

- Emile Roux contributed in the discovery of diphtheria toxin along with Alexander Yersin.
- Koch's bacilli is the common name given to Mycobaterium tuberculosis from the name of Robert Koch
- Alexander Yersin who discovered the bacilli along with Kitasato in 1894 from Hong Kong at the beginning of last epidemic, from its contribution genus **called Yersinia,** however Yersin bacilli word is not used for all species of genus but only for Yersinia pestis which also **called plague bacilli**

10) (b) }
11) (b) } Follow **table-2** for explanation

2 Taxonomy of microorganisms

Learning heading & subheadings

- Definition
- Components:

❖ **Definition:** Taxonomy is defined as description, identification, nomenclature & orderial classification of organisms according to their presumed natural relationships.

❖ **Components:** Three components

I. **Classification/ orderly arrangements**
II. **Identification of unknown with known unit**
III. **Nomenclature /naming of unit (bacteria)**

I. Classification /orderly arrangements

➢ **Five kingdom system of classification:** In 1969, R H Whittaker placed all organisms in five groups **called five kingdom system of classification.**

1. **Monera:** Prokaryote, unicellular. E.g. bacteria, blue green algae & archaebacteria
2. **Protista:** Eukaryote, unicellular. E.g. protozoa

Features	Prokaryotes	Eukaryotes
	General features	
Meaning	Pro = primitive/immature + Karyotes = nucleus	Eu = true/mature + Karyotes = nucleus
Organism's examples	Monera (bacteria, blue green algae)	Protista, fungi, plantae & animalia
	Anatomy	
Number(s) of cell	Unicellular	Uni & multicellular
Nucleus - Nuclear membrane - Nucleolus - Chromosome	 - - Single-circular	 + + Multiple-linear
Cytoplasm - Ribosomes - Plasmid, episomes, transposon - Golgi complex - Endoplasmic reticulum - Triglyceride fats - Mitochondria & lysosomes	 + 70S + - - - -	 + 80S - + + + +
	Physiology	
Site of respiration	Mesosome (contains respiratory enzymes)	Mitochondria
Reproduction	Mostly by binary fission	By meiosis or mitosis
Pinocytosis	-	+
Protoplasmic streaming	-	+
	Bio-chemistry	
Plasma membrane - Sterol - Phospholipid	 - (Except in *Mycoplasma* & *Ureaplasma*) +	 + (like cholesterol, ergosterol etc.) +
Cell wall - Muramic acid / peptidoglycan - Diaminopimelic acid - Others	 + Present in few GNB in pentapeptide bridge Lipid & protein	 - Absent Chitin, mannan, cellulose (green plants)

Table-1: Differences between Prokaryotes & Eukaryotes

- = Absent, + = Present

✓ **Notes:**

- **Ancient:** Prokaryotes are evolutionary ancient. Probably they are 1st organisms to evolve & eukaryotes evolving from prokaryotes like predecessors.
- **Viruses:** Viruses are neither classified as prokaryotes nor eukaryotes
- **Phospholipid:** Present in both

3. **Fungi:** Eukaryote, uni or multicellular. E.g. fungi
4. **Plantae:** Eukaryote, multicellular. E.g. plants
5. **Animalia:** Eukaryote, multicellular. E.g. metazoa (helminths/worms), birds, animals, human, reptiles, arthropod, molluscs & coelenterates.

- **Modification of five kingdoms system of classification:** Modified by Margulis & Schwartz, which includes two kingdoms like **Prokaryotes & Eukaryotes** as shown in **table-1** with differences
- **General scheme of classification:** Kingdom → Phylum (Division) → Class → Order → Family (Tribe) → Genus → Species (Specific Epithet) → Subspecies (Strain/type).
- **Phylogenetic classification:** The hierarchical classification represents a branching tree like arrangement based on evolutionary arrangement of species.
- **Adsonian classification:** Based on all features expressed at the time of study.
- **Molecular or genetic classification:** Based on genetic relatedness.
- **Abbreviation of species:** Species word is common for both singular & plural form, but abbreviation may be used as sp. & spp. for singular & plural form respectively.
- **Intraspecies classification:**

- **Useful for epidemiological purpose**
- **Classify unit up to subspecies / strain / type by using following method**

- **Biotypes:** Based on biochemical properties
- **Serotypes:** Based on serological properties
- **Bacteriophage types:** Based on susceptibility to Bacteriophage
- **Colicin types:** Based on production of bacteriocin

II. Identification of unknown with known unit

By using morphological, biochemical, genetic & other properties

III. Nomenclature/naming of unit (bacteria)

- **Order:** Labelled with suffix **"ales"**
- **Family:** Labelled with suffix **"aceae"**
- **Genus name:** Latin noun & start with capital letter. Scientific name includes genus & epithet / species with Italic pattern.
- **Species / epithet name:** Start with small letter & in Italic pattern irrespective of person or place name. It based on different properties of unit like

- *albus* meaning white
- *suis* meaning pig origin
- *pyogenes* meaning pus
- *welchii* meaning person who discovered it
- *tetani* meaning disease produce
- *australis* meaning place of origin

Question bank

Short notes

1) Differences between prokaryotes & eukaryotes

Short questions for theory/viva questions

1) What is protista?

MCQs for chapter review

Classification /orderly arrangements

1) **Prokaryotes are:** (PGI, May-10, 13)
(a) Bacteria (b) *Mycoplasma* (c) Fungi (d) Blue green algae (e) Protozoa
2) **Which is a eukaryotes** (PGI, Dec-08, May-10, Nov-13)
(a) *Mycoplasma* (b) Bacteria (c) Fungus (d) *Chlamydia*
3) **Fungi are** (AI-92)
(a) Prokaryotes (b) Eukaryotes (c) Plant (d) Animals
4) **Site of respiration in prokaryote is**
(a) Mitochondria (b) Mesosome (c) Endoplasmic reticulum (d) All of above
5) **Mesosomes are**
(a) Respiratory enzymes in bacteria (b) Cytoplasmic invagination (c) Destructive bodies (d) Protein forming bodies
6) **Prokaryotes are characterised by:** (AI-99)
(a) Absence of nuclear membrane (b) Presence of microvilli on its surface (c) Presence of smooth endoplasmic reticulum (d) All of above
7) **Which of the following is protista**
(a) Algae (b) Fungi (c) Protozoa (d) Bacteria
8) **Which of the following is bacterial taxonomy** (PGI, Dec-09, Nov-13)
(a) *Chlamydia* (b) *Rickettsia* (c) *Mycoplasma* (d) Prion (e) Bacteriophage
9) **True about bacteria** (PGI, Dec-00)
(a) Mitochondria always absent (b) Sterols always present in cell wall (c) Divide by binary fission (d) Can be seen only under electron microscope
10) **Eukaryotes are different in causing infection because**
(a) Divide by binary fission (b) Highly structure cell with organised cell organelles (c) Don't have all organelles (d) Evolutionary ancient

Answers of MCQs & explanation

1) **(a), (b) & (c)**
2) **(c)**
3) **(b)**
4) **(b)**
5) **(a)**
6) **(a)**
7) **(c)**

(1–7) Follow section, **classification / orderly arrangements (five kingdom system of classification & table-1)** for explanation

8) **(a), (b) & (c)**
- *Chlamydia. Rickettsia* & *Mycoplasma* are bacteria**.** Prion is proteinaceous infectious virus like-particle without nucleic acid
- Bacteriophage is a virus which eats bacteria
9) **(a) & (c)**
- Mitochondria always absent in bacteria & respiration is possible by presence of mesosome
- Sterols not present in all bacteria but only in *Mycoplasma*. Bacteria divide by binary fission & can be seen under all types of microscopy
10) **(b)**
- Eukaryotes are divides by meosis or mitosis. Eukaryotes have highly structured cell with all organelles.
- Prokaryotes are evolutionary ancient

3 Microscopy and staining

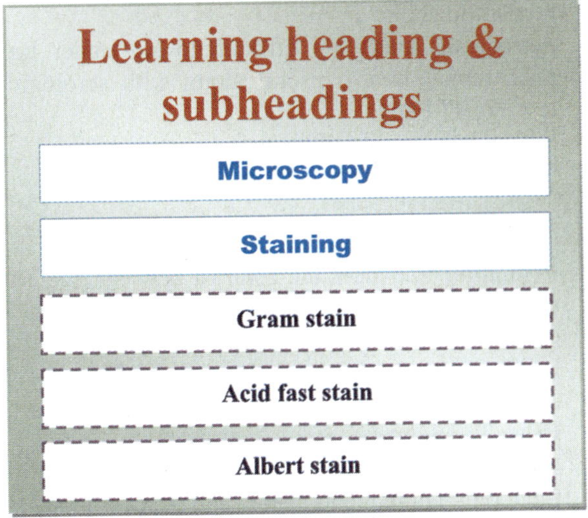

Microscopy

❖ **History:**

- In 1674 Antony van Leeuwenhoek, The Dutchman was draper, prepares the lenses & observes the diverse materials through it.
- In 1678, Robert Koch developed a compound microscope & confirmed Leeuwenhoek's observation.
- In 1931 Ernst Ruska & co invented the electron microscope for which he won the Nobel Prize in Physics in 1986

❖ **Types of microscope:** Commonly used microscope in Microbiology are as follows

I. Light microscope
II. Dark- Ground (field) Illumination Microscope (DGIM)
III. Phase-Contrast Microscope (PCM)
IV. Fluorescent Microscope (FM) & staining
V. Electron Microscope (EM)
VI. Others

I. Light microscope

➢ **Synonym:** Simple / compound / optical / bright-field microscope

➢ **Principle:** Produces a dark image against a bright background. Follow **fig.-1** for light transmission & image creation.

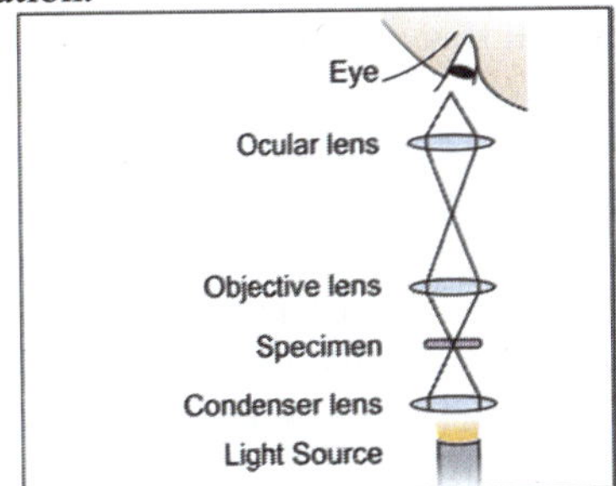

Figure-1: Principle of light microscopy

➢ **Parts:** Two parts **(fig.2).**

i. **Optical parts:** Two types of lenses

a. **Objective lenses:** They are attached to revolving nose piece with following three types

1. Low power (10X)
2. High power (40X)
3. Oil immersion lenses (100X)

b. **Ocular lenses (eye piece):** Eye piece have magnification of 10X, 12X or 15X

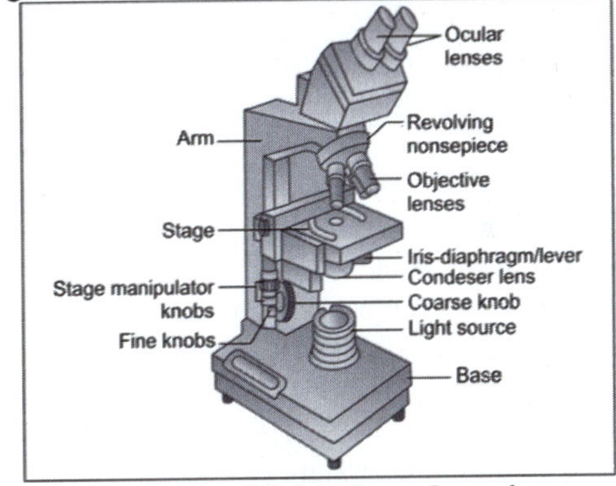

Figure-2: Parts of light binocular microscope

ii. **Mechanical parts:** It includes base (stand), diaphragm, stage etc. as shown in **fig.2**

➢ **Magnification power of microscope:**

- **Definition:** Degree of enlargement of image is **called magnification power of microscope.**
- **Example:** Eye lens (10X) x objective lens (10X) = Total Magnification (100X)

➢ **Resolution power of microscope:**

- **Definition:** Ability of a lens to distinguish two closely related structures **called resolution power of microscope.**
- **Unit:** It labelled as micron (μ) or micrometre (μm)
- **Limit of resolution with**

- Unaided eye is 200 µm (2,00,000 nm)
- Light microscope is 0.2µm (200nm)
- Electron microscope is 0.0005 µm (0.5 nm)

- **Effective factors:** It depends on the refractive index of the medium. Oil has a higher refractive index than air, hence use of the oil enhance the resolution power of microscope.

➤ **Technique of use:** The final magnification is the product of the magnification of the ocular and objective lenses. A slide is placed on the mechanical stage and is moved by rotating the stage control knobs. The height of the condenser may be varied (subjective variation) to give a bright, evenly illuminated field. Generally the condenser is used in its highest position for 100x & at lower level for 10x & 40x. A lever projects from the condenser and it is used to vary the opening of the condenser (or iris) diaphragm. For work with the scanning (4x) and low-power (10x) objectives, the condenser diaphragm should be wide open. For work with the high-dry (40x) and oil-immersion objectives (100x), however, the diaphragm should be closed slowly while looking at a sharply focused section until the level of illumination is just slightly reduced. This is the setting of the condenser diaphragm for optimum contrast and resolution. (From a theoretical point of view this is not quite correct. The diaphragm should be adjusted for each magnification. In most instances, however, it is much less critical at the lower magnifications).

➤ **Uses:**

1. **Scanner (4X):** To view a large area at a glance
2. **Low (10X) & high (40X) power:** For unstained preparations or wet mounts like KOH preparation, normal saline preparation, iodine preparation, hanging drop preparation, indicant ink preparation, peripheral smear etc.
3. **Oil immersion:** For stained preparations like gram stain, ZN stain, Albert stain, Giemsa stain etc.

➤ **Care:**

- **Do's**
  - Keep at room temperature
  - Keep it covered
  - Clean frequently with soft camel hair brush, fine tissue paper, muslin silk/cotton cloth
  - Clean the oil immersion lens with benzol/xylol
- **Don'ts**
  - Use gauze piece & cotton for cleaning lenses
  - Expose to direct sunlight
  - Use alcohol or acetone for cleaning lens

II. Dark- Ground (field) Illumination Microscope (DGIM)

➤ **Synonym:** Dark field microscope

➤ **Principle:** Produces a bright image of the object against a dark background. Dark field condenser with a central circular stop, which illuminates the object with a cone of light, without allowing any light ray to fall directly on the objective lens. Light rays fall on the object are scattered or reflected on the objective lens, resulting illumination of object against dark background

➤ **Uses:** To observe living organisms in unstained preparations like

1. Spirochetes very thin difficult to see under light microscope. It also useful along with serological test like TPI test
2. Flagella or motility of bacteria
3. Sheathed microfilaria

III. Phase Contrast Microscope (PCM)

➤ **Principle:** Enhances the contrast between bacterial cells & surrounding medium with difference in refractive index also creates contrast between intracellular structures with slight differences in refractive index

➤ **Uses:** To study

1. Intracellular structures
2. Bacterial components like endosome, inclusion body etc.
3. Microbial motility
4. Living cells & cell division

IV. Fluorescent Microscope (FM) & staining

➤ **Introduction:** Certain dyes **called fluors or fluorochrome** can be reached to high energy level from normal or low energy level after absorbing UV light. When dye back to normal or low energy level they release excess energy in form of visible light. This process **called fluorescence.**

➤ **Types:** Two types

i. **Fluorochroming:**

✪ **Principle:** Dyes combined with target bacteria & gives fluorescence **[fig.-3 (a)].**

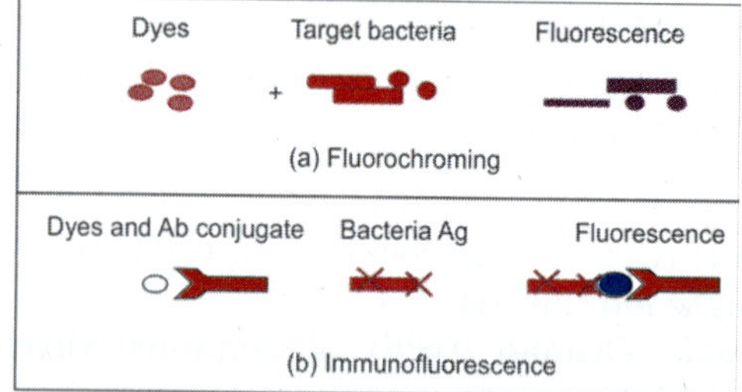

Figure-3: Types & principle of Fluorescence Microscope (FM)

✪ **Advantages:**

- Increase the contrast
- More sensitive (minimum concentration of organisms is 10^4/ml) than light microscopy (minimum concentration of organisms is 10^5/ml)

✪ **Dyes used are:**

a. **Acridine orange:**

1. It stains the nuclei of all cells in smear.

2. It does not discriminate between gram positive & gram negative cells.
3. It also stains the host cells

b. Auramine / Rhodamine: Used for *M. tuberculosis*

c. Calcofluor white stain: Used for fungus

ii. Immunofluorescence:

- **Principle:** Dyes is conjugated with antibody. This conjugate will combine with antigen of target bacteria & gives fluorescence **[fig.-3(b)].**
- **Advantage:** More sensitive
- **More detail:** **Follow chapter → Antigen – antibody (Ag-Ab) reactions.**

V. Electron Microscope (EM)

- **Principle:** Beams of electrons are used instead of light (as used in light microscope) to produce images.
- **Types:** Two types

i. Scanning Electron Microscope (SEM):

- It uses the electrons reflected from the surface of a specimen to create the image
- It produces a 3-dimensional image of specimen's surface features

ii. Transmission Electron Microscope (TEM):

- Electrons scatter when they pass through a specimen
- Transmitted electrons (those that do not scatter) are used to produce image
- Denser regions in specimen, scatter more electrons and appear darker

- **Uses:**

- For virus diagnosis
- Detailed study of cell structure

VI. Others

i. **Interference microscope**
ii. **Polarisation microscope**
iii. **Confocal microscopy**
iv. **Scanning probe microscopy**
v. **Stereoscopic microscope**
vi. **Dissection microscope**

Staining

- **Steps:** Three steps

I. **Smear preparation**
II. **Fixation**
III. **Staining**

I. Smear preparation

- Take the clean & dry slide
- **Label** the slide with patient name & number
- **Body fluid:** Take a drop with sterile loop over slide & spread evenly covering an area about 15-20 mm.
- **Tissue:** Hold the tissue with sterile forceps & rub over slide.
- **Swab:** Roll the swab on slide
- Keep the slide on rack for drying
- Avoid contact with dust, insect & sunlight during drying.

II. Fixation

- **Definition:** Process by which organism is killed and firmly attached to slide.
- **Aim:** To prevent the washing of microorganisms from smear during staining
- **Types:**

A. Heat fixation:

- **Steps:**

- Hold the smear with sterile forceps
- Pass 3-4 times through flame.
- Cool the slide & stain

- **Advantage:** Preserves overall morphology
- **Disadvantages:**

- Over heating will damage the organisms & alter the staining reaction
- It damages leucocytes & therefore unsuitable for fixing smear containing intracellular organisms like *N. gonorrhoea* & *N. meningitidis*.
- Sometimes heat may not kill some bacteria like *M. tuberculosis*.

B. Chemical fixation:

i. Alcohol fixation:

- **Steps:**

- Put 1-2 drops of ethanol/methanol on slide for 2 minutes or until the alcohol evaporates

- **Advantages:**

- Less damaging to microorganisms preserves morphology
- Does not damages leucocytes & therefore suitable for fixing smear containing intracellular organisms like *N. gonorrhoea* & *N. meningitidis* (absolute alcohol is used).
- Kill bacteria like *M. tuberculosis*. (70% alcohol is used)

ii. 40g/l $KMno_4$: For fixing *B. anthracis*

iii. Formaldehyde vapour: For *M. tuberculosis*

III. Staining

- **Types:** Two types

A. Vital stains:

- **Definition:** Stain which maintains the viability of organisms **called vital stain**.
- **Stains:** It is mostly unstained preparation as follows

i. Required emulsification: By using NS

a. Normal Saline (NS) wet mount:

- **Steps:**

- Take a drop of normal saline on slide
- Add the stool particles
- Mix with wooden stick
- Put cover slip

- Examine under low/high power
- **Uses:** For stool examination in parasite like *E. histolytica, T. vaginalis, G. lamblia* etc.

b. Hanging drop preparation from solid stool:

- **Steps: →Fig.4**
- Take a concavity slide & clean it.
- Take a drop of normal saline on cover slip
- Add the stool particles
- Mix with wooden stick

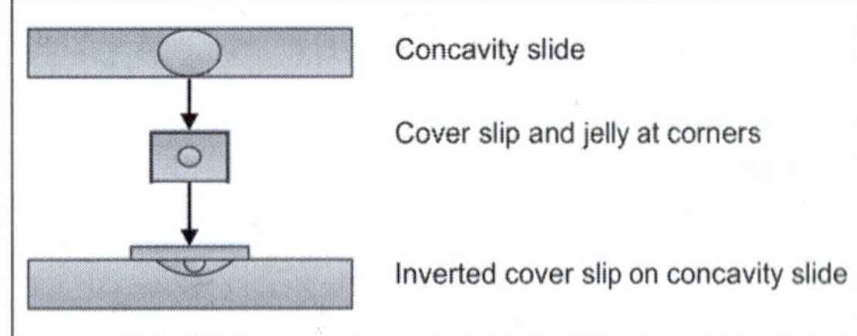

Figure-4: Hanging drop preparation

- Apply the adhesive jelly at all corner of cover slip.
- Invert the cover slip over concavity slide.
- Examine the edge of drop NS under low power & than focus the motility under high power
- **Use:** To detect motility of bacteria & parasites in solid stool

ii. Not required emulsification:

a. Direct wet mount:

- **Steps:**
- Take a drop of liquid culture or body fluid (e.g. urine) on slide **(called direct wet mount)**
- Put a cover slip & examined under low/high power
- **Use:** To examine inflammatory cells, deposits & motile organisms in body fluid

b. Hanging drop preparation (HDP) from liquid stool:

- **Steps:**
- Take a drop of liquid stool over cover slip
- Invert the cover slip over concavity slide
- Examine the edge of drop under low power & than focus the motility under high power
- **Uses:** To detect motile bacteria in liquid stool like *V. cholerae*

B. Supravital stains:

- **Definition:** Stain which does not maintains the viability of organisms **called supravital stain**.
- **Stains:** Different types are as follows

i. Simple staining (monochrome staining):

- **Principle:**
- Mostly one step staining
- It stain all organisms in same colour, however provides colour contrast between organisms & background
- **Stains & uses:**

a. Wet mount stain: Iodine preparation to examine the eggs of parasites.

b. Fix smear stain: Methyle violet or methylene blue or basic fuchsin for bacteria

ii. Negative staining (background staining):

- **Principle:** Background is stained & structures to be demonstrated are remain unstained
- **Stains & uses:** Indian ink, nigrosin stains are useful for bacterial capsule & spirochetes detection.

iii. Impregnation staining:

- **Principle:** Very thin organisms are difficult to see under light microscope & examined by increasing the thickness by applying the silver over surface.
- **Stains & use:** Fontana's stain (contains silver nitrate) for spirochetes like *Treponema, Borrelia & Leptospira*

iv. Fluorescent staining: → Vide supra

v. Differential staining:

- **Principle:** Utilize 2 different types of stains to distinguish between 2 different types of cells / organisms or different parts of cells / organisms.
- **Stains & uses:**

a. Histopathological stain:

- Giemsa stain, Haematoxylin & Eosin stain etc.
- For histological study of cells or tissues

b. Microbiological stains:

1. **Gram stain:** For gram + Ve & gram –Ve bacteria
2. **Acid fast stains:** For acid fast microbes like **Ziehl Neelsen (Z-N) stain**
3. **Others:**

- Stains for polar bodies, for fat globules, for spores & for flagella
- More details: Follow chapter → Morphology of bacteria

Gram stain

- **History & meaning:** So **called** because Hans Christian Gram, a histologist developed the technique to identify the bacteria in tissue in 1884.
- **Principle:** Certain bacteria stained with basic dyes (like methyl violet/crystal violet/gentian violet for 5 minutes) followed by staining with mordant (like Gram's iodine for 1 minute), which fix the dye in cell & prevent decolourisation on subsequent treatment with decolourising agent (like acetone for 1-2 seconds/alcohol for 20-30seconds / acetone-alcohol for 10 seconds). Decolourised cell are finally stain by counter stain (like basic fuchsin/safranin).
- **Modifications:** Following are the modifications in the original gram stain's method.

Kopeloff's & Beerman's (KB) method:

- Principle: It uses the methyl violet as primary stain & basic fuchsin as counter stain.
- Indication: Best useful method now a day for all bacteria & described in details as follows

Jensen's modification:

- Principle: It uses the absolute alcohol as decolouriser & neutral red as counter stain.

- Indications: For *N. meningitidis* & *N. gonorrhoea*

✪ **Weigert's modification:**
- Principle: It uses the aniline - xylol as decolouriser.
- Indications: Useful for staining of tissue sections

✪ **Preston & Morrell's modification:**
- Principle: It uses the iodine -acetone as decolouriser
- Indications: It is developed to overcome the irritating iodine in aerosols by reducing the iodine concentration to one-tenth & shortening the duration the duration of decolourisation to 10 seconds

✪ **Quick gram stain:**
- Principle: It includes the duration of 5 seconds for each primary stain, mordant & counter stain but 2 seconds for decolouriser.
- Indications: For single slide

✪ **Gram stain for multiple slide:**
- Principle: It includes the duration of 30 seconds for each step.
- Indications: For multiple slides (10-15) staining

Kopeloff's & Beerman's (KB) method

- **Full form:** Kopeloff's & Beerman's method
- **History:** Original gram stain was modified by Nicholas Kopeloff & Philip Beerman
- **Principle:** Vide supra
- **Steps:**
- Take clean & dry slide
- **Prepare** the smear & **fix** with heat
- Cover entire smear with **primary stain** like methyl violet/gentian violet/crystal violet & keep for 5 min.
- Apply the iodine as **mordant** for 2 minutes
- Wash & **decolourise** with 95-100% acetone (2-3 seconds) or ethanol (20-30 seconds) or acetone alcohol (10 seconds)
- **Wash** with tap water
- Apply the basic fuchsin (or safranin) as **counter stain** & keep over smear for 30 seconds.
- **Wash** with tap water
- **Dry** the slide
- **Add** a drop of cedar wood oil
- **Examine** under oil immersion lens
- **Precautions:** Cover the smear part with stain, not the entire slide.
- **Action of ingredients:**

1. **Methyl Violet:** It is primary stain (basic dye). It stains gram +Ve & gram -Ve organism in violet colour.
2. **Iodine solution:** Acts as a mordant. It fixes the primary stain in the cell.
3. **Acetone or ethanol or acetone alcohol:** Decolourising agent. It decolourise only gram -Ve organism. Gram +Ve retain the dye.
4. **Basic Fuchsin:** Acts as counter stain. Those organisms which are decolourised by acetone are counter stand by basic fuchsin.

- **Results:**

1. **Gram +Ve organisms:** Violet colour **(fig. 5 & 6)**
2. **Gram -Ve Organisms:** Pink colour **(fig. 7 & 8)**

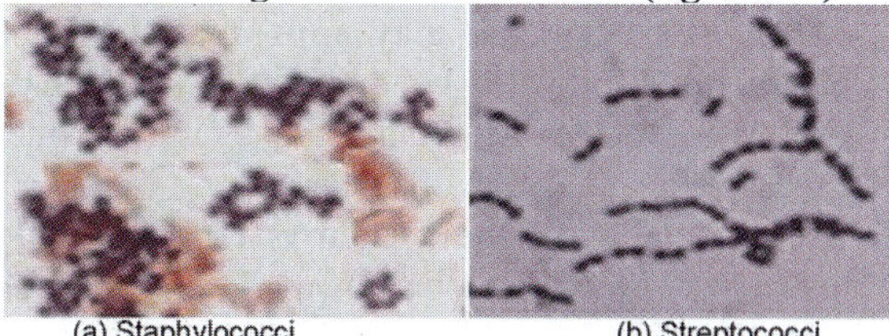

Figure-5: Gram Positive Cocci (GPC)

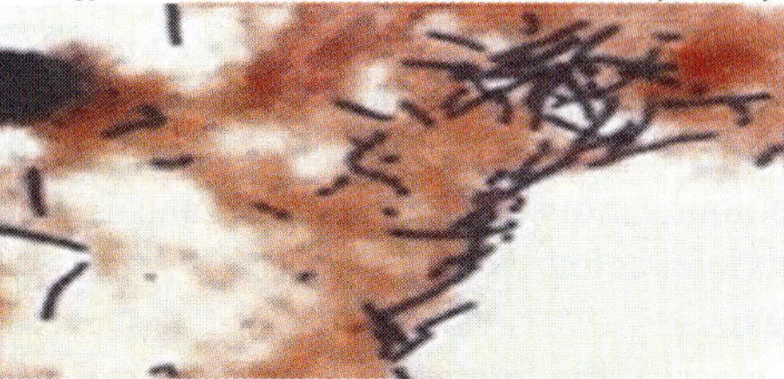
Figure-6: Gram Positive Bacilli (GPB)

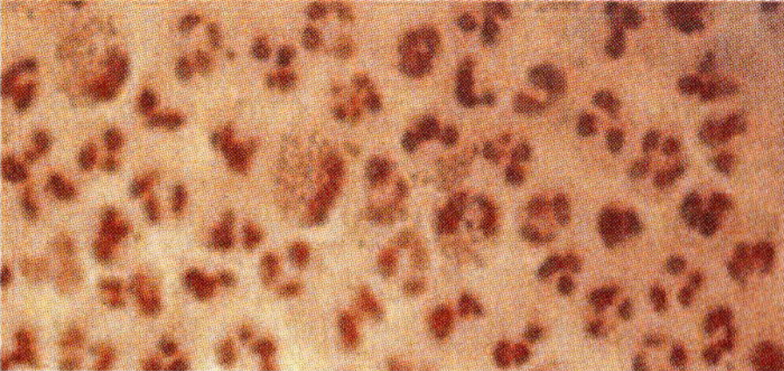
Figure-7: Gram Negative Cocci (GNC)

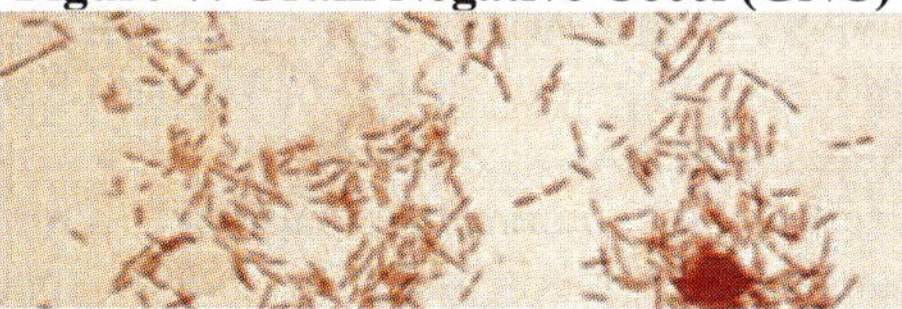
Figure-8: Gram Negative Bacilli (GNB)

- **Controls:** Always check new reagent with known Gram +Ve & Gram -Ve organisms.
- **Theories:** Exact reasons for violet colour in Gram +Ve & pink colour in gram –Ve organism are not known, but following theories are responsible.

1. **pH Theory:** Gram +Ve organisms has acidic pH & better stain with basic dye. Gram -Ve organism has basic pH not stain by basic dye.
2. **Lipopolysaccharide (LPS):** LPS is present in gram -Ve organism cell. LPS is dissolved by lipid solvent like acetone, resulting damage to cell wall of gram -Ve organism & primary stain will come out from cell, leaves the gram -Ve organism colourless.
3. **Thick Peptidoglycan:** In gram +Ve organisms & cell wall remain unaffected & retain the original colour of primary stain.
4. **Magnesium ribonuclease theory:** Magnesium ribonuclease enzyme is present in gram +Ve cell & makes dye-iodo-complex with dye & iodine. It is larger than the pores size of cell wall, hence not come out on treatment with acetone & maintains violet colour in gram +Ve cell. It is absent in gram –Ve cell & no dye- iodo complex formation. Dye

remains free in cytoplasm of gram –Ve cell & easily come out on treatment with acetone.

- **Gram variable reactions:**

1. **Gram +Ve organism may appear as Gram -Ve organism** in following conditions:
   - Cell wall damage due to antibiotic therapy or due to excessive heat fixation of smear
   - Use of iodine solution which is too old (yellow instead of brown colour, always store in brown glass bottle)
   - Over decolourisation of smear
   - Smear prepared from old culture like in *Cl tetani*
2. **Gram -Ve organism may appear as Gram +Ve organism:** Thick smear gives incomplete decolourisation of Gram -Ve organism & retained the violet colour.

- **Uses:**

1. **To classify the bacteria in gram +Ve & gram -Ve groups: →Table-1**
2. **To identify the bacteria:** From culture growth
3. **To identify the fungus:** Like *Candida* spp. or *Cryptococcus* spp.
4. **Early presumptive diagnosis:** It helps in early diagnosis of fastidious bacteria like *H. influenzae* which takes long time to grow on the culture
5. **To start the empirical therapy:** Broad spectrum antibiotic treatment can be started based on the shape, size & gram reaction of bacteria before the culture report will be available
6. **Selection of anaerobic culture:** Preliminary diagnosis of bacteria like *Clostridium* spp. under gram stain gives ideas to perform anaerobic culture.

Mnemonic: Follow table-1 for details

- **GPC:** S_4P_2EM
- **GNC:** MenGo MoVe
- **GPB:** MC DONALD
- **GNB:** EK LAVYA HE S_2P_2B2A (EK LAVYA HE with Sharp & Pointed Baw & Arrow

Types	Gram +Ve	Gram -Ve
Cocci	*Staphylococcus* *Streptococcus* *Strept. pneumoniae* *Stomatococcus* *Peptostreptococcus* *Peptococcus* *Enterococcus* *Micrococcus*	*N. meningitides* (**Men**ingococcus) *N. gonorrhoea* (**Go**nococcus) *Moraxella* *Veilonella*
Bacilli	*Mycobacterium* *Clostridium* *Corynebacterium* *(Diphtheria)* *Erysipelothrix,* *Bacillius (Others)* *Nocardia* *Actinomyces* *Listeria* *Lactobacilli* *(Doderlein's bacilli)*	*Escherichia, Klebsiella* *Legionella, Aeromonas* *Vibrio, Yersinia,* *Arcobacter, Haemophilus* *Enterobacter,* *Salmonella, Shigella,* *Proteus, Pseudomonas,* *Bordetella, Brucella* *Anaerobes (non-sporing)*

Table-1: Types of bacteria A/t gram stain

- **Limitations:**
  - Mycobacteria are not strict GPB: In gram stain gram +Ve bacteria gives violet colour following application of Methyl Violet, iodine, acetone & basic fuchsin. *Mycobacteria* resist decolourisation even without use of iodine & stains in violet colour. Hence *Mycobacteria* are not following the complete principle of gram stain & that's why strictly it's not correct to classify *Mycobacteria* as GPB.
  - Bacteria difficult to examine under the gram stain:

Mnemonic:
These Microbes May Lack Real Colour

- ***Treponema* & related genera like *Borrelia* & *Leptospira*:** To thin to be seen
- ***Mycobacteria:*** High lipid content in the cell wall & detected by acid fast stain
- ***Mycoplasma:*** Cell wall deficient bacteria
- ***Legionella:*** Primarily intracellular
- ***Rickettsia:*** Intracellular & examined under Giemsa or other stains
- ***Chlamydia:*** Intracellular

- **Summary of gram stain: →Table -2**

Acid fast stains

- **History:** Initially Ehrlich developed the acid fast stain in 1882 for tubercle bacilli with the use of aniline-gentian violet followed by nitric acid
- **Principle:** Stain acid-fast bacteria with basic dye (like carbol fuchsin/aniline gentil violet). Fix the dye by using physical (heat) or chemical mordant (carbolic acid) followed by decolourisation with acid (like nitric acid /sulphuric acid) or acid-alcohol. Decolourised organisms are counter stained by methylene blue or malachite green
- **Meaning:** Acid-fast bacteria once stain resist decolourisation even with the powerful solvent like acid or acid-alcohol so **called acid fast stain**
- **Modifications: Called modified acid fast stain**

- **ZN stain or Hot stain: → Vide infra**
- **Kinyoun's stain or Cold stain:**
  - It avoid the use of heating, so **called cold stain**
  - It uses the carbol fuchsin as primary stain with higher concentration of carbolic acid than hot stain. Carbolic acid act as chemical mordant
  - More duration than hot stain
- **Other modifications:**
  - Use of acid-alcohol as decolourising agent
  - Like use of malachite green as counter stain

ZN stain

- **Full form:** Ziehl-Neelsen stain
- **Synonym:** Hot stain because primary dye is fixed by using physical mordant like heat
- **History:**

Reagents	Time	Action	Gram +Ve colour	Gram -Ve colour
Methyl Violet	5 minutes	Primary stain	Violet	Violet
Iodine solution	2minutes	Mordant	Violet	Violet
Acetone 95-100%	2-3 seconds	Decolouriser	Violet	Colourless
Tap water		Washing		
Basic fuchsin	30seconds	Counter stain	Violet	Pink/red
Tap water		Washing		

Table-2: Summary of gram stain

- Initial Ehrlich technique was modified by Ziehl & Neelsen in 1882
- This method is widely used for acid fast bacteria
- **Principle:**
- Stain acid-fast bacteria with basic dye like carbol fuchsin with simultaneous application of heat which act as physical mordant & fix the dye in cell.
- Decolourisation is done by 25% H_2SO_4. Decolourised organisms are counter stained by methylene blue.
- **Steps:**
- Take clean & dry slide
- **Prepare** a thick smear from specimens
- Air dry and heat **fix**.
- Cover the entire smear with **basic dye** like carbol fuchsin (contains carbolic acid & basic fuchsin, so **called carbol fuchsin**). Simultaneously apply the heat for 5 minutes.
- Cool and **rinse** with water.
- **Decolourise** by 25% H_2SO_4 by allowing it to sit for 15 seconds on smear.
- **Wash** the top and bottom of slide with water and clean the slide bottom well.
- **Counter-stain** with Methylene Blue for 30 seconds to 1 minute.
- **Wash** and blot the slide with absorbing paper.
- **Add** a drop of cedar wood oil
- **Examine** under the oil immersion lens.
- **Precautions:**
- Apply the stain only on smear part, not on entire slide.
- Carbol fuchsin is a carcinogen. Wear gloves when working with it.
- Keep the stain steaming & do not boil.
- Add more stain if needed.
- **Action of ingredients:**

1. **Carbol fuchsin:** It is mixture of basic fuchsin & carbolic acid (phenol) hence **called carbol fuchsin**. Act as primary stain & stain all organisms in smear in pink colour
2. **Heat:** Act as physical mordant & fix the dye in cell.
3. **25% $H2SO_4$:** Decolouriser, remove colour from organisms except acid fast
4. **Methylene Blue:** Act as counter-stain & stain those organisms which are Decolourise by 25% $H2SO_4$.

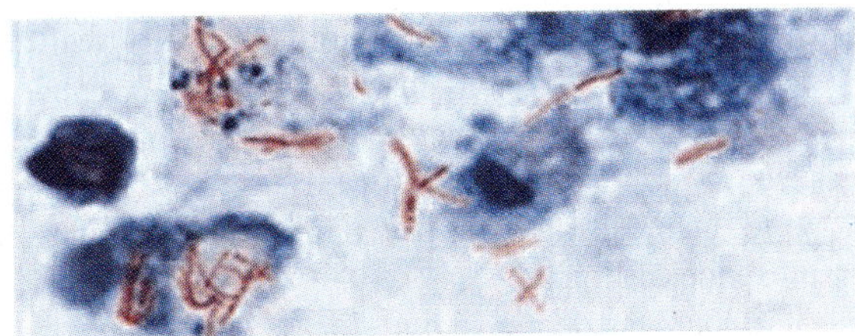

Figure-9: Acid fast bacilli in ZN stain

- **Results:** All acid fast organisms stain in pink colour while non acid fast & background stain in blue colour. **(fig.-9)**
- **Reporting/grading of smear:**
- Negative report should not be given before examining 100 fields or for 10 minutes
- Positive report can be given only if two or more bacilli have been seen
- *M. tuberculosis* appears as long, curved, beaded or barred form & not uniformly stained red coloured AFB
- *M. bovis* appears as short, straight, stout & uniformly stained red coloured AFB
- Smear should be graded as per RNTCP, India as shown in **table-3**

No. of AFB/fields	Fields to be examine	Result	Grading
No bacilli /100	Entire smear/ minimum 300 fields or 10 minutes	-Ve	0
1 – 9 /100	100	scanty	Report with exact numbers of bacilli
10 – 99/100	100	+Ve	1 +
1 – 10 /1	50	+Ve	2+
> 10/1	20	+Ve	3+

Table-3: Grading of smear as per RNTCP

- RNTCP grading is useful for

1. Monitoring the drug response
2. Assessing the severity of the disease
3. Assessing the infectiousness of the patient: Higher the grade more is the infectiousness. Smcar negative (< 10^4 bacilli per ml of sputum) are less infectious.

- **Controls:** Always check new reagent with known acid fast bacteria.
- **Theories of ZN stain:**

1. **Acid fastness theory:**
   - Definition: Bacteria once stain with primary dye resist decolourisation even with the powerful solvent like acid-alcohol **called acid fastness**
   - Reason for acid-fastness:
     - The acid fast genera have the unsaponifiable wax/lipid **called mycolic acid** in their cell walls. It is responsible for acid-fastness & prevents decolourisation by acid-alcohol.
     - Peptidoglycan-polysaccharide-mycolic acids complex forms the skeleton in cell wall of *Mycobacteria,* so acid fastness in *Mycobacteria* is not the property of mycolic acid alone, but depends also on the integrity of cell wall
   - Acid fastness increase by: Growing organisms in presence of lipid
   - Acid fastness decrease by:
     - Mechanical rupture of cell wall
     - Autolysis
     - Cell wall lysis by drug like isoniazide
     - Cell wall lysis by fat solvents

- **Further modifications in ZN stain:** It **called modified ZN stain** & can be done by modifying the concentration of sulphuric acid as follows
  - 0.25-0.5% sulphuric acid for bacterial spore
  - 0.5-1% sulphuric acid for sperm head
  - 1% sulphuric acid for *M. smegmatism* (Atypical mycobacteria), *Nocardia spp.* & for acid fast parasites
  - 5% sulphuric acid for *M. leprae*
- **Uses (acid-fast organisms):**

Bacteria	Concentration of H_2SO_4
Bacterial spores	0.25-0.5%
Atypical mycobacteria *Nocradia asteroids, N. brasiliensis, N. caviae*	1%
M. leprae	5%
M. tuberculosis	25%
Rhodococcus	-
L. micdadei	-

Table-4: Acid fast bacteria & concentration of H_2SO_4

Parasites	Diagnostic or Acid fast stage (1% H_2SO_4)
Isospora bellei	Oocyst
Cryptosporidium parvum	Oocyst
Cyclospora cayetanensis	Oocyst
Microsporidium	Spore
Taenia saginatum	Egg
Schistosoma intercalatum	Egg
Schistosoma mansoni	Egg
Schistosoma japonicum	Egg
Schistosoma mekongi	Egg

Table-5: Acid fast parasites

a. **Bacteria: → Table-4**
b. **Parasites: → Table-5**
c. **Human body cell:** Sperm head with 0.5-1%H_2SO_4

> **Mnemonic:**
> **Bacteria:** SAN MMR L **(table-4)**
> **Parasite:** TIC_2MS_3 **(table-5)**

- **Advantages of ZN stain:** Cheap, fast, easy to perform, high sensitivity > 90% & high specificity of 98%
- **Disadvantages of ZN stain:**
  - ZN stain is less sensitive than culture because at least 10,000 (10^4) bacilli should be present per ml of sputum for demonstration in direct smear, while culture can detect 10-100 bacilli per ml.
  - Rare useful in young children who may not produce sputum.
  - Beaded or barred forms frequently seen in *M. tuberculosis* under Z N stain as shown **in fig.-10.** *M bovis* stain more uniformly under ZN stain
  - Elder & HIV infected persons may not produce cavities & sputum containing AFB.

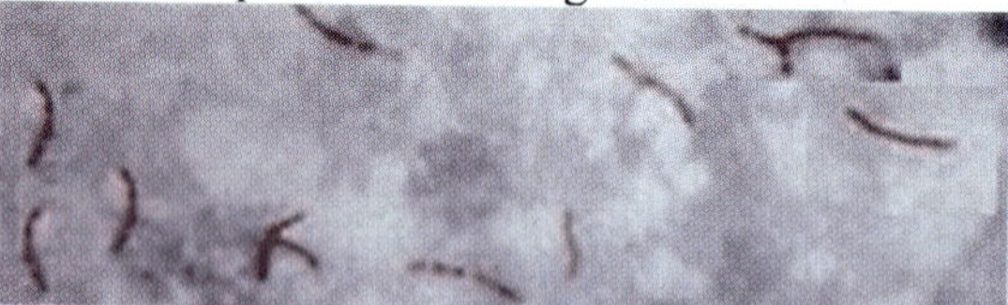

Figure-10: Beaded forms under ZN stain

- **Summary of ZN stain: →Table -6**

Albert stain

- **History & meaning:** So **called** because it was discovered by Albert (1878-1930), US Physician.
- **Principle:** Albert-A stains the polar bodies & bacilli followed by mordant effect of Albert-B
- **Reagent:**
  - Albert-A: Contain toludine blue & malachite green
  - Albert-B: Contain iodine
- **Steps:**
  - Cover the smear with Albert-A for 5 minutes.
  - Wash with water
  - Cover the smear with Albert-B for 1 minute
  - Wash and blot the slide with absorbing paper.
  - Apply a drop of cedar wood oil.
  - Focus under oil immersion lens
- **Action of ingredients & result:**

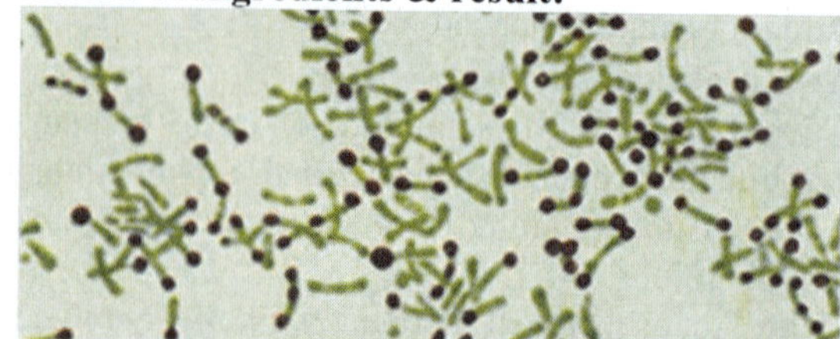

Figure-11: Polar bodies under Albert's stain

- Toludine blue stain the granules in bluish black & malachite green stains the bacillary body in green colour as shown in **fig.11**.
- Iodine act as mordant.

Reagents	Time	Action	Acid-fast organism	Non acid-fast organism
Carbol fuchsin & heat	5 minutes	Phenol in carbolic acid acts as chemical mordant & heat as physical mordant. Basic dye stain all cell in pink colour	Red/pink	Red/pink
Acid - alcohol / acid	15 seconds	Decolouriser	Red/pink	Colourless
Methylene blue	1 minute	Counter-stain	Red/pink	Blue

Table-6: Summary of ZN stain

- **Use:**
- To stain the polar bodies (Also **called metachromatic granules / volutin granules / Babes-Ernst granules**) in bacteria.
- Demonstration of polar bodies is done by Albert stain & other stains like Loeffler's methylene blue (Stain reddish violet), Neisser's stain & Ponder's stain.
- Bacteria contain polar bodies are *Corynebacterium diphtheriae* (causing diphtheria), *Corynebacterium xerosi, Mycobacterium leprae* (may be), *Bordetella pertusis, Gardnerella vaginalis,* & *Spirillum volutin.*

Question bank

Essay/Full question

1) Microscopy and staining in microbiology

Short notes

1) Light microscopy
2) Fluorescent microscopy
3) Gram stain
4) Acid fast stain
5) ZN stain
6) Acid fastness

Short questions for theory/viva questions

1) Define: Magnification power & resolution power of microscope.
2) Write the advantage of oil application on smear in microscopy
3) How you can take care of light microscope?
4) What is fluorescence?
5) What is vital & supravital stain? Write one example of each.
6) What is gram variable reaction?
7) Comment: Strictly it's not correct to classify *Mycobacteria* as GPB.
8) Name the physical & chemical mordant of ZN stain.
9) Name the four acid fast parasites.

MCQs for chapter review

Microscopy

1) **To see the bacteria, methods used are-** (PGI-97)
(a) Microscopy (b) Stained preparation (c) Both (d) None
2) **Arrangement of lens from eye to source of light, in light microscope**
(a) Ocular lens: Subjective lens: Condensor lens (b) Subjective lens: Ocular lens: Condensor lens (c) Condensor lens: Subjective lens: Ocular lens (d) Subjective lens: Condensor lens: Ocular lens
3) **Light microscopy resolution-** (PGI-, Dec-05, May-12)
(a) 200nm (b) 20nm (c) 0.2nm (d) 300nm
4) **Limit of resolution with unaided eye is**
(a) 2000 micron (b) 200 micron (c) 20 micron (d) 100 micron
5) **Dark ground microscopy is used to see-** (AI-95. AI-01)
(a) Refractile organisms (b) Flagella (c) Capsule (d) Fimbriae
6) **Dye used in fluorescent microscopy -** (PGI, Dec-04)
(a) Thioflavin T (b) Congo red (c) Brilliant blue (d) Eosin (e) Auramine

Staining

7) **One of the following staining method is an example of negative staining-** (PGI-99)
(a) Gram staining (b) Fontana's staining (c) Indian ink preparation (d) Ziehl-Neelsen staining
8) **In negative staining-** (AI-95)
(a) The structure to be demonstrated is stained (b) The structure to be demonstrated is not stained (c) The background is not stained (d) The background and structure are stained
9) **Wet Indian ink preparation is used for demonstration of-**
(a) Flagella (b) Capsule (c) Spirochetes (d) Fimbriae
10) **Sliver impregnation technique is used in the diagnosis of**
(a) Spirochetes (b) *Leptospira* (c) *Borrelia* (d) All of above
11) **Not used in gram staining**
(a) Methylene blue (b) Crystal violet (c) Iodine (d) Safranin
12) **Correct order of gram staining is**
(a) Methyl Violet → Iodine → Acetone (b) Methyl Violet → Acetone → Iodine (c) Methyl Violet → Basic fuchsin → Iodine (d) Methyl Violet → Iodine → Basic fuchsin
13) **Not a components of gram stain**
(a) Methylene blue (b) Ethanol (c) Iodine (d) Gentian Violet
14) **Gram negative stains in pink colour because of**
(a) Polysaccharide (b) Lipopolysaccharide (c) Techoic acid (d) None
15) **Following are gram negative cocci except-**
(a) Pneumococci (b) Meningococci (c) Gonococci (d) *Veillonella*
16) **H_2SO_4 concentration to stain *M. leprae* is-**
(a) 1% (b) 5% (c) 10% (d) 25%
17) ***Mycobacteria* can be diagnosed on microscopy when counts are-**
(a) 10,000 or more / ml (b) 1, 00,000 or more / ml (c) 1000 or more / ml (d) 10 or more / ml
18) **All of the following are acid fast except-**
(a) *Cryptosporidia* (b) *Mycoplasma* (c) *Mycobacteria* (d) *Nocardia*
19) **Acid fast structure is**
(a) *Vibrio* (b) *Nocardia* (c) *E coli* (d) *Bacillus anthracis*
20) **Albert stain is used for-**
(a) *Staphylococcus* (b) *Corynebacterium diphtheriae* (c) *Cl perfrigenes* (d) *Cl tetani*
21) **Metachromatic granules are found in -** (PGI-00)
(a) Diphtheria (b) *Mycoplasma* (c) *Gardnerella vaginalis* (d) *Staphylococcus*
22) **Metachromatic granules are stained by -**
(a) Ponder's stain (b) Negative stain (c) Gram's stain (d) Leishman stain

Answers of MCQs & explanation

1) **(a) & (b)**
- Bacteria are best visible by microscope with stained smear

2) **(a)**
- Follow section, **light microscope (fig.-1)** for explanation

3) **(a)** } Follow section light microscope (Resolution
4) **(b)** } power of microscope) for explanation
5) **(b)**
- Follow section, **dark ground (field) microscopy (uses)** for explanation

6) **(e)**
- Follow section fluorescent microscopy (types) for explanation

7) **(c)** }
8) **(b)** } Follow section, **staining (negative staining)**
9) **(b) & (c)** } for explanation
10) **(d)**
- Follow section, **staining (impregnation staining)** for explanation

11) **(a)**
- Follow section, **gram stain (principle)** for explanation

12) **(a)** } Follow **gram stain (KB method → steps)**
13) **(a)** } for explanation
14) **(b)**
- Follow **gram stain (theories)** for explanation

15) **(a)**
- Follow **table-1** for explanation

16) **(b)**
- Follow **table-4** for explanation

17) **(a)**
- Microscopy by ZN stain is less sensitive than culture for diagnosis of *Mycobacteria*, because at least 10,000 (10^4) bacilli should be present per ml of sputum for demonstration in direct smear, while culture can detect 10-100 bacilli per ml

18) **(b)** } Follow section, **ZN stain (uses & table-4 & 5)**
19) **(b)** } for explanation
20) **(b)** }
21) **(a) & (c)** } Follow section, **Albert stain (use)** for explanation
22) **(a)** }

4 Morphology of bacteria

Learning heading & subheadings

- Size of bacteria :
- Shape of bacteria:
- Arrangement of bacteria:
- Morphological parts (Anatomy) of bacteria:

Bacterial cell wall
Cytoplasmic / plasma membrane
Cytoplasm & cytoplasmic inclusions
Capsule & slime layer
Flagella
Fimbriae
Bacterial spores
Pleomorphism & involution forms

Size of bacteria:

➢ **Method to measure the size of bacteria:**

- Method to measure the size of bacteria **called micrometry.**
- Measuring unit **called micrometre** or **micron** (**µm** or **µ**).

➢ **Size of different bacteria:**

- **Coccus:** 0.5-1µm
- **Bacillus:** 0.2-0.5µm in breadth x 1-6 µm in length.
- **Coccobacillus:** 0.2-0.5µm in breadth x 0.5-1µm in length.
- **Spirochetes:** Very large up to 10 -20µm in length.
- **Pleomorphic bacteria:** Variable in size & shape.

Shape of bacteria: → Fig.-1

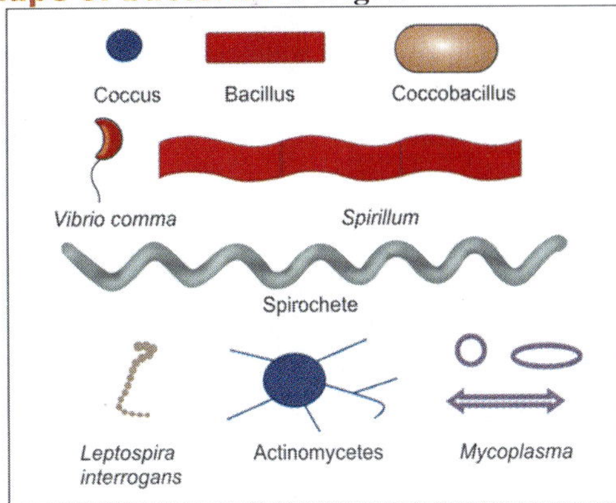

Figure-1: Shape of bacteria

1. **Coccus: From kokkos (Greek) = berry,** indicating spherical shape.
2. **Bacillus: From baculus (Latin) = rod,** indicating straight rod shape.
3. **Coccobacillus:** Indicating oval shape (intermediate between coccus & bacillus).
4. ***Vibrio comma*: Vibrio From vibrare = vibrating nature + comma = curved rods like comma** Indicating comma shaped & motile bacillus.
5. **Spirillum:** Rigid spiral forms
6. **Spirochete: From speira = coil + chaite = hair,** flexuous spiral forms.
7. ***Leptospira interrogans*:** Shape like interrogation mark or umbrella hook.
8. **Actinomycetes: Actino from actis = rays + mycetes from mykes (Greek) = branching like fungi.** It indicates the characteristic sun ray appearance & branching nature of bacterium.
9. ***Mycoplasma*:** Myco from **Mykes (Greek) = branching/filamentous form + Plasma = plasticity of nature.** Cell wall deficient bacteria & because of plasticity of nature assume any shape like spherical, oval, rod, balloon, filamentous etc.

Arrangement of bacteria:

A. Arrangement of cocci: → Fig.-2

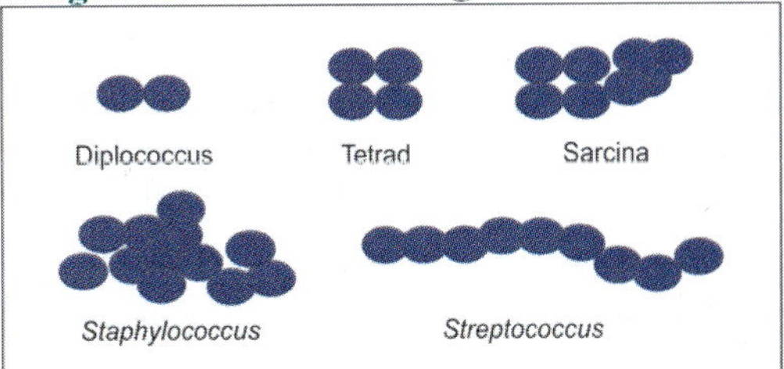

Figure-2: Arrangement of cocci

1. **Diplococcus:** In pair / group of two like pneumococci, meningococci, gonococci
2. **Tetrad:** Group of four
3. **Sarcina:** Group of eight
4. ***Staphylococcus*:** Grapes like cluster
5. ***Streptococcus*:** In chains

B. Arrangement of bacilli: →Fig.- 3

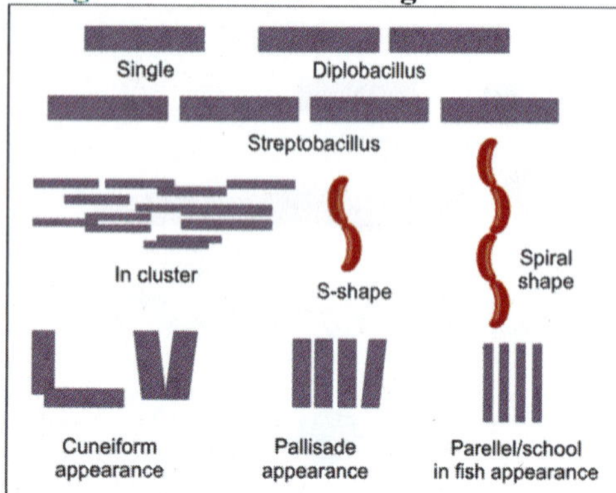

Figure-3: Arrangement of bacilli

1. **Singly:** Like *E. coli*
2. **Diplobacillus:** In pair like *Klebsiella pneumoniae & Moraxella lacunata*
3. **Streptobacillus:** In chain
4. **In group or in cluster:** Like *E. coli, S. typhi*
5. **S-shape:** Two comma shape bacilli arranged end-to end gives S-shape appearance in *V. cholerae* (*V comma*)
6. **Spiral shape:** Many comma shape bacilli arranged end-to end gives spiral-shape appearance in *V. cholerae* (*V comma*)
7. **Chinese latter or cuneiform pattern:** Bacilli arranged by making an angle to each other like Chinese letter V or L in *C. diphtheriae*
8. **Pallisade:** Like stakes of fence in *C. diphtheriae*
9. **Fish in stream/ school of fish:** Parallel to each other **called fish in stream** in *V. cholerae* and **school of fish** in *H. ducreyi*

Morphological parts (Anatomy) of bacteria:

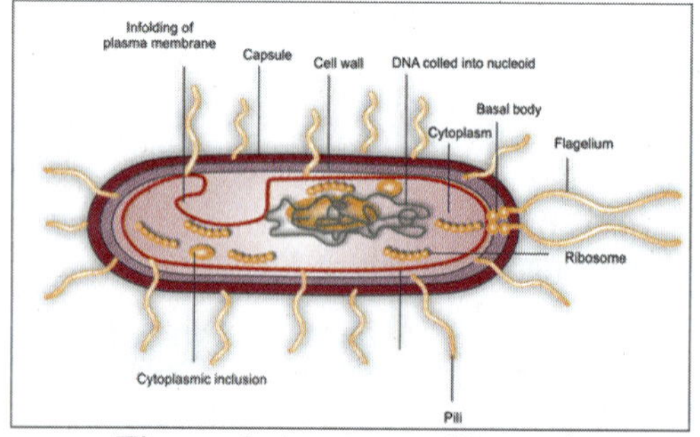

Figure-4: Anatomy of bacteria

It includes organs **(fig.-4)** like

◊ **Bacterial cell wall:**
◊ **Cytoplasmic / plasma membrane:**
} Collectively **called cell envelop** or **outer layer**

◊ **Protoplasm:**
◊ **capsule & slime layer:**
◊ **Flagella:**
} Appendages of cell wall
◊ **Fimbriae:**
◊ **Spores:**
◊ **Pleomorphism & involution forms:**

Bacterial cell wall

➢ **Properties:**
- Tough & rigid, surrounding the bacterium as like a shell.
- Size: 10-25 nm thick & hold the 20-30% of the dry weight of the cell.
- It is absent in some bacteria discussed later in this half

➢ **Cell wall antigen:**
- It **called somatic antigen**
- It is abbreviated as O-Ag, from **Ohne Hauch (German) = without film of breath.** It is opposite to **Hauch (German) = with film of breath** for flagellar antigen (Vide infra)

➢ **Functions of cell wall:**
1. Provide rigidity to cell
2. Maintain the bacterial shape
3. Plays fundamental role in vital activity of bacteria
4. Carries the bacterial antigen, play role in virulence & immunity
5. Provide mechanical support to cell membrane
6. Contain protein (**called porin protein**) which makes the porin channel for diffusion of material to & fro by bacteria
7. Helps to maintain osmotic pressure & protects cell against osmotic damage
8. Provide site for the phage absorption
9. Take part in cell division

➢ **Biochemistry of cell wall:**

A Cell wall of gram positive bacteria: → Fig.-5 & 6

✪ **Size:** Thick (80 nm)

✪ **Structure**

- **Layer:** Only one layer **called peptidoglycan** or **mucopeptide** or **mucoprotein** or **murein.** Thick peptidoglycan is composed of alternating unit of N-acetyl muramic acid (NAM) & N-acetyl glucosamine (NAG) linked together by beta-1-4 linkage & a set of tetra peptide side chain attached to N-acetyle muramic acid. Tetrapeptide chain attaches together by penta-peptide bridges as shown in **fig.-5.**
- **Teichoic acid:**
  - Types: Two types

1. **Cell wall teichoic acid:** Cell wall teichoic acid is polymer of ribitol (5-carbon) & covalently linked to peptidoglycan of cell wall as shown in **fig.-6.**
2. **Membrane teichoic acid:** Membrane teichoic acid is polymer of glycerol (3-carbon) & linked to

glycolipid of cytoplasmic membrane so also **called lipotechoic acid** as shown in **fig.-6.**

- Functions:
  - Teichoic acid helps to synthesize the peptidoglycan
  - Organ of adhesion: To adhere with host cell.
- **Surface proteins:** Like M,T, R proteins are useful for grouping the bacteria & for virulence

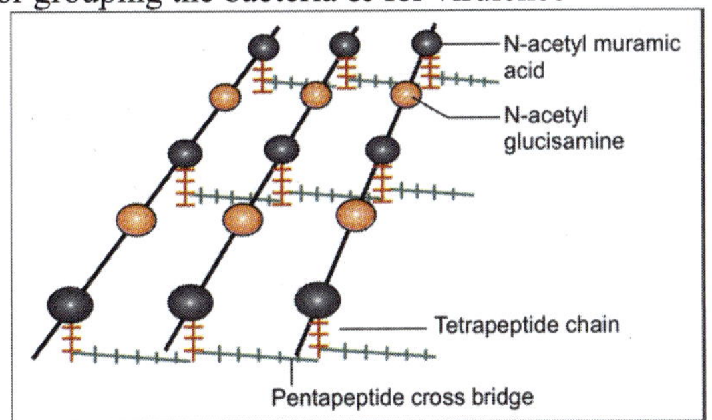

Figure-5: Peptidoglycan/murein

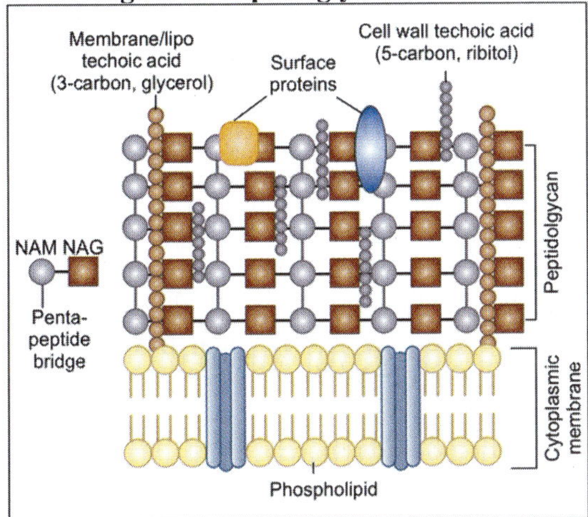

Figure-6: Gram positive cell wall

B Cell wall of gram negative bacteria: →Fig.-7 & 8

- **Size:** Thin (2nm)
- **Structure (layers):** Four layers from inner to outer are periplasmic space, thin peptidoglycan layer, Outer Membrane Protein (OMP) & Lipopolysaccharide (LPS) as shown in **fig.-7**.

i. **Periplasmic space:** Outer to plasma membrane contain enzymes

ii. **Peptidoglycan layer:** Very thin

iii. **Outer Membrane Protein (OMP):** Made up by phospholipids, surface proteins & lipoproteins.

- Phospholipids: Are similar to plasma membrane
- Surface proteins:
  - Synonym: Also **called major membrane protein or principal membrane protein.**
  - Types: Two types of proteins

1. **Porin protein:** Makes porin channel for diffusion of material to & fro by bacteria
2. **Non-porin protein:** Help as organ of adhesion, helps in production of exoenzymes & also provide receptors for antibiotic agents. e.g. Penicillin Binding Proteins (PBP)

- Lipoproteins: OMP attach to peptidoglycan by lipoproteins.

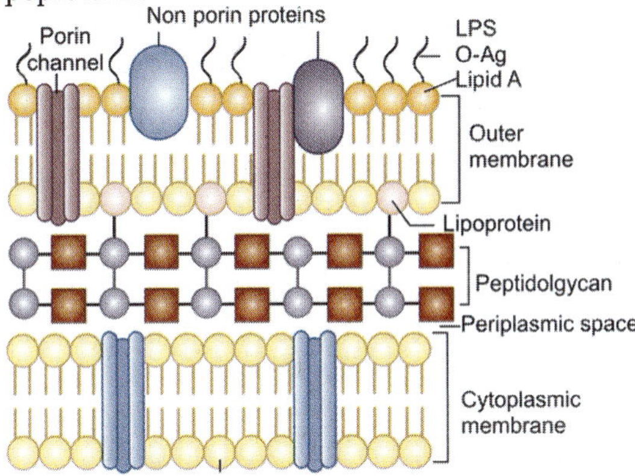

Figure-7: Gram negative cell wall

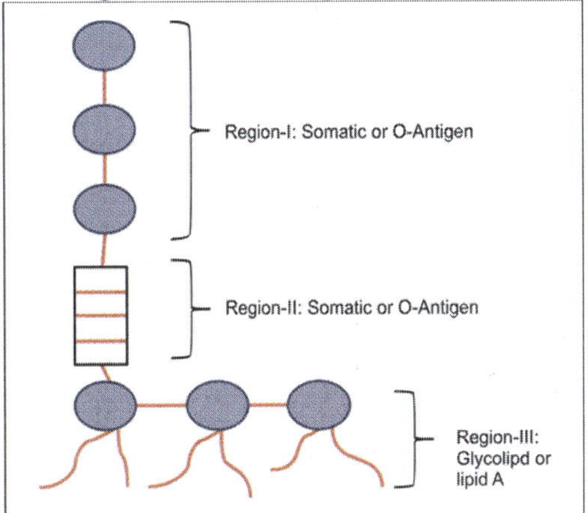

Figure-8: LPS structure

iv. **Lipopolysaccharide:** Three region as shown in **fig.-8**

1. **Region-I:**
   - Somatic/O-Antigen
   - Formerly **called Bovine-Ag**
   - It is responsible for O-Antigen specificity & typing
2. **Region-II:** Core polysaccharide
3. **Region-III:** Glycolipid or lipid A responsible for endotoxic activity like fever, shock, collapse, haemorrhage, necrosis, lethal effect, anticomplementary effect, B cell mitogenicity, antitumour activity.

C. Cell wall of acid-fast bacteria: Contains three layers (*Mycobacterium* spp. *Nocardia* spp. etc.) from inner to outer are peptidoglycan, polysaccharide & fatty acids (glycolipid).

i. **Peptidoglycan:** Similar to gram negative bacterial cell wall and link to polysaccharide layer by phosphodiester bond

ii. **Polysaccharide:** Layer **called arabinogalactan** & linked to mycolic acids

iii. **Fatty acid (glycolipid):**

- Responsible for acid fastness

- Glycolipid is the major part in cell wall which account 60% of the dry weight of cell wall
- It **called mycolic acid** in *Mycobacteria* & **nocardic acid** in *Nocardia* (unique mycolic / nocradic acid 6, 6 □ dimycolyltrehalose **called cord factor**)
- Mycolic acid or cord factor in *Mycobacteria* is act as virulence factor & responsible for cell membrane cytotoxicity, inhibition of PMNs migration, granuloma formation & activation of complement pathway
- Peptidoglycan-polysaccharide-mycolic acid complex forms the skeleton in cell wall of *Mycobacteria,* so acid fastness in *Mycobacteria* is not the property of mycolic acid alone, but depends also on the integrity of cell wall

✓ **Notes: Cell wall of *Corynebacterium***

- Some workers noticed the presence of acid fast cell wall in *Corynebacterium* with three layers as mentioned above where the glycolipid **called corynemycolenic acid.**

➢ **Differences between gram positive & negative bacterial cell wall: → Table-1**

Characteristics	Gram +Ve	Gram -Ve
Thickness	Thicker	Thin
Aminoacids (AA)	Few	Several
Aromatic & sulphur containing AA	-	+
Lipids	-, Or scanty	+
Techoic acid	+	-

Table-1: Differences between gram positive & negative bacterial cell wall

➢ **Demonstration of cell wall:**

- Plasmolysis: When bacteria placed in hypertonic solution it loss the cytoplasm **called plasmolysis** but cell wall retain it's size & shape such cell **called bacterial ghost**
- Micro dissection
- By mechanical rupture of cell wall
- Differential staining
- Reaction with antibody
- Electron microscopy

➢ **Inhibition of cell wall synthesis:** Bacteria without cell wall **called cell wall deficient bacteria**

✪ **Causes:** Cell wall synthesis is inhibited by

- Naturally cell wall absent: *Mycoplasma* spp.
- Antibiotics like penicillin
- Viruses like bacteriophage
- Enzymes like lysozyme or
- Spontaneously loss of cell wall

✪ **Clinical significances:** Absence of cell wall create following issues in bacterial infections

- Difficulty in diagnosis: They are difficult to cultivate & require agar containing solid medium having right osmotic strength.
- Difficulty in treatment: Cell wall deficient form of bacteria is ineffective to antibiotics. Sometimes it appears after treatment with penicillin.
- Persistence of infection: They are not causing the disease but causing persistence of certain chronic infection: such as pyelonephritis.
- Recurrence: Cause recurrence of infection

✪ **Types:** Four types of cell wall deficient bacteria as follows

A **Protoplast:**

- Produced artificially by allowing lysozyme action on gram positive bacteria in a hypertonic medium.
- Spherical in shape.
- Total loss of cell wall & cytoplasmic membrane hold the contents of cell.

B **Spheroplast:**

- Produced artificially by allowing lysozyme action on gram negative bacteria in a hypertonic medium.
- Spherical in shape.
- Partial loss of cell wall & some cell wall structures are retained.

C **L-forms:**

- **Meaning:** From Lister institute, London
- **History:** Kleinberger (Nobel Prize) while studying the culture of *Streptobacillus moniliformis* in the Lister institute, London, observed cell wall deficient, swollen, morphologically abnormal forms of the bacteria & named them L-forms after the Lister institute in 1941.
- **Types of L-forms:**

i. **According to induction:**

1. **Spontaneous type:** Sudden development
2. **Induced type:** By some agents like penicillin

ii. **According to durability:**

1. **Unstable:** Revert to original forms
2. **Stable:** Irreversible

- **Examples of bacteria showing L-forms:** *Staph. aureus, N. gonorrhoea, M. tuberculosis* & *Streptobacillus moniliformis*

D ***Mycoplasma*:** Follow chapter → Mycoplasmatales for more details

Cytoplasmic / plasma membrane

➢ **Properties:**

- Inner to cell wall
- It is elastic 5 -10 nm in size
- Semipermeable layer
- Always present in bacteria

➢ **Functions:**

- Acts as semipermeable layer & controls the inflow & outflow of metabolites
- It participates in active transport of selective nutrients by enzyme **permease**
- It contains enzymes required for respiratory activity to generate energy (ATP) by electron transport & oxidative phosphorylation

- Participate in synthesis of cell wall components like Peptidoglycan & OMP
- Function in synthesis of bacterial toxins & other bacterial enzymes
- Provide energy for flagellar movement & chromosomal mobilisation

➢ **Mesosomes (infolding of plasma membrane or Chondroids): →Figure-4**

✪ **Definition:**

- Invagination of the plasma membrane in to the cytoplasm **called condroids** or **mesosomes**
- They are more prominent in gram positive bacteria

✪ **Functions:**

1. Provide more surface area for anabolic & catabolic activity
2. Center for respiratory enzymes & helps in respiration
3. Act as an analogues for mitochondria in cell
4. Take part in DNA replication & cell division or binary division

➢ **Biochemistry of cytoplasmic membrane:**

- Shows the presence of phospholipids (30-60%), protein (50-70%) & carbohydrates.
- Sterol (cholesterol or ergosterol) is absent except in *Mycoplasma* spp. & *Ureaplasma urealyticum*.

➢ **Demonstration of cytoplasmic membrane:** Revealed by Electron Microscopy (EM)

Protoplasm

➢ **Definitions:**

✪ **Protoplasm:** Mixture of plasma membrane, cytoplasm, nucleus & nucleoplasm **called protoplasm.**

✪ **Cytoplasm:** Jelly like substance presents inner to plasma membrane but outer to nucleus **called cytoplasm.**

✪ **Nucleoplasm:** Jelly like substance presents inner to nucleus **called nucleoplasm.** Nucleus & nucleoplasm are absent in bacteria.

✓ **Notes: Eukaryotes & prokaryotes**

▪ In eukaryotes nucleus is present but in prokaryotes nucleus is absent, so we can say that nucleoplasm is absent or cytoplasm act as nucleoplasm which contains chromatin (chromosome, plasmid, episome & transposon).

Plasma membrane

Described above

Cytoplasm

- **Properties:**
- It is a colloidal system contains organic & inorganic solutes in a viscous watery solution
- Organelles like endoplasmic reticulum, mitochondria etc. are absent in bacteria.
- Cytoplasmic motility **called cytoplasmic (protoplasmic) streaming** is absent in bacteria unlike eukaryotic cell.
- Stains uniformly with basic dyes in young culture

- **Intracytoplasmic inclusion/ cytoplasmic matrix:**

a. Ribosomes:

- It is tiny granules scattered in cytoplasm.
- Made up of two subunit larger (50 s) & smaller (30s).
- Function: site for protein synthesis

b. Polar bodies:

○ Location in bacillar body: Situated at both poles of bacilli hence **called polar bodies.**

○ Synonym: Also

- **Called metachromatic granules:** Because they had the property of changing the colour of basic blue dyes used in light microscopy.
- **Called volutin granules:** Because they were 1st identified from *Spirillum volutans* by Meyer (1904)
- **Called Babes-Ernst granules**

○ Biochemistry:

- Composed of polymetaphosphate
- Strongly basophilic

○ Function: It act as energy & phosphate store house required in conditions with nutritional deficiency. It disappear when deficient nutrients are supplied.

○ Demonstration of polar bodies: For more details, **Follow chapter → Microscopy and staining (Albert stain → use)**

○ Bacteria contain polar bodies: For more details, **Follow chapter → Microscopy and staining (Albert stain → use)**

c. Polysaccharide granules: Stained by iodine. It act as storage product.

d. Fat globules/lipid globules:

- Act as energy storage product
- It contains lipid + poly metaphosphate (volition granules) + crystalline protein
- Present only in vegetative stage & makes confusion with spores
- Stains to differentiate spores & fat globules → **Table -2**

Staining method	Reagents	Spore	Fat globules
Ashby's method	Malachite green	Green spore & red bacilli	Unstained
Burdon's method	Sudan black B	Unstained	Blue-black
Holbrook & Anderson method	Malachite green + Sudan black B	Green spore & red bacilli	Blue-black
Modified acid fast	0.25 % H_2SO_4	Red spore & colour-less bacilli	Red

Table-2: Stains to differentiate spores & fat globules

e. Chomosome:
- Shape: Appear as oval or elongated body
- Numbers: Generally one percell or two or more
- Demonstration: By Acid hydrolysis or by EM
- Contains: Single-circular ds-DNA
- Functions:
- It controls the growth, multiplication & metabolism of cell.
- It controls the hereditary transmission of genetic information.

f. Plasmid:
- Extrachromosomal Intracytoplasmic DNA containing material **called plasmid**
- Serve for toxin production, drug resistance & other virulence purpose

g. Episomes: Type of plasmid which links with chromosomes

h. Jumping genes or transposons: Plasmid jump in-between chromosomal & extrachromosomal part **called jumping genes** or **transposons.**

Capsule & slime layer

➢ **Definitions:**
- **Capsule:** Many bacteria secrete the viscid materials around it which organize in a sharply defined structure **called capsule (fig.-9).**
- **Microcapsule:** Capsule is too thin to be seen under microscope **called microcapsule**
- **Slime layer:** Many bacteria secrete the viscid materials around it which remains loose, unorganise as ill-defined structure **called slime layer.**

➢ **Capsular antigen:** It abbreviated as K from Kapsel (**German** language for capsule)

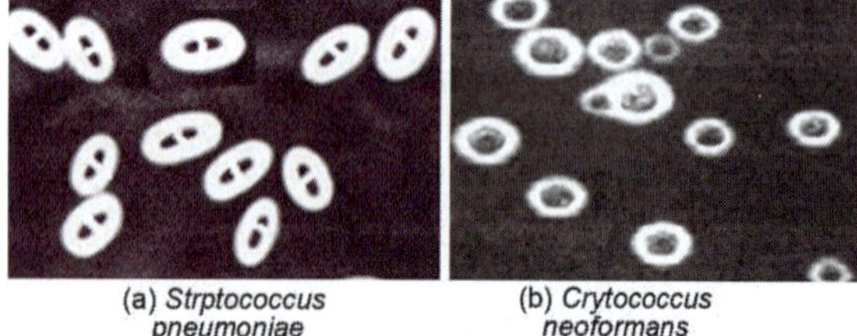

Figure-9: Capsule under Indian ink

➢ **Examples of microorganisms containing capsule & slime layer:**

i. Capsule:

a. Capsulated bacteria:
1. *Staph. aureus:* Some strains
2. *Streptcoccus* species:
- **α-Haemolytic (Viridans group):**
  - *Strept. mutans* (No Lancefield grouping)
  - Other species of viridans group are non capsulated
- **β-Haemolytic:**
  - *Strept. pyogenes* (Lancefield Group A)
  - *Strept. agalactiae* (Lancefield Group B)
  - *Strept. equisimilis* (Lancefield Group C)
- **Non haemolytic (Enterococcus group):**
  - *Enterococcus spp.* (Lancefield Group D)
3. *Strept. pneumoniae*
4. *Anthrax bacilli*
5. *Clostridium welchii*
6. *Neisseria meningitidis*
7. *E. coli:* In some strain
8. *Klebsiella pneumoniae, K. granulomatis* & other species.
9. *Enterobacter* spp.
10. *Yersinia enterocolitica:* In vivo but not in culture
11. *Aeromonas hydrophila*
12. *Vibrio cholerae* O139
13. *Haemophilus influenzae* & other species
14. *Pasteurella multocida*
15. *Bordetella pertusis* (No role in virulence)
16. *Bacteroides fragilis*

b. Capsulated fungus: *Cryptococcus neoformans*

ii. Slime layer containing bacteria:
1. *Leuconostoc*
2. *Pseudomonas aeruginosa*
3. *Yersinia pestis*
4. *Rickettsia* spp.

iii. Both capsule & slime layer containing bacteria:
1. *Strept. salivarius*

➢ **Biochemistry:**
- **Polysaccharides:** It is polysaccharides (glucan, dextran, levans) in nature in almost all bacteria
- **Polypeptide:** In *Anthrax bacillus* capsule is poly-peptide (d- glutamic acid) in nature
- **Protein:** In *Yersinia pestis* it is protein in nature
- **Hyaluronic acid:** In some strains of *Strept. pyogenes* (Lancefield Group A) & some strains of *Strept. equisimilis* (Lancefield Group C) capsule is hyaluronic acid in nature

➢ **Functions:**
1. **Inhibition of phagocytosis:** Enhance bacterial virulence by inhibiting phagocytosis, however capsule of *Bordetella pertusis* does not contribute in virulence.
2. **Protection:** Acts as protecting covering & protect bacteria against lysozyme, bacteriophages, colicins, antibodies, antibiotics, heavy metals, free radicals, complement action & also against desiccation.
3. **Breakdown of dietary fibres: →Flow chart-1**

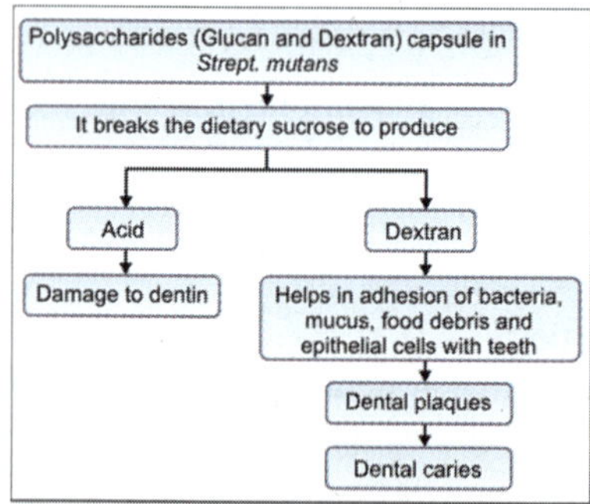

Flow chart-1: Breakdown of dietary sucrose

4. **Absscess formation:** Capsule of certain bacteria like *Bacteroides fragilis* is toxic in nature & responsible for abscess formation.
5. **Adhesion:** Helps in adhesion of bacteria with the host cells
6. **Source of energy & nutrition:** Attract the nutritional materials at cell surface because of polyanionic nature.
7. **Biofilms formation:** Help in colonisation of bacteria with hospital devices or instruments **called biofilms.**
8. **Vaccine preparation:** Capsule is antigenic in nature & produces protective antibodies. This principle helps to prepare the vaccine for pneumococci, meningococci & *H. influenzae* serotype-b.
9. **Diagnosis:** Antigenic in nature helps in identification & typing of bacteria.

➢ **Demonstration:** Very thin to see under the microscope **called microcapsule.** Following methods are useful.

a. **Microscopy:**
1. **Negative stains:** Like Indian ink (**fig.9**), nigrosin & Manveal stain.
2. **Gram stain:** Slime layer (even capsule also) has little affinity for basic dyes, so not visible under gram stain. Capsule is sometimes demonstrated under gram stain.
3. **Special stains:** For capsule of *Anthrax bacilli*

- **Giemsa stain:** Capsule appears in red color
- **Indian ink:** Capsule appears as clear halo around the bacilli
- **Methylene blue:** Capsule appears as purplish materials around the bacilli **called M'Fadyean's reaction.**

b. **Culture:** Mucoid colonies by capsulated bacteria.

c. **Serological test:** By **Quellung reaction or Capsular swelling**, Neufeld, 1902
- Mix capsulated strain with specific anti-capsular serum on slide & examined under microscope.
- Capsule becomes prominent & gets swell due to increase in refractivity.

➢ **Enhancement of capsule production**
1. **In *A. bacilli*:**
- In presence of 10-25% CO_2: When media contains biocarbonate
- In absence of CO_2: When media are enriched with serum, albumin, charcoal or starch.
2. **In *C. neoformans*:** By growing the fungus on chocolate agar at 37^0C in a CO_2 incubator

➢ **Inhibition of capsule synthesis (loss of capsule):**
- **Mechanisms:**
  - Due to mutation
  - Due to repeated subculture
- **Clinical significance:** Capsule has virulent property & loss of capsule change virulent strain to avirulent strain.

Flagella

➢ **Definition:** One or more, long, unbranched, wavy, filamentous structures for movement of organism **called flagella.**

➢ **Flagellar Ag:** It is abbreviated as H-Ag from **Hauch (German) = film of breath,** as growth of motile bacteria looks like film of breath on glass surface.

➢ **Properties:**
- 3-20 µm long & uniform diameter (0.1-0.013 µm)
- Terminate in square tip.

➢ **Types of bacteria according to location of flagella: →Flow chart-2 & fig.-10.**

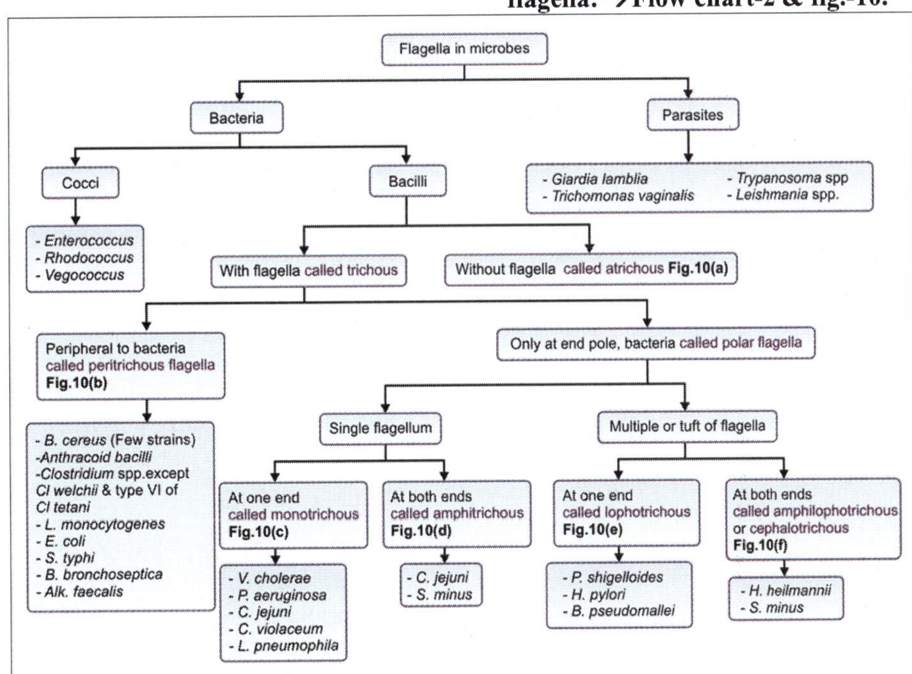

Flow chart-2: Types of bacteria according to location of flagella

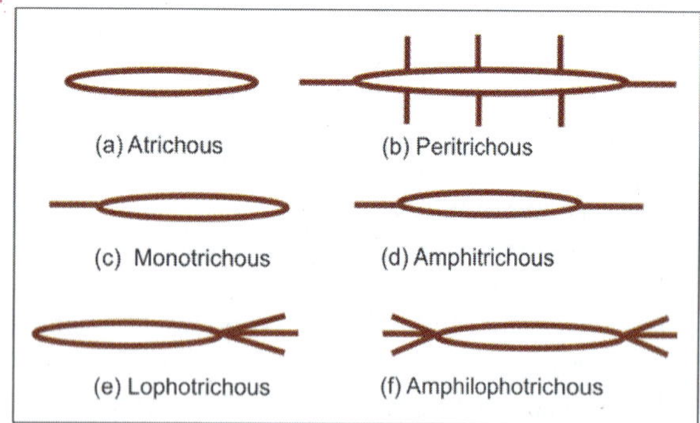

Figure-10: Types of bacteria according to location of flagella

- **Biochemistry:** Chemically flagella are composed of protein **called flagellin**, alike keratin & myosin. It has three parts **(fig.-11).**

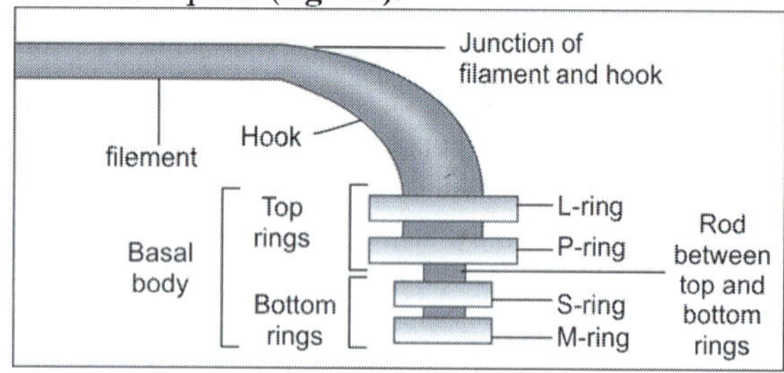

Figure-11: Parts of flagella

1. **Basal body:** It is a circular structure embedded in the cell envelope consist a central rod which bearing four rings like
   - M-ring: Embedded in the cell membrane.
   - S-ring: Embedded in the periplasmic space.
   - P-ring: Embedded in the peptidoglycan
   - L-ring: Embedded in the lipopolysaccharide.
2. **Hook:** is short curved structure connecting the filament & basal body. It is broader than the filament, protein in nature different from flagellin & embedded in cell envelop.
3. **Filament:** external to the cell & made up of flagellin.

- **Functions:**

1. **Organ of locomotion:**
   - Movement of bacterium towards nutrients **called chemotaxis**
   - Movement of bacterium towards air **called aerotaxis**
   - Movement of bacterium towards light **called phototaxis**
2. **Constitute the flagellar (H) antigen:** It produces the antibody which is useful for diagnosis & typing of bacteria.

- **Demonstration:**

i. Microscopy & staining methods:

a. Light microscopy:

1. **Wet mount:** Under low/high power
   - Hanging drop preparation by using concavity slide
   - Ryu's stain (Crystal violet & tannic acid as mordant)
2. **Impregnation technique:**
   - Thickness of the flagella are increased by coating them with mordants like tannic acid and potassium alum and staining them with
     - Basic fuchsin (**called Gray method**) or
     - Pararosaniline (**called Leifson method**) or
     - Silver nitrate (**called West method**) or
     - Crystal violet (**called Difco's method**).
   - Although flagella staining procedures are difficult to carry out, they often provide information about the presence and location of flagella which is of great value in bacterial identification.

b. Dark Ground Illumination Microscopy (DGIM)

c. Electron Microscope (EM)

ii. Culture methods:

a. Semi-solid media: (0.2-0.5% or 1% agar)

1. **Semisolid stab agar method:**
2. **By using Craigie's tube:**
3. **U-tube technique:**

} Follow chapter → Culture methods for more details

b. Solid media: (2-4% agar) →Spreading/swarming colony on solid agar

iii. Serological tests: By using specific antiserum

- **Different types of motility shown by bacteria:**

1. **Stately motility:** *Clostridium* spp. except. *Cl. welchii* & *Cl. tetani* type VI.
2. **Active motility:** *E. coli, Proteus bacilli, S. typhi* & *L. interrogans*
3. **Tumbling motility:** *L. monocytogenes* at 25^{0}C but not at 37^{0}C (**called differential motility** due to temperature dependent flagellar expression) & *C. jejuni.*
4. **Darting motility:** *V. cholerae, C. jejuni* & *S. minus*
5. **Flexion & extension:**
6. **Translatory motility:** } *T. pallidum*
7. **Cork screw motility:**
8. **Lashing motility:** *Borrelia* spp.
9. **Gliding motility:** *M. pneumoniae*
10. **Oscillatory motility:** *Cl. difficile*
11. **Swarming growth or Swarming motility:** *Proteus vulgaris, Proteus mirabilis* & *Cl. tetani*

- **Phase variation:**
  - Definition: Flagellar antigen (H-Ag) undergoes frequent antigenic variation **called phase variation.** 1ST observed in salmonella & later in other GNB.
  - Significance: It helps in bacterial typing.

✓ **Notes: Endo-flagella & bacteria showing motility without flagella**

- **Endo-flagella:** They are present in spirochetes like *T. pallidum* but not useful for motility and remain in periplasmic space between peptidoglycan and outer membrane.
- **Bacteria showing motility without flagella:**

1. **Brownian motility / movement:** Passive movement of bacteria not due to flagella but due to air current or by fluid movement.
2. **Sluggish motility:** *Moraxella lacunata* which are non flagellated but sluggishly motile.
3. **Jerking or twitching motility:** It occurs in *Eikenella corrodens,* not due to flagella but by contractile-fimbriae like filamentous appendages.
4. **Gliding motility:**

- *Capnocytophaga canimorsus* & other species of genus are lacking flagella but showing gliding motility, which is very difficult to observe.
- *Mycoplasma pneumoniae* is lacking flagella but showing gliding motility.

Fimbriae

➢ **Definition:** Very fine hair like surface appendages in gram negative bacteria **called fimbriae.**

➢ **Synonym:**

- Also **called pili** (singular → pilus) or **fibrillae**.
- The word sex pili are used only for fimbriae concerned with conjugation.

➢ **Fimbrial antigen** It is abbreviated as Fi Ag

➢ **Properties:**

- Shorter (0.5µm long) & thinner (0.001µm or 10 nm) & more in number than flagella as shown in **fig.-4.**
- They are unrelated to motility & are found on motile & nonmotile bacteria
- Originate from cell membrane
- Best develop in fresh culture & also in liquid media
- Loss following subculture in solid culture

➢ **Classification:**

i. **According to their function:** Fimbriae are named on basis of their function

a. **Sex pili:**

- Found in male bacterium & help to attach with female bacterium by forming a tube like structure **called conjugation tube.**
- Transfer of genetic information from one cell to other via conjugation tube **called conjugation.**
- Fimbriae help to make conjugation tube **called sex pili** & protein **called pilin**

b. **Fimbrial adhesin** or **pilus adhesin:** It is one type of adhesin, which helps the bacterium to attach with host cells & help in virulence. Following are different subtypes with special name.

1. **Colonisation Factor Antigens:** Present in ETEC & help to adhere with intestinal epithelial cells.
2. **Mannose resistant fimbriae:** Present in EHEC, specially in nephritogenic strain & help in attachment with uroepithelial cells.
3. **Toxin Co-regulated Pilus (TCP):** It present in *Vibrio cholerae* & constantly bind the *Vibrio* with host cell.
4. **Surface agglutinogen:** It favours the adhesion of *Bordetella pertusis* with respiratory epithelium.

c. **Haem Agglutinating pili (HA-pili):**

- Participation in haemagglutination reaction.
- Haemagglutination is affected by mannose & identify two subtypes
  - Type-I **called mannose sensitive:** Inhibition of haemagglutination by bacteria after incubation with mannose
  - Type-II **called mannose resistant**: No Inhibition of haemagglutination by bacteria after incubation with mannose e.g. gonococci

ii. **According to bacteriophage sensitivity:** Type F, type I etc.

➢ **Differences between flagella & fimbriae: → Table-3**

Features	Flagella	Fimbriae
Length	Long (3-20 µm)	Short (0.5µm)
Thickness	Thick (0.1-0.013 µm)	Thin (0.001µm or10 nm)
Made up by	Protein-flagellin	Protein-fimbrilin
Numbers	less	More
Organ of adhesion	No	Yes
Organ of conjugation	No	Yes
Organ of locomotion	Yes	No

Table-3: Differences between flagella & fimbriae

➢ **Biochemistry:** Made up by a protein **called fimbrilin** (*Neisseria gonorrhoea*) or by techoic acid (*Staphylococcus*) or by lipotechoic acid (*Enterococcus*) or by lipotechoic acid mixed with M protein (*Streptococcus*).

➢ **Functions:** Follow classification

➢ **Demonstration of fimbriae:** By

- Electron microscope (EM)
- By culture in liquid media: Pellicle formation
- Haemagglutination test is used for demonstration of pili in *E. coli, K. pneumoniae* etc.

➢ **Clinical significances:**

- **Antigenic** in nature & cross react with many related bacteria.
- Help to form **pellicle** in liquid media by adhering the bacteria on surface
- **Vaccine preparation:** *E. coli* diarrhoea in calves and piglets & gonorrhoea in humans are prevented by using vaccine prepared from fimbrial antigen.

Spores

➢ **Definition:** Highly resistance, resting & metabolically inactive stage of bacteria in unfavourable condition **called spores.**

➢ **Spore bearing or sporing bacteria:**

i. According to O_2 requirement of sporing bacteria:

a. Aerobic spore bearer:

1. **Cocci:** *Sporosarcina* spp. (GPC)
2. **Bacilli:** *Bacillus* spp. (GPB) & *Micromonosporum* spp. (GPB)

b. Anaerobic spore bearer:

1. **Bacilli:**
   - *Clostridium* spp. (GPB)
   - *Sporolactobacillus* spp. (GPB)

➢ **Properties:**

- Resistant to heat, chemicals, cold, desiccation & other abnormal environmental conditions.
- Spore is formed inside the bacterial cell **called endospore**
- Each bacterium forms one spore which on germination forms a single vegetative cell, hence it is not a method of reproduction.

ii. According to shape & location of spores: → Figure-12

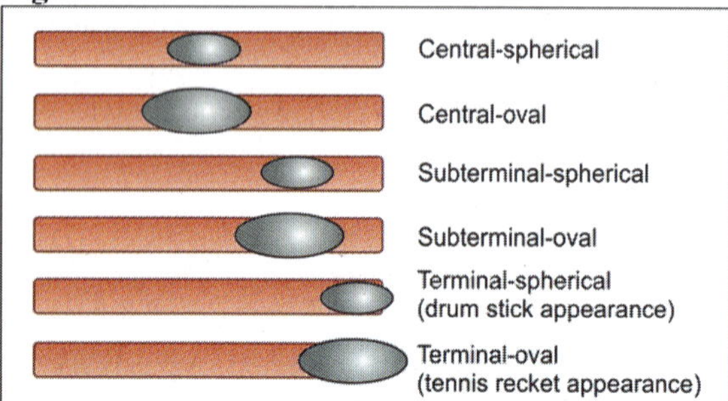

Figure-12: Shape & location of spores

a. Central/equatorial: Gives **spindle shape appearance** to bacilli like *Cl. bifermentans* & *Cl. sordelii* & *Bacillus* spp.

- Spherical (non-bulging): Same size of bacillary body like in *Bacillus* spp.
- Oval (bulging): Larger than size of bacillary body

b. Subterminal: Gives **club shape appearance** to bacilli like *Cl. perfringens* (*Cl. welchii*), *Cl. novyi, Cl. septicum, Cl. sordelii Cl. bifermentans*, *Cl. botulinum*, *Cl. sporogenes*, *Cl. histolyticum* & *Bacillus* spp.

- Spherical (non-bulging): Same size of bacillary body like in *Bacillus* spp.
- Oval (bulging): Larger than size of bacillary body

✓ **Notes: Mixed spores**

- *Cl. bifermentans* & *Cl. sordelii* produces both central & subterminal spores
- *Bacillus* spp. produces both central or subterminal, oval or elliptical spores & same in size of bacillary body (non-bulging).

c. Terminal: Two subtypes

- Spherical (non-bulging): It gives **drum stick appearance** to bacilli like *Cl. sphenoides, Cl. tetani* & *Cl. tetanomorphum*
- Oval (bulging): It gives **tennis racket appearance** to bacilli like *Cl. difficile, Cl. tertium* & *Cl. cochlearum*

➢ **Function:** Protect bacteria in unfavourable condition.

➢ **Sporicidal methods/agents:** Methods/agents which kills spores are **called sporicidal methods / agents** like

a. Physical methods (sterilisation):

1. Autoclave (121˚C at 15lbs for 15min.)
2. Hydroclaving
3. Hot air oven

b. Chemical methods (disinfection):

1. Formaldehyde
2. 2% Gluteraldehyde (Cidex): Slow action in 3-10 hrs
3. 1% Iodine (at higher concentration)
4. Chlorine tablets & sodium hypochlorite (at higher concentration)
5. Ethylene Oxide (EO)
6. H_2O_2
7. 4% $KMnO_4$
8. O-phthalic acid
9. Paracetic acid
10. Beta propiolactone
11. Ozone

c. Physical + chemical methods (Chemosterilisation):

1. Plasma sterilisation

➢ **Sporulation: →Figure-13**

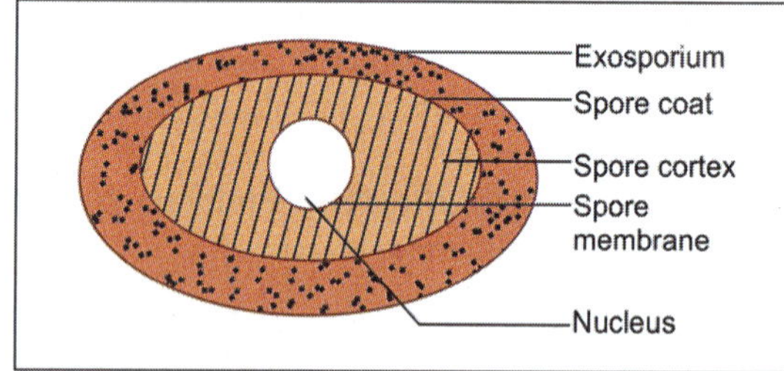

Figure-13: Spore structure

- Conversion of vegetative bacterium in to spore in unfavourable condition **called sporulation**
- Begins with appearance of clear area in the protoplasm of the cell that gradually opaque with condensation of nuclear material **called forespore or core.**
- The cell membrane grows to form **spore membrane or spore wall.**
- The cell wall grow around spore wall to form **cortex & multilayered tough spore coat.**
- Some spores have extra outer covering **called exosporium.**

➢ **Germination:** Occurs in favourable conditions Three stage involved

1. **Activation:** Occurs in nutritionally rich medium. Damage to spore coat is produced by heat, abrasion, acidity etc.

2. **Initiation:** During this stage a cortex peptidoglycan & a variety of other components are degraded, water is taking up & calcium dipiclonic acid is released.
3. **Outgrowth:** A new vegetative cell with spore protoplast emerges out. a period of active synthesis that terminates in cell division.

➢ **Use of spores:**

a. **Biological indicator:** Spores of certain species of bacteria are employed as biological indicator for proper sterilisation like
1. *Bacillus (Geobacillus) stearothermophilus:* For autoclave.
2. *Cl. tetani* (Non-toxigenic strain): For hot air oven.
3. *Bacillus subtilis* subspp. *niger:* For hot air oven.

b. **Bioterrorism:** Endospores of *Bacillus anthracis* were used in the 2001 in anthrax bioterrorism attack on USA.

➢ **Demonstration of spores:**

i. **Staining & microscopy:**

a. **Light microscopy:**
1. **Gram stain:** Coloured bacillary body with unstained spore
2. **Modified ZN stain:** Pink coloured spore

b. **Phase Contrast Microscopy:** By using wet mount

c. **Other staining & differential methods of spores with fat globules:** →**Follow Table -2**

ii. **Culture:**

a. **Culture methods for spores of *A. bacilli*:**
- **Enhancement of spore production (Sporulation):**
  - Naturally occur only in soil never in body.
  - Oxalated agar: Promoted by adding distilled water & 2% NaCl in to the medium followed by incubation at 25-30°C in presence of O_2.
- **Inhibition of sporulation:** By calcium chloride.

b. **Culture methods for spores of *Cl. welchii*:** Spores may develop in animal body. Following are the useful media
1. Phillips medium
2. Ellner's medium
3. Duncan & Strong's medium
4. Alkaline egg medium

✓ **Notes: Fungal spores**

- Spores are also present in fungus **called fungal spores**. They are exogenous **called conidia** or endogenous.

Pleomorphism & involution forms

➢ **Definitions:**

- **Pleomorphism:** Certain bacteria shows variation in size & shape **called pleomorphism.** e.g. *Cl. welchii, V. cholerae, Y. pestis, H. influenzae, B. pertusis, Mycoplasma* spp. etc.
- **Involution forms:** When variation in size & shape is present in high salt concentration medium **called involution forms.** E.g. *N. gonorrhoea, Y. pestis, Cl. welchii* etc.

➢ **Causes:** Involution forms occur in ageing culture especially due to high salt concentration. However, pleomorphism & involution forms also occur due to defective cell wall synthesis or by actions of autolytic enzymes.

Question bank

Essay/Full question

1) Morphology of bacteria

Short notes

1) Arrangement of bacteria
2) Bacterial cell wall
3) Cell wall appendages
4) Polar bodies
5) L-forms
6) Capsule / flagella / spores (Answer contains parasitic /fungal portion in addition to bacterial portion)
7) Bacterial capsule / bacterial flagella / bacterial spores (Answer contains only bacterial portion no parasitic / fungal portion)
8) Fimbriae

Short questions for theory/viva questions

1) Write the four functions of bacterial cell wall.
2) Write the four differences between gram positive & gram negative bacterial cell wall.
3) What is Bovine antigen?
4) Comment: Mycolic acid is not the alone reason for acid. fastness of *Mycobacteria.*
5) What is protoplast & spheroplast?
6) Name the four bacteria showing L-forms.
7) What are mesosomes or chondroides?
8) Write the four functions of cytoplasmic membrane.
9) Define: Protoplasm & cytoplasm
10) What are volutin granules?
11) Name the four stains for volutin granules.
12) Name the four bacteria contains volutin granules
13) Write four names of cytoplasmic inclusions.
14) What are fat globules? Name the methods used to differentiate it from bacterial spores.
15) Write the four functions of capsule.
16) Write the four examples of capsulated bacteria.
17) What is Quellung reaction or capsular swelling?
18) Write the four examples of bacteria with peritrichous flagella.
19) Write the four examples of flagellar parasites.
20) What are endoflagella?
21) Define flagella & bacterial spores.
22) Write the four examples of sporing bacteria.
23) Write the four examples of sporicidal methods.
24) What is pleomorphism & involution form?

MCQs for chapter review

MCQs

Cell wall

1) **Peptidoglycans are present in**
(a) Gram positive bacteria (b) Gram negative bacteria (c) Fungi (d) Protozoa
2) **Techoic acids**

(a) Found in gram positive bacteria (b) Make the outer wall of bacteria (c) Provide receptor for phage (d) Influence the permeability of phage

3) **Bacterial cell wall is composed of all except**
(a) Muramic acid (b) Techoic acid (c) Glucosamine (d) Mucopeptide

4) **The difference between gram +ve and gram –ve organism is that gram +ve organism contains (PGI-98)**
(a) Techoic acid (b) Muramic acid (c) N-acetyl neuramic acid (d) Aromatic amino acids

5) **Acid fastness of tubercle bacilli is attributed to-** (AIIMS 91)
(a) Presence of mycolic acid (b) Integrity of cell wall (c) Both of the above (d) None of the above

6) **Cell wall deficient organisms are-** (PGI-99)
(a) *Chlamydia* (b) *Mycoplasma* (c) *Streptococcus* (d) Anaerobes

7) **Cell wall structure found in all except-**
(a) *Staph aureus* (b) *Pseudomonas aeruginosa* (c) *Mycoplasma pneumoniae* (d) *Corynebacterium diphtheriae*

Cytoplasmic / Plasma membrane

8) **The cytoplasmic membrane of bacteria is responsible for -**
(a) Selective permeability (b) Motility (c) Cell division (d) Conjugation

9) **Which is always present in bacteria -**
(a) Cell wall (b) Cytoplasmic membrane (c) Mitochondria (d) Nucleoli

Capsule & slime layer

10) **All are capsulated bacteria except**
(a) *Neisseria* (b) *Corynebacterium* (c) *Haemophilus* (d) *Streptococcus salivarius*

11) **In which of the following organism capsule does not act as a virulence factor-** (AI-2011)
(a) *H influenzae* (b*) Strept pneumoniae* (c) *N meningitidis* (d) *Bordetella pertusis*

12) **Capsulated organism -** (AI-2011)
(a) *Candida* (b*) Klebsiella* (c) *Proteus* (d) *Cryptococcus* (e) *Histoplasma*

13) **True about bacterial capsule is following except -**
(a) Prevents phagocytosis (b) Stains by gram stain (c) Protects bacteria from lytic enzymes (d) Lost by repeated subculture

14) **Bacterial capsule id made up of**
(a) Monsaccharide (b) Polysaccharide (c) Long chain fatty acid (d) Small chain fatty acid

15) **Quellung reaction is useful to detect**
(a) Capsule (b) Flagella (c) Spores (d) Fimbriae

Flagella

16) **Bacteria with tuft of flagella at one end called** (PGI-95)
(a) Monotrichate (b) Peritrchate (c) Bipolar (d) lophotrichate

17) **Darting motility is shown by-**
(a) *L. monocytogenes* (b*) Proteus vulgaris* (c) *Borrelia* (d) *V cholerae*

18) **Darting motility occurs in *V cholerae* also found in-** (PGI, Dec-08)
(a) *Shigella* (b) *Campylobacter jejuni* (c) Pneumococcus (d) *Bacillus anthracis* (e) *Aeromonas*

19) **Following are motile organism except**
(a) *Proteus* (b) *Diphtheriae* (c) *T pallidum* (d) *Clostridia welchii*

20) **Tumbling motility is shown by-**
(a) *L. monocytogenes* (b) *Proteus vulgaris* (c) *Borrelia* (d) *Clostridia*

21) **Bacteria are motile due to**
(a) Flagella (b) Fimbriae (c) Both (d) None

22) **Flagella not true**
(a) Locomotion (b) Attachment (c) Protein in nature (d) Antigenic

23) **Bacterium with endoflagella is**
(a) S typhi (b) E coli (c) T pallidum (d) S minus

Bacterial spores

24) **Example of bacterium with central spore is**
(a) *Cl. tetani* (b) *Cl. bifermentans* (c) *Cl. welchii* (d) *Cl. tertium*

25) **Subterminal spores are found in-** (PGI, May-13 & Dec-08)
(a) *Clostridium sordelii* (b) *Clostridium sporogenes* (c) *Clostridium difficile* (d) *Clostridium tertium (e) Clostridium botulinum*

26) **Drum stick appearance is seen in-**
(a) *Cl. sphenoides* (b) *Cl. tetani* (b) *Cl. tetanomorphum* (d) *Clostridium tertium*

27) **Spores are formed by all except**
(a) *E. coli* (b) *B anthrax* (b) *B cereus* (d) None

28) **Bacterial spores are best destroyed by-** (PGI-98)
(a) UV rays (b) Autoclaving at 121°C for 20 min. (c) Hot air oven (d) Infrared rays

29) **Sporicidal agents are -** (PGI, June-09, 06)
(a) Gluteraldehyde (b) Ethylene oxide (c) Formaldehyde (d) Bezalkonium chloride (e) Chlorine

Answers of MCQs & explanation

1) **(a) & (b)**
- Peptidoglycan is present in gram positive (thick) & gram negative bacteria (thin), but not in fungi & protozoa

2) **(a)**
3) **(a), (b), (c) & (d)**
} Follow section, **bacterial cell wall (cell wall of gram positive bacteria & table-1** for explanation

4) **(a)**
- Follow **table-1** for explanation

5) **(c)**
- Peptidoglycan-polysaccharide-mycolic acids complex forms the skeleton in cell wall of *Mycobacteria,* so acid fastness in *Mycobacteria* is not the property of mycolic acid alone, but depends also on the integrity of cell wall
- For more explanation follow the section bacterial cell wall (cell wall of acid-fast bacteria)

6) **(b)**
7) **(c)**
} Follow section **bacterial cell wall (inhibition of cell wall synthesis)** for explanation

8) **(a)**
- Motility is a function of flagella, cell division is a function of reproductive system mostly by binary fission & conjugation is due to sex pili

9) **(b)**
- Follow section **cytoplasmic / plasma membrane (properties)** for explanation

10) **(b)**
11) **(d)**
12) **(b) & (d)**
13) **(b)**
14) **(b)**
15) **(a)**
} Follow section, **capsule** for explanation

16) **(d)**
- Follow **flow chart-2** for explanation

17) **(d)**
- *Vibrio cholerae* is actively motile with single sheathed polar flagellum **called darting motility**

18) **(b)**
- *Shigella,* pneumococcus & *Bacillus anthracis* are non motile while *Aeromonas* is motile in nature but showing motility other than darting

19) **(b) & (d)**
- Follow section, **flagella (flow chart-2) & notes** for explanation

20) (a)

21) (a)
22) (b)
Flagella is an organ of locomotion, it is made up by protein **called flagellin** & antigenic in nature. Fimbria is the organs of attachment.

23) (d)

- Follow section, **flagella (notes)** for explanation

24) (b)
25) (a), (b) & (e)
26) (a), (b) & (c)
27) (a)
Follow section, **bacterial spores (shape & location of spores)** for explanation

28) (b)
29) (a), (b), (c) & (e)
Follow section, **bacterial spores (sporicidal agents)** for explanation

5 Physiology of bacteria

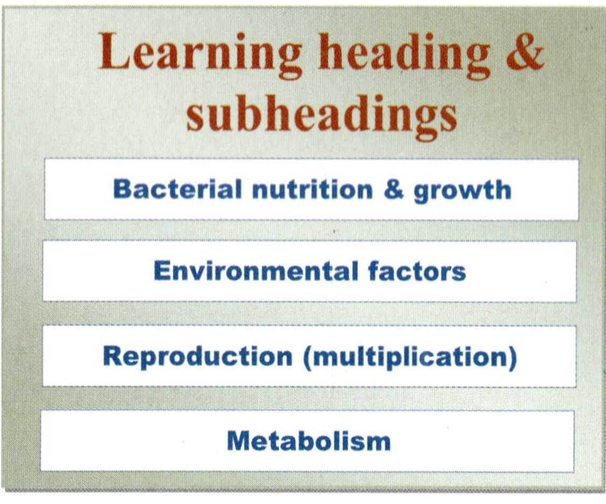

Physiology of bacteria is discussed with following headings

- ◊ **Bacterial nutrition & growth factors**
- ◊ **Environmental factors**
- ◊ **Reproduction (multiplication)**
- ◊ **Metabolism**

Bacterial nutrition & growth

❖ **Definition:** Nutrition is the process by which the organic & inorganic substances are obtained from surrounding environment & used for growth, metabolism & multiplication.

❖ Nutrients or growth factors:

➢ **Definition:** Organic & inorganic substances used for nutrition are **called nutrients.** Also **called growth factors.**

➢ **Types:** Two types of nutrients

A. **Macronutrients:** These are required in relatively large quantities and play important role in cell structure and metabolism.

B. **Micronutrients:** These are required in small quantities for functioning of certain enzyme systems.

➢ **Nutrients required for bacteria:**

A. **Water:**

- It holds 80% weight of total bacterial weight
- Act as vehicle to carry the nutrients to & fro from bacterial cell

B. **Carbon, nitrogen, energy:** Bacteria classified into 2 groups.

i. **Autotrophs** (or **lithotrophs):**

- This group of bacteria is able to utilize atmospheric CO_2 & N_2 for growth.
- Medically less important because they survive independently in soil and water (**called saprophytes**).
- They are concerned agriculture and with soil fertility. E.g. nitrogen fixing bacteria in soil.
- They required water, CO_2 & N_2 for growth.
- Two further group based on energy requirement

a. **Photolithotrophs:** Got energy from light.

b. **Chemolithotrophs:** Got energy from oxidation & reduction of chemicals like inorganic substances (Anions → phosphate, sulphate, Cations → sodium, potassium, magnesium, iron, manganese, calcium).

ii. **Heterotrophs (or organotrophs):**

- This group of bacteria is not able to utilise atmospheric CO_2 & N_2 for growth.
- These are bacteria which are unable to synthesize their own metabolites and depend on preformed **organic compounds such as** carbohydrates, amino acids, nucleotides, lipids, vitamins (B_1, B_2, B_4, B_6, folic acid, B_{12}) and co-enzymes for growth. Organic compound may be **essential** (no growth in their absence) or **accessory** (when they enhance growth).
- They are medically important cause disease.
- Two further group based on energy requirement

a. **Photoorganotrophs:** Got energy from light

b. **Chemoorganotrophs:** Got energy from oxidation & reduction of chemicals like inorganic substances.

C. **Bacterial vitamins:**

- Certain fastidious bacteria required essential nutrients for growth on media **called bacterial vitamins** as shown in **table-1**
- They are similar to mammalian vitamins

Vitamins	Bacteria
Biotin	*Leuconostoc* spp
B12	*Lactobacillus* spp.
Folic acid	*Enterococcus faecalis*
Pantothenic acid	*Morgnella morganii*
B6	*Lactobacillus* spp.
Niacin (Nicotinic acid)	*B. abortus* & *H. influenzae*
B2	*B. anthracis*

Table-1: Bacterial vitamins

Environmental factors

A. **Carbon dioxide:**

- All bacteria require small amounts (1-2%) of carbon dioxide for growth.
- This requirement is usually met by the carbon dioxide present in the **atmosphere**, or **produced endogenously** by cellular metabolism.
- Energy required for utilisation of CO_2 may come from light or from oxidation & reduction of chemicals like inorganic substances
- However, some bacteria require higher concentration (5-10%) of CO_2 **called capnophilic bacteria** like *Brucella abortus, Neisseria* spp., *Strept. pneumoniae, Listeria monocytogenes, Helicobacter pylori, Campylobacter jejuni, Gardnerella vaginalis, Actinobacillus actinomycetemcomitans, Eikenella corrodens, Capnocytophage* spp. *Legionella pneumophila* etc.

B. Oxygen: Based on oxygen requirements bacteria can be classified into 6 types.

i. Obligate or strict aerobes:

- **Definition:** Grow only in presence of O_2
- **Examples:** *Micrococci, Neisseria meningitidis, Moraxella lacunata, Acinetobacter baumanii, Corynebacterium jakeium, M. tuberculosis, Nocardia* spp., *Listeria monocytogenes, Serratia merscence, V. cholera, P. aeruginosa, Bukholderia pseudomallei, Bordetella pertusis, Brucella abortus, Francisell tularensis, Alkaligenes faecalis* etc.

ii. Obligate or strict anaerobes:

- **Definition:** Grow only in absence of O_2 (They die in presence of oxygen)
- **Types & examples:** Two subtypes

a. **Sporing anaerobes:** *Cl. botulinum, Cl. tetani & Cl. novyi*

b. **Non-sporing anaerobes:** For examples, Follow chapter → Non sporing anaerobes

- **Reasons of oxygen toxicity in anaerobic bacteria:**
  - In presence of oxygen, hydrogen peroxide and other toxic peroxides accumulate. The enzyme catalase which splits hydrogen peroxide is present in most aerobic bacteria but absent in anaerobes.
  - Some other enzymes like peroxidase & superoxide dismutase are also required to inactivate the oxygen products, but their deficiency in anaerobic bacteria makes the oxygen toxic for anaerobes.
  - Another reason is that obligate anaerobes possess essential enzymes that are active only in reduced state.

iii. Facultative anaerobes:

- **Definition:** They are aerobes but can grow in absence of O_2
- **Examples:** *Strept. pyogenes, Staph. aureus, Strept. pneumoniae, N. gonorrhea , E. coli, H. influenzae* etc.

iv. Facultative aerobes:

- **Definition:** They are anaerobes but can grow in presence of O_2
- **Examples:** *Lactobacillus* spp. etc.

v. Aerotolerant:

- **Definition:** They can tolerate oxygen for some times but can't grow in presence of O_2.
- **Examples:** *Cl. histolyticum, Propionibacterium acne, P avidum, P granulosum & Arcobaterium* spp.

vi. Microaerophilic:

- **Definition:** Require O_2 less than the environmental O_2 (About 5-10%)
- **Examples:** *Clostridium welchii, Mycobacterium bovis, Listeria monocytogenes, Erysipelothrix rhusiopathiae, Campylobacter jejuni, Helicobacter pylori, Streptobacillus moniliformis, Spirillum minus, Actinobacillus actinomycetemcomitans, Borrelia recurrentis, Borrelia bergdorferi, Leptospira interrogans* etc.

C. Temperature: Temperature affects growth and viability of bacteria.

i. Effect on growth:

- **Definition:**
  - For each species, there is a temperature range and growth does not occur above the **maximum temperature** or below the **minimum temperature**.
  - **Optimum temperature:** The temperature at which growth occurs best is **called the optimum temperature**.
- **Types of bacteria:** According to temperature effect bacteria are classified as follows

a. Psychrophilic (cryophilic) bacteria:

- Definition: Bacteria which can grow best at temperature below 20°C **are called psychrophilic (cryophilic) bacteria,** some of them even growing at temperature as low as -7°C.
- Examples: Saprophytes
- May cause spoilage of refrigerated food.

b. Mesophilic bacteria:

- Definition: Bacteria which grow best at temperature of 25-40°C are **called mesophilic bacteria.**
- Examples: All pathogenic bacteria are mesophilic bacteria & optimum temperature for such group is 37°C

c. Thermophilic bacteria:

- Definition: Bacteria which grow best at high temperature around 55-80°C are **called thermophilic bacteria**.
- Examples: *Bacillus steareothermophilus & Campylobacter* spp.
- They may cause spoilage of under processed canned food.

d. Extremely thermophilic bacteria:

- Definition: Bacteria which grow at higher temperature at 250°C are **called extremely thermophilic bacteria**.
- Examples: Bacterial spores.

✓ **Notes: Thermoduric bacteria**

- **Definition:** Bacteria which can survive but do not grow, to varying extents of the pasteurisation process or pasteurisation temperature **called thermoduric bacteria**
- **Examples:** *Bacillus*, *Clostridium, Micrococcus, Streptococcus, Lactobacillus*, *Enterococcus* & few gram negative rods.
- **Clinical significances:** The sources of contamination are poorly cleaned and sanitized utensils and equipment on farm and processing plants. These bacteria contribute to significantly higher Standard Plate Count on pasteurized milk.
- **Thermoduric count:** It has been used in the dairy industry primarily as a test of care employed in utensil sanitation and as a means of detecting sources of organisms responsible for high counts in the final product.

ii. Effect on viability:

- Heat is an important method for destruction of microorganisms.
- **Moist heat** causing coagulation and denaturation of proteins and **dry heat** causing oxidation and charring.
- Moist heat is more lethal than dry heat.
- **Thermal death point:** The lowest temperature that kills a bacterium under standard conditions in a given time is **called the thermal death point.**
- Under moist condition, most vegetative & hemophilic bacteria have a thermal death point is between 50°-65°C & for spores is between 100°-120°C.
- At low temperature some species die rapidly but most survive well.
- Storage in the refrigerator (3°-5°C) or deep freeze cabinet (-30° to -70°C) is used for preservation of cultures.
- Rapid freezing as with solid carbon dioxide or the use of a stabiliser such as glycerol, minimise the death of cells on freezing.

D. H-ion concentration (pH):

✪ **pH range:**

- Each species has a pH range, above and below which, it cannot survive.
- Bacteria are sensitive to variations in pH
- Strong solutions of acid or alkali (5% HCl) readily kill most bacteria, though *Mycobacteria* are exceptionally resistant to them.

✪ **Optimum pH:** pH at which, bacteria can grow best.

✪ **Pathogenic bacteria:** They can grow best at a neutral pH **(7.2-7.6)** or slightly alkaline pH **(>7.8)** and following are types

i. Acidic pH:

- Definition: Some bacteria grow at acidic pH (**<6.0**) are **called acidophilic bacteria**.
- Examples: *Lactobacillus* spp.

ii. Neutral pH: Most of the pathogenic bacteria grow at neutral pH (**7.2-7.6**).

iii. Alkaline pH: Some bacteria grow at alkaline pH (**>7.8**), like *V. cholerae.*

E. Moisture and drying:

- Moisture is absolute requirement for growth.
- The capacity to survive in dry environment varies from organism to organism.
  - *N. gonorrhoea* and *T. pallidum* die quickly in dry conditions.
  - *Staph. aureus* and *M. tuberculosis* can survive drying for weeks and months.
  - **Bacterial spores** can survive in drying for decades.
  - Drying in vacuum in the cold is a method for the preservation of bacteria, viruses and many labile biological materials **called freeze drying or lyophilisation**.

F. Light:

- Some bacteria required light for energy like **photolithotrophs/ photoorganotrophs**
- Light also required for certain bacterial functions e.g. pigment production.

i. Photochromogenic bacteria:

- Definition: Bacteria produce the pigment only in light, not in the dark **called photochromogenic bacteria**.
- Examples: *M. kansasii, M. marinum, M. simiae, M. asiaticum* etc.

ii. Scotochromogenic bacteria:

- Definition: Bacteria produce the pigment in light & in dark **called scotochromogenic bacteria**
- Examples: *M. scrofulaceum, M. gordonae* & *M. szulgai* (scotochromogen at 37°C & photochromogen at 25°C)

iii. Non-photochromogenic (non-chromogenic) bacteria:

- Definition: Bacteria which do not produce pigment in presence or absence of light **called non-photochromogenic (non-chromogenic) bacteria**
- Examples: *M. avium, M. intracellulare, M. xenopi* & *M. ulcerans.*

G. Osmotic effect:

- Bacteria more tolerate osmotic variation then most other cells due to the mechanical strength of their cell walls.
- Sudden exposure to hypertonic solutions may cause loss of water and shrinkage of cell **called plasmolysis.** More in gram-negative than in gram-positive bacteria.
- Sudden transfer to distilled water or any other hypotonic solution may cause water flow inside the cell & swelling and rupture of cell **called plasmoptysis**.

H. Mechanical & sonic stress: Though bacteria have tough cell walls, they may be ruptured by mechanical stress such as grinding, vigorous shaking with glass beads or ultrasonic vibration.

Reproduction (multiplication)

❖ Method of reproduction:

a. Binary fission:

- Bacteria multiply **by binary fission** after attaining certain size
- One mother cell gives two daughter cells
- Nuclear division occurs at 1st followed by cell division.
- Cell division initiated with formation of transverse septum across the cell.
- Normally daughter cells complete separated from mother cell, however in some it attaches to mother cell due **to incomplete binary fission.** E.g. *C. diphtheriae*

b. Budding:

- Some bacteria also reproduce **by budding** in which a small bud (small pouch like structure) develops from the mother cell and separates and grows further to form a new bacterium. E.g. *F. tularensis, M. pneumoniae*

c. Filamentous formation (?): E.g. *F. tularensis*

❖ Reproduction time: The interval of time between two cell divisions or the time required for a bacterium to give rise to two daughter cells under optimum conditions is **called generation time or population doubling time.**

- One bacterium gives 10^{21} progeny in 24 hrs.
- Generation time of few bacteria is shown in **table-2**

Organisms	Generation time
Cl welchii	10 minutes
Coliform bacilli (lactose fermenters like *E. coli* & *K. Pneumoniae*)	20 minutes
Leptospira spp.	12-16 hours in media & 4-8 hours in animals
M. tuberculosis	20 hours
T. pallidum	30-33 hours
M. leprae	13-15 days

Table-2: Generation time of different bacteria

❖ Effective factors on reproduction:

a. Nutrients & toxic products:

1. **Depletion of nutrients & accumulation of toxic products:** When bacteria are grown in artificial prepared nutritional media medium multiplication is arrested after a few cell divisions due to depletion of nutrients or accumulation of toxic products. Such culture **called batch culture**
2. **Replacement of nutrients & removal of toxic products: called continuous culture**

- **Special device:** Which replace nutrients & remove toxic products during cell division. It uses to maintain bacteria for industrial or research purposes.
- **Host tissue:** Which replace nutrients & remove toxic products during cell division, but bacteria have to compete with host defense. It is intermediate between batch culture and continuous culture

b. Inhibition of cell division: By certain drugs like Penicillin

❖ Bacterial count:

➢ **Definition:** Bacterial multiplication in number **called bacterial count**

➢ **Methods:** Two types of bacterial counts: Total counts and viable count.

a. Total count:

- **Definition:** Total number of cells in the sample irrespective of whether they are living or dead **called total count.**
- **Counting methods:** It can be obtained by,

1. Direct counting under the microscope using counting chambers,
2. Counting in an electronic device as in the coulter counter,
3. Using stained smears prepared by spreading a known volume of the culture over a measured area of a slide,
4. Comparing relative number, in a smears of the culture mixed with known numbers of other cells,
5. Opacity measurement using an absorptiometer or nephalometer,
6. Separation of cells by centrifugation or filtration & measuring their wet or dry weight
7. Chemical assay of cell components like nitrogen.

b. Viable count:

- **Definition:** number of living cells which are capable of multiply **called viable count**
- **Counting methods:** It can be obtained by,

1. Dilution:

- By using liquid media
- The suspension is diluted to a point beyond which unit quantities do not yield growth when inoculated in to suitable liquid media.
- Several tubes are incubated with varying dilutions and the viable count calculated statistically from the number of tubes showing growth.
- Disadvantage: does not give accurate values
- Use: for **water culture** to estimate the presumptive coliforms count in drinking water.

2. Plating methods:

- By using solid media
- Appropriate dilutions are inoculated on solid media, either on the surface of plates or as pour plates. Followed by incubation
- The number of colonies develop gives an estimate of the viable count.

- The method commonly employed is described by **Miles and Misra (1938)**.

❖ Bacterial growth curve:

✪ **Definition:** When a bacterium is inoculated into a suitable liquid medium & incubated, it under goes the multiplication. Count the bacteria at regular interval & plotted it against the time, a growth curve is obtained **called bacterial growth curve or kinetic of bacterial growth.**

✪ **Phases:** The curve shows the four phases during which morphological & physiological changes in cells are occurs as shown in **fig.-1**

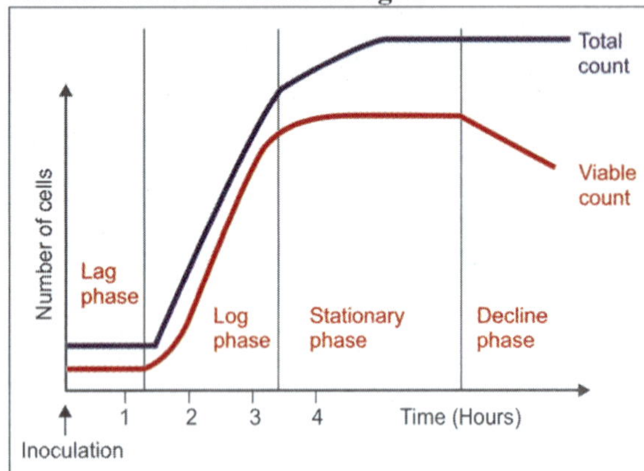

Figure-1: Bacterial growth curve

a. Lag phase:

- The initial period
- Required to adapt the new environment, to synthesize the necessary enzymes & metabolites for multiplication.
- Immediately following the seeding of a culture medium there is no increase in numbers, though there may be **an increase the size of a cell**.
- The duration of the lag phase varies from 1-4 hours with the type of species, size of the inoculum, nature of the medium, presence of growth factors & environmental factors like temperature, O_2, CO_2 etc.

b. Log /logarithmic/ exponential phase:

- As the time pass, cells start to divide & their numbers increase
- If the logarithm of the viable count is plotted against time a straight-ascending line will be obtained.
- **Smaller size & uniform staining occurs in this phase**

c. Stationary phase:

- After a varying period of exponential growth, cell division stops due to depletion of nutrients and accumulation of toxic products **(batch culture**).
- Progeny cells formed are enough to replace the number of cells that die.
- Viable count remains stationary as equilibrium exists between the dying & new cells.
- **Variable gram reaction, irregular staining due to storage granules & sporulation**

d. Decline phase:

- During this phase viable count decreases due to cell death.
- Cell death is due to nutritional exhaustion, accumulation of toxic products & by autolytic enzymes.
- Total count is runs parallel to viable count up to stationary phase, after that it continues steadily without any decline **till autolysis** will start.
- **After autolysis**, total count also decreases.
- Secondary metabolic products & **involution forms** occurs

✪ **Summary of bacterial growth curve: → Table-3**

> **Mnemonic:**
> - **SS:** Stationary phase & Sporulation
> - **In-in:** Involution form & phase of decline

Features	Lag	Log	Stationary	Decline
Bacterial division	No	Yes & high	Yes but low	Yes
Bacterial death	No	No	Yes	Yes
Total count	Flat	Increases	Increases	Flat
Viable count	Flat	Increase	Flat	decreases
Key features	- Synthesis of enzymes & meta-bolites - Size: Maximum	- Size: Small - Stain: Uniform	- Stain: Gram variable - Granules toxin & spores developed	-Auto lysis - Involu tion forms

Table-3: Summary of bacterial growth curve

Metabolism

❖ Steps:

- **Absorption** of food material
- **Breakdown & utilization**
- **Elimination** of metabolic end products

❖ **Metabolic pathway:** Bacteria are differs in the way of metabolism.

a. Aerobic bacteria:

- Obtain their energy by **oxidation (aerobic respiration)**
- Oxygen as the ultimate hydrogen (electron) acceptor.
- **Oxidation:** O_2 accept the carbon & energy to form CO_2 & H_2O. During this process energy rich phosphate bonds are released which convert ADP to ATP **called oxidative phosphorylation**.

b. Anaerobic bacteria:

- Obtain their energy by **fermentation (anaerobic respiration)**
- Nitrite or sulphite is hydrogen (electron) acceptor.

- Fermentation: it is an anaerobic utilisation of sugar to produce acids (like lactic acid, formic acid, pyruvic acid), alcohols & gases (CO_2, H_2)
- During this process energy rich phosphate bonds are released which convert ADP to ATP **called substrate level phosphorylation.**

c. **Facultative anaerobes** utilize both the pathways.

❖ Redox potential (oxidation-reduction potential or Eh):

- **Oxidizing agents** are substances, which are capable of **accepting electrons**.
- **Reducing agents** are substances that are able to **lose electrons**.
- The capability of substance to accept or to lose the electron is **called oxidation-reduction potential**
- It is abbreviated as ***Eh &*** measured in millivolts.
- It is **higher** in oxidized substances and **lower** in reducing agents.
- The strict anaerobes require **low** redox potential- **less than 0.2 volts**, however the redox potential of most of the media exposed to air is +0.2 to +0.4 volts.

Question bank

Essay/Full question

1) Physiology of bacteria
2) Environmental factors affecting growth of bacteria

Short notes

1) Effect of oxygen on bacteria
2) Effect of temperature on bacteria
3) Bacterial count
4) Bacterial growth curve

Short questions for theory/viva questions

1) What is a bacterial vitamin?
2) What are capnophilic bacteria?
3) Write four examples of capnophilic bacteria
4) Write four examples of strict aerobic bacteria
5) Write four examples of strict anaerobic bacteria
6) Write four examples of microaerophilic bacteria
7) Why oxygen is toxic for strict anaerobic bacteria
8) What is plasmolysis & plasmoptysis?
9) What is generation time?
10) Write the generation time for following bacterium
    - *E.coli*, - *M. leprae, M. tuberculosis* & *T. pallidum*
11) What are thermoduric bacteria? Write two examples
12) What is batch culture & continuous culture?
13) Name the four phases of bacterial growth curve
14) Name the phases of bacterial growth where sporulation & involution forms can develop
15) Name the two methods for multiplication (Reproduction) & two methods for metabolism in bacteria
16) What is Eh or Redox potential?

MCQs for chapter review

Environmental factors

1) **Obligate anaerobes cannot withstand oxygen because of absence of -**
   (a) Superoxide dismutase (b) Catalase (c) Peroxidase (d) Cytochrome oxidase
2) **Which of the following is bacteria classified facultative anaerobes** (AI -97)
   (a) *Pseudomonas* (b) *Bacteroides* (c) *Escherichia* (d) *Clostridia*
3) **Strict anaerobes is/are**
   (a) *Cl. novyi* (b) *Cl. botulinum* (c) a+b (d) None of above
4) **Obligate anaerobes are all except** (PGI -99)
   (a) *Cl. botulinum* (b) *Eikinella corrodens* (c) *Bacteroides* (d) *H pylori*
5) **Which of the following is microaerophilic** (AIIMS, May-09)
   (a) *Campylobacter* (b) *Vibrio* (c) *Bacteroides* (d) *Pseudomonas*
6) **Mesophilic organisms are those that grow best at temperature of -** (PGI -98)
   (a) -20°C to -7°C (b) -7°C to +20°C (c) 25°C to 40°C (d) 55°C to 80°C (e) 90°C to 120°C

Reproduction (Multiplication)

7) **Generation time for lepra bacilli is-**
   (a) 12 days (b) 5 minutes (c) 10 hours (d) 24 hours
8) **Correct sequence of bacterial growth curve-** (PGI, Dec -07)
   (a) Log phase – Lag phase – Stationary phase – Decline phase
   (b) Lag phase – Log phase – Stationary phase – Decline phase
   (c) Stationary phase – Lag phase – Log phase – Decline phase
   (d) Lag phase – Exponential phase –Log phase – Death phase
   (e) Exponential phase –Lag phase – Death phase – Stationary phase
9) **True regarding lag phase-**
   (a) Time taken to adopt in the new environment (b) Growth occurs exponentiallly (c) The plateau in lag phase is due to cell death (d) It is the 2nd phase in bacterial growth curve
10) **Sporulation occurs in-** (AI -98)
    (a) Lag phase (b) Log phase (c) Stationary phase (d) Decline phase

Answers of MCQs & explanation

1) **(a), (b) (c)**
- Follow section, **environmental factors (oxygen → Reasons of oxygen toxicity in anaerobic bacteria)** for explanation

2) **(c)**
- *Pseudomonas* is strict aerobes while *Bacteroides* & *Clostridia* are strict anaerobes

3) **(c)**
4) **(b) & (d)**
   } Follow section, **environmental factors (oxygen → obligate or strict anaerobes)** for explanation

5) **(a)**
- *Vibrio* & *Pseudomonas* are strict aerobes while *Bacteroides* is strict anaerobes

6) **(c)**
- Follow section, **environmental factors (temperature)** for explanation

7) **(a)**
- Generation time of different bacilli is given **table-2.**

8) **(b)**
9) **(a)**
10) **(c)**
   } Follow section, **reproduction (multiplication → Bacterial growth curve)** for explanation

6 Genetics of bacteria

Learning heading & subheadings

- Genetic structure
- Bacterial variation
  - Phenotypic variation
  - Genotypic variation
- Drug resistance mechanisms
- Molecular genetics

Genetic Structure

❖ **Definitions:**

➢ **Gene:** The unit or segment of DNA for heredity is called gene.

➢ **Genome:** Total component of genes in the cell called genome.

➢ **Genetics:** It is a study of heredity & variation.

❖ **Structure:** Two parts (**fig.-1**) of bacterial genome as described below

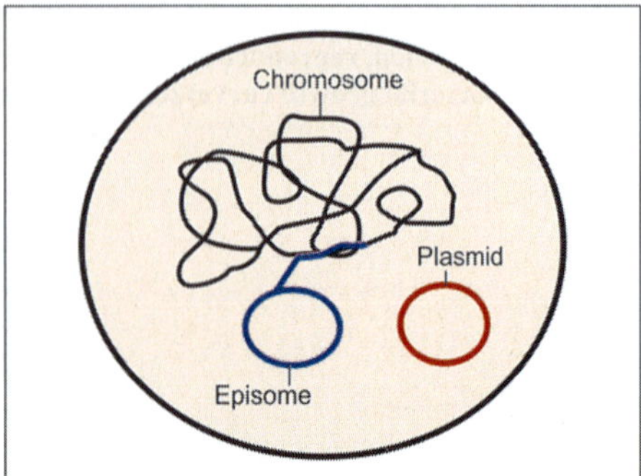

Figure-1: Bacterial genome

I. **Chromosomal parts:** It is a single (haploid), circular coiled body contains following two type's nucleic acid.

A. **DNA**

B. **RNA**

✓ **Note: Viral nucleic acid & meaning of haploid & diploid**

- **Viral nucleic acid:** Viruses contains either DNA or RNA, but not both
- **Meaning haploid & diploid:** Haploid indicates single (n) set of chromosome& diploid indicates double (2n) set of chromosome

II. **Extrachromosomal parts:** As below

A. **Plasmid**

B. **Episome**

C. **Transposon (Jumping gene)**

I. Chromosomal parts

➢ **Nucleic acid:** Following are the two types

A. **DNA:**

✪ **Full form:** Deoxyribo Nucleic Acid

✪ **History:** DNA model was described by James Watson & Francis Crick (Watson & Crick) in 1953

✪ **DNA Structure:**

- **DNA model: →Fig.-2(a)**

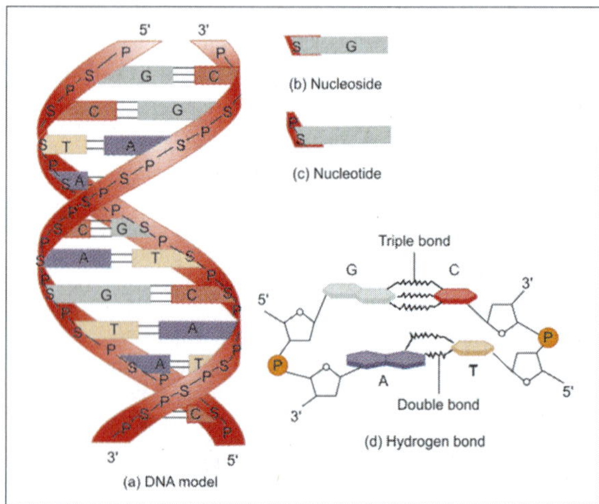

Figure-2: DNA structure

- <u>Number:</u> Single
- <u>Shape</u>: DNA is composed of two strand (double helix) with complimentary nucleotides that is arranged in the spiral form
- <u>Size</u>:

- Length: When straightened , it is about 1000μm in length
- Unit: It is expressed in kilobase (1kb = 1000 base pairs). Bacterial DNA is about 4000kb long while human DNA is about 3 million kb long

o Pattern:

- Circular: In loop form without ends (closed form) like in prokaryotes (like bacteria) & in few viruses like Poxviridae
- Linear: Straight with ends as in all eukaryotes & in few viruses like influenza virus

o Ladder:

- For the sake of simplicity it is denoted as a ladder
- Rungs of ladder is formed by nitrogen base united with phosphate bond
- Side of ladder formed by deoxyribose sugar & phosphate bond

• **Nucleoside & nucleotide:**

- Term nucleoside & nucleotide are frequently used in the DNA model
- Nucleoside **[Fig.-2(b)]**: Sugar + nitrogen base
- Nucleotide **[Fig.-2(c)]**: Nucleoside (sugar + nitrogen base) + phosphate bond.

• **Nitrogen bases:**

o Types: Two types of nitrogen bases in DNA

1. **Purine:** Adenine (A) & Guanine (G)
2. **Pyrimidine:** Thymine (T) & Cytosine (C)

o Ratio of nitrogen bases:

- Numbers of A are equal to that of T & also Numbers of G are equal to that of C
- Ration of A + T & G + C is constant for each species but varies widely from one species to another.

• **Hydrogen bond:** Both strands of DNA held together by the hydrogen bonds between the nitrogen base of opposite strand

• **Rule of bonding [Fig.-2(d)]:** Following two rules

1. **A-T bond:** Adenine (A) of one strand bound to the Thymine (T) of opposite strand by double hydrogen bonds.
2. **C-G bond:** Cytosine (C)) of one strand bound to the Guanine (G) of opposite strand by triple hydrogen bonds

✪ **Functions:**

1. **Replication:** Copying of DNA
2. **Transcription:** Synthesis of RNA from DNA

✪ **Segments of DNA (Gene):**

- Segment of DNA contains codon is specifying for particular polypeptide chain **called gene**
- Bacteria posses 1000-3000 genes which are codes for 1000-3000 polypeptide chains, as each gene is specify the particular polypeptide chain
- Each polypeptide chain made up of 1200 nucleotides & each nucleotide consists of 400 amino acids
- Chromosome contains 5×10^4 nucleotide pairs

✪ **Introns & exons in DNA:**

- In DNA there are several codons which do not function as gene **called introns** while codon which codes for particular gene are **called exons**
- During transcription the genome is copied entirely with introns & exons
- During translation the introns are excised from RNA before being translated in to the proteins

B. RNA:

✪ **Full form:** Ribo Nucleic Acid

✪ **RNA Structure:** Similar to DNA with minor differences as shown in **table-1**

Features	DNA	RNA
Acid	Phosphoric acid	Phosphoric acid
Purine bases	A & G	A & G
Pyrimidine bases	T & C	U & C
Sugar	D-2-Deoxyribose	D-Ribose

Table-1: Similarities & differences between DNA & RNA

✪ **Types:** Three types

1. **mRNA:** messenger RNA
2. **rRNA:** ribosomal RNA
3. **tRNA:** transfer RNA

✪ **Function:** Protein synthesis **called translation**

➤ **Genetic codons:**

- Sequence of genetic information stored in the DNA **called genetic codon.**
- It was described by Nirenberg & Khorana in 1968
- Each codon consists sequence of three nitrogen bases, so **called triplet codon** or **triplet**
- Each triplet codon codes for single amino acid. E.g. ACG codes for threonine
- Codon is the structural terminology & code is the functional terminology.
- Types:

1. **Sense codons:**
   - There are total 64 codons & out of which 61 codons are codes for 20 essential amino acids **called sense codons**
2. **Non-sense codons (stop codons):**
   - Out of 64 codons & 3 codons do not codes for any amino acid **called non-sense codons**
   - They terminate the elongation of polypeptide chain so **called stop codons**
   - Examples: UAA, UAG & UGA
3. **Start codon:**
   - First codon which start the amino acid synthesis **called start codon**
   - Example: AUG which codes for methionine in cukaryotcs & modified methionine [N-Formyl methionine (fMet)] prokaryotes
4. **Anti codon:** It is a set of three nucleotide bases present on tRNA that is complementary to the nucleotide bases of codon on mRNA.

II. Extrachromosomal parts

- **Nucleic acid:** Following are the three types

A. Plasmid:

- **Definition:** It is an extra-chromosomal intracytoplasmic DNA material (**fig.-1**).
- **Properties:**
  - **Numbers:** A bacterium can have no plasmids at all or have many plasmids (20-30) or multiple copies of a plasmid.
  - **Shape:** Usually they are closed circular molecules; however they occur as linear molecule in *Borrelia burgdorferi*.
  - **Size:** Vary from 1 kb to 400 kb.
  - **Replication:** Autonomous replication (independent replication)
  - **Present:** Present in bacteria & also in yeast
- **Types:**

i. **According to transmission:**

a. **Self transmissible/Conjugative:** Contains information for self transfer to other cell via conjugation. E.g. F factor

b. **Non-transmissible/Non- Conjugative:** Does not contain information for self transfer via conjugation (can be transduced).

ii. **According to functions:**

a. **Fertility (F) /sex factor or sex pili:**

- F factor is a plasmid codes for special fimbriae or sex pili which makes a conjugation tube between two cells & for necessary enzyme of conjugation.
- Those bacteria that possess F factor are **called F+**, such bacteria have sex pili on their surface & those are lacking **called F⁻.**
- The F factor plasmid is transferred to other cells through conjugation tube.
- A F⁻ cell will become F+ when it receives the fertility factor from another F+ cell.

b. **Resistance (R) Factor:** Responsible for drug resistance

c. **Colicinogenic (Col) factor:** Responsible for bacteriocins production.

iii. **According to restriction endonuclease enzyme fingerprinting:**

a. **Closely related plasmid:** Produces same or very similar fingerprinting

b. **Unrelated plasmid:** Produces different fingerprinting

iv. **Incompatibility typing:**

a. **Closely related plasmid:** Do not coexist stably in same bacterium

b. **Unrelated plasmid:** Coexist stably in same bacterium

- **Functions:** Transfer genetic information from one cell to another cell as below

1. **Virulence determinant:**
   - Fertility (F) factor is a plasmid codes for special fimbriae or sex pili which makes a conjugation tube between two cells & allow the transfer of genetic information from one cell to other **called conjugation**.
   - **Iron sequestering:** Plasmids carry virulence determinant genes like the plasmid Col V of *E. coli* contains genes for iron sequestering compounds.
   - **Capsule & toxin** in *B anthracis* are plasmid encoded. Removal of such plasmid makes the strain avirulent **called Sterne strain**, which used for vaccine production.
   - **Invasive property** in *Shigella* & EIEC is due to a special type of OMP **called VMA (Virulence Marker Antigen)** which is plasmid encoded, responsible for invasion, multiplication of bacilli & destruction of epithelial cells.
2. **Drug resistance:**
   - It codes for the drug resistance to several antibiotics **called Resistance Transfer Factor (RTF).**
   - Gram-negative bacteria carry plasmids that give resistance to antibiotics such as neomycin, kanamycin, streptomycin, chloramphenicol, tetracycline, penicillins and sulfonamides.
3. **Bacteriocins production:** Codes for the production of bacteriocins **called col factor**.
4. **Toxins production:** It codes **for the toxins production** in certain bacteria like
   - Enterotoxin production by *Staph. aureus*
   - Anthrax toxin by *B anthracis*
   - Tetanospasmin by *Cl. tetani.*
   - Labile toxin (LT) of *E. coli*
   - Stable toxin (ST) of *E. coli*
5. **Resistance to heavy metals:** Codes for resistance to heavy metals such as Hg, Ag, Cd, Pb etc.
6. **Resistance to UV light:** Codes for resistance to UV light (DNA repair enzymes are coded in the plasmid).
7. **Coding for enzymes:** Contains genes coding for enzymes that allow bacteria unique or unusual materials for carbon or energy sources. E. g. Urease synthesis in bacteria
8. **Metabolic plasmid:** They enables the bacteria in various metabolic activities like
   - Nitrogen fixation
   - Digestion of unusual substances: Toluene, salicylate, camphor etc.

- **Clinical applications of plasmid:**

1. **Used in genetic engineering as vectors:** Plasmid contains many sites for artificial insertion of genes by recombinant technology. Such plasmid can be used for various purposes such as protein production, gene therapy etc.
2. **Plasmid profiling is a useful genotyping method:** Useful tool for epidemiological study of microbes

B. Episome:

- Plasmid sometimes integrated with chromosomal part **called episome** (**fig.-1**) & such bacterial cells

are **called Hfr cells** (**H**igh **f**requency of **r**ecombination).
- Previously, it was considered as synonymous with plasmids.
- Jacob and Wollman coined the term episome.
- When it detaches with part of chromosome becomes free **called F prime (F/) factor**

C. **Transposons (Jumping gene):** It jumps between chromosomal & extra-chromosomal part, **so called jumping gene**

Bacterial variation

❖ **Types:** Two types like phenotypic variation & genotypic variation, as shown in **table-2**

Phenotypic variation	Genotypic variation
Reversible	Irreversible
Temporary (unstable)	Permanent (stable)
Not heritable	Heritable
Environment effect	No environment effect

Table-2: Differences between phenotypic & genotypic variation

Phenotypic variation

➢ **Meaning:** Phaeno = Display
➢ **Definition:** It is a physical expression of bacterial characteristics in given environment.
➢ **Examples of phenotypic variation:**

I. **Synthesis of flagella:** *S. typhi* are normally flagellated, but flagella are not synthesised when they grow in phenol agar. It reversed when subcultured in broth.

II. **Synthesis of enzyme:** β-galactosidase is the enzymes required for *E. coli* for lactose fermentation, but it produced when it grow in a lactose containing medium. It not synthesised when it grow in lactose free medium. Such enzyme which require the presence of substance **called induced enzyme** & opposite which does not require the presence of substance **called constitutive enzyme**

Genotypic variation

➢ **Meaning:** Geno = Related to gene
➢ **Definition:** It is a genetical expression of bacterial characteristics in given environment.
➢ **Examples of genotypic variation:**

I. **Mutation:**
II. **Gene transfer mechanisms/methods:**

I. Mutation

✪ **History:** Word "mutation (Latin)" was coined by Hugo de Vries, which means "to change".

✪ **Definitions:**
- **Mutation:** Change in the nucleotide sequence of DNA **called mutation**.
- **Wild type:** Organisms selected as reference (Normal) strains are **called wild type**
- **Mutants:** Yield of mutation **called mutants**
- **Mutagenesis:** The process of mutation **called mutagenesis**.
- **Mutagen:** The agent inducing mutations is **called mutagen**.

✪ **Type:** Two main types

A. **According to induction:**

i. **Spontaneous:**
- Occurs naturally about one in every million to one in every billion divisions.
- Occurs during DNA replication.

ii. **Induced:** By

a. **Chemical agents:**
- Alkylating agents
- Acridine dyes; nucleoside analogs that are similar in structure to nitrogenous bases
- Aflatoxin
- 2-amino purine
- 5-bromouracil
- Benzpyrene (from smoke and soot)
- Nitrous acid, which alters adenine to pair with cytosine instead of thymine.

b. **Physical agents:**
- X-rays & gamma rays have been shown to damage DNA.
- UV rays: UV light is responsible for the formation of thymine dimers in which covalent links are established between thethymine molecules. These links change the physical shape of the DNA preventing transcription and replication.

c. **Biological agents:** Viruses

B. **According to mechanisms:** → **Fig.-3**

i. **Point mutation:** Due to addition, deletion or substitution of single base.

A B C D E F	Normal (wild type)
A B X C D E F	Addition
A B D E F	Deletion
A B B C D E F	Duplication
A B X D E F	Substitution
A B C F E D	Inversion

Figure-3: Mutation according to mechanism

a. **Substitution of a nucleotide:**
- Involves the changing of single base in the DNA sequence.
- This mistake is copied during replication to produce a permanent change.
- This is the most common mechanism of mutation.
- Following are two subtypes

1. If a purine is replaced by a pyrimidine or vice-versa, the substitution is **called transversion.**
2. If one purine is replaced by the other purine or one pyrimidine is replaced by other pyrimidine, the substitution is **called transition**.

b. Deletion or addition of a nucleotide:

- Deletion or addition of a nucleotide during DNA replication.
- When a transposon (jumping gene) inserts itself into a gene, it leads to disruption of gene and is **called insertional mutation**.

ii. Frame shift mutation: Deletion or addition of a numbers of nucleotide.

iii. Multiple mutation: Cause extensive chromosomal rearrangement.

iv. Other types:

a. Missense mutation:

- Changes in the amino acid sequence due to change in triplet codon of the particular protein **called missense mutation**.
- This could be caused by a single point mutation or a series of mutations.

b. Nonsense mutation:

- Termination of polypeptide or protein synthesis due to formation of stop codon is **called a nonsense mutation**.
- It leads to incomplete or immature protein products.

c. Suppressor mutation:

- It is a reversal of a mutant phenotype by another mutation at a position on the DNA distinct from that of original mutation.
- True reversion or back mutation results in reversion of a mutant to original form, which occurs as a result of mutation occurring at the same spot once again.

d. Lethal mutation:

- Sometimes some mutations affect vital functions and the bacterial cell become nonviable.
- Hence those mutations that can kill the cell are **called lethal mutation.**

e. Conditional lethal mutation:

- Sometimes a mutation may affect an organism in such a way that the mutant can survive only in certain environmental condition **called conditional lethal mutation**.
- Examples: A temperature sensitive mutant (ts mutant) can survive at permissive temperature of 35°C but not at restrictive temperature of 39°C.

f. Inversion mutation: If a segment of DNA is removed and reinserted in a reverse direction, it is **called inversion mutation**.

g. Silent mutation: Sometimes a single substitution mutation change in the DNA base sequence results in a new codon still coding for the same amino acid. Since there is no change in the product, such mutations are **called silent mutation**.

✪ **Clinical significance of mutation:**

1. **Identification of the function of gene:** Discovery of a mutation in a gene can help in identifying the function of that gene.
2. **Vaccine production:** Mutations can be induced at a desired region to create a suitable mutant, especially to produce vaccines.
3. **Drug resistant:**
   - Spontaneous mutations can result in emergence of antibiotic resistance in bacteria.
   - Example: Drug resistance in *M. tuberculosis*
4. **Functional changes in bacteria:**
   - Mutation leads to functional changes.
   - Example: *E. coli* mutant loses the ability to ferment lactose. It can be detected on Mac Conkey's medium but not in nutrient agar.
5. **Survival advantage:**
   - It affects the vital function & confers survival advantage.
   - Example: Streptomycin resistant mutant to *M. tuberculosis* develop in a patients taking treatment. It multiplies & replaces initial drug sensitive bacteria & cause survival advantage. But patient who is not under treatment, it not causes any survival advantage.
6. **Change in phenotype:** Mutations can result in change in phenotypes such as
   - Appearance of novel surface antigen
   - Alternation in physiological properties
   - Change in colony morphology
   - Nutritional requirements
   - Biochemical reactions
   - Growth characteristics
   - Virulence
   - Host range.

✪ **Tests to detect the mutations:**

a. Fluctuation test:

✪ **History:** Developed by Luria & Delbruck in1943

✪ **Principle:** Bacteria undergoes to spontaneous mutation when they are challenged on agar plate contains growth limiting substances like streptomycin or bacteriophage. However the rate of mutation is wide, some bacteria mutate early while some late which leads to fluctuations. Fluctuations are wide (more frequent mutation) from small volume subcultures than large volume subcultures (less frequent mutation).

✪ **Disadvantages:** Not widely accepted due to complicated statistical evaluation.

✪ **Method:** Luria & Delbruck seeded the *E. coli* from small volume cultures & single large volume culture on media containing bacteriophage. The mutant bacteria formed the colonies. Colony count was compared. There was wide fluctuation in the numbers of resistant variant in small volume culture as compare to single large volume culture

b. Replica plating method:

✪ **History:** Developed by Lederberg in1952

- **Principle:** It based on differentiation between normal strain & auxotrophic mutants in which auxotrophic mutant can't grow in absence of particular nutrient. E.g. Lysin auxotroph can grow only on media contains lysin but not on lysin deficient media.

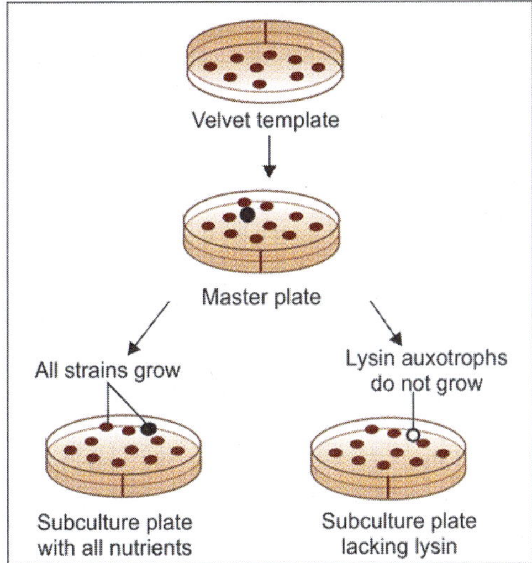

Figure-4: Replica plating method

- **Method (fig.-4):** Using velvet template, mixture of colonies (normal strain & auxotrophic mutants) of bacteria transferred from a master plate, on to two subculture plates where one plate is lacking with lysin. After incubation same colonies as master plate are obtained in subculture plates, except lysin auxotroph which do not grow on the media lacking lysin.

c. Ames test (Carcinigenicity testing):

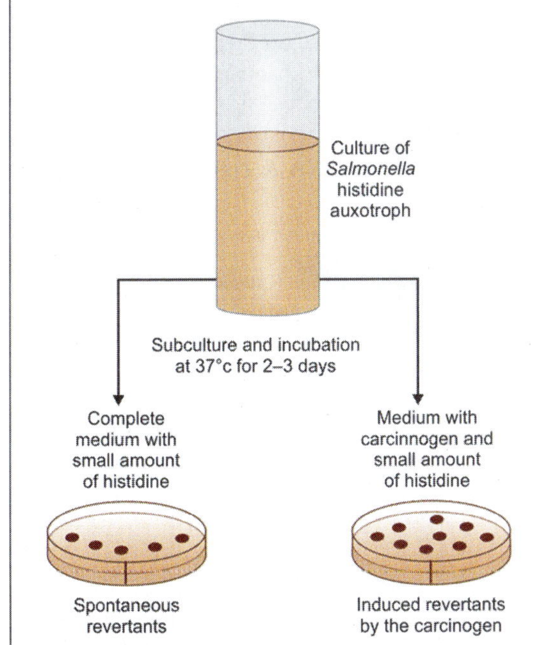

Figure-5: Ames test

- **History:** Developed by Bruce Ames in1970
- **Aim:** Used to identify the environmental carcinogens
- **Principle:** Based on mutational reversion by carcinogen
- **Method:** →**Fig.-5**
- Mutant strains (histidine auxotroph) of *Salmonella* which are subscribed on two agar plates containing small amount of histidine; one of the plate is added with the test mutagen.
- Incubate the plate at 37^0C for 2-3 days.
- All of the histidine auxotroph will grow for the first few hours until the histidine is depleted.
- Once the histidine source is exhausted, mutation revertant strain can grow by their ability to synthesize the histidine
- Reversed mutation may be induced by carcinogen (affect large numbers of strains) or occur spontaneously (affect only few strains)
- The relative mutagenicity of the carcinogen can be estimated by counting the colonies. More the number higher the carcinogenicity.

d. Penicilin enrichment:

II. Gene transfer mechanisms/methods

- **Definition:** Transfer of genetic materials or genetic information from one cell to other cell **called genetic recombination.** Cell donating the genetic materials or genetic information **called donor cell** to another cell **called recipient cell**.
- **Methods of gene transfer:** It is possible by two ways as follows
- **Vertical gene transfer:** Transmission of genes from parents to offspring. Not much important.
- **Horizontal gene transfer:** Transmission of genes from one bacterium to other. It is possible by following 5 methods

A. **Transformation**
B. **Transduction**
C. **Lysogenic conversion**
D. **Conjugation**
E. **Transposition**

A. Transformation:

- **Definition:** Transfer of genetic information from one cell to other cell through agency of free/naked DNA **called transformation**.
- **Mechanism:** → **Fig.-6**
- Transformation occurs in less than 1% of bacteria like *Bacillus, Haemophilus, Neisseria* and *Streptococcus.*
- When bacteria die, their DNA is released and it is referred to as naked DNA.
- Fragments of the naked DNA are taken in through the cell wall of another bacterial cell and incorporated into its chromosome

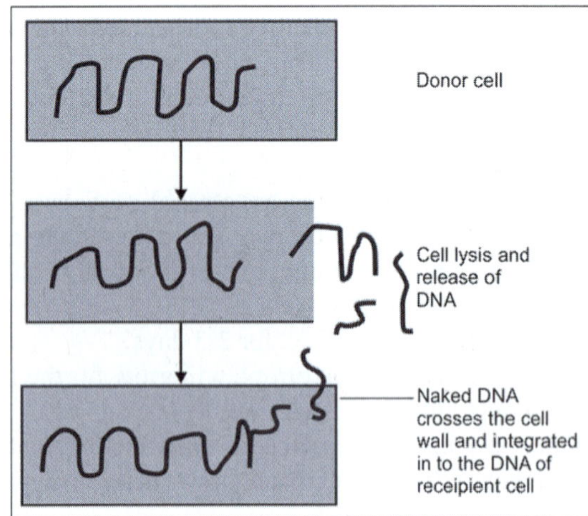

Figure-6: Mechanism of transformation

✪ **History: → Fig.-7**

- This was first demonstrated in an experiment conducted by Griffith in 1928
- Capsulated pneumococci give glistening, smooth (S) colonies while noncapsuled strains give rough (R) colonies.
- Pneumococci with a capsule (type I) are virulent and can kill a mouse while strains lacking it (type II) are harmless

  Griffith found that mice died when they were injected with a mixture of live non capsulated (R, type II) strains and heat killed capsulated (S, type I) strains. Neither of these two when injected alone could kill the mice, only the mixture of two proved fatal.
- Live S strains with capsule were isolated from the blood of the animal suggesting that some factor from the dead S cells converted the R strains into S type. The factor that transformed the other strain was found to be DNA by Avery, McLeod and McCarty in 1944.

✪ **Uptake of free DNA by bacteria:**

- Some bacteria are able to take up DNA naturally. However, these bacteria only take up DNA a particular time in their growth cycle (log phase) when they produce a specific protein **called a competence factor**.
- Gram +Ve bacteria take up single stranded DNA & the complementary strand is made in the recipient. Gram -Ve bacteria take up double stranded DNA.

✪ **Clinical significances:**

- Transformation occurs in nature and it can lead to increased virulence.
- Used in recombinant DNA technology.

B. Transduction:

✪ **Definition:** Transfer of genetic information from one cell to other cell through bacteriophage **called transduction**.

✪ **Bacteriophage:**

- **Definition:** Bacteriophage is a virus that eats bacterium & uses their machinery for their own replication.
- **Life cycle:** To understand the mechanism of transduction it is must to study the life cycle of bacteriophage as described below

* **Two cycle:**

i. **Lytic or virulent cycle: →Fig.-8 (A-G)**

- o <u>Definition</u>: Bacterial cell is killed with the release of mature phages **called lytic cycle**.
- o <u>Stages</u>: Following are the stages of transduction involving a lytic cycle:

a. **Adsorption:**

- Bacteriophage adsorbs to a bacterium surface by its tail.
- It is a complementary process between phage base plate & bacterial cell wall receptors.
- Cell wall receptors are present at different places like Vi Ag of *S. typhi*, on flagella or sex pili.
- Cell wall deficient bacteria cannot adsorb the phage.

b. **Penetration:**

- Release of phage DNA & entry in to the bacterium.

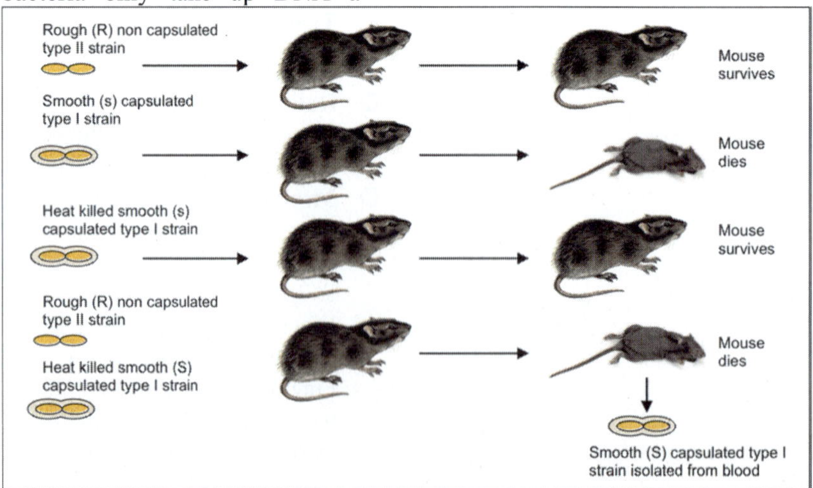

Figure-7: Transformation of Griffith

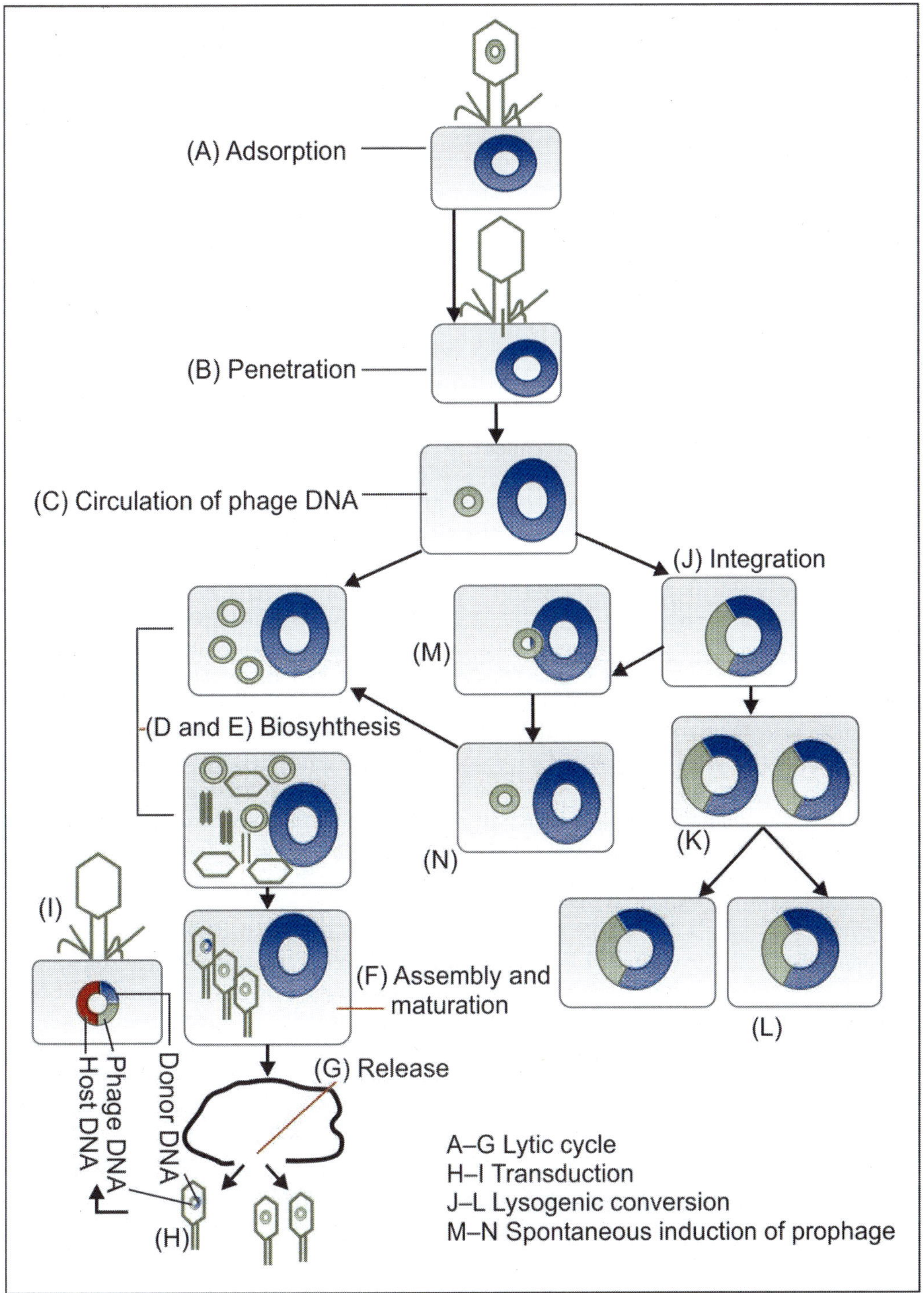

Figure-8: Life cycle of bacteriophage

- It is possible by formation of hollow core in cell wall by contractile tail sheath which derive energy from phage tail
- Hollow core formation facilitated by phage tail lysozyme.
- After penetration of phage DNA, head & tail sheath remain as ghost on surface.
- Penetration is also possible practically by direct injection of phage DNA.
- Infection of bacterium by naked phage DNA **called transfection**
- Sometimes bacterium is infected by multiple phage resulting multiple holes in cell wall & cell lysis without viral multiplication **called lysis from without**

c. **Biosynthesis:** Phage DNA directs the bacterium's metabolic machinery to manufacture bacteriophage components like head & tail & enzymes.

d. Maturation & assembly: Phage component synthesised in bacterium undergoes maturation & assembly

e. Release:

- After maturation bacterial cell wall gets weakened.
- Phage enzyme acts on weakened site & rupture the wall with the lysis of bacterium & release of progeny of bacteriophages.

o Eclipse phase:

- The interval between entry of phage DNA & appearance of 1st intracellular phage particle **called eclipse phase.**
- It is a time required for synthesis & assembly of phage particle.

o Latent period: The interval between infection of bacterium & 1st release of phage's progeny **called latent period**.

o Rise period: Immediately following latent period number of phage particle release are rise till it becomes maximum **called rise period.**

o Burst size: Average yield of progeny phage per infected bacterium **called burst size**.

o One step growth curve: It is estimated practically by infecting one bacterium with phage & count the release of phage particle over a period of time & plotted on a graph **called one step growth curve.**

ii. Lysogenic or temperate cycle: →Fig.-8 (J-L)

o Definitions:

- Phage DNA gets incorporated into the bacterial chromosome **called prophage**, behaves like additional segment of bacterial chromosome & multiplies along with it called **lysogenic or temperate cycle**.
- Bacterium undergoes to this cycle **called lysogenic bacterium**

o Synonym: This process or cycle also **called**

- **Lysogenic conversion** or
- **Phage conversion** or
- **Lysogenisation** or
- **Lysogeny**

o Clinical significances: Prophage confers certain new properties in lysogenic bacterium due to synthesis of new protein that are coded by prophage like

1. *C. diphtheriae* that have been lysogenised with β-prophage produce the diphtheria toxin. Elimination of β-prophage makes the strain non-toxigenic.
2. Lysogenic bacteria are resist to infection by same or related phages **called superinfection immunity**
3. It influences antigenic properties of bacterium.

iii. Variation in life cycle stage:

1. **Spontaneous induction of prophage: →Fig.-8(M-O)**

- The prophage sometimes excised from the host chromosome during multiplication of lysogenic bacteria & start lytic cycle with release of daughter phage **called spontaneous induction of prophage**
- It sometimes carries along with itself a fragment of bacterial chromosome; the subsequent phage progeny may have a piece of chromosomal DNA.
- When such phage infects another bacterium, newer characteristics coded by that chromosomal gene are conferred.

2. **Pseudolysogeny:** In certain bacteria prophage is not incorporated in host DNA but instead remains free as like plasmid **called pseudolysogeny.** E.g. *M. tuberculosis*
3. **Shifting of cycle:** Lysogenic cycle can be shift to Lytic cycle by exposure to UV light, H_2O_2 & nitrogen mustard
4. **Infection by two phages DNA:** If a bacterium simultaneously infected by two same or related phages, it releases two types of progeny. When this occurs many of the progeny are recombinants.

✪ **Mechanism of transduction: → Fig.8(H-I)**

- Occasionally during the assembly of bacteriophage's progeny inside the host bacterium, an error occurs **called packaging error** that resulting the incorporation of host DNA in to bacteriophage genome.
- The bacteriophage carrying the donor bacterium's DNA adhere on another bacterium & inserts the donor bacterium's DNA into the recipient cell.
- Transduction is not confirmed to transfer the chromosomal DNA only but episome & plasmid may also be transduced.

✪ **History:** Bacterial transduction was discovered by Norton Zinder & Joshua Lederberg in 1952 at the University of Wisconsin-Madison in *Salmonella.*

✪ **Types of transduction:** Two types

1. **Restricted (specialised) transduction:**

- Can transfer only those genes that lie adjacent to the prophage.
- Best studied by lambda phage. The lambda phage that infects *E. coli* always transfers gal^+ gene which is responsible for galactose fermentation.

2. **Generalised transduction:**

- Can transfer any bacterial gene.
- This process may occur with phages (lytic phages) that degrade their host DNA into pieces the size of viral genomes. If these pieces are erroneously packaged into phage particles, they can be delivered to another bacterium. Phage P22 of *S. typhimurium* and P1 and μ of *E. coli* carry out generalized transduction.

✪ **Clinical significances:**

1. **Transfer of extrachromosomal nucleic acid: --**

- Plasmid (R factor) & episome are also transfer by transduction.
- Example: Plasmid mediated penicillin resistant in *Staphylococci* is transfer from cell to cell by transduction

2. **Genetic mapping:** Most useful mechanism in prokaryotes for gene transfers & provide excellent tool for genetic mapping in bacteria.
3. **Treatment of metabolic disease:**
- It affects the eukaryotic cell & proposed method of genetic engineering in treatment of certain inborn error of metabolism.
- Example: Metabolic defect in fibroblast from galactosemic patients can be corrected by transduction using the lambda phage carrying the gal gene.

✪ **Differences between lytic/transduction & temperate cycle/lysogenic convesion: →Table-3**

Lytic cycle	Temperate cycle
Lysis of bacterium	Host bacterium is unharmed
Transfer of donor bacterium's DNA	Transfer of phage DNA
Phage is act as like vehicle or carrier between donor & recipient cell	Phage DNA behave like additional segment of bacterial chromosome & multiplies along with it & confers new properties

Table-3: Differences between lytic & temperate cycle

C. **Lysogenic conversion:** Follow lysogenic/temperate cycle of bacteriophage

D. **Conjugation:**

✪ **Definition:** Transfer of genetic information from one cell to other cell by formation of tube like structure between two cells **called conjugation** & such tube **called conjugation tube.**

✪ **History:** Conjugation was 1st discovered by Joshua Lederberg & Tatum in 1946 in *E. coli* K 12 strain.

✪ **Properties:**
- Conjugation is a process where male/donor bacterium mates or makes physical contact with female/recipient bacterium & transfer genetic information.
- It is like matting in higher organisms but following conjugation female bacterium is converted in to male bacterium.

✪ **Mechanisms:**
- It is due to formation of conjugation tube between two cells by **specialised fimbriae or sex pilus** present on cell surface.
- Such fimbriae are encoded by a plasmid **called sex or fertility (F) factor.**
- Such plasmid is multiply & act as donor (copy of it passes to recipient cell).
- Such plasmid is self transmissible or conjugative.
- Several such plasmids were discovered & acts as donor are collectively **called transfer factor**.

✪ **Clinical significances:** Conjugation allows transfer of genes (like plasmid, episome) or genetic information from one cell to other as below.

i. **Fertility (F)/sex factor conjugation: →Fig.-9**
- F factor is a plasmid codes for special fimbriae or sex pili which makes a conjugation tube between two cells & for necessary enzyme of conjugation.
- Those bacteria that possess F factor are **called F^+**, such bacteria have sex pili on their surface & those are lacking **called F^-.**
- It mediates it's own transfer.
- Vertical (**inheritance**) or horizontal (**transfer**) transmissions maintain plasmids.
- This results in the transfer of an F+ plasmid (coding only for a sex pilus) but not chromosomal DNA from a male donor bacterium to a female recipient bacterium.
- A F^-female cell will become F+ male when it receives the fertility factor from another F+ cell and can make a sex pilus.
- During conjugation, no cytoplasm or cell material except plasmid passes from donor to recipient.
- Two cell mates & form conjugation tube through which F factor can transfer

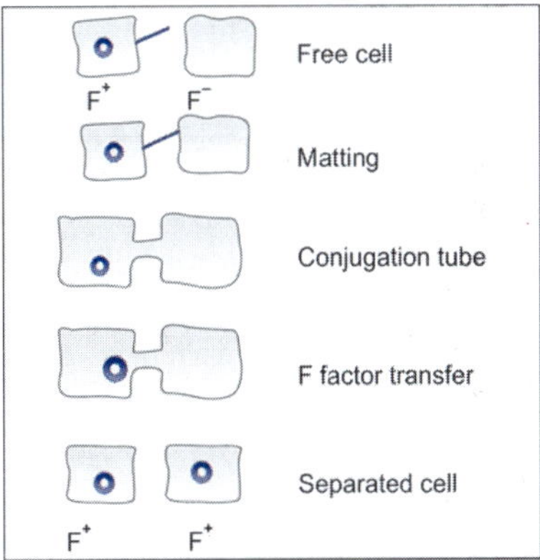

Figure-9: F/Sex factor conjugation

- The mating pairs can be separated by shear forces and conjugation can be interrupted. Consequently, the mating pairs remain associated for only a short time.
- After conjugation, the cells break apart.
- Following successful conjugation the recipient becomes F+ and the donor remains F+.

ii. **R factor conjugation: →Fig.-10**

o Properties of R factor:
- R factor is a plasmid
- responsible for drug resistance
- It present in gram –Ve bacteria

o Components: It has two components as follows
1. **RTF (Resistance Transfer Factor):** 1st that codes for self transfer (like F factor) & haemolysin-enterotoxin production in *E. coli* **called RTF**
2. **r determinant:** 2nd that codes for antibiotic resistance **called r determinant**

o Drug resistance by R factor:
- Transfer of drug resistance by R factor called **called transferable or episomal or infectious drug resistance**.

- R plasmids may confer resistance to as many as eight different antibiotics at once upon the cell and by conjugation it can be rapidly transfer to bacterial population.

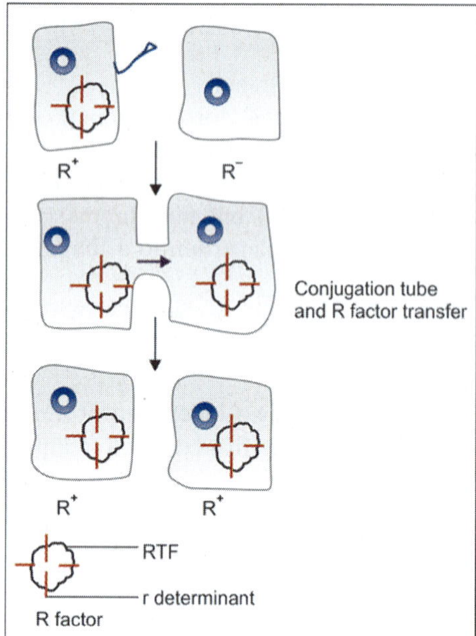

Figure-10: R factor conjugation

- Both F factor and R factor are self transferable but the differences are that the latter has additional genes coding for drug resistance & haemolysin-enterotoxin production.
- During conjugation there is transfer of resistance (R) factor from a donor bacterium to a recipient.
- The recipient becomes multiple antibiotic resistant and male, and is now able to transfer R-plasmids to other bacteria. When the recipient cells acquire entire R factor, it too expresses antibiotic resistance.
- Sometimes RTF may disassociate from the R determinant and the two components may exist as separate entities. In such cases the host cell remains resistant to antibiotics; it can't transfer this resistance to other cells.
- Transfer of multiple antibiotic resistances by conjugation has become a major problem in the treatment of certain bacterial diseases.

iii. Colicinogenic (Col) factor conjugation:

- Col factor is a plasmid
- Responsible for bacteriocins production can also transfer via conjugation.

iv. Episome conjugation/sex duction: →Fig.-11

- It includes the transfer of episome (plasmid integrated with chromosome).
- Cell carrying episome can transfer gene with high frequency hence **called Hfr cells.**
- Sometimes episome detached from chromosome along with some part of chromosome & becomes free **called F prime (F/) factor**
- When F prime (F/) factor cell mates to recipient cell (F−), it transfer F prime (F/) factor & host chromosome linked with it **called sexduction.** Following successful conjugation both cells becomes F/

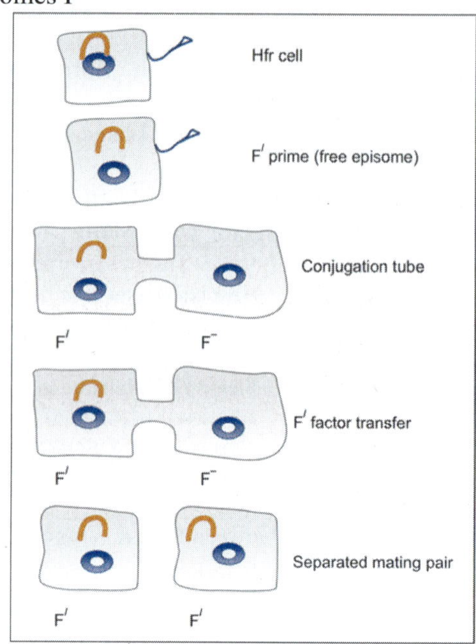

Figure-11: F/ factor conjugation (sex duction)

E. Transposons & transposition:

✪ **Definitions:**

- **Transposon:** Gene that jumps between chromosomal & extra-chromosomal part **called transposons**.
- **Transposition:** Transfer of genetic information from one cell to other cell via transposon **called transposition**.

✪ **Synonym:** Also called

- **Jumping gene:** Because of jumping nature **so called jumping gene**
- **Transposable genetic element:**

✪ **History:** It was discovered by Barbara Mc Clintock in plants during work in the 1940s & 50s for which she was awarded with Nobel Prize in 1983.

✪ **Properties:**

- **Random movement:** This mobile gene can move from one DNA to any DNA or even to another location on the same DNA. The movement is not totally random; there are preferred sites in a DNA molecule at which the transposable genetic element will insert.
- **Not capable of self replication:** Not self replicating & depends on plasmid or chromosomal DNA for replication.
- **Transposition can be accompanied by duplication:** In many instances transposition results in removal of the element from the original site and insertion at a new site. However, in some

cases the transposition event is accompanied by the duplication of thc transposable genetic element. One copy remains at the original site & the other is transposed to the new site.

- **Structural types & significance:**

i. **Insertion sequences (IS):**

- Structure:
  - Small segment of DNA about 1-2 kb without any essential genes **called IS**.
  - Such DNA is encodes for transposition
- Significances:

1. **Mutation:** The introduction of an insertion sequence into a bacterial gene will result in the inactivation of the gene.
2. **Selection of site for plasmid insertion in chromosome:** The sites at which plasmids insert into the bacterial chromosome are at or near insertion sequence in the chromosome.
3. **Phase variation:** In *Salmonella* there are two genes, which code for two antigenically different flagellar antigens. The expression of these genes is regulated by an insertion sequences.

ii. **Transposons:**

- Structure:→**Fig.12**

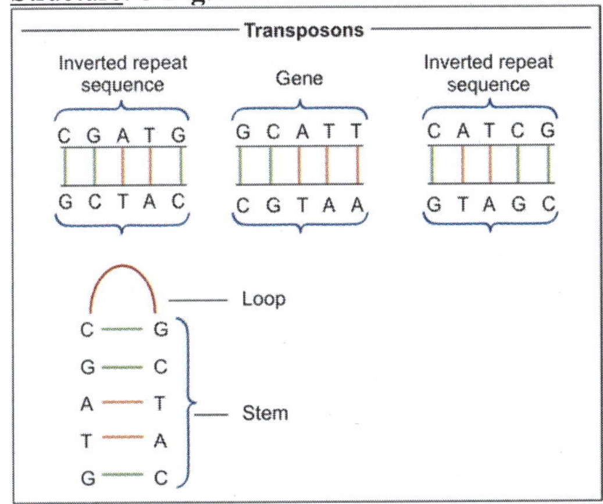

Figure-12: Structure of transposons

- Large segment of DNA about 4-25 kb with essential genes **called transposons**.
- It carries one or more genes in the centre & the two ends carrying inverted repeat sequences complementary to each other but in reverse order. Because of this two ends contains single stranded loop & centre contains double stranded stem formed by H_2 bonding between inverted repeat sequences.

- Significances:

1. **Drug resistance:** Many antibiotic resistance genes are located on transposons. When it jumps on a transferable plasmid it carries multiple drug resistance in a bacterium & causing major medical problem.
2. **Genetic engineering:** It is useful in laboratory for gene manipulation.

Drug resistance mechanisms

❖ **Definition:** Irresponsiveness of microorganisms against antibiotics is **called drug resistance**.

❖ **Types:** Two types

I. **Intrinsic (Natural / Primary / Pre-treatment / Initial) resistance:**

➢ **Definition:** Bacteria were resistant to the antibiotics even before the antibiotics were introduced.

➢ **Significance:** It does not cause any problems in prevention or in treatment of diseases.

➢ **Mechanisms:** Due to lack of
- metabolic process or
- target site required for drug action

➢ **Examples:**
- GNB are normally unaffected by penicillin
- *M. tuberculosis* are insensitive to tetracycline

II. **Acquired (Secondary / Post-treatment) resistance:**

➢ **Definition:** Bacteria were previously sensitive to the antibiotics become resistant after the introduction of antibiotics.

➢ **Significance:** It has great importance because it would result in
- Treatment failure
- Transfer of resistance to other bacteria.

➢ **Mechanisms, subtypes & examples:** Two subtypes

A. **Physiological & biochemical mechanisms:**

i. **Enzymatic inactivation of the antibiotics:** Bacteria produce many enzymes which inactivates or destroy the drugs.

a. **β- lactamase (penicillinase):**
- Destroy the β- lactam ring & inactivate the β-lactam antibiotic (Penicillin).
- Enzyme is inducible & it's production is controlled by plasmid. Such plasmid transmitted to other bacteria by conjugation or by transduction to make them resistant to penicillin.
- **Four types of penicillinase enzymes** are A to D. A is produced by hospital strain.
- **Example of penicillinase producing bacteria:** *Staph. aureus, E. coli, K. pneumoniae, S. typhi, P. mirabilis, N. gonorrhoea. H. influenzae* etc.

b. **Acetyl transferase:**
- Inactivate the chloramphenicol.
- **Examples of acetyl transferase producing bacteria:** *S. typhi, Haemophilus* spp. & *E. coli*

c. **Acetylase/adenylase/phoporylase:**
- Inactivate the aminoglycosides.

ii. **Decreases the permeability of drugs:**

- Many hydrophilic antibiotics enter in bacteria by specific channels formed by proteins **called porin channel** or need specific transport channel. Loss of these channels produce resistant.

- **Examples:**
- Low degree penicillin-resistant: Gonococci are less permeable to penicillin.
- Aminoglycosides resistance in GNB.

iii. Development of alternate metabolic pathway to bypass the action of antibiotic:

- **Examples:** Sulphonamide resistant bacteria like pneumococci, meningococci, gonococci, *E. coli, Staph. aureus, Shigella* spp., *Strept. pyogenes, Strept. viridans* etc. are utilise preformed folic acid from medium instead of synthesing it.

iv. Active efflux (pump out) of antibiotic:

- **Examples:** As in tetracycline, cephalosporin, fluoroquinolones & in macrolides group of drugs.

v. Cross resistance:

- **Definition:** Acquisition of resistance to one drug conferring resistance to other drug, to which organisms has not been exposed is **called cross resistance**.
- **Types:**

a. According to drug or group of drug:

1. Between related drug:

- **Complete resistance:**
  - Definition: Resistance to one drug may extend to other drug of same group
  - Examples:
    - Resistance to one sulphonamide means resistance to all other drug of sulphonamide group
    - Resistance to one tetracycline means resistance to all other drug of tetracycline group
- **Incomplete resistance**:
  - Definition: Resistance to one drug may not extend to other drug of same group
  - Example:
    - Resistance to one Aminoglycosides may not extend to other. E.g. bacteria resistance to gentamicin may sensitive to amikacin.

2. Between unrelated drugs:

- **Incomplete resistance only:**
  - Examples:
    - Tetracycline & chloramphenicol
    - Erythromycin & lincomycin

b. According to direction:

1. **Two ways:** Resistance to erythromycin extend to clindamycin & vice-versa.
2. **One way:** Neomycin resistance to Enterobactariceae extend to streptomycin but not vice-versa.

B. Genetic mechanisms:

i. Chromosomal: Only one method

a. Mutational resistance:

- **Mechanisms:**
  - Some antibiotic works after binding with certain protein
  - Mutation can alters such protein resulting in a protein with little or no affinity for the drug.
- **Types & examples:** Two subtypes

1. Step-wise mutations:

- **Definition:** High level of resistance is achieved by a series of small-step mutations.
- **Examples:**
  - Pn resistance in *Staph. aureus*:
    - Alteration in penicillin binding proteins of cell wall (PBP2a) & bacterial surface receptors in *Staph. aureus*, so antibiotic doesn't bind or binds with low affinity produce resistance to β-lactam antibiotics.
    - Such resistance extends to cover other β-lactam antibiotics like methicillin , cloxacillin or oxacillin **called Methicillin Resistance *Staph aureus* (MRSA)**.
  - Isoniazid & rifampin resistance in *M. tuberculosis*: Mutations in genes are associated with isoniazid & rifampin resistance in *M. tuberculosis*.

2. One-step mutation:

- **Definition:** Where single mutation is sufficient to produce resistance in the bacteria
- **Examples:**
  - Streptomycin resistance in *M. tuberculosis*:
    - Initially bacilli are sensitive to streptomycin but later resistant mutants develop which multiply unchecked & replace the sensitive ones resulting in treatment failure.
    - Presence of other drug can kill such mutant bacilli. For this reason multiple drugs are included in the treatment of tuberculosis.
    - In addition to all this inadequate or irregular treatment can develop Multiple Drug Resistance Tuberculosis (MDR TB) & extended resistance (XDT) strain.

ii. Extrachromosomal: By different methods of gene transfer **called transferable or infectious drug resistance.**

a. Transformation:

- **Definition:**
  - Resistance transferred by agency of free DNA
  - Resistance transfer by transformation is demonstrated experimentally, but not useful clinically.
- **Example:** Acquisition of altered PBP2a by pneumococci produces resistance against penicillin.

b. Transduction:

- **Definition:**
  - Resistance transferred by bacteriophage
  - Plasmid (R factor) is taken up by bacteriophage & transfer to other bacterium.
- **Examples:**
  - Plasmid mediated penicillin resistance in *Staphylococci.*
  - Plasmid mediated chloramphenicol resistance in *S. typhi.*
  - Erythromycin resistance is also phage mediated

c. Conjugation:

- **Definition:**

- Resistance transferred by conjugation tube
- Transfer of R factor plasmid by conjugation is the most important method of drug resistance.
- Acquisition of R factor confers resistance to several antibiotics.
- **Example:** Resistance to penicillin in gram negative bacteria due to beta-lactamase enzyme coded by plasmid.

❖ Prevention of drug resistance:

1. **Elimination of R factor:** By treating the bacteria with acridine dyes or ethidium bromide.
2. **Prefer narrow spectrum drug:** Avoid the use of broad spectrum antibiotics
3. **Combination therapy:** Use of combination therapy whenever long course is required. E.g. in tuberculosis, Sub Acute Bacterial Endocarditis (SABE)
4. **Avoid long term treatment:** This would minimize the selection pressure & time required for resistant strain to emerge.

❖ Differences between mutational & transferable drug resistance: →Table-4

Mutational	Transferable
Mediated by chromosomal part	Mediated by extra - chromosomal part
Low degree virulence	High degree virulence
One drug resistance	Multiple drug resistance
Treated by high dose	High dose is ineffective
Prevented by drug combination	Not prevented by drug combination
Mutants may be defective	Mutants may be not defective
Resistance does not spread	Resistance will spread to same or other species

Table-4: Differences between mutational & transferable drug resistance

Molecular genetics

❖ Introduction:
Development of molecular genetics has provided basis in diagnosis, prevention & treatment of disease over the conventional methods.

❖ Application of molecular genetics:

I. **Genetic engineering**
II. **DNA probe**
III. **Blotting techniques**
IV. **Molecular diagnostic application**

I. Genetic engineering

➢ **Synonym:** DNA recombinant (rDNA) technology or DNA cloning or genetic modification or genetic manipulation

➢ **Definition:** It is an artificial manipulation of DNA to identify & to obtain the gene or gene products.

➢ **Steps:** →**Fig.11**

a. **Developments of DNA fragment:** It is developed with the help of restriction endonuclease enzyme which cleaves the DNA in to nucleotide sequence specific fragment. → **Fig. 13 (a)**

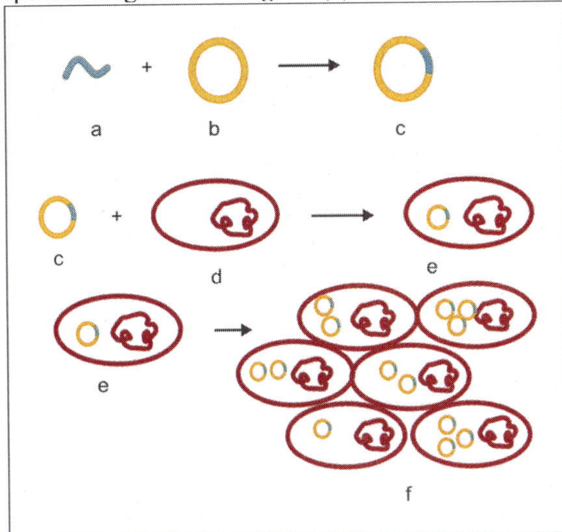

Figure-13: Steps or DNA cloning

b. **Cloning vector:**
- It is DNA molecule in which DNA fragment is inserted. → **Fig. 13(b)**
- Commonly used vectors are:
  - Plasmid e.g. R factor
  - Temperate bacteriophage
  - Cosmid - hybrid vector containing both plasmid & phage

c. **Ligation:** Combined DNA molecule (vector) & DNA fragment **called recombinant DNA**. → **Fig. 13(c).** This method is **called ligation** & it is cleaved by DNA ligase.

d. **Selection of host cell:** → **Fig. 13(d)**
- Commonly used host cell
  - Bacteria e.g. *E. coli*
  - Yeast cell
  - Virus e.g. Vaccinia virus

e. **Introduction of recombinant DNA in to host cell:** → **Fig. 13(e)**
- Recombinant DNA is introduced in to host cell by transformation

f. **Multiplication & obtaining desired product:** → **Fig. 13(f)**
- Host cell containing recombinant DNA is allowed to multiply in suitable medium to obtain desired protein or gene in large quantity.

➢ **Significances:**

a. **Production of hormones:**
1. Growth hormone
2. Somatostatin
3. Insulin
4. Thymosin used for lung & brain cancer

b. **Production of proteins:**

1. Enzymes: Urokinase used to dissolve the blood clots
2. Interleukin
3. Tumour Necrosis Factor (TNF)
4. Factor VIII

c. **Preparation of vaccine:**
1. HBV (Hepatitis B Virus)
2. Foot & mouth disease
3. Rabies vaccine
4. Malaria vaccine (Under trial)
5. HIV capsid protein (Under trial)

d. **Production of interferon:** Used to treat
1. Viral diseases
2. Cancer

e. **Production of antibiotics**

f. **Gene therapy** (Under trial)**:** To treat inherited disease like haemophilia, thalassaemia, sickle cell anaemia & some others diseases also.

g. **Extramedical uses are also possible:**

II. DNA probe

➢ **Definition:** It is a biotinylated or radiolaelled or chemiluminscent piece of single stranded DNA (ss DNA) for detection of homologous DNA by hybridisation method.

➢ **Production:**
- **In the past:** It was prepared by DNA recombinant or DNA cloning.
- **Now a day:** It is prepared by specific instrumentation.

➢ **Properties:**
- **Contains:** It contains unique nucleotide sequence for particular DNA (target DNA) of clinical samples or culture.
- **Labelling:** It is labelled with certain substances **called reporter molecules** such as
  - Biotin-avidin (biotinylated)
  - Radioactive substance (radiolabelled): Like ^{32}P, ^{125}I, ^{35}S
  - Chemicals/dyes (chemiluminscent): Like acridinium orange dye, Cy bromide green dye (PCR) etc.
- **Size:** Probe is about 100-1000 nucleotide base in length or oligonucleotide 20-25 base long.

➢ **Advantages:**
- High sensitivity
- High specificity
- Rapid result

➢ **Uses:**

1. In a hybridisation method to detect:
- Microbes that are difficult or impossible to culture
- Microbes without Ag
- Latent viral infection
- Cultured organisms
- Antibiotic resistance gene
- Epidemiological marker

2. It also used to differentiate virulent from avirulent strain.

➢ **Commercially available probes:** Probes are available for *M. tuberculosis, M. avium, M. intracellularae, E. coli, H. pylori*, Hepatitis B Virus, HSV (Herpes Simplex Virus), HIV, *Rotavirus*, *P. falciparum* etc.

III. Blotting techniques

➢ **Definition:** It is a method of separation (by gel electrophoresis) & transferring DNA, RNA or protein (like Ag) onto a carrier (like nylon or cellulose membrane) so they can be identified either by DNA probe or by enzyme immunoassay.

➢ **Types:** Three types

A. Southern blotting:
✪ **History:** Developed by E.M. Southern, hence the name

✪ **Steps:**
- **Fragmentation:** DNA molecule is fragmented by restriction endonuclease enzyme.
- **Separation:** DNA fragment is separated by gel electrophoresis.
- **Blotting or fixation:** Transfer separated piece on to nylon membrane or cellulose membrane & fixed.
- **Denaturation:** DNA bound to membrane is denatured in to ss DNA.
- **Hybridisation:** Membrane bound DNA is hybridised with radio labelled ss DNA probe.
- **Identification:** Hybridisation is detected on X-ray films

✪ **Use:** Used for identification of DNA

B. Northern blotting:
✪ **History:** Opposite (for RNA) to Southern blotting (for DNA) hence the name

✪ **Steps:** RNA is separated by gel electrophoresis, blotted & identified by labelled probe

✪ **Use:** Used for identification of RNA

C. Western (Immuno) blotting:
✪ **Steps:** Described below with example of HIV **(fig.-14)**

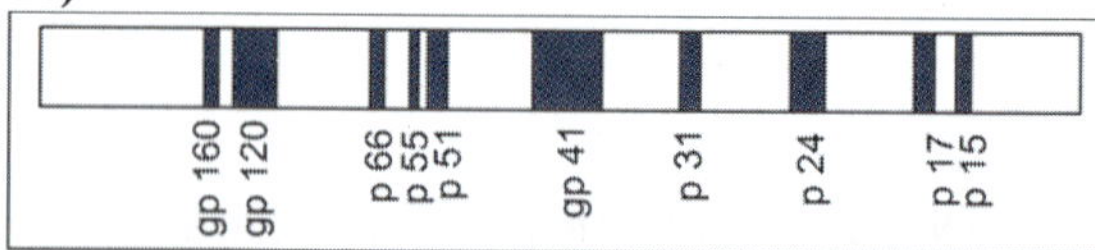

Figure-14: Western blot test for HIV-Ab

- **Separation:** Antigen (Ag) is separated by SDS-PAGE (Sodium Dodecyl Sulphate-Poly Acrylamide Gel Electrophoresis).
- **Blotting or fixation:** Transfer separated piece of Ag on to nylon membrane or cellulose membrane strip & fixed.
- **Reaction with test serum:** Strip is react with sera contains Ab (Antibody) & forms Ag-Ab complex

- **Conjugate step:** Strip then reacts with radio-labelled or enzyme labelled Ab (Anti human globulin).
- **Substrate:** Add the substrate in last, which produce colour band at the Ag site.
- **Result:** At least two band against any of following HIV-Ags like p24, gp41, gp120/160

✪ **Uses:**

- Used for detection of Ag
- Used for detection of Ab. E.g. Detection of HIV Ab against particular Ag like P24, GP120, GP41, gp36

✪ **Advantages:**

- 'Gold standard' for HIV diagnosis
- Confirmation of discordant result obtained by screening test
- Differentiate between HIV-1 & 2 infection

D. Eastern blotting: It is the modification of Western blotting for protein analysis for post translation modification by using probes to detect the lipids, carbohydrate & protein.

IV. Molecular diagnostic application

➢ **Uses:**

- To diagnose different bacterial, viral, fungal & parasitic infection
- To diagnose antimicrobial drug resistance
- To diagnose neoplastic disease
- Forensic investigation
- Examination of phylogenetic relationship in evolution
- Archaeological studies

➢ **Advantages over conventional methods:** Molecular methods have following advantages than conventional (microscopy, culture etc.) methods

- Fast & less labour intensive
- Highly sensitive
- Highly specific

➢ **Disadvantages:**

- High cost
- Required special instruments & infrastructure, so difficult to establish in peripheral set-up

➢ **Molecular diagnostic methods:** Three types of molecular diagnostic methods are

A. Hybridisation:

B. Amplification:

C. Sequencing & enzymatic digestion of nucleic acid:

A. Hybridisation:

✪ **Definition:** Method in which 2 complementary ss DNA come together to form one stable ds DNA molecule is **called hybridisation**.

✪ **Steps:** Five steps (**fig.-15**)

1. Production of target nucleic acid from the target cell: Target cell contains ds DNA which is denatured/cleaved by enzyme or chemical to ss DNA.
2. Production of DNA probe with reporter molecule: It is produced commercially & by instrumentation.
3. Mixture & hybridisation:
4. Separation of unbound labelled probe: It is done by using washer.
5. Identification of hybridisation according to reporter molecules used:

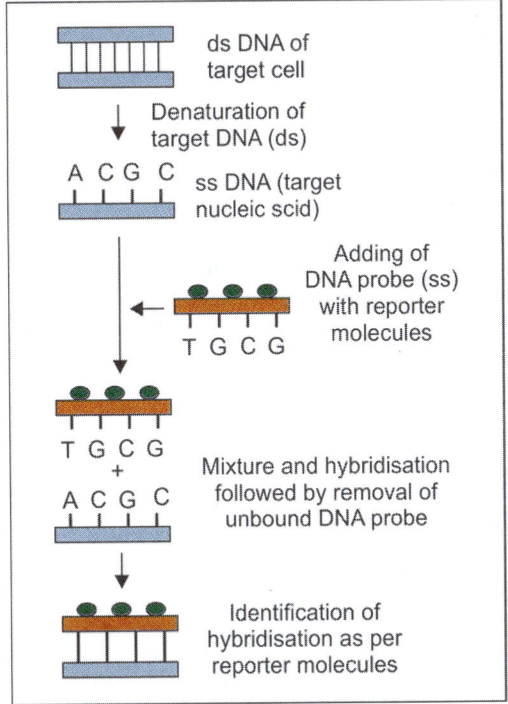

Figure-15: Steps of hybridisation

✪ **Types/format:** Hybridisation can be done in different format like

1. Liquid format
2. Solid support format

B. Amplification: Following four types of amplification methods:

i. PCR

✪ **Full form:** Polymerase Chain Reaction

✪ **Definition:** Rapid automated method for target nucleic acid amplification which combines the principles of hybridisation & replication.

✪ **History:** PCR was developed in 1983 by Kary B Mullis for which he won Nobel Prize in 1993.

✪ **Important features of PCR:**

- With this technique it is possible to make virtually unlimited copies of ss DNA & ds DNA.
- It is used to amplify a specific DNA (target) sequence lying between known positions (flanks) on a ds DNA molecule.
- In order to perform PCR, one must know at least a portion of the sequence of the target DNA molecule that has to be copied.
- PCR amplifies small DNA targets 100-1000 base pairs (bp) long. It is technically difficult to amplify targets >5000 bp long.

- A pair of single stranded oligonucleotide primers, which have DNA sequences complementary to the flanking regions of the target sequence, must be synthesized. The primers are complementary to either end of the target sequence but lie on opposite strands. The primers are usually 20-30 nucleotides long and bind to complementary flanking region.
- Single copy of a nucleic acid target is often undetected by hybridisation is multiplied to 10^7 or more copies in a short period.

✪ **Steps: → Fig.-16**

a. Extraction & denaturation:

- Extraction of ds DNA from clinical samples by heat, chemicals or by enzymatic digestion **called target nucleic acid**.
- Denaturation of ds DNA molecule to ss DNA by heating at 90-95°C for 20 seconds.
- The two strands separate due to breakage of the hydrogen bonds holding them together.

b. Annealing (primer–target duplex formation): Primer nucleic acid is selected specifically to hybridise **(anneal)** with target nucleic acid at 54°C.

c. Extension of primer –target duplex:

- It is extended by enzyme Taq polymerase by heating at 60-75°C for 30 seconds.
- Taq polymerase is not denatured by the high temp.
- It is usually obtained from *Thermus aquaticus*, a bacterium isolated from hot springs.

d. Detection of amplicon:

- The amplified product at the end of PCR is **called amplicon**.
- It is detected by following methods

1. **Probe/hybridisation based detection:** By using labelled probe with reporter molecules (vide supra).

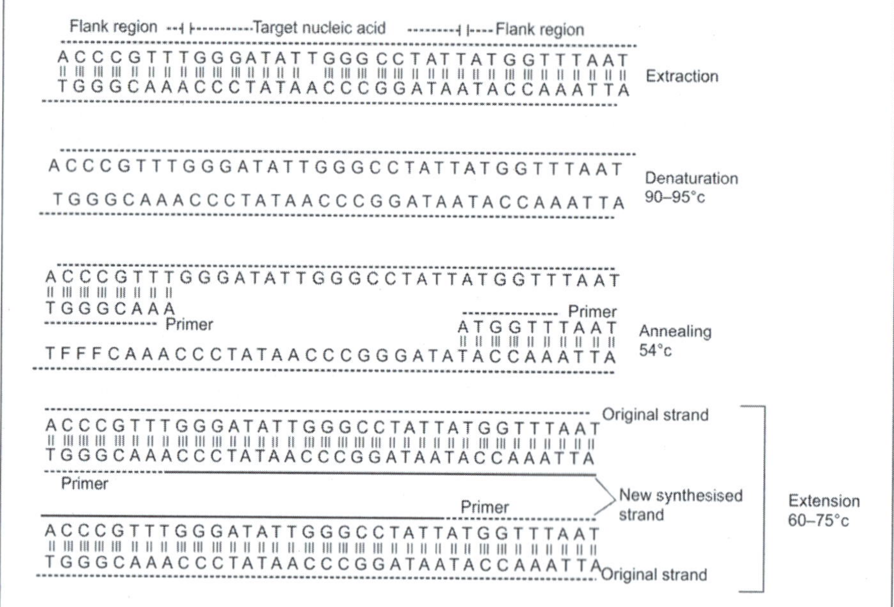

Figure-16: Steps of PCR

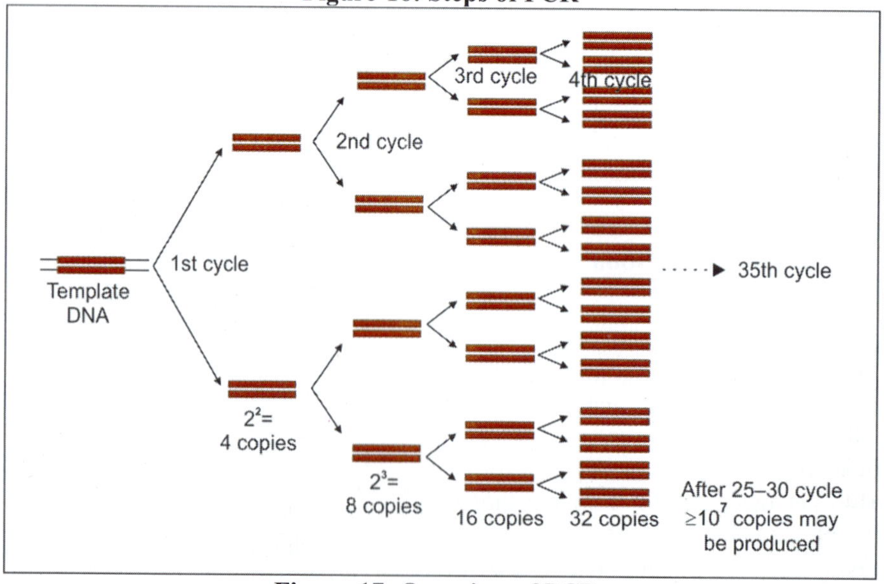

Figure-17: Overview of PCR

2. **Other methods:** Separation of amplicon by gel electrophoresis & stained with ethidium bromide to visualise the amplicon.

✪ **Overview of PCR (fig.-17):** After one cycle (initial three steps) two copies of target DNA are produced. After two cycle four copies, 3 cycle eight copies & after 25-30 successive cycle $\geq 10^7$ of target DNA copies are produced. The 1st three steps are repeated again & again to achieve the multiple copies of DNA.

✪ **Types:**

1. **Multiplex PCR:** Two primers are used. One as control/universal & second as test primer. Presence of control primer minimise the chances of invalid result. It detects two or more target simultaneously.
2. **Nested PCR:** two primer sets are used. 1st set is used to amplify target nucleic acid. Amplicon obtained is then used target nucleic acid for second amplification.
3. **Reverse transcriptase polymerase chain reaction** (**RT-PCR**):
   - For virus with RNA genome, like influenza virus, HIV etc.
   - RNA is converted to DNA (in vitro) by reverse transcriptase followed by routine PCR steps.
4. **Real time PCR (qPCR):**
   - Also **called quantitative real time polymerase chain reaction (qPCR) or real-time quantitative PCR** or **kinetic polymerase chain reaction**
   - RT-PCR is often confused with real time PCR (qPCR), but both are separate techniques. RT-PCR qualitatively detect the gene expression via creation of complementary DNA (cDNA) transcripts from RNA, qPCR quantitatively measure the DNA amplification by using fluorescent dyes.
5. **Real time reverse transcriptase polymerase chain reaction** (**qRT-PCR**):
   - In addition to the qualitative study of gene expression, qPCR can be utilized for quantification of RNA, in both relative and absolute terms, by incorporating qPCR into the technique. The mixed technique, **called quantitative reverse transcriptase polymerase chain reaction** (**qRT-PCR**) or **real-time reverse transcriptase polymerase chain reaction (real time RT-PCR)** or **quantitative real-time reverse transcriptase - PCR** (abbreviated as qRT-PCR, RT-qPCR, or RRT-PCR)
   - Compared to other RNA quantification methods, such as northern blot, qRT-PCR is considered to be the most powerful, sensitive, and quantitative assay for the detection of RNA levels.
6. **Other types:** Touchdown PCR, arbitrarily primed PCR, inverse PCR, allele specific PCR, asymmetric PCR, "Hot Start" PCR, core sample PCR, degenerate PCR and PCR-ELISA.

✪ **Limitations of PCR:**

1. **Contamination:**
   - From extraneous DNA leading to false positive results.
   - Cross-contamination between samples.
   - It is for this reason that sample preparation, running PCR & post-amplification detection must be carried out in separate rooms.
2. **Concentration of Mg:** Is very crucial as low Mg2+ leads to low yields (or no yield) and high Mg2+ leads to accumulation of nonspecific products.
3. **High cost:** Reagents and equipments are costly, hence can't be afforded by small laboratories.

ii. **TMA (Transcription Mediated Amplification):** Amplification of ribosomal RNA instead of DNA

iii. **NASBA (Nucleic Acid Sequence Based Amplification):** Similar to TMA. RNA is converted to DNA by reverse transcriptase & then RNA copies are synthesised by RNA polymerase

iv. **LCR (Ligase Chain Reaction):**
- Instead of target nucleic acid DNA probe (primer) is amplified
- Two probes are used.
- Once it anneals to target nucleic acid, space between two probes is closed by enzyme ligase **(ligation reaction)**.
- By heating joined probes released as single strand which is complementary to target nucleic acid.
- This newly synthesised strand is used for next cycle

C. Sequencing & enzymatic digestion of nucleic acid:

i. **Nucleic acid sequencing:** Determine exact nucleotide sequence of gene or gene fragment

ii. **High density DNA probe:** Based on hybridisation of a fluorescent- labelled nucleic acid target to large sets of oligonucleotide synthesised at precise location on a miniaturised glass substrate or chip.

iii. **Ribotyping:** Enzymatic digestion of chromosomal DNA followed by Southern hybridisation using probes that encodes for r RNA.

iv. **RFLP (Restriction Fragment Length Polymorphism):**
- After the digestion of nucleic acid it is separated by gel electrophoresis & nucleotide sequencing is analysed **called restriction pattern**.
- Difference between restriction patterns of microbes **called RFLP.**

v. **PFGE (Pulsed Field Gel Electrophoresis):** Electrophoresis device used to separate enzymatically digested chromosomal fragments of intact bacterial chromosomal DNA.

Question bank

Essay/Full question

1) Genetic structure of bacteria
2) Genotypic & phenotypic variation of bacteria

Short notes

1) Bacterial DNA
2) Plasmid
3) Transposons & transposition
4) Mutation
5) Gene transfer mechanisms
6) Transformation
7) Transduction
8) Bacterial conjugation
9) Drug resistance mechanisms
10) Blotting technique

Short questions for theory/viva questions

1) What is sense codon & non-sense codons?
2) What are introns & exons?
3) What is plasmid?
4) Name the two chromosomal & two extra chromosomal nucleic acids of bacteria
5) What is episome & transposons?
6) Write the four differences between phenotypic & genotypic variation
7) Write four differences between mutational & transferable drug resistance
8) Write four uses of genetic engineering

MCQs for chapter review

Genetic structure

1) Plasmid is
(a) Intracytoplasmic (b) Extrachromosomal (c) a+b (d) None

2) Plasmid (PGI-98)
(a) Involved in multiple drug resistance transfer (b) Involved in conjugation (c) Imparts capsule formation (d) Imparts pili formation

3) Jumping gene (PGI-98)
(a) Transposon (b) Episome (c) Cosmid (d) Plasmid

Bacterial variation

Genotypic variation

4) Natural method of horizontal gene transfer among bacteria includes (PGI, Nov-99)
(a) Electroporation (b) Transduction (c) Transformation (d) Conjugation (e) Mutation

5) Mechanism of direct transfer of free DNA-
(a) Transformation (b) Conjugation (c) Transduction (d) None

6) Virus mediated transfer of host DNA from one cell to another is known as (AI-05, AIIMS-93)
(a) Transduction (b) Transformation (c) Transcription (d) Integration

7) Lysogenic conversion is (PGI-96)
(a) New properties in a bacterium due to integration of phage genome (b) Transfer of DNA from one bacterium to another by a bacteriophage (c) Transfer of free DNA (d) transfer of genome during physical contact

8) The discovery of "gene transformation" came from the study of one of the following bacteria (PGI, Nov-99)
(a) *Bacillus subtilis* (b) *Streptococcus pyogenes* (c) *Streptococcus pneumoniae* (d) *Escherichia coli*

9) F factor integrated with bacterial chromosome to form (PGI -93)
(a) HFr (b) RTF+r (c) F^- (d) RTF

10) Conjugation does not involve
(a) Bacteriophage (b) HFr (c) F factor (d) Plasmid

11) The role of plasmid in conjugation was first described by Lenderberg and Tatum in (AIIMS -02)
(a) *H influenzae* (b) *Corynebacterium* (c) *Pseudomonas* (d) *Escherichia coli*

12) Bacteria may acquires characteristics by all of the following except
(a) Taking up soluble DNA fragments across their cell wall from other species (b) Incorporating part of host DNA (c) Through bacteriophage (d) Through conjugation

Drug resistance mechanisms

13) Multiple drug resistance is spread by
(a) Transformation (b) Conjugation (c) Transduction (d) Mutation

Molecular genetics

14) Cy bromide green dye is used for (AIIMS -06)
(a) HLPR (b) PCR (c) ELISA (d) Immunofluorescence

15) DNA is detected by
(a) Southern blot (b) Northern blot (c) Western blot (d) Eastern blot

16) PCR was discovered by
(a) Robert Koch (b) Kerry Mullis (c) Edward Jenner (d) Alexander Fleming

17) Taq polymerase is obtained from
(a) *E coli* (b) *Bacillus subtilis* (c) *Bacillus steriothermophilus* (d) *Thermus aquaticus*

18) Real time PCR is used for (AIIMS, May-13)
(a) Multiplication of RNA (b) Multiplication of specific segment of DNA (c) Multiplication of proteins (d) To know how much amplification of DNA has occurred

19) Reverse transcriptase polymerase chain reactions can be aid in diagnosis of all of the following viral infections except (AI-97)
(a) Adeno virus (b) *Astrovirus* (c) *Rotavirus* (d) Polio virus

Answers of MCQs & explanation

1) (c)
- Plasmid is an extra-chromosomal intracytoplasmic DNA material

2) (a), (b), (c) & (d)
- Plasmid is encode for multiple drug resistance transfer (RTF) conjugation or sex pili formation or F factor & capsule formation in *B anthracis*
- Follow section, **genetic structure (extra-chromosomal parts → plasmid)** for more detail

3) (a)
- Follow section, **genetic structure (extra-chromosomal parts → trasnposon)** for explanation

4) (b), (c) & (d)
- Follow section, **bacterial variation (genotypic variation → gene transfer mechanisms / methods)** for more detail

5) (a)
6) (c)
7) (a)
} Follow section, **bacterial variation (genotypic variation → gene transfer mechanisms / methods → lysogenic conversion)** for explanation

8) (c)
- Gene transformation came from the study of *Streptococcus pneumoniae* by Griffith

9) (a)
- F factor is plasmid but in question its written as 'integrated with bacterial chromosome" so it considered as episome. Cells

containing episome are transferring it with high frequency **called HFr cells** (<u>H</u>igh <u>f</u>requency of <u>r</u>ecombination), So option a is right answer

10) (a)

- Bacteriophage is involved in transduction

11) (d)

- Conjugation was 1st discovered by Joshua Lederberg & Tatum in 1946 in *E. coli* K 12 strain

12) (b)

- Bacteria are not acquiring any properties from host cell DNA but they may acquires characteristics by
  - Taking up soluble DNA fragments across their cell wall from other species **called transformation**
  - Through bacteriophage **called transduction**
  - Through conjugation tube **called conjugation**

13) (a), (b) & (c)

- Multiple drug resistance is mediated by extra-chromosomal part which is spread by transformation, conjugation & transduction while single drug resistance is mediated by chromosomal part which is spread by mutation

14) (b)

- Follow section, **molecular genetics (DNA probe → labelling)** for explanation

15) (a)

- Southern blot is used for DNA, Northern blot is used for RNA & Western (immuno) blot is for Ag/Ab detection. No Eastern blot technique is available. Follow section molecular genetics (Blotting technique) for more details.

16) (b) } Follow section, **molecular genetics (PCR)**
17) (d) } for more details

18) (d)

- Follow section, **molecular genetics (PCR → types →Real Time PCR)** for explanation

19) (a)

- Reverse transcriptase polymerase chain reactions is useful for RNS viruses, adenovirus is DNA virus while all other options are RNA viruses.

7 Sterilisation and disinfection

Learning heading & subheadings

Introduction

❖ **History:** Concept of sterilisation and disinfection was practised by Pasteur, Lister & Koch

❖ **Definitions:**

➢ **Sterilisation:**

- Method by which an article or surface or medium **completely** become free from all microorganisms including pathogenic, nonpathogenic & spores & organisms are incapable to give rise the reinfection.
- Done by using physical agents or methods so also **called physical sterilisation**

➢ **Disinfection:**

- Method by which an article or surface or medium **incomplete** become free from microorganisms including pathogenic & nonpathogenic except spores & organisms are capable to give rise the reinfection.
- Done by using chemical agents or methods, so also **called chemical sterilisation**
- As per definition of disinfection, spores are not killed by disinfectants; however some disinfectants have sporicidal action. For more details about sporicidal agent, **follow chapter → Morphology of bacteria**

➢ **Asepsis:** Prevention of infection by keeping the article or surface or medium away from the source of infection. It means absence of microbes.

➢ **Antisepsis:** Prevention of infection by inhibiting the growth of organisms.

➢ **Antiseptics:** Chemical agents used to prevent the infection or growths of microbes are **called antiseptics**. Few authors differentiated antiseptics from disinfectants by their use on skin or mucosa where later can use for inanimate objects. However antiseptics are also **called skin disinfectants**.

✪ **Common antiseptics / skin disinfectants:** As follows

1. Betadine (povidone iodine), Tincture iodine (iodine in 2% alcohol): Best skin disinfectants because less irritant & causes less staining
2. Spirit (ethyle alcohol/70% ethanol)
3. Isopropanol (isopropyl alcohol)
4. Hibitane (chlorhexidine)

✪ **Common hand disinfectants:** As follows

a. **Alcohol based: Sterilium or Bactilium**

- **Contains:** Both are same preparation but different brands with following contains in 500 ml solution
  - 1-propanol (*n*-propanol or propan-1-ol): 35 gm
  - 2-propanol (Isopropyl alcohol, isopropanol or propan-2-ol): 45gm
  - Macetronium ethyl sulfate (Ethyl-hetadecyl-dimethylammonium-ethysulphate): 0.2gm.
- **Contact time:**
  - For patient care hand wash is 3ml (2 push) for 30 seconds
  - For surgical hand wash is 9 ml (6 push) for 3 minutes for each hand.

b. **Chlorhexidine gluconate:**

- 2.5% hand rub & hand gel.
- Contact time: Same as sterilium

c. **Betadine (povidone iodine) solution:** It is high level disinfectants used for surgical hand scrub

➢ **Bacteriostatic agents:** Chemical agents capable of preventing / inhibiting multiplication of bacteria.

➢ **Bactericidal agents (germicides):** Chemical agents capable of killing the bacteria.

➢ **Sporicides or sporicidal agents:** Chemical agents capable of killing the spores. For more details about sporicidal agent, follow chapter → Morphology of bacteria

- **Cleaning:** Removal of all soil (e.g. organic and inorganic material) & other dirt from object or surfaces or medium by wiping or using water with detergent.
- **Decontaminations (sanitization):** Process of keeping article or area free from contaminants.

❖ **Differences between sterilisation & disinfection:** → Table-1

Sterilisation	Disinfection
By physical agents	By chemical agents
Kills all pathogenic, non-pathogenic microbes & spores	Kills all pathogenic & non-pathogenic microbes except spores
Complete killing of microbes, so no chances of reinfection	Incomplete killing (reduce the numbers) of microbes, so chances of reinfection

Table-1: Differences between sterilisation & disinfection

❖ **Order of resistance of microbes:** Decreasing order of resistance of microbes to the agents used for sterilisation & disinfection is mentioned in **flow chart-1**

Prion (Highest resistance) > *C. parvum* oocyst > Bacterial spores > *Mycobacteria* > Cyst of parasites (*G. lamblia*) > Small non-enveloped viruses > Trophozoites > Gram negative bacteria > Fungus > Large non-enveloped viruses > Gram positive bacteria > Enveloped viruses (Lowest resistance)

Flow chart-1: Order of resistance of microbes

Classification

Three types of methods as shown in **flow chart -2**

✓ **Note: Terminology**

- Physical methods & chemical methods are used as a synonym for sterilisation & disinfection respectively, but this practice is not correct because many physical methods are giving incomplete sterilisation & many chemical methods are giving complete disinfection with killing of spores.

I. Physical methods (sterilisation) or physical agents (sterilants)

❖ **Types:** Following three are the physical methods of sterilisation

A. Sunlight: Having bactericidal effect due to heat & UV rays. Rarely useful.

B. Drying:

- About 80% of bacterial weight is due to water & drying in air cause deleterious effect on bacteria.
- Unreliable & only theoretical value.

C. Heat: Method of choice for sterilization unless it is contraindicated.

- **Effective factors:**
  - Temperature of exposed heat.
  - Time of exposure.
  - Type of heat e.g. dry or moist heat
  - Presence of substances e.g. protein, starch, fats-oils, acids-alkalis
  - pH of medium
  - Type of organisms e.g. vegetative forms or spores forms
  - Numbers of organisms
  - Type of materials to be sterilized...
- **Thermal Death Time (TDT):** Minimum time required to killed organisms at given temperature called TDT
- **Types of heat:** Two main types of heat like

i. **Dry heat**

ii. **Moist heat**

i. Dry heat

✪ **Mechanism of action:** Killing effect due to

- Denaturation of protein
- Oxidative damage
- Toxic effect of elevated levels of electrolytes.

> **Mnemonic:** Mechanism of action
> - **Dry heat mechanisms:** DOT → Vide supra
> - **Moist heat mechanisms:** DC → Vide infra

✪ **Methods:** Following are three methods of dry heat

a. Red heat or red hot or flaming:

- **Principle:** Burning of article till it become red hot.
- **Articles to be sterilized are:** Nichrome wires, nichrome loops, tips of forceps

b. Incineration:

- **Principle:** Burning of article till it becomes ash.
- **Articles to be sterilized are:** Contaminated cloths, animal's carcasses, pathological materials, bio-medical waste and plastic items like PVC or polythene.

c. Hot air oven:

- **Principle:** Sterilisation by dry heat at 160°C for 2 hours.
- **Holding time & temperature:** → Table -2

Temperature (°C)	Time (minutes)
160	120
170	60
180	30

Table-2: Holding temperature & time of oven

✓ **Note:** British pharmacopoeia recommended 150°C for 1 hour for oils, glycerol & dusting powder.

- **Instrument's structure:** →Fig.-1
  - It is a bad conductor of heat.
  - Heating elements are heated by electricity & kept inside the wall.
  - It is fitted with fan for elimination of air & even distribution of air.

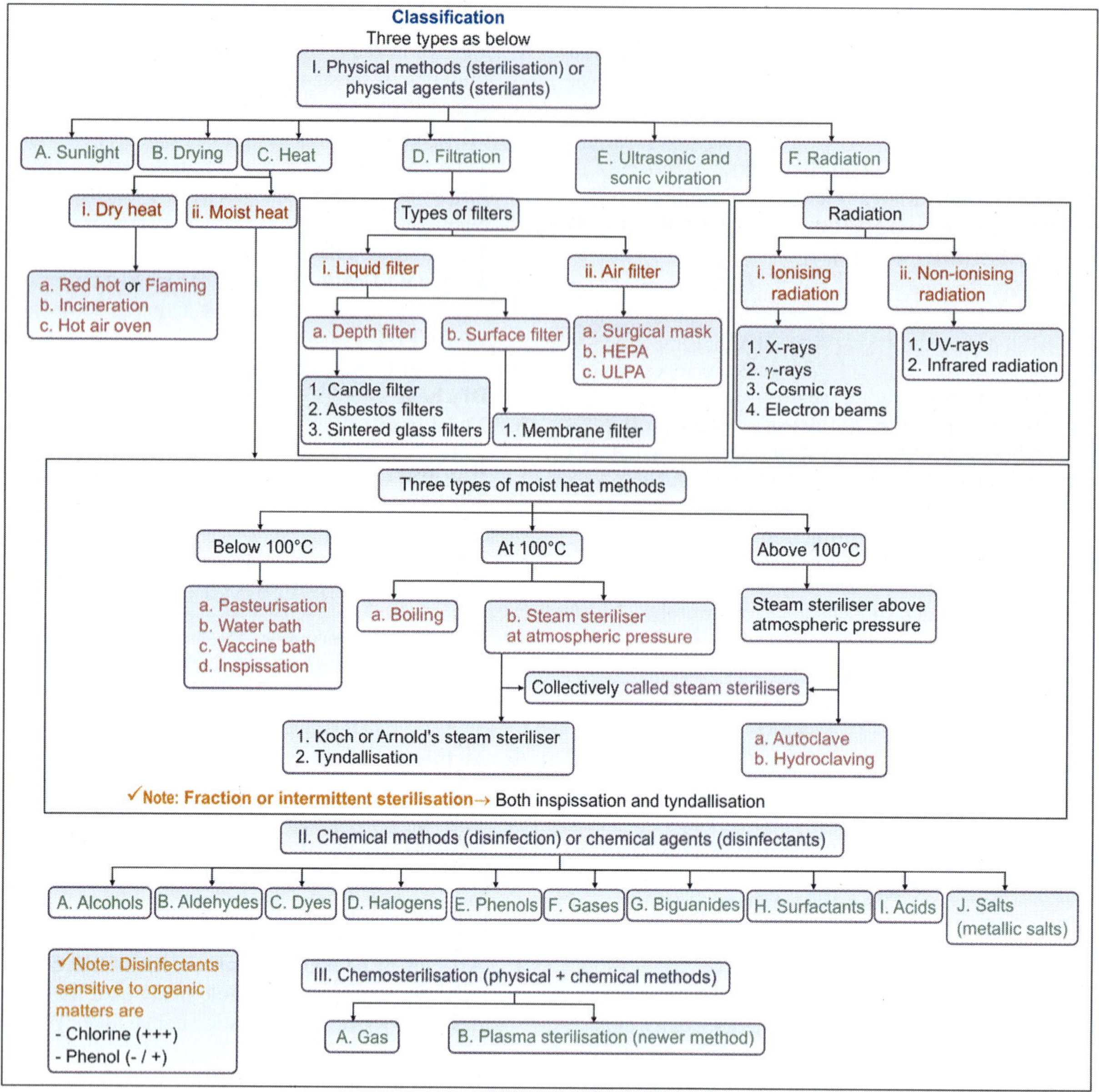

Flow chart-2: Classification of methods of sterilisation & disinfection

- **Articles to be sterilised:** All those which cannot be penetrated by steam & can tolerate high temperature like
  - Glass materials: Glass tubes, glass bottles, glass syringes etc.
  - Metal instruments: Forceps, scissors, scalpels etc.
  - Pharmaceutical products: Grease, liquid paraffin, fats, dusting powders etc.
- **Disadvantages:**
  - Long exposure time.
  - Temperature >185°C may destroy the instruments.
  - Higher temperature is corrosive, resulting loss of hardness.
- **Precautions:**
  - Should not be overloaded
  - Dry the glassware before putting in oven
  - Wrap the tubes or bottles in paper
  - Arrange articles in such a way which allow free circulation of air in between the articles.
  - Rubber except silicon rubber can't withstand the temperature, so don't put in oven.
  - Cotton plug may charred at 180°C, so don't put in oven.
  - After sterilisation, oven should be allowed to cool for 2 hours before opening the door to avoid the cracking of the glassware due to sudden or uneven cooling

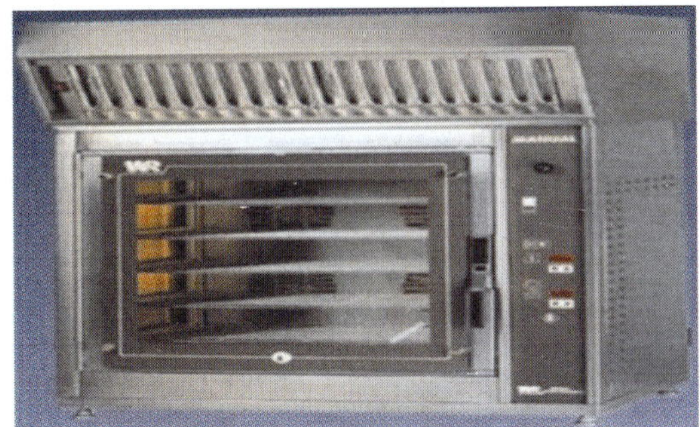

Figure-1: Hot air oven

- **Sterilisation control:** Three types
1. **Physical control:** Thermometer, thermocouple
2. **Chemical control:** Browne's tube or green spot which gives green colour after proper sterilisation.
3. **Biological control:**
- A strip containing 10^6 spores of *Cl. tetani* or *B. subtilis* subsp. *niger* is packed in envelops & putted in to oven.
- After proper sterilisation remove the strip & inoculated in thioglycolate broth or RCMM
- Incubate anaerobically at 36°C for 5 days for sterility testing.

✓ **Note: Microwave oven**

- **Principle:** It is basically radio wave (with 2500 MHz or 2.5GHz frequency) to cook the food. Radio waves are absorbed by fats, water & sugars of food to generate the heat.

ii. Moist heat

- **Mechanism of action:** Killing effect due to
  - Denaturation of protein
  - Coagulation
- **Moist heat is more advantageous than dry heat:** Because the steam of moist condenses over the surface of spores & other organisms which increases the temperature & water content of organisms. Later causes microbial death by hydrolysis & breaking down of bacterial proteins
- **Types of moist heat:** Three types of method as shown in **flow chart-3**

Below 100°C

- **Advantages:** Kills all mesophilic-vegetative bacteria, moulds, yeasts & some viruses.
- **Disadvantages:** Not able to kill spores & some heat resistant viruses like polio virus, HBV etc.
- **Methods:** Four types

a. Pasteurisation:

- Definition: Defined by WHO in 1970 as follows
  - Heating of milk to such temperature & for such periods of time as are required to destroy any pathogens that may be present while, causing minimal changes in the composition, flavour & nutritive value of milk **called pasteurisation**
- History: Invented by Louis Pasteur in 1863-65.
- Uses:
  1. For sterilisation of milk
  2. To control the microorganisms from beverages like beer, fruit juices & vegetable juices
- Methods:

1. **Holder method:** Milk is kept at 60°C for 30 minutes followed by rapid cooling at 5°C
2. **Flash (HTST-High Temperature & Short Time) method:**
   - Milk is heated at 72°C for 15-20 seconds followed by rapid cooling at 13°C or lower.
   - Rapid method
   - Most widely used method
   - Very large quantity of milk per hour can be pasteurised by this method
   - Relatively heat resistant bacteria like *Coxiella burnetii* may survive in Holder method but killed by Flash method

- Disadvantages:
  - Not destroy the bacterial spores, bacterial toxins & fungal toxins

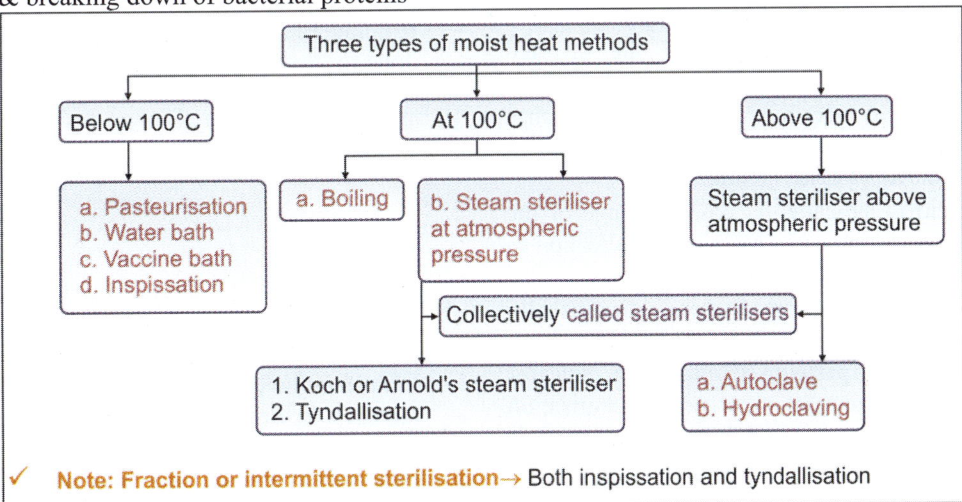

Flow chart-3: Types of moist heat methods

- Not kill the thermoduric bacteria: Follow chapter →Physiology of bacteria for more details
- Advantages: All non sporing bacteria like *Coxiella burnetii* (Q fever, survive under Holder method), *Mycobacteria* (tuberculosis), *Salmonella* (slamonellosis), *Brucella* (brucellosis) etc. are killed
- Tests of pasteurized milk:

1. **Phosphatase test:**

- **Principle:** Alkaline phosphatase enzyme breaks the phenyl disodium phosphate to release phenol (phenol is benzene derivatives & used as disinfectant. Also **called carbolic acid**).
- **Steps:** Add the solution contains phenyl disodium phosphate to milk in a sterile test tube. Later add the solution contains colour indicator. Incubate at 37^{0}C for 2 hours.
- **Result:** Change in colour occurs if free phenol is present. Phenol release is quantitated by measuring the absorbance of the colour developed by a spectrophotometer.
- **Interpretation:** Alkaline phosphatase enzyme present in milk is destroyed by heating the milk at 60°C for 30 minutes. Presence of enzyme indicates inadequate pasteurisation or later addition of raw milk.

✓ **Note: Phosphatase test *Staph aureus***
- **Follow chapter →Micrococcaceae**

2. **Standard plate count:**

- Bacteriological quality of milk is determined by culture technique **called standard plate count**. Most countries in the West enforce a limit of 30,000 bacterial count per ml of pasteurised milk

3. **Coliform count:**

- **Principle:** It based on fermentation of lactose of milk by coliform bacteria. Coliforms ferment the lactose of milk to produce acid and gas. Acid is indicated by colour change of the medium & gas is indicated by bubbles collection in the inverted Durham tube.
- **Steps:** Add the serially diluted milk to three tubes contains Mac Conkey's broth & inverted Durham tube. Incubate at 37^{0}C for 48 hours.
- **Result:** Acid is indicated by colour change of the medium & gas is indicated by bubbles collection in the inverted Durham tube.
- **Interpretation:** Coliform bacteria are usually completely destroyed by pasteurisation; therefore their presence in pasteurised milk is an indicator of inadequate pasteurisation or post-pasteurisation contamination. The standard in most countries is that coliform be absent in 1 ml of milk.

b. **Water bath: →Fig.-2**

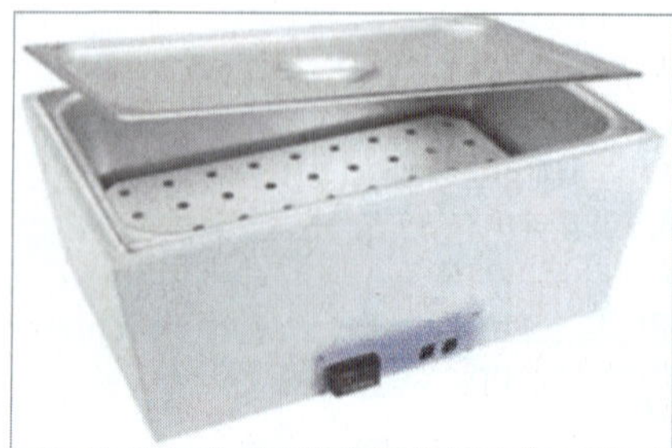

Figure-2: Water bath

- For serum/body fluid containing coagulable proteins.
- 56°C for 1 hour for several successive days.

c. **Vaccine bath:**

- For vaccine of non-sporing bacteria.
- 60°C for 1 hour.

d. **Inspissation: →Fig.-3**

- Synonym: Also **called fraction sterilisation** because it required three successive days for sterilisation of articles
- Principle: It sterilise the article by moist heat below 100°C for three successive days. 1st exposure kills all vegetative form & in the interval between the heating remaining spores germinates in to vegetative forms which are killed on subsequent heating.

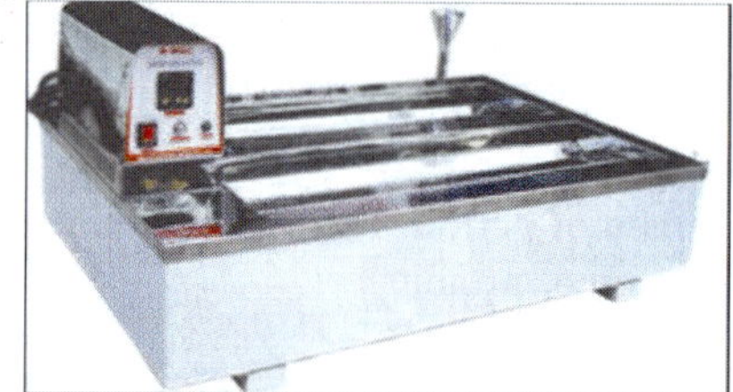

Figure-3: Inspissator

- Uses: For sterilisation of media contains serum & eggs which generally get destroyed at high temperature like LJ medium, Dorset egg medium & Loeffler's serum.
- Holding time & temperature: Sterilisation can be done for three successive days as follows
  1st day: 85°C for 1 hr
  2nd day: 75°C for 1 hr
  3rd day: 75°C for 1 hr

At 100°C

- **Methods:** Two types

a. **Boiling:**

- **Principle:** Heating in boiling water at 100° C for 5 minutes sufficient to kill all vegetative bacteria, HBV & some bacterial spore.
- **Articles to be sterilized are:** Medical & surgical equipment in emergencies like glass syringe.
- Heat labile articles and hollow or porous items where water will not penetrate in the lumen **cannot** be sterile by this way.

- Sterilisation may be **promoted** by adding 2% of sodium bicarbonate.

b. Steam steriliser at atmospheric pressure: Two categories

1. Koch or Arnold's steam steriliser:

- Principle: sterilisation by moist heat at 100°C for 90 minutes at atmospheric pressure.
- Instrument's structure:→**Figure-4**
  - **Cabinet:** Copper cabinet with walls suitably lagged.
  - **Lid:** Conical lid with central perforation for drainage of steam.
  - **Perforated tray** to put article to be sterilised.
  - **Water** at bottom with **heater.**
- Articles to be sterilized are: Selective heat labile media like DCA, XLD, TCBS and Selenite F broth.
- Disadvantage: Not kill the bacterial spores
- Advantages:
  - Inexpensive
  - No chances of explosion

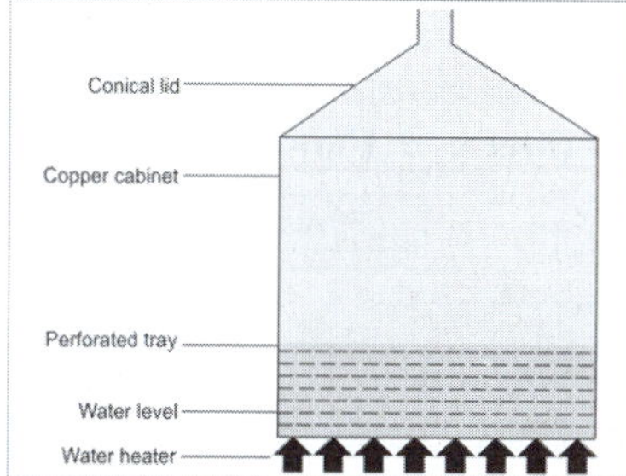

Figure-4: Koch or Arnold's steam steriliser

2. Tyndallisation:

- Synonym: Fraction sterilisation or intermittent sterilisation
- Principle: Sterilisation by moist heat at 100°C at atmospheric pressure for 20 min for 3 successive days. Hence **called fraction** or **intermittent sterilisation.** Kills the vegetative bacteria & spores will germinate in favourable condition will killed by successive sterilisation.
- Articles to be sterilized are: Media containing sugar or gelatin
- Advantage: Kills the bacterial spores

Above 100°C
(Steam steriliser above atmospheric pressure)

- **Methods:** Two types

a. Autoclave:

- Principle: Sterilisation by moist heat above 100°C above atmospheric pressure
- Instrument's structure: →**Figure-5**
  - **Cabinet/cylinder:** Horizontal or vertical cabinet made up from stainless steel or gunmetal with iron supporting sheet.
  - **Lid:** It is with
    - Screw clamps to make it airtight to prevent the leakage of steam.
    - Safety valve for drainage of steam.
    - Pressure & temperature gauge
  - **Perforated tray** to put an article to be sterilised.
  - **Water** at bottom of cabinet with heater
  - **Heater** operated by gas or electricity.

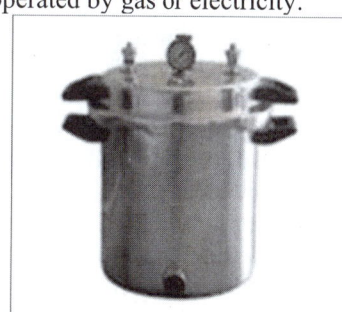

Figure-5: Autoclave

- Mechanism:
  - Enough amount of water is added
  - Place an article to be sterilised on tray & sterilisation control
  - Start the heater
  - Close the lid
  - Safety valve is set to the required pressure
  - Allow the steam-air mixture to escape till all air has been displaced from autoclave
  - Make the lid airtight by screw clamps
  - Steam start to collect in the cabinet and raise the pressure.
  - When pressure reach to desired level, safety valve open & remove excess steam.
  - Start to count the holding time from this point.
  - Off the heater when holding time is over
  - Allow the autoclave to cool till the pressure gauge indicates same pressure inside the cabinet & atmosphere.
- Articles to be sterilized are: Laboratory media, glassware, hospital dressing, cloths, apron, surgical instruments, pharmacological products, fluid in sealed container, biomedical waste before disposal etc.
- Holding time, temperature & pressure: →**Table 3**

Temperature (°C)	Time (minutes)	Pressure (lbs)
121	15	15
126	10	20
134	3	30

Table-3: Holding temperature, pressure & time of autoclave

- Types of autoclave:
  1. Laboratory autoclaves
  2. Hospital dressing steriliser
  3. Bowel & instrument steriliser
  4. Rapid cooling steriliser e.g. pressure cooker
  5. Others: gravity displacement & high vacuum sterilisers
- Advantages:
  - Non-toxic

- Cycle easy to control & monitor
- Inexpensive
- Least affected by organic/inorganic soils
- Bactericidal & Sporicidal
- Rapid cycle time
- Penetrates medical packing, device lumens

o Disadvantages:

- Deleterious for heat labile instruments
- Chances of explosion
- Required constant supervision during operation
- No facility for drying the load after the sterilisation
- Potential for burns
- No facility for air discharge & it is very difficult to judge the complete air removal. If air is not removed completely desired temperature & pressure can't be achieved.

o Sterilisation control: Three types

▫ **Physical:**

- Temperature & pressure monitoring gauge
- Thermocouple

▫ **Chemical:**

- Browne's tube or green spot: gives green colour after proper sterilisation.
- Autoclave tape: e.g. Bowie dick tapes

▫ **Biological:** A strip containing 10^6 spores of *Bacillus (Geobacillus) steriothermophilus* is packed in envelops & putted in to autoclave. After proper sterilisation remove the strip & inoculated in suitable medium& incubated at 55°C for 5 days for sterility testing

b. Hydroclaving:

o Principle: Sterilisation by indirect moist heat (no contact of article with steam) above 100°C under atmospheric pressure

o Mechanism: It is an expansion of autoclave method. Kept all article to be sterilised in inner jacket & steam is collected in outer jacket. Article turns mechanically with the help of a series of large rotating rods, which spin continuously rupturing the waste bags & ensuring complete exposure to heat.

Features	At atmospheric pressure	above atmospheric pressure
Examples	- Koch or Arnold's steam steriliser - Tyndallisation	Autoclave
Instrument's lid	Perforated, so no steam collection in cabinet	Not-perforated, so steam collection in cabinet
Temperature	At 100°C	>100°C
Pressure	Not rise in cabinet	Rise in cabinet due to steam collection
Supervision	Not required	Required

Table-4: Types of steam steriliser

o Articles to be sterilized are: Same as autoclave

o Advantages:

- Hydrolyse the organic matter
- No pretreatment of waste is required
- Reduction in volume & weight
- Easy to operate
- More heat penetrating than autoclave
- Economical

✓ **Note: Steam steriliser**

▪ **Types:** Two types with differences in **table-4**

D. Filtration:

➢ **Principle:** According to British pharmaceutical codex test pore size of filter prepared in such a way that retain the smallest bacteria like *S. marcescens*

➢ **Uses:**

1. Purification of water
2. To remove bacteria from heat labile liquids e.g. sera, sugar or antibiotics solution.
3. To separate exotoxin
4. To separate virus (viruses pass through the filters) from bacteria
5. To measure the size of virus
6. To separate bacteriophage

➢ **Control:** It is done by using smallest bacteria like *Serratia marcescens* & *Brevundimonas diminuta*

➢ **Types of filters:** → **Flow chart-4**

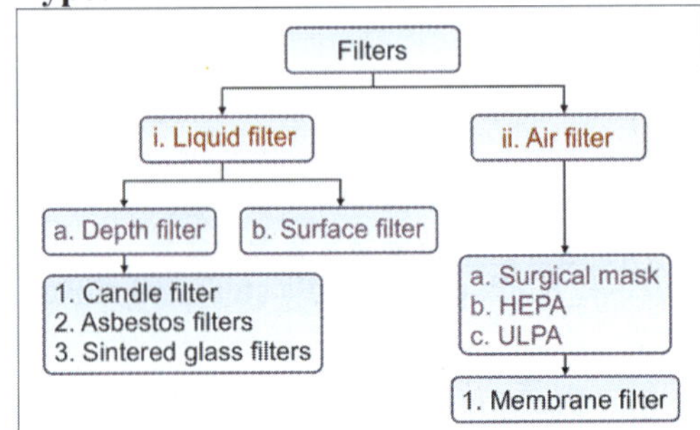

Flow chart-4: Types of filters

i. Liquid filter:

a. Depth filter:

✪ **Principle:** It is a porous filter that retain the particles throughout the depth of filter as shown in **fig.-6(a)**

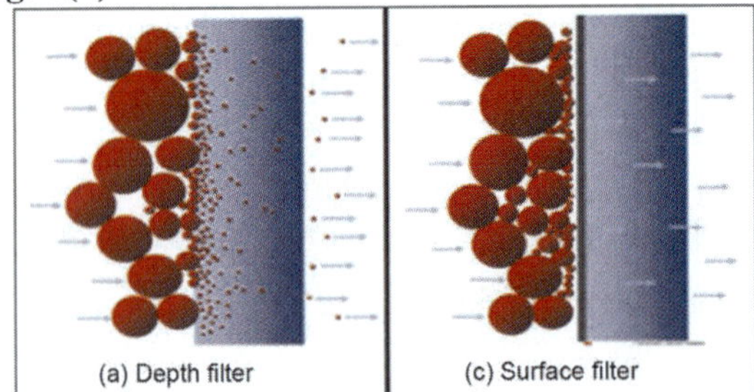

Figure-6: Principle of liquid filters

✪ **Composition:** Depth filters are composed of metals, polymer & inorganic materials.

✪ **Disadvantages:**

- Some of the particle still come out so not suitable for solution containing small size bacteria
- Composed of metals, which may be carcinogenic like asbestos filter

✪ **Advantages:**
- Retain the large mass of particle before becoming clogged
- Flow rate of fluid is high
- Low cost
- Useful when fluid to be filtered contains high load of particles like filtration of fluid, beverages or chemical in industries

✪ **Subtypes:** Three subtypes

1. **Candle filter: → Fig.-7**

- **Properties:**
  - Industrial & drinking water purification
  - Made up from special type of earth
- **Subtypes & examples:**
  - Unglazed ceramic filters like Chamberland filter & Doulton filter
  - Diatomaceous earth filters like Berkefeld filter & Mandler filter

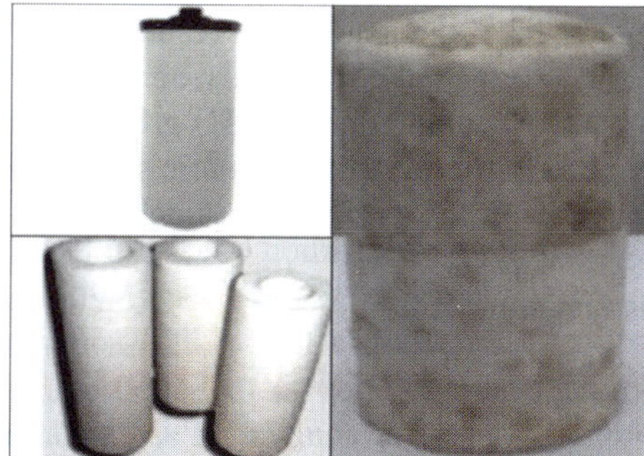

Figure-7: Different types of candle filter

2. **Asbestos filters:**

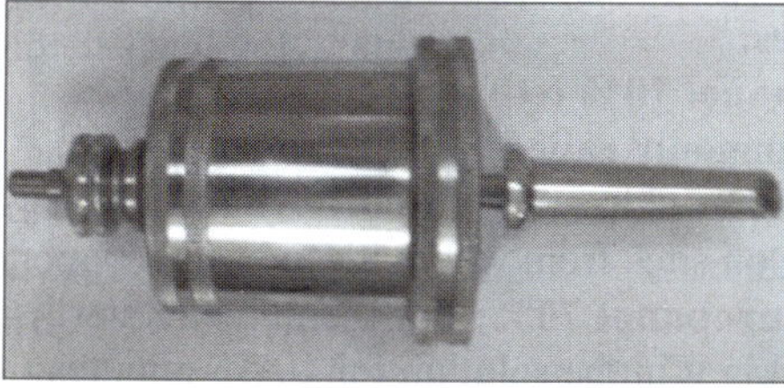

Figure-8: Seitz (Asbestos) filter

- **Properties:**
  - Disposable, single-used disc
  - High adsorbing capacity
  - Alkalinise the filtered liquid
  - Rarely useful because of carcinogenic property.
- **Examples:** Seitz filter (**fig.-8**) & Sterimat filters

3. **Sintered glass filter: →Fig.-9**

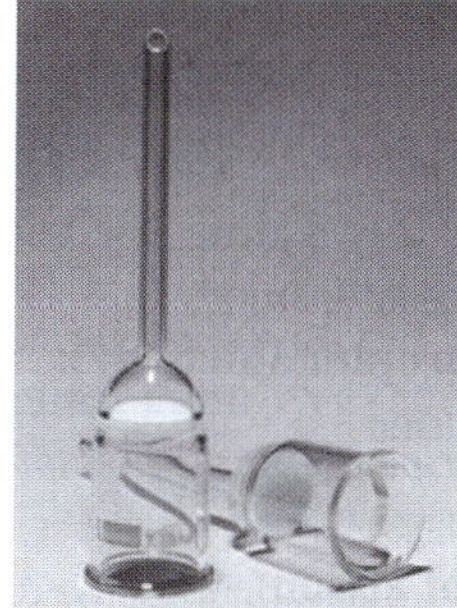

Figure-9: Sintered glass filter

- **Properties:**
  - Made up from heat fusing finely powered glass particles
  - Low absorptive properties
  - Brittle and expensive

b. Surface filter:

✪ **Principle:** It is a porous filter that retain all the particles on the surface as shown in **fig.-6(b)**

✪ **Composition: Made up from** cellulose acetate, cellulose nitrate, polycarbonate, polyvinylidene fluoride or other synthetic materials

✪ **Pore size:**
- Average of pores in membrane filter is 0.22µm which removes almost all bacteria but allowing viruses to pass
- 0.45µm size pores are useful to retain coliform bacteria in water
- 0.8µm size pores are useful to remove microbes from air to prevent air borne infection & to produces the bacteria free gases.

✪ **Subtypes & examples:**

1. **Membrane filters:**

- **Uses:**
  - For water purification and analysis
  - For sterilization and sterility testing
  - For preparation of solutions for parenteral use
- **Examples:**
  - Gradacol membrane filter
  - Modern membrane filter

ii. **Air filter:** Following are the examples to deliver bacteria free air

a. **Surgical mask:** It is the simplest example to deliver bacteria free air

b. **HEPA:**
- Full form: High Efficiency Particulate Air filter
- Pore size: ≥ 0.3µm
- Uses: In safety cabinet & remove 99.97% of pathogens from air

c. **ULPA**

.Full form: Ultra Low Particulate /Penetration Air
- Pore size: ≥ 0.12µm
- Uses: It remove 99.999% of dust, pollen, mold & pathogens from air

E. Radiation:

♣ **Types:** Two forms like ionising & non-ionising

i. Ionising radiation:

✪ **Methods:**
1. X-rays
2. γ- rays
3. Cosmic rays
4. Electron beams

✪ **Mechanism of action:**
- High penetrating power
- Lethal to DNA & other vital constitutes
- Sterile the articles without increasing the temperature **called cold sterilisation**.

- In allergic individual it cause rashes & systemic manifestation

ii. **Chlorine:**

✪ **Mechanism of action:** Protein denaturation by oxidative effect

✪ **Spectrum of activity:** Bactericidal, virucidal & sporicidal (at higher concentration), but not tuberculicidal

✪ **Uses:**

a. **Chlorine:** For chlorination of water by chlorine tablets

b. **Chlorophores:** Two types preparation

1. **Chlorinated lime (bleaching powder):** Obtained by action of chlorine on lime. Used for chlorination of drinking water, swimming pools, food and dairy industries.
2. **Sodium hypochlorite:**

- 1000 ppm for surface cleaning, 10,000 ppm for spillage (blood/body fluid), 2500ppm for discard container. 1000 ppm = 0.1% (1gm/litre) & ppm = parts per million
- For disinfection of equipment soiled with blood

✪ **Disadvantages:**

- Corrosive for metals & textiles
- Mixer with acid will liberate toxic gas
- Irritant
- Inactivated by organic matters

E. **Phenols or phenol group:** Obtained from distillation of coal tar between 170-270°C.

✪ **Mechanism of action:**

- Damage to cell membrane → releasing of cell contents → cell lysis so **called protoplasmic poison**
- Low concentration will precipitate proteins
- Bactericidal effect by inactivation of membrane bound enzymes (dehydrogenase, oxidase)

✪ **Spectrum of activity:** Bacteriostatic at 0.2% & Bactericidal at 1% but not sporicidal. Action does not affected by organic matter.

✪ **Uses:**

i. **Phenol (carbolic acid):**

- Carbolic acid was 1st used by Joseph Lister as antiseptic agents in surgery (1865).
- Earliest disinfectant, seldom use now.
- Very cheap
- For disinfection of urine, sputum, faeces of patients.
- Included in antipruritic lotion because of mild local anaesthetic action.

ii. **Methyl phenol or cresol:**

- Lysol: It contain 50% cresol
- It used for disinfection of utensils, excreta & hand wash

iii. **Chloroxylenol:** Following are the different preparation available

1. **Dettol:**

- It contain 4.8% Chloroxylenol + 9% terpeniol+13% alcohol
- Used as an antiseptic agent

2. **Dettolin:**

- It contain 1% chloroxylenol
- Used for mouthwash

3. **0.8% skin cream& soap**
4. **1.4% obstetric cream:** It used as an antiseptic during vaginal examination applied on forceps

iv. **Hexacholophane:** 2% is incorporated in soap, surgical scrub, deodorant, toilet product

v. **Orho-phenyl phenol (2- phenyl phenol or O-phenyl phenol or biphenol):** 0.1% in lysol for hard & soft surface.

✪ **Disadvantages:** Higher concentration cause skin burns

F. **Gases:**

i. **Ethylene oxide (EO):**

✪ **Mechanism of action:**

- Alkylating the amino, carboxyl, hydroxyl and sulphydryl groups in protein molecules.
- Also act on DNA and RNA.
- Explosive tendency of EO is decreased by 10% CO_2/ N_2 & water vapour increase its efficacy
- Two types of cycles for sterilisation by EO like

1. Cold cycle: 37±5°C
2. Warm cycle: 54±5°C

- In these cycles humidity is maintained by 40-50% & EO concentration is kept at 700mg per litre.

✪ **Spectrum of activity:** Bactericidal, fungicidal, tuberculicidal, virucidal, sporicidal

✪ **Uses:** It is a high level disinfectant used to sterilise the heat sensitive metal instrument (heart-lung machines, respirators, dental equipment,), glass, plastics (sutures, disposable syringe etc.), cloths, paper (books), soil, foods & tobacco items. Water vapour increases its efficacy.

✪ **Disadvantages: EO** is

- Inflammable& irritant
- Mutagenic & carcinogenic
- Explosive at concentration of >3%, which is overcome by mixing it with 10% CO_2/ N_2

ii. **Formaldehyde gas: → Vide supra**

iii. **BPL:** Product of ketane and formaldehyde with a boiling point of 163°C.

✪ **Spectrum of activity:** Capable of killing all microorganisms & very active against viruses.

✪ **Uses:** earlier it was use for fumigation

✪ **Disadvantages:** Carcinogenic.

iv. **H_2O_2 fogging:** Short cycle, non toxic & used for fumigation by using fogging machine.

G. **Biguanide:**

i. **Chlorhexidine (hibitane):**

✪ **Mechanism of action:**

- Disruption of bacterial cell membrane
- Protein denaturation

✪ **Spectrum of activity:** Against gram +Ve bacteria

✪ **Uses:**

✪ **Advantages:**
- Retain the large mass of particle before becoming clogged
- Flow rate of fluid is high
- Low cost
- Useful when fluid to be filtered contains high load of particles like filtration of fluid, beverages or chemical in industries

✪ **Subtypes:** Three subtypes

1. **Candle filter: → Fig.-7**

- **Properties:**
  - Industrial & drinking water purification
  - Made up from special type of earth
- **Subtypes & examples:**
  - Unglazed ceramic filters like Chamberland filter & Doulton filter
  - Diatomaceous earth filters like Berkefeld filter & Mandler filter

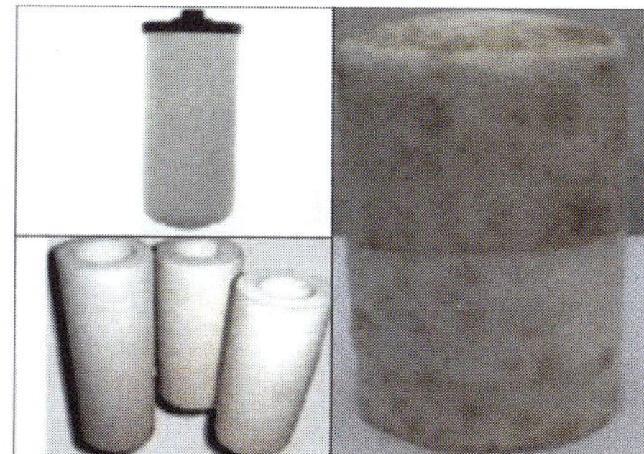

Figure-7: Different types of candle filter

2. **Asbestos filters:**

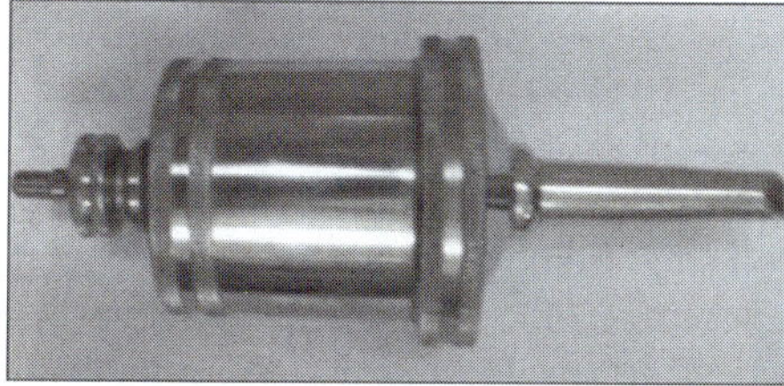

Figure-8: Seitz (Asbestos) filter

- **Properties:**
  - Disposable, single-used disc
  - High adsorbing capacity
  - Alkalinise the filtered liquid
  - Rarely useful because of carcinogenic property.
- **Examples:** Seitz filter **(fig.-8)** & Sterimat filters

3. **Sintered glass filter: →Fig.-9**

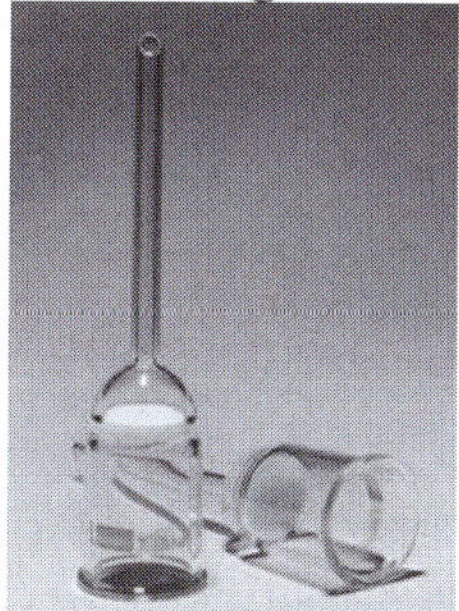

Figure-9: Sintered glass filter

- **Properties:**
  - Made up from heat fusing finely powered glass particles
  - Low absorptive properties
  - Brittle and expensive

b. Surface filter:

✪ **Principle:** It is a porous filter that retain all the particles on the surface as shown in **fig.-6(b)**

✪ **Composition: Made up from** cellulose acetate, cellulose nitrate, polycarbonate, polyvinylidene fluoride or other synthetic materials

✪ **Pore size:**
- Average of pores in membrane filter is 0.22µm which removes almost all bacteria but allowing viruses to pass
- 0.45µm size pores are useful to retain coliform bacteria in water
- 0.8µm size pores are useful to remove microbes from air to prevent air borne infection & to produces the bacteria free gases.

✪ **Subtypes & examples:**

1. **Membrane filters:**

- **Uses:**
  - For water purification and analysis
  - For sterilization and sterility testing
  - For preparation of solutions for parenteral use
- **Examples:**
  - Gradacol membrane filter
  - Modern membrane filter

ii. Air filter: Following are the examples to deliver bacteria free air

a. Surgical mask: It is the simplest example to deliver bacteria free air

b. HEPA:
- Full form: High Efficiency Particulate Air filter
- Pore size: ≥ 0.3µm
- Uses: In safety cabinet & remove 99.97% of pathogens from air

c. ULPA

.Full form: Ultra Low Particulate /Penetration Air
- Pore size: ≥ 0.12µm
- Uses: It remove 99.999% of dust, pollen, mold & pathogens from air

E. Radiation:

♣ **Types:** Two forms like ionising & non-ionising

i. Ionising radiation:

✪ **Methods:**
1. X-rays
2. γ- rays
3. Cosmic rays
4. Electron beams

✪ **Mechanism of action:**
- High penetrating power
- Lethal to DNA & other vital constitutes
- Sterile the articles without increasing the temperature **called cold sterilisation**.

- **Article to be sterilised (uses):** Exposing object to the radiation especially to ionising radiation **called irradiation**. γ- rays are best useful for this. Irradiation is done for
  - Disposable supplies **(plastic syringes, bandages, catheters and gloves)** and heat-sensitive pharmaceuticals products **(oils, grease, hormones, antibiotics etc.)**, cardboard, fabric & metal foils
  - Catgut suture, bone or tissue graft & adhesive dressing
  - Food, which is permitted in some countries.

ii. Non-ionising:

- **Methods:**

1. Ultraviolet/ UV rays (280-200 nm)
2. Infrared radiation

- **Mechanism of action:** Sterile the articles with increasing the temperature **called hot air sterilisation**.
- **Article to be sterilised (uses):**
  - Infrared radiation: Disposable supplies (syringes, bandages, catheters and gloves)
  - Ultraviolet/ UV rays(280-200 nm): For closed area like, hospital ward, Laboratory, operation theatre

✓ **Note: Cold sterilisation**

- **Definition:** Sterilisation of articles without increasing the temperature by radiation (ionising), chemicals (EO, formaldehyde etc.), membrane or by other measures **called cold sterilisation**.

♣ **Control in radiation:** Efficacy of ionising radiation is tested by *Bacillu pumilis*

F. Ultrasonic & sonic vibration: Have bactericidal power but variable sensitivity to microorganisms & survivors have been found after such treatment, hence practically not useful.

II. Chemical methods (disinfection) or chemical agents (disinfectants)

❖ **Definition of disinfection & disinfectant:**
→ **Vide supra**

❖ **Criteria for ideal disinfectants:** Ideal disinfectants should be

- Effective against all microorganisms e.g. bacteria, spores, virus, fungus
- Be active in presence of organic matter
- Equally effective in acid & in alkaline media
- Speedy action
- High penetrating power
- Compatible with other antiseptics & disinfectant
- Not corrode metals
- Not cause local irritation or sensitisation
- Not interfere with healing
- Not toxic if absorbed into circulation
- Inexpensive
- Easily available
- Safe
- Easy to use & stable

❖ **Effective factors:** Following factors determine the potency of disinfectants

- Numbers of organisms
- Nature/type of the organisms
- Time of exposure
- pH of the medium
- Temperature
- Presence of extraneous material
- Biofilm: It prevent the entry of disinfectant to act on microbes which are present inside the biofilms

❖ **Mechanisms of action:**

- Protein denaturation: (alcohols, phenols, aldehydes, oxidants)
- Protein coagulation (metallic salts)
- Damage to cell membrane resulting in loss of contents (surfactant compounds, alcohols)
- Removal of sulphhydryl (-SH) group required for enzymatic activities. (EO, metallic salts)
- Damage of RNA and DNA (aldehydes, oxidants, dyes)
- Substrate competition

❖ **Types & details of disinfectants:**

A. Alcohols:

- **Mechanism of action:** Protein denaturation
- **Spectrum of activity:** Bactericidal, fungicidal, tuberculicidal, virucidal but not sporicidal
- **Uses:**

i. Ethanol 70% (ethyl alcohol):

- Commonly **called spirit** (70%)
- Used as skin antiseptic befor injection. It is safe to use on sites from where it can easily evaporate.

ii. Isopropanol 70%: For themometer sterilisation by soakig it in the solution for 10-15 minutes

iii. Methanol (methyl alcohol):

- Treating cabinets & incubators.
- Wipe inside of chamber by methanol & than put a pad moistened with methanol & water at room temperature for few hours

- **Disadvantages:**
  - Methyl alcohol is toxic & inflammable.
  - It is not useful for cut skin because coagulate the protein under which bacteria can grow.
  - It has no sporicidal activity.

✓ **Note: See also**

- **Propranolol:** It is a drug used for reducing blood pressure and hand tremors.
- **Propanal (propionaldehyde):** It is a structural isomer of acetone

B. Aldehydes:

- **Mechanism of action:**
  - Protein denaturation

- Act as protoplasmic poison
- **Spectrum of activity:** Bactericidal, fungicidal, virucidal & sporicidal
- **Uses:**

i. Formalin:

- 37-40% aqueous solution of formalehyde **called formalin** or **formol**
- To preserve biological specimen or anatomical viscera.
- Used in mortuaries for embalming.
- To prepare toxoid from toxin
- To destroy the spores of *Bacillus anthracis* in hairs & wools

ii. Formalehyde gas:

- For sterilisation of instrument & heat sensitive catheter
- Fumigation: **Follow chapter → Microbiology of water, milk and air**

iii. Gluteralehyde (2% solution called cidex):

- Less irritating and more effective than formaldehyde.
- Bactericidal, tuberculicidal & virucidal in 10 minutes.
- Sporicidal in 3 to 10 hours (slow action).
- Commonly used to disinfect endoscopic instruments like bronchoscope, cystoscope, oesophagoscope etc. for 20 minutes. These instruments has lens which is heat sensitive so best sterilised by cidex.
- Used to treat corrugated rubber anaesthetic rubber, face masks, plastic endotracheal tubes, metal instruments and polythene tubing.

iv. Ortho-phthalalehyde:

- It is available as 0.55% solution
- Useful to sterile endoscopes & cystoscopes
- It is more advantageous than gluteraldehyde, because

1. High level disinfectant
2. Low exposure at ambient temperature
3. High mycrobactericidal activity
4. Does not required activation
5. Low vapour property
6. Better odour
7. Less toxic fumes
8. More stable during storage

C. Dyes: 2 groups of dyes like aniline dyes & acridine dyes

i. Aniline dyes:

- **Mechanism of action:** React with acid group of cells
- **Spectrum of activity:**
  - Bacteriostatic in high dilution but little bactericidal.
  - More active against gram +Ve (acidic pH)
  - Little or no effect on gram-Ve organisms (alkaline pH)
  - No effect on *Mycobacterium* spp.
- **Uses:**
  - Commonly useful aniline dyes are malachite green, brilliant green, crystal (gentian) violet etc.
  - Malachite green as selective agent in LJ medium.
  - Skin & wound antiseptic in boil, bed sore, Vincent's angina
- **Disadvantages:** Deep staining

ii. Acridine dyes:

- **Mechanism of action:** Impair the DNA of the organisms & thus kill the reproductive capacity of cell.
- **Spectrum of activity:**
  - Bacteriostatic in high dilution but little bactericidal.
  - More active against gram +Ve (acidic pH)
  - Little or no effect on gram-Ve organisms (alkaline pH)
  - Not selective as like aniline dyes.
- **Uses:**
  - Commonly useful acridine dyes are proflavine, acriflavine, euflavine, aminacrine etc.
  - Skin & wound antiseptic.
- **Disadvantages:** Loose efficacy on light exposure hence stored in amber colour bottle

✓ **Note: Triple dye lotion (Triple DY)**

- **Contains:** 0.25% brilliant green + 0.25%crystal violet + 0.1% acriflavine
- **Uses:** Used for burns & umbilical stump dressing

D. Halogens:

i. Iodine:

- **Mechanism of action:** Protein denaturation by oxidative effects
- **Spectrum of activity:** Bactericidal, fungicidal, tuberculicidal, virucidal & at higher concentration it is Sporicidal (It is more sporicidal than chlorine)
- **Uses:**

a. Iodine:

- Tincture iodine (iodine in 2% alcohol): Tincture means solution prepared by dissolving drug in alcohol
- Skin disinfectant in cuts/abrasion

b. Iodophores (iodine and surfactant like povidone) / Povidone iodine (Poly Vinyl Pyrrolidone & iodine : PVP-I):

- Surfactants like povidone will act as carrier & release the free iodine.
- As an antiseptics, disinfection of skin & small wounds, candidal/trichomonal/nonspecific vaginitis & degerming the skin before the operation
- Commercial preparation are:

1. **Betadine:** 5% cream/lotion, 7.5% scrub lotion, 200mg vaginal pessary
2. **Piodin:** 10% solution/cream, 1% mouth wash

- **Disadvantages:**
  - At higher concentration it cause burning & blistering of skin

- In allergic individual it cause rashes & systemic manifestation

ii. Chlorine:

- **Mechanism of action:** Protein denaturation by oxidative effect
- **Spectrum of activity:** Bactericidal, virucidal & sporicidal (at higher concentration), but not tuberculicidal
- **Uses:**

a. Chlorine: For chlorination of water by chlorine tablets

b. Chlorophores: Two types preparation

1. **Chlorinated lime (bleaching powder):** Obtained by action of chlorine on lime. Used for chlorination of drinking water, swimming pools, food and dairy industries.
2. **Sodium hypochlorite:**

- 1000 ppm for surface cleaning, 10,000 ppm for spillage (blood/body fluid), 2500ppm for discard container. 1000 ppm = 0.1% (1gm/litre) & ppm = parts per million
- For disinfection of equipment soiled with blood

- **Disadvantages:**

- Corrosive for metals & textiles
- Mixer with acid will liberate toxic gas
- Irritant
- Inactivated by organic matters

E. Phenols or phenol group: Obtained from distillation of coal tar between 170-270°C.

- **Mechanism of action:**

- Damage to cell membrane → releasing of cell contents → cell lysis so **called protoplasmic poison**
- Low concentration will precipitate proteins
- Bactericidal effect by inactivation of membrane bound enzymes (dehydrogenase, oxidase)

- **Spectrum of activity:** Bacteriostatic at 0.2% & Bactericidal at 1% but not sporicidal. Action does not affected by organic matter.
- **Uses:**

i. Phenol (carbolic acid):

- Carbolic acid was 1st used by Joseph Lister as antiseptic agents in surgery (1865).
- Earliest disinfectant, seldom use now.
- Very cheap
- For disinfection of urine, sputum, faeces of patients.
- Included in antipruritic lotion because of mild local anaesthetic action.

ii. Methyl phenol or cresol:

- Lysol: It contain 50% cresol
- It used for disinfection of utensils, excreta & hand wash

iii. Chloroxylenol: Following are the different preparation available

1. **Dettol:**

- It contain 4.8% Chloroxylenol + 9% terpeniol+13% alcohol
- Used as an antiseptic agent

2. **Dettolin:**

- It contain 1% chloroxylenol
- Used for mouthwash

3. **0.8% skin cream& soap**
4. **1.4% obstetric cream:** It used as an antiseptic during vaginal examination applied on forceps

iv. Hexacholophane: 2% is incorporated in soap, surgical scrub, deodorant, toilet product

v. Orho-phenyl phenol (2- phenyl phenol or O-phenyl phenol or biphenol): 0.1% in lysol for hard & soft surface.

- **Disadvantages:** Higher concentration cause skin burns

F. Gases:

i. Ethylene oxide (EO):

- **Mechanism of action:**

- Alkylating the amino, carboxyl, hydroxyl and sulphydryl groups in protein molecules.
- Also act on DNA and RNA.
- Explosive tendency of EO is decreased by 10% CO_2/ N_2 & water vapour increase its efficacy
- Two types of cycles for sterilisation by EO like

1. Cold cycle: 37±5°C
2. Warm cycle: 54±5°C

- In these cycles humidity is maintained by 40-50% & EO concentration is kept at 700mg per litre.

- **Spectrum of activity:** Bactericidal, fungicidal, tuberculicidal, virucidal, sporicidal
- **Uses:** It is a high level disinfectant used to sterilise the heat sensitive metal instrument (heart-lung machines, respirators, dental equipment,), glass, plastics (sutures, disposable syringe etc.), cloths, paper (books), soil, foods & tobacco items. Water vapour increases its efficacy.
- **Disadvantages: EO** is

- Inflammable& irritant
- Mutagenic & carcinogenic
- Explosive at concentration of >3%, which is overcome by mixing it with 10% CO_2/ N_2

ii. Formaldehyde gas: → Vide supra

iii. BPL: Product of ketane and formaldehyde with a boiling point of 163°C.

- **Spectrum of activity:** Capable of killing all microorganisms & very active against viruses.
- **Uses:** earlier it was use for fumigation
- **Disadvantages:** Carcinogenic.

iv. H_2O_2 fogging: Short cycle, non toxic & used for fumigation by using fogging machine.

G. Biguanide:

i. Chlorhexidine (hibitane):

- **Mechanism of action:**

- Disruption of bacterial cell membrane
- Protein denaturation

- **Spectrum of activity:** Against gram +Ve bacteria
- **Uses:**

- 0.5 -1% tooth paste: To prevent & to treat the gingivitis
- 0.12-0.2% oral rinse: Reduce & prevent the oral infection, even in AIDS patients
- Savlon (vide infra): Skin & obstetric antiseptic, surgical scrub, neonatal bath, mouth wash etc.

✪ **Disadvantage:** Brownish discolouration of teeth

H. Surface active agents:

➢ **Other name:** Also called **surfactants, tensides** or **detergents**

➢ **Definition:** Substances that alter the energy relationship at interfaces or reduce surface or interfacial tension are **called surface active agents.**

➢ **Types:** 4 main groups as follows

i. Cationic (quaternary ammonium compound):

✪ **Mechanism of action:**
- Protein denaturation
- Change in permeability of cell membrane by interfering with phosphate group.

✪ **Spectrum of activity:** Bactericidal (only for Gram +Ve), fungicidal but not virucidal, tuberculicidal, sporicidal & no effect on *Pseudomonas aeruginosa*

✪ **Uses:**

a. Cetrimide or acetyl trimethyl ammonium bromide:
- Used alone or along with chlorhexidine
- No effect on *Pseudomonas* & used as selective agent in cetrimide agar for isolation of *Pseudomonas*
- Antiseptic for surgical instrument, gloves, utensils, baths etc.
- Preparation are:

1. **Cetavlon:** 20% cetrimide
2. **Savlon liquid:** 3% cetrimide+1.5% chlorhexidine gluconate
3. **Savlon cream:** 0.5% cetrimide+0.1% chlorhexidine HCL
4. **Savlon hospital concentrate:** 15% cetrimide + 7.5% chlorhexidine gluconate

b. Benzalkonium chloride: Antiseptic for surgical instrument

✪ **Disadvantages:** Slow action & forms films on skin, porous material (cotton, poly ethylene) under which bacteria can grow.

ii. Anionic/soap:
- Soap can be prepared from other chemicals also.
- Soap prepared from saturated fatty acid (coconut oil) acts only on gram + Ve bacteria.
- Soap prepared from unsaturated fatty acid (oleic acid) acts only on gram - Ve & Neisseria.
- Cleaning effect & more effective in warm water.

iii. Amphoteric or ampholytic or Tego compounds: Acts on gram + Ve, gram -Ve bacteria & viruses but not in general use.

I. Acids:

✪ **Spectrum of activity:** Bacteriostatic.

✪ **Uses:**

i. Boric acid:
- 4% solution: For irrigation of eyes, mouth wash, douche
- 30% boroglycerine paint: For stomatitis & glossitis
- 10% ointment: For cuts, abrasion
- It is also included in prickly heat powder

ii. Acetic acid: 1-3% for douche & 5% to prevent *Pseudomonas* infection in burns

✪ **Disadvantages:** Systemic absorption causes vomiting, diarrhoea, abdominal pain, visual disturbances & kidney damage.

J. Metallic salts:

i. Mercury:

✪ **Mechanism of action:** React with sulphhydryl (-SH) group required for enzymatic action.

✪ **Spectrum of activity:** More bacteriostatic least bactericidal &fungicidal effect.

✪ **Uses**: Mercury compounds like mercury chloride, thiomersal, phenyl mercury nitrate & mercurochrome, merthiolate are acts as antiseptic agents.

✪ **Disadvantages:** Because of high toxicity & environmental hazards they are not suggested.

ii. Silver:

✪ **Mechanism of action:**
- Astringent effect (precipitation of protein)
- React with –SH, COOH, PO_4 & NH_2 groups of proteins.

✪ **Spectrum of activity:** *N. gonorrhoea* & *P. aeruginosa*

✪ **Uses:** Uses of silver compounds are like
- 1% silver nitrate solution in ophthalmia neonatorum (caused by *N. gonorrhoea*),
- 1% silver nitrate touch in aphthous ulcer & hypertrophied tonsillitis
- 1% silver sulfadiazine in burns (prevent *P. aeruginosa* infection)
- Water stored in silver vessels is said to become sterile, even at low Ag^+ ions concentration **called oligodynamic action** (Very tiny amounts are effective)

✪ **Disadvantages**: tissue gets black due to deposition of reduced silver

iii. Zinc:

✪ **Mechanism of action:**
- Astringent effect (precipitation of protein)

✪ **Uses:**

1. **Zinc sulphate:**
   - 0.1-1%% solution: for irrigation of eyes & eye/ear drops
   - White lotion: Contains 4% zinc sulphate + 4% sulfarated potash is used for acne & impetigo
2. **Zinc chloride:** For mouthwashes
3. **Zinc oxide:** It is used as antifungal agent in paints

iv. Copper: Copper sulfate is used to kill algae in pools and fish tanks.

v. **Selenium:** Kills fungi, fungal spores & prevent fungal infections. Also used in shampoos for dandruff.

vi. **Calamine:** dermal protective & adsorbent. Used in oily skin

❖ **Testing of disinfectants:** Various test are developed to know the efficacy/power of disinfectants, but none of them is satisfactory

i. **Rideal Walker (Phenol Coefficient) test:**

✪ **Method:**

- Suspensions containing various numbers of *S. typhi* are submitted to the action of varying concentration of phenol & test disinfectant.
- Concentration of test disinfectant which sterile the *S. typhi* is divided by corresponding concentration of phenol **called phenol coefficient (Phenol =1)**

✪ **Limitations:**

- Disinfectant is act directly without presence of any organic matter.
- Doesn't reflect the natural condition.

ii. **Chick Martin test:**

✪ **Method:**

- Modification of **Rideal Walker test.**
- Disinfectant acts in presence of organic matter as like yeast, faeces.

✪ **Limitation:** Doesn't reflect the natural condition.

iii. **Capacity (Kelsey-Sykes) test:** It tests the capacity of a disinfectant to retain its activity when repeatedly used microbiologically. (when microbiological load keeps increasing)

iv. **In-Use (Kelsey & Maurer) test:**

- It detects the capacity of disinfectants used in laboratory or in hospital.
- Efficiency is detected by the ability of disinfectants to inactivate the known number of standard strain of *Staphylococcus* on a given surface within a certain time

❖ **Level of disinfectants:**

- **Three categories:**

i. **High level disinfectant:** Kills all organisms & also spores if contact time is increased. Two types like

1. Heat resistant: E.g. Autoclave
2. Heat sensitive: E.g. Plasma sterilisation, H_2O_2 fogging, EO gas & gluteraldehyde

ii. **Intermediate level disinfectant:** Kills all organisms & *Mycobacteria*, naked (non-enveloped) viruses except spores. E.g. Alcohol, phenolic groups, iodophores

iii. **Low level disinfectant:** Kills vegetative bacteria, fungi & lipid enveloped viruses. E.g. Cationic

III. Chemosterilisation (physical & chemical methods)

❖ **Definition:** Sterilisation by chemical agents **called chemosterilisation** & such agent **called chemosterilizers**

❖ **Advantage:** Useful for heat sensitive articles

❖ **Methods:**

A. **Gases:** As described above

B. **Plasma sterilisation (Newer method):**

- **Principle:** Consist ions, electron or neutral particles. Radio frequency energy is applied to create an electromagnetic field. Later H_2O_2 vapour is introduced which generate a state of plasma containing free radicals of H_2 & O_2. This state sterilise the articles.
- **Biological control: → Table-5**
- **Use:** Arthroscope, bronchoscope, urethroscope etc.

Biological control or indicators

❖ **Aims:** Used to assess the efficacy of sterilisation method

❖ **List of indicators:** → **Table-5**

Methods	Control (Indicators)
Hot air oven	10^6 spores of *Cl. tetani* or *Bacillus subtilis* subsp. *niger*
Autoclave	10^6 spores of *Bacillus steriothermophilus*
Filtration	*Serratia marcescens* & *Brevundimonas diminuta*
Ionising radiation	*Bacillu pumilis*
Ethylene oxide	*Bacillu globigi* or *B. subtilis*
Plasma sterilisation	*Bacillus steriothermophilus* & *Bacillus subtilis* subsp. *niger*

Table-5: Biological indicators

❖ **Methods of use of indicators:**

- Put the indicator with the load in to the steriliser. During this process the organism are killed.
- After sterilisation , remove the indicators & inoculate in to different media
- No growth indicates the complete sterilisation

Selection of sterilisation & disinfection in health care setup

❖ **Aims:** Uses of contaminated equipments are act as source of infection, so they are completely sterilised & disinfected before use.

❖ **Splaundig's classification:** Splaundig classify such equipments in three categories & appropriate methods required for sterilisation & disinfection are shown in **table-6.**

Category of materials	Tissue affected	Equipments	Level of disinfectant	Sterilisation & disinfection method
Critical materials	Sterile tissues or vascular system	Cardiac catheter, implants	High level	Heat resistant - Autoclave
			High level	Heat sensitive - Plasma sterilisation, H_2O_2 fogging, EO gas
Semi-critical materials	Mucosa & non-intact skin	Endoscope	High level	2% Gluteraldehyde
		Thermometer	Intermediate level	Ethanol
Noncritical	Intact skin	BP cuffs	Low level	Cationic

Table-6: Splauding's classification

Question bank

Essay/Full question

1) Sterilisation & disinfection

Short notes

1) Types of methods of sterilisation & disinfection
2) Disinfection
3) Dry heat sterilisation
4) Hot air oven
5) Moist heat sterilisation
6) Moist heat sterilisation below 100^0C / at 100^0C / above 100^0C
7) Pasteurisation
8) Phosphatase test
9) Fractional sterilisation
10) Autoclave
11) Steam steriliser
12) Filtration

Short questions for theory/viva questions

1) Define: Sterilisation & disinfection
2) Write the differences between sterilisation & disinfection
3) Name the article sterilised by hot air oven
4) Comment: Moist heat is more advantageous than dry heat
5) Write two examples of fractional sterilisation methods
6) Name the biological control of hot air oven & autoclave, filtration & ionising radiation
7) What is pasteurisation? Name two methods of pasteurisation.
8) Why three successive days are required for sterilisation by inspissations (Or write the principle of inspissations)
9) What is cold sterilisation? Name two agents used in cold sterilisation
10) Write four examples of high level disinfectants.

MCQs for chapter review

Introduction

1) **'Disinfections' kills the following**
(a) All microorganisms except spore (b) Pathogenic microorganisms (c) Spores (d) Non-pathogenic microorganisms
2) **Asepsis means**
(a) Absence of microbes (b) Disinfection of surface (c) Prevention of infection (d) Destroying all forms of microbes
3) **An 'antiseptic' means** (AI-96)
(a) An agents applied on skin to eradicate pathogenic microbes (b) Used to sterilise inanimate objects (c) An agents which kills only bacteria but not spores (d) Kills all microorganisms
4) **The best skin disinfectant is -** (AIIMS -78)
(a) Alcohol (b) Savlon (c) Betadine (d) Phenol
5) **Which of the following can be readily used for hand washing** (PGI, Dec-00, June -01)
(a) Chlorhexidine (b) Isopropyl alcohol (c) Lysol (c) Cresol (d) Glutaraldehyde
6) **Agent which on addition to a colony inhibit its growth and on a removal the colony regrows is –** (AI-93, 96)
(a) Bacteriostatic (b) Bactericidal (c) Antibiotic (d) Antiseptic
7) **Which of the following is most resistant to sterilisation** (AI -08, 12)
(a) Cysts (b) Prions (c) Spores (c) Viruses
8) **Choose the correct ones for the decreasing order of resistant to sterilisation -** (PGI, Nov-13, Dec -07)
(a) Prions, Bacterial spores, Bacteria (b) Bacterial spores, Bacteria, Prions (c) Bacteria, Prions, Bacterial spores, (d) Prions, Bacteria, Bacterial spores (e) Bacterial spores, Prions, Bacteria

Classification

Physical methods (Sterilisation)

9) **All are methods of sterilisation by dry heat except** (PGI-90)
(a) Flaming (b) Incineration (c) Hot air oven (d) Autoclaving
10) **Tyndallisation is a type of**
(a) Intermittent sterilisation (b) Pasteurisation (c) Boiling (d) Autoclaving
11) **The best method of sterilisation of dusting powder is** (PGI-95)
(a) Autoclaving (b) Hot air oven (c) Inspissation (d) Tyndallisation
12) **Glass vessels and syringes are best sterilised by**
(a) Hot air oven (b) Autoclaving (c) Irradiation (d) Ethylene oxide
13) **Which of the following is true about pasteurisation** (AI-00)
(a) It kills all bacteria and spores (b) It kills all bacteria except thermoduric bacteria (c) It kills 95% of microorganisms (d) All bacteria are destroyed
14) **Holding temperature & time for pasteurisation by Holder method is**
(a) 60^0C for 30 seconds (b) 72^0C for 30 minutes (c) 72^0C for 15-20 seconds (d) 60^0C for 30 minutes
15) **Vaccines are best sterilised by**
(a) Seitz filtration (b) Hot air oven (c) Autoclaving (c) Heat inactivation
16) **Autoclaving is done in**
(a) Dry air at 121°C and 15 lbs pressure (b) Steam at 100°C for 30 minutes (c) Steam at 121°C for 15 minutes (d) Dry air at 160°C for 30 minutes
17) **Sterilisation by autoclave is work under principle of**
(a) Moist heat at 100^0C (b) Moist heat above 100^0C (c) Moist heat above 100^0C & above atmospheric pressure
(d) Moist heat below 100^0C
18) **Browne's tube is used for**
(a) Steam sterilisation (b) Radiation (c) Chemical sterilisation (d) Filtration

19) Out of the following the true statement regarding sterilisation is (AI-97)
(a) Dry heat is the best method of sterilisation of liquid paraffin (b) All glass wares are best sterilised by boiling at 100°C (c) Bacterial vaccines are best sterilised by ethylene oxide (d) Pasteurisation of milk by flash method is done by heating at 63°C for 30 minutes

20) Sterilisation of culture media containing serum is by
(a) Autoclaving (b) Micropore filter (c) Gamma radiation (d) Centrifugation

21) Which is a form of cold sterilisation -
(a) Gamma rays (b) Beta rays (c) Infrared rays (d) Autoclave

22) Irradiation can be used to sterilise A/E - (AIIMS, May -10)
A/E = All Except
(a) Bone graft (b) Suture (c) Artificial tissue graft (d) Bronchoscope

23) Sterilisation method for catgut suture - (PGI -11)
(a) Steam (b) Radiation (c) Boiling (d) Burning

Chemical methods (Disinfections)

24) False about alcohol in disinfection is (PGI, May-13, Dec-07)
(a) Ethanol is used (b) Isopropyl alcohol is used (c) Has sporicidal activity (d) Has bactericidal activity

25) 40% formalin is used to sterilise - (AI-94)
(a) Plastic syringe (b) All microbes + spores (c) Clothes (d) Stitches

26) Bronchoscope is sterilised by
(a) 2% Gluteraldehyde (b) Formaldehyde (c) Autoclave (d) Carbolic acid

27) Percentage of gluteraldehyde used-
(a) 1% (b) 2% (c) 3% (d) 4%

28) The operating temperature in an ethylene oxide sterilisation during a warm cycle is- (AIIMS, Nov-04)
(a) 20-35°C (b) 49-63°C (c) 68-88°C (d) 92-110°C

29) Heat labile instruments for use in surgical procedure can be best sterilised by - (AI -03)
(a) Absolute alcohol (b) Ultraviolet rays (c) Chlorine releasing compounds (d) Ethylene oxide gas

30) Which of the following is an important disinfectant on account of effectively destroying gram positive and gram negative bacteria, viruses and even spores at low pH level - (AIIMS-96)
(a) Phenol (b) Alcohol (c) Chlorine (d) Hexachorophene

31) Disinfection of sputum is done by (PGI, Dec-08)
(a) Boiling (b) Autoclaving (c) Sunlight (d) Burning (e) Airing

32) Phenolic disinfectants are (PGI-05)
(a) Dettol (b) Cresol (c) Lysol (d) Carbolic acid (e) Savlon

33) All of the sterilisation methods are properly matched except -
(a) Cat gut suture - Radiation (b) Culture media - Autoclaving (c) Bronchoscope - Autoclaving (d) Glassware & syringes – Hot air oven

34) Which of the following statements regarding disinfectants is not true – (AI-09)
(a) Hypochlorites are bactericidal and inactivated by organic matter (b) Gluteraldehyde is sporicidal and not inactivated by organic matter (c) Formaldehyde is bactericidal, sporicidal and virucidal (d) Phenol is bactericidal and readily inactivated by organic matter

35) All are true regarding disinfectants except (AIIMS, May-11)
(a) Gluteraldehyde is sporicidal (b) Hypochlorites are virucidal (c) Ethylene oxide is intermediate disinfectant (d) Phenol usually require organic matter to act

36) Disposable plastic syringe is sterilised by
(a) Ethylene oxide (b) Ionising radiation (c) Non-ionising radiation (d) Spirit

37) Operation theatre is sterilised by
(a) Carbolic acid spraying (b) Washing with soap and water (c) Formaldehyde (d) Ethylene oxide gas

38) Phenol Coefficient indicates
(a) Efficacy of a disinfectant (b) Dilution of a disinfectant (c) Quantity of a disinfectant (d) Purity of a disinfectant

39) Rideal –Walker (phenol test) Coefficient is related with
(a) Disinfectimg power (b) Parasitic clearance (c) Dietary equipment (d) Statistical correlation

Biological control or indicators

40) Indicator used in autoclave is
(a) *Clostridium tetani* (b) *Bacillus steriothermophilus* (c) *Bacillu pumilis* (d) *Bacillus subtilis* Var *niger*

41) Plasma sterilisation accuracy is assessed by using (AIIMS, Nov-10)
(a) *Bacillus subtilis* (b) *Bacillus steriothermophilus* (c) *Staphylococcus aureus* (d) *Clostridium tetani*

Selection of sterilisation & disinfection in health care setup

42) According to Splauding classification system of sterilisation, following is true except (AIIMS, Nov -10)
(a) "Non-critical devices" come in to contact with intact skin (b) Semi-critical equipment need low level sterilisation (c) "Semi-critical devices" come in to contact with non-sterile mucous membrane or non-intact skin (d) Cardiac catheter is critical equipment

43) Following is/are write about high level disinfectant
(a) Two subtypes like heat sensitive & heat resistant (b) Heat sensitive includes autoclave & heat resistant includes plasma sterilisation, H_2O_2 fogging & EO gas (c) Ethanol is high level disinfectant (d) None of above

Answers of MCQs & explanation

1) (b) & (c)
- Follow section, **introduction (definitions) & table-1** more explanation

2) (a)
- Follow section, **introduction (definitions → asepsis)** for explanation

3) (a)
- Antiseptic are also **called skin disinfectant** & can be applied on skin –mucosa to inhibit the growth of microbes

4) (c)
5) (a) & (b)
} Follow section, **introduction (definitions → antiseptics)** for explanation

6) (a)
- Bacteriostatic can inhibit the growth of microbes which is reversible & on removal organism can regrow while bactericidal can kill the microbes which is irreversible & on removal organis can't regrow

7) (b)
8) (a)
} Follow section, **introduction (order of resistance of microbes) & flow chart -1** for explanation

9) (d)
10) (a)
} Follow **flow chart-2** for more explanation

11) (b)
12) (a)
} Follow section, **physical methods (Dry heat → Hot air oven → articles to be sterilised)** for explanation

13) (b)
- Follow section, **physical methods (moist heat → pasteurisation →disadvantages)** for explanation

14) (d)
- Holding temperature & time for pasteurisation by Holder method is 60^0C for 30 minutes

15) (a)
- Vaccines are best sterilised by filtration & vaccine bath

16) (c)

- Follow **table-3** for more explanation

17) (c)
- Autoclave works under principle of sterilisation by moist heat above 100°C above atmospheric pressure

18) (a)
- Browne's tube is used for autoclave which is a type of steam steriliser

19) (a)
- All glass wares are best sterilised by hot air oven
- Bacterial vaccines are best sterilised by vaccine bath
- Pasteurisation of milk by flash method is done by heating at 72°C for 15-20seconds

20) (b)
- Heat labile liquids like sera, sugar or antibiotics solution are sterilised by filtration

21) (a)
- Follow section, **physical methods (Radiation → ionising radiation)** for explanation

22) (d)
- Bone graft, suture & artificial tissue graft are sterilised by irradiation. Follow section physical methods (Radiation → ionising radiation) for more explanation
- Bronchoscope is sterilised by cidex (2% Gluteraldehyde)

23) (b)
- Cat gut suture is sterilised by irradiation. Follow section physical methods (Radiation → ionising radiation) for more explanation

24) (c)
- Alcohol is bactericidal, fungicidal, tuberculicidal, virucidal but not sporicidal

25) (b)
- Formalin is bactericidal, fungicidal, virucidal & sporicidal

26) (a)
27) (b) } Follow section, **chemical methods (Aldehyde → Gluteraldehyde)** for explanation

28) (b)
29) (d) } Follow section, **chemical methods (Gases → Ethylene oxide)** for explanation

30) (c)
- Phenol, alcohol & hexachorophene are not sporicidal while chlorine is sporicidal

31) (a), (b) & (d)
- Sputum can be initially disinfected by 5% phenol followed by boiling, autoclaving or burning (incineration). All sterile materila should follow to deep burial.

32) (a), (b), (c) & (d)
- Follow section, **chemical methods (Phenol)** for explanation
- Savlon contains 3% cetrimide+1.5% chlorhexidine gluconate

33) (c)
- Bronchoscope is sterilised by cidex (2% Gluteraldehyde)

34) (d)
- Phenol is bactericidal and not inactivated by organic matter

35) (c) & (d)
- Ethylene oxide is high level disinfectant. Follow **table-6** for more explanation
- Phenol do not require organic matter to act

36) (b)
- Disposable plastic syringe is sterilised by ethylene oxide & ionising radiation

37) (c)
- Follow section, **chemical methods (gases → formaldehyde gas)** for explanation

38) (a)
39) (c) } Follow section **chemical methods (testing of disinfectant)** for explanation. Different tests are mentioned to test the efficacy/power of disinfectant

40) (b)
41) (b) } Follow **table-5** for more explanation

42) (b)
- Semi-critical equipment needs high or intermediate level sterilisation. Follow **table-6** for explanation

43) (a) & (b)
- Follow **table-6** for explanation.

8 Culture media

Learning heading & subheadings

- Definition:
- History:
- Ingredients / components:
- Classification of media:

- **Definition:** It is an artificial preparation of nutritional materials required for the growth of microorganisms.

- **History:**

- Robert Koch invented the culture method for pure isolation of bacteria over solid media. Earliest solid medium was **cooked cut potato** used by him, later he used gelatin for solidification of media, but gelatin is not satisfactory as it has tendency to get liquefy at 24^0C & by proteolytic bacteria.
- Use of agar in solidification of media was suggested by Frau Hesse, the wife of one investigator in Koch laboratory, who had seen her mother using agar to make jellies.

- **Ingredients / components:** Following materials are used for media preparation

➢ **Protein source:**

- **Peptone:**
  - Mixture of partially digested & uncoagulable proteins.
  - Available in powder form
- **Meat extract**
  - **Called "lab lemco"**
  - Semisolid in nature
- **Neopeptone & proteose peptone:**
  - Commercially available peptone brand
- **Other proteins sources are:**
  - Serum: Foetal calf serum which is sterilised by filtration.
  - Albumin:

➢ **Sugars:** Glucose, sucrose, lactose, maltose, mannitol, starch etc.

➢ **Electrolytes:** Sodium chloride.

➢ **Vitamins:** Like Vitamin K in thioglycollate broth

➢ **Water:**

- Essential for the growth of all microorganisms.
- Deionized or distilled water is used to prepare the media.
- Source of hydrogen and oxygen.

➢ **Blood:**

- Provide extra nutrition to the fastidious organisms & used in enriched media.
- 5-10% sheep blood is ideal. Horse or ox blood is also useful.
- Human blood can be used but contains inhibitory substances.
- Blood is collected with all aseptic precautions
- It is rendered non-coagulable by adding the anticoagulant (citrate or oxalate) or by defibrillation (by shaking the blood in a bottle contains sterile glass beads)

➢ **Agar: →Fig.-1 (a)**

✪ **Properties:**

- Also **called agar agar**
- Provides solidification to media.
- Agar agar has no nutrient property
- Polysaccharide obtained from sea-weeds like red algae of species *Gelidium* & *Gracilaria*
- Weed being dried & finally supplied as dried strands or as a powder.
- On heating becomes gelly at 45^0C & liquefy at 98^0 C. Thus once gelled the medium remains solid throughout the temperature growth range of all bacteria. Blood, serum etc., therefore can be added to nutrient agar at 55^0 C at which the medium is still fluid & the risk of denaturation of the serum proteins added is nil.

✪ **Concentration of agar in media:**

- **Semi-solid media:** 0.5%
- **Solid media:** Differ in properties from brand to brand
  - New Zealand agar: Yields gel at 1%
  - Japanese agar: Yields gel at 2%
- **Solid media to inhibit the *Proteus* swarming:** 3-4% or 6%

➢ **Buffer:**

- Contains carbonates & phosphates
- It resist in pH change of medium

➢ **Yeast extract:**

- From yeast cells like Baker's yeast
- Contains proteins, amino acids, vitamins carbohydrates, minerals (phosphate & potassium) etc.

➢ **Antibiotics:** Prevents the growth of unwanted organisms

➢ **Anticoagulants:** In a blood culture media like taurocholate broth, blood contains inhibitory or bactericidal substances which are obviated by four fold dilution of blood or by adding liquoid/anticoagulant like SPS (Sodium Polyanethol Sulphonate). Ration of blood to medium is 1:10

❖ **Classification of media:** It is very difficult to classify a particular medium in particular group, because it has many properties & many uses; however some types are described as below

I. According to physical form or concentration or consistency of agar:

A. Liquid media:
- Absence of agar
- Also **"called broth"** (e. g. nutrient broth).
- Available in test-tubes, bottles or flasks.
- Bacterial growth produce uniform turbidity, surface pellicle (e.g. aerobic bacteria) or deposit at bottom

B. Semi solid media:
- Contains 0.2-0.5% agar
- Soft, gelly like & flat surface at top
- Available in test tubes
- Use: → **Table -1**

C. Solid media:
- Contains 2% agar.
- Also **"called agar"** (e. g. nutrient agar).
- Available in petri-dish or as slant/slope in tubes.
- Most commonly used for isolation of organisms

D. Biphasic media: →Fig.-1 (b)

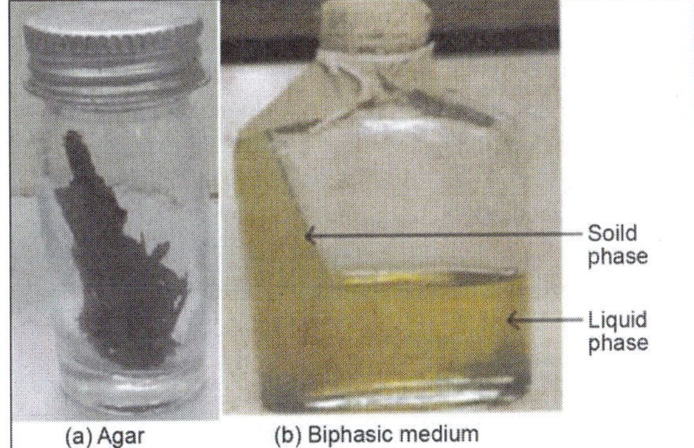

Figure-1: Agar & biphasic medium

- Media contains both liquid & solid phase are **called biphasic media**.
- Examples: Castaneda biphasic medium, Columbia biphasic medium etc.

II. According to nutritional components:

A. Simple/Basal media: →Table -1

B. Complex media/special media:
- Exact nutritional components are difficult to estimate
- All the media other than simple media are complex media. E.g. enriched media, selective media, transport media, enrichment media, differential media, sugar media, media for biochemical reactions

III. According to chemical composition:

A. Synthetic or defined medium:
- Prepared from pure chemical substances & the exact chemical composition (amount) is known.
- Used for various special studies such as metabolic requirements.
  E.g. Dubo's medium with Tween 80

B. Semi-synthetic or semi-defined medium: Chemical composition is approximately known.

IV. According to oxygen requirement:

A. Aerobic media: Media used for growth of bacteria other than obligate (strict) anaerobes are **called aerobic media**. E.g. basal media, enriched media etc.

B. Anaerobic media: Media used for growth of obligate (strict) anaerobes or to create the anaerobiosis are **called anaerobic media**. For more details, **Follow chapter → Culture methods**

V. According to uses or applications:

A. Simple/basal media:→ Table -1 & fig.-2

B. Enriched media: → Table -2 & fig.-3

C. Enrichment media: → Table -3 & fig.-4

D. Transport (holding) media: → Table-4 & fig.-5

E. Selective media: → Table -5 & fig.-6 & 7

F. Indicator media: Media contains substance (e.g. pH indicator) which indicates change in colour of medium. E.g. Sugar media, TCBS medium, Mac Conkey's medium etc.

G. Anaerobic media: For more details, **Follow chapter →Culture methods**

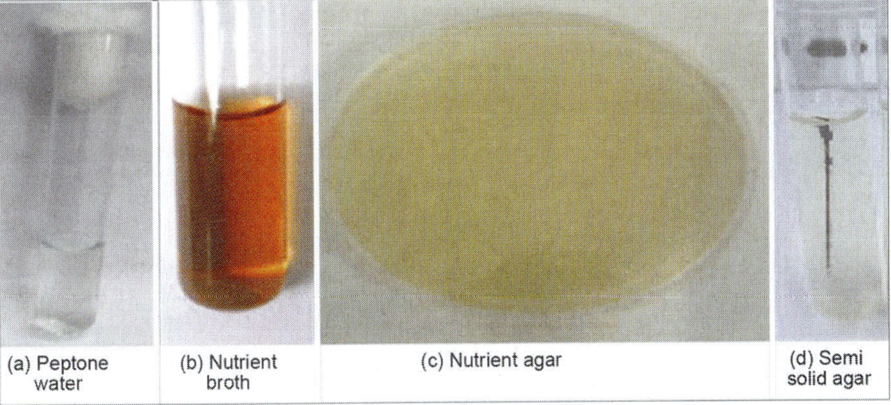

Figure -2: Simple / basal media

Definition: Media contains basic substances like meat extract, peptone, sodium chloride and water for growth of microorganisms are **called basal or simple media**. Exact nutritional components are known

No.	Name of medium	Important ingredients	Action of important ingredients	Method of sterilization	Uses
1	Peptone Water (PW)	Peptone, Salt, Water	Basic requirement for growth of microorganisms	Autoclaving	1. Used as a base for other media 2. Used for the growth of non- exacting microorganism
2	Nutrient Broth (N.B)	Peptone water & Meat extract	Do	Do	Do
3	Nutrient Agar (N.A.)	Nutrient broth & 2% agar	Do	Do	Do
4	Semisolid agar	Nutrient broth & 0.2-0.5% agar	Do	Do	1. To detect the motility of bacteria. 2. For growth of anaerobic and microaerophilic organisms. 3. Hugh-Leifson's (Oxidation – Fermentation / OF) test 4. Gelatin liquefaction test

Table -1: Simple / basal media

Definition: Media enriched with blood, serum, eggs, hydrocele fluid in addition to basic substances for growth of fastidious organisms are **called enriched media**

No.	Name of medium	Important ingredients	Action of important ingredients	Method of sterilization	Uses
1	Brain Heart Infusion Broth (BHIB) /Agar BHIA)	N.B./ Agar + Glucose +calf brain & cow heart	**Glucose, calf brain & cow heart** are enriching the organisms	Autoclaving	For growth of fastidious organisms.
2	Blood agar (BA)	N.A.+ 5–10% sheep or horse blood	**Blood** is enriching the organisms	Autoclave the N.A & when temperature comes down to 55^0C blood is added	1. To differentiate haemolytic from non-haemolytic organisms 2. For growth of *Staphylococcus* spp. & *Neisseria* spp. 3. For antibiogram of *Streptococcus* & pneumococcus
3	Chocolate agar (CA / heated blood agar)	BA+ heating	When blood is heated, RBCs will lysed & release **factor X (Haemin) & V (Vitamin)** free in medium	Keep BA in oven at 55^0C till become CA	To grow fastidious bacteria, like *H. influenzae, Staphylococcus* spp., *Neisseria* spp., *Streptococcus* spp. & pneumococcus
4	Loeffler's serum	N.B + Glucose + serum	**Serum& glucose** are enriching the medium	Inspissation	For growth of *C. diphtheriae*
5	Dorset's egg medium	N.B + egg (white+yellow)	**Egg** is enriching the medium	Inspissation	For growth of *M. tuberculosis* (Both human & bovine variety)

Table -2: Enriched media

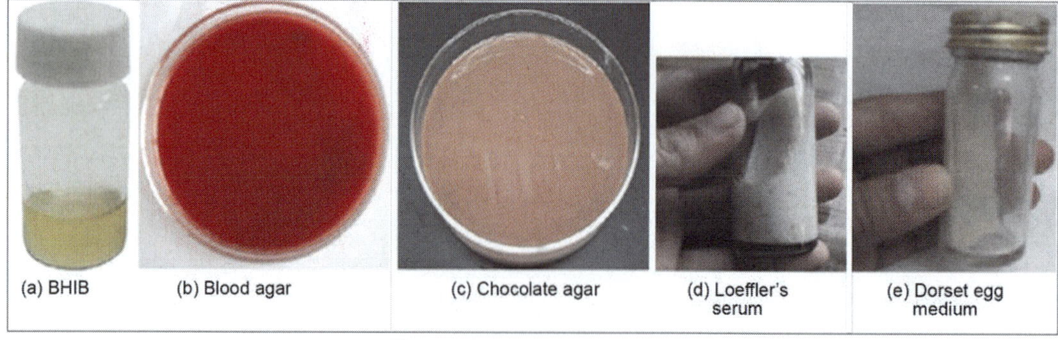
(a) BHIB (b) Blood agar (c) Chocolate agar (d) Loeffler's serum (e) Dorset egg medium

Figure-3: Enriched media

Definition: Media which favour the growth of particular organisms **called enrichment media**

No.	Name of medium	Important ingredients	Action of important ingredients	Method of sterilization	Uses
1	Glucose Broth (GB)	N.B.+ Glucose	**Glucose** is enriching the organisms	Tyndalli-sation	For pyogenic organisms & Sub Acute Bacterial Endocarditis **(SABE)**
2	Taurocholate broth	N.B.+ Sodium taurocholate	**Sodium taurocholate** is enriching the organisms	Autoclaving	For growth of *Salmonella* species from blood specimens
4	Tetrathionate broth	Tetrathionate + Potassium iodide + Brilliant green	**Tetrathionate** inhibits growth of Coliform bacilli & favour the growth of *Salmonella*	Tyndalli-sation	For growth of *Salmonella* species from faecal specimens
3	Selenite – F / broth	N.B + Lactose + selenite	**Selenite** is enriching the *Salmonella* species	Tyndalli-sation	For growth of *Salmonella* (more) & *Shigella* (less) species from faecal specimens
5	Alkaline Peptone Water (APW)	Peptone Water pH-8.6	**High pH** favours the *V. cholerae* growth	Autoclaving	For growth of *V. cholerae* from faecal specimens

Table -3: Enrichment media

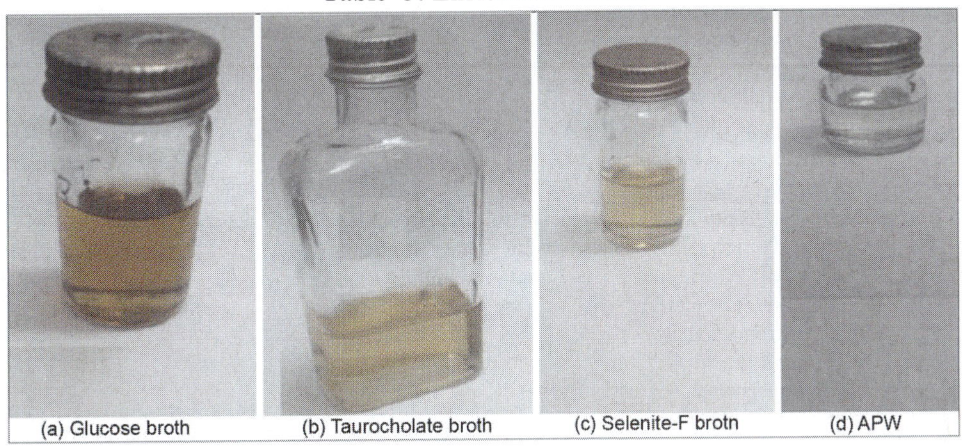

(a) Glucose broth (b) Taurocholate broth (c) Selenite-F brotn (d) APW

Figure-4: Enrichment media

Definition: Media which maintains the viability of the microorganisms without allowing the multiplication in specimens during transport to the laboratory **called transport** or **holding media**

No.	Name of medium	Important ingredients	Action of important ingredients	Method of sterilization	Uses
			Bacterial transport media (BTM)		
1	Pike's medium	Casein hydrosylate, tryptose, yeast extract, dextrose, crystal violet & sodium azide	Casein hydrosylate, Tryptose & yeast extract serve as nitrogen source. Dextrose as energy source. Crystal violet inhibits the gram +ve bacteria. Sodium azide inhibit the GNB plus non haemolytic streptococci	Autoclaving	- Selective, enrichment & transport medium for *Strept pyogenes* & other haemolytic streptococci from throat swab - It also preserve *Strept pneumoniae* & *H influenzae* from nasal & throat swabs
2	Stuart's medium	Charcoal, sodium thioglycolate (Reducing agent), inorganic phosphates, buffer	**Charcoal absorbs** the inhibitory substances **sodium thioglycolate** prevents oxidation during the transportation	Autoclaving	Provides viability of *Neisseria* spp.
3	Glycerol saline transport	Glycerol, sodium and potassium hydrogen	Prevents growth of intestinal commensals	Autoclaving	Preserves *Salmonella* & *Shigella* from faecal specimens

	medium	phosphate			
4	Gram negative broth	Tryptose, dextrose, mannitol, sodium citrate, sodium deoxycholate, monopotassium phosphate & dipotassium phosphate	Sodium citrate & sodium deoxycholate inhibit the growth of gram positive & coliforms	Autoclaving	Transport & selective medium for *Salmonella* & *Shigella* from clinical (faeces) & non clinical specimens
5	V. R. medium	P.W. + Crude sea salt, PH 8.6	High pH preserves viability of *V. cholerae*	Autoclaving	For transportation of *V. cholerae*
6	Alkaline Peptone Water (APW)				For transportation of *V. cholerae*
7	Autoclaved sea water				For transportation of *V. cholerae*
8	Cary Blair transport medium				For transportation of EHEC (O157:H7), *Salmonella, Shigella, V. cholerae* & *C jejuni*
	Viral transport media (VTM)				
1	Stuart's medium, Amie's medium, Leibovitz-Emory medium, Hank's balanced salt Solution (HBSS), Eagle's tissue culture medium	**Distilled water** + **Protein source** in this media are serum, albumin veal infusion (calf meat) & gelatin + **Antibiotics** like vancomycin gentamicin amphotericin B	**Protein** stabilise the virus. **Antibiotics** prevent bacterial and fungal contamination.	Filtration.	For collection of throat and nasal swabs from **human**
2	Modified Stuart's medium, Modified Amie's medium, Leibovitz-Emory medium			Filtration	For collection of respiratory & stool specimens from **human**
3	Transport medium 199	0.5% bovine serum albumin (BSA) + **Antibiotics** like benzylpenicillin, streptomycin, polymyxin B, nystatin & gentamicin	**Antibiotics** prevents bacterial and fungal contamination	Filtration	For collection of clinical specimens from all **animals** species for egg & tissue culture.
4	PBS-Glycerol transport medium	Phosphate-buffered saline (PBS) + **Antibiotics** as above	**Antibiotics** prevents the bacterial & fungal contamination	Auto-claving	For collection of specimens from all **animals** species for egg culture but not for tissue culture

Table -4: Transport or holding media

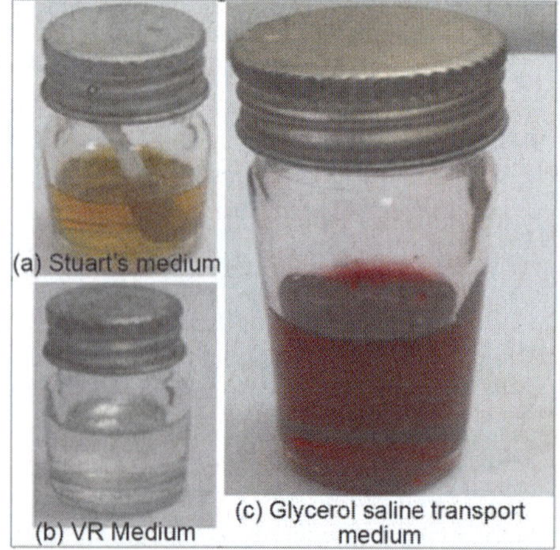

Figure-5: Transport or holding media

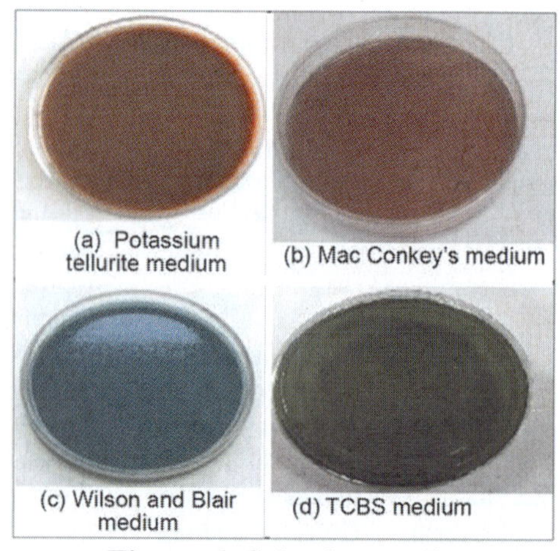

Figure-6: Selective media

Definition: Media contains inhibitory agents (e.g. antibiotics, chemicals) to prevent the growth of unwanted microbes called selective media

No.	Name of medium	Important ingredients	Action of important ingredients	Method of sterilization	Uses
1	Potassium tellurite medium	NA +blood + potassium tellurite	**Blood** to enrich the medium. **Potassium tellurite** is less inhibitory to *C. diphtheriae* compared to other throat commensals	Autoclave	-For the growth of *C. diphtheriae, Staph. aureus, E. faecalis, E. rhusiopathiae* -**Tellurite** is converted to metallic tellurium which gives black colour colonies.
2	Mac Conkey's agar	NA + Sodium taurocholate + lactose + neutral red	**Sodium Taurocholate** is inhibitory to non intestinal organisms. **Lactose** will be fermented by coliform bacilli with acid production & reduction in pH. **Neutral red** will give pink colour at acidic pH.	Autoclaving	1. For differentiating lactose fermenting organisms from non-lactose fermenting organisms 2. For growth of intestinal organisms
3	Wilson & Blair medium	NA +Glucose phosphate + Brilliant green +Bismuth sulphite + Ferric citrate	**Brilliant green** and **bismuth sulphite** inhibit intestinal organisms. Sulphite is converted to sulphide produces black colonies with **ferric citrate**	Autoclaving	For growth *Salmonella*
4	T.C.B.S (**T**hiosulph ate **C**itrate **B**ile salt **S**ucrose) agar	Thiosulphate + Citrate + Bile salt + Sucrose + Bromothymol Blue (B.B.)	**Sucrose** will be fermented by *V. cholerae* with acid production & reduction in pH of medium. **B.B.** gives yellow colour at acidic pH & green colour at alkaline pH (Sucrose non-fermenters).	Autoclaving	For growth of *V. cholerae* Ferments sucrose produces yellow colonies while sucrose non-fermenters give green colonies.
5	Lowen-stein Jensen (LJ) Medium	Egg + Malachite green+ mineral salts + glycerol	**Egg** to enrich the medium. **Malachite green** is least inhibitory for *M. tuberculosis*. **Glycerol** allows the growth of human variety.	Inspissation	For the growth of *M. tuberculosis*, human variety only
6	Sabou-raud's **D**extrose **A**gar (SDA)	Glucose +peptone + antibiotics like chloramphenicol, gentamicin & cycloheximide) + agar, pH: 5.4	**Acidic pH** and **high sugar** content make it selective for fungus. **Antibiotics** inhibit the bacterial growth.	Autoclaving	For cultivation of fungi
7	Thayer-Martin medium	CA+ Vancomycin Colistin + Nystatin	**CA** to enrich the *Neisseria* spp. & **antibiotics** inhibit the other bacterial growth.	Autoclaving	For the growth of the *Neisseria* spp.
8	Robertson's Cooked Meat Medium (RCMM): **Follow chapter →Culture methods**				For the growth of anaerobes
9	Deoxy Cholate Citrate agar (DCA)				For isolation of *Salmonella* & *Shigella* from stool
10	Xylose Lysine Deoxycholate (XLD) medium				

Table -5: Selective media

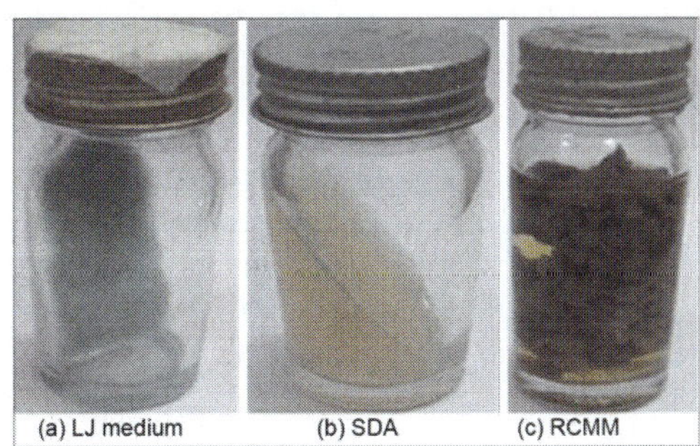

Figure-7: Selective media

✓ **Notes: Sorbitol Mac Conkey's medium / modified Mac Conkey's medium:** It contains sorbitol instead of lactose & useful to identify Entero Haemorrhagic *E coli* (EHEC)

H. Sugar media:

- **Definition:** Media contains fermentable substances (sugar)
- **Useful sugars are:**

a) **Monosaccharides:** Pentose (xylose, arabinose) & hexose (glucose, mannose)

b) **Disaccharides:** Lactose, saccharose

c) **Polysaccharides:** Starch, inulin
d) **Trisaccharides:** Raffinose
e) **Alcohol:** Sorbitol, glycerol
f) **Glucosides:** Salicin, esculin
g) **Non-carbohydrate substances:** Inositol

➢ **Media: → Fig.-8 & table-6**

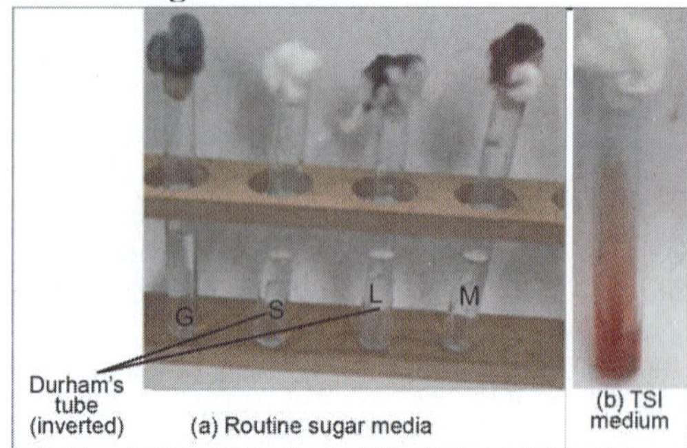

Figure-8: Sugar media

I. Differential media:

➢ **Synonym:** Some times differential media are defined as **indicator media**

➢ **Definition:** Media which distinguish particular characteristics of bacterial group from other group

➢ **Examples of differential media:**

Mnemonic: Differential media
TCBS + NBM (Nill By Mouth)

i. **TCBS medium:** It separate sucrose fermenter group (*V. cholerae*) from non- sucrose fermenter group

ii. **CLED:**

✪ **Full name:** Cysteine Lactose Electrolyte Deficient medium

✪ **History:** Previous culture methods used to inhibit the swarming of *Proteus* included adding chloral hydrate, alcohol, sodium azide, surface-active agents, boric acid, and sulfonamides to the medium. In the mid 1960s, Sandys and Mackey reported the laboratory diagnosis of urinary pathogens by lacking the medium with electrolyte (NaCl), which helps to prevent the swarming of *Proteus* spp.

✪ **Ingredients & action: → Table -7**

Ingredients	Weight	Actions
Lactose	10.0gm	To separate LF from NLF
Pancreatic Digest of Gelatin	4.0gm	Nitrogen, vitamins & carbon source for microbial growth
Pancreatic Digest of Casein	4.0gm	
Beef Extract	3.0gm	
L-Cystine	0.128gm	To enhance the growth of cystine-dependent "dwarf colony" coliforms
Bromothymol Blue	0.02gm	pH indicator
Agar	15.0gm	Solidifying agent
Final pH 7.3 +/- 0.2 at 25°C		

Table -7: Ingredients & action in CLED medium

✪ **Result: → Table -8 & fig.-9**

Microbes	Culture characteristics
E. coli	Opaque yellow colonies with a slightly deeper yellow centre
Klebsiella	Yellow to whitish-blue colonies, extremely mucoid
Proteus	Translucent blue colonies
P. aeruginosa	Green colonies with typical matted surface and rough periphery
Enterococcus	Small yellow colonies, about 0.5mm in size
Staph aureus	Deep yellow colonies, uniform in colour
CoNS	Pale yellow colonies, more opaque than *Enterococcus faecalis*

Table -8: Result in CLED medium

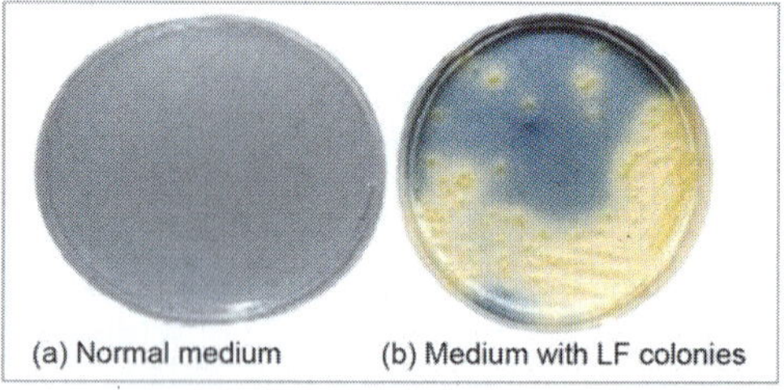

Figure-9: Result in CLED medium

✪ **Use:** For differentiate urinary pathogens LF from NLF, with controlling the swarming of *Proteus* spp. It also supports the growth of many pathogens like Enterobactericeae, *Pseudomonas, Staphylococcus, Enterococcus* and *Candida* and a number of contaminants such as diphtheroids, *Lactobacilli* & *Micrococci*.

No.	Name of medium	Important ingredients	Action of important ingredients	Method of sterilization	Uses
1	Routine sugar media like G, S, L & M	PW + 1 % sugar + Andrade's indicator + Durham's tube	Sugar fermentation gives **acid** which is indicated by pink colour & **gas** production by bubble formation in Durham's tube	Tynda-llisation	-For sugar fermentation test -Fo differentiation sugar fermenter (Enterobactericeae) & nonfermenters (*Pseudomonas*)
2	Hiss Serum	Sugar media + 3% serum	------------ Do -----------	----- Do -----	Sugar fermentation test in *C. diphtheriae* , *Neisseria* spp. & pneumococcus
3	TSI agar /composite medium: Follow chapter → Laboratory diagnosis of bacterial infections				
4	Kligler Iron Agar (KIA) Follow chapter →Laboratory diagnosis of bacterial infections				

Table -6: Sugar media

No.	Media	Important ingredients	Action of important ingredients	Method of sterilization	Uses
1	Gelatin liquefaction medium	NB+ Gelatin	Gelatin is liquefy by proteolytic organisms	Tyndallisation	To detect the proteolytic activity of organisms.

Table-9: Gelatin liquefaction medium

iii. **Blood Agar:** It separate haemolytic group from non-haemolytic group

iv. **Sugar media:** It separate sugar fermenter (Enterobacteriaceae) from non-fermenters group (*Pseudomonas*)

v. **Nagler's medium:** It differentiate between lecithinase activity of different bacterial group

vi. **Bile-Esculin agar:** It separate *Enterococcus* (*Streptococcus* group D) group from non-*Enterococcus* group

vii. **Mac Conkey's medium:** It separate lactose fermenter (*E. coli, K. pneumoniae*) group from non-lactose fermenter (*Salmonella, Shigella* etc.)

- **Advantages of differential media:**

1. It used in replacement of Mac Conkey's medium & blood agar for testing of urine sample
2. Separate lactose fermenter group from non- lactose fermenter
3. Advantage over Mac Conkey's agar: Less inhibitory than Mac Conkey's agar & support the growth of *Candida* spp. & gram positive bacteria except β-haemolytic *Streptococcus*
4. Advantage over blood agar: Prevent the *Proteus* swarming

J. **Media for biochemical reactions:**

1. **Sugar fermentation test:** Sugar media as described above
2. **Citrate test:** Bromothymol Blue as pH indicator
   - Koser's citrate broth:
   - Simmon's citrate agar:

   } Follow chapter → Laboratory diagnosis of bacterial infections
3. **Urease test:** Phenol red as pH indicator
   - Stuart's urea broth:
   - Christinsen's urea agar:

   } Follow chapter → Laboratory diagnosis of bacterial infections
4. **Gelatin liquefaction test:** Gelatin medium **(table-9)**

K. **Media for antibiogram:**

1. **Muller Hinton Agar (MHA):** Follow chapter →Laboratory diagnosis of bacterial infections

L. **Composite media:** Follow chapter → Laboratory diagnosis of bacterial infections

✓ **Note: Dehydrated media**

▪ **Preparation:**
- Available commercially
- Prepared by different companies from dehydrated materials which are mentioned on the label of the container.
- They are reconstituted in distilled water & sterilised before use in laboratory

▪ **Advantages:**
- Useful in peripheral laboratory
- Time saving & less labour intensive for preparation

VI. **According to ingredients:**

A **Chemically defined media or cell free media or artificially prepared nutritional media:**

✪ **Preparation:** Prepared by using different biochemical or chemical substances like protein source, carbohydrate source, lipid source, vitamins, minerals, antibiotics, agar etc.

✪ **Examples:** All earlier media discussed in this chapter are fall in this category

✪ **Uses:** They are not for viruses, but useful for
- Bacteria like *E coli, Staph aureus* etc.
- Fungi *C. albicans, Aspergillus* spp. etc.
- Few protozoa: Like *E histolytica, Trepanosoma* spp. *Leishmania* spp. etc.

✪ **Limitations:** Few microbes are not growing in cell free media are mentioned in **table-10.** Such microbes are **called viable but not cultivable.**

Bacteria	
Treponema pallidum	*Rickettsia* spp.
Mycobacterium leprae	*Orientia tsutsugamushi*
Chlymydiae spp	*Ehrlichia* spp.
Fungi	
Loboa loboi	*Pneumocystis jiroveci*
Parafungal agents	
Rhinosporidium seeberi	
Viruses	
All viruses	
Parasites	
Metazoa	

Table-10: Microbes can't grow in cell free media

B **Cell culture or tissue culture media:**

✪ **Preparation:** Prepared by using cells or tissues or bits of organ

✪ **Examples, uses & other details:** Follow chapter → Laboratory diagnosis of viral infections

✓ **Notes:** *Mycobacterium leprae*, pathogenic *Treponema pallidum* & *Lacazia loboi* are growing in animal culture.

Question bank

Essay/Full question

1) Culture media

Short notes

1) Components (Ingredients) used to prepare the media
2) Simple/Basal media
3) Enriched media
4) Enrichment media
5) Transport (holding) media
6) Selective media
7) Sugar media
8) Anaerobic media
9) Differential media
10) Composite media
11) Cell culture or tissue culture media

Short questions for theory/viva questions

1) Define media & name the person who introduced the cultivation technique on solid media.
2) Define biphasic media. Write two examples
3) What is agar? Write its role in preparation of media.
4) Mention the type of media according to their physical form with one example in each category.
5) Name the one medium useful for following laboratory tests: Citrate test, Urease test, Gelatin liquefaction test & antibiogram
6) Name the two green colour media
7) Write four examples of selective media
8) Write four examples of differential media
9) Name the pH indicator in following media Mac Conkey's medium, TCBS medium, Sugar medium & Stuart's urea broth
10) Name the two viral transport media
11) What is modified Mac Conkey's medium? Write its use.
12) Comment: Mac Conkey's medium is classified as both selective & differential medium.
13) Comment: Blood ager & TCBS are classified as differential media.
14) What is dehydrated media?
15) What is composite media? Write two examples.
16) Name four bacteria which can't grow on cell free media.

MCQs for chapter review

History

1) **Robert Koch was suggested to use agar in solidification of media by wife of one investigator of his laboratory, because**
(a) Gelatin liquefy at 24^0C (b) Gelatin liquefy by proteolytic bacteria. (c) Agar is cheap (d) Gelatin is costly
2) **Earliest solid medium used for bacterial cultivation was**
(a) Cooked cut potato medium (b) Blood agar (c) Mac Conkey's medium (d) Nutrient agar

Ingredients/Components

3) **Agar-agar is used in medium as**
(a) Nutritional agent (b) Solidifying agent (c) Selective agent (d) Preservative
4) **In nutrient agar, conc. of agar is**
(a) 1% (b) 2% (c) 3% (d) 4%
5) **Which anticoagulant is used when blood is sent for blood culture**
(a) Sodium citrate (b) EDTA (c) Oxalate (d) SPS
6) **In blood culture the ratio of blood to reagent is -**
(a) 1:5 (b) 1:20 (c) 1:10 (d) 1:100

Classification of media

7) **Which of the following is true** (AIIMS, Nov-06, AI-07)
(a) Agar has nutrient properties (b) Chocolate medium is selective medium (c) Addition of selective substance in a solid medium is called enrichment media (d) Nutrient broth is a basal medium
8) **Chocolate agar is an example of? -**
(a) Enriched medium (b) Enrichment medium (c) Selective medium (d) Transport medium
9) **Blood agar is an example of? -**
(a) Enriched medium (b) Indicator medium (c) Enrichment medium (d) Selective medium
10) **Which is an enrichment medium**
(a) Selenite F broth (b) Chocolate medium (c) Meat extract medium (d) Egg medium
11) **Selenite F broth is an enrichment medium for?**
(a) *Salmonella* (b) *Shigella* (c) *E. coli* (d) *Campylobacter*
12) **Lactose fermentation is seen in**
(a) Blood agar (b) Chocolate agar (c) Mac Conkey's agar (d) LJ medium
13) **Mac Conkey's agar is an example of? -**
(a) Enriched medium (b) Differential medium (c) Enrichment medium (d) Selective medium
14) **pH indicator in MacConkey's medium is**
(a) Phenol red (b) Andrade's indicator (c) Neutral red (d) Preservatives
15) **Recommended transport medium for stool specimen suspected to contain enteric pathogen is**
(a) Amies medium (b) Buffered glycerol saline medium (c) mac Conkey's medium (d) Stuart'smedium
16) **pH of SDA is adjusted to**
(a) 4-6 (b) 1-2 (c) 6-8 (d) 8-10
17) **In a patient with UTI, CLED (Cysteine Lactose Electrolyte Deficient) medium is preferred over Mac Conkey's medium because** (AIIMS, Nov-01, AI-01)
(a) It is a differential medium (b) It inhibit the swarming of *Proteus* (c) Promote growth of *Pseudomonas* (d) Promote growth of *Staph* and *Candida*
18) **Which organism cannot be cultured in cell free media** (PGI, May-13, Nov-11)
(a) *Klebsiella rhinoscleromatis* (b) *Klebsiella ozaenae* (c) *Treponema pallidum* (d) *Pneumocystis jiroveci* (e) *Rhinosporidium seeberi*
19) **The term "viable not cultivable" is used for** (PGI, Dec-07)
(a) *M leprae* (b) *M tuberculosis* (c) *Treponema pallidum* (d) *Salmonella* (e) *Staph*

Answers of MCQs & explanation

1) **(a) & (b)**
2) **(a)**
} Follow section, **history** for explanation
3) **(b)**
4) **(a) & (b)**
} Follow section, **ingredients/components (agar)** for explanation
5) **(d)**
6) **(c)**
} Follow section, **ingredients/components** for more explanation
7) **(d)**
- Agar has no nutrient properties
- Chocolate medium is enriched medium
- Addition of selective substance in a solid medium is called selective media

8) **(a)**
9) **(a)**
} Follow section, **classification of media (enriched media → table-2**) for explanation
10) **(a)**
11) **(a) & (b)**
} Follow section, **classification of media (enrichment media → table-3**) for explanation
12) **(c)**
- Mac Conkey's agar is a selective & differential medium. It contains lactose so it useful to differentiate LF from NLF

13) **(b) & (d)**
14) **(c)**
} Follow section **classification of media (selective media → table-5 & differential media)** for explanation
15) **(a)**
- Follow section, **classification of media (transport media → table-4**) for explanation

16) **(a)**

- Follow section, **classification of media (selective media → table-5)** for explanation

17) (b)

- As far as CLED medium is concerned all options are right but here case is of UTI, where it is more useful to inhibit the swarming of *Proteus* by its electrolyte deficient nature.

18) (c), d) & (e)
19) (a) & (c)
} Follow **table-10** for explanation

9 Culture methods

Learning heading & subheadings

Introduction

❖ **Definitions:**

➤ **Culture method:** Method used for growing (cultivation) of microorganisms in media **called culture method**.

➤ **Inoculum:** Liquid culture or suspension of microorganism used for cultivation **called inoculum**.

❖ **Aims of culture:** For

- Isolation of bacteria in pure culture: Isolation of bacteria is defined as separation of species/strain from clinical specimens/culture suspension, contains mixed population of microbes. (Identification of bacteria is defined as knowing the exact name of bacteria)
- Demonstration of bacterial properties.
- Preparation of the antigens & vaccine.
- Bacteriophage typing
- Bacteriocin typing.
- Antibiotic sensitivity testing
- Estimation of viable counts
- Maintenance of stock cultures

Classification

❖ **Methods:** Two types of culture methods

I. **Aerobic culture methods**

II. **Anaerobic culture methods**

I. Aerobic culture methods

➤ **Methods:** Four types as follows

A. **For solid media**

B. **For semi-solid media**

C. **For liquid media**

D. **For biphasic media**

A. **For solid media:**

i. **Streak culture (surface plating):**

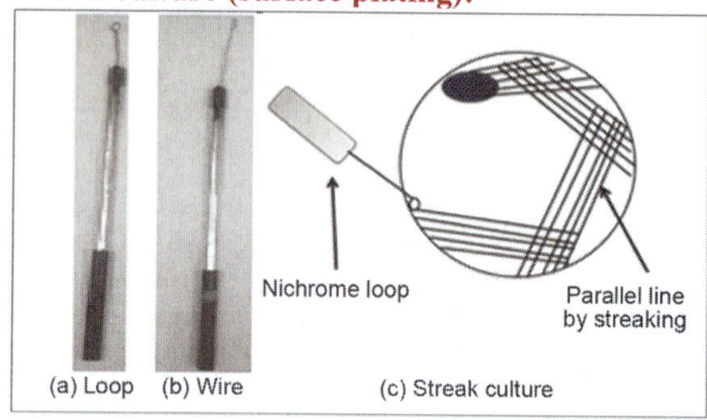

Figure-1: Nichrome loop, wire & streak culture

✪ **Steps:** →**Fig.-1**

- One loopful of culture is made as a primary inoculum & spread by streaking it with the nichrome loop (24 SWG) in a series of parallel lines in different segments of the plate.
- Loop flamed and cooled between the different sets of streaks.
- Incubate the plate for desired time & at desired temperature
- On incubation growth may be confluent at the site of the original inoculation but becomes progressively thinner and well separated colonies are obtained over the final series of streaks

✪ **Use:** For routine isolation of bacteria.

✪ **Advantage:** It provides the isolated growth from the mixed culture.

ii. **Lawn culture (carpet culture):**

✪ **Steps:** Different ways

a. **Flooding:** Flooding the surface of the plate with an inoculum.

b. **Pipetting:** Pipetting the surface of the plate with an inoculum.

c. **Swabbing:** Surface of the plate may be inoculated by applying a swab soaked in an inoculum.

✪ **Uses:**

- Useful for bacteriophage typing
- Antibiotic sensitivity testing (disc diffusion method).
- Also used in the preparation of bacterial antigens & vaccines.

✪ **Advantage:** Provides a uniform growth.

iii. Stroke culture: →**Fig.-2 (a)**

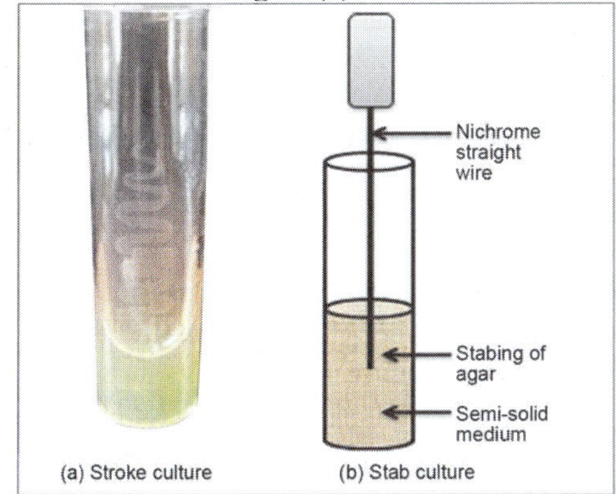

Figure-2: Stroke culture & stab culture

- **Steps:** Streaking of agar slope/slant in test tubes by using nichrome loop **[fig.-1(a)]** or straight wire **[fig.-1(b)]**
- **Use:** To identify biochemical properties like pigment production, citrate utilisation, sugar fermentation in TSI medium.
- **Advantage:** provides a pure growth of the bacterium.

iv. Pour plate culture:

- **Steps:**

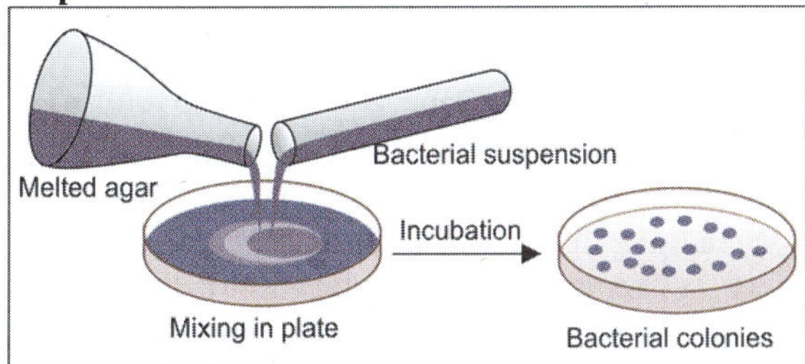

Figure-3: Pour plate culture

- Both agar & inoculum are plated simultaneously in petri-dish (**fig-3**)
- Tubes or flasks containing 15 ml of the agar medium are melted and left to cool in a water bath at 45-50 °C.
- Mix 1 ml of inoculum & melted agar in plate.
- Allowed to settle.
- After incubation colonies will be seen well distributed throughout the depth of the medium.
- Enumerated using colony counters.

- **Uses:**
- Used to estimate the viable bacterial count in a suspension.
- Used for quantitative urine cultures.

B. For semi-solid media:

i. Stab culture:

- **Steps:** Penetration of semi-solid agar medium (flat at top) in test tubes by using nichrome straight wire (not nichrome loop) as shown in **fig.-2(b).** Stop once the wire reaches 0.5 inches away from the bottom of the stab media.
- **Uses:**
- Motility detection test
- Gelatin liquefaction test
- O_2 requirement of the bacterium under research.
- In the maintenance of stock culture

C. For liquid media:

i. Liquid culture method:

- **Steps**: Liquid media are inoculated
- By touching with a loop dipped in inoculum or
- By adding the inoculum with pipettes or syringes.
- **Uses:**
- For blood & other body fluids culture
- Antibiotic sensitivity testing (dilution method)
- **Advantages:** Preferred when large yields are desired.
- **Disadvantages:** Does not provide pure growth from mixed culture

D. For biphasic media:

i. Biphasic/diphasic culture method: For more details, **Follow chapter → Culture media**

- **Steps:**
- Inoculum is inoculated in liquid part.
- Bottle is incubated at 37^0C for 24 hrs in upright position.
- Remove the bottle from the incubator
- Tilt the bottle, so liquid part will run over solid part.
- Bottle is re-incubated at 37^0C for 24 hrs in upright position.
- Next day examine the solid phase for growth.
- **Uses:** For isolation of bacteria like *N. meningitidis, S. typhi, B. abortus* etc.
- **Advantages:**
- Eliminate the chances of aerial contamination
- Less labour intensive

II. Anaerobic culture methods

- **Synonym:** Anaerobiosis
- **Definition:** Method to create an anaerobic condition **called anaerobiosis.**
- **Use:** For cultivation of anaerobic bacteria.
- **Classification of anaerobic bacteria:** **Follow chapter → Physiology of bacteria**
- **Methods:**

A **Physical methods:**
B **Chemical methods:**
C **Biological methods:**
D **By using reducing agents in anaerobic media:**
E **By using pre reduced systems:**

A. Physical methods:

i. Vacuum desiccators:

- **Steps:** Replacement of O_2 by vacuum.
- **Disadvantages:**
- Not useful because some O_2 left behind.
- Fluid culture may boil
- Solid media may detached from base of plate

ii. Candle (CO_2) jar:

- **Principle:** Replacement of O_2 by CO_2, generated from candle. Candle will burn till O_2 is present in jar, then after it extinguished.
- **Steps: →Fig.-4**
  - Put the culture plate in jar
  - Keep enlightened candle in jar
  - Put the lid & sealed the jar with vaseline.

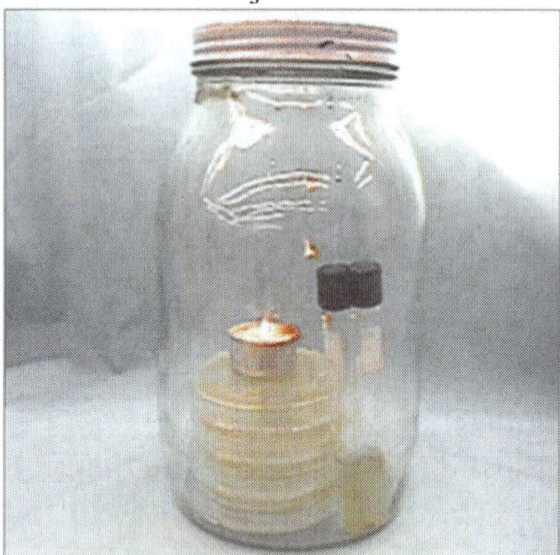

Figure-4: Candle jar

- **Advantage:** Provide CO_2 which stimulate the growth of most bacteria
- **Disadvantage:** Not useful because some O_2 left behind.

B. Chemical methods:

i. McIntosh & Filde's anaerobic jar:

- **Principle:** Based on **evacuation – replacement mechanism.** Evacuation of O_2 from jar by vacuum pump & residual O_2 combine with H_2 to form water in presence of catalyst. Hydrogen pump is act as source of H_2.
- **Structure:**
  - It consist metal **[fig.-5(a)]** or stout glass jar **[fig.-5(b)]** & metal lid
  - Lid has one inlet tube, one outlet tube, pressure gauge & electric terminal inner to which catalyst are attached

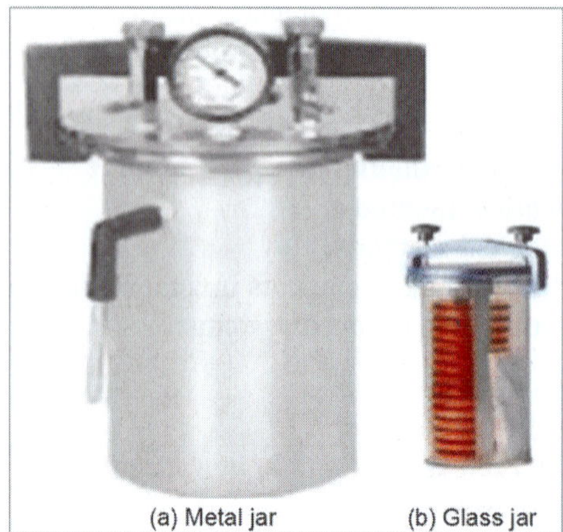

Figure-5: McIntosh & Filde's jar

- **Catalyst:**
  - Palladinised asbestos acts after heating
  - Alumina pellets coated with palladium: acts at room temp.
- **Steps:**
  - Put the inoculated test & control plates in a jar
  - Clamp the lid tightly.
  - Evacuate the air from jar by attaching outlet with vacuum pump
  - Close the outlet & attach the inlet with H_2 pump
  - Close the inlet when jar is filled with H_2
  - Connect the electric terminal & start the electric supply.
  - Palladinised asbestos catalysts are heated after electric supply & form water by combining the residual O_2 with H_2.
- **Advantage:** Complete anaerobiosis
- **Disadvantage:** Chances of explosion due to overheating if palladinised asbestos catalysts are used. That is overcome by using alumina pellets coated with palladium which acts at room temp.
- **Control:**

1. **Chemical control:** Colourless methylene blue gives blue colour if anaerobiosis is not maintained
2. **Biological control:**
   - **-Ve control:** *P. aeruginosa* (aerobic bacteria) will grow if anaerobiosis is not maintained
   - **+Ve control:** *Cl. tetani* (anaerobic bacteria) will grow if anaerobiosis is maintained

ii. Anoxomat:

- **Principle:** It is an automated method which based on **evacuation – replacement mechanism.** Evacuations of O_2 from jar & replace with H_2 gas from cylinder in presence of catalyst same as McIntosh & Filde's jar. Hydrogen cylinder is act as source of H_2.
- **Advantage:** More effective for anaerobiosis than McIntosh & Filde's jar

iii. Gas Pak method:

- **Principle:**
  Different chemicals generate H_2 & CO_2 on addition of water. H_2 combine with O_2 to form water in presence of cold catalyst & CO_2 favour the bacterial growth as shown in **fig.-6.**
- **Structure:** It is a plastic jar with chemical shown in **fig.-7.**
- **Catalyst:** Alumina pellets coated with palladium **called cold catalyst**
- **Steps:**
  - Put the inoculated test & control plates in a jar
  - Add the chemical (commercial available foil pack containing mixture: citric acid sodium borohydrate & sodium bicarbonate)
  - Add the water (about 10 ml) & screw tight the lid.
  - H_2 & CO_2 are generated from chemical after adding the water.

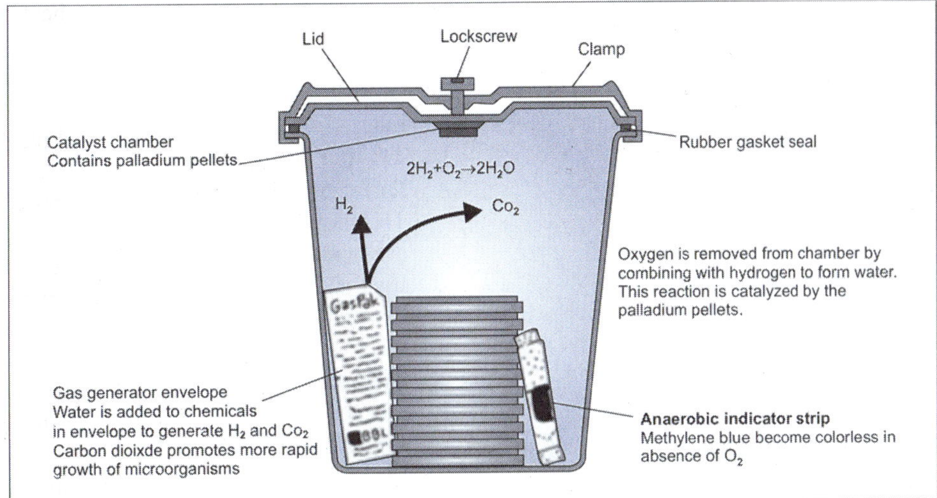

Figure-6: Principle of Gas Pak

- H_2 combines with O_2 to form water in presence of cold catalyst & gives anaerobic condition

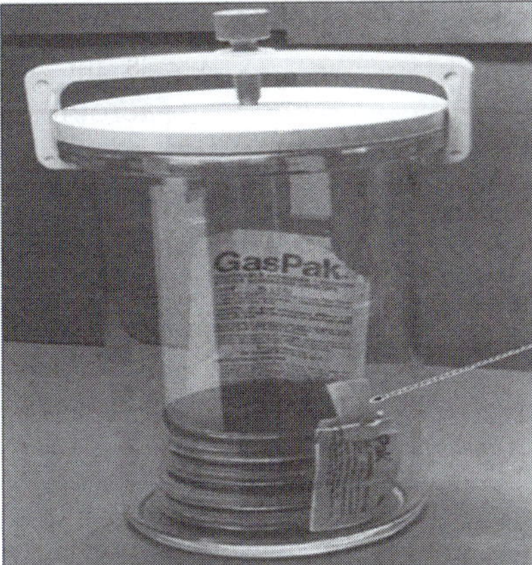

Figure-7: Gas pak method

✪ **Advantages:**
- Simple & effective
- Commercial available as disposable envelope
- No need of vacuum & H_2 pump
- Some gas pak do not need water

iv. Other chemicals used for anaerobiosis are:
1. Pyrogallol (Powder form, **By Buchner, 1888**)
2. Pyrogallic acid (liquid) + NaOH
3. Pyrogallol + sodium carbonate
4. Chromium + H2SO4 **(called Rosenthal method)**
5. Yellow phosphorous

C. Biological method:

✪ **Principle:** Replacement of O_2 by using biological materials like aerobic bacteria, germinating seeds or chopped vegetables

✪ **Steps:**
- Base of petri dish containing medium is inoculated with test organisms
- Top part of petri dish containing medium is inoculated with aerobic bacteria (*Pseudomonas*) & inverted over base part & sealed.

✪ **Disadvantage:** Slow & ineffective

D. By using reducing agents in anaerobic media:

i. RCMM: → **Fig.-8**

✪ **Full form:** Robertson's Cooked Meat Media

✪ **Principle:** Meat generates the **unsaturated fatty acids** & reducing substances **(glutathione)** which absorbed the O_2 & provide anaerobic condition (reduced Eh).

✪ **Ingredients:** N.B. & meat pieces

✪ **Method of sterilisation:** Autoclave

✪ **Steps:**
- Inoculate the test organism in RCMM.
- Anaerobes attack carbohydrates in meat (saccharolytic) turn meat in pink/red colour. E.g. *Cl. perfringens*
- Anaerobes attack protein in meat (proteolytic) turn meat in black. E.g. *Cl. tetani*

✪ **Uses:**
- To maintain the stock culture
- Widely used in routine practise for anaerobic organisms

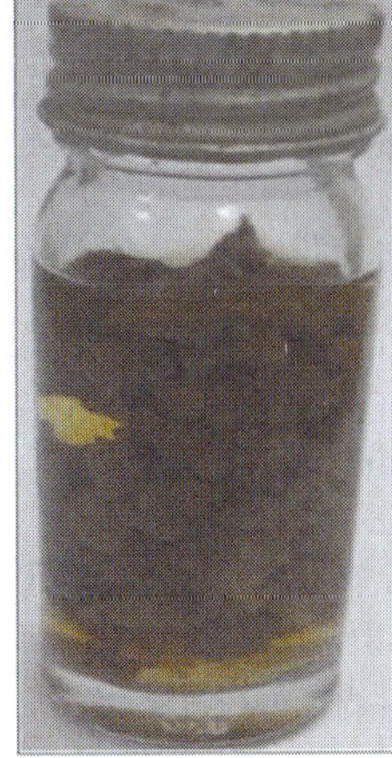

Figure-8: RCMM

ii. Smith- Noguchi medium (broth) or Noguchi medium (?):

- **Principle:** Replacement of O_2 by reducing agent generated from meat pieces.
- **Ingredients:** Broth is containing the meat pieces from rabbit kidney, heart, spleen or testes & red hot metallic ions
- **Steps:**
  - Inoculate the test organism in broth.
  - It is than layered over with sterile vaseline.
- **Use:** It support the growth of many bacteria like spirochetes

iii. 0.1% Thioglycollate broth:

- **Principle:**
  - Replacement of O_2 by thioglycollate (reducing agent) which absorbs oxygen.
  - There is gradation of O_2. O_2 being high at top & lower towards the bottom of medium. It allow the growth of aerobes (at surface) anaerobes (in bottom), microaerophilic (in middle)
- **Ingredients:** Casitone, NaCl, l-cystine, Thioglycollic acid, methylene blue, agar. pH 7.2. Broth is enriched with haemin & vitamin K
- **Steps:**
  - Boiled the broth to eliminate the O_2
  - Cool down & inoculate the test organism in broth.
  - Bacterial growth is identified by turbidity.
- **Use:** support the growth of anaerobes & microaerophilic bacteria
- **Modification**: addition of small quantity of agar (semisolid) in broth prevents the diffusion of O_2 & increase the anaerobic capacity.

iv. Other reducing agents: Are 1% glucose, 0.1% ascorbic acid, 0.05% cysteine etc.

E. By using pre reduced system:

i. Pre Reduced Anaerobic System (PRAS):

- For quantitative culture
- For fastidious bacteria

ii. Anaerobic chamber (glove box):

- Anaerobic chamber is an airtight, glass fronted cabinet filled with inert-gas.
- Entry lock for the introduction & removal of materials & gloves for the hands

Methods of pure culture isolation

- **Types:** Following are the different types of methods to obtain the pure growth of bacteria.

A. Surface plating: To isolate pure culture from mixed growth

B. Enrichment, selective & indicator media: To isolate pure culture from samples like faeces, urine etc. containing normal flora

C. Pre-treatment of specimens with bactericidal agents:

- Bactericidal agents like acid, alkali etc. kills the unwanted organisms(e.g. commensals) from specimens
- Used to isolate M. tuberculosis from sputum & other samples.

D. Temperature methods:

- **Different temperature incubation methods:**
  - Thermophilic can grow at 60^0C
  - Mesophilic can grow at 37^0C
  - Incubate a mixture of *N. meningitidis* & *N. catarrhalis* at 22^0C, where later can grow.
- **Heating method:** Heat a mixture of vegetative bacteria & spores 80^0C, where later can grow

E. Separation of motile from non motile bacteria:

1. **Craig's tube method: → Fig.-9**
   - Wide tube containing soft agar (0.2%) & both ended open narrow & small inner tube
   - Inoculate the strain in inner tube & after sufficient incubation subculture from agar surface outer to inner tube which yield the motile cell
2. **U- tube method:** Inoculate the strain from one end & S/C from opposite end will yield motile cells

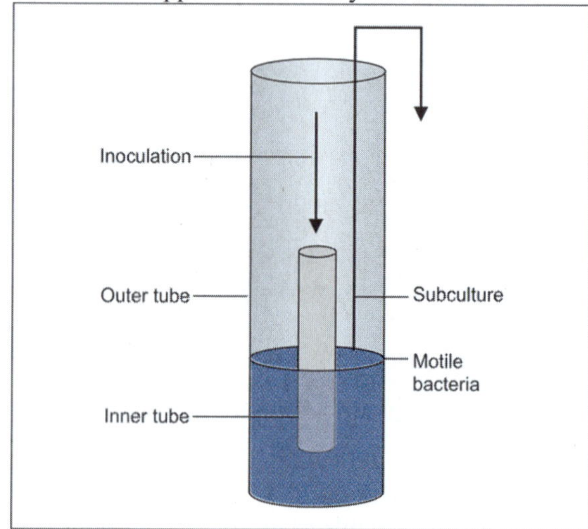

Figure-9: Craig's tube

F. Laboratory animal inoculation method: E.g. separation of *Anthrax bacilli* from aerobic spore bearer by inoculation in mice or guinea pigs. Produce fatal septicemia & *A. bacilli* is culture from heart blood.

G. Filtration methods:

- Separate the different size bacteria
- Separate the virus from bacteria

H. Anaerobiosis:

- It separate the aerobes from anaerobes
- Methods are described earlier

Methods of preservation of microorganisms

- **Introduction:** Preservation of microorganisms in microbiology is a tradition

❖ **Aims:** For
- Academic & research work
- Epidemiological purpose

❖ **Types:** Two types of methods like short term methods & long term methods

A. Short term methods: For weeks to months

✪ **Methods:**

i. Subculturing:
- Routine method for preservation by using different liquid & solid media specially nutrient agar slant
- RCMM is used for anaerobes.

ii. Freezing at -20^{0}C:

iii. Immersion method: Preservation by immersing the culture in mineral oil, glycerol, sterile distilled water etc.

iv. Drying: For fungus & spore bearing bacteria

✪ **Advantages:**
- Cheaper
- Easy to perform

✪ **Disadvantages:**
- Change in phenotypic properties like loss of capsule due to repeated subculture make virulent strain avirulent
- Change in genotypic properties due to mutation

B. Long term methods: Up to years

✪ **Methods:**

i. Ultra temperature freezing:
- Preservation of culture at -70^{0}C with mixture of preservatives like glycerol, skimmed milk, sucrose etc.
- Such preservatives are **called cryopreservatives**

ii. Freeze drying:
- Also **called lyophilisation**
- It involves the freezing of the liquid culture followed by dehydration to remove water from frozen bacterial suspension
- It gives stable & readily dehydrated culture
- Lyophilised culture is best store at 4^{0}C

iii. Drying: For fungus & spore bearing bacteria

✪ **Advantages:**
- Maintenance of phenotypic & genotypic properties
- Less space occupied by culture
- Maintain the viability of organisms
- Ideal method for preservation

✪ **Disadvantages:** High cost of equipments

Question bank

Essay/Full question

1) Culture methods

Short notes

1) Aerobic culture methods
2) Anaerobiosis
3) McIntosh & Filde's anaerobic jar
4) Gas Pak system or method
5) Methods to isolate the bacteria in pure culture
6) Methods for preservation of microorganisms.

Short questions for theory/viva questions

1) Write the four uses of culture methods
2) Write the principle of Gas Pak method / McIntosh & Filde's anaerobic jar method
3) What is Craig's tube?
4) What is lyophilisation?

MCQs for chapter review

Classification

1) **Stab culture method is useful for**
(a) Motility detection (b) Gelatin liquefaction test (c) a+b (d) None of above
2) **Medium for growth of anaerobic bacteria is**
(a) Smith Noguchi medium (b) LJ medium (c) Blood agar (d) Nutrient agar

Answers of MCQs & explanation

1) **(a)**
- Stab culture method is useful for motility detection & gelatin liquefaction test

2) **(a)**
- Follow section anaerobic culture methods (by using reducing agents in anaerobic media) for more explanation
- LJ medium is selective medium for M tuberculosis
- Blood agar is enriched & nutrient agar is simple (basal) medium

10 Laboratory diagnosis of bacterial infections

Learning heading & subheadings

Steps:

- Sample collection
- Transportation & storage
- Sample rejection criteria
- Pre-treatment of sample
- Testing methods
- Reference centres
- Summary of diagnosis

Steps: Following are the different steps employed for diagnosis of bacterial infections

◊ **Sample collection:**
◊ **Transportation & storage:**
◊ **Sample rejection criteria:**
◊ **Pre-treatment of samples:**
◊ **Testing methods:**

Sample collection

❖ **Precautions:** Following are the precautions to be taken before collecting the sample

- Collect the sample before administration of antimicrobial therapy.
- Take all the aseptic precautions
- Wearing the PPEs (Personal Protective Equipments) like disposable gloves, eye shields, apron, cap, mask & shoes cover.
- Selection of proper site.
- Collect at right time.
- Collect sufficient amount.
- Use disposable needle & syringe.
- Container should be sterile, leak proof & securely fastened.
- Collect two swabs one for direct smear & other for culture.
- For culture obtain material during acute stage of illness.
- Paired serum samples for serological tests one in acute stage & second 7-14 days later.
- Use appropriate transport medium whenever necessary.
- Filling the request form with complete data.
- If spillage of sample then wipe it with 10% sodium hypochlorite.
- Proper waste disposal of hazardous material.

❖ **Methods of collection:** All methods for collections of different samples are described in **table-1.**

Transportation & storage

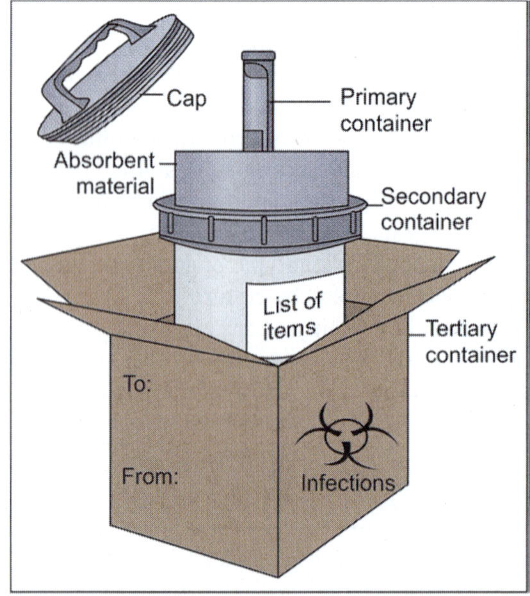

Figure-1: Triple layer packing

❖ **Transportation:** Transport the samples with **triple layer packing (fig.-1)** with biohazard symbol to the laboratory in desired time as described below.

- **Primary (inner) container:** It include container like test tubes, petri dishes, bottles, vials, etc. After putting specimen in the container, it should be capped tightly to prevent any leakage & labelled with patient details.
- **Secondary (middle) container:**
  - Secondary container can be rigid (with screw cap) or flexible (zip lock polythene bag).
  - Wrap the primary container by absorbent material & put in secondary container.
  - Do not put the requisition form in secondary container.
  - Enlist the secondary container at outside with all the samples it contains.
  - Many persons insist biohazard symbol on secondary container also.
- **Tertiary (outer) container:**
  - Outer container is leak proof & strong enough to withstand usual shocks, loadings and accidents during transportation like vaccine carrier.
  - Put the secondary container (contains primary container surrounded by absorbent material) in tertiary container.
  - Put the requisition form & other papers in tertiary container (outside the secondary container).
  - Label the tertiary container with name of sender, consignee & bio hazard symbol.

System	Specimen	Collection	Container	Transportation	Storage
Abscess, ulcer wound, pustules,	- Discharge - Tissue	- Small amount by nylon or dacron swab & large amount in syringe - Pick by forceps/biopsy	- Stuart's or Amies medium or anaerobic medium like RCMM - Sterile container	Within 24 hours room temp.	At room temperature
Blood system	Blood	By venepuncture	Glucose broth, BHIB, thioglycolate broth etc.	Within 2 hours at room temperature	Incubated at 37°C than subculture
CNS	CSF	Lumbar puncture	Sterile screw cap tube	At room temperature	at 37°C
GIT	Gastric aspirate	By Ryles tube	Sterile screw cap tube	Immediately at room temperature	Neutralised with $NaHCO_3$ within 1hr of collection
	Gastric Biopsy	By endoscopy	Sterile screw cap tube	Immediately 4°C	Must be set up immediately
	Rectal Swab	By swab	Transport medium (glycerol saline)	Within 24 hrs at 4°C	72 hrs at 4°C
	Stool culture	Manually	Clean, leak proof container. Transfer faeces in enteric transport medium if delay >1 hr.	Within 24 hrs at 4°C	72 hrs at 4°C
Genital tract	Discharge	Cervical, Vaginal or Urethral swab on Nylon/Dacron swab	Swab moistened with stuart's or Amies medium	Within 24 hours at room temperature	24 hours at room temperature
Respiratory system	Sputum	By coughing	Sterile screw top container	Within 24 hours at room temp.	24 hrs at 4°C.
	Throat or nasopharyngeal materials	Nylon/Dacron swab	Swab moistened with stuart's or Amies medium	Within 24 hours at room temperature.	24 hours at 4°C.
Urinary system	Urine	Midstream, catheter or suprapubic aspiration	Sterile, screw cap container	Within 2 hours/at 04°C.	24 hours at 04°C.
Ear/Eye	Conjunctiva/corneal discharge or scraping	By swab/ blade/ forceps	Aerobic swab moistened with Stuart's or Amies medium.	Beside inoculation , in 24 hours/room temperature	At room temperature
Nosocomial infection	IV catheters, ET tube, prosthetic valves etc.	With minimum air exposure	Sterile, screw cap Container	Immediately at room temp.	Plate as soon as received.
Others	Body fluids (amniotic, abdominal, ascitic, bile, joint / synovial, peritoneal, pericardial)		Sterile, screw cap, leak proof container	Immediately at room temp.	Glucose broth & urgent plating

Table-1: Sample collection (with containers), transport & storage

❖ **Storage:** If there is delay in transport of sample then it should be stored as mentioned in **table-1.**

Sample rejection criteria

❖ **Sample rejection criteria:** Sample should be rejected or disallowed for testing if anyone from following is noticed

- Unsterile container
- Leakage or breakage of container
- Patient's details on specimen are not match with request form
- Unlabeled specimen
- Dry swab
- Saliva mixed with sputum
- Sample mixed with disinfectant
- Contaminated by other materials

Pre-treatment of sample

➢ **CSF & urine:** Centrifuged at 1st & use sediment for testing.

➢ **Sputum:** It required digestion & decontamination, especially in case of tuberculosis.

Testing methods

Following are the different testing methods from **I - XI**

I. Microscopy & staining

A. Light microscopy:

i. Wet mount: Useful for identification of capsule (Indian ink mount), motility (hanging drop preparation) etc.

ii. Fixed smear & staining:

a. Differential stain:

1. **Gram staining:** To identify gram positive or gram negative nature, size, shape, arrangement, capsule, spore & other morphological features of bacteria.
2. **ZN stain:** For acid fast organism

b. Special staining for flagella:
c. Special staining for polar bodies:
d. Special staining for spores:
e. Special staining for fat globules:
} Follow chapter → Morphology of bacteria

f. Special staining for spirochetes: Silver impregnation stain like Fontana stain for culture and Levaditi stain for tissue section

g. Histopathological stain: Like Giemsa stain, Castaneda stains , Gimenez & Machiavello stain for *Rickettsia* & other bacteria which are poorly stain by gram stain.

B. DGIM:
C. PCM:
} For thin structure like flagella, spirochetes

D. EM: For detail study of bacteria

E. Fluorescent Microscopy (FM):

i. Fluorochrome staining:

a. Acridine orange:

- **Staining properties:** It stain the nucleic acid of gram positive & gram negative bacteria
- **Advantage:** Also stain cell wall deficient bacteria
- **Disadvantages:**
  - It also stain the nuclei of host cell
  - It does not differentiate between gram positive & gram negative bacteria

b. Auramine-o & Rhodamine-B: For *M. tuberculosis*

c. Calcofluor white stain: For fungus

ii. Immunofluorescent staining: Detection of antigens or antibodies by using a dye like FITC (Fluorescin Iso Thio Cyanate)

II. Culture

A. In artificial prepared (cell free) media: Three steps & four types of media.

i. Inoculation: Also **called culture methods** or **isolation methods of bacteria**

a. Liquid media: By using Pasteur pipette / syringe.

b. Semi-solid media: By using nichrome wire.

c. Solid media: By using nichrome loop/wire/swab.

d. Biphasic media: By tilting the bottle.

ii. Incubation:

- Temperature: Normally 37^{0}C for all bacteria
- Aerobic incubation:
- Anaerobic incubation: By using method of anaerobiosis
- Other type of incubation: 5-10% CO_2 for capnophilic bacteria & 5% O_2, +10% CO_2 + 85% nitrogen for *C. jejuni* & *H. pylori*

iii. Identification of growth:

a. Liquid media:

✪ **Growth properties:** Like

- **Pellicle** formation (aerobic bacteria)
- **Deposit at bottom** (anaerobic bacteria)
- **Uniform turbidity** (Facultative aerobes
- **Colour**
  - Pink by *Cl. perfringens* due to saccharolytic properties in RCMM
  - Black by *Cl. tetani* due to proteolytic properties in RCMM
- **Odour:** Foul smell by *Cl. tetani* due to proteolytic properties in RCMM

✪ **Disadvantage:** No pure growth

b. Semi-solid media: Motility detected by fine lines around the streaking line.

c. Solid media:

✪ **Cultural characteristics (C/Cs):** Size shape, elevation, margins, surface, edge, colour or pigment production, haemolysis, consistency, emulsification etc.

- **Advantage:** Gives pure growth

d. **Biphasic media:**

- **Growth properties:** Growth is examined over solid phase
- **Advantage:** Less chances of contamination & less labour intensive

B. **Automated culture method:**

1. **BACTEC system:**
- **Principle:** ^{14}C labelled palmitic acid is converted in to^{14} CO_2 by bacterial metabolism. $^{14}CO_2$ index is measured for interpretation of result

2. **MGIT** (Mycobacteria Growth Indicator Tube):
- **Principle:** *Mycobacteria* utilise the O_2 within the tube & growth is detected by O_2 quenched fluorescent dyes

3. **MB/ BacT system** (as like BacT/Alert):
- **Principle:** Based on colorimetric detection of CO_2

4. **ESP** (Extra Sensing Power) **culture system- II:**
- **Principle:** Detection of pressure change in a headspace of sealed culture bottle

C. **Egg culture:** Inoculation in yolk sac or CAM (Chorio Allantoic Membrane).

D. **Animal culture:** Laboratory animals used for bacterial cultivation are guinea pig, rabbit, rat, nine banded armadillo, mouse etc.

III. Biochemical reactions

A. **Sugar fermentation:** →Fig.-2

- **Commonly used sugars:** Are glucose, sucrose, lactose & mannitol abbreviated as GSLM respectively.
- **Other rarely used sugars:** Maltose, rhamnose etc.
- **Medium:** Peptone Water (PW) + 1% sugar + Andrade's indicator (NaOH & acid fuchsin) + Durham's tube
- **Principle:** Bacteria ferment sugar with production of only acid (A) or acid with gas (AG). pH (Andrade's) indicator converted in to pink colour at acidic pH & gas collected in Durham's tube.
- **Method:** Inoculate a loopful culture suspension in medium & incubate at 37^{0}C for 24 hrs. Examine for result after 24 hours.

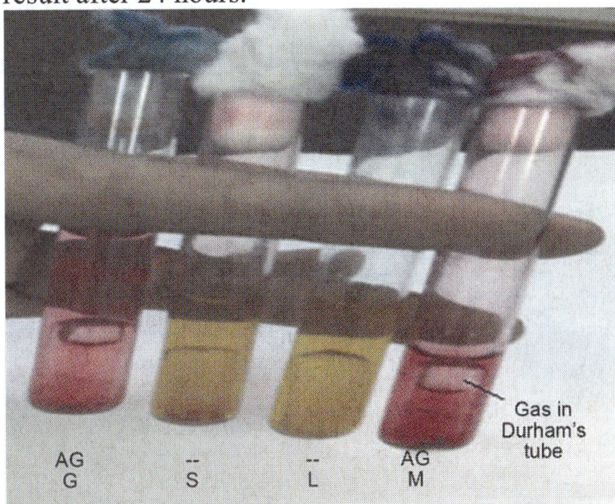

Figure-2: Sugar fermentation test

- **Result:**
  - **+Ve result:**
    - Only acid (A) production: Pink colour medium
    - Acid with gas (AG) production: Pink colour medium & gas collected in Durham's tube in form of bubbles.
  - **-Ve result:** No colour change of medium

B. **IMViC test:** Indole test, Methyle Red (MR) test, Voges-Proskauer (VP/Vi) test & Citrate test are in short **called IMViC test** & described in details in **table-2**.

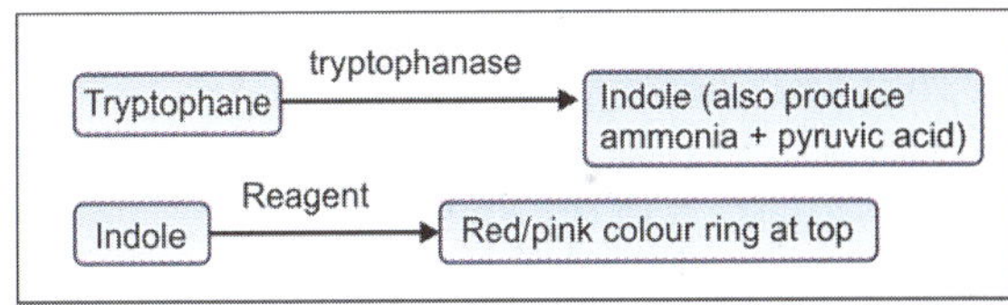

Flow chart-1: Principle of indole test

Particulars	Indole test	MR test	VP test	Citrate test
Principle	Indole produces from the degradation of tryptophan by enzyme tryptophanase (**flow chart-1**). When indole mixes with reagent it gives red colour ring at top due to reaction of indole with aldehydes group of PDAB.	Production of pyruvic acid from glucose by glycolysis (**EM-pathway**) which further metabolise to produce lactic acid, acetic acid & formic acid (**mixed acid pathway**). MR is a pH indicator which is yellow at pH 6.0 & red at acidic pH (pH=4.4) as shown in **flow chat-2.**	Production of pyruvic acid from glucose by glycolysis (**EM-pathway**) which further metabolise by mixed acid pathway to produce lactic acid, acetic acid & formic acid (**mixed acid pathway**). Sometimes instead of mixed acid pathway it pass by acetoin pathway (**butylene glycol pathway**) to produce acetoin (also **called AMC = Acetyl Methyl Carbinol**). Acetoin oxidized by KOH & environmental O_2 to produce diacetyl which gives red colour on contact with α-naphthol (**flow chat-2**).	- Citrate is salt of citric acid produced during Kreb's cycle in the form of citric acid. - Citrate is utilized by many bacteria as source of carbon to produce NH_3 which increase the pH of medium up to 7.6. - Bromothymol blue is a pH indicator which is green initially converted in blue colour at high pH & gives positive test.
Medium	PW rich in tryptophan.	Glucose	Same as MR test.	Citrate as sole source of

		Phosphate Broth (GPB) contains glucose, phosphate & peptone also **called MR broth or VP broth.**		energy. Bromothymol blue is pH indicator mixed in medium. Two types of media as follows **a. Solid medium: Called Simmon's citrate agar** which is available in test tube in slant form **b. Liquid medium: Called Koser's citrate broth**
Reagents	**a. Kovac's reagent:** - PDAB: 10g - Amyl/iso amyl alcohol: 150 ml - Concentrated HCL: 50 ml **b. Ehrlich's reagent:** - PDAB: 2g - Absolute ethyl alcohol: 190 ml - Concentrated HCL: 40 ml	MR reagent (pH indicator).	Contain 40% KOH + α-naphthol.	-
Control - + Ve control - – Ve control	 - *E. coli* - *K. pneumoniae*	 - *E. coli* - *E. aerogenes*	 - *Enterobacter aerogenes* - *E. coli*	 - *Enterobacter aerogenes* - *E. coli*
Methods	**a. Test tube method:** - Inoculate a loopful culture suspension in medium & incubate at 37^{0}C for 24 hrs. - After 24 hrs remove medium & add the reagent. - Examine for the result. **b. Filter paper strip method impregnated with PDAB** **c. In clinical practise Indole test is used in combination with other tests:** Like **1. SIM (Sulphide Indole Motility) test:** More sensitive than TSI for H_2S detection in *S. typhi* **2. MIO (Motile Indole Ornithine) test:** **3. IN (Indole Nitrate / Indoso Nitrate) test:** For *V. cholerae*	- Inoculate a loopful culture suspension in medium & incubate at 37^{0}C in incubator for 24 hrs. - After 24 hrs remove medium from incubator& add the reagent. - Examine for the result.	- Inoculate a loopful culture suspension in medium & incubate at 37^{0}C for 24 hrs. - After 24 hrs remove medium & add the reagent. - Examine for the result.	- Pick the colony from primary culture by nichrome loop/wire & inoculate the medium. - Incubate at 37^{0}C for 24 hrs & read the result.
Result (fig.-3) - +Ve test - -Ve test	 - Red/pink colour ring at top of medium - No colour change	 - Red/pink colour (Mostly upper half) in medium - No colour change	 - Red/pink colour in whole medium - No colour change	**Solid [fig.-3(d)] medium** - Blue colour in medium due to alkaline pH, also consider positive with growth without blue colour. - No change or original green colour of medium **Liquid medium** - Turbidity production - No change
Uses	To identify the indole positive bacteria like *E. coli. V. cholerae, P. vulgaris, E. tarda, Cl. tetani* etc.	To identify MR positive bacteria like *E. coli. S. typhi, Staph. aureus, Cl. welchii* etc.	To identify VP positive bacteria like *Staph. aureus, Enterobacter aerogenes, K. pneumoniae, Hafnia* spp., *Serratia marcescens* etc.	To identify the citrate positive bacteria like *Enterobacter aerogenes, Staph. aureus, S. typhi, K. pneumoniae, Hafnia* spp., *Serratia marcescens* etc.

Table-2: IMViC test

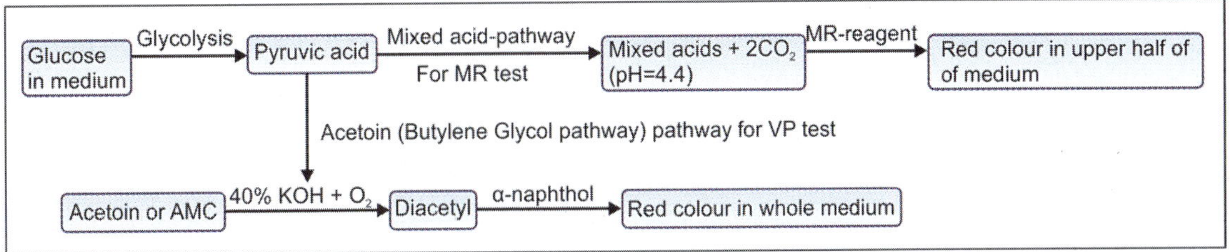

Flow chart -2: Principle of MR & VP test

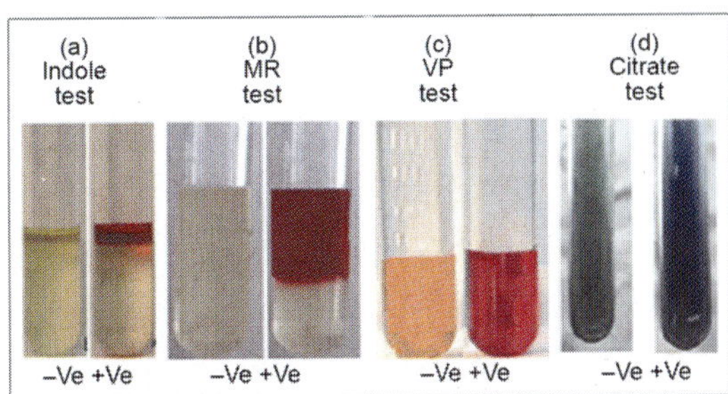

Figure-3: IMViC test

C. Oxidase test:

✪ **Principle:**

- Cytochrome oxidase enzyme present in aerobic bacteria. It takes part in aerobic respiration (Oxidation) by transferring electron (H_2) to O_2 to form H_2O.
- Cytochrome oxidase act as substitute (artificial electron acceptor) for O_2 & oxidise the dye (artificial electron donor) in purple/ violet colour

✪ **Reagent:**

- Name: Tetra methyl Para phenyl Di amine Hydro chloride.
- Colour variation: It is colourless in reduced state & purple/violet colour in oxidised state.

✪ **Control:**

- **+ Ve control:** *P. aeruginosa*
- **- Ve control:** *E. coli*

✪ **Methods:** Two type of methods

a. **Direct method / petri dish method:** 2-3 drops of reagent apply directly on colonies in petri dish.

b. **Indirect method / Kovac's method / filter paper strip method:**

- Take clean-sterile slide & add few drops of sterile saline
- Emulsify the reagent in saline
- Take a piece of filter paper & put over reagent containing slide (filter paper suck the reagent)
- Add colony over reagent containing filter paper
- Examine for the result.

✪ **Result: → Fig.-4(a)**

- **+Ve test:** Purple color development in 10 seconds
- **- Ve test:** No colour change
- **False +Ve:** Use of nichrome loop or wire may also give false +Ve reaction

✓ **Note: Kovac's reagent** → Used in indole test

✪ **Uses:**

- To identify oxidase positive bacteria (mostly belong to strict aerobic, facultative anaerobes & microaerophilic category) like
  - *Micrococci*
  - *Neisseria meningitidis*
  - *Moraxella lacunata*
  - *Acinetobacter baumanii*
  - *V. cholera*
  - *P. aeruginosa*
  - *Bordetella pertusis*
  - *Brucella abortus*
  - *Alkaligenes faecalis*

  } Strict aerobic

  - *Neisseria gonorrhea*
  - *H. influenzae*
  - *Pasteurella multocida*

  } Facultative anaerobes

  - *Campylobacter jejuni*
  - *Helicobacter pylori*

  } Microaerophilic

  - *Flavobacter meningosepticum*
  - *Moraxella catarrhalis*
- To differentiate from oxidase negative bacteria like *Enterobactariceae* family & anaerobic bacteria

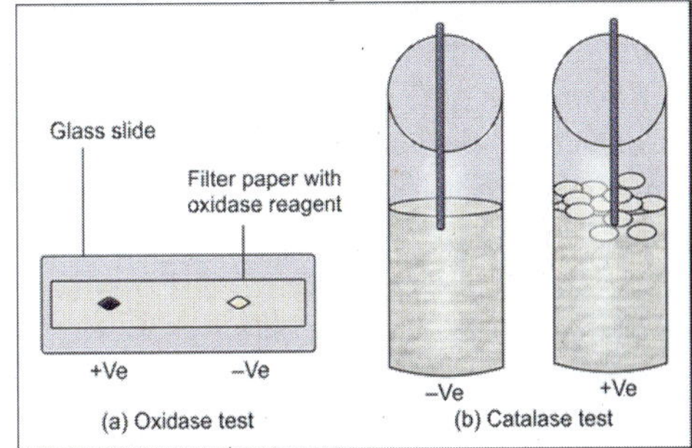

Figure-4: (a) Oxidase test (b) Catalase test

D. Catalase test:

✪ **Principle:** $2H_2O_2 \xrightarrow{Catalase} 2H_2O + O_2$ (produce bubbles)

✪ **Reagent:** 3% H_2O_2

✪ **Control:**

- **+ Ve control:** *Staph. aureus*.
- **- Ve control:** *Streptococcus pyogenes*.

✪ **Method:** Pick up the colony by using wooden stick and apply in 3% H_2O_2 solution either on slide or in tube. Examine for result.

✪ **Result: → Fig.- 4(b)**

- **+Ve test:** Produce bubbles. Few bacteria posses enzymes which can degrade the H_2O_2 & produce bubbles after 20-30 seconds but it is not consider as significant

- **-Ve test:** No bubbles
- **False +Ve:** False + Ve result can occur when it performed from blood agar, because RBCs contain catalase enzymes.

✪ **Uses:** To differentiate catalase positive & catalase negative bacteria from related families

- **Catalase –Ve bacteria:** O2 is the end product of catalase & anaerobes can't tolerate the O_2, so all *anaerobes like Clostridium, Actinomyces, Gardnerella vaginalis* & non-sporing anaerobes are catalase negative. However it's not absolute because some other members of different families like Streptococcaceae *(Streptococcus pyogenes) & Erysipelothrix rhusiopathiae* are also catalase negative
- **Catalase +Ve bacteria:** Catalase +Ve families/bacteria are
  - Micrococcaceae family bacteria like *Staph. aureus*
  - Neisseriae family like *N. meningitidis & N. gonorrhoea*
  - Moraxellaceae family ike *Moraxella catarrhalis & M. lcunata*
  - Mimeae like *Acenatobacter* spp.
  - *Corynebacterium diphtheriae*
  - Bacillaceae like *B. anthracis*
  - Non Tuberculous *Mycobacteria* (NTM) like *M. kansasi* & *M. xenopi* at 680C
  - *Listeria monocytogenes*
  - Actinomycetaceae like *Nocardia* spp.
  - Enterobactariceae family bacteria like *E. coli, K. pneumoniae, S. typhi, P. vulgaris, Shigella* except *Sh. dysenteriae* type I etc.
  - Vibrionaceae, *Aeromonas* and *Plesiomonas*
  - Campylobacterales like *C. jejuni*
  - Nonfermenters like *P. aeruginosa*
  - Pasteurellales like *H. influenza & P .multocida*
  - *Bordetella* spp.
  - *Brucella* spp.
  - Miscellaneous GNB *Francisella tularensis, Chromobacterium violaceum, Capnicytophaga canimorsu & L pneumophila*

E. Urease test:

✪ **Principle:** Urea is converted by enzyme urease in to NH_3 which increase the pH of medium >8.1. Phenol red (pH indicator) is converted from colourless (at pH<8.1) form to red/pink colour (at pH>8.1)

$$\text{Urea} \xrightarrow{\text{Ureaease}} NH_3 \xrightarrow{\text{Phenol red}} \text{red / pink colour}$$

(Alkaline pH)

✪ **Medium:** Urea & phenol red (pH indicator) are mixed in medium.

a. Solid medium:

- **Called Christensen's urea agar**
- Available in test tube in slant form: →**Fig.-4(a)**

b. Liquid medium: Called Stuart's urea broth [fig.-4(b)].

✪ **Control:**

- **+ Ve control:** *Proteus* spp.
- **– Ve control:** *E. coli*

✪ **Method:**

- Pick the colony from primary culture by nichrome loop/wire & inoculate the medium
- Incubate at 37^{0}C for 4 hrs & than after 24 hrs.

✪ **Result: →Fig.-5**

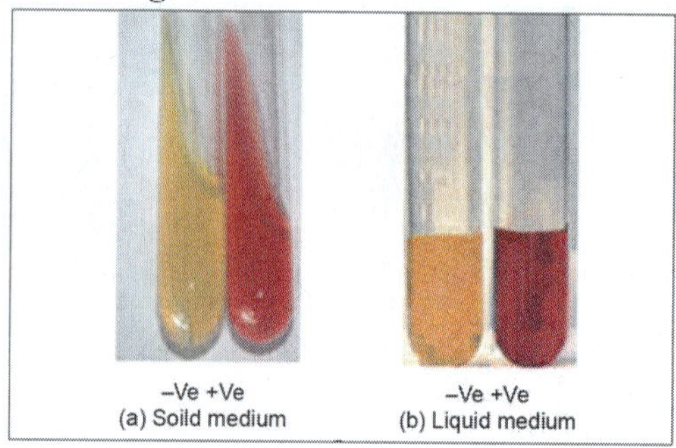

Figure-5: Urease test

- **+Ve test:** Red/pink colour in whole medium due to alkaline pH
- **-Ve test:** No change in original yellow colour of medium

✪ **Uses:** To identify the urease positive bacteria & fungi like

- ***K**lebsiella pneumoniae* **(slow urea splitters)**
- ***R**hodotorula mucinaginosa* **(fungus)**
- **E**nvironmental (Non-Tuberculous / Atypical) *Mycobacteria* like *M marinum & M. scrofulaceum*
- ***T**richophyton mentagrophytes* **(fungus)**
- ***Y**ersinia enterocolitica, Y. pseudotuberculosis*
- ***S**taph. aureus* **(slow urea splitters)**
- ***P**roteae family bacteria like Proteus, Providencia & Morgnella* **(slow urea splitters)**
- ***U**reaplasma urealyticum*
- ***N**ocardia asteroides, N. brasiliensis & N. caviae*
- ***C**ryptococcus neoformans* **(fungus)**
- ***H**elobacter pylori* **(rapid urea splitter):** Urease produced by *H pylori* is 100 times more active than produced by *Pr vulgaris.* Maximum (rapid) urease positive given by *H pylori*
- **S**ome strain of *V. parahaemolyticus*
- ***T**richosporon beigelii* **(fungus)**
- ***B**rucella abortus*
- ***C**orynebacterium* spp. *like C. ulcerans, C. psudodiphthericum & C. pseudotuberculosis*

> **Mnemonic:**
> **Urease +Ve bacteria & fungi: KRETY'S PUNCH**
> **S**top **T**he **B**us & **C**ar

F. Biochemical test by using composite media

➢ **Definition of composite media:**

- Media which define the multiple properties of a bacterium **called composite media.**
- Normally separate medium is required to define every property of bacterium, but composite media are defines many properties.
- Their use is increased now days for identification of bacteria.

➢ **Examples:**

i. TSI test:

✪ **Full form:** Triple Sugar Iron test, because contains three sugars (glucose, sucrose & lactose) & iron.

✪ **Advantages:**

- **Economical**
  - Most convenient & economical test
  - It is the most commonly used composite medium
- **It define many properties of bacterium:** Like
  - Fermentation of glucose
  - Fermentation of lactose
  - Fermentation of sucrose
  - Gas production
  - H_2S production

✪ **Disadvantage:** It cannot differentiate between lactose fermenter & sucrose fermenter, which is overcome by using KIA test

✪ **Principle:** Slant portion is constantly exposed to air, is aerobic & butt (deep) portion relatively less exposed to air, is anaerobic. **Four types of reaction occur as follows**

a. Non-fermenter: Non fermenter is not able to utilize the carbohydrates, so it utilize the peptone & produces NH3, which gives alkaline pH (red colour) of medium.

b. Glucose fermenter but Non-Lactose /Sucrose Fermenter (NLF or NSF): Utilize the glucose to produce acid (acidic (A) pH→yellow colour) but when glucose is exhausted it utilize peptones to produce NH3 (alkaline (K) pH →red colour).

c. Fermenter: Ferment all sugars to produce large amount of acid (acidic pH→yellow colour) in slant & butt. Sometimes gas produced which present as bubbles in bottom or in between the medium.

d. Glucose fermenter with H_2S production: Utilise the glucose to produce acid (acidic pH → yellow colour) but when glucose is exhausted it utilize peptones to produce NH3 (alkaline pH → red colour). Acid is required for H_2S production and due to presence of acid some bacteria utilize sodium thiosulfate to produce H_2S which react with ferrous sulfate & convert it in to ferrous sulfide to gives black colour.

✪ **Medium: Called TSI agar**

- **Parts of medium:** Two parts like slant & butt (but also **called deep**)
- **Ingredients:**
  - Three sugar:
    - G (0.1%), L (1%) & S (1%)
    - **G to L/S ratio 1:10)**
  - Four protein derivatives: Beef extract, yeast extract, peptone, proteose peptone
  - pH indicator: Phenol red (yellow at acidic pH & red/pink at alkaline pH)
  - Sodium thiosulfate: Source of sulfur atoms for H_2S production
  - Ferrous sulfate: As H_2S detector which gives black colour on combination with H_2S if produced
  - Agar: 2%
  - pH: 7.2

✪ **Sterilisation method:** Autoclave

✪ **Method:**

- Pick the colony from primary culture by nichrome wire & inoculate the medium up to the butt (deep) & than streaking over the slant.
- Incubate at 37^{0}C for 24 hrs & than examine for result

✪ **Result:**

- **End product of test are:**
  - Acid (A): Yellow colour
  - Alkaline (K): Red or pink colour
  - Gas (G): Bubbles
  - H_2S : Black colour
- **Types of result:** Four types

a. Non-Fermenter (NF) or no reaction:

- Red slant/red butt: K/K or K/Nil [→**fig.-6(a)]**
- Organisms: *Pseudomonas aeruginosa*

b. Glucose fermenter but (Non-Lactose / Sucrose Fermenter (NLF/NSF):

- Red slant/yellow butt: K/A [→**fig.-6(b)]**
- Organisms: *Shigella dysenteriae*

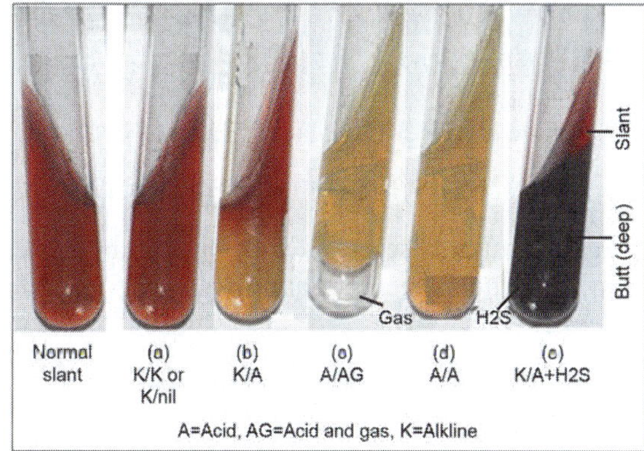

Figure-6: TSI test

c. Fermenter:

- Yellow slant & yellow butt with or without gas: A/AG [→**fig.-6(c)]** or A/A **[fig.-6(d)]**
- Organisms: Coliform bacilli like *E. coli, K. pneumonia* etc.

d. Glucose fermenter with H_2S production:

- Red slant/black butt: K/A+ H_2S [→**fig.-6(e)]**
- Organisms: These are glucose fermenter, but non lactose/ sucrose fermenter & H_2S producing bacteria like *Salmonella typhi, Proteus* spp., *Citrobacter frundi* etc.

- Acid is required for H_2S production & H_2S is present where acid is present, so yellow colour of acid is mask by black colour of H_2S, but it read as acid (yellow colour).

✪ **Uses:** To determine the carbohydrate fermenting & H_2S producing bacteria as above

ii. KIA test:

- **Full form:** Kligler Iron Agar test
- **Medium:** Similar medium to TSI but contains only glucose & lactose.
- **Uses:** Used to differentiate *Y. enterocolitica* (A/A in TSI, K/A in KIA) from *E. coli* (A/A in both), so by some microbiologist, KIA is preferred over TSI for faecal samples.

iii. Bile esculin agar:

- **Uses:**
- Used to differentiate *Enterococcous* (group D) group of *Streptococcus* from non enterococcus (*Strept mitis,* not group D) group
- Also used to know the growth of bacterium in presence of 40% bile, ability to hydrolyse the esculin to esculetin & glucose. Esculetin combine with ferric citrate to form dark brown or black colonies.

G. Other biochemical tests:

1. Nitrate reduction
2. Phenyl Pyruvic Acid (PPA) test
3. Aminoacid (lysine, arginine & ornithine) decarbo-xylation test
4. Coagulase test: } Follow chapter → Micrococcaceae
5. Phosphatase test:
6. Hugh-Leifson's (Oxidation –Fermentation / OF) test
7. Bile solubility test: Follow chapter →Pneumococcus
8. O-Nitro Phenyl- β-D-Galactosidase (ONPG) test

IV. Serological tests

Agglutination based tests, precipitation based tests, Toxin-antitoxin neutralisation tests, ELISA, Radio Immuno Assay(RIA) etc.

IV. Allergic (skin) tests

Tuberculin tests, Frei's test etc.

V. Molecular methods

PCR, Ligase Chain Reaction (LCR), Nucleic Acid Sequence Based Amplification (NASBA), Line Probe Assay (LPA) etc.

VI. Physiological methods

Gas Liquid Chromatography (GLC) & High Performance Liquid Chromatography (HPLC)

VII. Test to detect metabolic activities

1. Detection of tuberculo-stearic acid & Adenosine deaminase in *M. tuberculosis.*
2. Pigment production by *Staphylococcus* spp., *Pseudomonas aeruginosa* & other bacteria

VIII. Microbial typing

A Phenotyping methods:

i. Bacteriophage typing:

✪ **Synonym:** Phage typing

✪ **Principle:** It based on the susceptibility of bacterium to bacteriophage.

✪ **Typing method:** Method **called pattern method**

- **Steps:**
- Bacterium to be typed is inoculated in agar plate (Lawn culture), followed by application of phage in fixed dose
- Incubate the plate overnight at 37^0C
- **Result:**
- Result is lyses of bacteria by phage & produce clear zone **called plaque (fig.-7).**
- Bacterial typing will be done on the basis of size, shape & nature of plaque

✪ **Properties:**

- Genus specific: Affect all the genus of bacterium: like in *Salmonella*
- Species specific: Affect all the species of genus: like in *B. anthracis*
- Biotype or subspecies specific: Affect all the strain of subspecies: like Mukharjee phage –IV which lyses all strain of Classical Vibrio but not El Tor.

✪ **Uses:** For identification & epidemiological typing of bacteria which are difficult to distinguish by biochemical & serological methods. It is useful for following bacteria.

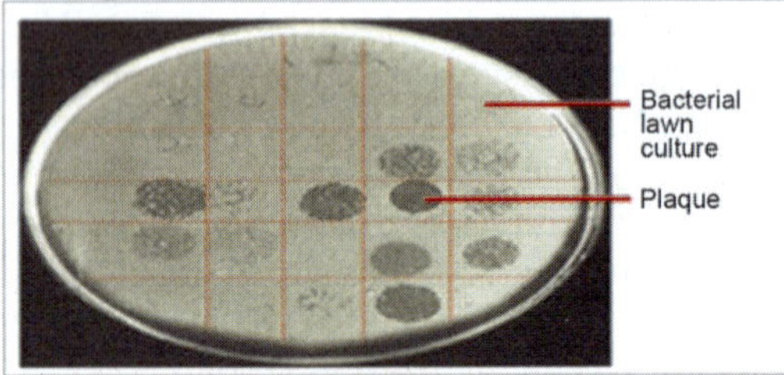

Figure-7: Phage typing

a. *Staph aureus:*

Lytic group of the phages	Designation of phages
Group I	29, 52, 52A, 79, 80
Group II	3A, 3C, 55, 71
Group III	6, 42E, 47, 53, 54, 75, 77, 83A, 84, 85
Group V	94, 96
Unclassified	81, 95

Table-3: Phage typing of *Staph aureus*

- If strain of *Staph aureus* is lysed by phages 52, 79 & 80 it is **called phage type 52/79/80**
- Phage type 80/81 is associated with outbreak in hospital & **called epidemic strain of *Staph aureus***

- International basic set of phages for typing of *Staph aureus* of human origin: → **Table-3**

b. *C. diphtheriae:* Bacteriophage **called corynephage**
- 15 bacteriophage typing identified.
- Type 1 & 3 are **mitis**, type 4 & 6 are **intermedius**, 7 avirulent & remainders virulent are **gravis.**

c. *M. tuberculosis:* Bacteriophage **called mycobacteriophage**
- Viral chromosome instead of being integrated in bacterial chromosome remain free like plasmid **called pseudolysogeny**
- Four types: A, B, C, I (I= Intermediate b/w A & B, common in India)

d. *Salmonella:*

1. **O-Ag variation:** Structural changes in O Ag of *Salmonella* can be induced by bacteriophage (lysogenisation) which results in new serotypes as shown in **flowchart-3**

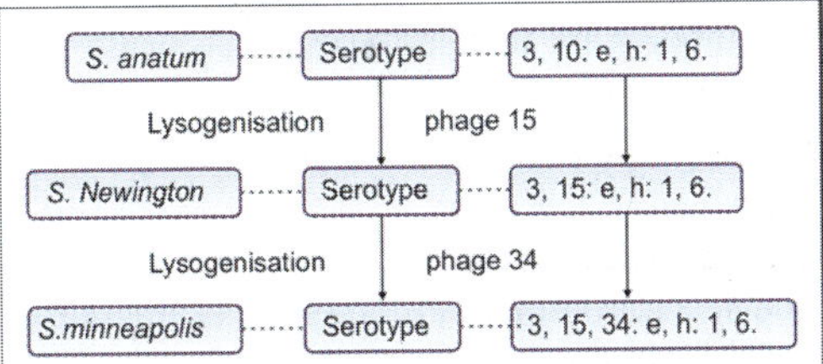

Flow chart-3: O-Ag variation by phage

2. **Vi phage type-II:**
- **Definition:** It act on Vi Ag of typhoid bacilli hence **called Vi phage type II**
- **History:** It was developed by Craigie & Yen in 1937
- **Significance:**
  - Useful for intraspecies classification of *Salmonella*
  - It also provides the information regarding trend & pattern of typhoid at local, national & international levels.
- **Common salmonella phage in India:**
  - *S typhi*: Phage A & phage E1
  - *S paratyphi A:* Type 1 & type 2
- **Limitations:**
  - Strain without Vi Ag are untypable
  - Not able to discriminate between the other species

3. **Nicole's complementary phage typing:** In some region one or more phage is available in such cases typing is done through Nicole's complementary phage like typing of type A strain in to 10 types

e. *Vibrio cholerae:* Bacteriophage **called vibriophage**
- **Significance:**
  - Useful epidemiological studies
  - Also useful to differentiate Classical *Vibrio* from El Tor *Vibrio*.
- **Phage typing:**

1. **Classical *Vibrio* typing:**
   - Classified in to five phage types by using Mukherjee's 4 phages (I-IV)
   - IVth phage lyses the all strains of Classical *Vibrio* but none of the strain of El Tor *Vibrio*
2. **El Tor *Vibrio* typing:**
   - Classified in to six phage types by using Basu & Mukherjee's phage 5
   - Vth phage lyses the all strains of El Tor *Vibrio* but none of the strain of Classical *Vibrio*
3. ***Vibrio cholerae* O1 typing:** Typing is done by Lee & Basu by using 14 phages

f. *Brucells spp.:*

1. **Tblisi (Tb) phage:**
   - Tb phage was isolated in former Soviet Union in 1950.
   - It is designated as reference phage.
   - *B. abortus* lysed at routine test dose (RTD) while *B. suis* lysed at 10, 000 RTD & *B melitensis* not lysed at all
   - Disadvantage: Less applicable because all the strains are not sensitive to Tb phage, so not identify all the strains
2. **Newer phages for typing:**
   - Numbers of newer phages are identified in last decades with wide host range.
   - Corbel defined 6 groups of *Brucella* on the bases of these newer phage in 1987

✪ **Bacteriophage typing centres for different bacteria:** → Follow section reference centres (Vide infra)

g. Other bacteria: Phage typing is done for few other bacteria s mentioned below but less useful.

1. ***P aeruginosa*:** Less useful because less discriminatory power
2. ***Proteus* spp.**
3. ***Anthrax bacilli***

ii. Bacteriocin typing: **Follow chapter → Bacterial growth products**

iii. Bio typing:

✪ **Principle:** It based on different biochemical properties of the organisms.

✪ **Uses:** It is useful for following bacteria

1. *C. diphtheriae:* It classifies the bacterium in to three biotypes like gravis, intermedius & mitis
2. *S. typhi:* Four subgenera from I-IV, are defined on the basis of biochemical properties
3. *Shigella* spp.: Four species on the basis of biochemical & serological properties.
4. *Vibrio cholerae:* It classifies the bacterium in to two biotypes like classical & El Tor
5. *Y. pestis:* It classifies the bacterium in to three biotypes like *Y. pestis var orientalis, Y. pestis var antigua & Y. pestis var medievalis*.
6. *H. influenzae:* It classifies the bacterium in to eight biotypes like from I-VIII.
7. *Brucella* spp.: Several biotypes are defined in *brucella* spp.

- **More details of biotypes of each bacterium:** Follow respective chapters

iv. Sero typing:

- **Principle:** It based on the serological properties of the organisms.
- **Uses:** It is useful for following bacteria

1. *Streptococcus* spp.*:* Lancefield grouping based on Carbohydrate antigen of cell wall
2. *E. coli, Shigell* spp., *Salmonella* spp. & *V. cholerae:* Grouping based on cell wall antigens
3. *Strept pneumoniae, H. influenzae, N. meningitidis:* Grouping based on capsular antigens

v. Antibiogram typing:

- **Principle:** It based on the susceptibility of the organisms to different antibiotics.
- **Uses:** It is done with antibiotic sensitivity testing for many bacteria & gives clue about occurrence of outbreak of resistant strain like
  - MRSA, VISA & VRSA in *Staphylococcus*
  - MDR-TB & XDR-TB in *Mycobacterium*
  - MDR strains in *Pseudomonas* & *Acinetobacter*
  - VRE
  - PPNG

vi. Auxo typing:

- **Principle:** It based on the nutritional requirement of the organisms.
- **Uses:** It is useful for following bacterium

1. *Neisseria gonorrhoea*

vii. Morpho typing:

- **Principle:** It based on the cultural characteristics of the organisms on different media.
- **Uses:** It is useful for following bacterium

1. *P. aeruginosa*

B Genotyping methods: Following are the genotyping methods

1. Plasmid profile analysis
2. RFLP: Restriction Fragment Length Polymorphisms
3. NASBA: Nucleic Acid Sequence Base Amplification
4. Ribotyping
5. PFGE: Pulsed Field Gel Electrophoresis
6. AFLP: Amplified Fragment Length Polymorphism

IX. Antibiotic sensitivity testing

➢ **Synonym:**

- Antibiotic susceptibility testing
- Antibiogram
- Resistogram

➢ **Definition:** Detection of sensitivity of microorganisms against antimicrobial agents (antibiotics) **called antibiotic sensitivity testing.**

➢ **Uses:**

a. Selection of antibiotics: To choose the antibiotics to treat the patient.

b. Diagnosis of organisms: To identify the organism & to differentiate one bacterium form other like

1. **Novobiocin** (5 mg) **sensitivity:** It is sensitive in *Staph aureus* & in *Staph epidermidis* while resistant in *Staph saprophyticus*, which helps in differentiation of these species.
2. **Bacitracin** (0.04 mg) **sensitivity:** It is sensitive in group A & resistant in group B, which helps in differentiation of two β- haemolytic *Streptococci.*
3. **Optochin (Ethyl hydrocuprein, 1/500,000) sensitivity:** Pneumococcus is sensitive to optochin while viridans group is resistant, which helps in differentiation between all these bacteria.

c. Bacterial typing: Called antibiogram typing → Vide supra

➢ **Methods or principles:** Two types of method or principles

i. By using liquid medium: Called dilution method & following are two subtypes

a. Macrodilution method:

- By using liquid media in large quantity
- Performed in test tube

b. Microdilution method:

- By using liquid media in very small quantity
- Performed in microtitre well

ii. By using solid medium: Called disc diffusion method & following are three subtypes

a. Rotary- plate method: Discovered by Pearson-Whitefield, 1974.

b. Comparative disc diffusion method: Discovered by Stokes & Flemington, 1972.

c. Kirby-Bauer method: It is the most commonly used method & described in detail as follows

Kirby-Bauer method

- **Materials required:**

1. **5ml Trypticase Soy Broth (TSB) or any other suitable broth:** To prepare the inoculum or culture suspension of test organisms.
2. **Muller Hinton Agar (MHA) plate:** Appropriately dried with pH= 7.2-7.6 & in 4mm thickness.
3. **0.5 Mac Farland standard inoculum:** To compare the turbidity of broth contains test organisms.
4. **Antibiotic disc:** Contains antibiotics for testing.
5. **Sterile forceps:** To hold the disc.
6. **Scale or calliper:** To measure the size of inhibition zone.

- **Steps:**
  - Inoculate few colonies from primary culture in TSB & incubate at 37^0C for few hrs.
  - Compare the TSB growth with 0.5 Mac Farland standard inoculums (1.5×10^8 cfu/ml).
  - Take the MHA plate & transfer TSB growth in it by swabbing or flooding method.
  - Allow the plate to dry for few minutes.

- Put the antibiotic disc by holding with sterile forceps.
- Incubate at 37^0C for 24 hrs & examine for sensitivity pattern.

✪ **Mechanisms during incubation:**

- During the incubation drug released from disc & diffuse in medium along with the growth of microorganisms.
- At a particular point drug met to bacteria & if bacteria are sensitive then there is a production of zone of inhibition around the disc.
- If bacteria are resistant to drug then they grow up to the margin of disc without producing the zone of inhibition.

✪ **Result (fig.-8):** Measure the size of zone of inhibition by using the scale or calliper.

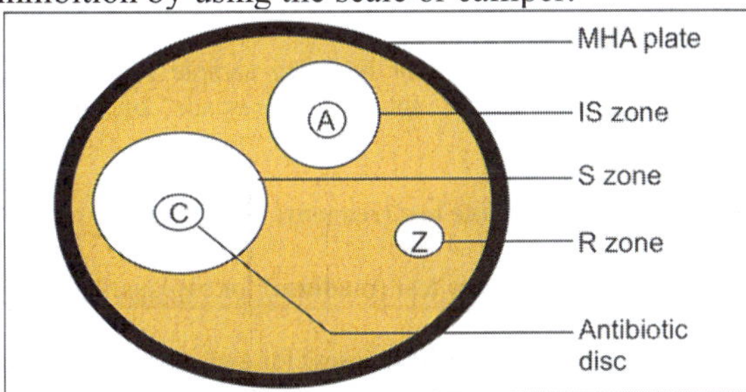

Figure-8: Antibiogram

1. **Sensitive (S) zone:** Organisms are susceptible to drug.
2. **Intermediate Sensitive (IS) zone:** Organisms are moderately susceptible to drug.
3. **Resistance (R) zone:** Organisms are not susceptible or resistant to drug.

Reference centres

Following are the reference centres for further diagnosis of bacteria up to strain or subspecies or type level in India

i. *Staphylococcus aureus*:

a. Bacteriophage typing centre: →Maulana Azad Medical College, New Delhi, India.

ii. *Streptococcus* spp.:

a. Lancefield grouping:

- **Reference laboratories:** →Streptococcal reference laboratories are
1. Lady Harding Medical College, New Delhi, India.
2. Christian Medical College, Vellore, India.
- **Data from reference laboratories:** Data showed that about 45% of haemolytic streptococcal isolates are from group A, 10-15% from group B & C each, 25% from group G while 5% from group F.

iii. *Salmonella typhi:*

a. Bacteriophage typing: National salmonella Vi phage typing centre: →Lady Harding Medical College, New Delhi, India.

b. Serotyping: National salmonella reference centre

1. **Human origin:** →Central Research Institute, Kasauli, India.
2. **Animal origin:** →Indian Veterinary Research Institute, Izzatnagar, India.

iv. *Vibrio cholerae:*

a. Bacteriophage typing: International reference centre for vibriophage → National institute of cholerae and enteric disease (NICED), Kolkata, India.

v. *Brucella:*

a. Biotyping: Central Veterinary Laboratory, New Haw, UK.

vi. *Mycobacteria:*

a. CLTRI

- **Full name:** Central Leprosy Teaching and Research Institute, Chengalpattu, Chennai, Tamil Nadu, India.
- **Aims & objectives:**
  - Research into the basic problems relating to the inception and spread of leprosy.
  - Field studies for controlling leprosy in the community.
  - Training of leprosy workers.
  - To give technical guidance and advice for the promotion of anti leprosy work.
  - Monitoring and evaluation of NLEP and providing technical support to central leprosy division, Govt of India.

b. NJILOMD

- **Full name:** National JALMA Institute for Leprosy & Other Mycobacterial Diseases, Agra, Uttar Pradesh, India.
- **Aims & objectives:** Nodal reference centre in all aspect of leprosy & research work in tuberculosis.

Summary of diagnosis

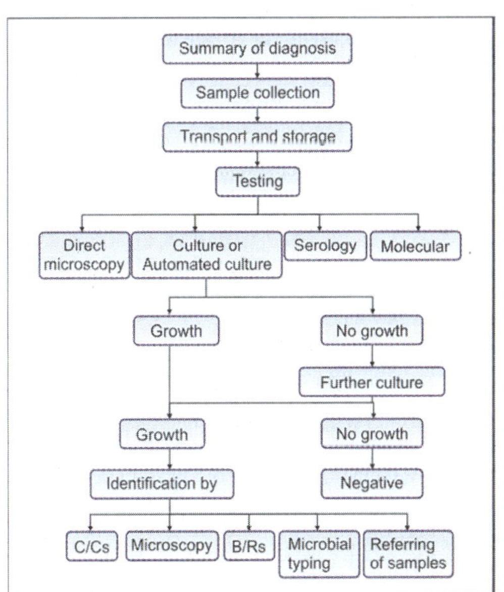

Flow chart-4: Summary of diagnosis

Question bank

Essay/Full question

1) Laboratory diagnosis of bacterial infections

Short notes

1) Triple layer packing of samples
2) IMViC test/ Catalase test / Oxidase test / Urease test/TSI test
3) Composite media
4) Microbial typing
5) Bacteriophage typing
6) Antibiogram

Short questions for theory/viva questions

1) What are composite media? Write two examples
2) Write two uses of antibiogram
3) Name the bacteriophage typing centre for following organisms: *Staph. aureus* & *S. typhi*
4) Name the sugar present in TSI medium & KIA medium
5) Write the principle of MR test & VP test
6) Write the clinical application of Kovac's reagent & Kovac's method.

MCQs for chapter review

Transportation

1) **In triple layer packing, the request form should be put in**
(a) In primary container (b) In secondary container (c) Outer to secondary container (d) In tertiary container

Sample rejection criteria

2) **Specific reason to disallow the sample for culture**
(a) Sample brought within 2 hr of collection (b) Sample brought in sterile plastic container (c) Sample brought in formalin (d) Sample obtained after cleaning the collection site

Testing methods

IMViC test

3) **Reagent(s) used in indole test is/are**
(a) Kovac's reagent (b) Ehrlich's reagent (c) a+b (d) None
4) **Medium (media) useful for citrate test is/are**
(a) Koser's broth (b) Simmon 's agar (c) a+b (d) None

Oxidase test

5) **Oxidase positive bacteria are -**
(a) *Vibrio* (b) *Pseudomonas* (c) *Clostridium* (d) *E coli*

Urease test

6) **Maximum urease positive is produced by-** (PGI, 2000)
(a) *H pylori* (b) *P mirabilis* (c) *K rhinomatis* (d) *Ureaplasma*
7) **Urease negative is -** (AI- 89)
(a) *E coli* (b) *Proteus* (c) *Klebsiella* (d) *Staphylococci*
8) **All of the following bacteria test "Urease positive" except** (AI- 98)
(a) *E coli* (b) *Proteus* (c) *Klebsiella* (d) *Staphylococci*
9) **Medium (media) useful for urease test is/are**
(a) Stuart's broth (b) Christensen 's agar (c) a+b (d) None

Microbial typing

10) **Lysis of bacterial colony in culture is seen bywhich virus**
(a) Pox (b) HSV (c) Bacteriophage (d) CMV
11) **Phage typing is useful as epidemiological tool in all except,**
(a) *Salmonella* (b) *Staph aureus* (c) *V cholerae* (d) *Shigella dysenteriae*
12) **Phage typing can be done for**
(a) *Salmonella* (b) *Streptococcus* (c) *Shigella* (d) *Pseudomonas*
13) **Phage typing is widely used for the intraspecies classification of one of the following bacteria**
(a) *Staphylococci* (b) *E coli* (c) *Klebsiella pneumoniae* (d) *Pseudomonas aeruginosa*

Antibiotic sensitivity testing

14) **Kirby-Bauer method is based on principle of**
(a) Dilution method (b) Disc diffusion method (c) a+b (d) None

Answers of MCQs & explanation

1. **(c) & (d)**
- Primary container contain specimen while secondary container contains primary container surrounded by absorbent. Request form should be put outer to secondary container & inner to tertiary container

2. **(c)**
- Reason for disallowing or rejecting sample for testing (like culture) from given option is presence of disinfectant (formalin)

3. **(c)**
- Follow section, **indole test (reagent)** for explanation

4. **(c)**
- Follow section, **citrate test (medium)** for explanation

5. **(c)**
- Follow section, **oxidase test (uses)** for explanation

6. **(a)**
- Urease produced by *H pylori* is 100 times more active than produced by *Pr vulgaris*. Maximum (rapid) urease positive given by *H pylori*

7. **(a)**
8. **(a)**
9. **(c)**

} Follow section, **urease test (uses)** for explanation

10. **(c)**
11. **(d)**

} Follow section, **microbial typing (bacteriophage typing)** for explanation

12. **(a) & (d)**
13. **(a)**
14. **(c)**
- Follow section, **antibiotic sensitivity testing (Methods or Principles)** for explanation.

11 Normal microbial flora of human body

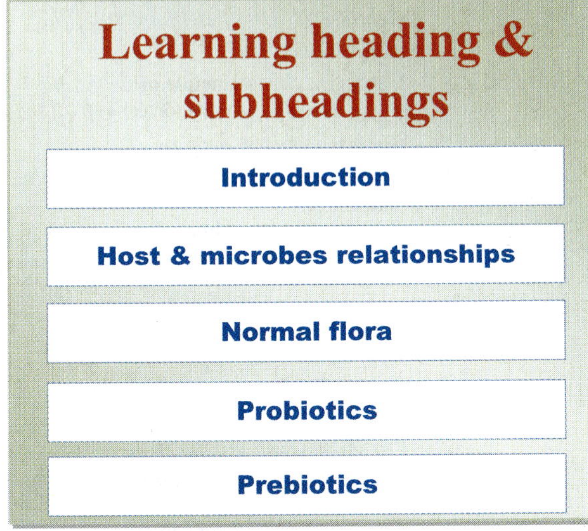

Introduction

According to habitat microbes have following types

a. **Saprophytes:**
- **Meaning:** Sapros (Greek) = decayed + Phyton (Greek) = Plant
- **Definition:** Free living microbes in/on dead or decaying organic matter such as soil & water. Incapable to multiply in living tissues except *B. subtilis*.

b. **Commensals: (Mostly normal flora)**
- **Meaning:** Com (Greek) = with + Mensa (Greek)= table
- **Definition:** Microbes live in complete harmony with the host without causing any damage (living together).

c. **Pathogens:**
- **Meaning:** Pathos (Greek) = suffering + Gen (Greek) = produce.
- **Definition:** Microorganism those are capable of producing disease in the host.

Host & microbes relationships

➢ **Types:** Normal floras are found in association with animals & also in the environment. Three types relationship between the host & microbes as follows.

a. **Symbiosis:**
- **History:** This theory was given by Lynn Margulis & widely accepted
- **Synonym:** Also **called endosymbiosis** or **called mutualism**
- **Definition:** Both are dependent on each other & both are getting benefit from each other without producing any harm to either partner.
- **Example:** Intestinal flora survives in gut produce Vitamins for host.

b. **Commensalism:**
- **Definition:** Association in which one partner getting benefits and other is unharmed.
- **Example:** Flora living on skin

c. **Parasitism:**
- **Definition:** Association in which one partner (Usually smaller **called parasite**) getting benefits with production of injuries to other partner (Usually larger **called host**).
- **Example:** Microbes get benefits at the expense of the host infection

✓ **Predation:**
- Association in which one animal (usually larger like tiger, lion) consume or kill the other (usually smaller like deer, rabbit) for food
- Larger is carnivorous **called predator**
- Smaller is herbivorous **called prey**

Normal flora

❖ **Synonym:** Microbiota, indigenous microbial population, microflora & microbial flora

❖ **Definition:** Mixture of microorganisms regularly found at any anatomical sites on or within the body of a healthy person.

❖ **Advantages:**

1. **Immunostimulation:** Raise the immunity of the body by sharing the common Ag.
2. **Endotoxin:** Liberates the endotoxin which triggers the alternative complement pathway as long as they are not produced in excessive amounts.
3. **Protection from external invaders:**
   - Normal flora occupies body's epithelial surfaces.
   - They prevent or interfere with colonisation or invasion by other bacteria by
     - Blocking receptors (attachment) sites

- Competing for essential nutrients
- Producing anti-bacteria substances like peroxides bacteriocins etc.

4. **Vitamins production:** Some of the intestinal floras like *E. coli* & *Bacteroides* are producing vitamin K, vitamin E & vitamin B in the gut which are available for use by host.
5. **Production of organic acids:** Like butyric acids & acetic acids which contributes in nutrition of host
6. **Digestion:** Intestinal flora degrades mucins, epithelial cells, carbohydrates & other dietary fiber & helps in digestion

❖ Disadvantages:

1. **Source of opportunistic infections**: E.g. In immunodeficient persons
2. **Entry in unusual sites cause infection:** E.g. intestinal flora may cause UTI
3. **Interference with antibiotics:** By producing some enzymes penicillinase which inactivates the penicillin & aggravates the infection
4. **Confusion in diagnosis:** It is difficult to differentiate between normal flora & pathogen by laboratory tests.
5. **Supra-infection:** Follow chapter → Infections and infectious diseases

❖ Types: Two types

I. Transient flora:

➢ **Properties:**

- Present for short (temporary) period not always.
- Includes non-pathogenic & pathogenic groups. Among the pathogenic group some examples are like meningococcus & pneumococcus from nasopharynx.
- In hospital patient may acquire the drug resistance organism as transient flora like MRSA from nose & skin & multi drug resistance gram negative bacteria which includes *E coli*, *Klebsiella*, *Pseudomonas*, *Acinetobacter* etc.
- Transient flora can be easily removed by improving the hygiene & taking infection control measures.

➢ **Transient flora in different organs: → Table-1**

Organ	Flora
Skin	- **Bacteria:** *Staph aureus, Strept pyogenes, Strept viridans, Enterococci, E. coli, Proteus, Klebsiella* - **Fungi:** *Candida spp., M. furfur, Trychophyton*
Eyes	- **Bacteria:** *Staph aureus, Strept pneumoniae, Strept viridans, Bacillus, Priopionibacterium*
Respiratory tract	- **Bacteria:** *Strept pneumoniae, Staph aureus, N. meningitidis, Moraxella*
Oral cavity	- **Bacteria:** *Strept pyogenes, Lactobacilli, N. meningitidis, Moraxella, E. corrodens,* - **Fungi:** *Candida* spp. - **Viruses:** CMV, HSV
GIT	**Stomach** - **Bacteria:** *H pylori, Streptococci, Lactobacilli* **Small intestine** - **Fungi:** *Candida* spp. - **Parasites:** *Entamoeba coli, Endolimax nana, Trichomonas hominis, Blastocystis hominis* **Large intestine** - **Bacteria:** *Corynebacterium, MAC, Pseudomonas* - **Fungi:** *Candida* spp. - **Parasites:** Same as small intestine
Urinary tract	- **Bacteria:** *Enterococci, Mycoplasma, M smegmatism, Bacteroides, Fusobacterium*
Genital tract	- **Bacteria:** *Strept pyogenes, Enterococci* - **Fungi:** *Candida* spp. - **Parasites:** *Trichomonas vaginalis*

Table-1: Transient flora in different organs

II. Resident flora:

➢ **Properties:**

- Constant flora or lifelong members
- Includes non-pathogenic groups which are harmless; infect beneficiary role.

➢ **Resident flora in different organs:** Described below

✪ Resident flora of skin:

- **Background:**

- Human adult has two square meters of skin
- Human skin is constantly attack by organisms present in environment & objects comes in contacts which are loaded with microbes.
- Skin floras are mostly transient in nature.

- **Effective factors:** The populations of normal flora over the skin depend on many factors like

- Differences in pH
- Oxygen
- Water
- Secretions
- Wearing cloths
- Occupation
- Environmental condition

- **List of flora of skin:**

A. Bacteria:

1. *Propionibacterium acne:*

- It is anaerobic *Corynebacterium*
- Children younger than 10 years are rarely colonized with it
- It present in areas rich in sebaceous gland.

2. Diphtheroids: (non-pathogenic *Corynebacterium*)
3. Anaerobic cocci
4. *Staph epidermidis*: Major inhabitant making up more than 90% of the flora
5. *Staph aureus:*

- Nose, perineum, vulval skin

- Occurrence in nasal passages varies with age being greatest in newborns, less in adults
- Penicillin resistant S. aureus present in hospital staff members
- Also present in hair follicles

6. *Micrococcus*
7. α haemolytic *Streptococci*:
8. *Enterococcus* & non entrococcus.
9. GNB like *E. coli, Proteus* spp.etc.
10. Non-pathogenic *Mycobacteria*

B. Fungi:

1. *Candida* spp.
2. *Pityrosporum ovale*
3. *Cryptococcus* spp.

✪ **Resident flora of eyes:**

- Conjunctiva normally free from microbes due to constant flushing action of tears which contains lysozyme.
- Conjunctival flora is scanty & occasionally present.
- Predominant organisms of the conjunctiva are –
  - *Corynebacterium xerosis*
  - *Staphylococci*
  - Non-haemolytic *Streptococci*
  - *Haemophilus* spp.
  - *Moraxella catarrhalis*

✪ **Resident flora of respiratory tract:**

A. Upper respiratory tract: It includes nose, ear, sinuses, pharynx & throat

- **Nose:** It includes the *Staphylococci, Streptococci (Strep. agalactiae), Corynebacteria, Haemophilus, & Moraxella.*
- **Nasopharynx:**

o Background: Often sterile at birth but may be contaminated within 2-3 days after birth by passage through the birth canal & by attendants.

o List of flora:

1. *Strept viridans* is established as the most prominent members of the resident flora & remain so for life.
2. Aerobic and anaerobic *Staphylococci*
3. Pneumococci
4. GNC: (Meningococci, *M. catarrhalis*)
5. *Diphtheroids*
6. *Lactobacilli*

- **Throat:** *Strept viridans, Moraxella catarrhalis*, pneumococci & certain GNB from intestine like *E. coli, P. aeruginosa*, paracolons & *Proteus* spp. are present in normal persons.

B. Lower respiratory tract: It includes trachea, bronchus & lungs

- Trachea contains organisms from pharynx or oral cavity
- Bronchus & alveoli are normally sterile

✪ **Resident flora of oral cavity:** Mouth is normally not sterile at birth it contains same organisms as present in birth canal as mentioned below.

A. Bacteria: *Staphylococci, Streptococcus mutans, Lactobacillus acidophilus, Corynebacteria, A. odontolyticus, Mycoplasma, Bacteroides*, anaerobic spirochetes, *Fusiform bacilli, Coliform bacilli, Proteus, Vibrio* (comma-shaped bacteria) etc.

B. Fungi: *Candida* spp. & *Geotrichum candidum*

✪ **Resident flora of Gastro-Intestinal Tract (GIT):**

- **In children:**
  - At birth the intestine is sterile but organisms are soon introduced with food.
  - Bowels of newborns in intensive care nurseries tend to be colonized by Enterobacteriaceae like *Klebsiella, Citrobacter & Enterobacter.*
  - In breast-fed children the intestine contains large numbers of *Streptococci & Lactobacilli* (*L. bifidus* constitutes 99% of total organisms in faeces).
  - In bottle-fed children a more mixed flora exists in the bowel and lactobacilli are less prominent.
- **In normal adult:**

* **Effective factors:**

i. Diet:

- As food habits develop toward the adult pattern which changes the bowel flora.
- Diet has a marked influence on the relative composition of the intestinal & faecal flora.

ii. pH:

o Oesophagus: Contains microorganisms arriving with saliva and food.

o Acidic pH of stomach:

- Acidity of stomach keeps the number of microbes at a minimum (10^3–10^5/g of contents) unless obstruction at the pylorus favours the proliferation of gram-positive cocci and bacilli.
- The normal acidic pH of the stomach markedly protects against infection with some enteric pathogens. E.g. *V. cholerae.*
- Administration of cimetidine for peptic ulcer leads to a great increase in microbial flora of the stomach,

o Alkaline pH of intestine: As the pH of intestinal contents becomes alkaline the resident flora gradually increases.

iii. Oral administration of antibiotics:

- Antimicrobial drugs taken orally can temporarily suppress the faecal flora. E.g.

1. **Neomycin plus erythromycin can suppress aerobes in 1–2 days.**
2. **Metronidazole can suppress the anaerobes.**

- The drug-susceptible microorganisms are replaced by drug-resistant ones, particularly *Staphylococci, Enterobacters, Enterococci, Clostridium difficile Pseudomonas, Proteus* spp. & yeasts.
- The feeding of large quantities of *Lactobacillus acidophilus* may result in the temporary establishment of this organism in the gut and the concomitant partial suppression of other gut flora.

iv. **Minor trauma:** Minr trauma during sigmoido-scopy, barium enema may induce transient bacteraemia in about 10% of procedures.

* **List of intestinal flora in adult:** More than 100 distinct types of organisms occur regularly in normal faecal flora as follows

A. Anaerobes:
- Mostly present in lower intestine.
- Anaerobes outnumber facultative aerobes organisms by 1000-fold. (1000:1)
- 96–99% of the resident bacterial flora consists of anaerobes: like *B. fragilis* (Most common), *fusobacterium* spp., *Lactobacilli (L. Bifidus or bifidobacteria), Cl. perfringens, Cl. difficile* and anaerobic gram-positive cocci (*Peptostreptococcus* spp.*)*.

B. Facultative aerobes:
- Mostly present in upper intestine
- 1–4% are facultative aerobes: Like gram-negative coliform bacteria (*E. coli*), *Enterococci, Proteus spp., Pseudomonas, Lactobacilli* etc.

C. Fungi: *Candida* spp.

* **Density of flora in different intestinal part: →Table-2**

Location (adult)	Bacteria/gram contents
Stomach	10^3- 10^5
Duodenum	10^3-10^6
Jejunum and ileum	10^5-10^8
Cecum & transverse colon	10^8-10^{10}
Sigmoid colon and rectum	10^{11} (10-30% of faecal flora)

Table-2: Density of flora in different intestinal part

* **Clinical significances:**
1. Intestinal bacteria are important in **synthesis** of vitamin K
2. Role in **conversion** of bile pigments and bile acids
3. Role in **absorption** of nutrients and breakdown products
4. Role in d **antagonism** to microbial pathogens.
5. The intestinal flora **produces ammonia** and other breakdown products that are absorbed and can contribute to hepatic coma.
6. **Abscess formation:**
   - The anaerobic flora of the colon, including *B. fragilis, Clostridia & Peptostreptococci* plays a main role in abscess formation after bowel perforation.
   - *Prevotella bivia & P. disiens* are important in abscesses of the pelvis originating in the female genital organs.
7. **Drug resistant:** *B. fragilis* are penicillin-resistant; therefore, another agent should be used.
8. **Superinfection or suprainfection:** **Follow chapter → Infections and infectious diseases**

✪ **Resident flora of urinary tract:**

A. Upper urinary tract:
- It includes kidneys, ureters, bladder
- These organs are usually sterile

B. Urethra:
- Usually sterile or may contains same flora as skin & intestinal flora like α-haemolytic *Streptococci, Enterococcus, Lactobacilli, Bacteroides, G. vaginalis, U. urealyticum & C. trachomatis.*
- The urine of a healthy individual is sterile but can become contaminated due to transfer of microbes from the GIT or genital tract.
- Normal flora in urine: 10^2–10^4/ ml.

✪ **Resident flora of genital tract:**

A. Male genital organs:
- *M. smegmatism* can be found on the penis or genital secretion of both sexes.
- It's presence in urine creates confusion in diagnosis renal tuberculosis.

B. Female genital organs:
- Norma vaginal secretion contains 10^8 bacteria / ml.
- Also showing presence of *M. smegmatism.*
- Vagina: Complex microbiota

1. **At birth:** Sterile at birth but after 24 hrs acquire microbes from vagina, skin & intestines.
2. **In 24 hrs**: Invaded by *Micrococci, Enterococci & Diphtheroides.*
3. **In 2-3 days:**
   - Maternal estrin induce deposition of glycogen in vaginal epithelium. This favour the growth of *Lactobacilli* (also **called Doderlein's bacilli**) & flora similar to adult stage. *Lactobacilli* convert glycogen in to acid. Acidic pH prevents the vaginal colonisation by foreign bacteria.
   - After that estrin & *Lactobacilli* are disappears, pH becomes alkaline & vagina return to normal flora.
4. **At pre-puberty:** Flora includes anaerobic cocci, *Listeria, Streptococci,* Mimeae, *Mycoplasma, G. vaginalis, Neisseria,* Spirochetes & *Candida* spp.
5. **At puberty/adult:** *Lactobacillus* reappear, pH becomes acidic. Normal flora includes anaerobes like *Gardnerella vaginalis, Bacteroides, Mobiluncus, Prevotella* & rare like *M. hominis*
6. **At pregnancy:** Increase *Staph. epidermidis*, Doderlein's bacilli & *Candida*
7. **At menopause:** Return to pre-puberty flora

✪ **Resident flora of blood & tissues:** Microbes are invades from GIT, mouth, nasopharynx & some other body parts, but they are eliminated by defence system of body.

Probiotics

➢ **Definition:** Live microorganisms which are administered for treatment or prevention of diseases.

- **Properties:**
  - Probiotics are the part of normal flora of body
  - They are useful when normal flora are suppressed
  - They are available commercially in the form of capsule or sachet
  - Capsule or sachet contains *Bacillus coagulus, Bifidobacterium longum, Lactobacillus acidophilus, Saccharomyces boulardii* etc.
- **Uses:** Probiotics are used in following clinical conditions

1. **Infectious diseases:**
   - *H. pylori* infection
   - Bacterial vaginosis: To restore the vaginal pH by using lactobacilli which produce the acidic pH
   - To prevent the infections
   - Antibiotic associated diarrhoea
2. **Inflammatory diseases:**
   - Gastroenteritis
   - Colitis
   - Necrotising enteritis
   - Irritable bowel syndrome
   - Modulatory response in inflammation
3. **Hypersensitivity reactions:** Modulatory response in eczema, dermatitis & other allergic disorders.
4. **Immunodeficiency diseases:** To restore the immunity
5. **High lipid profile:** It reduce the serum cholesterol by breaking the bile in the gut, thus inhibiting the reabsorption
6. **Hypertension:** It reduce the high blood pressure by producing the Acetyl Choline Esterase (ACE) inhibitors like peptides during fermentation

- **Limitations:** Live organisms present in probiotics produce their action only after their establishment in intestine for that they have to compete with normal flora of intestine to establish them self. So, now a days probiotics are more useful instead of probiotics.

Prebiotics

- **Definition:** Preparation contains dietary fibers which when administered stimulate the growth & activity of normal flora.

Question bank

Essay/Full question

1) Normal flora of human body

Short notes

1) Normal flora of skin
2) Normal flora of GIT
3) Normal flora of genital tract
4) Probiotics

Short questions for theory/viva questions

1) Define: Saprophytes & commensals
2) Mention the two differences between resident & transient flora of human body
3) Mention the different types of relationship between host & microbes
4) Write two advantages & two disadvantages of normal flora
5) What is Doderlein's bacilli
6) How probiotics are differentiated from prebiotcs

MCQs for chapter review

Normal flora

1) **Transient colonisation is caused by** (PGI, Dec-08)
   (a) HSV (b) *Trichomonas vaginalis* (c) *H influenzae* (d) *N gonorrhea* (e) *Staphylococcus aureus*
2) **It is true regarding the normal microbial flora present on the skin and mucous membrane that-** (AI-05)
   (a) It cannot be eradicated by antimicrobial agents (b) It is absent in the stomach due to the acidic pH (c) It establishes in the body only after the neonatal period (d)The flora in the small bronchi is similar to that of trachea
3) **Common natural floras of skin are** (PGI, June-09)
   (a) *Streptococcus* (b) *Staphylococcus aureus* (c) *Candida albicans* (d) *Bacteroides fragilis* (e) *Propionibacterium acne*
4) **Normal commensal of skin** (PGI, June-08)
   (a) *Staphylococcus aureus* (b) *Candida albicans* (c) *Bacteroides fragilis* (d) *Propionibacterium acne* (e) *Corynebacterium*
5) **Which of the following is the main coloniser of sebaceous gland** (PGI, June-07)
   (a) *Propionibacterium acne* (b) Diphtheria (c) *Strept pyogenes* (d) *Staph aureus* (e) *Candida*
6) **In the gut, anaerobic bacteria outnumber the aerobes by ratio of-** (AIIMS, May-06)
   (a) 10:1 (b) 100:1 (c) 1,000:1 (d) 10,000:1
7) **Most common commensals gut flora in adult-** (PGI-00)
   (a) *Lactobacilli* (b) *Bacteroides* (c) *E coli* (d) *Klebsiella*
8) **Most dominant colonic bacterium is**
   (a) *E coli* (b) *Bacteroides* (c) *Clostridium* (d) *Veilonella*
9) **The predominant colonic bacteria are** (PGI-88)
   (a) *Largely aerobic* (b) *Largely anaerobic* (c) *Bacteroides* (d) *Staphylococci*
10) **Bacterial count in duodenum-**
    (a) 10^5 per gram (b) 10^8 per gram (c) 10^{10} per gram (d) 10^{12} per gram
11) **Doderlein's bacilli word associated with**
    (a) *Lactobacilli* (b) Mimeae (c) *Listeria* (d) *Gardnella*
12) **Normal commensal in female genital tract**
    (a) *Gardnerella vaginalis* (b) *Bifidobacterium* (c) *Proteus* (d) *Neisseria*

Probiotics & prebiotics

13) **Probiotics are useful for** (AI-08)
    (a) Necrotising enterocolitis (b) Breast milk jaundice (c) Hospital acquired pneumonia (d) Neonatal seizures
14) **Probiotics are differentiated from prebiotcs**
    (a) Probiotics contain microbes while prebiotcs contains dietary fibres (b) Probiotics contain dietary fibres while prebiotcs contains microbes (c) Probiotics are prepared from animal products while prebiotcs are prepared from human products (d) None

Answers of MCQs & explanation

1) **(a), (b) & (e)**
   - Follow section, **transient flora → table-1** for explanation
2) **(a)**

- Resident flora are permanent & can't be eradicated by antimicrobial agents

3) **(a), (b), (c) & (e)**
4) **(a), (b), (d) & (e)**
5) **(a)**

} Follow section, **resident flora of skin** for explanation

6) **(c)**
7) **(b)**
8) **(b)**
9) **(b)**
10) **(a)**

} Follow section, **resident flora of GIT & table-2** for explanation

11) **(a)**
12) **(a)**

} Follow section, **resident flora of genital tract → Female genital organs** for explanation

13) **(a)**

- Follow sections, **probiotics (uses)** for explanation.

14) **(a)**

- Follow sections, **probiotics & prebiotcs (definition)** for explanation.

12 Infections and infectious diseases

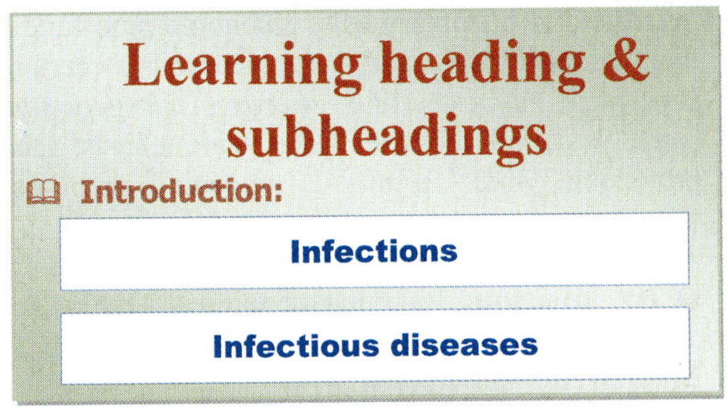

Introduction: Infection is an interaction between microbes & host.

Infections

❖ Definitions:

➢ **Infestation:**

- The lodgment and multiplication of infectious agents on the body surfaces or on the cloths of a host constitute infestation.
- Lodgment & multiplication over the surfaces but no entry in body

➢ **Contamination:**

- Only presence of infectious agents on surface or inside the body or inanimate object like fluid, food, clothes or soil but no multiplication
- Lodgment over surfaces / entry in body + no multiplication.
- Example: Bacteremia means entry of bacteria in blood & no multiplication. (Only detectable bacteria in blood)

➢ **Infection:**

- The entry and multiplication of infectious agents in the body of a host constitute infection.
- Entry in body + multiplication + no sign-symptoms

➢ **Infectious disease:**

- The entry, multiplication & production of clinical sign-symptoms **called infectious disease**.
- Entry in body + multiplication + sign & symptoms
- Examples:

1. **Septicemia:** Means entry of bacteria in blood, multiplication & clinical sign-symptoms.
2. **Toxemia:** Means entry of bacteria in blood, multiplication & clinical sign-symptoms are due to toxin production. It is one type septicemia.
3. **Pyemia:** Septicemia + abscess in organs like liver, spleen & other tissues

➢ **Contagious disease:** A disease that can be transmitted from one host to another by direct contact.

➢ **Communicable disease:** A disease that can be transmitted from one host to another either direct or indirect mode of transmission.

➢ **Non-communicable disease:** A disease that is not transmitted from one host to another

❖ Types of infection:

A. According to causative agents:

i. **Bacterial infection**
ii. **Viral infection**
iii. **Fungal infection**
iv. **Parasitic infection**
v. **Mixed infection:** When more than one organism causes infection simultaneously.
vi. **Co-infection or symbiotic infection:** Concomitant infection by combination of microbes **called co-infection**. Following are the examples

1. **Gas gangrene:** Follow chapter → Clostridium (Sporing anaerobe)
2. **Vincent's angina or fusospirochetosis:** Follow chapter → Spirochetales
3. **Adeno Associated Virus (AAV) & adeno virus:** Exact infection by AAV is not known but it always required adenovirus as a helper virus to produce the infection
4. **HDV & HBV:** Follow chapter → Hepatitis viruses
5. **Fournier gangrene:** Follow chapter → Systemic infections

B. According to nature of onset & progress:

1. **Acute infection:** Infection characterized by sudden onset, rapid progression & often with severe symptoms.
2. **Chronic infection:** Infection characterized by gradual onset and slow progression.

C. According to host involvement:

1. **Primary infection:** Initial infection in a host by organisms.
2. **Re-infection:** Subsequent infection in a same host by same parasite.
3. **Opportunistic infection:** Infection in an immunodeficient host by pathogen.

D. According to site/location:

1. **Local or focal infection (focal sepsis):** Infection that is restricted to a specific location within the body of the host.
2. **Systemic or generalised infection:** Infection that has been spread to several organs or areas in the body of the host.

E. According to source of infection:

i. If source is human body itself or outer source:

1. **Endogenous infection:**
- Organisms are originated from host itself. These are mostly normal flora from different parts of body.
- Example: Meningitis by *N. meningitidis* from nasopharynx
2. **Exogenous infection:**
- Organisms are originated from outside.
- Mostly from environment, soil, water etc.

ii. If source is hospital itself or outer source:

1. **Nosocomial (hospital acquired or health care associated) infection:** **Follow chapter → Health Care Associated Infections (HCAIs)**
2. **Community acquired infection:** Infection originated from outside the hospital environment.
3. **Iatrogenic (physician induced) infection:** Infection acquired by patients from physician during diagnosis, treatment or prevention of disease.

iii. If source is animal/animal products, human body or nonliving objects:

a. Anthoponoses / cross infections:
- Definition: Entry of infection from one human host to another human host.
- Meaning: Anthrópos (Greek) = man + nosos (Greek) = disease
- Examples include rubella, smallpox, diphtheria, gonorrhea, ringworm (*Trichophyton rubrum*), and trichomoniasis

b. Anthropozoonoses / zoonotic infections (disease) / zoonosis:
- Definition: Infection of human from animal or animal products.
- Meaning: Anthrópos (Greek) = man + zoon (animal) + nosos (Greek) = disease
- Examples & more details: **Follow chapter → Systemic infections**

c. Zooanthroponoses / reverse zoonosis:
- Definition: Infection of animal from human.
- Examples:
1. Leishmaniasis: Both zoonotic & reverse zoonotic
2. Influenza, measles, pneumonia & other pathogens are reverse zoonotic for many type of primates.
3. Tuberculosis: - Both zoonotic & reverse zoonotic, with birds, cows, elephants, meerkats, mongooses, monkeys, and pigs known to have been affected.
- This word is abandoned & no much significant

d. Sapronoses:
- Definition: Entry of infection from abiotic / nonliving substrate like soil, water, decaying plants, or animal corpses, excreta, and others.
- Meaning: Sapros (Greek) = decaying + nosos (Greek) = disease
- Examples: "Dimorphic fungi" like coccidioido-mycosis and histoplasmosis, "monomorphic fungi" like aspergillosis and cryptococcosis, certain superficial mycoses like *Microsporum gypseum*, some bacterial diseases like legionellosis, and protozoan like primary amoebic meningo-encephalitis

F. According to clinical presentation:

i. Overt infection: Presence of clinical features of disease

ii. Inapparent / subclinical:
- Clinical features (C/Fs) are not apparent.
- It includes inapparent, missed or abortive cases.
- Can be detected by lab test like recovery of organism, antibody response, biochemical & skin tests.

iii. Atypical: Infection in which the typical clinical manifestation of disease are not present.

iv. Latent (recrudescence):
- Following primary infection parasites remain in the body in silent/latent form for a very long period & again proliferating & producing the clinical disease in a later part of life when the host resistance is lowered or by specific stimulation **called latent infection**.
- Example: Zoster/zona/shingles by Varicella Zoster Virus (VZV)

v. Relapse:
- It is the primary infection with on-off features
- Example:
1. **Relapsing fever:** Caused by bacteria from *Borrelia* spp. Sudden onset of fever (bacteria are in blood) which last for 3-5 days followed by afebrile period (bacteria are in brain). After afebrile period of 3-5 days another bouts of fever.
2. **Relapses in malaria:** In the initial infection patient feel fever during erythrocytic phase & another episode of fever during exo-erythocytic phase in case of *P vivax, P malariae* & *P ovale* but in *P falciparum* there is no exo-erythocytic phase, so there is no relapse or subsequent attack of fever.

G. Other types:

i. Superinfection:
- **Synonym:** Suprainfection
- **Definition:** Appearance of new infection as a result of antimicrobial therapy.
- **Mechanisms:**
- Normal flora are contributes to host defence by production of bacteriocins or nutritional competition with pathogens.
- Use of antibiotics may result in alteration of such flora, loss of competition & other useful function,

which allows other flora (e.g. *Candida*) to predominate, to invade & to produce superinfection.
- More commonly superinfection is due to use of broad spectrum Anti Microbial Agents (AMAs) like tetracycline, chloramphenicol, ampicillin, cephalosporins.
- It is more common with combination therapy.

➢ **Precipitating factors:** Superinfection is more common in patients with immunocompromised status like
- Steroid therapy
- Malignancies e.g. leukemia
- AIDS
- Agranulocytosis
- Diabetes Mellitus (DM)

➢ **Sites:** Which harbour the normal flora like nasopharynx, GIT, upper respiratory tract, genital tract, urinary tract & occasionally skin

➢ **Organisms, manifestation & treatment of superinfection: →Table-1**

Organisms	Manifestations	Treatment
C. albicans	Diarrhoea, thrush etc.	Clotrimazole, nystatin
Staphylococcus	Enteritis	Cloxacillin
Proteus	UTI, enteritis	Cephalosporin or gentamicin
Pseudomonas	UTI, enteritis	Carbenicillin or pipericillin or gentamicin
Cl. difficile	Antibiotic Associated Colitis (AAC): Follow chapter → Clostridium (Sporing anaerobe)	

Table-1: Organisms, manifestations & treatment of superinfection

➢ **Prevention:**

✪ **Don'ts:**
- Avoid to use broad spectrum AMAs
- Avoid long term therapy
- Avoid AMAs for self limiting disease like viral infection or for untreatable disease.

✪ **Do:** Use narrow spectrum AMAs

✓ **Note:** Infection by Hepatitis D Virus (HDV) in patients already infected with Hepatitis B Virus (HBV) also **called superinfection**.

ii. Emerging & re-emerging infections:

➢ **Definitions:**

✪ **Emerging infection:** Are those
- Newly identified
- Previously unknown
- Spreading to new geographical areas
- Cause public health problems nationally or Internationally
- Increased incidence in last 2-3 decades.

✪ **Re-emerging infection:** Are those
- Which were previously under controlled
- Now re-appearing due to

1. AMAs resistance
2. Breakdown of public health measures: Epidemic of Chikungunya virus in 2005 was the great example.

- Cause major public health problems often in epidemic proportion

➢ **Risk factors:** Three types

1. **Microbial factors:** Antibiotics & insecticides resistance which allows new strain to arise like
   - Multi Drug Resistance Tuberculosis (MDR-TB)
   - Extended Drug Resistance Tuberculosis (XDR-TB)
   - Methicillin Resistant *Staph aureus* (MRSA)
   - Vancomycin Intermediate *Staph aureus* (VISA)
   - Vancomycin Resistant *Staph aureus* (VRSA)
   - Penicillinase Producing *N. gonorrhoea* (PPNG)
   - Vancomycin Resistant *Enterococcus* (VRE)
   - β-Lactamase producers like Extended Spectrum β-Lactamase (ESBL) producers, Carbapenemase producers & Amp C β-Lactamase producers
2. **Host factors:**
   - Immunosuppressive status
   - Malnutrition:
   - Behavior changes like drug abuse or sex
   - Illiteracy & ignorance
3. **Environmental factors:**
   - High population
   - Technology, industrial & economic development, land use, unplanned urbanisation
   - International travel
   - Poor or breakdown of public health measures
   - Natural disasters

➢ **Emerging infections in the World since 1973: →Table-2**

➢ **Re-emerging infections:**
- MDR-TB
- Malaria
- Cholera
- Dengue
- Chikungunya
- Plague
- Meningococcal meningitis

➢ **Prevention:**
- Epidemiological surveillance
- Laboratory surveillance
- Ecological surveillance
- Anthrapological surveillance
- Early diagnosis, treatment & implementation of control measures
- Constant monitoring & evaluation under the supervision of global outbreak & response network to control the infection & further spread

➢ **Indian scenario:** Following are the emerging & re-emerging infections in India

✪ **Bacterial diseases:**
- Plague
- Leptospirosis
- Brucellosis

- Anthrax
- Cholera

✪ **Viral diseases:**

- Iinfluenza
- Chikungunya
- Chandipura
- Dengue
- Japanese encephalitis
- SARS-CoV
- Hantavirus
- Human enterovirus 71

Year	Mibrobes	Disease
1973	*Rotavirus*	Enteritis/Diarrhoea
1976	*Cryptosporidium parvum*	Enteritis/Diarrhea
1977	*Ebola virus*	VHF
1977	*Legionella pneumophilla*	Legionnaire's disease
1977	Hantaan virus	VHF , renal failure
1977	*Campylobacter*	Enteritis/Diarrhoea
1980	HTLV-1	Lymphoma
1981	Toxin producing *Staph aureus*	Toxic Shock Syndrome
1982	*E. coli* 0157:H7	HUS
1982	HTLV-II	Leukemia
1982	*Borrelia burgdorferi*	Lyme disease
1983	HIV	AIDS
1983	*Helicobacter pylori*	Peptic ulcer
1988	Hepatitis E	Hepatitis
1989	Hepatitis C	Hepatitis
1990	Guanarito virus	VHF
1991	Encephalitozoon	Disseminated disease
1992	*Vibrio cholerae* 0139	Cholera
1992	*Bartonella henselae*	Cat scratch disease
1993	Sin Nombre virus	Hanta Pulmonary Synd.
1994	Sabia virus	VHF
1994	Hendra virus	Respiratory dz
1995	Hepatitis G	Hepatitis
1995	Herpesvirus-8	Kaposi sarcoma
1996	vCJD prion	Variant CJD
1997	Avian influenza (H5N1)	Influenza
1999	Nipah virus	Encephalitis
1999	West Nile virus	Encephalitis
2003	SARS-CoV	SARS
2009	H1N1	Pandemic swine flu
2011	CCHF virus	Haemorrhagic fever
2012	MERS-CoV	Middle East Respiratory Syndrome
2013	H7N9	Influenza
2016	Zika virus	Zika fever

Table-2: Emerging infections in the World since 1973

iii. Autoinfection:

- Common in parasites
- More details: Follow chapter → Miscellaneous topics in Parasitology

iv. Opportunistic infection: Follow chapter → Systemic infections

❖ Reservoirs of infection:

➢ **Definition:**

- Person, animal, insect, plant or inanimate objects like water, soil (or combination of all these) in which infectious agents can live, multiply & pass to susceptible host.
- Survival + multiplication + transmission

➢ **Types:** Reservoirs for different agents are described in respective chapters. Few are described below in two different categories.

A. According to living or non living object which act as reservoir:

i. Living reservoir:

a. Human reservoir:

- It includes human case or carrier
- Example: *M tuberculosis* (tuberculosis), *S typhi* (typhoid), *V. cholerae* (cholera), *B recurrentis* (louse borne relapsing fever), *N gonorrhoea* (gonorrhoea), *Cl tetani* (tetanus, it also has non living reservoir), *T pallidum* (syphilis), measles etc.

b. Animal reservoir:

- It includes zoonotic disease
- Example: *M bovis* (bovine tuberculosis), rabies, yellow fever, swine flu, bird flu etc.

ii. Non-living reservoir:

- Soil & inanimate matter can also act as reservoir
- Example: Soil is reservoir for *Cl tetani* (tetanus), *B anthracis* (anthrax), *C immitis* (coccidioido-mycosis), agents causing mycetoma etc.

✓ **Note: Multiple reservoirs**

- *Cl tetani* (tetanus): Human & soil reservoirs
- *E coli:* Human & animal reservoir

B. Other types:

1. Homologous reservoir:

- When reservoir & susceptible host are from same species.
- Example: *V. cholerae* where reservoir is man & susceptible host is man

2. Heterologous reservoir:

- When reservoir & susceptible host are from different species.
- Example: Typhoid where reservoir is man & susceptible host is bird/animal

❖ Sources of infection:

➢ **Definition:**

- Person, animal, insect, plant or inanimate object like water, soil (or combination of all these) from which infectious agents can pass to susceptible host.
- Survival only, no multiplication + transmission.

- **Confusion with reservoir of infection:**
- Sometimes it seems that reservoir & source of infection are synonyms but in fact both are different.
- Examples:

1. **Hook worm:** Reservoir of infection is man but source of infection is soil
2. **Tetanus:** Reservoir of infection & source of infection is soil

- **Types of source:** Source for different agents are described in respective chapters. Following are types (also reservoir)

A. **Humans:** Commonest source. Human may be case (patient) or carrier.

i. **Case (patient):** It is person who harbours the pathogens with sign-symptoms of disease & serves as potential source of infection for others.

ii. **Carrier:**

- **Definition:** It is person who harbors the pathogens without any sign-symptoms of disease & serves as potential source of infection for others.
- **Types of carrier:**

a. **According to clinical status:**

1. **Healthy carrier:** Harbours the pathogens but never suffered from the disease. E.g. polio, meningococcal meningitis, cholera, diphtheria etc.
2. **Convalescent carrier:** Recovered from the disease & continue to harbour the pathogens in his body. E.g. Typhoid fever, bacillary & amoebic dysentery, cholera, diphtheria etc.
3. **Incubatory carrier:** Shed pathogens during the incubation period of infection. E.g. measles, mumps, HBV, polio, pertussis etc.

b. **According to duration:**

1. **Temporary carrier:** Carrier state last < 6 months. E.g. it may be healthy or convalescent or incubatory carrier
2. **Chronic carrier:** Carrier state last for several years or may for rest of life. E.g. typhoid fever, HBV, gonorrhea etc.

c. **According to portal of exit:**

1. **Urinary:** E.g. typhoid fever
2. **Intestinal (Faecal):** E.g. typhoid fever
3. **Respiratory:** E.g. Influenza
4. **Nasal:** E.g. Influenza
5. Skin eruption, open wound & blood are also a carrier:

d. **Other type:**

1. **Contact carrier:** Person who acquire the pathogen from carrier.
2. **Paradoxical carrier:** Carrier who acquire pathogen from another carrier

B. **Animals & birds:**

- May act as case or carrier.
- Infectious disease transmitted from animals to human is **called zoonoses.**
- **Examples:**

1. **Cattle:** Anthrax, brucellosis, bovine tuberculosis
2. **Goat:** Brucellosis
3. **Sheep:** Anthrax
4. **Dogs:** Rabies, hydatid disease
5. **Horse:** Glanders
6. **Rats:** Rat bite fever, Weil's disease, plague
7. **Pigs:** Swine flu
8. **Birds:** Bird flu, ornithosis (psittacosis from parrot)

C. **Insects:** Diseases transmitted by insects are **called arthropod borne disease** & that insects are **called vectors**. It may also acts as source of infection

D. **Soil:** Spores of tetanus bacilli, fungi (*Histoplasma capsulatum*), *Nocardia asteroids*, Larvae of round worm & hookworm are found on soil.

E. **Water:** *Vibrio cholerae*, infective hepatitis viruses (HAV) are found in water.

F. **Food:** May contains

1. **Preformed toxin:** Food poisoning by –
   - *Staphylococcus aureus*
   - *B. cereus*
   - *Salmonella* species
   - *Cl. botulinum* (botulism)
   - *Cl. perfrigenes*
2. **Preexisting infectious agents in food:** E.g. meat (beef tape worm, pork tape worm).

❖ Modes of transmission of infection: Two categories as below

I. **Direct transmission:** Not required the mediator/vehicle for transmission of infection

A. **Droplet infection:**

- Droplet nuclei/particles of saliva or nasopharyngeal secretion arise during coughing, sneezing, speaking, talking or invasive procedure (bronchoscopy) enter in to other host directly who is in close contact.
- Such particles are ≥ 5 μm in diameter & spread to short distance (< 3 feet) & directly enter in other host. However such larger particle can be filtered by nose.
- Particles ≤ 5 μm in diameter are traverse to long distance & produces the air borne (indirect) infection described later in this chapter.
- Infection by droplet nuclei is increased in close contact, overcrowding & lack of ventilation.
- **Bacteria** transmitted by droplet nuclei are *Strept pyogenes, N meningitidis, C diphtheriae, H influenzae* type b, *B pertusis, Y pestis* & *M pneumoniae*
- **Viruses** transmitted by droplet nuclei are influenza virus, rubella virus, mumps virus, adeno virus & parvo virus B 19

B. **Inoculation/injection under skin or mucosa:** By contaminated needle or syringe like, HBV, HCV, HIV etc.

C. **Contact with skin/mucosa:** Examples are

- Sexually Transmitted Diseases/Infections (STDs or STIs): Follow chapter → Systemic infections
- Direct skin-to-skin contact transmitted disease like scabies, fungal & viral infection like HHV-1 & 2 (HSV-1 & 2 respectively), HHV-3 (VZV) pox virus, molluscum contagiosum etc.)

D. Contact with soil:

- **Bacteria:**
  - **Direct soil contact:** *Cl tetani* spores are present on soil & deposition of such soil on wounded skin allows the transmission. Anthrax spores are present in soil & in dead animal products. Animal acquired the anthrax by ingestion of spores present in soil, but human infection direct from soil spore is query. Transmission of anthrax to human occurs from animal products.
  - **Man (faeces)-soil-man (water/food):** *V cholerae, Salmonella* spp., hepatitis A etc.
- **Fungi (better to consider as source than mode of transmission):** Spores of many systemic (dimorphic) fungi are present in soil & spores are transmitted to man by air like *Histoplasma capsulatum* (histoplasmosis), *Coccidioides immitis* (coccidioidomycosis), *Blastomyces dermatitidis* (blastomycosis) & *Paracoccidioides brasiliensis* (paracoccidioidomycosis)
- **Parasites:** By walking with bare foot on contaminated soil like *Ancyclostoma duodenale* & *Strogyloides stercoralis*

E. Vertical: → **Table-3**

Time	Infections
Antenatal / before birth / congenital / transplacental / teratogenic Commonly **called TORCH agents**	- T: Toxoplasmosis - O: Others like syphilis (congenital syphilis), zika virus, parvovirus B19, Chikungunya virus, *P falciparum* etc. - R: Rubella (congenital rubella syndrome) - C: CMV (congenital cytomegalovirus infection) - H: Herpesviruses (HSV causing congenital herpes simplex while VZV causing foetal varicella syndrome & congenital /neonatal varicella), HBV, HIV-AIDS
Intranatal / during birth (transcervical)	- Candidiasis - Gonorrhoea (ophthalmia neonatorum) - Listeriosis (neonatal listeriosis) - *Strept agalactiae* (neonatal meningitis) - HSV - CMV - HPV
Postnatal / after birth by breast feeding	- Tuberculosis - CMV - HIV

Table-3: Vertical infections

II. Indirect transmission: Required the mediator/vehicle for transmission of infection

A. Inhalation (air borne):

- Particles arise during coughing, sneezing, talking or invasive procedure from patient & ≤ 5 µm in diameter are traverse to long distance & produces the air borne infection
- Some droplet nuclei settle over different object & become part of dust & cause air borne infection
- **Bacteria** transmitted by air borne route is *M tuberculosis* (open/active pulmonary tuberculosis)
- **Viruses** transmitted by air borne route are measles virus, VZV, influenza virus and haemorrhagic fever viruses with pneumonia.

B. Ingestion (food & water borne): Like *E. coli*, *V. cholerae*, polio virus, *Rotavirus* etc.

C. Vector borne:

- **Definition:** Arthropod or any living carrier (e.g. snail) which transports an infectious agent to susceptible host **called vector**.
- **Epidemiological types of vector borne disease:** following types

i. Method in which vectors are involved in transmission, multiplication & development:

a. Mechanical transmission:

- By crawling or flying through soiling of feet or proboscis or sometimes pass through GIT & passively excreted without development or multiplication in or on the body.
- E.g. amoebic & bacillary dysentery by house fly which settle from one food to other.

b. Biological transmission:

- Pathogen undergoes development or multiplication or both in the body of vector.
- The interval between the entry of the pathogen into the vector and the vector become infective is **called extrinsic incubation period.**
- Three types:

1. **Propagative:** Only multiplication, no development of pathogen. E.g. plague bacilli in rat fleas
2. **Cyclo-developmental:** No multiplication & only development of pathogen. E.g. microfilariae in mosquito.
3. **Cyclo-propagative:** Multiplication & development of pathogen. E.g. *Plamodium* spp. in mosquito.

ii. According to host involvement:

a. Invertebrate type:

1. Diptera: Flies & mosquitoes
2. Sphinonaptera: Fleas
3. Orthoptera: Cockroaches
4. Hemiptera: Bugs including kissing bugs
5. Anoplura: Lice
6. Acarina: Ticks & mites
7. Copepoda: Cyclops

b. Vertebrate type: Mice, rodents & bats

iii. By transmission channel:

a. Man & no vertebrate host:

1. Man-arthropod-man: Malaria
2. Man-snail-man: *S. haematobium*

b. Man & another vertebrate host & non-vertebrate host:
1. Mammal-arthropod-man: Plague
2. Bird-arthropod-man: Encephalitis

c. Man & two intermediate host:
1. Man-cyclops-fish-man: Fish tape worm
2. Man-snail-fish-man: *C. sinensis*
3. Man-snail-crab-man: *P. westermanii*

iv. According to deposition of agents in host by vectors:
1. Biting: E.g. *Plasmodium* spp. by mosquito bite
2. Regurgitation:
3. Scratching of infective faeces of vectors against abraded skin: *Borrelia* in relapsing fever

✪ **Inheritance transmission:**

a. Trans-ovarial transmission: Infected mother to progeny

b. Trans-stadial transmission: One stage of life cycle to other stage: E. g. nymph to adult

✪ **Effective factors of vector borne disease:**
- Feeding preference
- Infectivity: ability to transmit the agent
- Susceptibility: ability to become infected
- Survival of vectors in environment
- Domesticity: degree of association with man
- Seasonal: like malaria more in monsoon season

D. Blood borne: By transfusion of blood or blood products following organisms are transmitted
- **Bacteria:** *T. pallidum*
- **Viruses:** HHV-4 (EBV), HHV-5 (CMV), HHV-8 (KSHV), HBV, HCV, HDV, HGV (GB/G Baker virus C) HTLV-I, HTLV-II, HTLV-III (HIV), Parvovirus B19, zika virus etc.
- **Parasites:** *Trypanosoma cruzi*, *Leishmania donovani*, *Plasmodium* spp., *Babesia* spp., *Toxoplasma gondii* etc.

E. Saliva borne:

✪ **From human saliva (human bite):**
- **Viruses:** Like HHV-4 (EBV), HHV-6 (HBLV), HHV-7 (RK virus), ECHO virus, mumps virus etc.
- **Bacteria:**
- Bites by children rarely gets infected while bites from adults get infected in 15-20% cases
- Human bits carry aerobes (44%) & anaerobes (55%)
- Common aerobes transmitted by human bite are: *Streptococcus*, *Staphylococcus* & *Eikenella corrodens*
- Common anaerobes transmitted by human bite are: *Anaerobic streptococci*, *Prevotella* & *Fusobacterium*

✪ **From monkey bite:** Herpes virus simiae or B virus

✪ **From dog's bite:** Like rabies virus

✪ **From cat bite:** Like *Bartonella henselae*

✪ **Both by dog & cat bite:** *Pasteurella multocida*

F. Fomites borne: Contamination of fomites like towel, handkerchief, pen, pencils, clothes, cups, spoon, keys etc may transmit the infection like eye disease (trachoma), ear infection, diphtheria, dysentery & hepatitis A etc.

G. Unclean hand & fingers: May transmit the infection like dysentery, trachoma etc.

Infectious diseases

❖ **Definition:** → **Vide supra**

❖ **Types:**

A. According to location:

i. Generalised:

ii. Localised: it may be superficial or deep

B. According to spread in community:

i. Endemic disease:
- **Meaning:** En= in + demos = people
- **Definition:** constant presence of a disease within a given geographic area or population group without importation from outside.

ii. Epidemic disease:
- **Meaning:** Epi= upon + demos = people
- **Definition:** Sudden onset of disease clearly in excess of "expected occurance"

iii. Outbreak: Small, usually localised epidemic in the interest of minimising public alarm, unless the number of cases is indeed large.

iv. Sporadic:
- **Meaning:** Means scattered about
- **Definition:** Few cases occurs irregularly, haphazardly from time to time & separated widely in space neither identifiable common source of infection nor or little connection with each other.
- It is a starting point of epidemic when conditional are favourable for it's spread.

v. Pandemic: Epidemic that spreads in many areas of the world & affecting large population.

vi. Prosodemic diseases: Some pandemic disease (like water or air borne) spread very rapidly while some spread very slowly by person to person contact **called prosodemic diseases**. E.g. cerebrospinal fever.

vii. Exotic: Disease is imported in to country in which, it do not occur otherwise.

Question bank

Short notes

1) Types of infections
2) Suprainfection / superinfection
3) Emerging & re-emerging infections
4) Sources of infection
5) Carrier
6) Modes of transmission of infection

7) Vector borne infectious diseases
8) Types of infectious diseases

Short questions for theory/viva questions

1) Define infestation & infection
2) What is contact carrier & paradoxical carrier
3) Define case & carrier
4) What is TORCH agents
5) What is extrinsic incubation period
6) Define co-infection & write four examples.

MCQs for chapter review

Infections

1) **Septicemia is-** (AIIMS,May-06)
(a) Bacteria in blood (b) Toxin in blood (c) Pus in blood (d) Multiplication of bacteria & toxin in blood
2) **Emergence or resurgence, seen in which of the following organisms-** (PGI, Dec-04)
(a) Polio virus (b) Measles virus (c) Nipah virus (d) West Nile virus (e) hepatitis B virus
3) **New infectious agents are-** (PGI, Dec-07)
(a) Nipah virus (b) *Pneumocystis jiroveci* (c) Corona virus (d) SARS (e) Prion
4) **Which of the following does not have non human reservoir** (PGI, June-09, Nov-09, May-13)
(a) *Salmonella typhi* (b) *N gonorrhoea* (c) *E coli* (d) *Clostridium tetani* (e) *Treponema pallidum*
5) **Man is the only reservoir of** (AIIMS-90)
(a) Rabies (b) Measles (c) Typhoid (d) Japanese encephalitis
6) **Which of the following is not transmitted by soil** (AI-08)
(a) Coccidioidomycosis (b) Tetanus (c) Brucella (d) Anthrax
7) **Vertically transmitted disease caused by all except**
(a) *Toxoplasma* (b) CMV (c) HIV (d) *Treponema pertenue*
8) **Which of the following are transmitted by blood** (PGI-01)
(a) Toxoplasma (b) Syphilis (c) CMV (d) Hepatitis B and C (e) Hepatitis A
9) **All of the following infections may be transmitted via blood transfusion except** (AI-02)
(a) Parvo B-19 (b) Dengue virus (c) CMV (d) Hepatitis G virus
10) **Most common agents responsible for human bite infections are** (AI-98)
(a) Gram –ve bacilli (b) Gram +ve bacilli (c) Sporochetes (d) Anaerobic *Streptococci*

Answers of MCQs & explanation

1) **(d)**
- Multiplication of bacteria & toxin in blood **called toxaemia**, which is one type septicemia

2) **(c)**
3) **(a), (c) & (d)**
} Follow section, **emerging & re-emerging infections (table-2)** for explanation

4) **(a), (b) & (e)**
5) **(b) & (c)**
} Follow section, **reservoirs of infection** for explanation. Also follow respective chapters for more explanation.

6) **(c) & (d)**
- Follow section, **mode of transmission (direct → contact with soil)** for explanation.

7) **(d)**
- Follow section, **table-3 & respective chapters** for more explanation.

8) **(a), (b) (c) & (d)**
9) **(b)**
} Follow section, **mode of transmission (indirect → blood borne)** for explanation.

10) **(d)**
- Follow section, **mode of transmission (indirect → saliva borne)** for explanation.

13 Pathogenicity or virulence of microbes

Learning heading & subheadings

- Pathogenicity:
- Virulence:

- **Pathogenicity**: Ability of a microbial species to produce the disease **called pathogenicity**
- **Virulence**: Ability of microbial strain to produce the disease **called virulence**.

➢ **Exaltation:**
- Enhancement of virulence **called exaltation.**
- Demonstrated by serial passage in susceptible individual.

➢ **Attenuation:**
- Reduction of virulence **called attenuation**.
- Demonstrated by serial passage in unfavorable host, repeated subculture, growth in high temperature, desiccation, long storage in culture or by using antiseptics like formalin.

➢ **Precipitating factors (epidemiological determinants):** Virulence of microbes is affected by following three factors **called precipitating factors** or **epidemiological determinants**

I. **Agent factors (virulence factors** or **determinants of virulence):**
II. **Host factors:**
III. **Environmental factors:**

I. Agent factors (virulence factors or determinants of virulence)

♣ **Factors:** Following are the three types

A. **Intracellular or cell associated:**

i. **Adhesion:**

✪ **Definitions:**
- It is a process of attachment of pathogens with host cells.
- Organ used for adhesion is **called adhesin**

✪ **Organs of adhesion:** Following are the different type of organs used for adhesion (adhesins)

a. **Fimbrial adhesion** or **pilus adhesin** (From pili, synonym for fimbriae): **Follow chapter → Morphology of bacteria**

b. **Non fimbrial adhesins** or **non pilus adhesins:**

1. **Protein receptors in *Staphylococci*:** *Staphylococci* have receptors for many mammalian proteins like fibronectin, fibrinogen, IgG and C1q. Help in adhesion with host cells.
2. **Protein F in *Streptococcus pyogenes*:** Helps in attachment with pharyngeal wall.
3. **Extracellular surface protein in *Enterococcus*:** Help in adhesion.
4. **Glycocalayx:** Extracellular polysaccharide matrix, having ability to bind with plastic material of medical devices like catheter, suture materials, pacemakers, implants, Ryle's tube etc. **called biofilms**. Present in few bacteria like *Staph. albus* (*Staph epidermidis*), *P. aeruginosa* etc.
5. **D-galactose:** Present in *Listeria monocytogenes* help to bound with D-galactose receptors on macrophage's polysaccharides of payer's patches & epithelial cells.
6. **Internalins (A & B are subtypes):** Present in *L. monocytogenes* help to attach with phagocytic cells
7. **Outer membrane proteins (OMP) Ag:** Present in *H influenzae* which contributes in adhesion & invasion.
8. **Filamentous Haem Agglutinin (FHA):** Appear as filamentous structure under electron microscope, hence the name. It adhere the *B pertusis* with cilia of respiratory epithelium. It also favour adhesion of other bacteria like *H. influenzae* & *Strept pneumoniae* to respiratory epithelium **called piracy of adhesion**
9. **P_1 or cytadhesin or protein Ag:** It present in *Mycoplasma pneumoniae* which helps in adhesion to respiratory epithelium & block the ciliary movement **called ciliostasis**.
10. **Glycolipid Ag:** It also present in *Mycoplasma pneumoniae* which helps in adhesion to RBCs & responsible for haemolytic anaemia

11. **Hook of *Leptospira*:** Hooks on the ends of *Leptospira* allow them to attach & latch on to host tissues.
12. **Adhesin proteins in *Yersinia* spp.:** Different types like MyF Ag, pH6 Ag, inv (invasive) protein, ail (attachment & invasive locus) protein & Yad A (*Yersinia* adhesin A → it binds with collagen & fibronectin to aid the invasion of tissue by organism & also it inactivate the complement)
13. **Cell surface lectin:** E.g. *Chlamydia*

✪ **Clinical significances:**

- Adhesin may account for tissue trophism and host specificity.
- As it used for virulence, loss of adhesion makes the strain avirulent.
- Adhesin is usually protein & antigenic. It produce antibody which is protective, hence it can be used as method of prophylaxis. e.g. *E. coli* diarrhoea in calves and piglets & gonorrhoea in humans are prevented by using vaccine prepared from fimbrial antigen.

ii. Cell wall components:

a. **Peptidoglycan:** Provide rigidity & structural integrity to cell.

b. **Proteins Antigens:** M protein in *Streptococci.*

c. **Somatic (carbohydrate) Ag:** In *Streptococci* play role in non-suppurative lesions.

d. **Endotoxin (lipopolysaccharide / LPS):** LPS is present in gram negative not in gram positive bacteria & responsible for endotoxic activities as mentioned below. However LPS of *V cholerae* has no role in the pathogenesis of disease (**called cholera**) in human, but intraperitoneal inoculation in mice cause fatal effect

- Pyrogenicity
- Activation of complement
- Leucocytosis
- Macrophage inhibition
- Lethal action
- Inhibition of glucose & glycogen synthesis in the liver
- Interferon release
- Depression of blood pressure
- Leucopenia
- Stimulation of B lymphocyte
- Induction of prostaglandin synthesis
- Protect the bacilli from phagocytosis (in *E. coli*)
- Protect the bacilli from serum complement (in *Klebsiella* spp.)
- DIC, septic shock (endotoxic shock) & possible death in *P aeruginosa*

✓ **Note: Endotoxin (LPS) & *Listeria***

▪ An early study suggested that *L. monocytogenes* is unique among Gram-positive bacteria in that it might possess LPS, which serves as an endotoxin. Later, it was found to not be a true endotoxin. *Listeria* cell walls consistently contain lipoteichoic acids resemble the LPS of Gram-negative bacteria in both structure & function.

iii. Other components related to bacterial cell:

a. **Capsular (K) Ag:** Capsular (K) antigen present in different bacteria & fungus inhibit the phagocytosis.

b. **Slime layer:** It inhibit the phagocytosis

c. **Vi antigen:**

- Present in *S. typhi*
- Inhibit the phagocytosis
- Resist complement activity
- Resist bacterial lysis by alternative pathway & by peroxidase killing
- Bacilli with Vi Ag are causing more consistent disease than those are lacking

d. **Antigenic cross reactivity:** Cytoplasmic membrane & vascular intima in *Streptococci.*

iv. Genetical factors:

a. **Plasmid:** It is coding for some virulence properties of bacterial like

- Codes for surface antigen for colonization of *E. coli*
- Enterotoxin production by *E. coli* & *Staph. aureus*
- Drug resistance in many bacteria is plasmid borne.

b. **Tox^{+} gene:** E.g. in diphtheria bacilli gene for toxin production is present in beta or other tox+ corynephages.

v. Invasiveness:

- Defined as ability of a pathogen to spread in the host tissue. E.g. *Streptococcus* is highly invasive producing septicemia whereas *Staphylococcus* is less invasive producing localized lesion.
- However some pathogen are less invasive although produce fatal diseases. E. g *Cl. tetani* confirmed to site of entry & produce fatal disease by elaborating the toxin.

vi. Communicability:

- Defined as ability of parasite to spread from one host to another host.
- Play major role in development of epidemic or pandemic.
- Role in interruption of disease. E.g. in hydrophobia & in H. cyst human infection represents the dead end host.

vii. Infecting dose & lethal dose:

✪ **Definitions:**

- **Infectious dose (ID):** It is the amount of pathogen (measured in number of microorganisms) required to cause an infection in the host.
- **Lethal dose:** It is the amount of pathogen (measured in number of microorganisms) required to cause death in the host.
- **MID (minimum infecting dose) or MLD (minimum lethal dose):** It is minimum numbers of bacteria require producing clinical evidence of infection or death respectively.

- **ID_{50} or LD_{50}:** Dose required to infect or to kill 50 percent of animal under standard condition.

✪ **Effective factors over infective dose:**

1. **Age:** Low dose in lower age
2. **Gastric acidity:**
   - Many microbes are susceptible to gastric acidity (like *Salmonella, Vibrio cholerae* etc.) required high dose while many resist gastric acidity (like *Shigella,* etc.) required low dose
   - Factors like use of antacids, presence of local disease like hypochlorhydria, achlorhydria etc. can alter the gastric acidity are also effective over ID
3. **Use of antibiotics:** It reduce the competition between pathogens & normal flora, so it decrease the ID
4. **Local surgery**
5. **IDDs**

✪ **Infective dose by different bacteria: →Table-1**

Bacteria	Infective dose (ID)
Low infective dose	
Mycobacterium tuberculosis	< 10 bacilli
***Escherichia coli* O157:H7**	< 10 bacilli
Shigella	10-100 bacilli
Francisella tularensis	10-50 bacilli
Campylobacter jejuni	500 - 10^3 bacilli
Cryptosporidium parvum	10 to 30 oocysts
Entamoeba coli	1 cyst
Giardia lamblia	Few cysts
High infective dose	
Bacillus anthracis	10^4 spores
Escherichia coli	10^6 - 10^8 bacilli
Salmonella	10^3-10^6 bacilli
Vibrio cholerae	10^4 - 10^6bacilli

Table-1: Infective dose by different bacteria

viii. **Route of infection:** Initiation of infection depends on route of entry. E.g. *V cholerae* are infective orally only while *Streptococci* are infective by any mode.

ix. **Site of infection:** Bacteria differ in their site of selection in host and their ability to damage different organs. E.g. *M. tuberculosis* injected in rabbits damages kidneys & infrequently to liver & spleen while in guinea pigs lesions are mainly in liver & spleen & sparing the kidneys.

B. Extracellular:

i. Enzymes:

1. **Coagulase:** Production by *Staphylococci* form fibrin barrier around bacteria & produce localised infection.
2. **Hyaluronidase**: Split component of intracellular connective tissue.
3. **Fibrinolysin:**
4. **Proteases:**
5. **Nucleases (DNAse):**

   (3–5: Initiation & spread of infection by breaking the fibrin barrier)
6. **Lipase:** Help to infect skin & subcutaneous tissues.
7. **Enzymatic inactivation of the antibiotics:** Follow chapter → Genetics of bacteria.
8. **Ig A protease:**
   - Produce by *N. meningitidis, N, gonorrhoea, H. influenzae & Strept pneumoniae*
   - It destroy the IgA & reduces the local immunity
9. **Amidase:** In pneumococci, this autolytic amidase activated by surface-active agents such as bile or bile salts, cleaves bond between alanine and muramic acid in peptidoglycan of cell wall, resulting in lysis of organisms & released of bacterial product in medium.
10. **Neuraminidase (receptor destroying enzyme):** Present in *V. cholerae*. It destroys the receptors on RBCs & releases the bounded bacteria & favours its spread to other part of intestine.
11. **Other diagnostically useful enzymes are:** Catalase, phosphatase, urease, oxidase, etc.

ii. Exotoxin: Bacteria produce two types of toxin

a. Endotoxin (Lipopolysaccharide): →Vide supra

b. Exotoxin:

✪ **Properties:**

- Exotoxins are heat labile or heat stable

1. **Heat labile toxin producing bacteria:** LT (labile) of ETEC, *Cl perfringens* (*Cl welchii*), *V cholerae*, diarrhoeal illness producing toxin of *B cereus*
2. **Heat stable toxin producing bacteria:** *Staph. aureus, Y enterocolitica,* ST (stable) of ETEC, emetic illness producing toxin of *B cereus*

- In contrast to endotoxins, which are integral part of bacteria; exotoxins are actively synthesized and released free in medium.
- Exotoxins are produced by a variety of bacteria including gram-positive and gram-negative bacilli
- They are antigenic and can be toxoided.
- Their activity can be neutralized by antitoxins.
- Most of the toxins have enzymatic activity.
- Many toxins are extraordinarily powerful, small amounts can be lethal.
- Toxins can be separated from the culture broth by filtration.

✪ **Exotoxin producing bacteria:** Exotoxin is mostly produced by gram positive bacteria & rarely by gram negative bacteria.

- **Gram positive bacteria:** *Staph. aureus, Strept. pyogenes, Strept pneumoniae, B. anthracis, B. cereus, Cl. welchii, Cl. tetani, Cl. botulinum, C. diphtheriae, M. ulcerans (M. buruli)* etc.
- **Gram negative bacilli:** ETEC, EIEC, EHEC, *Shigella* spp., *Y. enterocolitica, V. cholerae, P. aeruginosa, C. jejuni, H pylori B. pertusis, F. fusiforme* etc.

✪ **Nomenclature of exotoxins:**

1. **According to targeted cell/organ:** Exotoxins which attack a variety of cell types are **called cytotoxins** whereas exotoxins that attack specific cell/organ types are named according to the cell type or organ they damage such as haemolysin, leucocidin, neurotoxin, enterotoxin etc.
2. **According to the species, which produces them and from the disease with which they are associated:** Like cholera toxin from *Vibrio cholerae*, causes cholera & tetanus toxin from *Clostridium tetani*, causes tetanus.
3. **According to activities:** Like adenylate cyclase or exotoxin A of *Pseudomonas aeruginosa*.

✪ **Biological actions of exotoxin:**

- **Cytotoxicity:** Causing cell lysis

1. Haemolysin: E.g. lysis of RBCs in *Staph. aureus*
2. Leucocidin: E.g. damage to polymorphonuclear leucocyte in *Staph. aureus*
3. Verotoxin/verocytotoxin:
   - It includes Shiga toxin & Shiga Like Toxin (SLT).
   - Shiga toxin of *Shigella dysenteriae*
   - SLT of Enterohaemorrhagic *E. coli, V. cholerae, Aeromonas hydrophila* & *Campylobacter jejuni*
   - In vitro effect: Both Shiga toxin & Shiga Like Toxin (SLT) causing cytotoxicity to the cultured Vero cells (Afrcian monkey kidney cells used for cell culture are **called Vero cells**).
   - In vivo effect: Toxin consists two sub units like binding (B) & active (A). Sub unit A divided in to two fragments like A1 & A2. B helps in adhesion with host cells. A2 links A1 to B. A1 inactivate the host cell 60S ribosome & inhibit the protein synthesis leading to cell death. Cell death resulting discontinuity of mucosa & haemorrhage (bloody diarrhoea)
4. Diphtheria toxin:
   - Produced by *C. diphtheriae, C. ulcerans* & *C. pseudotuberculosis*
   - It inhibit protein synthesis by inactivating elongation factor (EF-2) & causing cell death
5. Vacuolating cytotoxin produced by *H pylori* producing injury to host cells
6. Exotoxin A
   - Released from *P. aeruginosa,*
   - Same actions as like diphtheria toxin

- **Enterotoxicity:** Causing outpouring of electrolytes & fluid in to intestinal lumen responsible for watery diarrhoea like

1. LT and ST produced by Enterotoxigenic *E. coli*
2. Verotoxin/verocytotoxin
3. Enterotoxin of *Y. enterocolitica*
4. Cholera toxin produced by *Vibrio cholerae*
5. Enterotoxin of *P. aeruginosa*
6. Enterotoxin of *C. jejuni*

- **Neurotoxicity:** Toxin act on nerve system

1. Enterotoxin of *Staph aureus:* It causing food poisoning features by vagal stimulation
2. Tetanospasmin from *Cl tetani*: Locks synaptic inhibition (pre-syneptic) in spinal cord by blocking the release of inhibitory neurotransmitters like glycine & Gamma Amino Butyric Acid (GABA) → Resulting in uncontrolled spread of impulses → Tonic muscle rigidity & spasm
3. Botulinum from *Cl botulinum:* Block the production or release of acetylcholine & causing descending flaccid paralysis (arflexia)
4. Shiga like toxin/SLT (having cytotoxic, enterotoxic & neurotoxic properties): Shiga like toxin causing paralysis & death on injection in mice/rabbit. Not act directly on CNS but on the blood vessels, neurotoxic effect is secondary.
5. Shiga (having cytotoxic, enterotoxic & neurotoxic properties) toxin: Shiga toxin causing paralysis & death on injection in mice/rabbit. Not act directly on CNS but on the blood vessels, neurotoxic effect is secondary.

- **Enzyme based actions:** Exotoxins produced by *Cl welchii* have enzyme based actions
- **Connective tissues action:** Toxin act on the extracellular matrix of connective tissue & aid in spreading the infection by breaking down extracellular matrix of connective tissue. Like

1. Kappa toxin (collagenase) produced by *Cl. welchii*
2. Exfoliative toxin produced by *Staph. aureus*

- **Hormonal:** Pertusis toxin of *B. pertusis* activate the intracellular cAMP in pancreatic islet & increase the insulin secretion in animal not in human
- **Immune mediated action:**
  - Lymphocytosis: Like
    - Pertusis toxin of *B. pertusis*
  - Superantigen: Like
    - Staphylococcal enterotoxins
    - Staphylococcal toxic shock syndrome toxin (TSST-1)
    - Streptococcal pyrogenic exotoxins (exotoxin A and exotoxin B)

✓ **Note: Superantigen**

▪ **More details:** **Follow chapter → Antigen (Ag)**

✪ **Regulatory genes:** Three types as below.

1. **Chrmosome mediated:**
   - Staphylococcal exfoliative toxin A (heat stable).
   - Streptococcal pyrogenic exotoxins B
   - Shiga toxin
2. **Plasmid mediated:**
   - Enterotoxin production by *staph. aureus*
   - Staphylococcal exfoliative toxin type B (heat labile)
   - Anthrax toxin by *B. anthracis*.
   - Tetanospasmin by *Cl. tetani.*
   - Labile toxin (LT) of *E. coli*
   - Stable toxin (ST) of *E. coli*

3. **Bacteriophage mediated:**
- Staphylococcal toxic shock syndrome toxin
- Streptococcal pyrogenic exotoxins A & C
- Botulinum type C & D
- Diphtheria toxin
- Shiga like toxin (SLT)
- Labile toxin (LT) of *V. cholerae*

✪ **Detection of exotoxins:**

1. **Culture:**
- **In Vivo:** By using laboratory animals
- **In Vitro:** By using cell/tissue culture, like Vero cell culture for verotoxin

2. **Serological tests:** Precipitation (like Elek's gel precipitation test for diphtheria toxin), agglutination, ELISA, RIA etc. can be used.
3. **Molecular tests:** DNA probe

✪ **Clinical uses:** Uses & other details of different toxins are described in respective chapters

✪ **Differences between two toxin: →Table-2**

iii. **Biological active substances:** E.g. released by *Cl. perfringens* in gas gangrene like

1. **Haemagglutinin:** Active against RBCs of human & animals in gas gangrene
2. **Bursting factor:** For muscle lesion in gas gangrene
3. **Circulating factor:** Increase sensitivity to capillary bed & also inhibit phagocytosis
4. **Histamine:**

iv. **Pigments:** For more details Follow chapter → Bacterial growth products

Exotoxin	Endotoxin
Produce by gram +Ve bacteria & also by GNB	Produce by GNB
Converted in toxoid with formalin treatment	Not converted in toxoid
Proteins	Lipopolysaccharide
Heat labile (gets denatured on boiling) & few are heat stable	Heat stable (Not denatured on boiling)
MW: 50-1000kDa	MW: 10 kDa
Actively secreted by cell & diffuse into surrounding medium	Part of cell wall & do not diffuse into surrounding medium
Separated by filtration	By cell lysis
Enzymatic	Non enzymatic
Specific pharmacological effect for each toxin	Nonspecific
Specific tissue affinity	No specific tissue affinity
Active in very minute doses (<1µg)	Active only in very large doses (>100µg)
Highly antigenic	Weakly antigenic
Action specifically neutralised by antibody	Neutralization by antibody is ineffective
Detected by different tests as described earlier in text	Detected by limulus lysate assay

Table-2: Differences between two exotoxin & endotoxin

Obligate intracellular	Facultative intracellular
Definition	
These microbes are not able to synthesize their own ATP & remain dependent on host cells	These microbes are able to synthesize their own ATP & remain dependent on host cells & can live extracellularly
Bacteria	
M. leprae *Rickettsia* spp. *Chlamydia* spp. *C. burnetii*	*M. tuberculosis, S. typhi* *Y. pestis, N. meningitidis* *Nocardia* spp., *Brucella* spp., *L. pneumophilla, Francisella tularensis, L. monocytogenes* etc.
Viruses	
All viruses	
Fungi	
P. jirovecii	*H. capsulatum* & *C. neoformans*
Parasites	
T. gondii, C. parvum, Plasmodium spp., *Leishmania* spp., *Babesia* spp., *Trypanosoma* spp.	

Table-3: Intracellular location of microbes

C. **Others:**

i. **Intracellular location of microbes:**
- Organisms survive intracellularly.
- Intracellular location of the organisms helps to escape the host defence & the effect of antibiotics.
- Types: Two types like obligate & facultative as shown in **table-3.**

ii. **Bacterial secretory system:** Bacteria utilize particular strategies to release the virulence factors **called bacterial secretory system.** It is the important mechanism in bacterial survival & pathogenesis. There are six types of secretory system from type I to type VI.

♣ **Regulatory genes:** Above all virulence factors of bacteria, responsible for pathogenicity are under control of specific genes located on the chromosome **called pathogenicity islands.** Removal of such genes makes the bacterium avirulent. Pathogenicity islands have been detected in many bacteria like *Staphylococcus aureus, Escherichia, Shigella, Salmonella, Vibrio cholerae Helicobacter* etc.

II. Host factors

i. **Age:** Certain infection are common at particular age like *H. influenzae B*, Thread worm in paediatric age group

ii. **Sex:** UTI is more common in female due to close proximity of genital to anus allow the faecal contamination

iii. **Religion:** Infection by *T. saginata* is common in Mohmedian population due to custom of eating beef

iv. **Immune status:** Immunodeficiency status favour certain infection like *S. typhi, M. tuberculosis* etc.

v. **Blood groups:**
- *N. gonorrhoea* infection is common in group O
- *V. cholerae* infection is common in blood group B & least in blood group AB.
- Exact reasons for all these are not known

vi. **Deficiency of complement components:** E.g. deficiency of C_5-C_9 components favour the meningococcal infection

vii. **Occupation:** Like laboratory infection in laboratory workers

viii. **Gastric acidity:** It affect over the infective dose of bacteria

III. Environmental factors

i. **Overcrowding:**
ii. **Water reservoir:**
iii. **Humidity:**
iv. **Presence of reservoir or source or transmitting agents of infection (e.g. vectors) in environment:**

Question bank

Essay/Full question

1) Virulence of microbes

Short notes

1) Determinants of virulence
2) Bacterial adhesins
3) Determinants of virulence
4) Bacterial exotoxin
5) Differences between exotoxin & endotoxin

Short questions for theory/viva questions

1) Write four examples of bacterial adhesions.
2) What is attenuation & exaltation?
3) Name the blood group in which, infection by following bacteria is common
   N. gonorrhoea & *V. cholerae*
4) Name the four bacteria producing IgA protease
5) Comment: IgA protease is known to reduce local immunity
6) Write the four functions of endotoxin
7) Name the four GNB producing the exotoxin
8) Name the four bacteria producing the neurotoxin
9) How following toxins are showing neurotoxicity.
   Tetanospasmin, Botulinum, Shiga toxin & Shiga like toxin
10) What is biofilms?
11) What is Pathogenicity Island?

MCQs for chapter review

1) **Exaltation is**
   (a) Decreased virulence (b) Increased virulence (c) No change (d) None
2) **Adhesin is useful in-** (PGI -98)
   (a) Motility (b) Bacterial attachment (c) Toxigenicity (d) Bacterial division
3) **The endotoxin which leads to endotoxic shock is actually-** (AIIMS -00)
   (a) Lipoprotein (b) Lipopolysaccharide (c) Polysaccharide (d) Polyamide
4) ***Salmonella typhi* is the causative agent of typhoid fever. The infective dose of *S. typhi* -** (AI -12, AIIMS-06)
   (a) One bacillus (b) 10^8-10^{10} bacilli (c) 10^2-10^5 bacilli (d) 1-10 bacillus
5) **All are true except-**
   (a) Exotoxin has enzymatic action (b) Endotoxin has enzymatic action(c) Exotoxin is highly antigenic (d) Endotoxin is weakly antigenic
6) **Endotoxin from gram negative organism is** (AIIMS-00)
   (a) Polysaccharide (b) Glycoprotein (c) Lipoprotein (d) Lipopolysaccharide
7) **True about exotoxins-**
   (a) Lipopolysaccharide (b) Not antigenic (c) Can be toxoided (d) Heat stable
8) **Exotoxins are** (AIIMS-95)
   (a) Lipopolysaccharide in nature (b) Produced by gram -ve bacilli (c) Highly antigenic (d) Very stable and resistant to chemical agents
9) **Septic shock is due to-**
   (a) Protein (b) Lipopolysaccharide (c) Techoic acid (d) Peptidoglycan
10) **Heat stable enterotoxin causing food poisoning is caused by all the following except**
   (a) *Bacillus cereus* (b) *Yersinia enterocolitica* (c) *Staphylococcus* (d) *Clostridium perfringens*
11) **Gram negative bacterium producing exotoxin is**
   (a) *V. cholerae* (b) *Sh. dysenteriae* (c) *C. jejuni* (d) All of above
12) **True about mechanism of bacterial toxins** (PGI, May-13)
   (a) Cholera toxin acts by inhibition of guanyl cyclase (b) Botulinum toxin inhibits Ach release (c) Shiga toxin of *Shigella dysenteriae* act by inhibiting protein synthesis (d) Diphtheria toxin act by inhibiting protein synthesis
13) **Endotoxin of following gram negative bacteria does not play any part in the pathogenesis of the natural disease-** (AIIMSN, Nov -12, 06, AI-12)
   (a) *E. coli* (b) *Klebsiella* (c) *Vibrio cholerae* (d) *Pseudomonas*
14) **Enterotoxin is produced by all except -** (AI -89)
   (a) *Clostridium perfringens* (b) *Staphylococcus aureus* (c) *Streptococcus pyogenes* (d) *Bacillus cereus*
15) **All of the following organisms are known to survive intracellularly except -** (AI -05)
   (a) *Neisseria meningitidis* (b) *Salmonella typhi* (c) *Streptococcus pyogenes* (d) *Legionella pneumophila*
16) **Which of the following are intracellular** (AI -00)
   (a) Viruses (b) *Chlamydiae* (c) *Mycoplasma* (d) *Rickettsia*
17) **Obligate intracellularly organisms is -**
   (a) *Mycoplasma* (b) *Chlamydiae* (c) *Cryptococcus* (d) *H. pylori*
18) **All are intracellularly parasites, except -**
   (a) *Leishmania* (b) *Plasmodium* (c) *Toxoplasma* (d) None of above

Answers of MCQs & explanation

1) **(b)**
- Decreased virulence **called attenuation** & increased virulence **called exaltation**

2) **(b)**
- Adhesin is the organ of adhesion & useful in bacterial attachment with host cells

3) **(b)**
- Endotoxic shock is due to endotoxin which is lipopolysaccharide in nature while exotoxin is protein in nature

4) (c)
- Infective dose of different bacilli is mentioned in **table-1**

5) (b)
6) (d)
7) (c) & (d)
8) (b) & (c)

Follow **table-2** for explanation

9) (b)
- Septic shock is also **called endotoxic shock**, which is due to endotoxin which is lipopolysaccharide in nature

10) (d)
- Follow section, **exotoxin (properties)** for explanation

11) (d)
- Follow section, **exotoxin (exotoxin producing bacteria → Gram negative bacilli)** for explanation

12) (b), (c) & (d)
- Follow section, **exotoxin (biological actions of exotoxins)** for explanation

13) (c)
- Follow section, **endotoxin (Lipopolysaccharide / LPS)** for explanation

14) (c)
- *Streptococcus pyogenes* produces the pyrogenic exotoxin & haemolysin (**called streptolysin**) but not the enterotoxin.

15) (c)
16) (a), (b) & (d)
17) (b)
18) (d)

Follow **table-3** for explanation

14 Bacterial growth products

Learning heading & subheadings

- ❖ Definition:
- ❖ Types:

❖ **Definition:** During the growth, bacteria secrete the several products **called bacterial growth products**.

❖ **Types:** Following are the types

A. Vitamins: Vitamin K, E & B are produce by intestinal flora like *Bacteroides* spp. & *E. coli.*

B. Chemicals/ Drugs:

i. Chemicals: Acetone & butanol from *Cl. acetobutylicum*

ii. Toxins: Intramuscular injection of ***Cl. botulinum*** **toxin type A** 1st used for strabismus, is now recognised as safe & effective for many neuromuscular diseases.

iii. Enzymes:

1. **Streptokinase:** Useful for myocardial infarction & other thomboembolic diseases.
2. **Streptodornase:** Useful for empyema to liquefy thick pus.

iv. Antibiotics: Following are the examples

a. Chloramphenicol: Initially it was prepared from *Streptomyces venezuelae* in 1947. But now a days all the commercial products of chloramphenicol are prepared synthetically.

b. Aminoglycosides: Two categories are as follows

1. **Obtained from *Streptomyces* spp.:** Drugs are labelled with suffix “mycin”. Following are the examples
   - Streptomycin (1944): From *Streptomyces griseus*
   - Kanamycin(1957): From *Streptomyces kanamyceticus*
   - Tobramycin(1970): From *Streptomyces tenebrarius*
   - Neomycin: From *Streptomyces fradiae*
   - Framyctin: From *Streptomyces lavendulae*
2. **Obtained from *Micromonosporum* spp.:** Drugs are labelled with suffix “micin”. Following are the examples
   - Gentamicin(1964): From *Micromonosporum purpurea*
   - Sisomicin(1980): From *Micromonosporum inoyoensis*

c. Others:

- Erythromycin (1952): From *Streptomyces erythreus*
- Mupirocin: From *Pseudomonas* spp.
- Polymyxin B(1940): From *Bacillus polymexa*
- Colistin (1940): From *Bacillus colistinus*
- Bacitracin: From *Bacillus subtilis*
- Tyrothricin: From *Bacillus bravis*
- Rifampicin (Rifampin): From *Streptomyces mediterranei* (suffix “micin”)

v. Insectisides: Useful to prevent the food crops from disease & prepared from *B. thuringenesis*

C. Spores: **Follow chapter → Morphology of bacteria**

D. Bacteriocins:

✪ **Definition:** Specific antibacterial substances produce by bacteria **called bacteriocins**.

✪ **History:** Bacteriocins production was 1st observed by Gratia in 1952 from *E. coli*

✪ **List of bacteriocins & producing bacteria:**

- Colicins: *E. coli, Sh. sonnei*
- Diphthericin: *C. diphtheriae*
- Megacins: *B. megaterium*
- Proticin: *Proteus* spp.
- Aeroginosin (Pyocins): *P. aeruginosa (P. pyocyanea)*
- Pesticins: *Y. pestis*

Mnemonic: List of bacteriocins

- **Indian states like Chhatisgargh, Delhi, Madhya Pradesh & Andhra Pradesh**

✪ **Synthesis**:

- Determined by specific plasmid **called col factor.**
- Col factor is transfers from one cell to other cell by **conjugation** or by **transduction.**
- Its production is stimulated by physical (UV rays) & chemical agents (nitrogen mustard).

✪ **Properties:**

- Proteins while some are LPS in nature
- It resemble like phage. E.g. pyocins appears like tail of phages under electron microscopy
- Bacteria produce bacteriocins are immune to it, but they are susceptible to other bacteriocins.
- It adsorb on surface of susceptible cell as like phage

✪ **Bacteriocins typing:**

- **Principle:** Based on ability of bacteriocins producing strain to kill standard indicator strain.
- **Method:**
  - Name: Plate diffusion technique.
  - Steps:
    - Inoculate the test bacterium as broad streak in centre of culture plates.
    - Standard indicator strain is inoculated at right angle to original inoculum.
    - Incubate the plate at required temperature & time.
  - Result: Pattern of inhibition of standard indicator strain represent the type of bacteriocins
- **Use:** Useful in epidemiological typing of bacterial strain

E. Pigments:

- **Definition:** These are coloured substances produce by bacteria.
- **Role of pigments in virulence:** Exact role is not know but may produces the following effects which increases the virulence of bacterium
  - Stop ciliary movement of respiratory epithelium & protect the bacteria from host defense.
  - Inhibit growth of other bacteria & makes the bacteria dominant in mixed infection.
  - Catalyses production of superoxide & H_2O_2.
- **List of bacteria & pigments produced by them:**

1. ***Staphylococcus* spp.:**
   - Types of *Staphylococcus* according to pigment production: } **Follow chapter → Micrococcaceae**
   - Properties of pigments: }
2. ***Streptococcus agalactiae* (Group B, β-haemolytic *Streptococci*):** **Follow chapter → Streptococcaceae**
3. ***Neisseria* spp.:** Commensal *Neisseria* like *N. flavescens* (yellow pigment) & *N. flava*
4. **Photochromogens:** Produces the yellow-orange pigment in light only.
5. **Scotochromogens:** Produce the yellow-orange-red pigment in light & in dark.
6. ***Nocardia* spp.:** Also producing the pigments
7. ***Serratia marcescens* (*S. prodigiosus*):**
   - Red colour pigment **called prodigiosin**
   - Best produced at room/ low temp-20^{0}C
   - Its presence in sputum simulating presence of blood **called pseudo-haemoptysis**
8. ***Erwinia* spp.:** Yellow pigment
9. ***Yersinia pestis:*** Absorb the haemin & produces the dark brown pigmented colonies in blood agar & other haemin containing media. Pigment production is essential for biofilm formation & flea blocking.
10. ***Pseudomonas*:**
    - Type & Properties of pigments } **Follow chapter → Non-fermenters**
    - Media for production & identification of pigment }
11. ***Flavobacterium meningosepticum*:** **Follow chapter → Non-fermenters**
12. ***Bordetella parapertusis:*** It produces the brown diffusible pigments on nutrient agar after two days of incubation
13. ***Chromobacterium violaceum*:** **Follow chapter → Miscellaneous GNB**
14. ***Capnocytophaga canimorsus* & other species:** Believed to produces yellow or orange pigment on blood agar
15. ***Legionella pneumophila:*** Diffusible brown pigment is produced on Feeley Gorman (FG) agar, which fluoresces in dull yellow colour on UV light exposure. This may be enhanced by addition of tyrosine in medium.
16. ***Porphyromonas* spp.:** Also have ability to produce the pigment
17. ***Prevotella melaninogenica:*** It produce the hemin derived black or brown pigment

F. Exotoxin: } **Follow chapter → Pathogenicity or virulence of microbes**

G. Enzymes: }

H. Acids (by fermentation) & alkalis:

I. Gases: Like NH_3, H_2S etc.

J. Cell wall components: Like antigens, proteins etc. are released free in medium during infection or growth of bacteria.

Question bank

Short notes

1) Bacterial growth products
2) Bacteriocin
3) Pigment producing bacteria

Short questions for theory/viva questions

1) Name the four bacteria producing the bacteriocins
2) Name the four pigment producing bacteria
3) What is the role of pigments in virulence of bacteria

MCQs for chapter review

1) **Following is/are the bacteriocins producing bacterium/bacteria:**
   (a) *E. coli* (b) *Sh. sonnei* (c) *C. diphtheriae* (d) *B. megaterium*
2) **Pigment producing bacterium is:**
   (a) *Streptococcus pyogenes* (b) *Streptococcus agalactiae* (c) *Streptococcus mutans* (d) *Streptococcus pneumoniae*
3) **Pigment producing colonies are seen in**
   (a) *Pseudomonas* (b) Atypical *mycobacteria* (c) *Serratia marcescens* (d) All of the above

Answers of MCQs & explanation

1) **(a), (b), (c) & (d)**
   - Follow section, **types (bacteriocin → list of bacteriocins & producing bacteria)** for explanation
2) **(a)** } Follow section, **types (pigments → list of bacteria & pigments produced by them)** for explanation
3) **(d)** }

15 Bio-Medical Waste (BMW) management

Learning heading & subheadings

- ❖ Definitions:
- ❖ Objectives of management:
- ❖ Sources of waste:
- ❖ Quantification of waste:
- ❖ Health hazards:
- ❖ BMW, regulation:
- ❖ Classification:
- ❖ Waste disposal:

❖ Definitions:

- ➢ **Hospital waste:** All waste coming out of hospital.
- ➢ **Bio-Medical Waste (BMW):** Solid or liquid waste including its container, generated during the diagnosis, treatment, prevention or research activities in human beings or animals by healthcare set up or research facility or slaughter house **called bio-medical waste**.

❖ Objectives of management:

To prevent the injuries & accidental transmission of infection to:

- Hospital staff & workers
- Patients
- Attendants or visitors
- Patient's relatives
- Person working with waste disposal

❖ Sources of waste:

- All hospitals like government, private, dental clinic, clinician's office, dispensaries, PHC etc.
- Medical research & training centres
- Blood banks & laboratories
- Animal & Slaughter houses
- Vaccination centres
- Mortuaries
- Biotechnologies units.

❖ Quantification of waste:

Different survey says that waste generation in India is 1/2-4 kg/bed/day in Government hospital, 1/2-2 kg/bed/day in private hospital & 1/2-1 kg/bed/day in nursing homes.

❖ Health hazards:

1. Public sensitivity
2. Infection: HBV infection, HCV infection, HIV-AIDS
3. Allow breeding of rodents & vectors
4. Genotoxic: Affect the genetic materials
5. Trauma: From sharp items
6. Corrosion from chemicals
7. Radiation (dizziness, vomiting, headache): From X-ray, MRI plates.

❖ BMW, regulation:

Legal aspect of BMW is mentioned below

- The air (control of pollution and prevention) act, 1981.
- The environment (protection) act, 1986.
- The hazardous waste (management and handling) rules, 1989.
- The national environmental tribunal act, 1995.
- Bio-medical waste (management and handling) rules, 1998: They were published vide notification number S.O. 630(E) dated 2oth July. 1998, by the Government of India in the erstwhile Ministry of Environment and Forests (MoEF), provided a regulatory framework for management of bio-medical waste generated in country
- Bio-medical waste rule (draft), 2011: The Ministry of Environment and Forests (MoEF) had proposed a revised draft of bio-medical waste rules 2011. It is simpler & containing 8 categories of BMW, each has to be collected & segregated in different colour coded bag, thus clears the confusion over the colour coding of containers used for disposal of BMW rules, 1998. However still it is under consideration & not enforced yet.
- Bio-medical waste management rules, 2016: They were published in the Gazette of India, Extraordinary, Part-II, Section 3, Subsection (i), Government of India, Ministry of Environment, Forests and Climate Change as a notification on March 2016 (detail available at http://mpcb.gov.in/bomedical/pdf/BMW_Rules_2016). The major changes are in the segregation in the colour coded bags as mentioned in **table-2 & fig.-1**

❖ Classification:

A. According to risk associated:

i. Non-hazardous waste: 85% of total waste

- Mostly coming from housekeeping & administrative function of hospital.
- Examples: General kitchen waste & office waste like food, papers, files etc.

Category	Waste type	Treatment & disposal
1	**Human anatomical waste** (human tissues, organs, body parts)	Incineration & deep burial
2	**Animal waste** (animal carcasses)	Incineration &deep burial
3	**Microbiology & biotechnology waste** (Wastes from Microbiology laboratory e.g. cultures)	local autoclaving, microwaving & incineration
4	**Sharp waste** (needles, syringes, scalpels, blade, glass, etc.)	Disinfection, autoclaving, microwaving & mutilation/shredding
5	**Discarded medicines & cytotoxic drugs** (outdated & contaminated medicines)	Incineration, destruction &drugs disposal in secured landfills
6	**Solid waste** (soiled waste contaminated with blood & body fluids including cotton, dressings, clothes bedding)	Autoclaving, microwaving & incineration
7	**Solid waste** (other than the sharps such as tubing, catheters, intravenous sets etc.)	Disinfection, autoclaving microwaving & mutilation, shredding
8	**Liquid waste** (generated from washing, cleaning, housekeeping and disinfecting activities)	Disinfection & discharge into drains
9	**Incineration ash** (Ash from incineration of any hospital waste)	Disposal in municipal landfill
10	**Chemical waste**	Chemical treatment, discharge into drains for liquids & secured landfill for solids

Table-1: Categories according to bio-medical waste management & handling rules, 1998

Color of bag	Type of waste
Yellow bag **[fig.-1(a)]**	- Body organs (human + animal) - Microbiology waste - Items contaminated with blood/body fluid like cotton etc. - Glass or plastic items like vials, ampoules etc. contaminated with cytotoxic drugs or antibiotics - Chemical waste
Red bag **[fig.-1(b)]**	Plastic wastes (recyclable) like tubes, catheter, syringe without needle etc.
Black bag **[fig.-1(c)]**	Paper, foods etc.
White puncture proof box (translucent) **[fig.-1(d)]**	Sharp metal items like needle, syringe fixed with needle, scalpel, blade etc,
Blue cardboard box **[fig.-1(e)]**	- Glass items like vials, ampoules etc. contaminated with drugs except cytotoxic drugs - Metallic body implant
Green bag/container **[fig.-1(f)]**	Household waste

Table-2: Type of waste containers

ii. Hazardous waste: It includes 15% of total waste with following two categories.

a. Non-infectious but hazardous: 5% of total waste

- This includes radioactive (X-ray plates), chemicals (corrosive), & pharmaceuticals (expired drugs) etc.

b. Infectious & hazardous: 10% of total waste

- Mostly generated during diagnosis, treatment or prevention of diseases
- Examples: Sharps (needles, syringes, glass test tubes), non sharps (body tissues, organs, dressing materials), plastics disposables (plastic syringes, ryles tubes, catheter etc), liquid waste (body fluid) etc.

B. Total 10 categories according to bio-medical waste (management & handling) rules, 1998: → **Table-1**

❖ **Waste disposal:** With following steps:

A. Volume reduction: Reduction of volume by proper planning & using reusable items.

B. Collection & segregation:

- Biomedical waste should not be mixed with any other kind of waste.
- It should be collected & separated /segregated (duty of generator) at the point of generation in different colour coded bags/boxes/containers as suggested in **table-2 & fig.-1** before storage or transport.

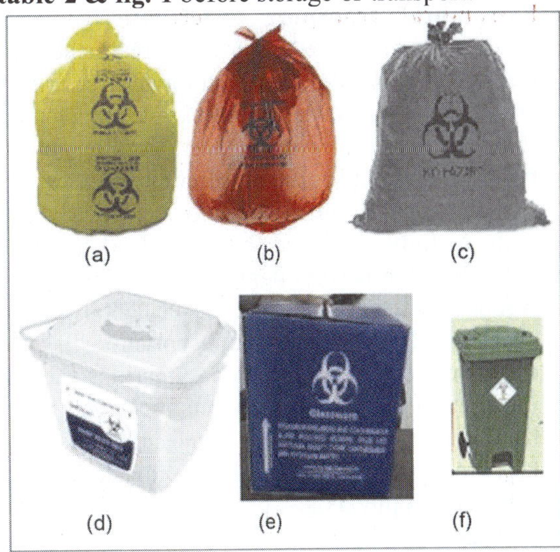

Figure-1: Different colour containers/bag

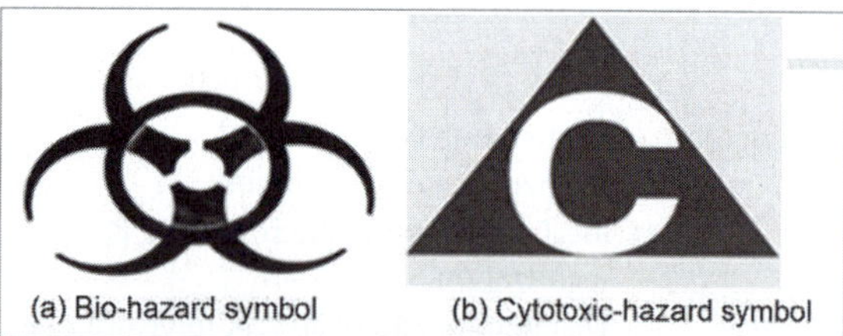

Figure-2: Bio-hazard symbol & cytotoxic-hazard symbol

- Bag should be sealed once filled ¾ & labeled with symbol of bio-hazard **[fig.-2(a)]** or cytotoxic drugs **[fig.-2(b)]** & with other details as shown in **table-3**

Day:__, Month ___, Year___	
Waste Category No.	Date of generation.
Waste Description: (E.g. wt in kg)	
Sender's Name & Address Phone No: Fax No.	Receiver's Name & Address Phone No. Fax No.
In case of emergency please Contact: Name & Address & Phone No.	

Table-3: Label for transport of bio-medical waste containers/bags

✓ **Note:** Label shall be non-washable and prominently visible

C. **Handling & transportation:** There are two types of transport

i. **Intramural transport (internal):** It involves the movement of waste bag inside the hospital premises. Separate closed type; cleaned & disinfected trolleys with bio-hazard symbol shall be used & it is not used for any other purposes. There must be a selection waste transportation route & low activity timings (like post OPD, post round in wards etc.) to avoid contact with patients. General waste shall not be transported with BMW.

ii. **Extramural transport (external):** It involves movement of waste for offsite treatment and/or disposal. The contractor is authorized for transport and disposal of waste. Handling and transfer leads to closer contact with wastes, leading to high hazards. The transportation of clinical waste offsite shall be carried out in specially designed vehicles with a fully enclosed body and a bulk head separating the drivers compartment from the local compartment vehicle trolley. Accidental exposure chances are more during transportation, if proper care is not taken. Appropriate authorities should be informed in case of accidents occurring during handling or transportation. The authorities should take the needful action like provision of post exposure prophylaxis.

D. **Storage:**

- No waste should be stored in the place of generation for more than two days, if needed one should take permission from competent authority
- The storage area shall be, in a secured hospital location, limited access, cleaned, roofed, properly drained, rodent proof, insect proof with water supply, good lighting and passive ventilation.
- It shall not be situated near the food stores or food preparation areas or public places & marked with a biohazard symbol.
- This area shall be kept locked with key available to staff throughout 24 hours. Only authorized personnel are allowed to enter.

E. **Treatment & disposal:** The duration of generation of bio-medical waste to the final disposal shall not exceed 48 hours including the temporary storage. Several methods are available but choice of method depends on type of waste.

i. **Disinfection:** Add chemical to kill the microbes it contain.

ii. **Moist heat sterilisation:**

- **Method:** By autoclaving or hydroclaving.
- **Advantages:** It reduce the volume & weight

iii. **Dry heat sterilisation:**

- **Method:** Incineration
- **Use:** It burns waste like paper, clothes, plastics, anatomical waste till it becomes ash.
- **Advantage:** Complete disposal of waste
- **Disadvantages:**
  - Ideally not useful for sharp items
  - Generate toxic gases from plastics like PVC
  - Expensive to maintain & to operate

iv. **Microwaving:** Electromagnetic sterilisation of small volume waste at the point of generation.

v. **Deep burial:**

- **Use:** For sharp
- **Area selected is:** Very large in a unhabited land
- **Method:** After disinfection wastes are placed in deep trenches, covered with lime & filled with soil.

vi. **Inertization:** Mixing 65% pharmaceutical waste with 15% cement + 15% lime + 5% water in order to minimise the risk of toxic substances contained in waste.

vii. **Liquid waste:** Treat with disinfectants (e.g. sodium hypochlorite) & drain in to sewer.

Question bank

Short notes

1) Bio medical waste management

Short questions for theory/viva questions

1) Draw the bio hazards symbol & cytotoxic-hazard symbol
2) Name the different types of bags for collection of biomedical waster & type of waste collected in it.

MCQs for chapter review

1) **Microbiological waste is collected in:**

(a) Yellow bag (b) Blue bag (c) Black bag (d) Green container

2) **Following is true method of disposal for plastic syringe without needle & plastic syringe with needle:**
(a) Syringe without needle in yellow bag & syringe with needle in white puncture proof box (b) Syringe without needle in red bag & syringe with needle in white puncture proof box (c) Syringe without needle in black bag & syringe with needle in white puncture proof box (d) Syringe without needle in red bag & syringe with needle in blue box

Answers of MCQs & explanation

1) **(a)** } Follow section, **waste disposal** (**table-2**) for explanation
2) **(b)** }

17 Miscellaneous topics

(World days, Health care related symbols)

Learning heading & subheadings

- World days
- Health care related symbols

World days

Table-1

Diseases	World day	Comment
Tuber-culosis	24th March of every year	*M. tuberculosis* was identified & described on 24th March 1882 by Robert Koch
Leprosy	Last Sunday of January in each year	This day was chosen in commemoration of the death of Gandhi, the leader of India who understood the importance of leprosy
Polio	24th Oct. of every year	It was fixed by Rotary International over a decade ago to commemorate the birth of Jonas Salk, who led the first team to develop a vaccine against poliomyelitis.
HIV-AIDS	1st Dec. of every year	Since 1988, 1st Dec is celebrated as an AIDS day to raising awareness of the AIDS pandemic caused by HIV by Josh Lowe & mourning those who have died of the disease
Rabies	28th Sept of every year	It is the anniversary of the death of Louis Pasteur who, with his colleagues, developed the 1st effective rabies vaccine
Hepatitis	28th July of every year	It aims to raise global awareness & to encourage the prevention, diagnosis & treatment of hepatitis A, B, C, D & E
Malaria	25th April of every year	It aims the control of malaria
Health	7th April of every year	It is celebrated under the sponsorship of the WHO, as well as other related organisations

Table-1: World days

✓ **Note:** World health day is one of eight official global health campaigns marked by WHO, along with World tuberculosis day, World immunization week, World malaria day, World no tobacco day, World AIDS day, World blood donor day, and World hepatitis day.

Health care related symbols

Figures-1 to 7

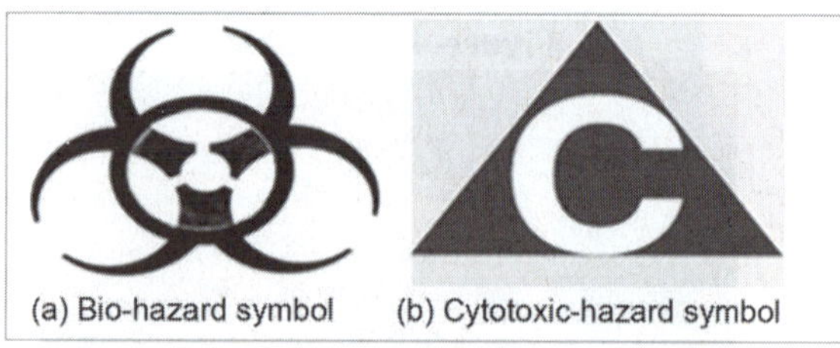

Figure-1: Bio-hazard symbol & Cytotoxic-hazard symbol

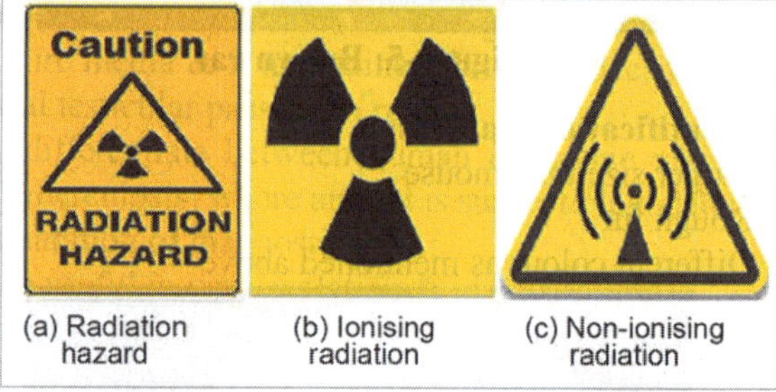

Figure-2: Radiation hazard symbols

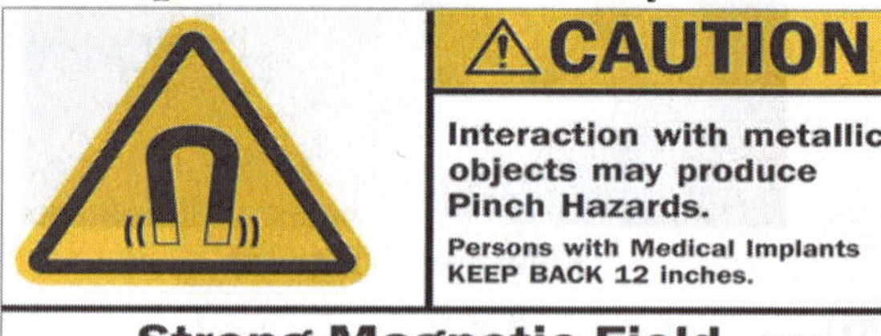

Figure-3: Magnetic field symbol

Figure-4: Gas hazard symbols

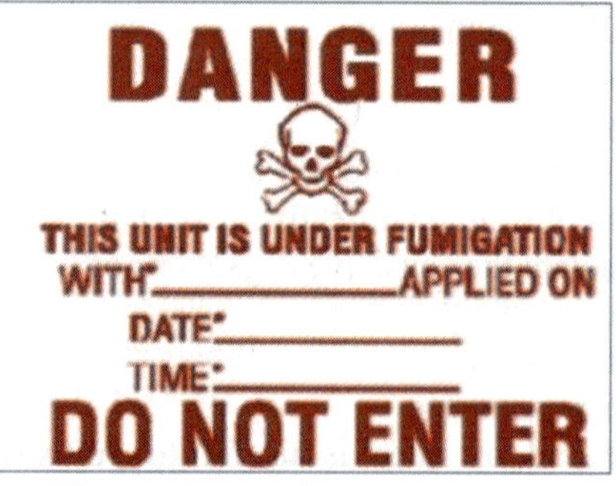

Figure-5: Fumigation symbol

(a) Yellow bag (b) Blue bag (c) Black bag (d) Green container

2) **Following is true method of disposal for plastic syringe without needle & plastic syringe with needle:**
(a) Syringe without needle in yellow bag & syringe with needle in white puncture proof box (b) Syringe without needle in red bag & syringe with needle in white puncture proof box (c) Syringe without needle in black bag & syringe with needle in white puncture proof box (d) Syringe without needle in red bag & syringe with needle in blue box

Answers of MCQs & explanation

1) (a)
2) (b)
} Follow section, **waste disposal** (**table-2**) for explanation

16 Laboratory animals

Learning heading & subheadings

- ❖ Common uses of animals:
- ❖ Disadvantages for uses of animals:
- ❖ Animals & specific uses:

❖ Common uses of animals:

1. Isolation of microorganisms
2. Identification of microorganisms
3. Preparation of immune sera or therapeutic sera or vaccine
4. Preparation of diagnostic sera/ antigens

❖ Disadvantages for uses of animals:

1. Ethical issues regarding uses of animal. Required to take permission from the animal ethical committee of institute.
2. Time consuming about 6-9 months
3. May not give desired result due to interference by animal immunity

❖ Animals & specific uses:

A Nine banded armadillo: →Fig.-1

- **Synonym:** Long nosed armadillo
- **Scientific name:** *Dasypus novemcinctus*
- **Identification features:** There are nine (sometimes fewer) narrow, jointed armor bands on its midsection that let it bend.

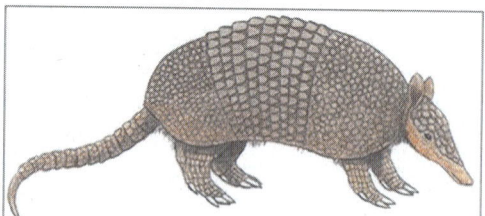

Figure-1: Nine banded armadillo

- **Uses:**

- It develops generalised lepromatous leprosy following inoculation of lepra bacilli.
- It act as reservoir of infection in *T. cruzi*
- Naturally infected in *P. braziliensis* & may provide clue to understand the patho-physiology of fungus

B. Rabbit: →Fig.-2

- **Scientific name:** Many genus & species like *Oryctolagus cuniculus* (Europian rabbit)

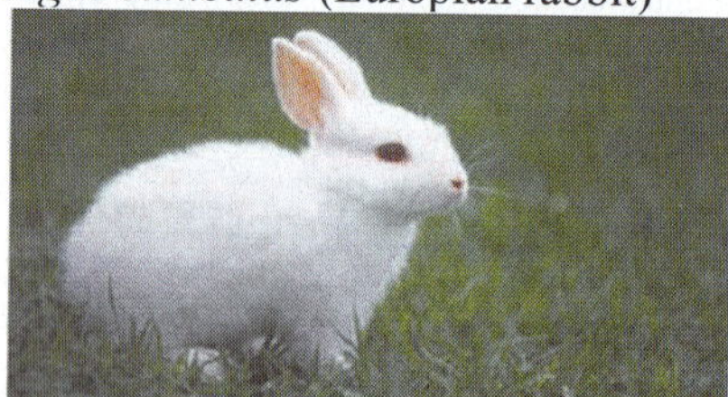

Figure-2: Rabbit

- **Uses:**

1. Pathogenic *Treponema* do not grow in artificial culture media & it maintained for many decades by serial testicular passage in rabbits
2. To differentiate between human & bovine variety of tuberculosis, where animal is susceptible to later
3. Preparation of diagnostic sera.
4. Also useful in virus isolation & identification

C. Guinea pig: →Fig.-3

- **Scientific name:** Many species like *Cavia porcelus*

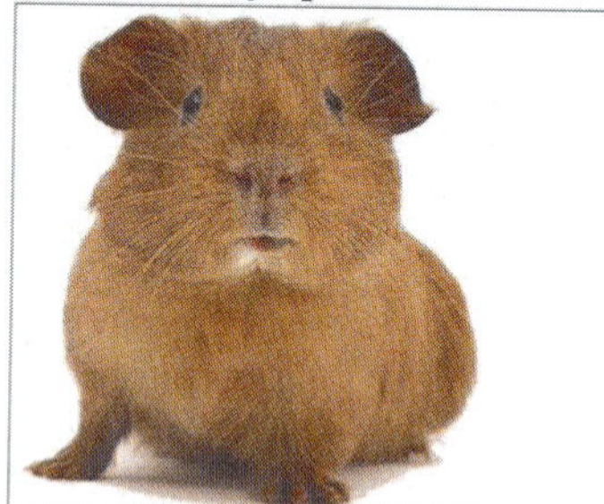

Figure-3: Guinea pig

- **Uses:**

1. To isolate human & bovine variety of tuberculosis & animal is susceptible to both
2. Virulence test in diphtheria & tetanus
3. It was used to establish many theory like
   - Germ theory by Pasteur
   - Pfiffer's phenomenon
   - Theobald Smith phenomenon
4. To obtain the complement for CFT.
5. To investigate the typhus fever
6. To investigate the Entero Invasive *Escherichia coli* (EICE) **called Sereny test**
7. Also useful in virus isolation & identification
8. Guinea pig is the highly susceptible animal to diagnose the anaphylaxis

D. Rat:

- **Scientific name:** Different types

- **Black rat (fig.-4):** *Rattus rattus*
- **Brown rat (fig.-5):** *Rattus norvegicus*
- **White rat or albino rat (fig.-6):** *Rattus albus*

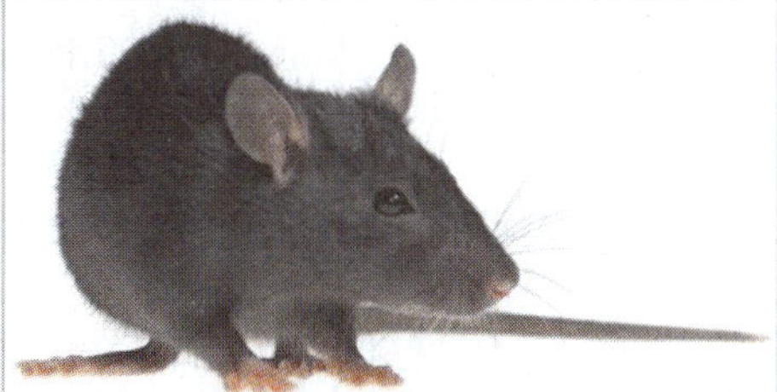

Figure-4: Black rat

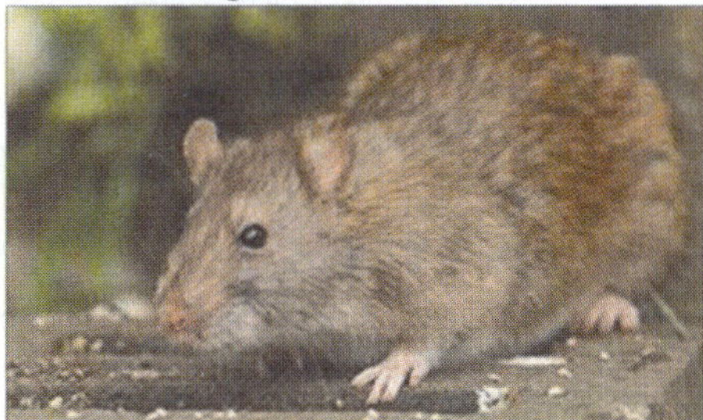

Figure-5: Brown rat

➢ **Identification features:**
- Larger size than mouse
- Rough fur
- Different colour as mentioned above

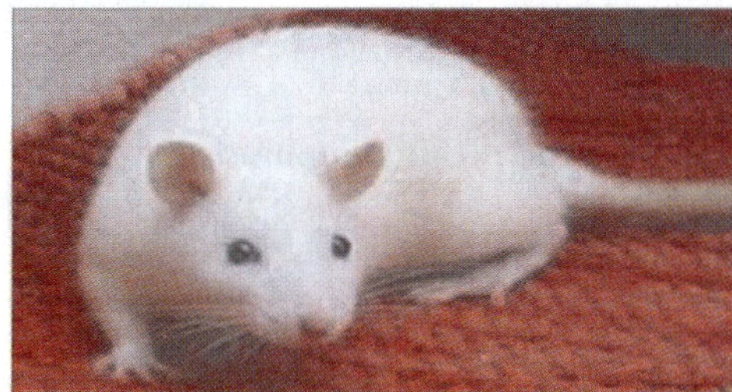

Figure-6: White rat

➢ **Uses:**
1. To differentiate between *Yersinia pseudotuberculosis* & *Yersinia pestis*
2. It also associated with other zoonotic pathogen like
- *Leptospira*
- *T. gondii*
- *C. jejuni*

E. Mouse (Singular)/ Mice(Plural): →Fig.-7

➢ **Scientific name:** *Mus musculus*

➢ **Identification features:**
- Smaller size than rat
- Smooth fur

➢ **Uses:**
1. It is very susceptible to Pneumococcus & useful to isolate it from the infective materials
2. To isolate the causative organisms of
- Relapsing fever
- Rat bite fever
- Trypanosomiasis
3. Foot pad of mice is useful to cultivate the *M. leprae*.
4. To demonstrate the ascending & descending tetanus
5. To demonstrate the influenza virus & Chlamydiae
6. Infant suckling mice is useful in virus isolation & identification

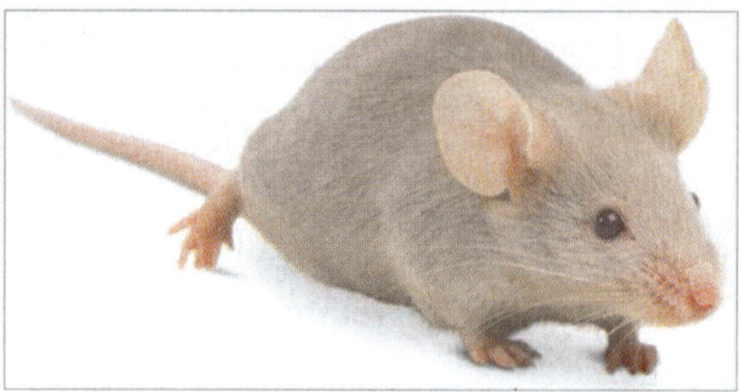

Figure-7: Mouse

F. Sheep:

➢ **Uses:**
1. Sheep blood is useful to prepare the blood agar
2. RBCs of sheep are useful in
- CFT
- Paul Bunnel test
- SRBC (Sheep Red Blood Cells) rosette or E (Erythrocyte) rosette formation with CD2 cells
- EAC (Erythrocyte Antibody Complement) rosette formation with CR2 (Complement Receptor-2)

G. Monkey:

➢ **Use:** Monkey kidney cells **called Vero cells** are useful for viral culture

Question bank

Short notes

1) Animals in microbiology laboratory

Short questions for theory/viva questions

1) Write the two uses of nine banded armadillo/rabbit/guinea pig
2) Name the parasite in which armadillo act as reservoir of infection
3) Write the scientific name of following animals
   Nine banded armadillo, rabbit, guinea pig & black rat

MCQs for chapter review

1) **Scientific name of nine banded armadillo**
   (a) Oryctolagus cuniculus (b) Dasypus novemcinctus (c) Cavia porcelus (d) Rattus rattus
2) **Animal used to demonstrate the anaphylaxis in the lab is** (JIPMER 98)
   (a) Rabbit (b) Adult mice (c) Monkey (d) Guinea pig

Answers of MCQs & explanation

1) **(b)**
- Scientific name of all animals are described in the text.

2) **(b)**
- Guinea pig is the highly susceptible animal to diagnose the anaphylaxis.

17 Miscellaneous topics (World days, Health care related symbols)

Learning heading & subheadings

- World days
- Health care related symbols

World days

Table-1

Diseases	World day	Comment
Tuberculosis	24th March of every year	*M. tuberculosis* was identified & described on 24th March 1882 by Robert Koch
Leprosy	Last Sunday of January in each year	This day was chosen in commemoration of the death of Gandhi, the leader of India who understood the importance of leprosy
Polio	24th Oct. of every year	It was fixed by Rotary International over a decade ago to commemorate the birth of Jonas Salk, who led the first team to develop a vaccine against poliomyelitis.
HIV-AIDS	1st Dec. of every year	Since 1988, 1st Dec is celebrated as an AIDS day to raising awareness of the AIDS pandemic caused by HIV by Josh Lowe & mourning those who have died of the disease
Rabies	28th Sept of every year	It is the anniversary of the death of Louis Pasteur who, with his colleagues, developed the 1st effective rabies vaccine
Hepatitis	28th July of every year	It aims to raise global awareness & to encourage the prevention, diagnosis & treatment of hepatitis A, B, C, D & E
Malaria	25th April of every year	It aims the control of malaria
Health	7th April of every year	It is celebrated under the sponsorship of the WHO, as well as other related organisations

Table-1: World days

✓ **Note:** World health day is one of eight official global health campaigns marked by WHO, along with World tuberculosis day, World immunization week, World malaria day, World no tobacco day, World AIDS day, World blood donor day, and World hepatitis day.

Health care related symbols

Figures-1 to 7

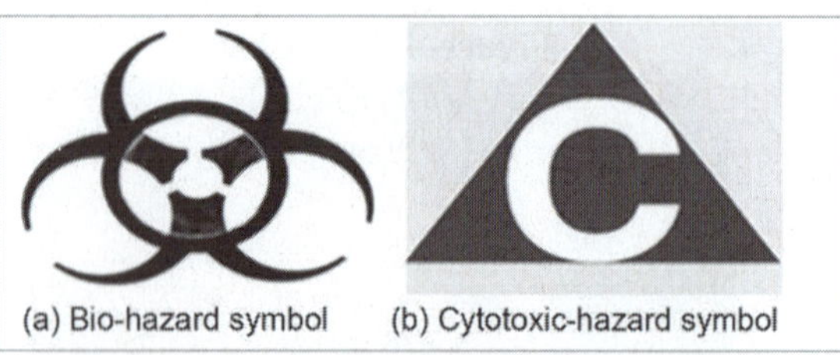
(a) Bio-hazard symbol (b) Cytotoxic-hazard symbol

Figure-1: Bio-hazard symbol & Cytotoxic-hazard symbol

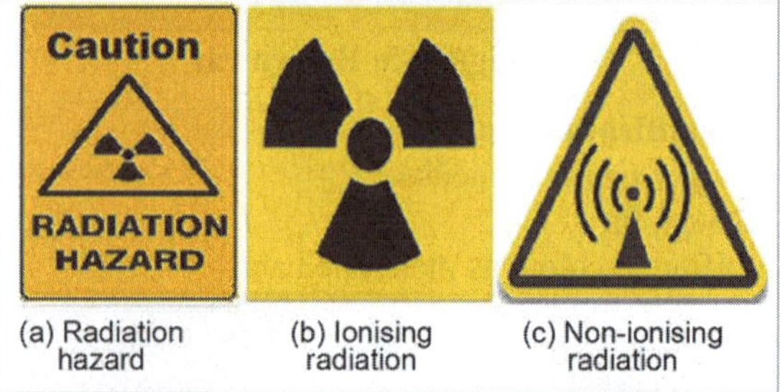

(a) Radiation hazard (b) Ionising radiation (c) Non-ionising radiation

Figure-2: Radiation hazard symbols

Figure-3: Magnetic field symbol

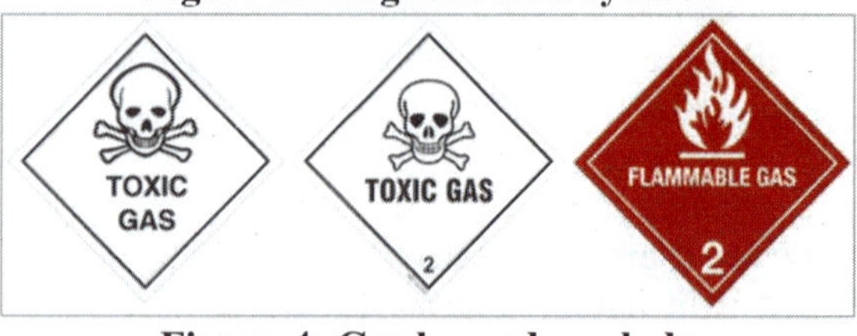

Figure-4: Gas hazard symbols

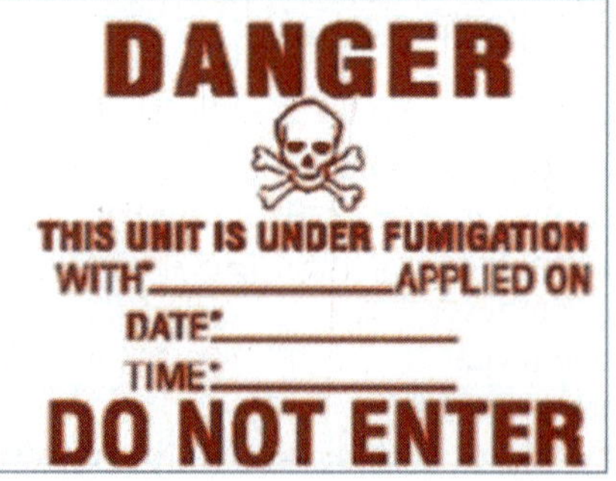

Figure-5: Fumigation symbol

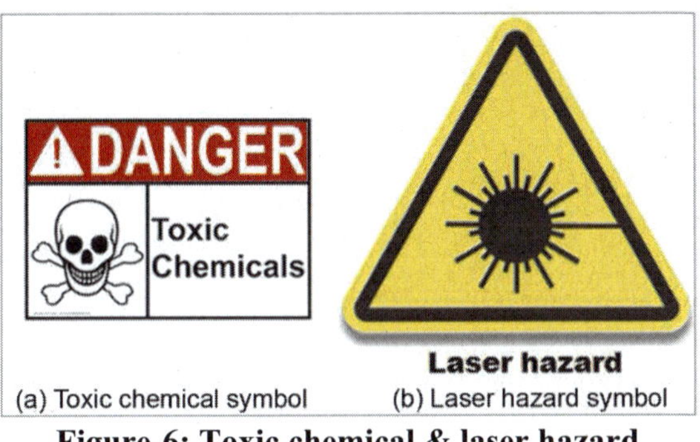

(a) Toxic chemical symbol (b) Laser hazard symbol

Figure-6: Toxic chemical & laser hazard symbols

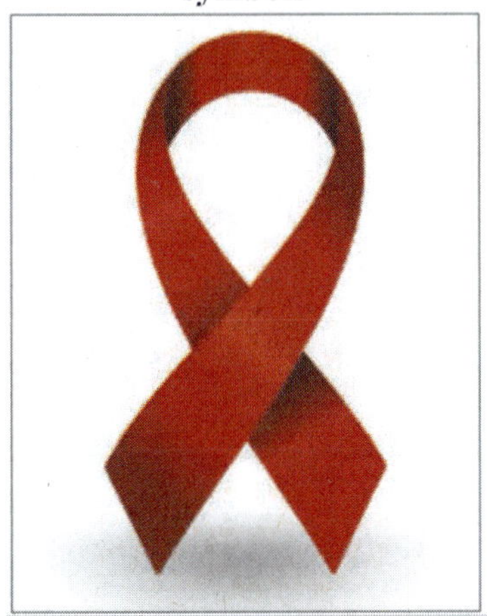

Figure-7: Red ribbon symbol of HIV-AIDS

Question bank

Short questions for theory/viva questions

1) Mention the day/date on which following diseases are celebrated as world day.
- Tuberculosis
- Leprosy
- Rabies
- Malaria

MCQs for chapter review

World days

1) **24th March of every year is celebrated as**
(a) World tuberculosis day (b) World leprosy day (c) World rabies day (d) World malaria day

Health care related symbols

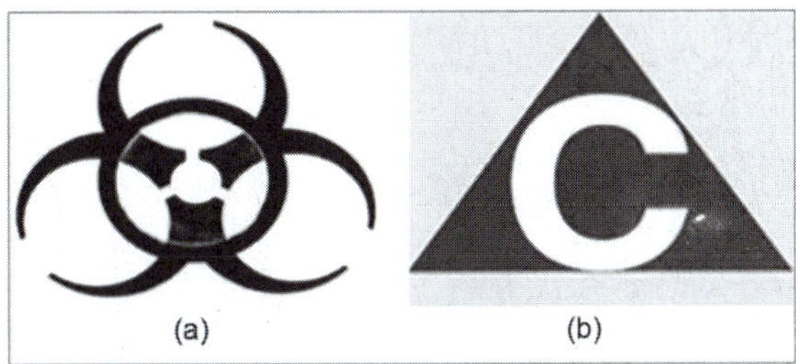
(a) (b)

2) **Symbol shown in above image represent**
(a) a: radiation hazard & b: cytotoxic hazard (b) a: radiation hazard & b: bio hazard (c) a: bio medical waste & b: cytotoxic hazard (d) a: cytotoxic & b: bio medical waste

Answers of MCQs & explanation

1) **(a)**
- Follow section **world days** ***(table-1)*** for explanation

2) **(c)**
- Follow section **health care related symbols (fig.-1 to 7)** for explanation

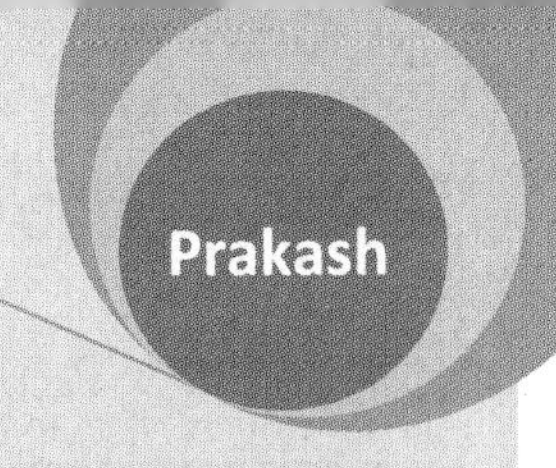

Section II

Immunology

Preview of Immunology

Almost all the serological tests are mentioned by using following common headings & subheadings

- **History:**
- **Principle:**
- **Antigen(s):**
- **Other materials:**
- **Methods / steps:** With test, control & all necessary figures.
- **Result:**
  - **+Ve test:**
  - **-Ve test:**
- **Interpretation:**
- **Uses:**

18 Immunity

Learning heading & subheadings

- ❖ Meaning:
- ❖ Definitions:
- ❖ Types:
- ❖ Measurement of immunity:

❖ **Meaning:** Immunity word originated from **immuntans (latin) = Freedom from disease**.

❖ **Definition:** Resistance exhibited by host towards injury produced by microorganisms and/or their products.

❖ **Types:**

I. Innate (native) immunity:
II. Acquired (adaptive) Immunity:
III. Other types:

I. Innate (native) immunity

➢ **Definition:** Resistance to infection that an individual possesses by virtue of his/her genetic or constitutional make –up.

➢ **Properties:**

- It is the 1st line defence
- No prior contact with microbes (already present before contact with antigen)
- Immunological memory absent
- Active against limited numbers of antigens

➢ **Classification:**

A. Non-specific: Resistance is in general
i. Species:
ii. Racial:
iii. Individual:

B. Specific: Resistance is against the particular agent.
i. Species:
ii. Racial:
iii. Individual:

➢ **Innate immunity at the level of species, racial & individual:**

✪ **Species level:**

- **Definition:** Total or relative resistance to a pathogen shown by all members of species. E.g. human shows resistance to plant pathogens.
- **Mechanisms:** Due to physiological & biochemical differences in between tissues of different species.

✪ **Racial level:**

- **Definition:** Resistance to a pathogen shown by different races of particular species.
- **Examples:**
  - Anthrax resistance in Algerian sheep
  - Peoples of African origin are more susceptible to tuberculosis than Caucasians.
  - Genetic resistance to *P. falciparum* in some parts of Africa & Mediterranean coast.
  - Genetical abnormalities in RBCs (sickle cell anaemia) provide protection against malaria.
- **Mechanisms:** It is genetic origin

✪ **Individual level:**

- **Definition:** Resistance to a pathogen shown by different individuals of particular races.
- **Examples:** Homozygous twins are resistant or susceptible to lepromatous leprosy / tuberculosis. Such correlation is not seen heterozygous twins.
- **Mechanisms:** It is genetic origin

➢ **Effective factors:**

a. Age: Paediatric & old age are more susceptible to infection than adults.

- **Fetus** is protected by placental barrier but some pathogens **(like TORCH agents)** can cross this barrier & cause fetal death.
- HBV infection in **new born** is usually asymptomatic, because of absence of adequate immune response which required setting up the clinical disease.
- **Pre-pubertal girls** are sensitive to Gonococcal infection due to lack of protection in vaginal epithelium.
- Poliomyelitis & chickenpox are more common in **adult stage** due to well developed immune system which causes hypersensitivity & more tissues damage.
- **Older age** are more vulnerable to infection due to waning of immunity & deformities like enlarge prostate which obstruct the urinary flow & favour the UTI.

b. Hormones: Endocrine dysfunctions increase the chances of infection.

- **Diabetes mellitus:** Sugar deposition in tissues favours the *Staphylococcus* infection.
- **Corticosteroids:** It decreases the immunity by
  - Anti phagocytic effect
  - Anti-inflammatory effect
  - Hypersensitivity
  - Reduction of antibodies formation (However steroid neutralise the bacterial products & minimise the damage)

c. Nutrition:

- Malnutrition reduces the CMI & AMI (HI).

- False negative Mantoux test in protein deficiency diseases like kwashiorkor.

➢ **Mechanisms or components of innate immunity:**

A. Anatomical (mechanical) barrier

i. Skin:

- **Mechanical barrier**: Skin acts as barrier to invasion of microbes
- **Chemical barrier:**
  - Skin acts as chemical barrier & provides bactericidal activity due to presence of high salts in dry sweat, sebaceous secretion, long chain fatty acids, acidic pH (5.2-5.9, acidic pH present in vagina, stomach, urine & skin) & soaps.
  - Detection of bactericidal activities of skin:

1. *S. typhi* die in a few minutes when culture placed on skin & cultured at regular interval while *S. typhi* remain unaffected when placed simultaneously on glass surfaces.
2. Frequent washing of hands in soapy water for long periods at occupation leads to pyogenic & mycotic infection.

ii. Mucosa:

- **Mechanical barrier:** Can trap pathogens & prevent the entry.
- Secrete **mucus** which is a protective barrier.
- Mucosal secretion contains **lysozyme**
  - It present in all body secretion/body fluid except CSF, urine & sweats
  - It has powerful digestive abilities that render antigens harmless.
  - It splits the polysaccharide components of bacterial cell wall & provides bactericidal effect.
  - Helps in phagocytosis to form phagolysosome.
- It also secretes **IgA,** which provides local immunity
- **Respiratory mucosa:**
  - If pathogen inhaled they are then sneezed or coughed out or swallowed.
  - Cough reflex is an important defence mechanism.
  - Ciliary movement can propel the particles upward.
  - Mucopolysaccharides in nasal & respiratory epithelium can combine with influenza & other viruses.
  - If microbes reach to alveoli, can killed by phagocytic cells **called Pulmonary Alveolar Microphages (PAMs)**.
- **GIT & genitourinary mucosa:** Also have protective role.

B. Physiological:

i. Hairs: Nasal hairs can trap the pathogens.

ii. Eyes:

- Flushing action of tears (lachrymal secretion) makes the conjunctiva free from foreign particles.
- Tears also contain lysozyme.

iii. Mouth: Saliva, which constantly bathed the mouth, has inhibitory effect on microbes. Also contains lysozyme.

iv. Stomach: Acidity destroys pathogens

v. Urine: Flushing action of urine eliminates the bacteria from urethra.

vi. Semen: Contain antibacterial substances like spermine & zinc.

C. Biochemical: Following are biochemical substances present in blood & tissues having antimicrobial actions

1. **Lysozyme:** →Vide supra
2. **B-lysin:** Active against anthrax & related bacilli
3. **Leukins:** Derived from leucocytes
4. **Plakins:** Derived from platelets
5. **Lactic acid:** Present in muscles, tissues & at inflammatory sites.
6. **Lactoperoxidase:** Present in milk
7. **Properdin:** Present in serum
8. **Integrins:** Present in host cells & help to attach the host cell with extra cellular matrix like attachment of host cell with adenovirus, HFMD virus, ECHO virus & hantavirus
9. **Interferon (IFN):**
   - Antiviral properties
   - More details: **Follow chapter → Viral-Host interections**
10. **Others like:** Lactoferrin, transferrin, Tumour Necrosis Factors-α (TNF-α), fibronectin, oligosaccharides, Antibodies etc.

D. Microbiological

i. Normal microbial flora of vagina: Acidic pH due to glycogen fermentation by Doderlein's bacilli (*Lactobacillus*) in vagina keeps vagina healthy.

ii. Normal flora in GIT: *E. coli* & other intestinal flora can prevent the microbial colonisation by competing with pathogens for nutrition & adhesion.

E. Immunological

i. Complement system

- It act by activation of alternative pathway by bacterial endotoxin & Lectin pathway or Mannose Binding Lectin (MBL) pathway by combination with mannose residues present on microbial surface (like *Salmonella, Neisseria, Listeria, C. neoformans* & *C. albicans*)
- Following activation complement mediated lysis is take place by formation of pores on bacterial surface or by secretion of inflammatory mediators.

ii. Reticulo Endothelial (RE) system (RE cells): **Follow chapter → Structure and functions of immune system**

iii. Null cell or **Large Granular Lymphocyte (LGL):** **Follow chapter → Structure and functions of immune system**

iv. Pattern Recognition Receptors (PRRs):

- **Definitions:** Receptors on different cells recognise the unique molecular pattern of pathogens **called Pathogen Associated Molecular Patterns**

(PAMPs) & such receptors **called Pattern Recognition Receptors (PRRs).**

- **Types:** Three types of PRPs

1. **Toll-Like Receptors (TLRs):**
- Certain cell associated receptors involved in innate immunity have ability to recognise & to destroy the unique molecules of microbes and prevent the microbial invasion **called Toll-like receptors**.
- They are present on phagocytic cells like dendritic cells & macrophages & helps in phagocytosis.
- There are 13 TLRs.

2. **Scavenger receptors:**
- Bind with LPS, peptidoglycan of bacterial cell wall & also with infected, injured or apoptotic cells.
- Includes CD-36, CD-68 & SRB-1

3. **Mannose receptors:** Present on phagocytic cells & binds with mannose rich glycans of microbes

F. Pathological

i. Inflammation: Inflammation starts following biological or any other types of injuries & it provides defence by

a. Outpouring of plasma: It dilutes the toxic products.

b. Increase blood flow: Improving blood flow at the site by vascular constriction & dilatation.

c. Fibrin barrier: Formation of fibrin barrier which localise the infection

d. Phagocytosis: Recruiting phagocytes at the site, leading to phagocytosis of microbes

e. Acute phase response (acute phase reaction):

- **Definitions:** Change in the concentration of many proteins following inflammation **called acute phase proteins** or **acute phase reactants** and this response **called acute phase response** or **acute phase reaction**
- **Properties:**
- Synthesises mostly by liver & rare by endothelial cells, fibroblasts, monocytes & adipocytes.
- All these acute phase proteins have antimicrobial & anti-inflammatory actions.
- They also have chelating action for iron, copper making them unavailable for bacteria.
- **Types & examples:** Two types with increasing synthesis **called positive acute phase proteins** & decreasing synthesis **called negative acute phase proteins**

1. **Positive acute phase proteins:** Like
- C - reactive protein (CRP): **Follow chapter → Pneumococcus**
- Mannose binding protein
- Serum amyloid P components
- α-1-acid glycoprotein
- α-2 microglobulin
- Coagulation proteins: fibrinogen, prothrombin, von Willebrand factor, factor VIII
- Hepatoglobin
- D-dimer protein
- Ferritin
- Ceruloplasmin
- Complement factors

2. **Negative acute phase proteins:** Like
- Albumin & prealbumin
- Transferin
- Transthyretin
- Transcortin
- Antithrombin
- Retinol binding protein

- **Synthesis of acute phase proteins: → Flow chart-1**

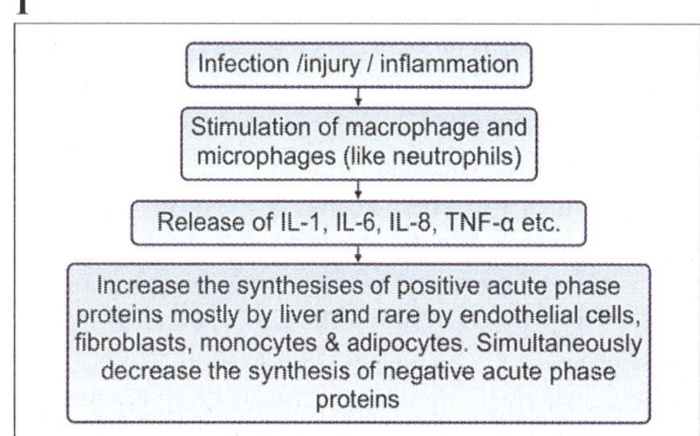

Flow chart-1: Synthesis of acute phase proteins

ii. Fever: Rise in temperature following injuries provides defence by
- Acceleration of physiological process
- Antiviral action: Increase interferon production
- Antibacterial action over certain bacteria like *T. pallidum* (Therapeutic fever induction was used to treat syphilis before penicillin became available)

II. Acquired (adaptive) immunity

- **Definition:** Resistance to infection that an individual acquire during life.
- **Properties:**
- It is the 2nd line defence
- Developed after contact with antigens
- Antigenic specificity: Differentiation between two different proteins or antigens.
- Immunological memory present: It remember the previous type of antigenic attack which helps to elicit strong immune response in subsequent antigenic attack
- Active against wide range of antigens
- Differentiation between self & non-self: It eliminates the foreign particle without disturbing the self particles. Self tolerance is the unique properties of immune system. Failure to this can cause autoimmune diseases.
- **Mechanisms or components of acquired immunity:**

1. **Antibody Mediated Immunity(AMI) / Humoral Immunity(HI):** By production of antibody from B cells (plasma cells)

2. **Cell Mediated Immunity(CMI):** By cell stimulation & production of cytokines (lymphokines) from T cells
3. **Classical complement pathway:** Follow chapter → Complement system
4. **Antigen presenting cells (APCs):** Follow chapter → Structure and functions of immune system

✓ **Notes:** Many components of innate & acquired immunity like APC, complement, null cell (ADCC) etc. are interconnected in both types of immunity & make the bridge between two.

➢ **Classification:**

✪ **Types:** Three types

A. **Active immunity:**

B. **Passive immunity:**

C. **Combined immunity:**

✪ **Differences between active & passive immunity:** As shown in **table-1**

Active immunity	Passive immunity
More effective & better protection	Less effective & less protective
Produced actively by host's immune system	Transferred passively, no active participation by host's immune system
Induced by infection or vaccination	Readymade Ab is transferred
Immunity developed after effective lag period	Immediate protection
Immunological memory present & booster effect in subsequent dose (secondary response)	No memory & subsequent dose is less effective (no secondary response)
Long lasting immunity	Transient immunity
-Ve phase may occur	No -Ve phase
Not applicable in immunodeficient persons	Applicable in immunodeficient persons

Table-1: Differences between active & passive immunity

A. **Active immunity:**

- **Definition:** Resistance developed due to antigenic stimulation.
- **Sub types:** Two subtypes as described below

a. **Natural:**

- o Definition: Resistance developed due to infection.
- o Examples:

1. **Viral infection:** Some viral infection provide long lasting or lifelong immunity like polio, measles, chickenpox while some viral infection provide short lived immunity like Influenzae.
2. **Bacterial infection:** Immunity following bacterial infection is short lived unlike viral infection; however some bacteria like *S. typhi* provide durable protection.
3. **Parasitic infection:** High level of Ig is found in some parasitic infection is protective & helps in recovery of diseases.
4. **Fungal infection:** In most of the fungal infection protection is achieved by CMI while AMI little or rare useful.

b. **Artificial:**

- o Definition: Resistance developed by administration of immunising agents (immunisation).
- o Examples:
  - Vaccine
  - Toxoids

B. **Passive immunity:**

- **Definition:** Resistance transmitted in readymade form.
- **Sub types:** Two subtypes as described below

a. **Natural:**

- o Definition: Resistance transmitted from mother to baby
- o Examples:

1. **Colostrum:** Rich in IgA & provides protection to neonate.
2. **Maternal antibodies:**
   - **IgG:** can transfer through placenta & provides passive protection to foetus against virus or toxin.
   - **IgM** develops at 22nd week of gestational age but it is not able to give protection. Infant immune system start to develop at 3rd month of life until then infant is passively protected by maternal antibodies.
   - Injection of **Tetanus Toxoid (TT)** to mother during pregnancy minimise the chances of neonatal tetanus due to passive transfer of antibodies. It is recommended in communities in which neonatal tetanus is common.

b. **Artificial:**

- o Definition: Resistance transmitted to recipient by administration of antibodies.
- o Examples:
  - Development of immunity after administration of antisera, antitoxin & Ig.
  - For more details: Follow chapter → Immunising agents and National immunisation schedule

C. **Combined immunity:**

- **Definition:** It is a combination of active & passive immunisation.
- **Uses:** In some disease like tetanus where TIG (Tetanus Immuno Globulin) is injected in one arm & TT in other arm followed by full course of TT. TIG provides passive protection till the active immunity will start by TT.

III. Other types

A. **Adoptive immunity:**

✪ **Definition:** Passive transfer of CMI achieved by administration of viable immunological competent lymphocytes **called adoptive immunity**.

✪ **Transfer factor:**

- Instead of whole immunological competent lymphocyte, only it's extract is used for administration **called transfer factor**.
- For more details: **Follow chapter → Immune response (Ir)**

B. Local (mucosal) immunity:

- **History:** Concept of local immunity was 1st proposed by Besredka
- **Definition:** When particular cells or tissues are targeted by certain pathogens, they produce the immunity against such pathogens **called local immunity**
- **Principle:** It based on production of IgA **called secretory IgA**, by plasma cells present in mucosa & by secretory glands in breast.
- **Uses:** For immunisation in some diseases.

1. **Poliomyelitis:**
   - Injectable (killed) polio vaccine provides systemic immunity & prevents the blood stream infection but it does not provide local (intestinal) immunity and not able to prevents the virus multiplication in GIT mucosa & faecal shedding of virus.
   - Local (intestinal) immunity is achieved by administration of oral (live) polio vaccine or by natural infection
2. **Influenza:**
   - Injectable (killed) vaccine provides systemic immunity and prevents the blood stream infection but it does not provide local (respiratory) immunity and not able to prevents the virus multiplication in respiratory mucosa.
   - Local (respiratory) immunity is achieved by administration of intranasal (live) vaccine or by natural infection

C. Herd immunity:

- **Definition:** Mass immunity in community to prevent the epidemic diseases.
- **Effective factors:**

1. **Immunisation to herd:**
2. **Herd structure:** It includes population, animals, vectors & all those environmental & social factors which favour or inhibit the spread of infection.
3. **Infection:** Occurrence of clinical/subclinical infection in herd

- **Uses:**

1. **Prevention of epidemic diseases:** When herd immunity is high, spread of epidemic diseases is less & it is in mild form or **vice –versa**.
2. **Eradication of diseases:** Development of high level of herd immunity by means of active artificial immunisation helps to eradicate the certain diseases like polio, diphtheria.

D. Premunition:

- **Synonym:** Infection immunity or concomitant immunity
- **Definition:** "Relative resistance offered by host to re-infection already harbouring the microbes."
- **Properties:** Immunity to re-infection lasts as long as active infection is present, once active infection cured patients become susceptible to subsequent infection by same organisms.
- **Infection in which premunition occurs:** It occurs in syphilis, malaria & schistosomiasis

E. Ring immunity:

- **Synonym:** Ring vaccination
- **Definition:** The vaccination of all susceptible individuals in a prescribed area around an outbreak of an infectious disease.
- **Principle:** The idea is to form a buffer of immune individuals to prevent the spread of the disease.
- **Uses:**

a. **Monitoring a ring of people around each infected individual.**

b. **In control of outbreak of following diseases:**

1. **Small pox:** Ring vaccination was used to control smallpox until the last naturally occurring case in 1977. When an infection was diagnosed, all people who were or may have been exposed were identified and vaccinated. Then, a second "ring" of people who may have been exposed to the first ring were also identified and vaccinated. Ring vaccination was also recommended by the American Academy of Paediatrics (IAP) in 2002 for smallpox, should there be another outbreak (from terrorism or whatever).
2. **Foot-and-mouth disease** in livestock in the UK. Also known as surveillance & containment
3. **Polio:** When a case of polio is detected all children less than 5 years of age within a radius of 5 km are immunized within 24-48 hours. The repeat extra dose is given to the same children after one month. The ring immunization drive arrests the spread of wild virus and creates a film of vaccine virus in the community.

F. Tolerance: Cessation of clinical phenomenon despite infection by microbes (Infection to host without any adverse effect & host become resistant to reinfection)

❖ **Measurement of immunity:** It is very difficult to measure the exact level of immunity, but some useful methods for AMI & CMI detection are described in chapter of immune response (Ir)

Question bank

Essay/Full question

1) Immunity

Short notes

1) Mechanisms of innate immunity
2) Acquired immunity

Short questions for theory/viva questions

1) Write the four differences between active & passive immunity
2) What is local immunity / herd immunity / ring immunity?
3) What is premonition?

MCQs for chapter review

Innate immunity

1) **All of the following are part of the innate immunity except-** (AIIMS, May-05)
(a) Complement (b) NK cells (c) Macrophages (d) T cells
2) **Lysozyme is present in the following secretion of the body all except-** (PGI-94)
(a) Lacrimal secretion (b) CSF (c) Saliva (d) Respiratory tract secretions
3) **All are true about innate immunity except-**
(a) Non-specific (b) First line of defence (c) Not affected genetically (d) Include complement
4) **Components of innate immunity are-** (PGI, Noc-10)
(a) T lymphocytes (b) Complement proteins (c) B lymphocytes (d) NK cells (e) Integrins
5) **First chemical barrier encountered by microorganisms for common exposed sites-** (AIIMS, Noc-11)
(a) Lysozyme (b) Acidic pH (c) Skin (d) Lactose
6) **Acute phase reactions in acute inflammation are-** (PGI, June-03)
(a) Albumin (b) Fibrinogen (c) Hepatoglobulin (d) Gammaglobulin
7) **Acute phase reactants are except-** (PGI, June-03)
(a) C-reactive protein (b) Hepatoglobulin (c) Endothelium (d) Fibrinogen
8) **Pro-inflammatory cytokines includes all except**
(a) IL-1 (b) IL-2 (c) IL-6 (d) TNF-α

Acquired (adaptive) immunity

9) **Active immunity is not acquired by:**
(a) Infection (b) Vaccination (c) Ig transfer (d) Subclinical infection
10) **Active immunity can be induced by** (PGI, May-13)
(a) Toxoids (b) Subclinical infection (c) Antitoxin (d) Immunoglobulin (e) Antigen exposure
11) **Type immunity conferred on an individual by vaccination is**
(a) Artificial active (b) Artificial passive (c) Natural active (d) Natural passive
12) **True about active immunity:** (AI -93)
(a) Less effective (b) Can be given in immunodeficient person (c) Immunological memory present (d) No lag period
13) **True about passive immunity:** (AI -93)
(a) Cannot b given with active immunity (b) Last for 4-5 days (c) It can be given before disease occurrence (d) Can be transferred by antibodies from another host (e) Takes long time to develop

Answers of MCQs & explanation

1) **(d)**
- Alternative pathway & lectin pathway of complement, NK cells (one type of null cell) & macrophages (one type of phagocytic cell) are part of innate immunity while T cells is responsible for CMI & part of acquired immunity

2) **(b)**
- Lysozyme is present in all body secretion/body fluid except CSF, urine & sweats

3) **(c)**
- Innate immunity is due to genetic or constitutional make –up of an individual

4) **(b), (d) & (e)**
- Follow section, **innate immunity (Mechanisms or components of innate immunity)** for explanation

5) **(b)**
- Skin acts as chemical barrier & provides bactericidal activity due to presence of high salts in dry sweat, sebaceous secretion, long chain fatty acids, acidic pH (5.2-5.9, acidic pH present in vagina, stomach, urine & skin) & soaps.

6) **(a), (b) & (c)**
7) **(c)**

} Follow section **innate immunity [Mechanisms or components of innate immunity → Acute phase response (acute phase reaction)]** for explanation

8) **(b)**
- Follow section, **acute phase response (flow chart-1)** for more explanation.

9) **(c)**
- Ig transfer provide an artificial passive immunity

10) **(a), (b) & (e)**
- Introduction of
  - Toxoids induced artificial active immunity
  - Subclinical infection induced natural active immunity
  - Antitoxin & Immunoglobulin induced artificial passive immunity
  - Antigen exposure like vaccine induced artificial active immunity

11) **(a)**
- Artificialmactive immunity is achieved by administration of vaccine & toxoids.

12) **(c)**
13) **(c) & (d)**

} Follow section, **acquired immunity [table-1]** for explanation

19 Immunising agents and National immunisation schedule

Learning heading & subheadings

Immunising agents

National immunisation schedule

Immunising agents

❖ **Types:** Two types of immunising agents

I. **Used for artificial active immunisation (Immunoprophylaxis)**

II. **Used for artificial passive immunisation (Immunotherapy)**

III. **Used for combined immunisation**

I. Used for artificial active immunisation (Immunoprophylaxis)

A. Vaccines:

- **Definition:** Biological products, acts by reinforcing the immunological defence of the body against foreign particles.
- **History:** Vaccine word derived from **Vacca (Latin) = cow**, because 1st such biological product (prophylactic preparation) was prepared by **Edward Jenner** for smallpox disease from pox lesion in cow. Later **Louis Pasteur** coined term vaccine for such biological product (prophylactic preparation).
- **Principle:** After the primary immune response to the pathogen, B cells are differentiated to plasma cells & memory cells. Memory cells lie dormant in immune system; they detect the same pathogen later on & mount strong & rapid immune response. This makes the basis of vaccine development. Vaccine contains antigen/pathogen which induces the production of memory cells & provide strong & rapid protection if same antigen/pathogen encountered later on.
- **Types:** Following are the different types

i. Live attenuated vaccines:

✪ **Preparation:**

- Vaccines contain a living microbe that has been weakened (attenuated) in the laboratory, so it can't cause disease.
- Vaccine is prepared
  - From natural virus (Jenner's smallpox vaccine) or
  - By serial passage in cells/tissues (yellow fever) or
  - By plaque selection (OPV)
  - From ts mutant (influenza)
  - By recombination technique (influenza)

✪ **Advantages:**

1. Vaccine is the closest thing to a natural infection; these vaccines are good "teachers" of the immune system: They elicit strong AMI & CMI.
2. Confer strong & lifelong immunity with only one or two doses, except OPV where three or more doses are required.
3. Administered by natural route of infection, so provide both systemic & local immunity. E.g. oral polio vaccine, intranasal polio vaccine
4. Used for mass immunisation (Herd immunity)
5. Given in combination (MMR vaccine)

✪ **Disadvantages:**

1. But they may not be safe for use in immunocompromised individuals
2. Live attenuated organisms may rarely mutate to a virulent form and cause disease. (disease to contact)
3. Heat labile & inactivated if temperature is not maintained during storage & transportation.
4. More difficult to create for bacteria because they have thousands of genes, thus hard to control, while

easy for viruses because viruses are simple microbes containing a small number of genes.

5. Cause immediate (local & systemic) & remote complications.

✪ **Contraindications:**

1. Person with immunodeficiency status
2. Pregnancy

ii. Killed/ inactivated vaccines:

✪ **Preparation:**

- Microbes are inactivated by treatment with chemicals [Phenol, BPL (Beta Propio Lactone), formaldehyde or formalin], heat or radiation.
- However UV-radiation is unsatisfactory because of risk of multiplicity reactivation.

✪ **Advantages:**

1. More stable &safe than live vaccines because the dead microbes can't mutate back to their disease-causing state.
2. No disease to contact
3. Don't require refrigeration, can be easily stored and transported.
4. Given in combination with polyvalent vaccine

✪ **Disadvantages:**

1. Not or poor induction of CMI.
2. Weaker immune response than live vaccines. So it would likely take several additional dose or booster dose to maintain a person's immunity.
3. Short lived immunity
4. Provides only systemic but not local immunity.

✪ **Contraindication:** If severe local or systemic side effect to previous doses

✪ **Differences between live & killed vaccine:** → **Table-1**

Features	Killed	live vaccine
Numbers of dose	Multiple	Mostly single
Need of adjuvant	Yes	No
Immunity	Short lived	Long lived
Protection	Less	More
Ig produced	IgG	IgA & IgG
Local (Mucosal) immunity	No	Yes
CMI	Poor/no	Yes
Reversion to virulence	No	Yes
Excretion of vaccine microbes & transmission to non-immune contacts	No	Yes
Interference by other virus in host	No	Yes
Heat stability	No	Yes
Temp. maintenance during storage & transport	No	Yes

Table-1: Differences between live & killed vaccine

iii. Toxoid vaccines:

✪ **Preparation:**

- These vaccines are used when a bacterial toxin like *Cl. tetani, C. diphtheriae* etc. is the causative agent.
- Detoxification of toxins (exotoxin) by treating with formalin **called toxoid**.
- When the immune system receives a toxoid, it learns how to fight off the natural toxin. The immune system produces antibodies that lock onto and block the toxin.

✪ **Advantages:** Safe & effective protection

✪ **Differences between toxins & toxoid:** Toxin has toxicity & antigenicity while toxoid has no toxicity but only antigenicity.

iv. Cellular fraction/subunit /acellular vaccines:

✪ **Definition:** Instead of the entire microbe (whole-agent vaccine), a fragment (subunit) of it can create an immune response.

✪ **Preparation:**

- It prepared by growing the microbe in the laboratory & then uses chemicals to break it apart and gather the important antigens.
- Subunit vaccines include only the antigens or epitope (the very specific parts of the antigen) which best stimulate the immune system.
- Subunit vaccines may be
  - Monovalent contain one antigen (single strain)
  - Polyvalent contains 20 or more antigens (multiple strains). Of course, identifying which antigens best stimulate the immune system is a tricky & time-consuming process.
- Cellular parts/antigens used are:
  - PRP Ag (capsular polysaccharide type b Ag/Hib PRP) in *H. influenzae*
  - Pertusis vaccine (combine with DPT)
  - Capsular polysaccharide Ag in pneumococci
  - Capsular polysaccharide Ag in meningococci
  - Hemagglutinin and neuraminidase subunits of the *Influenzavirus*.
  - Capsid protein in Human Papilloma Virus (HPV).
  - All antigenic components of HBsAg (Pre-S1, Pre-S2 & S) in HBV

✪ **Advantage:** Because subunit vaccines contain only the essential antigens & not the entire microbe, the chances of adverse reactions to the vaccine are less.

v. Conjugate vaccines:

✪ **Preparation:**

- Sometimes bacterial polysaccharide is poorly immunogenic in children below 2 years, it's immunogenicity is increased by coupling with protein carrier like toxin, toxoid or antigen.
- PRP Ag in Hib is conjugated with diphtheria toxoid or tetanus toxoid or with meningococcal Outer Membrane Protein (OMP) Ag.

vi. Recombinant (cloned) vaccines:

✪ **Preparation:**

- Cloning the desired antigen or gene in bacteria (e.g. *E. coli*) or in yeast (Baker's yeast) is the new concept of recombinant technology (genetic engineering) to prepare the vaccine.

- Cloned vaccine currently used is HBV vaccine, prepared by cloning the S gene in Baker's yeast.
- Also prepared in Influenza virus by hybridisation of antigen of newer strain &established strain

✪ **Advantages:**

1. Couldn't cause the disease because it wouldn't contain the microbe, just copies of a few of its genes.
2. Strong antibody response.

✪ **Disadvantage:** Expensive

vii. Future prospects of vaccines:

Types	Examples
Live attenuated vaccines	**Bacterial vaccines:** BCG Typhoid oral Epidemic typhus **Viral vaccines:** Oral Polio Vaccine (OPV/Sabin), Measles Mumps Rubella Chickenpox Influenza (nasal spray) Rotavirus Yellow fever (17D)
Inactivated or killed vaccines	**Bacterial vaccines:** Typhoid Cholera Pertusis Meningococcal meningitis Plague **Viral vaccines:** Injectable Polio Vaccine(IPV/Salk) Hepatitis A Hepatitis B Influenza Kyasnur Forest Disease Japanese Encephalitis (JE) HDCV of rabies
Toxoid (inactivated toxin)	Diphtheria Tetanus
Cellular fraction / subunit / acellular vaccines	**Bacterial vaccines:** *H. influenzae* type b (Hib PRP vaccine) Pertussis (part of DTP combined immunization) Pneumococcal (capsular vaccine) Meningococcal (capsular vaccine) **Viral vaccines:** *Influenzavirus* (injection), HBV & HPV
Conjugate vaccines	*H. influenzae* type b (Hib)
Recombinant (Cloned) vaccine	Hepatitis B Influenza virus

Table-2: Types & examples of vaccine

✪ **Naked DNA vaccines:** Naked DNA is injected in body

➢ **Examples of different types vaccine: →Table-2**

➢ **Administration of vaccines:** The method of introduction of vaccine **called vaccination** while the protection offered to body after vaccination **called immunisation**. Vaccination does not guarantee immunisation. Vaccines are available & administered as plain or in mixed form, as follows

i. Plain / single / monovalent / univalent vaccines:

✪ **Definition:** It is designed to immunize against a single antigen (serotype) or single strain or single microorganism

✪ **Examples:** TT, BCG vaccine, monovalent meningococcal vaccine contains single capsular polysaccharide of group A or C etc.

ii. Mixed / combined / polyvalent / multivalent vaccines:

✪ **Definition:** It is designed to immunize against two or more strains of the same microorganism or two or more antigens (serotypes) of the same microorganism or against two or more microorganisms

✪ **Examples:**

- **Double / bivalent vaccine:** DT, DP etc.
- **Triple / trivalent / tetravalent vaccine:** DPT (DTP), MMR etc.
- **Quadruple / quadrivalent vaccine:** DPT (DTP) with Hib etc.
- **Pentavalent vaccine:** Two type of preparations

- **Pentvac** contains Diphtheria, Pertusis, Tetanus, HBV, H. influenza type b (Hib)
- **Pentaxim** contains D, P, T, IPV & Hib

✪ **Advantages of mixed vaccine over plain vaccine:**

- Simple administration
- Low cost
- Minimise the hospital visit

➢ **Adjuvant:**

- **Meaning:** From Latin adiuvare – to help
- **Definition:** Adjuvants are substances that are added to vaccine to increase the antigenicity / immune response.
- **Advantages:** Less amount of Ag & less number of doses are required.
- **Common adjuvants**:

o <u>Aluminium adjuvants:</u> Aluminium phosphate, aluminium hydroxide & aluminium sulphate

o <u>Freund's incomplete adjuvant:</u> Water-in-oil → incorporation of protein Ag in water phase of water-in-oil emulsion.

o <u>Bacteria</u>: Like

- *Propionibacterium acne*
- *B. pertusis*: Used in DPT (antibody response to toxoid is potentiated by *B. pertusis*).

o <u>BCG:</u>

o <u>Adjuvants for laboratory animals:</u>

- Freund's complete adjuvant: water-in-oil with *Nocardia* Ag or *Mycobacteria* Ag.
- Bacterial endotoxin (LPS)
- Vitamin A in toxic dose
- Fungal polysaccharide
- **Mechanisms for immune enhancement by adjuvants:** Exact mechanisms are not known but it may be as below
  - Protection of Ag: Provide protection to Ag, which allow slow releases antigen for loner time. (depot generation)
  - Recruitment of APCs: By recruiting of professional Antigen-Presenting Cells (APCs) to the site of antigen exposure., which enhance the immunogenicity leading to improve the immune response
  - Enhancement of innate & acquired (adaptive) immunity:
- Adjuvants are interfere with Pattern Recognition Receptors (PRRs) specially Toll-Like receptors to increase the innate immunity
- Immunomodulation by local granuloma formation leads to cytokine production which attract T & B cells at the site of infection to increase the acquired (adaptive) immunity
- Innate & acquired (adaptive) immunity are linked with each others, so adjuvant mediate enhance of one can encourage the other immunity.

➢ **Adverse reactions:** Two types

a. **Local:** Pain, swelling/induration, ulceration, scar etc.

b. **Systemic:**

1. **Hypersensitivity:** Like anaphylaxis, serum sickness etc.
2. **General symptoms:** Fever, headache, acute flaccid paralysis by polio vaccine, anxiety etc.

II. Used for artificial passive immunisation (Immunotherapy)

➢ **Types, preparation & example of passive immunising agents:**

A. **Antisera (antiserum):**

✪ **Preparation:** Prepared by injecting (hyperimmune sera) the specific antigen in animal like horse or in human that leads to antibody formation.

✪ **Example:** Rabies antiserum

B. **Antitoxin:**

✪ **Preparation:** Prepared by injecting (hyperimmune sera) the toxin or toxoid in animal like horse or in human that leads to formation of antitoxin.

✪ **Examples:** ATS (Anti tetanus Serum), ADS (Anti Diphtheria Serum), AGS (Anti Gas gangrene Serum), ASV (Anti Snake Venom)

C. **Immunoglobulin (Ig):**

✪ **Ig subtypes:** Two subtypes

i. **Normal human Ig (non specific human Ig):**

- **Preparation:** Prepared from pooled sera of at least thousand healthy adults.
- **Example:** Ig for measles & HAV.

ii. **Specific human Ig:**

- **Preparation:** Prepared by two ways

1. **Convalescent sera:** Prepared from patients recovered from infectious diseases.
2. **Hyperimmune sera:** Prepared from hyperimmune animal like horse or from human

- **Examples:** Rabies Ig, HBV Ig, Tetanus Ig, Diphtheria Ig, Rh-D Ig,

✪ **Ig administration:**

- Route: By IM or IV route
- Dose: 5ml, if more than divided in 4-6 intragluteal sites.
- IM injection is painful, overcome by mixing 1 part of procaine with 10 parts of Ig.

➢ **Indication of passive immunising agents:**

1. **Instant passive immunity:** In emergencies where immediate & temporary protection is needed in some clinical conditions like tetanus, diphtheria, snake bite, rabies, HAV, HBV, measles etc.
2. **Suppression of active immunity:** E.g. in Rh –Ve mother with Rh +Ve babies
3. **Immunodeficiency diseases:**

➢ **Disadvantages of passive immunising agents:**

1. **Immune elimination:** Which limits the passive immunisation
2. **Hypersensitivity reaction:** Like serum sickness, anaphylaxis mostly with animal preparation, overcome by using human preparation.

III. Combined immunisation

➢ **Combination of active (immunoprophylaxis) & passive (immunotherapy) immunisation:** In some disease like diphtheria, tetanus, snake bite, rabies, HAV, HBV, measles etc. passive immunisation is prescribed with active immunisation with aim to start instant immunity till the active immunity will develop.

➢ **Examples:**

- In some disease like tetanus where TIG (Tetanus Immuno Globulin) is injected in one arm & TT in other arm followed by full course of TT.
- TIG provides passive protection till the active immunity will start by TT.

National immunisation schedule

❖ **Introduction:**

- In May 1974 WHO launched the global immunisation programme **called Expanded Programme on Immunisation (EPI)** against 6 Vaccine Preventable Diseases (VPDs) like Diphtheria, Pertusis (Whooping cough), Tetanus, Polio, Tuberculosis and Measles.

- Different countries employ the immunization schedule according to their priorities

❖ **Routine immunisation:** EPI was launched in India in January 1978 **called Indian national immunisation schedule** as shown in **table-3**

Age	Vaccines
Birth	BCG, OPV-0
6 weeks	BCG (if not given at birth) DPT-1,OPV-1, Hepatitis B -1
10 weeks	DPT-2, OPV-2, Hepatitis B -2
14 weeks	DPT-3, OPV-3, Hepatitis B-3
9 months	Measles
18-24 months	DPT & OPV
5-6 years	DT (second dose of DT after 1 month if not previously immunized by DPT)
10-16 years	TT (second dose of TT after 1 month if not previously immunized by DPT, DT or TT)
For pregnant women	TT1 or booster in early pregnancy TT2 one month after

Table-3: Indian national immunisation schedule

✓ Notes:

1. Interval between DPT,OPV, Hepatitis B should not be less1 month
2. Minor cough, fever, colds are not the contraindication of vaccine
3. In some state combined vaccine **(Pentvac)** contains Diphtheria, Pertusis, Tetanus, HBV, H. influenza type b (Hib) is given at 6th weeks, 10th weeks & 14th weeks with OPV. Other same preparation is **Pentaxim** contains D, P, T, IPV & Hib given with OPV & HBV.
4. After primary immunisation of DPT at 6, 10 & 14 weeks, 1st booster of DPT is given at 18-24 months followed by 2nd booster dose (DT only) at 5-6 year (school entry age)
5. Severity of pertusis is decrease with age, so DPT vaccine is usually not recommended after 5 year, but only double (DT) vaccine is advised.
6. Vitamin A given at 9th, 18th, 24th, 30th, 36th month.

❖ **Individual Immunisation:**

- Some vaccines are available but they are not the part of immunisation schedule due to high cost. These are **called newer vaccines.**
- They are prescribed after consultation with parents.
- Examples: Following are the examples of vaccine given as an individual immunisation

1. **Varicella:** 15 months or after 1 year
2. **HAV:** High risk infant, 18 months & 6 months later
3. **Pneumococcal conjugate vaccine:** 6 weeks
4. **Influenza vaccine:**
5. **Typhoid vaccine:**
6. **MMR vaccine:**

❖ **Immunisation schedule by IAP:** The Indian Academy of Paediatrics (IAP) recommends inclusion of more vaccines in the immunisation schedule. These vaccines are not includes in national immunisation schedule due to high cost. Immunisation schedule approved by IAP is as follows.

- **BCG:** At birth-2weeks
- **OPV:** At 6th weeks, 10th weeks, 14th weeks, 16-18 months & 5 years
- **DPT:** At 6th weeks, 10th weeks, 14th weeks, 16-18 months & 5 years
- **Hepatitis B:** At 6th weeks, 10th weeks & 14th weeks or birth, 6th weeks & 14th weeks.
- **Hib Conjugate:** At 6th, 10th & 14th weeks
- **Measles:** At 9 months
- **MMR:** At 15 months
- **Typhoid:** At 2 years, 5 years, 8 years & 12 years
- **TT:** At 10 or 16 years (second dose of TT after 1 month if not previously immunized by DPT, DT or TT & 1st booster dose after 1 year)
- **TT:** 2 doses at 1 month interval in pregnant women or booster in early pregnancy if immunised earlier.

Question bank

Essay/Full question

1) Immunising agents

Short notes

1) Vaccine
2) National immunisation schedule

Short questions for theory/viva questions

1) Write the two examples of each, live attenuated bacterial & viral vaccines.
2) Write four differences between live & killed vaccine
3) What is toxin & toxoid?
4) What is adjuvant?

MCQs for chapter review

Immunising agents

1) **Vaccination is based on the principle of** (AI-12)
(a) Agglutination (b) Phagocytosis (c) Immunological memory (d) Clonal detection
2) **BCG vaccine is a type of**
(a) Killed vaccine (b) Conjugate (c) Live attenuated (d) Recombinant
3) **Cell fraction derived vaccine is**
(a) Hepatitis B (b) Measles (c) Mumps (d) Rubella
4) **Which of the following is killed vaccine**
(a) Hepatitis B (b) Measles (c) Yellow fever (d) Japanese encephalitis
5) **Which of the following is not a killed vaccine**
(a) Yellow fever (17D) (b) Salk (polio) (c) Hepatitis B (d) Human diploid cell rabies vaccine
6) **The main aim of adjuvant is to increase-**
(a) Distribution (b) Absorption (c) Antigenicity (d) Metabolism
7) **Role of adjuvant in vaccine is are-** (PGI, NovI-11)
(a) Stimulation of Toll-Like receptors (b) Activate B lymphocyte only (c) Increase both adaptive and innate immune

response (d) Activate both B and T lymphocytes (e) Ensure prolonged delivery of antigen

Answers of MCQs & explanation

1) **(c)**
- Follow section, **vaccines (principle)** for explanation

2) **(c)**
3) **(a)**
4) **(a) & (d)**
5) **(a)**

(2–5) Follow **table-2** for explanation

6) **(c)**
- Adjuvant is a substance that added to the vaccine to increase antigenicity or immune response.

7) **(a), (c), (d) & (e)**
- Follow section, **vaccines (adjuvant)** for explanation

20 Antigen (Ag)

Learning heading & subheadings

- Antigen (Ag)
- Other related terms to antigen

Antigen (Ag)

❖ **Meaning:** Antigen = **Anti**body **gen**erator

❖ **Definitions:**

➢ **Antigen:** Any substance (self/foreign, protein/lipid/carbohydrate) which when enter into the body by any route produces

1. AMI/HI or
2. CMI or
3. Hypersensitivity / autoimmunity or
4. Tolerance.

➢ **Immunogen:** Any substance which when enter into the body by any route, must produces immune response (AMI or CMI or hypersensitivity / autoimmunity) but no tolerance.

❖ **All immunogens are antigens but all antigens are not antigens:**

- Antigen is considers as particle enters in body like dust, pollen or microbes. It may induce immune response (AMI, CMI etc.) or no immune response (tolerance)
- Immunogen is considers as particle which must induce an immune response. So immunogens contains all properties of antigens but not vice versa, hence it's safe to say that all immunogens are antigens but all antigens are not immunogens.

❖ **Attributes of antigenicity:** Antigenicity means ability of an antigen to combine specifically with TCR, whether immunogenic or non immunogenic. Antigenicity has following two attributes.

a. **Immunogenicity:** Ability of an antigen to induce an immune response (like AMI or CMI) **called immunogenicity**.

b. **Immunological reactivity:** Specific reaction of Ag with Ab or sensitised cells **called immunological reactivity**.

✓ **Note: Confusing terms**

- **Immunological reactivity:** Few author defined it as a synonym for antigenicity while few defined it as part (attribute) of antigenicity as mentioned above.
- **Immunological reaction:** It is an in vivo Ag-Ab reaction

❖ **Classification:** Following are the different types of antigens

I. **Functional classification:** Two types.

A. **Complete Ag:**

- **Synonym:** Immunogen
- **Definition:** Complete Ag is a substance that is capable to induce an immune response (immunogenic) by itself & also react specifically & in observable manner with products (like Ab) of immune response.
- **Attributes:** Having both attributes of antigenicity

B. **Incomplete Ag:**

- **Synonym:** Hapten.
- **Meaning:** From **Haptein (Greek) = To fasten**
- **Definition:** Hapten is a substance that is incapable to induce an immune response (not immunogenic) by itself, but can react specifically with products (like Ab) of immune response.
- **Attributes:**
  - Having attribute like immunological reactivity but no immunogenicity
  - Haptens become immunogenic on combining with a larger molecule **called carrier molecule**.
  - Haptens are generally low molecular weight lipids & carbohydrates, while carrier molecules are proteins like albumin, globulin or synthetic polypeptide.
- **Types:** Two types like simple & complex as mentioned in **table-1**

Simple hapten	Complex hapten
Simple chemical substance	Relatively complex & large
Monovalent	Polyvalent
Can react with Ab, but unable to precipitate the reaction.	React with specific Ab & able to precipitate reaction

Table-1: Types of hapten

- **Examples of haptens:**

1. **Bacterial haptens:** Polysaccharide capsule of pneumococcus, C (Carbohydrate) - Ag of *Streptococcus*
2. **Drugs:** Allergen causing contact dermatitis
3. **Blood group substances:** Glycoproteins in ABO blood group
4. **Lipids:** Cardiolipin Ag released from heart tissue in syphilis, Forssmann Ag, transplantation Ag etc.

II. According to infectious agents:

A. Bacterial antigens:

- **Flagellar (H) Ag:**
  - H from **Hauch (German) = film of breath**.
  - As motile bacteria produce thin film on agar, resembling the mist produced by breathing on glass
- **Capsular (K) Ag:** K from Kapsel, German language for capsule
- **Somatic (O) Ag:**
  - O from **Ohne Hauch (German) = without film of breath**.
  - Nonmotile bacteria will grow without surface film on agar.
- **Fimbrial (F) Ag:**

B. Viral Ag:

- **Envelop Ag:** gp120, gp 41, neuraminidase Ag, haemagglutinating Ag are the examples.
- **Capsid Ag:** p24, p15, p55
- **Nucleic acid Ag:**

C. Fungal Ag: Mannan in *C. albicans*, capsular Ag in *Cryptococcus neoformans*, gp43 in *P. brasiliensis*

D. Parasitic Ag: Histidine Rich Protein (HRP) & Merozoite Surface Protein (MSP) in *Plasmodium* spp., K39 & Witebusky Klingstein Kuhn (W.K.K.) Ag in *L. donovani*.

III. Biological classification: Antigen which require T cell participation for antibody production from B cell is **called T cell dependent antigen (TD Ag),** while antigen which can directly stimulate B cell for antibody production without participation by T cell is **called T cell independent antigen (TI Ag)**. Differences between two are mentioned in **table-2.**

Features	TD Ag	TI Ag
T cells cooperation	Yes	No
Preliminary process by macrophages	Yes	No
Type of Ag	Soluble protein	Type I: LPS Type II: Capsular polysaccharide of pneumococci, flagellin
Degradation	Rapid	Slowly
Complement activation	No	By type II
Immunological memory	Yes	No
Polyclonal activation	No	By type-I
Ab production	Full range IgM, IgG, IgA &IgE	Limited to IgM and IgG3.
Tolerance	Do not cause tolerance	High dose results in tolerance.

Table-2: Differences between TD & TI Ag

IV. According to mode of origin:

A. Exogenous antigen: Antigen that entered the body from the outside, for example by inhalation ingestion or injection.

B. Endogenous antigen: Antigen that originated from body, for example fragment of normal cell generated by metabolism or infection.

❖ Antigenic determinant:

- **Synonym:** Epitope
- **Definition:** Whole antigen is not responsible for antigenicity but smaller area on it, usually contains four or five amino acid or monosaccharide residues is responsible for antigenicity **called epitope.**
- **Properties:**
  - Molecular Weight (MW): 400-1000
  - Specific chemical structure
  - Electrical charge
  - Steric configuration
  - Capable of sensitising an immunocytes
  - React with specific complimentary site on the specific antibody **called paratope** or on T cell receptors.
  - Epitope and paratopes determine the specificity of immunological reaction.
  - The presence of the same or similar epitopes on the different antigens accounts for one type of antigenic cross-reaction.
  - Antigenic determinants are usually limited to those portions of the antigen that are accessible to antibodies.
  - T cell recognises linear epitope while B cell recognises conformational epitope.
- **Types: →Fig-1**

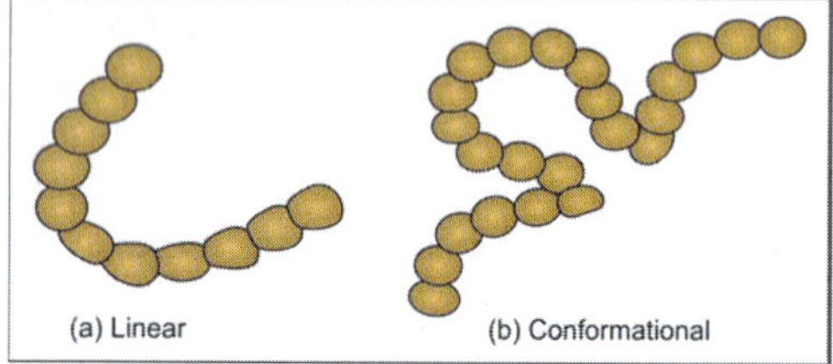

Figure-1: Types of antigen

A. Linear/Sequential: Epitope may be present as a linear segment of primary sequence

B. Conformational: Epitope may be formed by bringing together on the surface residue from different site of peptide chain during its folding into tertiary structure.

❖ Factors influencing antigenicity or immunogenicity: Also **called determinants of antigenicity**

➢ **Size: Antigenicity is related to molecular size.**

- Antigen with High Molecular Weight (HMW) is highly antigenic. E.g. haemocyanins

- Antigen with Low Molecular Weight (LMW) is less antigenic.
- LMW substances may be rendered antigenic by adsorbing them on large inert particles like bentonite or kaolin.

➢ **Foreignness:**
- An individual does not normally mount immune response against his or her own normal constituent antigens.
- Tolerance of self antigens is conditioned by contact with them during the development of immune system. Breakdown of this homeostatic mechanism leads to autoimmunisation & auto immune disease.

➢ **Biochemical nature:**
- **Proteins:**
- The vast majority of immunogens are proteins.
- These may be pure proteins or they may be glycoproteins or lipoproteins.
- In general, proteins are usually very good immunogens, as protein made of different 20 or more amino acid residues.
- Not all proteins are antigenic like gelatin, histones & protamines
- **Polysaccharides & carbohydrates:**
- Pure polysaccharides and lipopolysaccharides are good immunogens, but weaker than protein & stronger than nucleic acid & lipids
- Natural proteins, composed of 20 different amino acids, are better antigens than polysaccharides composed of 4-5 monosaccharide units.
- Carbohydrate are weaker immunogen
- **Nucleic acids:** Nucleic acids are usually poorly immunogenic. However, they may become immunogenic when single stranded or when complexed with proteins.
- **Lipids:** In general lipids are non-immunogenic, although they may be haptens.
- **Immunogenic nature:** Proteins (except gelatin) > polysaccharides & carbohydrates > nucleic acids & lipids

➢ **Susceptibility to tissue enzymes:**
- Substances which are metabolized and are susceptible to the action of tissue enzyme behave as antigen.
- Antigens introduced into the body are degraded by the host into fragment of appropriate size containing antigenic determinants.
- Substances not metabolized by tissue enzymes are not antigenic. E.g. polystyrene latex and synthetic polypeptide contains D-amino acids.
- Substances metabolized by tissue enzymes are antigenic. E.g. polypeptide contains L-amino acids.

➢ **Methods of administration:**
- **Dose:** The dose of administration of an immunogen can influence its immunogenicity. There is a dose of antigen above or below which the immune response will not be optimal.
- **Route:** Generally the subcutaneous route is better than the intravenous or intragastric routes. The route of antigen administration can also alter the nature of the response
- **Adjuvants:** Substances that can enhance the immune response to an immunogen are **called adjuvants**. The use of adjuvants, however, is often hampered by undesirable side effects such as fever and inflammation. E.g. adjuvants used in vaccines.

➢ **Host factors:**
- **Genetic factors:**
- Some substances are immunogenic in one species but not in another, similarly, some substances are immunogenic in one individual but not in others of same species (*i.e.* responders and non-responders).
- The species or individuals may lack or have altered genes that code for the receptors for antigen on B cells and T cells or they may not have the appropriate genes needed for the APC to present antigen to the helper T cells.
- **Age:**
- Age can also influence immunogenicity.
- Usually the very young and the very old have a diminished ability to mount and immune response in response to an immunogen.

❖ Antigenic specificity:

➢ **History:** The basis of antigenic specificity is stereo chemical was first demonstrated by Obermayer and Pick and later confirmed by Landsteiner.

➢ **Basis of antigenic specificity:**
- The importance of the position of the antigenic determinant group in the antigen molecules was evidenced by the difference in specificity in compound with the group attached at the ortho, meta or para position
- The influence of spatial configuration of the determinant group was shown by difference in antigenic specificity of the dextro, levo & meso isomers of substance such as tartaric acid.
- Antigenic specificity is not absolute & cross reactions can occur between antigens that bear stereo chemical similarities.

➢ **Types:** Natural tissue antigens shows the following types of specificity

i. **Species specificity:**
- **Definition:** Tissues of all individual in a species contain species-specific antigens.
- **Clinical applications**:

1. **Forensic science:** It has forensic applications in the identification of the species from blood & seminal stains.
2. **Phylogenetic study:** It has been used in tracing phylogenetic (evolutionary) relationship between species.

ii. **Isospecificity:**

- **Definition:** Isoantigens are antigens found in some but not all members of a species.
- **Clinical applications:**

1. **Grouping of species:**
   - Isoantigens on human RBCs are used for blood grouping & Blood Transfusion (BT).
   - Isoantigens on human WBCs are used for HLA typing & organ transplantation.
2. **Paternity test:** Providing valuable evidence in disputed paternity.
3. **Isoimmunisation:** Helpful during pregnancy.

iii. **Autospecificity:**

- **Definition:** Autologous or self antigen are ordinarily non antigenic, however some are exception **called self antigens**, as below
- **Clinical applications:**
  - Some sequestrated antigens that are not normally found free in circulation or tissues fluid like eye lens protein, sperm antigen & other antigens which are not exposed during embryonic life.
  - When such antigens are found free in circulation, body identifies them as foreign antigens & produces autoimmune diseases.

iv. **Organ specificity:**

- **Definition:** Some organs such as the brain, kidney and lens protein of different species, sharing the same antigens **called organ-specific antigens**.
- **Clinical applications:** The neuroparalytic complication following anti-rabies vaccination using sheep brain vaccines are a consequence of brain-specific antigens shared by sheep & human being. The sheep brain antigen of the vaccine induces immunological response which damages the nervous tissue of human.

v. **Heterogenetic (heterophile) specificity:**

- **Definition:** The same or closely related antigens may sometime occur in different biological species, classes and kingdoms. They are **called heterogenetic** or **heterophile antigens**.
- **Clinical applications:**

1. **Forssmann antigen:** It is a lipid carbohydrate complex widely distributed among animals, birds, plants & bacteria but absent in rabbits, so anti-Forssmann antibody can be prepared in rabbits.
2. **Other heterophile antigen:** Used in serological test to diagnose the diseases in which antigen unrelated to etiological agents are employed.
   - Weil Felix reaction in typhus fever.
   - Paul Bunnel test in infectious mononucleosis.
   - Cold agglutinin test in primary atypical pneumonia.
   - Streptococci MG test in primary atypical pneumonia.

Other related terms to antigen

❖ Superantigen:

- **Definition:** Some antigen can polyclonally activate a large numbers of T cells irrespective of their antigenic specificity **called superantigen**.
- **Properties:**
  - Medium sized protein: 22-29 kDa
  - High resistance to protease & denaturation by CD4+
  - Produced intracellularly by bacteria & released upon infection as extracellular mature toxins
  - Normal antigen activates 0.0001-0.001% of the body's T-cells while superantigen activate 20% of the body's T-cells.
  - Anti-CD3 & Anti-CD28 antibodies are also identified as highly potent superantigens & can activate up to 100% of T cells
- **Mechanism of action: → Flow chart-1**

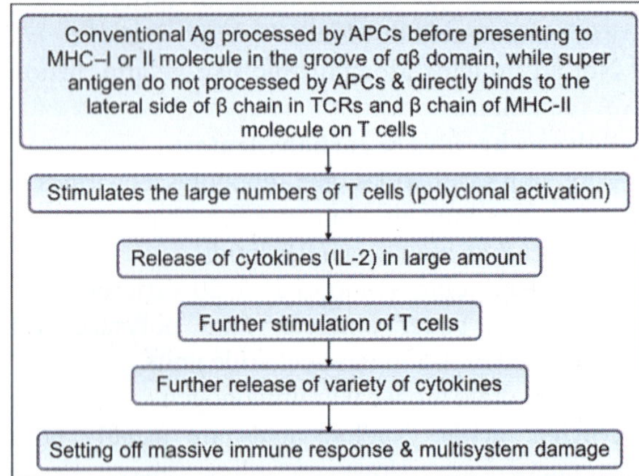

Flow chart-1: Mechanism of action of superantigen

- **Examples of superantigens:**
- **Bacterial**
  - Staphylococcal enterotoxins
  - Staphylococcal toxic shock syndrome toxin-1 (TSST-1)
  - Streptococcal pyrogenic exotoxin (exotoxin A & C)
  - Others: Released by *Mycobacterium tuberculosis*
  - *Yersinia pseudotuberculosis*
- **Viral**
  - Nef (Negative regulatory factor) in HIV
  - Nucleocapsid in rabies virus
  - Mouse mammary tumor virus (retrovirus)
  - EBV (Epstein Barr Virus)
- **Fungal:** *Malassezia furfur*

❖ Mitogen:

- **Definition:** Substance that induces the division of immune cells **called mitogen**.

- **Examples:**

1. **Pneumococcal polysaccharide:** Stimulate the B cell, causing polyclonal activation & production of large number of IgM.
2. **Lectin glycoprotein:** Bind with cells having sugar on surface & causing polyclonal activation.
3. **LPS (bacterial endotoxin):** Activate the B cells

❖ **Allergen:** A Substance capable of causing an allergic/hypersensitivity reaction **called allergen** like dust, pollen, ovalbumin etc.

❖ **Tolerogen:** A substances not capable to produce immune response due to low molecular weight (LMW) **called tolerogen.** If it's molecular weight is changed, it becomes immunogen.

Question bank

Essay/Full question

1) Antigen (Ag)

Short notes

1) Hapten
2) Antigenic determinant
3) Superantigen

Short questions for theory/viva questions

1) Define: Antigen & immunogen
2) Comment: All immunogens are antigens but all antigens are not immunogens.
3) What is epitope?
4) What is heterophile antigen? Write two examples.
5) Name four serological tests based on the use of heterophile antigen
6) What is superantigen? Write two examples.
7) What is mitogen? Write two examples.

MCQs for chapter review

Antigen (Ag)

1) **Following are the features of antigen**
(a) Produce antibody (b) Produce lymphokine (c) Produce hypersensitivity (d) All of above
2) **Meaning of hapten is**
(a) Fasten (b) Antibody (c) Toxin (d) None of above
3) **Hapten is** (AI -98)
(a) Same as epitope (b) Small molecular weight protein (c) Require carrier for specific antibody production (d) Simple haptens are precipitate
4) **Which of the following statement is true about hapten** (AI-04)
(a) It induce brisk immune response (b) It needs carrier to induce immune response (c) It is a T independent antigen (d) It has no association to MHC
5) **The exact part of the antigen that reacts with the immune system is called as-**
(a) Clone (b) Epitope (c) Idiotope (d) Effector
6) **Which of the following is very difficult to induce antibody**
(a) Carbohydrate (b) Protein (c) Ag (d) Repeated infections
7) **Which of the following chemical nature makes a better Ag?**
(a) Lipids (b) Nucleic acids (c) Polysaccharides (d) Proteins
8) **Which of the following T cell independent Ag acts through**
(a) T cells (b) B-cells (c) Macrophages (d) $CD8^+$ cells
9) **Isoantigens**
(a) Found in some but all members of a species (b) Found in some but not all members of a species (c) Occurs in different biological species, class and kingdom (d) All individual in particular species
10) **Auto antigen is**
(a) Blood group Ag (b) Forssmann Ag (c) Both (d) None
11) **Which is not a heterophile agglutination test** (PGI-01)
(a) Weil Felix test (b) Widal test (c) Paul Bunnel test (d) Streptococci MG test
12) **Heterophile antibody is found in**
(a) Weil Felix reaction (b) Widal test (c) VDRL test (d) All

Other related terms to antigen

13) **A super antigen is a bacterial product that** (AI -08)
(a) Binds to B7 and CD28 costimulatory molecules (b) Binds to the beta chain of TCR and MHC class II molecule of APC stimulating T cell activation (c) Binds to the CD4+ molecule causing T cell activation (d) Is presented by macrophages to a larger than normal number of T helper CD4+ T lymphocytes
14) **Super antigen causes**
(a) Polyclonal activation of T cells (b) Stimulation of B cells (c) Enhancement of phagocytosis (d) Activation of complement
15) **Super antigens are** (PGI, June -05)
(a) Erythrotoxin of *Staph aureus* (b) *Cl difficile* toxin (c) Staphylococcal toxic shock syndrome toxin (d) Cholera toxin

Answers of MCQs & explanation

1) **(d)**
- Ag produces AMI/HI (Ab production) or CMI (lymphokine production) or hypersensitivity / autoimmunity or tolerance.
- Follow section **definition** for more explanation

2) **(a)**
- Follow section, **functional classification (incomplete antigen → meaning)** for explanation

3) **(c)**
- Option a → Follow section, **antigenic determinant (definition)** for explanation
- Haptens are generally low molecular weight lipids & carbohydrates & not able to synthesise the Ab
- It combine with carrier molecules mainly proteins like albumin, globulin or synthetic polypeptide to produce the Ab
- Simple haptens are not precipitate

4) **(b)**
- Haptens are generally low molecular weight lipids & carbohydrates & not able to synthesise the Ab
- It combine with carrier molecules mainly proteins like albumin, globulin or synthetic polypeptide to produce the Ab

5) **(b)**
- Follow section, **antigenic determinant (definition)** for explanation

6) **(a)**
- Carbohydrate is less immunogenic than proteins & induce Ab synthesis with great difficulties

7) **(d)**
- TI Ag can directly stimulate B cell for antibody production without participation by T cell

8) **(b)**
- Descending order of chemical substance according to their antigenicity is: Proteins (except gelatin) > polysaccharides & carbohydrates > nucleic acids & lipids

9) **(d)**
- Follow section, **antigenic specificity (Isospecificity)** for explanation

10) **(d)**
- Autoantigens are sperm Ag & lens Ag

11) (b) } Follow section, **antigenic specificity [heterogenetic**
12) (a) } **(heterophile) specificity]** for explanation
13) (b) } Follow section, **super antigen (mechanism of action**
14) (a) } **of superantigen)** for explanation
15) (c)

- Follow section, **super antigen (examples of superantigen)** for explanation.
- Erythrotoxin is not the property of *Staph aureus*

21 Antibody (Ab) - Immunoglobulin (Ig)

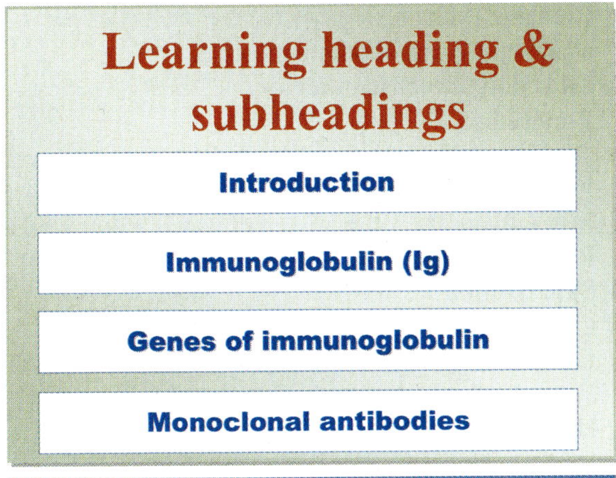

Learning heading & subheadings
Introduction
Immunoglobulin (Ig)
Genes of immunoglobulin
Monoclonal antibodies

Introduction

❖ **Definition:** Protein (Glycoprotein) substance produced after antigenic stimulation & reacts specifically (not absolute, because of cross reactivity) with responsible antigen & in some observable manner **called antibody (Ab)**.

❖ **Immune sera:** Antisera containing antibody **called immune sera**.

❖ **Hyperimmune sera:** Antisera containing high titre of antibody **called hyperimmune sera**.

❖ **Fractionation of immune sera:** Done by following methods

➢ **Half saturation** with ammonium sulphate separates proteins into soluble albumin & insoluble globulins. Globulin can be separated in to water soluble pseudoglobulin & insoluble euglobulins.

➢ **Sedimentation coefficient (S) studies** divides them into molecules that sediments at 7S (MW - 150000) & some heavier molecules that sediments at 19S (MW-900000), designated as M or macroglobulins.

➢ **Electrophoretic mobilities:**

- In 1937 plasma protein was separated by Tiselius as shown in **flow chart-1**
- In 1938 Tiselius & Kabat found that antibody activity was associated with γ-globulins **called immunoglobulin (Ig)**.
- The confusion about the indiscriminate use of various terms was resolved when, in 1964, WHO endorsed internationally accepted term "Immunoglobulins" for proteins of animal origin endowed with known antibody activity & for certain other proteins same by chemical structure.

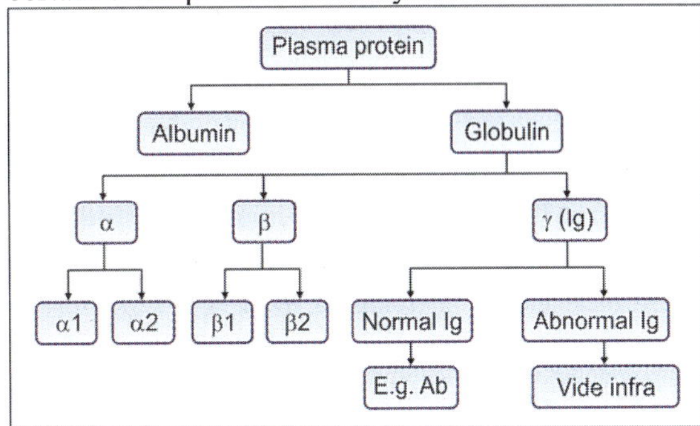

Flow chart-1: Parts of plasma protein

❖ **All antibodies are immunoglobulins, but all immunoglobulins may not be antibodies:** Because

- Besides antibody globulins, Ig also includes the abnormal proteins founds in myeloma, macroglobulinemia, cryoglobulinemia & naturally occurring subunits of immunoglobulins.
- Immunoglobulins (abnormal Ig) are synthesized by plasma cells & to some extent by lymphocytes while antibodies are synthesized by plasma cells only.
- Immunoglobulins provide a structural & chemical concept, while the term 'Antibody' is a biological & functional concept.

❖ **Properties of antibody:**

- Immunoglobulins constitute 20-25% of total serum proteins.
- It contains proteins & sugar residues hence **called glycoprotein** (gp).
- Heat labile & denatured at 70^0 C for 1 hour.
- Activity also affected by pH of medium.

Immunoglobulin (Ig)

❖ **Structure of Ig:** →**Fig.-1**

➢ **Polypeptides chains:** Each molecule consisting of two light (short) & two heavy (long) chains (total four) of polypeptides chains of different sizes. Total MW approx. >1, 50, 000 Da.

a. Light (L) chains:

- Smaller
- MW: Approx. 25, 000 Da.
- Light chains are similar in all classes of Ig
- Two varieties: kappa (k from Korngold) & lambda (l from Lapari).

- A molecule of Ig may have either kappa or lambda chains, but never both together.
- In human sera 60% are kappa and 40% are lambda chains occur.

b. Heavy (H) chains:

- Larger
- MW: Approx. 50, 000 Da.
- Heavy chains are structurally & antigenically distinct for each classes of Ig.
- Five varieties: According to H chain five varieties of Ig designated as IgG, IgA, IgM, IgD & IgE from Greek letters like Gamma (γ), Alpha (α), mu (μ), Delta (δ) & Epsilon (ε) respectively. This order also suggests the descending order of concentration in serum. All classes are differentiated in **table-1.**

➢ **Two ends:**

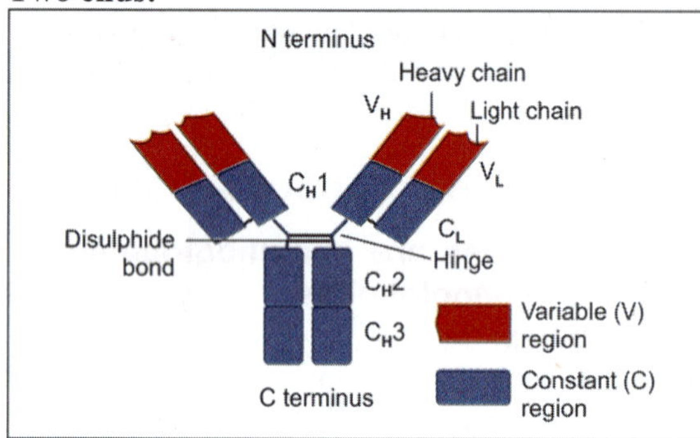

Figure-1: Structure of Ig

a. Aminoterminus (N terminal/Fab fraction) end:

- **Properties:**
- Contains both H & L chain
- Made up by amino acids & 1st 110 amino acids are quite variable **called variable (V) region**, thus the variable light chain (V_L) & variable heavy chain (V_H) regions are defined.
- Sequence of amino acid beyond the variable region is relatively constant throughout the rest of molecule **called constant region**, thus the constant light chain (C_L) & constant heavy chain (C_H) regions are defined.
- **Function:** It is the antigen binding site
- **Hypervariable region:**
- Aminoacid sequence in the variable region is sometimes hypervariable **called hypervariable (HV) region (also called hot spot)** & sometimes less variable **called framework (FV) region.**
- Hypervariable (HV) regions actual makes contact with epitope **called Complemantarity Determining Regions (CDRs) or paratopes.**
- **Valency:**
- Normally antigenic determinant (epitope) binds with antigen binding site (paratope) on Ig.
- Monomer Ig has two antigen binding sites
- Valency is defines as number of antigenic determinants (epitopes) bind with antigen binding sites (paratopes) on an individual Ig
- Follow table-1 for number of valency of different classes of Ig
- **Fd piece:** The portion of the H chain present in the Fab fragment is **called Fd piece**.

b. Carboxyterminus (C terminal/ Fc fraction) end:

- **Properties:**
- Contains H chain
- Made up by carbohydrate moieties.
- Linked to the constant region.
- **Functions:**

1. Complement fixation: IgM > IgG1 > IgG3 & rarely IgG2 activate the classical pathway while IgG4 & IgA activate the alternative pathway
2. Placental transfer
3. Skin fixation
4. Catabolic rate
5. Formation of Ag- Ab complex by combining with Fc receptors present on host cells

➢ **Disulfide (s-s) bonds & Ig domain:**

- Both H chains are links by internal disulfide bonds
- H & L chains are links together by interchain / intrachain disulfide bonds.
- These intrachain disulfide bonds form loops in peptide chain, & each of the loops is compactly folded to form a globular domain (Ig fold).
- L chain has one domain in variable region (V_L) & one domain in constant region (C_L)
- H chain has one domain in variable region (V_H) & 3-4 domains in constant region (C_H1, C_H2, C_H3, C_H4) depends on Ig class
- Each domain has a separate function.
- The variable region domains V_L & V_H are responsible for the formation of a specific **antigen binding site**.
- The C_H2 region binds C1q in the classical complement sequence.
- C_H3 domain mediates adherence to monocyte surface.

➢ **Hinge region:**

- **Definition:** The area of the H chain in the C region between the 1st & 2nd C region domains (C_H1 & C_H2) is **called hinge region**.
- **Functions:**
- It is more flexible & is more exposed to enzymes & chemicals.
- Papain acts here to produce 1 Fc & 2 Fab fractions.

❖ Digestion or degradation of Ig:

➢ **Aim:** To understand the detailed structure of Ig

➢ **History:** Porter, Edelman, Nisonoff & colleagues have digested the rabbit IgG antibody developed against egg albumin, by papain & pepsin & they obtained the following results.

➢ **Papain digestion:** Produces the three parts (**fig.-2).**

- **One part of Fc or crystallisable fraction:** An insoluble fraction which is crystallized in cold.

- **Two parts of Fab or antigen binding fraction:** A soluble fraction which binds to egg albumin, but unable to precipitate with it.
- **Having a sedimentation coefficient of 3.5S.**

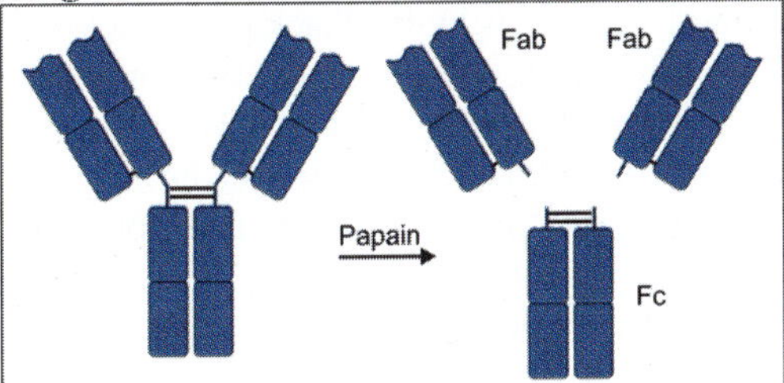

Figure-2: Papain digestion

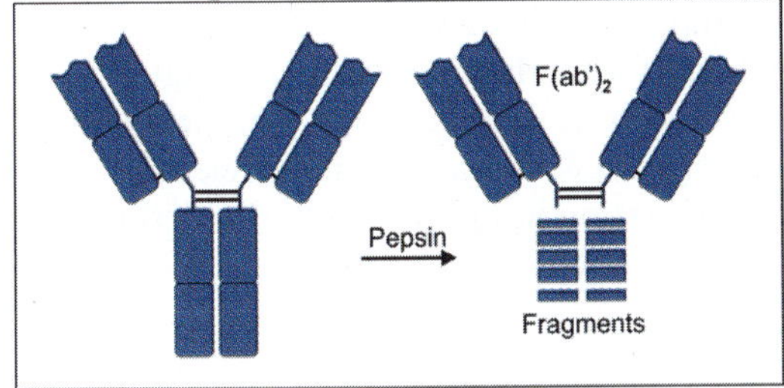

Figure-3: Pepsin digestion

Thus each molecule of IgG is split by Papain into 1 Fc piece & 2 Fab pieces,

➢ **Pepsin digestion:** Produces following parts **(fig.-3).**

- **Two Fab fragments:**
  - Held together in position by disulphide bond.
  - It is bivalent & precipitates with the antigen.
  - This fragment is **called F(ab')$_2$**
- **The Fc portion:** Digested into smaller fragments.
- **Having a sedimentation coefficient of 5S.**

➢ **Chemical treatment by mercaptoethanol:** It cleaves the disulphide bonds in to four subunits structure **(fig.-4).**

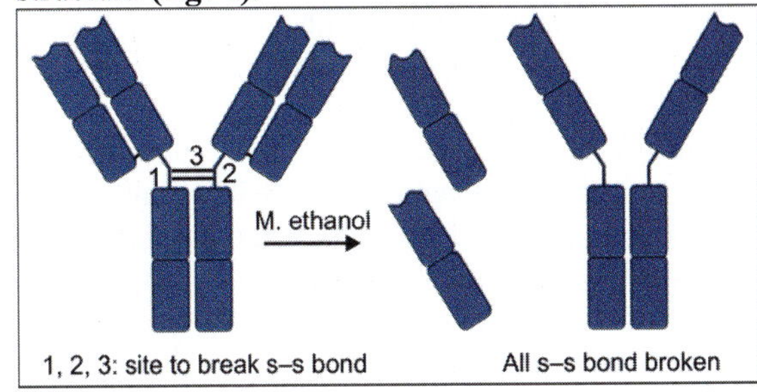

Figure-4: Digestion by mercaptoethanol

❖ **Classification of Ig:** Two ways to classify the Ig like structural & physical classification as below

I. Structural classification

Features	IgG	IgA	IgM	IgD	IgE
Subclasses	IgG1, IgG2, IgG3 & IgG4	- Serum & secretory IgA - IgA1 & IgA2	- Membrane IgM - Soluble IgM	None	None
Structure	Monomer	Monomer, Dimer	Monomer, Pentamer	Monomer	Monomer
Valency	2	2, 4	2, 10	2	2
Type of heavy chain	γ	α	μ	δ	ε
Sedimentation co-efficient	7	7	19	7	8
Additional unit	-	S & J pieces	J piece	-	-
MW	150000	160000	9,00,000-10,00,000 **(called millionaire molecule)**	180000	190000
Serum concentration (mg/ml)	12	2	1.2	0.03	0.00004
Half life(days)	23	6	5	2-8	1-5
Production (mg/kg/day)	34	24	3.3	0.4	0.0023
Intravascular distribution	45	42	80	75	50
Carbohydrate content (%)	3	8	12	13	12
Complement fixation Classical pathway Alternative pathway	 ++ -	 - +	 +++ -	 - +	 - -
Placental transfer	+	-	-	-	-
Present in the milk	+	+	-	-	-
Selective secretion by secretory/mucus glands	-	+	-	-	-
Heat stability (56 °C)	+	+	+	+	-
Participation in agglutination	+	++	+++	-	-
Participation in precipitation	+++	Variable	+	-	-
Fixation to mast cells & basophils	-	-	-	-	-
Primary Ab response	-	-	+	-	-

Table-1: Differences between each classes of Ig

- **Five classes:** Based on physiochemical & antigenic variation in H chain (in constant region), 5 classes of Igs have been recognized like IgG, IgA, IgM, IgD & IgE.
- **Differences between each classes of Ig:→Table-1**
- **Individual types:**

A. IgG:

✪ **Properties:**

- Major serum immunoglobulin
- Constitutes 70-80% of the total Ig.
- Molecular weight is 150,000 (7 S).
- Half life is ~ 23 days.
- Normal serum concentration is 8-16 mg/ml
- Equally distributed between intravascular & extra vascular compartment.
- Catabolism of IgG is unique in that it varies with its serum concentration.

✪ **Structure: →Fig.-5**

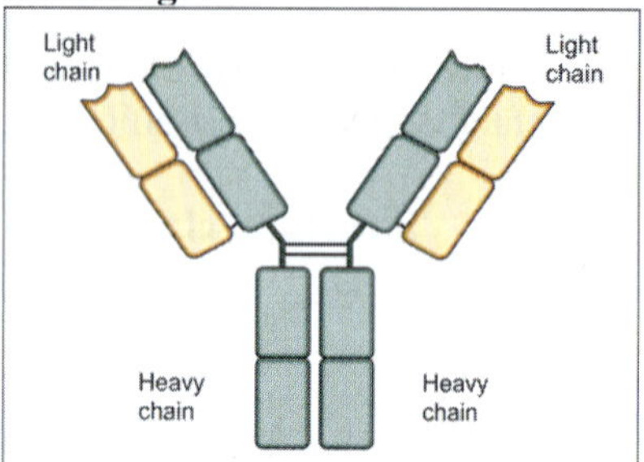

Figure-5: Structure of IgG

- Occasionally exist in polymerised form.
- Contains less carbohydrate than other Ig.
- Each heavy chain has V_H & three C_H domains.

✪ **Subclasses:**

- Four subclasses has been recognized like IgG1, IgG2, IgG3 & IgG4
- Each possessing a distinct type of gamma chain like γ1, γ2, γ3 & γ4 respectively.
- Each IgG subclass is different from other by size of hinge region & numbers-location of interchain s-s bonds.
- Having approximate proportion of 65%, 23%, 8% and 4% respectively.

✪ **Clinical significances:**

1. **Diagnostic:**
   - Its level is raised in some chronic condition like malaria, kala azar and myeloma.
   - With most antigens, IgG is a late antibody & makes its appearance after the initial immune response which is IgM in nature.
2. **Protective:** It may consider a general purpose antibody, protective against infectious agents which are active in blood & tissues.
3. **Therapeutic:** To treat hypogammaglobulinemia.
4. **Natural passive immunity:**
   - Maternal IgG can transport by placenta & provides natural passive immunity to fetus.
   - Not synthesized by fetus in any significant amount.
5. **Isoimmunisation or artificial passive immunity:**
   - Passively administered IgG suppresses homologous antibody synthesis by feedback process.
   - This principle is utilized in the isoimmunisation of Rh -Ve women who delivered Rh +Ve baby, by administration of anti-Rh (D) IgG during delivery.
6. **Phagocytosis:** IgG binds to microorganisms & enhances their phagocytosis.
7. **Extracellular killing:** of the target cells coated with IgG is mediated through recognition of the surface Fc fragment by K cells bearing the appropriate receptor.
8. **Platelets function:** interaction of IgG complexes with platelet Fc receptors probably leads to aggregation & vasoactive amine release.
9. **Participation in immunological reactions:** Like
   - Complement fixation: IgG1, IgG3 & rarely IgG2 activate the classical pathway & IgG4 activate the alternative pathway
   - Coagglutination: IgG except IgG3 bind with protein A of *Staph aureus* (Cowan I strain) to mediate the coagglutination reaction
   - Others: Precipitation & neutralization of toxins & viruses.

B. IgA:

✪ **Properties:**

- 2nd most abundant class of Ig after IgG.
- Constitutes about 10-13% of serum Ig.
- Half-life: 6 days
- Normal serum level is 0.6-4.2 mg/ml.

✪ **Structure & subclasses:**

i. According to numbers of Y shaped structure (H & L chains joined by s-s bond) & distribution: Two classes

a. Serum IgA:

- Mostly monomer: Single Y shaped structure
- MW about 160,000 (7S).
- In humans over 80% of serum IgA is a monomer of the four chains (2 H & 2 L chains), but in most mammals it is predominantly polymeric, occurs mostly as a dimer.

b. Secretory IgA (SIgA): →Fig.-6

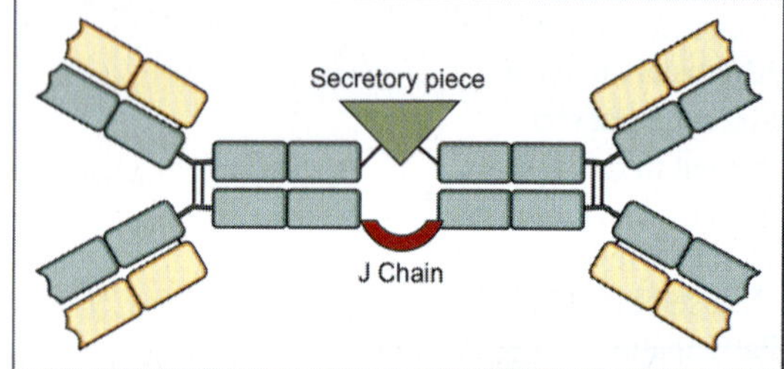

Figure-6: Structure of SIgA

- Mostly dimer: Electron micrographs of IgA dimers show double Y shaped structures, suggesting that the monomeric subunits are linked end-to-end by J chain at the C terminal Ca3 regions as shown in **fig.-6**

- SIgA is much larger molecule than serum IgA.
- It is the exocrine secretion (Secretion on epithelial surfaces by glands/cells through duct **called exocrine secretion** & such glands or cells **called exocrine glands/cells**) & synthesized by plasma cells situated near mucosal or granular epithelium.
- SIgA is relatively resistant to the digestive enzymes & reducing agents.
- **J- chain:** It is a dimer formed by two monomer units joined together at their carboxyterminals by a glycopeptide **called the J chain (J for joining).** J chain is also produced by plasma cells situated near mucosal or granular epithelium.
- **Secretory (S) component or piece:** SIgA contains other glycine rich polypeptide **called the secretory component or secretory piece.** It is produced by mucosal or granular epithelial cells. Dimeric IgA binds to a receptor on the surface of the epithelial cells & is endocytosed & transported across the cell to the luminal surface. During this process, a part of the receptor remains attached to the IgA dimer, which serve secretory component. This secretory component is believed to protect IgA from denaturation by bacterial proteases.

✓ **Note: Origin of**

- **SIgA & J chain:** By plasma cells situated near mucosal or granular epithelium
- **Secretory (S) component or piece:** By mucosal or granular epithelial cells

ii. According to amino acid sequences on the constant region of H chain: Two IgA subclasses like IgA1 & IgA2.

a. IgA1:

- The hinge of IgA1 is extended & bears O-linked oligosaccharides while hinge of IgA2 is truncated.
- Both heavy chains bear N-linked oligosaccharides.
- It is dominant subclass in serum IgA (90%)

b. IgA2:

- IgA2 lacks interchain/intrachain disulfide bonds between the heavy & light chains.
- Though IgA2 is a minor component of serum IgA, it is the dominant form in the secretory IgA.
- It holds the minor part in serum IgA (10%) but dominant subclass in secretory IgA. IgA2 range from 10-20% in nasal & male genital secretions, 40% in saliva, 60% in colonic & female genital secretions.
- Polysaccharide Ags induce more IgA2 synthesis than protein Ags.

✪ **Clinical significances:**

1. **Immunological reactions:** Serum IgA combine with Fc receptor on immune cells & takes part in ADCC & degranulation.
2. **Local (Mucosal) immunity:** Secretory IgA is the major Ig in colostrum, saliva, milk, tears, respiratory, intestinal & genitourinary secretion. SIgA is selectively concentrated in secretions & on the mucus surface forming a layer '**called antibody paste**' & thereby preventing the entry of microbes in the body tissues & provides local immunity against respiratory & intestinal pathogens.
3. **Complement activation:** Does not fix complement but can activate alternative complement pathway.
4. **Phagocytosis:** It promotes phagocytosis & intracellular killing of microorganisms.

C. IgM:

✪ **Properties:**

- Constitutes 5-8% of total serum Ig.
- It is a heavy molecule (19S; MW 9,00,000-10,00,000), hence **called the millionaire molecule.**
- Half life of about 5 days.
- Normal serum level is 0.5-2 mg/ml
- Most of IgM (80%) is intravascular in distribution.
- Treatment of serum with 0.12 M 2-mercaptoethanol selectively destroys IgM, hence it is a simple method for differential estimation of IgG & IgM antibodies.

✪ **Structure & subclasses:** Two physical forms like

i. Membrane or **surface Ig:** It is monomer & expressed in bound form with B cell receptor (BCR) on the surface of B cells

ii. Soluble form: →**Fig.-7**

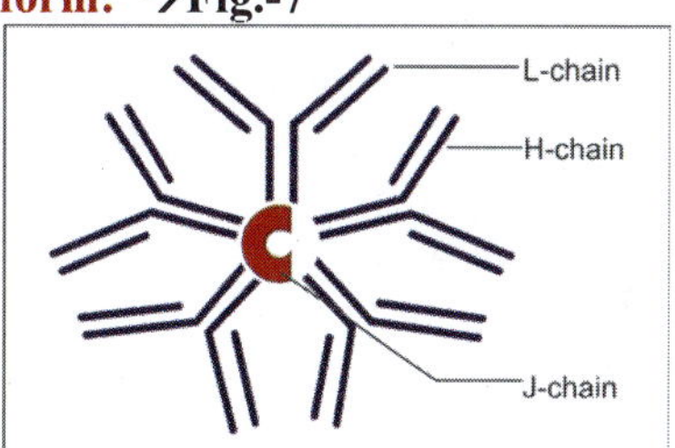

Figure-7: Structure of soluble IgM

- It is a pentamer of basic five chain structure, formation of which is aided by inclusion of the J polypeptide chain of mass ~15 KDa.
- Each heavy chain has V_H & four C_H domains & no hinge region.
- Theoretical valency is ten, but this is observed only with small haptens. With larger antigens, the effective valency falls to five, probably because of steric hindrance.
- Available free in blood/plasma

✪ **Clinical significances:**

a. Phylogenetic importance: Phylogenetically it is the oldest Ig class. It is also the earliest Ig to be synthesized by fetus, beginning by about 20 weeks of age.

b. Diagnostic role:

1. **Diagnosis of intrauterine infection:** As it is not transported by placenta & synthesised after 20

weeks of gestational age, its presence in the fetus or newborn indicates intrauterine infection & its detection is useful in diagnosis of congenital infection like TORCH agents.

2. **Acute (recent) infection:** They are relatively short lived, disappearing earlier than IgG; hence their demonstration in serum indicates recent infection.

c. **Immune haemolysis:** A single molecule of IgM can bring about immune haemolysis, where as 1000 IgG molecules are required for the same effect.

d. **Opsonisation:** It is also 500-1000 times more effective than IgG in opsonisation.

e. **Bactericidal action:** 100 times more effective in bactericidal action than IgG.

f. **Bacterial agglutination:** 20 times more effective in bacterial agglutination than IgG.

g. **Activation of classical path way of complement:** IgM (+++) is more effective than IgG (++)

h. **Immunological reactions:**
- **Neutralisation:** It neutralise the toxins & viruses but less effective than IgG.
- **Precipitation:** Useful but less effective than IgG

i. **Protective role:** It is distributed in to the intravascular space, it is believed to responsible for protection against blood invasion by microorganisms; hence its deficiency is often associated with septicemia.

j. **Ag recognition:** Monomeric IgM is the major antibody receptor on the surface of B lymphocytes for antigen recognition.

k. **Natural Abs:** Most natural Abs are IgM type like
- Isohaemagglutinin (Anti-A, Anti-B)
- Reagin Ab to syphilis
- Ab to *S. typhi* O Ag
- Ab to other microbes are IgM in nature in primary or acute infections

✓ **Note: IgM & IgG comparison**

- **IgG:** IgG is more effective than IgM, in
  - Neutralisation
  - Precipitation
- **IgM:** IgM is more effective than IgG, in
  - Immune haemolysis
  - Opsonisation
  - Bactericidal action
  - Bacterial agglutination
  - Activation of classical path way of complement

D. IgD:

✪ **Properties:**
- Constitutes less than 1% of the serum Ig.
- MW: 180000
- Half life is about 3 days.
- Normal serum level is 3 mg/100 ml.
- Mostly intravascular in distribution.
- Least important Ig in human beings.

✪ **Structure:**
- It resembles IgG structurally.
- Each heavy chain has V_H & three C_H domains with an extended hinge region that is susceptible to proteolysis, at least on purification.

✪ **Clinical significances:**

1. **Antigen recognition:** It is a transmembrane monomeric form present as a antigen-specific receptor on unstimulated mature B cells & serve as recognition receptors for Ag.
2. **Antibody production:** Combination of this IgD molecule with its corresponding antigen leads to specific stimulation of the B cells- either activation or cloning to produce antibody or suppression.

E. IgE:

✪ **History:** It was discovered in 1966 by Ishizaka during the investigation of atopic reagin antibodies.

✪ **Properties:**
- It is estimated that serum IgE accounts for 50% of total body IgE, with the rest being bound to mast cells & basophils through their high-affinity IgE Fcε receptor.
- It is an 8S molecule with MW about 190,000.
- Half life is about 2 days.
- Serum level is very low (< 0.05 mg/ml).
- It is susceptible to mercaptoethanol.
- It does not pass the placenta or fix complement.
- It is mostly extravascular in distribution.
- Heat labile: Inactivated at 56°C in one hour
- Affinity for the surface of the tissue cells (particularly mast cells) of the same species (homocytotropism).
- IgE is chiefly produced in lining of the respiratory & intestinal tract.
- Its production increased following exposure of allergen like ovalbumin

✪ **Structure:**
- It resembles IgG structurally.
- Each heavy chain has V_H & four C_H domains & no hinge region.

✪ **Clinical significance:**

a. **Diagnostic role:**

1. **Allergic diseases.** Its level is greatly elevated in atopic (type 1 allergic) condition such as asthma, hay fever & eczema.
2. **Parasitic diseases:** Children living in insanitary conditions, with high load of intestinal parasites, have high serum levels of IgE.

b. **IgE deficiency:** It increases the susceptibility to infections.

c. **Anaphylactic reaction:** It is responsible for anaphylactic reaction.

d. **Prausnitz-Kustner reaction:** It mediates the Prausnitz-Kustner reaction.

e. **Protective role:** The physiological role of IgE appears to be protection against pathogens like helminthic infections, by mast cell degranulation & release of inflammatory mediators.

II. Physical classification

- **Two classes:** Based on availability, like free form in blood or bound form with receptors on B cells.

A. **Membrane** or **surface Igs:** IgD & IgM (secretory IgA?) are bound on B cell receptors (BCR) on surface hence **called membrane** or **surface Ig.** BCR is found only on the surface of B cells & facilitates the activation of these cells & their subsequent differentiation into either antibody producing plasma cells (antibody producing cells) or memory B cells that will survive in the body and remember that same antigen, so the B cells can respond faster upon future exposure.

B. **Free** or **soluble Igs:** IgG, IgA & IgE are secreted from the cells to be free in the blood / plasma.

❖ Age of Ig production: →Fig.-8

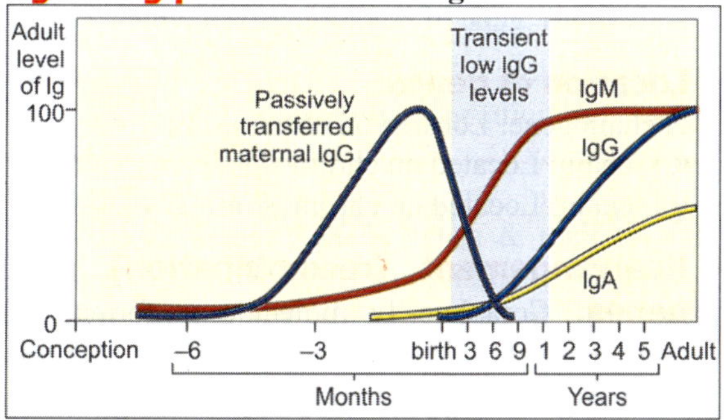

Figure-8: Age of Ig production

- **IgG:**
  - It is the only Ig which can cross the placenta.
  - New born has high level of passively transferred IgG, immediately after birth which start to fall after birth as shown in dark blue line in **fig.-8**.
  - Light blue line in **fig.-8** suggest that immune system of new born start to produce the IgG in 2-6 months following birth & reaches at peak in 1 year.
- **IgM:** It is the earliest Ig synthesise during foetal life between 3-6 months (approx 20 weeks), however it is immature & at very low level. Peak level achieved after birth in 1 year.

❖ Factors affecting concentration of Ig:

- **Increase concentration:** In diseases like leprosy, kala azar, malaria, syphilis, tuberculosis, Sub-Acute Bacterial Endocarditis (SABE) & some other chronic infection
- **Decrease concentration:** Due to
  - Congenital diseases
  - Delayed production
  - Secondary to diseases like myeloma, leukemia or drug induced.
- **Deficiency:** In nephritic syndrome

❖ Ig specificities:

A. **Idiotype specificity:**

- **Definition:**
  - The specific antigenic determinants on the antigen binding sites (paratopes, variable region) are **called idiotopes.**
  - The sum totals of idiotopes on an immunoglobulins molecule are **called idiotype specificities**.
- **Clinical significance:** →Vaccine production
  - By immunization with Fab fragments, anti-idiotype antibodies can be produced.
  - These resemble the epitopes of the original antigen.
  - Used as a vaccine, these show protection against the original antigen (pathogen or tumour) in experimental animals.
  - Sequential anti-idiotypic antibody formation is the basis of **Jerne's network hypothesis** of immune regulation.

B. **Isotype specificity:**

- **Definition:** Five classes of Ig (IgG, IgA, IgM, IgD & IgE) their subclasses **called isotype specificities.**
- It is due to genetical or structural differences in constant region of H chain. All individuals of one species have same isotype or same constant region. However different species have different isotype or different constant region. When such isotype or constant region of one species is injected in to other, it will be identified as foreign, resulting Ab production

C. **Allotype specificity:**

- **Definition:** Antigenic specificities which distinguish immunoglobulins of the same class, between different groups of individuals in the same species are **called allotype specificities.**
- It is not found in all member but some member of species **called allotype.**
- **Clinical significance:** In paternity testing & in population genetics

❖ Abnormal Ig:

- **Definition:** apart from antibodies, other structurally similar proteins are seen in serum in many pathological conditions & sometime even in healthy persons **called abnormal Ig.**
- **Types:**

A. **Light chains diseases:**

i. **Bence Jones proteins:**

- **History:** The earliest description of an abnormal Ig was given by Bence Jones (1847), who found protein in multiple myeloma.
- **Clinical significance:**
  - It is the excessive production of light chains.
  - Bence Jones proteins are the light chains of the Ig & so may occur as either K or γ forms in any one patient, but never both, being uniform in all other respect.

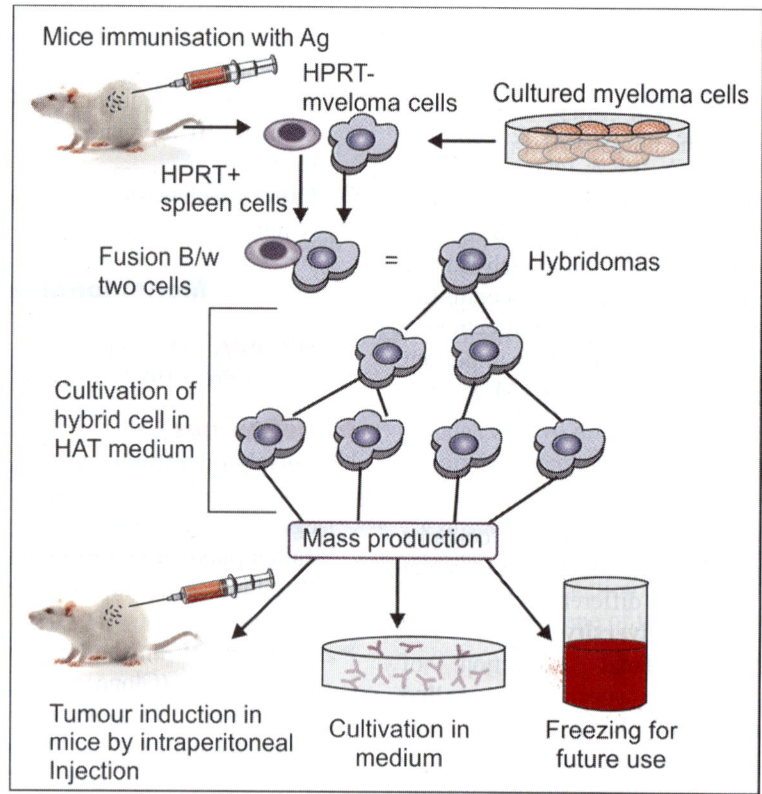

Figure-9: Production of monoclonal Ab

- To grow on HAT medium cells required to synthesize the purine which is possible by either *de novo* pathway or salvage pathway. Aminopterin blocks the *de novo* pathway while for salvage pathway cells required HGPRTase & thymidine kinase. Myeloma cells are HGPRTase deficient, so salvage pathway & ultimately purine synthesis is not possible by myeloma cells on HAT medium & they can't grow.
- It allows the growth of spleen cells contains HGPRTse, but it do not last longer as the cells are not immortal
- It allows the growth of only hybrid cells which last longer.

✪ **Mass production of monoclonal antibodies :**

- These hybridomas are clone & examined for production of Abs.
- Such clones are selected and used for **mass production** of Abs by following ways.

1. By growing in culture
2. By growing as tumour by injecting intraperitoneally in mice & monoclonal Abs are harvested from ascetic fluid.
3. Freeze for future use

❖ Uses:

a. Diagnostic:

1. **Isolation & identification of protein:** Monoclonal Ab is useful to isolate & to identify the interferon & coagulation factor VIII from the mixture, if present even in low concentration
2. **Identification of cells:** Identification of CD4 & CD8 cells by using anti CD4 & anti CD8 monoclonal antibodies respectively.
3. **Identification of antigens:** Like

- HBV, HIV etc
- Human chorionic gonadotropin by using anti human chorionic gonadotropin
- Blood group antigen by using anti-A & anti-B monoclonal antibodies.
- Tumour antigens: They secreted by tumour cells & diagnosed by imaging technique like prostate specific antigen.
- HLA: useful in tissue typing & can be done by anti-HLA monoclonal Ab.

Used in ELISA & IF kits

b. Prophylactic: Vaccine preparation

c. Therapeutic (immunotherapy):

- For monitoring drug & protein level in serum
- In treatment of cancer, inflammatory & allergic disease. Monoclonal antibody act by suppressing immune system, killing/inhibiting the tumour cells or by inhibiting the angiogenesis.
- Monoclonal antibody is used as post exposure prophylaxis in rabies, HBV etc.
- Immunotoxin: Monoclonal antibody is conjugated with specific toxin (like diphtheria toxin), where it combine with specific surface receptors & allowing toxin to kill target cells such as cancer cells.

helminthic infections, by mast cell degranulation & release of inflammatory mediators.

II. Physical classification

- **Two classes:** Based on availability, like free form in blood or bound form with receptors on B cells.

A. **Membrane** or **surface Igs:** IgD & IgM (secretory IgA?) are bound on B cell receptors (BCR) on surface hence **called membrane** or **surface Ig**. BCR is found only on the surface of B cells & facilitates the activation of these cells & their subsequent differentiation into either antibody producing plasma cells (antibody producing cells) or memory B cells that will survive in the body and remember that same antigen, so the B cells can respond faster upon future exposure.

B. **Free** or **soluble Igs:** IgG, IgA & IgE are secreted from the cells to be free in the blood / plasma.

❖ Age of Ig production: →Fig.-8

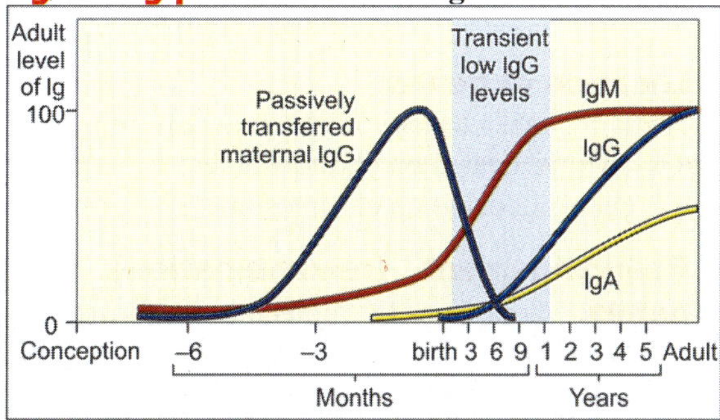

Figure-8: Age of Ig production

- **IgG:**
  - It is the only Ig which can cross the placenta.
  - New born has high level of passively transferred IgG, immediately after birth which start to fall after birth as shown in dark blue line in **fig.-8**.
  - Light blue line in **fig.-8** suggest that immune system of new born start to produce the IgG in 2-6 months following birth & reaches at peak in 1 year.
- **IgM:** It is the earliest Ig synthesise during foetal life between 3-6 months (approx 20 weeks), however it is immature & at very low level. Peak level achieved after birth in 1 year.

❖ Factors affecting concentration of Ig:

- **Increase concentration:** In diseases like leprosy, kala azar, malaria, syphilis, tuberculosis, Sub-Acute Bacterial Endocarditis (SABE) & some other chronic infection
- **Decrease concentration:** Due to
  - Congenital diseases
  - Delayed production
  - Secondary to diseases like myeloma, leukemia or drug induced.
- **Deficiency:** In nephritic syndrome

❖ Ig specificities:

A. **Idiotype specificity:**

- **Definition:**
  - The specific antigenic determinants on the antigen binding sites (paratopes, variable region) are **called idiotopes.**
  - The sum totals of idiotopes on an immunoglobulins molecule are **called idiotype specificities**.
- **Clinical significance:** →Vaccine production
  - By immunization with Fab fragments, anti-idiotype antibodies can be produced.
  - These resemble the epitopes of the original antigen.
  - Used as a vaccine, these show protection against the original antigen (pathogen or tumour) in experimental animals.
  - Sequential anti-idiotypic antibody formation is the basis of **Jerne's network hypothesis** of immune regulation.

B. **Isotype specificity:**

- **Definition:** Five classes of Ig (IgG, IgA, IgM, IgD & IgE) their subclasses **called isotype specificities.**
- It is due to genetical or structural differences in constant region of H chain. All individuals of one species have same isotype or same constant region. However different species have different isotype or different constant region. When such isotype or constant region of one species is injected in to other, it will be identified as foreign, resulting Ab production

C. **Allotype specificity:**

- **Definition:** Antigenic specificities which distinguish immunoglobulins of the same class, between different groups of individuals in the same species are **called allotype specificities.**
- It is not found in all member but some member of species **called allotype.**
- **Clinical significance:** In paternity testing & in population genetics

❖ Abnormal Ig:

- **Definition:** apart from antibodies, other structurally similar proteins are seen in serum in many pathological conditions & sometime even in healthy persons **called abnormal Ig.**
- **Types:**

A. **Light chains diseases:**

i. **Bence Jones proteins:**

- **History:** The earliest description of an abnormal Ig was given by Bence Jones (1847), who found protein in multiple myeloma.
- **Clinical significance:**
  - It is the excessive production of light chains.
  - Bence Jones proteins are the light chains of the Ig & so may occur as either K or γ forms in any one patient, but never both, being uniform in all other respect.

- This is because myeloma, a plasma cell dyscrasia in which there is unchecked proliferation of one clone of plasma cells, resulting in excessive production of the particular Ig synthesized by the clone. Such Ig **called monoclonal.**
- Multiple myeloma may affect plasma cells synthesising IgG, IgA, IgD or IgE.
- Because of the monoclonal nature, they have been valuable models for the understanding of immunoglobulin structure & function.

- **Diagnosis:** It can be identified in the urine by its characteristic property of coagulation when heated to 50°C but redissolving at 70°C.

ii. Waldenstrom's macroglobulinemia /M proteins:

- Similar involvement of IgM producing cells **called Waldenstrom's macroglobulinemia**.
- In this condition there is excessive production of the respective myeloma proteins (M proteins) & of their light chain (Bence Jones proteins).

B. Heavy Chain Disease (HCD):

- Characterized by the overproduction of the Fc parts of the Ig heavy chain due to lymphoid neoplasia.
- Three types of HCD are recognised based on class of heavy chain produced by malignant cells like α, γ &μ

C. Cryoglobulinemia:

- It is a condition in which a gel or precipitate is formed on cooling the serum, which redissolves on warming. It may not always be associated with disease but is often found in myeloma, macroglobulinemia & autoimmune condition such as SLE.
- Most cryoglobulins consist of IgG, IgM or their mixed precipitates.

❖ **Important aspects of Ig:** In general

- **IgG:** Protects the body fluids.
- **IgA:** Protects the body surfaces.
- **IgM:** Protects the bloodstream.
- **IgE:** Mediates the hypersensitivity.
- **IgD:** It is a recognition molecule on B cell surface.

✓ **Note:** All Igs are bifunctional except IgD because IgD is found only in bound form, so its Fc region remains attached to the B cells & not available for effectors function which all other Igs mediate.

Genes of immunoglobulin

❖ **History:** Ig chains are coded by more than one gene, this concept was 1st introduced by Dreyer & Bennett. Later it was proved by Tonegawa & Hozumi in 1975, for which they were awarded Nobel Prize in 1987.

❖ **Names of gene:**

- **Genes for H & L chain:** Two H & two L chains of an Ig are coded by separate genes, later all they are joined.

✪ **H chain's genes:** It is coded by four genes (gene segments), of which 3 are for V region & one is for C region

- Variable region: V (variable, V_H) gene, D (Diversity, D_H) gene & J (Joining, J_H) gene
- Constant region: C (Constant, C_H) gene, which consist 9 segments like Cα, Cβ, Cμ, Cδ etc.

✪ **L chain's genes:** It is coded by three genes (gene segments), of which 2 are for variable region & one is for constant region. Kappa & Lambda chains are coded by two different sets of V, J & C genes.

- Variable region: V (variable, V_H) gene & J (Joining, J_H) gene. D (Diversity, D_H) gene is absent.
- Constant region: C (Constant, C_H) gene.

- **Other genes:** It includes gene of enzyme, necessary for Ig formation like RAC (recombination activation) gene of recombinase enzyme

❖ **Location of genes:**

- H chain gene: Located on chromosome 14
- K L chain: Located on chromosome 2
- γ L chain: Located on chromosome 22

❖ **Rearrangement (recombination) of Ig genes:** Complete Ig molecule is formed after rearrangement between genes, which occurs at DNA & RNA level

- **Rearrangement at DNA level:**
  - It includes the rearrangement & joining of V, D & J genes of H & L chains
  - C genes of H & L chains are not undergoes for rearrangement at DNA level
  - Rearrangement occurs 1st in H chain followed by L chain genes
  - In H chain V-D joining occurs 1st followed by J joining **called V-D-J joining**
  - In L chain only V-J joining occurs
  - Rearrangement & joining of different genes is mediated by recombinase enzyme
- **Rearrangement at RNA level:**
  - V, D, J & C genes are transcribed to produce primary RNA like V region RNA, D region RNA, J region RNA & C region RNA respectively.
  - C region RNA combines with V region RNA to form complete H & L chains.
  - The whole C region RNA does not transcribed at a time but 1st Cμ & Cδ genes are transcribed & combined with V region RNA to form complete molecule of Ig like IgM, IgD respectively
- **Ig class switching:**

- **Synonym:** Ig isotype switching
- **Definition:** It is a biological process, which allows the synthesis of other classes or other isotypes of Ig (like IgA, IgE & IgG) after synthesis of IgM & IgD.

- **Mechanism:**
- Only the C_H region changes during class switching; the variable regions, and therefore antigen specificity, remain unchanged.
- Different C_H region gene transcribed & combine with other gene to form IgA, IgE & IgG
- **Clinical significance:** Absence of class switching does not allow the synthesis of IgA, IgE & IgG or may cause the hyper IgM syndrome, which lead to increased mucosal ulcer, diarrhoea & susceptibility of skin plus respiratory tract to bacterial infections.
- **Differential Ig RNA processing:** It is important for synthesis of membrane bound Ig (IgM & IgD) or secretory Ig.

Antibody diversity:

- **Definitions:**
- **Antibody diversity:** Human body contains enormous numbers ($\geq 10^8$) of structurally distinct antibodies, each with different specificity (paratope) **called antibody diversity**.
- **Antibody repertoire:** Total collection of antibodies with different specificities **called antibody repertoire**.
- **Mechanisms:** Genetic diversity is due to availability of plenty of Ig genes & their genetic rearrangement by following possible mechanisms.
- **Multiple genes for each region of Ig:** Large number of different genes are exist for each region of Ig such as $51V_H$ genes for H chain & each H chain would have one out of $51V_H$ genes. Follow **table-2** for other genes of H & L chain

Gene	Numbers of genes		
	H chain	κ L chain	γ L chain
V	51	40	30
D	27	0	0
J	6	5	4
C	9	1	4

Table-2: Multiple genes of H & L chain

- **Antigenic variation of genes:** It also responsible for antibody diversity
- **Multiple rearrangements (recombinations) of genes:** Multiple recombinations of genes of variable region allow the formation of multiple IgG classes. Follow **table-3** for multiple recombinations of V genes.

Type of joining	Possible recombinations
VDJ combination in H chain	$51V_H \times 27D_H \times 6J_H = 8262$
VJ combination in κ L chain	$40V_k \times 5J_k = 200$
VJ combination in γ L chain	$30V_\gamma \times 4J_\gamma = 120$
Combination in H & L chains	$8262 \times 200 \times 120 = 2.64 \times 10^6$

Table-3: Multiple recombinations of V genes

- **Mutation/Hypermutation:** After formation of Ig molecule, further changes occur in the nucleotide sequence of V region. It is due to point mutation with high frequency (10^{-3}/bp/generation then normal 10^{-8}/bp/generation), so **called hyper-mutation**.
- **Other mechanisms:** It includes junctional diversity & junctional flexbility.

Monoclonal antibodies

History:
Developed by Kohler and Milstein (Nobel Prize 1984) by using Hybridoma technique.

Definitions:

- **Polyclonal antibodies:**
- Antibodies produce in natural infection are usually against many epitope or antigenic determinant **called polyclonal antibodies**.
- Resulting antisera contains Ab with different classes.
- **Monoclonal antibodies:** Antibodies produce by single clone (Clone = single Ab producing cell) against single epitope or antigenic determinant **called monoclonal antibodies**.
- **Hybridomas (Hybrid cell):** Cell produced by fusion between mouse myeloma cells (ability to multiply indefinitely) & spleen cells (ability to produce Ab) **called hybrid cell or hybridomas**.

Technique:

- **Principle:**
- To produce the monoclonal antibody, cells required following two properties

1. Ability to produce the large number of Abs like splenic B cell
2. Ability to multiply indefinitely like myeloma cells (cancerous plasma cells)

- Take these two cells & prepare a hybrid cell
- Proliferate the hybrid cell in particular medium to produce large numbers of monoclonal Ab.
- **Steps: →Fig.-9**
- **Preparation of hybrid cells/hybridomas:**
- Immunise the mice with Ag, against which monoclonal Ab is required to produce.
- Cultivates the mouse myeloma cells which multiply indefinitely, do not form the Ig & deficient in enzyme HGPRTase (Hypoxanthine Guanine Phospho Ribosyl Transferase)
- Take the spleen cells contain HGPRTase from immunised mice & fuse with mouse myeloma cells to produce hybrid cells.
- **Growth of hybrid cells in HAT medium:**
- HAT medium contains <u>H</u>ypoxanthine, <u>A</u>minopterin and <u>T</u>hymidine

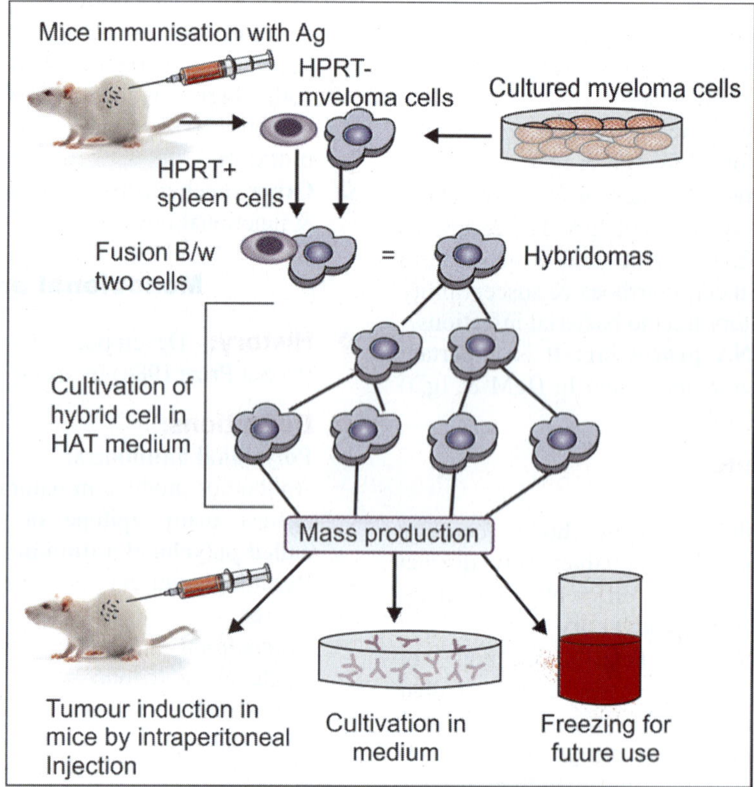

Figure-9: Production of monoclonal Ab

- To grow on HAT medium cells required to synthesize the purine which is possible by either *de novo* pathway or salvage pathway. Aminopterin blocks the *de novo* pathway while for salvage pathway cells required HGPRTase & thymidine kinase. Myeloma cells are HGPRTase deficient, so salvage pathway & ultimately purine synthesis is not possible by myeloma cells on HAT medium & they can't grow.
- It allows the growth of spleen cells contains HGPRTse, but it do not last longer as the cells are not immortal
- It allows the growth of only hybrid cells which last longer.

✪ **Mass production of monoclonal antibodies :**

- These hybridomas are clone & examined for production of Abs.
- Such clones are selected and used for **mass production** of Abs by following ways.

1. By growing in culture
2. By growing as tumour by injecting intraperitoneally in mice & monoclonal Abs are harvested from ascetic fluid.
3. Freeze for future use

❖ Uses:

a. Diagnostic:

1. **Isolation & identification of protein:** Monoclonal Ab is useful to isolate & to identify the interferon & coagulation factor VIII from the mixture, if present even in low concentration
2. **Identification of cells:** Identification of CD4 & CD8 cells by using anti CD4 & anti CD8 monoclonal antibodies respectively.
3. **Identification of antigens:** Like
   - HBV, HIV etc
   - Human chorionic gonadotropin by using anti human chorionic gonadotropin
   - Blood group antigen by using anti-A & anti-B monoclonal antibodies.
   - Tumour antigens: They secreted by tumour cells & diagnosed by imaging technique like prostate specific antigen.
   - HLA: useful in tissue typing & can be done by anti-HLA monoclonal Ab.

   Used in ELISA & IF kits

b. Prophylactic: Vaccine preparation

c. Therapeutic (immunotherapy):

- For monitoring drug & protein level in serum
- In treatment of cancer, inflammatory & allergic disease. Monoclonal antibody act by suppressing immune system, killing/inhibiting the tumour cells or by inhibiting the angiogenesis.
- Monoclonal antibody is used as post exposure prophylaxis in rabies, HBV etc.
- Immunotoxin: Monoclonal antibody is conjugated with specific toxin (like diphtheria toxin), where it combine with specific surface receptors & allowing toxin to kill target cells such as cancer cells.

d. **Research applications:**

e. **Other uses:** Abzyme is a monoclonal antibody with catalytic activity

❖ **Disadvantages:** Mice monoclonal Ab is unsuitable for humans use because of

- Development of anti mouse immune response in human or
- Fc piece of mice Ab could not elicit effective defensive mechanisms.

❖ **Overcoming of disadvantages:** All the disadvantages of mice monoclonal Ab for human use are corrected by following ways, so it is suitable for human use.

1. **Coupling method:** Coupling of Fab piece of Ig with active substances like toxins, enzymes, drugs or radiological substances.
2. **Genetic method:** (Chimeric antibodies production): by using murine variable region & human constant region.
3. **Grafting method:** Grafting of murine monoclonal Ab on CDR (Complementary Determining Region) loops on human Ig.
4. **Bacteriophage method:** Genes for monoclonal Ab production are fused in bacteriophage, which later allow infecting the bacteria & production of large quantity of Ab.

Question bank

Essay/Full question

1) Immunoglobulin (Ig)

Short notes

2) Structure of Ig
3) Differences between different classes of Ig
4) IgG
5) IgA
6) IgM
7) Clinical significances of IgG, IgA, IgM, IgD & IgE
8) Abnormal Ig
9) Genes of Ig
10) Monoclonal antibody

Short questions for theory/viva questions

1) Comment: All antibodies are immunoglobulins, but all immunoglobulins may not be antibodies.
2) Write the end result of digestion of Ig by papain & pepsin
3) What is hypervariable region in Ig?
4) Write the four functions of C-terminal of Ig
5) What is membrane Ig? Write two examples.
6) What is epitope & paratopes?
7) What is the hinge region? Write its function.
8) What is the valence in IgG? Write the valence numbers for IgG, IgA, IgM, IgD & IgE.
9) Write the two names of gene, each for H & L chain of Ig.
10) What is class switching in Ig? Write its clinical significance.
11) Define: Monoclonal antibodies & Polyclonal antibodies
12) Comment: Myeloma cells can't grow in HAT medium

MCQs for chapter review

Introduction

1) **Electrophoretic analysis of plasma protein was done by**
(a) Tiselius (b) Emil A Behring (c) Charles Richet (d) Peyton Rous

Immunoglobulin (Ig)

2) **Papain acts on gamma globulin to form**
(a) 2 Fc fragments (b) 2 Fab fragments (c) 1 Fab fragment (d) None
3) **Portion of immunoglobulin molecule with molecular weight of 50,000**
(a) Secretory piece (b) H chain (c) L chain (d) J piece
4) **A single immunoglobulin molecule contains** (AI-95)
(a) 1 light chain, 1 heavy chain (b) 2 heavy chain, 1 light chain (c) 2 light chain, 2 heavy chain (d) 2 light chain, 1 heavy chain
5) **A single immunoglobulin molecule contains** (AI-95)
(a) Single peptide chain (b) Two peptide chain (c) Non sulphur amino acid (d) 2 long and 2 short peptide chains
6) **Numbers of variable regions on each light & heavy chain of an antibody**
(a) 1 (b) 2 (c) 3 (d) 4
7) **Different classes of Ig are determined by**
(a) L chain (b) J chain (c) H chain (d) None
8) **Antigen binding site on antibody is-** (PGI, June -02)
(a) Hinge region (b) Constant region (c) Variable region (d) Hypervariable region (e) Idiotype region
9) **Antigen combing site of antibody**
(a) Idiotype (b) Paratope (c) Epitope (d) Hapten
10) **Complement attaches to immunoglobulin at**
(a) Aminoterminal (b) Fab region (c) Variable region (d) Fc fragment
11) **A variable portion of antibody molecule is**
(a) C-terminal (b) N-terminal (c) CHO moiety (d) None
12) **The following is constitute approximately 75% of total Ig in human**
(a) IgA (b) IgG (c) IgM (d) IgD (e) IgE
13) **The most abundant Ig in human body**
(a) IgM (b) IgG1 (c) IgG2 (d) IgG3
14) **Antibody transfer mother to foetus is**
(a) IgG (b) IgA (c) IgM (d) IgD (e) IgE
15) **Which immunoglobulin is scarce in human serum** (PGI, June-05)
(a) IgA (b) IgG (c) IgM (d) IgD (e) IgE
16) **Heat labile immunoglobulin**
(a) IgA (b) IgG (c) IgE (d) IgM
17) **True about immunoglobulin**
(a) IgE has maximum concentration (b) IgG has maximum concentration (c) IgA has minimum concentration (d) IgM has minimum concentration
18) **True of the following is/are** (PGI, June-01)
(a) IgA crosses placenta (b) Half life of IgG is 23 days (c) IgD is heat stable (d) IgE has highest carbohydrate content (e) IgG induce leukotrienes release during inflammation
19) **Which of the following Ig can cross the placenta**
(a) IgA (b) IgM (c) IgG (d) IgD
20) **Maximum half life**
(a) IgA (b) IgM (c) IgG (d) IgD
21) **Pentamer immunoglobulin is**
(a) IgA (b) IgG (c) IgM (d) IgE
22) **Antibody known as millionaire molecule is**
(a) IgA (b) IgM (c) IgG (d) IgE
23) **Activation of classical complement pathway**
(a) IgA (b) IgG (c) IgM (d) IgD
24) **The most avidly complement fixing antibody is** (AIIMS, May-02)
(a) IgA (b) IgG (c) IgM (d) IgE

25) J chain is a structural part of
(a) IgA (b) IgM (c) IgG (d) a+b

26) The serum concentration of which of the following human Ig subclass is maximum (AI-05)
(a) IgG1 (b) IgG2 (c) IgG3 (d) IgG4

27) The commonest IgG with maximum individual variation is (PGI-96)
(a) IgG1 (b) IgG2 (c) IgG3 (d) IgG4

28) Function of IgA is
(a) Act as mucosal barrier for infection (b) Circulating antibody (c) Kills virus infected cell (d) Activates macrophages (e) Causes delayed hypersensitivity

29) Antibody responsible for local immunity is
(a) IgA (b) IgM (c) IgG (d) IgE

30) In respiratory and GIT infections, which is the most affected immunoglobulin (AI-94)
(a) IgA (b) IgG (c) IgM (d) IgD

31) The secretory component of immunoglobulin molecules is (PGI-01)
(a) Formed by epithelial cells of lining mucosa (b) Formed by plasma cells (c)) Formed by epithelial cells and plasma cells (d) Secreted by bone marrow

32) Secretory piece is a structural part of
(a) IgA (b) IgM (c) IgG (d) a+b

33) Which of the following Ig is responsible for opsonisation
(a) IgA (b) IgG (c) IgM (d) IgE

34) Haemagglutinis (anti-A & anti-B) are which type of antibodies
(a) IgG (b) IgM (c) IgA (d) IgE

35) Which of the immunoglobulin is associated with allergic disorders?
(a) IgG (b) IgM (c) IgA (d) IgE

36) Antibody elevated in parasitic infection
(a) IgA (b) IgE (c) IgG (d) IgM

37) Ovalbumin was injected in to a rabbit. Which of the following classes of antibodies are likely to be produced initially (AI-11)
(a) IgG (b) IgM (c) IgE (d) IgD

38) IgE is secreted by (PGI-02)
(a) Mast cells (b) Basophils (c) Eosinophils (d) Plasma cells (e) Neutrophils

39) Ig are produced by
(a) Macrophages (b) B-cells (c) T-cells (d) NK cells

40) Plasma cells are derived from (AI-99)
(a) T-cells (b) B-cells (c) Macrophages (d) Neutrophils

41) True about immunoglobulin is (AIIMS, Feb-97)
(a) IgE fixes complement (b) IgM fixes complement (c) IgG found in minimum concentration (d) IgG is elevated in primary immune response

42) Which of the following statement concerning immunoglobulin is wrong (AI-97)
(a) IgM does not cross the placenta (b) IgE increased in parasitic infection (c) IgM increased in primary response (d) Foetal infection is characterised by increased in IgG

43) Capacity of producing IgG start at which age
(a) 6th month (c) 1st year (d) 2nd year (e) 3rd year

44) The earliest Ig to be synthesised by the foetus is- (AI-03)
(a) IgA (b) IgG (c) IgE (d) IgM

45) Which immunoglobulin is least important in human being
(a) IgE (b) IgD (c) IgG (d) IgA

46) Which of the following immunoglobulins constitutes the antigen binding component of B cell receptor
(a) IgA (b) IgD (c) IgM (d) IgG

47) Antigen idiotype is related to
(a) Fc fragment (b) Hinge region (c) C-terminal (d) N-terminal

48) Ig change in variable region is
(a) Idiotype (b) Isotype (c) Allotype (d) Autotype

49) Isotype specificity in Ig is due to
(a) Changes in constant region of L chain (b) Changes in constant region of H chain (c) Changes in variable region of L chain (d) Changes in variable region of H chain

50) Which of the following statements is true about isotypic variation? (AIIMS, Nov-08)
(a) These result due to subtle amino acid changes resulting from allelic differences (b) These result due to changes in amino acid in heavy chain and light chain at variable region (c) Changes in heavy and light chain in constant region is responsible for class and subclass of immunoglobulin (d) These are areas in antigen that bind specifically to antibody

51) Which precipitates at 50^0C-60^0C, but disappears on heating (AI-96)
(a) Heavy chain (b) Light chain (c) Both (d) None of the above

52) Bence Jones proteins are best described as (AI-96)
(a) α chain (b) γ chain (c) Kappa & Lambda chains (d) Fibrin split products

Genes of immunoglobulin

53) Which of the following statement is true regarding kappa, lambda and heavy chain immunoglobulin (PGI-01)
(a) Coded on the same site of chromosome (b) Coded on the different sites of same chromosome (c) The chains are formed by genetic rearrangement after maturation (d) Different chains of same immunoglobulins are coded by different chromosomes (e) Different chains of same immunoglobulins are coded by same chromosomes

54) Class switching is required for synthesis of following immunoglobulin
(a) IgA (b) IgM (c) IgG (d) IgD

55) Synthesis of an immunoglobulin in membrane bound or secretory form is determined by (AIIMS, May-12)
(a) One turn to two turn joining rule (b) Class switching (c) Differential RNA processing (d) Allelic exclusion

56) Antibody diversity is due to (PGI, Dec-08, Nov -13)
(a) Gene rearrangement (b) Gene translocation (c) Antigenic variation (d) CD40 molecule (e) Mutation

Monoclonal antibody

57) Theory of monoclonal antibody was developed by
(a) Theobald Smith (b) Kohler & Milstein (c) Richet (d) Paul Ehrlich

58) Hybridoma technique is used to obtain
(a) Specific antigen (b) Complement (c) Specific antibody (d) Interleukins

59) Medium for monoclonal antibody production is
(a) HAT medium (b) Kelly's medium (c) Pike's medium (d) Islam's medium

60) All of the following statements about Hybridoma technology are true except (AIIMS, Nov-08)
(a) Specific antibody producing cells are integrated with myeloma cells (b) Myeloma cells with mutation pathway grows well in HAT medium (c) Aminopterin a folate antagonis, inhibit the de novo pathway (d) HGPRTase and thymidine synthetase are required for salvage pathway.

61) Use of monoclonal antibody is
(a) Immunotherapy (b) Immunological identification of cells & tissues (c) Radio immuno imaging (d) All of above

Answers of MCQs & explanation

1) (a)
- Emil A Behring: Developed antitoxin to Diphtheria
- Charles Richet: Discovered the anaphylaxis
- Peyton Rous: Discovered viral oncogenesis

2) (b)
- Follow section, **digestion or degradation of Ig & fig.-1** for explanation

3) (b)
4) (c) Follow section, **structure of Ig** & **fig.-4** for explanation
5) (d)
6) (a)
7) (c)
- Different classes/isotypes of Ig are determined by different type of H chain. Different types L chain like kappa & lambda are also available but not significant as like H chain. J chain has joining function between different Ig molecules.

8) (d) Follow section, **structure of Ig [Aminoterminus (N**
9) (b) **terminal/Fab fraction) end → hypervariable region]** for explanation
10) (d) Follow section, **structure of Ig [Carboxyterminus**
11) (b) **(C terminal/ Fc fraction) end →]** for explanation
12) (b)
- IgG constitutes 70-80% of the total Ig.

13) (b)
- IgG constitutes 70-80% of the total Ig. There are four subclasses of IgG like IgG1, IgG2, IgG3 & IgG4 with approximate proportion is 65%, 23%, 8% & 4% respectively.

14) (A)
- IgG can cross the placenta & it transfer from mother to foetus.

15) (e)
16) (c)
17) (b)
18) (b) & (c)
19) (c)
20) (c) Follow **table-1** for explanation
21) (c)
22) (b)
23) (b) & (c)
24) (c)
25) (d)
26) (a) Approximate proportion of IgG1, IgG2, IgG3 & IgG4
27) (a) is 65%, 23%, 8% & 4% respectively.
28) (a)
29) (a) Follow section, **IgA (clinical significances)**
30) (a) for explanation
31) (a) Follow section, **IgA (structure & subclasses**
32) (a) **→ Secretory IgA)** & **fig.-6** for explanation
33) (b) & (c)
- IgM is more effective than IgG in opsonisation

34) (b)
- Follow section, **IgM (clinical significances → natural Abs)** for explanation

35) (d)
36) (b) IgE is elevated in allergic reaction & parasitic infection
37) (c)
- IgE production increased following exposure of allergen like ovalbumin

38) (d) After antigenic stimulation B cells are differentiated in to
39) (b) plasma cells & memory cells. Plasma cells are the Ab
40) (b) producing cells & kown to produce the all kinds of Ig
41) (b)
- IgE does not fixes complement
- IgM (+++) & IgG (++) fixes classical pathway of complement while IgA fixes the alternative pathway
- IgG found in maximum concentration
- IgM is elevated in primary immune response, while IgG is elevated in primary immune response

42) (d)
- Foetal infection is characterised by increased in IgM

43) (a) Follow section, **age of Ig production &**
44) (d) **fig.-8** for explanation
45) (b)
- IgD is the least important Ig in human being

46) (b) & (c)
- IgD & IgM are the surface Igs and they are fixed with B cells by specific receptors **called B cell receptor (BCR)**

47) (d)
- Idiotype of Ig are due to change in variable region of H chain, which is present at aminoterminus end or N terminal

48) (a) Idiotypes are due to change in variable region,
49) (b) isotypes are due to change in constant region of H chain. Allotype are present in some members of species. Follow section, Ig specificities for more explanation.
50) (c) **→ Partially correct**
- Isotypes of Ig are due to change in constant region of H chain only, not due to change in L chain

51) (b)
- Difficult to judge the answer, but light chain is the correct answer
- Bence Jones protein is an abnormal Ig, formed due to excessive production of L chain (either kappa or lambda forms in any one patient, but never both). It is detected from urine by coagulation (precipitation) when heated to 50°C but redissolving at 70°C

52) (c)
- Follow section, **abnormal Ig (Bence Jones protein)** for explanation

53) (c) & (d)
- Genes for H chain, K L chain & γ L chain are located not on same chromosome but on different chromosome like number 14, 2 & 22 respectively
- Different chains of Ig are formed by genetic rearrangement
- Follow section, **genes of Ig** for more explanation

54) (a) & (c)
- Follow section, **genes of Ig (Ig class switching)** for explanation

55) (c)
- Follow section, **genes of Ig (Differential Ig RNA processing)** for explanation

56) (a), (c) & (e)
- Follow section, **genes of Ig (antibody diversity → mechanisms)** for explanation

57) (b)
- Follow section, **monoclonal antibody** (**history**) for explanation

58) (c)
- Hybridoma technique is used to obtain specific antibody not for specific antigen, complement or for interleukins

59) (b)
- Follow section, **monoclonal antibody** for explanation

60) (b)
- Myeloma cells are deficient with HGPRTase so they can't grow on HAT medium. Follow section, **monoclonal antibody** for more explanation

61) (d)
- Follow section, **monoclonal antibody (uses)** for explanation

22 Antigen-antibody (Ag-Ab) reactions

Learning heading & subheadings

Introduction

❖ **Combination:** Antigen & antibody combine with each other specifically & in observable manner.

❖ **Types:** →Flow chart-1

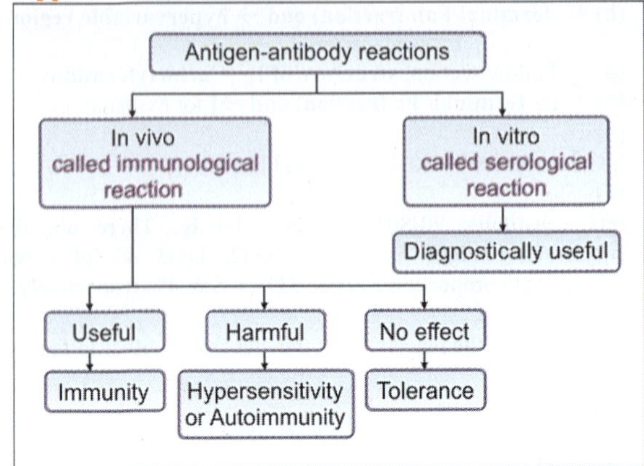

Flow chart-1: Antigen-antibody reactions

❖ **Stages of Ag-Ab reactions:** Three stages.

A. Primary stage:

- Initial interaction, without any visible effects.
- Reaction is rapid, occurs even at low temperatures and reversible.
- Ag-Ab complex formation is possible by weaker intermolecular forces like ionic (electrostatic) bonds, Van der Waal's forces & hydrogen bonds
- **Detection of reactions:** By estimating free and bound antigens or antibodies separately in reaction mixture by use of markers such as radioactive isotopes, fluorescent dyes or ferritin

B. Secondary stage:

- Occur in most instances, but not at all times.
- Demonstrable events (in vitro) such as precipitation, agglutination, lysis of cells, killing of live antigens, neutralisation of toxins and other biologically active antigens, compliment fixation, immobilisation of motile organisms and enhancement of phagocytosis.
- Name of Ag & Ab as per reaction: →**Table-1**

Reaction	Ag	Ab
Precipitation	Precipitinogen	Precipitin
Agglutination	Agglutinogen	Agglutinin

Table-1: Name of Ag & Ab as per reaction

- Participation by different antibodies in different reaction is mentioned in table-1 of chapter Antibody (Ab) –Immunoglobulin (Ig).

C. Tertiary stage (In vivo): In vivo type Ag-Ab reactions initiate chain reactions that lead to tissue protection (immunity by neutralisation or destruction of antigens) or lead to tissue damage (hypersensitivity or autoimmunity).

❖ General features:

1. **Reactions are specific:**
- Antigen combines only with its homologous antibody and vice versa.
- However specificity is not absolute & cross-reactions may occur due to antigenic similarity.
2. **Participation in reaction:**
- Entire molecules and not fragments react. When an antigenic determinant which is present in large molecule or on 'carrier' particle reacts with its antibody, whole molecules or particles are agglutinated.
- Both antigens & antibodies participate in the formation of agglutinates or precipitates.
3. **No denaturation:** No denaturation of antigen or antibody during reaction.
4. **Combination between Ag-Ab:**
- **Nature:**
  - Occurs at surface.
  - Reversible.
  - Firm but influenced by affinity and avidity of reaction.
- **Affinity:**
  - Intensity of attraction between Ag-Ab.
  - Depend on closeness between epitope & paratope.
  - It is a quantitative measurement.
  - Low affinity→ weak binding→ early dissociation
  - High affinity→ strong binding→ long association
- **Avidity:**
  - Strength of bond to remain together after formation of Ag-Ab complex.
  - IgM has low affinity than IgG, but high avidity enables it to bind very effectively with Ag.
5. **Proportions of Ag-Ab combination:**
- Ag-Ab can combine in varying proportions.
- Both antigens and antibodies are multivalent.
- Antibodies are generally bivalent, though IgM molecules may have five or ten combining sites.
- Antigens may have valences up to hundreds.

❖ Measurement:

➢ **Unit:** In terms of mass or units or titre.

➢ **Titre:**
- **Definition:** Highest dilution of serum that shows an observable reaction in particular test.
- **Influenced:** It is done for both Ag & Ab & influenced by
  - Nature of antigen.
  - Quantity of antigen.
  - Type of test.
  - Conditions of tcst.

➢ **Sensitivity:**
- Ability of a test to detect even very minute quantities of Ag or Ab from sample.
- High sensitive of test minimise the false negative result.

➢ **Specificity**
- Ability of test to detect reactions between homologous Ag and Ab only.
- High specificity of test minimise the false positive result.

➢ **Proportion:** Sensitivity and specificity of test are in inverse proportion.

Serological reactions

Following are the different types of serological reactions or tests

- ◊ **Precipitation**
- ◊ **Agglutination**
- ◊ **Complement Fixation Test (CFT)**
- ◊ **Neutralisation**
- ◊ **Opsonisation**
- ◊ **Radio Immuno Assay (RIA)**
- ◊ **Enzyme Immuno Assay (EIA)**
- ◊ **Immuno Fluorescence Assay (IFA)**
- ◊ **Immuno Electroblot Technique**
- ◊ **Immuno Chromatographic Test (ICT)**
- ◊ **Immuno concentration test**
- ◊ **Tests by using Electron Microscopy**

Precipitation reaction

❖ Definitions:

➢ **Precipitation:** Formation of an insoluble precipitate due to soluble Ag-Ab complex in presence of electrolytes (NaCl) at suitable temperature and pH **called precipitation**.

➢ **Flocculation:** When precipitate remains suspended as floccules instead of sedimentation, reaction is **called flocculation**.

❖ Properties:

- Precipitation occurs at the bottom of tube
- Medium of reaction: Liquid media or in gels such as polyacrylamide, agar or agarose.

❖ Zone phenomenon:

- Amount of precipitate/agglutinate formed is influenced by relative proportions of Ags & Abs.
- Increasing quantities of antigens are added to same amount of antiserum in different tubes, precipitation will be found to occur most rapidly & abundantly in one of the middle tubes in which antigens & antibodies are present in optimal or equivalent proportions **called zone of equivalence**.
- In preceding tubes in which antibodies are in excess **called prozone (Ab excess) phenomenon** and in later tubes in which antigens are in excess **called postzone (Ag excess) phenomenon**, precipitation will be weak or even absent.
- For given antigen-antibody system, optimal or equivalent ratio will be constant, irrespective of quantity of reactants.

- **Clinical significance:** Sera rich in antibody may sometimes give false negative precipitation or agglutination result, unless several dilutions are tested.
- **Correction of prozone/post zone phenomenon:** By serial dilution of serum

❖ Mechanism of precipitation (Lattice hypothesis): →Fig.-1

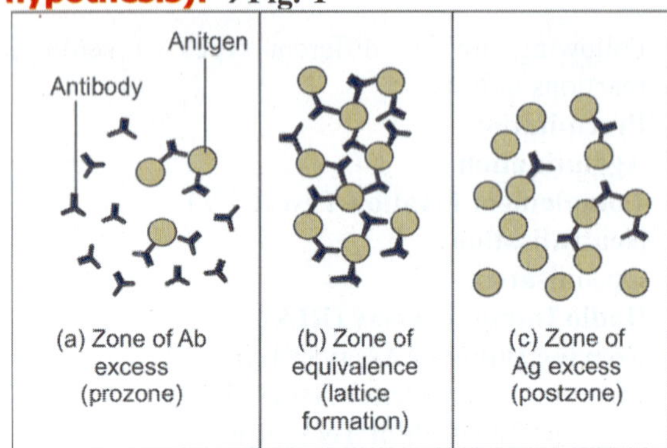

Figure-1: Lattice hypothesis

- In 1934 Marrack proposed the lattice hypothesis to explain the mechanism of precipitation (also related to agglutination).
- According to him precipitates (agglutinate) results when large lattice formed between Ag & Ab.
- It is possible in zone of equivalence while in zones of Ab or Ag excess lattice does not enlarge.

❖ Uses or applications of precipitation reaction:

a. **Diagnostic:**
1. Detection of antigens
2. Toxigenicity testing in *C. diphtheriae*.
3. VDRL testing in syphilis

b. **Forensic application:** In identification of blood & seminal stains

c. **Testing for food adulterants:**

d. **Typing or grouping of bacteria:** E.g. Lancefield grouping of *Streptococci*

❖ Testing method or procedures: Two types

1. **Qualitative test:** It detect the presence or absence of Ag/Ab
2. **Quantitative test:** It detect the exact titre of Ag/Ab

❖ Serological test based on precipitation or flocculation:

✓ **Note: Differences between precipitation & flocculation**

- **Precipitation:** Ag-Ab complex sediment at bottom of mixture. Mostly done in tube.
- **Flocculation:** Ag-Ab complex float at top of mixture. Done in tube & slide.

I. Ring test

➢ **Method:** Layering antigen solution over a column of antiserum in a narrow tube. A precipitate forms at junction of two liquids.

➢ **Examples:**

1. Ascoli's thermoprecipitin test.
2. Lancefield grouping of *Streptococci*.

II. Slide test

➢ **Method:** Drop of antigen and antiserum are placed on slide and mixed by shaking, floccules appear.

➢ **Examples:**

A **VDRL test:**

B **RPR test:**

A. VDRL test

✪ **History:**

- Initial test was developed by August Paul Von Wasserman with the aid of Albert Neisser in 1906
- VDRL test done today was developed by Harris, Rosenberg & Riedel in 1946.

✪ **Full name:** Venereal Disease Research Laboratory, New York, where the test was developed

✪ **Principle:** It is the non-specific (non treponemal) test, based on slide flocculation test

✪ **Ag:** It is prepared from bovine heart & lipid in nature hence **called cardiolipin** (cardia for heart & lipin for lipid) & added with lecithin & cholesterol hence also **called cholelecithin** Ag. It standardised by Pangborn in 1945. In India it is prepared by Institute of serology, Kolkata.

✪ **Ab: Called reagin Ab** present in patient's serum which is IgG or rarely IgM in nature. IgE antibody of type-I hypersensitivity (atopy) also **called reagin antibody**, however there is no correlation between two.

✪ **Procedures:** Two methods

i. **Qualitative method:**

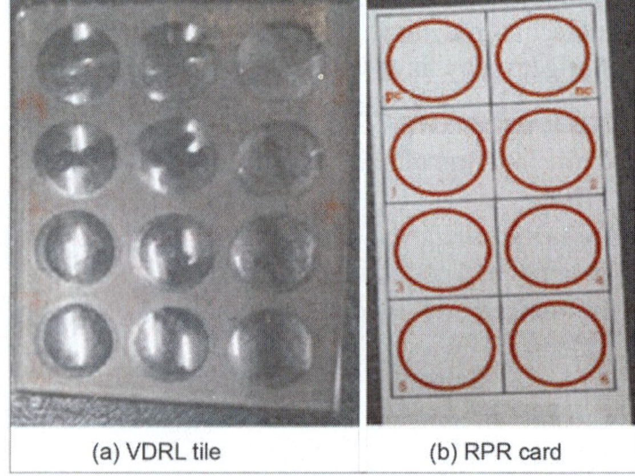

Figure-2: VDRL tile & RPR card

- Performed on VDRL tile/slide [**fig.-2(a)**] contains 12 concavities/circles.
- Put 1 drop of heat inactivated serum (56 °C for 30 minutes) in one circle. Heating is required to remove non specific inhibitors.

- Mixed serum with one drop of cardiolipin antigen solution.
- Put –Ve & +Ve control on separate circles.
- Rotate manually or on VDRL rotator at 180 rpm for 4 min.
- Read the result under a low power microscope.

ii. Quantitative method:

- All samples reactive by qualitative method are subjected to the quantitative method
- Put one drop of normal saline (ns) in circle numbered 1, 2, 3, 4…
- Place one drop of serum in 1st circle
- Prepare the serial dilution by transferring the drop of serum from 1st to 2nd, 2nd to 3rd and so…..
- Add one drop of Ag in each circle & mix properly
- Rotate manually or on VDRL rotator at 180 rpm for 4 min
- Read the result under a low power microscope.

✪ **Results: →Table-2 & fig.3**

Result/report	Reading
Non-reactive (NR)	No floccules
Weakly reactive (W)	Small floccules
Reactive (R)	Medium/large floccules

Table-2: Result of qualitative VDRL test

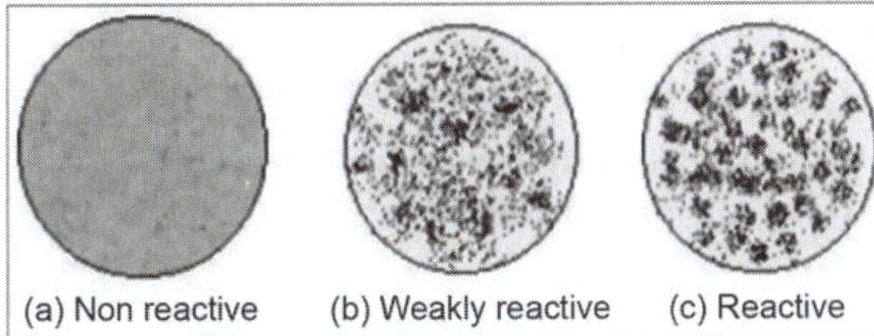

Figure-3: Result of qualitative VDRL test

✪ **Interpretation:**

1. **Positive:** Indicating syphilis. Significant titre is 1:8
2. **Negative:** No syphilis

✪ **Uses:**

- **Diagnostic:**
  - Useful for diagnosis of syphilis
  - Useful for diagnosis of neurosyphilis: It be performed from CSF **called VDRL-CSF**, where prior heating is not required
- **Therapeutic:** Useful to monitor the treatment of syphilis where titre decline following successful therapy

✪ **Advantages:** Simple, rapid & most widely used

✪ **Disadvantages:** Chances of Biological False Positive (BFP)

- **Definition:** Positive reaction with non-treponemal tests & negative result with treponemal tests in absence of past/present infection & not due to technical faults **called Biological False Positive (BFP)**
- **Properties:**
  - **Frequency:** Occurs in 1% normal serum
  - **Type of Ab:** BFP antibody is mainly IgM type
- **Aetiology:** Cardiolipin Ag present in treponemal and also in mammalian host tissue which induces reagin Ab production. BFP result is due to cross reaction of cardiolipin Ag with non specific antibodies produced by other infections or diseases.
- **Types:** Following types

1. **Acute:** Antibodies are last for few weeks/months
   - Infection
   - Inflammation
   - Trauma
2. **Chronic:** Antibodies last for > 6 months
   - Autoimmune disease like Systemic Lupus Erythematosus (SLE)
   - Lepromatous leprosy (LL), hepatitis, infectious mononucleosis, malaria, tropical eosinophilia.
3. **Others:**
   - All serological tests of syphilis are false positive in endemic treponematoses like yaws, pinta & endemic syphilis
   - BFP also occurs in HIV, genital herpes, measles, *M pneumoniae*, relapsing fever, parenteral drugs etc.

✪ **Differences between VDRL test & RPR test: → Table-3**

Features	VDRL test	RPR test
Samples	- Heated serum - No plasma - CSF	- Unheated serum - Plasma - No CSF
Preheating of serum	Required to remove non specific inhibitors	Not required as choline chloride is used to remove inhibitors
Material required	Glass slide with 12 concavities or depression with 14mm size **called tile** [fig.2(a)]	Plastic disposable slide with 10 circles with 18mm size **called RPR card** [fig.2(b)]
Nature of Ag	- Freshly made & should be used within 24 hours.	- Ag can be stabilised by EDTA, stored at 4-10^{0}C for 4-6 months & can be used long
Rotation of slide	4 minutes	8 minutes
Clumps	Clumps are small & white. Uncoated Ag.	Large & black because Ag coated with carbon particles
Reading of result	By microscope	By naked eyes
Sensitivity in primary syphilis	78%	86%
Cost	Cheaper & 250 tests can be performed from1 vial, so used as screening tests	Expensive & preferred when sample size is less

Table-3: Differences between VDRL & RPR test

B. RPR test

- **Full name:** Rapid Plasma Reagin test
- **Principle:** Based on slide flocculation test
- **It is similar to VDRL test, but some differences are listed in table-3**
- **Use:** Useful for diagnosis of syphilis

III. Tube test

- **Examples:**

1. **Kahn test:** Useful for diagnosis of syphilis.
2. **Quantitative tube flocculation test:**

- Serial dilutions of toxin / toxoid added to tubes containing fixed quantity of antitoxin.
- Amount of toxin or toxoid that flocculates optimally with 1 unit of antitoxin **called Lf dose.**

IV. Immunodiffusion (precipitation in gel)

- **Advantages of allowing precipitation in gel than liquid medium:**
  - Reaction is visible as distinct band of precipitation, which is stable and can be stained for preservation.
  - Each antigen-antibody reaction gives line of precipitation, number of different antigens in mixture can be observed.
  - Indicates identity, nonidentity & cross-reaction between different the antigens.
- **Medium:** Performed in soft (1%) agar or agarose gel.
- **Examples of immunodiffusion (modification of immunodiffusion test):**

A. Single diffusion in single dimension (Oudin procedure):

- **Steps: →Fig.-4(a)**
  - Incorporate the Ab in agar gel in test tube.
  - Add the Ag solution over it.
  - Ag diffuses downward through agar gel & forms the line of precipitation.

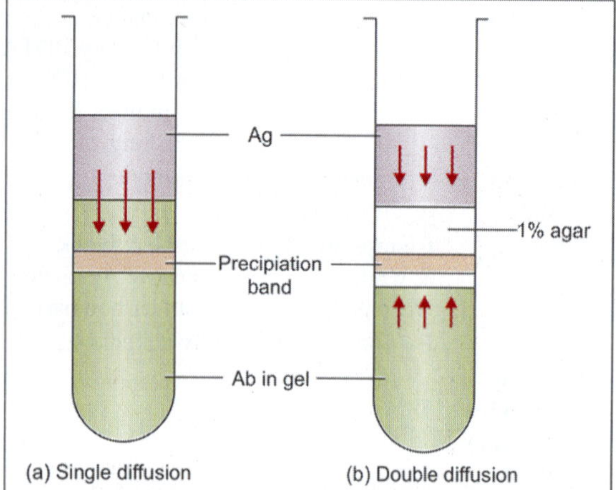

Figure-4: Oudin & Oakley-Fulthorpe procedure

B. Double diffusion in single dimension (Oakley-Fulthorpe procedure):

- **Steps: →Fig.-4(b)**
  - Incorporate the Ab in agar gel in test tube.
  - Place the column of plain agar above Ab solution.
  - Ag is layered on top of this.
  - Ag- Ab move towards each other through column of plain agar and form band of precipitate where they meet at optimum proportion.

C. Single diffusion in double dimensions (radial immunodiffusion):

- **Steps: →Fig.-5**
  - Ab is incorporated in agar gel poured on flat surface (slide or petri dish).
  - Ag is added to wells cut on surface of gel.
  - It diffuses radially from well and forms ring-shaped bands of precipitation (halos) concentrically around the well.
- **Uses:**
  - Diameter of halo gives estimate of antigen concentration (Ag estimation).
  - To estimate of Ig classes in sera
  - Screening sera for antibodies to influenza viruses.

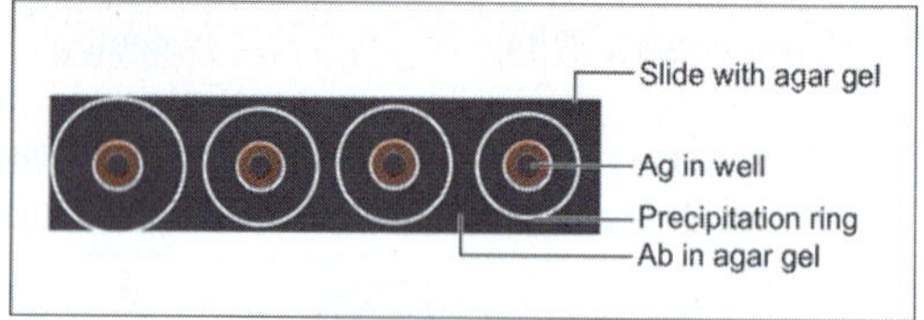

Figure-5: Radial immunodiffusion

D. Double diffusion in double dimensions (Ouchterlony procedure):

- **Steps: →Fig.-6**

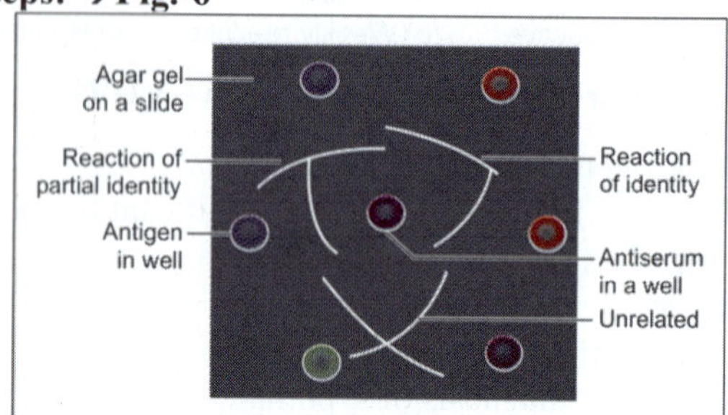

Figure-6: Ouchterlony procedure

- Agar gel is poured on slide and wells are cut.
- Ab is placed in central well and different antigens in surrounding wells.
- If two adjacent antigens are identical, lines of precipitate formed by them will fuse.
- If they are unrelated, lines will cross each other.
- Cross-reaction or partial identity characterised by spur formation.

- **Uses:**
  - Compare different antigens and antisera directly.
  - Toxigenicity testing. E.g. Elek's gel precipitation test in *C. diphtheriae*

E. Immunoelectrophoresis:

- **Principle:** Involves electrophoretic separation of composite antigen (serum) into its constituent proteins, followed by immunodiffusion against its antiserum, resulting in separate precipitin lines, indicating reaction between each individual protein with its antibody.

- **Steps: →Fig.-7**
- Incorporate agar or agarose gel on a slide
- Made an Ag well & an Ab trough cut on it.
- Place the antigen in well and separate by electrophoresis.
- Place Ab in trough cut
- Allow the diffusion.
- Resulting formation of precipitin line can be photographed & slides dried, stained and preserved.

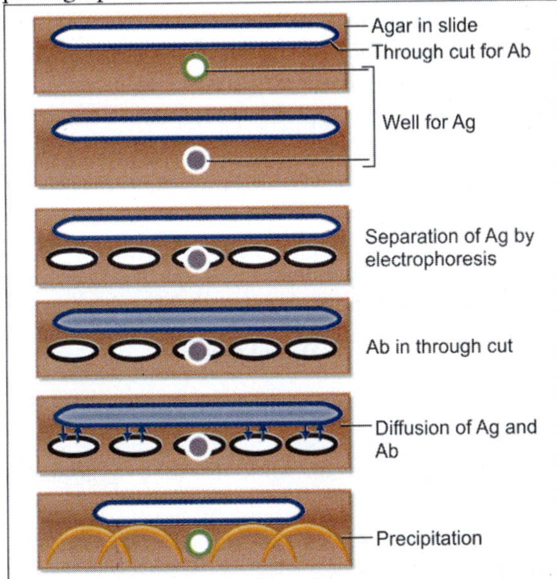

Figure-7: Immunoelectrophoresis

- **Uses:** Identification & approximate quantitation of various normal & abnormal proteins (heavy chain diseases) of serum.

V. Electroimmunodiffusion

- **Method:** Developments of precipitin lines can be speeded up by electrically driving antigen and antibody.
- **Examples or types of tests:** Following are the different types of tests based on electroimmunodiffusion tests

i. Counter Immuno Electrophoresis (CIE, counter-current immunoelectrophoresis):

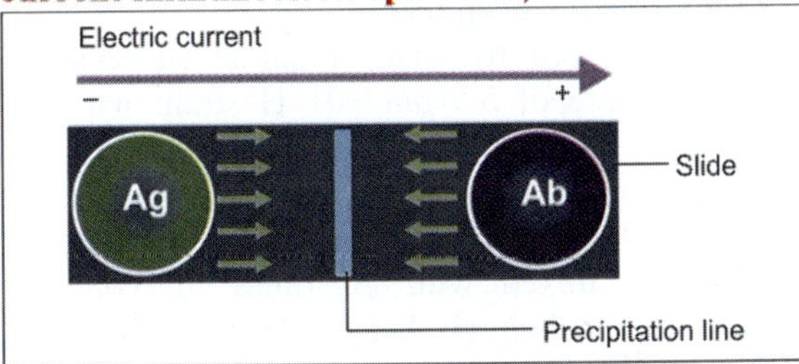

Figure-8: CIE

- **Steps:** Simultaneous electrophoresis of antigen and antibody in gel in opposite directions resulting in precipitation at mid-point between them as shown in **fig.-8**
- **Uses:** Clinical applications to detect the various antigens: such as
- Alpha Feto Protein (AFP) in serum
- Specific antigens of C. *neoformans* in CSF.
- Ag of *N. meningitidis* in CSF.

ii. One-dimensional single electroimmunodiffusion (rocket electrophoresis):

- **Steps: →Fig.-9**
- Place the agar gel on glass slide
- Incorporate the antiserum in to agar
- Antigen, in increasing concentrations, is placed in wells punched in set gel.
- Ag is electrophoresed into an Ab containing agarose.
- Formation of rocket like pattern of immunoprecipitation.
- **Use:** For quantitative estimation of antigens.

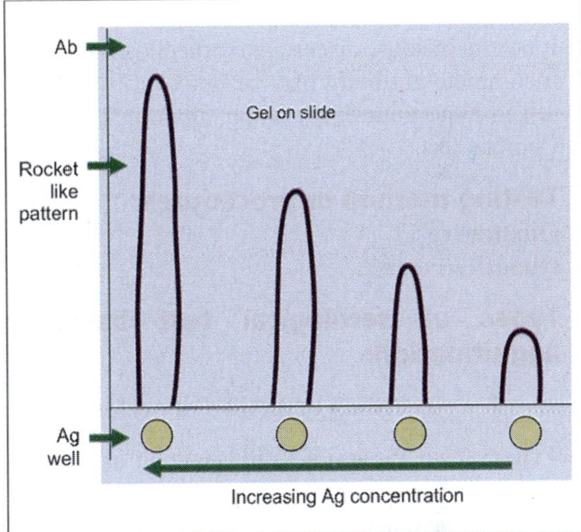

Figure-9: Rocket electrophoresis

iii. Laurell's two-dimensional electrophoresis:

- **Steps:** Ag mixture is electrophoretically separated in direction perpendicular to that of final rocket stage as shown in **fig.-10.**

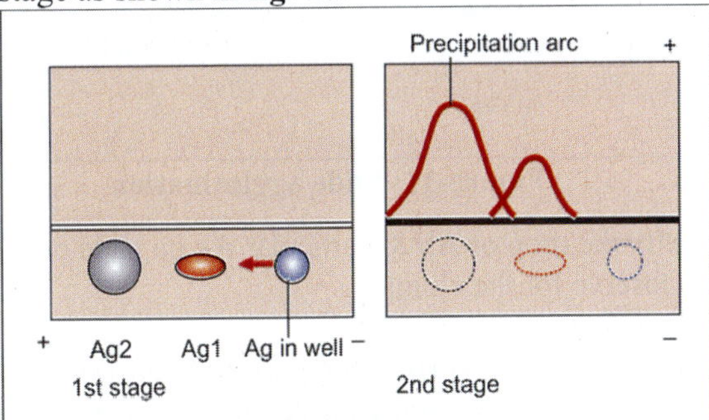

Figure-10: Laurell's two-dimensional electrophoresis

- **Use:** To quantitate each of several antigens in mixture.

Agglutination reaction

❖ **Definition:** When particular Ag is mixed with its Ab in presence of electrolytes at suitable temperature and pH, particles are clumped or agglutinated **called agglutination**.

❖ **Properties:**

- More sensitive than precipitation for detection of antibodies.
- It also following the zone phenomenon.
- Agglutination occurs optimally in zone of equivalence.
- It sediments at bottom of tube.
- **Blocking antibodies (incomplete antibodies):**
  - Incomplete or monovalent antibodies do not cause agglutination, though they combine with antigen.
  - They may act as **'blocking' antibodies,** inhibiting agglutination by complete antibody added subsequently.
  - It occurs in some disease like brucellosis.
  - Incomplete antibody may be detected by doing the test in hypertonic (5%) saline, albumin saline or by Coombs test.

❖ **Testing method or procedures:** Two types

1. **Qualitative**
2. **Quantitative test.**

❖ **Types of serological test based on agglutination:**

I. According to method of performance

➢ **Types:** Two types like slide & tube as described below.

A. Slide agglutination:

✪ **Steps:**

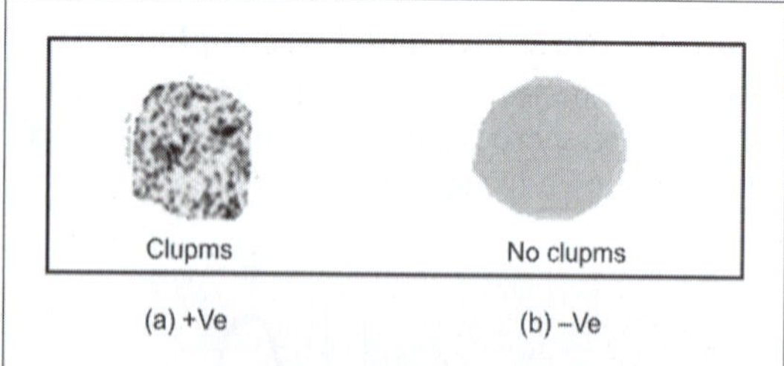

Figure-11: Slide agglutination

- Mix the drop of Ab & particular Ag on slide or tile
- Observe for the clumps.

✪ **Results:**

- Positive [**fig.-11(a)**]: Clumps formation (visible to naked eye, may require microscopic confirmation.)
- Negative [**fig.-11(b)**]: No clumps

✪ **Uses:**

1. Identification of bacterial isolates: Like serotyping of *S. typhi, Shigella* spp. & *V. cholerae*
2. Slide Widal test for *S. typhi* & *S. paratyphi*
3. RF (Rheumatoid Factor) test: For RA factor
4. ASO test: For streptococcal infection.
5. Blood grouping and cross-matching.

B. Tube agglutination:

✪ **Advantage:** Standard quantitative method for measurement of antibodies.

✪ **Uses:** In diagnosis of following diseases.

i. **Enteric fever:** By tube Widal test (vide infra)

ii. **Brucellosis:** Quantitative Ab diagnosis.

iii. **Heterophile Ag detection:**

a. **Weil-Felix reaction:** For typhus fever (vide infra).

b. **Paul Bunnel test:**
- For infectious mononucleosis.
- More details: **Follow chapter → Herpesviridae**

c. **Streptococcus MG agglutination test:**
- For primary atypical pneumonia caused by *Mycoplasma pneumoniae*
- More details: **Follow chapter → Mycoplasmatales**

d. **Cold agglutination test:**
- For primary atypical pneumonia caused by *Mycoplasma pneumoniae*
- More details: **Follow chapter → Mycoplasmatales**

Widal test

♣ **History:** It was developed by Fernand Widal in 1896

♣ **Principle:** Based on slide & tube agglutination reaction.

♣ **Antigen used:**

- ***S. typhi* antigens:**
  - Somatic Ag: O- Ag
  - Flagellar Ag: H-Ag
- ***S. paratyphi* antigens:** Somatic Ag / O- Ag (group specific) of *S. paratyphi* can cross react with O-Ag of *S. typhi* hence only flagellar (species specific) Ag of *S. paratyphi* is included in the widal reaction.
  - AH-Ag
  - BH-Ag

♣ **Preparation of Ag:**

- **Principle for preparation:**
  - H-Ag: Heat labile destroyed by boiling or by treatment with alcohol but not by formaldehyde.
  - O-Ag: Heat stable, alcohol stable but formaldehyde labile.
- **Technique for preparation:**
  - H-Ag prepared by treating saline suspension or broth culture of *S typhi* 901 H strain with 0.1% formalin.
  - O-Ag prepared by growing the *S typhi* 901 O strain on phenol agar (to inhibit H Ag) → scrapped of in saline → mixed with 20 times its volume of absolute alcohol → heated at 40-50^{0}C for 30 minutes → centrifuged → re-suspend the deposit in saline → add the preservative like chloroform

♣ **Antibodies:** Patient serum contains antibodies.

♣ **Other materials:** Normal saline (ns)

♣ **Methods:** Two types as follows

a. Slide (rapid/screening/qualitative) Widal test:

- **Steps:**
- **Figure-12** shows the different types of slides available commercially for slide Widal test
- Mix one drop of serum & one drop of Ag (O, H, AH, BH) in respective circle on slide.
- Mix properly & rotate for one min. & examine for clumps
- Put –Ve & +Ve controls also

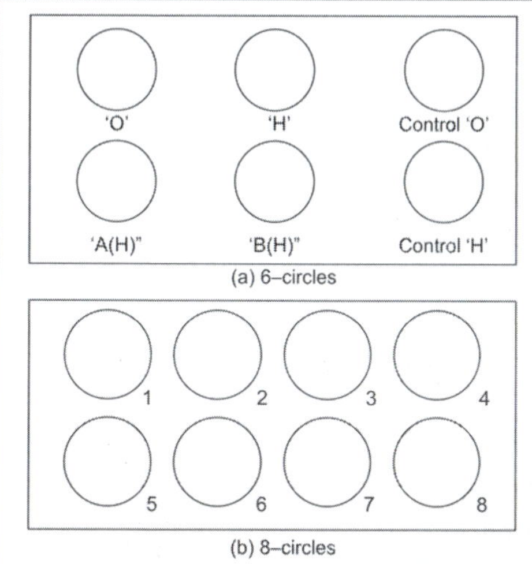

Figure-12: Slides for Widal test

- **Result:**
- +Ve: Clumps
- –Ve: No clumps

b. Tube (quantitative) Widal test:

- **Steps:** Following are the four main steps

1. **Master dilution:**
- Take one test tube & prepare 1:10 dilution of serum **called master dilution**.
- E.g. 2000 µl (2ml) includes 1800 µl of ns + 200 µl of serum

2. **Serial dilution:**
- Take total 16 test tubes & arrange in 4-rows
- Conical bottom tube (**Dreyer'e tube**) for H-Ag & round bottom tube (**Felix tube**) for 0-Ag
- Add 500 µl ns in each test tube
- Add 500 µl master diluted serum in 1st vertical row only
- Do the serial dilution by transferring the 500 µl serum from 1st to 2nd vertical row, 2nd to 3rd, 3rd to 4th & from 4th it will discarded
- So, dilution in 1st, 2nd, 3rd & 4th vertical row is 1:20. 1:40, 1:80, 1:160 respectively.

3. **Final dilution:**
- Add 500 µl O, H, AH & BH Ag in 1st, 2nd, 3rd & 4th horizontal row respectively.
- So, final dilution in 1st, 2nd, 3rd & 4th vertical row is 1:40, 1:80, 1:160 and 1:320 respectively.
- Put –Ve & +Ve controls also

4. **Incubation:** For 24 hrs at 37^{0}

- **Results:**
- Positive O agglutination: Disc like clumps or chalky granular clumps at bottom of tube with clear supernatant fluid
- Positive H agglutination: Spherical, granular, cotton woolly clumps at the bottom of test tube with clear supernatant fluid
- Negative O & H agglutination: Button formation at the bottom of tube due to deposition of antigens & lazy supernatant fluid

♣ **Interpretation:**

1. **Positive: → Table-4**

Rising titre	Interpretation
O & H	Typhoid fever
O & AH	Paratyphoid fever A
O & BH	Paratyphoid fever B
O (Only)	Group specific (Typhoidal group/Enteric fever group)
H (Only)	Species specific, convalescent phase or cross reaction by other related bacteria **called anamnestic reaction** or **false positive result**
H, AH & BH	TAB vaccination

Table-4: Differences between VDRL & RPR test

2. **Negative:** No enteric fever
3. **Significant titre:**
- The maximum dilution of serum at which agglutination occurs **called significant titre** of antibody**.**
- Significant titre for O is ≥1:100 & for H is ≥1:200

4. **Rising titre:**
- Ab appears after 1st week, so test may be negative in 1st week and become positive in 2nd week.
- Titre rise in 3rd or 4th week (four fold rise) after which it decline gradually.
- If sample is taken in late stage, rising titre may not be demonstrated.

5. **False +Ve result:**

- **Definition:** Rising titre of O & H agglutinins may encountered in condition other than enteric fever **called anamnestic reaction** or **false positive result.**
- **Causes:** It occurs in following conditions
- In normal serum
- Repeated subclinical infection
- Immunization with TAB vaccine: Immunisation with TAB vaccine shows high titre against *S. typhi. S. paratyphi A* & *S. paratyphi B*, while case shows high titre only against infecting species.
- Past history of enteric fever Healthy carrier
- Fimbrial Ag
- Tuberculosis
- Malaria
- Dengue
- Brucellosis
- Influenza

- Nephritic syndrome
- Infection with related bacterium from Enterobactericeae family
- Person with immunological diseases like RA, RF
- Also in person from endemic area: Base line titre may be affected by endemicity of disease & antibody may be present due to inapparent infection, immunisation or prior infection, especially in high endemic areas. So, distribution of agglutinin in normal sera is different in different areas.

- **Differentiation between false positive result & true case (fourfold rise):** Rising titre due to anamnestic reaction may fall after 1 week while titre due to true case remains increased by four fold after 1 week, so repeated testing of paired sera at 1 week interval is more significant than single high titre.

6. **False -Ve result:** May encountered following antibiotic treatment or by masking of O Ag by Vi Ag
7. **Non-specific Widal activity:** It may occur in narcotics addict, lipemic serum, haemolysed samples & contaminated serum.
8. **No response to *Salmonella* antibodies:** 5-10% patient don't show any response in Widal test even though *S. typhi* infection documented

♣ **Use:** To diagnose the enteric fever [typhoid fever + paratyphoid fever A & B].

Weil-Felix reaction

♣ **History:** Developed by Weil & Felix in 1916

♣ **Principle:** Based on tube agglutination reaction

♣ **Antigens (Ags):**

- **Heterophile Ags** like OX 19, OX2 and OX K (O antigens) of certain nonmotile *Proteus* spp.
- Sharing of a common alkali-stable carbohydrate antigen by *Rickettsia* & *Proteus* is makes the basis of test.
- Antigens are prepared from *Proteus* strain which is isolated from urine of patient.

♣ **Other materials required:** Serum, ns

♣ **Antibody response in patient serum:**

- The antibody appears rapidly during the course of the disease
- Reaches peak titre of up to 1:1000 or 1:5000 by the second week
- Declines rapidly during convalescence phase

♣ **Method:**

1. **Master dilution:**
- Take one test tube & prepare 1:10 dilution of serum **called master dilution**.
- E.g. 2000 µl (2ml) includes 1800 µl of NS + 200 µl of serum

2. **Serial dilution:**
- Take total 12 test tubes & arrange in 3-rows
- Add 500 µl ns in each test tube
- Add 500 µl master diluted serum in 1st vertical row only
- Do the serial dilution by transferring the 500 µl serum from 1st to 2nd vertical row, 2nd to 3rd, 3rd to 4th & from 4th it will discarded
- So dilution in 1st, 2nd, 3rd & 4th vertical row is 1:20. 1:40, 1:80, 1:160 respectively.

3. **Final dilution:**
- Add 500 µl OX 19, OX2 & OX K Ag in 1st, 2nd & 3rd horizontal row respectively.
- So final dilution in 1st, 2nd, 3rd & 4th vertical row is 1:40, 1:80, 1:160, and 1: 320 respectively.
- Put –Ve & +Ve control also

4. **Incubation:** For 24 hrs at 37^0

♣ **Result:**

- +Ve: Agglutination→ Disc like clumps at the bottom of test tube.
- -Ve: No clumps

♣ **Interpretation: → Table-5**

Disease	Agglutination pattern		
	OX 19	OX 2	OX K
Epidemic typhus	+++	+	-
Brill Zinsser disease	-Ve/weak +Ve	-	-
Endemic typhus	+++	+/-	-
Spotted fever	++	++	-
Scrub typhus	-	-	+++

Table-5: Interpretation of Weil-Felix reaction

1. **Positive:**
- Sera from epidemic and endemic typhus agglutinate OX 19 & sometimes OX 2
- OX K agglutinins are found only in scrub typhus
- In tick borne spotted fever both OX 19 and OX2 are agglutinated

2. **Negative:**
- The test is negative or only weakly positive in Brill-Zinsser disease
- The test is not diagnostic (negative) in Rickettsial pox, trench fever & Q fever

3. **Significant titre:** 1:80
4. **False positive reaction:** May occur in some cases of urinary or other infections by *Proteus*, in typhoid fever and liver diseases

♣ **Use:** For the diagnosis & differentiation of some Rickettsial diseases as shown in **table-4**

II. According to free Ag/Ab or fixed Ag/Ab with carrier particle

According to free Ag/Ab

➢ **Types of tests**: Here antiserum is mixed with whole pathogen/cell. In this type of reaction whole pathogen/cell is used as an Ag & not coated with any carrier particle, hence **called active (direct)**

agglutination. Following are the different type of tests.

i. **Active (direct) agglutination**:

- **Principle:** When antiserum is mixed with whole pathogen it **called active (direct) agglutination.** In this type of reaction whole pathogen is used as an Ag & not coated with any carrier particle.
- **Use:** Identification of bacterial isolates: Like serotyping of *S. typhi, Shigella* spp. & *V. cholerae*

ii. **Active (direct) haemagglutination**:

- **Principle:** When antiserum is mixed with whole RBC **called active (direct) haemagglutination.** In this type of reaction whole RBC is used as an Ag & not coated with any carrier particle.
- **Uses:**

1. **Blood grouping test:** Whole RBCs (free) are mixed with anti-A, anti-B & anti-O sera to detect the blood group
2. **Cold agglutination test:**
   - Positive in primary atypical pneumonia which is caused by *M. pneumoniae*
   - Patient's sera agglutinate human O group erythrocytes at 4 °C **hence called cold agglutination**. Clumps are dissociated at 37 °C.

According to fixed Ag/Ab with carrier particle

➢ **Carrier particles:** Following are the different types of carrier particle used to fix Ag or Ab.

A. **Latex particles (latex agglutination test):**
- Structure: Made up from polystyrene latex
- Shape: Spherical
- Size: 0.8-1.0 µm

B. **Protein A of *Staph. aureus* (Co- agglutination)**

C. **RBCs (Haem-agglutination test):**

D. **Bentonite**

E. **Carbon particle:** Not for agglutination but for flocculation like RPR test **(vide supra)**

➢ **Types of tests:** Here Ag/Ab is not free but fixed with carrier particle hence **called passive (indirect) agglutination**. Following are the different type of tests according to carrier particle used.

A. **Latex agglutination test:** Ag/Ab is fixed with latex particle. Subtypes are as follows

i. **Passive (indirect) agglutination:**

- **Principle:** By attaching antigen with latex particle antibody is detected.
- **Advantages:** High sensitive
- **Disadvantages:** Less specific, so false +Ve result may occur.
- **Uses:**

a. **Modified Rose Waaler test**

- **Synonym:** RA (Rheumatoid Arthritis) factor test or RF (Rheumatoid Factor) test.
- **Principle:**
  - Rheumatoid arthritis is an autoimmune diseases characterised by presence of autoantibody **called Rheumatoid Factor (RF) or RA (Rheumatoid Arthritis) factor**.
  - RF is actually anti-globulin.
  - RF (Ab) is detected by attaching globulin (Ag) with latex particle.
  - White clumps are visible against black background of slide
- **Steps:**
  - Mix one drop of serum contains Ab with one drop of reagent (Ag attached to latex particle) on a slide.
  - Rotate for 1 minutes & examine for the result
- **Result:** → Fig.-13

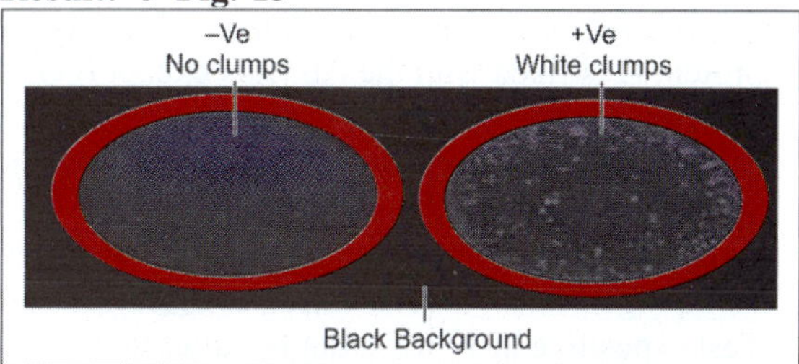

Figure-13: Latex agglutination test

- +Ve test: White clumps against black background.
- -Ve test: No clumps
- **Interpretation:**
  - Positive test: Indicates the RA
  - Negative: No RA
  - Significant titre is ≥8 IU/ml
- **Disadvantage:** Non-specific because it also found in other connective tissue disorders.
- **Uses:** Used to diagnose the rheumatoid arthritis

b. **ASO (Anti-Streptolysin -O) test**

- **Principle:**
  - Used in Acute Rheumatic Fever (ARF) caused by *Streptococci*.
  - *Streptococci* released the exotoxin **called streptolysin-O** (Ag) which produce specific antibody **called Anti Streptolysin-O (ASO)**.
  - ASO (Ab) is detected by attaching streptolysin-O (Ag) with latex particles
  - White clumps are visible against black background of slide
- **Steps & result:** Same as modified Rose Waaler test
- **Interpretation:**
  - Positive test: Indicates the streptococcal infection
  - Negative: No streptococcal infection
  - Significant titre is ≥200 IU/ml
- **Uses:** Used to diagnose the ARF

c. **Capillus test to detect HIV-Ab**

d. **Also used for detection of CRP, HCG etc.**

ii. **Reverse passive agglutination:**

- **Principle:** Instead of antigen, antibody is adsorbed to latex particle to detect the antigen.

- **Advantage:** Test is rapid, sensitive & specific
- **Use:** HBsAg detection in HBV infection

B. Agglutination by using protein A of *Staph. aureus* as carrier particle:

i. Co-agglutination:

- **Principle:**
  - Instead of antigen, antibody is adsorbed to carrier particle like protein A of *Staph aureus* to detect the antigen.
  - It is similar or subtype of reverse passive agglutination, only difference is in carrier particles.
- **Advantage:** Test is rapid, sensitive & specific
- **Uses:**

a. *S. typhi* detection:

- *Staph aureus* (Cowan I strain) which contain protein A is fixed with the Ab (IgG except IgG3) of *S. typhi*
- Mixed such sensitised *Staph aureus* with patient's serum containing Ag
- Typhoid Ag combines with *S. typhi* Ab & produce clumping of *Staph aureus* **called coagglutination**.
- Test is positive in 1st week but not after that.

b. Other infections: Also used for Ag detection in *Legionella pneumophilla, N. gonorrhoea & Strept pyogenes* infection.

C. Agglutination by using RBCs as carrier particle: Test **called haemagglutination test** when carrier particle is RBC

- **Types:** Three subtypes of haemagglutination

i. Active (direct) haemagglutination: → vide supra

ii. Passive (indirect) haemagglutination:

- **Principle:** RBC is coated with Ag from other organism to detect the Ab of that organism.
- **Uses:**

1. **Rose Waaler test:**
   - Used for RF or RA factor.
   - Sheep RBCs coated with anti-erythrocyte Abs are used as Ag
2. **TPHA (*Treponema pallidum* Haem Agglutination) test:** Used to detect the specific Ab of *T. pallidum,* where RBCs are coated with antigen of *T. pallidum.*

iii. Reverse passive haemagglutination (RPHA):

- **Principle:** Instead of antigen, RBC is coated with antibody to detect the antigen. **Figure-14** shows the RPHA microtitre plate with fixed wells (differentiated from ELISA microtitre plate where wells are free).
- **Use:** RPHA test to detect the HBsAg of HBV.

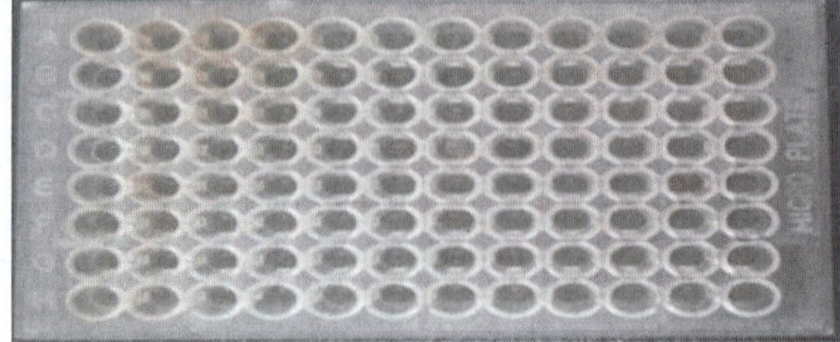

Figure-14: RPHA microtitre plate

III. Anti-globulin test

- **Synonym:** Coombs test
- **History:** It was invented by Coombs, Mourant & Race in 1945.
- **Principle:**
  - Detection of anti-Rh antibodies that do not agglutinate the Rh-positive RBCs in saline.
  - When sera containing incomplete (blocking) anti-Rh antibodies are mixed with Rh-positive red cells, antibody globulin coats surface of erythrocytes, though they are not agglutinated.
  - Such RBCs coated with Ab globulin are washed free of all unattached protein and treated with rabbit antiserum against human γ-globulin (anti-globulin or Coombs serum), cells are agglutinated.
- **Types:** Coombs test may be direct or indirect.

a. Direct (In vivo) Coombs test:

- **Steps: →Fig.-15**
  - Sensitisation of RBCs with incomplete antibodies takes place in vivo (immune mediated haemolytic anaemia of newborn due to Rh incompatibility).
  - When RBCs of case with immune mediated haemolytic anaemia are washed free of unattached protein and mixed with drop of Coombs serum, agglutination results.
  - Test is often negative in hemolytic disease due to ABO incompatibility.
- **Use:** To detect the immune mediated haemolytic anaemia of newborn due to Rh incompatibility

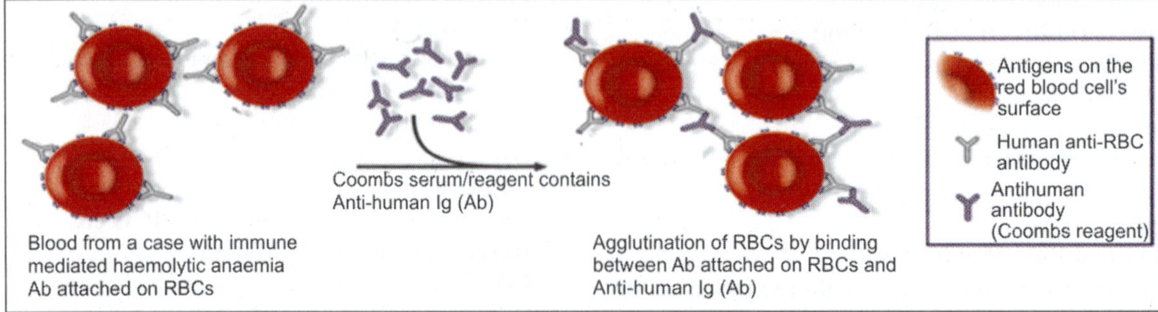

Figure-15: Direct/ In vivo Coombs test

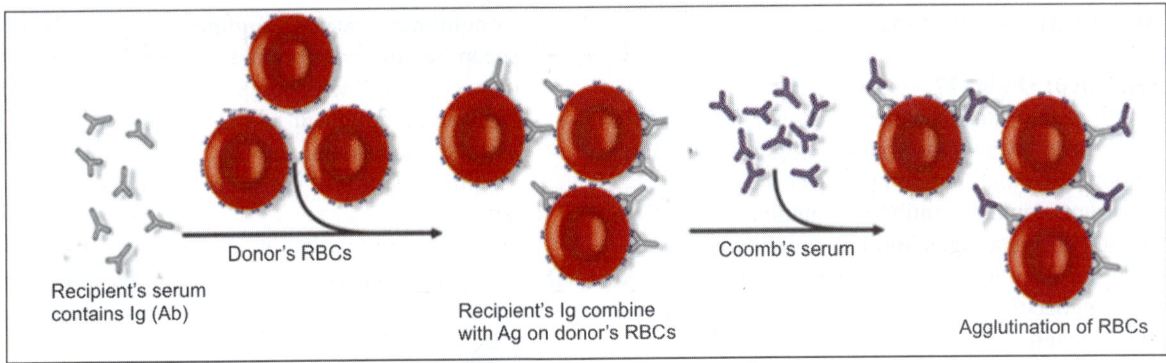

Figure-16: Indirect/ in vitro Coombs test

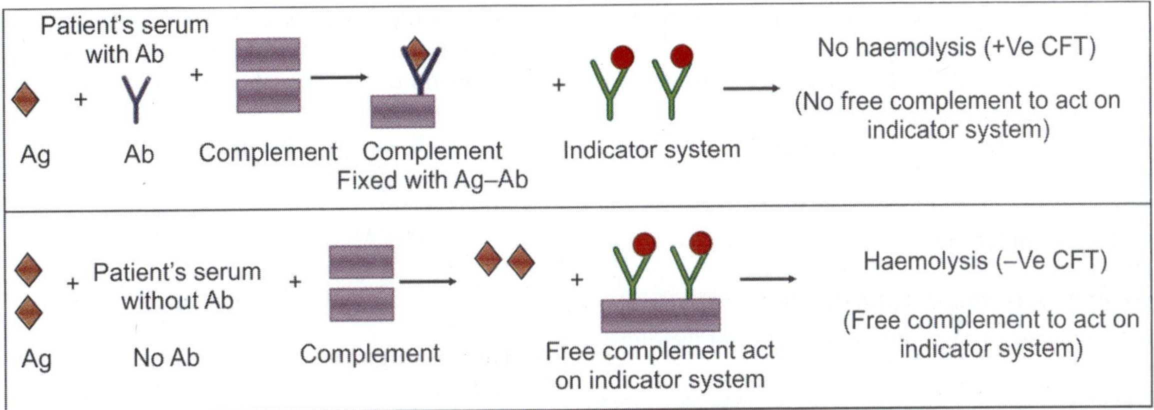

Figure-17: Wassermann reaction

a. Indirect (In vitro) Coombs test:

- **Steps (fig.-16):** Sensitisation of red cells with antibody globulin is performed in vitro. Other steps are same as direct test.
- **Uses:**

1. For demonstrating any type of incomplete (non-agglutinating) antibody, like in brucellosis
2. To detect the anti-Rh Ab (free) in patient's serum.

Complement Fixation Test (CFT)

- **History:** Bordet & Gengou (1901) described the complement fixation test using the hemolytic indicator system.
- **Introduction:** Complement is a system of different factors of serum which takes part in many immunological reactions and is absorbed during combination of antigens with antibodies.
- **Role of complement:**
  - Takes part in Ag-Ab reaction.
  - In presence of appropriate antibodies, complement lyses erythrocytes, kills bacteria, immobilise the motile organisms, promotes phagocytosis and immune adherence and contributes to tissue damage in certain types of hypersensitivity.
- **Sensitivity of CFT:** Very versatile and capable of detecting as little as 0.04 mg of Ab & 0.1 mg of Ag.
- **Reagents of CFT:** As mentioned below

1. **Ag:** May be soluble or particulate
2. **Ab:** Antiserum should be heated at 56 °C (inactivated serum) for half an hour to destroy the any complement activity if serum may have and also to remove nonspecific inhibitors of complement present in sera (anti-complementary activity).
3. **Complement:**
   - Obtained from the guinea pig serum.
   - As complement is heat labile, serum should be freshly drawn or lyophilized or frozen or preserve by Richardson's method.
4. **Indicator system:** It includes sensitised sheep RBC with amboceptor (amboceptor = rabbit Ab to sheep RBC)

- **Use of CFT:** To diagnose the various bacterial, viral, fungal & parasitic infections
- **Serological tests based on CFT:**

A. Wassermann reaction:

- **Principle:** It based on complement fixation
- **Reagents:** As described above

- **Steps:** Test consists of two steps.

i. **First step:** →**Fig.-17**
- Inactivated serum of patient is incubated at 37 °C for 1 hour with Wassermann antigen and a fixed amount (two units) of guinea pig complement.
- If serum contains antibody complement will be utilised during antigen-antibody interaction.
- If serum does not contain the antibody, no Ag-Ab reaction occurs & complement will remain free.

ii. **Second step:**
- Add sensitised cells (sheep erythrocytes coated with amboceptor) & incubating at 37 °C for 30 minutes.
- Examine the result.

- **Control:** Also put control tube along with the test. It has following advantages.
- Ag & serum control: To know that they are not anti-complementary.
- Complement control: To know that desired amount of complement is added.
- RBCs: To know that sensitised RBCs are not lysed without complement.

- **Result:**
- **Positive test:** Absence of RBCs lysis indicates that complement was used up in first step and therefore, serum contained the antibody.
- **Negative test:** Lysis of RBCs indicates that complement was not fixed in first step and therefore, serum did not have antibody.

- **Use:** For the sero-diagnosis of syphilis.

B. **Indirect Complement Fixation Test:**
- **Advantage:** Certain avian (duck, turkey, parrot) and mammalian (horse, cat) sera do not fix guinea pig complement.
- **Steps:**
- Here the test is set up in duplicate and after the first step; the standard antiserum known to fix the complement is added to one set.
- If test serum contained antibody, antigen would have been used up in the first step and therefore standard antiserum added subsequently would not be able to fix complement.
- **Result:** Haemolysis indicates a positive result.

C. **Conglutinating Complement Fixation Test (Conglutination):**
- **Advantage:** For systems which do not fix guinea pig complement.
- **Reagent, steps & result in brief:**
- Horse complement which is non-haemolytic.
- Indicator system is sensitised sheep erythrocytes mixed with bovine serum.
- Bovine serum contains beta globulin component **called conglutinin**, acts as antibody to complement.
- Conglutinin causes agglutination of sensitised sheep erythrocytes **called conglutination** if they have combined with complement.
- If horse complement had been used up by antigen-antibody interaction in first step, agglutination of sensitised cells will not occur will indicates positive test.
- Here no agglutination indicates the negative test.

D. **Immune adherence:** When some bacteria (like *V. cholerae, T. pallidum* etc.) react with specific Ab in presence of complement & particulate materials RBCs, platelets or bacteria are aggregated and adhere to the cells **called immune adherence**.

E. ***Treponema pallidum* Immobilisation (TPI) test:** Mix motile suspension of *T. pallidum* with specific antiserum in the presence of complement. On incubation, specific Ab inhibits motility of *T. pallidum.*

F. **Cytolytic or cytocidal tests:** When bacterium like *V. cholerae*, is mixed with its Ab in presence of complement, bacterium is killed and lysed (vibriocidal Ab test).

Neutalisation reaction

- **Disadvantage:** Historical value & less useful now a days.

- **Types:** As follows

A. **Virus neutralisation tests:**
- **Principle:** Neutralisation of virus by specific antiserum.
- **Uses:**

1. **Plaque inhibition test:**
- Bacteriophages seeded in appropriate dilution on lawn cultures of susceptible bacteria
- It lyses the bacteria & forms the lytic zone **called plaques.**
- Inhibition of plaque formation by using specific antiphage serum **called plaque inhibition**.

2. **Haemagglutination inhibition test:** Useful to diagnose the influenza
3. **Other method:** Virus neutralisation test can be performed in animals, chick embryo or in tissue/cell culture

B. **Toxin neutralisation tests:**
- **Principle:** Bacterial exotoxin is good antigen & induce neutralising antibody (antitoxin), important clinically, in protection & recovery from diseases.

✓ **Note:** Toxicity of endotoxin is not neutralised by antisera.

- **Types:** Two types

a. **In vivo:**

1. **Schick test:**
- Used to detect the immunity or susceptibility to diphtheria toxin

- When diphtheria toxin is injected intradermally in patients, no reaction at injection site due to neutralisation of diphtheria toxin.

2. **Toxigenicity testing in *C. diphtheria* in animals:** More details: Follow chapter→ *Corynebacterium*
3. **Toxigenicity testing in *Cl. tetani* in animals like guinea pig or mice:** More details Follow chapter → *Clostridium* (sporing anaerobe)

b. In vitro test:

1. **Nagler's reaction:**
   - For *Cl. Perfringens*.
   - More details: Follow chapter → *Clostridium* (sporing anaerobe)
2. **Toxigenicity testing in *Cl. tetani* in blood agar:** More details, Follow chapter → *Clostridium* (sporing anaerobe)
3. **ASO test:** Described earlier also based on neutralisation test, as Streptolysin (Haemolysin/Haemolytic exotoxin)-O is neutralised by ASO.

Opsonisation

❖ Definitions

➢ **Bacteriotropin:**
- It is a heat stable serum factor which facilitate the phagocytosis
- It was **called 'bacteriotropin'.**

➢ **Opsonin:**
- It is heat labile substance present in fresh normal sera which facilitate the phagocytosis
- Term opsonin is now used to refer to both these factors.

❖ Opsonic index:

➢ **Definition:** Ratio of phagocytic activity of patient's blood for a given bacterium, to phagocytic activity of normal individual's blood.

➢ **Measurement:** Measured by incubating fresh citrated blood with bacterial suspension at 37 °C for 15 minutes & estimating average number of phagocytosed bacteria per polymorphonuclear leucocyte (phagocytic index) from stained blood films.

➢ **Use:** To study the progress of resistance of host against the progress of illness.

Radio Immuno Assay (RIA)

❖ **History:** it was 1st described by Berson & Yellow in1959 & later Nobel Prize was awarded to Yallow IN 1977.

❖ Definitions:

➢ **Reaction: Called binder-ligand-assay**

➢ **Analyte or Ligand:** Substance (Ag) whose concentration is to be determined **called analyte** or **ligand**.

➢ **Binder:** Binding protein (antibody) which binds to the ligand **called binder**.

❖ **Sensitivity of test:** Permits the measurement of analytes up to picogram (10^{-12} g).

❖ Methods:

- RIA is competitive binding assay, fixed amounts of antibody and radiolabelled antigen react in presence of unlabeled antigen.
- Labeled and unlabeled antigens compete for limited binding sites on antibody; this competition is determined by level of unlabeled (test) antigen present in reacting system.
- After the reaction, antigen is separated into 'free' and 'bound' fractions and their radioactive counts measured.
- Concentration of test antigen calculated from ratio of bound and total antigen labels, using a standard dose response curve.

❖ **Use:** In quantitation of hormones, drugs, tumour markers, IgE and viral antigens.

❖ **Disadvantages:** Radiation hazard

Enzyme Immuno Assay (EIA)

❖ Advantages:

- No radiation hazard
- Versatile
- Sensitive
- Specific
- Economical

❖ Disadvantages:

- Time consuming about 3-4 hours
- Labour intensive
- Require special instruments like reader & washer

❖ **Types:** Two types

A. Homogeneous EIA:

➢ **Properties:**
- No need to separate bound and free fractions
- Single step test.

➢ **Example: EMIT** → described below

EMIT

✪ **Full form:** Enzyme Multiplied Immunoassay Technique

✪ **Uses:** Only for assay of haptens such as drugs (opiates, cocaine, barbiturates, amphetamine) and not for microbial antigens and antibodies.

B. Heterogeneous EIA:

➢ **Properties:**
- Required separation of free and bound fractions either by centrifugation or by absorption on solid surfaces and washing.

- Multistep test.
- **Example: ELISA →** described below

ELISA

- **Full form:** Enzyme Linked Immuno Sorbent Assay
- **Meaning of immuno sorbent:** Antigens or antibodies are not free but absorbed on cellulose membrane, agarose or solid phase like tubes or microtitre plates made up from polyvinyl or polystyrene or polycarbonate.
- **Equipments required:**

1. Microtitre plate (12x8 wells=96 wells)
2. Single channel & multichannel pipette
3. Micropipette tips
4. Kit with all reagent ready to use
5. ELISA Washer
6. ELISA Reader
7. Other common laboratory equipment like centrifuge, timer etc.

- **Types of ELISA:** It is classified in to several types on different basis.

i. On the basis of solid phase used:

a. Micro- ELISA: Performed in microtitre plates with 96 wells

b. Macro- ELISA: Performed in tubes

ii. On the basis of Ag utilised:

a. 1st generation: Infected cell lysates are used as an antigen

b. 2nd generation: Glycopeptide (recombinant Ag) used as an antigen.

c. 3rd generation: Synthetic peptide used as an antigen.

d. 4th generation: Simultaneously recombinant & synthetic peptide used as antigen for the detection of antibody

iii. On the basis of principle:

a. Indirect (non-competitive) ELISA:

- **Principle:** If sample contains HIV-Ab, it is fixed to the Ag coated wells & makes the Ag-Ab complex. When conjugate (enzyme labeled antibody: Ab-E) is added subsequently, it fix with Ag-Ab complex. Subsequently add the substrate which is split by enzyme of conjugate to yield yellow compound indicates the positive result. **[fig.-18(a) & flow chart-2]**

> Ag in well + Ab in serum = Ag -Ab complex
> Ag -Ab complex + Ab-E + substrate = Colour product

Flow chart-2: Principle of indirect ELISA

- **Reagents: → Fig.-19(a)**

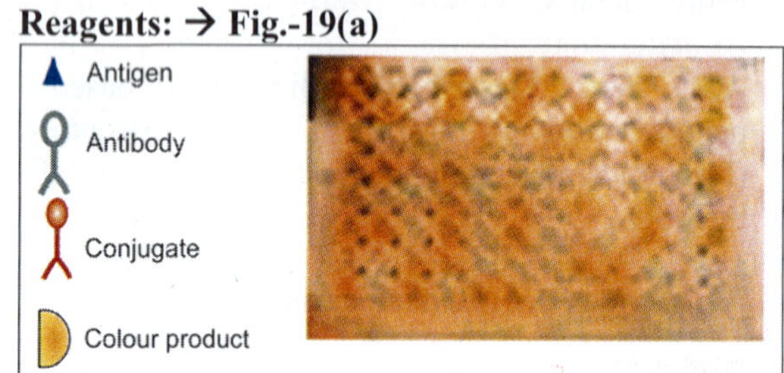

Figure-19: (a) Reagents (b) colour plate of ELISA

1. **Well:** Contains HIV-Ag
2. **Sample:** Contains HIV-Ab
3. **Conjugate:**

- Contains Anti Human Globulin (AHG) fixed with Horse Radish Peroxidase (HRP) or AHG+HRP (from horse)
- Other enzyme used: Alkaline phosphatase from *E. coli*, β-galactosidase from *E. coli* & urease

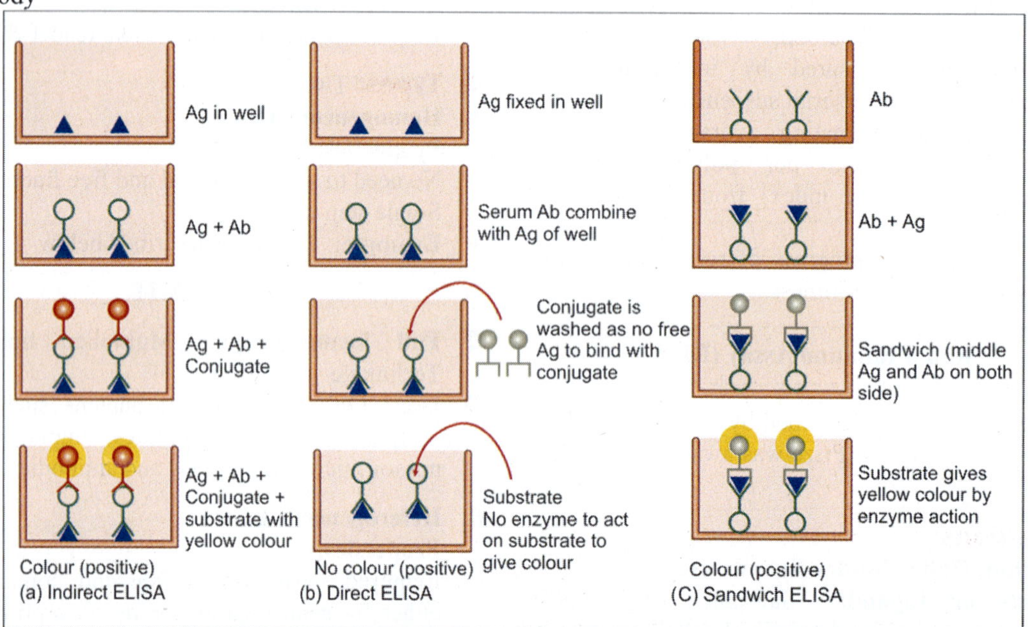

Figure-18: Principle of (a) indirect, (b) direct & (c) sandwich ELISA

4. **Substrate or colour reagent or chromogen:**
- Contains chemical like Tetra Methyle Benzidine (TMB) or peroxidase or Para Nitro Phenyl Phosphate (PNPP) or O-phenylene diamine dihydrochloride.
- It is colourless substance & when come in contact with light it produce colour & gives false positive result, so store it in dark area to avoid the contact with light
5. **Stop solution:** Contains acid like phosphoric acid or mineral acid etc.

♣ **Steps:**
- **Preparation of microtitre plate:** Remove the excess wells from microtitre plate & arrange the required numbers of wells in to the plates.
- **Control:** Put –Ve & +Ve controls
- **Adding the sample:**
  - Add samples in to the wells according to scheme on the work sheet
  - Cover the plate and incubate at 37^0C for few hours.
- **Adding the conjugate:**
  - Take out the plate from incubator after recommended time & wash the plate with ELISA plate washer to remove the unbounded Ag & Ab.
  - Dry the plate after washing
  - Add the conjugate with multichannel pipette
  - Incubate the plate at room temperature for the recommended time.
- **Adding the substrate or colour reagent:**
  - Remove the unbounded conjugate materials by washing the plates with ELISA plate washer.
  - Dry the plate after washing
  - Add the substrate by using multichannel pipette.
  - Incubate in the dark area for the recommended time.
- **Add the stop solution:**
  - Take out the plate from dark area after the recommended time & add the stop solution.
  - It stops all reaction between the Ag & Ab before taking the result.

♣ **Result:** Result is taken by two ways
1. **Naked eye:**
- +Ve: Development of colour in well **[fig.-19 (b)].**
- -Ve: Colourless well
2. **ELISA Reader:** Which measure the Optical Density (OD) in each well

b. Direct (competitive) ELISA:

♣ **Principle:** Both sample's Ab & enzyme labeled Ab of conjugate competes (**hence called competitive ELISA**) with Ag of well. Sample's Ab will combine with Ag of well while enzyme labeled antibody of conjugate remains unbound & removed by washing, so enzymes is not available to split the substrate in colour compound, so colourless well indicates the positive result. **[fig.-18(b) & flow chart-3]**

Ag in well + Ab in serum = Ag -Ab complex Ag -Ab complex + substrate = No colour product

Flow chart-3: Principle of direct ELISA

♣ **Steps:**
- **Preparation of microtitre plate:** Remove the excess wells from microtitre plate & arrange the required numbers of wells in to plate.
- **Adding the sample & conjugate simultaneously** followed by same step as like indirect ELISA.

♣ **Result:**
- +Ve: Colourless well
- -Ve: Development of colour in well

c. Sandwich ELISA: Called sandwich ELISA, because Ag is sandwich on either side by antibodies.

♣ **Principle:** Add serum contains Ag to well, fixed with polyclonal Ab. Incubate the plate, followed by washing which removes unbound Ag & Ab. Later add the conjugate contains monoclonal Ab with enzymes (HRP). After sufficient time of incubation wash the plate to removes unbound conjugate materials. Fixation of conjugate to Ag-Ab complex is identifying by adding substrate, which produce colour on reacting with enzyme indicates positive result. Finally add the stop solution & read the result. **[fig.-18(c) & flow chart-4]**

Ab in well + Ag in serum = Ab -Ag complex Ab-Ag complex + Ab-E + substrate = Colour product

Flow chart-4: Principle of sandwich ELISA

d. Antigen/antibody capture ELISA: It capture particular type of Ab like IgG, IgM etc. hence **called capture ELISA.**

e. Rapid ELISA (cylinder or cassette ELISA):

♣ **Advantages:**
- Each specimen is tested in a separate disposable cassette.
- Test is rapid (36 minutes).
- No need for microtitre plate washers or readers.
- Result is read visually.
- Inbuilt positive & negative controls usually provided.
- It separates the HIV-1 & 2 infection.

♣ **Example:**
1. Immunocomb HIV 1 & 2 bispot.
- **Reagent: →Fig.-20**
- **Result: →Fig.-21**

f. ELISPOT test:

♣ **Advantages:** It quantitatively measures the cells producing antibodies (plasma cells) & cytokines (macrophage)

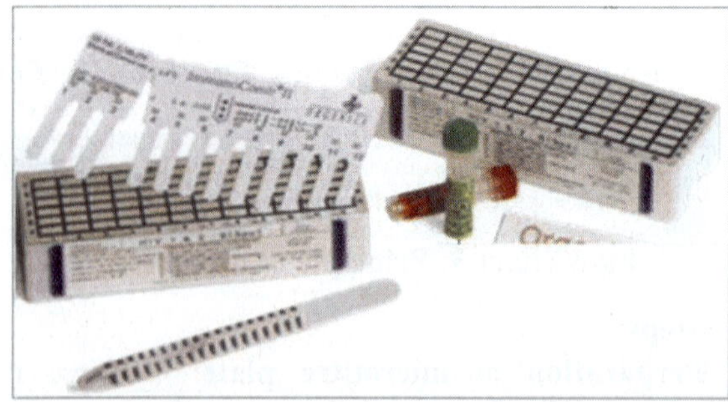

Figure-20: Reagents of immunocomb HIV 1 & 2 bispot

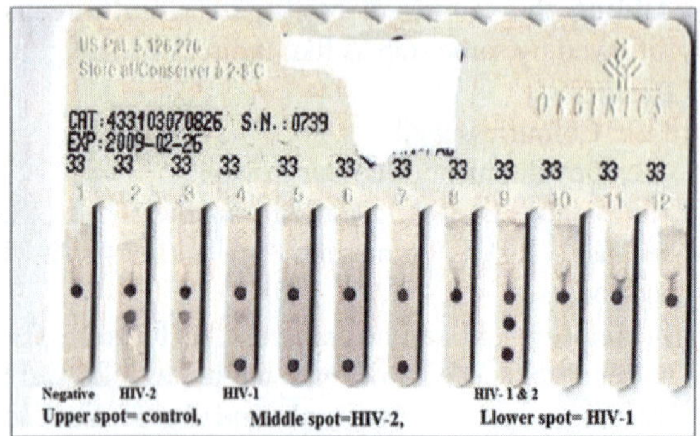

Figure-21: Result of immunocomb HIV 1 & 2 bispot

♣ **Principle: → Flow chart-5**

Cytokine's Ab in well + cytokine (Ag) in sample = Ab -Ag complex
Ab -Ag complex + Anti –cytokine Ab-E + substrate = Colour product

Flow chart-5: Principle of ELISPOT test

♣ **Steps:**
- Microtitre well is fixed with antibodies to cytokines
- Add the sample contains cytokine or cytokine producing cells & incubated. During this time cytokine or cytokine producing cells are attached to the antibodies fixed with microtitre well.
- Remove the plate from incubation & wash it to remove unbound cytokines.
- Dry the plate after washing
- Add the conjugate contains anti-cytokine antibody labelled with enzyme with multichannel pipette.
- Incubate the plate at room temperature for the recommended time.
- Remove the unbounded conjugate materials by washing the plates with ELISA plate washer.
- Dry the plate after washing
- Add the substrate by using multichannel pipette.
- Incubate in the dark area for the recommended time.
- Take out the plate from dark area after the recommended time & add the stop solution.
- It stops all reaction between the Ag & Ab before taking the result.

♣ **Result:** Result is taken by two ways

1. **Naked eye:**
- +Ve: Development of colour in well.
- -Ve: Colourless well
2. **ELISA Reader:** Which measure the Optical Density (OD) in each well

✪ **Uses of ELISA:** It is universal test used for several purposes

a. **To detect Ag & Ab in infectious diseases like,**
1. **Bacterial:** *M. tuberculosis, E. coli, S. typhi* etc.
2. **Viral:** HBV, HIV, HCV, Dengue virus, Chikungunya virus etc.
3. **Fungal:** *C. albicans, C. neoformans* etc.
4. **Parasitic:** *Plasmodium* spp., Filarial parasite, *E. histolytica* etc.

b. **Diagnosis of human allergen:** Specially by capture ELISA

c. **Food toxin:** Like aflatoxin

d. **Food adulterants detection.**

e. **Measuring hormone level:**
- HCG (as a test for pregnancy)
- LH (determining the time of ovulation)
- TSH, T3 and T4 (for thyroid function)

f. Measuring "rheumatoid factors" and other autoantibody in **autoimmune diseases** like lupus erythematosus.

g. **Detecting drugs:** E.g., cocaine, opiates

Immuno Fluorescence Assay (IFA)

❖ **Introduction:**
- Fluorescent dye used is **called Fluorescein Iso Thio Cyanate (FITC)** (Blue-green fluorescence) or lissamine rhodamine (orange-red fluorescence).
- It absorbed the UV light & illuminates in visible light **called fluorescence**.

❖ **History:** In 1942 Coons & his colleague conjugate the dye with Ab & such 'labeled' Ab can be used to locate & identify Ag in tissues.

❖ **Uses:** For detection of
1. Infectious agents like bacteria, viruses, fungus & parasites
2. Auto- antibody
3. Hormones
4. Tumour markers
5. Enzymes
6. Organs & tissues antigens

❖ **Types:**

A. **Direct immunofluorescence test:**
- ➢ **Principle:** Ag combined with 'labeled' Ab & produce visible light on UV exposure. **[fig.-22(a)]**
- ➢ **Disadvantage:** Separate fluorescent labelled Ab have to be prepared against each Ag to be tested.

B. **Indirect immunofluorescence test:**
- ➢ **Principle:** Ag combined with sample's Ab & produce Ag-Ab complex which later combines with

conjugate (dye + anti-globulin) & produce visible light on UV exposure. **[fig.-22(b)].**

- **Advantage:** Overcomes the disadvantage of direct method by using an antiglobulin fluorescent conjugate.

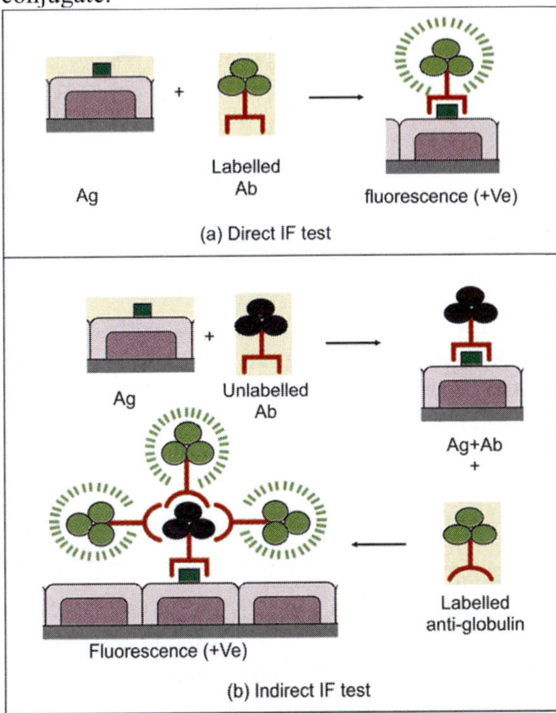

Figure-22: Principle of IFA

- **Steps:** Discussed with example of fluorescent treponemal antibody test for syphilis.
  - Drop of test serum is placed on a slide contains the smear of *T pallidum* & incubate the smear.
  - Slide is washed well to remove all the free serum, leaving behind only antibody globulin, if present, coated on the surface of treponemas.
  - Smear is then treated with a fluorescent labeled antiserum to human gamma globulin.
  - Fluorescent conjugate reacts with antibody globulin bound to treponemas.
- **Result:** After washing away unbound fluorescent conjugate, slide is examined under ultraviolet illumination
  - **+Ve result:** Bright objects against the dark background.
  - **-Ve result:** If sample does not contain Ab & it will not bind the conjugate & no illumination in the end
- **Other modifications:**
  - Single antihuman globulin fluorescent conjugate can be employed for detecting human antibodies to any antigen.
  - Fluorescent dyes may also be conjugated with the complement. Labeled complement is a versatile tool and can be employed for the detection of antigen or antibody.
  - Antigens also take fluorescent labeling but not as well as antibodies do.

C. Sandwich IF test:

- **Principle:** Unlabeled Ab is allowed to react with Ag. Ag-Ab complex is then treated with fluorescent labeled Ab. Sandwich is formed, Ag is in middle while labeled & unlabeled Abs are on either side **(fig.-23).**
- **Use:** Detection of antibodies

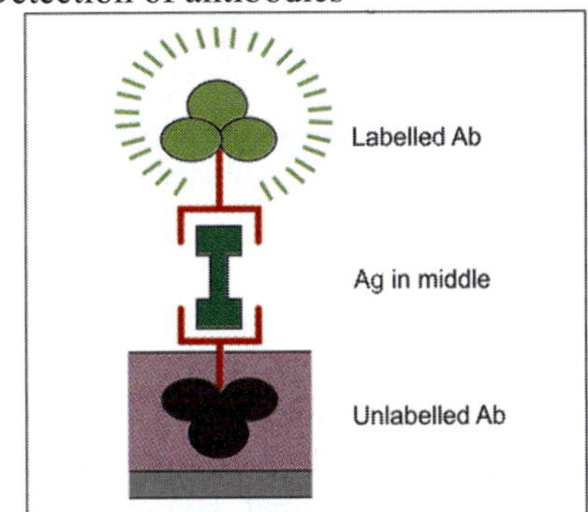

Figure-23: Principle of sandwich IF test

D. Immunohistochemical test:

- It is the combine technique of serology & histology.
- It detects the Ag-Ab reaction in tissue (In -situ), hence **called immunohistochemical test**
- Commonly used dye is FITC or rhodamine.
- Disadvantage: Non-specific fluorescence in tissue

E. Flow cytometry:

- **Principle:** Suspending the fluorescent labelled cell in a stream of fluid & passing them through an electronic detection apparatus.
- **Uses:**
  - To identify cells bearing particular Ag or surface marker like CD_4 & CD_8 cells in HIV patients.
  - Size, granularity, DNA or RNA content of cells.
  - Cell counting like differential leucocyte count (DLC)
  - For diagnosis, treatment & prognosis of cancer specially leukemia.
  - To study the cell cycle & apoptosis
  - For research purpose.

Chemiluminescence Linked Immuno Assay (CLIA)

- **Principle:** Like RIA, EIA & IFA some chemicals are used as label to provides the signal of Ag-Ab reaction. Produce signal in the form of light which can be amplified, measured & concentration of analyte can be calculated.
- **Commonly used Chemical:** Luminol or acridinium esters
- **Advantage:** it is fully automated & used in laboratories where volume of work is large.

Immunoelectroblot technique

- **Synonym:** Western Blot (WB) test
- **Advantages:**
  - High sensitivity like EIA

- Greater specificity than EIA.
- **Steps:** Three steps
1. **Separation of ligand (Ag):** By PAGE
2. **Blotting (fixation):** Separated Ags particle are blotted or transfer electrophoretically from PAGE to nitrocellulose membrane strip.
3. **EIA or RIA:** After blotting, steps are similar to indirect ELISA
- Strip contain Ag is exposed to serum contains Ab.
- Followed by conjugate & substrate step.
- **Result:**
- **+Ve test:** If serum contains specific Ab to strip Ag, it produces the colour band indicates the positive result.
- **–Ve test:** No band indicates the negative result.
- **Use:** Definitive or confirmatory test for detection of antibody against particular HIV-Ags like gp-120, gp-41, P-24, P-15, P-55 etc.

Immuno Chromatographic Test (ICT)

- **Synonym:** Also **called lateral flow assay** because serum moves laterally or parallel to the long axis of strip or biscuit/card as shown in **fig.-24**.
- **Types of test:** Test device is available either in the form of strip or in the form of biscuit (card). Both types are discussed as below.

a. **Strip form:** Discussed with example of HBsAg.

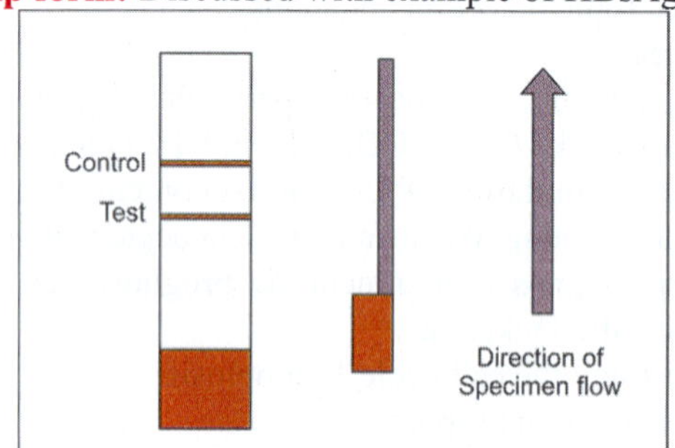

Figure-24: Structure of strip & direction of specimen flow in ICT

- **Structure of strip:** It is impregnated with reagents at two sites like test site (T) & control site (C) as shown in **fig.25**.
1. **Test site:** With anti-HBsAg antibody with colloidal gold dye conjugate
2. **Control site:** Anti-globulin
- **Method:**
- Put the strip in test tube contains serum.
- Strip absorb the serum & if serum contains HBsAg it combine with anti-HBsAg antibody-colloidal gold dye conjugate to produce visible band **called test band**.
- Control band produce at the control site.
- **Result: →Fig.-25**
- **–Ve test:** Control band, no test band
- **+Ve test:** Control band & test band
- **Invalid test:** No control band with or without test band.

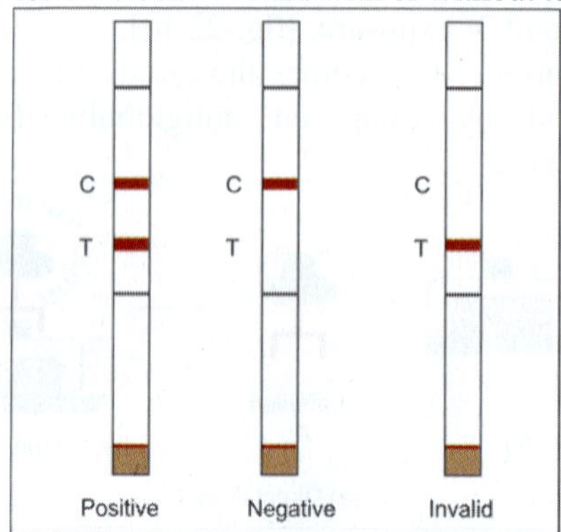

Figure-25: Result of ICT in strip form.

b. **Biscuit (card) form:** Discussed with example of HBsAg as shown in **fig.-26**.

- **Structure of biscuit (card):** Biscuit has two separate windows like sample window & result window. Result window is impregnated with reagents at different sites as follows
1. **Test site:** With anti-HBsAg antibody with colloidal gold dye conjugate.
2. **Control site:** Anti-globulin
- **Method:**
- Put the 2-3 drops of serum in sample window.
- Serum runs along the long axis of biscuit towards the result window.
- Read the result after 15-20 minutes.
- Test (T) site absorb the serum & if serum contains HBsAg it combine with anti-HBsAg antibody-colloidal gold dye conjugate to produce visible band **called test band**.
- Control band produce at the control (C) site.
- **Result: →Fig.-26**
- **–Ve test:** Control band, no test band
- **+Ve test:** Control band & test band
- **Invalid test:** No control band with or without test band.

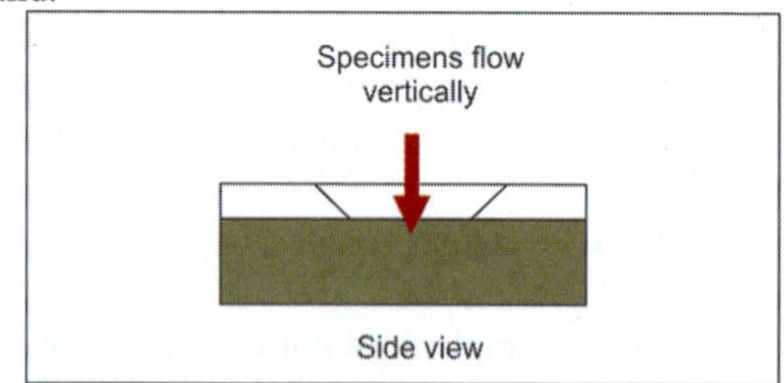

Figure-26: Principle & result of ICT in biscuit form

- **Advantages:**
- Simple & one step (rapid) testing, because colour reagent (colloidal gold) already attached to device, so no need to add separately.
- Economical
- Nearly as sensitive and specific as EIA test.
- **Disadvantages:** It is qualitative not a quantitative method.

➢ **Uses:** For detection of
- HBsAg.
- HCV antibodies
- HIV1 & 2 antibodies

Immuno concentration test

➢ **Synonym:** Also **called vertical flow** or **dot blot assay** or **flow through assay**, because serum moves vertically or perpendicular to the long axis of device **(fig.-27).**

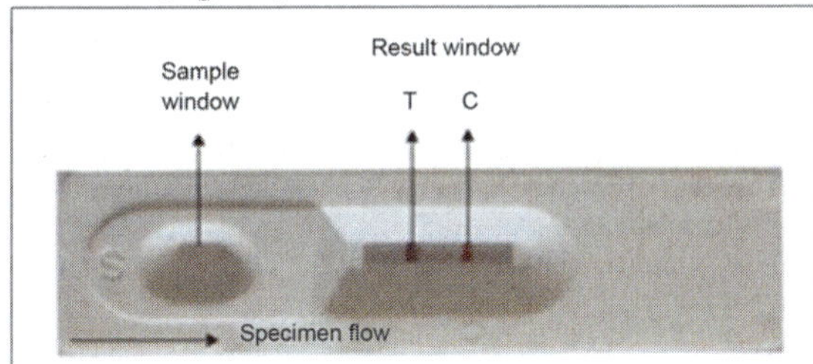

Figure-27: Vertical flow

➢ **Types of test:** Test device is available either in the form of biscuit/card (mostly with single window) or in the form of comb. Both types are discussed as below.

a. Biscuit / card form: Discussed with the example of HIV tridot for HIV-1 & 2 antibodies detection

✪ **Structure of biscuit (card):** Device is impregnated at three sites

1. HIV-1 test site: With HIV-1-Ag (gp120 & gp41)
2. HIV-2 test site: With HIV-2-Ag (gp36)
3. Control site: With anti-globulin

✪ **Method:**
- Add the sample contains HIV antibodies
- Later add the buffer
- Add the signal reagent (Protein A conjugate)
- Again add the buffer
- Read the result within few (around 10) minutes.

✪ **Result: → Fig.28**

- **+Ve test:**
  - If serum contains Ab, it bind with Ag of test site & produce colour dot indicates positive result
  - Control dot produce at control site.
- **-Ve test:** No dot at test site, only dot at control site
- **Invalid:** No control dot with or without test dot.

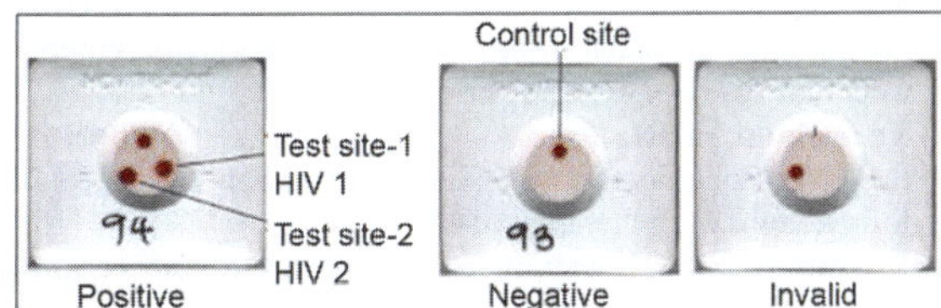

Figure-28: Result of immunoconcentration test (HIV tridot) in biscuit/card form.

b. Comb form: Discussed with the example of HIV comb AIDS-RS for HIV antibodies detection

✪ **Structure of comb:** Device is impregnated at two sites
- Test site: With HIV-1 & 2-Ag (gp41 & gp36)
- Control site: With anti-globulin

✪ **Method:**
- Treat the comb with sample contains HIV antibodies in microtitre well as shown in **fig.-29(a)**.
- Later treat the comb with buffer
- Treat the comb with signal reagent (Protein A conjugate)
- Again treat the comb with buffer
- Read the result within few (around 10) minutes.

✪ **Result: → Fig.29(b)**

- **+Ve test:**
  - If serum contains Ab, it bind with Ag of test site & produce colour dot on comb.
  - Control dot produce at control site
- **-Ve test:** No dot at test site, only dot at control site
- **Invalid:** No control dot with or without test dot.

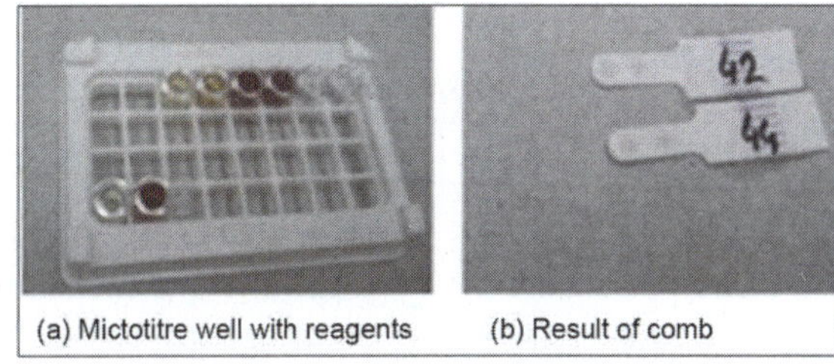

Figure-29: Result of immunoconcentration test (HIV Comb AIDS-RS) in biscuit/card form.

➢ **Advantage:**
- It is a simple & rapid test.
- Qualitative
- Economical
- Nearly as sensitive and specific as EIA test

➢ **Disadvantage:**
- Two step testing than ICT, because colour reagent (Protein A conjugate) is not attached to device, so need to add separately in the form of signal reagent.
- It is qualitative not a quantitative method.

➢ **Uses:** For detection of
- HBsAg
- HCV antibodies
- HIV1 & 2 antibodies

✓ **Note: Comb assay or comb type device of test**
- Comb type device is used in ELISA based serological test (rapid ELISA) like immunocomb HIV 1 & 2 bispot test & immunoconcentration based serological test like HIV Comb AIDS-RS.

Tests by using Electron Microscopy (EM)

A. Immunoelectronmicroscopy:

➢ **Principle:** When viral particles mixed with specific antisera are observed under the Electron Microscope (EM), they are seemed to be clumped.

➢ **Use:** To study some virus like HAV.

B. Immunoferritin test (IFT):

- **Principle:** Ferritin can be conjugated with Ab & such labeled Ab reacting with an Ag can be viewed under the EM.

C. Immunoenzyme test (IET):

- **Principle:** Some stable enzymes like peroxidase can be conjugated with Ab. Tissue section carrying the corresponding Ag is treated with peroxidase labeled Ab. Formation of labelled Ab –Ag complex can be visualised under the EM, by microhistochemical methods.
- **Other enzymes**: Such as glucose oxidase, phosphatase and tyrosinase may be used.

Comparison of immunoassays

Table-6

Test / Assay	Molecule used for labelling	Visible effect	Detection method
RIA	Radioactive isotope	Emits β & γ rays	β & γ counter
ELISA	Enzyme	Colour	ELISA reader
IFA	Dyes	Light	FM
CLIA	Luminol or acridinium esters	Light	Luminometer
WB	Enzyme	Colour band	Naked eye
ICT	Colloidal gold	Colour band	Naked eye
Vertical flow	Protein A conjugate	Colour dot/band	Naked eye
IFT	Ferritin	Black dot	EM
IET	Antibody	Dot	EM

Table-6: Comparison of immunoassay

Question bank

Essay/Full question

1) Antigen-antibody reactions

Short notes

1) VDRL test
2) RPR test
3) Precipitation in gel (Immuno diffusion)
4) Electroimmuno diffusion
5) Widal test
6) Weil-Felix test
7) Paul Bunnell test
8) Anti-globulin (Coomb's) test
9) Modifies Rose Waller test
10) Indirect (passive) agglutination test
11) CFT
12) Neutralisation tests
13) Radio Immuno Assay (RIA)
14) ELISA
15) Immuno Fluorescent Assay (IFA)
16) ICT

Short questions for theory/viva questions

1) Write the difference between immunological reaction & serological reaction
2) What is zone phenomenon?
3) Define titre of serological reactions
4) What is affinity & avidity of serological reactions?
5) What is sensitivity & specificity of serological reactions?
6) What is biological false positive test in treponema infection?
7) Write two uses of CIE.
8) What is blocking (incomplete) antibody?
9) Name the four serological tests based on agglutination principle.
10) What is anamnestic reaction in Widal test?
11) What are carrier particles in serological test?
12) Write the difference between Rose Waaler & modified Rose Waaler test.
13) What is amboceptor?
14) What is coagglutination & conglutination?
15) What is ELISPOT test?

MCQs for chapter review

Introduction

1) **All of the following forces are involved in antigen-antibody reaction except-** (AI-98, AIIMS, Sept-96)
(a) Van der Waal's forces (b) Electrostatic bond (c) Hydrogen bond (d) Covalent bond

2) **Which of the following statement is true-** (AIIMS, Dec-94)
(a) Paul Bunnel test is used to diagnose measles (b) Rose Waller test is complement fixation test (c) Indirect haemagglutination test is less sensitive than gel diffusion test (d) Antigen-antibody reaction cannot occur in the absence of electrolytes

Precipitation reaction

3) **The reaction between antibody and soluble antigen is demonstrated by** (AI-94)
(a) Agglutination (b) Precipitation (c) Complement Fixation Test (d) Haemagglutination test

4) **Prozone phenomenon is due to**
(a) Excess antigen (b) Excess antibody (c) Hyperimmune reaction (d) Disproportionate antigen-antibody levels

5) **Antigen antibody precipitation is maximally seen in which of the following?** (AIIMS, May-05)
(a) Excess of antibody (b) Excess of antigen (c) Equivalence of antibody and antigen (d) Antigen hapten interaction

6) **False positive VDRL, is seen in all except-** (AI-2000)
(a) Lepromatous leprosy (b) Infectious mononucleosis (c) HIV (d) Pregnancy

7) **False positive nontreponemal serological test for syphilis, are seen in -** (PGI, Dec-08)
(a) HIV (b) Collagen disorders (c) Paediatric age group (d) Tuberculosis (e) Chronic liver disease

8) **True about VDRL test** (AIIMS-2001)
(a) Non-specific test (b) Slide flocculation test (c) Best followed for drug therapy (d) All

9) **Reason for black colour clump in RPR test is antigen coating with**
(a) Carbon particle (b) Latex particle (c) Bentonite particle (d) RBCs

Agglutination reaction

10) **Widal test is based on**
(a) Precipitation (b) Flocculation (c) Slide agglutination (d) Tube agglutination (e) Complement Fixation Test

11) **All are correct regarding Widal test, except –** (AIIMS, Nov-99)
(a) Baseline titre differ depending upon the endemicity of the disease (b) High titre value in a single widal test is not confirmative (c) O antibody last longer and hence is not indicative of recent infection (d) H antibody cannot differentiate between types

12) **Coombs test is**
(a) Precipitation test (b) Agglutination test (c) CFT (d) Neutralisation test

13) **Weil-Felix reaction is based on the principle of sharing common antigen between**
(a) *Streptococcus* & *Staphylococcus* (b) *Rickettsia* & *Chlamydia* (c) *Rickettsia* & *Proteus* (d) *Rickettsia* & *Pseudomonas*

14) **A man came from Nagaland and shows positive test with OXK antigen. Diagnosis is**
(a) Trench fever (b) Scrub typhus (c) Endemic typhus (d) Epidemic typhus

Radio Immuno Assay (RIA)

15) **Most sensitive test for antigen detection is** (PGI-97)
(a) RIA (b) ELISA (c) Immunofluorescence (d) Passive haemagglutination

16) **Hormones are best diagnosed by** (PGI-98)
(a) Flow cytometry (b) Electrophoresis (c) ELISA (d) RIA

Comparison of assays

17) **The following methods of diagnosis utilise labelled antibodies except-** (AIIMS, May-05)
(a) ELISA (Enzyme Linked Immuno Sorbent Assay) (b) Haemagglutination inhibition test (c) Radio Immuno Assay (d) Immunofluorescence

Answers of MCQs & explanation

1) **(d)**
- Ag-Ab complex formation is possible by weaker intermolecular forces like ionic (electrostatic) bonds, Van der Waal's forces & hydrogen bonds

2) **(d)**
- Paul Bunnel test is used to diagnose infectious mononucleosis
- Rose Waller test is passive agglutination test
- Indirect haemagglutination test is more sensitive than gel diffusion test

3) **(b)**
- In given question antigen is soluble, which is detected by precipitation

4) **(b)** Follow section, **precipitation reaction**
5) **(c)** **(Zone phenomenon)** for explanation
6) **(d)**
7) **(a) & (b)** } Follow section. VDRL test for explanation
8) **(d)**
9) **(a)**
- Follow **table-3** for explanation

10) **(c) & (d)**
- Widal test is based on agglutination principle which may be both slide as well as tube type

11) **(c)**
- Base line titre of widal is different according to endemicity of areas
- High titre value in a single widal test is may be due to anamnestic reaction, so it is not confirmative. It is confirmed by retesting after 1 week, so repeated testing of paired sera at 1 week interval is more meaningful than single high titre.
- O antigen is less immunogenic. Antibody is not long lasting, so indicate the recent infection.
- In Widal test, separate H antigens for *S. typhi, S. paratyphi A* & *S. paratyphi B* are included so it can differentiate between types

12) **(b)**
- Coombs test fall in anti globulin category of agglutination reaction

13) **(c)**
- Follow section, **Weil-Felix reaction [Antigens (Ags)]** for explanation

14) **(b)**
- Follow section, **Weil-Felix reaction (table-5)** for explanation

15) **(a)**
- RIA is the most sensitive test for detection of Ag from given options
- Sensitivity of different test for Ag detection is
  - RIA: 0.5-1 IU/ml
  - ELISA: 1-2 mIU/ml
  - Direct agglutination: 0.2 IU/ml
  - Agglutination inhibition: 0.5-1 IU/ml

16) **(d)**
- RIA is useful in quantitation of hormones, drugs, tumour markers, IgE and viral antigens

17) **(a) & (c)**
- Follow **table-6** to know the name the tests in which Ag/Ab is labelled

23 Complement system

Learning heading & subheadings

- History:
- Definitions:
- Properties:
- Components:
- Fraction of complement components:
- Biosynthesis of complement components:
- Model of C - activity:
- Complement activation:
- Complement pathways:
- Highlights of complement pathways:
- Regulation of complement pathway:
- Biological effects of complement:
- Measurement of complement system:
- Deficiencies of complement components:

History:

- **Hans Ernst August Buchner (1889):** Who 1st observed that bactericidal effect of serum was destroyed by heating at 55^0C for 1 hour.
- **Pfiffer(1894):** He discovered that *V. cholera* were lysed when injected intraperitoneally into specifically immunised guinea pigs **called bacteriolysis in vivo or Pfirffer's phenomenon.**
- **Jules Bordet (1895):** He observed that serum has two factors like heat stable Ab & heat labile **called alexine**
- **Paul Ehrlich:** He replaced the term alexine with complement, because having complementary action like Ab.

Definition:
System of normal serum factors which are activated by Ag-Ab reaction & takes part in many biological activities.

Properties:

- **Contains:** It comprise around 30 serum proteins (glycoprotein), together constituting nearly 5% of the total serum proteins.
- **Concentration** will not rise by immunisation
- **Present:** In mammals, animals, birds, fish & amphibians.
- **Temperature effect:** Heat labile, inactivated at 56^0C in 30 minutes.
- **Abbreviation:** It is abbreviated as "C"
- **Binding/fixation/consumption:**
  - It binds with Ag-Ab complex, not to free Ag or Ab.
  - Fixation is affected by Ab type: E.g. IgM & IgG 3, 1 & 2 (in that order) are the only immunoglobulin capable of activating C, but not IgG4, IgA, IgD or IgE.
  - Fixation is not affected by Ag type
  - It binds with Fc piece of Ig.

Components:
It comprise 20-30 different serum proteins, which includes

1. Complement components: C1-C9
2. Properdin system:
3. Regulatory proteins:

Fraction of complement components:

- **Complement proteins:**
  - It shows nine distinct proteins from C1 to C9 separated by Electrophoresis.
  - All they are come in sequence, except C4 comes after C1 but before C2.
- **C1:**
  - It is heat labile & forms the main bulk of the component.
  - It is Ca^{+2} dependent & on chelation with EDTA it forms three protein subunits **called C1q, r, s.**

Biosynthesis of complement components:

- C1: In intestinal epithelium
- C2 & C4: In macrophages
- C5 & C8: In spleen
- C3,C6 & C9: In liver

Model of C - activity:

- It is explained by RBCs lysis with Ab.
- Erythrocyte (E) makes complex with Antibody (A) **called EA.**
- When C components are attached **called EAC** followed by their numbers like **EAC14235** or **EAC1-5.**
- Biological (like enzymatic) activity is shown as bar ($C\bar{1}$) over components.
- Fragments cleaved during cascade are indicated by small letters like C3a, C3b etc.
- Inactivated components are presented by using prefix 'i' like iC3b.

Complement activation:

- Normally present in the body in an inactive form
- Its activity induced by Ag-Ab combination or other stimuli.
- C components react in a specific sequence as a cascade.
- Cascade is a series of reaction in which the preceding components act as enzymes on the succeeding components, cleaving in to dissimilar fragments.
- The larger fragments usually join the cascade.
- The smaller fragments which are released often posses biological effects **(as described in later part of this chapter)** which contribute to defence mechanisms.

❖ **Complement pathways:** Three pathways & final step is identical in all 3 pathways.

A. Classical pathway:

➢ **Definition:** The chain of events in which C components react in specific sequence following activation of C1 & typically culminate in immune cytolysis is **called the classical pathway**.

➢ **Properties:**

- Initiated by formation of an Ag-Ab complex (Ab dependent). Antibodies useful are IgG (++, IgG1, IgG3 & rarely IgG2) & IgM (+++).
- Also initiated by other stimuli like DNA, CRP, trypsin like enzymes or by retroviruses.
- It was identified at first.
- Useful in active immunity.

➢ **Steps: →Flow chart-1**

✪ **C1:**

- Classical pathway is initiated by binding of C1to Ag-Ab complex.
- It begins with the binding of C1 to the Ag-Ab complex.
- The recognition unit of C1 is C1q, which reacts with the Fc piece of bounded IgM or IgG.
- C1q has six combining sites.
- Effective activation occurs only when C1q is attached to Ig by at least 2 of its binding sites.

C1q binds in the presence of calcium ions leads to sequential activation of C1r & s (Cqrs = C) **called Ag-Ab C** or **C1qrscomplex** or **C1s esterase**

✪ **C4:**

- It cleaved by C1s esterase, into two fragments

1. **C4a:** Which is an anaphylatoxin
2. **C4b:** Which bind to cell membrane along with C1qrs & forms the complex **called Ag-AbC4b** or **Ag-AbCqrs4b** or **C4b**

✪ **C2:**

- C4b in the presence of magnesium ions cleaves C2 into two fragments

1. **C2a:** Which remains linked to cell- bound C4b
2. **C2b:** Which released into the fluid phase, having kinin like activity & increase vascular permeability

- C4b2a has enzymatic activity & **called C3 convertase**.

✪ **C3:**

- C3 convertase splits C3 into two fragments

1. **C3a:** Anaphylatoxin
2. **C3b:** Remains cell-bound along with C4b2a to form a trimolecular complex **called C4b2a3b** which has enzymatic activity & is **called C5 convertase**

✪ **C5:**

- Membrane attack phase start at this level.
- C5 convertase cleaves C5 into

1. **C5a:** Released into the medium & having anaphylatoxic & chemotactic activities (chemoattractant)
2. **C5b:** Which continue with cascade

✪ **C6 & C7:**

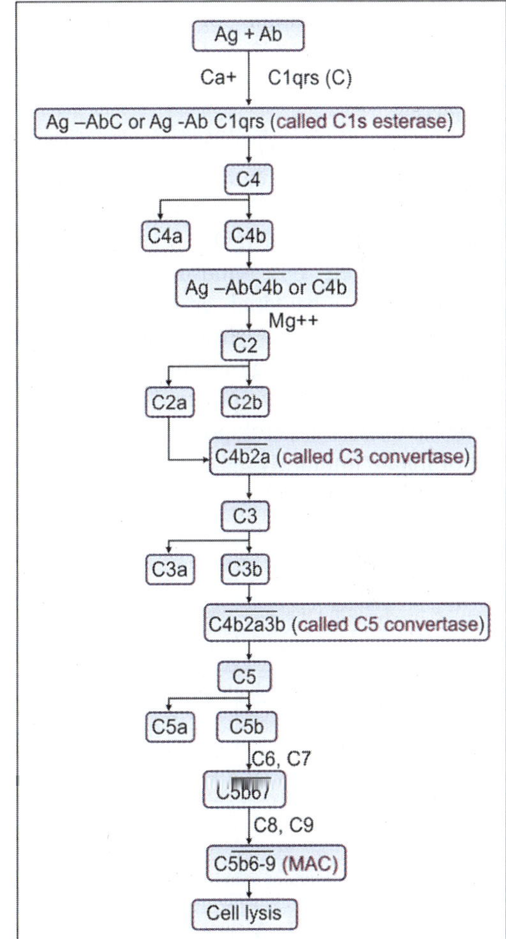

Flow chart-1: Classical pathway

- Join together with C5b & forms the heat trimolecular complex C5b67, which have two functions.

1. Bystander cells**:** Most of C5b67 escape & serve to amplify the reaction by adsorbing on to unsensitised '**bystander cells**'& rendering them susceptible to lysis by C8 &C9.

2. Bind to cell membrane & prepare it for lysis by C8 & C9

- **C8 & C9:** Bind with C5b67, which bounded to the cell membrane & form C5b6-9 complex **called Membrane Attack Complex (MAC)** causing lysis.
- **Chemotaxis & cell lysis:**
  - The unbound C5b67 has chemotactic activity, though the effect is transient due to its rapid inactivation.
  - The mechanism of compliment mediated cytolysis is the production of holes approximately 100°A in diameter on the cell membrane; this disrupts the osmotic integrity of the membrane, leading to the release of the cell contents (increase permeability).

B. Alternative or properdin pathway:

- **History:** 1st described by **Pillemer** in 1954 (antimicrobial protein present in serum)
- **Definition:** Activation of C3 without prior participation of C1, C4 & C2 is **called alternate pathway**.
- **Properties:**
  - The alternate pathway bypasses participation of C4b2a (C3convertase) & activates C3 directly.
  - Antibody-independent, but some Ab can stimulate the pathway like IgA & IgD.
  - It is stimulated by zymosan (yeast cell wall polysaccharide), bacterial endotoxin, IgG4, IgA, IgD, cobra venom, nephritic factor (present in patient with acute glomerulo nephritis-AGN), teichoic acid from Gram positive cell walls, certain viruses, parasites, heterologous red cells etc.
  - Part of innate immunity
- **Steps: →Flow chart-2**

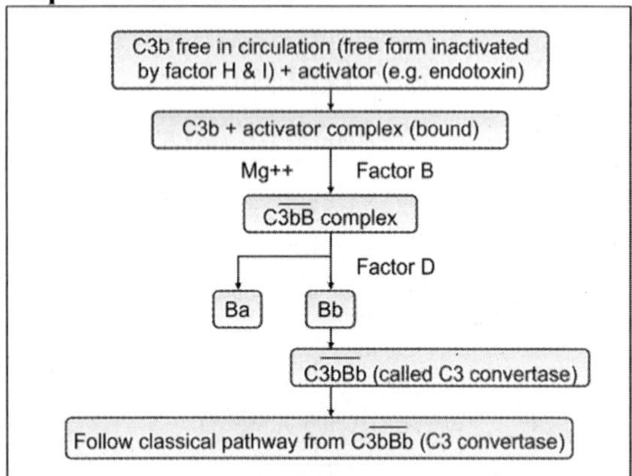

Flow chart-2: Alternative pathway

- **C3b:**
  - Continuously generated in serum, but free form is inactivated by **factors H &I.**
  - It is protected from such inactivation by **factor B** also **called C3B proactivator**.
  - C3b binds with factor B in presence of Mg^{++} to form C3bB complex.
  - Factor B is cleaved by **Factor D** (also called **C3B proactivator convertase**) in to two fragments.

1. **Ba:** Released into the medium
2. **Bb:** Binds with c3b to form C3bBb complex.
   - C3bBb complex is as like C3 convertase (C4b2a) activity but it is extremely labile & loses its activity; but binding with properdin it formsPC3bBb complex & becomes stable.

- **After formation of C3 convertase further steps are like classical pathway.**

C. Lectin or Mannose Binding Lectin (MBL) pathway:

- **Definition:** C4 activation can be achieved by lectin without Ab & C1 participation **called lectin pathway**
- **Properties:**
  - Stimulated by combination of mannose residues present on microbial surface (like *Salmonella, Neisseria, Listeria, C. neoformans & C. albicans*) with MBL of serum & later combination with two specific protease like MASP1 (**Mannan-binding lectin-Associated Serine Proteases**) & MASP2.
  - Antibody-independent
  - Part of innate immunity
  - **Mannose Binding Lectin (MBL):** is an acute phase protein, present in serum & produced in inflammatory responses.
- **Steps: →Flow chart-3**

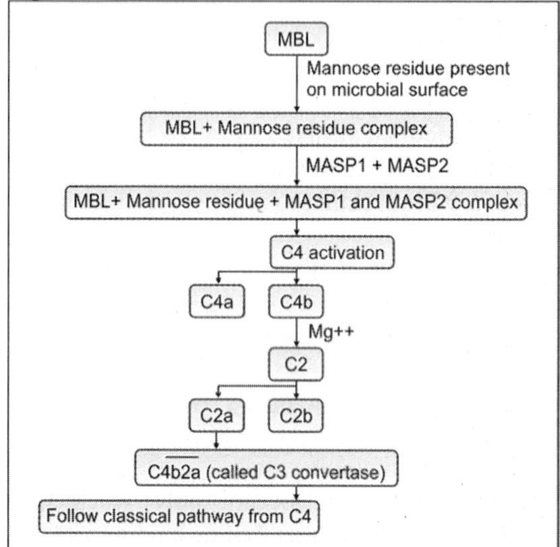

Flow chart-3: MBL pathway

- **C4:**
  - In this pathway MBL binds to certain mannose residues present on many microbial surfaces and subsequently interacts with MASP and MASP2.
  - The Mannose residues-MBL-MASP1-MASP2 complex is similar to Ab-C1qrs complex (of classical pathway) and leads to activation of C4 & cleaved it in to two fraction

1. **C4a:** It is an anaphylatoxin.
2. **C4b:**

- **C2:**
  - C4b in the presence of magnesium ions cleaves C2 into two fragments

1. **C2a:** It remains linked to C4b & form C4b2a
2. **C2b:** It released into the fluid phase.

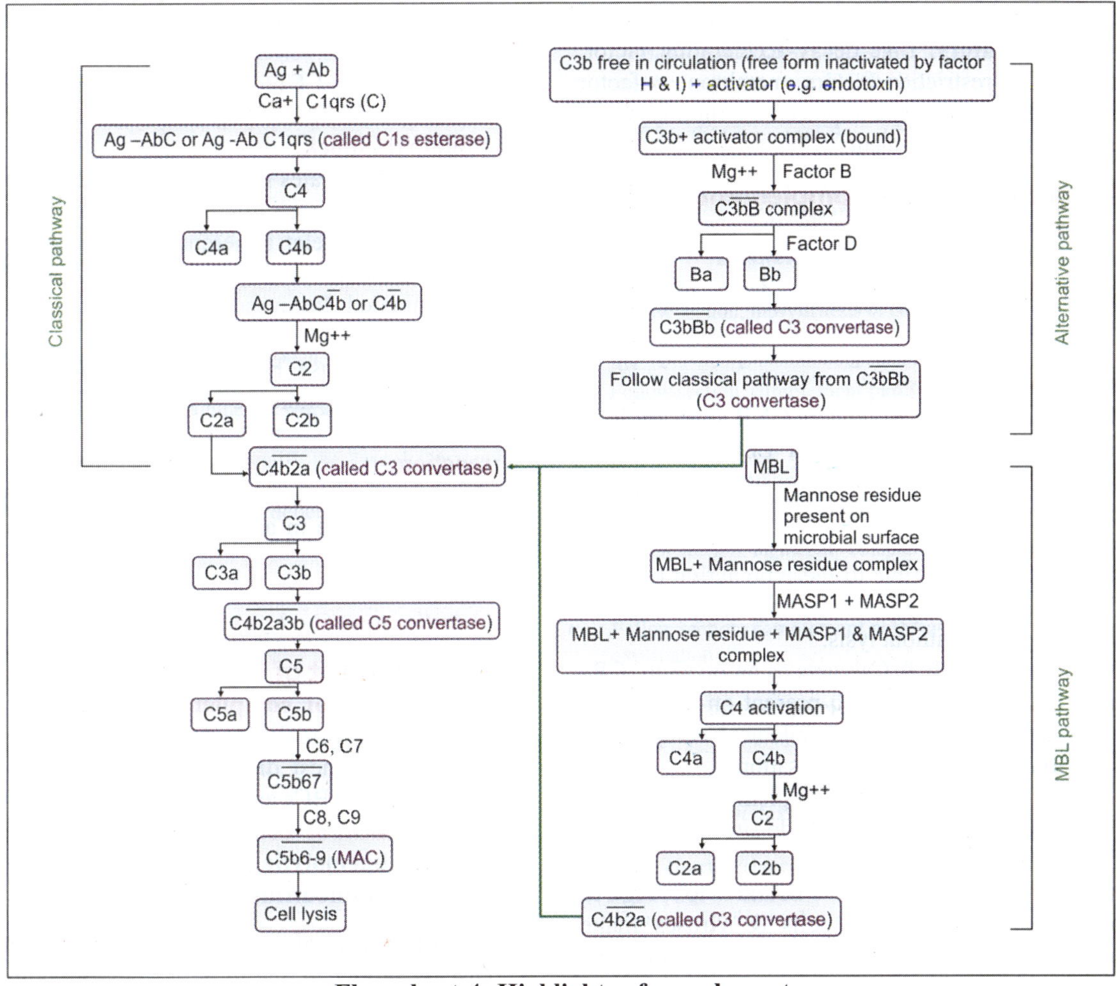

Flow chart-4: Highlights of complement

- C4b2a has enzymatic activity & is referred to as the classical pathway C3 convertase.

✪ **The rest follows as in classical pathway:**

❖ Highlights of complement pathways: → Flow chart-4

- Three pathways converge at the **Membrane Attack Complex (MAC)**, which includes C5b-9.
- C5b-9 makes holes or channels in cell membrane of pathogens or target cell through which cell contents are come out & resulting cell death
- C3 is the major components. It is common in both classical & alternative pathways & also acts as centre for complement pathways.

❖ Regulation of complement pathway:

➢ **Unchecked complement activation may cause:**

- Exhaustion of the complement system
- Serious damage to tissues hence, regulation of complement activation is necessary.

➢ **Control mechanisms:** Two types

a. **Inhibitors:** They bind to C components & halt the further functions.

1. **C1 esterase inhibitors (C1s INH):**

- Heat labile
- α- neuroaminoglycoprotein in nature.
- This does not prevent the normal progress of the complement cascade but check autolytic prolongation.
- It also inhibits the other esterase found in serum like kininogen, plasmin & hageman factor.

2. **S protein:**

- Present in serum
- Binds to C67 & prevents their insertion into cell membrane modulating the cytolytic activity of the MAC.

b. **Inactivators:** These are the enzymes that destroy the complement proteins

1. **Factor-I:** It is a serum β-globulin that control C3 activation, particularly by the alternate pathway. It also cleaves & inactivates C3b & C4b.
2. **Factor-H:** It is a another β-globulin that acts in cooperation with factor-I & modulate C3 activation
3. **C4 binding protein:** It controls the activity of cell bound C4b
4. **Anaphylatoxin inactivators:** It is an α-globulin that enzymatically degrades C3a, C4a & C5a which

24 Structure and functions of immune system

Learning heading & subheadings

- Introduction
- Classification of immune system
  - I. Specific immune system / lymphoid system
  - II. Non specific immune system
- Major Histocompatibility Complex (MHC)

Introduction

❖ **Synonym:** Lymphoreticular system

❖ **Definition:** It is a complex organization of cells of diverse morphology distributed widely in different organs and tissues of the body responsible for immunity.

Classification of immune system

❖ **Parts:** Two parts

I. **Specific immune system / lymphoid system:** It includes lymphoid organs & lymphoid cells. It produces the specific immune response **called acquired immunity**, which may be either AMI or CMI.

II. **Non specific immune system:** Like

- **Reticulo Endothelial (RE) system & RE cells:** It produces the non-specific immune response **called phagocytosis**.
- **Ir by cells without TCRs**
- **Complement system:** Follow chapter → Complement system
- **Neutralisation:** Follow chapter → Antigen – Antibody (Ag-Ab) reactions

I. Specific immune system / lymphoid system

➢ **Components:** Two components like organs & cells

A **Lymphoid organs:** →**Flow chart-1**

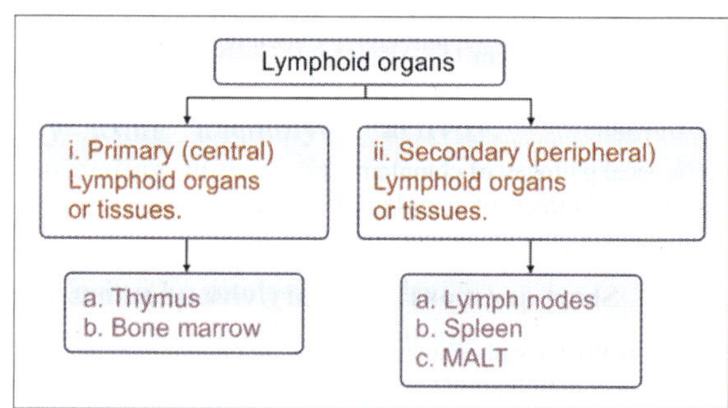

Flow chart-1: Lymphoid organs

B. **Lymphoid cells:**

i. **Cells with T - Cell Receptors (TCRs): Called lymphocytes**

a. **T-cells**

b. **B-cells (plasma cells)**

ii. **Cells without TCRs: Called null cells** or **large granular lymphocytes (LGLs).** They produce non specific immune response.

a. **Natural Killer (NK) cells.**

b. **Antibody Dependent Cytotoxic Cells (ADCCs)**

c. **Lymphokine Activated Killer (LAK) cells**

iii. **APCs (Antigen Presenting Cells):**

a. **Major cells or professional cells:**

b. **Minor cells or non-professional cells:**

A. **Lymphoid organs:**

i. **Primary (central) lymphoid organs or tissues:**

a. **Bone marrow: (Bursa of fabricius in birds):**

✪ **Origin of all blood cells:**

- All the blood cells are originated from the haematopoietic stem cell of bone marrow by the process **called haematopoiesis (vide infra)**.
- In early foetal life cells are derived from liver & yolk sac, which gradually migrate to bone marrow.

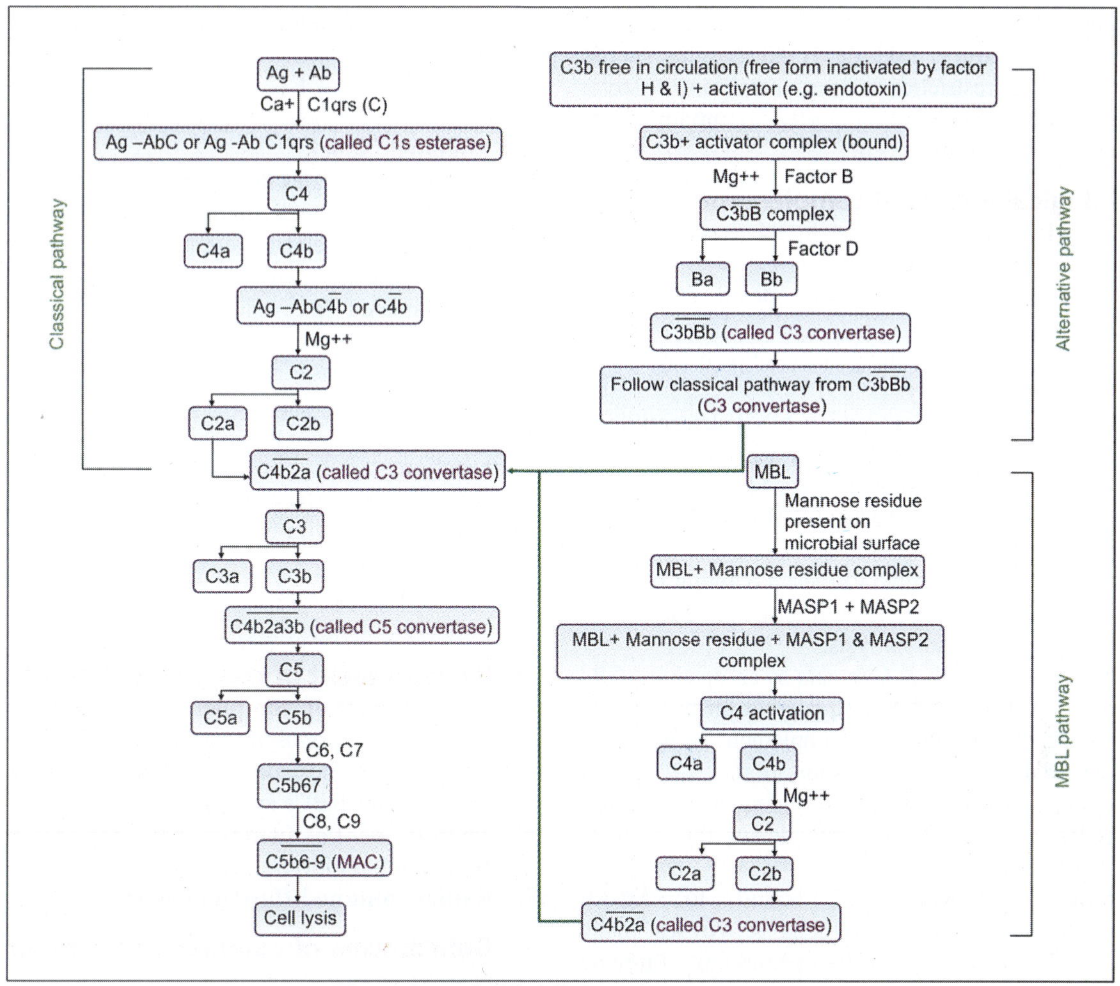

Flow chart-4: Highlights of complement

- C4b2a has enzymatic activity & is referred to as the classical pathway C3 convertase.

✪ **The rest follows as in classical pathway:**

❖ Highlights of complement pathways: → Flow chart-4

- Three pathways converge at the **Membrane Attack Complex (MAC)**, which includes C5b-9.
- C5b-9 makes holes or channels in cell membrane of pathogens or target cell through which cell contents are come out & resulting cell death
- C3 is the major components. It is common in both classical & alternative pathways & also acts as centre for complement pathways.

❖ Regulation of complement pathway:

➢ **Unchecked complement activation may cause:**

- Exhaustion of the complement system
- Serious damage to tissues hence, regulation of complement activation is necessary.

➢ **Control mechanisms:** Two types

a. **Inhibitors:** They bind to C components & halt the further functions.

1. **C1 esterase inhibitors (C1s INH):**
   - Heat labile
   - α- neuroaminoglycoprotein in nature.
   - This does not prevent the normal progress of the complement cascade but check autolytic prolongation.
   - It also inhibits the other esterase found in serum like kininogen, plasmin & hageman factor.
2. **S protein:**
   - Present in serum
   - Binds to C67 & prevents their insertion into cell membrane modulating the cytolytic activity of the MAC.

b. **Inactivators:** These are the enzymes that destroy the complement proteins

1. **Factor-I:** It is a serum β-globulin that control C3 activation, particularly by the alternate pathway. It also cleaves & inactivates C3b & C4b.
2. **Factor-H:** It is a another β-globulin that acts in cooperation with factor-I & modulate C3 activation
3. **C4 binding protein:** It controls the activity of cell bound C4b
4. **Anaphylatoxin inactivators:** It is an α-globulin that enzymatically degrades C3a, C4a & C5a which

are anaphylatoxins released during the complement cascade.

5. **Other regulators:** Like decay-accelerating factor, homologous restriction factors, membrane cofactor protein, etc. have been reported to modulate the activity of the complement.

❖ Biological effects of complement:

a. **Neutralisation of viruses:** In the early stage of infection by either pathway.

b. **Anticancer activity:** Causing death of tumour cells.

c. **Haemolysis:** By activating classical pathway

d. **Bactericidal activity:**

- GNB: The complement renders GNB susceptible to lysozyme by binding holes in LPS layer which protects inner lysozyme sensitive layer of peptidoglycan & thus makes GNB sensitive to lysis (bacteriolysis).
- GPC are not susceptible to the lytic action because of their cell wall composition, however they killed by complement without lysis.

e. **Phagocytosis:** C3b & C4b acts as an opsonin. CRs like C1, C4, C2, C3 & C1q present on phagocytic cells are the receptors for complement components like C3b & C4b helps in opsonisation.

f. **Pathogenesis of diseases:** Complement Receptors-2 (CRs2/CD21on B cells) provide site for adhesion of Epstein- Barr Virus (EBV)

g. **Immune adherence:** C bound to Ag-Ab complexes, Ab sensitized cells & viruses make them to adhere to cells possessing immune adherence receptors (macrophages, B-lymphocytes, primate RBCs etc.) & increase susceptibility to phagocytosis & increase the body defence.

h. **Inflammatory:** C2b kinin released during cascade, which increase the increases vascular permeability

i. **Hypersensitivity reaction:**

1. **Anaphylatoxin activity:** C4a, C3a & C5a stimulate the release of histamine from mast cells that causes constriction of smooth muscles, increases vascular permeability &vasodilatation.
2. **Type II hypersensitivity reaction:** e.g. RBCs destruction following incompitable transfusion.
3. **Type III hypersensitivity reaction:**

- C is required for serum sickness & Arthus reaction.
- E.g. Kidney damage in nephrotoxic nephritis

j. **Autoimmune disease:** C components are decrease in SLE & RA. It play major role in auto immune haemolytic anaemia.

k. **Conglutination:**

- Bovine serum contains β-globulin component **called conglutinin (K)**, which causes clumping of particles or cells coated with complement **called conglutination.**
- It reacts with bound C3 in presence of Ca^{+2}. It is not Ab, but when K coated with C is injected, it produces Ab **called immunoconglutinin (IK)**. It may occur as autoantibody in human & acts on fixed C.
- Conglutinating CFT: More details, **Follow chapter →Antigen-antibody (Ag-Ab) reactions.**

l. **Endotoxic shock:**

- Endotoxin activates the alternative pathway.
- In endotoxic shock there is large amount of C-fixation & platelet adherence, resulting release of large amount of platelet factors causing Disseminated Intravascular Coagulation (DIC) & thrombocytopenia.
- E.g. Water-house Friderichsen syndrome, dengue haemorrhagic syndrome

m. Depletion of C protects against **Shwartzman reaction:**

n. **Rise in acute infection:** It is an acute phase protein & it's level rise in acute infection particularly C3, C4, C5 & C6.

o. **In serological test:** E.g. CFT, **Follow chapter →Antigen-antibody (Ag-Ab) reactions.**

❖ Measurement of complement system:

a. **Measurement of complement activity:**

1. **By using haemolytic activity:** measured by estimating highest dilution of serum sheep RBCs lysed by anti-RBCs antibody.

b. **Measurement of complement components:**

1. **By using haemolytic activity:**
2. **Radial immunodiffusion in agar:**

❖ Deficiencies of complement components:

Disease produced due to deficiency of complement components are shown in **table-1**

Deficiency	Disease
C1inhibitor	Hereditary angioedema
C1s, C2, C4	SLE & other collagen diseases
C3, regulatory proteins & C3b inactivator	Pyogenic infections
C5-8	GN-bacteremia & toxoplasmosis
C9	No particular disease
C5-9	*Neisseria* like meningococcus & gonococcus

Table-1: Disease due to deficiency of complement components

➢ **Hereditary angioedema:**

✪ **Mechanism:**

- Reduced amount of C1inhibitor leads to autolytic activation of C1 & uncontrolled breakdown of C4 &C2.
- Main mediators for oedema is released of C2b

✪ **Clinical features:**

- Angioedema of subcutaneous tissues or mucosa of GIT or respiratory tract
- Death

Treatment:

- Infusion of fresh plasma as source of inhibitors.
- Administration of epsilon amino caproic acid or its analogue: inhibits the activation of plasma enzymes & sparing the small amount of the C1 inhibitor present.

Question bank

Case study

1) A 8 years male child brought to skin OPD with history of pyogenic infection like boil in nose. He completed the antibiotic course & maintaining the hygiene, in spite of all this recurrence is there. Serum investigation reported the deficiency of complement component. Identify the case & answer the following
a) Name the complement component deficient in given case
b) Name the complement components & disease produced due to their deficiency
c) Write biological effects of complement

Essay/Full question

1) Complement system

Short notes

1) Classical pathway of complement
2) Biological effects of complement
3) Regulation of complement

Short questions for theory/viva questions

1) What is Pfiffer's phenomenon?
2) What is conglutination?
3) Write the origin for following complement components C1, C2, C3 & C4
4) Name complement components & related disease produced due to their deficiency.
5) Name the C3 convertase for classical, alternate & MBL pathways of complement.

MCQs for chapter review

1) **Complement formed in liver-**
(a) C2, C4 (b) C3, C6, C9 (c) C5, C8 (d) C1
2) **C3 convertase acts on**
(a) C4b2b (b) C4b2B3a (c) C4b (d) C3
3) **Which complement component is involved in both classical and alternative pathways** (AI-11)
(a) C1 (b) C2 (c) C3 (d) C4
4) **Centre for complement pathway**
(a) C3 (b) C1 (c) C5 (d) C2
5) **C3 convertase in alternative complement pathway-**
(a) C4b2a (b) C3b (c) C3bBb (d) C3a
6) **Chemoattractant is** (PGI-89)
(a) C5a (b) C1 (c) C3 (d) C2
7) **In cell lysis by complement**
(a) They activate cyclise (b) Inhibits elongator factor p (c) Destruction of P (d) Increased permeability of cell membrane
8) **Which of the following best denotes classical complement pathway activation in immuno-inflammatory condition?**
(a) C2, C4 and C3 decreased (b) C2 and C4 normal, C3 decreased (c) C3 normal, C2 and C4 decreased (d) C2, C4 and C3 all are elevated
9) **Deficiency of C1 inhibitor in complement system produce**
(a) Hereditary angioedema (b) Toxoplasmosis (c) Bacteremia (d) Collagen disease
10) **Hereditary angioneurotic oedema is due to**
(a) Deficiency of C1 inhibitors (b) Deficiency of NADPH oxidase (c) Deficiency of MPO (d) Deficiency of properdin
11) **Which deficiency would cause *Neisseria* infection-**
(a) C5 (b) C6 (c) C9 (d) C7 (e) C8
12) **Deficiency of C5-C9 complement components predispose to which infection?**
(a) Meningococci (b) Pneumococcal (c) Pseudomonas (d) All

Answers of MCQs & explanation

1) **(b)**
- Follow section, **biosynthesis of complement components** for the explanation
2) **(d)**
- Follow section, **complement pathways (flow chart-1)** for the explanation
3) **(c)**
- Follow section, **complement pathways (flow chart-1 & flow chart-2)** for the explanation
4) **(a)**
- Follow section, **highlights complement pathways (flow chart-4)** for the explanation
5) **(c)**
- Follow section, **complement pathways (flow chart-2)** for the explanation
6) **(a)**
- Follow section, **complement pathways (classical pathway → steps)** for the explanation
7) **(d)**
- Follow section, **complement pathways (classical pathway → steps → Chemotaxis & cell lysis)** for the explanation
8) **(a)**
- **Flow chart -4** showing all the pathways of complement. In classical pathway C1-C9 are utilised & decreased while in alternative pathway all are decrease except C1,C2 &C4

9) **(a)**
10) **(a)**
11) **(a) to (e)**
12) **(a)**

} Follow **table-1** for the explanation

24 Structure and functions of immune system

Learning heading & subheadings

Introduction

❖ **Synonym:** Lymphoreticular system

❖ **Definition:** It is a complex organization of cells of diverse morphology distributed widely in different organs and tissues of the body responsible for immunity.

Classification of immune system

❖ **Parts:** Two parts

I. **Specific immune system / lymphoid system:** It includes lymphoid organs & lymphoid cells. It produces the specific immune response **called acquired immunity**, which may be either AMI or CMI.

II. **Non specific immune system:** Like

- **Reticulo Endothelial (RE) system & RE cells:** It produces the non-specific immune response **called phagocytosis**.
- **Ir by cells without TCRs**
- **Complement system:** Follow chapter → Complement system
- **Neutralisation:** Follow chapter → Antigen – Antibody (Ag-Ab) reactions

I. Specific immune system / lymphoid system

➢ **Components:** Two components like organs & cells

A **Lymphoid organs:** →**Flow chart-1**

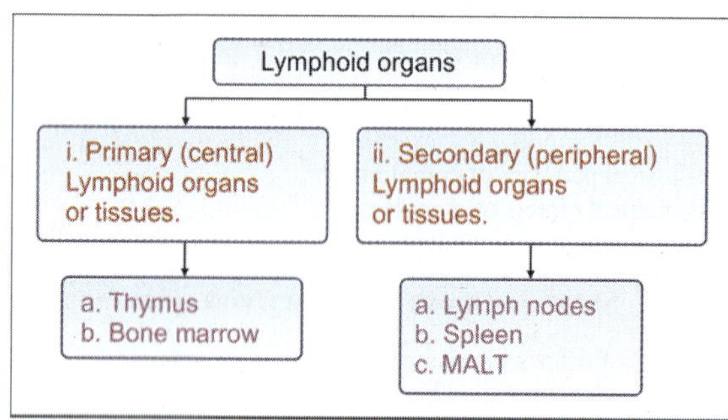

Flow chart-1: Lymphoid organs

B. **Lymphoid cells:**

i. **Cells with T - Cell Receptors (TCRs): Called lymphocytes**

a. **T-cells**

b. **B-cells (plasma cells)**

ii. **Cells without TCRs: Called null cells** or **large granular lymphocytes (LGLs).** They produce non specific immune response.

a. **Natural Killer (NK) cells.**

b. **Antibody Dependent Cytotoxic Cells (ADCCs)**

c. **Lymphokine Activated Killer (LAK) cells**

iii. **APCs (Antigen Presenting Cells):**

a. **Major cells or professional cells:**

b. **Minor cells or non-professional cells:**

A. **Lymphoid organs:**

i. **Primary (central) lymphoid organs or tissues:**

a. **Bone marrow: (Bursa of fabricius in birds):**

✪ **Origin of all blood cells:**

- All the blood cells are originated from the haematopoietic stem cell of bone marrow by the process **called haematopoiesis (vide infra)**.
- In early foetal life cells are derived from liver & yolk sac, which gradually migrate to bone marrow.

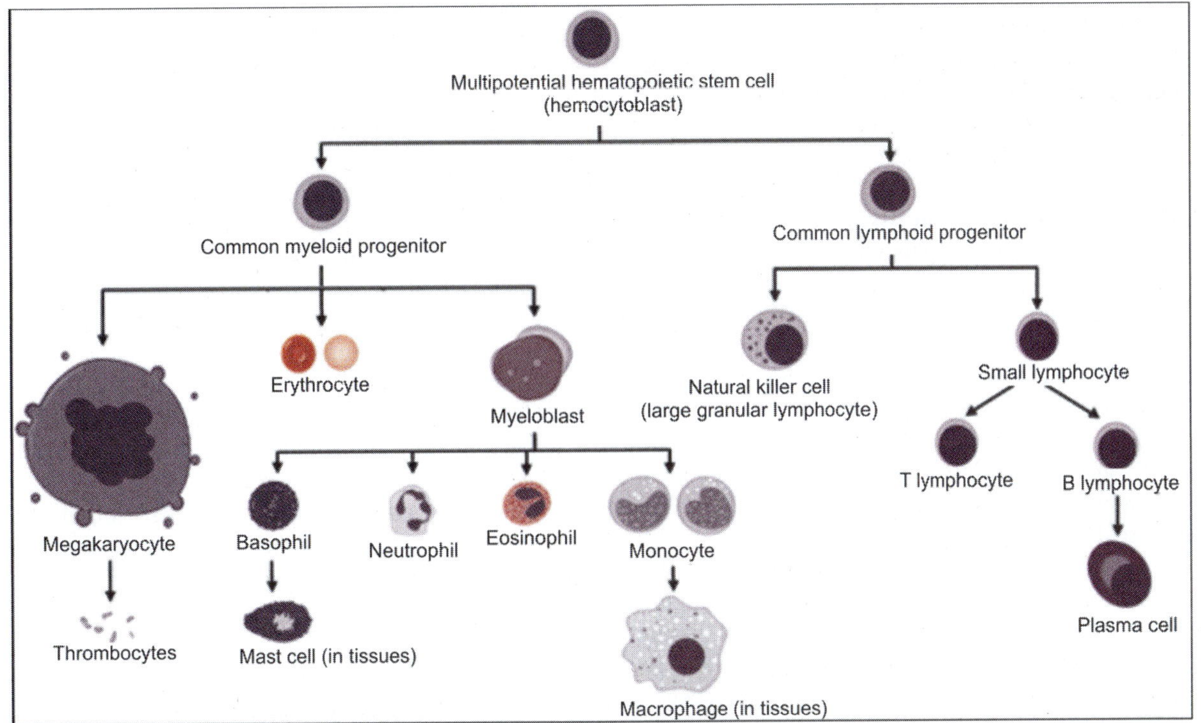

Figure-1: Haematopoiesis

- By the birth, almost all stem cells occupy the position in bone marrow of large bones.
- With advancing age haematopoietic activity of large bones is decrease & after puberty haematopoiesis is mostly confirmed to axial bones like pelvis, vertebrate, skull, sternum & ribs.

✪ **Maturation of cells in bone marrow:** The precursors of B-cell enter in to bone marrow from fetal liver, yolk sac & mature in B-cells (B= Bursa of fabricius in birds or Bone marrow in human).

✪ **Function:** Allow the maturation of B-cells responsible for AMI.

Haematopoiesis

- **Meaning:** Haema (Greek) = Blood + Poiesis = To make up
- **Synonym:** Haemopoiesis
- **Definition:** It is a process of formation of blood cells components.
- **Haemapoietic stem cells:** This are the cells reside in the medulla of the bone **called bone marrow** & have the ability to form the all blood cells as shown in **fig-1**.

b. Thymus:

✪ **Embryology:**

- It develop from the epithelium of the 3rd & 4th pharyngeal pouches at about 6th week of gestation.
- It is thus the first organ in all animal species to become predominantly lymphoid.

✪ **Anatomy:**

- **Location:** It located behind the upper part of sternum in the thoracic cavity overlying heart & major blood vessels.
- **Lobes:** It has two lobes surrounded by fibrous capsule.
- **Parts:** Septa arising from capsule divide the gland into an outer cortex & inner medulla as shown in **fig.-2**

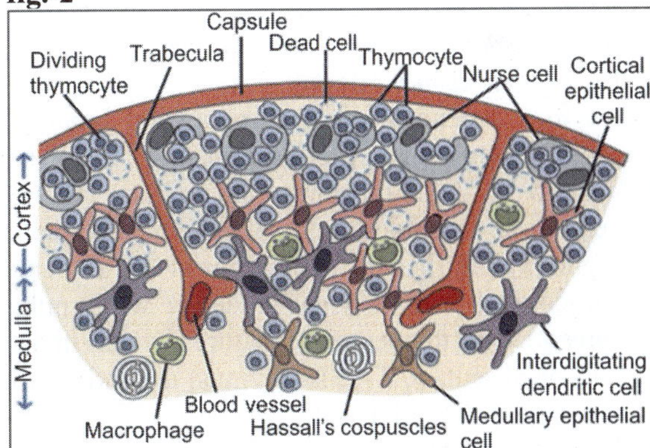

Figure-2: Cross section of thymus

1. **Outer cortex:** Contains
- T-cells: Immature T cells present in thymus are **called thymocytes.** These cells are plenty in numbers
- Nurse cells: Special type of epithelial cells that surround the thymocytes
- Cortical epithelial cell: Looks like star shape

2. **Inner medulla:** Contains

- T-cells: Thymocytes are less in number but relatively mature
- Degenerated epithelial cells: Aggregated in whorls like pattern **called Hassall's corpuscles.**
- Medullary epithelial cell: Looks like star shape
- Interdigitating dendritic cells

✪ **Functions:**

1. **Maturation of T-cells in thymus:**
- The precursors of lymphocytes enter in to thymus from bone marrow, fetal liver, yolk sac & mature in cortex, acquire surface properties of T-lymphocytes (T = Thymus dependent) & than migrate in to medulla, where the completely mature & exit in to blood as mature T-cells.
- In thymus the cells becomes educated to mount CMI against appropriate Ags & seeded in to secondary lymphoid organs.
2. **Central tolerance:** About 95% cell entered in thymus are died & 5% released in circulation. The cells died are, may be not efficient to recognise MHC or believed to be self reacting in nature. Destruction of self reacting T cells prevents the development of autoimmunity. Such tolerance to self antigen mediated by thymus **called central tolerance**
3. **Synthesis of hormones:** Thymus hormones like thymulin, thymosin & thymopoietin are produced by epithelial cells & role in attraction of precursor T cells from bone marrow.

✪ **Clinical significances:**

1. **Di George syndrome:** Congenital aplasia of the thymus leads to deficiency of CMI in human **called Di George syndrome** & in mice **called nude mice.**
2. **Runt disease:** Deficiency of CMI evident from lymphopenia, deficient graft rejection.
3. **Post-thymectomy effect:**
- Thymus dependent areas in peripheral organs are grossly depleted. After originating from bone marrow & getting maturity in thymus, mature T cells enter in certain areas of peripheral lymphoid organs **called thymus dependent areas.** It includes paracortical area in lymph nodes & while pulp in spleen. After thymectomy, mature T cells (thymus) will be absent, so T cells (thymus) dependent areas will be depleted of T cell.
- Decreasing CMI
- Decreasing AMI for thymus dependent Ag.

ii. Secondary (peripheral) lymphoid organs or tissues:

a. Lymph nodes:

✪ **Anatomy: →Fig.-3**

- **Location:** They are placed along the course of lymphatic vessels.
- **Capsule:** They are surrounded by a fibrous capsule
- **Trabecula:** penetrated part of capsule into the nodes **called trabecula.**
- **Parts:**

1. **Outer: Called cortex**
- In the cortex, are accumulation of lymphocytes (primary lymphoid follicles) within which germinal centre (secondary follicles) develop during antigenic stimulation.
- Follicles also contains dendritic macrophages, which capture and process the antigen
2. **Middle between cortex & medulla: Called paracortical area**
- Contains T-lymphocytes & interdigitating cells. It is a **thymus dependent area.**
3. **Inner: called medulla.**
- Contains B-lymphocytes, plasma cells & macrophages are arranged as elongated branching bands **called medullary cords.**

- **Bursa dependent areas:** Cortical follicles and medullary cords contain B- lymphocytes and constitute the bursa dependent areas.

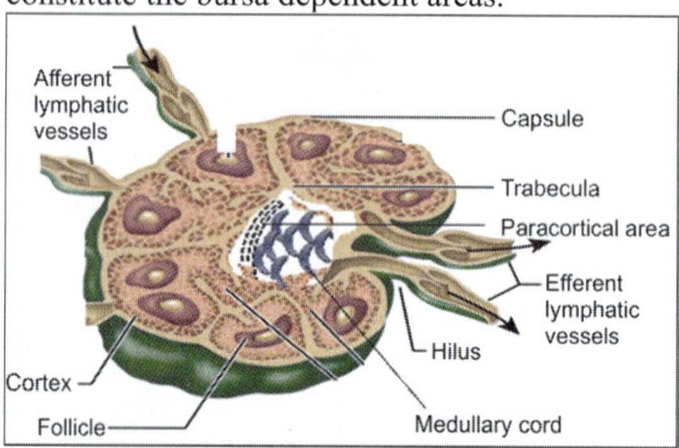

Figure-3: Cross section of lymph nodes

✪ **Functions:**

1. Act as a filter for foreign particles
2. They phagocytose the foreign materials including microorganisms and help in development, proliferation and circulation of T and B cells.
3. They enlarge following local antigenic stimulation.

b. Spleen:

✪ **Anatomy: →Fig.-4**

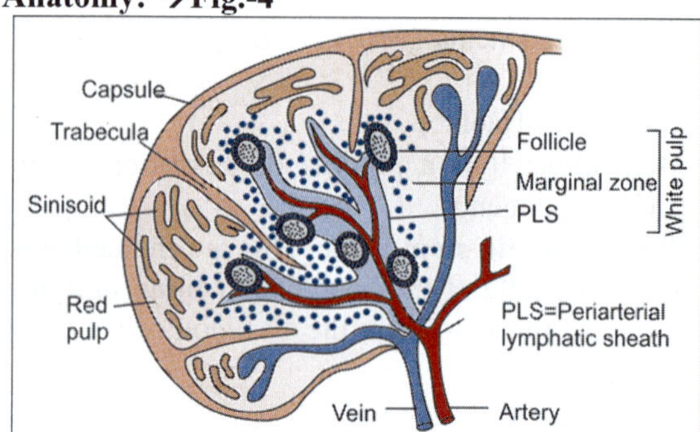

Figure-4: Cross section of spleen

- **Feature:** It is the largest lymphoid organ
- **Capsule:** They are surrounded by a fibrous capsule
- **Trabecula:** Penetrated part of capsule into the spleen **called trabecula** which divides the organ into several interconnected compartments.

- **Parts:** Two parts

1. **White pup:**

- The branches of the splenic artery travel along the trabecula & on leaving them branch again to form central arterioles, which are surrounded by a sheath of the lymphoid tissue contains T-lymphocytes **called white pulp**.
- It is a **thymus dependent area**
- The periarterial lymphoid collection in the white pulp of spleen is **called malpighian corpuscles** or **follicles**.

2. **Red pulp:** The central arterioles proceed into the red pulp, so called because of the abundance of RBCs in it.

✪ **Functions:**

- Ab synthesis against blood borne antigens.
- Filtering of blood borne antigens.

✪ **Clinical significance:**

1. **Post-splenectomy effect:** It leads to bacteremia with *S. pyogenes*, *N. meningitidis*, *H. influenzae* etc.

c. Mucosa Associated Lymphoid Tissue (MALT):

✪ **Definition:** Mucosa lining the alimentary, respiratory, genitourinary & other surfaces is constantly exposed to numerous antigens. So, these areas are endowed with a rich collection of lymphoid cells or follicles which are collectively **called MALT**.

✪ **Cells:** It consist mixture of T- cells, B-cells & phagocytes

✪ **Types:**

1. **Gut Associated Lymphoid Tissue (GALT):** Lymphoid tissue lining the intestinal mucosa **called GALT**. It has following structure & functions.

- **Epithelial layer:** In includes following cells

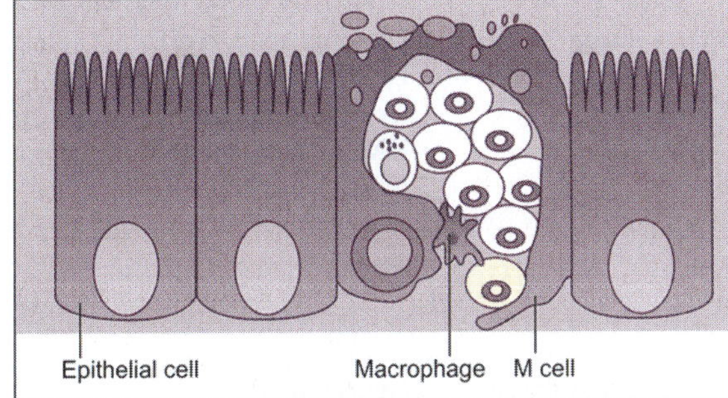

Figure-5: M cells

- CD 7 2 3 γδ TCR cells: Also **called intra epithelial lymphocytes**
- B cells: Present in lining epithelium, lamina propria & submucosa. They secrete the secretory type of IgA which provide the local immunity
- Epithelial cells with microvilli
- Epithelial cells without microvilli **called M cells.** They do not have microvilli on surface but having pockets or Invagination on basolateral side that contains T cell, B cells & macrophages as shown in **fig.-5**. Invading microbes like *Vibrio, Salmonella, Shigella,* Polio virus etc. are taken up by M cell by endocytosis.

- **Lamina propria:** Contains B cell, Th cells & plasma cells
- **Submucosa:** Contains peripheral lymphoid tissue **called peyer's patches**

2. **Tonsils:** Lingual, palatine & pharyngeal type
3. **Bronchus Associated Lymphoid Tissue (BALT):**

- Lymphoid tissue of respiratory tract **called BALT**.

✪ **Function:** MALT serves for Ig production. The predominant Ig produced in the mucosa is secretory IgA & others are IgG, IgM and IgE provide local immunity.

d. Skin associated lymphoid Tissue: Skin also has few loose lymphocytes **called Langerhans cell**, act as APC. Few authors described that Langerhans cells are the type of immature dendritic cells. (Described later in this chapter under the section of APCs).

B. Lymphoid Cells: These cells provide efficient, specific & long-lasting immunity against microbes & are responsible for acquired immunity. They have following three types.

i. Cells with T-Cell Receptors (TCRs): Called Lymphocytes

✪ **Morphology:**

- **Constitutes:** 20-40% of WBCs & 99% cells in lymph
- **Shape:** Round
- **Nucleus:** Round with prominent chromatin materials
- **Cytoplasm:** Thin rim with scattered ribosomes, but without endoplasmic reticulum, Golgi apparatus & other organelles.
- **Motility:** Slow motile & assume a **hand mirror like appearance** with nucleus in front & cytoplasmic tail

✪ **Subtypes:**

a. Based on size:

1. **Small:** 5-8μ
2. **Medium:** 8-12μ
3. **Large:** 12-15μ

b. Based on life span:

1. **Short lived:**

- About 2 weeks
- Generate immune response
- Includes regulatory cells & effector cells

2. **Long lived:**

- About 3 years or whole life
- Generate immune memory
- Includes memory cells.

c. Based on site of maturation:

1. **Thymus-dependent cells or T lymphocytes:** Secrete lymphokines (lymphotoxin) useful in CMI & AMI

2. **Bursa of fabricius (Bone marrow) dependent cells or B lymphocytes:** Differentiate into plasma cells to secrete antibodies & produce AMI

d. **Based on functions:**

1. **Regulatory cells:** These cells are involved in immune regulation
- **Subtypes:**
  - Helper/inducer **(CD4)** cells
  - Suppressor cells **(CD8)**: Not includes cytotoxicity
- **Clinical significance:** To regulate the Ir
  - Increase inducer cells & decrease suppressor cells function: Autoimmunity
  - Decrease inducer cells & increase suppressor cells function: Immuno Deficiency Diseases (IDDs)
2. **Effector cells:** These are active cells involved in immune response.
- **Subtypes & clinical significance:**
  - Cytotoxic **(CD8)**: Not includes suppression function. Role in CMI
  - Plasma cells **(CD19,** B-cells): Role in AMI
3. **Memory cells:** Role in immunological memory.

e. **Based on Cluster of Differentiation (CD marker):**

- **Types:**
  - Numbers of surface Ags or surface markers have been identified on lymphocytes & leucocytes by using monoclonal Abs **called CD markers**
  - When cluster of monoclonal Ab react against particular Ag defined as separate Ag or surface markers then separate CD number is given.
  - CD marker or antigens are useful for differentiation of leucocytes & also to know the functional properties of cell.
  - Around 364 CD markers have been identified
  - Few are, as shown in **table-1**
- **Count of CD4 & CD8 cells in healthy person:**
  - Normal CD4 range is 400 – 1600 cells/ cmm.
  - Normal CD8 range is from 150 to 800 cells/ cmm

CD number	Cell type association	Former designation
CD1	- Present on cortical thymocytes (in early stage only) & Langerhans cells - Composed on 3-polypeptide chain & β-globin	T6, Leu 6
CD2	- Receptors for sheep RBCs (SRBC). - Persist in all stage of maturation & in all mature T cell	T11, Leu 5
CD3	- Present on all T cells, so **called pan CD marker** - Makes TCR-CD3 complex with TCR & transmit the signal interior to the cell following Ag binding on TCR	T3, Leu 4
CD4	Helper/inducer cells (HIV & HHV-7 receptors)	T4, Leu 3
CD8	Suppressor/cytotoxic cells	T8, Leu 2
CD19	B cells	B4, Leu 12

Table-1: CD markers

Features	T- cell	B- cell
Origin (same lineage)	All blood cells from bone marrow (also from liver & yolk sac in foetus)	
Site of maturation	Thymus	Bursa of fabricius/bone marrow
Amount	70-80% of blood lymphocytes	10-20% of blood lymphocytes
Rosette formation	Binding with sheep RBC (Erythrocytes = E) to form SRBC or E-rosette by CD2 receptor	Binding with sheep Erythrocytes (E) coated with Ab (A) & Complement (C) to form EAC-rosette due to C3 receptors (CR2) on B cell surface.
CR2 (CD 21) as a receptors for EBV	-	+
Receptors for Fc piece of Ig	-	+
Thymus specific Ag	+	-
Microvilli on surface	-	+
Recognition of Ag by APCs before binding to surface receptors	Required (except in superantigen)	Not required
Function	Lymphokine (lymphotoxin) production which contributes in CMI	Antibody production which contributes in AMI
Lymphoblast transformation (multiplication)		
• Anti-CD3	+	-
• Phytohaemagglutinin	+	-
• Concanavalin A (Con A)	+	-
• Anti-Ig	-	+
• Endotoxin	-	+
• *Staph. aureus* Cowan-I strain	-	+
• EBV	-	+

Table-2: Differences b/w T- cells & B- cells

- **Ratio of CD4 & CD8 cells in healthy person:**
- In normal adults & children CD4 to CD8 ratio is 2:1, it means CD4 constitute 65% & CD8 constitute 35% of total T cells or it means that there are about 2 CD4 cells for every CD8 cell out of total T cells.
- However, in new born infants more CD4 & less CD8 cells. CD4 to CD8 ratio is 3.4-4:1, it means CD4 constitute 75-80% & CD8 constitute 20% of total T cells or it means that there are about 3.4-4 CD4 cells for every CD8 cell out of total T cells.

✪ **Lymphocytic recirculation:**
- There is constant circulation of lymphocytes in the blood, lymph, lymphatic organs & tissues, so produce immune response when Ag enters.
- Lymphocytic complete one cycle of recirculation in about 1-2 days.
- Recirculating lymphocytes can be recruited by lymphoid tissues.
- It is more in T-cells, while B-cells are more sessile (immobile).

✪ **Differences b/w T - cells & B- cells: →Table-2**

✪ **Maturation of lymphocytes:**

a. **T- cell maturation: →Fig.-6**

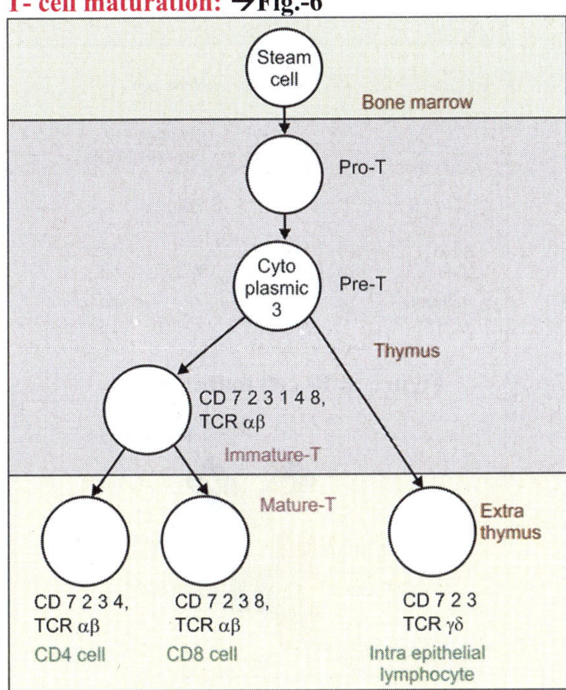

Figure-6: T- cell maturation

- **Pro-T cells:** Lymphocyte precursors **called pro-T cells** are develop in the fetal liver, bone marrow & yolk sac and in to thymus for maturation.
- **Pre-T cells:**
  - o Earliest identifiable lineage is CD7+ pro-T cells, which acquire CD2 on surface & CD3 in cytoplasm on entering thymus and becomes pre-T cells.
  - o TCR (T- Cell Receptor) synthesis also takes place.

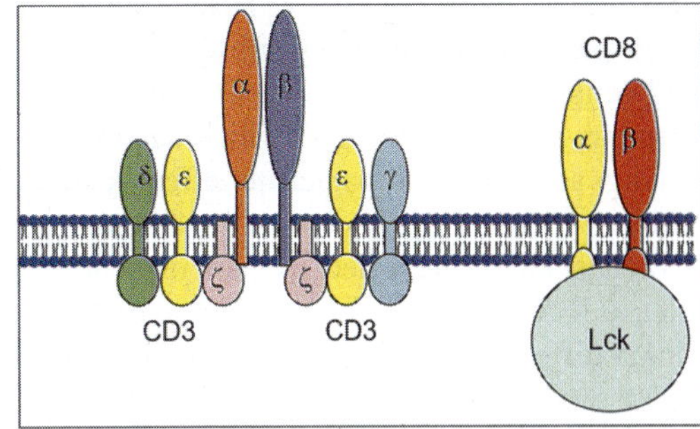

Figure-7: Structure of T- cell receptor (TCR)

- TCR is a glycoprotein chain (**fig.-7**). Occurs in two pairs of chain like αβ or γδ, which differentiate pre-T cells in to two lineages like αβ TCR (present in 95% T cells) or γδ TCR (present in 5% T cells).
- TCR has three domains like extracellular αβ domain (with variable & constant region in α & β chains), transmembrane domain (γε chains & δε chains) & cytoplasmic tail [CD3 molecule plus ζζ (zeta) chains]. Transmembrane domain plus cytoplasmic tail **called CD3 complex** while TCR with CD3 complex **called TCR-CD3 complex**.
- Function of TCR: It is the site for binding of Ag. Following binding between Ag & TCR, a signal is generated that is transmitted through CD3 complex to activate the T cells. It allows the binding of only Ag recognised by APCs (except super antigen which binds directly to lateral side of β chain of TCR without earlier recognition by APCs).
- TCR is an analogous to Ig on B-cell surface. Unlike TCR, Ag binds directly on B cell receptor without earlier recognition by APCs.

o HLA (MHC restriction) synthesis also takes place to respond to foreign Ag.
- CD4→ React to MHC class-II molecule
- CD8→ React to MHC class-I molecule

- **Immature T- cells:** Immature cells in thymus contains CD 7 2 3 1 4 8 in addition to TCR & HLA
- **Mature T- cells:** They form outside the thymus. Immature cells differentiated in to following type mature cells.

1. **Naive cells:** Mostly stimulated by IL-1 of APCs like mature dendritic cells. Mature T-cell before undergoes to immune response (resting T cells) **called Naive cells**, have following functions.
   - Recognition of Ag.
   - Storage of immunological memory.
2. **CD 7 2 3 4 αβ TCR cells: Called CD4 cells:**

* **Common name:**
- Also **called helper (Th) cells** because helps in CMI by producing lymphokines & **called inducer cells** because induce differentiation of B- cells & proliferation of CD8 cells

* **Properties:**
- They also regulate the erythropoiesis.
- Constitute 55-70% of the total T-cells.

- Contains receptors for HIV & HHV-7 adhesion.

* **Subtypes:** Th has following subsets

o <u>Th0 cells</u>:

- Original mature CD 4 cell which secrete the IL-2 having autocrine & paracrine effect **called Th0 cells.**
- IL-2 has autocrine effect & act on Th0 cells to release IFN-γ, IL-4 & further release of IL-2. Later Th0 is differentiated in to effector cells (Th1 & Th2 cells) & memory cells. One new type Th17 also identified recently.

o <u>Th1 cells</u>: Driven by IFN-γ. Th1has following functions

- AMI: Activation of B cells
- CMI: Activation of CD8 cells (by endocytic pathway). Intracellular killing of bacteria (*M tuberculosis, M leprae* etc.) & protozoa by release of free radical like NOx
- Phagocytosis: Activation of macrophages
- DTH: Over activity of T_h1 cells against autoantigens will cause Type 4 delayed-type hypersensitivity like tuberculin reaction
- Autoimmunity: Over activity of T_h1 cells against autoantigens will also cause type 1 diabetes

o <u>Th2 cells</u>: Driven by IL-4. Th2 has following functions

- For B-cell proliferation.
- Also in granuloma formation in infection by *M tuberculosis.*

o <u>Th17 cells</u>: It is the new subtype of Th cell, identified recently. It releases IL-17 which promote inflammation & autoimmune diseases like SLE & RA.

o <u>Memory cells</u>: Concerned with recall phenomenon

3. **CD 7 2 3 8 αβ TCR cells: Called CD8 cells**

* **Common name:**

- Also **called cytotoxic cells,** as they release cytokines which kill target cells like virus infected cells, tumour cell & allograft cells in transplanted tissues by endocytic or cytosolic pathway.
- Also **called suppressor cells** because suppress Ab synthesis by B- cells.

* **Properties:**

- Some cells are converted in to **memory cells**.
- Constitute 25-40% of the total T-cells.

4. **CD 7 2 3 γδ TCR cells: Called intra epithelial lymphocytes.** Exact role is uncertain but may be for

- Immune surveillance on epithelial surface (like intestinal epithelium)
- Defence against intracellular bacteria (Innate immunity)

b. B- cell maturation: →Fig.-8

- **Pro-B cells:** Lymphocyte precursors **called pro-B cells** are develop in the fetal liver and than in bone marrow continuous for life.
- **Pre-B cells:** With synthesis of cytoplasmic IgM pro-B cells are converted in to the pre-B cells.
- **Immature B- cells:** Pre-B cells converted in to immature B- cells in bone marrow with synthesis of IgM & BCR on the cell surface. IgM molecule complexed with transmembrane molecule like Igα & Igβ to form BCR as shown in **fig.-9.** [In mature B cells, after combination of Ag on Fab region of Ig molecule, α & β molecule generate the signal to activate & to differentiate the B cells]

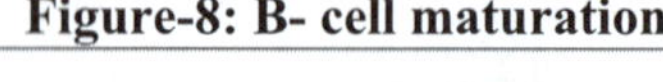

Figure-8: B- cell maturation

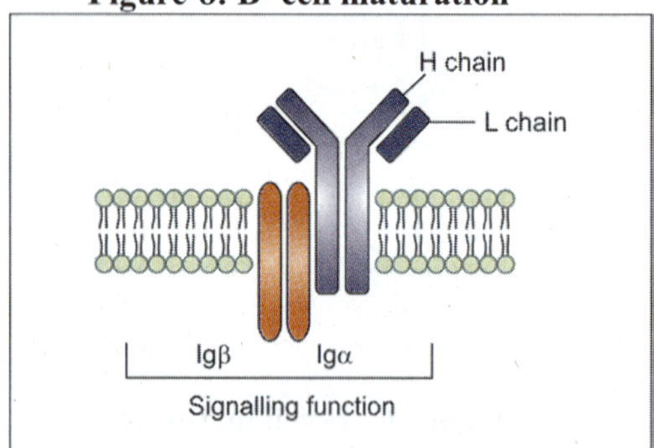

Figure-9: Structure of B- cell receptor (BCR)

- **Mature B- cells:**

o They are forms outside the bone marrow in peripheral organs.

o Immature cells converted in to mature cells with synthesis of other Ig classes like IgG, IgD, IgA and IgE on surface.

o Immature cells differentiated in to following type mature cells.

1. **Naive cells:** Mature B-cell before undergoes to immune response (resting B cells) **called Naive cells,** have following functions.
- Recognition of Ag (APC= Ag Presenting Cell).
- Storage of immunological memory.

2. **Memory cells:**
- On contact with appropriate antigen, the mature B cell undergoes clonal proliferation.
- **Role:** Some activated B cells become long-lived memory cells responsible for the **recall phenomenon** seen on subsequent contact with the same antigen.
- The majority of activated B cells transformed into plasma cells.

3. **Plasma cells:**
- **Role:** Secrete the antibodies & produces the AMI.
- **Shape:** Oval
- **Size:** About twice the size of small lymphocyte
- **Nucleus:** Eccentrically placed oval nucleus containing large blocks of chromatin located peripherally (**called cartwheel appearance**).
- **Cytoplasm**: Is large & contains abundant endoplasmic reticulum & a well developed golgi apparatus.
- **Life span:** Plasma cells are end cells and have a short life span of two or three days.
- **Other Ab producing cells:** plasma cell is the best antibody producing cell, but lymphocytes, lymphoblast and transitional cells may also synthesize the Ab to some extent.

c. B1 (CD5) cell:

- **Properties:**
  - Separate lineages of B cells, which are predominant in fetal & early neonatal life, express the T cell marker CD5 on their surface and have been **called B1 cells**.
  - Their progenitor cells move from the fetal liver to the peritoneal cavity where they multiply. They secrete low affinity polyreactive IgM antibodies, many of them auto-antibodies.
- **Functions:**
  - They are responsible for the T-independent 'natural' IgM antibacterial antibodies which appear in neonates seemingly without antigenic stimulus.
  - CD5+ B cells may be relevant in the causation of autoimmune conditions.

ii. Cells without TCRs: Called null cells or Large Granular Lymphocytes (LGLs)

✪ **Synonym:** Large Granular Lymphocyte (LGL), because contains large azurophilic cytoplasmic granules.

✪ **Properties:**
- About 5 to 10% of total lymphoid cells.
- These are lymphocytes but produces non specific immune response.
- Heterogeneous group of cells with difference in their functional and surface marker features.

✪ **Morphology:**
- **Size:** nearly double the size of the small lymphocytes
- **Nucleus:** indented nuclei
- **Cytoplasm:** abundant cytoplasm containing several azurophilic granules, mitochondria, ribosomes, endoplasmic reticulum & Golgi apparatus.

✪ **Types & function:**

a. Natural Killer (NK) cells:

- **Properties:**
  - They possess spontaneous cytotoxicity (cytotoxic / cytolytic / Type – II hypersensitivity) towards various target cells like malignant & virus infected cells.
  - Their cytotoxicity is not antibody dependent or MHC restricted.
  - Their activity is 'natural' or 'nonimmune' & not required sensitization by prior antigenic contact & therefore they form a part of the innate immunity.
  - They belong to a different lineage from T and B cells and are therefore normally active in 'severe combined immunodeficiency diseases', in which mature T and B cells are absent.
  - They have CD16 & CD56 on their surface.
  - NK cell activity is augmented by interferon & IL-2.
  - Ab induced proliferation does not occurs in NK cells
  - They mature in the bone marrow instead of the thymus unlike other T cells.
  - Their cytoplasm has granules **called azurophilic granules**.

✓ **Note: Azurophilic granules**
- **Meaning: Azure = blue,** as the granules stain bluish in colour by Romanowsky stain
- **Synonym:** Also **called "primary granules"**
- **Contains:** Granules contain proteins such as perforin & proteases enzymes **called granzymes** Granzymes includes serine protease like myeloperoxidase, phospholipase A2, elastase, acid hydrolases, defensins, neutral serine proteases, bactericidal/permeability-increasing protein, lysozyme, cathepsin G, proteinase 3 & proteoglycans.

- **Differences & similarities between NK cells & Tc cells:** Tc cells & NK cells are similar in function. NK cells acts against virus infected cells & tumour cells till Tc cells are activated & carry on the function. However Tc cells are differ from NK cells by many ways as shown in **table-3**
- **Function:** Nk cells bind to the glycoprotein receptors on the surface of autologous as well as allogenic target cells & release several cytolytic factors like

1. Perforin: It is a compliment like substance & resembles the complement component C9, causes trans-membrane pores through which cytotoxic factors such as the TNF (Tumour Necrosis Factor) -β & granzymes enter the cell & destroy it by apoptosis.
2. TNF (Tumour necrosis Factor)
3. Lymphotoxin

Features	NK cells	Tc cells
	Differences	
CD marker	CD16 & CD56	CD3 & CD8
Ab role	Independent	Dependent by endocytic pathway
MHC molecule	MHC restricted	MHC-1
Immune memory	No	Yes
Immunity	Innate	Acquired
	Similarities	
Target cells	Virus infected & tumour cells	
Mechanisms	Perforins, TNF & lymphotoxin	

Table-3: Differences & similarities between NK cells & Tc cells

✓ **Note: Ab role in Tc cells**

- **More details:** **Follow chapter → Immune response (Ir) (section → endocytic pathway)**

b. Antibody dependent cytotoxic cells (ADCCs):

- This type of LGLs possesses surface receptors for the Fc part of Ig. Antigen is attached at Fab region.
- They are capable of killing target cells sensitized with IgG like tumour cells, parasites or graft rejection.
- It is mostly IgG mediate. In certain instances IgE is useful like eosinophilic mediated killing of parasites
- This antibody dependent cellular cytotoxicity is distinct from the action of cytotoxic T cells, which is independent of antibody.

c. Lymphokine activated killer (LAK) cells:

- LAK cells are treated with IL-2, which are cytotoxic to tumor cells without affecting normal cells.
- Used in treatment of some tumors such as renal cell carcinoma.

iii. APCs (Antigen Presenting Cells):

- **Definition:** Any antigen presented to lymphocytes is prior presented & processed by a special type of cells **called APCs**.
- **Types:** Two types like major & minor cells

a. Major cells or professional cells:

1. Dendritic cells:

- **Meaning:** So called because having long membranous cytoplasmic extension like dendrites of neuron.
- **Origin:** From bone marrow
- **Morphology:** → **Fig.-10**
  - Highly pleomorphic
  - Oval/spherical nucleus
  - Small central body and many long niddle-like processes **called dendritic process**
- **Location:** Present in the peripheral blood and in the peripheral lymphoid organs, particularly in the germinal areas of the spleen and lymph nodes.
- **Types of dendritic cells:** Following two types
  - Immature dendritic cells: **Called Langerhans cells.** Present in epidermis & after making contact with Ag releases the cytokines which cause loss of adhesiveness of Langerhans cells & migrate the cells free in blood **called mature dendritic cells**
  - Mature dendritic cells: They are known to stimulate the naïve cells
- **Significances:**
  - They possess MHC class-2 antigens but not Fc or sheep RBC receptors or surface Igs.
  - Dendritic cells are involved in the presentation of antigens to T cells during the primary immune response.
  - They also posses the B7 & CD28 which are required for Th cell activation

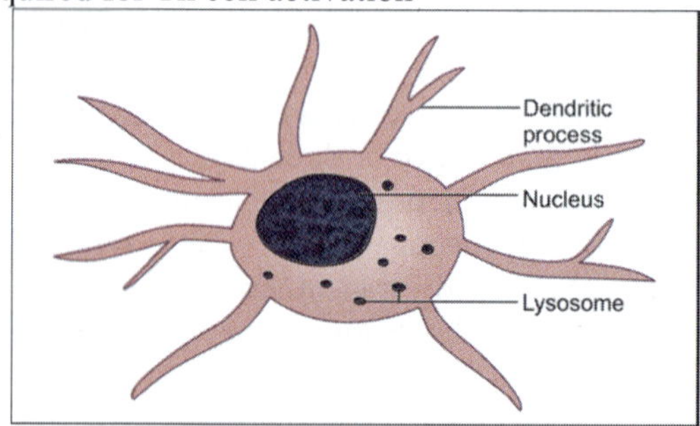

Figure-10: Dendritic cell

2. B-cells: Another antigen presenting cells, particularly during the secondary immune response.

3. Macrophages:

- Any Ag presented to lymphocytes is prior presented & processed by macrophages
- They trap the antigen and provide it in optimal concentration to the lymphocytes.
- It is possible by presence of common surface Ag on both the cells **called MHC-antigen**.
- When macrophage contains different MHC-antigens, it does not participate in Ag processing & presentation to lymphocytes **called MHC-restriction.**
- If too high concentration of antigen is presented, it produces tolerance, and too low concentration may not be immunogenic.

4. Langerhans cells:

- **Location:** In the skin
- **Significances:**
  - Possess features of macrophages & immature dendritic cells.
  - They process & present the Ag that reaches to the dermis.

b. **Minor cells or nonprofessional cells:** It includes
- Fibroblasts (skin)
- Thymic epithelial cells
- Pancreatic beta cells
- Vascular endothelial cells
- Glial cells (brain)
- Thyroid epithelial cells

✪ **Functions of lymphocytes:**

♣ **Types of lymphocytes A/t functions:** Vide supra

♣ **Functions of individual lymphocytes:**

- Naive cells:
- CD4 (CD 7 2 3 4 αβ TCR) cells:
- CD8 (CD 7 2 3 8 αβ TCR) cells:
- Intra epithelial lymphocytes (CD 7 2 3 γδ TCR cells):
- Memory cells
- Plasma cells
- B1 (CD5) cells
- Null cells (LGLs)
- Langerhans cells

} Vide supra

II. Non specific immune system

Reticulo Endothelial (RE) system & RE cells

➢ **Introduction:**
- Phagocytosis is an oldest defence mechanism in animals.
- Originating in protozoa as a combined mechanism for nutrition & defence, along the course of evolution, the phagocyte lost its nutrition function with the development of digestive enzymes.
- In higher organisms it specialized in the removal of foreign particles.

➢ **Definition:** Cells that are responsible for engulfment & digestion of foreign particles, often with the help of Ab & C (complement) **called RE cells** or **phagocytic cell** & this mechanism of defence **called phagocytosis**.

➢ **History:** 1st described by Metchnikoff in 1883

➢ **Types & properties of RE cells:** Two types

A. **Macrophages** (mononuclear cells):

✪ **Subtypes: → Flow chart-2**

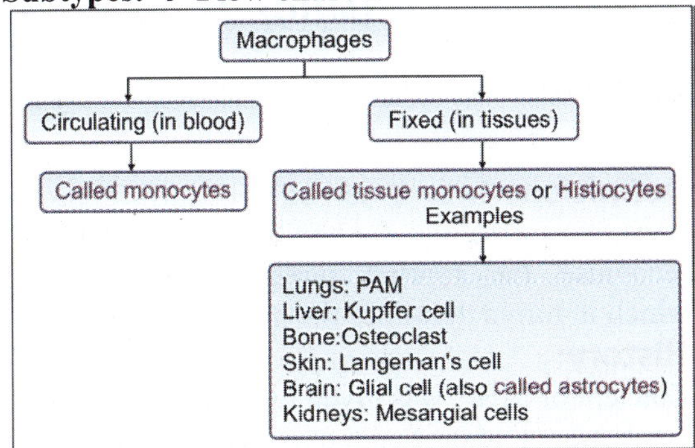

Flow chart-2: Subtypes of macrophages

✪ **Properties of macrophages:**
- Blood macrophages (**called monocytes**) are the largest of the lymphoid cells (12-15μm).
- Tissue macrophages (**called histiocytes**) are larger (15-20μm).
- Monocytes in circulation have an approximate half life of 3 day
- Tissue macrophages survive for months.
- Macrophages are originating from bone marrow from precursor cells & become mature in 6 days.
- Multinucleated cells & epitheloid cells seen in granulomatous inflammatory lesions such as tuberculosis, originate from mononuclear macrophage
- Macrophages may be activated by lymphokines, compliment components or interferon.
- Activated macrophages are not antigen-specific.
- Activated macrophages show morphological and functional changes as compared with unstimulated quiescent macrophages. They are larger, adhere better, spread faster & are more phagocytic.

B. **Microphages (PMNs** = polymorphonuclear cells**):**

✪ **Subtypes: → Flow chart -3**

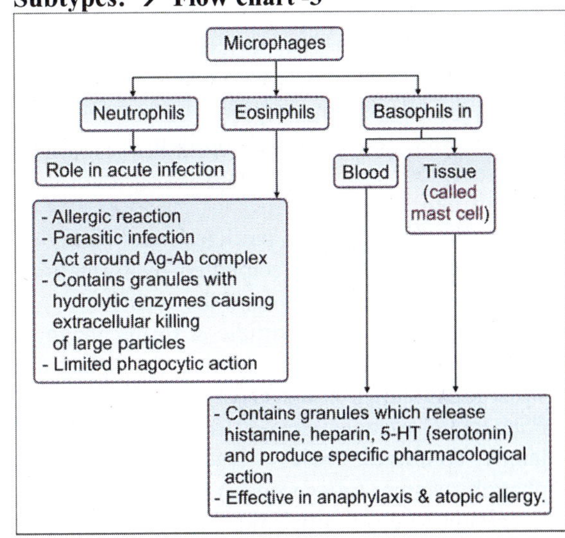

Flow chart-3: Subtypes of microphages

✪ **Properties of microphages:**
- Microphages are originating from bone marrow from precursor cells & become mature & finally released in circulation.
- They are short lived with half life about 2 days & few hours in tissue after penetration.

➢ **Functions:**

i. **Phagocytosis:**

✪ **Definition:** Engulfment & digestion of foreign particles by single cell, often with the help of Ab & C **called phagocytosis**. (**Scavanger cell role**)

✪ **Steps:** Following 5 steps

a. **Opsonisation: →Fig.-11(a)**
- After entry of foreign particles in the body, it combines with opsonin (Factor present in serum).

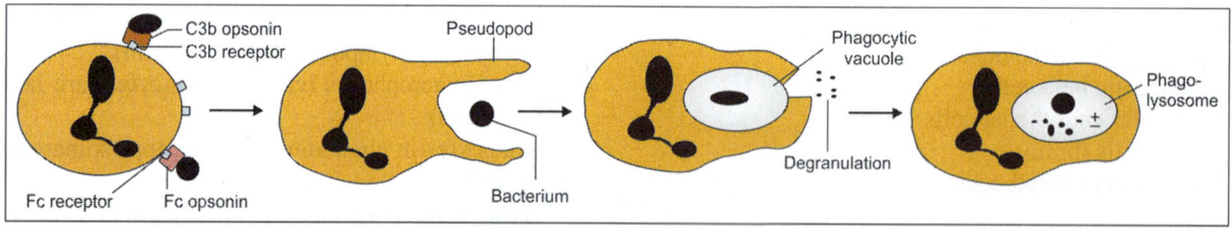

Figure-11: Steps of phagocytosis

- Opsonisation is defined as coating of foreign material or antigens by substance present in serum.
- Types of opsonin:
  - Antibody (Fc opsonin): IgM & IgG act as opsonin from the Ab category. IgM is also 500-1000 times more effective than IgG in opsonisation. IgM & IgG bind with Fc end to the specific opsonin receptors present on the phagocytic cell, so such opsonin **called Fc opsonin** & receptors **called Fc receptors.**
  - Complement: Like C3b & C4b (C-fragments)
  - Fibronectin

b. Attachment: →Fig.-11(a)

- Corresponding receptors for opsonin are present on the surface of phagocytic cells, through which opsonised particle adhere with phagocytic cell.
- Two types of opsonin receptors:
  - Fc receptors: For IgM & IgG opsonin
  - C3b receptors: For C3b opsonin

c. Engulfment:

- After an attachment, particles are ready for engulfment, which is precipitated by formation of pseudopod [**fig.-11(b)**] around the particle.
- Pseudopod engulfs the particle & forms phagocytic vacuole (pseudopod + particle = phagocytic vacuole) as shown in **fig.-11(c)**
- Phagocytic vacuole remains free in cytoplasm & later combines with lysosomes to form phagolysosomes (phagosomes) [**fig.-11(d)]**

d. Secretion or degranulation:

- Secretion of metabolites from preformed stored granule's (e.g. lysosomes) which kills the foreign particle
- There is also new synthesis & secretion of other metabolites like IL-2, TNF, arachnoid acid metabolites (e.g. prostglandins, leukotreins & platelets activating factors) & O_2 metabolites (e.g. Superoxide O_2, H_2O_2, Hypochlorous acid)

e. Killing or degradation: After killing of particles, they are degraded by certain metabolites, which are following 3-types

1. O_2 dependent mechanisms:

- It is bactericidal
- O_2 dependent metabolites are HOCl, HOI, HOBr, OH, O_2, H_2O_2

2. O_2 independent mechanisms:

- It is bactericidal
- O_2 independent metabolites are lysosomal hydrolase, permeability increasing factor, defensins & cationic proteins

3. Nitric oxide mechanisms: It is fungicidal or having anti-parasitic action

ii. Act as APC (Antigen Presenting Cell) & helps in specific immune response: Vide supra

iii. Antitumour activity & graft rejection:

- When stimulated by cytophilic antibodies and certain lymphokines, macrophages become 'armed'.
- Such armed macrophages are capable of antigen-specific cytotoxicity, which is important in anti-tumour activity and graft rejection

iv. M_1 marker:

- Mac 1 is a protein Ag found on mouse macrophages.
- A similar protein on human macrophages has been named the M1 marker.
- This appears closely related to CR3, a cell receptor for C3 components.

v. Release of biologically active substances: Macrophages secrete a number of biologically active substances like

- Hydrolytic enzymes
- Binding proteins(fibronectin , transferrin)
- TNF (cachectin)
- Colony Stimulating Factor(CSF)
- IL-1 (leucocyte activating factor): It acts as an endogenous pyrogen and also induces synthesis of interleukin-2 by T cells.

vi. Functions of microphages: → Flow chart -3

Major Histocompatibility Complex (MHC)

❖ **Synonym:** HLAs (Human Leucocyte Antigens) complex

❖ **Definition:** It is a set of cell surface proteins (receptors) essential for the acquired immunity to recognise the foreign molecules in vertebrate, which in turn determines the histocompatibility.

❖ **History:**

- Concept of MHC was given by Peter Gorer in 1936
- George Snell identified the tissue compatibility upon transplantation & MHC locus (genes), for

which he got Nobel Prize in 1980 along with Baruj Bena cerraf & Jean Dausset.

❖ **Components of MHC:** Two components

A. **MHC antigens** or **MHC molecules** or **HLAs:**

➢ **Definition:** Ag present on leucocytes surface, induce immune response & responsible for allograft rejection **called MHC antigen** or **MHC molecule** or **HLAs**.

➢ **Properties:** MHC antigens are 2 chain glycoprotein molecules anchored on the surface membrane of cells.

➢ **Types:** MHC antigens has following three types

i. **MHC class-I antigens / MHC class-I molecules / HLAs class-I: →Fig.-12(a)**

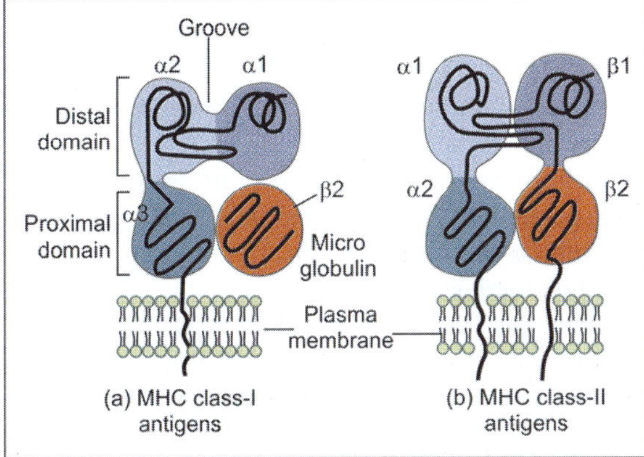

Figure-12: MHC antigens / MHC-molecules / HLAs

- These are consist of a heavy peptide chain (alpha chain) non-covalently linked to a much smaller peptide **called beta 2-microglobulin** (beta chain).
- The beta chain has a constant amino acid sequence & is coded for by a gene on chromosome 15.
- The alpha chain consist of three globoid domains (alpha 1, 2 & 3) which protrude from the cell membrane and a small length of transmembrane C terminals reaching into the cytoplasm.
- The distal domains (alpha 1& 2) have highly variable amino acid sequences and are folded to form a cavity or groove between them.
- Protein antigens processed by macrophages or dendritic cells to form small peptides are bound to this groove for presentation to CD8 T cells.
- The T cell will recognize the antigen only when presented as a complex with MHC class 1 molecule. T cell will not recognize the other antigens which are not presented with MHC class 1 molecule **called MHC restriction**. When so presented, the CD 8 cytotoxic killer cell destroys the target cell (for example virus infected cells).
- MHC class 1 antigens (A, B & C) are **found on the surface of virtually all nucleated cells.**
- They are the principal antigens involved in graft rejection & cell mediated cytolysis.
- Class 1 molecules may function as components of hormone receptors.

ii. **MHC class-II antigens / MHC class-II molecules / HLAs class-II: →Fig.-12(b)**

- These antigens are more restricted in distribution, being **found only on cells of immune system** like macrophages, dendritic cells, activated T cells & particularly on B cells.
- Class 2 antigens are heterodimers, consisting of an alpha and a beta chain.
- Each chain has 2 domains, the proximal domain being the constant region & the distal being the variable region.
- The 2 distal domains (alpha 1, beta 1) constitute the antigen binding site, for recognition by CD 4 lymphocytes, in a fashion similar to the recognition of class 1 antigen peptide complex by CD 8 T cells.
- MHC class 2 molecules are primarily responsible for the graft versus host response and mixed leucocyte reaction (MLR).
- Both class 1 & 2 molecules are members of the immunoglobulin gene superfamily.
- The immune response (Ir) genes which control immunological responses to specific antigens are believed to be situated in the MHC class 2 regions, probably associated with the DR locus.
- Ir genes have been studied extensively in mice and located in the I region of mouse MHC. They code for Ia (I region associated) antigens consisting of 1A and 1E proteins. However, the relevance of Ir genes in human is not clear.

iii. **MHC class-III antigens / MHC class-III molecules / HLAs class-III:**

- These are heterogenous molecules.
- They include complement components linked to the formation of C3 convertases, heat shock proteins and tumor necrosis factors.
- They also display polymorphism.
- The MHC system was originally identified in the context of transplantation, which is an artificial event.
- In the natural state, besides serving as cell surface markers that help infected cells to signal cytotoxic and helper T cells, the enormous polymorphism of the MHC helps maximise protection against microbial infection.
- By increasing the specificity of self-antigens, the MHC prevents microbes with related antigen make up sneaking past host immune defenses by molecular mimicry.
- The primary aim of the MHC may be defense against microbes and not against the graft.
- MHC has been implicated in a number of nonimmunological phenomena such as individual odour, body weight in mice and egg laying in chickens.

➢ **Pleomorphism in HLA system:**
- HLA loci are multiallelic.
- HLA system is very pleomorphic for example at least 24 distinct alleles have been identified at HLA locus A & 50 at B.
- Each allele determines distinct Ag.

B. Genes of MHC or **genes of HLA complex:**

➢ **Definition:** MHC Ag are regulated (encoded) by specific genes **called genes of MHC** or **genes of HLA complex**

➢ **Location:** MHC genes are present on short arm of chromosome-6

➢ **Types of genes:** Similar complex of genes present in different species, with following three different classes of genes **(fig.-13).**

i. Class 1 genes:
- That determines histocompatibility and acceptance or rejection of allografts.
- Compromising A,B & C loci

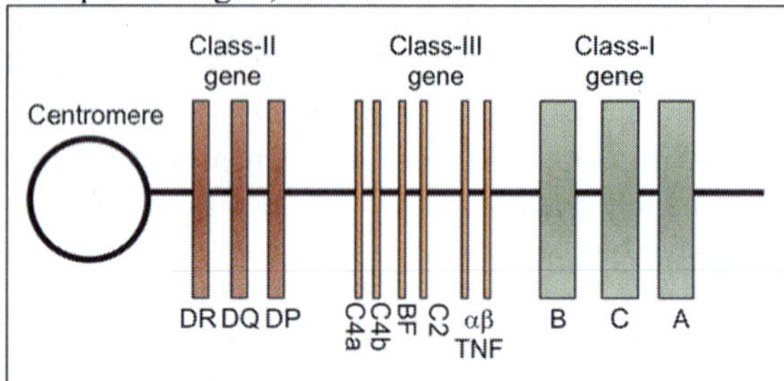

Figure-13: Genes of MHC or genes of HLA complex

ii. Class 2 genes (D region):
- That regulates the immune response.
- Consisting of DR, DQ & DP loci

iii. Class 3 genes (complement region):
- That determines the complement components C2 & C4 of the classical pathway, properdin factor B of the alternative pathway, heat shock proteins & tumor necrosis factors alpha & beta.

❖ HLA typing:

➢ **Definition:** Typing of HLA by using specific monoclonal Ab (antisera) **called HLA typing**.

➢ **Preparation of antisera:** Antisera for HLA typing were obtained principally from multiparous women as they tend to have antibodies to the HLA antigens of their husbands, due to sensitization during pregnancy.

➢ **Typing methods:**

a. Serological method:

✪ **Principle:** based on microcytotoxicity, in which there is complement mediated lysis of peripheral blood lymphocytes with standard set of tying sera.

✪ **Limitation:** It is not possible for HLA DR antigens.

b. Mixed leucocyte reaction and primary lymphocyte typing: For HLA DR antigen.

c. Genetic methods:
- Used in advanced centers.
- Typing methods:

1. Restriction Fragment Length Polymorphism(RFLP)
2. Gene sequence-specific oligonucleotide probe typing.

➢ **Clinical significance:**

a. Organ or tissue transplantation: HLA typing is used primarily for testing compatibility between recipient & potential donors before transplantation.

b. Paternity: It also applications in disputed paternity.

c. Anthropological studies: as the prevalence of HLA types varies widely between different human races and ethnic groups, HLA typing is used in anthropological studies.

d. Association between HLA type and certain diseases:
- An association has been observed between HLA type and certain diseases.
- Such diseases are generally of uncertain origin, associated with immunological abnormalities and exhibit a hereditary tendency.
- For examples

1. Ankylosing spondylitis and HLA-B27
2. Rheumatoid arthritis and HLA-DR4
3. Many autoimmune conditions and HLA-DR3.

❖ **MHC restriction:** →**Vide supra**

Question bank

Essay/Full question

1) Structure & function of immune system

Short notes

1) Lymphoid organs
2) Types & functions of lymphocytes
3) Antigen Presenting Cells (APCs)
4) RE system or RE cells
5) Phagocytosis
6) MHC complex

Short questions for theory/viva questions

1) Write the two example of each primary & secondary lymphoid organs
2) What is thymus dependent area? Write two examples.
3) Comment: Thymus dependent areas will be depleted after thymectomy.
4) What is TCR? or Describe in brief about structure & function of TCR
5) What is BCR? or Describe in brief about structure & function of BCR
6) What is naive cell?
7) Write the functions of following Th (T helper) lymphocytes Th0 cells, Th1 cells, Th2 cells & Th17 cells
8) Write the functions of following immune cells Intra epithelial lymphocytes. NK cells, Astroytes & Dendritic cells
9) What is opsonisation? Write two examples of opsonin.

10) Write two examples of each microphage & macrophage type phagocytic cells
11) What is MHC restriction?

MCQs for chapter review

Classification of immune system

Lymphoid system

1) **Lymphoreticular system includes-** (PGI, June-08)
(a) T-cells (b) B-cells (c) Platelets (d) Macrophages (e) Neutrophils
2) **All are peripheral lymphoid organs except** (PGI, May-10, 13)
(a) Lymph nodes (b) Spleen (c) Mucosa associated lymphoid tissue (d) Thymus
3) **Apart from B cell and T cell, there is a 3rd distinct type of lymphocyte. This is** (PGI -02)
(a) MHC cell (b) NK cell (c) Macrophage (d) Neutrophil (e) Microglia
4) **Which of the following cell is known as Large Granular Lymphocytes (LGLs)**
(a) Plasma cell (b) NK cell (c) T cell (d) K cell
5) **Common between B and T cells-** (PGI, June-07, Nov-13)
(a) Origin from same lineage (b) Site differentiation (c) Antigenic marker (d) Both humoral and cellular immunity (e) Further differentiation seen
6) **B cells maturation take place in-** (PGI -98)
(a) Thymus (b) Lymph nodes (c) Bone marrow (d) Spleen
7) **T cells mature in-**
(a) Peyer's patch (b) Lymph nodes (c) Thymus (d) Bursa of fabricus
8) **Neonatal thymectomy leads to** (AI-02)
(a) Decreased size of germinal centre (b) Decreased size of paracortical areas (c) Increased antibody production by B cells (d) Increased bone marrow production of lymphocytes
9) **T cell dependent region is**
(a) Cortical follicles of lymph node (b) Medullary cords (c) Mantle layer (d) Paracortical area
10) **Apart from T & B lymphocytes, the other class of lymphocyte is** (PGI -02)
(a) Macrophages (b) Astrocytes (c) NK cells (d) Langerhans cells
11) **Type of receptors present on T cells are** (AI-93)
(a) IgA (b) IgG (c) Prostaglandin (d) CD4
12) **Which of the following is pan T lymphocytes marker**
(a) CD2 (b) CD3 (c) CD19 (d) CD25
13) **Group B cell lymphocyte belongs to**
(a) CD19 (b) CD69 (c) CD59 (d) CD68
14) **The following are true except for T lymphocytes except**
(a) Constitute about 70-80% of circulating pool of lymphocytes (b) Release macrophage inhibition factor (c) Secrete specific antibodies (d) Release lymphotoxin
15) **Normal % of CD4 cells in a new born** (JIPMER 11)
(a) 35% of T cells (b) 45% of T cells (c) 55% of T cells (d) 65% of T cells
16) **Which cells cause rosette formation with sheep RBCs**
(a) T cells (b) NK cells (c) Monocytes (d) B cells
17) **EAC rosette formation is the property of following immune cells**
(a) T cells (b) B cells (c) Macrophages (d) All of the above
18) **What enhances multiplication of T cells in culture**
(a) Phytohaemagglutinin (b) Chemotactic factor (c) Leukotrienes (d) Prostaglandin
19) **T cells are identified by**
(a) Rosette formation with sheep RBCs (b) Immunoglobulin on their surface (c) EAC rosette with sheep erythrocytes (d) Have filamentous projection on their surface
20) **Helper cells belong to** (AI-93, 96)
(a) T cells (b) Macrophages (c) B cells (d) Monocytes
21) **All of the following are functions of CD4 helper cells, except** (AI-09)
(a) Immunological memory (b) Produce immunoglobulin (c) Activate macrophages (d) Activate cytotoxic cells
22) **Cellular immunity is induced by**
(a) NK cells (b) Dendritic cells (c) Th1 cells (d) Th2 cells
23) **NK cells are-**
(a) Activated macrophages (b) Ab activated T cells (c) Null cells activated by complement (d) Derived from plasma cells (e) Independent of antibody
24) **Regarding NK cells, false statement is-** (AI-01)
(a) It is activated by IL-2 (b) Express CD3 receptor (c) It is a variant of large lymphocytes (d) There is antibody induced proliferation of NK cells
25) **NK cells activity is enhanced by**
(a) IL-1 (b) TNF (c) IL-2 (d) TGP-β
26) **All are true regarding NK cells** (PGI, Nov-10)
(a) CD 16 positive (b) CD 56 positive (c) Secrete compliment like substance (d) Important role in viral infected cell
27) **Perforins are produced by** (PGI-01)
(a) Cytotoxic T cells (b) Suppressor T cells (c) Memory helper T cells (d) Plasma cells (e) NK cells
28) **NK cells provide immunity against**
(a) Virus (b) Bacteria (c) Fungus (d) *Chlamydia*
29) **NK cells & cytotoxic T cells are differentiated by**
(a) Interferon reduces NK cells activity (b) Antibody specificity (c) Receptor for IgG (d) Presence in spleen
30) **Killer cells & helper cells are part of** (PGI, Nov-97)
(a) B cells (b) T cells (c) Monocytes (d) Macrophages
31) **Most potent stimulator of naïve T cells -** (AII-11, AIIMS, Nov-08, 05)
(a) Mature dendritic cells (b) Pigment producing cells (c) Macrophages (d) B cells
32) **All these are antigen presenting cells (APCs) except-** (PGI-02)
(a) T cells (b) B cells (c) Fibroblast (d) Dendritic cells (e) Langerhans cells
33) **Most efficient antigen presenting cell in the skin -**
(a) Dendritic cell (b) Macrophage (c) Langerhans cell (d) Kupffer cell

Reticulo Endothelial (RE) system & RE cells

34) **All are mononuclear-macrophages except**
(a) Histiocytes (b) Microglia (c) Kupffer cells (d) B cells
35) **The function common to neutrophils, monocytes & macrophages is**
(a) Immune response (b) Phagocytosis (c) Liberation of histamine (d) Destruction of old lymphocytes
36) **The process increasing the ability for phagocytosis of foreign bodies by body is called**
(a) Cross reactivity (b) Opsonisation (c) Immune tolerance (d) Immune surveillance
37) **Opsonisation occurs due to all except** (PGI -99)
(a) Endotoxin (b) Complement (c) IgM (d) IgD
38) **Opsonisation take place through**
(a) C3a (b) C3b (c) C5a (d) C5b
39) **Bacteria coated with complement and Ig; phagocytosis is enhanced by** (AIIMS, Nov-11)
(a) Receptor mediate endocytosis (b) Pseudopod formation (c) Myeloperoxidase mediated destruction (d) C3b-Fc mediated destruction

Haematopoiesis

40) **Mononuclear phagocyte are produced by**
(a) Thymus (b) Spleen (c) Bone marrow (d) Liver

Major Histocompatibility Complex (MHC)

41) **HLA-I is present on**
(a) All nucleated cells (b) Only on cells of immune system (c) Only on B-cells (d) Only on T-cells

42) **MHC II are presented by** (PGI, May -13, Nov-10)
(a) Macrophages (b) Dendritic cells (c) lymphocytes (d) Eosinophils (e) Platelets

43) **Cell type which lacks HLA antigen is** (AIIMS, May-05)
(a) Monocyte (b) Thrombocyte (c) Neutrophil (d) Red blood cell

44) **Peptide binding site on class I MHC molecules for presenting processed antigens to CD8 T cells is formed by** (AI –10)
(a) Proximal domain of α subunits (b) Distal domain of α subunit (c) Proximal domains of α and β subunit (d) Distal domains of α & β subunit

45) **T helper cells recognises** (PGI -02)
(a) MHC class I (b) MHC class II (c) Processed peptides (d) Surface Ig

46) **True about MHC**
(a) Present on chromosome 4 (b) Class II comprises A, B C loci (c) Class III has complement (d) Class I is involved in mixed leucocyte reaction

47) **HLA complex is on chromosome**
(a) 6 (b) 7 (c) 8 (d) 4

48) **Gene components of HLA class I includes**
(a) A, B, C (b) DR (c) DQ (d) DP

49) **MHC class III genes encode-** (AI -03)
(a) Complement component C3 (b) Tumour necrosis factor (c) Interleukin 2 (d) Beta 2 microglobulin

50) **HLA III gene codes in graft rejection-**
(a) Immunological reaction in graft rejection (b) Complement (c) Graft versus host reaction (d) Immunoglobulin

51) **The role played by Major Histocompatibility Complex-1 and 2 is to** (AIIMS -03)
(a) Transduce the signal to T cells following antigen recognition (b) Mediate the immunogenic class switching (c) Present antigens for recognition by T cell antigen receptors (d) Enhance the secretion of cytokines

Answers of MCQs & explanation

1) **(a), (b), (d) & (e)**
- Lymphoreticular system includes lymphoid system & RE system. T-cells & B-cells are parts of lymphoid system while macrophages & neutrophils are parts of RE system.

2) **(d)**
- Thymus is central lymphoid organ

3) **(b)**
4) **(b)**
} Follow section, **Specific immune system / lymphoid system (components →lymphoid cell → Cells without TCRs)** for the explanation

5) **(a) & (e)**
- B cells & T cells has same origin from bone marrow. In early foetal life cells are derived from liver & yolk sac.
- B cells differentiation/maturation takes place in bone marrow while of T cells in thymus
- Bothe have different antigenic markers
- B cells are for humoral and T cells are for cellular immunity

6) **(c)**
7) **(c)**
} Both B & T cells are originated from bone marrow. B cells differentiation/maturation takes place in bone marrow, while of T cells in thymus

8) **(b)**
9) **(d)**
} Follow section, **thymus (Clinical significances →Post-thymectomy effect)** for explanation

10) **(c) & (d)**
- Macrophages& astrocytes (glial cell of brain) are RE cells
- NK cells are lymphocytes but without TCR
- Langerhans cells are one type of lymphocytes present in skin & acts like APCs

11) **(d)**
- T cells carry CD markers, TCR & MHC receptors on the surface. CD4 present on helper/inducer cells.

12) **(b)**
13) **(a)**
} Follow, **table-1** for the explanation

14) **(b) & (c)**
- T cells releases macrophage activating factors not the macrophage inhibition factor.
- For explanation of other options follow **table-2**

15) **All options are wrong**
- CD4 count in new born in 75-80% of total T cells.

16) **(a)**
17) **(b)**
18) **(a)**
19) **(a)**
} Both T & B cells can make rosette with SRBC, but T cell binds directly while B cell bind with the cell which is coated with Ab & C (complement). Follow, **table-2** for more explanation

20) **(a)**
- CD4 T cells are known as helper cell also **called inducer cells**.
- CD8 T cells are known as cytotoxic cell also **called suppressor cells**.

21) **(b)**
22) **(c)**
} Follow section, **T cell maturation (CD 7 2 3 4 αβ TCR cells)** for the explanation

23) **(d)**
24) **(d)**
25) **(c)**
26) **(a), (b), (c) & (d)**
27) **(e)**
28) **(a)**
} Follow section, **Natural killer (NK)** cells for the explanation.

29) **(b)**
- Follow **table-3** for explanation

30) **(b)**
- Both Killer cells & helper cells are T cell but killer cells are without TCR while helper cells are with TCR

31) **(a)**
32) **(a) & (c)**
} Follow section, **APCs (Antigen Presenting Cells)** for the explanation

33) **(c)**
- From the all given option Langerhans cell is the only APC located in skin

34) **(b)**
- Follow section, **phagocytosis (flow chart-2)** for the explanation

35) **(b)**
- Follow section, **phagocytosis (flow chart-2 & flow chart-3)** for the explanation

36) **(b)**
37) **(a) & (d)**
38) **(b)**
} Follow section, **phagocytosis (opsonisation)** for the explanation

39) **(d)**
- C3b & Fc are the opsonins. Required for the opsonisation in phagocytosis

40) **(c)**
- Mononuclear phagocytes are **called macrophages** which are present in blood (**called monocytes**) & in tissues (**called histiocytes**) as shown in **flow chart-2** & all they are originated from bone marrow as shown in **fig.-1**

41) **(a)**
42) **(a), (b) (c) & (e)**
43) **(d)**
} MHC I are present on nucleated cell (Not on RBCs, as it is non nucleated) while MHC II are present immune cells, which does not include platelets

44) **(b)**
- Protein antigens processed by macrophages or dendritic cells to form small peptides are bound to the groove between distal domains like α1 & α2 of α subunit

45) **(b)**
- T helper cells are CD4 cells which recognise the MHC class II molecule while MHC class I molecule is recognise by cytotoxic T cells which are CD8 cells

46) (c)

- MHC genes are present on short arm of chromosome 6
- Class II comprises DR, DQ & DP loci
- Class III determines the complement components C2 & C4 of the classical pathway, properdin factor B of the alternative pathway, heat shock proteins & tumor necrosis factors alpha & beta
- Mixed leucocyte reaction is determined by DR gene of MHC class II gene.

47) (a)

- MHC genes are present on short arm of chromosome 6

48) (a)

- Follow **fig.-13** for the explanation

49) (b)
50) (b)

} Class III gene determines the complement components C2 & C4 of the classical pathway, properdin factor B of the alternative pathway, heat shock proteins & tumour necrosis factors alpha & beta.

51) (c)

- After the entry of antigen, it recognise according to MHC molecule. Those processed by MHC-I can presented to CD8 cells & those processed by MHC-II can presented to CD4 cells.

25 Immune response (Ir)

Learning heading & subheadings

Introduction

❖ **Definition:** Specific reactivity of host to the antigenic stimulation **called immune response.**

❖ **Types:** → **Flow chart-1**

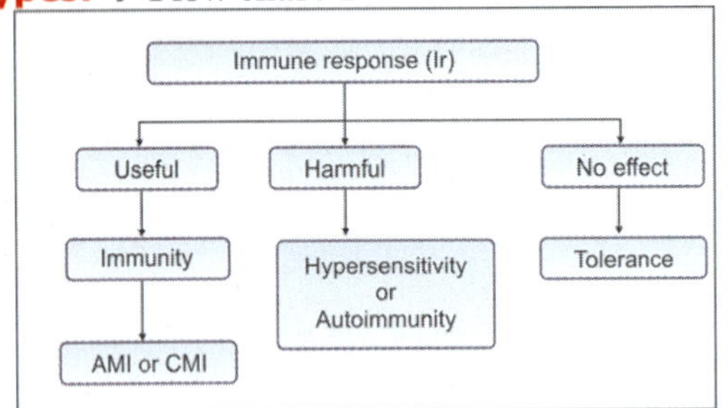

Flow chart-1: Types of Ir

❖ **AMI &CMI:** Both may work together, but in opposite way. One may be more active than other.

AMI

❖ **Full form:** Antibody Mediated Immunity

❖ **Synonym:** Humoral Immunity (HI)

❖ **Meaning:** Humoral from **humor = body fluid** (old term), as Ab present free in blood & other body fluid.

❖ **Definition:** Resistance exhibited by host towards the injury produce by microorganism and/or their product by production of Ab from plasma cell (B cell) **called AMI**.

❖ **Origin:** Ab is originated from plasma cells (B cells), however its required participation by other immune cells.

❖ **Clinical significances:** Participates in

1. Infection by extra cellular pathogens like bacteria, fungus etc.
2. Type 1, 2 & 3 (Immediate) hypersensitivity reactions
3. Auto immune disorders

❖ **Stages of production of Ab:** Contain three stages

1. **Afferent limb:** Entry of Ag, its distribution, fate in the tissues & its contact with appropriate immunocompetent cells.
2. **Central limb:** Processing of Ag by cells and the control of the antibody forming process.
3. **Efferent limb:** Secretion of antibody, its distribution in tissues & body fluids & manifestations due to its effects.

❖ **Pattern of production of Ab:**

1. **Lag Phase:** Stage immediately after Ag stimulation
2. **Log Phase:** Raise antibody titre.
3. **Plateau or steady phase:** Equilibrium between Ab synthesis & catabolism.
4. **Decline phase:** Increase catabolism of Ab than production.

❖ **Antigenic dose:** Two types

a. **Priming dose:** Initial antigenic stimulation **called priming dose.** It is Sensitising dose.

b. **Booster dose:** Subsequent antigenic stimulation **called booster dose.** Subsequent dose is more effective.

❖ **Primary (fig.-1)& secondary Ir (fig.-2):**

✪ **Definitions:**

- **Primary Ir:** Ab response to initial antigenic (**Priming dose**) stimulation **called primary Ir**
- **Secondary Ir:** Ab response to subsequent antigenic (**booster dose**) stimulation **called secondary Ir**

- **Negative phase:** When Ag is injected in to animals already carrying the Ab, temporary fall in Ab concentration due to combination of Ab with newly injected Ag **called negative phase**.

✪ **Differences b/w primary & secondary Ir: → Table-1**

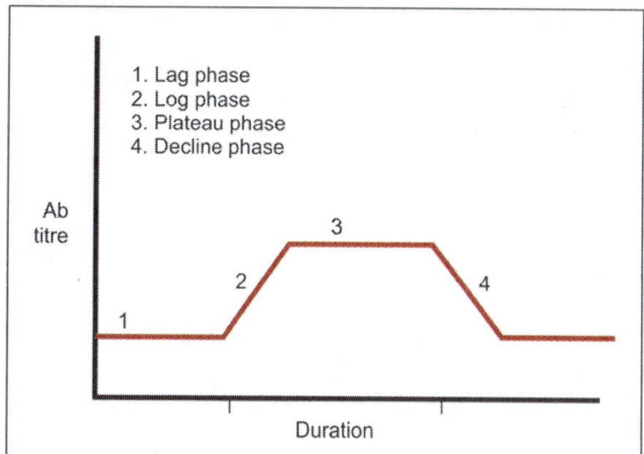

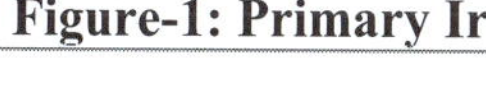
Figure-1: Primary Ir

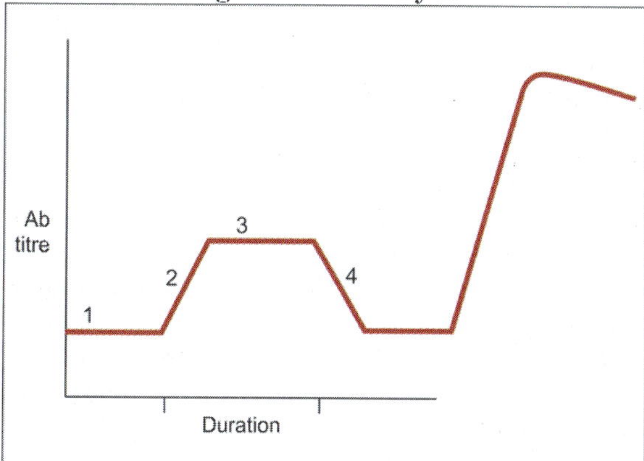

Figure-2: Secondary Ir

Primary Ir	Secondary Ir
Slow	Prompt
Sluggish	Powerful
Short lived	Long lived
Lag phase: Long (4-10 days) & slow Ab production	Lag phase: Short (1-3 days) & rapid Ab production
Low titre of Ab	High titre of Ab
Ab lasting for short duration	Ab lasting for log duration
IgM type of Ab appear 1st following injuries or in primary infection	IgG type of Ab appear late or in secondary infection
Low affinity of Ab	High affinity of Ab
Involve memory B cell: Few B- cells are converted in to Ab producing cell, majority of cell converted in to memory cell.	Involve Plasma cell: B-cells are converted in to Ab producing cells (plasma cells).
Adjuvant is needed	Adjuvant not needed
No negative phase	Negative phase occur:

Table-1: Differences b/w primary & secondary Ir

❖ Fate of antigens:

➢ **Effective factors:**

✪ **Physical and biochemical nature of Ag:**

- Proteins Ag: Eliminated in few days to weeks
- Polysaccharide: Slowly metabolised, persist for months or weeks. E. g. Pneumococcal polysaccharide Ag persist for 20 years in human after single injection

✪ **Dose of Ag:** Whether induced primarily or secondarily

✪ **Route of entry of Ag:**

- **Introduced by IV route:**
  - Rapidly localized in the spleen, liver, bone marrow kidney and lungs.
  - Broken down by RE cells & excreted in urine.
  - About 70 – 80 % eliminated in one or two days.
- **Introduced by subcutaneous route:**
  - Mainly localized in the draining lymph nodes only small amounts being found in the spleen

➢ **Elimination:** The antigens are removed from circulation in two phase:

✪ **Non-immune phase:** By phagocytosis

✪ **Immune phase:** Destruction by Ab.

❖ Induction of AMI (Production of antibodies):

➢ **Participation by cells:** Three types of cells are involved in Ab production:

1. Antigen Presenting Cells (APCs): Follow chapter → Structure and functions of immune system.
2. T lymphocytes.
3. B lymphocytes.

➢ **Role of MHC molecules:**

- Capture & recognition of Ag by APCs in accordance to MHC molecules & their presentation to T cells.
- Ag with MHC- II molecules are presented to CD4 (Helper-Th) cells while Ag with MHC- I molecules are presented to CD8 (Cytotoxic-Tc) cells
- B cells also carrying Ig & MHC-II molecules, can present Ag to T-cells particularly during secondary Ir.

➢ **Steps:** Depends on type's of antigen

a. **T-cell dependent (TD) Ag: Called endocytic pathway** as shown in **fig.-3**

- Entry of Ag
- Ag + APC complex formation in accordance to MHC –II molecules.
- Such complex is presented to the naïve cells of Th-cells (CD4) as they carry TCR
  - Formation of Ag + APC + Th/CD4 (TCR) complex
  - APC also secretes IL-1, which stimulate the naïve cells of CD4 type to differentiate in to effector cells like Th0 cells. Th0 cells liberate IL-2.
  - IL-2 has autocrine effect & act on Th0 cells to release IFN-γ, IL-4 & further release of IL-2. Later

Th0 is differentiated in to effector cells (Th1 & Th2 cells) & memory cells.

- Th1 can activate the B cells. It also capable to activate the Tc (CD8) cells for CMI by endocytic pathway.
- Th2 cells release IL-4, IL-5, IL-6 & other cytokines acts as BCGF (B Cell Growth Factors) & BCDF (B Cell Differentiation Factors) & activates the B-cells
- Now, B- cells are differentiated in to memory cells & plasma cell.
- Memory cells responsible for recall phenomenon & plasma cell secrete Ab which kills the Ag by opsonisation (phagocytosis), complement activation, neutralisation or by antibody dependent cellular cytotoxicity (ADCCs).

b. T-cell independent (TI) Ag:

- Ag directly presented to B-cells, which stimulate the mature & immature B cells to produce limited classes of antibodies (IgG3 & IgM). No memory cells formation.
- More details of TI Ag: **Follow chapter → Antigen (Ag)**

❖ Factors influencing antibody production:

i. Genetic factors:

- Ir is under controlled of genes **called Ir genes**.
- Individual may be of two types:

1. **Responder:** The individual who respond to antigenic stimulation **called responder.**
2. **Non responder:** The individual who not respond to antigenic stimulation **called non responder**.

ii. Age:

- Embryos is immunologically immature
- Immunity starts with development & differention of lymphoid organs & cells.
- During the embryonic life, if any foreign Ag comes in contact with the developing lymphoid cells, it leads to **tolerance**.
- During the embryonic life, if any self Ag comes in contact with the developing lymphoid cells, which is released by cellular breakdown, leads to **non-antigenicity of self antigens**.
- Infant is protected by maternal antibodies up to 3-6 months.
- Immunity develops as the infant grows, mostly after 3-6 months
- Full immunity developed for Ig G at 5-7 years & at 10-15 years for IgA.

iii. Nutrition: Deficiencies of vitamins, amino acids, proteins & fat reduced THE both, CMI & AMI.

iv. Routes of administration:

- AMI is better by parenteral route than oral or nasal route.
- Large particles like bacteria, RBCs are more antigenic when introduced by parenteral route.
- IgA produced by oral or nasal route.
- IgE produced by inhalation of pollen.
- Protein injection in to mesenteric vein or intrathymically induce tolerance.

v. Site of administration: HBV vaccine is more effective following injection in deltoid than gluteal injection, because of paucity of APC in gluteal region, delaying the presentation of Ag to T & B cells.

vi. Size & dose of Ag:

- Very small dose of Ag is ineffective.
- Ag is effective above certain level, further increase in dose also increase the Ir.
- However beyond certain level Ag is ineffective & instead of increasing the Ir, it swamp & cause paralysis of the immune system **called immunological paralysis by Felton** (1949).

vii. Multiple antigens: When more than two Ags are administered simultaneously, antibody response by one may affect the other **called antigenic competition**.

- **Two bacterial vaccines:** Like typhoid & cholera are given in mixed form, the antibody response has no effect on each other.
- **Two toxoid vaccines:** Like diphtheria & tetanus are given together with one in excess, Ir to other is inhibited
- **Triple antigen (DPT):**
  - Ab response to diphtheria & tetanus toxoid is potentiated by *B. pertusis* vaccine
  - When DPT given to a patient had earlier immunisation with diphtheria toxoid, Ir to tetanus & pertusis is decreased.

viii. Adjuvants: **Follow chapter → Immunising agents & National immunisation schedule**

ix. Immunosuppressive agents: Use of Immunosuppressive agents may suppress the Ir as mentioned below

1. **Radiation:** X- rays
2. **Alkylating agents:** Cyclophosphamide & nitrogen mustard
3. **Anti-inflammatory:** Corticosteroids which may
   - Reduce the lymphocytes from circulation & lymphoid organs
   - Reduces the release of histamine → anti-inflammatory effect
   - Inhibit the induction of DTH.
4. **Anti metabolites:**

- **Mechanism:** they inhibit the synthesis of DNA, RNA or both & thus inhibit the cell division & differention which required for CMI & AMI.
- **Commonly used anti metabolites:**
  - Folic acid antagonist: Methotrexate
  - Purine analogues: 6-mercaptopurine & azathioprine
  - Uracil analogues: 5-fluorouracil
  - Cytosine analogues: Cytosine arabinoside
  - Alkylating agent: Cyclophosphamide

5. **Cyclosporine:** Immunosuppressive drug derived from fungus *Tolypocladium inflatum*. It inhibits the Th cell activity. Other related drug is rapamycin.
6. **ALS (Anti-Lymphocyte Serum):**

- **Properties:**
  - It is an antiserum against lymphocyte.
  - It acts against lymphocyte of circulation, not against the lymphocytes in lymphoid organs.
- **Others similar anti-serum:**
  - ALG: Anti-Lymphocyte Globulin
  - ATS: Anti-Thymocyte Serum
  - ATG: Anti- Thymocyte Globulin

x. **Effect of Ab:**

- Ab production is inhibited by passive administration of homologous Ab. It act by following ways
  - Feedback mechanisms.
  - Prevention of Ag presentation to immunocompetent cells
- This concept used in treatment of many clinical conditions
  - Anti Rh Ab injection in Rh-Ve women with Rh +Ve child.
  - Passive immunisation in diphtheria & tetanus.
- IV administration of Ig has immunomodulatory effect, which used in treatment of following diseases.
  - Autoimmune haemolytic anaemia
  - Thrombocytopenia

❖ **Detection of AMI:**

1. **Non-specific (in general) test:** Detection of Ab to several antigens present in host by agglutination test, ELISA, Precipitation test, CFT & Neutralisation test
2. **Specific test:** Detection of Ab to particular Ag present in host. E. g Ab to diphtheria Ag (toxin) is detected by Schick test (in vivo & in vitro type)

❖ **Limitation of AMI:** AMI is effective only against the antigens/microbes which are extracellular, free in circulation or bound on cell surface. It is not effective against antigens/microbes which are intracellular.

CMI

❖ **Full form:** Cell Mediated Immunity

❖ **Definition:** Resistance exhibited by host towards the injury produce by microorganism and/or their product by production of lymphokines (cytokines) from sensitised T-cell **called CMI**.

❖ **Origin:** CMI is originated mostly from Tc cells (Type of T lymphocytes), but also dependent on other immune cells

❖ **Clinical significances:** Participates in

1. Infection by intra cellular pathogens like **bacteria** (tuberculosis, leprosy, listeriosis, brucellosis,), **virus** (measles, mumps), **fungus** (histoplasmosis, cocccidioidomysosis, blastomycosis) & **parasite** (trypanosomiasis, leishmaniasis).
2. Type 4 (delayed type) hypersensitivity
3. Auto immune disorders like thyroiditis, encephalomyelitis etc,
4. Immunology in transplantation & graft versus host reaction.
5. Immunology in malignancy.
6. Immunological surveillance.

❖ **Induction of CMI:**

➢ **Effective factors:**
- Depends on type of antigenic stimulation
- Only T cell dependent antigens induce CMI.
- Best developed by intracellular pathogens.
- Live vaccine is highly stimulating
- Killed vaccine is not very effective, but effective if contains **Freund type adjuvant**.

➢ **Role of MHC molecules & mechanisms:** CMI is induced by two types of pathways (signals) as follows

A. **Cytosolic pathway: → Fig.-3**

- Entry of Ag
- Ag + APC complex formation in accordance to MHC –I molecules.
- Such complex is presented to the naïve cells of cytotoxic T(Tc)/CD8 - cells as they carry TCR
  - Formation of Ag + APC + Tc/CD8 (TCR) complex
  - Naïve cells differention in to cytotoxic T (Tc) cells & memory T cells. Tc cells undergo blast transformation & clonal proliferation.
  - Tc cells release cytokines like
    1. Perforins that makes pores in the target cell membrane (contains intracellular microbes or antigens) like virus infected cell, tumour cell & allograft cell in transplanted tissues, release its all contents & destroy the cell.
    2. Serine protease: It induce cell death by apoptosis

    Memory cells are useful for recall phenomenon
  - Tc effect is similar to NK cells. NK cells acts against virus infected cells & tumour cells till Tc cells are activated & carry on the function.
  - Cytokines may contribute in the effects of LAK cells

B. **Endocytic pathway: → Fig.-3**

- Entry of Ag
- Ag + APC complex formation in accordance to MHC II molecules.
- Such complex is presented to the naïve cells of Th-cells (CD4) as they carry TCR
  - Formation of Ag + APC + Th/CD4 (TCR) complex

- APC also secretes IL-1, which stimulate the naïve cells of CD4 type to differentiate in to effector cells like Th0 cells. Th0 cells liberate IL-2.
- IL-2 has autocrine effect & act on Th0 cells to release IFN-γ, IL-4 & further release of IL-2. Later Th0 is differentiated in to effector cells (Th1 & Th2 cells) & memory cells.
- Th1 can activate the Tc (CD8) cells for CMI by endocytic pathway. It also capable to activate the B cells.
- Tc cells undergo blast transformation, clonal proliferation & differention in to cytotoxic T (Tc) cells & memory T cells.
- Tc cells release cytokines like perforins & Serine protease. Later steps are same as described in cytosolic pathway

❖ Cytokines:

➢ **Definitions:**

- **Cytokines:** Biologically active substance released by activated immune cells.
- **Lymhokines**: Biologically active substance released by activated T- lymphocytes. It also **called lymphotoxin**
- **Monokines:** Biologically active substance released by monocytes and macrophages
- **Interleukins (IL):** Biologically active substance released by leucocytes.
- **Chemokines:** Included in chemotaxis & other leucocyte behavior

➢ **Properties:**

✪ **Biochemistry:** Soluble polypeptide (protein)

✪ **Hormonal properties:**

- **Unlike hormones:**
  - Not secreted by endocrine gland but secreted by widely distributed cells like lymphocytes, macrophages, platelets & fibroblasts.
  - Hormones are independent in actions while cytokines are work together & showing interaction with each other
- **Like hormones:** They are like hormones because
  - Active at femtomolar (10^{-15}M) concentration
  - Acts on cell present at distant sites.

✪ **Actions:** Different types of effect

1. **Autocrine:** Cytokine acts on the cell that secretes it.
2. **Paracrine:** Cytokine acts on the surrounding cells.
3. **Endocrine effect:** Acts on cell present at distant sites
4. **Pleotrophic effects:** Multiple effects by same cytokine on various cells.
5. **Redudancy effects:** Same effects by different cytokine on same cell.

✪ **Interactions:** Cytokines are showing various types interactions as mentioned below

1. **Synergism:** Two cytokines may augment each other's actions.
2. **Antagonism:** Two cytokines may inhibit each other's actions.
3. **Cascade action:** It is the serial action by multiple cytokines, where one cytokine act on a target cell to release cytokine which act on subsequent cell and so on.

➢ **Types of cytokines:**

A. Interleukin (IL):

i. IL-1:

- **Nomenclature**: Initially it was described as LAF (Leucocyte Activating Factor) & BAF (B-cell Activating Factor), but in 1979 it renamed as IL-I.
- **Two subset**: Alpha and Beta
- **Secretion:** By APCs.
- **Stimulation for production:** By Ag, toxins, injury & inflammation,
- **Inhibition of production:** By cyclosporins, corticosteiods & prostaglandins (PG).
- **Functions:**

1. **Sensitisation of Th cells:**
   - Sensitise the Th cells to liberate IL-2 & other cytokines.
   - IL-2 & other cytokines acts as BCGF (B Cell Growth Factors) & BCDF (B cell differentiation Factors) which are activates & differentiate the B-cells in to memory cells & plasma cell.
   - Memory cells responsible for recall phenomenon & plasma cell secrete Ab which kills the Ag.
2. **Sensitisation of Tc cells:**
   - Sensitise the Tc cells to liberate cytokines that destroy the Ag (target cells).
   - Differentiate some T- cells in to memory cells
3. **Chemotaxis:** Helps neutrophils in chemotaxis
4. **Phagocytosis:** Promotes phagocytosis
5. **Others:** Promotes metabolic, physiological, inflammatory & haematological effect by acting on bone marrow, epithelial, synovial cells, osteoclasts, fibroblasts, hepatocytes, vascular endothelial cells & other target cells.
6. **Role as pyrogen:** Crucial in promoting fever and so **called pyrogen**.
7. **Role in infections:** With the help of TNF causes hematological changes in septicemias, shock and bacterial meningitis.

- **Use:** Beneficial effect in immunocompromised host.

ii. IL-2:

- **Secretion:** By activated Th0-cells (type of CD4 lymphocytes).
- **Functions:**
  - Modulates the immune response
  - Major activator of T and B Lymphocytes
  - Stimulates cytotoxic T cells and NK cells
- **Use:** It converts LGLs in to LAK cells, which can destroy NK-resistant tumour cells. This property used in treatment of tumour cells

iii. **IL-3:**

- **Secretion:** By activated T-cell.
- **Function:** Stimulates multilineage cells of the haematopoietic system, hence **called multi-colony stimulating factor (multi-CSF)**

iv. **IL-4:**

- **Secretion:** By Th2-cells (type of CD4 lymphocytes.
- **Functions:**

- Acts as BCGF & BCDF
- Also act as TCGF (T Cell Growth Factor) & mast cells growth factor.
- Increase the action of Tc cells
- Role in atopic hypersensitivity, as it augment IgE synthesis.

v. **IL-5:**

- **Secretion:** By Th2-cells
- **Functions:**

- Proliferation of activated B Lymphocytes.
- Induce maturation of eosinophils

vi. **IL-6:**

- **Secretion:** By Th2-cells, B-cells, macrophages & fibroblasts
- **Functions:**

- Differentiation of B Lymphocytes.
- Induces the production of Ig.
- Stimulates the hepatocytes, nerve cells & hematopoietic cells
- Inflammatory response mediator in host defence against infections.
- Pyrogen

vii. **Other IL (IL-7 to IL-13 & IL-17): →Table-2**

B. **CSF (Colony Stimulating Factor): →Table-2**

C. **TNF(Tumour Necrosis Factor): →Table-2**

D. **IFN (Interferon): Follow chapter →Virus-host interactions (viral infections).**

E. **Other cytokines: →Table-2**

➢ **Therapeutic uses of cytokines:** IL1, 2, 3 and CSF are used in

- Inflammatory diseases
- Infections
- Immunocompromised host
- Autoimmune diseases (IL17)
- Haematopoietic dysfunction
- Neoplastic diseases

➢ **Regulation of cytokines:**

a. **Exogenous stimuli:** Like antigens & mitogens

b. **Endogenous stimuli:**

1. **Hormones:** Corticosteroids, endorphins
2. Lipo-oxygenase & cyclo-oxygenase pathways

c. **Regulation of each other by +Ve & -Ve feedback mechanisms**

❖ **Detection of CMI:** Two types of test

Cytokines	Sources	Functions
Other IL		
IL-7	Spleen, marrow stromal cells	BCGF & TCGF
IL-8	Macrophages, other cells	Neutrophil chemotactic factor
IL-9	Th cells	TCGF & proliferation.
IL-10	Th2 cells, B cells, macrophages	Inhibit IFN production & mononuclear cell function
IL-11	Marrow stromal cells	Induce acute phase proteins
IL-12	T cells	Activate NK cells
IL-13	Th2 cell	Inhibit mononuclear cell function
IL-17	Th17 cell	Pro inflammatory marker
CSF (Colony Stimulating Factor)		
GM (Granulocyte, Mononuclear) -CSF	T cell, macrophages, fibroblasts	TCGF & macrophage growth stimulation
G (Granulocyte) - CSF	Fibroblasts, endothelium	Granulocyte growth stimulation
M (Mononuclear) -CSF	Fibroblasts, endothelium	Macrophage growth stimulation
TNF(Tumour Necrosis Factor): Induce haemorrhagic necrosis in certain tumour hence the name		
TNF-α	Macrophages & monocytes	Tumour cytotoxicity, wasting syndrome (**cachexia, so called cachectin**), lipolysis, acute phase proteins, antiviral & anti-parasitic effect, phagocytic cell activation, pyrogen, endotoxic shock
TNF-β	T cells	Induce other cytokines & other action are similar to TNF-α
Other cytokines		
TGF-β	T cell & B cells	Transform the fibroblast, hence **called TGF-β** (Transforming Growth Factor Beta), promote wound healing, down regulation of haematological & immunological process
LIF	T cells	LIF (Leukemia Inhibitory Factor) helps in stem cell proliferation & eosinophil chemotaxis

Table-2: Sources & functions of cytokines

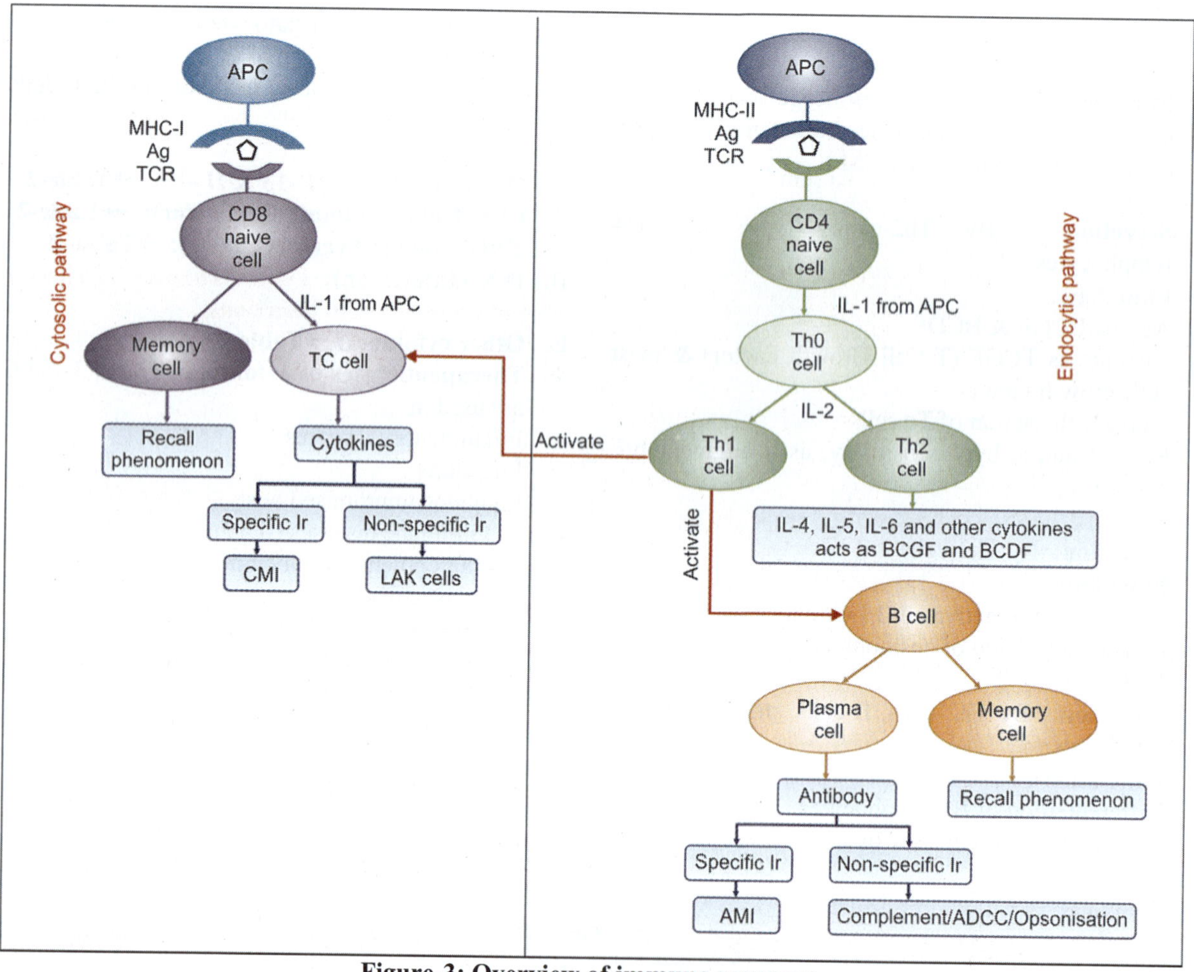

Figure-3: Overview of immune response

a. **In vivo test:**

1. **Skin test:**

- **Principle:** Based on DTH
- **Example:** Tuberculin test, Lepromin test

b. **In vitro tests:**

1. **Lymphocyte transformation test:**

- **Principle:** Transformation of culture sensitised T-Lymphocyte on contact with Ag.

2. **Target cell destruction test:**

- **Principle:** destruction of target cell of culture by T-lymphocyte sensitised against them.

3. **Migration inhibiting factor test:**

- **Principle:** Macrophages packed in capillary tube when placed in a tissue culture medium in a chamber; they migrate out, spread over the glass walls of the chamber & form lacy fan like appearance. If macrophages are from sensitised guinea pig, addition of Ag to the culture chamber will inhibit the migration.
- **Use:** Human peripheral leucocytes packed in capillary tube & placed in a tissue culture medium in a chamber. Add the specific Ag which inhibits the migration of leucocytes.
- **Result:** By comparing with control test, a semi-quantitative assessment of migration inhibition is possible.

4. **Detection of T cells by SRBC rosette test**
5. **Immunofluorescence test:**

❖ Passive transfer of CMI or adoptive immunity:

➢ **Definitions:**

- **Adoptive immunity:** Passive transfer of CMI achieved by administration of viable immunological competent lymphocytes **called adoptive immunity**.
- **Transfer factor (TF):** Instead of whole immunological competent lymphocytes only it's extract is used for administration **called transfer factor.**

➢ **Properties of TF:**

- **Non-antigenic**
- **Biochemistry:** Polypeptide-polynucleotide
- **Dialysable**
- **Low Molecular Weight (LMW):** 2000-4000
- **Resistant to:** Trypsin, DNAase, RNAase, freeze thawing (stable for several years at -20^{0}C)

- **Sensitive:** To heat at 56^0C in 30 minutes
- **Potency:** Highly potent, 0.1ml dose is effective

➢ **Limitation of TF:**

- It does not induce AMI
- It induces only systemic CMI but not the local CMI.

➢ **Clinical significance of TF:**

1. In treatment of some disease like Lepromatous Leprosy (LL), tuberculosis, mucocutaneous candidiasis
2. In treatment of malignant malenoma & other cancer.
3. In treatment of autoimmune diseases like SLE, RA & some other diseases like sarcoidosis, multiple sclerosis
4. To restore the immunity in patients with T-cell deficiency (Wiskott-Aldrich syndrome).

Interconnections of Ir

➢ **Specific immune response:** Like AMI & CMI cannot work individually because

- Both required initial participation by APCs & Th cells
- Th cells which are part of CMI, secrete the IL-2 which allows the proliferation & differentiation of B cells in to plasma cells (Ab producing cells) & memory cells

➢ **Non specific immune response:** Like complement system, phagocytosis, antibody dependent cellular cytotoxicity & LAK cells are also inter connected with specific immune response as follows

- Complement system: It acts after formation of Ag – Ab complex which required Ab synthesis by AMI
- Phagocytosis: Opsonisation in phagocytosis is dependent to IgM & IgG of AMI
- Antibody dependent cellular cytotoxicity: It uses antibodies as a receptors to identify & to kill the target cells
- LAK cells: Required lymphokines from CMI

➢ **Overview of immune response: → Fig.-3**

Immunological tolerance

❖ **Synonym:** Immunological unresponsiveness

❖ **Definition:** Inability of immune system to mount an immune response against particular Ag when administered subsequently **called immunological tolerance**.

❖ **Historical concept:**

- In 1949, **Burnet & Fenner** suggested that, if substance comes in contact with immature immunological system during embryonic life, it will be considered as self-antigen & there is no Ir.
- Hence all **body Ags** are considered as self -Ags & there is no Ir & all **foreign Ags** comes in contact with immature immunological system during embryonic life are also considered as self -Ags & there is no Ir.
- This was proved experimentally in 1953 by **Medawar & colleagues** by using two strains of syngenic mice as described below.

- Skin graft from strain of mice (B) in applied on another strain (A), it is rejected. When cells from strain-B are injected in strain-A in embryonic life, strain-A will not reject the graft in later part of life.
- Concept of self-Ag is enlarged by contact with foreign Ag during embryonic life **called specific immunological tolerance**.

❖ **Types:**

a. According to quantity:

1. Total
2. Partial

b. According to duration:

1. Short lived: example
   - Tolerance induced by using immunosuppressive agents in adult is temporary.
   - Tolerance to bovine albumin in rabbit is overcome by injection of human albumin
2. Long lived: example
   - Tolerance by living substances like rubella & cyto megalo virus (CMV) infection, in which persistent viremia reduce Ab production **called persistent tolerant infection**

❖ **Effective factors:** Induction, degree & duration of tolerance depends on following factors.

a. Species of animal: More common in rabbits & mice than chickens & guinea pigs

b. Immonocompetence of host: It is very difficult to induce tolerance in host with high immonocompetence. Tolerance is induced temporary by using immunosuppressive agents.

c. Nature of Ag:

- Soluble Ag & haptens are more tolerogenic than particulate Ag.
- Tolerogenicity of Ag is modified by certain procedures.
  - **Heat:** Heat aggregated human Igs are more immunogenic, while disaggregated Igs are tolerogenic.
  - **Centrifugation:** Centrifugation of serum proteins at high speed separate the tolerogenic supernatant & immunogenic sediment

d. Dose of Ag:

- Larger dose is required, also further increase in dose increase the duration.
- Types of tolerance according to dose:
  - **High dose**: High zone tolerance like immunological paralysis by Felton.

- **Low dose:** Low zone tolerance
- **Intermediate dose:** No tolerance, but induce immunity.

e. Route of Ag administration:

- Certain Ags are immunogenic in guinea pigs by intradermal route & tolerogenic by IV or oral route.
- Tolerance is induced best by the route which equilibrated the Ag between intra & extra vascular compartment.

❖ **Mechanisms:** Following are the possible ways for tolerance.

1. **Contact of Ag in embryonic life:** Vide supra
2. **Afferent mechanisms:** Contact of Ag to immune cell is interfered
3. **Efferent mechanisms:** Ab produced is inhibited or neutralised or blocked.
4. **Central mechanisms (Helplessness of B cell):** elimination of Th will prevent the activation of B cell.
5. **Split tolerance:** Tolerance to either AMI or CMI but not to both. E.g. in guinea pig DTH to tuberculin Ag is blocked without interference to Ab production.
6. **Lack of genes:** Which are required for development of Ir

❖ **Artificial induction of tolerance:** Following are the possible ways to induce tolerance artificially.

1. Administration of antisera or Ab.
2. Cytotoxic drugs
3. Surgical ablation.

Theories of Ir

❖ **Introduction:** Numbers of theories have been proposed as described below, but none of them is satisfactory

❖ **Theories:**

A. Instructive theory: According to this, Immuno Competent Cell (ICC) can synthesise Ab of any specificity. Ag encounters the ICC & instructs it to produce the complementary Ab.

i. Direct template theory:

- According to this theory Ag (epitope) enters in to the cell & act as template against which Ab molecules are synthesised by cell.
- Such Ab are complementary to Ag (epitope)

ii. Indirect template theory:

- According to this theory not the Ag (epitope) but it's genocopy (indirect template) enters in to the cell & Ab molecules are synthesised by cell.
- It makes the genetic changes in cell & transmitted to progeny cells.
- **Advantage:** It explains the specificity, secondary Ir & non antigenicity to self
- **Disadvantages:** Becomes challenging with advance molecular biology

B. Selective theory: According to this theory, selective synthesise of Ab by ICC on antigenic stimulation.

i. Natural selection theory:

- **History:** Proposed by Jerne in 1955
- **Synonym:** Jerne's theory
- **Hypothesis:**
  - According to this theory, numbers of Abs are synthesised during the embryonic life.
  - This Abs acts as receptors & combines with complementary Ag.
  - This complex settles in cell & stimulates the cell to produce large numbers of Abs.
- **Drawback:** It is not accepted because it not explains the immunological memory.

ii. Clonal selection theory: →**Figure-4**

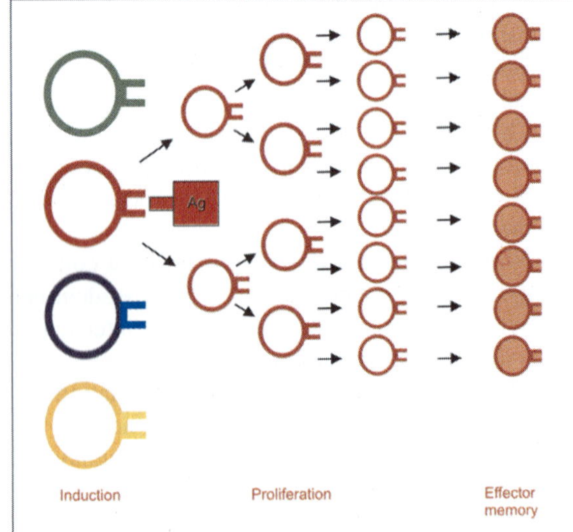

Figure-4: Clonal selection model

- **History:** Proposed by Burnet in 1957
- **Hypothesis:**
  - According to this theory numbers of ICC were synthesised during embryonic life by somatic mutation.
  - The cells that react with self antigens are eliminated & **called forbidden clones**.
  - Their persistence & development in later life by mutation leads to autoimmune process.
  - ICC will recognise & combine with Ag & undergoes the proliferation to produce Ab.
  - Some of the progeny cell acts as memory cell.
- **Advantage:** It is accepted than other theories
- **Drawback:** Not explains the all features of Ir.

C. Side chain theory:

- Proposed by Ehrlich in 1900

- According to this theory cell have side chain (receptors) for assimilation of nutrients.
- Sometimes complementary Ag enters & combines with such side chain leading to interference in absorption of nutrients.
- By compensatory mechanisms cell start to overproduce same receptors which are circulate as Ab.
- **Drawback:** It is not accepted because it not explains the secondary Ir, tolerance & autoimmunity.

Regulation of Ir

❖ Jerne's network hypothesis:

- **Theory:**
  - It explains the mechanism of Ab response
  - The variable region of an immunoglobulin molecule carrying the antigen combining site is different in different antibodies
  - The distinct aminoacid sequence at antigen combing site (paratope) and the adjacent parts of the variable regions are termed as idiotype
  - Produce antiidotypic antibodies
  - Forms a idiotype network
  - The above process controls the amount of antibodies
- **Nobel Prize:** The above theory was given by Niels K. Jerne & he was awarded with Nobel Prize of Medicine in 1984.

❖ Genetic basis:

- Individual has capacity to produce 10^8 different Abs.
- Each Ab required separate gene.
- Discovery of split-gene theory, demolished the **'one gene-one protein'** concept.
- It has important implication in biology & immunology.
- **Nobel Prize:** The above theory was discovered by Susumu Tonegawa & he was awarded with Nobel Prize of Medicine in 1987.

Question bank

Case study

1) A 40 year male has chronic cough & cavitary lesion in the lungs. His sputum is positive for AFB. Identify the clinical conditions & answer the following
a) Which type of immunity required to this patient to fight against this infection.
b) Write the clinical significance of immunity, which patient required in given case.
c) How you diagnose the immunity, which patient required in given case.
d) Describe in general about the steps/mechanisms of induction of required immunity of given case.

Essay/Full question

1) Immune response (Ir)

Short notes

1) AMI
2) Factors influencing the antibody production
3) CMI
4) Cytokines

Short questions for theory/viva questions

1) What is priming dose & booster dose of antigen?
2) What is antigenic competition?
3) Comment: Cytokines are like hormones.
4) Comment: All the immunes responses are interconnected
5) What is adoptive immunity?
6) What is transfer factor?

MCQs for chapter review

AMI

1) Cells involved in humoral immunity:
(a) B cells (b) T cells (c) Helper cells (d) Dendritic cells

2) First immunoglobulin to appear following infection
(a) IgG (b) IgM (c) IgA (d) IgE

3) Primary immune response is mediated by – (PGI-94)
(a) IgE (b) IgM (c) IgA (d) IgD

4) Secondary immune response is mediated by –
(a) IgG (b) IgA (c) IgE (d) IgM

5) True about secondary immune response is– (PGI-98)
(a) Long latent period (b) Usually of low titre (c) Antibodies appear in short time (d) Persist for long

6) Possible source of "second signal" to a B cell bound by specific antigen include (PGI -81)
(a) EB virus (b) Endotoxin (c) Antigen specific T cells (d) Plasma cells

CMI

7) Which is concerned with cell mediated immunity: (AI -98)
(a) B lymphocytes (b) T lymphocytes (c) Eosinophils (d) Monocytes

8) CMI is seen in (PGI-05)
(a) Histoplasmosis (b) Leprosy (c) Tetanus (d) Measles

9) Adoptive immunity is by (PGI, May-10)
(a) Infection (b) Injection of antibodies (c) Injection of lymphocytes (d) Immunisation

10) Cell mediated immunity is transferred by
(a) Antibody (b) Transfer factor (c) Interferon (d) Toxoid

11) When transfer factor is given as treatment result in:
(a) Natural active immunity (b) Artificial active immunity (c) Artificial passive immunity (d) Adoptive immunity

12) True about cytokines is (AIIMS -97)
(a) It is always a polypeptide (b) It acts on protein target (c) It takes part in intrinsic enzymatic reactions (d) Chemotactic

13) IL-1 produces (AI -02)
(a) T lymphocytes activation (b) Delayed wound healing (c) Increased pain perception (d) Decreased PMN release from bone marrow

14) Interleukin I primarily act on
(a) T lymphocytes (b) B lymphocytes (c) Neutrophils (d) Macrophages

15) IL-1 is produced by (PGI-00)
(a) Macrophages (b) Helper T lymphocytes (c) B cells (d) Cytotoxic T cells

16) **IL-2 is produced by** (AIIMS, Feb-97, AI-00, 97)
(a) CD4 lymphocytes (b) CD8 cells (c) Macrophages (d) Neutrophils

17) **Cachectin is produced by**
(a) Neutrophils (b) Eosinophils (c) Macrophages (d) Basophils

18) **IL-7 is produced by**
(a) Macrophages (b) B cells (c) T cells (d) Dendritic cells (e) Stromal cells

19) **T cells functions are assessed by** (AIIMS -92)
(a) Phagocytic index (b) T cell count (c) Migration inhibition test (d) Immunoglobulin index

20) **Which is not pyrogenic**
(a) IL-1 (b) TNF-α (c) IL-4 (d) IL-6

21) **Fever is caused by**
(a) IL-3 (b) IL-6 (c) IL-5 (d) IL-9

Immunological tolerance

22) **Specific immunological unresponsiveness is called tolerance. Which one of the following statements best describes immunological tolerance.**
(a) Immunological maturity of the host does not play a major role (b) It occurs only with polysaccharide antigens (c) It is related to the concentration of the antibody (d) It is prolonged by administration of immunosuppressive drugs

Answers of MCQs & explanation

1) **(a)**
- Follow section, **AMI (origin)** for explanation.

2) **(b)**
3) **(b)**
4) **(a)**
5) **(c) & (d)**

} Follow section, **AMI (table-1)** for explanation

6) **(c)**
- In AMI T (Th) cells participation required. Follow section, **AMI (induction of AMI/Production of antibodies → steps)** for explanation.

7) **(b)**
- Follow section, **CMI (origin)** for explanation.

8) **(a), (b) & (d)**
- Follow section, **CMI (clinical significances)** for explanation.

9) **(c)**
10) **(b)**
11) **(d)**

} Follow section, **CMI (Passive transfer of CMI or adoptive immunity → definitions)** for explanation.

12) **(a)**
- Cytokines are soluble polypeptides (proteins)

13) **(a)**
14) **(a)**
15) **(a)**

} Follow section, **CMI (Cytokines→ IL-1)** for explanation

16) **(a)**
- Follow section, **CMI (Cytokines→ IL-2)** for explanation.

17) **(c)**
18) **(e)**

} Follow section, **CMI (Table-2)** for explanation.

19) **(c)**
- Follow section, **CMI (detection of CMI)** for explanation.

20) **(c)**
21) **(b)**

} IL-1, TNF-α & IL-6 are pyrogens & they are known to induce fever

22) **(d)**
- Follow section, **immunological tolerance (types→ according to duration)** for explanation.

26 Hypersensitivity

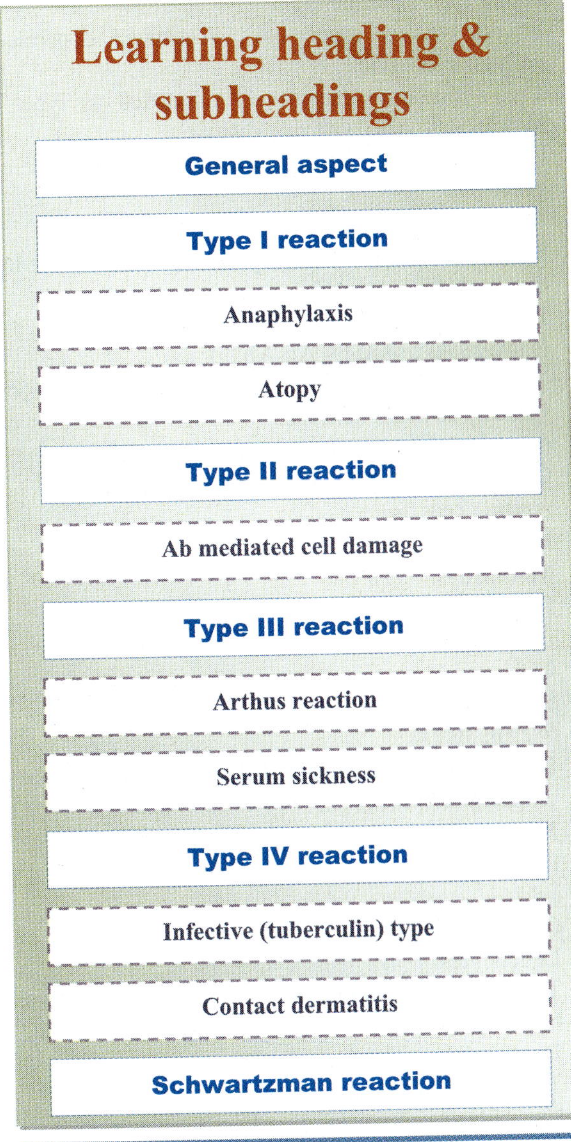

Learning heading & subheadings
General aspect
Type I reaction
Anaphylaxis
Atopy
Type II reaction
Ab mediated cell damage
Type III reaction
Arthus reaction
Serum sickness
Type IV reaction
Infective (tuberculin) type
Contact dermatitis
Schwartzman reaction

General aspect

❖ Definitions:

a. **Hypersensitivity:** Excessive or exaggerated immune response in sensitised host due to contact with particular Ag leading to tissue damage, disease or even death **called hypersensitivity**.

b. **Allergy:**
- Word used by Von Pirquet & it is most confusing
- Sometimes it used to refer the alter state of reactivity to antigen which includes both protective (immunity) & harmful (hypersensitivity & autoimmunity) immune response
- Sometimes it used only injurious immune response (hypersensitivity & autoimmunity)
- Most commonly used as a synonym of hypersensitivity (no autoimmunity).
- Sometimes it used to refer to only one type of hypersensitivity namely **atopy**.

c. **Allergen:** A substances capable of causing an allergic or hypersensitivity reaction.

d. **Antigenic dose:** Two types
1. **Priming or sensitising dose:** Initial antigenic stimulation **called priming** or **sensitising dose.**
2. **Booster or shocking dose:** Subsequent antigenic stimulation **called booster dose** or **shocking dose.** Subsequent dose is more effective, because it cause all manifestation of hypersensitivity.

e. **Humoral amplification system:** Thc pathology & clinical outcome of hypersensitivity is influenced by immune & non-immune body mechanisms like complement (C), fibrinolytic system, kininogenic system, inflammation & coagulation **called humoral amplification system.**

❖ Classification:

I. **According to time required by sensitised host to respond to the shocking dose of antigen:**

➢ **Types:** Two major types like immediate & delayed

A. **Immediate**

✪ **Definition:**
- Start in few minutes to few hours
- B cell or Ab mediated
- Induced by hapten or Ag by any route
- Passive transfer is possible with serum
- Desensitisation is easy, but short lived

✪ **Subtypes:**
i. **Anaphylaxis**
ii. **Atopy**
iii. **Ab-mediated cell damage**
iv. **Arthus reaction**
v. **Serum sickness**

B. **Delayed**

✪ **Definition:**
- Start in 24 hours, reaches peak in 48 -72 hrs.
- T cell mediated. No circulating Ab.
- Induced by hapten or Ag or by Freund's adjuvant by intradermal route or by skin contact.
- Passive transfer is not possible by serum but by Transfer Factor (TF).
- Desensitisation is difficult, but long lived

✪ **Subtypes:**
i. **Infection or tuberculin type**
ii. **Contact dermatitis type**

➢ **Differences between immediate & delayed type of hypersensitivity: →Table-1**

Features	Immediate	Delayed
Appearance	Rapid	Slow
Duration	Short	Longer
Induction	By Ag / Hapten by any route	By Ag / Hapten by ID route or by skin contact or by Freund's adjuvant
Mediators	Ab mediated	Cell mediated
Passive transfer	Possible by serum	Rarely by Transfer factor
Desensiti-sation	Easy & transient	Difficult but long lasting

Table-1: Differences between immediate & delayed type of hypersensitivity

II. Coombs and Gel's classification (1963):

➢ **Types:** Following are the major types

A. Type I (anaphylactic, IgE or reagin dependent hypersensitivity):

✪ **Properties:** Antibodies (cytotropic IgE) are fixed on surface of tissue cells in sensitised individual. The antigen combines with cell fixed antibody, leading to release of pharmacologically active substances (vasoactive amines) which produce the clinical reaction.

✪ **Clinical syndromes & mediators:**

i. **Anaphylaxis:**

- **Examples of diseases:** Occurs following exposure of allergens like honey bee bite etc.
- **Mediators:**
  - IgE fixed with tissue basophils (mast cells) & blood basophils (Free IgE is not useful)
  - Histamine & pharmacological agents.

ii. **Atopy**

- **Examples of diseases:**
  - Allergic asthma
  - Allergic conjunctivitis
  - Allergic rhinitis (Hay Fever)
  - Dermatitis
- **Mediators:**
  - Overproduction of IgE

B. Type II (cytotoxic or cytolytic hypersensitivity, IgG or rarely IgM dependent hypersensitivity):

✪ **Properties:**

- This type of reaction is initiated by IgG or rarely IgM/IgE.
- Ab react either with the cell surface or tissue antigen.
- Ab produces cell/tissue damage in presence of complement or mononuclear cells.
- Sometimes stimulates the cell (Type-V) or inhibit the cell.
- Type 2 reactions are intermediate between hypersensitivity and autoimmunity.

✪ **Clinical syndromes & mediators:**

i. **Ab mediated damage**

- **Examples of diseases:** The antibody could be
  - Lytic for cell: Thrombocytopenia, agranulocytosis (agrnulosis or granulopenia), autoimmune haemolytic anaemia etc.
  - Supportive to other cell: Antibody dependent cellular cytotoxicity
  - Cell stimulatory (separately classified as type V hypersensitivity): Grave's disease
  - Cell inhibitory: Pernicious anaemia, myasthenia gravis etc.
- **Mediators:** Autoantibodies

C. Type III (immune complex or toxic complex disease):

✪ **Properties:**

- Damage is caused by Ag-Ab complex.
- These may precipitate in & around the small blood vessels, causing damages to cell secondarily or on membranes interfering with their functions.

✪ **Clinical syndromes & mediators:**

i. **Arthus reaction**

- **Examples of diseases:** Like farmer's lung
- **Mediators:**
  - IgG
  - IgM
  - C
  - Leucocytes

ii. **Serum sickness**

- **Examples of diseases:** Like post streptococcal glomerulonephritis
- **Mediators:**
  - IgG
  - IgM
  - C
  - Leucocytes

D. Type IV (delayed or cell mediated hypersensitivity):

✪ **Properties:**

- This is cell mediated response.
- The antigen activates specifically sensitised T4 & T8 cells, leading to the secretion of lymphokines with fluid & phagocytes accumulation.

✪ **Clinical syndromes & mediators:**

i. **Infection or tuberculin type**

- **Examples of diseases:** Infective, autoimmune conditions & allograft rejection
- **Mediators:**
  - T cells
  - Lymphokines
  - Macrophages

ii. **Contact dermatitis type**

- **Examples of diseases:** Dermatitis due to contact with allergens
- **Mediators:**
  - T cells
  - Lymphokines
  - Macrophages

E. Type V hypersensitivity (stimulatory type):

Features	Type I	Type II	Type III	Type IV
Type	Immediate	Immediate	Immediate	Delayed
Response	Humoral	Humoral	Humoral	Cellular
Period between onset of symptoms & Ag contact	2-30 minutes	5-8 hours	2-8 hours	24-72 hours
Antigen	Soluble	Cell surface bound	Soluble	Soluble or cell surface bound
Mediators	IgE, histamine & pharmacological agents	IgG IgM C or phagocytic cells	IgG IgM C or Leucocytes	T cells Lymphokines Macrophages
Desensitisation	Easy but short lasting	Easy but short lasting	Easy but short lasting	Difficult but long lasting
Syndrome	Anaphylaxis Atopy	Ab-mediated cell damage	Arthus reaction Serum sickness	Infection or tuberculin type Contact dermatitis type

Table-2: Comparison between all types of hypersensitivity

✪ **Properties:**
- Ab mediated
- Ab causes stimulation instead of damages.

✪ **Clinical syndromes:**

i. **Grave's disease**
- LATS (Long Acting Thyroid Stimulator), an antibody against some determinant of thyroid cells, which stimulate excessive secretion of thyroid hormones leading to Grave's disease.
- Sometimes it is considered as a part of Type II hypersensitivity.

ii. **Stevens-Johnson syndrome**

iii. **Sulphonamide induced Morbilliform rash**

✪ **Mediators:** Autoantibodies like IgG or IgM

➢ **Comparison between all types of hypersensitivity:** →Table-2

Type-I reaction

❖ **Common terminology:** Anaphylactic, IgE or reagin dependent hypersensitivity

❖ **Properties:** Antibodies (cytotrophic IgE) are fixed on surface of tissue cells in sensitised individual. The antigen combines with cell fixed antibody, leading to release of pharmacologically active substances (vasoactive amines) which produce the clinical reaction

❖ **Clinical syndromes:** Two types like anaphylaxis & atopy as follows

Anaphylaxis

It is discussed with following four types

A. **Systemic anaphylaxis:**

➢ **History:**

✪ **Richet:** Term was given by Richet in 1902, who observed that dogs had survived with sublethal dose of toxic extract from sea anemones, were rendered susceptible to minute dose given days or weeks later.

✪ **Theobald Smith:** He observed similar thing in guinea pigs, **Ehrlich** named it as **Theobald smith phenomenon.**

➢ **Meaning:** Ana = without + Phylaxis = protection.

➢ **Definition:** It is an acute & potentially fatal form of type-I hypersensitivity

➢ **Properties:** It is possible only by cell fixed IgE **called cytotrophic Ab** but not possible by free IgE.

➢ **Agents inducing systemic anaphylaxis:**
- Heterologous serum therapy like ATS, AGS or ADS
- Injection of drugs like penicillin (Pn) or insulin
- Insect bite like honey bee, ant sting or wasp
- Ingestion of sea foods
- Nuts

➢ **Factors influencing anaphylaxis:**

1. **Sensitisation:** Injection, inhalation or contact.
2. **Shocking dose:**
   - Most effective when parenteral administration, less by intraperitoneal or subcutaneous & least by intradermal.
   - Shocking Ag is identical with or related to sensitising Ag.
3. **Waiting period:** An interval of 2-3 weeks between sensitising & shocking dose is required.

➢ **Mechanism:**

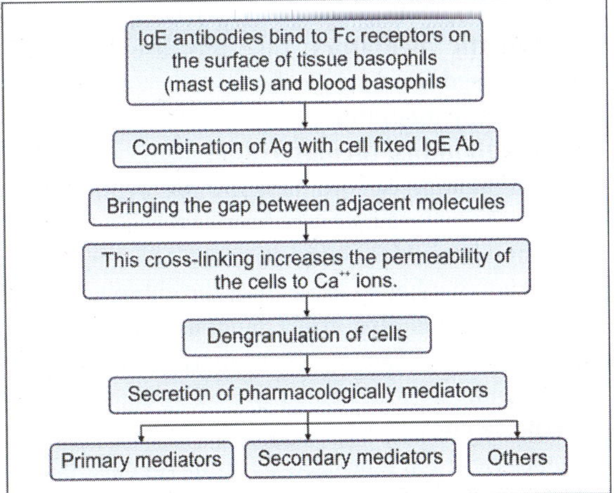

Flow chart-1: Mechanism of anaphylaxis

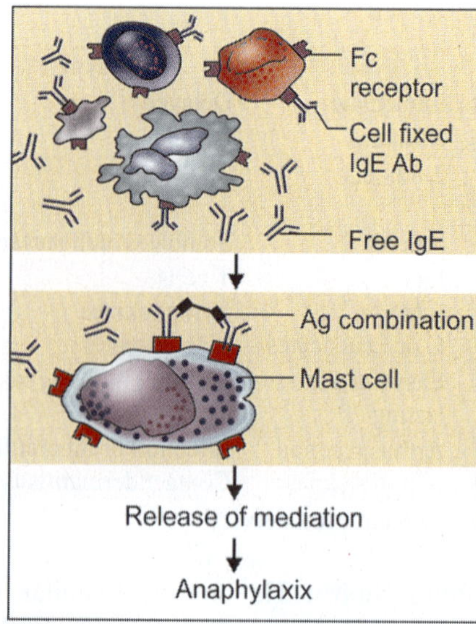

Figure-1: Mechanisms of anaphylaxis

- **Steps: →Fig.-1 & flow chart-1**
- **Primary mediators:**

i. **Histamine:**
- Formed by decarboxylation of histidine from granules of mast cells, basophils & platelets.
- Released in to skin & stimulates the nerves to produce itching & burning sensation.
- It cause vasodilatation, hyperaemia (flare effect) & oedema by increasing the capillary permeability (Wheal effect)
- Induce smooth muscle contraction.

ii. **5-HT (5-Hydroxy Tryptamine) / serotonin:**
- Formed by decarboxylation of tryptophane.
- Present in intestinal tissues, brain & platelets.
- It cause vasoconstriction & increase the capillary permeability
- Induce smooth muscle contraction.

iii. **Eosinophil Chemotactic Factor of Anaphylaxis (ECF-A):**
- Released from granules of mast cells.
- Attract the eosinophils & causing the eosinophilia.

iv. **Neutrophil Chemotactic Factor (NCF):**
- High Molecular Weight (HMW) substances.
- Attract the neutrophils

v. **Enzymatic mediators:** Like protease & hydrolase are released from mast cells

- **Secondary mediators:**

i. **Prostaglandins, thromboxane:**
- Prostaglandins & thromboxane are synthesised by cyclo-oxygenase pathway from arachidonic acid
- Causing bronchial constriction.
- Common mediators are F2α & thromboxane A_2.
- Prostaglandins also affect mucous gland secretion, platelets adhesion, capillary permeability & pain threshold.

ii. **Leukotrienes:**
- Leukotrienes synthesised by lipoxygenase pathway from arachidonic acid.
- Induce slow, sustained smooth muscle contraction, hence called <u>S</u>low <u>R</u>eacting <u>S</u>ubstances of <u>A</u>naphylaxis (SRS-A).
- Common lLeukotrienes are LTB4 (It has high affinity receptor for neutrophils), C4, D4, E4

iii. **Platelets Activating Factors (PAF):**
- LMW
- Released from basophils
- Causing platelets aggregation & release of vasoactive amines.

- **Other mediators:**

i. **Anaphylactoid:** Released from C-activation

ii. **Kinins:** Like bradykinin & other kinins from plasma kininogens

➢ **Clinical features:** Organs involved in anaphylaxis are **called target tissues or shock organs** with following features
- Fever
- Itching
- Flushing of skin or oedema
- Nausea, vomiting, abdominal pain, diarrhoea & sometimes blood in stool
- Dyspnoea due to bronchial spasm.
- Low Blood Pressure (BP)
- Loss of consciousness
- Blood pictures shows decrease coagulability, leucopenia, thrombocytopenia
- Death

➢ **Diagnosis:**

a. **Animal inoculation:** Guinea pig is the highly susceptible animal to diagnose the anaphylaxis.

b. **Radioimmunosorbent test:**

- **Advantages:**

1. It quantitatively measure the serum IgE up to nanogram level
2. Highly sensitive test

- **Principle:** Patient serum contains IgE is made to react with paper disk/beads contains anti-IgE. After washing the disk/beads, it allows to react with radiolabelled anti-IgE. Radioactivity of the disk/beads is measured by gamma counter

c. **Radioallergosorbent test:**

- **Advantages:** Same as above test

1. It quantitatively measure the allergen specific serum IgE
2. Highly sensitive test

- **Principle:** Patient serum contains IgE is made to react with paper disk/beads contains allergen, so only allergen specific IgE would bound. After washing the disk/beads it allows to react with radiolabelled anti-IgE. Radioactivity of the disk/beads is measured by gamma counter

➢ **Prevention:**

a. **Avoidance of contact with known allergen:** Difficult task

b. Desensitisation: By following two methods

1. Acute desensitisation:

- **Method:**
  - Small amount of Ag is administered at 15 minutes interval for 1 hour to 2 hour
  - Ag-Ab complex is formed which release the chemical mediators but not enough to produce the major reaction
  - This technique is adopted on the subsequent entry of allergen like ATS or Pn
- **Disadvantage:** Short lasting & hypersensitivity may return after few days or months

2. Chronic desensitisation:

- **Method:**
  - Small amount of Ag is administered at weekly interval to the hypersensitive individual
  - Ag stimulates the IgE blocking Ab production which prevents the contact of allergen with IgE - Ab present on mast cell.
- **Advantage:** It is a long lasting procedure

➢ **Treatment:** Prompt treatment with adrenaline (0.5ml, 1-in-1000solution) by IM or SC route.

B. Local anaphylaxis: It has following three subtypes

i. Cutaneous anaphylaxis:

✪ **Definition:**
- Intradermal introduction of small shocking dose of Ag in sensitised individual, produce local wheal & flare effect **called cutaneous anaphylaxis**.
- It also developed on ingestion of allergen followed by absorption & characterised by utricaria or angio-neurotic oedema

✪ **Mechanisms: Called wheal & flare effect**
- **Wheal effect:** Central pale area due to oedema by increasing the capillary permeability.
- **Flare effect:** Peripheral red (erythema) area due to hyperaemia by vasodilatation.

✪ **Diagnosis:** By skin test with following methods

1. Intradermal injection:
- **Method:** 0.1ml antigen is introduced intradermally in one forearm **called test arm** with normal saline in other arm **called control arm**.
- **Result:** Wheal & flare response in test arm & no response in control arm suggest the positive reaction
- **Disadvantages:**
  - Risk of anaphylaxis by test antigen
  - Negative test does not rule the possibility of IgE mediated hypersensitivity because it is positive in about 60% of sensitive individual
- **Example of test:** Casoni's test

2. Prick method:

3. Patch method:

ii. Mucosal anaphylaxis:

✪ **Definition:** Entry of small shocking dose of Ag in conjunctiva, nasal mucosa or in respiratory mucosa of sensitised individual produce conjunctivitis, rhinorrhoea or bronchospasm respectively

✪ **Diagnosis:** By conjunctival test with following methods

1. Conjunctival test:
- **Method:** One drop of antigen is instilled in to the one eye **called test eye** with normal saline in other eye **called control eye**.
- **Result:** Conjunctivitis (redness, lacrimation with itching) in test eye & no response in control eye suggest the positive reaction

iii. Passive Cutaneous Anaphylaxis (PCA):

✪ **History:** Developed by Ovary in1952.

✪ **Mechanisms:** Intradermal (ID) injection of Ab, followed by IV injection of Ag fixed with dye like Evans blue, 4-24 hrs afterwards will produce vasodilatation & hyperaemia at ID site. It is a wheal-flare effect.

✪ **Use:** Extremely sensitive method for detection of antibodies. PCA can be used to detect human IgG antibody which is heterocytotropic (capable of fixing the cells of other species) but not IgE which is homocytotropic (capable of fixing the cells of homologues species only).

C. Anaphylaxis in vitro:

✪ **Synonym:** Schultz-Dale phenomenon

✪ **Mechanisms:**
- Isolated tissues strip like intestinal or uterine muscle from sensitised guinea pigs, held in bath of the Ringer's solution, will contract on addition of the specific Ag to the bath.
- Reaction is specific and elicited only by Ag to which animals is sensitive.

D. Anaphylactoid reaction:
- IV injection of certain substances like trypsin, peptone provokes the reaction like anaphylaxis **called anaphylactoid reaction**.
- It is mostly produce due to release of biological substances from C-activation.

Atopy

➢ **History:** Was first coined by Coca 1923

➢ **Meaning:** Out of place or strangeness

➢ **Definition:** It is type-I hypersensitivity reaction that occurs naturally, spontaneously in response to substances encountered in the environment in everyday life.

➢ **Properties:**
- It is very difficult to induce atopy artificially.
- It produces local effect, but sometimes remote effect also occurs. E.g. utricaria following ingestants.
- Atopens are generally not good antigens when introduced parenterally.

- It occur in human beings, it is not induced experimentally (artificially) in animals.
- **Agents causing atopy: Called atopens** as mentioned below
- Inhalants: Pollen, dust
- Ingestants: Milk, egg
- Contact allergen to skin & conjunctiva
- **Mechanism:**
- About 10% populations are prone to develop sensitization to various environmental atopens such as pollen or dust.
- Small amount of IgE is produced by individual but atopy is due to overproduction of IgE **called reagin antibody** with simultaneous deficiency of IgA. When atopens enter in to body it is prevented by IgA to produce damage, but due to deficiency of IgA it combines with cell fixed IgE & release the mediators producing allergic reaction.
- It shows marked familial distribution and it is suspected that the sensitisation is inherited probably MHC genotype.
- Inheritance is not sensitivity to particular Ag, but tendency to develop IgE.
- **Clinical features:** Depends on route of entry of atopens.
- Allergic asthma
- Allergic conjunctivitis
- Allergic rhinitis (hay Fever)
- Dermatitis
- **Diagnosis:** IgE is detected by

a. **Passive agglutination**
b. **ELISA**

- **Prevention:** Avoidance of contact with known allergen, but difficult
- **Treatment:** Desensitisation by injecting serum or repeated injection of Ag.
- **Praunitz-Kustner reaction (PK reaction)**
- **History:** It was 1st reported by Prausnitz & Kustner in 1921.
- **Principle:**
- IgE is homocytotrophic, which is species specific. Only human IgE can fix to the surface of human cells.
- This is the basis of Prausnitz- Kustner (PK) reaction which was the original method for detecting atopic antibodies.
- **Method:**
- **Steps:**
- Serum is collected from Kustner (atopic hypersensitive to certain species of cooked fish)
- Inject in to Prausnitz by Intracutaneous (IC) route.
- After 24 hrs small dose of cooked fish Ag is injected in to Prausnitz by intracutaneous route at same site.
- **Result:** Local wheal-flare effect at IC injection site
- **Disadvantage:** It carries the risk of transmission of infection so no longer is used.

Type-II reaction

Common terminology:

- Cytotoxic or cytolytic hypersensitivity
- IgG or rarely IgM dependent hypersensitivity

Properties:

- This type of reaction is initiated by IgG or rarely IgM/IgE.
- Ab react either with the cell surface or tissue antigen.
- Ab produces cell/tissue damage in presence of complement or mononuclear cells.
- Sometimes stimulates the cell (Type-V) or inhibit the cell.
- Type 2 reactions are intermediate between hypersensitivity and autoimmunity.

Clinical syndromes: It includes Ab mediated cell damage

Ab mediated cell damage

- **Types of antigens:** Two types

i. **Intrinsic Ag:** "Self" antigen, part of the host cells.
ii. **Extrinsic Ag:** Adsorbed on to the cells & arise from pathogens or by drugs.

- **Mechanisms:** Ab damage the cell by following four ways

i. **Ab mediated cell lysis:**

- **Steps**
- Antigens are adsorbed on to the cells
- The antibodies produced by the immune response mostly IgG & rarely IgM are binds to antigens on the patient's own cell surfaces.
- Such cells with Ag-Ab complex on surfaces are killed by phagocytic cells or by C-activation as shown in **fig.2**.
- **Clinical syndrome:**
- Thrombocytopenia: Destruction of platelets by cell fixed antigens & antibodies.
- Agranulocytosis or agranulosis or granulopenia: Destruction of WBCs (specially neutrophils → Neutropenia) by cell fixed antigens & antibodies.
- Autoimmune haemolytic anaemia: Destruction of RBCs by cell fixed antigens & antibodies.
- Rh incompatibility (Erythroblastosis foetalis): It is due to Rh incompatibility, where Rh –Ve mother have anti-Rh antibodies due to earlier pregnancy with Rh+Ve foetus. Such antibodies can cross the placenta & destroy the Rh+Ve foetal RBCs **called erythroblastosis foetalis.**

- ABO incompatibility (transfusion reaction): Donor's RBCs are lysed by recipient anti RBCs antibodies due to incompatible blood transfusion.
- Drug induced haemolytic anaemia: Drug or its products, absorbed on RBC surface. Synthesis of antibody to drug or its products lyses the attached RBCs by complement activation.
- Pemphigus vulgaris: Autoantibody against desmosomal protein that lead to disruption of epidermal intracellular junction.

✪ **Mediators:**
- IgG
- IgM
- C (Complement) or phagocytic cells

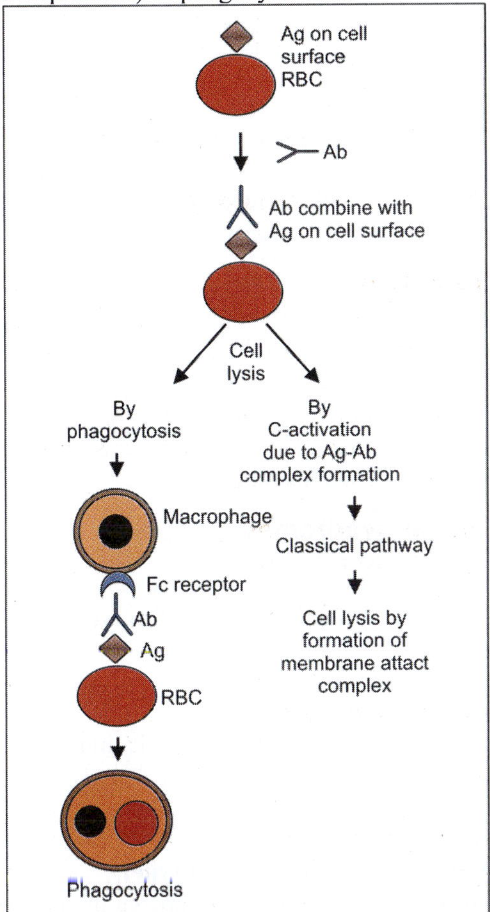

Figure-2: Cell lysis by type –II hypersensitivity

ii. Antibody dependent cytotoxic cells (ADCCs):
- It is possible by LGLs (Large Granular Lymphocytes)
- This type of LGLs possesses surface receptors for the Fc part of Ig. Antigen is attached at Fab region.
- They are capable of killing target cells sensitized with IgG likc tumour cells, parasites or graft rejection.
- It is mostly IgG mediate. In certain instances IgE is useful like eosinophilic mediated killing of parasites
- This antibody dependent cellular cytotoxicity is distinct from the action of cytotoxic T cells, which is independent of antibody.

iii. Cell stimulatory: It is separately classified as type V hypersensitivity, discussed earlier

iv. Cell inhibitory: Antibody produces is inhibitory in nature instead of stimulatory like in
- Pernicious anemia: Where antibodies against parietal cells of gastric mucosa decrease the secretion of acid leads to achlorhydria & atrophic gastritis.
- Myasthenia gravis: Where antibody present against acetylcholine (Ach) receptors at neuromuscular junction in striated muscle. It prevents the combination of Ach with its receptor & impairs the muscle contraction.

✓ **Note: Cell stimulatory & cell inhibitory hypersensitivity**

- **More details:** Both are better classified as autoimmunity. For more details follow chapter → Autoimmunity.

Type-III reaction

❖ **Common terminology:** Immune complex or toxic complex disease

❖ **Properties:**
- Damage is caused by Ag-Ab complex.
- These may precipitate in & around the small blood vessels, causing damages to cell secondarily or on membranes interfering with their functions.

❖ **Clinical syndromes:** Two types like arthus reaction & serum sickness as follows

Arthus reaction

➢ **History:**
- Reported by Arthus in 1903
- He observed that when rabbits were repeatedly injected subcutaneously with normal horse serum, the initial injection had no local effect but with later injections, there is a production of intense local edema, indurations & haemorrhagic necrosis. This is **called arthus reaction**.

➢ **Definition:** It is a **local manifestation** of generalized hypersensitivity.

➢ **Passive transfer:** Passively transferred with sera containing precipitating (IgG, IgM) Abs in high titers.

- **Mechanism: →Flow chart-2**

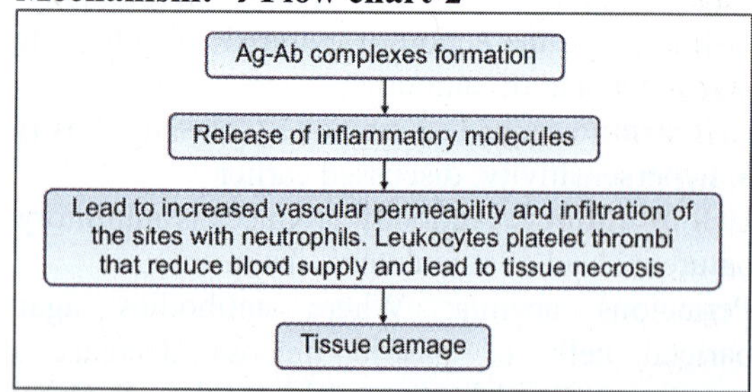

Flow chart-2: Mechanism of arthus reaction

- **Examples of diseases:** Arthus reaction is seen in some clinical conditions like

1. Farmer's lung: Thermophilic actinomycetes from mouldy hay or grain cause **farmers lung** and other types of hypersensitive pneumonitis
2. Allergic bronchopulmonary aspergillosis
3. Allergic fungal rhionosinusitis
4. Bagassosis

- **Mediators:**
  - IgG
  - IgM
  - C (Complement)
  - Leucocytes

Serum sickness

- **History:** Originally it was described by Von Pirquet and Shick in1905.
- **Properties:**
  - It is a **systemic manifestation** of type-III hypersensitivity.
  - Single injection can serve both as the sensitising dose and shocking dose.
  - It appeared a 7-12 days **following a single injection** of high concentration of foreign serum such as diphtheria antitoxin.
  - As heterologous serum injections are not used now a days the syndrome is more commonly seen with injection of Pn or other antibiotics
- **Mechanism: →Flow chart-3**

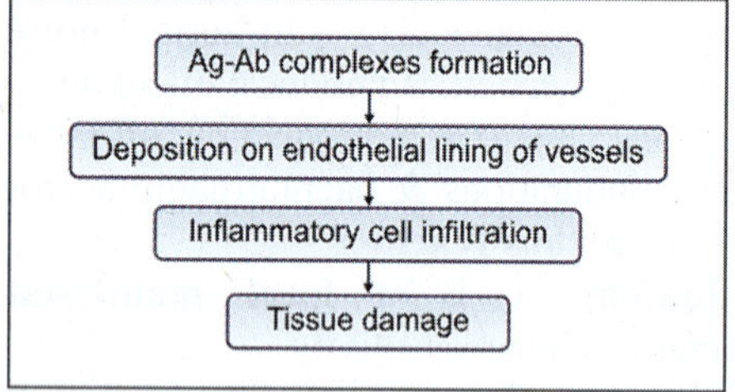

Flow chart-3: Mechanism of serum sickness

- **Clinical features:**
  - Fever, lymphadenopathy, splenomegaly, arthritis, glomerulonephritis, endocarditis, vasculitis, urticarial rashes, abdominal pain, nausea, vomiting.
  - It is self limiting disease.
  - With continued rise in Ab production the immune complex become larger and more susceptible to phagocytosis and immune elimination. When all antigens are thus eliminated and free antibodies appear the symptoms clear.
- **Examples of diseases:**

1. Rheumatoid Arthritis: Autoantibody (IgM) against Fc piece of IgG to form IgM-IgG complex
2. Acute Post Streptococcal Glomerulo Nephritis (APSGN): It is type III hypersensitivity reaction due to immune complex formation between streptococcal antigens & respective antibodies, which later deposited in renal glomeruli.
3. PAN (polyartritis nodosa): Immune complex formation but exact nature of autoantibody is unknown
4. SLE: Autoantibody against nuclear material which makes immune complex & deposited in PMN cell **called LE cell**

Type-IV reaction

❖ **Common terminology:** Delayed or cell mediated hypersensitivity

❖ **Properties:**

- It is not Ab mediated, but by sensitised T cells.
- In unsensitised individual the injection of Ag provokes no response.
- It differs from type I hypersensitivity not only in longer interval of appearance but also in its morphology and histology.

❖ **Clinical syndromes:** Two types like infective & contact dermatitis type

Infective (tuberculin) type

- **Causes (allergens):** As follows

i. **Infective conditions:**
- Mostly seen in subacute or chronic infections
- Pathogens are intracellular
- Examples:

a. **Bacterial infections:**

1. ***M. tuberculosis*** **(Tuberculin type):**
   - When a small dose of tuberculin is injected intradermally in individual sensitised to tuberculo protein by prior infection or immunization, an indurated inflammatory reaction develops within 48-72 hours.
   - Tuberculin test (More details Follow chapter → *Mycobacterium tuberculosis*) therefore provides a useful indication of the state of delayed hypersensitivity (cell mediated immunity to the bacilli)
2. ***M. leprae***: Lepromin test (More details Follow chapter →*Mycobacterium leprae*)
3. ***L. monocytogenes***
4. ***B. abortus***

b. Viral infections:
1. **Small pox virus**
2. **HSV (Herpes Simplex Virus)**
3. **Measles virus**

c. Fungal infections:
1. ***P. carinii***
2. ***C. albicans***
3. ***C. neoformans***
4. ***H. capsulatum***

d. Parasitic infections:
1. ***L. donovani***

ii. Allograft rejection:

iii. Autoimmune diseases: Multiple sclerosis

- **Mechanism: → Flow chart-4**

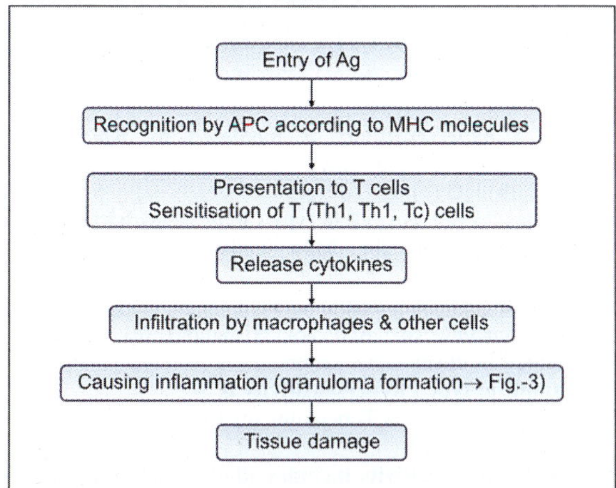

Flow chart-4: Mechanism of infective type hypersensitivity

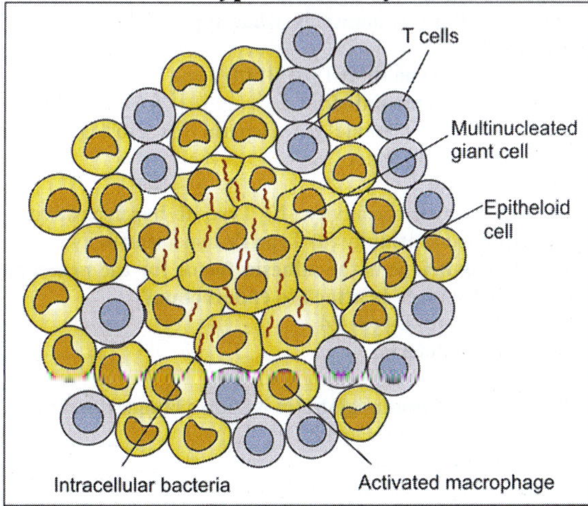

Figure-3: Granuloma formation

- **Mediators:** T cells, lymphokines & macrophages
- **Clinical features:** Characterised by granuloma formation in tissues.
- **Diagnosis:** By **skin test** like tuberculin test, lepromin test etc.

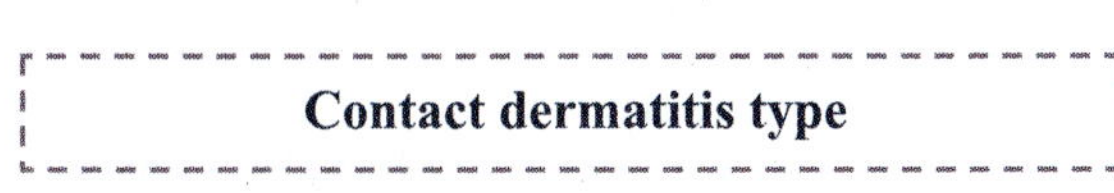

Contact dermatitis type

- **Causes (Allergens):** As follows

1. **Chemicals:** Dyes, picryl chloride & dinitrochlorobenzene,
2. **Metals:** Like nickel, chromium etc.
3. **Drugs:** Penicillin
4. **Plant allergens:** Parthenin from perthenium.

- **Mechanisms: →Flow chart-5**
- **Mediators:** T cells, lymphokines & macrophages
- **Clinical features:** Contact with allergen in sensitised individual lead to contact dermatitis, the lesions varying from macule and papule to vesicle that break down, leaving behind raw weeping areas typical of acute eczematous dermatitis.
- **Diagnosis:** By **patch test,** in which allergen is applied to the skin under an adherent dressing. Sensitivity is detected by itching, erythema (redness) after 4-5 hrs & vesicle to blister formation after 24-48 hrs.

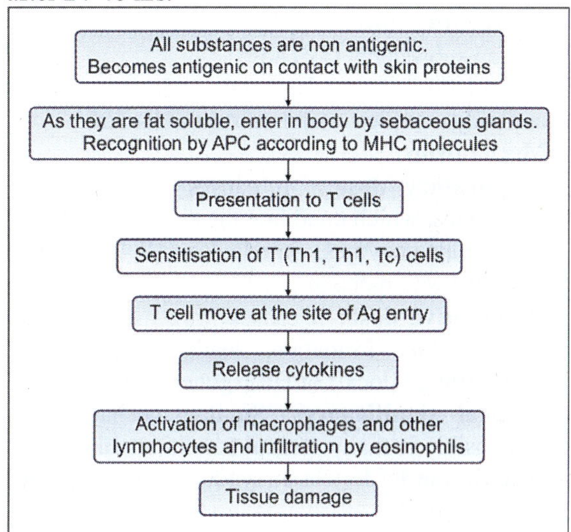

Flow chart-5: Mechanism of contact dermatitis type hypersensitivity

✓ **Note: Cutaneous basophil hypersensitivity**

- Intradermal injection of some protein leads to basophilic infiltration.
- Formerly it was known as Jones-Mote reaction
- It is like tuberculin reaction but differ histological by basophilic infiltration.
- It differs from DTH, passive transferred by serum.
- Clinically not significant

Schwartzman reaction

- **Synonym:** Shwartzman phenomenon
- **Definition:** It is an overwhelming non-immune response with multisystem involvement leading to local or systemic vasculitis.
- **History:** Reported by Gregory Shwartzman in 1928
- **Types:**

1. **Local Shwartzman reaction.**

- It based on development local vasculitis (local haemorrhage & necrosis)

- Shwartzman observed that when rabbits were injected intradermally with culture filtrate (endotoxin) of *S. typhi*, with 24 hrs later IV injections by same filtrate, there is a production of intense local haemorrhagic necrosis at the site of intradermal injection. This is **called Shwartzman reaction**.

2. **Generalised Shwartzman reaction:**
- It based on development systemic vasculitis (DIC)
- If both the injection are given by IV route, animal will die 12-24 hrs after second injection.
- Similar reaction observed by Sanarelli in Cholera in 1924 so **called Sanarelli –Shwartzman reaction**.

➢ **Antigenic doses:**
- **Preparatory dose:**
- It is an initial dose
- It includes some bacterial endotoxin
- **Provocative dose:**
- It is an subsequent (IV) dose
- It includes some bacterial endotoxin, antigen antibody complex, starch, serum or kaolin

➢ **Mechanisms:**
- **Preparatory dose:** It causes accumulation of leucocytes, which condition the site by releasing the lysosomal enzymes, interleukin (IL-1 & 6) & capillary wall damage.
- **Provocative dose:** It causes intravascular clotting & thrombus formation, leads to necrosis & haemorrhage (local) or DIC (generalised).

➢ **Clinical significances:** Similar mechanisms are responsible in many clinical conditions like
- Waterhouse Friderichsen syndrome in infection by *N. meningitidis*
- Infection by *Staph aureus*

Question bank

Case study

1) A 28 years male patient brought to the medical emergency with history of honey bee bite with complains of coughing & dyspnoea. Identify the hypersensitivity & answer the following
a) Name the clinical condition
b) Write mechanisms & diagnosis of given clinical condition
c) Write treatment of given clinical condition

2) A 28 years female patient visited the skin OPD with history of skin rash on forehead, 2 days after the application of hair dyes. A case of hypersensitivity was diagnosed. Identify the clinical the type of hypersensitivity & answer the following
a) Name the type of hypersensitivity
b) Name the allergic test useful to diagnose the hypersensitivity
c) Write mechanisms of hypersensitivity in given case
d) Write the classification of hypersensitivity

Essay/Full question

1) Hypersensitivity

Short notes

1) Classification of hypersensitivity
2) Systemic anaphylaxis
3) Type II hypersensitivity
4) Atopy
5) Arthus reaction
6) Serum sickness
7) Delayed type hypersensitivity

Short questions for theory/viva questions

1) Differences between immediate & delayed type of hypersensitivity
2) Define: Immunity & Hypersensitivity
3) What is Theobald Smith phenomenon
4) What is anaphylactoid reaction
5) What is Schultz Dale phenomenon
6) What is Schrwartzman reaction

MCQs for chapter review

Type I reaction

1) **Type I hypersensitivity is mediated by which of the following immunoglobulin** (AI-05)
(a) IgA (b) IgG (c) IgM (d) IgE
2) **The most important cell in type I hypersensitivity** (AI-92)
(a) Macrophages (b) Mast cells (c) Neutrophils (d) Lymphocytes
3) **Mast cell synthesize and/or secrete** (PGI, June -03)
(a) Adrenaline (b) Ach (c) Histamine (d) Heparin (e) Neutrophilic chemotactic factor
4) **Example of type I hypersensitivity is** (AI-98)
a) Lepromin test (b) Tuberculin (c) Casoni's test (d) Arthus reaction
5) **Type I hypersensitivity includes all of the following except-** (PGI-00)
(a) Autoimmune haemolytic anaemia (b) Anaphylaxis (c) Extrinsic asthama (d) Hay fever
6) **Wheal & flare response is what type of hypersensitivity reaction?**
(a) Type I (b) Type II (c) Type III (d) Type IV
7) **Anaphylaxis is mediated by** (PGI, May-13)
(a) 5-hydrpxytryptamine (b) Heparin (c) Prostaglandin (d) Platelet activating factor
8) **Casoni's test is**
(a) Type I hypersensitivity (b) Type II hypersensitivity (c) Type III hypersensitivity (d) Type IV hypersensitivity
9) **Which leukotriene is the adhesin factor for the neutrophils on the cell surface to attach to endothelium?**
(a) B4 (b) C4 (c) D4 (d) E4
10) **PK reaction detects**
(a) IgG (b) IgA (c) IgE (d) IgM
11) **Which of the immunoglobulin is shows homocytotropism**
(a) IgG (b) IgA (c) IgE (d) IgD
12) **Atopy is mediated by**
(a) IgE (b) IgD (c) IgM (d) IgA

Type II reaction

13) **True about type II hypersensitivity reaction is?**
(a) May be complement mediated (b) Schultz dale phenomenon is a type 2 hypersensitivity (c) Antibody independent (d) Role of IgE
14) **Prototype of type II hypersensitivity reaction is?**
(a) Arthus reaction (b) SLE (c) Autoimmune haemolytic anaemia (d) Contact dermatitis
15) **Grave's disease is an example of which type of immunological response?** (PGI 91)
(a) Type I (b) Type II (c) Type III (d) Type IV (e) Type V
16) **Erythroblastosis foetalis is an example of which type of hypersensitivity reaction**

(a) Type I (b) Type II (c) Type III (d) Type IV

17) **Myasthenia gravis is which type of hypersensitivity**
(a) Type I (b) Type II (c) Type III (d) Type IV

18) **All are type II hypersensitivity reaction except**
(a) Haemorrhagic disease of new born (b) Grave's disease (c) Autoimmune disease (d) Haemolytic anaemia

Type III reaction

19) **Type III reaction is** (AI-93)
(a) Antibody mediated (b) Immune complex mediated (c) Cell mediated (d) None

20) **Which is an example of type III hypersensitivity reaction**
(a) Contact dermatitis (b) Haemolytic anaemia (c) Serum sickness (d) Good pasture syndrome

21) **Arthus phenomenon is an example of which hypersensitivity**
(a) Type I (b) Type II (c) Type III (d) Type IV

22) **All of the following are immune complex disease except**
(a) Serum sickness (b) Farmer's lung (c) SLE (d) Graft rejection

Type IV reaction

23) **Delayed hypersensitivity involves** (AIIMS-92)
(a) Neutrophils (b) Monocytes (c) Eosinophils (d) Lymphocytes

24) **Which of the following is type IV hypersensitivity**
(a) Arthus reaction (b) Serum sickness (c) Schwartzman reaction (d) Granulomatous reaction

25) **Not a delayed type hypersensitivity reactions**
(a) Arthus reaction (b) Bronchial asthama (c) Haemolytic anaemia (d) Multiple sclerosis

26) **Contact dermatitis is** (AI-94)
(a) Type I hypersensitivity (b) Type II hypersensitivity (c) Type III hypersensitivity (d) Type IV hypersensitivity

27) **In contact dermatitis which cell play a major role** (PGI, June -08)
(a) T-cells (b) B-cells (c) Langerhans cells (d) Macrophages

28) **Skin tests are used for which hypersensitivity reactions?** (PGI, June -07)
(a) I (b) II (c) III (d) IV (e) V

29) **Which of the following is false** (AI-95)
(a) Theo bald smith phenomenon is a type I hypersensitivity reaction (b) Serum sickness is a type II hypersensitivity reaction (c) Allograft rejection is type IV hypersensitivity reaction (d) Transfusion reaction a type II hypersensitivity reaction

30) **Tuberculin test is reaction of**
(a) Anaphylaxis mediated (b) Cell mediated (c) Antibody mediated (d) Immune complex mediated

31) **Type IV hypersensitivity reaction include all except**
(a) Paul Bunnel test test (b) Lepromin test (c) Tuberculin test (d) Granulomatous reaction

Answers of MCQs & explanation

1) **(d)**
2) **(b)**
3) **(c), (d) & (e)**
4) **(c)**
5) **(a)**
6) **(a)**
7) **(a), (b), (c) & (d)**
8) **(a)**
9) **(a)**

(1–9) Follow section, **type I hypersensitivity** for explanation

10) **(c)**
11) **(c)**
12) **(a)**

(10–12) Follow section, **type I hypersensitivity (atopy)** for explanation

13) **(a) & (c)**
- Type II hypersensitivity mediated by autoantibody & damage to target cell occurs by phagocytes, complement, ADCC, cell stimulation or cell inhibition

14) **(b)**
15) **(c)**
16) **(b)**
17) **(b)**

(14–17) Follow section, **type II hypersensitivity** for explanation

18) **(a)**
- Haemorrhagic disease of new born is due to vitamin K deficiency
- Grave's disease is an autoimmune disease, where Ab is stimulatory type & it is classified separately as type V hypersensitivity
- Haemolytic anaemia & other autoimmune disease are part of type II hypersensitivity

19) **(b)**
20) **(c)**
21) **(c)**
22) **(d)**

(19–22) Type III hypersensitivity is immune complex or toxic complex disease in nature which includes arthus reaction & serum sickness

23) **(b) & (d)**
- Type IV hypersensitivity is mediated by lymphocytes, lymphokines & macrophages (monocytes)

24) **(d)**
- Type IV hypersensitivity, specially tuberculin type present with granulomatous reaction

25) **(a), (b) & (c)**
- Arthus reaction → Type III hypersensitivity
- Bronchial asthama →Type I hypersensitivity
- Haemolytic anaemia → Type II hypersensitivity

26) **(d)**
- Type IV hypersensitivity includes infective (tuberculin) & contact dermatitis varieties

27) **(a)**
- Follow section, **type IV hypersensitivity (contact dermatitis)** for explanation

28) **(a) & (d)**
- Skin tests are based on immediate (Type I) hypersensitivity like Casoni's test & delayed (Type IV) hypersensitivity like tuberculin test

29) **(b)**
- Serum sickness is a type III hypersensitivity reaction

30) **(b)**
- Tuberculin test is type IV hypersensitivity, which cell mediated

31) **(a)**
- Paul Bunnel test test → based on agglutination reaction
- Lepromin test, tuberculin test & granulomatous reaction are based on Type IV or delayed type hypersensitivity

27 Immuno Deficiency Diseases (IDDs)

Learning heading & subheadings

- Definition
- Classification:

Primary IDDs

Secondary IDDs

- **Definition:** Conditions with impairment of defence mechanisms of body resulting susceptibility to infections & malignancies **called Immuno Deficiency Diseases (IDDs).**
- **Classification:** Two types according to etiological factors & involvement of immune system like primary IDDs & secondary IDDs.

Primary IDDs

- **Definition:** Immunodeficiency due to abnormalities in development of immune mechanisms or immune organs.
- **Etiological factors:** Congenital or genetical
- **Subtypes:**

A. Deficiency of specific immune system:
i. Deficiency of AMI
ii. Deficiency of CMI
iii. Combined deficiency of AMI & CMI
B. Deficiency of non-specific immune system:
i. Deficiency of phagocytosis
ii. Complement (C) deficiency

A. Deficiency of specific immune system:
i. Deficiency of AMI (HI)
a. X-linked agammaglobulinemia:

- **History:** 1st IDD identified by Bruton in 1952, so **called Bruton's disease**.
- **Pathogenesis:** Defective AMI but normal CMI. Failure of B cells to mature beyond the pre-B cell stage in the bone marrow because of mutations or deletions in the gene encoding B cell tyrosine kinase or Bruton's tyrosine kinase (BTK).
- **Clinical features:**
  - Occurs in male infants
  - Child is protected by maternal Abs up to 6 months. Symptoms start afterward.
  - Atrophy of tonsils & adenoids.
  - Recurrent serious infection by *Strept pyogenes*, *N. meningitidis*, *H. influenzae*, *S. pneumoniae*, *P. aeruginosa* etc.
  - Patients respond normally to viral infection like measles, chicken pox, though patients develop poliomyelitis or progressive encephalitis following OPV or wild virus entry.
  - Autoimmune diseases develop in ~20% of patients
  - Haemolytic anaemia, arthritis & atopic manifestation are observed.
- **Diagnosis:**
- **Blood picture:**
  - Low levels or absence of all classes of Abs in the blood. IgG level is less than tenth & IgA plus IgM less than hundredth of the normal level
  - Reduced or absent B cells in the peripheral blood
- **Lymph node biopsy**
  - Depletion of bursa dependent areas
  - No plasma cells & germinal centres in lymph nodes even after antigenic stimulation.
  - Maturation, numbers and functions of T cells are usually normal
- **Other features:** Tonsils & adenoids are atrophic
- **Skin tests:**
  - **For immediate type hypersensitivity:** Wheal-flare effect is not demonstrated
  - **For DTH:** CMI is not affected, so all skin tests based on DTH are normal
  - **Allograft rejection:** Normal
- **Treatment:**
  - Live microbial vaccine are contraindicated

- Initial administration of 300 mg Ig/kg of body weight in three doses followed by 100 mg Ig/kg/ month.
- Commercial preparation contains only IgA & IgM, therefore whole plasma have been infused.

b. Transient hypergammaglobulinemia of infant:

✪ **Pathogenesis:** Maternal Ab catabolise at 2 months. IgG start to develop at this age. Delay in synthesis of IgG produces IDD.

✪ **Clinical features:**
- Occurs in infants of both sexes.
- Recurrent otitis media & respiratory infection.
- Spontaneous recover y occurs in 18-30 months.

✪ **Treatment**: Transient, so treatment is not required usually.

c. Common Variable Immuno Deficiency Disease (CVIDD):

✪ **Synonym:** It occurs at 15-35 years of age so **called late onset hypo γ-globulinemia**.

✪ **Pathogenesis:**
- B cells normal in numbers, but fail to differentiate in to plasma cells, so reduced total Ig level.
- Increased Tc cell activity & decreased Th cell activity may cause the disease.

✪ **Clinical features:**
- Recurrent pyogenic infection
- Malabsorption
- Giardiasis
- Increased incidence of autoimmune diseases

✪ **Diagnosis:** Low levels of antibodies in blood

✪ **Treatment:** Administration of IM or IV Ig

d. Selective Ig deficiency:

✪ **Pathogenesis:**
- Selective deficiency of one or more Ab while others are remains normal or elevated, so also **called dysgammaglobulinemia**
- May be presence of Ab to Ig like IgA- Ab.

✪ **Clinical features:**

- **IgA deficiency:**
  - Most common primary IDD
  - Respiratory infection present with rhinitis, common cold, cough, fever etc.
  - Steatorrhoea
  - Atopic type of allergy
- **IgM deficiency:** Septicemia
- **IgG deficiency:** Chronic progressive bronchiectasis

✪ **Treatment**: Antibiotics to prevent recurrent infection.

e. Combined deficiencies of IgA & IgG (IgG2):

✪ **Pathogenesis:** It includes deficiency of IgA & IgG2

✪ **Clinical features:** Deficiency of IgG2 favours the infection by bacteria with polysaccharide capsule. Such infection is more common if associated with deficiency of IgA.

f. X-linked hyper IgM syndrome:

✪ **Pathogenesis:**
- Deficiency of IgG, IgA, and IgE – elevated levels of IgM
- Normal numbers of B cells
- Both X-linked & acquired

✪ **Clinical features:**
- Recurrent infection
- Autoimmune diseases like neutropenia, thrombocytopenia, haemolytic anaemia & renal lesions

✪ **Treatment**: Ig therapy by IV route

g. Bloom syndrome:

✪ **Synonym:** Congenital telangiectetic erythema

✪ **Pathogenesis:** Decreased IgA & IgM with or without IgG changes

✪ **Clinical features:**
- Telangiectatic erythema appears as macules or papules in butter fly fashion on face & other areas.
- Photosensitivity
- Repeated respiratory & GIT infections
- Delay in growth, which encourage the parents to seek medical advices.
- 150-300 times increased risk of malignancy

h. Nucleotidase deficiency:

✪ **Pathogenesis:** Ecto-5 nucleotidase deficiency is an alteration in purine metabolism that produces deficiency of B cells, which is responsible for AMI.

i. Transcobalamin-II deficiency:

✪ **Pathogenesis:**
- Inherited autosomal recessive trait.
- Vitamin B12 deficiency due to defective metabolism.
- Associated immunological defect of phagocytosis, plasma cells & low Ig level

✪ **Clinical features:**
- Villous atrophy
- Megaloblastic anaemia

✪ **Treatment**: Vitamin B12 therapy

ii. Deficiency of CMI

a. Di George syndrome:

✪ **Synonym:** Congenital thymic aplasia

✪ **Etio-pathogenesis:**
- In 90% cases, it occurs due to deletion of chromosome 22q11 resulting malformation of 3rd & 4th pharyngeal pouches, so all the structure developed from 3rd & 4th pharyngeal pouches like thymus, parathyroid gland (congenital aplasia or hypoplasia of thymus & parathyroid gland), portions of face & aortic arch are defective.
- It is not inheritance, but may be due to intrauterine infection

✪ **Clinical features:**

- **Parathyroid defect:** Hypocalcemic tetani is evident within 24 hrs of birth due to a deficiency of parathormone or parathyroid hormone which is normally produced by the parathyroid and regulates K+ & Ca+2 metabolisms.

- **Thymus defect:**
- Defect in T cell maturation due to defect or absence of thymus, resulting depression of CMI which leads to repeated infections by bacteria, viruses & fungi (*Candida* spp. & *P. jirovecii*) & protozoa
- Thymus dependant area of lymph nodes & spleen are depleted.
- T-cells are reduced in numbers with normal B cells
- DTH & graft rejection is depleted.
- **Normal AMI:** AMI remains unaffected. B cells & Ig levels are normal.
- **Other features**
- Fallot's tetrology.
- Characteristic facial appearance

✪ **Treatment:** Foetal thymus transplantation.

b. Chronic Mucocutaneous Candidiasis (CMC):

✪ **Pathogenesis:**
- Abnormal Ir to *C. albicans*.
- CMI, DTH & phagocytosis to *Candida* are defective.
- Circulating antibodies to *Candida* are in high titre

✪ **Clinical features:** Chronic Candidiasis of skin, mucosa & nail.

✪ **Treatment:** Transfer Factor (TF) with Amphotericin B (AMB) is effective.

c. Purine Nucleoside Phosphorylase (PNP) deficiency:

✪ **Pathogenesis:**
- This enzyme degrade purine to hypoxanthine & finally in to uric acid.
- Deficiency of enzyme as an autosomal recessive trait shows decreased CMI & recurrent or chronic infection.

✪ **Clinical features:**
- Hypoplastic anaemia, diarrhoea, chronic candidiasis, pneumonia etc.

✪ **Diagnosis:** Low serum uric acid.

✪ **Treatment:** Haematopoietic stem cell transplantation to restore the immune function.

iii. Combined immunodeficiency of AMI & CMI

a. Nezelof syndrome:

✪ **Pathogenesis:** Depressed CMI with decreased, elevated or normal Ig (Cellular immunodeficiency with abnormal Ig synthesis)

✪ **Clinical features:** Autoimmune haemolytic anaemia, diarrhoea, chronic candidiasis, pneumonia & recurrent infection by bacteria, virus, fungi & protozoa.

✪ **Diagnosis:**
- Abudant plasma cells in lymph nodes, spleen, intestine & in other body tissues.
- Thymic dysplasia

✪ **Treatment:**
- Bone marrow, thymus & TF transplantation
- Antibiotic to infection.

b. Ataxia telangiectasia:

✪ **Pathogenesis:** Autosomal recessive disease with chromosomal abnormalities characterized by
- Depressed CMI resulting impairment of DTH & graft rejection.
- Decreased IgE level
- Lack of serum & secretory IgA & also presence of Ab to IgA.

✪ **Clinical features:**
- Cerebral ataxia
- Telangiectasia in conjunctiva, face & other parts of body usually at 5 or 6 years of life.
- Ovarian dysgenesis
- Death in early life due to sinopulmonary infection or in 1st or 2nd decade of life due to malignancy.

✪ **Treatment:** Thymus or transfer factor transplantation

c. Good's syndrome (Immunodeficiency with thymoma):
- Occurs in adults
- Thymic tumour
- Depressed CMI
- Agammaglobulinemia
- Present with aplastic anaemia.

d. Immunodeficiency with short limbed dwarfism:
- Autosomal recessive defect
- Short limb dwarfism
- Ectodermal dysplasia
- Thymic defect
- Increased susceptibility to infection

e. Episodic lymphopenia with lymphocytotoxin:
- Lymphocytotoxin is actual an Ab to lymphocyte
- Familial disease
- Patient present with lack of immunological memory & secondary Ab response is abolished.

f. SCID (Severe combined immunodeficiency):

✪ **Synonym:** Known with multiple names as follows
- Alymphocytosis
- Glanzmann–Riniker syndrome
- Severe mixed immunodeficiency syndrome
- Thymic alymphoplasia
- Bubble boy disease / bubble baby disease because its victims are extremely vulnerable to infections & become famous for living in a sterile environment.

✪ **Definition:** Genetic disorder characterized by the disturbed development of functional T & B cells due to mutation in different genes that result in heterogeneous clinical presentations.

✪ **Pathogenic subtypes:**
- In SCID immune system is highly compromised or considered as almost absent due to defective Ab response due to either direct involvement of B cells or improper B cells activation due to non-functional Th cells.
- Consequently, both "arms" (B & T cells) of the adaptive immune system are impaired due to

mutation in one of several possible genes. There are now at least nine different known genes in which mutations lead to a form SCID.

- Pathogenic subtypes according to mutation in different gens are mentioned in **table-1**

✪ **Clinical features:**

- SCID patients are usually affected by severe bacterial, viral, or fungal infections early in life and often present with interstitial lung disease, chronic diarrhoea, and failure to thrive.
- Ear infections, recurrent *Pneumocystis jirovecii* (previously *carinii*) pneumonia, and profuse oral candidiasis commonly occur.
- These babies, if untreated, usually die within one year due to severe, recurrent infections unless they have undergone successful hematopoietic stem cell transplantation.

✪ **Diagnosis:**

- Real time PCR to measure the concentration of T-cell receptor excision circles
- Genetic tests to detect the mutant genes
- Blood lymphocyte count

✪ **Treatment:** Bone marrow transplantation & gene therapy

g. Wiskott –Aldrich syndrome (WAS):

✪ **Pathogenesis:** X-linked disease characterized by Depressed CMI due to depletion of T lymphocytes in peripheral blood & also in T cell zones of lymph nodes.

Type	Description
X linked severe combined deficiency (X-SCID)	- Most common type - It is due to mutations in the gene encoding the common gamma chain , a protein that is shared by the receptors for IL-2, IL-4, IL-7, IL-9, IL-15 and IL-21. These IL and their receptors are involved in the development and differentiation of T and B cells. Because the common γ chain is shared by many IL receptors, mutations that result in a non-functional common gamma chain cause widespread defects in IL signalling. The result is a near complete failure of the immune system to develop and function, with low or absent T cells and NK cells and non-functional B cells. - The common γ chain is encoded by the gene IL-2 receptor gamma (IL-2Rγ), which is located on the X-chromosome. For this reason, immunodeficiency caused by mutations in IL-2Rγ is **called X-linked severe combined immunodeficiency**. The condition is inherited in an X-linked recessive pattern.
Adenosine deaminase (ADA) deficiency	- The second most common form of SCID after X-SCID - It is caused by a defective ADA enzyme, necessary for the breakdown of purines. - Lack of ADA causes accumulation of dATP, which inhibit the activity of ribonucleotide reductase, the enzyme that reduces ribonucleotides to generate deoxyribonucleotides. The effectiveness of the immune system depends upon lymphocyte proliferation & hence dRNTP synthesis. Without functional ribonucleotide reductase, lymphocyte proliferation is inhibited & the immune system is compromised. - Present with complete absence to mild abnormal T & B cells. - Associated with chondrocyte abnormalities.
Purine nucleoside phosphorylase deficiency	- An autosomal recessive disorder involving mutations of the purine nucleoside phosphorylase (PNP gene. PNP is a key enzyme in the purine salvage pathway. Impairment of this enzyme causes elevated dGTP levels resulting in T-cell toxicity and deficiency.
Reticular dysgenesis of De Vaal	- Inability of granulocyte precursors to form granules secondary to mitochondrial adenylate kinase 2 malfunction. - Defect at multipotent haemopoietic stem cells level resulting anaemia, thrombocytopenia, neutropenia, Lymphopenia, bone marrow aplasia, death in few weeks of life.
Omenn syndrome	- The manufacture of immunoglobulins requires recombinase enzymes derived from the recombination activating genes RAG-1 and RAG-2. These enzymes are involved in the first stage of V(D)J recombination, the process by which segments of a B cell or T cell's DNA are rearranged to create a new T or B cell receptor (and, in the B cell's case, the template for antibodies). - Certain mutations of the RAG-1 or RAG-2 genes prevent V(D)J recombination, causing SCID.
Bare lymphocyte syndrome	- **Type 1:** MHC class I is not expressed on the cell surface. The defect is caused by defective TAP proteins, not the MHC-I protein. - **Type 2:** MHC class II is not expressed on the cell surface of all APCs. Autosomal recessive. The MHC-II gene regulatory proteins are what is altered, not the MHC-II protein itself.
JAK3	Janus kinase-3 (JAK3) is an enzyme that mediates transduction downstream of the γ chain signal. Mutation of its gene causes SCID.
Artemis / DCLRE1C	Although researchers have identified about a dozen genes that cause SCID, the Navajo and Apache population has the most severe form of the disorder. This is due to the lack of a gene **called artemis**. Without the gene, children's bodies are unable to repair DNA or develop disease-fighting cells.
Swiss type agamma-globulinemia	Defect at lymphoid stem cell level

Table-1: Pathogenic types of SCID

- B cell count is normal: Normal IgG & IgA. Decreased IgM & raised IgE
- Inability to respond to polysaccharide Ag, due to defect in AMI.
- Cellular depletion of thymus.

✪ **Clinical features:**
- Recurrent infection
- Eczema
- Thrombocytopenic purpura
- Death of affected patient is occurs in 1st decade of life due to infection, haemorrhage or lymphoreticular malignancy.

✪ **Treatment:** Bone marrow & TF transplantation

B. Deficiency of non-specific immune system:

i. Deficiency of phagocytosis

* **Introduction:** Two types of defect

1. **Intrinsic:** Defect in cell. E. g. enzyme deficiency
2. **Extrinsic:** Due to deficiency of opsonin, effect of drugs or by presence of anti-neutrophil Ab.

* **Common diseases due to deficiency of phagocytosis are described below**

a. Chronic Granulomatous Disease (CGD):

✪ **Pathogenesis:**
- Familiar disease
- X-linked (70%) in boys and autosomal recessive (30%) in girls.
- Associated with defect inH_2O_2 production (due to defect in NADPH oxidase) that kills bacteria, O_2 consumption, hexose monophosphate pathway & myloperoxidase release.

✪ **Clinical features:**
- Recurrent infection by catalase positive bacteria like *Staphylococci*, coliforms etc.
- Catalase -Ve bacteria are handled normally.
- Chronic granulomatous lesion in skin, lymph nodes, lungs & in bones with hepatosplenomegaly

✪ **Diagnosis:** By following tests

1. **Nitroblue Tetrazolium (NBT) reduction test:**

• **Principle:**
- In normal patient phagocytic cells (microphages & macrophages) produces the enzyme NADPH oxidase which is responsible for production of H_2O_2 & other free radicals. These free radicals reduce NBT to formazan.
- In patient with CGD, NADPH oxidase is not produced so no production of H_2O_2 & other free radicals & no reduction of NBT to formazan.

• **Result:**
- **+Ve test:** Reduction of NBT to formazan, means CGD is absent
- **-Ve test:** No reduction of NBT to formazan, means CGD is present

• **Uses:** Screening test for CGD

2. **Di Hydro Rhodamine (DHR) test:**
3. **Immunoblot test for NADPH production:**

b. Myeloperoxidase deficiency: Deficiency of myeloperoxidase in leucocytes increases the chances of *C. albicans* infection.

c. Chediak-Higashi syndrome:

✪ **Pathogenesis & clinical features:**

• **Defective LYST gene:**
- Autosomal recessive disease due to defect/mutation in LYST gene, which is encodes for lysosome of phagocytic cells.
- Lysosome contains many enzymes required to kill the bacteria. During phagocytosis lysosome fuse with phagosome to form phagolysosome. Once phagolysosome has been formed lysosome secrete the all necessary enzymes.
- Due to defect in LYST gene, structure & functions of lysosome are disturbed & it is not able to fuse with phagosome to form phagolysosome, resulting impaired bacteriolysis leads to persistent infections in infancy & early childhood which may be life threatening

• **Other defects:** Beside lysosomal fusion defect , it also associated with other cellular defect like
- Melanocytes: Contains large melanosome → reduced melanin production → albinism, characterised by decreased pigmentation of skin, eyes & hair
- Granules in Schwann cells: Peripheral neuropathy
- Abnormal platelets: Bleeding disorders.
- Giant peroxidise positive granules / inclusions in leucocytes. Peroxidise positive inclusion is result of autophagocytic activity
- Eye: Photophobia & nystagmus
- Accelerated phase defect: WBCs divide uncontrollably & invade many organs leading to fever, bleeding disorders, overwhelming infections, organs failure & may be death.

d. Leucocyte G6PD deficiency:
- Deficiency of G6PD reduce bactericidal effect of phagocytes
- It is like CGD in reduced myeloperoxidase activity and increases the chances of infection.
- NBT test is normal.

e. Job's syndrome:

✪ **Pathogenesis:**
- Not clear but due to defect in phagocytic activity.
- Little inflammatory response
- Serum Ig is normal but increased IgE.

✪ **Clinical features:**
- Multiple, recurrent cold *Staphylococci* abscess in skin & other organs.
- Otitis media
- Atopic eczema
- Chronic nasal discharge

f. Tuftsin deficiency:

- Tuftsin is a leukokinin discovered in Tufts University, Boston
- It is tetrapeptide (Thr-Lys-Arg)
- It stimulates the phagocytic activity.
- Deficiency of Tuftsin increases the chances of local & systemic infections.

g. Lazy leucocyte syndrome:

✪ **Pathogenesis:**
- Bone marrow has normal numbers of neutrophils, but due to defect in chemotaxis & mobility peripheral neutropenia occurs.
- Poor response to inflammatory & chemical stimulation.

✪ **Clinical features:**
- Increased susceptibility to bacterial infections
- Otitis media
- Gingivitis
- Recurrent stomatitis.

h. Hyper IgE syndrome:

✪ **Pathogenesis:** AMI & CMI are normal but increased ten times level of IgE.

✪ **Clinical features:**
- Early onset of eczema
- Recurrent *Staph aureus* & *Strept. pyogenes* infection with abscess & pneumonia

i. Actin binding protein deficiency:
- Frequent infection
- Slow mobility of leucocytes

j. Shwachman's disease:
- Frequent infection
- Slow mobility of neutrophils
- Pancreatic malfunction
- Bone abnormalities

ii. Complement (C) deficiency: **Follow chapter → Complement system**

Secondary IDDs

➢ **Definition:** Immunodeficiencies due to factors interfere with functions of immune system.

➢ **Etiological factors:** Due to
- Physical agents: Like radiation
- Chemical agents: Like immunosuppressive drugs
- Biological agents: Like diseases such as AIDS
- Malnutrition or
- Other process like old age

➢ **Subtypes:**

i. AMI (HI) deficiency:
- B-cell deficiency in chronic lymphatic leukemia
- Ig catabolism in nephritic syndrome
- Excessive loss of serum proteins in exfoliative skin disease & protein loosing enteropathies.
- Over production of Ig in multiple myeloma

ii. CMI deficiency:
- CMI deficiency in Hodgkin's disease
- Obstruction of lymph circulation.
- Thymus dependant area is infiltrated with non-lymphoid cells in Lepromatous Leprosy (LL)
- Viral infection like measles

iii. Combined deficiency of AMI & CMI:
- Old age
- Malnutrition
- Immunosuppressive drugs
- Disease: Like AIDS
- Radiation
- Anti lymphocyte antibody.

Question bank

Case study

1) A 11 month old male child is brought to the hospital with history of fever & dyspnoea. Mother reported attack of measles with full recovery in previous month. Lymph node biopsy revealed depleted bursa dependent areas. IgA, IgM & IgG are less than normal level. Identify the clinical conditions & answer the following
a) Name the clinical condition or syndrome
b) Write clinical features & diagnosis of clinical condition
c) Write treatment of clinical condition

2) A 10 year old girl child is brought to the paediatric OPD with history of cough, common cold & fever since a very long time. Identify the clinical conditions & answer the following
d) Name the Ig deficient in given clinical condition
e) Draw the structure of Ig deficient in given case
f) Describe in detail about IDDs due to deficiency of AMI

Essay/Full question

1) Immunodeficiency diseases (IDDs)

Short notes

1) Define & classify the immunodeficiency diseases
2) Primary immunodeficiency diseases
3) Secondary immunodeficiency diseases

Short questions for theory/viva questions

1) Define primary immunodeficiency diseases
2) Define secondary immunodeficiency diseases

MCQs for chapter review

Primary IDDs

Deficiency of AMI

1) **The commonest primary immunodeficiency** is (AI-94, PGI, June-05)
(a) Common variable immunodeficiency (b) Isolated IgA immunodeficiency (c) Wiskott – Aldrich syndrome (d) AIDS

2) **All are true regarding agammaglobulinemia except** (PGI-01)
(a) Loss of germinal centre in lymph node (b) Normal cortical lymphocytes (c) Normal cortical lymphocytes in paracortex and medulla (d) Decreased red pulp in spleen (e) Immunodeficiency (cell mediated)

3) **A child present with recurrent episode of sinopulmonary infection by bacteria with polysaccharide rich capsule. Deficiency of which of the following immunoglobulin subclasses should be investigated** (AI-12, AIIMS, May -12)
(a) IgA (b) IgG1 (c) IgG2 (d) IgA + IgG2

4) **True about Bloom syndrome**
a) Decreased IgG (b) Decreased IgM (c) IgA absent (d) Increased IgE

5) **Nucleotidase deficiency**
a) Humoral immunity deficiency (b) Acquired immunity deficiency (c) SCIDs (d) Cell mediated immunity deficiency

6) **Giardiasis is associated with** (AIIMS, Feb-97, Nov-02)
a) Common variable immuno deficiency (b) C_1 esterase deficiency (c) C_8 deficiency (d) Anaemia

Deficiency of CMI

7) **Which is found in Di George syndrome** (PGI-01)
(a) Tetany (b) Eczema (c) Mucocutaneous candidiasis (d) Absent B and T cells (e) Total absence of T cells

8) **Di George syndrome is characterised by all except**
(a) Congenital thymic aplasia (b) Abnormal development of 3rd and 4th pouch (c) Hypothyroidism (d) Hypocalcemic tetany

9) **Which fungal infection is commonest occur in neutropenia** (AIIMS, June-99)
(a) *Candida* (b) *Histoplasma* (c) *Aspergillus niger* (d) *Aspergillus fumigatus*

Combined deficiency of AMI & CMI

10) **Adenosine deaminase deficiency is seen in the following** (AI-01, 05)
(a) Common variable immunodeficiency (b) Severe combined immunodeficiency (c) Chronic granulomatous disease (d) Nezelof syndrome

11) **Which of the following about SCID is false**
(a) Due to malfunction of adenylate kinase-2 (b) Peyer's patches are present and normal (c) X-linked type is the most common (d) Gene therapy is used

12) **Wiskott – Aldrich not true is** (AIIMS 97)
(a) Raised IgE (b) Raised IgM (c) Reduced IgA (d) CD4 and CD8 defect

13) **A patient present with thrombocytopenia, eczema and recurrent infection**
(a) Wiskott – Aldrich syndrome (b) Di George syndrome (c) Agammaglobulinemia (d) SCID

Deficiency of phagocytosis

14) **Which of the following statement is correct regarding chronic granulomatous disease** (AIIMS, Nov-04)
(a) It is an autosomal dominant disease (b) It is characterised by abnormal bacterial phagocytosis (c) Recurrent streptococcal infections are usual in this disease (d) Nitroblue tetrazolium test is useful for screening

15) **Chronic granulomatous disorder is due to defect in**
(a) B cell (b) NADPH oxidase (c) IgA (d) T cell

16) **Most common cause of chronic granulomatous disease in children is** (AI-98)
(a) Myeloperoxidase deficiency (b) Defective phagocytosis (c) Defective H_2O_2 production (d) Job's disease

17) **The NBT (Nitroblue tetrazolium) reduction assay is used to**
(a) Evaluate granulocyte function (b) Evaluate T cell function (c) Determine whether polymorphonuclear leucocytes can produce superoxide (d) Stain B lymphocytes

18) **Candida infection is common in**
(a) Chronic granulomatous disease (b) Chediak-Higashi syndrome (c) Myeloperoxidase deficiency (d) Lazy leucocyte syndrome

19) **Chediak-Higashi syndrome, defect is**
(a) Fusion of lysosome (b) T cells (c) B cells (d) Complement

20) **Chediak-Higashi syndrome , true is**
(a) Defect in phagocytosis (b) Neutropenia (c) Agammaglobulinemia (d) IgA deficiency

21) **Job's syndrome is the following type of immunodeficiency diseases?**
(a) Humoral immunodeficiency (b) Cellular immunodeficiency (c) Disorder of complement (d) Disorder of phagocytosis

Answers of MCQs & explanation

1) **(b)**
- Selective IgA immunodeficiency is the most common primary IDD

2) **(b), (c), (d) & (e)**
- Follow section, **deficiency of AMI (X-linked agammaglobulinemia)** for explanation

3) **(d)**
- Follow section, **deficiency of AMI [Combined deficiencies of IgA & IgG (IgG2)]** for explanation

4) **(b)**
- Follow section, **deficiency of AMI (Bloom syndrome)** for explanation

5) **(a)**
- Follow section, **deficiency of AMI (Nucleotidase deficiency)** for explanation

6) **(a)**
- Follow section, **deficiency of AMI (Combined variable immuno deficiency)** for explanation

7) **(a) & (c)**
8) **(c)**
} Follow section, **deficiency of CMI (Di George syndrome)** for explanation

9) **(a)**
- Follow section, **deficiency of CMI (Chronic Mucocutaneous Candidiasis)** for explanation

10) **(b)**
11) **(b)**
} Follow section, **combined deficiency of AMI & CMI (SCID & table-1)** for explanation

12) **(b) & (c)**
13) **(a)**
} Follow section, **Combined deficiency of AMI & CMI (Wiskott – Aldrich syndrome)** for explanation

14) **(d)**
15) **(b)**
16) **(c)**
17) **(c)**
} Follow section, **phagocytosis (chronic granulomatous disease)** for explanation

18) **(c)**
- Deficiency of myeloperoxidase in leucocytes increases the chances of *C. albicans* infection
- *Candida* infection is also common in syndrome where CMI is deficient as described in text.

19) **(a)**
20) **(a)**
} Follow section, **phagocytosis (Chediak-Higashi syndrome)** for explanation

21) **(d)**
- Follow section, **phagocytosis (Job's syndrome)** for explanation

28 Autoimmunity

Learning heading & subheadings

- History:
- Meaning:
- Definition:
- Common features of autoimmune diseases:
- Mechanisms/ steps:
- Classification:
- Diagnosis:
- Treatment:

❖ **History:** Paul Ehrlich gives the concept of 'horror autotoxicus' means horror of self toxicity.

❖ **Meaning:**

- Literally meaning "protection against self" but actually it is an "injury to self."
- Normally immune system shows tolerance to self
- It is a condition in which tolerance or unresponsiveness to self is breakdown & production of autoimmune diseases.

❖ **Definition:** Abnormal immune response in which antibodies or sensitized lymphocytes are capable of reacting with self components **called autoimmunity**.

❖ **Common features of autoimmune diseases:**

- Increased level of antibodies **called autoantibodies**
- Autoantibodies are demonstrable
- Accumulation of Abs, plasma cells & lymphocytes at target site like renal glomeruli.
- More in females
- Chronic
- Non-reversible
- Occurrence of more than one lesion in patients.
- Benefit after steroid therapy.

❖ **Mechanisms / steps:** Autoimmunity developed in two steps

Step-I: Formation of autoantibody or sensitisation of lymphocyte

Step-II: Action of formed autoantibody or sensitised lymphocyte

Step-I: Formation of autoantibody or sensitisation of lymphocyte

➢ **Mechanisms:** By following ways

i. Neo-antigen:

✪ **Definition:** Native cell or tissue antigen may undergo antigenic alteration by different factors and assume a new antigenic specificity **called neo-antigen or altered antigen.** This altered antigen stimulates immune reaction and cause tissue injury.

✪ **Factors:**

- **Physical:** Irradiation, photosensitivity, cold-allergy
- **Chemical:**
  - Contact dermatitis due to contact of chemical with skin protein.
  - Drug induced anaemia, leucopenia & thrombocytopenia
- **Biological:**
  - Infectious mononucleosis in Epstein-Barr Virus (EBV)
  - Many bacteria acts on RBCs & releasing T-Ag
- **Genetic:** Mutation

ii. Release of hidden or sequestered antigen:

✪ **Definition:**

- **Self Antigen:** Tissue antigen which is unable to induce immune response because exposed to lympho-reticular system during embryonic life & identified as self antigen.
- **Sequestered antigen:** Tissue antigen anatomically confined to site which is not access by lympho-reticular system & it is unable to induce immune response but when it exposed free in circulation it is identified as foreign & induce immune response. This tissue Ag **called sequestered antigen**.

✪ **Examples:**

- Eye lens protein
- Brain tissue protein
- Thyroglobulin
- Sperm

iii. Cross reaction with microbial antigens or molecular mimicry:

✪ **Definition:** Antigenic similarities between foreign antigen (**called heterophile antigen** or **cross reacting antigen**) & self antigen are the basis of this theory. Antibody formed in response to foreign antigen may cross react with self antigen of to produce tissue damage.

✪ **Examples:** Cross reaction between

1. **Human & sheep brain antigens:** Anti-rabies vaccine prepared from sheep brain when injected in human it produce antibody which may cause neurological injury in human due to antigenic cross reactivity between human brain & sheep brain antigens.
2. **Streptococcal antigens & human tissue:** Like

- Plasma membrane and vascular intima/glomeruli (**called nephritogenic strain**): Causing glomerulonephritis
- Peptidoglycan and skin Ag
- Group A carbohydrate and cardiac valves
- Protein M Ag and myocardium: Repeated streptococcal infection can therefore damage the heart to produces the rheumatic fever
- Hyaluronic acid capsule and human synovial fluid

3. **Cornea & HSV- I:** Causing stromal keratitis
4. **Joint membrane & *M. Tuberculosis*:**
5. **Myocardium & Coxsackie B virus:**
6. **HLA-B27 & arthritogenic *Sh. flexneri*:**

iv. Polyclonal B-lymphocyte activation:

✪ **Definition:** Instead of normal specific stimulation of B-cells by Ag, there is abnormal, non-specific stimulation of B-cells by antigen resulting multiple non specific Abs are formed. Polyclonal Ab is IgM in nature & produced by CD5+ B cells.

✪ **Examples of agents causing polyclonal activation:**

- **Chemical:**
  - Nystatin
  - 2-mercaptoethanol
- **Biological:**
  - Virus: EBV which produces anti-sheep erythrocyte antibodies
  - Bacteria: *Mycoplasma pneumoniae* which produces anti-human erythrocyte cold antibodies & bacterial products like PPD, LPS
  - Parasites: Malaria
- **Enzymes:** Trypsin

v. Forbidden clones:

✪ **Definition:** It is due breakdown of tolerance to self - Ag & production of Ir to self-Ag

✪ **Examples:** Injection of self-Ag with Freund's adjuvants

vi. Loss of immunoregulation:

✪ **Examples:**

- Increased activity of T helper cells & decreased activity of T suppressor cells
- Defects in development of stem cells in the thymus
- Defect in macrophages function.
- Defect in idiotype-anti-idiotype of network

vii. Genetic factors:

a. Defect in genes of Ig or Ir

b. Association between HLA type and certain diseases:

- An association has been observed between HLA type and certain diseases.
- Such diseases are generally of uncertain origin, associated with immunological abnormalities and exhibit a hereditary tendency.
- For example
  - Ankylosing spondylitis and HLA-B27
  - Rheumatoid arthritis and HLA-DR4
  - Many autoimmune conditions and HLA-DR3.

Step-II: Action of formed autoantibody or sensitised lymphocyte

➢ **Mechanisms:** Exact mechanisms are unknown, but may cause damage by hypersensitivity reaction, as described below

a. Type II (cytotoxic or cytolytic): Damage or destruction of cell by Ab. The antibody could be

- Lytic for cell: Thrombocytopenia, Agranulocytosis (agrnulosis or granulopenia), autoimmune haemolytic anaemia etc.
- Supportive to other cell: Antibody dependent cellular cytotoxicity
- Cell stimulatory (separately classified as type V hypersensitivity): Grave's disease
- Cell inhibitory: Pernicious anaemia, myasthenia gravis etc.

b. Type III (immune complex or toxic complex disease):

- Damage or destruction of cell by Ag-Ab complex.
- Mostly seen in RA, SLE, PAN, post streptococcal glomerulonephritis etc.

c. Type IV (delayed or cell mediated hypersensitivity):

- Damage or destruction of cell by T-cells.
- Mostly seen in multiple sclerosis.

d. Type V (stimulatory hypersensitivity):

- No damage or destruction of cell but stimulation of cell by Ab & which increase the secretion.
- Mostly seen in Grave's disease

e. Combined effect by Ab & T-cells: Mostly seen in experimental orchitis.

❖ **Classification:** Based on location & nature of lesion, autoimmune diseases are classified as follows.

A. **Haemocytolytic autoimmune diseases:**
B. **Organ specific (localized) autoimmune diseases:**
C. **Non-organ specific (systemic) autoimmune diseases:**
D. **Transitory autoimmune diseases:**

A. Haemocytolytic autoimmune diseases:

i. Autoimmune thrombocytopenia:

✪ **Definition:** Presence of Ab to platelets

✪ **Examples:**

- Idiopathic thrombocytopenic purpura
- Sedormid purpura: It is drug induced

ii. Autoimmune leucopenia:

✪ **Definition:** Presence of Ab to leucocytes

✪ **Examples:**

- SLE
- RA

iii. Autoimmune hemolytic anemia:

✪ **Definition:** Presence of Ab to RBCs.

- ✪ **RBC destruction:** RBCs coated by Abs are prematurely killed by spleen & liver in haemolytic anaemia.
- ✪ **Examples:** Two groups are identified
- • **Cold antibodies**:
  - Complete, agglutinating IgM Abs which agglunatinate erythrocytes at 4° C but not at 37° C.
  - Produced in primary atypical pneumonia caused by *Mycoplasma pneumoniae*, black water fever & Trypanosomiasis.
  - Detected by cold agglutination test.
- • **Warm antibodies:**
  - Incomplete, non-agglutinating IgG Abs
  - Produced due to sulphonamides, alpha-methyldopa etc
  - Detected by direct Coombs test.

B. Organ specific (localized) autoimmune diseases:

i. Myasthenia gravis:

✪ **Pathogenesis:**
- Abs against acetylcholine (Ach) receptors at neuromuscular junction in striated muscles.
- It prevents the combination of Ach with its receptor & impairs the muscle contraction.
- Child born from affected mother shows the symptoms & gets clear with increasing age, which indicates that autoantibodies are passively acquired from mother.

ii. Hashimoto's disease:

✪ **Synonym:** Lymhadenoid goitre

✪ **Pathogenesis:**
- Cytotoxic autoantibody are produced which react mainly with thyroglobulin & also with acinar colloid, microsomal antigen & thyroid cell surface component & cause enlargement of thyroid gland.
- Symptoms of hypothyroidism or frank myxoedema.
- Frequently seen in females.

iii. Grave's disease:

✪ **Synonym:** Thyrotoxicosis or Hyperthyroidism

✪ **Pathogenesis:**
- IgG type **auto-antibodies called Long Acting Thyroid Stimulator (LATS)**, against some determinant of thyroid cells, which stimulate excessive secretion of thyroid hormones leading to Grave's disease.
- Sometime it considered as part of Type II hypersensitivity.

iv. Pernicious anemia:

✪ **Pathogenesis:** Two types of antibodies are produced :

1. Against parietal cells of gastric mucosa which cause achlorhydria & atrophic gastritis.
2. Against the intrinsic factor which prevents the absorption of vitamin B12 & cause megaloblastic anaemia.

v. Addison's disease:

✪ **Pathogenesis:** Lymphocytic infiltration of adrenal glands & antibodies against zona glomerulosa are seen

vi. Insulin dependent diabetes mellitus:

✪ **Pathogenesis:**
- Auto-reactive T cell attack on islet cell enzyme glutamic acid decarboxylase.
- Antibodies against various antigens of β- cells also are produced but major damage by T cells that destroy the islet cells of pancreas.
- Coxsackie virus B4 triggers the disease because a six amino acid sequence is common between Coxsackie virus B4 & glutamic acid decarboxylase.

vii. Celiac disease:

✪ **Pathogenesis:** Gliadin is the antigen that stimulates cytotoxic T-cells which attack on enterocytes, resulting in villous atrophy.

viii. Autoimmune diseases of nervous system:

a. Multiple sclerosis:

✪ **Pathogenesis:**
- autorective T cells & activated macrophages causes demyelination of the white matter of brain.
- Viral infection like EBV triggers the disease mostly in people with HLA DR2 positive.

b. Guillain-Barre syndrome:

✪ **Pathogenesis:**
- Ab against myelin protein are formed which result in demyelinating polyneuropathy.
- Occurs in infection by C. jejuni & in some viral infections also

c. Neuroparalysis: Occurs following rabies vaccination due to cross reaction between human & sheep brain antigens.

ix. Autoimmune diseases of eye:

a. Phacoanaphylaxis: Intraocular inflammation due to autoimmune response to lens proteins following cataract surgery

b. Perforating injury: Involve the iris or ciliary bodies following the sympathetic opnthalmia in the opposite eye.

x. Autoimmune diseases of skin:

a. Pemphigus vulgaris: Abs against desmoglein are formed which result in disruption of tight junctions between epithelial cells & formation of bullae all over the body.

b. Bullous pephigoid: Abs against dermal epithelial junction has been noticed.

c. Dermatitis herpetiformis: Specific Ab is not identified

C. Non-organ specific (systemic) autoimmune diseases:

i. Rheumatoid Arthritis (RA):

✪ **Pathogenesis:**
- In this disease, IgM type autoantibodies against Fc portion of IgG are produced **called Rheumatoid Factor** (RF).

- Other classes of Abs like IgA, IgE & IgG are also noticed.
- Autoantibody (IgM) bind with circulating IgG & makes an IgM-IgG complex (Type III hypersensitivity → immune complex disease →serum sickness) which deposited in the joint & stimulates compliment system to destroy the cells & to recruits neutrophils.

✪ **Clinical features:**
- More in women
- Polyartritis, muscle wasting, subcutaneous nodules, serositis, myocarditis, vasculitis & other disseminated lesions.

✪ **Diagnosis:**
1. Rose Waaler test:
2. Modified Rose Waaler test:

} **Follow chapter → Antigen-antibody (Ag-Ab) reactions**

ii. Systemic Lupus Erythematosus (SLE):

✪ **Meaning:**
- Word systemic indicates the wide range of distribution
- Lupus: **Lupus (Latin) = "wolf"**, the disease was so-named in the 13th century as the rash was thought to appear like a wolf's bite.
- Erythematosus because of development of red rash across the nose and upper cheeks on both side

✪ **Synonym:** Simply **called lupus.**

✪ **Etiology:** The Exact cause of SLE is not clear. It is due to genetics, environmental or by following precipitating factors.
1. **Age:** Women of childbearing age are affected about nine times more often than men. It most commonly begins between the ages of 15 and 45.
2. **Races:** African, Caribbean, & Chinese descent are at higher risk than white people
3. **Others:** Female sex hormones, sunlight, smoking, vitamin D deficiency &certain infections, are also believed to increase the risk.

✪ **Pathogenesis:**
- A variety of auto-antibodies directed against cell nuclei (antinuclear Ab), intracytoplasmic cell constituents, thyroid, RBCs, WBCs & other unknown antigens are produced.
- The important immunological feature is **LE cell phenomenon**. The **LE cell** is a PMN- leucocyte with ingested nuclear material complexed with anti-nuclear antibody (type III hypersensitivity → immune complex disease →serum sickness).

✪ **Clinical features:**
- Patient present with a red rash across the nose and upper cheeks on both sides gives butterfly appearance as shown in **fig.-1**.
- Other symptoms are painful & swollen joints, fever, chest pain, hair loss, mouth ulcers, swollen lymph nodes & feeling tired
- Often there are periods of illness, **called flares**, and periods of remission during which there are few symptoms.

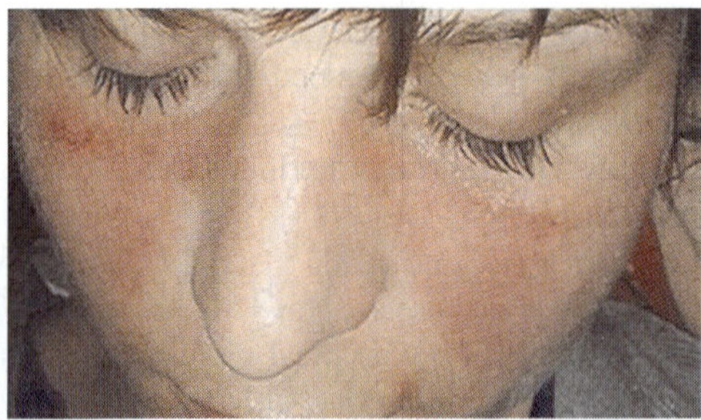

Figure-1: "Butterfly rash" found in lupus

- Haemolytic anaemia, thrombocytopenia, leucopenia, lesion in kidneys, vascular tissues, joints, spleen & heart are seen.

✪ **Diagnosis:**
- **Detection of LE cells**
  - By incubating patient's blood or bone-marrow at 37° C & then observing for LE cells.
  - **Giemsa stained** smear can demonstrate LE cells but less sensitive.
- **Detection of antinuclear Ab:**
  - By Immunofluorescence test
  - Sensitive but less specific
- **Anti-DNA antibodies detection:**
  - Types: Three types of anti-DNA antibodies
    - Ab to ss-DNA
    - Ab to ds-DNA
    - Ab to ss & ds -DNA
  - Tests: Tested by RIA or ELISA.
  - Interpretation: High titer of anti-ds DNA antibody is relatively specific for SLE.
- Another SLE specific Ab is anti-sm antibody.

✪ **Treatment:**
- NSAIDs
- Corticosteroids
- Immunosuppressants: Hydroxychloroquine, and methotrexate.

✪ **Prognosis:**
- Life expectancy is lower among people with SLE.
- SLE significantly increases the risk of cardiovascular disease with this being the most common cause of death.
- With modern treatment about 80% of those affected survive more than 15 years.
- Women with lupus have pregnancies that are higher risk but are mostly successful

iii. Sjogren's syndrome:

✪ **Pathogenesis:** Varieties of antibodies are formed like antinuclear antibodies, RF, antibodies against salivary duct, lacrimal glands, smooth muscle, mitochondria, thyroid gland etc.

✪ **Clinical features:** Triad of kerato-conjunctivitis sicca, xerostomia with or without salivary gland enlargement & RA.

iv. Polyarteritis Nodosa (PAN):

✪ **Pathogenesis:**

- It is a component of serum sickness & other immune complex diseases (Type III hypersensitivity).
- Autoimmune disease but autoantibody is not identified.

✪ **Clinical features:**
- It is a necrotizing angitis involves the small and medium sized arteries.
- The disease end fatally due to coronary thrombosis, cerebral haemorrhage or gastro-intestinal bleeding.
- It is more commonly seen in males.

v. Wegener's granulomatosis:
- It is a necrotizing granulomatous vasculitis that primarily affects the upper and lower respiratory tracts & kidneys.
- Diagnosed by finding antineutrophil cytoplasmic antibodies (ANCA) in patient's serum.

vi. Reiter's syndrome: Follow chapter → Neisseriae, Moraxellaceae and Mimeae for more details

vii. Goodpasture's syndrome:
- Antibodies against collagen in basement membranes of the kidneys & lungs are formed.
- It affects young men & those with HLA-DR2 genes positive.
- Diagnosed by detection of Ab & compliment C5a bound to basement membranes in fluorescent-antibody test.

D. Transitory autoimmune diseases:

✪ **Etiological factor:** Certain microbial infections or drug therapy.

✪ **Pathogenesis:** The infecting agent or drug induces antigenic alteration in some self-Ag that initiates an Ir leading to tissue damage.

✪ **Clinical features:** Anaemia, thrombocytopenia or nephritis

✪ **Treatment:** It is transient & recovery occurs following removal of causative factors.

❖ **Diagnosis: General tests** [(CRP, autoantibody titers (anti DNA, anti phospholipids, presence of RF)] & **disease specific tests**

❖ **Treatment:**
1. **T-cell vaccination:** Suppresses the autoimmune cells.
2. **Synthetic blocking peptide:** Compete with autoantigen for binding to MHC molecules
3. **Immunosuppressive drugs:**
4. **Thymectomy:** Removal of thymus
5. **Plasmapheresis:** Removes Ag-Ab complexes & reduction in symptoms for a short-term.

Question bank

Case study

1) A 40 year female visited the orthopaedic OPD with history of pain in wrist joint. Physical examination revealed subcutaneous nodule. Autoantibody is diagnosed by serological test. Identify the clinical conditions & answer the following
a) Name the clinical condition & one serological test useful to diagnose it.
b) Write the mechanisms of autoimmunisation
c) Classify the autoimmune diseases.

2) A 30 year female visited the skin OPD with history of red rash across the nose and upper cheeks on both sides in butterfly fashion. Anti nuclear antibody is diagnosed by serological test. Patient is responsive to immunosuppressive drugs. Identify the clinical conditions & answer the following
a) Name the clinical condition & one serological test useful to diagnose it.
b) Write the etio-pathogenesis of given case.
c) Write the diagnosis of given case.

Essay/Full question

1) Autoimmunity

Short notes

1) Mechanisms of autoimmunity
2) Types of autoimmunity
3) SLE

Short questions for theory/viva questions

1) Define autoimmunity
2) What is neo-antigen?
3) What is LE cell?

MCQs for chapter review

1) **Epstein Barr virus causes autoimmunity by-** (AI-12)
(a) Molecular mimicry (b) Release of sequestrated antigen (c) Inappropriate expression of MHC class II molecules (d) Polyclonal Bb cell activation

2) **All are true about autoimmune disease except**
(a) T cell recognise the auto antigen (b) Polyclonal B cell activation (c) Higher incidence in male (d) Hashimoto;s thyroiditis is an example of autoimmune disease

3) **Example of sequestrated antigen is**
(a) Eye lens protein (b) Liver cell antigen (c) Intestinal epithelial cell (d) Macrophage cell

Answers of MCQs & explanation

1) **(d)**
- Epstein Barr virus causes autoimmunity by polyclonal B cell activation

2) **(c)**
- Autoimmune diseases are more common in female

3) **(a)**
- Follow section, **mechanism/steps (release of sequestered antigen) for explanation.**

29 Immunology of transplantation and malignancy

Learning heading & subheadings

- Immunology of transplantation
- Immunology of malignancy

Immunology of transplantation

❖ Definitions:

➢ **Transplant or graft:** Tissue or organs selected for transplantation is **called transplant** or **graft**.

➢ **Donor:** Individual from whom transplant or graft is obtained **called donor**.

➢ **Recipient:** Individual to whom transplant or graft is applied **called recipient**.

❖ Classification of transplant or graft:

A. Based on organ or tissues transplanted: Kidney, heart, liver, skin transplant etc.

B. Based on anatomical site of origin & placement:

1. **Orthotropic:** Both sites are same like skin graft
2. **Heterotropic:** Both sites are different like Thyroid tissue placed in subcutaneous pocket.

C. Based on duration after receiving the graft:

1. **Fresh graft:**
2. **Stored graft:**

D. Based on viability

1. **Vital graft:** Living graft like kidney, heart, liver or skin transplant.
2. **Structural/static:** Non-living graft like bone/artery.

E. Based on genetic & antigenic relationship between donor & recipient:

1. **Autograft:**
   - Definition: Transplantation in the same individual.
   - Example: Skin graft from one site of patient to other site of same patient (donor & recipient are same).
2. **Isograft:**
   - Definition: Transplantation between genetically identical individuals & same species.
   - Example: Twins (donor & recipient are synergic member).
3. **Allograft or homograft:**
   - Definition: Transplantation between two genetically non-identical members but same species.
   - Skin graft from cadaver (human donor) to patient (human recipient).
4. **Xenograft or heterograft:**
   - Definition: Transplantation between genetically un-identical members & different species.
   - Baboon heart (animal donor) to human (human recipient).

❖ Allograft rejection:

➢ **Basis of allograft rejection:**

- When a graft is applied to genetically unrelated animal of same species, it looks health & seems to be accepted initially.
- Approximately on 4th day, graft is invaded by lymphocytes & macrophages, occlusion of blood vessels by thrombi & necrosis of graft.
- Graft becomes scab-like & sloughs off by 10th day **called 1st set rejection or reaction or response**.
- If another graft is applied from same donor, it is rejected in accelerated fashion **called 2nd set rejection or reaction or response**.
- If another graft is applied from other donor, it is rejected by 1st set rejection.
- Allograft is accepted if animal is immunologically tolerant.

➢ **Mechanisms of allograft rejection:** Graft is rejected by lymphocytes and/ or by antibodies.

✪ **Rejection by lymphocytes:** Play major role in graft rejection-

- Directly by Tc cells.
- Directly by NK cells.
- Indirectly by releasing lymphokines.
- By ADCC.

✪ **Rejection by antibodies:**

- Antibodies are formed more rapidly & abundantly during 2nd set response & play important role with CMI in 2nd set response.
- Antibodies formed are detected by serological tests.
- It deposited along the vascular endothelium & activates the complement & coagulation system which result in
- Inflammatory cells infiltration.
- Platelets thrombi.
- Fibrin deposition.
- Coagulative necrosis.
- Play role in graft rejection by ADCC.
- When graft is applied to recipient with high Ab titre, **hyperacute rejection** take place. Graft becomes pale & rejected immediately in hours **called white graft response**.
- High Abs titre present prior transplantation, pregnancy, transfusion.
- Hyperacute rejection take place sometimes following kidney transplant.

❖ Measures to prevent graft rejection:

➢ **MHC testing:**
- Graft is rejected due to presence of Ags in graft tissue, which are absent in donor.
- Graft is not rejected, if same Ags are present in donor & recipient.
- Following methods are employed to match the Ags of donor & recipient.
  - o ABO blood grouping.
  - o HLA typing by
  - Micro-cytotoxicity testing.
  - Molecular methods like RFLP, PCR, Southern blotting etc.
  - Tissue matching: MLR (Mixed Leucocytes Reaction) or MLC (Mixed Leucocytes Culture).

➢ **Uses of immunosuppressive agents:** **Follow chapter → Immune response (Ir)**

➢ **Immunological enhancement:**

✪ **Definition:** Abs produced may act opposite to CMI & prevent the graft rejection **called immunological enhancement.**

✪ **History:** 1st described by Kaliss in tumour transplant.

✪ **Method:** It happens when recipient is pre-treated with one or more injection of killed donor tissue & than graft is applied, the graft survival is increased.

✪ **Mechanisms of action:** Abs act by following three possible ways.

a. **Afferent inhibition:** Abs are combines with Ags released from graft & prevent the induction of Ir.

b. **Central inhibition:** Abs are combines with specific lymphoid cells, make them incapable to generate Ir to graft Ags.

c. **Efferent inhibition:** Abs are coating the cells of graft & prevent their contact with sensitised lymphoid cells.

➢ **Privileged sites:** These are sites where allograft are permitted to survive & safe from immunological attack.

a. **Foetus in uterus:** foetus is protected from maternal immunological attack by
- Immunological barrier of placenta.
- Relative resistance of cell membrane of trophoblastic cell to T or K cells.
- Low density of MHC-Ags on trophoblastic cell.
- Muco-polysaccharide barrier rich in sialic acid in trophoblastic cell protect them from Tc cells.
- High level of α-feto protein which protect foetus from immunological damage by maternal leucocytes entering in foetal circulation.
- Shedding of foetal Ags, which blocks the Abs or T cells by enhancement effect.

b. **Cartilage:** Less accessible by immunocompetent cells (ICC).

c. **Brain or hamster cheek pouch:** Absent of lymphatic drainage.

d. **Testes:** Lymphatic drainage is ineffective.

e. **Cornea:** Low vascularity.

❖ Histocompatibility reaction:

➢ **Definition:** Reaction between grafted tissue & host **called histocompatibility reaction.**

➢ **Participation of cells:** It is due to participation by T cells, both Th cells & Tc cells. When antigen presented to MHC-I molecule Tc cells are involved & when antigen presented to MHC-II molecule Th cells are involved.

➢ **Types:** Following two types.

A. **Host versus graft reaction or response:**

✪ **Definition:** Reaction of host to the graft tissue **called host versus graft reaction or response**.

✪ **Clinical features:** Graft rejection.

B. **Graft versus host reaction or response:**

✪ **Definition:**
- Graft mounts an Ir against the Ags of host **called graft versus host reaction or response.**
- Opposite to host versus graft reaction.

✪ **Reasons:**
- It is due to the presence of immunocompetent T cells in the graft.
- Recipient possesses Ags that are absent in graft.
- Recipient must not reject the graft.
- Recipient is immunodeficient.

✪ **Mechanisms:** It is predominantly by CMI.

✪ **Clinical features:** Syndrome **called runt disease**
- Retardation of growth.
- Emaciation.
- Diarrhoea.
- Hepatosplenomegaly.
- Lymphoid atrophy.

- Anaemia.
- Death.

Immunology of malignancy

❖ Introduction:
- When cell undergoes malignant transformation it loose normal Ags & acquired new Ags on surface.
- It makes the tumour antigenically different from normal tissues & tumour is considered as allograft & expected to induce Ir.

❖ Clinical evidence of Ir in malignancy:
- **Spontaneous regression:** of malignant melanoma & neuroblastoma indicates Ir against malignancy as like Ir against infection.
- **Cures by chemotherapy:** cancer like Burkit's lymphoma & choriocarcinoma are cleared by cytotoxic drugs.
- **Overcome immunity:** certain cancers are observed by autopsy finding, indicated that they are clinically controlled by body defence.
- **Cellular response:** indicated by presence of lymphocytes, plasma cells & macrophages in tumour.
- **Immunodeficiency state:** It favours the development of cancer, like Kaposi sarcoma, Hodgkin's lymphoma are common in AIDS.

❖ Tumour Ags: Two types of tumour Ags

A. Tumour specific antigen (TSTA) or Tumour Associated Transplant Antigen (TATA):

- **Definition:** These are the Ags present on tumour cells not on normal cells.
- **Properties:**
  - They induce Ir when tumour is transplanted in to syngeneic animals, finally tumour is rejected.
  - Specificity:
    - If tumour is induced by chemical they are tumour (cell) specific.
    - If tumour is induced by virus they are virus specific.

B. Tumour associated Ags:

- **Definition:** These are the Ags present on tumour cells & on normal cells.
- **Examples:**
  - **α-feto protein:**
    - α-globulin.
    - Produced by hepatocytes.
    - It found in embryonic life & in carcinoma of liver.
    - High level in adults indicates hepatic carcinoma.
    - It's level drop after birth & never found in normal adult.
  - **Carcino Embryonic Ag (CEA):**
    - Glycoprotein.
    - High level in serum indicates carcinoma of colon.
    - High level in serum found in alcoholic cirrhosis, hence less diagnostic value.
  - **Prostate Specific Ag (PSA):**
    - High level in serum indicates carcinoma of prostate.
  - **Ca 125 Ag:**
    - Cancer/Carbohydrate 125 Ag.
    - High level in serum indicates ovarian cancer.

❖ Detection of Ir in malignancy:
- Body produces both humoral & cellular response against malignancy.
- CMI is protective while AMI favours the tumour growth by process of immunological enhancement.

a. **Detection of humoral response:** By detecting Anti-TSTA abs.

b. **Detection of cellular response:**

1. **Detection of DTH:** By skin test by using tumour cell extract as an Ag.
2. **Detection of CMI:**
   - By stimulating the synthesis of lymphokines & DNA by using patient's leucocytes on exposure to tumour Ag.
   - Culture method: destruction of tumour cells by patient's Tc cell.

❖ Immunological surveillance in malignancy:
- **Introduction:**
  - Concept was given by Lewis Thomas in 1950.
  - He postulates that CMI 'seek & destroy' the malignant cell.
- **Mechanisms:** Immunological surveillance includes all mechanisms that favour the growth of cancer, as mentioned below.
  - **IDDs:** May allow the growth of cancer.
  - **Larger size of tumour:** May escape the body defence.
  - **Tumour Ag:**
    - Act as smoke screen.
    - Covers the lymphoid cells & prevent their attack on tumour cells.
  - **Neutral substances of body:** Cover the tumour cells & makes them inaccessible by lymphoid cells.
  - **Immunological enhancement:** AMI favours the tumour growth by suppressing the CMI.
  - **Low immunogenicity of tumour**
  - **Cytokines formation:** [ike Tumour Growth Factor-β which suppresses the CMI.
  - **Low level of MHC-I molecules:** Minimise the chances of recognition & destruction by Tc cells.

❖ Immunotherapy in malignancy:
- **Aim:** To augment antitumour defence of body.
- **Types of therapy:**

A. Non specific (active) therapy:

i. Live agent:

- **BCG vaccine:** It augments antitumour response by:

- Activation of T-lymphocytes.
- Increasing macrophages cytotoxicity.

ii. **Non living agents:**

- ***Corynebacterium parvum*:**
  - Glycan (glucose polymer) derived from organism is protective.
  - Immunomodulator.
- **Levamisole (anthelminthic drug) & DNC (Di Nitro Chlorobenzene):** Stimulate the CMI & macrophage activity.

B. **Specific therapy:**

i. **Active:** By injecting following types of vaccine.

- **Vaccine contains tumour cell antigens:** Not productive.
- **Vaccine contains tumour cell membrane antigens & tumour cells treated with neuraminidase:** Increase immune potential.

ii. **Passive:**

- **Specific antisera:** Neutralise circulating tumour Ags & allow sensitised ICC to acts on tumour cells.
- **Monoclonal Abs:** Acts as carrier & transport the cytotoxic & radioactive drugs to the tumour cells.

iii. **Adoptive:**

- **By using lymphocytes, Transfer Factor (TF) & -immune RNA:**
  - All they are boost up the immunity.
  - Prepared from persons who recovered from cancer or who is immunised against the patient's tumour.
- **LAK cells:**
  - Useful in renal carcinoma.
  - Prevents the metastasis.
  - Prepared treatment with NK cells with IL-2.
- **Thymosin:**
  - Also have antitumour activity.
  - Prepared from human or bovine thymus.

C. **Combined therapy:** Best result is obtained by combining the

- Radio therapy.
- Chemotherapy.
- Immunotherapy.

Surgery.

Question bank

Case study

1) A woman with infertility receives an ovary transplant from her sister who is an identical twin. Identify the type of graft & answer the following
a) Which type of graft it is?
b) Mentioned the different types of grafts.
c) Write the mechanism & ways of prevention of allograft rejection.
d) Describe histocompatibility reaction in details.

2) A 50 year male patient with renal failure received a kidney from genetically un-identical donor. Identify the type of graft & answer the following
a) Which type of graft it is?
b) Mention the pre-transplantation tests to know the compatibility of transplant.
c) Describe in details, about immunological enhancement.

Short notes

1) Classification of transplant or graft.
2) Graft versus host reaction.

Short questions for theory/viva questions

1) Define: Autograft, Isograft, homograft & heterograft.
2) What is white graft response?
3) What is runt disease?

MCQs for chapter review

Immunology of transplantation

1) **Transplantation of host's own tissue is known as**
(a) Isograft (b) Allograft (c) Xenograft (d) Autograft
2) **Allograft is defined as**
(a) Graft from one self (b) Graft from identical twin (c) Graft from member of same species (d) Graft from other species
3) **Types of graft, best suited for renal transplantation** (AI-99)
(a) Allograft (b) Autograft (c) Xenograft (d) Isograft
4) **Graft versus host reaction is caused by** (PGI-86)
(a) B lymphocytes (b) T lymphocytes (c) Macrophages (d) Complement
5) **Type of T lymphocyte responsible for histocompatibility reaction** (AIIMS-89)
(a) Suppressor T cell (b) Activator T cell (c) Effector T cell (d) Helper T cell
6) **Runt disease**
(a) Graft rejection (b) Graft versus host reaction (c) Deficient function (d) Complement deficiency
7) **Antibodies are most responsive to**
(a) Recipient tissue (b) Donor tissue (c) Isograft (d) Autograft

Answers of MCQs & explanation

1) **(b)**
2) **(d)**
} Follow section, **classification of transplant or graft (Based on genetic & antigenic relationship between donor & recipient)** for explanation.

3) **(d)**
- Best graft is autograft, but not possible for renal transplantation, so best answer is isograft.

4) **(b)**
5) **(a), (c) & (d)**
} Follow section, **histocompatibility reaction (Participation of cells)** for explanation.

6) **(b)**
- Follow section, **histocompatibility reaction (Types → Graft versus host reaction or response → reasons)** for explanation.

7) **(b)**
- In graft rejection antibodies are formed against donor tissue.

30 Immunohaematology

Learning heading & subheadings

- History:
- ABO blood group system:
- H Ag:
- Rh blood group:
- Other blood group system:
- Clinical significance of blood group:

❖ **History:** Landsteiner 1st proposed the human blood group in 1900 & he was awarded the Nobel Prize late in 1930.

❖ **ABO blood group system:** Typing is done according to Ag on RBCs surface as shown in **table-1**

Group	Ag on RBCs	Ab in Serum
A	A	Anti-B (mostly IgM type)
B	B	Anti-A (mostly IgM type)
AB	AB	None
O	None	Anti-A & Anti-B

Table-1: ABO blood group system

❖ **H Ag:**
- RBCs of all ABO blood group posses common H Ag, which is a precursor of A & B Ags.
- Amount of H Ag is related with ABO group of cell, AB group has least & O group has most amounts.
- Due to it's universal distribution, it less useful in blood grouping & blood transfusion (BT).
- Bhende et al., from Bombay define the blood group in which there is A, B & H were absent on RBCs surface **called Bombay or OH blood group**.
- Serum of such person contains Anti-A, Anti-B & Anti-H antibodies and their sera are incompatible to all RBCs except of same group.

❖ **Rh blood group:**

➢ **History:** In 1939, Philip Levine and Rufus Stetson demonstrated new type of Ab in serum of mother received ABO compatible blood from her husband. She had just delivered a stillbirth foetus with haemolytic disease. It indicates that woman had sensitised by Ag from foetus inherited from its father. This newer Ab **called Anti-Rh** (from Rhesus monkey) or **Anti-D Ab**, it was a cause of **Haemolytic Disease of New born (HDN)**.

➢ **Rh typing:**
- Based on D Ag on RBCs surface & corresponding Ab **called Anti-D** or **Anti-Rh antibody**.
- Person with D antigen **called Rh +Ve** & without **called Rh –Ve**.

❖ **Other blood group system:** Less clinical significance.

➢ **Lewis blood group system:** It consist two Ags like Le^a Le^b. It differs from other blood group system, as Ags are present in plasma & saliva.

➢ **MN system:**
- Different groups are identified like M, N & MN
- Later S-Ag was added to the list.
- Total 28 different Ags are identified.

❖ **Clinical significances of blood group:**

A. Blood Transfusion (BT):

➢ **Condition to be satisfied are:**
- Recipient's plasma should not contain any Abs which damage the donor's cell & vice-versa.
- Donor RBCs should not have any Ag that is lacking in recipient. If transfused cells possess a foreign Ags, it mounts Ir in recipient.

➢ **Universal donor:**
- Group O is transfused to any group, as it does not contain Ag like A or B, so **called universal donor**.
- Group O contain anti-A & anti-B isoantibodies which are diluted by recipient's plasma.
- However sometimes donor's plasma contain high titre of isoantibodies, which damage the recipient's cells **called dangerous O group**.

➢ **Universal recipient:** Group AB does not contain any isoantibodies, so transfused by any group **called Universal recipient.**

➢ **Rh compatibility is important when recipient is Rh negative:**

➢ **Complications:**

✪ **By incompatible transfusion:**

- **Pathogenesis:**
  - Clumping & intravascular haemolysis of RBCs
  - RBCs are coated by antibodies & phagocytosed.
  - Removal of RBCs from circulation & extravascular lysis
- **Clinical features:**
  - Shivering, tingling sensation, headache, lumbar pain, hypotension, cold-calmmy skin, cyanosis, feeble, collapse, jaundice, haematuria, oliguria, anuria etc.
  - Hypersensitivity reaction like utricaria, rigor due to presence of allergen in donor's blood.
  - Serious reaction occurs due to haemolysed BT
- **Diagnosis:** ABO blood group substances are present in high concentration in saliva, semen, vaginal secretion & gastric juices while in low concentration in sweat, tears & urine. They are also

present in tissues but not in CSF. So above mentioned samples except CSF are used for diagnosis of ABO blood group substances.

- **By infectious transfusion:**
- **Bacteria:**
  - *Treponema pallidum*
  - *Leptospira* spp.
  - *Pseudomonas aeruginosa*: If donor blood contains *P. aeruginosa*, it unmasks hidden Ag of RBCs **called T-Ag**, produce anti-T Ab which agglutinates the RBCs by all blood group sera & by normal sera also. This phenomenon **called Thomsen-Freidenrich phenomenon**.
- **Viruses:** HBV, HCV, HDV, HIV, CJD (Creutzfeldt-Jacob Disease), CMV etc.
- **Parasites:**
  - *Leishmania donovani*
  - *Plasmodium* spp.
  - *Toxoplasma gondii*

B. Haemolytic Disease of New born (HDN):

- **Pathogenesis:** When Rh-Ve women carry the Rh +Ve foetus, Foetal RBCs enter in to maternal circulation & produce anti Rh-Ab. This Abs is IgG in nature & can pass through placenta. However 1st child escape the damage, during subsequent pregnancy the maternal IgG pass through placenta & damage the RBCs of foetus **called erythroblastosis of foetalis**.
- **Clinical features:**
- **Symptoms and signs in the foetus:** Enlarged liver, spleen or heart and fluid build up in the foetus abdomen seen via ultrasound.
- **Symptoms and signs in the newborn:**
  - Anaemia: pale appearance
  - Jaundice or yellow discoloration of the newborn's skin, sclera or mucous membrane. This may be evident right after birth or after 24–48 hours after birth.
  - Enlargement liver and spleen.
  - Severe oedema of the entire body.
  - Dyspnoea
- **Diagnosis:** Anti Rh-Ab, which is IgG in nature & incomplete, is detected by
  - Indirect Coombs test
  - By using colloid medium like 20% bovine serum albumin.
  - Using RBCs treated with enzymes like trypsin, pepsin, ficin or bromelin.
- **Prevention:**
- **Early diagnosis:** Identification of Anti Rh-Ab by ICT at 32-34 weeks & every months thereafter
- **Antepartum intrauterine Rh-Ve blood transfusion:** When disease is diagnosed in antenatal stage
- **Introduction of RBCs in foetal peritoneal cavity:** RBCs will survive & find their way in to circulation
- **Premature delivery with transfusion**
- **Isoimmunisation or artificial passive immunity:**
  - Passively administered IgG suppresses homologous antibody synthesis by feedback process.
  - This principle is utilized in the isoimmunisation of Rh -Ve women who delivered Rh +Ve baby, by administration of anti-Rh (D) IgG during delivery.

C. ABO haemolytic disease:

- **Pathogenesis:** Occurs in O group mother with A or B group foetus, due to presence of natural isoantibodies like Anti-A & Anti-B in maternal circulation.
- **Clinical features:** It is mild than HDN due to Rh incompatibility.

D. Blood group & susceptibility to diseases or infections:

- Duodenal ulcer is common in O group.
- Stomach cancer is common in group A.
- Gonococci is common in group B
- Vibrio is common in group O, less in group AB.

Exact reasons for such association are unclear.

Question bank

Short notes

1) Clinical significance of blood grouping

Short questions for theory/viva questions

1) What is Bombay blood group?
2) What is universal donor & universal recipient?
3) What is Thomsen-Freidenrich phenomenon?
4) Name the bacterial infection common in following blood group
   - Group O - Group B

MCQs for chapter review

History

1) **AB blood group antigens are known as..........factor**
   (a) Duffy (b) Landsteiner (c) Rhesus (d) Lutheran (e) Kidd

Clinical significance of blood group

2) **Diagnosis of ABO incompatibility can be from all of the following except** (AI-94, 97)
   (a) Sweat (b) Saliva (c) Semen (d) CSF
3) **Thomsen-Freidenrich phenomenon is**
   (a) Red cell infection by CMV (b) Red cell agglutination by all blood group sera (c) Haemolysis of transfused blood (d) Due to B antigen

Answers of MCQs & explanation

1) **(b)**
   - Landsteiner 1st proposed the human blood group in 1900 & he was awarded the Nobel Prize late in 1930.
2) **(d)**
   - Follow section, **clinical significances of blood group ((blood transfusion→complications → by incompatible transfusion → diagnosis)** for explanation
3) **(b)**

- Follow section, **clinical significances of blood group (blood transfusion→complications → by infectious transfusion)** for explanation

Section III
Systemic Bacteriology

Prakash

Preview of Systemic Bacteriology

Prakash

Almost all the bacteria are written with following headings & subheadings

- **Meaning / Common name / Synonym / Uses:**
- **Classification:**
- **History:**
- **Morphology:** With appropriate figures
  - **Type according to gram stain:**
  - **Size:**
  - **Shape:**
  - **Arrangement:**
  - **Motility :**
  - **Capsule:**
  - **Spore:**
  - **Other features:** Like fimbriae, L-form or polar bodies, L-forms etc.
- **Culture characteristics (C/Cs):**
  - **Effective factors:**
    - O_2/ Co_2 effect:
    - Temperature:
    - pH:
  - **Culture in media:**

    A. **Liquid Media:**

    B. **Solid media:**

    C. **Selective media:**
  - **Culture in animals:** In few bacteria
  - **Culture in egg:** In few bacteria
- **Biochemical reaction (B/Rs):**

  i. **Sugar fermentation:** G S L M

  ii. **I M Vi C test:**

  iii. **Catalase test:**

  iv. **Oxidase test:**

  v. **Urease test:**

  vi. **Other tests:** Like nitrate test, TSI test, Coagulase test etc.
- **Resistance:**
- **Immunity:**
- **Pathogenicity:**
  - **Disease name:**
  - **Synonym:**
  - **Nature & history of disease:**
  - **Reservoir of infection:**
  - **Source of infection:**
  - **Mode of transmission:**
  - **Incubation period:**
  - **Portal of entry:**
  - **Sites:**
  - **Precipitating factors (epidemiological determinants):**

    I. **Agent factors (virulence factors)**

    II. **Host factors**

    III. **Environmental factors**
  - **Pathogenesis:**
  - **Clinical features:**
  - **Complications:**
- **Laboratory diagnosis:**
  - **Specimens:**
  - **Testing methods:**

    A. **Microscopy:**

    B. **Culture:**

    C. **Biochemical reactions (B/Rs)**

    D. **Serological tests:**

    E. **Molecular methods:**

    F. **Other methods:** Like typing method, physiological method, toxigenicity testing etc.
- **Prevention:**
  - **General measures:**
  - **Chemoprophylaxis:**
  - **Immunoprophylaxis:**
- **Treatment:**

31 Micrococcaceae

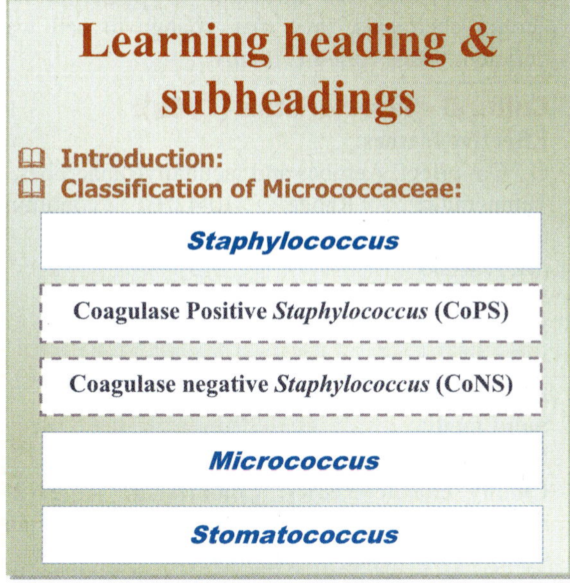

Learning heading & subheadings
Introduction:
Classification of Micrococcaceae:
Staphylococcus
Coagulase Positive Staphylococcus (CoPS)
Coagulase negative Staphylococcus (CoNS)
Micrococcus
Stomatococcus

Introduction:

GPC are classified under two families like **Micrococcaceae** & **Streptococcaceae**.

Features	Micrococcaceae	Streptococcaceae
Catalase test	+	-
Arrangement	Tetrads / cluster due to multiple planes division	Pair / chain due to single plane division

Table-1: Families of GPC

Types of Micrococcaceae: → Flow chart-1

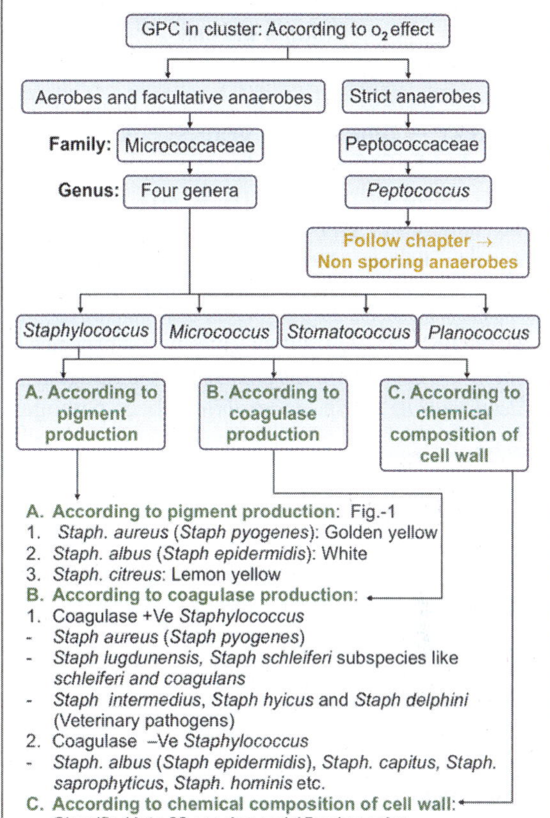

Flow chart-1: Pigment producing *Staphylococci*

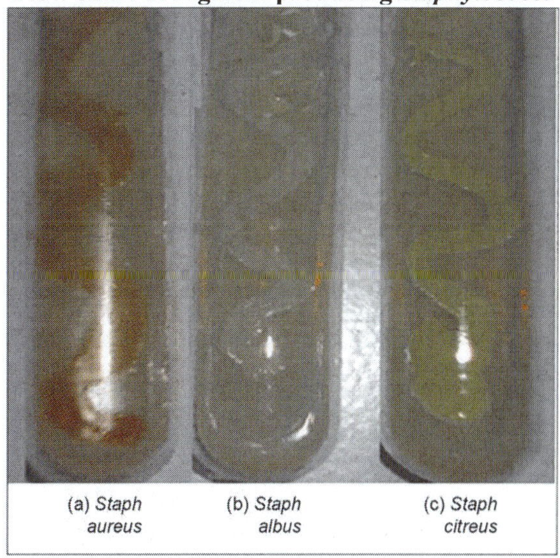

Figure-1: Pigment producing *Staphylococci*

Staphylococcus

Coagulase Positive *Staphylococcus* (CoPS)

Staph aureus

❖ Meaning:

- **Genus name: Staphylo** derived from **Staphyle (Greek) = bunches of grapes + Cocci** derived from **kokkos (Greek) = berry**, as the bacteria are spherical in shape like berry & arranged in cluster like bunches of grapes hence the name is given.
- **Species name: Aureus** from **aurum (Latin) = gold**, because of golden yellow pigment production.

❖ Subspecies: Few author gives two subspecies like

- *Staph aureus* subsp. *aureus*: Human pathogen.
- *Staph aureus* subsp. *anaerobius*: Sheep pathogen.

❖ Synonym: *Staph pyogenes*

❖ Uses of *Staph aureus*:

1. **CAMP test:**
   - Haemolytic toxin of *Staph aureus* gives synergistic haemolysis with *Strept agalactiae* **called CAMP test.**
   - More details: **Follow chapter → Streptococcaceae**
2. **Co-agglutination test:**
   - More details: **Follow chapter → Antigen - antibody (Ag-Ab) reactions**
3. **Satellitism:**
   - More details: **Follow chapter → *Pasteurellales***

❖ Morphology: →Fig. 2.

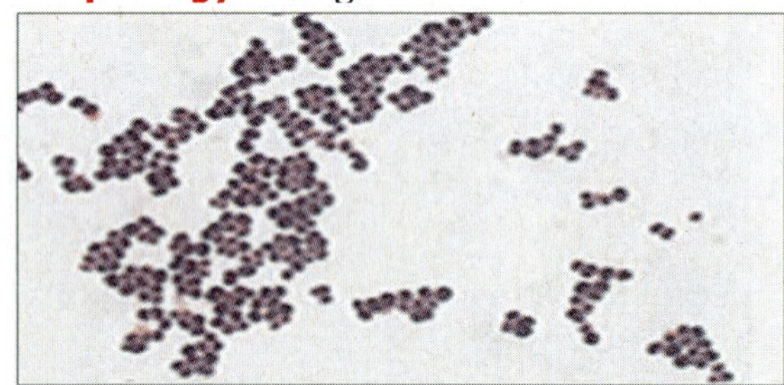

Figure-2: *Staph aureus* under Gram stain

- **Type according to gram stain:** Gram positive cocci.
- **Size:** 1 μm in diameter.
- **Shape:** Spherical / oval.
- **Arrangement:**
  - Characteristically arranged in grape like clusters due to cell division occurs in three planes & daughter cells remain in close proximity to mother cells.
  - Also found in pairs, tetrads and short chains especially when examined from liquid culture.
- **Motility:** Non motile.
- **Capsule:** Few strains with polysaccharide capsule.
- **Spore:** Non-sporing.
- **Fimbriae:** Organ of adhesion made up by teichoic acid.
- **L-form:** Under the influence of penicillin and certain chemicals, they may change to cell wall deficient forms **called L forms.**

❖ Cultural characteristics (C/Cs):

- **Effective factors:**
  - O_2/ Co_2 effect: Aerobes and facultative anaerobes.
  - Temperature: Range 10-42°C; optimum temperature is 37°C.
  - pH: 7.4-7.6
- **Culture in media:**

A. Liquid media:

- Like peptone water & nutrient broth.
- Producing uniform turbidity.

B. Solid media:

1. **Nutrient agar plate or slope/slant:**

- **Colony characteristics:** Colonies are large (2-4 mm), circular, convex, smooth, shiny, opaque and easily emulsifiable and **pigmented.**
- **Properties of pigments:**
  - Colour: Most strains produce golden yellow/orange pigment as shown in **fig.-1(a).**
  - Optimum production: At 22°C & in aerobic culture.
  - Increased production: By incorporating 1% glycerol monoacetate or milk in medium.
  - Chemically pigments are lipoprotein allied to carotene.
  - Pigment does not diffuse into medium (non diffusible in nature). Because of non diffusible nature, pigment remains at the site of inoculation and confluent growth presents a characteristic "oil-paint appearance" as shown in **fig.-1.**

✓ **Note: Differentiation from the pigment of *Pseudomonas***

- Pigment of *Pseudomonas* is diffusible in nature hence spread throughout the depth of nutrient agar slant & entire slant becomes pigmented.

2. **Blood agar:**
   - Most strains are β-haemolysis **[fig.-3(a)]**, especially when incubated under 20-25% CO_2.
   - Haemolysis is marked on rabbit and sheep blood and weak on horse blood agar.

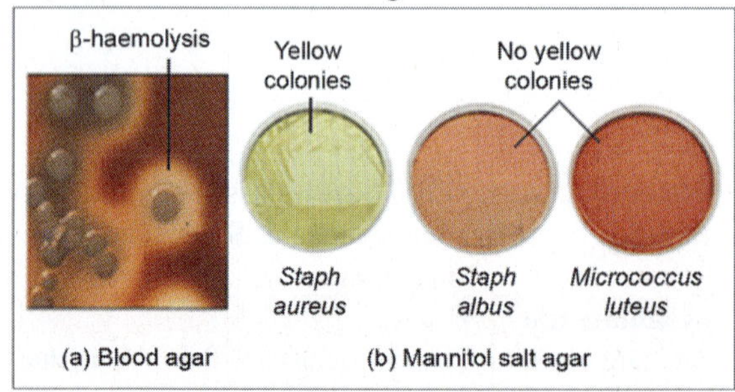

Figure-3: Colonies by *Staph aureus*

3. **MacConkey's agar:** May produce small pink (pinkish-white) colonies due to lactose fermentation.

C. **Selective media:**

i. **Liquid selective media:** Contains 8-10% NaCl like

1. **Salt broth.**
2. **Salt cooked meat broth.**

ii. **Solid selective media:**

1. **Ludlam's medium:**
- Containing lithium chloride and tellurite.
- Black colonies on potassium tellurite medium.
2. **Mannitol salt agar:** Producing the yellow colonies as shown in **fig.-3(b).**
3. **Salt milk agar**
4. **Media containing polymyxin B.**

✓ **Note: Selection of blood for blood agar**
- For primary isolation, sheep blood agar is used.
- Human blood is not recommended as it may contain antibodies and other inhibitors.

❖ Biochemical reaction (B/Rs):

i. **Sugar fermentation:**
- Ferment number of sugars producing acid only.
- Mannitol fermented anaerobically with production of acid only which gives pink colour to the medium as shown in **fig.-4(a).**
- Mannitol fermentation is diagnostically useful & helps in differentiation of species, as it is fermented by *Staph aureus* only & not by other species of *Staphylococcus*.

ii. **I M Vi C test:** - + + -

iii. **Catalase test:** Positive

iv. **Oxidase test:** Negative

v. **Urease test:** Positive

vi. **Nitrate test:** Positive (reduce nitrate to nitrite)

vii. **Phosphatase test:** Positive

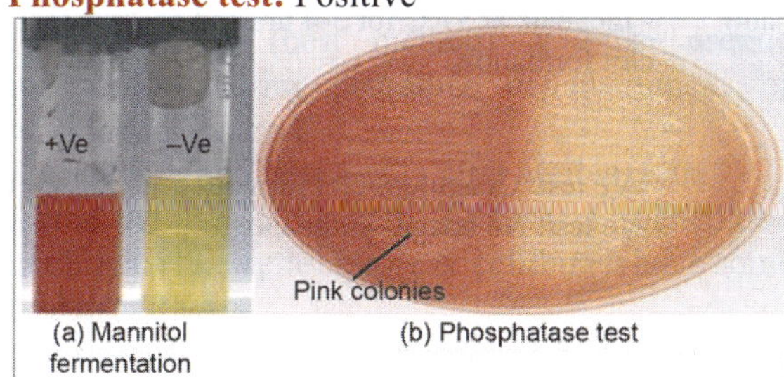

Figure-4: (a) Mannitol fermentation test (b) Phosphatase test

- **Principle:** Based on production of phosphatase enzyme, which break the phenolphthalein diphosphate to release the free phenolphthalein, which change the colonies to pink colour on exposure of ammonia. Phenolphthalein is quinone derivative & used as pH indicator, which turns pink at alkaline pH by ammonia.
- **Method:** Inoculate *Staph aureus* in phenolphthalein diphosphate agar. After growth expose culture to ammonia vapour & check for the result.
- **Result:** Positive result is indicated by pink colour colonies due to presence of free phenolphthalein as shown in **fig.-4(b).**
- **Interpretation:** It is positive in *Staph aureus, Staph epidermidis* & *Staph xylosus.*

viii. **Coagulase test:** Positive

➤ **Background with coagulase enzyme:**
- Coagulase is an enzyme (protein) of unknown chemical composition.
- Having prothrombin like activity to convert fibrinogen in to fibrin, resulting clot formation in a suitable test system.
- It produces fibrin barrier at the site of *Staphylococcus* infections causing localised abscess (carbuncle, boil etc.).
- Two forms of enzymes like bound & free coagulase as shown in **table-2.**

Bound coagulase (Clumping factor)	Free coagulase
Detected by slide test	Detected by tube test
Heat stable	Heat labile
Attached to cell wall (Cell surface protein)	Enzyme secreted into medium
Independent of Coagulase Reacting Factor (CRF)	Dependent to CRF
Only 1 serotype	8 sero-types

Table-2: Differences between bound & free coagulase enzyme

➤ **Coagulase test: →Table -3 & fig.-5.**

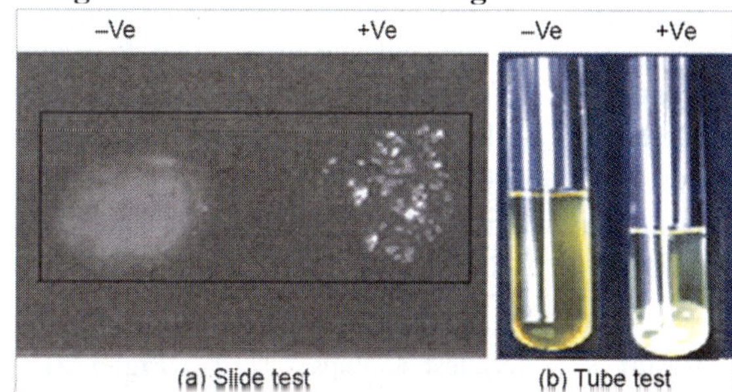

Figure-5: Coagulase test

ix. **Lysostaphin sensitivity:** Sensitive to lysostaphin **(mixture of enzymes produced by *Staph epidermidis*).**

x. **Gelatin Liquefaction test:** Positive

xi. **Lipase production test:** Most strains are lipolytic producing dense opacity when grown on egg yolk containing media due to lipase production.

xii. **Heat stable thermo nuclease test:** Positive
- Based on production of thermo stable nuclease.
- Demonstrated by the ability of boiled culture to degrade DNA.

➢ **Mode of transmission:**
- **Endogenous infection:** Most common mode & occurs following disturbances of normal flora.
- **Exogenous infection:** It occurs by direct contact (from the hand of hospital staff), air borne, dust borne, fomites borne.

➢ **Portal of entry:** Respiratory tract, skin or mucosa.

➢ **Sites:** Multisystem or organs are infected.

➢ **Precipitating factors (epidemiological determinants):** Three types

I. Agent factors (virulence factors)

Two types like intra cellular & extracellular.

A. Intracellular (cell wall associated) factors:

1. Peptidoglycan:
- Provide rigidity and integrity to cell.
- Activate complement & induce release of inflammatory cytokines.

2. Adhesins:
- **Fimbrial adhesin (techoic acid):**
  - Organ of adhesion.
  - Protects from opsonisation.
- **Protein receptors:** *Staphylococci* have receptors for many mammalian proteins like fibronectin, fibrinogen, IgG and C1q. Help in adhesion with host cells.

3. Capsular polysaccharides: Inhibits phagocytosis.

4. Protein A:

✪ **Biological actions:**
- Chemotactic.
- Antiphagocytic.
- Anti-complementary effect.
- Causing platelet damage.
- Causing hypersensitivity.
- Coagglutination.
- It binds to Fc portion of IgG (except IgG3) leaving Fab site free to combine with specific Ag present in samples.
- When protein A bearing *Staphylococci* will mixed with IgG antiserum will be agglutinated **called coagglutination**.
- Used for streptococcal typing, gonococcal typing and ligand for isolation of IgG.

✪ **Properties:**
- It is a B cell mitogen.
- It is found in 90% strain of *Staph aureus* **called Cowan 1 strain.**
- It absent in coagulase –Ve *Staphylococci*.

5. Clumping Factor:
- Surface protein also **called bound coagulase enzyme**.
- Responsible for "slide coagulase test".
- Routinely used for identification of *Staph aureus*.

B. Extracellular factors: Two types like enzymes & toxins as mentioned below.

i. Enzymes:

1. Free coagulase:
- Protein of unknown chemical composition.
- Having prothrombin like activity to convert fibrinogen in to fibrin, resulting clot formation in a suitable test system.
- Fibrin barrier at the site of *Staph aureus* infection causing localize abscess (carbuncle, boil etc.).

2. Hyaluronidase: Breaks the connective tissues and help in spread of infection.

3. Penicillinase (β-lactamase): As discussed above

4. Nucleases (DNAse):
5. Proteases:
6. Staphylokinase (fibrinolysin):
} All will help in initiation & spread of infection

7. Lipase: Helps to infect skin & subcutaneous tissues.

8. Other diagnostically useful enzymes are: Catalase, phosphatase, urease etc.

ii. Toxins:

a. Haemolysin (staphylolysin, cytolytic category): 4 types like α, β, γ & δ

1. α Haemolysin:
- It is a protein inactivated at 70°C but reactivated paradoxically at 100°C.
- It lyses rabbit RBCs, less active against sheep & human RBCs.
- It is leucocidal, cytotoxic, dermonecrotic after intradermal inoculation in rabbits, neurotoxic & lethal after intravenous inoculation in rabbits.
- It is toxic to macrophages, lysosomes, muscles, renal cortex & CVS.

2. β Haemolysin:
- Sphingomyelinase.
- Hemolytic for sheep RBCs but not for human & rabbit RBCs.
- It initiate the haemolysis at 37^0C but evident after chilling **called hot-cold phenomenon.**

3. γ Haemolysin: Composed of 2 proteins both are essential for haemolytic action.

4. δ Haemolysin: It has detergent like action on membrane of RBCs, WBCs, macrophages & platelets.

b. Leucocidin [PVL (Panton-Valentine toxin)]:
- It is a cytolytic toxin.
- It has two-component like S & L (S=slow and F=fast) similar to gamma haemolysin.
- γ- haemolysin & leucocodin are bicomponent membrane active toxins grouped as **synergohymenotropic** toxins.

c. Enterotoxin:

✪ **Properties:**
- Heat stable (resisting 100°C for 10-40 minutes).
- Bacteria can grow best at 37°C, which may be the optimum temperature for toxin production.
- Very potent & microgram (μg) amounts can cause illness.
- Transmitted by meat, fish, milk & milk products.

3. **MacConkey's agar:** May produce small pink (pinkish-white) colonies due to lactose fermentation.

C. Selective media:

i. Liquid selective media: Contains 8-10% NaCl like

1. **Salt broth.**
2. **Salt cooked meat broth.**

ii. Solid selective media:

1. **Ludlam's medium:**
   - Containing lithium chloride and tellurite.
   - Black colonies on potassium tellurite medium.
2. **Mannitol salt agar:** Producing the yellow colonies as shown in **fig.-3(b).**
3. **Salt milk agar**
4. **Media containing polymyxin B.**

✓ **Note: Selection of blood for blood agar**

- For primary isolation, sheep blood agar is used.
- Human blood is not recommended as it may contain antibodies and other inhibitors.

❖ Biochemical reaction (B/Rs):

i. Sugar fermentation:

- Ferment number of sugars producing acid only.
- Mannitol fermented anaerobically with production of acid only which gives pink colour to the medium as shown in **fig.-4(a).**
- Mannitol fermentation is diagnostically useful & helps in differentiation of species, as it is fermented by *Staph aureus* only & not by other species of *Staphylococcus*.

ii. I M Vi C test: - + + -

iii. Catalase test: Positive

iv. Oxidase test: Negative

v. Urease test: Positive

vi. Nitrate test: Positive (reduce nitrate to nitrite)

vii. Phosphatase test: Positive

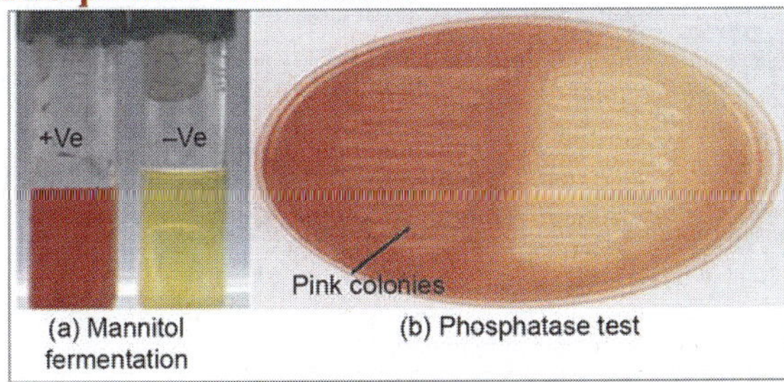

Figure-4: (a) Mannitol fermentation test (b) Phosphatase test

- **Principle:** Based on production of phosphatase enzyme, which break the phenolphthalein diphosphate to release the free phenolphthalein, which change the colonies to pink colour on exposure of ammonia. Phenolphthalein is quinone derivative & used as pH indicator, which turns pink at alkaline pH by ammonia.
- **Method:** Inoculate *Staph aureus* in phenolphthalein diphosphate agar. After growth expose culture to ammonia vapour & check for the result.
- **Result:** Positive result is indicated by pink colour colonies due to presence of free phenolphthalein as shown in **fig.-4(b).**
- **Interpretation:** It is positive in *Staph aureus, Staph epidermidis & Staph xylosus.*

viii. Coagulase test: Positive

➢ **Background with coagulase enzyme:**

- Coagulase is an enzyme (protein) of unknown chemical composition.
- Having prothrombin like activity to convert fibrinogen in to fibrin, resulting clot formation in a suitable test system.
- It produces fibrin barrier at the site of *Staphylococcus* infections causing localised abscess (carbuncle, boil etc.).
- Two forms of enzymes like bound & free coagulase as shown in **table-2.**

Bound coagulase (Clumping factor)	Free coagulase
Detected by slide test	Detected by tube test
Heat stable	Heat labile
Attached to cell wall (Cell surface protein)	Enzyme secreted into medium
Independent of Coagulase Reacting Factor (CRF)	Dependent to CRF
Only 1 serotype	8 sero-types

Table-2: Differences between bound & free coagulase enzyme

➢ **Coagulase test: →Table -3 & fig.-5.**

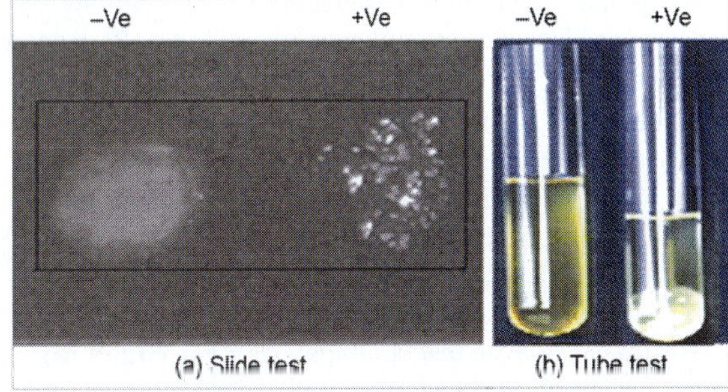

Figure-5: Coagulase test

ix. Lysostaphin sensitivity: Sensitive to lysostaphin **(mixture of enzymes produced by *Staph epidermidis*).**

x. Gelatin Liquefaction test: Positive

xi. Lipase production test: Most strains are lipolytic producing dense opacity when grown on egg yolk containing media due to lipase production.

xii. Heat stable thermo nuclease test: Positive

- Based on production of thermo stable nuclease.
- Demonstrated by the ability of boiled culture to degrade DNA.

❖ Resistance:

- Resist drying for 3-6 months, 60°C for 30 minutes & 1% phenol for 15 minutes.
- Grow in presence of 10-15% NaCl. Clinically it is important in food preservation.
- Resistant to lysozymes.
- Thermal death point is 62°C for 30 minutes.
- Killed by 1% mercury perchloride in 10 minutes.
- Aniline dyes like crystal violet (1 in 500,000) & brilliant green (1 in 10,000,000) are lethal.
- Sensitive to **lysostaphin (mixture of enzymes produced by *Staph epidermidis*).**
- **Drug resistance in *Staph aureus*:** It is discussed with resistance to β-lactam antibiotics (penicillin), vancomycin & few other drugs as follows.

A. Resistance to β-lactam antibiotics (penicillin)

- **Background:** Initially *Staphylococci* are uniformly sensitive to penicillin, but resistant strains began to emerge, 1st in hospitals then in community.
- **Mechanisms:** *Staphylococci* develop resistance to β-lactam antibiotics (penicillin) by following ways.

i. Plasmid mediated resistance or resistance due to β- lactamase (penicillinase) production:

- By production of β- lactamase (penicillinase) enzyme which cleaves the β-lactam ring & produces the resistance.
- Enzyme is inducible & it's production is controlled by plasmid. Such plasmid transmitted to other bacteria by transduction (more common) or by conjugation to make them resistant to penicillin.
- About 90% of strains of *Staph aureus* are penicillinase producer.
- **Types of penicillinase enzymes:** Four types from A to D. A is produced by hospital strain.
- **β- Lactamase (penicillinase) producing bacteria:** *Staph aureus, N. gonorrhea, M. catarrhalis, Acenatobacter* spp., *E. coli, K. pneumoniae, Salmonella* spp., *P. mirabilis, Bacteroides* spp. etc.

ii. Chromosomal mediated (mutational) resistance or MRSA:

- **Mechanisms:** Chromosomal mediated gene **called mec A gene** (Staphylococcal cassette chromosomal mec gene) alters the penicillin binding proteins of cell membrane (PBP2a) & bacterial surface receptors.
- **Definition:** Such resistance extends to cover other β-lactam antibiotics like methicillin, cloxacillin or oxacillin **called Methicillin Resistance *Staph Aureus* (MRSA).**
- **Epidemiology:**
  - There is increasing trend of MRSA in last few decades.
  - It varies from place to place.
  - Around 30-40% strains of *Staph aureus* are MRSA.

Features	Slide test	Tube test
Principle	Bound coagulase is present in cell wall, not in a culture filtrate. Fibrin strands are formed between the bacterial cells causing them to clump together.	Free coagulase having prothrombin like activity. React with CRF of plasma to convert fibrinogen in to fibrin to form visible clot.
Reagents	- Rabbit or human plasma containing EDTA, heparin, oxalate as anticoagulant. - Citrate utilising bacteria (**e.g. *Pseudomonas***) giving false +Ve result, so citrate plasma is not useful.	
Control	**+Ve control:** *Staph aureus* & **- Ve control:** *Staph albus*	
Method	- Place a drop of sterile water or saline on two ends of clean & dry slide. - Emulsify the colony of test organism in one end, add one drop of plasma and mix with wooden stick. - Leave the other end as control. - Rock the slide back-forth & read for the clumps.	- Mix a 0.1 ml of organism culture suspension with 0.5 ml of human or rabbit plasma. - Incubate at 37°C for 3-4 hrs and observe for clot formation.
Result	+Ve test: Clumps -Ve test: No clumps } **Fig.-5 (a)**	+Ve test: Coagulum/clot formation -Ve test: No coagulum/no clot } **Fig.-5 (b)**
Interpre-tation	**a. +Ve test:** **1. Only slide positive:** *Staph lugdunensis.* **2. Only tube positive:** *Staph intermedius, Staph hyicus* & *Staph schleferi* subspecies *coagulans.* **3. Both slide & tube positive:** - *Staphylococcus: Staph aureus, Staph delphini* & some strains of *Staph schleferi* subspecies *schleferi.* - Other groups: *E. rhusiopathiae* (tube and/or slide tests are +Ve with rabbit and/or bovine serum) & *Y. pestis* (exactly not defined about variation in slide & tube positivity). **b. -Ve test:** Coagulase –Ve *Staphylococcus* are mentioned in **flow chart-1.** **c. False +Ve test:** Citrate is used by many bacteria like *Pseudomonas*, so if citrate plasma is used for testing will give false positive result. **d. False –Ve test:** 1. Positive tube test become negative after longer incubation, because of clot lysed by **fibrinolysin (staphylokinase)** produce by *staph. aureus.* 2. Slide test may become false negative by **capsulated strains**, because capsule mask the clumping factor.	

Table-3: Coagulase test

- **Types:** Two types of MRSA.

1. **Hospital Acquired (HA MRSA):**
- Also **called hospital strain.**
- Some time resistance extended to antibiotics like erythromycins, tetracycline, aminoglycosides, heavy metals & produce epidemic of hospital cross infection **called epidemic strain or epidemic MRSA.**
- Resistance expressed by mec A gene subtype I, II & III.
- Less virulent & multidrug resistant.
- Produces post operative wound infections & other hospital acquired infections.

2. **Community Acquired (CA MRSA):**
- Resistance expressed by mec A gene subtype IV, V & VI.
- More virulent & produces the PVT (**vide infra**).
- It produces the soft tissues infections like necrotising fasciitis.

- **Diagnosis of MRSA:**

a. **Antibiogram:**

1. **Disc diffusion based method**
- It is done by using cefoxitin or oxacillin (6µl/ml) discs.
- Reduced temperature: Oxacillin required 24 hours incubation at 30°C with supplementation of 2-4% NaCl in medium.

2. **Dilution based method:** By using microdilution method.

b. **Culture:** By using following media
- Chromogenic media for MRSA.
- Mannitol oxacillin agar.

c. **Serological test:** Latex agglutination test to detect PBP2a by using antibody fixed with latex particles.

d. **Molecular method:** PCR to detect mec A gene.

- **Prevention of MRSA:**
- Hand washing (best method) & other aseptic precautions during handling of instrument or working in hospital.
- Selection of antibiotics only after antibiogram.
- Avoid the use of β-lactam, however 5th generation antibiotics like ceftobiprole & ceftibuten have some role in MRSA.

- **Treatment of MRSA:** Antibiogram is necessary before treatment.

a. **Local treatment:**

1. **Skin lesions:** 2% Mupirocin oinment TDS for 5 days.
2. **Nares lesion:** 2% Mupirocin ointment TDs for 1 week. (Applied anterior part of inside of each nostrils).
3. **Skin carriers:**
- 4% Chlorhexidine
- 2% Triclosan
- 7.5% Povidone iodine –daily for 1 week.
- Apply solution on face, nose, axilla, umbilicus, groin & perineum.

b. **Systemic treatment:**

1. **1st line drugs:**
- Vancomycin: Drug of choice
- Linezolid
- Deptomycin
- Teicolpanin
- Tigacycline
- Quinupristin/dalfopristin

2. **2nd line drugs:** In non life threatening infections
- Rifampin with fusidic acid.
- Cotrimoxazole
- Gentamicin / erythromycin
- Tetracycline

iii. **Development of tolerance to penicillin:** Bacterium is only inhibited but not killed.

B. **Resistance to vancomycin**

- **Types:** Overuse of vancomycin produces two types of resistant strains like low grade & high grade.

1. **Low grade resistance:**
- **Called VISA** (Vancomycin Intermediate *Staph aureus*).
- It is due to increase in cell wall thickness.
- More common in India.

2. **High grade resistance:**
- **Called VRSA** (Vancomycin Resistant *Staph aureus*).
- It is due to transfer of Van A gene by horizontal conjugation mechanism from *E. faecalis.*
- Rare common in India & reported from Hyderabad, Kolkata & Lucknow.

- **Treatment:** VRSA is treated by linezoild, telavancin, daptomycin & quinupristin/dalfopristin.

C. **Resistance to other drugs:** *Staphylococci* also exhibit the plasmid borne resistance to other antibiotics like erythromycins, tetracycline, aminoglycosides & almost all clinically used antibiotics.

Pathogenicity:

- **Nature of disease:** Outbreak is common in hospital.
- **Reservoir of infection:**
  - Normal flora of human skin, nose (10-30%), vagina (5-10%), perineum (10%), axilla, respiratory tract, skin glands, hair & mucosa.
  - Vaginal carriage is increased during menses which is responsible for TSS.
  - Newborn colonised the bacteria in skin or nose from mother, hospital staff or environment. Umbilical stump is contaminated in hospital born babies which act as carrier **called shedders**, which sheds the cocci in handkerchief, blankets & bed sheets for days or weeks.
- **Source of infection:** Case, carrier (like hospital staff), animals (like cow) or inanimate objects.

➢ **Mode of transmission:**
- **Endogenous infection:** Most common mode & occurs following disturbances of normal flora.
- **Exogenous infection:** It occurs by direct contact (from the hand of hospital staff), air borne, dust borne, fomites borne.

➢ **Portal of entry:** Respiratory tract, skin or mucosa.
➢ **Sites:** Multisystem or organs are infected.
➢ **Precipitating factors (epidemiological determinants):** Three types

I. Agent factors (virulence factors)

Two types like intra cellular & extracellular.

A. Intracellular (cell wall associated) factors:

1. **Peptidoglycan:**
- Provide rigidity and integrity to cell.
- Activate complement & induce release of inflammatory cytokines.
2. **Adhesins:**
- **Fimbrial adhesin (techoic acid):**
- Organ of adhesion.
- Protects from opsonisation.
- **Protein receptors:** *Staphylococci* have receptors for many mammalian proteins like fibronectin, fibrinogen, IgG and C1q. Help in adhesion with host cells.
3. **Capsular polysaccharides:** Inhibits phagocytosis.
4. **Protein A:**

✪ **Biological actions:**
- Chemotactic.
- Antiphagocytic.
- Anti-complementary effect.
- Causing platelet damage.
- Causing hypersensitivity.
- Coagglutination.
- It binds to Fc portion of IgG (except IgG3) leaving Fab site free to combine with specific Ag present in samples.
- When protein A bearing *Staphylococci* will mixed with IgG antiserum will be agglutinated **called coagglutination**.
- Used for streptococcal typing, gonococcal typing and ligand for isolation of IgG.

✪ **Properties:**
- It is a B cell mitogen.
- It is found in 90% strain of *Staph aureus* **called Cowan 1 strain.**
- It absent in coagulase –Ve *Staphylococci.*

5. **Clumping Factor:**
- Surface protein also **called bound coagulase enzyme**.
- Responsible for "slide coagulase test".
- Routinely used for identification of *Staph aureus*.

B. Extracellular factors: Two types like enzymes & toxins as mentioned below.

i. Enzymes:

1. **Free coagulase:**
- Protein of unknown chemical composition.
- Having prothrombin like activity to convert fibrinogen in to fibrin, resulting clot formation in a suitable test system.
- Fibrin barrier at the site of *Staph aureus* infection causing localize abscess (carbuncle, boil etc.).
2. **Hyaluronidase:** Breaks the connective tissues and help in spread of infection.
3. **Penicillinase (β-lactamase):** As discussed above
4. **Nucleases (DNAse):**
5. **Proteases:**
6. **Staphylokinase (fibrinolysin):**

   } All will help in initiation & spread of infection
7. **Lipase:** Helps to infect skin & subcutaneous tissues.
8. **Other diagnostically useful enzymes are:** Catalase, phosphatase, urease etc.

ii. Toxins:

a. Haemolysin (staphylolysin, cytolytic category): 4 types like α, β, γ & δ

1. **α Haemolysin:**
- It is a protein inactivated at 70°C but reactivated paradoxically at 100°C.
- It lyses rabbit RBCs, less active against sheep & human RBCs.
- It is leucocidal, cytotoxic, dermonecrotic after intradermal inoculation in rabbits, neurotoxic & lethal after intravenous inoculation in rabbits.
- It is toxic to macrophages, lysosomes, muscles, renal cortex & CVS.
2. **β Haemolysin:**
- Sphingomyelinase.
- Hemolytic for sheep RBCs but not for human & rabbit RBCs.
- It initiate the haemolysis at 37^0C but evident after chilling **called hot-cold phenomenon.**
3. **γ Haemolysin:** Composed of 2 proteins both are essential for haemolytic action.
4. **δ Haemolysin:** It has detergent like action on membrane of RBCs, WBCs, macrophages & platelets.

b. Leucocidin [PVL (Panton-Valentine toxin)]:
- It is a cytolytic toxin.
- It has two-component like S & L (S=slow and F=fast) similar to gamma haemolysin.
- γ- haemolysin & leucocodin are bicomponent membrane active toxins grouped as **synergohymenotropic** toxins.

c. Enterotoxin:

✪ **Properties:**
- Heat stable (resisting 100°C for 10-40 minutes).
- Bacteria can grow best at 37°C, which may be the optimum temperature for toxin production.
- Very potent & microgram (μg) amounts can cause illness.
- Transmitted by meat, fish, milk & milk products.

- Source of infection is usually a food handler, who is a carrier.
- It is plasmid mediated.
- Self-limiting illness, with recovery in a day or so.
- It is antigenic & neutralised by specific antitoxin.

✪ **Biological effects:**
- It is a **superantigen** causing multisystem disease.
- Acts on autonomic nervous system (neurotoxic) rather than on Gastro Intestinal (GI) mucosa. It stimulates the vagus nerve & vomiting center. It also knows to stimulate the peristaltic activity.
- Causing **food poisoning**- nausea, vomiting, diarrhoea, 2-6 hrs after consumption of contaminated food containing preformed toxins **called intradietic toxin**. Fever is absent.
- Incubation period is very short about 2-6 hours, because it is the preformed toxin.
- Other effects of toxin: Pyrogenic, mitogenic, hypotensive, thrombocytopenic & cytotoxic.

✪ **Antigenic types:** 8 types like A, B, C1-3, D, E & H. Type A is responsible for most cases.

✪ **Detection:** Latex agglutination test & ELISA.

d. **Toxic shock syndrome toxin (TSST):** Produced by *Staph aureus* usually belongs to bacteriophage group 1. Initially **called enterotoxin F** or **pyrogenic exotoxin C.** TSST also caused by enterotoxin B & C of *Staph aureus* very rarely.

✪ **Types:** Like TSST-1 (by *Staph aureus*) & TSST-2.

✪ **Biological effects:** It is a **superantigen** stimulates the large numbers of T cells irrespective of its antigenicity, which release cytokines, IL-1, IL-2, TNF & interferon (IFN) $-\gamma$ leads to multisystem disease.

✪ **Risk factors:**
- It was 1st detected from women using highly absorbent vaginal tampons.
- It also reported from men & non-menstruating women due to pre-existing staphylococcal infection.
- Now tampons related disease is rare & now it is common infection of skin, mucosa & surgical wound.
- Absence of TSST-1 antibodies which formed in convalescents.

✪ **Clinical features:** Causing **Toxic Shock Syndrome (TSS) called staphylococcal toxic shock syndrome.**
- Multisystem disease which is fatal in nature.
- Present with fever, hypotension, myalgia, vomiting, diarrhoea, mucosal hyperemia & an erythematous rash which desquamates subsequently.
- Later includes liver, kidneys, GIT, CNS etc.

✪ **Diagnosis:** TSST is detected by latex agglutination & its gene by PCR.

✪ **Treatment:** Clindamycin (reduce the toxin production) is the drug of choice given with semisynthetic Pn or vancomycin.

e. **Exfoliative toxin / exfoliatin / epidermolytic toxin / epidermolysin:**

- **Mechanism of action:** Causing Staphylococcal Scalded Skin Syndrome (SSSS) characterized by separation of outer layer of the epidermis from the underlying tissue as shown in **fig.-6**. Also **called exfoliative skin disease.** It usually occurs in infants. Exfoliatin is glutamate-specific serine proteases highly specific to the cadherin desmoglein I, an adhesion protein in the desmosomes of the stratum corneum facilitates intracellular adhesion between keratinocytes. Exfoliatin (protease) cleaves the desmoglein I resulting separation of skin layer. A very similar non-infectious condition is seen in the autoimmune skin disorder pemphigua in which there is an IgG antibody against the cadherin desmoglein III.

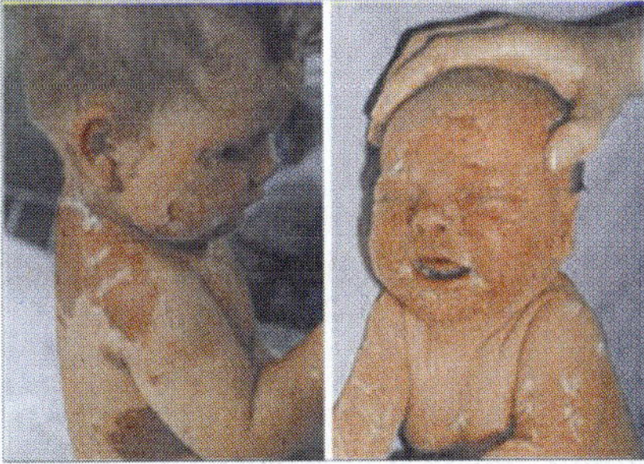

Figure-6: Exfoliative skin disease

- **Severe form:**
  - In newborn **called Ritter's disease.** It was 1st described in 1878 by Baron Gottfried Ritter von Rittershain, who observed 297 cases among children in a single Czechoslovakian children's home over a 10-year period.
  - In older **called toxic epidermal necrolysis.**
- **Mild form:** Pemphigus neonatorum & bullous impetigo.

✓ **Notes:**
- **Reiter's syndrome:** Follow chapter → Neisseriae, Moraxellaceae and Mimeae
- **Epidermolysin is not a superantigen:** Follow link →https://www.ncbi.nlm.nih.gov/pmc/articles/PMC97528/

II. Host factors

1. **Age:** Human colonisation of *Staphylococci* start in new born life in umbilical stump from hospital environment.
2. **Sex:** Vaginal carriage increase in menses which contribute in pathogenesis of TSS.

III. Environmental factors

1. **Hospital environment:** Infections are common from hospital environment or staff.

➢ **Clinical features:** 2 types of diseases like intoxications and infections.

a. **Intoxications:** Due to toxin production
1. **Food poisoning: → Vide supra**
2. **TSS: → Vide supra**
3. **SSSS/ Exfoliative skin disease: → Vide supra**

b. **Infections:** *Staphylococci* produce the enzyme coagulase which makes the fibrin barrier around the lesions & makes them localise in contrast to spreading lesions of *Streptococci.*

1. **Skin & soft tissue:**
- Folliculitis: Infection/inflammation of hair follicle present as a pin point red spot.
- Furuncle (boil): It is a deep folliculitis infecting hair follicle which present with painful swelling due to collection of pus & dead tissues in hair follicle.
- Carbuncle: It is the cluster of boils that are connected with each other beneath the skin.
- Sycosis barbae: An infection of hair follicles in the beard area due to *Staph aureus.* It also **called folliculitis barbae** & leads to scarring & permanent hair loss. It occurs in men due to or not due to shaving & infection acquired from infected razors or towels.
- Cellulitis:
- Impetigo:
- Ecthyma:

} **Follow chapter → Streptococcaceae** for more details

- Paronychia: Word is originated from **Para (Greek) = around & Onyx (Greek) = nail.** It is the bacterial infection around finger nail regions.
- Others: Like abscess & wound infection.

✓ **Note: Pseudofolliculitis barbae**
- Inflammatory foreign body (non-infective) reaction surrounding in grown facial hairs, which results from close shaving. It can also occur on any site of body, where hair is shaved or plucked, including axilla, pubic area & legs. It is also **called shaving rash** or **razor bumps**.
- Folliculitis barbae and pseudofolliculitis barbae can co-exist.
- It occurs mainly in person with curly hair because sharp pointed end of a recently shaved hair comes out from the skin and re-enters the skin & causing a foreign body inflammatory reaction.

✓ **Note: Hiradenitis suppurative** → Few authors mentioned that it is caused by *Staph aureus*, but in fact it's neither having infective aetiology nor having contagious nature & in contrarily infection occurs as secondary complication.

2. **Organs:**
- Postoperative parotitis.
- Pneumatocele: **Follow chapter → Systemic infections**

3. **Musculoskeletal:** Osteomyelitis, arthritis, bursitis, pyomyositis (also **called tropical pyomyositis** or **myositis tropicans** → Abscess in skeletal muscles) & botryomycosis.

Botryomycosis

- **Definition:** It is a chronic granulomatous mycetoma like lesion caused by *Staph aureus* & other pyrogenic bacteria.
- **Synonym:** It is resemble to mycetoma, so **called pseudomycosis.**
- **Meaning & history:** Word is originated from **Botryo (Latin) = grapes & Mycosis (Greek, mykes = fungus) = fungal disease.** The disease was originally discovered by Otto Bollinger in 1870, and its name was coined by Sebastiano Rivolta in 1884. Initially mistaken as fungal disease, later in 1919 it is identified as bacterial origin, however name is still persisting.
- **Etiological agents:** It is the bacterial infection caused by *Staph aureus* & other pyrogenic bacteria like *P. aeruginosa*, *E. coli* & *Proteus* spp.
- **Pathogenicity:**
  - Sites:
    - It involves the subcutaneous tissues, muscles & bones.
    - Rarely affect internal organs. Lungs are the most commonly infected and usually there is a predisposing factor such as surgery or impaired immunity.
  - Precipitating factors:
    - Trauma, surgery or the presence of a foreign body usually precedes infection.
    - Common in HIV-AIDS.
    - Alcoholism.
    - Cystic fibrosis.
    - Prolonged corticosteroid use.
    - Diabetes mellitus.
  - Clinical features:
    - Botryomycosis most commonly affects the skin and presents as subcutaneous nodules, abscesses, large verrucouslesions, ulcers, fistulae and sinuses with purulent discharge.
    - The lesions generally develop over several months and may drain pus.
    - The pus may contain small yellow "grains" similar to the sulphur granules of actinomycosis.
- **Laboratory diagnosis:**
  - Specimens: Skin biopsy, discharge like pus or granules.
  - Testing methods:
    - Microscopy: The sulfur granules seen in botryomycosis contain bacteria surrounded by an eosinophilic matrix with club-like projections. This histologic appearance is commonly referred to as the Splendore-Hoeppli phenomeno and can be seen using gram stain, giemsa stain or silver stain.
    - Culture: Also a useful method.
- **Treatment:**
  - Long-term antibiotics: The choice of antibiotics depends on the bacteria identified and includes

trimethoprim-sulfamethoxazole, oral clindamycin, cephalexin, doxycycline and erythromycin.
- Surgical drainage and debridement.
- Laser vapourisation.

4. **Central nervous system:** Abscess, meningitis, encephalitis & intracranial thrombophlebitis.
5. **Respiratory:** Tonsillitis, pharyngitis, sinusitis, otitis media, bronchopneumonia (most common cause), lung abscess & empyema.
6. **Haematogenous:** Bacteremia, septicemia & pyemia.
7. **Endovascular:**

- Endocarditis to the native valve is caused by *Staph aureus*. It is common in IV drug abusers & specially involves the tricuspid valve (right side valve). Few authors suggested that right side valves are commonly infected by *Staph aureus* while left side valves are infected by *Staph aureus, enterococcus* & other bacteria.
- Endocarditis is a manifestation with prosthetic valve up to 12 months (**called early onset prosthetic valve endoarditis**) by *Staph epidermidis* & after 12 months (**called late onset prosthetic valve endoarditis**) by viridans group of bacteria.

8. **Urinary:** Due to local catheterisation, implants or diabetes.
9. **Eyes:** Conjunctivitis, keratitis, corneal ulcer, uveitis, blepharitis, stye (hordeolum externum), chalazion (hordeolum internum) etc.

❖ Carrier: Following are the types.

➢ **Types of carriers:**

a. **New born carrier or shedders:** Colonisation of *Staphylococcus* start early in a life, like umbilical stump in new born baby in hospital. Some carrier **called shedders**. It sheds the cocci in handkerchief, blankets & bed sheets for days or weeks.
b. **Healthy carrier:** Healthy persons (like hospital staff) carry *Staphylococci* in nose (10-30%), in perineum (10%) & also on the hair.
c. **Vaginal carrier:** About 5-10% vaginal carrier, rises greatly during menses, a relevant factor in pathogenesis of TSS related to menstruation.

❖ Laboratory diagnosis:

➢ **Specimens collection: → Table-4**

System involved	Specimens
Skin, soft tissue & musculoskeletal	Pus/discharge on swab, If available in large amount than collect by using sterile syringe
Respiratory:	Sputum or BAL
CNS	C.S.F
Haematogenous & CVS	Blood
Urinary system	Mid stream urine samples

Table-4: Specimens collection

➢ **Testing methods:**

I. **Microscopy: → Follow morphology**
II. **Culture: → Follow C/Cs**
III. **Biochemical reaction: → Follow B/Rs**
IV. **Serological tests:** Anti staphylolysin test.
V. **Molecular method:** PCR
VI. **Typing method:**

A. **Phenotyping methods:**

i. **Bacteriophage typing:** More details, Follow chapter → Laboratory diagnosis of bacterial infections
ii. **Typing by antibiogram pattern**

B. **Genotyping methods:** Following are the methods.

i. **Pulsed Field Gel Electrophoresis**
ii. **DNA fingerprinting**
iii. **Ribotyping**
iv. **Sequence based typing method**
v. **Plasmid profile**

❖ Prevention: Hospital infection is controlled by

- Isolation of patients with open staphylococcal lesion.
- Identification of staphylococcal infection in hospital staff person & keeping them away from work till the infection will cure.
- Strict aseptic precautions like hand washing & use of disinfectant to prevent the spread of hospital strains.
- Diagnosis of **hospital carrier** & treated with local application of mupirocin or chlorhexidine & allow to work after complete recovery.
- Selection of antibiotics only after antibiogram.

❖ Treatment:

a. **Treatment of case:**

1. **Local:** Sometimes topical use of antibiotics like bacitracin, chlorhexidine or mupirocin is sufficient without systemic use of drugs.
2. **Systemic:** Drug resistance is common problem in staphylococci, the appropriate antibiotic should be chosen based on Penicillin (Pn) antibiotic sensitivity pattern as shown in **flow chart-2.**

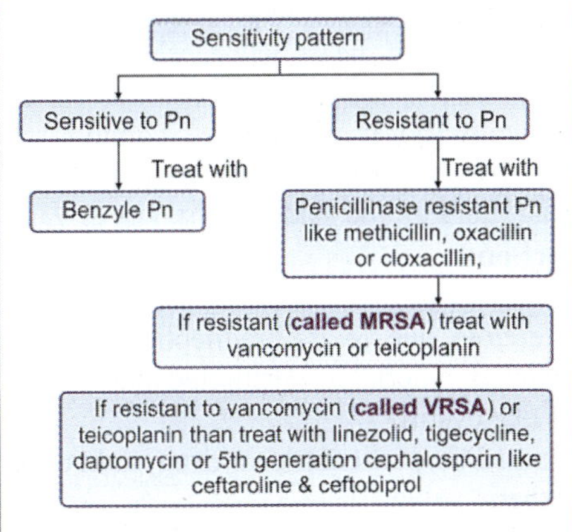

Flow chart-2: Systemic treatment of *Staph aureus*

b. **Treatment of carrier:**

1. **Local:** Treated with local application of mupirocin or chlorhexidine.
2. **Systemic:** If resistant develop than treated with rifampicin with other oral antibiotics.

Other CoPS

1. **Only slide positive:** *Staph lugdunensis.*
- Rapidly established itself as human pathogen.
- It causes catheter related bacteraemia, native valve endocarditis, osteomyelitis & shunt associated meningitis.
2. **Only tube positive:** *Staph intermedius, Staph hyicus* & *Staph schleferi* subspecies *coagulans* (dog). All are animal pathogens.
3. **Both slide & tube positive:**
- *Staph aureus:* Described above.
- *Staph delphini:* Causing purulent skin lesions in dolphins.
- Some strains of *Staph schleferi* subspecies *schleferi:* Native valve endocarditis, osteomyelitis, nosocomial UTI & other infections associated with implanted medical devices.
- *Y. pestis:* Follow chapter → Enterobactericeae-IV(Yersinia)
- *E. rhusiopathiae:* Follow chapter → *Listeria* and *Erysipelothrix*

✓ **Note:** ***Y. pestis & E. rhusiopathiae***
- Exactly not defined about variation in slide & tube coagulase positivity.

Coagulase Negative *Staphylococcus* (CoNS)

❖ **Species:**

1) ***Staph. capitus:***
2) ***Staph. hominis:***
3) ***Staph. haemolyticus:***

} All are normal flora of skin

4) ***Staph. albus (Staph epidermidis)***

➢ **Precipitating factors:**
- Immunodeficiency disease.
- Drug addiction.
- Implantation of foreign bodies (indwelling prosthesis) like heart valve, shunt, intravascular catheter etc.

➢ **Pathogenicity:** It is the most common (75-80%) isolated CoNS from clinical samples. It present as normal flora on the skin, oropharynx & vagina.

- **Infections:**
- Stitch abscess.
- Bacteremia due to its predilection for growth on implanted material as mentioned above.
- UTI like cystitis.
- Endocarditis particularly in drug addicts & having prosthetic valve.
- Central line associated blood stream infection. Identified as gram positive cocci under gram stain & positive blood culture & catalase test with negative coagulase test.
- Normal flora in lid & conjunctiva & may kwon to produce the blapharoconjunctivitis.
- **Biofilms formation:** Colonisation of bacteria over different materials (medical devices like implants, catheter etc.) **called biofilm**. It is due to
- Drug resistance.
- Extracellular polysaccharide matrix, having ability to bind with plastic material of medical devices.

➢ **Diagnosis:** Mannitol non fermenter, so no yellow colour production on mannitol salt agar as shown in **fig.-3(b)**.

➢ **Treatment:** Hospital strains are multiple drug resistant.

5) ***Staph. saprophyticus:***

➢ **Precipitating factors:**
- Age and sex: Common in sexually active young girls and older males.

➢ **Pathogenicity:** Upper UTI in sexually active young girls. It is due to its enhanced capacity to adhere with uroepithelial cells by presence of 160 KDa haemagglutinin adhesin proteins.

➢ **Treatment:** It is sensitive to common antibiotics except nalidixic acid & novobiocin.

❖ **Laboratory diagnosis of CoNS:** → Table-5

Test	*Staph aureus*	*Staph epidermidis (albus)*	*Staph saprophyticus*
Mannitol fermentation	Acid, no gas	-	-
Phosphatase test	+	+	-
Coagulase test	+	-	-
Novobiocin (5µg) sensitivity	S	S	R
Thermonuclease test	+	-	-
Pigments / colonies in NA	Golden yellow	White	No pigment production

Table -5: Diagnosis of CoNS

❖ **Treatment:** Same as *Staph aureus.*

Micrococcus

➢ **Common species:** *M. luteus* & *M. roseus*

➢ **Morphology:** → **Fig.-7**
- GPC looks like *Staphylococci* but larger in size & gram variable.
- Arranged in pairs, tetrads or irregular cluster.

➢ **Culture:**
- Strict aerobes.
- Smaller colonies in culture.

➢ **Differences with *Staphylococci*:** → **Table-6**

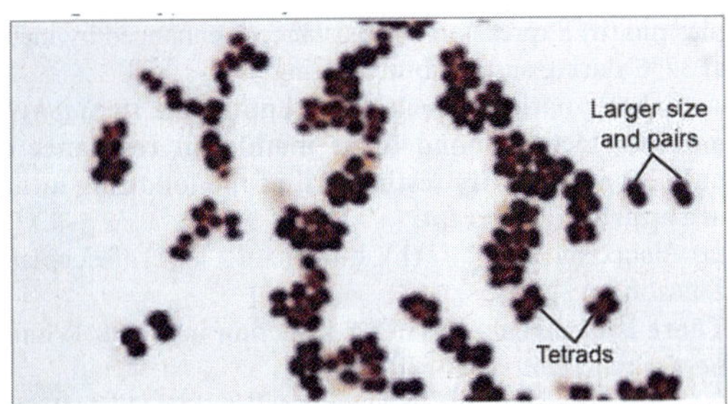

Figure-7: *Micrococcus* under gram stain

Features	*Staphylococcus*	*Micrococcus*	*Stomatococcus*
Anaerobic growth	+	-	+
O-F test (most useful)	F	O	F
Catalase	+	+	Weak
Oxidase	-	+	-
Bacitracin	R	S	S
Furazolidone	S	R	R
Lysostaphin	S	R	R
Agar adherence	-	-	+

Table-6: Differences between genera of Micrococcaceae

+ = Positive, - = Negative, O - F test = Oxidation-Fermentation test, S = Sensitive, R = Resistant

Stomatococcus

- **Common species:** *S. mucilaginosus*
- **Morphology:**
  - GPC
  - Arranged in pairs, tetrads or irregular cluster.
- **Culture:**
  - Aerobes & facultative anaerobes.
  - Produces the small, dome shaped, greyish brown colonies. Colony is with rubbery consistency & adherent to agar, so string is produced when loop attached to colony followed by its withdrawal.
- **Differences with *Staphylococci*: → Table-6**

✓ **Note: Common sensitivity pattern for diagnosis of bacteria:**

- *Staph aureus:* Novobiocin (5µg) sensitive
- *Staph epidermidis:* Novobiocin (5µg) sensitive
- *Strept pyogenes:* Bacitracin sensitive
- *Strept pneumoniae:* Optochin sensitive
- Classical *V. cholerae:* Polymixin B sensitive (50 U)
- *C. jejuni, C. coli & C. curvus:* Nalidixic acid sensitive
- *C. fetus:* Cephalothin sensitivity
- *H. pylori:* Cephalothin sensitivity

✓ **Note: Basic steps to diagnose GPC: → Flow chart-3**

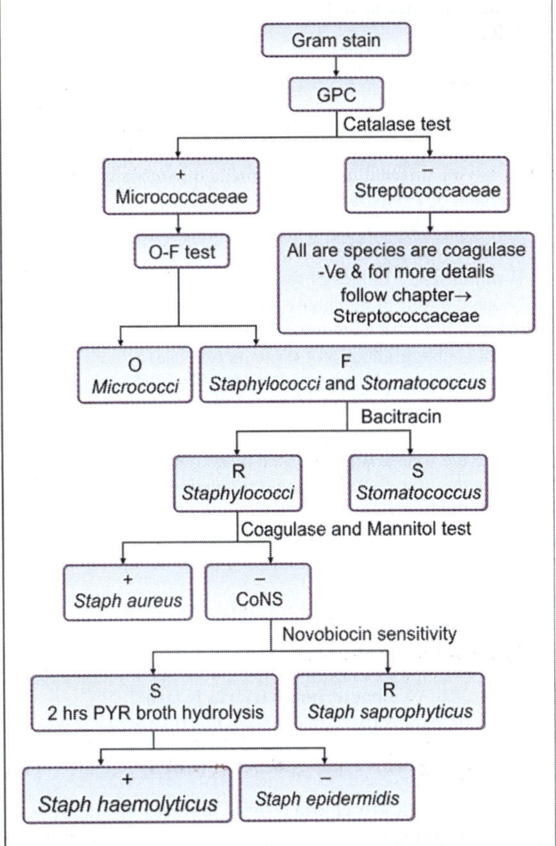

Flow chart-3: Diagnosis of GPC

Question bank

Case study

1) A 28 years female patient visited the hospital with pus discharging swelling on the hand. Gram stain of discharge shows the presence of GPC in cluster. Culture shows the β-haemolysis on blood agar. Bacteria ferments mannitol with acid only. Identify the organism & answer the following
   a) Name the causative agent & describe the morphology of causative agent
   b) Write the pathogenicity of causative agent
   c) Describe the lab. diagnosis of causative agent
2) A child present with diarrhoea in 1-5 hours after consumption of food in party prepared from milk.
   a) Name the causative agent. Enumerate the four toxins & four enzymes produced by causative agent
   b) Write the B/Rs useful in diagnosis of causative agent
   c) Describe in detail about food poisoning (in general)

Essay/Full question

1) *Staph aureus*

Short notes

1) Classification of *Micrococcaceae*
2) Cultural characteristics/ Biochemical reactions/ Pathogenicity/ Lab. diagnosis of *Staph aureus*
3) Toxins of *Staph aureus*
4) Phosphatase test in *Staph aureus*
5) Coagulase test

6) Drug resistance in *Staph aureus*
7) MRSA
8) CoNS
9) Botryomycosis

Short questions for theory/viva questions

1) How you differentiate the pigment of *Staphylococci* from the pigment of *Pseudomonas?*
2) Write the effect of lysozyme & lysostaphin on *Staph aureus.*
3) What is lysostaphin?
4) Write different modes of resistant to penicillin in *Staph aureus.*
5) Name the four β- lactamase (penicillinase) producing bacteria
6) What is hot-cold phenomenon?
7) What is coagglutination? Write its two uses.
8) Name the four enzymes produced by *Staphylococci.*
9) Write the four differences between bound & free coagulase enzyme.
10) Name the four toxins produced by *Staphylococci.*
11) Name the four CoPS or coagulase positive bacteria.
12) Name the four CoNS.
13) Write the principle of phosphatase tests, used in *Staph aureus* & in pasteurisation.

MCQs for chapter review

Types of *Micrococcaceae*

1) **Coagulase +Ve bacterium/bacteria is /are**
(a) *Staph aureus* (b) *Staph intermedius* (c) *Staph hyicus* (d) All

Coagulase Positive *Staphylococcus* (CoPS)

2) **The following are characteristic features of staphylococcal food poisoning except-** (AIIMS -04)
(a) Optimum temperature for toxin production is 37^{0}C (b) Intradietic toxin is responsible for intestinal symptoms (c) Toxin can be destroyed by boiling for 30 minutes (d) Incubation period is 1-6 hours
3) **All the following statements about *Staphylococci* are true, except -** (AI-10)
(a) Most common source of infection is cross infection from infected people (b) About 30% of general population is healthy nasal carrier (c) Epidermolysin & TSS toxin are superantigen (d) Methicilin resistance is chromosomally mediated
4) **Synergohymenotropic toxins of *Staphylococcus* consist of-**
(a) α-haemolysin (b) β-haemolysin (c) γ-haemolysin (d) δ-haemolysin (e) Leucocidin
5) **Staphylococcal toxic shock syndrome is due to -**
(a) Enterotoxin A (b) Enterotoxin B (c) Enterotoxin C (d) Enterotoxin D
6) **Toxic shock syndrome was 1st discovered in**
(a) Tampon users (b) Diabetic septicemia (c) Drug addicts (d) None
7) **In *Staphylococcus* drug resistance has been transferred by**
(a) Transformation (b) Transduction
(c) Conjugation (d) Transfection
8) **All the following statements are true regarding *Staphylococci*, except -** (AIIMS Nov-04)
(a) A majority of infections caused by coagulase negative *Staphylococci* are due to *Staphylococcus epidermidis* (b) β-Lactamase production in *Staphylococci* is under plasmid control (c) Expression of methicillin resistance in *Staphylococcus aureus* increases when it is incubated at 37°C on blood agar (d) Methicillin resistance in *Staphylococcus aureus* is independent of β- Lactamase production
9) **Which of the following statements is most correct regarding resistance to methicillin in MRSA** (AI-11)
(a) Resistance is produced as a result of alteration in Penicillin Binding Proteins (PBP) (b) Resistance is produced by production beta- lactamase (c) Resistance is mediated by plasmid (d) Expression of resistance is enhanced by incubating at 37°C during susceptibility testing
10) **A diabetic patient developed cellulitis due to *Staphylococci aureus* which is found to be methicillin resistance on the antibiotic sensitivity testing. All of the following antibiotics are appropriate except,** (AI-06)
(a) Vancomycin (b) Imipenam (c) Teicoplanin (d) Linezolid
11) **There is outbreak of MRSA infection in ward. What is the best way to control the infection**
(a) Vancomycin given empirically to all patients (b) Fumigation of ward frequently (c) Washing hand before & after attending patient (d) Wearing mask before any invasive procedure in ICU
12) **Which of the following organisms is implicated in causation of botryomycosis** (PGI, Dec-01)
(a) *Staphylococcus aureus* (b) *Staphylococcus albus* (c) *Pseudomonas aeruginosa* (d) *Streptococcus pneumoniae* (e) *Streptococcus pyogenes*

Coagulase Negative *Staphylococcus* (CoNS)

13) ***Staphylococcus aureus* differs from *Staphylococcus epidermidis* by** (AI-02)
(a) Is coagulase positive (b) Forms white colonies (c) A common cause of UTI (d) Causes endocarditis in drug addicts
14) **A patient in an ICU is on a CVP line. His blood culture shows the growth of gram positive cocci which are catalase positive and coagulase negative. The most likely agent is** (AIIMS, May-03)
(a) *Staphylococcus aureus* (b) *Staphylococcus epidermidis* (c) *Streptococcus pyogenes* (d) *Enterococcus faecalis*
15) **Which of the following gram positive organism is most common cause of UTI among sexually active women?** (AIIMS-04)
(a) *Staphylococcus epidermidis* (b) *Staphylococcus aureus* (c) *Staphylococcus saprophyticus* (d) *Enterococcus*
16) **Food poisoning is seen with.**
(a) *Staph aureus* (b) *Staph epidermidis* (c) *Staph pyogenes* (d) *Staph saprophyticus*

Answers of MCQs & explanation

1) **(d)**
- Follow section, **type of Micrococcaceae** (**flow chart-1**) for explanation

2) **(c)**
- Bacteria can grow best at 37°C, which may be the optimum temperature for toxin production.
- Food poisoning occurs after consumption of contaminated food containing preformed toxins **called intradietic toxin**.
- Toxin is heat resistant
- Symptoms start 2-6 hrs after ingestion of toxin

3) **(a)**
- It is the endogenous infection & most common source is hospital personnel
- Healthy persons (like hospital staff) carry *Staphylococci* in nose (10-30%)
- Option c is partially correct because epidermolysin is not superantigen only TSS toxin is superantigen
- Methicilin resistance is mediated by chromosomes while β-Lactamase (penicillinase) production is plasmid mediated

4) **(c) & (e)**
- γ- haemolysin is haemolytic in nature.
- Leucocidin is a cytolytic toxin also **called Panton-Valentine toxin**
- γ- haemolysin & leucocodin are composed of two proteins like S & L (S=slow and F=fast), these bicomponent membrane active toxins are grouped as **synergohymenotropic** toxins

5) **(b) & (c)** } Follow section, **pathogenicity [Toxic shock**
6) **(a)** } **syndrome toxins (TSST)]** for explanation
7) **(b) & (c)**
- Three types of drug resistance occurs in *Staphylococcus* as mentioned earlier in text, of which β- lactamase (penicillinase) production is mediated by plasmid which is transmitted from one cell to other by transduction (more common) & conjugation

8) **(c)**
- A majority of infections caused by CoNS are due to *Staphylococcus epidermidis* & it is the most commonly (75-80%) isolated CoNS from clinical samples.
- β- Lactamase production in *Staphylococci* is under plasmid control while MRSA is chromosome mediated
- Expression of methicillin resistance in *Staphylococcus aureus* increases when it is incubated at reduced temperature (< 37°C, at 30°C) on blood agar
- Methicillin resistance having or any correlation with β-Lactamase production

9) **(a)**
- MRSA is due to alteration in Penicillin Binding Proteins (PBP) of cell membrane by chromosomes (mec A gene)
- MRSA is not beta- lactamase
- Resistance is mediated by chromosome
- Expression of resistance is enhanced at reduced temperature & diagnosed best by using cefoxitin or oxacillin (6μl/ml) discs. Oxacillin required 24 hours incubation at 30^0C with supplementation of 2-4% NaCl in medium.

10) **(b)**
- First line drugs for MRSA are
  - Vancomycin (drug of choice)
  - Linezolid
  - Deptomycin
  - Teicolpanin
  - Tigacycline
  - Quinupristin/dalfopristin
- Imipenam is useful in methicillin sensitive *Staphylococcus aureus* but not for MRSA

11) **(c)**
- Follow section, ***Staph aureus*** **(resistance → chromosomal mediated resistance or MRSA → prevention)** for explanation

12) **(a)**
- Botryomycosis is caused by *Staph aureus*

13) **(a)**
- Differences between *Staphylococcus aureus* & *Staphylococcus epidermidis* is shown in **table-5**

14) **(b)**
- *Staph. aures* is catalase & coagulase positive
- Following are the features of *Staph. albus* (*Staph epidermidis*)
  - Causing central line associated blood stream infection.
  - Identified as gram positive cocci under gram stain & positive blood culture with catalase positive & negative coagulase test.
- *Streptococcus pyogenes* & *Enterococcus faecalis* are catalase & coagulase negative.
- More points for differentiation between GPC are shown in **table-5 & flow chart-3**

15) **(c)**
- Follow section, **CoNS (*Staph saprophyticus*)** for explanation

16) **(a) & (c)**
- Follow section, **coagulase Positive *Staphylococcus* (CoPS) (pathogenicity → enterotoxin)** for explanation.

32 Streptococcaceae

Learning heading & subheadings

Introduction: Organism belongs to Streptococcaceae family has following features.

- Catalase negative.
- Arranged in pair or chain due to single plane division.

Meaning: Strepto from **Streptos (Greek) = easily twisted / coiled/curved/bent like a chain (twisted chain)** + **Cocci** from **kokkos (Greek) = berry**, as the bacteria are spherical in shape like berry & arranged in chain hence the name.

Reference centres:

- **Reference laboratories for Lancefield grouping:**

1. Lady Harding Medical College, New Delhi, India.
2. Christian Medical College, Vellore, India.

- **Data from reference laboratories:** Data showed that about 45% of haemolytic streptococcal isolates are from group A, 10-15% from group B & C each, 25% from group G while 5% from group F.

Uses of Streptococci:

1. **Streptodornase (DNAase):** Enzyme produced by *Strept. pyogenes* (group A) is used for empyema to liquefy the thick pus.
2. **Reverse CAMP test:**
   - CAMP factor produced by *Strept. agalactiae* (group B) is used for the detection of α-toxin of *Clostridium perfringens.*
   - More details: Follow chapter → *Clostridium* (Sporing anaerobe)
3. **Streptokinase (fibrinolysin):** Enzyme produced by *Strept. equisimilis* (group C) is used for thrombolytic therapy in myocardial infarction & other thomboembolic diseases.

Classification of Streptococcaceae: → **Flow chart-1**

α-Haemolytic *Streptococci*

➢ **Two groups identified (1)** *Pneumoniae* group **(2)** Viridans group

Pneumoniae group

Follow chapter → Pneumococcus

Viridans group

➢ **Meaning:** Viridans derived from **viridis** = **green,** because of produces the α-haemolytic colonies which is appear in green colour.

➢ **Cultural characteristics:** Green colour α-haemolysis on blood agar **(fig.1)** due to production of H_2O_2 by bacteria which oxidise the Hb to green colour methemoglobin.

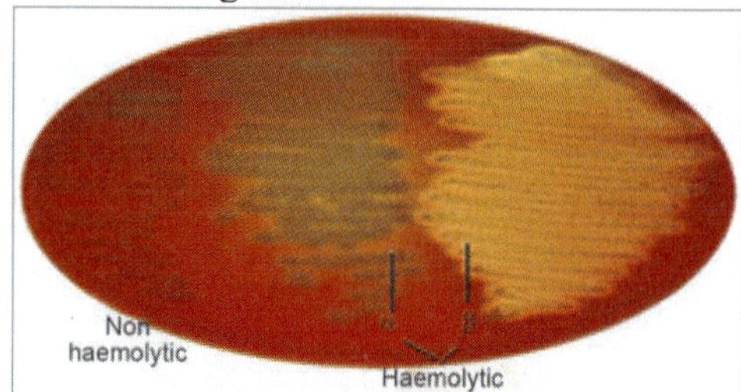

Figure-1: Haemolysis on blood agar

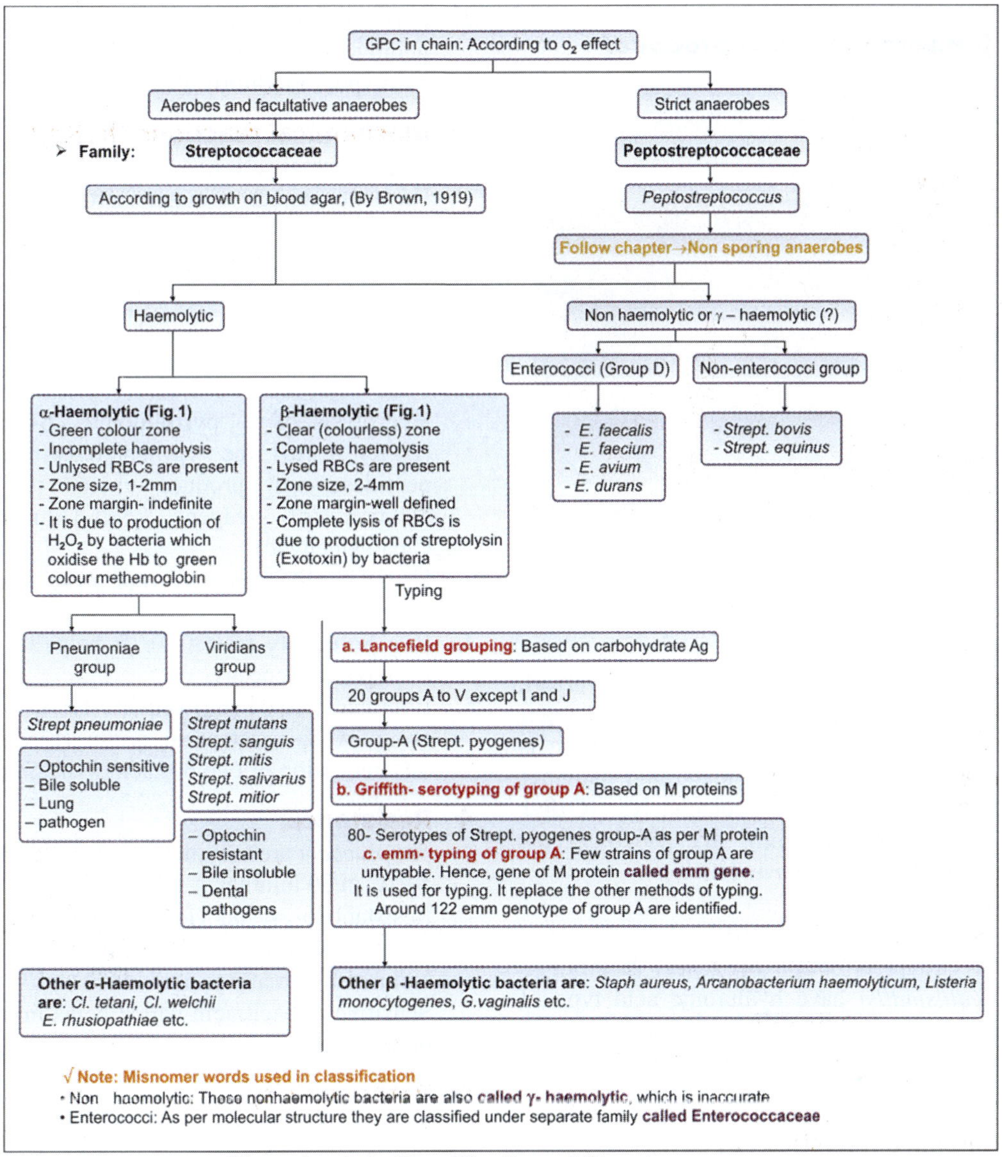

GPC in chain: According to o_2 effect
Aerobes and facultative anaerobes
Strict anaerobes
Family:
Streptococcaceae
Peptostreptococcaceae
According to growth on blood agar, (By Brown, 1919)
Peptostreptococcus
Follow chapter→Non sporing anaerobes
Haemolytic
Non haemolytic or γ – haemolytic (?)
Enterococci (Group D)
Non-enterococci group
α-Haemolytic (Fig.1)
- Green colour zone
- Incomplete haemolysis
- Unlysed RBCs are present
- Zone size, 1-2mm
- Zone margin- indefinite
- It is due to production of H_2O_2 by bacteria which oxidise the Hb to green colour methemoglobin
β-Haemolytic (Fig.1)
- Clear (colourless) zone
- Complete haemolysis
- Lysed RBCs are present
- Zone size, 2-4mm
- Zone margin-well defined
- Complete lysis of RBCs is due to production of streptolysin (Exotoxin) by bacteria
- E. faecalis
- E. faecium
- E. avium
- E. durans
- Strept. bovis
- Strept. equinus
Typing
Pneumoniae group
Viridians group
Strept pneumoniae
Strept mutans
Strept. sanguis
Strept. mitis
Strept. salivarius
Strept. mitior
– Optochin sensitive
– Bile soluble
– Lung
– pathogen
– Optochin resistant
– Bile insoluble
– Dental pathogens
a. Lancefield grouping: Based on carbohydrate Ag
20 groups A to V except I and J
Group-A (Strept. pyogenes)
b. Griffith- serotyping of group A: Based on M proteins
80- Serotypes of Strept. pyogenes group-A as per M protein
c. emm- typing of group A: Few strains of group A are untypable. Hence, gene of M protein called emm gene.
It is used for typing. It replace the other methods of typing.
Around 122 emm genotype of group A are identified.
Other α-Haemolytic bacteria are: Cl. tetani, Cl. welchii E. rhusiopathiae etc.
Other β -Haemolytic bacteria are: Staph aureus, Arcanobacterium haemolyticum, Listeria monocytogenes, G.vaginalis etc.
√ Note: Misnomer words used in classification
• Non haemolytic: These nonhaemolytic bacteria are also called γ- haemolytic, which is inaccurate
• Enterococci: As per molecular structure they are classified under separate family called Enterococcaceae

Flow chart-1: Classification of Streptococcaceae

➢ **Pathogenicity:** Non pathogenic, occasionally cause diseases.

1. ***Strept. mutans*: →Flow chart-2**

Polysaccharides (glucan & dextran) capsule in Strept mutans
It breaks the dietary sucrose to produce
Acid
Dextran (extracellular polysaccharide)
Damage to dentin
Helps in adhesion of bacteria, mucus, food debris & epithelial cells with teeth
Dental caries
Dental plaques

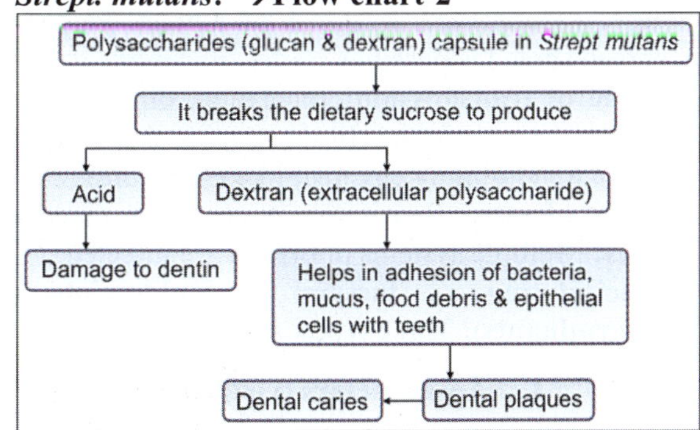

Flow chart-2: Breakdown of dietary sucrose

2. ***Strept sanguis*:**
- Normal flora of oral cavity.
- Enter in blood following chewing, tooth brushing & dental procedures to causing transient bacteraemia & SABE with prosthetic, damaged & congenitally diseased valves.

3. ***Strept milleri* group:**
- It includes the *Strept. intermedius, Strept. angiosus* & *Strept. constellatus.*
- Produces brain abscess & suppurative lesions in other organs.

4. **Others species:** *Strept. mitis, Strept. salivarius, Strept. mitior* etc.

➢ **Laboratory diagnosis:**

A Gram stain: GPC

B Culture:
- Three blood samples are taken at interval of 1 hour for SABE.
- Bacteria produce α –haemolysis on blood agar.

C Tests to differentiate pneumoniae group from viridians group: Follow chapter → Pneumococcus (section →table-1)

β-Haemolytic *Streptococci*

Group A / *Strept pyogenes*

❖ Morphology: → Fig.-2

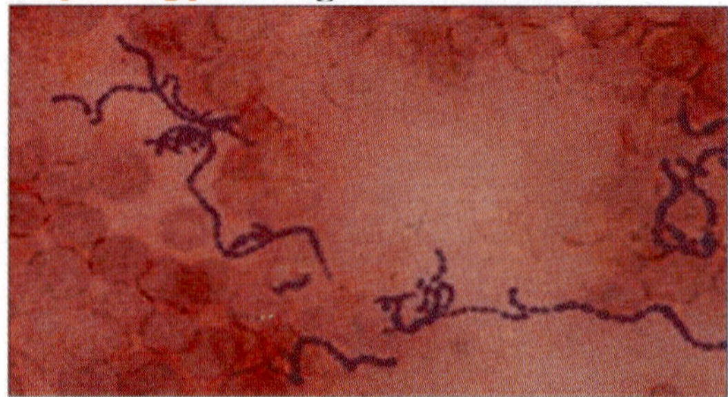

Figure-2: ***Strept pyogenes* under gram stain**

- **Type according to gram stain:** Gram positive cocci.
- **Size:** 0.5-1 µm.
- **Shape:** Spherical or oval.
- **Arrangement:** Arranged in chains (length varies), and influenced by nature of culture medium, longer in liquid than in solid media. Chain formation is due to cocci dividing in one plane and daughter cells failing to separate completely. (**Other bacteria arranged in chain are** *Enterococcus*, *Peptostreptococcus* & *Anthrax bacilli*).
- **Motility:** Non-motile.
- **Spore:** Non-sporing.
- **Capsule:** Group-A (*Strept. pyogenes*) & group-C (*Strept. equisimilis*) have hyaluronic acid type of capsule while groups B (*Strept. agalactiae*) and D (*Enterococcus* spp.) having polysaccharide capsules. Best observed in young culture.

❖ Cultural characteristics (C/Cs):

- **Effective factors:**
- Temperature: 37 °C (22-42 °C).
- pH: Neutral pH
- O_2 effect: Aerobes & facultative anaerobes.
- Co_2 effect: Growth & haemolysis are promoted by 10 % CO_2.
- Enriching substances: Exacting in nutritive requirements, growth occurs only in media enriched with fermentable carbohydrates, blood or serum.
- **Culture in media:**

A. Liquid media:

1. **Glucose broth:**
2. **Serum broth:**

} Granular turbidity with powdery deposit type colony occurs.

B. Solid medium:

1. **Blood agar:** Produces β-haemolysis **(fig.-1).**

C. Selective media:

1. **Blood agar with** crystal violet, nalidixic acid & colistin is selective medium for *S. pyogenes* and *S. pneumoniae*.
2. **PNF medium:** Blood agar with **p**olymixin B, **n**eomycin & **f**usidic acid.

D. Transport medium: Pikes medium is useful.

❖ Biochemical reactions (B/Rs):

1. **Sugar fermentation:**
   - Ferment number of sugars, producing acid but no gas.
   - Ribose fermentation: -Ve, Help to differentiate *Strept. pyogenes* from other *Streptococci*.
2. **Catalase test:** -Ve & helps to differentiate from *Staphylococci*
3. **PYR test:** +Ve
   - Hydrolysis of L- pyrrolidonyl β-naphthylamide (PYR) in to free β-naphthylamide by amino peptidase will produce cherry red colour on addition of reagent (N,N-Dimethyl Amino Cinamaldehyde).
   - Useful to differentiate *Strept. pyogenes* from other *Streptococci*.
4. **Bile Solubility test:** -Ve & helps to differentiate from pneumococcus.
5. **Bacitracin** (0.04 mg) **sensitivity:** It is sensitive in group A & resistant in group B, which help in differentiation of two β- haemolytic *Streptococci*.

❖ Resistance:

- *Streptococci* are very delicate & killed by heating at 54 ^{0}C in 30 minutes.
- Resistant to crystal violet which used as selective agent in media.
- Not resistant many to antibiotics.
- Sensitive to bacitracin which helps in identification of *Strept. pyogenes*.

❖ Pathogenicity:

- **Nature of disease:** Outbreak is common in closed communities like army camp, school boarding etc.
- **Reservoir of infection:** They are present as normal flora in the nose, nasopharynx & throat of human. Asymptomatic human carrier/case is the reservoir.
- **Source of infection:** Sources are droplets from nose, nasopharynx & throat of human. Person to person spread is possible.
- **Mode of transmission:** Inhalation, direct contact, dust or fomites borne. In the tropics skin infection is due to non-biting eny gnat like *Hippelates.*
- **Portal of entry:** Respiratory tract, skin & mucosa.
- **Sites:** Multiple systems or organs are infected.
- **Precipitating factors (epidemiological determinants):** Three types

I. Agent factors (virulence factors)

Two types like intra cellular & extracellular.

A. Intracellular (cell wall associated) factors:

i. Cell wall layers: It include three cell wall layers from inner to outer as below **(fig.-3)**.

a. **Peptidoglycan:** Provide rigidity to cell & also having pyrogenic & thrombolytic properties.

b. **Group specific carbohydrate Ag (C- Ag):**

- Help in Lancefield grouping.
- Play important role in non-suppurative lesion.
- Carbohydrate Ag is detected by capillary precipitation test or by agar gel precipitation test with specific antisera.
- Organisms are grown in Todd- Hewitt broth & extracted by HCl (**Lancefield's acid extraction method**), by formamide (**Fuller's method**), by enzyme of *Streptomyces albus* (**Maxted's method**) or by autoclaving (**Rantz & Randall's method**).

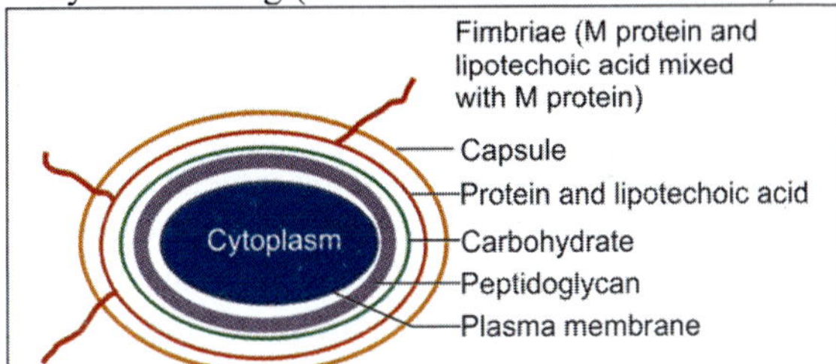

Figure-3: Cell wall layers of *Streptococcus*

c. **Protein Ags:** Three types like M, T & R proteins.

1. **M protein:**

- It is heat & acid stable but susceptible to tryptic digestion.
- It useful for Griffith- serotyping of *Streptococcus.*
- M proteins is extracted by Lancefield's acid extraction method & based on this, 80 serotypes of *Strept. pyogenes* group-A are identified.
- It act as virulence factor & inhibits the phagocytosis.
- It is antigenic & antibody to M protein phagocytoses the cocci, hence it is protective.
- It also mixed with lipotechoic acid as a structure of fimbriae.
- A non type protein associated with M protein is also identified **called M associated protein.**

2. **T protein:**

- It is acid labile & trypsin resistant.
- T proteins is extracted by trypsin treatment to *Streptococci* & demonstrated by slide agglutination test.
- It is non-virulent.

3. **R protein:**

- It is present in *Strept. pyogenes* group-A (2,3,28 & 48), B, C & G.
- It is non-virulent.

ii. **Capsular Ag:**

- Inhibit phagocytosis. It is not antigenic in human beings.
- More detail: Vide supra (morphology → capsule).

iii. **Fimbria:** Hair like (**fig.-3**) structure consist lipotechoic acid & mixed with M protein is helpful in attachment of *Streptococci* with epithelial cells.

iv. **Other protein Ags:**

- **M associated protein:** Described above.
- **Protein F:** Helps in attachment with pharyngeal wall.
- **Protein G:** It binds with Fc portion of IgG, which hinds the Ab binding site over phagocytic cell and prevent the phagocytosis.

v. **Antigenic cross reactivity with human tissues:** Streptococcal antigens which are cross reactivity with human tissues are mentioned **table-1.** Such cross reactivity is responsible for autoimmunity.

Streptococcal Ag	Human tissue
Plasma membrane	Vascular intima/gomeruli
Peptidoglycan	Skin Ag
Group A carbohydrate	Cardiac valves
Protein M Ag	Myocardium
Hyaluronic acid capsule	Synovial fluid

Table-1: Streptococcal antigenic cross reactivity

B. **Extracellular factors:** Two types like enzymes & toxins as mentioned below.

i. **Enzymes:**

1. **Streptokinase (fibrinolysin):**

- Acts like plasminogen and break fibrin to spread the infection. It is produced by group A, C & K.
- **Use:** It given intravenously to treat myocardial infarction and thromboembolic disorders.

2. **Streptodornase (DNAase):**

- It degrades the DNA from neutrophils which is collected as pus.
- **Use:** It helps to liquefy thick pus (serous character). This property is useful to liquefy thick pus in empyema. A preparation containing streptokinase & streptodornase is available for this purpose.
- Four types A, B, C & D.
- B is most common

3. **NADase / DPNase (Nicotinamide Adanine Dinucleotidase / Diphospho Pyridine Nucleotidase):** It is leucotoxic.
4. **Proteinase:** It destroys the protein.
5. **Hyaluronidase:** It splits the hyaluronic acid which binds the connective tissues together and helps in spread of infection.
6. **Lipoproteinase (Serum Opacity factor/SOF):** Produce opacity when applies to agar gel containing horse or swine serum.
7. **Other enzymes:** Phosphatase, esterase, amylase, N acetyl glucosaminase and neuraminidase, but their exact role is not known.

ii. **Toxins:**

a. **Haemolysin (streptolysin):** Two types O & S.

1. **Streptolysin O:**

- O_2 labile, so active in absence of O_2 (reduced state).
- Heat labile.
- Leucotoxic & cardiotoxic.
- Responsible for haemolysis by pour plate culture under anaerobic incubation.

- It resembles to haemolysin of *Cl. welchii*, *Cl. tetani*, *Strept. pneumoniae* & *Cl. novyi*.
- Diagnosis: By Anti Streptolysin O (ASO) test. ASO appears in serum after streptococcal infection. ASO titre >200 units is considered significant titre.

2. **Streptolysin S:**

- O_2 stable.
- Heat stable.
- Soluble in serum, so **called streptolysin S**.
- Leucocidal activity.
- Responsible for haemolysis by surface culture.

b. **Erythrogenic toxin [Dick toxin, scarletinal toxin, SPE (Streptococcal Pyrogenic Exotoxin)]:**

- **Dick test:** Intradermal inoculation in susceptible individual causes erythematous reaction hence toxin **called Erythrogenic toxin** & test **called "Dick test"**. This test is used to identify the children susceptible of scarlet fever, so **called "scarletinal toxin"**.
- It induces fever so **called SPE.**
- In addition to erythema & fever it also induces the necrotising fasciitis & toxic shock syndrome (**called streptococcal toxic shock syndrome**).
- Three types like A, B & C. A & C are bacteriophage coded while B is chromosome coded.
- Type A & C are superantigens & T cell mitogens - release large numbers of inflammatory cytokines causing fever, shock and tissue damage.

II. Host factors

1. **Age:** Common between 5-8 years of age. Less below 2 years & in adults.
2. **Immunity:** Immunity is type specific & reinfection is possible because of multiple serotypes.

III. Environmental factors

1. **Season:** Common in winter in temperate countries while seasonal distribution has not been identified in tropical countries.
2. **Overcrowding:** Major factor in transmission is due to close contact. Outbreak occurs in closed communities like army camp, school boarding etc.

➢ **Clinical features:** Two types of infection like suppurative & non-suppurative.

a. **Suppurative lesions:**

1. **Respiratory tract infections:**

- Sore throat, pharyngitis & tonsillitis.
- Scarlet fever: Acute pharyngitis with erythematous rash.
- Streptococcal pneumonia occurs secondary to viral & influenza infection.

2. **Skin & soft tissue infections:**

- **Common infections:** Infection of minor abrasion, traumatic or burn wounds.
- **Cellulitis [fig.-4(a)]:** It is the infection of skin (dermis) & subcutaneous tissues. It present with redness (generally not sharp), pain, swelling & warmth of the affected area. More common due to *Strept. pyogenes* than *Staph. aureus*.

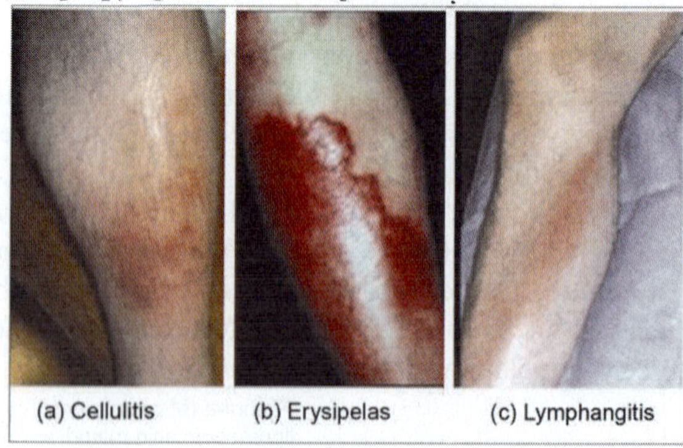
(a) Cellulitis (b) Erysipelas (c) Lymphangitis

Figure-4: Skin & soft tissue infections

- **Erysipelas [fig.-4(b)]:** It is the infection of skin & superficial lymphatics. Affected skin becomes red (sharply defined from surrounding health skin), swollen & indurated. It found mainly in older patients.
- **Lymphangitis [fig.-4(c)]:** It is the infection of lymphatic vessels. It present with redness which run along the course of lymphatic vessels, pain & swelling.
- **Pyoderma:**
  - Meaning: Pyon (Greek) = pus & derma (Greek) = skin.
  - Definition: It is the skin infection present with pus.
  - Types: It includes different type clinical conditions like impetigo, folliculitis, boil (furuncle), carbuncle, tropical ulcer, pyoderma gangrenosum (autoimmune) etc., but of them impetigo is streptococcal origin has following features.

Impetigo

- It is the superficial skin infection which begins with red spot, then change to blister (pustule), eventually break up, ooze fluid & develop yellowish-brown crust.
- It may be itchy or painful. Fever is uncommon.
- Mostly present on face, neck & also on hands or legs.
- It found mainly in young child. Impetigo & streptococcal lesion of scabies are the main cause of acute glomerulonephritis in children in tropics.
- It is further classified as non-bullous (also **called contagious impetigo**) & bullous impetigo as mentioned in **table-2.**

○ Diagnosis of pyoderma:

- Moderate ASO titre (not high) & don't have significant role, however ASO test is much important in pharyngeal infection.
- Anti DNAase B titre antibody to hyaluronidase are elevated, help in diagnosis of pyoderma antecedent to acute glomerulonephritis.

Features	Non-bullous impetigo [fig.5(a)]	Bullous impetigo [fig.5(b)]
Etiology	*Staph. aureus* & *Strept. pyogenes*	*Staph. aureus*
Sites	It starts around the nose & face, but rarely affect the arms & legs	Appear in various skin areas, especially the buttocks & trunk.
Features	- It starts as small red papules like insect bites which rapidly evolve to small blisters & then to pustules that finally scab over with a characteristic honey-colored crust. This entire process usually takes about one week. - At times, there may be non-tender but swollen lymph nodes (glands) nearby.	- Bacteria produce a toxin that reduces cell to cell stickiness, causing separation between the top skin layer (epidermis) & the lower layer (dermis). This leads to the formation of a blister. (In medical terminology, blister is **called bulla**) -These bullae are fragile & contain a clear yellow-colored fluid. The bullae are delicate & often break with the overlying "roof" of skin lost, leaving red, raw skin with a ragged edge. A dark crust will commonly develop during the final stages of development. With healing, this crust will resolve.

Table-2: Types of impetigo

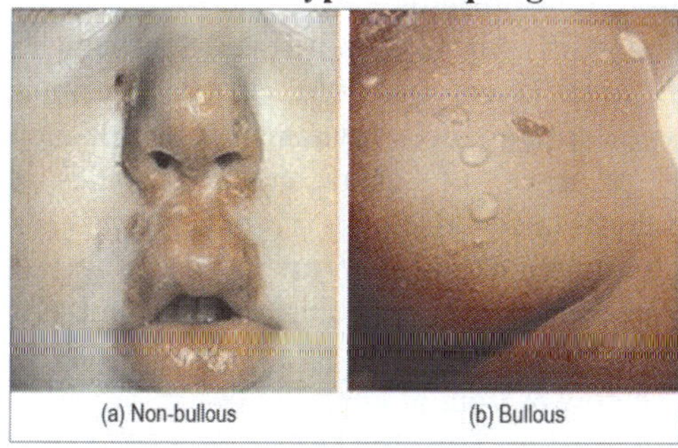

(a) Non-bullous (b) Bullous

Figure-5: Types of impetigo

- **Ecthyma (deep impetigo):** It is the extension of impetigo from the epidermis to dermis. It also **called deep impetigo.** It present with deeper erosion of dermis. It is caused by *Strept. pyogenes* alone or with *Staph. aureus.*

✓ **Note: Related terminology to ecthyma**

- **Erythrasma:** It is the localised infection of the stratum corneum affecting axilla & groin. It is caused by *C. minutissimum.*
- **Ecthyma gangrenosum:** Caused by *P.aeruginosa.*
- **Erythrasma migrans:** Caused by *B.bergdorferi.*
- **Ecthyma contagiosum:** Caused by orf virus.

- **Necrotising fasciitis (fig.-6):**
    - Synonym: Also **called flesh-eating disease** or **flesh-eating bacteria syndrome** or **necrotizing soft tissue infection.**
    - Definition: It is the rapidly progressive necrosis of subcutaneous tissues, muscle & fascia.

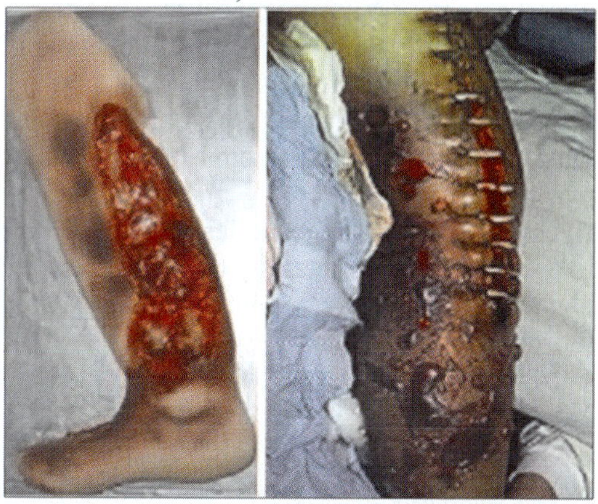

Figure-6: Necrotising fasciitis

- Etiology & types: It is mixed infection by aerobic & anaerobic bacteria. M types 1 & 3 of *Strept. pyogenes* may alone be responsible for this condition which **called flesh eating bacteria.** Recent knowledge on the disease classified it in to following four categories depending on the infecting organism.
    - Type I: Most common type is caused by a mixture of bacterial types, and commonly occurs at sites of surgery or trauma, usually in abdominal or perineal areas and accounts for 70 to 80% of cases.
    - Type II: It is caused by Group A *Streptococci* alone or often with a co-infection of *S. aureus*, and usually occurs on the head, neck, arm or legs. It is less often associated with predisposing risk factors such as surgery or a compromised immune system.
    - Type III: It is caused by *Vibrio vulnificus*, which enters the skin via puncture wounds from fish or insects in seawater.
    - Type IV: It is due to a fungal infection.
- Diagnosis of necrotising fasciitis:
    - Isolation of *Strept. pyogenes* from the lesion.
    - ASO titre: High
    - Anti DNAase B titre: High
- Treatment of necrotising fasciitis:
    - Surgical debridement.
    - Isolates are sensitive to penicillin in vitro but less effective. Combined intravenous drugs like piperacillin/tazobactam, clindamycin & vancomycin are effective.

3. **Streptococcal toxic shock syndrome**
    - It is characterised by DIC & multisystem failure.

- **Caused** by strain 1, 3, 12 & 28 of M types of *Strept. pyogenes.*
- Sometimes it may present with necrotising fasciitis
- It may resemble to staphylococcal TSS.
- Streptococcal Toxic Shock Syndrome & necrotising fasciitis occurs in person not immune to the infecting M types.

4. **Genital infection:**
- Puerpural sepsis & puerpural fever.
- Exogenous by hospital staff & instrumentation.
- Endogenous by anaerobic streptococci.

5. **Cardio Vascular System (CVS):** Endocarditis
6. **Haematogenous:** Bacteremia, septicemia & pyaemia.
7. **Eyes:** It produces the same lesion as *Staph aureus* like conjunctivitis, keratitis, corneal ulcer, uveitis, blepharitis, stye (hordeolum externum), chalazion (hordeolum internum) etc.
8. **Other suppurative:** Abscess of brain, liver, kidney, lungs etc.

b. **Non-suppurative lesions:** ARF & APSGN are the two non-suppurative lesions described below with differences in **table-3.**

1. **Acute rheumatic fever (ARF):**

- **Meaning:** Rheumatic word came from **rheum (Greek) = flow,** as this disease flow/spread from one connective tissue to the other.
- **Definition:** It is an autoimmune disease of heart, skin, joints & brain characterised by fever, multiple painful joints, involuntary muscles movements & occasionally a characteristic non-itchy rash (**called erythema marginatum**). Basically it is the lesion of connective tissues around the arterioles.
- **Onset:** Develops 2-3 weeks following repeated or persistent throat infection by any serotype of Group A, β-haemolytic streptococci (*Strept pyogenes*).
- **Pathogenesis:** It is an autoimmunity / type II hypersensitivity reaction due to cross-reactions between antigens of heart, joint tissues and *Streptococci* (M protein). Antigenic similarities between streptococci & human tissues are listed earlier in this chapter. When antibody develop against such streptococcal antigen it may produces the cytotoxic (type II hypersensitivity) damage to the heart & joint tissues.
- **Predisposing factors:**
  - Age: Common in children between 5-15 years of age. Occurs in 20% adults. It rarely present in children below 4 years & adults above 40 years.
  - Socio-economical factors: Poverty & overcrowding are also the contributory factors.
  - Genetic predisposition: Due to their genetics, some people are more likely to get the disease when exposed to the bacteria than others.
  - Diseases: Dental problems, bacterial endocarditis, heart transplant, artificial heart valves or congenital heart defects are also the risk factors.

Features	ARF	APSGN
Earlier infection	Throat	Skin or throat
Repeated attack	Common	Absent
Prior sensitisation	Required	Not required
Serotypes	Any M serotype of *Strept pyogenes*	49, 53-55, 59-61 after skin infection. 1 & 12 after pharyngitis
Pathogenesis	Type II	Type III
Immune response	Marked	Moderate
Risk factors		
- Age	- Child age	- Any age
- Genetic	- Present	- Absent
Diagnosis		
- ASO titre	- Raised	- Normal
- Anti-DNAase	- Raised	- Raised
- Complement	- Normal	- Lowered
Penicillin prophylaxis	Indicated	Not indicated
Course	Progressive	Self limited
Prognosis	Poor/variable	Good

Table-3: Differences between ARF & APSGN

- **Features (Jone's diagnostic criteria):** It was 1st published by T. Duckett Jones in 1944 in two categories like major & minor criteria.
  - Major criteria:
    - **Migratory polyarthritis (up to 75%):** Inflammation of large joints, usually begins from legs & flow upwards.
    - **Pancarditis (up to 35%):** It is the inflammation of all three layers of heart. It most common in myocardium **called myocarditis** & characterised by presence of characteristic nodules **called Aschoff's nodules**.
    - **Subcutaneous nodules (up to 10%):** It is due to collection of collagen fibres. It present on bony prominences or tendon like back of wrist, outside the elbow & front of knee.
    - **Skin rashes (up to 10%):** It **called erythema marginatum**. Red rash begins as macules on the trunk or arms spread outward & clear in the middle to form rings. It spares the face.
    - **Sydenham's chorea (up to 10%):** It is also **called St. Vitus dance**. It is the random, rapid & involuntary movement of the face & arms. It occurs very late in the disease mostly 3 months after the infection.
  - Minor criteria:
    - **Fever:** Temperature is 38.2-38.9^{0}C (101-102^{0}F)
    - **Arthralgia:** Joint pain without swelling & not the part of Polyarthritis which is the major criteria.

- **Increased acute phase reactants:** Increased CRP & ESR
- **TLC:** Leucocytosis (neutrophilia)
- **ECG features:** It suggest the 1st degree heart block, such as prolonged PR interval. This minor cannot be included if major pancarditis is present.
- **History:** Previous episode of rheumatic fever or inactive rheumatic heart disease.

✓ **Note: Aschoff's nodule**

- **Onset of Aschoff's nodule:** It develops after several weeks after the onset of symptoms.
- **Stages of Aschoff's nodule:** Three phases
  - Early/exudative/degenerative phase: Characterised by swelling of collagen fibres around the blood vessels & last up to the 4th week.
  - Intermediate/proliferative/granulomatous phase: Characterised by granulomatous reaction & occurs between 4th-13th weeks.
  - Late/fibrous/healing phase: Eventually nodule is replaced by scar.
- **Macroscopy of Aschoff's nodule:**
  - **Shape:** It is elliptical or fusiform in shape.
  - **Location:** It present in any layer of the heart. Occasionally present in the pericardium. It also identified from the adventitia of the aorta.
- **Microscopy of Aschoff's nodule [fig. 7(a) & (b)]:** It is composed of swollen eosinophilic collagen fibres with central fibrinoid necrosis surrounded by macrophages (**called Anitschkow's cells**), lymphocytes, plasma cells & multinucleated giant cells (giant cell **called Aschoff's cells**).
- **Aschoff's body:** Fusion of multiple Aschoff's nodules form the giant stricture **called Aschoff's body**. It located over bony prominences & over the tendon.
- **Anitschkow's cells (fig.-8):**
  - These are the macrophages present in heart, so **called cardiac macrophages.**
  - These cells are participating in formation of Aschoff's nodules.
  - Nuclei of these cells contains central band of clumped chromatin, that gives caterpillar like appearance in longitudinal section, hence **called caterpillar cells** & **owl-eye appearance** in cross section.

- **Complications of ARF:** The heart is involved in about half of cases. Damage to the heart valves, **called Rheumatic Heart Disease (RHD)**, usually occurs after repeated attacks but can sometimes occur after one. The damaged valves may result in heart failure, atrial fibrillation & infection of the valves
- **Diagnosis of ARF:** According to revised Jone's criteria by American Heart Association, diagnosis of ARF is based on two major or one major with two minor criteria supported by laboratory evidence like
  - ASO titre: Raised > 200.
  - Raised Anti-DNAase.
  - Normal complement level.
  - Positive streptococcal culture (history of sore throat).

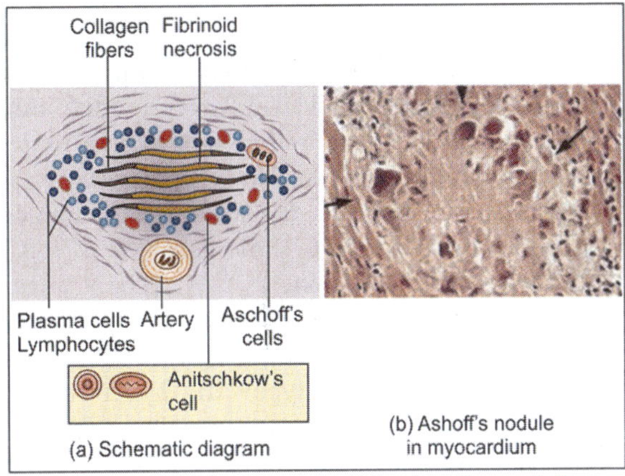

Figure-7: Microscopy of Aschoff's nodule

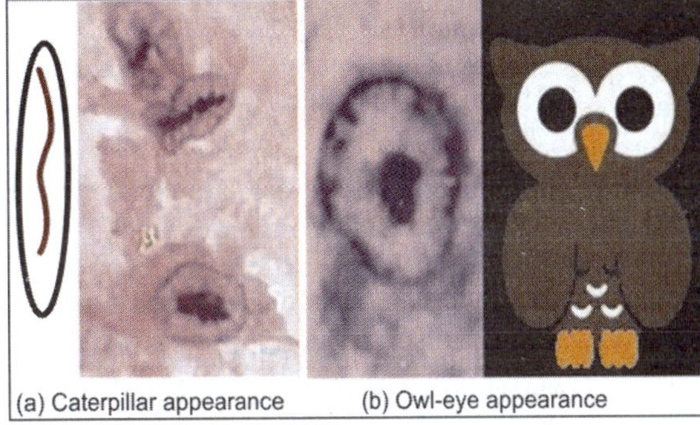

Figure-8: Anitschkow's cell

- **Prevention of ARF:**
  - General measures: Improvement in dental health & personal hygiene.
  - Chemoprophylaxis: Penicillin is given to the patient with streptococcal sore throat infection. Long term antibiotics are also recommended in patients with underlying disease like dental problems, bacterial endocarditis, heart transplant, artificial heart valves or congenital heart defects.
  - Immunoprophylaxis: No vaccines are currently available to protect against *Strept pyogenes* infection.
- **Treatment of ARF:**
  - Antibiotics: Monthly injections of long-acting penicillin for five years in patients having one attack of rheumatic fever. If there is evidence of carditis, the length of therapy may be up to 40 years. It also required the continual use of low-dose antibiotics like Pn, sulfadiazine or erythromycin.
  - Anti-inflammatory: Like steroids or aspirin are required to reduce the inflammation.
- **Prognosis of ARF:** Poor.

2. **Acute Post-Streptococcal Glomerulo Nephritis (APSGN):**

- **Onset:**
- Develops 2-6 weeks following skin infection (impetigo), rarely but 1-3 weeks after throat infection (pharyngitis) by M serotype of Group A, β-haemolytic streptococci (*Strept pyogenes*).
- Common M serotypes are (**called nephritogenic strains**) 49, 53-55, 59-61 following skin & 1 & 12 following throat infection.
- Prior sensitisation is not necessary, it mean single infection can produces the damage.
- **Pathogenesis:** It is type III hypersensitivity reaction due to immune complex formation between streptococcal antigens & respective antibodies, which later deposited in renal glomeruli.
- **Predisposing factors:**
- Age: Occurs at any age, but common in children between 2-14 years of age & only 10% patients are above 40 years.
- Socio-economical factors: Common in developing countries due to poverty & overcrowding.
- Genetic predisposition: Not significant.
- Diseases: Nothing particular.
- **Features:** It present with hypertension, haematuria, oliguria, periorbital puffiness, anaemia & flank pain.
- **Complication of APSGN:** Acute renal failure
- **Diagnosis of APSGN:**
- ASO titre raised moderately or may be normal.
- Anti DNAase titre is elevated.
- Antibody to hyaluronidase is elevated.
- Complement level lowered.
- Urine analysis: Haematuria
- **Prevention of APSGN:**
- General measures: Improvement in personal hygiene.
- Chemoprophylaxis: Antibiotics are given to treat skin infections.
- Immunoprophylaxis: No vaccines are currently available to protect against *Strept. pyogenes* infection.
- **Treatment of APSGN:** Self limited disease. Only conservative treatment is given & can heal without any permanent damage.
- **Prognosis of APSGN:** Good prognosis.

➢ **Complications:**
- Respiratory infection produce otitis media, peritonsillar abscess, quinsy, mastoiditis, suppurative adenitis, Ludwig's angina, meningitis, cervical lymphadenitis etc.
- Skin & soft tissues infection may lead to fatal septicemia.

❖ Laboratory diagnosis:

➢ **Samples collection: → Table-4**

System involved	Specimens
Respiratory	Throat swab, sputum
Skin & Soft tissue	Pus/discharge by swab/syringe
Genital infection	Pus/discharge by swab, urine
CNS	CSF
Haematogenous & endovascular	In SABE three blood samples are collected at 1 hr interval

Table-4: Specimens collection

➢ **Testing methods:**

I. **Microscopy: → Follow morphology**
II. **Culture: → Follow C/Cs**
III. **Biochemical reactions: → Follow B/Rs**
IV. **Serological tests:**

1. **Anti Streptolysin-O (ASO) test:** Passive agglutination, significant titre >200 IU/ml in ARF.
2. **Anti DNAase B test:** Passive agglutination, significant titre >300 IU/ml, for APSGN.
3. **Anti-hyaluronidase test:** For retrospective streptococcal infection.
4. **Streptozyme test:** Passive haemagglutination type test.

V. **Molecular methods:** PCR & DNA probe.

❖ Prophylaxis:
- Long term benzyl Pn is given to children to prevent rheumatic fever & reinfection.
- Prophylaxis is not useful for glomerulonephritis.

❖ Treatment:
Benzyl Pn is given. If allergy to Pn than erythromycin or cephalexin may be used. Common modes of treatment are as follows.
- Cellulitis, erysipelas, impetigo, ecthyma & pneumonia: Local antiseptic plus systemic Pn.
- Pharyngitis: Pn
- Empyema: Pn + drainage.
- Streptococcal toxic shock syndrome: Pn + clindamycin + Intravenous Ig.

Group B / *Strept. agalactiae*

➢ **Morphology:**
- Gram +Ve cocci present in pairs or short chains.
- Contains polysaccharide capsule.

➢ **Cultural characteristics (C/Cs):**

a. **Blood agar:** Produces β-haemolysis & colonies is larger about 2mm in size with mucoid consistency.
b. **Pigment producing media:** Three media as below.

✪ **Properties of pigment of group B *Streptococci:***
- It was first noted by Lancefield in 1934 in nine of twenty-four strains grown anaerobically. However about 95-99% strains of group B can produces the pigment with modification in Islam agar.
- Biochemically it is carotenoid.
- Produced under anaerobic incubation.
- Bright-red in colour.
- Pigment production is increased by co-trimoxazole.

✪ **Media to detect the pigment production:**

1. **Islam agar:**

- **History:** This medium was designed by Islam in 1977, hence the name.
- **Uses:**
  - It is useful to detect the pigment production properties of *Strept agalactiae.*
  - Other organisms like anaerobic *Streptococci, Bacteroides* & *Clostridium* species are able to grow on this medium but do not produce the pigment.
- **Growth properties:** Colonies of Group B *Streptococci* are 0.5-1mm in diameter, round and pigmented orange/red after 24-48 hours under anaerobic incubation.

2. **Columbia agar:**
3. **Starch serum agar:**

➢ **Biochemical reactions (B/Rs):**

1. **Hippurate hydrolysis test:** +Ve
2. **Bacitracin sensitivity test:** Resistant
3. **PYR test:** Negative
4. **CAMP test:** +Ve

- **Full form:**
  - CAMP is an acronym for "Christie–Atkins–Munch-Petersen" test, for the 3 persons who invented the test.
  - It is often incorrectly reported as the product of four people (counting Munch-Petersen as two people).
  - The true relationship (three people) is the reason for two en dashes & then one hyphen in "Christie–Atkins–Munch-Petersen".
  - The name has no relationship to cyclic adenosine monophosphate(cAMP).
- **Principle:** *Strept. agalactiae* produce extracellular protein **called CAMP factor** which act synergistically with β-haemolysin of *Staph aureus* to cause lysis of RBCs.
- **Properties of CAMP factor:**
  - It is encoded by CAMP factor gene.
- A similar factor has been identified in *Bartonella henselae.*
- **Method:**
  - Single streak of *Streptococcus* to be tested and a *Staph. aureus* are made perpendicular to each other
  - Left 3-5 mm distance between two streaks.
  - Incubate the plate.
- **Control:** Make the control line by using the Group A *Streptococci.*
- **Result:** A positive result appear as an arrowhead shaped zone (**fig.-9**) of complete haemolysis.
- **Interpretation:**
  - *Strept. agalactiae* is CAMP test positive while non group B *Streptococci* are negative.
  - *Listeria monocytogenes* is also CAMP test positive.

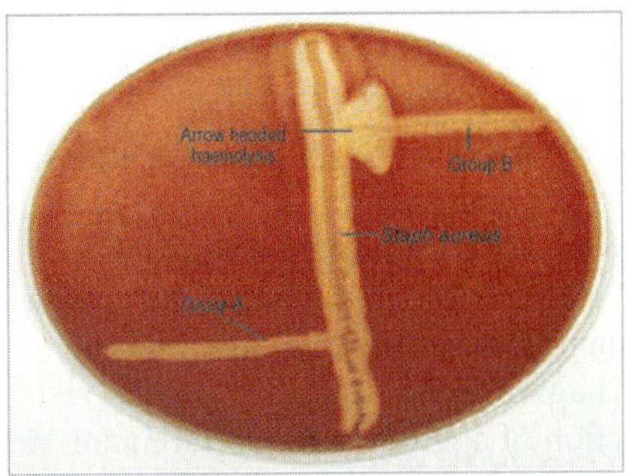

Figure-9: CAMP test

➢ **Pathogenicity:**

✪ **Virulence factors:** Polysaccharide capsule has virulent property. Nine capsular serotypes are identified each provide the type specific protection.

✪ **Clinical features:** Normal flora of the vagina causing following two types of infection.

A. **In new born:**

i. **Septicemia & neonatal meningitis:** Two forms

a. **Early onset type:** Occur in 1st week after birth.

✪ **Causative serotypes:** Mostly by1a, 1b, 2, 3 & 5.

✪ **Mode of transmission:** From infected birth canal.

✪ **Clinical features:** Present as meningitis & septicemia.

✪ **Case fatality:** 4.7%

b. **Late onset type:** Occur between 2nd to 12th weeks of life.

✪ **Causative serotypes:** Mostly by serotype 3.

✪ **Mode of transmission:** From the environment.

✪ **Clinical features:** Present as septicemia.

✪ **Case fatality:** 2.8%

ii. **Other infections:** It includes arthritis, osteomyelitis, conjunctivitis, respiratory infections, peritonitis, omphalitis, endocarditis etc.

B. **In adult:** Pneumonia & puerpural sepsis.

➢ **Diagnosis:**

✪ **Specimens:** Blood, CSF & genital discharge.

✪ **Testing methods:** By microscopy (morphology), C/Cs & B/Rs as described earlier.

➢ **Treatment:** Pn is the drug of choice for all group B infection.

Group C / *Strept. equisimilis*

➢ Animal pathogen & in human habitat in throat.

➢ Source of **streptokinase, used for thrombolytic therapy.**

➢ Ferment ribose & trehalose.

➢ Produce Upper Respiratory Tract Infection (**URTI**), endocarditis, osteomyelitis, brain abscess, pneumonia, puerperal sepsis & other infections.

➢ It produces streptokinase & streptolysin O, which are antigenically distinct from that produce by *Strept. pyogenes.*

➢ Resistant to Pn, addition of gentamicin is recommended in serious cases.

Group F / *Strept. angiosus*

- Grow very poorly on blood agar unless incubated under CO_2 atmosphere.
- They are **called minute streptococci.**
- One member of this group is ***Streptococcus* MG**, causing **primary atypical pneumonia.**
- It is diagnosed by streptococcus MG test based on detection of agglutinin by agglutination reaction.

Other groups

- **Group G:** *Strept. dysgalactiae.*
  - Normal flora of throat in human, monkeys & dogs.
  - In human it causes UTI, Endocarditis & tonsillitis.
- **Group H:** *Strept. sanguis*, may cause endocarditis.
- **Group K:** *Strept. salivarius*, may cause endocarditis.
- **Group L:** *Strept. dysgalactiae* (?)
- **Group M &O:** *Strept mitior*
- **Group N:** *Lactococcus lactis*
- **Group R & S:** *Strept suis*
- Other *Streptococcus* species are classified as 'non-Lancefield streptococci'.

Non haemolytic *Streptococci*

Features	*Entero-coccus*	Non *Enterococcus* group
C/Cs		
Growth in presence of 6-5% salt, 45°C temp., high pH (9.6) & 40% bile	Yes	No
Growth on blood agar	No or α or β haemolysis	Non haemolysis
B /Rs		
Esculin hydrolysis	Yes	No
PYR test	Yes	No
Pathogenicity		
Intestinal flora	More	Less
Pathogenicity	More	Less
Treatment		
Drug resistance	More	Less

Table-5: Differences between *Enterococcus* & Non *Enterococcus* group

- **Introduction:** Two groups identified like **(1)** faecal *Streptococci* which are classified under a separate genus **called *Enterococcus*** & **(2)** non-faecal *Streptococci* which are classified under streptococcal category **called Group D *Streptococcus*.**
- **Differences between two groups: →Table-5.**

Enterococcus

- **Species:** *E. faecalis, E. faecium, E. avium, E. durans* etc.
- **Morphology:** Oval shape, arranged in pair, at angle to each other or in short chain **(fig.-10).**
- **Culture characteristics (C/Cs):** Grow in presence of high salt concentration (6.5%), high temperature (45 °C), high pH (9.6) & 40% bile.
  - MacConkey's agar: Pin point pink colonies.
  - Blood agar: Non haemolytic. Some strains could be α or β haemolytic.
  - Potassium tellurite: Black colonies.
  - Bile esculin agar: Black colonies.

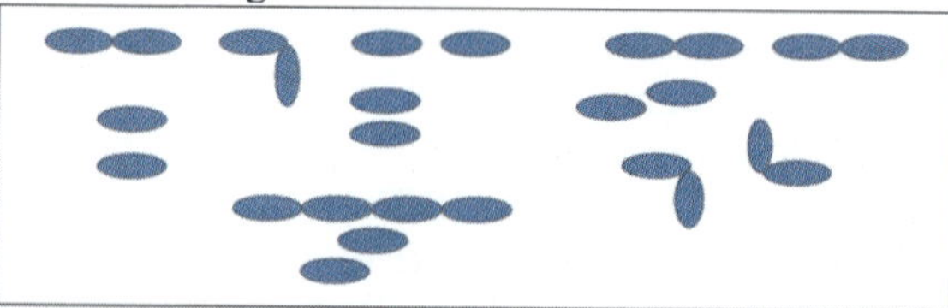

Figure-10: Morphology of *Enterococcus*

- **Biochemical reactions (B/Rs):**
  - Sugar fermentation: Ferments the sucrose, lactose, Mannitol & sorbitol.
  - Esculin hydrolysis: +Ve
  - PYR test: +Ve
- **Pathogenicity:**
- **Virulence factors:**
1. **Lipotechoic acid:** It has many functions like adhesion with host cells, regulation of autolytic enzymes of cell wall (muramidase), induction of release of cytokines (TNFα) etc.
2. **Haemolysin:** It lyses the RBCs in sheep & human.
3. **Extracellular surface protein:** Help in adhesion.
4. **Coccolysin:** It is a vasoactive peptide which inactivates the endothelium.
5. **Aggregation substances:** They help in clumping of adjacent cells to transfer the gene like plasmid responsible for drug resistance.

- **Clinical features:**
  - Normal flora in intestine, genital tract & saliva.
  - Causing UTI, septicemia, endocarditis, peritonitis, SABE, billiary tract infection, intra abdominal abscesses, wound infection & suppurative infection.
- **Diagnosis:**
- **Specimens:** Urine, blood, faeces, pus/discharge from local lesions etc.
- **Testing methods:** By microscopy (morphology), C/Cs & B/Rs as described earlier.
- **Treatment:**
  - *Enterococci* are intrinsically resistant to Pn, cephalosporin & aminoglycosides.
  - Vancomycin is the drug of choice in resistant strain, however **Vancomycin Resistant *Enterococci* (VRE)** are emerged due to alteration / elimination of target site like D-alanyl-D-alanine chain.

Group D / Non *Enterococcus* group

- **Lancefield grouping:** It is included in group D of β-haemolytic *Streptococci.*
- **Species**: *Strept. bovis & Strept. equinus*
- Inhibited at high salt & 40% bile.
- **Pathogenicity:** Causing UTI & endocarditis.
- **Treatment:** Susceptible to penicillin.

Comparison of *Streptococci*

Table-6

Group	Scientific name	Habitat	Colony	Tests
α-Haemolytic *Streptococci*				
Pneumoniae group	*Strept pneumoniae*	Lungs	α-haemolytic	Optochin: S & Bile solubility test: +Ve
β-Haemolytic *Streptococci*				
A	*Strept pyogenes*	Throat & skin	β-haemolytic	Bacitracin: S, PYR: +Ve & Trehalose: -Ve
B	*Strept agalactiae*	Genitals	β-haemolytic	Bacitracin: R, CAMP test: +Ve & Hippurate hydrolysis: +Ve
C	*Strept equisimilis*	Throat	β-haemolytic	Ribose & Trehalose fermentation: +Ve
Non-Haemolytic *Streptococci*				
	Enterococcus	Colon	No or α or β haemolysis	Grow at high salt, temperature, bile & pH. PYR: +Ve & Esculin hydrolysis: +Ve
D	Non *Enterococcus*	Less in colon	No haemolysis	No growth at high salt, temperature, bile & pH. PYR: -Ve & Esculin hydrolysis: -Ve

Table-6: Comparison of *Streptococci*

Question bank

Case study

1) A child present with infective skin lesion on the leg. Culture shows β-haemolysis in blood agar. Biochemically organism is bacitracin sensitive. Identify the organism & answer the following
a) Name the causative agent & describe the C/Cs of causative agent
b) Describe the B/Rs & serological tests useful in diagnosis of causative agent
c) Write the virulence factors of causative agent

2) A 10 year old girl visited the hospital with complain of sore throat. Oral examination diagnosed the pharyngitis clinically. Throat swab examination shows the GPC in chain under gram stain & β-haemolysis in blood agar. Identify the organism & answer the following
a) Name the causative agent & describe the morphology of causative agent
b) Write the pathogenicity of causative agent
c) Describe the lab. diagnosis of causative agent

Essay/Full question

1) *Strept pyogenes*

Short notes

1) Classification of *Streptococcaceae*
2) Pathogenicity/ Lab. diagnosis of *Strept pyogenes*
3) Non-suppurative complications of *Strept pyogenes*
4) *Strept agalactiae*
5) *Enterococcus*

Short questions for theory/viva questions

1) Write two uses of each, *Staph aureus & S pyogenes.*
2) Write four differences between α & β haemolysis.
3) Write four examples of α haemolytic bacteria.
4) Write two uses of *Streptococci.*
5) What is Lancefield grouping & Griffith typing of *Streptococci.*
6) Comment: *Streptococci* are arranged in chain & *Staphylococci* are in cluster.
7) Write four examples of bacteria arranged in chain.
8) Write the biochemical nature of capsule of following bacteria: *Strept pyogenes, Strept agalactiae, Strept equisimilis & E. faecalis*
9) Name the two bacteria (from different genera) causing toxic shock syndrome.
10) What is CAMP test?

MCQs for chapter review

Classification of Streptococcaceae

1) **Lancefield grouping of *Streptococci* is done by using** (AIIMS Nov-07)
(a) M protein (b) Group C peptidoglycan cell wall (c) Group C carbohydrate antigen (d) Staining properties

Viridans group

2) **A patient of RHD developed infective endocarditis after dental extraction. Most likely organism causing this is** (AIIMS, Nov-01)
(a) *Strept viridans* (b) *Streptococcus pneumoniae* (c) *Streptococcus pyogenes* (d) *Staphylococcus aureus*

Group A / *Strept pyogenes*

3) ***Streptococcus pyogenes* is-**
(a) GPC (b) GPB (c) GNC (d) GNB
4) **Catalase negative β-haemolytic *Streptococci* is -**
(a) *Strept mutans* (b) *Streptococcus pneumoniae* (c) *Streptococcus pyogenes* (d) *Strept mitior*
5) **Toxin involved in streptococcal toxic shock syndrome is -** (AI-01)
(a) Pyrogenic exotoxin (b) Erythrogenic exotoxin (c) Haemolysin (d) Neurotoxin
6) **Which of the following streptococcal antigen cross react with synovial fluid?** (AI-08)
(a) Carbohydrate (Group A) (b) Cell wall protein (c) Capsular hyaluronic acid (d) Peptidoglycan
7) **Streptococcus all are true except-** (AIIMS May-11, 10)
(a) Streptodornase cleaves DNA (b) Streptolysin O is active in reduced state (c) Streptokinase is produced from serotype A,C,K (d) Pyrogenic exotoxin is plasmid mediated

8) **The commonest organism causing cellulitis is-** (AIIMS Nov-02)
(a) *Streptococcus pyogenes* (b) *Streptococcus faecalis* (c) *Streptococcus viridans* (d) Microaerophilic *Streptococci*

Group B / *Strept. agalactiae*

9) **Scientific name for group-B, β-haemolytic streptococci**
(a) *Strept agalactiae* (b) *Strept pyogenes* (c) *Strept equisimilis* (d) *Strept angiosus*

10) **A child present with sepsis. Bacteria isolated showed beta haemolysis on blood agar, resistance to bacitracin, and a positive CAMP test. The most probable organism causing infection is-** (AI-10)
(a) *Strept pyogenes* (b) *Strept agalactiae* (c) *Enterococcus* (d) *Strept pneumoniae*

Group D / *Enterococcus*

11) **A beta haemolytic bacteria resistant to vancomycin shows growth in 6.5% NaCl, is non bile sensitive. It is likely to be** (AI-01)
(a) *Strept agalactiae* (b) *Strept pneumoniae* (c) *Enterococcus* (d) *Strept bovis*

Answers of MCQs & explanation

1) **(c)**
- Follow section, **classification of Streptococcaceae (flow chart-1)** for explanation.

2) **(a)**
- Viridans group include many species like *Strept mutans, Strept. sanguis, Strept. mitis, Strept. salivarius, Strept. mitior etc. of which S. sanguis* is the normal flora of oral cavity & it enter in blood following chewing, tooth brushing & dental procedures to causing transient bacteraemia & SABE (Sub Acute Bacterial Endocarditis) with prosthetic, damaged & congenitally disease valves.

3) **(a)**
- *Streptococcus pyogenes* is GPC arranged in chain. Follow section, **group A / *Strept. pyogenes* (morphology)** for more explanation

4) **(c)**
- All the bacteria belong to *Streptococcaceae* family are catalase negative & from the given option all are α-haemolytic except *Streptococcus pyogenes* which is β-haemolytic. More explanation is given in **flow chart-1** of this chapter.

5) **(a) & (b)**
- Pyrogenic exotoxin & erythrogenic exotoxin are the synonym for one toxin
- It has some other name also as mentioned earlier in text in this chapter.
- In addition to erythema & fever it also induces the necrotising fasciitis & streptococcal toxic shock syndrome

6) **(c)**
- Follow section, **group A / *Strept. pyogenes* (pathogenicity →table-1)** for explanation.

7) **(d)**
- Streptodornase (DNAase) degrade the DNA from neutrophils which is collected as pus
- Streptolysin O is O_2 labile & active in absence of O_2 (reduced state)
- Streptokinase (Fibrinolysin) is plasminogen & break fibrin to spread the infection. It is produced by group A, C & K. It given intravenously to treat myocardial infarction & thromboembolic disorders
- Three types of streptococcal pyrogenic exotoxin, such as A, B & C. A & C are bacteriophage coded while B is chromosomal mediated

8) **(a)**
- Cellulitis is caused mostly by haemolytic bacteria
- Option b: Follow section, **group D / *Enterococcus* (pathogenicity)** for explanation
- Option c: Follow section, **viridans group (pathogenicity & flow chart-2)** for explanation

9) **(a)**
- Follow section, **comparison of *Streptococci* (table-5)** for explanation.

10) **(b)**
- *S. agalactiae* is causing septicemia & neonatal meningitis, giving CAMP test +Ve & bacitracin resistant. Differentiation with other streptococcal species is given in **table-5**

11) **(c)**
- *Enterococcus*
  - Can grow in presence of high salt concentration (6.5%), high temperature (45 ^{o}C), high pH (9.6) & 40% bile
  - Are non haemolytic but some strains could be α or β haemolytic
  - Are intrinsically resistant to Pn, cephalosporin & aminoglycosides. Vancomycin is the drug of choice in resistant strain; however Vancomycin Resistant *Enterococci* (VRE) are emerged due to alteration of D-alanyl-D-alanine chain in the cell wall.

33 Pneumococcus

Learning heading & subheadings

- Scientific name:
- Morphology:
- Cultural characteristics (C/Cs):
- Biochemical reaction (B/Rs):
- Resistance:
- Antigenic variation:
- Pathogenicity:
- Laboratory diagnosis
- Prevention:
- Treatment:

Scientific name:

- *Diplococcus pneumoniae* because arranged in pair & causing pneumonia.
- *Streptococcus pneumoniae.*

Morphology:

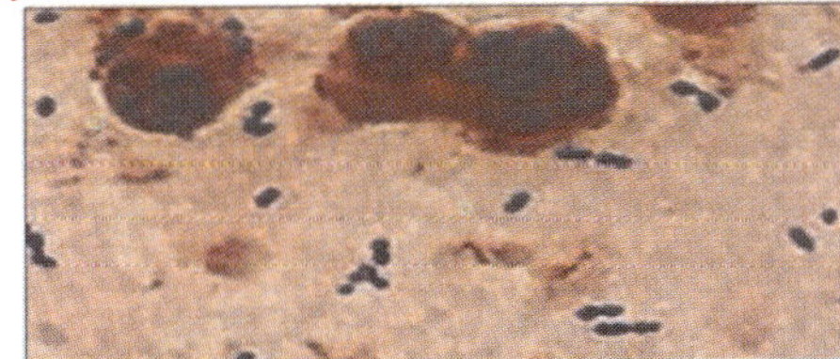

Figure-1: Pneumococcus under Gram stain

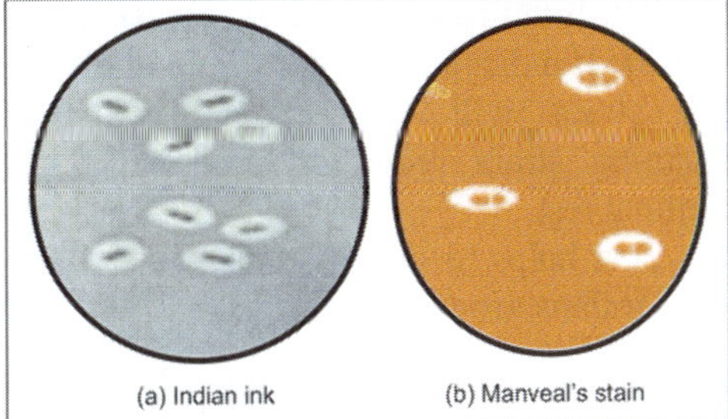

Figure-2: Capsular stains of pneumococcus

- **Type according to gram stain:** GPC.
- **Size:** 1 μm.
- **Shape:** Flame or lanceolate in shape.
- **Arrangement:** In pair with broad ends are apposite.
- **Motility:** Nonmotile.
- **Spore:** Nonsporing.
- **Capsule:** Polysaccharide in nature & tested by

1. **Gram stain:→ Fig.1**
2. **Negative stains:** Like India ink **[fig.-2(a)]**, Manveal's stain **[fig.-2(b)]** & Nigrosin stain.
3. **Quellung reaction:**

- Also **called capsular swelling.**
- Described by Neufeld in 1902.
- Take a loopful pneumococcal suspension on a slide.
- Add a drop of type specific antiserum.
- Add loopful of methylene blue solution.
- Observe under the microscope.
- Capsule appears swollen, sharply delineated, refractile & clear halo around blue stained cocci.
- Methylene blue stains the cocci blue.
- It can be performed directly from sputum of acute pneumonia case.
- In the past it was performed bedside by using specific antiserum, used to treat pneumonia.

Cultural characteristics (C/Cs):

- **Effective factors:**
  - O_2 effect: Aerobes and facultative anaerobes.
  - Co_2 effect: Growth facilitated by 5–10 % CO_2 **called capnophilic bacteria.**
  - Temperature: 37 °C (25-42 °C).
  - pH: 7.8
  - Exacting in nutritional requirements, growth occurs on media enriched with carbohydrates, blood or serum.
- **Culture in media:**

A. Liquid media:

i. Glucose broth: Produces uniform turbidity.

B. Solid media:

i. Blood agar:

a. Aerobic incubation:

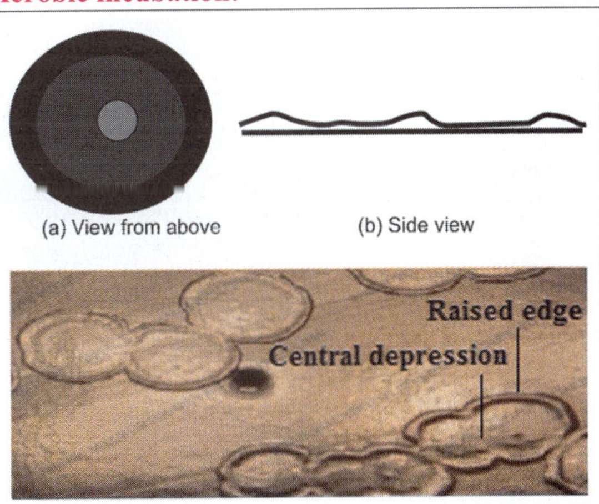

Figure-3: Draughtsman appearance

- **After 18 hrs:** Colonies are small (0.5-1.0 mm), dome-shaped, glistening, α-hemolytic like viridans group of *Streptococci.*
- **After longer incubation:** Colonies become flat with raised edges and central depression or

umbilication like concentric rings. When viewed from top giving **Draughtsman or Carrom coin appearance as shown in fig.-3(a).**

- Central depression or umbilication is due to autolytic enzymes (amidase, autolysin).
- Some strains like 3 & 7 develops abundant capsular materials give large mucoid colonies.

b. Anaerobic incubation: Produces β-haemolysis due to oxygen labile haemolysin O.

ii. Chocolate agar: Produce greenish discoloration

C. Selective medium: Blood agar with crystal violet+ nalidixic acid +colistin.

➢ **Culture in animal:** Intraperitoneal inoculation of *Strept pneumoniae* in mice causes the death in 1-3 days. It helps to differentiate the *Strept pneumoniae* from the viridans group where animal can survive in later.

❖ Biochemical reaction (B/Rs):

i. Sugar fermentation: :→ Fig.4(a)

- Ferment number of sugars, producing acid only.
- Fermentation tested in Hiss's serum broths / Hiss's serum agar slopes.
- **Inulin fermentation:** Ferments with acid only & help to differentiate from viridans group.

ii. Bile Solubility test: → Fig.4(b)

✪ **Principles:**

- *Strept pneumoniae* produces autolytic enzymes (autolysin, amidase) which cleave the bond between alanine & muramic acid in peptidoglycan and causing lysis of bacteria.
- Bile salts (sodium deoxycholate, sodium taurocholate) activate the amidase and accelerate the lysis in culture.
- Test should be carried out at neutral pH because sodium deoxycholate may precipitate at pH ≤6.5

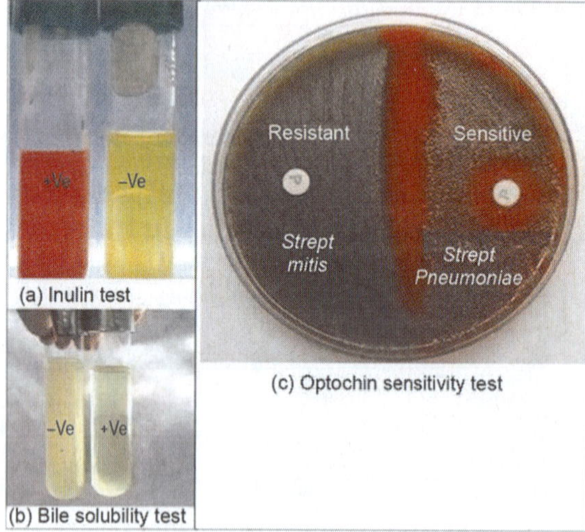

Figure-4: B/Rs of Pneumococcus

✪ **Media & reagents:**

a. For tube (broth) test:

- Culture suspension of *Strept pneumoniae* in test tube.
- 10% sodium deoxycholate.

b. For culture plate test:

- Culture of *Strept pneumoniae* in blood agar.
- 2% sodium deoxycholate.

✪ **Control:**

- **+Ve control:** *Strept pneumoniae.*
- **–Ve control:** Viridians group bacteria like *Strept mitis.*

✪ **Methods:**

a. Tube (broth) test:

- Take 0.5-1 ml overnight broth culture in two test tubes.
- Add 0.5 ml 10% sodium deoxycholate in one tube.
- Add 0.5 ml sterile normal saline in other tube as a control.
- Incubate at 37^0C in incubator for 2-3 hrs and read the result.

b. Culture plate test:

- Take two pneumococcal blood agar plates.
- Add 0.5 ml 2% sodium deoxycholate in plate.
- Add 0.5 ml sterile normal saline in other plate as a control.
- Incubate at 37^0C for 30 min in incubator (without inverting the plate) and read the results.

✪ **Results:**

a. Tube (broth) test:

- **+Ve test:** Clearing of suspension in tube containing 10% sodium deoxycholate & no change in control tube.
- **-Ve test:** No change in turbidity of both tubes.

b. Culture plate test:

- **+Ve test:** Clearing of colonies in plate containing 2% sodium deoxycholate & no change in control plate.
- **-Ve test:** No change in colonies in either of plate.

✪ **Interpretation:**

- **+Ve test:** It indicates the *Strept pneumoniae.*
- **-Ve test:** It indicates viridans group like *Strept mitis*
- 86% strain will lyses completely while for remaining strain required additional testing like Quellung test.

✪ **Use:** Test helps to differentiate *Strept pneumoniae* from viridans group.

iii. Optochin (ethyl hydrocuprein, 1/500,000) sensitivity: About 98% isolates of pneumococcus are sensitive to optochin [**fig.4(c)],** while viridans group like *Strept mitis* is resistant, which help in differentiation of all these bacteria.

iv. Catalase test: -Ve

v. Oxidase test: -Ve

❖ Resistance:

- Pneumococci are sensitive to heat. **Thermal Death Point (TDP)** is 52^0C for 15 minutes.

- Die in culture on prolonged incubation due to accumulation of toxic products.
- Strain maintained by lyophilisation or on semisolid blood agar.
- Sensitive β-lactam antibiotics, however resistant strain start to appear since 1967.
- Sensitive to optochin.

❖ **Antigenic variation:** Capsulated strain produce smooth (S) colonies & strain is virulent, on subculture it loose capsule & becomes rough (R), avirulent & autoagglutinable.

❖ **Pathogenicity:**

➢ **Disease name: Called pneumonia.**

➢ **Nature of disease:** In India, it occurs as sporadic or epidemic in close communities like army camp.

➢ **Reservoir of infection:** Carrier or rarely case.

➢ **Source of infection:** About 50% of human carry the pneumococci in the throat / nasopharynx (respiratory tract). Human is the source & person to person spread is possible.

➢ **Mode of transmission:**

- **Endogenous infection**

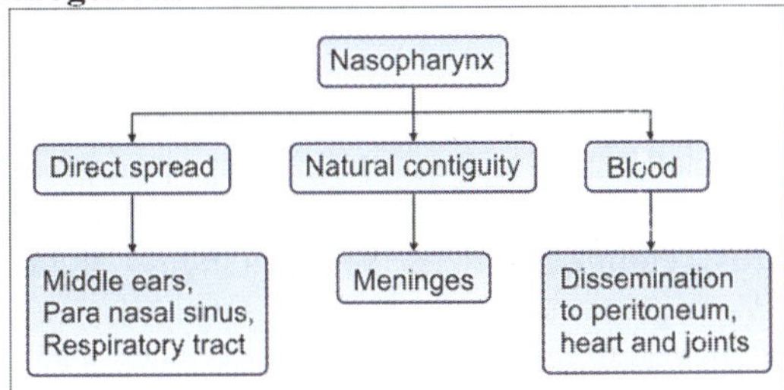

Flow chart-1: Spread of pneumococcus

- Colonise the human nasopharynx.
- Usually **endogenous infection** precipitated by viral infection, anaesthesia, chilling, stress, malnutrition, alcoholism, old age, over-crowding, splenectomy, immunodeficiency disease, sickle cell disease etc.
- Spread: →**Flow chart-1**

- **Exogenous infection:** It occurs by inhalation of nasopharyngeal/respiratory droplets.

➢ **Portal of entry:** Respiratory tract.

➢ **Sites:** Chiefly lungs but also infect other organs are or tissues.

➢ **Precipitating factors (epidemiological determinants):** Three types

I. Agent factors (virulence factors)

Two types like intra cellular & extracellular.

A. Intracellular (cell wall associated) factors:

1. **Peptidoglycan:** It activate alternative pathway of complement system.
2. **Capsular Ag:**
- Diffuse into culture medium & tissue **called SSS (Specific Soluble Substance).**
- Inhibit the phagocytosis.
- 90 serotypes.
- **Typing** is done by agglutination, precipitation or Quellung reaction (capsular swelling).
- Case fatality is depends on virulence & sero type of bacteria. Type 3 is most virulent.
- Serotype 6, 14, 19F &23F are most common in West in patient with local disease.
- In adults types 1-8 are responsible for 75% cases of pneumonia with 50% fatalities.
- In children types 6, 14, 19 & 23 are the major cause of disease.
- Anticapsular antibodies are serotype specific.

3. **Techoic acid:** It is the organ of adhesion.
4. **Somatic C (Carbohydrate) Ag:** It stimulates the hepatocytes to produces an abnormal protein (β-globulin) which precipitates somatic C (Carbohydrate) Ag of pneumococcus **called C-reactive protein (CRP).**

CRP

- **Meaning:** So called because it precipitates somatic C (Carbohydrate) Ag.
- **History:** Discovered by Tillett and Francis in 1930.
- **Properties:**
- It is not an Ab but an abnormal, non specific, inflammatory protein which increased in concentration following acute inflammation, bacterial infection (like *Strept pneumoniae*), tissue destruction, malignancy & in some other pathological conditions.
- Interferon-α (produced following viral infection) inhibits CRP production from liver cells which may explain the relatively low levels of CRP found during viral infections compared to bacterial infections.
- It is classified as positive acute phase protein or positive acute phase reactant.
- It is β-globulin (β1 & β2?) but many workers considered it between β & γ zone.
- Present in acute phase & disappear in convalescence phase.
- Activates the classical complement pathway.
- Used as index of response in treatment of rheumatic fever and certain other conditions.

- **Production of CRP: → Flow chart-2**

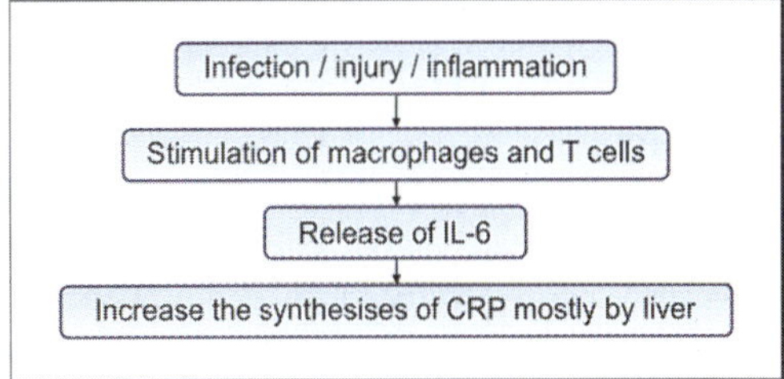

Flow chart-2: Production of CRP

- **CRP level:**
- Normal: 0.2mg/dl.

- Mild (insignificant) increase: 0.2 - <1 mg /dl in pregnancy, heavy exercise & common cold.
- Moderate increase: >1-10 mg /dl in pancreatitis, bronchitis, cystitis, myocardial infarction & cancer.
- Marked increase: >10 mg /dl in acute bacterial infection, major trauma & systemic vasculitis.

- **Diagnosis**: It is one of the most common markers of acute inflammation & detected by
- Capillary precipitation test: Out dated method.
- Latex (passive) agglutination test: It detects CRP up to 0.6mg/dl & most widely used test.
- ELISA & nephelometry: Most sensitive & useful to monitor the cardiovascular disease.

B. Extracellular factors: Two types like enzymes & toxins as mentioned below.

i. Enzymes:

1. **Autolytic enzymes:** Autolytic amidase activated by surface-active agents such as bile/bile salts, cleaves bond between alanine & muramic acid in peptidoglycan of cell wall, resulting lysis of organisms & release of bacterial products, which contribute in the pathogenesis of disease.
2. **IgA proteases:** Cleaves IgA & reduce the local immunity of respiratory mucosa. (Other bacteria producing IgA protease are *N. miningitidis, N. gonorrhea* & *H. influenzae*).

ii. Toxins:

1. **Haemolysin:**
- O_2 labile **called pneumolysin.**
- Weak & thiol-activated toxin.
- It effects on ciliary cell & PMNs (cytotoxic) & activates the classical pathway of complement by direct binding with C1q.
2. **Leucocidin:** Act on WBCs.

II. Host factors

1. **Age:**
- In adults, types 1-8 are responsible for 75% cases of pneumonia with 50% fatalities.
- In children types 6, 14, 19 & 23 are the major cause of disease.
2. **Immunity:** Infection is favoured by local & systemic factors like

- **Local:** Respiratory viral infections, respiratory congestion (pulmonary or mucosal), allergic disease etc.
- **Systemic:**

- **Splenectomy:**
  - Spleen & microbes: Spleen is required to inhibits the infection by capsulated bacteria like *Strept pneumoniae*, *H. influenzae*, members of Enterobactariceae family & parasite like *Babesia.* No risk of viral infection after splenectomy.
  - Role of spleen in immunity: Absence of spleen predispose the pneumococcal infection due to
    - Deficiency of opsonin antibody or inability to induce the specific antibody response.
    - Interference in bacterial clearance from the blood, which is done by slow passage of blood through the splenic sinuses & prolonged contact with RE cells in the cord of Billroth.
    - Deficiency of tuftsin, a tetrapeptide secreted by spleen & plays a role in combating pneumococcal sepsis.
  - Indication of vaccine: Post splenectomy patient required pneumococcal vaccine to prevent the infection.
- **Others:** Alcoholism, malnutrition, stress. IDDs, sickle cell disease etc.

III. Environmental factors

1. **Season:** Common in winter.
2. **Overcrowding:** Mostly by close contact & infection is common in army camp.

➢ **Clinical features:**

1. **Ear & para nasal sinuses:** Commonest pneumococcal infections are acute otitis media (most common cause) & sinusitis.
2. **Meninges**:
- It causes very serious (fulminant) meningitis especially in patient of splenectomy **called pneumococcal meningitis** (mortality is 20%).
- Most common causes for meningitis in adults: *Strept. pneumoniae* from gram positive category & *N. meningitidis* from gram negative category.
3. **Respiratory tract**
- Lobar pneumonia: Pneumococcus is the most common cause for lobar pneumonia & community acquired pneumonia.
- Bronchopneumonia Most common cause is *Staphylococcus*. Also caused by pneumococcus.
- Acute trachea-bronchitis.
- Acute exacerbation of chronic bronchitis which is associated with *H. influenzae.*
4. **Disseminated infection:**
- Bacteraemia, pericarditis, peritonitis, conjunctivitis, arthritis & endocarditis in previously damaged heart valves.
- **Austrian syndrome** is a medical condition first described by Robert Austrian in 1957. It is the classical triad of pneumococcal pneumonia, endocarditis & meningitis, all caused by *Strept pneumoniae*. It is common in alcoholic person due to reduced splenic function, and in males between 40-60 years.

➢ **Complications:**

- Empyema is the most common complication, characterised by collection of pus in pleural cavity. It also **called pyothorax** or **purulent pleuritis.**
- Mortality is 20% in pneumococcal meningitis, while 50% of survival develops acute or chronic

complications like deafness, hydrocephalus & mental retardation.

✓ **Note: Most common causes for pneumonia**

- Pneumatocele: *Staphylococcus aureus.*
- Bronchopneumonia: *Staphylococcus aureus.*
- Lobar pneumonia: *Strept. pneumoniae.*
- Primary atypical pneumonia: *Mycoplasma pneumoniae.*

❖ Laboratory diagnosis:

➢ **Specimens:** Ear discharge, laryngeal swab, sputum, CSF & blood.

➢ **Testing methods:**

I. Microscopy: → Follow morphology

II. Culture: → Follow C/Cs

III. Biochemical reactions: → Follow B/Rs

IV. Serological tests:

1. **Quellung reaction:** → Vide supra
2. **Ag detection:** Capsular polysaccharide antigens (SSS) detected from blood, CSF, urine by CIE (precipitation), latex agglutination, coagglutination & immunochromatographic test.
3. **Ab detection:** From blood by agglutination, precipitation, Radio Immuno Assay (RIA), Indirect Haem Agglutination (IHA) & Indirect Fluorescent Antibody (IFA) tests.

Features	Pneumoniae group	Viridans group
Microscopy		
-Shape **-Arrangements** **-Capsule**	- Lancet/ flame - In pair **(fig.-1)** - Present **(fig.-2)**	- Spherical/oval - In chain - Variable
C/Cs		
-Liquid media (Glucose broth) **- Solid media (Blood agar)**	- Uniform turbidity - Initially dome shape & α-haemolytic later carrom coin / draughts-man appearance **(fig.-3).**	- Granular turbidity - Dome shape & α-haemolytic
-Intraperitoneal inoculation in mice	- Fatal (mice die in1-3 days)	- Non-fatal
B /Rs: →Fig. 4		
-Inulin fermentation **-Bile solubility test** **-Optochin sensitivity test**	- Ferments with acid no gas - Positive - Sensitive	- Non-fermentative - Negative - Resistance
Serological test		
Quellung test	Positive	Negative

Table-1: Differences between pneumoniae group & viridians group

V. Molecular: PCR

VI. Biomarker:

1. **CRP** by latex agglutination test.
2. **Procalcitonin** is useful to determine the prognosis & response of treatment.

VII. Tests to differentiate between pneumoniae group & viridians group: →Table-1

❖ **Prevention:** Type specific Ab required according to capsular type. Practically it is not possible to make complete polyvalent vaccine due to existence 90 serotypes. Two types of pneumococcal vaccines are described below.

a. Polyvalent (23-valent) Polysaccharide Vaccine (PPV):

- **Preparation:** It is prepared by using capsular polysaccharide antigen of 23 most prevalent serotypes of *Strept. pneumoniae,* so also **called 23 valent pneumococcal vaccine.**
- **Indications:** It is not in general use but indicated to protect the high-risk individuals like
  - Absent or dysfunctional spleen.
  - Sickle cell disease.
  - Chronic renal (nephrotic syndrome), lungs, liver & heart disease.
  - Coeliac disease.
  - Diabetes Mellitus (DM).
  - Immuno Deficiency Diseases (IDDs) like HIV.
  - CSF leak due to meningeal disruption or dural tear.

➢ **Advantages:** It provides 80-90% protections which last for 5 years.

➢ **Contraindications:**

- < 2 year of age.
- Lymphoreticular malignancy.
- Immunosuppressive therapy .

b. Polyvalent (7-valent) conjugated vaccine

- **Preparation:** It is prepared by using capsular polysaccharide antigen of 7 most common serotypes of *Strept. pneumoniae,* which are conjugated to the CRM 197 protein (toxoid) of *C. diphtheriae*, so also **called 7 valent conjugated vaccine.**
- **Indication:** < 2 year of age, however protection depends on serotype included in vaccine & infective serotype.
- **Contraindications:** < 6 weeks.

❖ Treatment:

➢ **β -lactam antibiotics:** *Strept pneumoniae* are sensitive to β -lactam antibiotics. Parenteral Pn is given in severe cases, while mild cases are treated with amoxycillin. However β -lactam resistant strains start to appear since 1967, due to **alteration in penicillin binding protein.**

➢ **Other antibiotics:** β -lactam resistant strain are also resistant to other antibiotic like erythromycin & tetracycline. Such type of resistance strains are identified in **Spain called Drug Resistant S. Pneumoniae (DRSP)** & later spread to other country. It is due to **mutation** or by **other mechanism of gene transfer.** 3rd generation cephalosporin is indicated in such cases while vancomycin is the reserve drug.

- **Commonly used antibiotics:**
  - Otitis media, sinusitis & pneumonia: Amoxicillin
  - Meningitis: Ceftriaxone + Vancomycin.
  - Endocarditis: Ceftriaxone/cefotaxime + Vancomycin.

Question bank

Case study

1) A female patient presents with history of fever & neck rigidity. CSF examination revealed presence of lancet shape GPC in pairs. Culture shows the α-haemolysis on blood agar. Identify the organism & answer the following

a) Name the causative agent & describe the morphology of causative agent

b) Describe the pathogenicity of causative agent

c) Write the laboratory diagnosis of causative agent

Essay/Full question

1) Pneumococcus

Short notes

1) Tests to differentiate between pneumoniae group & viridians group of *Streptococcus.*
2) Bile solubility test.
3) Biochemical reactions of *Strept. pneumoniae*
4) Pathogenicity of *Strept. pneumoniae*
5) Lab. diagnosis of *Strept. pneumoniae*

Short questions for theory/viva questions

1) What is capsular swelling (Quellung reaction)?
2) What is carom coin appearance?
3) Write the principle of bile solubility test.
4) Name the four bacteria producing the IgA protease.
5) What is Austrian syndrome?

MCQs for chapter review

1) An infant had high grade fever and respiratory distress at the time of presentation to the emergency room. The sample collected for blood culture was subsequently positive showing growth of α-haemolytic colonies. On gram staining these were gram positive cocci. In the screening test for identification, the suspected pathogen is likely to be susceptible to the following agent- (AIIMS, May-06)
(a) Bacitracin (b) Novobiocin (c) Optochin (d) Oxacillin

2) A patient present with sign of pneumonia. The bacterium obtained from sputum was gram positive cocci which showed alpha haemolysis on sheep agar. Which of the following test will help to confirm the diagnosis - (AI-11)
(a) Bile solubility (b) Coagulase test (c) Bacitracin test (d) CAMP test

3) The sputum specimen of a 70 year old male was cultured on a 5% sheep blood agar. The culture showed α-haemolytic colonies next day. The processing of this organism is most likely to yield- (AIIMS, Nov-05)
(a) Gram positive cocci in short chains, catalase negative and bile resistant (b) Gram positive cocci in pairs, catalase negative and bile soluble (c) Gram positive cocci in clusters, catalase positive and coagulase positive (d) Gram negative coccobacilli, catalase positive and oxidase positive

4) True statements about pneumococcus are all except- (AI-98)
(a) Pneumolysin a thiol activated toxin, exerts a variety of effect on ciliary cell & PMNs (b) Autolysin may contribute to the pathogenesis of pneumococcal disease by lysing the bacteria (c) Anticapsular antibodies are serotype specific (d) The virulence of pneumococci is dependent only on the production of the capsular polysaccharide

5) True statements regarding pneumococcus is- (AI-99)
(a) Virulence is due to polysaccharide capsule (b) Capsule is protein in nature (c) Antibodies against capsule are not protective (d) Resistance to antibiotics has not yet reported

6) Risk of pneumococcal meningitis is seen in - (AIIMS-99)
(a) Post splenectomy patient (b) Patient undergoes neurological intervention (c) Patient following cardiac surgery (d) Patient with hypoplasia of lung

7) In a splenectomised patient, there is increase of infection by all the organisms except
(a) *Salmonella* (b) *Klebsiella* (c) *Streptococcus pneumoniae* (d) *Haemophilus influenzae*

8) Which of the following statements about pneumococcus is false - (AI-11)
(a) Capsule aids in virulence (b) Commonest cause of otitis media (c) Causes mild form of meningitis (d) Respiratory tract of carriers is the most important source of infection

9) Most common causative organism for lobar pneumonia is- (AIIMS 04)
(a) *Staphylococcus aureus* (b) *Streptococcus pyogenes* (c) *Streptococcus pneumoniae* (d) *Haemophilus influenzae*

10) An eight year old with history of pain and discharge from right ear present with fever, neck rigidity, and a positive Kerning's sign. Discharge was stained with gram stain which revealed gram positive cocci. Which of the is most likely organism (AI-11)
(a) *H. influenzae* (b) *Staphylococcus* (c) Pneumococcus (d) *Pseudomonas*

11) C-reactive protein stand for- (AI-11)
(a) Capsular polysaccharide in pneumococcus (b) Concanavalin-a (c) Calretin (d) Cellular

12) C-reactive proteins are- (PGI, Dec-00)
(a) Alpha-globulin (b) Beta-1 globulin (c) Beta-2 globulin (d) Non specific inflammatory protein

13) Following is true about C-reactive protein (AIIMS-95)
(a) Detected by precipitation with carbohydrate (b) Raised in acute pneumococcal infection (c) It is an antibody (d) Detected by agglutination test

14) C-reactive protein is- (AIIMS-91)
(a) Produced by pneumococcus (b) A marker of septicemia (c) Raised in acute inflammation (d) Low in rheumatoid arthritis

15) The 23 valent vaccine is recommended in all except-
(a) CSF leak (b) Chronic cardiac disease (c) Children less than 2 years (d) Nephrotic syndrome

Answers of MCQs & explanation

1) (c)

- In given case, organism is gram positive cocci & producing alpha haemolysis on sheep agar, which includes two groups like viridans group (*Strept mutans, Strept. sanguis, Strept. mitis, Strept. salivarius, Strept. mitior etc.*) & pneumoniae group (*Streptococcus pneumoniae*). But patient present with high grade fever and respiratory distress, so infective agent is

Strept pneumoniae & it is confirmed by optochin (Ethyl hydrocuprein, 1/500,000) sensitivity test. It is also confirmed by bile solubility test, but this option is not given in question.

2) **(a)**
- In given case, organism is gram positive cocci & producing alpha haemolysis on sheep agar, which includes two groups like viridans group (*Strept mutans, Strept. sanguis, Strept. mitis, Strept. salivarius, Strept. mitior etc.*) & pneumoniae group (*Streptococcus pneumoniae*). But patient present with sign of pneumonia, so infective agent is *Strept pneumoniae* & it is confirmed by bile solubility test. It is also confirmed by optochin (Ethyl hydrocuprein, 1/500,000) sensitivity test, but this option is not given in question.

3) **(b)**
- Culture showing the α-haemolysis (greenish colonies due to incomplete haemolysis) on 5% sheep blood agar, which is given by viridans group (*Strept mutans, Strept. sanguis, Strept. mitis, Strept. salivarius, Strept. mitior* etc.) & pneumoniae group (*Streptococcus pneumoniae*). Both are gram positive cocci & catalase negative but later is arranged in pairs & bile soluble.

4) **(d)**
- Pneumolysin a thiolactivated toxin. It is cytotoxic &, exerts a variety of effect on ciliary cell & PMNs
- Autolysin (autolytic enzyme): Follow text
- Anticapsular antibodies are serotype specific
- The virulence of pneumococci is not dependent only on the production of the capsular polysaccharide but also on other factors like peptidoglycan, somatic C Ag, amidase, IgA protease, haemolysin & leucocidin as described earlier in text.

5) **(d)**
- Most important virulence factors is polysaccharide capsule, however it has other virulence factors as described earlier in text.
- Capsule is not in protein, but polysaccharide in nature
- Antibodies against capsular antigens are protective, hence such antigens are used in vaccine preparation
- Resistance to antibiotics has been reported, as described earlier in text under the section of treatment

6) **(a)** } Follow section, **pathogenicity (host factors)**
7) **(a)** } for explanation

8) **(c)**
- Capsule is the most important virulence factor
- Commonest pneumococcal infections are otitis media & sinusitis
- It causes not mild but very serious (fulminant) meningitis
- About 50% of human carry the pneumococci in the throat/nasopharynx (respiratory tract). Respiratory tract of carriers is the most important source of infection

9) **(c)**
- Follow section, **pathogenicity (clinical features) & notes (most common causes of pneumonia)** for explanation

10) **(c)**
- In given case patient is suffered with otitis media & meningitis, where most likely organism is Pneumococcus. Explanation is given in text under the section of clinical features.

11) **All options are wrong**
- In CRP, C is stands for carbohydrate antigen of cell wall of pneumococcus, neither the capsular polysaccharide Ag nor other

12) **(d)**
- Few authors mentioned it as β -1 globulin, few as β -2 globulin while few considered it between β & γ zone.

13) **(a), (b) & (d)**
- CRP is detected by precipitation reaction (Out dated method) with carbohydrate Ag & by agglutination test.
- It is not an antibody but it is a non specific inflammatory protein.
- Its concentration raised in acute inflammation, bacterial infection (like *Strept pneumoniae*), tissue destruction, malignancy & in some other pathological condition

14) **(c)**
- CRP is produced by liver not by pneumococcus

15) **(c)**
- Follow section, **prevention** for explanation.

34 Neisseriae, Moraxellaceae and Mimeae

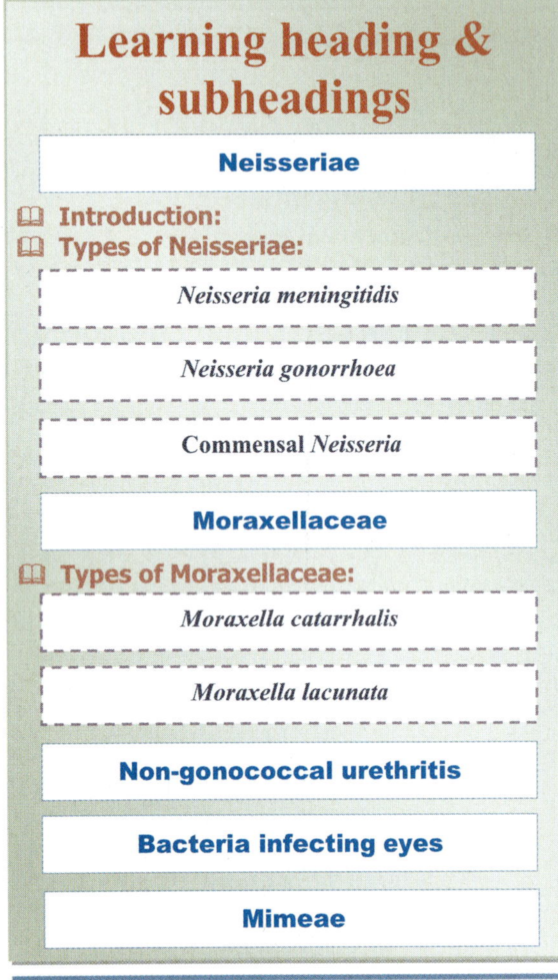

Learning heading & subheadings

Neisseriae

❖ **Introduction:** GNC are classified under the family *Neisseriae* which are catalase positive, oxidase positive, arranged in pairs & fastidious in growth requirements.

❖ **Types of Neisseriae:** → **Flow chart-1**

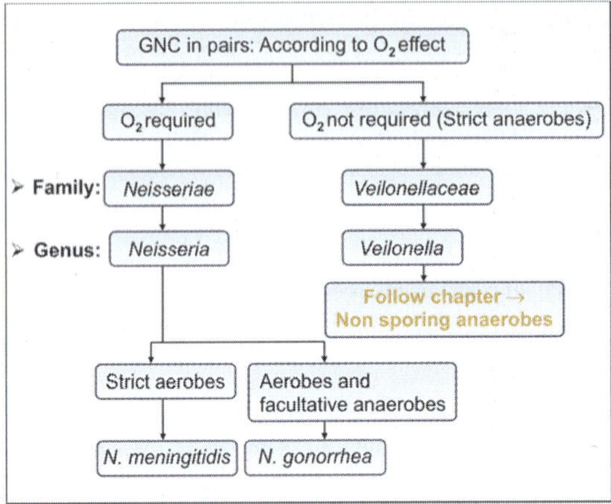

Flow chart-1: Types of Neisseriae

Neisseria meningitidis

❖ **Common name:** Meningococcus

❖ **Morphology:** →**Figure-1**

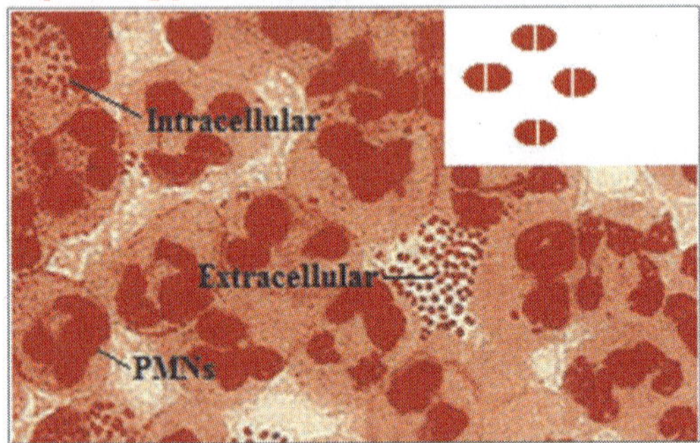

Figure-1: ***N. meningitidis*** **under gram stain**

- **Type according to gram stain:** GNC.
- **Size:** 0.6–0.8 µm.
- **Shape:** Half moon shape.
- **Arrangement:** Pairs, with adjacent sides flattened. Cocci are found intracellularly in CSF in leucocytes & often extracellularly.
- **Motility:** Nonmotile.
- **Spore:** Nonsporing.
- **Capsule:** Fresh isolates are capsulated.

❖ **Culture characteristic (C/Cs):**

- **Effective factors:**
  - O_2 effect: Strict aerobes.

- CO_2 effect: Growth is facilitated by 5–10 % CO_2 **called capnophilic bacteria** and by high humidity.
- Temperature: 35 – 36 °C.
- pH: 7.4 – 7.6.
- Exacting in nutritional requirements. Growth occurs on media enriched with blood, serum or ascitic fluid.

➢ **Culture in media:**

A. **Liquid media:** Poor growth in liquid media, producing a granular turbidity with little or no surface growth.

B. **Solid media:**

1. **Blood agar:** Weak haemolytic colonies.
2. **Chocolate agar:** Also a useful medium.
3. **Mueller-Hinton starch casein hydrolysate agar:**

C. **Selective media:**

1. **Thayer-Martin medium:** Chocolate agar (heat lysed human/horse blood) + vancomycin + colistin + nystatin.
2. **Modified Thayer-Martin Medium (MTMM):** Chocolate agar + vancomycin + colistin + nystatin + trimethoprim.
3. **Martin Lewis Medium:** Chocolate agar + Vancomycin (higher concentration) + colistin + anisomycin + trimethoprim.

➢ **Growth properties:** Colonies are small (1 mm dia.) translucent, round, convex, bluish grey, with smooth glistening surface, lenticular shape, butyrous consistency and easy emulsification.

❖ Bio-chemical reaction (B/Rs):

1. **Sugar fermentation tests (fig.-2):** Meningococcus is oxidative, hence sugar fermentation occurs very weak which is best tested in peptone serum agar slopes contains agar & pH indicator. It ferments glucose & maltose with acid production only but do not ferments lactose, sucrose & mannitol.

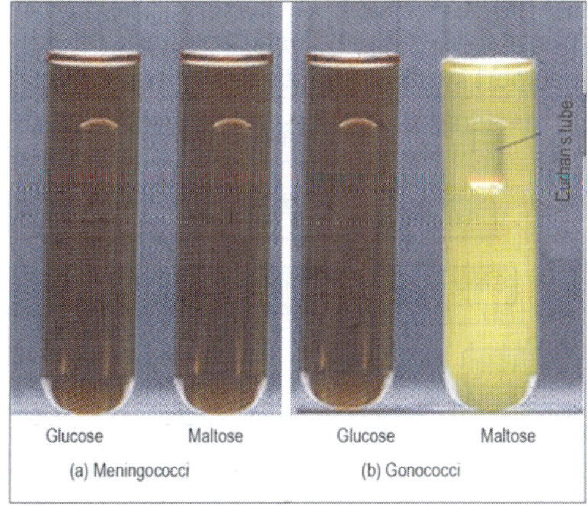

Figure-2: Sugar fermentation tests

2. **I M Vi C test:** Not useful.
3. **Catalase test:** +Ve
4. **Oxidase test:** Prompt oxidase positive by meningococcus & gonococcus help in identification of these species.

❖ Resistance:

- Easily killed by heat, drying, alteration in pH and antiseptics.
- They were uniformly sensitive to penicillin (Pn) & other antibiotics but now resistant strains are common.

❖ Pathogenicity:

➢ **Disease name:** Infection (inflammation) of meninges **called meningitis.**

➢ **Nature & history of disease:** Natural infection occurs only in human. It occurs in epidemic & endemic form.

✪ **World:** It is highest in Africa from Ethiopia to Senegal **called meningitis belt of Africa**. Frequent epidemics are occurring at here. Largest was in 1996, when 1, 50, 000 cases were reported with 15,000 deaths.

✪ **India:** Type A is the major cause of endemic infection.

➢ **Reservoir of infection:** Carrier not case. Carrier rate is 5-10% & may increase up to 90% during epidemic.

➢ **Source of infection:** Meningococcus present as normal flora in nasopharynx. Nasopharyngeal droplet of human carrier is the source & person to person spread is possible. Case is present as a negligible source of infection.

➢ **Mode of transmission:**

- **Endogenous infection:**
  - Organisms are located as normal flora in nasopharynx.
  - Spread: Exact route for meninges involvement from nasopharynx is unknown, but possibly routes are mentioned in **flow-chart -2.**

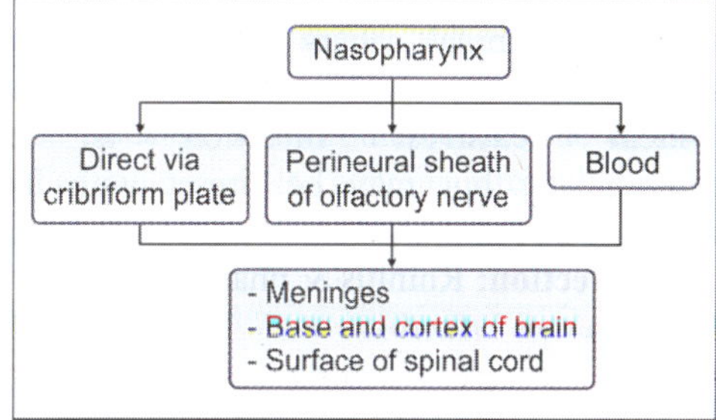

Flow chart-2: Spread of meningococcus

- **Exogenous infection:** By inhalation of nasopharyngeal/respiratory droplets or by fomites borne.

➢ **Incubation period:** 3-4 days.

➢ **Portal of entry:** Respiratory tract.

➢ **Sites:** Chiefly damages the meninges but also infect other organs or tissues.

➢ **Precipitating factors (epidemiological determinants):** Three types

I. **Agent factors (virulence factors)**

- **Capsule:** Non-capsulated.
- **Fimbriae:** Facilitate adhesion of cocci to mucosal surfaces & inhibiting phagocytosis. It agglutinates the human RBC **called haemagglutination**.
- **L-form:** Cell wall deficient form also present but not identified by routine test.
- **Fluorescent microscopy:** Highly sensitive & specific.

❖ Cultural characteristics (C/C):

- **Effective factors:**

- O_2 effect: Aerobes & facultative anaerobes.
- Co_2 effect: Growth is facilitated by 5–10 % CO_2 **called capnophilic bacteria**.
- Temperature: 35 – 36°C.
- pH: 7.4 – 7.6
- Exacting in nutritional requirements & more difficult to grow than meningococci.

- **Media:**

A. Liquid media:

1. **Glucose broth:**
2. **Blood culture broth:**

} Poor growth in liquid media

B. Solid media:

1. **Chocolate agar:**
2. **Muller- Hinton agar:**

C. Selective media:

1. **Thayer-Martin medium:** Chocolate agar (heat lysed human/horse blood) + vancomycin + colistin + nystatin.
2. **Modified Thayer-Martin Medium (MTMM):** Chocolate agar (heat lysed human/horse blood) vancomycin + colistin + nystatin + trimethoprim.
3. **New York City Medium (NYCM):** Saponin lysed human / horse blood + yeast dialysate + same antibiotics as MTMM.
4. **Modified New York City Medium (MNYCM):** Saponin lysed human / horse blood+ yeast dialysate + lincomycin + colistin + amphotericin b + trimithoprim.

T_1 and T_2	T_3 and T_4
Small	Large
Brown	Non-pigmented
Piliated cocci	Non-piliated cocci
Autoagglutinable cocci	Non- agglutinable
Virulent cocci	Avirulent cocci
Fresh cocci	On serial subculture
T_1 called P^+ & T_2 called P^{++}	**Both called P^-**

Table-1: Colonies of gonococci

- **Growth properties:** Small, round, translucent, convex or slightly umbonate with finely granular surface, lobate margins, soft and easily emulsifiable colonies. Four types of colonies identified as described in **table-1.**

D. Transport media:

- If no delay in testing (< 6 hours) of specimens then it should be collected & transported in
  - Charcoal coated swab kept in Stuart's medium.
  - Charcoal containing Amie's medium.
- If delay in testing (> 6 hours) of specimens then it should be collected & transported in commercially available transport system like
  - JEMBEC system.
  - Gono-Pak system.

❖ Biochemical reaction (B/Rs):

1. **Sugar fermentation tests [fig.-2(b)]:** Gonococci have same properties as meningococci, except only glucose (no maltose) fermentation.

Glucose	Maltose
A	-

2. **Rapid Carbohydrate Utilisation Test (RCUT):** Based on presence of preformed enzymes in bacteria. Not dependent on growth of bacteria in sugar media. Rapid & more sensitive.
3. **Catalase test:** +Ve
4. **Oxidase test:** Prompt +Ve

❖ Resistance:

- Easily killed by heat, drying and antiseptics.
- Cocci die very rapidly outside the human body so fomite borne infection is the rare possibility.
- Resistant to Pn occurs by two ways.

1. Plasmid mediated: Due to penicillinase enzyme.
2. Chromosome mediated: By mutation.

- Resistant to fluoroquinolones occurs by two ways

1. Alteration in DNA gyrase.
2. Topoisomerase.

- Plasmid mediated resistance also occurs in tetracycline & sulfonamides.

❖ Typing of gonococcus:

a. **Serotyping:** As shown in **flow chart-4.**

b. **Auxotyping:**

- It based on nutritional requirement of gonococci.
- AHU auxotype needs arginine, hypoxanthine & uracil.

❖ Pathogenicity:

- **Disease name:** Natural disease occurs only in human (exclusive human pathogen) **called gonorrhoea** (rrhoea = discharge/flow of seeds). No natural infection in animals. Mouse is infected by intracerebral inoculation & chimpanzee by urethral inoculation.
- **Nature & history of disease:** Incidence of gonorrhoea has been rise all over the world. WHO estimated 106 million cases globally in 2008, which was 21% higher than 2005, however actually cases may be higher due to under-reporting & asymptomatic infections. It may be due to increase in drug resistance.
- **Reservoir of infection:** Asymptomatic (10% men & 50% women) carrier or case is the reservoir.

- **Source of infection:** Infected genitals or discharge from genitals act as source of infection.
- **Mode of transmission:**
  - Venereal infection: By sexual intercourse.
  - Non-venereal infection: From infected birth canal to the newborn.
- **Incubation period:** 2-8 days.
- **Portal of entry:** Genital tract in case of venereal infection & ocular organs (ophthalmia neonatorum) in case of non-venereal infection.
- **Sites:** Chiefly genitals & eyes in case of non-venereal infection.
- **Precipitating factors (epidemiological determinants):** Three types

I. Agent factors (virulence factors)

Two types like intra cellular & extracellular.

A. Intracellular (cell wall associated) factors:

1. **Outer Membrane Protein (OMP):** Helpful for **serotyping** as shown in **flow chart-4.**

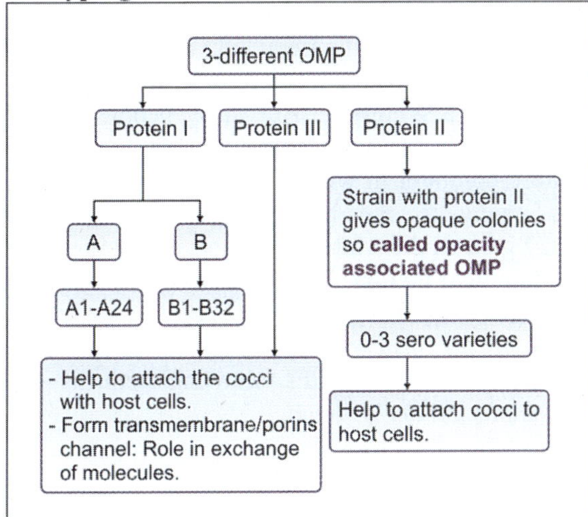

Flowchart-4: Outer Membrane Protein

2. **Pili (fimbriae):** Organs of adhesion & made up by pilin protein.
3. **Lipopolysaccharide (LPS):** For endotoxic activity.

B. Extracellular factors:

1. **IgA proteases:** Cleaves IgA which reduce the mucosal immunity.
2. **Penicillinase (β-lactamase):** Inactivate the β-lactam antibiotics & produces the resistance to β-lactam antibiotics.

II. Host factors

1. **Age:** Incidence is high between 20-24 years.
2. **Sex:** Carrier rate is high in women (50%) than men (10%).
3. **Blood group:** Common in blood group B, exact reason is not known.
4. **Sexual behaviour:** Unsafe sexual practise like no use of condom increases the chances of infection.
5. **Associated disease:** Global burden of gonorrhoea is increase due to increase the cases of HIV.
6. **Others:** Like lack of health education, poor hygiene etc. are also the contributory factors.

III. Environmental factors

1. **Location:** WHO noticed highest incidence in Africa & Western pacific (China & Australia).

- **Pathogenesis:** → **Flowchart-5**

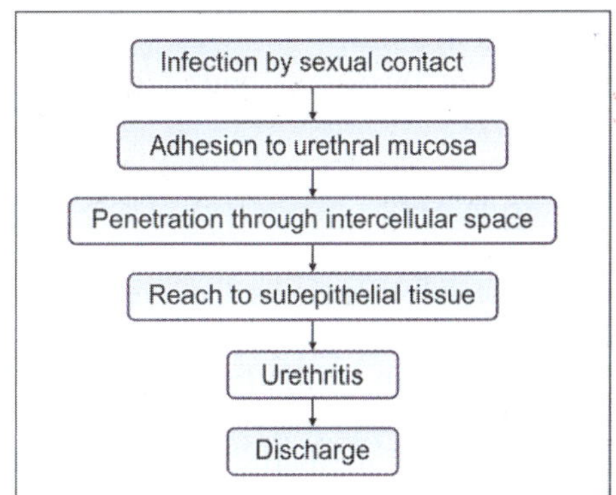

Flowchart-5: Pathogenesis of gonorrhoea

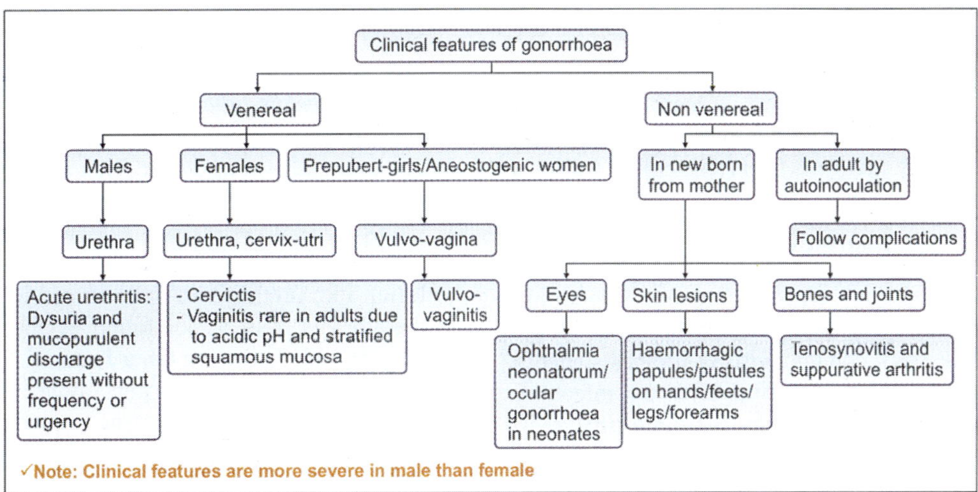

Flow chart-6: Clinical features of gonorrhea

Clinical features: → Flow chart-6

➢ **Complications:**

a. **Local spread:** By natural contiguity of mucosa.

1. **Male:**
- Urethritis may extends to prostate, seminal vesicles and epididymis.
- Chronic urethritis may lead to stricture formation.
- Extends to periurethral tissues, causing abscesses & multiple discharging sinuses **called 'water can perineum'**.

2. **Female:**
- Cervictis may extend to Bartholin's glands, endometrium and fallopian tubes.
- Pelvic inflammatory disease and salpingitis may lead to sterility.
- Sometimes peritonitis with perihepatic inflammation **called Fitz-Hugh-Curtis syndrome.**
- Proctitis

b. **Blood spread (metastasis):** Few strain like Por 1A, disseminated in to other organs by blood **called disseminated gonococcal infections** & causing arthritis, ulcerative endocarditis & rarely meningitis. It occurs in 3-5% of untreated cases.

c. **Self spread (autoinoculation/autoinfection):** Autoinoculation by contaminated finger in eyes in adult leads to conjunctivitis with profuse purulent discharge, swollen eye lids, chemosis, corneal ulceration & rarely perforation **called ocular gonorrhoea in adult.**

d. **Spread from pregnant lady (gonorrhoea in pregnancy):**
- Foetal damage: It may lead foetal loss, abortion or premature delivery.
- New born eyes damage: Infected birth canal may transmit the infection in to the eyes of new born during parturition **called ocular gonorrhoea in neonates** or **called ophthalmia neonatorum.** It is prevented by instillation of 1% silver nitrate solution in eye of newborns (**Crede's method**) or by using ophthalmic preparation contains erythromycin or tetracycline.
- Other damage to new born: In joints & skin as mentioned in **flow chart-6.**

e. **Physical:** By anal sex in males leads to proctitis

f. **Reiter's syndrome:** Some times L-form of gonococcus is persist for long time causing arthritis, conjunctivitis & urethritis / cervictis **called Reiter's syndrome.**

Reiter's syndrome

✪ **Definition:** It is an autoimmune condition characterised by classic triad of arthritis (large joints like knees), conjunctivitis & urethritis (male) / cervictis (female) occurring after an infection, particularly from urogenital or gastrointestinal tract

✪ **Synonym:**
- **Reactive arthritis:** Because arthritis in this condition is usually the result of an infection affecting another body part.
- **Reiter's arthritis:** From the name of Hans Conard Julius Reiter & clinical features
- **Reiter's disease:** From the name of Hans Conard Julius Reiter

✪ **History:** It was 1st described by a German military physician & Leader of Nazi party, Hans Conard Julius Reiter in 1918. He discovered this disease as he was examining a World War I Prussian soldier who was recuperating from a bout of diarrhoea.

✪ **Incubation period:** Symptoms generally appear within 1–3 weeks but can range from 4 to 35 days from the onset of the inciting episode of the disease.

✪ **Precipitating factors:** It can occur in epidemic form. Following are the contributory factors.

1. **Age:** 20–40 years of age.
2. **Sex:** More common in men than in women.
3. **Immune status:** High risk in HIV patient.
4. **Genetic factors:**
- HLA-B27: It is located on chromosome 6. People with reactive arthritis frequently have the HLA-B27 gene.HLA-B27 is identified in 70-80% of patients of Reiter's syndrome. But many people have this gene without getting reactive arthritis.
- More common in white than in black people. This is owing to the high frequency of the HLA-B27 gene in the white population.

✪ **Etiological factors:** Two types like

1. **Urogenital pathogens:**
- *Chlamydia trachomatis:* It is the most common cause of reactive arthritis following urethritis
- *Ureaplasma urealyticum*
- *Neisseria gonorrhoea*

2. **Gastrointestinal pathogens:**
- *Shigella flexneri:* It is the most common organism causing reactive arthritis following diarrhoea.
- *Salmonella typhimurium, Salmonella enteritidis* & *Salmonella haldar.*
- *Campylobacter jejuni* & *C coli.*

3. **Others rare causes:**
- *Strept pyogenes* & viridans group.
- *Mycoplasma pneumoniae.*
- *Mycobacterium tuberculosis.*
- *Cyclospora.*
- *Yersinia enterocolitica* and *pseudotuberculosis.*
- *Clostridium difficile.*

✪ **Clinical features:** It is a classic triad of arthritis (large joints like knees), conjunctivitis & mucosal lesion like urethritis in male or cervictis in female, though this triad is not found in all cases. It also present with following other features.
- When arthritis & urethritis alone are present (conjunctivitis absent) the condition **called abortive Reiter's syndrome.**

- Spinal inflammation (spondyloarthropathy).
- Lesions are also present in musculoskeletal system, skin, nails, eyes (anterior uveitis, keratitis, scleritis etc.), CVS, kidney etc.

✪ **Diagnosis:** The diagnosis is based on clinical, history & physical examination. No laboratory study or imaging finding is diagnostic.

○ Specimens: The urethra, cervix and the throat may be swabbed in an attempt to culture the causative organisms. Cultures may also be carried out on urine and stool samples or on fluid obtained by arthrocentesis.

○ Testing methods:
- C-reactive protein.
- ESR.
- Gene detection: A blood test for the genetic marker HLA-B27 may also be performed. About 75 percent of all the patients with Reiter's arthritis have this gene.
- Molecular tests: PCR assay to detect *C trachomatis* DNA in synovial samples. It may be a good method for establishing the diagnosis of *Chlamydia* induced arthritis.
- Radiological like CT, MRI etc.

✪ **Treatment:** The main goal of treatment is to identify and eradicate the underlying infectious source with the appropriate antibiotics if still present. Otherwise, treatment is symptomatic for each problem.
- Antibiotics as per causative agent.
- NSAID.
- Steroids.
- Immunosuppressants.
- Local corticosteroids are useful in the case of iritis
- Exercise to strengthen muscles and improve joint function.

✪ **Prognosis:** Most people with reactive arthritis can expect to live normal life spans and maintain a near-normal lifestyle with modest adaptations to protect the involved organs. Prognosis is variable; 15% to 20% of patients may develop severe chronic sequelae.

✓ **Notes: Reiter's syndrome, Ritter's disease & Reiter's strain**

- **Reiter's syndrome: Vide supra**
- **Ritter's disease:**
  - Don't get confuse with the word **Ritter's disease** with different spelling & different causative agent like exfoliative toxin of *Staph aureus.*
  - More details: Follow chapter → Micrococcaceae
- **Reiter's strain:** Follow chapter → Spirochetales

❖ Laboratory diagnosis:

➢ **Specimens:**

1) **Acute urethritis:** Urethral discharge (50% sensitivity in culture) is collected. 1st clean the meatus with sterile gauze saline then collect the discharge
   - Directly on slide.
   - By using loop.
   - By using rayon/dacron swab (don't use cotton swab because it contain inhibitory fatty acids).
2) **Chronic urethritis:** Urethral discharge is not available, so following samples are collected.
   - Morning drop of urethral secretion.
   - Exudates collection after prostatic massage.
   - Urine: Gonococci are identified from centrifuged deposits.
3) **Asymptomatic gonorrhoea:** Asymptomatic carrier of gonococcus is rare in men while clinical disease is less sever in women, many of them carry gonococci in the cervix, so swab from endocervix is the best specimens for asymptomatic gonorrhoea. It has 80-90% sensitivity in culture.
4) **Eye lesions:** Purulent discharge.
5) **Other:** Cervical swab, vaginal swab from posterior vault, anal swab, conjunctival swab, blood & synovial fluid. Rectal swab in case of anal sex.

➢ **Transport:**
- All swabs in Amies transport medium.
- Blood & synovial fluid in trypticase soy broth.

➢ **Testing methods:**

I. **Microscopy: → Follow morphology**
II. **Culture: → Follow C/Cs**
III. **Biochemical reaction: → Follow B/Rs**
IV. **Serological:** Ab detection by using polyvalent antigens with following test.
   - CFT.
   - Passive (latex) agglutination.
   - Precipitation.
   - Radio Immuno Assay (RIA).

❖ Prophylaxis:

➢ **General measures:** Early detection of cases & follow up, contact tracing, health education, good hygiene, safe sex, use of barrier contraceptives & reduction of miss use of antimicrobials.

➢ **Chemoprophylaxis:** Instillation of 1% silver nitrate solution in eye of newborns to prevent opthalmia neonatorum (**Crede's method**).

➢ **Immnoprophylaxis:** Not useful & even clinical case does not provide any protection.

❖ Treatment:

➢ **Penicillin (Pn):** Pn was drug of choice since 1957, thereafter strain develop resistant to Pn. Such strain treated with high dose, 2.4-4.8 million unit of Pn.

➢ **Regime recommended by Centre for Disease Control & Prevention (CDC), USA, 1993:**

a. **If sensitive to ciprofloxacin:** **Ceftriaxone** (3rd generation cephalosporin like ceftriaxone or cefixime is the drug of choice) 125mg single IM or **ciprofloxacin** 500mg single oral dose or **ofloxacin** 400mg single oral dose.

b. **If resistant to ciprofloxacin:** **Ceftriaxone** 125mg single IM with **azithromycin** 1gm single oral dose or with **doxycycline** 100mg twice daily for 7 days.

❖ **Differences between meningococci & gonococci:** → Table-2

Features	Meningococci	Gonococci
Morphology **- Shape** **- Capsule**	**Fig.1** Half moon +	**Fig.4** Kidney/Bean --
O_2 effect	Strict aerobes	Aerobes & facultative anaerobes
C/Cs	Easy growth	Difficult to grow
B/Rs (Fig.2) Glucose Maltose	 A A	 A -
Habitat	Nasopharynx	Genitals
Transmission	Endogenous	Exogenous
Location	Intra & extracellular	Predominant intracellular
Pathogenicity	Brain & respiratory lesions	Genital lesions
Plasmid	Rarely present	Present & coded for drug resistance

Table-2: Differences between meningococci & gonococci

Commensal *Neisseria*

➢ **General properties:**
- Normal flora of nasopharynx/respiratory tract.
- Non- pathogenic but can cause the disease.
- Few are rod shaped: *N. elongate* & *N. weaver.*
- Few are capsulated: *N. mucosa.*
- Can grow at lower temperature: 22^0C.
- Not required CO_2 (not a capnophilic).
- Can grow on simple media like nutrient agar.
- Can't grow on selective media except *N. lactamica.*
- Some are pigmented: *N. flava* & *N. flavescens.*
- Ferment numbers of sugars.
- ONPG test is positive in *N. lactamica.*
- Other common features are shown in **table-3.**

Species	*N. flavescen*	*N. sicca*	*M. catarrhalis*
Colonies in nutrient agar	Yellow pigment	Small, wrinkled, dry, opaque & brittle	Smooth & transparent or opaque & adherent, not easily emulsifiable
Glucose **Maltose**	- -	A A	- -
Serology	Homoge-nous Ags	Autoaggl-utinable	Autoagglu-tinable

Table-3: Features of commensal *Neisseria*

➢ **Pathogenic role:**
1. ***N. flavescens*:**
- Resemble to meningococcus.
- Reported as causative agent of meningitis.
- Produces the yellow pigment.
2. ***N. sicca*:** Avirulent & closely related to meningococcus.
3. ***N. lactamica*:**
- Avirulent & closely related to meningococcus.
- Differentiated from meningococcus by positive ONPG test for beta –galactosidase.
- Their presence in nasopharynx of children provides protection to meningococcus.

Moraxellaceae

🕮 **Types of Moraxellaceae:** → Flow chart-7

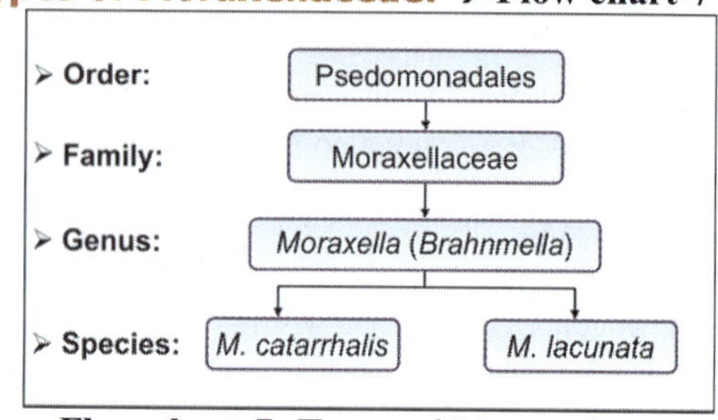

Flow chart-7: Types of Moraxellacae

Moraxella catarrhalis

❖ **Synonym:**
- *B. catarrhalis.*
- Previously it was know with some other names like *N. branhmenalis* or *N. catarrhalis.*

❖ **Morphology:** → Fig.-5(a)
- GNC.
- 0.6-1μm in size.
- Oval in shape.
- Arranged in pair with flat adjacent surface.

❖ **Culture characteristics (C/Cs):**

➢ **Effective factors:**
- Co_2 effect: Growth is facilitated by 5% CO_2 **called capnophilic bacteria.**
- Temperature: 18–42 °C.

➢ **Media:**
1. **Nutrient agar (table-3):** Grow on nutrient agar at 18-42^{0}C & producing non-pigmented colonies.
2. **Modified Thayer-Martin medium:** Produces the typical colonies.

❖ **Biochemical reactions (B/Rs):**
- Non fermenter.
- Catalase test: +Ve
- Oxidase test: +Ve
- Tributyrin hydrolysis test: +Ve
- DNAase test: +Ve

❖ **Pathogenicity:**

➢ **Mode of transmission:** Normal flora of respiratory tract & causes the endogenous infections.

- **Virulence factors:** It secrets the **β-lactamase** which make the bacteria resistant to β-lactam antibiotics.
- **Clinical features:** Opportunistic pathogen & causing tracheobronchitis, bronchopneumonia, laryngitis, meningitis, sinusitis & otitis media. It is a more common cause of respiratory disease in person with COPD & old age.

❖ Laboratory diagnosis:

- **Specimens:** Sputum
- **Testing methods:**

I. **Microscopy: → Follow morphology**
II. **Culture: → Follow C/Cs**
III. **Biochemical reaction: → Follow B/Rs**
IV. **Molecular:** PCR

❖ Treatment:

Don't use β-lactam antibiotic or if prescribed than only in combination with sulbactam or clavulanate.

Moraxella lacunata

❖ Synonym:

Also **called Morax-Axenfeld bacillus** or **called Morax-Axenfeld diplobacillus** because it was 1st reported by Victor Morax & Theodor Axenfeld from the case of angular conjunctivitis in 1897.

❖ Morphology: → Fig.-6(b)

- GNB & rod shaped, but becomes shorter & loose gram staining properties if culture left out for 5 days.
- Non flagellated but sluggishly motile.
- Arranged in pair (diplobacilli).

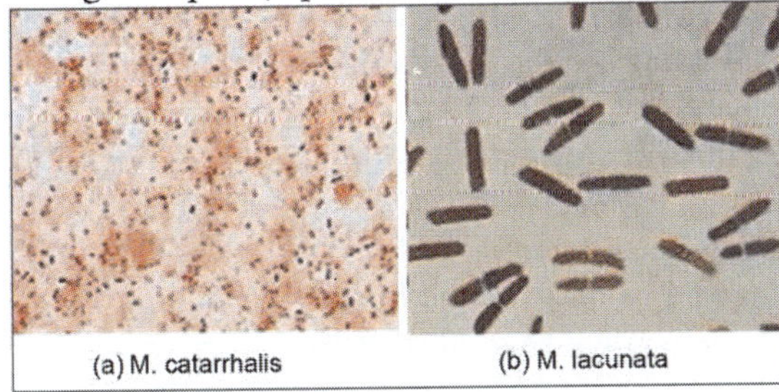

Figure-6: Morphology of *Moraxella* spp.

❖ Culture characteristics (C/Cs):

- **Effective factors:** Strict aerobes.
- **Media:** Grow on routine media like blood agar.

❖ Biochemical reactions (B/Rs):

- Non fermenter.
- Catalase test: +Ve
- Oxidase test: +Ve
- Indole test: -Ve
- H_2S production: -Ve

❖ Pathogenicity:

- **Disease name:** It causes eye lesion mainly in adults, but can occur at any age **called Angular conjunctivitis** or **called catarrhal conjunctivitis** or **called "Morax-Axenfeld conjunctivitis"**.
- **Clinical features:** Infection is characterized by
  - Chronic, mild angular blepharo-conjunctivitis frequently localized on the lid at the outer canthus.
  - Typical erythema of the edges of the lids.
  - Slight maceration of the skin, most marked at the angles, especially the outer canthus.
  - Superficial infiltration of the cornea is not uncommon.
  - The discharge is greyish yellow, adherent to the lashes and accumulates mainly at the angles.

❖ Laboratory diagnosis:

- **Specimens:** Eye discharge.
- **Testing methods:**

I. **Microscopy: → Follow morphology**
II. **Culture: → Follow C/Cs**
III. **Biochemical reaction: → Follow B/Rs**
IV. **Molecular:** PCR.

Non-gonococcal urethritis

❖ Synonym:

Nonspecific urethritis.

❖ Definition:

Chronic urethritis where gonococci are not identified as etiological agents **called non Gonococcal urethritis**.

❖ Etiological agents:

a. **Bacteria:**
1. *Chlamydia trachomatis:* Most common cause in 23-55% cases.
2. *Ureaplasma urealyticum.*
3. *Mycoplasma hominis.*
4. *Gardnerella vaginalis.*
5. *Acinetobacter lwoffi.*
6. *Acinetobacter calcoaceticus.*

b. **Viruses:**
1. Herpes virus.
2. Adenovirus.
3. Cyto Megalo Virus (CMV).

c. **Fungus:** *Candida albicans.*

d. **Parasite:** *Trichomonas vaginalis.*

e. **Others:**
1. Mechanical irritation: By catheter, cystoscope etc.
2. Chemical irritation: Like spermicides.

❖ Pathogenicity:

- **Mode of transmission:** NGU is transmitted by touching the mouth, penis, vagina or anus by penis, vagina or anus of a person who has NGU. NGU is more common in men than women.
- **Clinical features:**

✪ **Common symptoms:**
- Onset: Longer (>1 week).
- Pain or burning sensation upon urination (dysuria).
- White/cloudy discharge.
- Feeling to pass urine frequently.

✪ **Male:**
- Discharge from the penis.
- Burning or pain when urinating.
- Itching, irritation or tenderness.

✪ **Female:**
- Discharge from vagina.
- Burning or pain when urinating.

➢ **Complication:** Pelvic inflammatory disease.

❖ **Laboratory diagnosis:**

➢ **Specimens:**
- Urethral discharge.
- Urine.

➢ **Testing methods:**

1. Gram stain:
- Pus cells: > 4 / oil immersion field in urethritis & > 30 in urethritis.
- Bacteria: Above bacteria are difficult to identify under gram stain but useful to differentiate from gonococci which are stained as GNC.

2. Other specific test: As per etiological agents.

❖ **Differential diagnosis:** It should be differentiated from Gonococcal Urethritis (GU) as shown in **table-4.**

Features	GU	NGU
Onset	48 hours	Longer, >1 week
Discharge	Purulent (Flow like seed)	White/cloudy discharge
Gram stain	GNC in pair	Rare useful

Table-4: Differences between GU & NGU

❖ **Treatment:** As per etiological agents.

Bacteria infecting eyes

1. *N, gonorrhoea:* Disease **called ophthalmia neonatorum.**
2. *M. lacunata:* Disease **called Angular conjunctivitis** or **called catarrhal conjunctivitis** or **called "Morax-Axenfeld conjunctivitis".**
3. *H. aegyptius:* Disease **called pink eye.**
4. *C. trachomatis:* Two type's diseases **called trachoma** (serovars A-C) & **called inclusion conjunctivitis** (derovars D-K).

Mimeae

❖ **Meaning:** Tribe/family Mimeae, because mimicking GNC like Neisseriae **.**

❖ **Classification:** → **Flow chart-8**

❖ **Morphology:**
- GNB or gram negative coccobacilli or gram negative diplococci like Neisseriae.
- Size: 1–1.5 µm x 1.6–2.5 µm.
- Shape: Short-stout.
- Capsulated.
- Non motile.

❖ **Biochemical reaction (B/Rs):**
- Catalase +Ve
- Oxidase -Ve but some strains are +Ve.
- TSI test: Red slant/red butt → K/K or K/Nil.

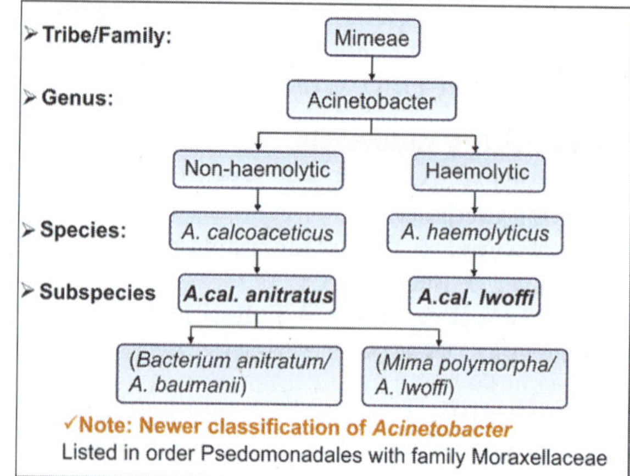

Flow chart-8: Classification of Mimeae

❖ **Differentiating features of species:**

i. ***A baumanii:*** (*A. cal. anitratus, bacterium anitratum*).

- **Cultural characteristics (C/Cs):**
  - Strict aerobes.
  - Grow at 44°C.
  - Non-haemolytic.
  - A pink colony on Mac Conkey's medium.
- **Biochemical reactions (B/Rs):**
  1. **Sugar fermentation test:** Ferments glucose, xylose, arabinose, rhamnose, 10% lactose (but not 1% lactose) with acid without gas.
  2. **Citrate test:** +Ve
  3. **OF test:** Oxidative pattern.

ii. ***A. lwoffi:*** (*A. cal. lwoffi, Mima polymorpha*)

- **Cultural characteristics (C/Cs):**
  - No growth at 44°C.
  - Non-haemolytic.
  - A pale colony on Mac Conkey's medium.
- **Biochemical reactions (B/Rs):**
  1. **Sugar fermentation test:** Non fermenter.
  2. **Citrate test:** -Ve
  3. **OF test:** Non fermentative pattern.

iii. ***A. haemolyticus:*** Haemolytic colonies.

❖ **Pathogenicity:**

➢ **Mode of transmission:**

✪ **Endogenous infection:** These are the normal flora of skin, oral cavity & intestine. Activated in immunosuppressive conditions.

✪ **Exogenous infection:**
- They are also the saprophytes in soil, water & phytosphere. Heavily available in hospital environment.
- Transmitted by contact with contaminated hands of hospital staff.

➢ **Precipitating factors:**

1. Prolonged hospitalization.
2. Immunosuppressive conditions.
3. Unhygienic practice in hospital by contaminated hands of staff.
4. Warm atmosphere of hospital.

➢ **Virulence factors:**

1. **OMP antigen**
2. **LPS:** Showing endotoxic activities.
3. **Ability to form biofilm:**
4. **Siderophores:** Helps in iron acquisition.
5. **Drug resistant:**

- Common in hospital strains.
- It produces resistant to many drugs like β-lactam, aminoglycosides & quinolones.
- β-Lactam resistance is due to production of metallo β-lactamase (MBL). Amp C β-lactamase & OXA type β-lactamase.

➢ **Clinical features:**

1. Non Gonococcal Urethritis (NGU).
2. Conjunctivitis.
3. Opportunistic infection & Nosocomial infection: It causes infection in patients with prolonged hospitalisation like ventilator associated pneumonia, meningitis, UTI, septicemia, traumatic wound infection, infection in burns patients etc.

❖ **Lab. diagnosis:** From CSF, urine, blood by using microscopy, culture & biochemical tests.

❖ **Prevention:** Strong aseptic precautions like improvement in hand hygiene to prevent the nosocomial infections.

❖ **Treatment:** Effective antibiotics are fluoroquinolones, carbapenems, amikacin, tigecycline & colistin.

Question bank

Case study

1) A 8 year old boy carried to emergency department with fever since 1 days along with headache, vomiting & disorientation. CSF is collected & examined by gram stain which shows the capsulated gram negative cocci in pair. Identify the organism & answer the following

a) Name the causative agent & describe the morphology of causative agent
b) Write the pathogenicity of causative agent
c) Describe the immunoprophylaxis of causative agent

2) A male patient visited the STD clinic with complain of urethral discharge. History ruled out the sexually activity with many partners. Urethral discharge is collected & examined microscopically under gram stain which shows the gram negative diplococci. Identify the organism & answer the following

a) Name the causative agent & describe the morphology of causative agent
b) Write the pathogenicity of causative agent
c) Describe the lab. diagnosis of causative agent

3) A man present with complain of redness, lacrimation & discharge from his left eye. Later he developed perforation. Gram stain from discharge revealed non capsulated gram negative cocci which are oxidase positive. Identify the organism & answer the following

d) Name the causative agent & describe the B/Rs of causative agent
e) Write the pathogenicity of causative agent
f) Mention the bacteria infecting eyes with the name of disease.

Essay/Full question

1) *N. meningitidis*
2) *N. gonorrhoea*

Short notes

1) Pathogenicity/Lab. diagnosis of *N. meningitidis*
2) Pathogenicity/Lab. diagnosis of *N. gonorrhoea*
3) Non Gonococcal Urethritis (NGU)
4) Acinetobacter

Short questions for theory/viva questions

1) Write the two morphological differences between meningococcus & gonococcus.
2) What is Ritter's disease & Reiter's syndrome?
3) Name four bacteria causing Reiter's syndrome.
4) Name the four bacteria causing Non Gonococcal Urethritis (NGU).
5) Name the four eye infecting bacteria with disease name.

MCQs for chapter review

Neisseria meningitidis

1) **Following is/are true about *N. meningitidis***
(a) Arranged in pairs (b) Capsulated (c) Flat apposition surface (d) a+b+c

2) **Following statements about meningococcal meningitis are true except-** (AI-03)
(a) Source of infection is mainly clinical cases (b) The disease is more common in dry and cold months of the year (c) Chemoprophylaxis of close contact of cases is recommended (d) The vaccine is not effective in children below 2 years of age

3) **Xavier and Yogender stay in the same hostel of same university. Xavier develops infection due to group B meningococcus. After few days Yogender develops infection due to group C meningococcus. All of the following statements are true except -** (AI-02)
(a) Educate students about meningococcal transmission and take preventive measures
(b) Chemoprophylaxis to all against both group B and group C
(c) Vaccine prophylaxis of contacts of Xavier
(d) Vaccine prophylaxis of contacts of Yogender

4) **Conjugate vaccines are available for the prevention of invasive disease caused by all of the following statements except -** (AIIMS-04)
(a) *H. influenzae* (b) *Strept pneumoniae* (c) *N. meningitidis* (group C) (d) *N. meningitidis* (group B)

5) **Treatment of choice for meningococcal infection is-** (AI -99)
(a) Tetracycline (b) Clindamycin (c) Gentamicin (d) Cephalosporin

6) **Young female with 3 day fever present with headache, BP 90/60 mmHg, heart rate of 140/min, and pin point spots developed distal to BP cuff. Most likely organism is -** (AIIMS May-13)
(a) *Burcella abortus* (b) *Burcella suis* (c) *N. meningitidis* (d) *Staphylococcus aureus*

Neisseria gonorrhoea

7) **Which of the following statement is not true about *Neisseria gonorrhoea* -** (AIIMS, Nov- 09)
(a) It is an exclusive human pathogen (b) Some strains may cause disseminated disease (c) Acute urethritis is the most common manifestation in males (d) All strains are highly sensitive to penicillin

8) **The virulence factors for *Neisseria gonorrhoea* includes all of the following except-** (AIIMS-03)
(a) Outer membrane proteins (b) IgA protease (c) M protein (d) Pilli

9) **Which of the following literally means "flow of seed"** (AIIMS-80)
(a) *Anthrax* (b) *Clostridia* (c) Gonorrhoea (d) *Proteus*

10) **True statement for Gonococcal urethritis is-**
(a) Rectum & prostate are not infected (b) Symptoms are more severe in female than male (c) Most patients are present with symptoms of dysuria (d) Single dose of ciprofloxacin is effective in treatment (e) Commonly leads to arthritis

11) **The best site to obtain a swab in asymptomatic gonorrhoea is** (AI-95, 02)
(a) Endocervix (b) Urethra (c) Lateral vaginal wall (d) Posterior fornix

12) **Differentiation between *Neisseria gonorrhoea* and *Neisseria meningitidis* is by-** (AI-90)
(a) Glucose fermentation (b) Maltose fermentation (c) VP reaction (d) Indole test

Reiter's syndrome

13) **Triad of Reiter's syndrome** (PGI-07)
(a) Conjunctivitis (b) Uveitis (c) Polyarthritis (d) Mucosal lesions (e) Glaucoma

14) **Following is true regarding Reiter's syndrome except-**
(a) It is an allergic disease (b) Most common in patient with HLA B27 (c) Most common uro-pathogen responsible is *Chlamydia trachomatis* (d) Most common gastrointestinal pathogen responsible is *Shigella*

15) **Reactive arthritis is caused by** (AIIMS-08)
(a) *Staphylococcus* (b) *H influenzae* (c) *N gonorrhoea* (d) *C trachomatis*

Non gonococcal urethritis

16) **Non-Gonococcal Urethritis (NGU) is caused by**
(a) *N. gonococci* (b) *C. albicans* (c) *C. trachomatis* (d) b+c

17) **Most common cause of non-gonococcal urethritis is** (AIIMS, May-93, AI-96)
(a) Menigococci (b) *E coli* (c) *Chlamydiae trachomatis* (d) *Mycoplasma*

18) **A 28 year old sexually active male presents with burning micturation. On clinical examination no ulcer in the genitals. Urine examination shows 50WBCs/HPF, no RBCs, leucocyte esterase positive, Gonococcal culture negative. What could be the most probable organism?** (AIIMS, Nov-07)
(a) *Treponema pallidum* (b) *Neisseria* (c) *Chlamydiae trachomatis* (d) *H ducreyi*

Answers of MCQs & explanation

1) **(d)**
- *N. meningitidis* are capsulated, arranged in pairs with flat apposition surface.

2) **(a)**
- Source of infection is mainly carrier not the case.
- Other options are explained in text

3) **(c)**
- Xavier develops infection due to group B meningococcus which is less immunogenic and vaccine is not available

4) **(d)**
- Conjugate vaccine is not available for group B meningococcus

5) **(d)**
- 3rd generation cephalosporin (ceftriaxone, ceftazidime) is the drug of choice for case & it may be used for initial treatment (first 2 days)
- Rifampicin is the drug of choice to remove the nasopharyngeal carrier & in person who is in close contact to carrier

6) **(c)**
- It is a case of septic shock (hypotension & tachycardia) along with meningitis (headache). Patient also develop skin lesion, so organism is *N. meningitidis* because only meningococcal meningitis present with skin lesions.

7) **(d)**
- It is an exclusive human pathogen & human disease **called gonorrhoea** (Rrhoea = discharge/flow of seeds).
- Some strain like Por 1A, may cause disseminated diseases like arthritis, ulcerative endocarditis & rarely meningitis
- Acute urethritis is the most common manifestation in males while in female the most common manifestation is cervictis & in prepubertal girls (Aneostogenic women) the most common manifestation is vulvovginitis or vaginitis as mentioned in **flow chart-6**
- All strains are not sensitive to penicillin & resistance has been developed to many drugs as explained in text under the section resistance

8) **(c)**
- M protein is the virulence factor in *Streptococci* not in gonococci.
- Follow section, ***Neisseria gonorrhoea* [pathogenicity → agent factors (virulence factors)]** for explanation

9) **(c)**
- Follow section, ***Neisseria gonorrhoea* (pathogenicity → meaning)** for explanation

10) **(c) & (d)**
- Proctitis (inflammation of rectum) occurs after anal sex & prostitis occurs due to extension from urethritis (inflammation of prostate)
- Symptoms are more severe in male than female
- Dysuria & mucopurulent discharge present without frequency or urgency
- Single dose of ciprofloxacin or other fluoroquinolones like ofloxacin / levofloxacin is effective in treatment.
- Arthritis is not occurs commonly but occurs in 3-5% of untreated cases.

11) **(a)**
- Follow section, ***Neisseria gonorrhoea* (laboratory diagnosis → specimens→ asymptomatic gonorrhoea)** for explanation

12) **(b)**
- Differentiation between *Neisseria gonorrhoea* and *Neisseria meningitidis* is explained in **table-2**

13) **(a), (c) & (d)**
14) **(a)**
15) **(c) & (d)**
} Follow section **Reiter's syndrome** for explanation

16) **(d)**
17) **(c)**
} Follow section **Non-Gonococcal Urethritis (etiological agents)** for explanation.

18) **(c)**
- It is a case of NGU, because gonococcal culture is negative
- Absence of **ulcer in the genitals is rule out the possibilities of** *Treponema pallidum* & *H ducreyi*
- Pus cells in urine is a feature of *Chlamydiae trachomatis*

35 Corynebacterium

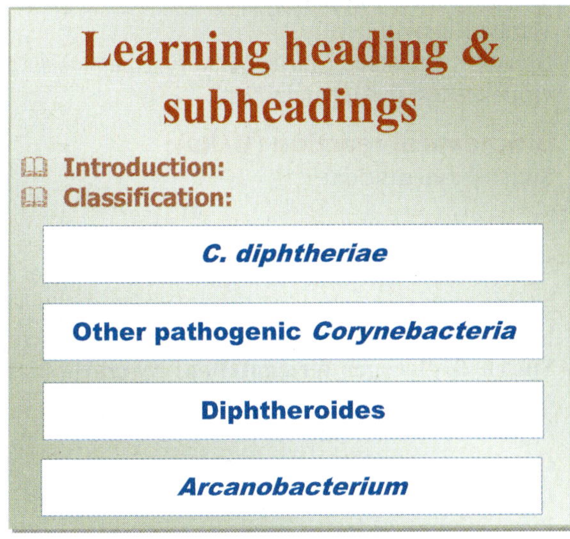

Introduction:

- Meaning: Derived from word **Coryne = Club** as showing club shaped swelling due to presence of metachromatic granules at the ends.
- *Corynebacteria* containing peptidoglycan, polysaccharide, fatty acids (glycolipid) in cell wall closely related to *Mycobacteria, Nocardia* so **called CMN group.**
- *Corynebacterium* composed of > 59 species of which 36 are medically important.
- They define together on genetic basis (16S rRNA, 16Sr DNA sequencing, nucleic acid hybridisation)
- Nonpathogenic **called coryneform or diphtheroids.**

Classification:

A. Pathogenic: Produce toxin.

i. Genus: *Corynebacterium*

1. *C. diphtheriae* [Kleb-Loeffler's Bacilli (KLB)]
2. Other pathogenic *Corynebacterium:*
   - *C. ulcerans*
   - *C. pseudotuberculosis* (*C. ovis*)
   - *C. minutissimum*
   - *C. tenuis*
   - *C. jakeium* (formerly JK group)
   - *C. urealyticum*

B. Non-pathogenic: Called coryneform or diphtheroids

i. Genus: *Corynebacterium*

1. *C. pseudodiphtheriticum*
2. *C. xerosis*
3. *C. parvum*

ii. Genus: *Propionibacterium:* More details, **Follow chapter → Non sporing anaerobes**

iii. Genus: *Arcanobacterium:*

1. *A. haemolyticum:* Earlier **called *C. haemolyticum***

iv. Genus: *Brevibacterium*

v. Genus: *Oerskovia*

vi. Genus: *Turicella*

vii. Genus: *Rhodococcus:* Formerly called *Corynebacterium.*

viii. Genus: *Rothia*

C. diphtheriae

Synonyms & history:

- *C. diphtheriae* was 1st identified by **Klebs** in 1883 but 1st cultivated by **Loeffler** in 1884 hence commonly **called Klebs- Loeffler Bacillus (KLB).**
- Diphtheria bacilli, as the disease produced.

Morphology:

- **Type according to gram stain:** GPB **[fig.-1(a)]**
- **Size:** 3–6 μm x 0.6–0.8 μm.
- **Shape:** Slender rod with clubbing at one or both ends.
- **Arrangement:**
  - In pairs, palisades (resembling stakes of a fence) or in small groups.
  - Sometimes arranged end to end by making an angle to each other, resembling letters V or L **called Chinese letter appearance or Cuneiform arrangement**. It is due to incomplete separation of daughter cells after binary fission.
- Nonmotile, nonsporing & non capsulated.

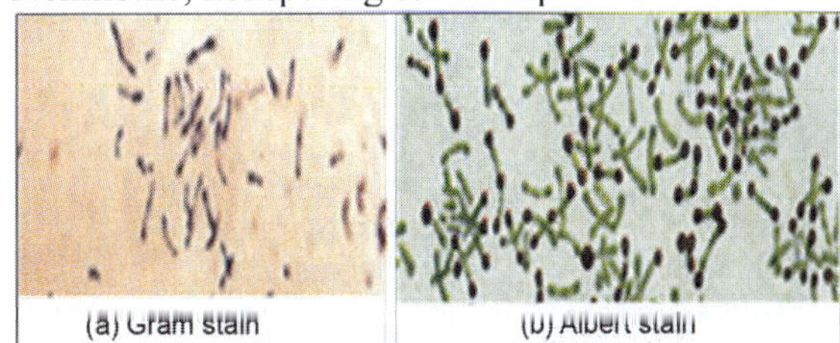

Figure-1: Morphology of *C. diphtheriae*

- **Polar bodies [fig.-1(b)]:** More details, **Follow chapter → Morphology of bacteria**
- **Immunofluorescence microscopy:** Also useful

Cultural characteristics [C/Cs]:

- **Effective factors:**
  - O_2 effect: Aerobes and facultative anaerobes.
  - Temperature: 37°C (15–40°C).
  - pH: 7.2
  - Growth occurs on enriched media with blood, serum or eggs.
- **Culture in Media:**

A. Liquid media: →Follow table 1

B. Solid media:

1. Loeffler's serum :

- Grow very rapidly within 6-8 hours.
- Colonies are small, circular & white become large & yellowish on longer incubation.

2. Blood agar: Some strains are haemolytic while some are non haemolytic.

C. Selective media:

1. Potassium tellurite (PT) medium:

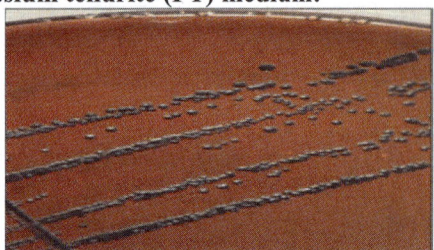

Figure-2: *C diphtheriae* in PT medium

- Containing heat lysed blood & potassium tellurite.
- Slow growth (48 Hrs).
- 0.04% tellurite inhibits growth of other bacteria & acts as selective agents.
- Colonies are grayish or black (**fig.-2**) due to reduction of potassium tellurite to metallic tellurium.
- Incubated at least for 2 days before giving –Ve report.
- Other bacteria producing black colonies in PT medium are: *Staph aureus, Enterococcus faecalis* & *Erysipelothrix rhusiopathiae.*

2. McLeod's & Hoyle's medium: Containing saponin lysed blood.

3. Cystine Tellurite agar: Containing potassium tellurite + cysteine.

4. Tinsdales medium: Containing cystine tellurite agar + sodium thiosulphate.

➢ **Culture in animal:**

- It is done by using the guinea pigs to differentiate the toxigenic / virulent strain from no toxigenic / avirulent strain.
- Broadly described in laboratory diagnosis as virulence test (toxigenicity test).

❖ Biochemical reaction (B/Rs):

1. Sugar fermentation:

G	S	L	M
A	-	-	-

- Other sugars fermented are galactose, maltose & dextrin with acid only.
- Sugar fermentation is tested in Hiss's serum water.
- **Starch & glycogen fermentation:** By gravis strain only but not by intermedius and mitis strains.

2. Nitrate reduction test: +Ve

3. Catalase test: + Ve

4. Oxidase test: - Ve

5. Pyrazinamidase test: +Ve

6. Urease test: It is -Ve & helps to differentiate from *C. ulcerans* & *C. pseudotuberculosis* where it is positive.

❖ Resistance:

- Destroyed by heat at 58^{0}C in 10 minutes & at 100^{0}C in 1 minute. It survives for 14 weeks on dried piece of pseudomembrane.
- Sensitive to routinely used disinfectants. It dies rapidly by treatment with 0.85% NaCl solution.

❖ Typing: Two types of typing methods.

i. Phenotyping:

a. Biotyping:

- Given by McLeod & Anderson as shown in **table 1.**
- Based on colony morphology on PT medium & other properties.

Features	Gravis	Intermedius	Mitis
		Morphology	
Length **Granules** **Pleomorphism**	-Short rods -Few/no granules -Less pleomorphic	-Long rods -Poor granulation -Very pleomorphic	-Long –curved -Prominent granules -Pleomorphic
		C/ Cs	
Liquid media	-Surface pellicle -No turbidity -Granular deposit	-Turbid in 24 hrs, clear in 48hrs -Granular deposit	-Diffuse turbidity & soft pellicle
Blood agar	Variable	Nonhaemolytic	Haemolytic
PT medium/agar	Daisy Head colony	Frog's Egg colony	Poached Egg colony
Consistency	'Cold margarine' brittle, not easily emulsifiable	Intermediate between gravis and mitis	Soft, buttery, easily emulsifiable
		B/Rs	
Glycogen + starch	Fermentation	Non-fermentation	Non-fermentation
		Pathogenicity	
Virulence	Severe	Moderate	Mild
Nature of disease	Epidemic	Epidemic	Endemic
Complication	Paralytic	Haemorrhagic	Obstructive

Table-1: Biotypes of *C. diphtheriae*

b. **Serotyping:**

- **Antigenic structure:** Bacilli are antigenically heterogeneous & posses following three antigens.

1. **Deep seated antigen:** Found in all *Corynebacterium* species & in *M. tuberculosis*.
2. **K antigen:** It is a heat labile protein.
3. **O Ag:** It is a heat stable polysaccharide antigen.

- **Typing:**
  - By agglutination, **gravis** has 13, **intermedius** has 4 & **mitis** has 40 serotypes.
  - Gravis type 2 is common worldwide.
  - No connection has been established between antigenic type & other features.

c. **Bacteriophage Typing:** Follow chapter → Laboratory diagnosis of bacterial infections

d. **Bacteriocin (Diphthericin) typing:** Gibson & Colman demonstrated 10 pattern of bacteriocin.

ii. **Genotyping:** Molecular techniques are

1. Bacterial polypeptide analysis.
2. DNA restriction patterns.
3. Hybridisation.
4. DNA probe.

Pathogenicity:

- **Disease name:** Disease **called diphtheria.**
- **Meaning:** Word derived from **Diphtheros (Greek) = leather,** because of leathery pseudomembrane formation.
- **Definition:** It is a toxemia & locally characterized by pseudomembrane formation.
- **Nature & history of disease:** It occurs as endemic or epidemic form. The disease was 1st recognised by Bretonneau in 1826, who **called it diphtherite** from **Diphtheros (Greek) = leather.**
  - **World:** Epidemic was occurred in Soviet Union in 1990 involving thousands of case with 20% mortality.
  - **India:** Condition is under controlled due to effective immunisation.
- **Reservoir of infection:** Human & animals like cows are reservoirs. In human bacteria are present in nose or throat & in animal they are present in udder & transmitted via milkers by milk ingestion.
- **Source of infection:** Respiratory droplets arise from nose or throat of human & the milk (may be tissue from udder) of infected animal are the sources of infection.
- **Mode of transmission:**

1. Air borne (inhalation).
2. Fomites borne (toys and pencils).
3. By milk of infected cows.

- **Incubation period:** 3-4 days.
- **Portal of entry:** Respiratory tract & also by skin.
- **Sites:** Different sites like faucial (throat), nasal, conjunctival, otitic, laryngeal, genital, vulval, vaginal or prepucial & cutaneous.
- **Precipitating factors (epidemiological determinants):** Three types

I. Agent factors (virulence factors)

Bacilli do not penetrate deep in to the mucosal tissues & bacteremia do not occurs. Diphtheria is a toxemia & all clinical manifestations are due to productions of powerful exotoxin **called diphtheria toxin.** Salient features of diphtheria toxin are described below.

- **History:**
  - Loeffler studied the effect of bacilli in animals & concluded that the illness is not due to bacilli itself but by its diffusible product.
  - Emile Roux & Alexander Yersin identified the diffusible product in 1888 which **called diphtheria toxin** & established its pathogenic effects.
  - Diphtheria antitoxin was discovered by von Behring in 1890.
- **Properties:**
  - "Park -Williams 8" Strain of *C. diphtheriae* widely used for toxin production.
  - 90-95% gravis & intermedius strains are toxigenic.
  - 80-85% mitis are toxigenic.
  - Heat-labile.
  - Toxin is produced locally & it spread to distant organs by blood (exotoxemia) with special affinity for certain tissues like myocardium, adrenals glands & nerve endings.
  - It is phage coded.
  - Lethal dose and effects: It is highly potent. The lethal dose for humans is about 0.1 μg of toxin per kg of body weight. Death occurs through necrosis of the heart and liver. Diphtheria toxin has also been associated with the development of myocarditis. Myocarditis secondary to diphtheria toxin is considered one of the biggest risks to unimmunized children.
- **Lf unit:**
  - It is defined as Loeffler's flocculating unit.
  - 1 Lf unit is defined as the amount of diphtheria toxin which flocculates very rapidly with one unit of antitoxin.
- **Other bacteria producing diphtheria toxin:**
  - *C. ulcerans*
  - *C. pseudotuberculosis*
- **Structure:**
  - Biochemical nature: Protein
  - MW: 62,000
  - Two fragments: A (MW 24,000) & B (MW 38,000)
  - A is active fragment while fragment B is for binding of toxin to cells.
  - Antibody to fragment B protects by preventing binding of toxin to cells.
- **Mechanism of action:**

- Fragment A inhibits polypeptide chain elongation in presence of NAD by inactivating elongation factor (EF-2).
- Toxin acts by inhibiting protein synthesis.

✓ **Notes: Toxins act by inhibiting the protein synthesis**

- Diphtheria toxin: } By inactivation of EF-2
- *Pseudomonas* toxin:
- Shiga like toxin (SLT): } By inactivation of 60S ribosome
- Shiga toxin:

✪ **Factor affecting the toxin production:**

- **Iron**
- Minimum concentration is 0.1 mg/l.
- Higher concentration (0.5mg/l) decreases the production.
- **Tox$^+$ phage/ β prophage**
- Bacteriophage infecting *Corynebacterium* is **called corynephage.**
- It introduces new nucleic acid in to bacterial chromosome **called Tox$^+$ phage/ β prophage.**
- Bacterium with **Tox$^+$ phage/ β prophage** is **called lysogenic bacterium.**
- **Tox$^+$ phage/ β prophage** multiplies along with bacterial chromosomes. This phenomenon is **called lysogeny.**
- In presence of new **Tox$^+$ phage/ β prophage,** bacteria acquired certain new properties [like toxin production] **called phage conversion** or **lysogenic conversion.**
- Elimination of **Tox$^+$ phage/ β prophage** makes the organism non-toxigenic.

✪ **Uses:**

1. **Toxoid:**
- Prolonged storage, incubation at 37 °C for 4-6 weeks, treatment with 0.2-0.4 per cent formalin or acid pH converts it to toxoid.
- Having antigenicity but no toxicity
- It is capable of inducing antitoxin and reacting specifically with it.
- Used in prevention of diphtheria
2. **Antineoplastic agent:**
- The drug denileukin diftitox uses diphtheria toxin as an antineoplastic agent.
- Resimmune is an immunotoxin which uses diphtheria toxin is used clinical trials in cutaneous T cell lymphoma patients.

II. Host factors

1. **Age:**
- It is rare below one year of age due to passive protection from maternal antibodies.
- It is maximum between 2-5 years & less between 5-10 years. Very low afterward due to repeated subclinical infections.
2. **Immunity:**
- Single attack of disease or inapparent infection provides lifelong immunity (usually, not always), so child recovered from disease does not required active immunisation.
- It is less in developing countries due to proper immunisation while more in countries not following proper immunisation.

III. Environmental factors

1. **Temperate regions:** Carriage is more in nose & throat. Nasal carriage harbours the bacilli for longer period.
2. **Tropical regions:** Bacilli are found more in skin & causing cutaneous diphtheria. Bacilli lasting for 3 years in skin. Cutaneous diphtheria may stimulate the natural immunity & also faucial diphtheria in non-immune individual.

➢ **Pathogenesis:** It is explained in **flow chart-1.** It is good to remember that non toxigenic strain can produces only local lesion (in skin/nasopharynx) not the systemic lesion, while toxigenic strain can produces both local & systemic lesions. To produces the local lesion toxigenic strain is not necessary.

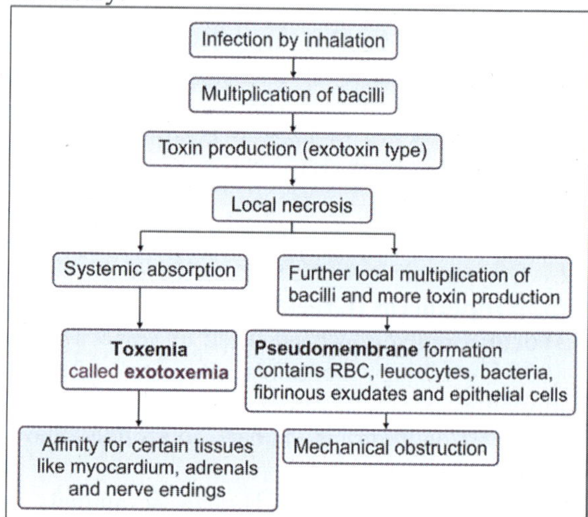

Flow chart-1: Pathogenesis of diphtheria

➢ **Clinical features:** Clinically different types.

a. **Based on site of infection:**

1 **Nasal:**
- Mildest & toxemia is minimal.
- Present with unilateral or bilateral nasal discharge.

2 **Faucial (tonsilo pharyngeal):**
- Commonest variety involving throat/ nasopharynx.
- More severe (moderate) than nasal diphtheria.
- It causes localized infection of throat, tonsils (white patch present over tonsil in child), pharynx, larynx and adjacent surface.
- Clinically it present with mild grade fever, sore throat, malaise & pseudomembrane (gray or white) in throat as show in **fig.-3(a).**
- Removal of pseudomembrane leads to bleeding.

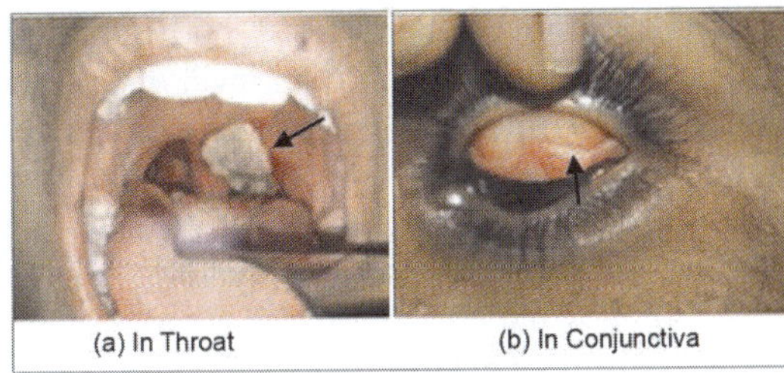

Figure-3: Pseudomembrane

3 **Laryngeal:**
- Most severe with highest mortality, so immediately required tracheostomy; however tracheostomy is not mandatory in all cases.
- Present with hoarseness & cough.

4 **Conjunctival:** Also shows the presence of pseudomembrane [**fig.-3(b)**].

5 **Otitic:** Otitis media

6 **Genital:** Vulval, vaginal or prepucial.

7 **Cutaneous:**
- Secondary infection due to pre-existing skin lesions.
- Present as ulcer **called ecythema diphtheriticum** or **diphtheritic whitlow.**
- Commonly caused by nontoxigenic strains.

b. Based on clinical severity:

1. **Malignant or hypertoxic:** Cervical lymph nodes are enlarge (severe adenitis) due to oedema **called bull neck diphtheria.**
2. **Septic:** Causing ulceration, cellulitis & gangrene around pseudomembrane.
3. **Haemorrhagic:** Bleeding from the edge of membrane, conjunctiva, nasal mucosa (epistaxis), cutaneous and generalised bleeding.

➢ **Complications:**

a. Local / mechanical: Due to pseudomembrane formation. It extends up in nasal mucosa & down in to larynx causing suffocation & respiratory obstruction **called mechanical asphyxia.**

b. Systemic: Due to toxin production.

1 **Cardio vascular:**
- Myocarditis: Cardiac damage occurs at the end of 1st week or in the beginning of 2nd week. It is irreversible (recovery of nerve damage is rule but not the cardiac damage)
- Endocarditis.
- Central or peripheral circulatory failure.
- Death is due to circulatory failure.

2 **Neurological:**
- Palatine and cilliary (not pupillary) paralysis occurs in 3-4 wks of disease which recovered spontaneously.
- Neuropathy.

3 **Others:**
- Respiratory: Pneumonia.
- Degenerative change in liver, adrenal glands & kidneys (renal failure).

❖ Laboratory diagnosis

➢ **Key points before moving to laboratory diagnosis:**
- Diagnosis based on clinical ground & start treatment without waiting for laboratory report.
- Laboratory help needs for
  - Confirmation of disease.
  - Epidemiological & research purpose.
  - Differentiation of other cause of pseudomembrane like acids/alkalis injuries, Vincent's angina & infectious mononucleosis.
  - Control measure.

➢ **Specimens:**
- 2 throat swabs: One is for microscopy & 2nd is for culture.
- Swab also collected from nose, larynx, pseudomembrane, skin lesion or any other site where diphtheria is suspected.

➢ **Collection:**
- Collect before antibiotics & antiseptic mouth wash.
- Rayon/Dacron swab is preferred over cotton swab.
- Swabs are collected by using tongue depressor.
- Swab rubbed over affected area and pseudomembrane.

➢ **Transport:** If swab cannot be inoculated promptly it should be kept moistened with sterile serum.

➢ **Testing methods:**

I. Microscopy: → Follow morphology

II. Culture: → Follow C/Cs

III. Biochemical reaction: → Follow B/Rs

IV. Virulence test (toxigenicity test): Two types

a. In vivo test:

1. Subcutaneous test:

➢ **Steps: →Flow chart-2**

➢ **Disadvantage:** Wastage of unprotected animal.

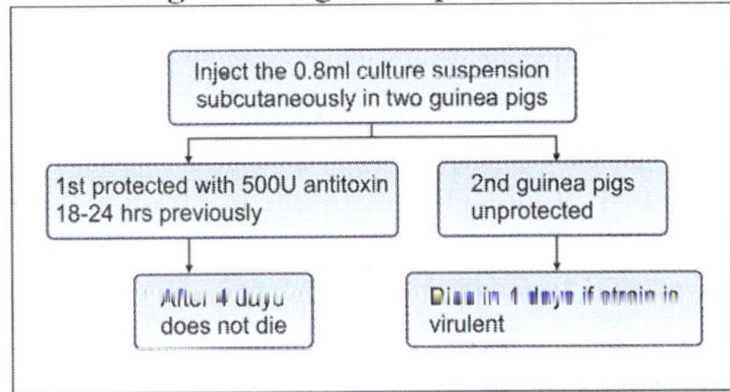

Flow chart-2: Subcutaneous test

2. Intracutaneous test:

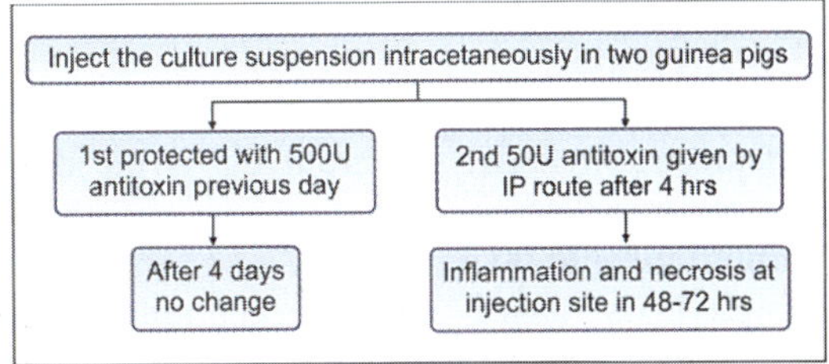

Flow chart-3: Intracutaneous test

➢ **Steps: →Flow chart-3**

➢ **Advantage:** No wastage of unprotected animal.

b. In vitro test:

1. Tissue culture:

➢ **Steps: →Flow chart-4**

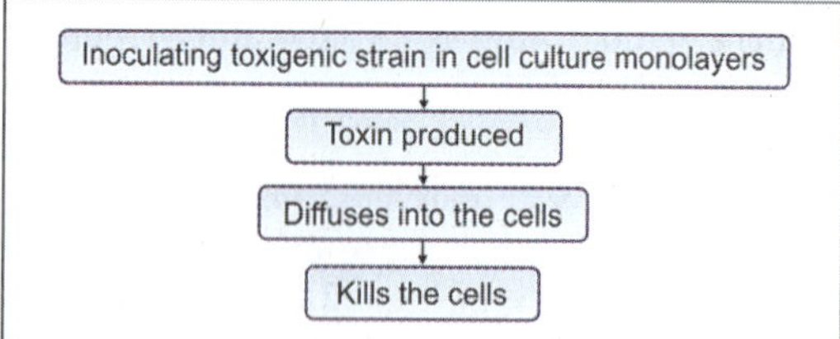

Flow chart-4: Tissue culture test

2. **Molecular:** PCR to detect the tox gene.
3. **Toxin detection:** By ELISA & ICT.
4. **Elek's gel precipitation test:**

✪ **Principle:** Based on precipitation reaction.

✪ **Method: → Fig.-4.**

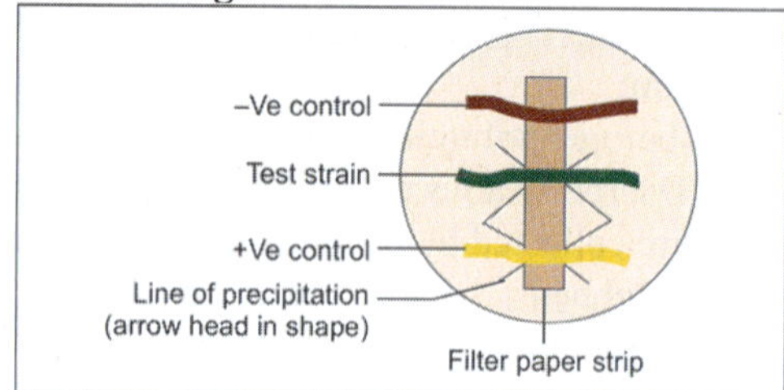

Figure-4: Elek's gel precipitation test

- Rectangular filter paper strip impregnated with diphtheria antitoxin (1000 u/ml) is placed in 20% normal horse serum agar.
- Inoculate the strain at right angle to paper strip.
- Also set the positive and negative controls.
- Incubate the plate at 37 °C for 24-48 hours.

✪ **Result:**

- **+Ve test:** Toxins produced by bacteria will diffuse in agar & meets with antitoxin to produce the arrow head line of precipitation.
- **-Ve test:** No line of precipitation.

✪ **Interpretation:**

- **+Ve test:** It indicates the toxigenic strain.
- **-Ve test:** It indicates the nontoxigenic strain.

V. Bacterial typing: → Vide supra

✓ **Note: No serological tests**

- *C. diphtheriae* confirmed to the site of entry & does not invade the blood stream, so no antibodies formation & no role of serological tests.

❖ Prophylaxis:

➢ **General measures:** Avoid contact with carrier.

➢ **Chemoprophylaxis:** Erythromycin is the drug of choice for carrier.

➢ **Immunoprophylaxis:**

✪ **Prophylaxis based on:** Susceptibility test for assaying circulatory antitoxin level.

1. Schick test: No longer in use.
2. Passive haemagglutination test.
3. Neutralisation in cell culture.

✪ **Index of immunity:** Antitoxin level of 0.01unit or more per ml of blood is considered as index of immunity.

✪ **Types of immunoprophylaxis:**

A. Active immunisation: It includes diphtheria toxoid. Following types of toxoid are available.

i. APT (Alum Precipitated Toxoid): It gives reaction so not useful.

ii. FT (Formal Toxoid / Fluid Toxoid) or plain toxoid): Prepared by incubating the toxin with formalin.

iii. Adsorbed (purified) toxoid: It is purified toxoid adsorbed on to insoluble aluminium compound usually aluminium phosphate (**called Purified Toxoid Aluminium Phosphate/PTAP**) or less often aluminium hydroxide (**called Purified Toxoid Aluminium Hydroxide PTAH**). Study shows that adsorption by using aluminium compound act as an adjuvant & it increase the immunological effectiveness of vaccine.

✪ **Advantages of adsorbed toxoid:**

- It is much more immunogenic than fluid toxoid.
- It is preferred now days.
- Efficacy is approximately 95%.

✪ **Disadvantage of adsorbed toxoid:** Toxoid is against the toxin not against the organism, so it can prevent the case not the carrier.

✪ **Storage:** Adsorbed toxoid should be stored between 4-10^{0}C & no freezing at any time.

✪ **Administration of adsorbed toxoid:** WHO recommended to use purified toxoid in national schedule. It is used as a single vaccine or in the form of combined vaccine as follows.

a. Single / plain / monovalent / univalent vaccine:

- APT, FT, PTAP & PTAH are available but not in wide use as single vaccine.
- For young children, diphtheria toxoid is given in a dose of 10-25 Loeffler (Lf) units. Smaller dose (1-2 Lf units) used for older children and adults.

b. Mixed / combined / molyvalent / multivalent vaccines: Adsorbed diphtheria toxoid is used in combination with following vaccines.

- **Double / bivalent vaccine:** DT (contains Diphtheria + Tetanus) & DP (contains Diphtheria, + Pertusis)
- **Triple / trivalent / tetravalent vaccine:** DPT/DTP contains Diphtheria, Pertusis & Tetanus.
- **Quaduple / quadrivalent vaccine:** DPT (DTP) with Hib etc.
- **Pentavalent vaccine:** Two type of preparations

1. **Pentvac** contains Diphtheria, Pertusis, Tetanus, HBV, *H. influenzae* type b (Hib).
2. **Pentaxim** contains D, P, T, IPV & Hib.

- **Dosing schedule of triple (DPT) vaccine, pentavalent vaccine & double (DT) vaccine as per national immunisation schedule:**

Triple (DPT) vaccine

- Three (Primary) doses of DPT, each with 0.5 ml amount by deep IM route, are given at 6th weeks, 10th week & 14th week of age.
- After primary immunisation of DPT at 6, 10 & 14 weeks, 1st booster of DPT is given at 18-24 months followed by 2nd booster dose (DT only) at 5-6 year (school entry age).

Pentavalent vaccine

- In some states instead of DPT, pentavalent vaccine (**Pentvac**) contains Diphtheria, Pertusis, Tetanus, HBV, H. influenza type b (Hib) is given at 6th weeks, 10th weeks & 14th weeks with OPV. Other same preparation is **Pentaxim** contains D, P, T, IPV & Hib given with OPV & HBV.

Double (DT) vaccine

Double (DT) vaccine is given at 5-6 years /school entry age (Second dose of DT after 1 month if not previously immunized by DPT/pentavalent vaccine)

- **Storage:** DPT/DT should be stored between 4-10^{0}C & no freezing at any time.
- **Adverse reactions of DPT vaccine:**
- Local reactions (erythema / induration).
- Exaggerated local reactions (Arthus-type).
- Fever and systemic symptoms not common.
- Severe systemic reactions rare.
- **Contraindications and precautions of DPT vaccine:**
- Severe allergic reaction to vaccine component or following a prior dose.
- Moderate or severe acute illness.
- **Efficacy of DPT vaccine:** It is 70%.

B. Passive immunisation:

- It is used when susceptible is exposed to infection and in case of diphtheria patient.
- It consists of SC injection of 500-1000 U of antitoxin **called Anti Diphtheritic Serum (ADS).**
- **Adverse reaction:** Hypersensitivity.

C. Combined immunisation:

- It consists of administration of the first dose of adsorbed toxoid on one arm **(active immunisation)** & ADS to the other arm **(passive immunisation)** followed by the full course of active immunisation.

✓ **Note: Schick test**

- **Principle:** Based on toxin-antitoxin neutralisation & hypersensitivity reaction.
- **Indication:** Test was indicated to judge the susceptibility (immune status) & hypersensitivity to diphtheria toxin before immunisation.
- **Limitations:**
- Test is no longer in use, because toxoid is available which is free from hypersensitivity.
- Level of antitoxin (immune status) is also assessed by passive haemagglutination or by neutralisation in cell culture. Antitoxin level of ≥0.01 unit / ml of blood is considered as an index of immunity.
- **Method:**
- Intradermal injection of diphtheria toxin in one forearm (**called test arm**) & diphtheria toxoid in other forearm (**called control arm**).
- Observe the result 1st after 24-48 hours & 2nd after 5-7 days.
- **Result, observation & interpretation: → Table-2**

Observation	Interpretation
Negative result	
No reaction in any arm	- No susceptibility (Toxin neutralise by specific antitoxin) - No hypersensitivity
Positive result	
- Erythematous reaction in test arm that persist - No reaction in control arm	- Patient is susceptible to diphtheria (No antitoxin in patient to neutralise the toxin due to absence of vaccination) - No hypersensitivity
Combined result	
- Erythematous reaction in both arms but reaction persist only in test arm	- Patient is susceptible to diphtheria (No antitoxin in patient to neutralise the toxin due to absence of vaccination) - Hypersensitivity
Pseudo positive result (Schick's negative)	
Diffuse erythematous reaction in both arms appear in 24 hrs & disappear in 4 days	

Table-2: Schick test

❖ Treatment:

➢ **Treatment of case:** Consist of ADS & antibiotic therapy.

1. **ADS:** 20, 000-1, 00, 000 U by SC route in serious case. Half dose by IV route.
2. **Antibiotic therapy:** Pn (procaine pn) is drug of choice. Other options are clindamycin, rifampicin or erythromycin.

➢ **Treatment of carrier:** Erythromycin.

➢ **Treatment of contact:** Three categories.

- **Primary immunisation or booster dose received in last two years:**
- No further treatment.
- **Primary immunisation or booster dose received in before two years:**
- Only booster dose of toxoid.
- **No immunisation:**
- Prophylactic Pn or erythromycin.
- ADS.
- Active immunisation.

Other pathogenic *Corynebacteria*

❖ *C. ulcerans*:

➢ **Similarities with *C. diphtheriae*:**
- Causes diphtheria like lesion.
- Resemble to gravis variety of diphtheria bacillus.
- Black colonies on Tinsdales medium.

➢ **Difference with *C. diphtheriae*:**
- Liquefy gelatin.
- Ferment trehalose.
- Does not reduce nitrate to nitrite.
- Urease test positive.

➢ **Pathogenicity:**
- **Mode of transmission:** Human infection transmitted by cow's milk.
- **Toxin:** Produce 2 type of toxin one is identical to diphtheria toxin and other to toxin of *C. pseudodiphthericum* (phospholipase-D) affect sphingomyelin.
- **Clinical features:**
  - Produce infection in cows.
  - In human it produces the ulcer in throat.

➢ **Treatment:** Erythromycin is effective.

❖ *C. pseudotuberculosis*:

➢ **Synonym:** Commonly **called Preisz-Nocard bacillus.**

➢ **Similarities with *C. diphtheriae*:**
- Black colonies on Tinsdales medium.
- Reverse CAMP test is positive.

➢ **Difference with *C. diphtheriae*:** Urease positive.

➢ **Pathogenicity:**
- **Toxin:** Produce diphtheria toxin.
- **Clinical features:**
  - Produce infection in pseudotuberculosis in sheep & suppurative lymphadenitis in horses.
  - In human it produces the ulcer in throat.

❖ *C. minutissimum:*

- Lipophilic & grow in media containing 20% fetal calf serum.
- It produces the localised infection of the stratum corneum **called erythrasma**, affecting axilla and groin.
- On Wood's lamp examination it gives coral red colour.

❖ *C. tenuis:*

It produces the pigmented nodules around the axillary & pubic hair shaft **called trichomycosis axillaris.**

❖ *C. jakeium:*

- Earlier **called JK group.**
- Lipophilic species.
- Strictly aerobic.
- Pyrizinamide and alkaline phosphatase test positive.
- Multiple antibiotic resistant, responding only to vancomycin.
- Opportunistic pathogen causing bacteremia, endocarditis, meningitis & skin features.

❖ *C. urealyticum:*

- Normal flora of skin.
- Causes UTI like pyelonephritis, cystitis in patient with IDDs & renal transplant.
- It is a strong urease producer; infection of urinary tract may lead to formation of stones.

Diphtheroides

❖ **Definition:** Bacilli resemble to *Corynebacterium* are **called diphtheroides.** They are the normal flora of skin, throat, conjunctiva & other areas.

❖ **Differences B/W *C. diphtheriae* & diphtheroides:** →Table 3

Features	*C. diphtheriae*	Diphtheroids
Morphology		
-Gram stain	Weak gram +Ve	Strong gram +Ve
-Size	Thin	Thick
-Arrangement	Cuneiform	Pallisade
-Granules	Present	Few/absent
-Pleomorphism	More	Little
C/Cs	Growth on enriched media	Growth on ordinary media
Biochemical reaction	Sucrose non ferments	Ferments sucrose
Toxin production	Toxigenic	Nontoxigenic
Virulence test	+Ve	-Ve

Table-3: Differences between *C. diphtheriae* & diphtheroides

❖ Species:

1. ***C. psudodiphthericum:***
- Synonym: *C. hofmannii.*
- Found in throat.
- Biochemically it is urease & pyrazinamidae positive & glucose non fermenters.
- Causes pharyngitis, endocarditis in patient with IDDs.

2. ***C. xerosis:***
- Found in conjunctival sac.
- Biochemically it is pyrazinamidae positive, urease negative & glucose fermenters.

3. ***C. parvum:***
- Used as an immunomodulator.
- It is a mixture of *Propionibacterium* spp.

Arcanobacterium

- Species: *A. haemolyticun.*
- Formerly **called *C. haemolyticum.***
- Produces the β-haemolysis on blood agar.
- Reverse CAMP test positive.
- Causes pharyngitis & skin ulcer.

Question bank

Case study

1) A six year old patient present with complain of throat pain & high grade fever. Clinical examination indicates the cervical lymphadenopathy & pseudomembrane in throat. Throat swab microscopy identifies GPB under gram stain. Identify the organism & answer the following
a) Name the causative agent & describe the morphology of causative agent
b) Describe the pathogenicity of causative agent
c) Write the laboratory diagnosis of causative agent

Essay/Full question

1) *C. diphtheriae*

Short notes

1) Pathogenicity/Lab. diagnosis of *C. diphtheriae.*
2) Virulence test in of *C. diphtheriae.*
3) Elek's gel precipitation test.

Short questions for theory/viva questions

1) Name the four bacteria producing black colonies in PT medium.
2) Write the use of Albert stain. Draw the labelled diagram of appearance of organism under Albert stain.
3) Write the four differences between *C. diphtheriae* & diphtheroides.

MCQs for chapter review

Introduction

1) **Meaning of Corynebacterium**
(a) Club shape (b) Pigment production (c) Leathery pseudomembrane formation (d) Causing diphtheria

C. diphtheriae

2) **Wrong about *C. diphtheriae* -** (AIIMS-95)
(a) Capsulated bacteria causes infection (b) Gram negative (c) Babes Ernst granules are seen (d) Chinese latter pattern (e) Nonmotile
3) **A 12 years child present with fever and cervical lymphadenopathy. Oral examination shows a gray membrane on the right tonsil extending to the anterior pillar. Which of the following medium will be ideal for the culture of the throat swab for a rapid identification of the pathogen-** (AIIMS Nov-02, 99)
(a) Nutrient agar (b) Blood agar (c) Loeffler's serum slope (d) LJ medium
4) **A child present with white patch over the tonsils. Diagnosis is best made by culture in-** (AI-04)
(a Loeffler's medium (b) LJ medium (c) Blood agar (d) Tellurite medium
5) **Daisy head colonies are seen with following strain of *C. diphtheriae* -**
a) Nontoxigenic strain (b) Mitis (c) Intermedius (d) Gravis
6) **True statement about diphtheria toxin is -** (AI-99)
(a) Toxin is phage mediated (b) Toxin is required for local infections (c) Endotoxemia causes systemic manifestation (d) Toxin act by inhibiting synthesis of capsule
7) **Which of the following statement (s) is/are not true about diphtheria toxin -**
(a) Heat stable (b) Toxin production is dependent on iron (c) Inhibit the cAMP (d) All types produce the toxin
8) **True about *Corynebacterium. diphtheriae* is all except-** (AIIMS May-07 & Nov-07)
(a) Deep invasion is not seen (b) Elek's test is done for toxigenicity (c) Metachromatic granules are seen (d) Toxin is mediated by chromosomal change
9) **Positive Schick's test indicates that person is-** (AI-02, AIIMS Nov-07)
(a) Immune to diphtheria (b) Hypersensitive to diphtheria (c) Susceptible to diphtheria (d) Carrier to diphtheria
10) **Drug of choice for diphtheria carrier is-**
(a) Pn (b) Erythromycin (c) Tetracycline (d) Septran

Other pathogenic *Corynebacteria*

11) **Erythrasma is caused by-**
(a) *C. minutissimum* (b) *C. ulcerans* (c) *C. pseudotuberculosis* (b) *C diphtheriae*

Answers of MCQs & explanation

1) **(a)**
- Follow section, **introduction (meaning)** for explanation

2) **(a) & (b)**
- Follow section, ***C. diphtheriae* (morphology)** for explanation

3) **(c)**
- Pathogen is *C. diphtheriae* which grow very rapidly within 6-8 hours in Loeffler's serum slope
- Nutrient agar & blood agar are not useful rapid identification
- LJ is the selective medium for M. tuberculosis

4) **(d)**
- Best diagnosis of any pathogen is made by using the selective medium. For *C. diphtheriae* selective medium is tellurite medium. Loeffler's medium is useful for the rapid diagnosis not for best diagnosis.

5) **(d)**
- C/Cs on PT medium by various biotype of *C. diphtheriae* like gravis, intermedius & mitis is described in **table-1**

6) **(a)**
- Toxin is phage (tox+ phagee or β-phage) mediated
- Toxin does not required for local infections, it is required for systemic manifestation & even non toxigenic strain can cause local lesions in skin & nasopharynx
- Systemic manifestations are due to exotoxemia not due to endotoxemia
- Toxin act by inhibiting the protein synthesis

7) **(a), (c) &(d)**
- Toxin is heat labile
- Toxin production is dependent on iron as mentioned earlier in text
- Toxin does not inhibit the cAMP but inhibiting the protein synthesis
- All types produces the toxin: Partially not correct because all types means toxigenic strain which produces the toxin & nontoxigenic strain which does not produces the toxin, but on a contrary all types means all biotypes, which are produces the toxin

8) **(d)**
- Deep invasion is not seen by bacilli & all systemic manifestations are due to systemic absorption of toxin not due to bacilli itself
- Elek's test is done for toxigenicity detection
- Metachromatic granules are seen in bacilli
- Toxin is mediated by phage not by chromosomal change

9) **(c)**
- Follow section, ***C. diphtheriae* (Schick's test & table-2)** for explanation.

10) **(b)**
- Follow section, ***C. diphtheriae* (treatment)** for explanation.

11) **(a)**
- Follow section, **other pathogenic *Corynebacteria* (*C. minutissimum*)** for explanation.

36 Bacillaceae

(sporing aerobe)

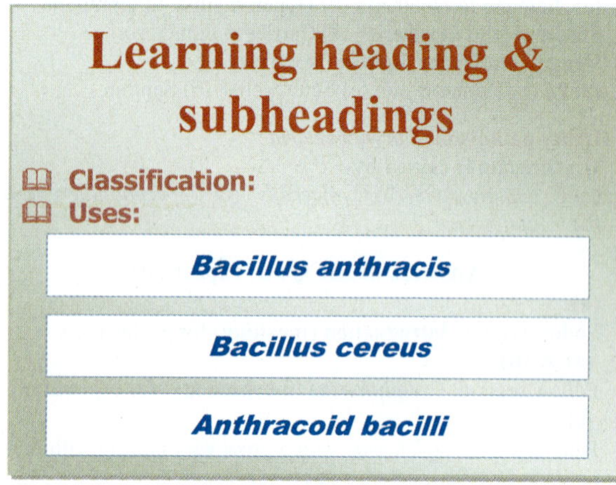

Classification: → Flow chart-1

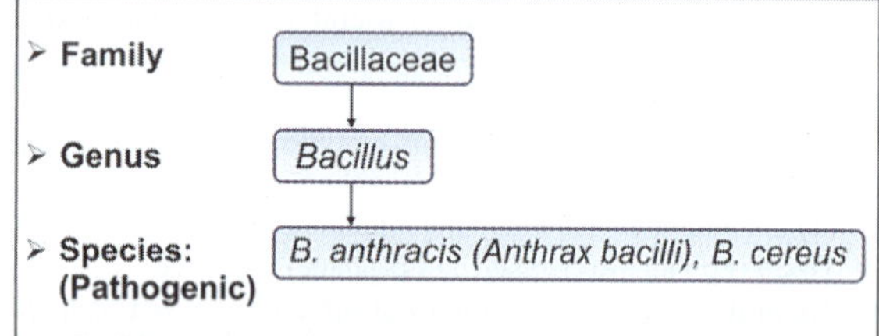

Flow chart-1: Classification of Bacillaceae

Uses:

a. **Bioterrorism:** Endospores of *B. anthrcis* were used for this purpose in USA in 2001. It is a category A (highest priority) pathogen for bioterrorism.

b. **Antibiotics production:**

- Polymyxin B(1940): From *Bacillus polymexa.*
- Colistin (1940): From *Bacillus colistinus.*
- Bacitracin: From *Bacillus subtilis.*
- Tyrothricin: From *Bacillus bravis.*

c. **Genetic model:** *B. subtilis* is used as genetic model for bacterial study.

d. **Insecticide preparation:** Prepared from *B. thuringenesis* to prevent the food crops from disease.

e. **Historical importance:** *B. anthrcis* was the 1st bacterium used to

1 Identify under microscope (by Pollender, 1849).
2 Isolate in pure culture (by Robert Koch, 1876).
3 Prepare 1st live attenuated bacterial vaccine (by Louis Pasteur, 1881).
4 Establish germ theory of disease.
5 Know the blood transmitted infection.

f. **Biological sterilisation controls:**

1 **Hot air oven:** Strip contains spores of *B. subtilis* subsp. *niger.*
2 **Autoclave:** Strip contains spores of *B. (Geobacillus) stearothermophilus.*
3 **Ionising radiation:** *B. pumilis.*
4 **Ethyle oxide:** *Bacillu globigi* or *B. subtilis.*
5 **Plasma sterilisation:** *Bacillus steriothermophilus* & *Bacillus subtilis* subsp. *niger.*

Bacillus anthracis

❖ **Synonym:** *Anthrax bacilli*

❖ **Meaning:** From **Anthrax = coal** because of production of **black scar called eschar.**

❖ **History:** Isolated in pure culture (by Robert Koch, 1876).

❖ **Morphology:**

➢ **Type according to gram stain:** GPB
➢ **Size:** 3–10 μm x 1-1.6 μm.
➢ **Shape:** Slender rod.
➢ **Arrangement:**

- In tissue: In long chain or singly or in pairs.
- In culture: Swollen end giving **"Bamboo-stick" appearance** as shown in **fig.-1.**
- **Motility:** Nonmotile.

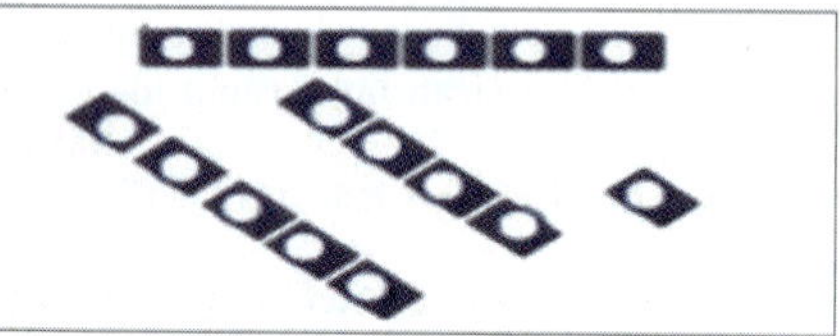

Figure-1: "Bamboo-stick appearance"

➢ **Capsule:** Polypeptide capsule is present which is stained by

- Giemsa stain: Red color.
- Indian ink: Clear halo around the bacilli.
- Polychrome methylene blue: Purplish materials around bacilli **called M'Fadyean (McFadyean) reaction.**

Staining method	Reagents	Spore	Fat globules
Ashby's method	Malachite green	Green spore & red bacilli	Unstained
Burdon's method	Sudan black B	Unstained	Blue-black
Holbrook & Anderson method	Malachite green + Sudan black B	Green spore & red bacilli	Blue-black
Modified acid fast	0.25 % H_2SO_4	Red spore & colourless bacilli	Red

Table-1: Stains to differentiate spores & fat globules

- **Spore:** Central or subterminal, oval or elliptical spore. Same in size of bacillary body (non-bulging).
- **Fat/lipid globules:**
  - It contains lipid + poly metaphosphate (volutin granules) + crystalline protein.
  - Act as an energy store product.
  - Present only in vegetative stage & makes confusion with spores.
- **Stains to differentiate spores & fat globules: → Table-1**
- **Fluorescent microscopy:** Highly sensitive & specific

❖ Cultural characteristics (C/Cs):

- **Effective factors:**
  - O_2 effect: Aerobes and facultative anaerobes.
  - Temperature: 35-37 °C.
  - pH: 7.0- 7.4
  - **Enhancement of capsule production:**
    - In presence of 10-25% CO_2: When media contains biocarbonate **called bicarbonate agar.**
    - In absence of CO_2: When media are enriched with serum, albumin, charcoal or starch.
  - **Enhancement of spore production (sporulation):**
    - Sporulation occurs only in soil, in culture or in products of infected animals like dead tissues or hairs where bacilli turns to spore on air exposure, but never in animal body during life.
    - Medium **called oxalated agar** & sporulation is promoted by adding distilled water & 2% NaCl in to the medium followed by incubation at 25-30°C in presence of O_2.
  - **Inhibition of sporulation:** By Calcium chloride.
- **Culture in media:**

A. Liquid Media: Producing floccular deposit with little or no turbidity.

B. Semi solid media:

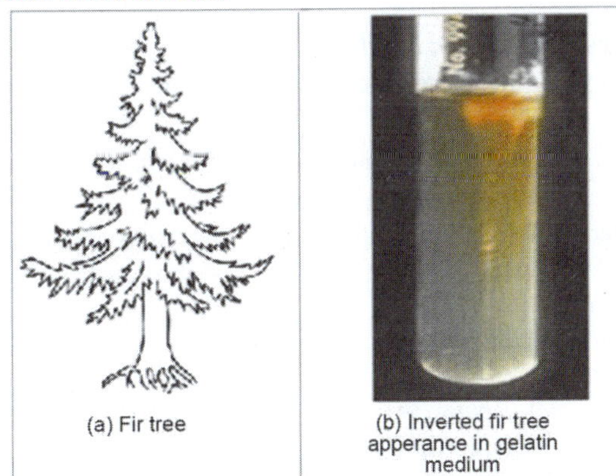

(a) Fir tree
(b) Inverted fir tree apperance in gelatin medium

Figure-2: Inverted free tree appearance

1. **Gelatin medium:** Maximum liquefaction of gelatin occurs at the surface than the bottom which gives **"inverted fir tree" appearance** as shown in **fig.-2.**

C. Solid media:

1. **Nutrient Agar plate:**
   - Colonies are gray-white.
   - Examination of colonies under the low power microscope gives **"frosted glass appearance"** and edge of colony gives **"medusa head appearance"** due to interlacing of bacilli like interlacing of long, curly hair as shown in **fig.-3.**

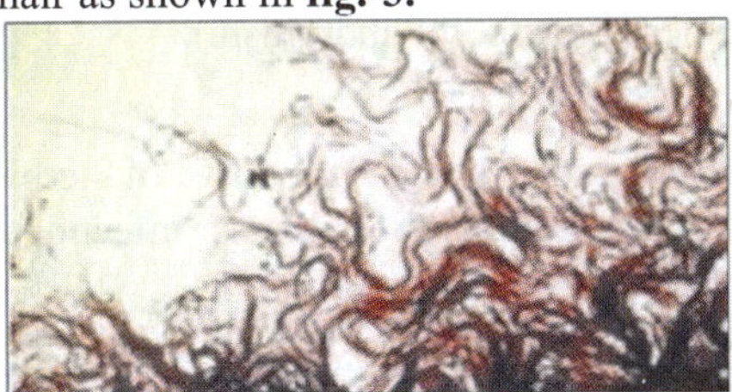

Figure-3: "Medusa head appearance"

2. **Blood agar:** Some strains are haemolytic while some are non-haemolytic.
3. **0.25% Chloral hydrate agar:**
   - Growth of *Anthrax bacilli* is inhibited.
   - Other bacilli like *B. cereus* & *B. mycoides* can grow. Helps to differentiate *Anthrax bacilli* from other bacillus.

D. Selective media:

1. **Penicillin agar:**
   - Solid media with 0.05-0.5 U Pn/ ml (**no growth at 10U Pn /ml**).
   - Bacilli become large, spherical & arranged in chain **called "string of pearl appearance".**
2. **Knisely's PLET medium:** BHIA+ Polymyxin, Lysozyme, EDTA & Thallous acetate.

E. Capsule producing media: → Vide supra

F. Spore producing media: → Vide supra

- **Culture in animal:**
  - Rabbit, guinea pig, mice are sensitive.
  - Subcutaneous injection in guinea pig leads **locally** haemorrhagic oedema & **systemically** enlarged, dark red spleen. Guinea pig dies within 24-72 hrs.

❖ Biochemical reaction s(B/Rs):

1. **Sugar fermentation:** Glucose, sucrose & maltose are fermented with acid production only.
2. **Nitrate reduction test:** + Ve
3. **Catalase test:** + Ve

❖ Resistance:

- Vegetative bacilli are killed by heating at 60°C in 30 minutes.
- Spores are highly resistant to physical agents like heat. Resist dry heat at 140°C for 2-3 hrs & boiling for 10 minutes.
- They are also highly resistant to chemical agents like 5% phenol for weeks & $HgCl_2$.
- **Sporicidal agents:**
  - Agents used to kill the spores are **called sporicidal agents.**

- More details: Follow chapter → Morphology of bacteria (section →spore).

❖ **Molecular typing:** Methods are

➢ **Indication:** For epidemiological studies & strain characterisation.

➢ **Methods:** MLVA (Multi Locus Variable number tandem repeat Analysis) & AFLP (Amplified Fragment Length Polymorphism).

❖ **Pathogenicity:**

➢ **Disease name:** It is a zoonosis of herbivores & human are relatively resistant to infection. Disease **called anthrax.**

➢ **Meaning: Anthrax (Greek) = Coal,** because of formation of characteristic black scar **called eschar**, which looks like coal.

➢ **Nature & history of disease:**

✪ **World:** Rare

✪ **India:** It is enzootic in India. Epizootic of anthrax is common in sheep in Andhra Pradesh-Tamil Nadu border causing many cutaneous & meningo-encephalitis type human infections with high mortality. Few outbreaks noticed in Karnataka & West Bengal.

➢ **Reservoir of infection:** Herbivores animals like sheep, cattle, horses, swine etc. It is more common in herbivores than carnivores.

➢ **Source of infection:**

- Bacilli are discharge in animal products like saliva, nasal secretion, intestinal materials, hide, bone, blood, hairs etc., which sporulate on exposure to air & serve as the source of infection.
- Soil is also the source of infection, which gets contaminated from animal products. Soil is also contaminated by vulture which spread the organism from one area to another after feeding on the anthrax infected carcasses.
- Dried or processed hide of infected animals may harbours the spores for the years which may be serve as the source of infection. Use of shaving brushes made from hair of infected animals also the source of infection.
- LD_{50} (Lethal dose 50): 10,000 spores are required to produce the lethal disease in 50% animals **called LD_{50}.** However sometimes 1-3 spores are enough to produce the disease.

➢ **Mode of transmission: → Table-2**

➢ **Incubation period: → Table-2**

➢ **Portal of entry:** Skin, respiratory tract & GIT.

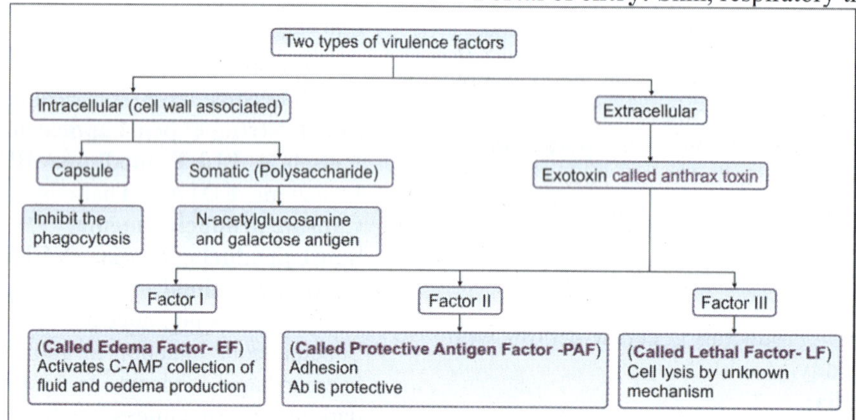

Flow chart-2: Virulence factors of *Anthrax bacilli*

✓ **Note:** Capsule & toxin are plasmid encoded. Removal of such plasmid makes the strain avirulent **called Sterne strain**, which used for vaccine production.

Features	Cutaneous anthrax	Pulmonary anthrax	Intestinal anthrax
Synonym	Hide porters disease	Wool sorter's disease	-
Mode of trans-mission	- By direct contact by carrying hides & skins of infected animals on backs. - Use of shaving brushes made from hair of infected animals. -Mechanically by biting insect like *Stomoxys calcitrans.*	Inhalation of spores of infected wool	Ingestion of poorly cooked meat
IP	1-3 days	1-3 days	2-7 days
Clinical features	- Most common type nowadays. - Painless vesicle skin lesion **called malignant pustules** & healed with black scar **called eschar** surrounded by non pitting indurated oedema.	Haemorrhagic pneumonia	Haemorrhagic diarrhoea
Prognosis	Resolved spontaneously, though 10-20% develops fatal septicemia or meningitis.	100% fatal, though survival is possible with prompt treatment	High mortality

Table-2: Clinical types of anthrax

- **Sites:** Skin (face, neck, hands, arms & back are usually infected) respiratory tract, GIT, blood, meninges etc.
- **Precipitating factors (epidemiological determinants):** Three types

I. Agent factors (virulence factors)

- Follow **flow chart-2**

II. Host factors

1. **Age:** In adults who are industrial workers.
2. **Immunity:** Single attack provides lifelong immunity so second attack is very rare.
3. **Occupations:** Two types like industrial & non-industrial.

- **Industrial:**
  - Cutaneous anthrax is common in dock workers / abattoir workers / slaughter house workers, who are regularly touching the infected meat or carrying loads of hides & skins on their bare back.
  - Pulmonary anthrax is common in workers of wool industry due to inhalation of dust from infected wool.
- **Non-industrial:** Common in persons frequently dealing with animals like butchers, veterinarians, farmers, forest workers etc.

4. **Community:** Common in communities who eat the carcasses of animal dying due to anthrax.

III. Environmental factors

1. **Soil:** More than 70 species of *Bacillus* are found in soil & water. Spores are found in soil, dead animal products or hair of infected animals.

- **Clinical features:**

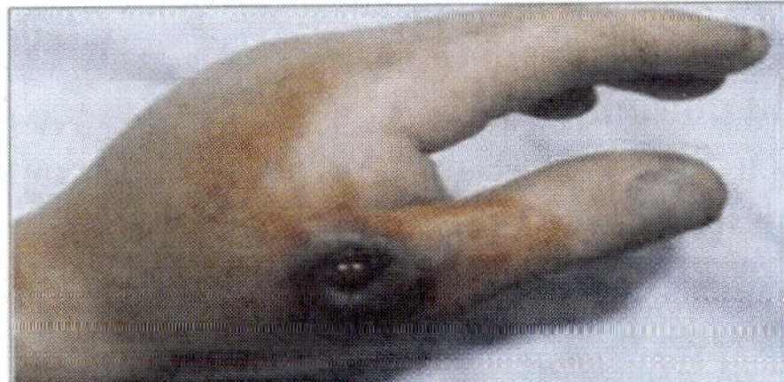

Figure-4: Malignant pustule

i. **Animal infection:**
  - In animals it is transmitted by ingestion of spore from soil. Animal to animal spread occurs very rarely.
  - It is more common in herbivores than carnivores.
  - It causes septicemia & rarely skin lesions. Bacilli are especially present in animal's spleen, which is enlarged & soft, giving rise to fever **called spleenic fever in ox** & German name for the organism is **Milzbrand bazillus (spleen destroying bacillus).**

ii. **Human infection:** Animal acquired the anthrax by ingestion of spores present in soil & but human infection direct from soil spore is query. Three clinical types as shown in **table-2 & fig.-4.**

- **Complications:**
  - Septicemia.
  - Haemorrhagic meningitis.

Laboratory diagnosis:

- **Specimens:**
  - **Human specimens:** Blood, CSF, stool, vomitus, sputum, pus or discharge from pustules.
  - **Animal specimens:** Animal carcass like cut ear piece. Autopsy can't be performed in animal died due to suspected anthrax due to risk of soil contamination.
- **Testing methods:**

I. **Microscopy: → Follow morphology**

II. **Culture: → Follow C/Cs**

III. **Biochemical reaction: → Follow B/Rs**

IV. **Serological tests:**

- **Ag detection:**
  - CFT.
  - Gel diffusion.
  - Haemagglutination.
  - ELISA.
  - Animal inoculation technique: Done by using animal samples. Apply organism over shaven skin of guinea pigs, later organism will enter in tissue by minor abrasion. Ag is detected by **Ascoli's thermo precipitation test from tissues.**
- **Ab detection:** ELISA.

V. **γ – Phage sensitivity:**
  - Spread the *Anthrax bacilli* on BHIA.
  - Inoculate γ – Phage on such plate, Incubate at 37^0C & observe for reaction.
  - Clear area due to lysis of bacilli.

VI. **Molecular method:** PCR.

Prophylaxis:

A. **General measures:**
  - Improvement of factory hygiene.
  - Sterilisation of animal products like hides & wool.
  - Carcasses of animal died due to anthrax are buried deep in quicklime or cremated to prevent soil contamination.

B. **Chemoprophylaxis:** Doxycycline & ciprofloxacin are useful.

C. **Immunoprophylaxis:**

i. **Prepared from vegetative bacilli:**
  - **Called Pasteur's anthrax vaccine.**
  - Prepared by attenuating anthrax bacilli at 42^0C-43^0C. Only historical value.

ii. **Prepared from spores:**
  - **Advantage:** Used for animals & single injection can give protection for a year.
  - **Disadvantage:** Not safe for human use.
  - **Types:**

1. **Sterne vaccine:** Prepared from spore of non-capsulated, avirulent, mutant strain **called Sterne strain**.
2. **Mazzucchi vaccine:** Prepared from spore of stable attenuated Carbazzo strain in 2% saponin.

iii. Alum precipitated toxoid:

- **Advantages:** Safe & effective for human.
- **Preparation:** Prepared from protective Ag of *Anthrax bacilli.*
- **Administration:**
  - Three doses are given by IM route.
  - Six weeks interval between 1st & 2nd dose and six months interval between 2nd & 3rd doses.
  - Booster dose given after a year if necessary.

❖ Treatment:

- Pn is the drug of choice, but resistant strains have been seen.
- Bacilli are susceptible to sulphonamide, erythromycin, doxycycline, ciprofloxacin & chloramphenicol.
- Antibiotic have no role after the toxin production.

Bacillus cereus

❖ Morphology:

- **Type according to gram stain:** GPB
- **Motility:** Motile by peritrichous flagella but some strains are nonmotile.
- **Spore:** Central & non-bulging.
- **Capsule:** Non-capsulated.

❖ Cultural characteristics (C/Cs):

A. Semi solid media: In gelatin medium it produces fast liquefaction in 4-7 days at 20 °C.

B. Solid media:

1. **Nutrient Agar plate:** Colonies are gray-white like *B anthracis* but less membranous consistency.
2. **Blood agar:** Haemolytic.
3. **Egg-yolk agar:** Opacity around colonies indicating lecithinase production.
4. **0.25% Chloral hydrate agar:** Anthrax growth is inhibited but others like *B. cereus* & *B. mycoides* can grow which helps to differentiate *Anthrax bacilli* from other bacillus.

C. Selective media:

1. **Baker's MYPA** (Mannitol-egg Yolk Phenol red polymyxin Agar) **medium:** Showing **clear zone** around **pink colonies** due to lecithinase production & mannitol nonfermentation. Polymyxin is selective agent.
2. **Holbrook & Anderson's PEMBA** (Polymyxin Egg yolk Mannitol Bromothymol blue Agar) **medium:** Showing **clear zone** around **blue colonies** due to lecithinase production & mannitol nonfermentation.

❖ Biochemical reactions(B/Rs):

1. **Sugar fermentation:**

G	S	L	M	Maltose
A	-	-	-	-

❖ Pathogenicity:

- **Virulence factors:** →**Flow chart-3**

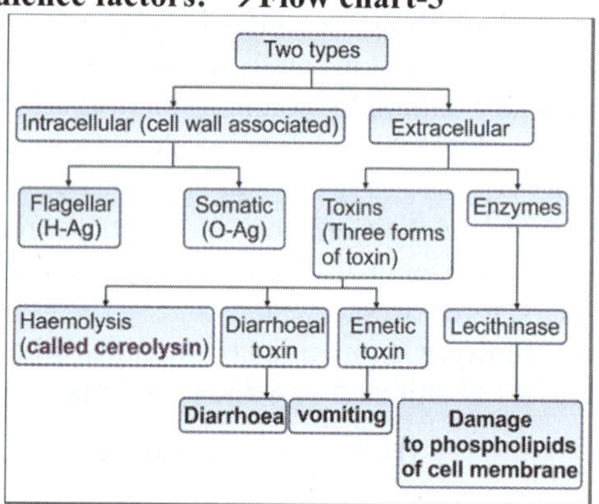

Flow chart-3: Virulence factors of *B. cereus*

- **Clinical features:**

1. **Opportunistic infection:** Septicemia, meningitis, endocarditis, pneumonia, wound & other suppurative infections.
2. **Food poisoning:**
   - When food stored at warm temperature spore will germinate & produce toxin causing food poisoning.
   - Types of food poisoning: Two types of illness like diarrhoeal & emetic are mentioned in **table-3** with differences.

Features	Diarrhoeal illness	Emetic illness
Type of food	Vegetable & cooked meat	Rice (Chinese restaurant)
Incubation period	8-16 hrs after meal	1-5 hrs after meal
Predominant features	Diarrhoea & abdominal pain	Nausea & vomiting
Less features	Nausea, vomiting & fever	Diarrhoea, abdominal pain & no fever (?)
Serotype	2,6,8,9, 10 or 12	1,3 or 5
Bacilli in stool	Less	More
Toxin nature	Heat labile & formed inside the intestine (no preformed or intradietic toxin)	Heat stable & preformed (intradietic)
Mechanism of action of toxin	Activation of C-AMP → Fluid collection in intestine	Unknown
Toxin resembling	Enterotoxin of *E.coli*	Enterotoxin of *Staphylococci*

Table-3: Types of food poisoning of *B. cereus*

Features	*Anthrax bacilli*	*Anthracoid bacilli*
	Morphology	
Arrangement:	Long chain	Short chain
Motility:	Non-motile	Motile by peritrichous flagella
Capsule	Present	Absent
M'fadyean reaction	+Ve	-Ve
	Cultural characteristics (C/Cs)	
Growth at 45°C	No growth	Grow
Liquid media	Floccular deposit	Turbidity
Gelatin medium	Slow liquefaction	Fast liquefaction
Nutrient agar plate	Medusa head colony	Not typical
Blood agar	Weak haemolytic	Strong haemolytic
Penicillin (Pn) agar	No growth at 10U Pn /ml	Growth at 10U Pn /ml
0.25% Chloral hydrate agar	Growth is inhibited	Not inhibited
Animal inoculation	Pathogenic	Non-pathogenic
	Others	
γ – Phage sensitivity	Sensitivity	Not sensitivity
Salicin fermentation	-Ve	+Ve

Table-4: Differences between *Anthracoid bacilli* & *Anthrax bacilli*

❖ **Laboratory diagnosis:**

➤ **Specimens:** Blood, stool, vomitus & food materials.

➤ **Testing methods:**

I. **Microscopy: → Follow morphology**

II. **Culture: → Follow C/Cs**

III. **Biochemical reaction: → Follow B/Rs**

Anthracoid bacilli

❖ **Synonym:** *Pseudoanthrax bacilli*

❖ **Definition:** Contaminants of culture resembling the *Anthrax bacilli* are **called *anthracoid bacilli*.**

❖ **Differences B/W *Anthracoid bacilli* & *Anthrax bacilli*: → Table 4**

Question bank

Case study

1) A female patient with history of malignant pustules with healed black scar admitted in medical ward. Identify the organism & answer the following

a) Name the causative agent & describe the morphology of causative agent

b) Describe the pathogenicity of causative agent

c) Write the lab. diagnosis of causative agent

Essay/Full question

1) *B. anthracis*

Short notes

1) Pathogenicity/Lab. diagnosis of *B. anthracis*

2) *B. cereus*

Short questions for theory/viva questions

1) What is M'Fadyean reaction?

2) Name the four staining methods used to differentiate bacterial spores from fat globules.

3) What are malignant pustules & eschar?

MCQs for chapter review

Bacillus anthracis

1) **Meaning of Anthrax**
(a) Black eschar formation (b) Pseudomembrane formation (c) Susceptibility to γ phage (d) Typical colony characteristic

2) **'Bamboo stick' appearance is characteristic of**
(a) *B. anthracis* (b) *Clostidium spp.* (c) *H. influenzae* (d) *Lactobacilli*

3) **An abattoir worker developed pustule which later progress to necrotic ulcer. Which of the following stain is useful for demonstration of organism from smear made from pustule?** (AI-06 & 07, AIIMS May-12)
(a) Polychrome methylene blue (b) Calcofluor white (c) Giemsa (d) Modified kinyoun stain

4) **A man, after skinning a dead animal, developed pustule on his hand. A smear prepared from the lesion showed the gram positive bacilli in long chain which were positive for McFadyean reaction. The most likely aetiological agent is:** (AI -04)
(a) *Clostridium tetani* (b) *Listeria monicytogenes* (c) *Bacillus anthracis* (d) *Actinomyces* sp

5) **A malignant pustule is a term used for:** (AIIMS -03)
(a) An infected malignant melanoma (b) A carbuncle (c) A rapidly spreading rodent ulcer (d) Anthrax of skin

6) **A malignant pustule is caused by:** (AIIMS Nov-10)
a) *B. anthracis* (b) Leishmaniasis (c) Basal cell carcinoma (d) All

7) **True regarding anthrax is all except-** (AIIMS Dec -97)
(a) Caused by insect bite (b) Caused by rubbing of skin (c) Cutaneous types is rare nowadays (d) Pulmonary infection occurs by inhalation

8) **Which of the following statement is true regarding anthrax:** (PGI-01)
(a) McFadyean reaction shows capsule (b) Human are usually resistant to infections (c) Less than 100 spores can cause pulmonary infection (d) Gram stain shows organism with bulging spores (e) Sputum microscopy helps in diagnosis

9) **True about anthrax:** (PGI June-09)
(a) Causes gram positive bacilli (b) Soil reservoir (c) Spore formation takes place (d) It is more common in carnivores than herbivores (e) Pn is the drug of choice

10) All of the followings are true regarding *Bacillus anthracis* except- (AI -98)
(a) Plasmid is responsible for toxin production (b) Cutaneous anthrax generally resolve spontaneously (c) Capsular polysaccharide aids virulence by inhibiting phagocytosis (d) Toxin is a complex of two fractions

Bacillus cereus

11) Characteristic of *Bacillus cereus* food poisoning is? (AIIMS Nov-10)
(a) Presence of fever (b) Presence of pain in abdomen (c) Absence of vomiting (b) Absence of diarrhoea

Anthacoid bacilli

12) *Anthrax bacilli* differs from *Anthracoid bacilli* by being-
(a) Non-capsulated (b) Strict aerobes (c) Non-motile (d) Haemolytic colonies on blood agar

Answers of MCQs & explanation

1) (a)
- Follow section, ***Bacillus anthracis* (meaning)** for explanation

2) (a)
- Follow section, ***Bacillus anthracis* (morphology)** for explanation

3) (a) & (c)
- It is a case of cutaneous anthrax (hide porters disease), where malignant pustule is the characteristic features & commonly present in abattoir workers (slaughter house workers) due to direct contact with infected meat or carrying the infected skin on back. Organism is *Bacillus anthracis* which is capsulated in nature & stains useful to demonstrate the capsule are explained in text under the section of morphology.
- Calcofluor white: Fluorescent stain for fungus
- Modified kinyoun stain: Useful for *M. tuberculosis*

4) (c)
- It is a case of cutaneous anthrax (hide porters disease), where malignant pustule is the characteristic features & commonly present in abattoir workers (slaughter house workers) due to direct contact with infected meat or carrying the infected skin on back. Organism is *Bacillus anthracis* which is gram positive bacilli, arranged in long chain in tissue & capsulated. Capsule appears as Purplish materials around bacilli under Polychrome methylene blue **called M'Fadyean reaction.**

5) (d)
6) (a)
7) (c)
} Follow section, ***Bacillus anthracis* (pathogenicity & table-2)** for explanation

8) (a), (b), (c) & (e)
- Option a: Follow section, ***Bacillus anthracis* (morphology)** for explanation
- Option b: Anthrax is a zoonosis & human are relatively resistant to infection
- Option c: Follow section, ***Bacillus anthracis* [pathogenicity → source of infection** (LD_{50})] for explanation
- Option d: Bacilli contain spores, but it is equal to the breadth of bacillary body so there is nobulging. Bulging spores is a feature of *Clostridium* spp.
- Option e: Sputum microscopy helps in diagnosis of pulmonary anthrax

9) (a), (c) & (e)
- Soil is the source, not the reservoir
- Anthrax is more common in herbivores than carnivores

10) (a), (b) & (c)
- Capsule & toxin are plasmid encoded. Removal of such plasmid makes the strain avirulent **called Sterne strain**, which used for vaccine production.
- Resolved spontaneously, though 10-20% develop fatal septicemia or meningitis
- Capsular polysaccharide aids virulence by inhibiting phagocytosis
- Toxin is a complex of not two but three fractions

11) (b)
- Follow section, ***Bacillus cereus* (pathogenicity → clinical features & table-3)** for explanation.

12) (c)
- Follow section, ***Anthacoid bacilli* (table-4)** for explanation.

37 Clostridium

(sporing anaerobe)

Learning heading & subheadings

- Meaning:
- Uses:
- Classification:
  - *Cl. perfringens*
  - *Cl. tetani*
  - *Cl. bitulinum*
  - *Cl. difficicile*
  - Other *Clostridium* spp.
    - *Clostridium septicum*
    - *Clostridium novyi*
    - *Clostridium histolyticum*
    - *Clostridium tertium*

Meaning: Word derived from **Kloster =Spindle,** because containing spore larger than the bacillary body & giving bacilli **a spindle shape appearance.**

Uses:

1. **Chemical production:** Used for production chemicals like acetone & butanol from *Cl. acetobutyricum.*
2. **Biological control:** Spores of non toxigenic strain of *Cl tetani* are employed as biological indicator for hot air oven.
3. **Decomposition:** *Cl. perfringens* & *Cl. tetani* are the intestinal flora in human & animals. They invade the blood & tissues after death to initiate the decomposition of body.
4. **Bioterrorism:** *Cl. botulinum* is used as category A (highest priority) pathogen for bioterrorism.
5. **Therapeutic:** Intramuscular injection of type A toxin of *Cl. botulinum* was 1st used for strabismus, is now recognised as safe & effective for many neuromuscular diseases as shown in **table-1.**

Muscular diseases	Plastic surgery
- Myoclonus - Palatal myoclonus - Focal dystonias - Fascial spasm - Painful muscle spasm - Tremor - Parkinson's progressive supranuclear palsy	- Masseter hypertrophy - Facial asymmetry (post Bells) - Wrinkles - Muscles flap paralysis during healing
Ophthalmic diseases	**ENT diseases**
- Strabismus - Lower lid entropion - Acquired nystagmus - Hyperlacrimation - Thyroid ophthalmology	- Stittering - Vocal cord polyps - Hypersalivation
Genitourinary diseases	**GIT diseases**
- Detrusor sphincter dyssynergia - Vaginismus	- Achalasia - Cricopharyngeal spasm - Rectal fissure
Rehabilitation	
Painful muscle spasm, tympanomandibular related muscle spasm & focal myofascial pain	

Table-1: Therapeutic uses of botulinum

Classification:

I. Morphological classification:

A. According (A/C) to spore shape & location: Follow chapter → Morphology of bacteria

B. A/C to motility:

1. **Non-motile:** *Cl. perfringens* & *Cl. tetani* type VI.
2. **Motile by peritrichous flagella:** Others are motile.

C. A/C to capsules properties:

1. **Capsulated:** *Cl. perfringens* & *Cl. butyricum.*
2. **Non- capsulated:** All others are non-capsulated.

II. According to morphological & biochemical nature: →**Table-2**

III. According to existence:

A Always present: *Cl. sporogenes.*

B Rarely present: *Cl. perfringens.*

IV. According to O_2 effect:

1. **Strict anaerobes:** *Cl. botulinum, Cl. tetani* & *Cl. novyi.*
2. **Aerotolerant:** *Cl. histolyticum.*
3. **Microaerophilic:** *Cl. perfringens.*

Spore	Both P & S		Either P or S		Neither P nor S
	Predominant P	Predominant S	Slightly P	Slightly S	
Central or Subterminal	*Cl. bifermentans* *Cl. botulinum* A, B & F *Cl. sporogenes* *Cl. histolyticum*	*Cl. perfringens* *Cl. septicum* *Cl. novyi*	-	*Cl. fallax* *Cl. botulinum* C, D & E	-
Terminal -oval	-	*Cl. difficle*	-	*Cl. tertium*	*Cl. cochlearum*
Terminal-spherical	-	-	*Cl. tetani*	*Cl.tetanomorphum*	-

Table-2: Morphological & biochemical classification of *Clostridium*

P=Proteolytic → turns meat in black colour with foul smelling, **S** = Saccharolytic →turns meat in pink colour

V. Clinical:

A. Gas gangrene:

1. **Established pathogen:** *Cl. perfrigens, Cl. septicum* & *Cl. novyi.*
2. **Less pathogenic:** *Cl. histolyticum* & *Cl. fallax.*
3. **Doubtful pathogen:** *Cl. bifermentans* & *Cl. sporogenes.*

B. Food poisoning:

1. **Gastroenteritis:** *Cl. perfrigens* type A.
2. **Necrotising enteritis:** *Cl. perfrigens* type C.
3. **Botulism:** *Cl. botulinum.*

C. Tetanus: *Cl. tetani.*

D. Acute colitis: *Cl. difficile.*

✓ **Note:** Spores of *Anthrax bacilli* are never formed in animal body during life, while of *Clostridium* spp. developed in animal body during life.

Cl. perfringens

❖ History & synonyms:

- *Cl. welchii:* 1st isolated & described by Welch & Nuttall in 1892 from the blood & organs of cadaver.
- Bacillus aerogenes capsulatus.
- Bacillus phlegmonis emphysematosa.

❖ Morphology: →Fig. 1

- **Type according to gram stain:** GPB.
- **Size:** 4-6µm × 1µm.

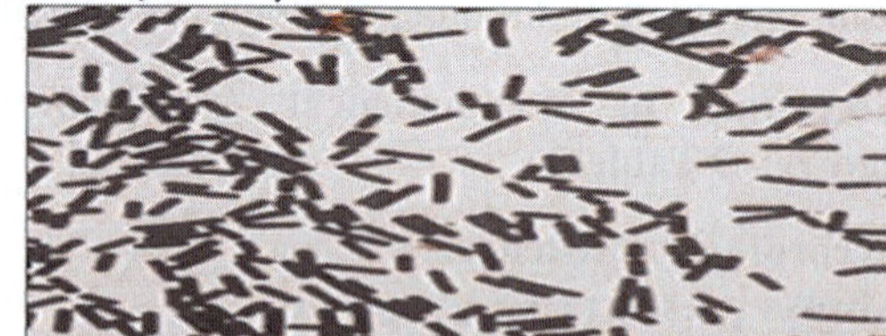

Figure-1: *Cl. welchii* under Gram stain

- **Shape:** Elongated, straight rod with rounded or truncated ends **called boxcar appearance.** (Boxcar = railway wagon with sliding doors on sides).
- **Arrangement:** Singly or in chains or in small bundles.
- **Spores:** Sub-terminal but rarely seen in culture / tissues which is the characteristic feature of bacilli.
- **Motility:** Non-motile.
- **Capsule:** Capsulated.
- It is pleomorphic, filamentous and showing involution form.

❖ Cultural characteristics (C/Cs):

- **Effective factors:**
  - O_2 effect: Strict anaerobe & microaerophilic.
  - Optimum temperature: 45°C (20–50°C).
  - pH: 5.5-8.0.
  - Generation time: 10 minutes (utilized to obtain pure culture).
  - Bacilli present in intestine so isolation from the faeces except in large number is not significant. Isolation from the food is meaningful.
- **Culture in media:**

A. Robertson's Cooked Meat Medium (RCMM): It grows rapidly and the meat turns pink due to saccharolytic properties. Sub culture from this will yield pure growth.

B. Blood agar: Produce narrow zone of complete haemolysis by α toxins & a much wider zone of incomplete haemolysis by α toxin **called target haemolysis.**

C. Selective medium: Blood agar with neomycin.

D. Spore producing media:

1. Phillips medium.
2. Ellner's medium.
3. Duncan & Strong's medium.
4. Alkaline egg medium.

- **Culture in animals:** Guinea pig is used for detection of virulence & typing.

❖ Biochemical reaction (B/Rs):

1. **Predominant saccharolytic & slightly proteolytic**
2. **Sugar fermentation:** It ferments glucose, sucrose, lactose & maltose with production of acid & gas.
3. **Stormy fermentation (litmus milk test):**
   - Test performed in litmus milk medium.
   - Lactose fermented with acid & gas production.
   - Acid change litmus from blue to red & coagulates. the casein **(acid clot).**
   - Gas will disrupt the clotted milk.
   - Paraffin plug is pushed up and shreds of clot are seen sticking to sides of the tube **called "stormy fermentation".**
4. **I M Vi C tests:** - + - -

5. **Nitrate reduction:** + Ve
6. **H_2S test:** + Ve
7. **Nagler reaction (Nagler effect):**

- **Introduction:** Nagler reaction occurs due to α-toxin, which has following features.
  - Produced by all types of *Cl. perfringens* **(predominantly by type A).**
  - It is a lecithinase C (phospholipidase) which split lecithin in to phosphoryl choline & diglyceride in presence of Ca^{+2} & Mg^{+2}. This reaction is seen in egg yolk or serum media & specifically neutralised by antitoxin.
  - Responsible for profound toxemia of gas gangrene.
  - Lethal & dermonecrotic.
  - Haemolytic (**hot-cold variety**) in most species because of presence of phospholipids on RBC cell wall.
  - Relatively heat stable.
- **Principle:** In-vitro toxin- antitoxin neutralization test.
- **Medium:**
  - Agar medium with 6 % agar + 5% fildes peptic digest sheep blood + 20% human serum + antitoxin spread on half of plate.
  - 20% human serum will be replaced by 5% egg yolk.
  - Add neomycin to makes the medium selective which inhibit coliforms (lactose fermenters) & aerobic spore bearers.
- **Method:** Test bacteria are inoculated in whole medium with antitoxin in 1 half. Incubate the plate at 37°C for 24 hrs.
- **Result (fig.-2):** Clear haloes around colonies in area without antitoxins due to lecithinase activity of toxin & no haloes around colonies in area with antitoxin due to neutralisation of alpha toxin.

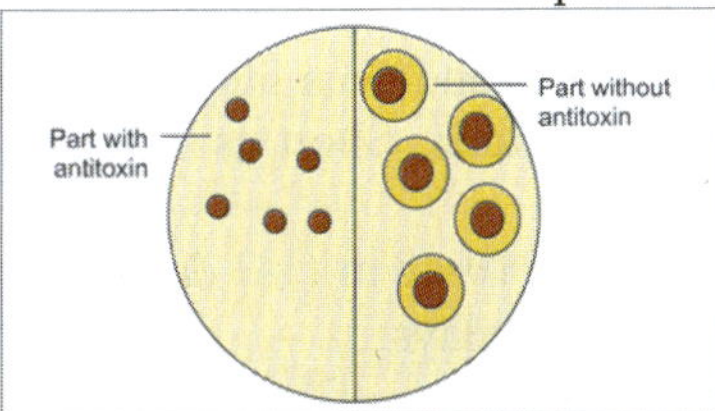

Figure-2: Nagler reaction

- **Use:** For rapid detection of *Cl. welchii.*
- **Interpretation:** +Ve reactions by other bacteria like *Cl novyi, Cl bifermentans*, *Vibrio* & aerobic spore bearers.

8. **Reverse CAMP test:**

- **Meaning:**
  - Original CAMP test is used to detect the CAMP factor produced by *Strept agalactiae* by using *Staph aureus.*
  - The test is **called reverse CAMP test** because CAMP factor produced by *S. agalactiae* is used for the detection of α-toxin of *Clostridium perfringens* from other *Clostridium* species.
- **History:** Hansen developed the test by using the synergistic relationship between the two microbes.
- **Principle:** It based on synergistic relationship between the two microbes. Enhancement of haemolysis by α-toxin of *Clostridium perfringens* with synergistic action by CAMP factor of *Strept agalactiae* (Group B *Streptococcus*).
- **Method:**
  - A CAMP positive *Strept agalactiae* is streaked in the centre of sheep blood agar.
  - Streak the *Clostridium perfringens* at right angle to it without touching.
  - Incubation the plate at 37°C for 24-48 hours in anaerobic conditions.
- **Result:** "Bow-tie" zone of enhanced haemolysis **(fig. 3)** pointing towards *Streptococcus agalactiae* is seen. This is because of alpha toxin produced by Clostridium perfringens interacts with CAMP factor and produce synergistic haemolysis.
- **Bacteria giving reverse CAMP test positive:**
  - *Cl. welchii.*
  - *C. pseudotuberculosis.*
  - *A haemolyticum.*
  - *Listeria monocytogenes.*

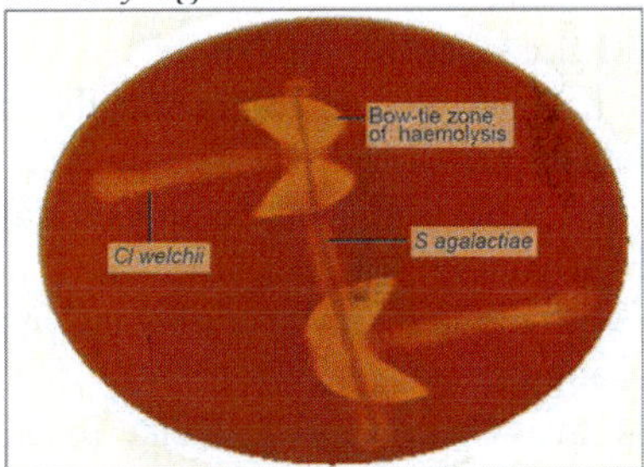

Figure-3: Reverse CAMP test

Resistance:

- Spores of gas gangrene causing strains of *Cl. perfringens* specially type A, are inactivated by boiling in few minutes while spores of food causing strains of *Cl. perfringens* are heat resistant & can survive boiling for few hours.
- Spores are sensitive to different physical & chemical agents **called sporicidal agents,** as described in chapter → **Morphology of bacteria** (section → spore).

Typing:

- Based on **in-vivo** toxin- antitoxin neutralization test.
- Typing is done by intracutaneous injection in guinea pigs or intravenous in mice.
- Five types like A, B, C, D & E.

Pathogenicity:

- **Disease name:** Causing different disease like gas gangrene, food poisoning etc., as described below.
- **Reservoir of infection:** *Cl. perfringens* (Type A is predominant) is a normal flora of large intestine of

human & animal. It is found in feces and it contaminates the skin of perineum, buttock and thigh via faeces. The spores commonly found in soil, dust & air.

- **Source of infection:** Spores are present in faeces of human & animals, soil, dust, clothes & hospital articles which serve as source of infection.
- **Mode of transmission:**
- **Incubation period:**
- **Portal of entry:**
- **Sites:**

(Mode of transmission, Incubation period, Portal of entry, Sites:) Different in gas gangrene & food poisoning, described below in respective sections

- **Precipitating factors (epidemiological determinants):** Three types

I. Agent factors (virulence factors)

Cl. perfringens is invasive; it can spread in tissues & produces following type virulence factors.

1. **Toxin:** 12 distinct toxins.

✪ **Major toxins:**

- **Alpha (phospholipase / lecithinase C): → Vide supra in Nagler rection**
- **Others are Beta, Epsilon and Iota:** Are lethal, necrotising & increasing the capillary permeability.

✪ **Minor toxins:**

- **Theta (Like streptolysin O):**
  - It is haemolytic & antigenically related to **streptolysin O.**
  - It is a thiol activated cytolysin also **called perfringolysin O.**
  - Along with alpha toxin theta play an important role in gas gangrene.
- **Others are** Gamma, **Eta,** Delta (haemolytic for RBCs of sheep, goat & pig), Kappa (collagenase), Lambda (proteinase & gelatinase), Mu (hyaluronidase) & Nu (deoxyribonuclease).

2. **Enzymes:** Neuraminidase, fibrinolysin & hyaluronidase (break the intracellular cement substances & allow the spread of infection).
3. **Biological active substances:**
   - Haemagglutinin.
   - Haemolysin: Different from alpha, theta & delta.
   - Histamine.
   - Circulating factor.
   - Bursting factor: Responsible for muscles damage.

II. Host factors

1. **Road accidents:** Injury involving crushing of large muscles.
2. **War:** Extensive wound with heavy contamination.
3. **Surgery:** Especially amputation for vascular disease.

III. Environmental factors

1. **Distribution of spores:** They are present in soil, dust, clothes & hospital articles.

- **Diseases:**

A. Gas gangrene:

✪ **Synonym:** Malignant oedema, anaerobic myositis, clostridial myonecrosis & clostridial myositis.

✪ **Definition (fig.-4):** Rapidly spreading, edematous, myonecrosis occurs due to severe contamination of wound especially by *Cl. perfringens* **called gas gangrene.**

✪ **History:** It was defined by Oakley in 1954.

✪ **Bacteriology:** Gas gangrene rarely occurs by single bacterium. It is a co-infection of *Clostridia* with other bacteria.

- **Clostridial species:** *Cl. perfringens* most frequent cause (responsible for 60-80% cases of gas gangrene) followed by *Cl. novyi* & *Cl. septicum* (20-40% cases of gas gangrene by both) & less often by *Cl. histolyticum, Cl. sporogenes, Cl. fallax & Cl. bifermentans.*
- **Other bacteria:** *Staphylococci*, anaerobic *Streptococci*, *E. coli*, *Proteus* spp. etc.

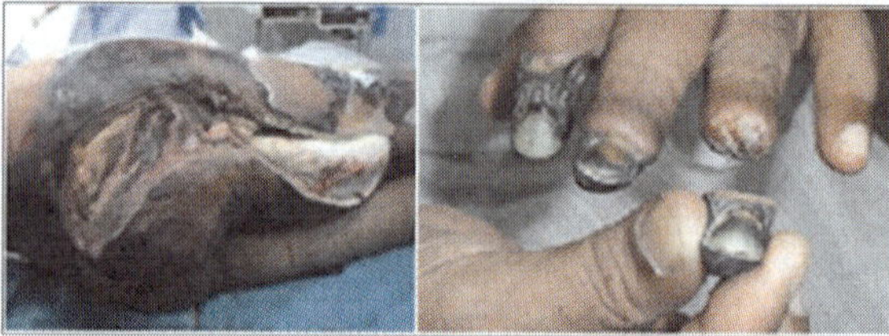

Figure-4: Gas gangrene in different sites

✪ **Mode of transmission:**

- **Endogenous:** From contaminated skin of perineum, buttock & thighs via faeces.
- **Exogenous:**
  - By contamination of wound through soil, road dust, bits of clothing. Gas gangrene may occasionally follow clean surgical procedures (amputation for vascular disease) and even injections (adrenalin).

✪ **Incubation period:** Short as 7 hr or long up to 6 weeks.

- *Cl. perfringens*: 10-48 hr (1-2 days).
- *Cl. septicum*: 2-3 days.
- *Cl. novyi*: 5-6 days.

✪ **Portal of entry:** Wounded skin.

✪ **Sites:** Muscles & other soft tissues.

✪ **Pathogenesis:** Condition that produce low oxygen tension will favour the disease.

- Ca^{+2} & silicic acid in the soil allow multiplication of *Clostridia* & causing necrosis.
- α- toxin (Phospholipidase) damages the phospholipids of cell membrane and increase permeability leading to extravasations of blood and increased tension on vessels & affected muscles which reduce the blood supply & causing further anoxic damage.
- α- toxin (phospholipidase) damages the phospholipids of cell membrane in RBC causing

hemolytic anemia & extravasated haemoglobin & myohaemoglobinemia cease to act as an O_2 carrier.

- Abundant production of gas reduces the blood supply by pressure effect, causing further anoxic damage.
- Reduction of Eh (oxidation – reduction potential) & pH allow further proliferation of bacteria.
- Break down of carbohydrate and liberation of amino acids from protein provide ideal platform for proliferation of anaerobes.
- Collagenase breaks the collagen fiber & hyaluronidase breaks the intercellular substance, helps *Clostridia* to spread further.

✪ **Clinical types given by MacLenan:**

i. Simple contamination of wound:

- Small numbers of bacteria with low virulence.
- Do not invade underlying tissue but causing delayed wound healing.

ii. Anaerobic cellulitis:

- Invade fascia but not the muscle tissue.
- Toxin production is minimal.
- Limited gas production & good prognosis.

iii. Gas gangrene: Invades the healthy muscle tissue and abundant toxin production.

✪ **Clinical features:**

i. Local:

- Swelling & oedema of infected area.
- Pain & tenderness.
- Crepitation due to gas collection.
- Foul smelling & watery discharge.
- Rapidly spreading necrosis.

ii. General:

- High grade fever
- Toxaemia
- Prostration

✪ **Complications:** Shock & death due to circulatory failure.

✪ **Laboratory diagnosis of gas gangrene:** Diagnosis based on clinical parameters & laboratory help required for confirmation.

- **Specimens:**
  - Direct smear preparation from edge of muscle.
  - Exudates/pus/ discharge collected by swab/ capillary pipette.
  - Necrotic tissue and muscle fragments.
- **Transportation:** All samples collected & transported in RCMM / thioglycollate broth.
- **Testing methods:**

i. Microscopy: By Gram stain

- *Cl. perfringens*: Follow morphology
- *Cl. novyi:* Large bacilli, oval subterminal spore
- *Cl. septicum*: Citron bodies & Leaf-boat shape bacilli, central/subterminal spore

ii. Culture: Follow C/Cs

iii. Biochemical reaction: Follow B/Rs

iv. Physiological method: By Gas Liquid Chromatography (GLC).

✪ **Prophylaxis of gas gangrene:**

1. **General measures:** Keeping the wound clean.
2. **Surgery:** Removal of necrosed tissue, blood clots & foreign materials from wound.
3. **Chemoprophylaxis:** Metronidazole, gentamicin & amoxicillin are useful.
4. **Immunoprophylaxis:** Anti Gas gangrene Serum (AGS) contain equine polyvalent antitoxin in a dose of 10,000IU for *Cl. perfringens*, 10,000IU for *Cl. novyi* and 5, 000 IU for *Cl. septicum* given IM (in emergencies IV) used for prophylaxis.

✪ **Treatment of gas gangrene:**

1. **Surgery:** Excision of all affected parts (**amputation**) with antibiotics cover is life saving.
2. **Hyperbaric O2:** It also beneficial in treatment.
3. **Antibiotics:** Metronidazole, gentamicin & amoxicillin are useful.
4. **Passive immunisation with AGS (anti gas gangrene serum):** It has not yields any useful result, so it is not advised. AGS contains *Cl. perfringens* (10, 000 IU), *Cl. septicum* (10, 000 IU) & *Cl. novyi* (5, 000 IU) & given by IM / IV.

B. Food poisoning: By enterotoxin production.

✪ **Properties of enterotoxin:**

- Produce by some strains of type A.
- Heat labile.
- Similar to enterotoxin of *ETEC* & *V. cholerae* leads to fluid accumulation in the rabbit ileal loop.
- Food poisoning strains also producing the alpha & theta toxins.

✪ **Mechanism of action of enterotoxin:** Activation of C-AMP → collection of fluid in intestine.

✪ **Mode of transmission:**

- By ingestion of contaminated meat (like beef & poultry meat) & legumes.
- When contaminated meat is cooked, spores in interior may survive. During storage or warming they germinate & multiply in anaerobic condition.
- Large numbers of *Clostridia* thus consumed, pass unharmed by gastric acid due to high protein in meal & reach intestines where they produce toxin. (no preformed or intra-dietic toxin).

✪ **Incubation period:** 8-24 hours.

✪ **Portal of entry:** GIT.

✪ **Sites:** GIT.

✪ **Clinical features:** Abdominal pain/cramps, diarrhoea & vomiting. These features are self-limited & recover in 24-48 hrs.

✪ **Laboratory diagnosis of food poisoning:**

- **Specimens:** Stool & suspected food particles.
- **Transportation:** All samples collected & transported in RCMM/ Thioglycollate broth.
- **Testing methods:**

i. Microscopy: Gram stain → Follow morphology

ii. **Culture:** → Follow C/Cs
iii. **Biochemical reaction:** Follow B/Rs

C. **Necrotising enteritis or enteritis necroticans or pigbel:**
- Due to ingestion of pig meat with trypsin inhibitor like sweet potatoes. It occurs in susceptible host having limited proteolytic activity.
- It occurs due to beta toxin produced by Type C of *Cl. perfringens.*
- Source of organism is patient own intestinal flora.
- It present with intestinal features.

D. **Gangrenous appendicitis:**
E. **Gas gangrene of abdominal wall:** Endogenous origin from intestine during abdominal surgery.
F. **Biliary tract infection:** Two types are reported
- Acute emphysematous cholecystitis.
- Post cholecystectomy septicemia.

G. **Urogenital infection:** Following nephrectomy or septic abortion.
H. **Thoracic infection:** More in war due to thoracic injuries.
I. **Panophthalmitis:** Following penetrating injury of eyes.
J. **Brain abscess and meningitis:**
K. **Septicemia and endocarditis:**

Cl. tetani

❖ **Synonym:** Nicolaier's bacillus, who 1st discovered the tetanus toxin.

❖ **History:** Bacilli were 1st isolated by Kitasato Shibasaburō in 1889 in pure culture & reproduced the disease in animals by inoculation of pure culture. He also noticed that toxin could be neutralized by specific antibodies.

❖ **Morphology:** →**Fig. 5**
- **Type according to gram stain:** Strong **GPB** in young culture but old culture gives gram variable staining & probably **GNB.**
- **Size:** 0.5 µm x 4–8 µm.
- **Shape:** Slender rod, straight axis, parallel sides and rounded ends.
- **Arrangement:** Singly or chains.
- **Capsule:** Noncapsulated.
- **Motile:** By peritrichate flagella except *Cl. tetani* type VI.
- **Spores:** Terminal & spherical giving **drumstick appearance &fig.-5**).

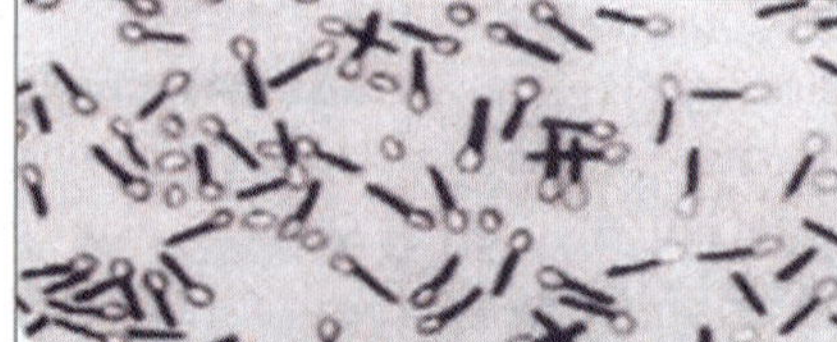

Figure-5: ***Cl. tetani*** **under Gram stain**

❖ **Cultural characteristics (C/Cs):**
- **Effective factors:**
  - O_2 effect: Strict anaerobe.
  - Optimum temperature: 37°C.
  - pH: 7.4
  - Grow on ordinary media & enriched media contains blood or serum but not glucose.
- **Culture in media:**

✪ **Swarming growth:** Occurs in moist media & interfere with isolation of pure culture.

✪ **Fildes' technique:**
- It overcome the disadvantage of swarming growth & helps to isolate the bacilli in pure culture.
- Water of condensation at bottom of slope of nutrient agar is inoculated with mixed cell culture, after anaerobic incubation for 24 hours, subcultures from top of tube yield pure growth of tetanus bacillus.

A. **Liquid media:**
1. **Thioglycollate broth:** Turbidity in the bottom.
2. **RCMM:**
- Gas production & turbidity. Meat turned black on prolonged incubation due to slightly proteolytic activity.
- Three RCMM bottles are used:
  1st bottle: Heated at 80 °c for 15 min.
  2nd bottle: Heated at 80 °c for 5 min. and
  3rd bottle: Left unheated.
- Purpose of heating is to kill vegetative forms & leaving the spores undamaged.
- Incubated at 37°c for 24-48 hr.
- Subculture on blood agar daily upto 4 days and observed for growth.

B. **Semi-solid media: Gelatin stab culture** → Fir-tree growth with slow liquefaction.

C. **Solid media:**
1. **Blood agar:**
- Initialy **α haemolysis (incomplete)** followed by **β (complete)** due to production of haemolysin (**tetanolysin**).
- Produce swarming growth on opposite half of plate after 1-2 dys anaerobic incubation.

2. **Mac Conkey's medium:** Green flourescence is produced.

D. **Selective media:** Blood agar + polymyxin B.
- **Culture in animals:** Widely described below in lab. diagnosis under the heading of toxigenicity testing (in vivo).

❖ **Biochemical reaction (B/Rs):**
1. **No saccharolytic, but slightly proteolytic**
2. **Not ferments any sugar**
3. **I M Vi C tests:** + - - -
4. **Nitrate reduction:** - Ve
5. **H_2S test:** -Ve

❖ **Resistance:**

- Spores of some strains of *Cl. tetani* are destroyed by boiling in 5 minutes while spores of few strains are heat resistant & can survive boiling for 15-90 minutes. Spores can survive in soil (dry earth) for several years.
- They resist killing by 5% phenol or o.1% mercury chloride.
- Spores are sensitive to different physical & chemical agents **called sporicidal agents,** as described in chapter → **Morphology of bacteria** (section → spore).

❖ Classification:

- Based on flagellar (H) Ag, it is classified into 1-10 serotypes by agglutination reaction.
- Type 6 is non flagellar strain.
- All the types produce the same toxin which is neutralised by antitoxin of other type.

❖ Pathogenicity:

➢ **Disease name: Called tetanus.** Tetanus is toxaemia occurs due to powerful neurotoxin (exotoxin) **called tetanospasmin.**

➢ **Definition**: Tonic muscular spasm which is initially local followed by whole of the somatic muscular system.

➢ **Nature & history of disease:** Tetanus is known from the time of Hippocrates & Aretaeus.

➢ **Reservoir & source of infection:** Spores are ubiquitous, present in soil, intestine of human-animals (mainly herbivorous), hospital environment, plaster of paris, bandage, cotton, catgut, talc granules, cloths, stitch materials, syringe & needles. All these serve as reservoir & source of infection.

➢ **Mode of transmission:**

- **Spores are transmitted by:**
  - Injury.
  - Suppurative infection e.g. otitis media.
  - Unsterile injection.
  - Septic abortion.
  - Unhygienic practices like application of cow dung, soil or ashes on the umbilical stump.
  - Rituals such as ear boring or circumcision.
- **Not transmitted:** From person to person.
- **Spores are destroyed** by phagocytes & harmless in contaminated wound.
- **Germination & toxin production:** Occurs in favourable conditions like
  - Reduced Eh potential.
  - Co- infection by anaerobes.
  - Necrosed & devitalized tissues.
  - Presence of foreign body.

➢ **Incubation period:** It is 6-12 days; however it may be short as 1 day & long as a month. It is influenced by

- Site & nature of wound.
- Immune status of patient.
- Dose and toxigenicity of contaminating organism.

➢ **Portal of entry:** Wounded skin or tissues.

➢ **Sites:** Toxin targets muscles by pre-syneptic action.

➢ **Precipitating factors (epidemiological determinants):** Three types

I. Agent factors (virulence factors)

Cl. tetani is little invasive, remain at the site of lodgment & produces two type powerful exotoxins as follows.

1. **Tetanolysin (haemolysin):**
   - Heat labile & oxygen labile.
   - Antigenically related haemolysin produce by *Cl. perfringens, Cl. novyi* & *S. pyogenes.*
   - Not relevant in pathogenesis.
2. **Tetanospasmin (neurotoxin)**

- **History:** Arthur Nicolaier isolated the tetanus toxin from free-living, anaerobic soil bacteria in 1884.
- **Properties:**
  - Heat labile & oxygen stable.
  - Two chains: H-chain (MW 93, 000) & L- chain (MW 52, 000) joined by disulphide bond.
  - Change to toxoid by treatment with low concentrations of formaldehyde.
  - Plasmid coded.
  - Good antigenic & neutralised by specific antitoxin.
  - Purified toxin is active in extremely small amounts.
  - MLD is different in different species. For human MLD is 130 nanogram.
- **Effective factors over toxicity:** Influenced by route of administration.
  - Orally: Destroyed by digestive enzymes, so not effect.
  - Subcutaneous, intramuscular and intravenous injections: Equally effective.
  - Intraneural injections: More lethal.
  - Injections directly into CNS: Very much more lethal.
- **Site of action:** Strychnine like action but acts pre-syneptically while strychnine acts post-syneptically.

✓ **Note: Examples of neurotoxins**

- Enterotoxin of *Staph aureus.*
- Tetanospasmin from *Cl tetani.*
- Botulinum from *Cl botulinum.*
- Shigal like toxin: (Having cytotoxic, enterotoxic & neurotoxic properties) from *E. coli* & *V. cholerae.*
- Shiga (having cytotoxic, enterotoxic & neurotoxic properties) toxin from *Shigella* spp.

II. Host factors

1. **Age:**
   - Tetanus is the disease of 5-15 years of age, which is most vulnerable for trauma.

- Neonatal tetanus is common with unhygienic practices like application of cow dung, soil or ashes on the umbilical stump.

2. **Sex:**
- Men are more susceptible to tetanus toxin than women.
- In wcmen it is common due to septic abortion of delivery, **called uterine tetanus.**

3. **Occupation:** Agriculture workers are more prone to infection due to repeated contact with soil.
4. **Immunity:** No age is immune, unless protected by previous immunisation. Immunity can be transferred from mother to the baby, if mother is immunised or having high immunity during pregnancy.
5. **Other factors:** Host factors which favours the transmission of spores are like
- Injury.
- Suppurative infection like otitis media.
- Unsterile injection.
- Rituals such as ear boring or circumcision.

III. Environmental factors

1. **Distribution of spores:** Spores are ubiquitous, present everywhere as described earlier.
2. **Seasonal:** Tetanus is common in developing countries where the climate is warm in summer months & in rural areas where soil is fertile by bacteria from the animal/human faeces.

➢ **Pathogenesis: → Flow chart-1**

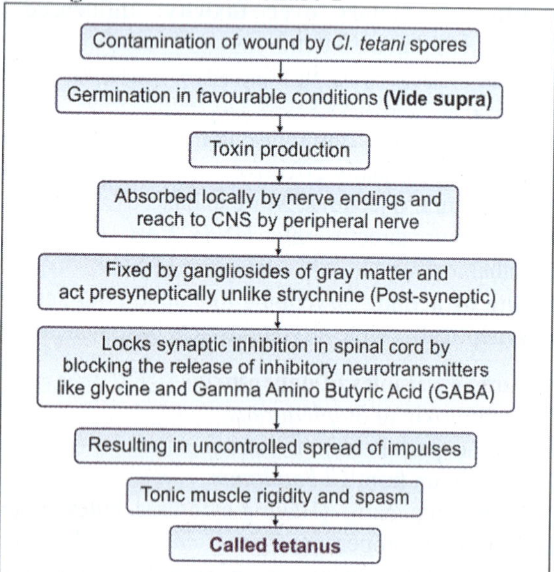

Flow chart-1: Pathogenesis of tetanus

➢ **Clinical types & clinical features:**

✪ **Clinical types of tetanus:** Tetanus is classified in different ways.

a. **Experimental types:**

1. **Local tetanus:** Toxin inoculated by IM route in one of hind limbs followed by tonic muscles spasms of inoculated limb. Manifestations are limited to the muscles near the wound.
2. **Ascending tetanus:** Toxin inoculated by IM route in one of hind limbs spread up in to spinal cord & involved opposite hind limbs, trunk & forelimbs in ascending fashion.
3. **Descending tetanus:** Toxin is injected intravenously; spasticity develops first in muscles of head and neck and then spreads downward, like natural tetanus.

b. **According to mode of onset:**

1. **Otogenic tetanus:** It develops after ear infection. Mortality rate is less.
2. **Cephalic tetanus:** It follows the head injury.
3. **Uterine tetanus:** May be due to aseptic abortion. Mortality rate is 70-100%.
4. **Tetanus neonatorum:** It follows the unsterile treatment of the umbilical cord stump. Mortality rate is 70-100%.

✪ **Clinical features:**

- Increased muscle tone with generalised/neck/back rigidity/stiffness.
- Tonic muscular spasms 1st local & later involving whole of somatic muscular system [**fig.-6(a)**]. Slightest stimulation can produce generalised muscle spasm, but not seizure. Muscle spasm is very painful. It can threaten the respiration by laryngospasm or by sustained contraction of respiratory muscles.
- Trismus (lock jaw) is the characteristic feature [**fig.-6(b)**].
- Back muscles are more powerful, so creating backward arc **called opisthotonus,** noticed by Sir Charles Bell in1809 as shown in **fig.-6(c).**
- Clinical findings: **Electromyogram** shows continuous discharge of motor units & shortening/absence of silent interval normally seen after an action potential.

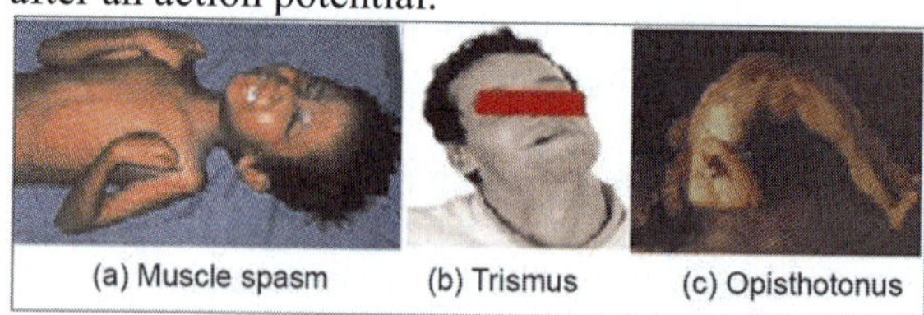

(a) Muscle spasm (b) Trismus (c) Opisthotonus

Figure-6: Features in tetanus

➢ **Complications:**

- High mortality
  - Before specific treatment 80-90%
  - With specific treatment 15-50-%

❖ **Laboratory diagnosis:**

➢ Tetanus is diagnosed on clinical ground with history of injury & introduction of soil/faeces in wound. Laboratory help is required for confirmation.

➢ **Specimens:**
- Wound swab.
- Exudates/discharge from wound.
- Necrotic tissue from the depth of wound.

➢ **Transport:** All samples are collected & transported in RCMM.

➢ **Testing methods:**

I. **Microscopy:** Gram stain is not reliable because,
- Bacilli may present in wound without tetanus.
- Not differentiate *Cl. tetani* from *Cl. tetanomorphum* & *Cl. sphenoides*.

II. **Culture:** Most reliable→ Follow C/Cs

III. **Biochemical reaction:** →Follow B/Rs

IV. **Blood picture:** Leucocytosis & raised muscle's enzymes level.

V. **Toxigenicity testing:** Two types.

A. **In vitro in blood agar: (4% agar to prevent swarming)**
- Take one blood agar plate with antitoxin in one half & other half without antitoxin.
- Inoculate *Cl. tetani* on both half.
- Incubate the plate anaerobically for 24-48 hrs and observed for haemolysis around colony.
- The half which contains antitoxin does not show any haemolysis.
- **Limitation:** Detect only tetanolysin not tetanospasmin which is pathogenic toxin.

B. **In vivo in laboratory animal:**
- Inoculate 0.2 ml culture in root of tail in two different mice.
- One is protected with 1000 U of tetanus antitoxin before 1 hr act as control animal.
- After 12-24 hrs test animal showing stiffness of tail & dies within two days.
- Control animal does not show any features due to neutralisation of toxin by antitoxin.
- **Advantage:** Detect tetanospasmin.

❖ Prophylaxis:

I. **General measures:** Keeping the wound clean.

II. **Surgery:** Removal of necrosed tissue, blood clots & foreign materials to prevent the development of anaerobic environment.

III. **Chemoprophylaxis:**
- Antibiotics are useful when given in 4 hrs before toxin production.
- It kills the bacilli & prevents the toxin production.
- **Systemic antibiotics:** Pn & tetracycline.
- **Local antibiotics:** Bacitracin or neomycin.

IV. **Immunoprophylaxis:** Three types

A. **Active immunisation:** It includes tetanus toxoid (TT). Following types of toxoid are available

i. **APT (Alum Precipitated Toxoid):** It gives reaction so not useful

ii. **FT (Formal Toxoid / Fluid Toxoid) or plain toxoid:** Prepared by incubating the toxin with formalin.

iii. **Adsorbed (purified) toxoid:** It is purified toxoid adsorbed on to insoluble aluminium compound usually aluminium phosphate (**called Purified Toxoid Aluminium Phosphate/PTAP**).

✪ **History:** Tetanus toxoid vaccine was developed by P. Descombey in 1924.

✪ **Advantages of adsorbed TT:** The adsorbed toxoid provides higher & long lasting immunity than plain toxoid.

✪ **Storage:** Adsorbed TT should be stored between 4-10^{0}C & no freezing at any time.

✪ **Adverse reactions:** Frequent injection of TT cause hypersensitivity.

✪ **Administration of adsorbed TT:** Adsorbed TT is used as single or combined (mixed) vaccine.

a. **Single / plain / monovalent / univalent vaccine:**
- It is given in the dose of 0.5 ml by IM route in to the arm at 10 or 16 years (second dose of TT after 1 month if not previously immunized by DPT, DT or TT & 1st booster dose after 1 year).
- TT in pregnant women: 2 doses at 1 month interval in pregnant women or booster in early pregnancy if immunised earlier.
- Immunity last for 10 year. Booster dose is given every 10 year or if wound occur.
- Avoid frequent booster doses.
- TT does not provide herd immunity.

b. **Mixed / combined / polyvalent / multivalent vaccines:** Adsorbed Tetanus Toxoid (TT) is used in combination with following vaccines.

- **Double / bivalent vaccine:** DT (contains Diphtheria + Tetanus).
- **Triple / trivalent / tetravalent vaccine:** DPT/DTP contains Diphtheria, Pertusis & Tetanus.
- **Quaduple / guadrivalent vaccine:** DPT (DTP) with Hib etc.
- **Pentavalent vaccine:** Two type of preparations.

1. **Pentvac** contains Diphtheria, Pertusis, Tetanus, HBV, *H. influenzae* type b (Hib).
2. **Pentaxim** contains D, P, T, IPV & Hib.

- **Dosing schedule of triple (DPT) vaccine, pentavalent vaccine & double (DT) vaccine as per national immunisation schedule:**

Triple (DPT) vaccine
- Three (Primary) doses of DPT, each with 0.5 ml amount by deep IM route, are given at 6th weeks, 10th week & 14th week of age.
- After primary immunisation by DPT at 6, 10 & 14 weeks, 1st booster of DPT is given at 18-24 months followed by 2nd booster dose (DT only) at 5-6 year (school entry age).

Pentavalent vaccine
- In some states instead of DPT, pentavalent vaccine (**Pentvac**) contains Diphtheria, Pertusis, Tetanus, HBV, *H. influenzae* type b (Hib) is given at 6th weeks, 10th weeks & 14th weeks with OPV. Other

same preparation is **Pentaxim** contains D, P, T, IPV & Hib given with OPV & HBV.

Double (DT) vaccine

Double (DT) vaccine is given at 5-6 years /school entry age (Second dose of DT after 1 month if not previously immunized by DPT/pentavalent vaccine)

- **Storage:** DPT/DT should be stored between 4-10^{0}C & no freezing at any time.
- **Adverse reactions of DPT vaccine:**
  - Local reactions (erythema / induration).
  - Exaggerated local reactions (arthus-type).
  - Fever and systemic symptoms not common.
  - Severe systemic reactions rare.
- **Contraindications and precautions of DPT vaccine:**
  - Severe allergic reaction to vaccine component or following a prior dose.
  - Moderate or severe acute illness.
- **Efficacy of DPT vaccine:** It is 70%.

B. Passive immunisation:

- **History:** Edmond Nocard showed that tetanus antitoxin induced passive immunity in humans & could be used for prophylaxis & treatment (1897).
- **Indication:** Passive immunization recommended only in non immune persons and only once.
- **Types:** Two types.

i. Anti – tetanus serum (ATS):

- **Dose:** 1500 IU given subcutaneously or intramuscularly in non immune persons soon after receiving any tetanus prone injury.
- **Disadvantages of ATS:**
  - Immune elimination.
  - Hypersensitivity.

ii. Tetanus immunoglobulin (TIG) of human:

- **Aim:** It is the preparation of choice to neutralise the toxin.
- **Dose:** 250 IU has longer half life.

C. Combined immunisation:

- TIG on one hand & TT on other hand followed by 2nd & 3rd dose of TT at one month interval.
- Use adsorbed toxoid, because immune response to plain toxoid may be inhibited by TIG.

V. Integrated prophylaxis of tetanus following injury: It depends on the type of wound & immune status of patient as shown in **table-3.**

❖ Treatment:

1. **General measures:**
   - Isolation of patients from noise & light.
   - Maintenance of airway, breathing & circulation.
2. **Immunisation:**
   - TIG followed by full course of active immunisation.
   - TIG may not neutralise toxin already bound to nervous tissue, it can inactivate unbound toxin and any further toxin that may be produced.
   - Patients recovering from tetanus should receive full course of active immunisation, as an attack of the disease does not confer immunity.
3. **Antibacterial therapy:**
   - **Aim:** To eradicate the source of toxin by removing the vegetative cells.
   - **Drugs:**
     - Penicillin & metronidazole are drugs of choice.
     - Clindamycin & erythromycin are useful in patient allergic to penicillin.
     - Tetracycline is not used.
4. **Other medication:**
   - Control of muscle spasm: Many agents as alone or in combination are used. **Benzodizepines** (dizepam, lorazepam, midazolam etc.) are most commonly used drugs. **Barbiturates** & **chlorpromazine** are the alternative agents.
   - Autonomic dystunctions: For sympathetic over activity labetalol, esmolol or clonidine are used.
5. **Mechanical ventilation:** If spasm is unresponsive to medication, then it could be controlled by mechanical ventilation with non depolarizing neuromuscular blocking agents. Other agents useful are propofol, dantrolene, intrathecal baclofen, succinyl choline & magnesium sulphate.
6. **Surgery:** Tracheostomy to maintain airway.

Cl. botulinum

❖ **Meaning:** Word derived from **botulus = sausage** a type of food prepared from meat**.** Sausage word used for food item in the form of cylindrical length **[fig. -7(a)]** of minced pork or other meat.

❖ **History:** Bacilli was 1st isolated by van Ermengem from the piece of ham that caused an outbreak of botulism in 1896.

Category	Immune status	Wound: < 6 hrs, non-penetrating, clean, no/negligible tissue damage	Wound: Contaminated
A	Completely immune in < 5 yrs	Nothing	Nothing
B	Completely immune in > 5 - < 10 yrs	1 dose of TT	1 dose of TT
C	Completely immune in > 10 yrs	1 dose of TT	1 dose of TT + TIG
D	Incompletely or immune status is unknown	Complete course of TT	Complete course of TT + TIG

Table-3: Integrated prophylaxis of tetanus following injury

✓ **Note:** Completely immune: Patient had full course of 3 injections of toxoid.

❖ **Classification:**

- Eight types of *Cl. botulinum* have been identified (A, B, C1, C2, D, E, F & G) based on immunological difference in toxins produced by them.
- C2 is cytotoxic, while all the others are neurotoxic.

❖ **Morphology:** →**Fig. -7(b)**

➢ **Type according to gram stain:** GPB.
➢ **Size:** 1µm × 5 µm.
➢ **Shape:** Straight or curve rod.
➢ **Arrangement:** Single, pair or in short chain.
➢ **Motility:** Motile with peritrichate flagella.
➢ **Spores:** Spores are subterminal & oval (bulging).
➢ **Capsule:** Non capsulated.

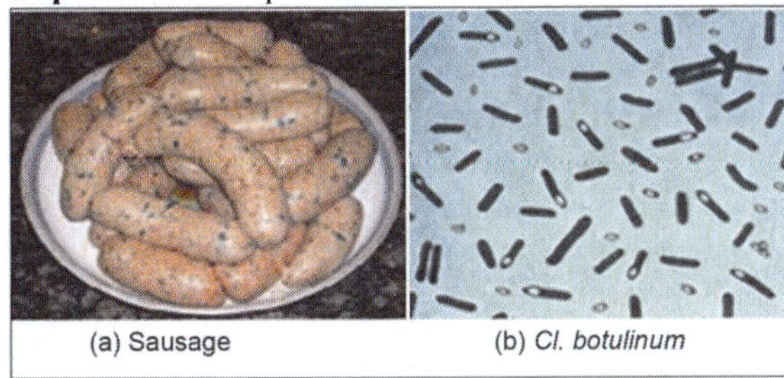

(a) Sausage (b) *Cl. botulinum*

Figure-7: Images of botulism

❖ **Cultural characteristics (C/Cs):**

➢ **Effective factors:**
- O_2 effect: Strict anaerobe.
- Temperature: 35°C, but it can grow at 1-5°C.

➢ **Culture in media:**

A. Routine media:

1. **Nutrient agar:** 3-8mm, semitransparent colonies with a fimbriated border.
2. **RCMM:** Type A, B & F are predominant proteolytic causing blackening of meat & C, D & E are saccharolytic turn meat in to pink colour.
3. **Alkaline glucose gelatin media:** Produces spore at 20-25°C.
4. **Egg yolk agar:** Produces opalescence & pearly lipolytic effect.

B. Selective medium: Egg yolk agar + cycloserine + sulfamethoxazole + trimithoprim.

➢ **Culture in animals:**
- Food or feces macerated in saline and filtered – extracted is used.
- Inoculation into two mice or two guinea pig (one as control & other as test animal) intraperitoneally.
- Test animal die if toxin present.
- Controlled animal protected with antitoxin --remain healthy.

❖ **Biochemical reaction (B/Rs):**

1. **Type C, D & E are saccharolytic while A, B & F are predominant proteolytic.**
2. **Sugar fermentation:** It ferments glucose & maltose with production of acid & gas but not sucrose & lactose.
3. **H_2S test:** + Ve

❖ **Resistance:**

- Spores of *Cl. botulinum* are survives boiling after 3-4 hours even at 105^{0}C they are not killed completely in less than 100 minutes.
- They resist killing by 5% phenol or o.1% mercury chloride.
- **Sporicidal agents:** Follow chapter → Morphology of bacteria (section →spore)

❖ **Pathogenicity:**

➢ **Disease:** It causes food poisoning **called botulism.**
➢ **Nature & history of disease:**
- It is the most serious type of food poisoning but occurs very rare. It kills two third of its victims.
- Infant botulism can occurs as sporadic cases but not as an epidemic. Outbreak/epidemic of food borne botulism has been reported from UK in 1989 with 27 cases & one death.

➢ **Reservoir of infection:** Spores are widely distributed in soil, dust & intestines of animals.
➢ **Source of infection:** Preserved food-meat or meat product, fish, sea foods & canned vegetables.
➢ **Mode of transmission:** } **Follow clinical types**
➢ **Incubation period:** } **(vide infra)**
➢ **Portal of entry:** GIT & skin (wound).
➢ **Sites:** Synapse (presyneptic), neuromuscular junction, parasympathetic nerve endings & peripheral ganglia. CNS is not involved. No sensory features except blurred vision.
➢ **Precipitating factors (epidemiological determinants):** Three types

I. Agent factors (virulence factors)

Cl. botulinum is non invasive & produces powerful exotoxin in food (preformed toxin/intradietic toxin) **called botulinum** which is responsible for food poisoning. Toxin has following properties.

- Produced intracellularly & released in medium only after death or autolysis of organism not during the life of organism.
- Initially inactive as protoxin or progenitor toxin, convert to active form by trypsin and other proteolytic enzyme.
- Heat labile (relatively heat stable), inactivated at 80°C in 30-40 minutes & at 100°C after 10 minutes
- Resistant to intestinal digestion and absorbed through small intestine in active form.
- MW: 70,000
- Lethal Dose (LD): Most lethal toxin & lethal dose for human being is 1-2 µg. Botulinum toxin once bound leads to permanent dysfunction of that neuron. Recovery takes usually 3 months when

dysfunctioned nerve terminal are replaced as a result of sprouting.

- Pure crystalline protein.
- It **is neurotoxin** and acts slowly, except C2 which is cytotoxic (enterotoxic).
- Human disease is caused by type A, B, E & F, however few authors mentioned that all types can cause human disease.
- Toxin production is determined by bacteriophage at least in type C & D.
- Botulinum is also produced by other species like *Cl. butyrocum* & *Cl .baratti*

II. Host factors

Wound & infantile age are favouring factors.

III. Environmental factors

Spores are widely distributed in soil & dust.

➢ **Pathogenesis of botulism: → Flow chart-2 & fig.-8**

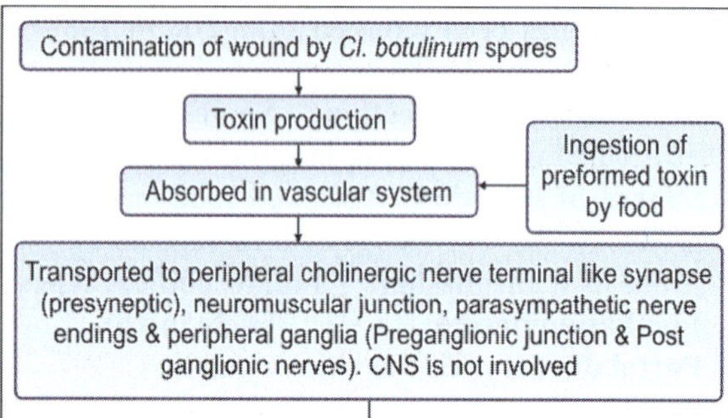

Contamination of wound by *Cl. botulinum* spores
Toxin production
Ingestion of preformed toxin by food
Absorbed in vascular system
Transported to peripheral cholinergic nerve terminal like synapse (presyneptic), neuromuscular junction, parasympathetic nerve endings & peripheral ganglia (Preganglionic junction & Post ganglionic nerves). CNS is not involved

Block the production or release of acetylcholine and causing descending flaccid paralysis (arflexia) **called botulism**.

- **Onset:** It start within 18-24 hours and it is marked by diplopia, dysphagia and dysarthria
- **Other features:** It includes dyspnoea, dizziness, dry mouth (thirst), ptosis **[fig.8(a)]**, blurred vision (only sensory deficit), ocular paresis, nausea, vomiting, abdominal pain, severe constipation/paralytic ileus (no diarrhoea), urinary retention, upper and lower limb weakness and quadriplegia due to bilateral cranial nerve involvement.
- **Reflexes:** Following reflexes are suppressed (arflexia)
  - Gag reflex may be suppressed
  - Deep tendon reflex may be normal/decreased
  - Pupillary reflex may be depressed or fixed **called non reactive pupil** as shown in **fig.8(b)**
- **End stage:**
  - Symmetric descending paralysis is characteristic pattern.
  - Death due respiratory paralysis or cardiac failure.

√ **Notes: Points to be remember in botulism**

- **Botulism** is present with symmetric descending paralysis while **polio** present with asymmetric descending paralysis
- No CNS involvement
- No sensory involvement except blurred vision
- No fever. Normal or slow heart rate. Patient is responsive
- No loss of deep tendon reflex in early stage
- No papillary reflex in **botulism** while **polio**, **diphtheria** and **porphyria** are present with papillary reflex

Flow chart-2: Pathogenesis of botulism

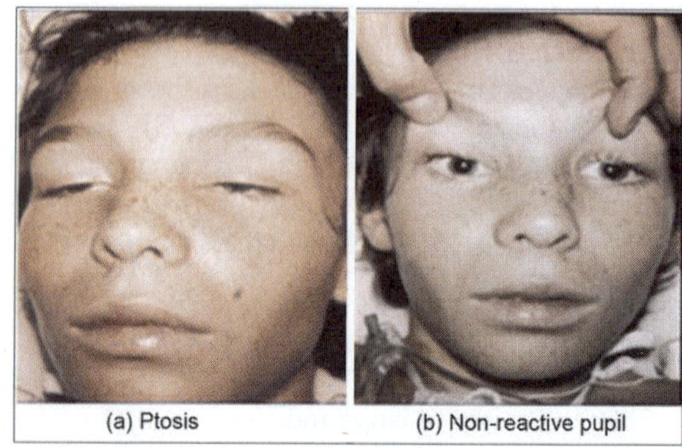

Figure-8: Eye features in botulism

➢ **Clinical types:** Three main types of botulism with two newer types (total five types) as per mode of transmission.

a. Food borne botulism:

- **Mode of transmission:**
  - By ingestion of preformed toxin in preserved food-meat or meat product, fish, sea foods & canned vegetables. Type F outbreak occurs especially with fish products.
  - Spores contaminate the food, germinate and form toxin **[preformed /intradietic toxin]**.
- **Incubation period:** 12-36 hrs following ingestion of food.
- **Clinical features:** Vomiting, thirst, constipation, ocular paresis, difficulty in swallowing, difficulty in speaking & difficulty in breathing are common features.
- **Complication:** Death **(20-70 % cases)** due to respiratory failure in 1-7 days.

b. Wound botulism:

- **Mode of transmission:** Wound contamination by spores → germination → toxin production → absorption. Most cases are due to type A.
- **Clinical features:** Same as food borne botulism except GIT features.

c. Infant botulism:

- **Mode of transmission:**
  - It is the most common types of botulism. It also **called floppy baby syndrome**. It was first recognized in 1976, and is the most common form of botulism in the United States.
  - It occurs in infant below 6 months.
  - It occurs due to ingestion of food like honey contaminated by spores → ingestion in gut → germination → toxin. For this reason honey is not recommended for infants less than one year of age.
- **Incubation period:** Symptoms of infant botulism begin between 3 to 30 days after an infant ingests the spores.

- **Clinical features:**
- Constipation, poor feeding, lethargy, weakness, pooled oral secretion, altered cry, floppiness and loss of head control (**fig.9**).
- Patient excretes toxins and spores in their faeces.
- Most of the patient recovered with supportive therapy.

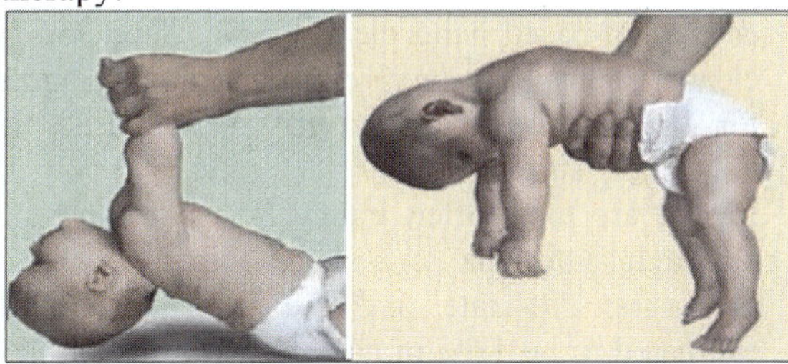

Figure-9: Loss of head control in botulism

d. **Adult intestinal toxemia botulism:**

- **Mode of transmission:** Result from absorption of toxin produced in situ after rarely occurring intestinal colonisation with toxigenic clostridia.

e. **Iatrogenic botulism:**

- **Mode of transmission:** Result from injection of botulinum.

❖ Laboratory diagnosis:

➢ **Specimens:** Food, vomitus, feces or gastric fluid.

➢ **Testing methods:**

I. **Demonstration of bacilli:**

A **Microscopy:** Follow morphology.

B **Culture:** Follow C/Cs.

C **Biochemical reaction:** Follow B/Rs.

II. **Demonstration of toxin:** Toxin is detected from food, feces, blood or in the liver postmortem.

III. **Demonstration of antitoxin:** Retrospective diagnosis can be made by detecting the antitoxin from the patient's serum, but not seen in all cases.

❖ Prophylaxis:

A. **General measures:** Proper canning and preservation of food.

B. **Antitoxin:** When an outbreak occurs, prophylactic dose of antitoxin should be given IM to all who consumed food.

C. **Active immunisation:** To laboratory workers exposed to risk. Total 2 injections of aluminium sulphate adsorbed toxoid are given at interval of 10 weeks, followed by booster dose 1 year later.

❖ Treatment:

1. **General measures:** Supportive therapy to maintain respiration.
2. **Antitoxin:** Polyvalent antitoxin to type A, B & E may be administered immediately after diagnosis.

Cl. difficile

❖ **Meaning:** Difficult to isolate, hence **called *difficle*.**

❖ **History:** Bacilli were 1st isolated in 1935 from the stool of new born infant.

❖ Morphology:

➢ **Type according to gram stain:** GPB but GNB in old culture.

➢ **Size:** 0.5-1μm × 4-8 μm.

➢ **Shape:** Rod shape.

➢ **Motile:** Oscillating motility by peritrichate flagella.

➢ **Spores:** Terminal & oval.

❖ **Cultural characteristics (C/C):** Diagnosis of *Cl. difficile* by culture is the most sensitive method.

➢ **Effective factors:**

- O_2 effect: Strict anaerobe.
- Temperature: 37°C.

➢ **Culture in media:**

A. **Blood agar:** Non haemolytic colony.

B. **Selective media:**

1. Cefoxitine Cycloserine Fructose Agar (CCFA).
2. Cefoxitine Cycloserine Egg yolk Agar (CCEA).

➢ **Culture in cells:** Hep-2 & human diploid cell are used for toxin demonstration. It is the most specific method for diagnosis of *Cl. difficile.*

❖ Biochemical reaction (B/Rs):

1. Predominant saccharolytic and weakly proteolytic.
2. Fermentation of glucose, fructose & mannitol.
3. Aesculin hydrolysis test: +Ve
4. Gelatin liquefaction test: +Ve

❖ Pathogenicity:

➢ **Disease name:** **Called Antibiotic Associated Diarrhoea (AAD) or *Clostridium difficile* Associated Diarrhoea (AAD) or Antibiotic Associated Colitis (AAC) or Pseudo Membranous colitis (PMC).**

➢ **Nature & history of disease:**

Outbreak with plenty of deaths has been reported from the different part of world.

- Pseudomembranous colitis was 1st described as a complication of *Cl. difficile* infection in 1978.

➢ **Reservoir of infection:** Spores are present as normal flora in the colon of neonate during initial 6 months. Spores are excreted in faeces. It is present in 2–5% of the adult population, but studies have shown that colonise individual have a less risk to disease (no endogenous infection) & never become sick, though they may still spread the infection.

➢ **Source of infection:** Infected hands or food.

➢ **Mode of transmission:** Spores present in the faeces which may contaminate the food or surface. Infection is exogenous.

- Infection occurs by swallowing of infected hands especially by health care workers, which gets infected from the surface or food contact.
- *C. difficile* is transmitted from person to person by the faecal-oral route. Once spores are ingested, their acid-resistance allows them to pass through the stomach unscathed. Upon exposure to bile acids, they germinate and multiply into vegetative cells in the colon. It is the most common bacterial cause of nosocomial diarrhoea.

➢ **Incubation period:** Clinical features usually develop within 5-10 days after starting antibiotics, but may occur as soon as the 1st day or up to 2 months later.

➢ **Portal of entry:** GIT

➢ **Sites:** Colon

➢ **Precipitating factors (epidemiological determinants):** Three types.

I. Agent factors (virulence factors)

It produces two types of toxin. Both these toxins are glucosyltransferases that target and inactivate the Rho family of GTPases.

1. **Toxin A:** It is histotoxic (cytotoxic?) causing tissue damage & enterotoxic allowing accumulation of fluid in colon to produce the bloody diarrhoea.
2. **Toxin B:** It is cytotoxin which damages the gut mucosa causing acute colitis with/without pseudomembrane formation.

II. Host factors

1. **Age:** Older age.
2. **Sex:** Women are more prone to disease than men.
3. **Drugs:**

- **Antibiotics:**
  - Use of antibiotics like ampicillin/amoxicillin, tetracycline, chloramphenicol, lincomycin, clindamycin, cephalosporin (cefotaxime, ceftriaxone, cefuroxime & ceftazidime) etc., will disturb the normal flora & reduces the nutritional competition with other remaining bacteria which allow the colonisation of *Cl. difficile.*
  - Pipericillin/tazobactam & ticarcillin/clavulanate are posses less risk for AAD.
- **Antacids or proton pump inhibitors:** H2-receptor antagonists increased the risk 1.5-fold & proton pump inhibitors like pantoprazole by 1.7 with once-daily use and 2.4 with more than once-daily use.

4. **Prolonged hospitalization:** *Cl. difficile* are more encountered in hospital environment & prolong stay in hospital increase the chances of infection.
5. **Malignancy:** Acute myeloid leukemia & acute lymphocytic leukemia are the risk factors following chemotherapy.
6. **Other health problems:**

- Use of electric rectal thermometer.
- Central tube feeding.
- Gastrointestinal surgery.
- Presence of other chronic diseases.

III. Environmental factors

1. **Hospital environment:**

- The organism forms spores that are resistant to heat & alcohol-based hand cleansers or routine surface cleaner. Thus, they survive in clinical environments for long periods & they may be cultured from almost any surface.
- People are most often infected from the hospitals although infection outside medical settings is increasing. The rate of *Cl. difficile* acquisition is estimated to be 13% in patients with hospital stays of up to two weeks & 50% with stay longer than four weeks.

➢ **Pathogenesis: → Flow chart-3**

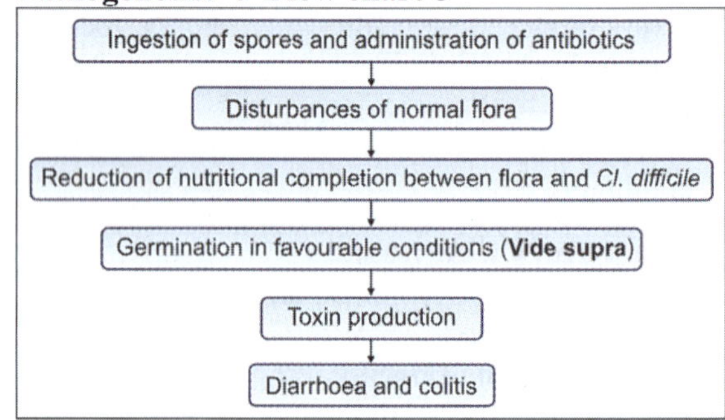

Flow chart-3: Pathogenesis of AAC

➢ **Clinical feature:**

- Diarrhoea: Watery diarrhoea ≥ 3times/day for ≥ 2 days. Presence of blood in stool (dysentery) is uncommon.
- Other associated features: Fever, nausea, and abdominal pain.

➢ **Complications:**

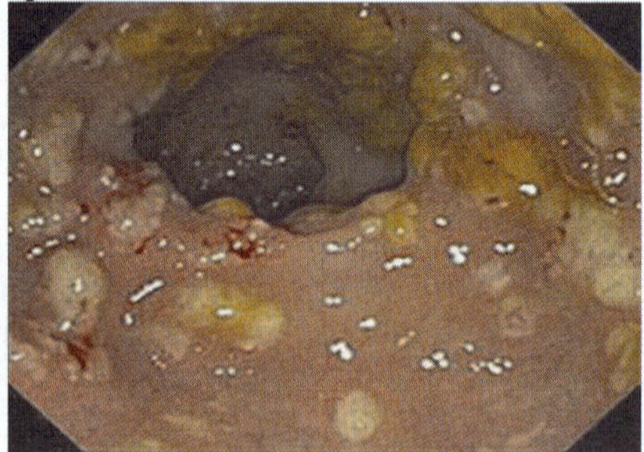

Figure-10: Endoscopic image of pseudomembranous colitis, with yellow plaque seen on the wall of the sigmoid colon

- Damage to the gut mucosa causing acute colitis **called Antibiotic Associated Colitis (AAC).**
- Colitis may present with pseudomembrane **called Pseudo Membranous colitis (PMC).** It is composed of inflammatory cells, fibrin, mucus &

necrotic cells. It attach to the underlying mucosa. It appear as whitish yellow plaque under the endoscopic examination (**fig.10**) and ranging from 1-2 mm to large enough to cover entire colonic mucosa. It causing problems in treatment against the effect of antibiotics.

- Toxic megacolon.
- Perforation of the colon.
- Sepsis.

❖ Laboratory diagnosis:

➢ **Specimens:** Faeces.

➢ **Testing methods:**

I. Demonstration of bacilli:

A. Microscopy: Follow morphology.

B. Culture: Follow C/Cs.

C. Biochemical reaction: Follow B/Rs.

D. Gas liquid chromatography (GLC):

II. Toxin Demonstration: From feces by

- **Cell culture** like Hep-2 & human diploid cell culture.
- **ELISA.**

III. Toxin neutralisation: By antitoxin of *Cl. sordelli.*

IV. Histological findings: In the earliest stage of disease tiny superficial encryptal erosions may be found **called summit lesions.**

V. Sigmoidoscopy: It is the most specific method along with toxin demonstration by cell culture.

VI. Molecular testing: Real time PCR aids in the diagnosis.

❖ Prevention:

- Limiting antibiotics use.
- Improvement of hand hygiene.
- Cleaning in hospital.
- No specific vaccine is available.

❖ Treatment:

1. **Discontinuation of antibiotics:** It may result in resolution of symptoms within three days in about 20% of those infected.
2. **Antibiotics:**
   - Antibiotic treatment may be difficult, due to resistance & physiological factors of the bacteria like spore formation plus protective effects of the pseudomembrane
   - Metronidazole is drug of choice. Vancomycin, fidaxomi & bacitracin are other options.
   - Relapse after treatment is common & seen in 15-30% cases.
3. **Probiotics:** Less significant but may decrease the risk of relapse.
4. **Faecal microbiota transplantation or faecal bacteriotherapy or stool transplant:**
   - It is approximately 85% to 90% effective in those for whom antibiotics have not worked.
   - It involves infusion of bacterial flora acquired from the faeces of a healthy donor to reverse the bacterial imbalance responsible for the recurring nature of the infection.
   - Procedure replaces normal healthy colonic flora that had been wiped out by antibiotics & re-establishes resistance to colonization by *Cl. difficile*
   - There is evidence that looks hopeful that fecal transplant can be delivered in the form of a pill.
   - They are available in the United States but are not FDA-approved as of 2015.
5. **Surgery:** Colectomy may improve the outcomes in colitis patients.

Other *Clostridium* spp.

Clostridium septicum

➢ **History:** It was first described by Pasteur & Joubert in1887 and **called *vibrion septique*.**

➢ **Morphology:**

- **Type according to gram stain:** GPB.
- **Size & shape:** It is a pleomorphic bacillus, about 3-8 × 0.6 μmin size.
- **Spore:** Oval, central or subterminal spores.
- **Motility:** It is motile by peritrichate flagella.

➢ **Cultural characteristics (C/Cs):**

- Growth occurs anaerobically on ordinary media.
- Colonies are irregular and transparent initially, turning opaque on long time incubation.
- Haemolysis occurs on horse blood agar.

➢ **Biochemical reactions (B/Rs):** Saccharolytic & produces the gas.

➢ **Classifications:** Six types on based on flagellar antigen.

➢ **Pathogenicity:**

- **Sources:** It found soil & in animal intestine.
- **Virulence factors:** Two types

a. Toxins: Four toxins

1. **α-toxin:** Hemolytic, dermonecrotic & lethal.
2. **β-toxin:** Leucotoxic and deoxyribonuclease.
3. **γ- toxin:** Hyaluronidase.
4. **δ- toxin:** Oxygen labile haemolysin.

b. Enzymes: Fibrinolysin.

- **Clinical features:** It is associated with gas gangrene in human being, usually with other *Clostridia.*

Clostridium novyi

➢ **Morphology:**

- **Type according to gram stain:** GPB.
- **Size & shape:** It is a pleomorphic bacillus.
- **Spore:** Large, oval & subterminal spores.
- **Motility:** It is motile by peritrichate flagella.

➢ **Cultural characteristics (C/Cs):** Strict anaerobes & killed on exposure of O_2.

- **Biochemical reactions (B/Rs):** Predominant saccharolytic.
- **Classifications:** Four types based on toxins production. Only type A cause gas gangrene.
- **Pathogenicity:**
  - **Sources:** It is widely distributed in soil.
  - **Virulence factors:** Produces the four different types of toxins.
  - **Clinical features:** It is associated with gas gangrene (Mostly by Type A) characterised by high mortality & large amount of oedema fluid with little or no gas.

Clostridium histolyticum

- **Morphology:**
  - **Type according to gram stain:** GPB.
  - **Spore:** Oval, subterminal spores or bulging spores.
  - **Motility:** It is motile by peritrichate flagella.
- **Cultural characteristics (C/Cs):** It is aerotolerant and may grow in aerobic culture.
- **Biochemical reactions (B/Rs):** Predominant proteolytic.
- **Pathogenicity:**
  - **Virulence factors:** Produces the five different types of toxins.
  - **Clinical features:** It is infrequently associated with gas gangrene.

Clostridium tertium

- GPB; often gram variable.
- Having terminal-oval spore which gives tennis racket appearance.
- It does not produce the exotoxin.
- It causes bacteraemia, meningitis, septic arthritis, enterocolitis, spontaneous bacterial peritonitis, post-traumatic brain abscess etc.

Question bank

Case study

1) A truck driver admitted in hospital with accidental wound on his left lower limb after 5 days of accident. Wound is present with oedema, severe contamination by blood & soil & with watery discharge. Local examination of wound revealed tenderness on palpation & crepitation on auscultation. Discharge is collected & examined under gram stain which noticed the GPB mixed with GPC. Identify the organism & answer the following
   a) Name the clinical disease & describe the morphology of causative agent
   b) Write the pathogenicity of causative agent
   c) Describe the lab. diagnosis of causative agent

2) An adult patient admitted in hospital 5-7 following traumatic wound which is severely contaminated. Patient having features of lock jaw & muscle spasm. Tissue biopsy from the wound identified the GPB with terminal spores.
   a) Name the clinical condition & causative agent
   b) Describe the morphology & C/Cs of causative agent
   c) Write the pathogenicity of causative agent
   d) Describe the prophylaxis of given case.

3) A patient of chronic myeloid leukemia presents with diarrhoea & fever following amoxicillin therapy. He is improved with Metronidazole therapy.
   a) Name the causative agent
   b) Describe the morphology & C/Cs of causative agent
   c) Write the pathogenicity of causative agent
   d) Describe the lab. diagnosis of causative agent

Essay/Full question

1) *Cl. welchii*
2) *Cl. tetani*

Short notes

1) Uses of *Clostridia*
2) Classification of *Clostridia*
3) Nagler reaction
4) CAMP test & reverse CAMP test
5) Pathogenicity of *Cl welchii*
6) Laboratory diagnosis of *Cl welchii*
7) Gas gangrene
8) Tetanus
9) Tetanus toxoid
10) DPT vaccine
11) Botulism
12) Antibiotic associated diarrhoea
13) *Cl. difficile*

Short questions for theory/viva questions

1) What is target haemolysis?
2) What is stormy fermentation?
3) Write four examples of neurotoxins & bacteria producing it
4) How does infant botulism differ from foodborne botulism?

MCQs for chapter review

Classification

1) **Saccharolytic species of *Clostridium* is**
   (a) *Cl. tertium* (b) *Cl. cochlearum* (c) *Cl. tetani* (d) *Cl. tetanomorphum*

Clostridium perfrigens

2) **Boxcar appearance is the feature of**
   (a) *Cl. tertium* (b) *Cl. cochlearum* (c) *Cl. tetani* (d) *Cl. perfrigens*
3) **Gas gangrene is due to:** (PGI June-08)
   (a) Alpha toxin (b) Theta toxin (c) Beta toxin (d) Delta toxin (e) Epsilon toxin
4) **Regarding gas gangrene one of the following is correct:** (AI -04)
   (a) It is due to *Clostridium botulinum* infection (b) *Clostridium* species are gram negative spore forming anaerobes (c) The clinical features are due to release of protein endotoxin (d) Gas is invariable present in muscles compartments
5) **Following statements are true regarding *Clostridium perfringens* except:** (AI-05)
   (a) It is the commonest cause of gas gangrene (b) It is normally presents in human faeces (c) The principle toxin of the *Clostridium perfringens* is alpha toxin (d) Gas gangrene producing strains of *Clostridium perfringens* produce heat resistant spores

6) **Opacity around colonies of *Clostridium perfringens* is due to:** (PGI-94)
a) Theta toxin (b) Lecithinase (c) Desmolase (d) Cytokinin

7) **Incubation period of gas gangrene is:** (PGI-94) (PGI June-09)
(a) 1-3 days (b) 4-6 days (c) 7-10 days (d) 10-15 days.

8) **Gas gangrene is/are caused by all except-** (PGI, May -11)
(a) *Cl. novyi* (b) *Cl. septicum* (c) *Cl. histolyticum,* (d) *Cl. perfringens* (e) *Cl. tetani*

9) **True about gas gangrene** (PGI, May -13)
(a) Underlying skin and muscles are normal (b) Caused by tetanospasmin toxin (c) Most common organism implicated is *Clostridium perfringens* (d) Passive immunisation does not help

Clostridium tetani

10) **All are true regarding tetanus except-** (AIIMS, Nov-10)
(a) Transmission through contaminated wound and injuries (b) Most common in winter and dry weather (c) Reservoir in soil and intestine of humans and animals (d) No herd immunity or lifelong immunity

11) **True about tetanus-** (PGI, May -13 & Dec-14)
(a) Gram –Ve spore forming organism (b) Produces tetanolysin and tetanospasmin (c) Trismus and neck stiffness are early sign (d) Generalised tonic-clonic seizures occurs on hyperstimulation (e) Wound debridement is necessary

12) **Mechanism of action of tetanospasmin-**
(a) Inhibition of release of GABA (b) Inhibition of C-AMP (c) Inactivation of Ach receptors (d) Inhibition of c-GMP

13) **Which of the followings are true regarding tetanus -** (PGI, Nov-13, 09)
(a) Gram -Ve spore forming aerobes (b) Because of tetanospasmin (c) Muscle enzymes are normal (d) Vegetative cell will die with tetracycline (e) Muscle spasm seen

14) **Toxigenicity of *Clostridium tetani* is tested in**
(a) Rabbit (b) Horse (c) Mouse (b) Guinea pig

15) **A person received complete immunisation against tetanus 10 years ago. Now he present with a clean wound without any laceration from an injury sustained 2.5 hours ago. He should be now be given** (AI-01)
(a) Full course of tetanus toxoid (b) Single dose of tetanus toxoid (c) Human tetanus globulin (b) Human tetanus globulin and single dose of tetanus toxoid

16) **A 10 year old boy following to the road traffic accident present to the casualty with a contaminated wound over left leg. He has received his complete primary immunisation before preschool age and received a boosted doseof DT at school entry age. All of the following can be done except** (AIIMS-01)
(a) Injection of TT (b) Injection of human antiserum (c) Broad spectrum antibiotics (b) Wound debridement and cleaning

17) **All of the following statements regarding *Clostridium tetani* are true, except-** (AI-11)
(a) Spores are resistant to heat (b) Primary immunisation consists three doses (c) Incubation period is 6-10 days (d) Man to man transmission is seen

Clostridium botulinum

18) **Botulism is a disease of-**
(a) Neural transmission caused by the toxin of the bacterium *Clostridium botulinum* (b) Muscular transmission caused by the toxin of the bacterium *Clostridium botulinum* (c) Neuromuscular transmission caused by the toxin of the bacterium *Clostridium botulinum* (d) Non-neuromuscular transmission caused by the toxin of the bacterium *Clostridium botulinum*

19) **Botulinum toxin acts on-**
(a) Sympathetic system (b) Parasympathetic system (c) Amygdala (d) Motor cortex

20) **Botulinum affects all except-** (AI-07)
(a) Neuromuscular junction (b) Preganglionic junction (c) Post ganglionic nerves (d) CNS

21) **Among the toxin produced by *Clostridium botulinum,* the non neurotoxic one is -**
(a) A (b) B (c) C1 (d) C2 (e) D

22) **All of the following statements are true regarding botulism except-** (AIIMS, May-03)
(a) Infant botulism is caused by preformed toxin (b) *Clostridium botulinum* A, B, C and F causes human disease (c) Gene for botulinum toxin is encoded by a bacteriophage (d) *Clostridium baratti* may cause botulism

23) **Botulism is most commonly due to-**
(a) Egg (b) Milk (c) Meat (d) Dysarthria

24) **All occurs in botulism except-** (AIIMS, Dec-97)
(a) Diplopia (b) Diarrhoea (c) Dysphagia (d) Dysarthria

25) **Botulinum causes-** (PGI, May-13 & Dec-07)
(a) Descending flaccid paralysis (b) Ascending flaccid paralysis (c) Ascending paralysis (d) Ascending spastic paralysis

26) **All of the following statements about botulism are true except-** (AI -97)
(a) Botulism is caused by endotoxin (b) Honey ingestion caused infant botulism (c) Constipation is seen (d) Detection of antitoxin in the serum can aid in the diagnosis

27) **A 18 year old male presented with acute onset descending paralysis of 3 days duration. There is also history of blurring of vision for the same duration. On examination, the patient quadriparesis with areflexia. Both the pupils are non-reactive. The most probable diagnosis is-** (AIIMS, -06)
(a) Poliomyelitis (b) Botulism (c) Diphtheria (d) Porphyria

28) **Not true about botulinum toxin-** (PGI, May-13 & Dec-07)
(a) Short life span (b) Increased acetylcholine release (c) Used for the treatment of blepharospasm, static & dynamic wrinkles (d) Irreversible decrease acetylcholine in neuromuscular junction

Clostridium difficile

29) ***Clostridium difficile* infection occurs after-** (PGI, Nov-13 & June-07)
(a) After prolong antibiotic therapy (b) Pantoprazole increase the risk (c) Associated with rectal thermometer (d) Increased with proportion of hospital stay

30) **Pseudo Membranous colitis, all are true except-** (AIIMS, May-07)
(a) Toxin A is responsible for clinical manifestation (b) Toxin B is responsible for clinical manifestation (c) Blood in stool is common feature (d) Summit lesion is early histopathological finding

31) **True regarding Pseudo Membranous colitis are all, except-** (AI -00)
(a) It is caused by *Clostridium difficile* (b) Organism is normal commensal of gut (c) It is due to production of phospholipsae A (d) It is treated by vancomycin

Clostridium tertium

32) **True about *Clostridium tertium*-** (PGI-08)
(a) Gram variable (b) Terminal spores (c) Produces the exotoxin (d) Causes septic arthritis

Answers of MCQs & explanation

1) **(a) & (d)**
- Follow section, **classification (table-2)** for explanation

2) **(d)**
- Follow section, ***Cl. perfringens*(morphology)** for explanation

3) **(a) & (b)**
- Along with alpha toxin theta toxin play an important role in gas gangrene

4) (d)
- Gas gangrene is not due to *Clostridium botulinum* infection but due to *Clostridium perfringens*
- *Clostridium* species are not gram negative spore forming anaerobes, but they are gram positive spore forming anaerobes
- The clinical features are not due to release of protein endotoxin but due to due to release of enxotoxin
- Gas is invariable present in muscles compartments

5) (a) (b) & (c)
- *Clostridium perfringens* is causing gas gangrene in 60-80% cases
- It is the normal flora of human & animal intestine & normally present in human faeces
- *Clostridium perfringens* produces 12 distinct toxins, but the principle toxin is alpha toxin
- Option d: Follow section, ***Clostridium perfringens*** **(resistance)** for explanation

6) (b)
- It is due to alpha toxin, which is lecithinase

7) (a) & (b)
- IP of different bacteria causing gas gangrene is
  - *Cl. perfringens*: 10-48 hr (1-2 days)
  - *Cl. septicum*: 2-3 days
  - *Cl. novyi*: 5-6 days.
- If one option is required to choose, than go with 10-48 hr/1-2 days (option a), because 60-80% of gas gangrene is caused by *Cl. perfringens*

8) (a), (b), (c) & (d)
- Follow section, ***Clostridium perfringens*** **(pathogenicity → gas gangrene → bacteriology)** for explanation

9) (c) & (d)
- Underlying skin and muscles are also infected in gas gangrene
- Caused by alpha & theta toxins of *Clostridium perfringens* while tetanospasmin is produced by *Cl. tetani* which is responsible for tetanus
- Passive immunisation does not help & it is not advised

10) (b)
- Tetanus is common in developing countries where the climate is warm in summer months & in rural areas where soil is fertile by bacteria from the animal/human faeces
- Other options are already explained in text

11) (b), (c) & (e)
- *Cl. tetani* is gram +Ve spore forming anaerobes
- Slightest stimulation can produce generalised muscle spasm, but not seizure.

12) (a)
- Follow section, ***Clostridium tetani*** **(pathogenicity → pathogenesis & flow chart-1)** for explanation.

13) (b) & (e)
- Gram +Ve spore forming anaerobe
- Muscle enzymes are elevated
- Vegetative cell will die with metronidazole (drug of choice). Vancomycin, fidaxomi & bacitracin are other options

14) (c)
- Follow section, ***Clostridium tetani*** **[laboratory diagnosis → toxigenicity testing (in vivo)]** for explanation.

15) (b)
- Follow section, ***Clostridium tetani*** **(prophylaxis & table-3)** for explanation

16) (b)
- Patient is of category B. Follow section, ***Clostridium tetani*** **(prophylaxis & table-3)** for explanation

17) (d)
- Spores of some strains of *Cl. tetani* are destroyed by boiling in 5 minutes while spores of few strains are heat resistant & can survive boiling for 15-90 minutes. Spores can survive in soil (dry earth) for several years.
- After primary immunisation by DPT at 6, 10 & 14 weeks, 1st booster of DPT is given at 18-24 months followed by 2nd booster dose (DT only) at 5-6 year (school entry age).

18) (c)
19) (c)
20) (b)
} Follow section, *Clostridium botulinum* (pathogenesis & **flow chart-2)** for explanation

21) (d)
- Follow section, *Clostridium botulinum* **(pathogenicity → virulence factors)** for explanation

22) (a)
- Infant botulism is not caused by preformed toxin because spores 1st enters in gut by food specially via honey, germinate to vegetative form in gut to produce the toxin, so toxin is not preformed
- Other options: Follow section, *Clostridium botulinum* **(pathogenicity → virulence factors)** for explanation

23) (b)
- Botulism occurs by ingestion of preformed toxin in preserved food- meat or meat product, fish, sea foods, canned vegetables. Type F outbreak occurs specially with fish products.

24) (b)
25) (a)
} Other options: Follow section, *Clostridium botulinum* **(pathogenicity → pathogenesis & flow chart-2)** for explanation.

26) (a)
- Botulism is caused by exotoxin not by endotoxin
- For explanation of option b follow infant botulism
- For explanation of option c follow **flow chart-2**
- Retrospective diagnosis of botulism can be made by detecting the antitoxin from the patient's serum, but not seen in all cases

27) (b)
- Descending paralysis, blurring of vision, quadriparesis with areflexia & non-reactive pupilsare features of botulism due to bilateral cranial nerve involvement
- For more explanation follow **flow chart-2**.
- In poliomyelitis, diphtheria & porphyria pupil is reactive

28) (a) & (b)
- It block the release of acetylcholine
- Follow **table-1** for uses of toxin
- Botulinum toxin once bound leads to permanent dysfunction of that neuron. Recovery takes usually 3 months when dysfunctioned nerve terminal are replaced as a result of sprouting.

29) (a), (b) (c) & (d)
- Follow section, ***Clostridium difficile*** **(pathogenicity →host factors)** for explanation

30) (c)
- In pseudo membranous colitis, presence of blood in stool is uncommon feature

31) (c)
- Pseudo Membranous colitis is caused by*Clostridium difficile*
- Organism is normal commensal in gut of infant < 6 months & 2–5% of the adult population, but studies have shown that infection is not endogenous it is exogenous
- It is due to production of toxin A & toxin B as described earlier not due to phospholipsae A
- Metronidazole is the drug of choice & vancomycin is the other option

32) (a), (b) & (d)
- Follow section, ***Clostridium tertium*** for explanation

38 Mycobacterium tuberculosis

Learning heading & subheadings

- Meaning of mycobacteria:
- Synonym of mycobacteria:
- Classification of mycobacteria:

M. tuberculosis

Meaning of mycobacteria: **Myco** word derived from **mykes (greek) = mushroom (types of edible fungus),** because this bacterium has branching or filamentous pattern as like fungus.

Synonym of mycobacteria: All mycobacteria **called Acid Fast Bacilli** (AFB) because once stained resist decolourization with acid also.

Classification of mycobacteria:

A. ***Mycobacterium tuberculosis*** **complex / tubercle bacilli:** All species are know to cause tuberculosis in human or in animals.
1. **Human:** *M. tuberculosis.*
2. **Bovine:** *M. bovis* (in cattle).
3. **Human in West Africa:** *M. africanum,* intermediate between human & bovine & causing tuberculosis in West Africans by air borne route. Pathogenicity is lower than *M. tuberculosis.*
4. **Avian:** *M. avium* (in birds).
5. **Cold blooded** (fish, frog, lizard etc.): *M. marinum.*
6. **Murine:** *M. microti* (in voles = mouse like animal)
7. **Other cattle pathogen:** *M. caprae.*
8. **Seals pathogen:** *M. pinnipedii.*
9. **Others:** *M. canetti* similar to *M. africanum.*

B. **Lepra bacilli :** All species are know to cause leprosy in human or in animals.
1. **Human leprosy:** *M. leprae.*
2. **Rat leprosy:** *M. leprae murium.*

C. **Atypical mycobacteria:** (By Runyon, 1959): Not causing tuberculosis but tuberculosis like lesion (hence **called atypical mycobacteria**)
1. **Group-I: Called photochromogens.**
2. **Group-II: Called scotochromogens** .
3. **Group-III: Called nonphotochromogens (nonchromogens).**
4. **Group-IV: Called rapid growers.**

D. **Saprophytic mycobacteria:** Non pathogenic & living free in water, soil or over decaying materials.
1. **In smegma:** *M. smegmatism.*
2. **In butter:** *M. butyricum.*
3. **In grass:** *M. phlei.*
4. **In dung:** *M. stercoris.*

E. **Johne's bacillus:** *M. paratuberculosis* (chronic specific enteritis, paratuberculosis or Johne's disease).

F. **Causing skin ulcer (skin pathogens):**
1. *M. ulcerans* (*M buruli*).
2. *M. balnei* (*M. marinum*).

M. tuberculosis

❖ **History:** *M. tuberculosis* was identified & described on 24th March, 1882 by Robert Koch, for this reason the **world tuberculosis day** is fixed on 24th March. Robert Koch received the Nobel Prize in physiology or medicine in 1905 for this discovery.

❖ **Synonym (common name):** Also **called Koch's bacilli**, from the name of Dr. Robert Koch, who discovered the bacilli in 1882.

❖ **Morphology:**

➢ **Staining properties:** Following are the different stains used to stain the AFB.

✪ **Gram stain: Mycobacteria are GPB** but strictly not correct, because after primary staining with methyl violet they resist decolourisation with alcohol without iodine (no mean to use iodine & not following complete principle or all steps of gram stain hence strictly not considered as GPB).

✪ **Acid fast stains:**
- **ZN / hot (fig.-1) stain:**
- **Kinyoun's / cold stain:**

} Follow chapter → Microscopy and staining

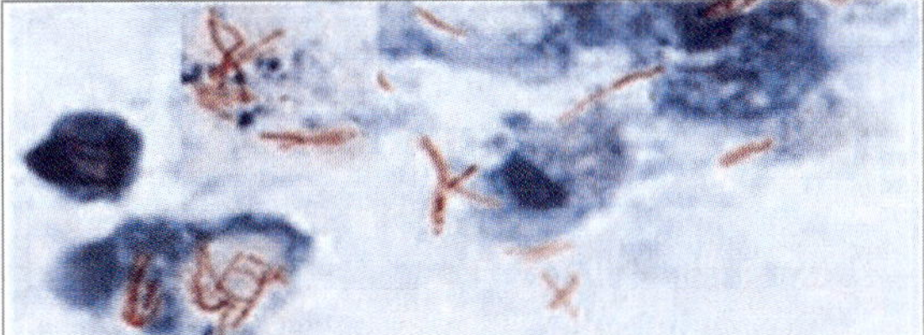

Figure-1: ***M tuberculosis*** **under ZN stain**

✪ **Fluorescent stain:**

- **Principle:** It uses the auramine phenol (mixture of auramine-O + phenol) stain as primary stain, acid alcohol as decolouriser & potassium permanganate as counter stain.
- **Steps:**
- Smears are prepared just like that for ZN staining.
- Stain with auramine-phenol for 20 minutes (other dye used is rhodamine).
- Rinse with water.
- Decolourise in acid alcohol.
- Rinse with water.
- Counter stain with 0.1% potassium permanganate for 30 seconds.
- Rinse and air dry.
- Examine the smear under fluorescent microscope.
- **Result:** Bacilli stain yellow rods in dark field as shown in **fig.-2.**

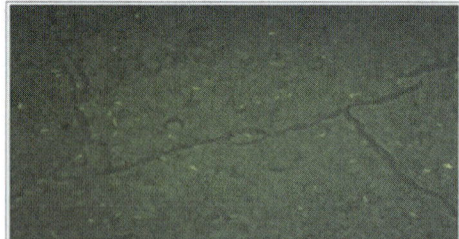

Figure-2: *M tuberculosis* under fluorescent stain

- **Advantages:** More sensitive & rapid than acid fast stains.
- **Disadvantages:** Hazards of dye toxicity & more expensive.

➢ **Size:** 3μm × 0.3μm.
➢ **Shape:** Straight or slightly curved club & branching shape.
➢ **Arrangement:** Singly, pair or in group.
➢ Nonmotile, nonsporing & non-capsulated.
➢ **Protoplast** forms in presence of lysozyme **& L-forms** are also present.
➢ **Cell wall:** Follow chapter → Morphology of bacteria.
➢ It is very important to **differentiate** *M. tuberculosis* from *M. bovis* as mentioned in **table-1.**

❖ Cultural characteristics (C/Cs):

➢ **Effective factors:**
- O_2 effect, 0.5% glycerol effect & type of growth: **Table 1**
- Optimum temperature: 37°C
- Optimum pH -6.4 – 7.0
- Time: Grow very slowly in 2-8 weeks & generation time is 20 hrs.

➢ **Culture in media:**

✪ **Advantages of culture:**
- It is more sensitive than microscopy as it can detect up to 10-100 bacilli per ml of sputum while for microscopy to be positive, sputum should contai10^4 bacilli/ml.
- It maintains the viability of microbes.

Features		*M. tuberculosis*	*M. bovis*
Morphology under ZN stain	Length	Long	Short
	Shape	Curved	Straight
	Strength	Beaded or barred	Stout
	Staining property	No uniform stain. Beaded or barred forms can be seen	Uniform stain
	Fast to	Acid (25%) & alcohol (95%)	Only acid
Cultural characteristic	O_2 effect	Obligate aerobe.	Microaerophilic on primary isolation, become aerobic on subculture.
	0.5% glycerol	Improve the growth	No effect / impair the growth
	Type of growth	Grow luxuriously on media hence **called 'eugonic'**	Grow sparsely on media hence **called 'dysgonic'**
	C/Cs on solid media	Dry, rough, raised, irregular, creamy-white colonies (**fig.-3**) become buff/yellow on longer incubation	Moist, smooth, flat, regular, white colonies which easily break-up when touched
B/ Rs	Nitrate reduction	+Ve	-Ve
	Niacin test	+Ve	-Ve
	TCH/T_2H test	Resistance	Sensitive
	Tween 80 hydrolysis	Variable	Always -Ve
Mode of transmission		- Inhalation - Ingestion - Inoculation - Congenital (by placenta)	- Ingestion of raw milk from infected cattle
Reservoir of infection		Human	Animal like cattle
Source of infection		Respiratory droplet	Infected milk of cattle
Animal pathogenicity		Pathogenic to guinea pig	Pathogenic to guinea pig & rabbit
Infectivity to human		Both are equally pathogenic for human	

Table 1: Differences between *M. tuberculosis* & *M. bovis*

- **Disadvantages of culture:** It is a time consuming method & required 8-12 weeks incubation before giving negative report.
- **Media:** Three type's media like liquid, solid & selective.

A. Liquid media:

- **Name of liquid media:**

1. Beck's medium
2. Dubo's medium
3. Middlebrook 7H9 and 7H12 media
4. Proskauer medium
5. Sula's medium
6. Sauton's medium

- **Uses of liquid media:**

1. Sensitivity testing.
2. Biochemical reactions.
3. Antigen preparation.
4. Vaccine preparation.

- **C/Cs in liquid media: →Flow chart-1**

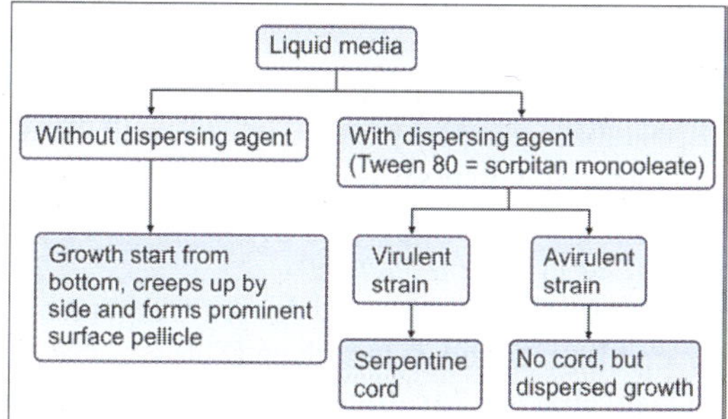

Flow chart-1: C/Cs in liquid media

B. Solid media:

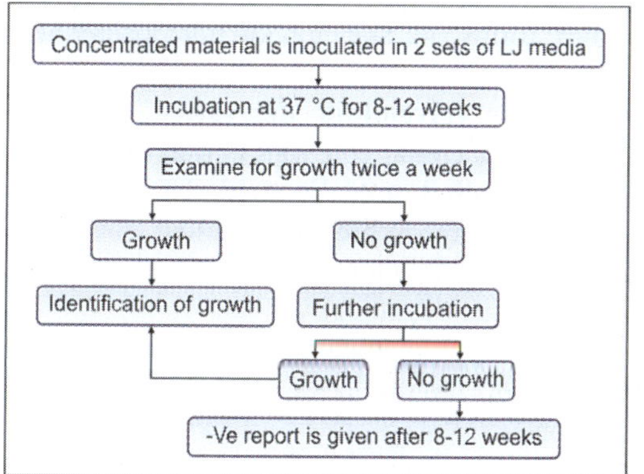

Flow chart-2: Cultivation technique in solid media

- **Name of solid media:**

1. Egg based media
   - Lowenstein-Jensen (LJ) medium.
   - Petragnini medium.
   - Dorset egg medium.
2. Blood based: Tarshis medium.
3. Potato based: Pawlowsky medium.
4. Serum based: Loeffler medium.
5. Agar based: Middlebrook7H10 & 7H11 media.

- **Use of solid media:** LJ medium is most useful & selective medium & recommended by IUAT (International Union Against Tuberculosis) for culture.
- **Cultivation technique in solid media: → Flow chart-2**
- **C/Cs in solid media:→ Table 1**

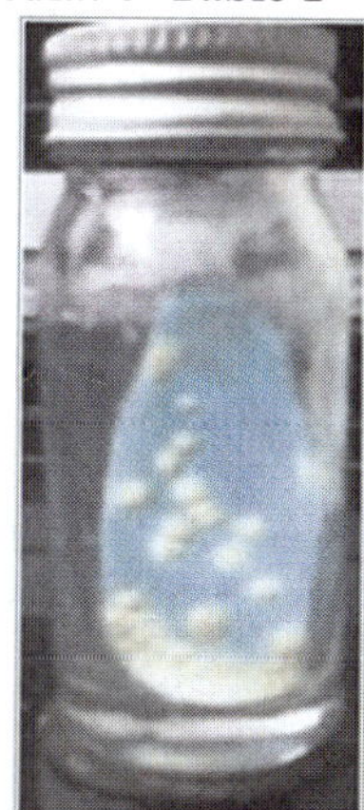

Figure-3: *M tuberculosis* in LJ medium

C. Selective media: Prepared by adding antibiotics in liquid/solid media like polymyxin B, amphotericin B, nalidixic acid, trimethoprim & azlocillin.

➢ **Automated (newer) culture technique:**

1. **BACTEC system: Principle →** ^{14}C labelled palmitic acid is converted in to^{14} CO_2 by bacterial metabolism. $^{14}CO_2$ index is measured for interpretation of result.
2. **MGIT** (Mycobacteria Growth Indicator Tube): **Principle →** Mycobacteria utilise the O_2 within the tube & growth is detected by O_2 quenched fluorescent dyes.
3. **MB/BacT system** (as like BacT/Alert)**: Principle →** Based on colorimetric detection of CO_2.
4. **BacT/Alert system: Principle →** Based on colorimetric detection of pH change due to CO_2 production by *M tuberculosis.*
5. **ESP** (Extra Sensing Power) **culture system-II: Principle →** Detection of pressure change in a headspace of sealed culture bottle.

➢ **Culture in animals:**

1. **Guinea pig:**

- **Pathogenicity testing:**
  - Both *M. tuberculosis* & *M. bovis* both are pathogenic for guinea pig.
  - Inoculate concentrated material intramuscularly into thigh of 2-guinea pigs (12 wks age).
  - The animals are weighed before inoculation and at intervals thereafter, progressive loss of weight and positive tuberculin test indicate the infection.
  - One animal is killed after 4 weeks and autopsied. If it shows no evidence of tuberculosis, another is autopsied after 8 weeks.
- **Autopsy findings of animal:**

- Draining and internal lymph nodes are enlarged.
- Tubercles seen in peritoneum, lung, at site of inoculation but not in kidney.
- Autopsy lesions have to be confirmed by acid fast staining.

2. **Rabbit:** *M. bovis* is pathogenic to rabbit but not the *M. tuberculosis.*

❖ Biochemical reaction (B/Rs):

➢ **Tests to differentiate *M tuberculosis* from *M bovis:***

1. Nitrate reduction
2. Niacin
3. TCH/T_2H (Thiopen$_2$ Carboxylic acid Hydrazine)
4. Tween 80 hydrolysis:

(1–4: Follow **table -1**)

➢ **Tests to differentiate *M tuberculosis* from atypical mycobacteria: → Table -2**

Tests	*M. tuberculosis*	Atypical *Mycobacteria*
Catalase	Weak +Ve	Strong +Ve
Peroxidase test	Strong +Ve	Weak +Ve
Amidase test	-Ve	+Ve
Aryl sulphatase test	-Ve	+Ve

Table -2: Tests to differentiate *M tuberculosis* from atypical mycobacteria

❖ Resistance:

- Bacteria remain viable in sputum for 20-30 hr, in droplet nuclei for 8-10 days & in culture for 6-8 months.
- They are relatively resistance to disinfectant like 5% phenol, 15% H_2SO_4, 3% nitric acid, 5% oxalic acid & 4% NaOH.
- Killed by heat at 60^0C in 15-20 minutes, sunlight after 2 hours exposure, 80% ethanol in 2-10 min, tincture iodine in 5 minutes, formaldehyde & gluteraldehyde.

❖ Epidemiological typing:

A Phenotyping methods:

i. Bacteriophage typing: Follow chapter → Laboratory diagnosis of bacterial infections

ii. Bacteriocin typing:

B Genotyping methods:

1. **RFLP:** Done by using IS (Insertion Sequence) 6110.
2. **Spoligotyping (spacer oligotyping):** Based on polymorphism in the direct repeat locus.
3. **PFGE**
4. **DNA sequencing**

❖ Pathogenicity:

➢ **Disease :**

- **Called tuberculosis / Koch's disease.**
- About 1/3 of world's population is died due to tuberculosis, so **called 'the captain of the men death'.**
- It has been termed as **white plague.**

➢ **Nature & history of disease:**

- Tuberculosis has been present in humans since the time of Hippocrates.
- About one-third of the world's population has been infected with *M. tuberculosis* of which 90–95% remains asymptomatic while 5-10% progress to clinical disease.
- India carries 25% cases out of total global cases.
- In India, 2 deaths/minute, >1000 deaths/day & 0.37 million deaths/year occurs due to tuberculosis.

➢ **Reservoir & source of infection: →Table-1**

➢ **Mode of transmission: → Table 1**

➢ **Incubation period:** 3-8 weeks.

➢ **Portal of entry:** Respiratory system.

➢ **Sites:** Pulmonary & extra pulmonary organs.

➢ **Precipitating factors (epidemiological determinants):** Three types as follows.

I. Agent factors (virulence factors)

a. Intracellular location: Ability of *Mycobacterium* to survive & to multiply in the macrophage helps to escape the effect of antibiotics & host immunity. Lipoarabinogalactan present in cell wall, facilitate the intracellular survival of *M. tuberculosis.*

b. Antigens: Following three types of antigens are identified in *Mycobacteria.*

1. **Proteins:** Group specific is Ag responsible for tuberculin reaction & to induce DTH.
2. **Polysaccharide (arabinogalactan):** Type specific Ag. Exact role in pathogenesis is uncertain but induce immediate type of hypersensitivity (ITH). Peptidoglycan-polysaccharide-mycolic acid complex forms the skeleton of mycobacterial cell wall.
3. **Cord factor (glycolipid derivative or mycolic acid):** Mycobacterial cell wall is rich in long chain fatty acids **called mycolic acid.** Unique mycolic acid 6,6 □ dimycolyltrehalose **called cord factor** which is responsible for
   - Cell membrane cytotoxicity.
   - Activation of complement pathway.
   - Inhibition of migration of PMNs → granuloma formation.
   - Inhibition of phagolysosome formation→ inhibition of lysis by macrophage.
   - Development of immunity.
   - Bacilli to grow in serpentine cord (parallel arrangement of bacilli).

c. Drug resistance: Resistance to antituberculous drugs is due to point mutation in regulatory genes. It occurs at a rate of once in 10^8 cell divisions. Drugs & related genes responsible for resistance are mentioned in **table-3.**

d. Regulatory genes:

1. **Drug resistance genes: → Table-3**

2. **rpo V:** The main sigma factor initiating the transcription of many genes.
3. **erp gene:** It encodes for production of proteins necessary for bacterial multiplication.
4. **RD-1 (Region of difference-1):** Encodes for early secretory antigen target-6 (ESAT-6) & culture filtrate protein -10 (CFP-10).
5. **Other genes:** Leu D, Pan CD, Sig C (Sigma factor C), Sig H (Sigma factor H) & Car D genes.

Drugs	Genes
Isoniazide (H)	**Kat G** (Catalase & oxidase) **inhA** (Enoyl ACP reductase) **Ahpc** (Alkyl hydroperoxide reductase)
Rifampicin (R)	**rpo B** (RNA polymerase subunit B)
Pyrazinamide (Z)	**pncA** (pyrazinamidase)
Ethambutol (E)	**rpsL** (Ribosomal protein subunit 12)
Streptomycin (S)	**rpsL** (Ribosomal protein subunit 12) **rrs** (16s ribosomal RNA) **strA** (Aminoglycoside phosphotransferase gene)
Fluoroquinolones	**gyr A & B** (DNA gyrase)

Table-3: Drug resistance genes in *M tuberculosis*

II. Host factors

1. **Age:** Common in all ages.
2. **Sex:** Common in male than females.
3. **Heredity:** Tuberculosis is not a hereditary disease but study shows that inherited susceptibility is a risk factor.
4. **Nutrition:** Widely prevalent in malnourished individual.
5. **Immunity:** IDDs like HIV-AIDS is the major risk factor for increasing the incidence & prevalence of tuberculosis. Association between tuberculosis & HIV is described below in details.
6. **Others:** Smoking, drug abuse, poor hygiene, lack of education etc.

III. Socio-economical factors

- Overcrowding, poverty, large family, population exposure etc.

➢ **Types & pathological aspects of tuberculosis: → Flow chart-3**

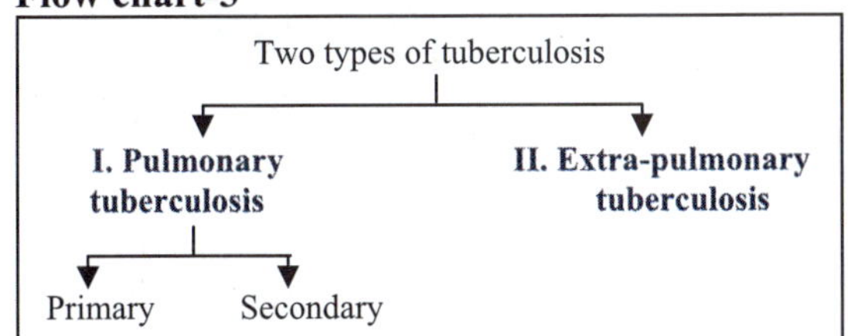

Flow chart-3: Types of tuberculosis

I. Pulmonary tuberculosis

A. Primary tuberculosis / Ghon's complex / childhood tuberculosis:

✪ **Definition:** Initial infection in host who has not been previously infected / sensitised **called primary tuberculosis.**

✪ **Sites:** Lower lobe / lower part of upper lobe, tonsils, cervical & mesenteric lymph nodes & small intestine.

✪ **Pathogenesis:**

i. Pathogenesis of *M. tuberculosis*:

- Generally tubercle bacilli survive in the macrophages. They lyse the macrophages & later infect the other macrophages.
- Humoral immunity has no role but CMI plays the major role to interact with the infected macrophages. CD4+ helper cells differentiate in Th1 cells & Th2 cells.
- Th1 releases the cytokines which activates the pulmonary alveolar macrophages to kill the intracellular bacilli of macrophages while Th2 releases the cytokines that are responsible for DTH & progression of tuberculosis as shown in **flow chart-4 & fig.-4.**

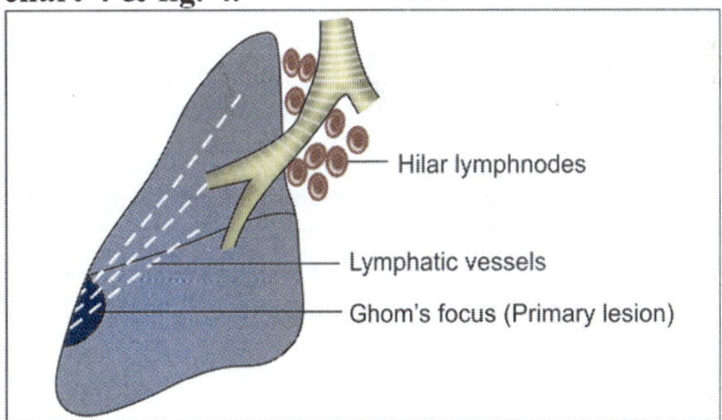

Figure-4: Ghon's complex

ii. Pathogenesis of *M. bovis*: →Flow chart-5

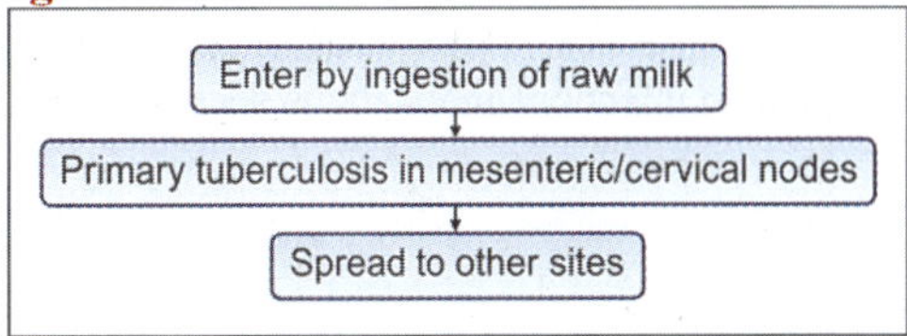

Flow chart-5: Pathogenesis of *M bovis*

B. Secondary tuberculosis / reinfection / chronic tuberculosis / adult type tuberculosis:

✪ **Definition:** Infection in host who has been previously infected / sensitised **called secondary tuberculosis.**

✪ **Sites:** Apical lungs & other sites are like tonsils, pharynx, larynx, small intestine & skin.

✪ **Pathogenesis: → Flow chart-6**

➢ **Differences between primary & secondary tuberculosis: → Table-4**

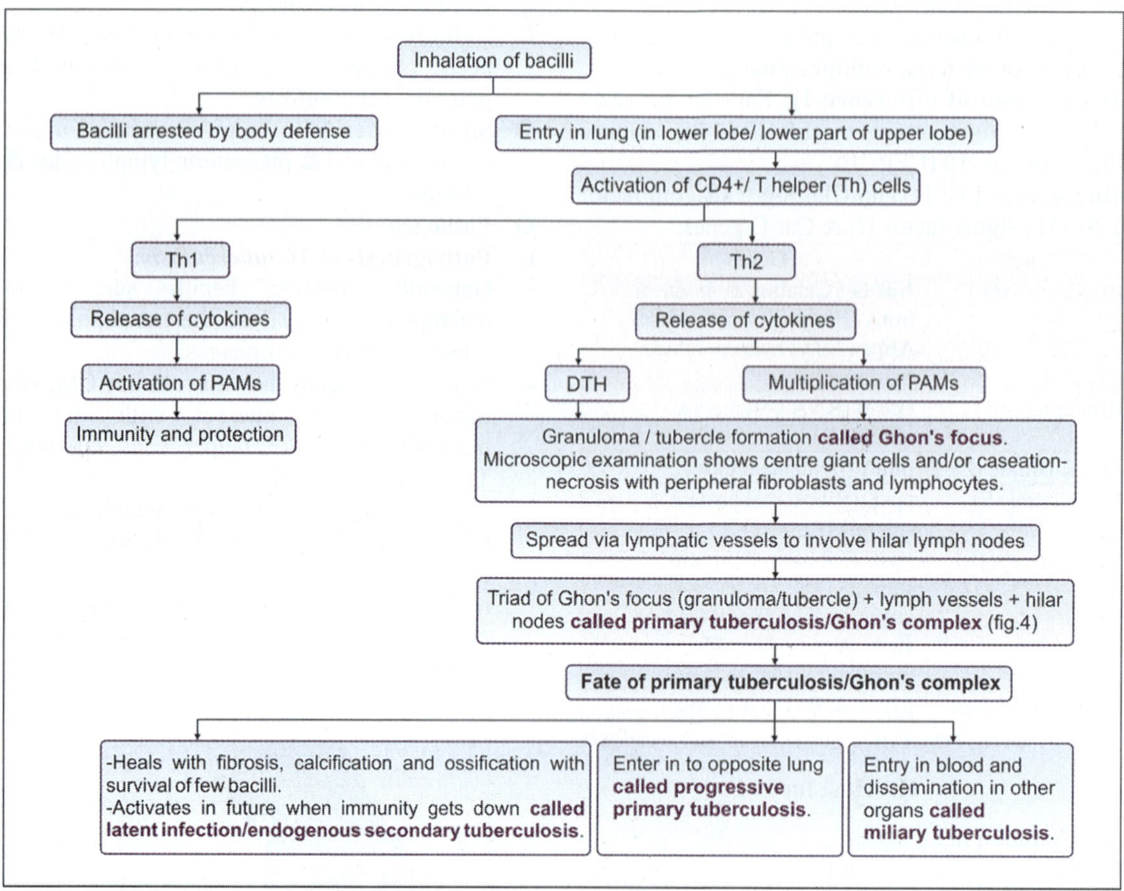

Flow chart-4: Pathogenesis of *M tuberculosis*

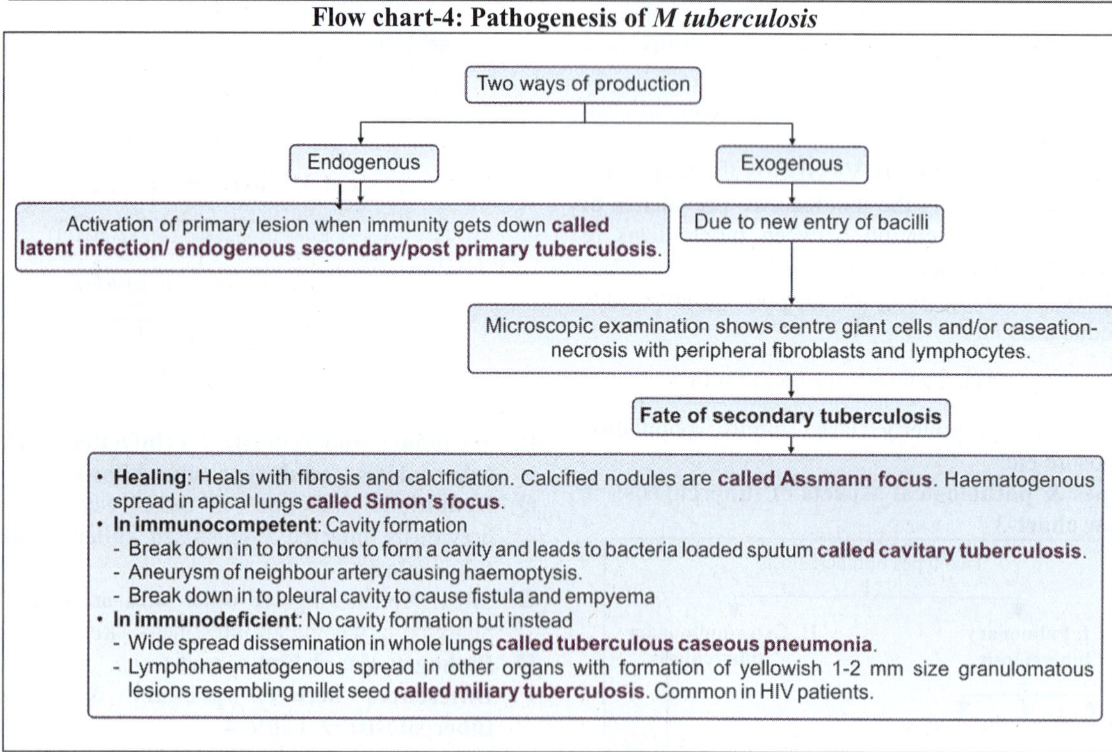

Flow chart-6: Pathogenesis of secondary tuberculosis

Features	Primary tuberculosis	Secondary tuberculosis
Other name	Ghon's complex / Childhood tuberculosis	Reinfection / chronic / adult type tuberculosis
Past infection	No	Yes
Age	In children	In adults
Mode of entry	Exogenous	Exogenous & endogenous
Sites	Affects middle & lower lobe / lower part of upper lobe	Affects apical lungs
Lesion	Small	Large
Lymph node involvement	Common (hilar nodes)	Rare
Cavity formation	Rare	Common
Local spread	Rare	Common
Tuberculin test	-Ve in initial stage	+Ve
Clinical features	• **Respiratory:** - Asymptomatic - Productive cough with or without haemoptysis - Pleural effusion - Dyspnoea & - Orthopnoea • **General:** Low grade evening rise fever, weight loss, fatigue, anorexia & night sweat.	Symptoms are same but more pronounced

Table -4: Differences between primary & secondary tuberculosis

II. Extra-pulmonary tuberculosis

✪ **Incidence:** Extra-pulmonary tuberculosis occurs in 15-20% of all cases of pulmonary tuberculosis. In HIV patient it is 20-50%.

✪ **Origin & spread:** → **Flow chart-7**

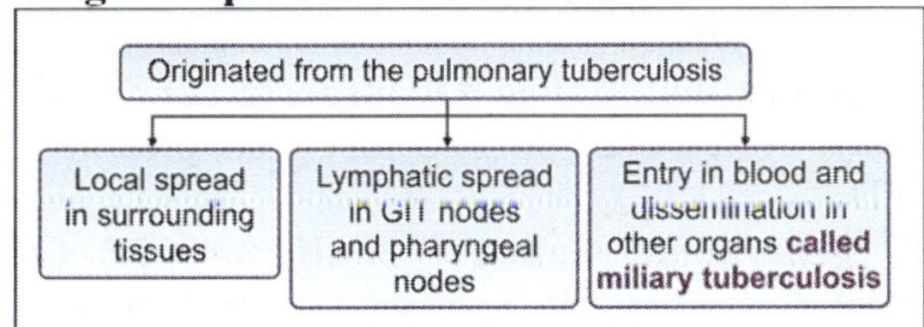

Flow chart-7: Pathogenesis of extra-pulmonary tuberculosis

✪ **Sites:** It can affect any organs but clinically significant sites are mentioned below.

- **Most common sites:**
  - Lymph node (35%) is the most common site for extra-pulmonary tuberculosis.
  - It mostly affects the cervical & supraclavicular lymphnodes **called scrofula / scrophula / King's evil.**
  - Scrofula is caused by *M. tuberculosis* as well as by atypical mycobacteria.
  - It preset as painless swelling without warmth or colour changes. The nodes are usually discrete in early stage but inflamed & produce fistula or sinus which drains the caseous materials.
- **Other sites:**
  - <u>Pleural cavity:</u> It occurs in 20% cases & present with pleural effusion.
  - <u>Pericardium:</u> It occurs due to direct spread from adjacent nodes or by haematogenous spread. Common in older age group.
  - <u>Urinary system:</u> **Called renal tuberculosis.**
  - <u>Genital system:</u> Epididymis in male & fallopian tube in female are the most commonly infected organs.
  - <u>Skin:</u> Different verities of cutaneous tuberculosis are mentioned below.
    1. Lupus vulgaris (55%): It is the most common variety of cutaneous tuberculosis & it is present with caseation necrosis.
    2. Scrofuloderma (27%): It is the 2nd most common variety of cutaneous tuberculosis resulting from extension of scrofula which involves the cervical & supraclavicular lymph nodes with skin. It also **called tuberculosis cutis colliquativa.**
    3. Tuberculids (7%).
    4. Tuberculosis verucosis (6%).
    5. Tubercular gumma (5%).
  - <u>Skeletal</u>:
    1. Pott's disease or tuberculous spondylitis: It is the infection in spine.
    2. Other skeletal organs: Hips & knee are also infected. With advanced disease, collapse of vertebral bodies result in kyphosis (gibbus) & a paravertebral cold abscess may also form.
  - <u>Meninges:</u> Common in children. Tuberculous meningitis (low grade fever, headache, vomiting, neck stiffness etc.) & tuberculoma are the common forms.
  - <u>GIT:</u>
    - Caused by both *M. tuberculosis* & *M. bovis.*
    - *M. bovis* is transmitted by ingestion of milk of infected cow (in developing countries).
    - *M. tuberculosis* is transmitted by swallowing of sputum (common in children) or by haematogenous spread.
    - Terminal ileum & caecum are the commonest sites to be infected.
  - <u>Oral cavity:</u>
    - Irregular, painful tuberculous ulcer mostly present on tongue followed by palate, buccal mucosa, lips, gingival & floor of oral cavity. Sometimes diffuse inflammatory lesions or fissures are also present.
    - Haematogenous spread from oral lesions causing tuberculous osteomyelitis in mandible & maxilla in later stage of disease.

- Bacilli are diagnosed from biopsy lesion, however numbers are very less tough to diagnose by microscopy while culture gives good results.

➢ **Complications:** Death usually due to pulmonary insufficiency, pulmonary haemorrhage, secondary amyloidosis, cor-pulmonale or sepsis by miliary tuberculosis.

❖ **Laboratory diagnosis:** It is discussed separately for pulmonary & extra pulmonary cases as below.

Diagnosis of pulmonary tuberculosis

➢ **Specimens:**
- Two sputum samples: Spot & next day early morning before meal.
- Bronchial washing & laryngeal swab are collected when sputum is not available.
- Gastric aspiration in child & in adult patient who swallow the sputum.

➢ **Transport of specimens:**
- If delay about more than 2 hour is expected then refrigerated the samples to prevent multiplication of flora.
- If more delay is expected equal volume of CPC (cetyl pyridium chloride)-NaCl solution is added to sputum. It liquefies the sputum, prevent the growth of other bacteria & also maintain the viability up to 8 days.
- Pleural fluid should be collected in citrated bulb.

➢ **Preparation of specimens:** Methods used to prepare the specimens **called concentration / homogenisation / digestion-decontamination methods** which are of following two types.

a. Preparation of specimens for microscopy:
- Required killed bacilli without alteration of morphology or staining reaction.
- **Methods:** Treat the specimens with

1. Sodium carbonate or hypochlorite.
2. Antiformin.
3. Detergents like tergitol.
4. Autoclave method.
5. Flotation methods by using hydrocarbons.

b. Preparation of specimens for culture & animal inoculation:
- Required live bacilli.
- **Methods:**

1. **Petroff's method:** Mix sputum + equal volume of 4% NAOH → Incubation at 37^0C & frequent shaking for 20 min → Centrifuge at 3000rpm, 20 min. → discard the supertant & neutralised the sediment with 0.1 N HCL and used for culture & animal inoculation.
2. **Cetrimonium bromide method**: Mix sputum with equal volume of sterile solution (containing 20 g cetrimonium bromide + 40 g of NaOH per litre of distilled water) → mixed with a cotton swab; stand for 5 min. → 0.2 ml of mixture is smeared firmly with swab over LJ medium. Same swab is used for inoculating second slope after stirring contents again.
3. **Other homogenisation methods:**
   - N- Acetyl L-Cysteine (NALC).
   - Pancreatin.
   - Cetrimide.
   - By treatment with dilute acids (6% H_2SO_4, 3% HCL or 5% oxalic acid).

➢ **Testing methods:**

I. **Microscopy: →Follow morphology**
II. **Culture: → Follow C/Cs**
III. **Biochemical reaction:→ Follow B/Rs**
IV. **Serological test:** Three types of test.

A Detection of Ag:
- Various antigens like lipoarabinomannan & Ag-5 are detected by ELISA, dip stick & latex agglutination tests from clinical samples like sputum, urine etc.
- Tests are less useful because of low sensitivity (40-50%).

B Detection of Ab:
- Less useful because of cross reactivity by atypical mycobacteria & also by other antigens.
- In 2013 WHO banned IgM ELISA because of high rate of false positivity.

C Interferon Gamma Release Assay (IGRA):

✪ **Principle:** Based on detection of γ-interferon released by sensitised T lymphocytes.

✪ **Methods:**
- Sensitised T lymphocytes are collected from suspected case, are exposed to ESAT-6 & CFP-10, which leads to release of γ-interferon from the sensitised T lymphocytes. This γ-interferon is detected by ELISA, which is classified in following three categories.

i. **1st generation: Called Quantiferon –TB (QFT) assay.** It responds to one tuberculo protein like PPD.

ii. **2nd generation: Called Quantiferon –TB Gold (QFT-G) assay.** It responds to two tuberculo proteins like (1) early secretory antigen target-6 (ESAT-6) & (2) culture filtrate protein -10 (CFP-10). Both are secreted by *M. tuberculosis, M. bovis, M. kansasi, M. szulgai* & *M. marinum*, hence test can not differentiate between these organisms.

iii. **3rd generation: Called Quantiferon –TB Gold In Tube (QFT-GIT) assay.** It responds to three tuberculo proteins like (1) ESAT-6, (2) CFP-10 & (3) TB 7.7.

✪ **Advantages:** Highly specific & no chances of false positive result.

V. **Molecular:** PCR, LCR, LPA, TMA, SDA, NASBA etc.

VI. **Epidemiological typing:** → Vide supra

VII. **Chromatography:** GLC & HPLC for mycolic acid detection.

VIII. **Allergic test: Called tuberculin test.**

- **History:** It was discovered by Von Pirquet in 1907.
- **Principle:** Based on DTH (Delayed Type Hypersensitivity).
- **Antigens:**
- **Types:** Two types.

1. **OT (Old Tuberculin):** It is a crude preparation of tubercle bacilli. It was used in past. It was described by Robert Koch.
2. **PPD (Purified Protein Derivative):** OT is replaced by PPD.

- **Preparation:**
  - PPD is prepared by Siebert in 1941 by growing the human strain of *M. tuberculosis* (PPD-S) in semisynthetic medium.
  - It also prepared from other *Mycobacteria* like Batty bacilli (PPD-B), *M. kansasi* (PPD-Y), *M. scrofulaceum* (scrofulin) etc. However they may cross react.
- **Standardisation:** It is standardised in terms of tuberculin unit (TU). International standardisation is maintained by WHO. One TU is equal to 0.01ml of OT or 0.00002mg PPD. The WHO advocates a PPD tuberculin known as PPD-RT-23 with tween 80.

- **Methods:** Two methods.

a. Single puncture method:

1. Mantoux test

- **Steps:**
  - Inject 0.1 ml-PPD, intradermally (inbetween the layers of skin not subcutaneously) on flexor aspect of forearm with tuberculin syringe.
  - Site examined after 48-72 hours.
- **Result:**
  - Don't consider the erythema as it is difficult to measure. Measure only induration at its widest point transversely to long axis of forearm by ruler or caliper (in terms of length not breadth).
  - Negative: ≤ 5 mm.
  - Doubtful/equivocal (false positive?): 6-9 mm.
  - Positive: ≥ 10 mm.
  - Strong reactor: ≥ 20 mm.
- **Interpretation:**
  - False -Ve test: Overwhelming (fulminant) tuberculosis including miliary tuberculosis, convalescence from some viral infections (like measles, chickenpox, glandular fever), lymphoreticular malignancy, sarcoidosis, malnutrition, immunosuppressive disease or therapy (steroids), impaired CMI, inactive PPD preparations or faulty technique.
  - -Ve test: Never contacted with tubercle bacilli & at more risk to develop tuberculosis than 6-9 mm group.
  - False +Ve test (doubtful/equivocal): Infections by related mycobacteria (atypical mycobacteria).
  - +Ve test:
    - Positive result in adult (Type IV Hypersensitivity to tuberculoprotein) indicates the exposure of bacilli either recently or in past due to infection or vaccination with or without active tuberculosis, so adult who had never contacted to tubercle bacilli are gives negative result.
    - Positive result in children below 2 years is an indirect evidence of active tuberculosis even if it is not manifest.
    - Test becomes positive 4-6 weeks after infection & 8-14 weeks after immunisation.
    - Positive result may revert to negative result (occasionally) on isoniazide treatment.
  - Strong reactor: At greater risk to develop tuberculosis ≥ 10 mm group.
- **Uses:** Mantoux test is useful
  - To diagnose the infection in infant & young child.
  - To detect the successful vaccination.
  - To know the prevalence of tuberculosis, this is calculated by counting all tuberculin reactors in a community.
  - To know the incidence of tuberculosis, this is calculated by counting new converter to tuberculin test in a community.
  - To know the prognosis: Strong reactors (≥ 20 mm) are at greater risk to develop tuberculosis than ≥ 10 mm group, while tuberculin negative (≤ 5 mm) have more risk of developing tuberculosis than 6-9 mm group. In short, ≤ 5 mm & ≥ 20 mm are at high risk to develop tuberculosis. Studies indicate that among the new cases, around 92% are strong reactors. These findings justify the prognostic significance of the test.
- **Repeated (two steps) tuberculin testing:** It will not cause positive reaction in non infected person, but may enhance intensity (**called booster effect**) of response in reactive individuals, so another tuberculin test following 1-2 weeks later will give strong reactor.
- **Tuberculin conversion:** It is a condition at where negative result (≤ 5 mm) turns to positive result (≥ 10 mm) within a 24 months period. It indicates the latent tuberculosis infection which may turn to active disease.
- **Limitations:** Despite following limitations tuberculin test is the only tool to measure the prevalence of tuberculosis.

1. **Validity of test:** It is variable due to faulty technique, errors in reading the result, test materials used etc.

2. **Lack of specificity & sensitivity:** Due to cross reaction by other mycobacteria & also by booster effect.
3. **DTH:** DTH measured by tuberculin test is irrelevant to combat the disease. It does not indicate whether the person is able to mount an immune response to tubercle bacilli or not (as in lepromin test).
4. **Susceptibility:** It does not indicate the resistance or susceptibility to tubercle bacilli (as in Schick test).

b. **Multiple puncture method:**

1. **Heaf test:**
- Used for screening & survey in large group but not for diagnosis.
- It is quick, cheap, reliable & easy to perform.
2. **Tine test:** Used for individual testing, but not reliable so not recommended.

IX. **Drug sensitivity testing:**

- **Absolute concentration method:** Media containing serial concentrations of drugs are inoculated and Minimum Inhibitory Concentrations (MIC) is calculated.
- **Resistance ratio method:** Two sets of media containing graded concentrations of drugs are inoculated. 1st with test strain and 2nd with standard strain of known sensitivity.
- **Proportion method:** Numbers of colonies growing on LJ media with or without drug is compared. Strain is resistant if more than 1% of the bacteria grow on LJ with drug.
- **Automated method by using BACTEC MGIT**
- **Molecular methods:** PCR based assay, line probe assay & DNA microarray.

X. **Other tests:** Detection of tuberculo-stearic acid & adenosine deaminase (ADA) are also useful method.

✓ **Note: Methods of diagnosis of latent tuberculosis**

- Tuberculin test } Vide supra
- IGRA }

Diagnosis of extra-pulmonary tuberculosis

➢ **Specimens:**

- CSF in tuberculous meningitis: CSF shows the cobweb coagulum on standing, elevated CSF pressure, raised proteins, raised chloride, increased lymphocytes count & decreased glucose level.
- Urine in renal tuberculosis: Bacilli are shedding very intermittently in urine, hence 3-6 consecutive early morning urine samples are collected, centrifuged & use sediment for processing. Acid alcohol is used as decolouriser.
- Blood
- Pleural fluid
- Pus in cold abscess
- Bone & joint fluid
- Lymph node aspirate.

➢ **Testing methods:**

I. **Microscopy:** Extra pulmonary specimens are containing less numbers of bacilli so less useful.
II. **Culture:** Also a useful method.
III. **Serological test:** IGRA is best method.
IV. **Molecular:** Best useful method.
V. **Other method:** Adenosine deaminase (ADA) detection.

❖ Prevention:

A. **General measures:** Adequate nutrition, good housing and health education.
B. **Immunoprophylaxis:** Active immunisation by using BCG vaccine.

✪ **Full name:** Bacille Calmette Guerin vaccine.

✪ **History:** Developed by Calmette and Guerin in 1921 in France.

✪ **Preparation:**

- It is live attenuated vaccine prepared from strain of *M. bovis* attenuated by 239 serial subcultures in glycerine-bile-potato medium over period of 13 years. It is available in 0.5-1.0mg dry powder form in ampules containing 1-2.5 × 10^7 Colony Forming Units (CFU).
- In India, WHO recommended **Danish 1331** strain of BCG for preparation of vaccine. It is prepared in BCG laboratory, Guindy, Chennai, India.

✪ **Types:** Two forms are available.

1. Liquid (fresh) form: Less stable form.
2. Lyophilised (freeze dries) form: Most stable & widely used form.

✪ **Administration & dose:**

- Lyophilised form is suspended in 1ml sterile water. Don't use distilled water, as it is irritant.
- Once reconstituted, it should be used in 1 hour, not later.
- Don't sterile skin by using the alcohol.
- 0.05ml in neonate & 1 ml in older children, injected intradermally just above the insertion of left deltoid by using 26 swg tuberculin syringe.
- It is given immediately after birth or as early as possible before 12 month. If not given than vaccine can be given maximum up to 2 year of age.
- Direct BCG: Given to new born immediately after birth in developing countries including India.
- Indirect BCG: Given after tuberculin testing.

✪ **Changes following proper BCG vaccination:** → **Flow chart-8**

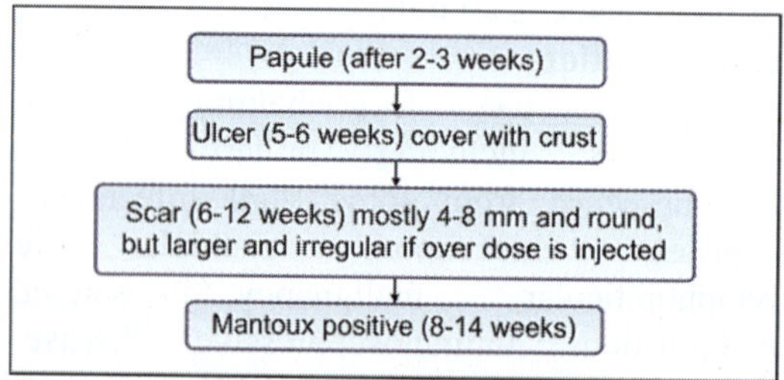

Flow chart-8: Changes following proper BCG vaccination

- **Efficacy:** Variable efficacy from 0-80%. Immunity may last for 15-20 years.
- **Complications:** Three types

1. **Local:** Abscess, indolent ulcer, keloid, tuberculides, confluent lesions, lupoid lesions or lupus vulgaris.
2. **Regional:** Enlargement and suppuration of draining lymph nodes.
3. **General:** Fever, mediastinal adenitis, erythema nodosum, progressive tuberculosis, disseminated BCG infection (BCGitis) or rarely nonfatal meningitis.

- **Uses:**

1. BCG vaccine does not protect the person from TB, but give protection to infant and children against serious type of infection like disseminated tuberculosis & tubercular meningitis.
2. Provide protection against leprosy and leukemia by non-specific stimulation.
3. Adjuvant therapy: Multiple injection of BCG vaccine (**called Onco TICE strain of BCG**) has been tried in bladder cancer & in other diseases as an adjuvant therapy.
4. Some research suggests that it is superior for tuberculin testing than PPD.

- **Contraindications:**

1. Pregnancy.
2. Infant & children with AIDS.
3. Baby born by AFB positive mother.
4. Tuberculin test positive person.

C. Chemoprophylaxis:

- **Aim:** To prevent the progression of latent tuberculosis to active disease.
- **Indications:**
  - Persons with latent tuberculosis.
  - Persons at high risk.
  - Neonate of tubercular mother.
  - Child with Mantoux positive & TB patient in family.
  - Patients with leukemia, diabetes, silicosis, AIDS, who are Mantoux positive.
  - Patients with old inactive disease who received inadequate therapy.
- **Regime (monoherapy):**
  - Isoniazide (H) 10 mg/kg for 6-12 months.
  - Patients resistant to H: H with rifampicin (R) 10mg/kg for 6 months.
- **Drawbacks of monotherapy:** Development of resistance.

D. "Stop TB strategies" of WHO:

WHO launched stop TB strategies in 2006 which aims at

- **By 2005:** > 70% of sputum smear positive cases will be diagnosed with >85% cure rate.
- **By 2015:** Global burden of tuberculosis including prevalence & death rate will be reduced by 50%.
- **By 2050:** Global incidence of tuberculosis will be <1/million population/year.

Treatment:

a. Chemotherapy:

- **Classification of drugs:** Antituberculous drugs are classified as follows.

1. **1st line drugs:** These drugs have high antitubercular efficacy, low toxicity & used routinely.
   - **Bactericidal:** Isoniazide (H), Rifampicin (R), Pyrazinamide (Z) & Streptomycin (S).
   - **Bacteriostatic:** Ethambutol (E)
2. **2nd line drugs:** These drugs have low antitubercular efficacy, high toxicity or both & used in special cases.
   - **Bacteriostatic:** Thiacetazone (Tzn), Paraaminosalicylic acid (PAS), Ethionamide (Etm), Cycloserine (Cys), Kanamycin (Kmc), Amikacin (Am), Capreomycin (Cpr).
3. **Newer drugs:** Ciprofloxacin, Ofloxacin, Clarithromycin, Azithromycin & Rifabutin.

- **Revised National Tuberculosis Control Programme (RNTCP).**
  - **History:** It is introduced in 1993 in India in collaboration with WHO & World Bank.

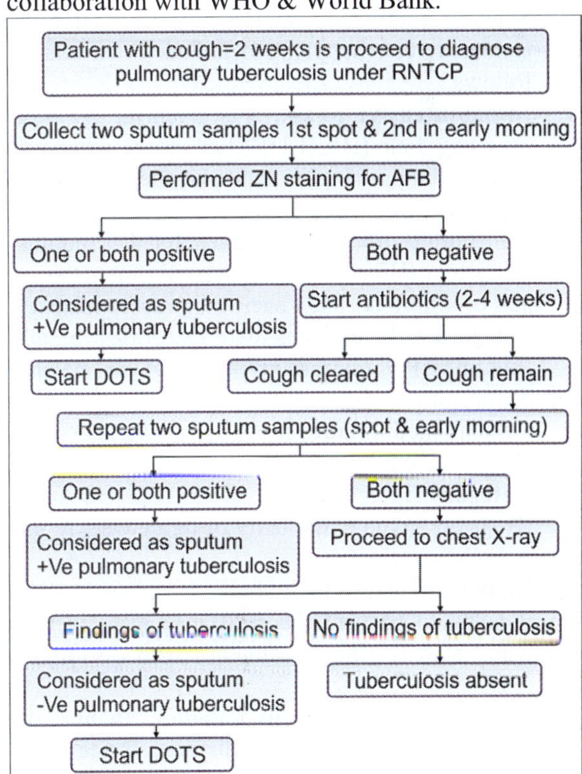

Flow chart-9: Diagnosis of pulmonary tuberculosis under RNTCP

- **Strategies:**
  - Diagnosis of >70% estimated cased by sputum smear microscopy.
  - Treatment **called DOTS**. It is done under supervision.
  - Implementing **DOTS PLUS** for MDR-TB cases.
  - Cure rate not <85%.

Category	Indications	Intensive phase	Continuous phase	Duration
I (New patient)	- Sputum smear +Ve - Sputum smear –Ve - New extra pulmonary	2HRZE	4HR	6 months
II (Old patient)	- Previously treated - Sputum smear +Ve like relapse, treatment failure or return after default - Awaiting drug sensitivity report	2HRZES+ 1 HRZE	5HRE	8 months (with low risk of MDR-TB)
		Empirical MDR regime	Empirical MDR regime	18-24 months or tills DST results (with high risk of MDR-TB)

Table-5: Categories of tuberculosis as per RNTCP & WHO guideline, 2010

- Involvement of NGOs (Non Government Organisations).

- **Diagnosis: → Flow chart-9**
- **Treatment (DOTS):**
  - Full form: Direct Observed Treatment, Short course chemotherapy, **so called** because whole course of therapy is supervised to improve the result.
  - Other features of DOTS:
    - It is recommended by RNTCP & WHO.
    - Treatment response is monitored by periodic sputum microscopy.
  - Short chemotherapy: DOTS rely on 1st line drugs isoniazide & rifampicin. It includes two phases as follows

1. **Initial/intensive phase:** It is given for 2-3 months by using four (HRZE) 1st line drugs with aim of rapid killing of bacilli to make the patient smear negative.
2. **Continuous phase:** It is given for 4-5 months by using two (HR) or three (HRE) 1st line drugs with aim of killing dormant bacilli to prevent relapse.

- Categories: It includes two categories based on sputum AFB microscopy (positive or negative), history of past treatment, sites & severity of disease as mentioned in **table-5**.
- Dosing schedule:

1. **Category I:**
   - Drugs are given either daily or thrice weekly in one or both phases.
   - Daily treatment in both phases is advisable because it helps to prevent the resistance even in patient who started the treatment with primary H resistance.
   - However keeping in mind about drugs administration & cost reduction thrice weekly therapy is accepted in continuous phase with supervision. If constraints are still pressing then thrice weekly therapy in intensive phase is also recommended with keeping in mind about HIV co-infection or risk of HIV infection during therapy.
   - WHO suggest inclusion of E with H & R in areas where primary H resistance is present.
2. **Category II:**
   - 5 Drugs (HRZES) are given daily for 2 months & 4 drugs (HRZE) are given daily for 1 month in intensive phase followed by continuous phase with 3 drugs (HRE) for 5 months.
   - Outcome of regime is monitored by clinical status, microscopy & culture report.

✪ **Types of resistance to antituberculous drugs:** Due to mutation. Different terminology for drug resistance are

- **Primary (pre-treatment, initial) resistance:** Defined as person infected with the strain that is already resistant.
- **Secondary (post-treatment, acquired) resistance:** Defined as person infected with the strain which was sensitive become resistant.
- **Multi drug- resistant tuberculosis (MDR-TB):**
  - Definition: Defined as resistant to Isoniazide (I) & Rifampicin (R) with or without resistance to other 1st line antituberculous drugs.
  - Epidemiological features: MDR-TB cases are identified by WHO in BRICS (Brazil, Russia, India, China & South Africa) countries. However these cases may be more because drug sensitivity facilities are not available everywhere.
  - Diagnosis: MDR-strains are diagnosed by drug sensitivity testing.
  - Treatment: DOTS plus regime is recommended by RNTCP in 2000 for MDR-TB cases as shown in **table-6**.

Intensive phase (6 drugs for 6-9 months)	Continuous phase (4 drugs for 18 months)
Kanamycin	Ofloxacin/levofloxacin
Ofloxacin/levofloxacin	Ethionamide
Ethionamide	Cycloserine
Cycloserine	Ethambutol
Pyrazinamide	
Ethambutol	

Table-6: DOTS plus regime for MDR-TB

- **Extended drug- resistant tuberculosis (XDR-TB):**
  - Definition: Defined as MDR-TB plus resistant to fluoroquinolones (ciprofloxacin, ofloxacin) & one of the second line injectable drugs like Kanamycin (Kmc), Amikacin (Am) or Capreomycin (Cpr). MDR-TB treatment failure cases are presumed to be XDR-TB.

- Epidemiological features: About 3% of MDR-TB cases have been found as XDR-TB in USA. Exact incidence of XDR-TB in India is not found.
- Diagnosis: XDR-strains are diagnosed by drug sensitivity testing.
- Treatment: XDR-TB cases are difficult to treat. They have a rapid progress of disease with high mortality.

✪ **Genes of resistance to antituberculous drugs: → Table-3**

b. Treatment for restoration of CMI:

1. **Transfer factor:** Help for recovery in immunodeficient persons.
2. **Vaccine:** Contain heat killed *M. vaccae*, an environmental mycobacterium. Act as an immunomodulator for stimulation of Th-1 cells which promote the protective immunity.

✓ **Note: Tuberculosis and HIV**

- **Introduction:** Deficiency of CMI is a major contributory factor for infection. Tuberculosis is most commonly present opportunistic infection in HIV. It present in 70-80% cases of HIV.
- **Mode of onset:** Following are possible mode of onset of tuberculosis in HIV patients.

a. Primary infection: It is the infection in HIV patient who is not previously infected by tuberculosis. Risk is high in immunodeficient person than immunocompetent.

b. Secondary infection: Two subtypes.

1. **Post primary infection / endogenous reinfection / reactivation of latent infection:** Bacilli remain in latent form, after healing of primary infection. They are under control by immune system but once immunity down by HIV, latent infection reactivated to develop the tuberculosis.
2. **Exogenous reinfection:** New infection in HIV patient who is previously infected by tuberculosis.

- **Pathology:** More frequency in extra pulmonary pathology than pulmonary.
  - Lungs: Patient is with CMI deficiency, so no granuloma formation & no cavitary lesions. Wide spread dissemination of bacilli in whole lungs **called tuberculous caseous pneumonia.**
  - Lymph node: Biopsy showing poor or no granuloma in HIV positive patient but bacillary load is more than HIV negative individual.
- **Clinical features:** Features are same as of Tuberculosis without HIV.
- **Diagnosis:**

1. **Microscopy:** No cavity formation, so bacilli are less in sputum & there is high frequency of negative sputum smear.
2. **Culture:** Best useful method as described earlier. It detects the bacilli up to 10-110/ml of sputum.
3. **Tuberculin test:** False negative because of poor or no CMI.
4. **Chest X-ray:** No cavitation but instead widespread dissemination in lungs. Less useful.

- **Treatment:** Tuberculosis can be cured if diagnosed early & prompt treatment had been given. DOTS can control & extend the life of patient with HIV.

Question bank

Case study

1) A 40 year old male patient visited the medical OPD with history of low grade evening rise fever, weight loss & productive coughing since 1 month. Sputum examination revealed AFB. Tuberculin test is positive. Identify the organism & answer the following
a) Name the causative agent & describe the morphology of causative agent.
b) Write the pathogenicity of causative agent.
c) Describe the lab. diagnosis of causative agent.
d) Write treatment of clinical condition.

2) A 10 year old boy admitted in hospital with history of low grade fever, headache, vomiting & neck stiffness. CSF examination shows the cobweb coagulum on standing, raised proteins, increased lymphocytes count & decreased glucose level. Identify the case & answer the following
a) Name the clinical condition in given case & its causative agent.
b) Describe the lab. diagnosis of extra pulmonary manifestation causative agent.
c) Write the immunoprophylaxis of causative agent.

Essay/Full question

1) *M. tuberculosis*

Short notes

1) Classification of mycobacteria.
2) Differences between *M. tuberculosis* & *M. bovis*.
3) C/Cs or pathogenicity or lab. diagnosis of *M. tuberculosis*.
4) Newer laboratory methods for diagnosis of *M. tuberculosis*.
5) Tuberculin test
6) Tuberculosis & HIV.
7) BCG vaccine
8) Treatment of tuberculosis / RNTCP
9) MDR TB

Short questions for theory/viva questions

1) Comment: Strictly it's not correct to classify mycobacteria as GPB.
2) Name four automated methods for cultivation of *M. tuberculosis*.
3) What is Ghon's focus & Ghon's complex?
4) Define primary & secondary tuberculosis.
5) Role of BCG vaccine.
6) How you diagnose the pulmonary tuberculosis under RNTCP?
7) What is MDR-TB & XDR-TB?

MCQs for chapter review

Classification

1) Tuberculosis complex include all except-
(a) *M. tuberculosis* (b) *M. microti* (c) *M. kansasi* (d) *M. bovis*

2) John's bacillus is
(a) *M. tuberculosis* (b) *M. paratuberculosis* (c) *M. kansasi* (d) *M. bovis*

M. tuberculosis

3) ***Mycobacterium tuberculosis* was discovered by**
(a) Robert koch (b) Louis pastuer (c) Alexander (d) Vircho

4) **Rapid examination of tubercle bacilli is possible with-** (AI 96)
(a) Ziehl-Neelsen stain (b) Kinyoun stain (c) Auramin – rhodamine stain (d) Giemsa stain

5) **True regarding *Mycobacterium tuberculosis* is -** (PGI 02)
(a) Produces visible colonies in 1 week time on Lowenstein Jenson medium (b) Decolourise by 20% sulphuric acid (c) Facultative aerobe (d) Niacin positive

6) **Reactivation tuberculosis is almost exclusively a disease of**
(a) Lungs (b) Bones (c) Brain (d) Lymph nodes

7) **Cavitation is most often seen in** (AI 11)
(a) Mycoplasma pneumonia (b) Tuberculous pneumonia (c) Streptococcal pneumonia (d) Staphylococcal pneumonia

8) **In which types of cutaneous tuberculosis caseation necrosis is present**
(a) Tuberculosis verucosis (b) Scrofuloderma (c) Tuberculids (d) Lupus vulgaris

9) **The most common focus of scrofuloderma is** (AI 96, 04)
(a) Lung (b) Lymph node (c) Larynx (d) Skin

10) **Collection of a urine sample of a patient of TB/Kidney is done** (AIIMS, May 06)
(a) 24 hrs urine (b) 12 hrs urine (c) In early morning (d) Any time

11) **Which is used in digestion and decontamination of sputum in smear preparation** (PGI, June-03)
(a) NaOH (b) KOH (c) NaCl (d) KCl (e) N-acetyl L cysteine

12) **Drug resistance in tuberculosis is due to**
(a) Transformation (b) Transduction (c) Conjugation (d) Mutation

13) **Tuberculin test is positive if induration is**
(a) >2mm (b) >5 mm (c) >7mm (d) >10 mm

14) **Tuberculin test positive is dependent on –** (AI-96)
(a) Erythema (b) Nodule formation (c) Induration (d) Ulcerative change

15) **True about Mantoux is –** (PGI, June-01)
(a) False negative in fulminant disease (b) If once done, next time it is always positive (c) Results are given in terms of negative & positive (d) Induration given in terms of length & breadth (e) Always indicate active TB infection

16) **True about Mantoux is –** (PGI, June-03)
(a) < 5cm always positive (b) Usually –Ve after treatment (c) Positive reaction in children < 2 yrs is not important than adult (d) Usually read after 48-72b hours (e) False +Ve in post measles state

17) **Which of the following statements regarding Gamma – Release - Assay for diagnosis of tuberculosis is true-** (AI-12)
(a) First generation Quantiferon –TB assay used ESAT-6 (b) Second generation Quantiferon –TB (Gold) assay used ESAT & CFP-10 (c) These tests can distinguish between *M. tuberculosis* & *M. bovis* (d) None of the *Mycobacteria* give a positive reaction with the test

18) **All of the following is true about tuberculosis except –** (AI-12)
(a) For sputum to be positive bacilli should be > 10^4 / ml (b) Niacin test differentiate *M tuberculosis* and *M bovis* (c) Pathogenicity to rabbit differentiate *M tuberculosis* and *M bovis* (d) Culture technique has low sensitivity

19) **In tuberculosis immunity is provided by –**
(a) CD4+ (b) CD8+ (c) IgG (d) IgM

20) **True about BCG vaccine is -**
(a) Killed vaccine (b) Subcutaneously given (c) Given in positive tuberculin patient (d) Live vaccine

21) **BCG vaccine in HIV positive new born is-**
(a) Contraindicated (b) Double dilution (c) Half dilution (d) Dose double

22) **In a patient, the lymphnode shows necrosis with poor granuloma formation with plenty of AFB. Diagnosis suggest-**
(a) Tuberculosis in immunocompetent patient (b) Tuberculosis in HIV patient (c) Sarcoidosis (d) Infection by *M. bovis*

Answers of MCQs & explanation

1) **(c)**
2) **(b)** } Follow section, **classification of *Mycobacteria*** for explanation

3) **(a)**
- *M. tuberculosis* was identified and described on 24 March 1882 by Robert Koch, for this reason the world tuberculosis day was established on 24 March & bacilli **called koch's bacilli**

4) **(c)**
- Follow section, ***M. tuberculosis* (morphology)** for explanation

5) **(d)**
- *M. tuberculosis* visible colonies in 8-12 weeks time on Lowenstein Jenson medium
- Initially 20% sulphuric acid was used for decolourisation, but now a days it is 25%
- It is not facultative aerobe, but strict aerobe
- It is niacin positive

6) **(a)**
- Reactivation tuberculosis is present in apical lungs & other sites are like tonsils, pharynx, larynx, small intestine & skin

7) **(b)**
- Following types of pathological lesions in lungs are produced by different microbes
  - Cavity: *Mycobaterium tuberculosis*
  - Lobar: *Strept. Pneumoniae*
  - Interstial pneumonia (primary atypical pneumonia): *Mycoplasma pneumoniae, Pneumocystic jirovecii* etc.

8) **(d)**
- Lupus vulgaris present with caseation necrosis

9) **(b) & (d)**
- Scrofula / scrophula / King's evil affects the cervical & supraclavicular lymphnodes
- Scrofuloderma: It is the 2nd most common variety of cutaneous tuberculosis resulting from extension of scrofula which involve the cervical & supraclavicular lymphnodes with skin. It also **called tuberculosis cutis colliquativa.**

10) **(c)**
- Bacilli are shedding very intermittently in urine, hence 3-6 consecutive early morning urine samples are collected, centrifuged & use sediment for processing. Acid alcohol is used as decolouriser.

11) **(a) & (e)**
- Follow section, **diagnosis of pulmonary tuberculosis (preparation of specimens)** for explanation

12) **(d)**
- Follow section, **pathogenicity [agent factors (virulence factors) → drug resisatance)]** for explanation.

13) **(d)**
14) **(c)** } Follow section, **diagnosis of pulmonary tuberculosis [tuberculin test / Mantoux (result)]** for explanation.

15) **(a)**
- False negative occurs in overwhelming (fulminant) tuberculosis including miliary tuberculosis, convalescence from some viral infections (like measles, chickenpox, glandular fever), lymphoreticular malignancy, sarcoidosis, malnutrition, immunosuppressive disease or therapy (steroids), impaired CMI, inactive PPD preparations or faulty technique.
- If once done, next time it is not positive, however booster effect can occurs following (two steps) testing
- Results are given in terms of negative, positive, doubtful (equivocal) & strong reactors

- Induration given in terms of length not breadth. It is measured at its widest point transversely to long axis of forearm by ruler or caliper.
- It indicates active TB infection, latent infection, immunisation etc.

16) (d)
- < 5cm always negative
- Positive result may revert to negative result (occasionally) on isoniazide treatment
- Positive reaction in children < 2 yrs is important & indicates the active infection
- Read the result usually read after 48-72b hours
- False -Ve result occurs in post measles state not false +Ve

17) (b)
- First generation Quantiferon –TB assay used PPD but not ESAT-6
- Second generation Quantiferon –TB (Gold) assay used ESAT & CFP-10. ESAT & CFP-10 are produced by *M. tuberculosis* & *M. bovis,* so the tests can distinguish between the two
- Follow section, **Interferon Gamma Release Assay (IGRA)** for more explanation

18) (d)
- Culture is more sensitive than microscopy as it can detect up to 10-100 bacilli per ml of sputum while for microscopy to be positive, sputum should contains 10^4 bacilli/ml
- Niacin test is positive in *M. tuberculosis* & negative in *M. bovis* so useful for differentiation *M tuberculosis* and *M bovis*
- *M. bovis* is pathogenic to rabbit but not the *M. tuberculosis,* so useful for differentiation between two

19) (a)
- In tuberculosis immunity is cell mediated specially by CD4 cells & humoral immunity (IgG & IgM) is not significant

20) (d) } Follow section, **immunoprophylaxis (BCG vaccine)**
21) (a) } for explanation

22) (b)
- Follow section, **tuberculosis in HIV** for explanation

39 Mycobacterium leprae

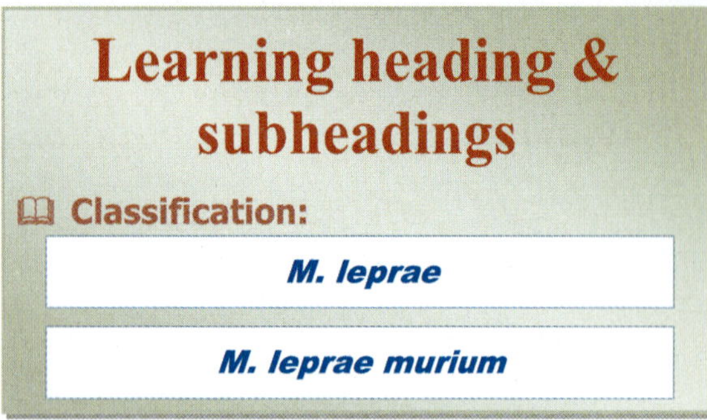

Classification: Two types of lepra bacilli

1. **Human leprosy:** *M. leprae.*
2. **Rat leprosy:** *M. leprae murium.*

M. leprae

❖ Synonym (common name) & history:

a. **Hansen's bacilli:** From the name of Gerard H Armauer Hansen, who 1st discovered the bacilli in 1868.

b. **Lepra bacilli:** Because producing the disease **called leprosy**.

❖ Morphology:

➢ **Staining properties:**

✪ **Type according to gram stain:** GPB & stain more readily than *M. tuberculosis.*

✪ **Acid fast stain:** Less acid fast than *M. tuberculosis*, need 5% sulphuric acid. Differences between *M. tuberculosis* & *M. leprae* are shown in **table-1.**

Features	*M. tuberculosis*	*M. leprae*
Staining technique		
Acid fastness	25%	5%
Alcohol fast	Yes	No
Culture		
Generation time	14-15 hrs	12-15 days
Media	Growth	No growth

Table-1: Differences between *M. tuberculosis* & *M. leprae*

✪ **Morphological index (MI):**

- Live bacilli in smear stain more uniformly than dead bacilli.
- Dead bacilli in smear are stain less uniformly & may give granular appearance.
- The percentage of uniformly stained bacilli in tissue **called Morphological Index (MI).**
- It helps to monitor antibiotics response.
- Continued fall in MI indicates response to treatment while rise indicates drug resistance.
- Solid fragmented granular rod percentage: Percentage of solid fragmented granular bacilli is counted separately, as it gives more ideas about treatment response & better useful than MI.

✪ **Bacteriological Index (BI):**

- **Bacteriological index:** It is the total numbers of pluses in all smears divided by numbers of smear.
- Count the total no. of bacilli (live or dead) & grade the smear as shown in **table-2.**
- For calculation minimum 4 skin smears, 1 nasal smear & smears from both ear lobules should be examined.

BI/grade	Number of AFB / oil immersion field
1+	1-10 /100 fields
2+	1-10/ 10 fields
3+	1-10/ field
4+	10-100/ field
5+	100-1000/ field
6+	> 1000, globi / field

Table-2: Grading of *M. leprae*

➢ **Size:** 1-8 μm × 0.2-0.5 μm (length is five times of breadth).

➢ **Shape:** Straight rod, slightly curved, clubbed, lateral buds or branching forms.

➢ **Arrangement:**

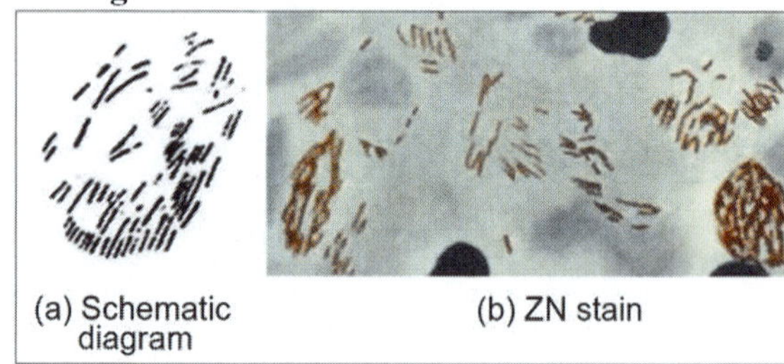

Figure-1: Morphology of *M leprae*

- Located extra or intra cellular in tissue monocytes (histiocytes). They also lying extra-cellularly.
- Intracellular bacilli arranged parallel & bound together by lipid like substance **called glia** & giving appearance **called globi or cigar in bundle appearance** as shown in **fig.-1 (a) & fig.-1 (b).**

- Histiocytes containing globi are **called foamy / Virchow's / lepra cells.**
- Non motile, non-sporing, non capsulated.
- **Polar bodies or other intracellular elements:** May be present.

Cultural characteristics (C/Cs):

- **Effective factors:**
- Bacilli are not cultivable in media & cultivation technique was developed by Shepard in 1960 in foot pad of mice at 20^{0}C.
- Generation time in laboratory animal: 12-15 days.
- **Media:**
- It is not growing on artificial prepared media, however several successful report of growth of lepra bacilli [**called ICRC bacilli**] from leprosy patient on human foetal spinal ganglion cell culture has been given by **ICRC [Indian Cancer Research Centre],** Bombay in1962.
- ICRC bacilli are growing on LJ medium.
- Its relation to lepra bacilli is uncertain.
- **Animal culture:**
- **Animals:** Following animals are used.

a. **Mice:**

- Technique was discovered by Shepard in 1960 as shown in **fig.-2.**
- Inoculate the lepra bacilli by intradermal in footpad of mice & keep it at low temperature about 20^{0}C.

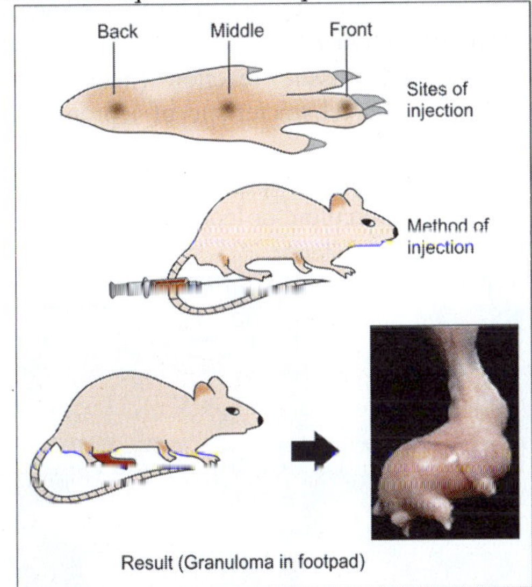

Figure-2: Inoculation of *M leprae* in foot pad of mice

- Result: → **Flow chart-1**

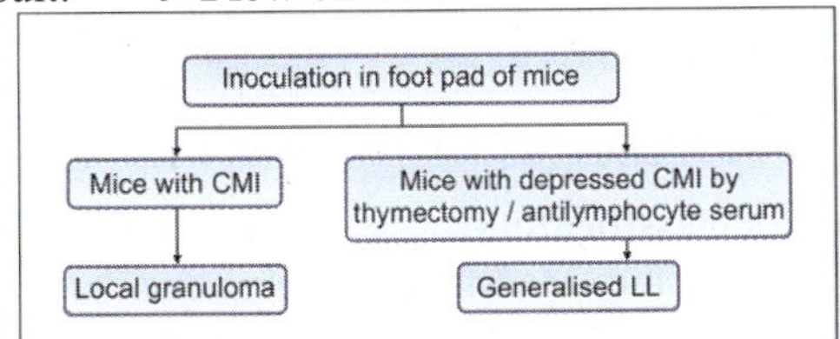

Flow chart-1: Mice culture

- Bacilli replicate very slowly in armadillo (10^6 bacilli / gram of tissue after 6-8 hours), so it is the best animal for culture & for determination of sensitivity of antileprosy drugs.

b. **Nine banded armadillo: (*Dasypus novemcinctus*):** → **Fig.-3**

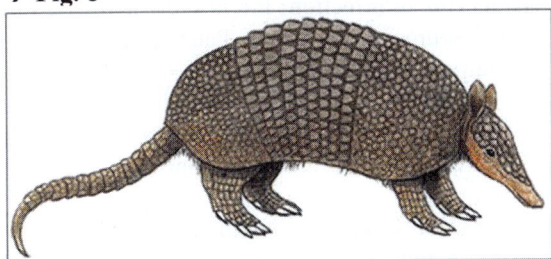

Figure-3: Nine banded armadillo

- Following inoculation of lepra bacilli generalised LL is developed.
- Natural disease occurs in some wild armadillo.
- Bacilli replicate very extensively in armadillo (10^{10} bacilli / gram of tissue), so it provide sufficient bacilli for study purpose/experimental work & for preparation of skin test reagent (lepromin A).
- **Other uses of animals:**

1. To isolate & to study the bacilli. It is 10 times more sensitive than microscopy.
2. To prepare the antigen.
3. To prepare the vaccine.
4. To see the sensitivity pattern to antileprosy drugs.

- **Problems with the uses of animals:**

1. Ethical issues regarding uses of animal. Required to take permission from the animal ethical committee of institute.
2. Time consuming about 6-9 months.

Resistance:

- Bacilli remain viable in a warm humid environment for 9-16 days & in moist soil for 46 days.
- Resist to direct sunlight for 2 hrs & Ultra Violet light (UV) for 30 minutes.

Pathogenicity:

- **Disease name:** Disease **called leprosy.**
- **Synonym: Hansen's disease,** because bacilli 1st observed by Armauer Hansen (1868).
- **Definition:** Chronic granulomatous disease of human primarily affecting skin, peripheral nerves and nasal mucosa but capable to affect any tissue or organ.
- **Nature & history of disease:**
- Leprosy is a disease of antiquity & bacilli are 1st identified by Hansen in 1868.
- It is recognised since
- The time of Vedic in India (**called Kustha Roga**, in Sushruta Samhita, 600BC.
- The time of Biblic in Middle East.
- The time of Hipocrates, 460BC.

- **Scenario of leprosy in India:** It is distributed worldwide, but maximum in India. It present in all states highest prevalence in Orissa (>5 per 1000 population) & least in Haryana (<0.1 per 1000 population).

➢ **Reservoir of infection:** Exclusively human disease, only source is human. Paucibacillary leprosy contains less numbers of bacilli, so having less risk of transmission & can transmit the infection after longer contact. Multibacillary leprosy contains large numbers of bacilli & must be considered infectious.

➢ **Source of infection:** Nasal secretion. A sneeze from an untreated LL patient may contain > 10^{10} bacilli.

➢ **Mode of transmission:** Exactly unknown but may be by
- Inhalation/droplet nuclei: Very large numbers of bacilli are discharged in to nasal secretion.
- Skin to skin/skin to mucosa contact.
- Contact with soil or with fomites like clothes, linen etc.
- Congenital via placenta.
- Via milk of leprosy patient to infant.
- Other rare possibilities routes are by tattooing with infected needles or by insect vectors.

➢ **Incubation period:**
- Very long from few months to as long as 30 years (2- 5 years).
- It is long because of slow generation of bacilli.
- It is longer in LL than TT.

➢ **Portal of entry:** Nasal mucosa or skin.

➢ **Sites:**
- Bacilli can grow better in cooler tissues like skin, peripheral nerves, anterior chamber of eye, upper respiratory tract & testis & sparing the warms areas like axilla, groin, scalp & midline of back.
- Bacilli have affinity for Schwann cells & RE cells.
- Median nerve & ovaries are never involved in TT.

➢ **Precipitating factors (epidemiological determinants):** Three types as follows

I. Agent factors (virulence factors)

1. **Phenolic glycolipid -1:** It acts as virulence factor.
2. **Intracellular location:** Help the bacilli to evade the host defence & effect of antibiotics.

II. Host factors

1. **Age:** Occurs at any age.
2. **Sex:** Double in male than female. Disease occurs more likely if contact occurs during childhood.
3. **Genetic:** Immune response in leprosy may matter the type of HLA antigens.
4. **Immunity:** CMI is needed to develop the resistance to lepra bacilli.
5. **Close contact:** It is not highly communicable. Required longer contact for transmission & only 5% of spouse living with leprosy patient can acquired the infection.

III. Environmental & socio-economical factors

1. **Humidity:** It favours the survival of bacilli. Bacilli remain viable for 9 days in dry condition while for 46 days in moist area.
2. **Overcrowding:** It favours the transmission of disease.
3. **Location:** LL is common in rural areas but now spread to urban population due to migration of patients.
4. **Social stigma:** Leprosy remains as a social stigma because of lack of knowledge, fear, superstition beliefs, complications, deformities & disfigurement of disease.

➢ **Classification of leprosy:**

A. **Madrid / Polar classification, 1953:** Four types

i. **TT(Tuberculoid Type)** } → Table-3

ii. **LL(Lepromatous Leprosy / Lepromata)** }

iii. **BL [Borderline (Dimorphous) Leprosy]:**
- Lesions possessing characteristics of both tuberculoid and lepromatous types.
- It may shift to LL or TT depending on response to chemotherapy or alterations in host resistance.

iv. **Intermediate leprosy:**
- Early unstable tissue reaction (macular lesion) which is neither characteristic of lepromatous nor tuberculoid type.
- Lesions may undergo spontaneous healing or may progress to tuberculoid or lepromatous types.
- Bacteriologically sterile.

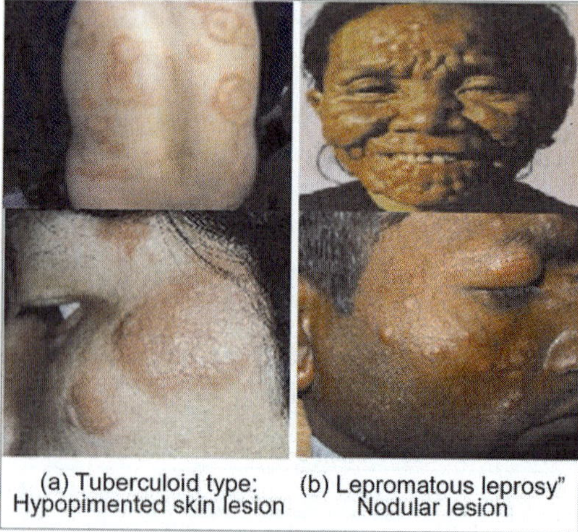

(a) Tuberculoid type: Hypopimented skin lesion (b) Lepromatous leprosy" Nodular lesion

Figure-4: Skin lesions in leprosy

B. **Indian classification:**
- It includes four Madrid's types and one more type (total five types) **called Indian (I) type / Pure neuritic.**

- Extra type in Indian classification is bacteriologically sterile & shows nerve involvement without skin lesion.

C. **Ridley & Jopling classification, 1966:**

✪ **Types:** Five types as differentiated in **table-4.**

i. **TT (Tuberculoid Type)**
ii. **BT (Borderline tuberculoid)**
iii. **BB (Borderline)**
iv. **BL (Borderline Lepromatous)**
v. **LL (Lepromatous Leprosy)**

✪ **Spectrum of disease:** It is from TT → BT → BB →BL → LL, which is associated with asymmetrical localised maules & papules to nodular, indurated symmetrical lesions with increasing numbers of lesions, increasing bacterial load & decreasing or loss of CMI.

D. **Therapeutic types:** Two types like paucibacillary & multibacillary as shown in **table-5.**

Features	TT	LL (Lepromata)
	Bacteriology	
Bacterial load	Paucibacillary (bacilli are less or absent), in destroyed nerve as beaded or granular forms.	Multibacillary (bacilli are multiple), bacilli are inside the lepra cells as globi.
Bacterial index	0-1+	4-6+
Infectivity	Low	High, because of more bacilli in lesions
	Pathology	
Sites	Skin & peripheral nerves like ulnar, post auricular, peroneal & posterior tibial	All organs except lungs & CNS
Macroscopic pathology	Granulomatous lesion with predominance of CD4+ cells, IL-2, IF-γ & IL-12 Granulomatous lesion in dermis erodes the basal layer of epidermis. No clear zone.	No granuloma with predominance of CD8+ cells, IL-4, IL-5 & IL-10 Collection of lepra cells in dermis separated from epidermis. Clear zone
Microscopic pathology Granuloma formation Plasma cell infiltration Lymphocyte infiltration	 Common Poor Common	 Absent Common Not present
	Clinical features	
Skin lesions	- Asymmetrical - Single/few lesion - Sharp margin - Dry, scaly hypopigmented macular lesion **[(fig.-4(a)]**	- Symmetrical - Multiple lesions - Irregular margin - Shiny maculopapular/nodular **[(fig.-4(b)].** Coalesce together to give **leonine facies** appearance
Nerve involvement	- Due to external compression by granuloma - Early, more sensory loss (Early hyposthesia or anaesthesia)	- Due to direct bacillay invasion - Late, little or no loss of sensation (late hyposthesia)
	Immunology	
Host resistance	High	Low
CMI	Good	Deficient/ absent
Lepromin test	Positive	Negative
AMI	Normal	Exaggerated, with hyper γ- globulinemia & reverse albumin/globulin ratio
Ab to PGL-1	60%	95%
Autoimmunity	Autoantibodies are rare	Autoantibodies are more
Type II lepra reaction	Negative	Positive
Phagocytic cells	Mature epitheloid	Macrophage
Giant cells	Absent	Langhans type
HLA association	HLA DR-2	HLA MT-1 & HLA DQ-1
VDRL test	-Ve	Biological false positive
Lymphocyte transformation test	+Ve	-Ve
	Cytology	
CD4+:CD8+ ration	Normal (2:1)	Reversed (1:2)
	Others	
Prognosis	Good	Poor

Table-3: Differences between TT & LL

Features	TT	BT	BB	BL	LL
Bacilli seen in skin	-	-/+	+	++	+++
Bacilli in nasal secretion	-	-	-	+	++
Granuloma formation	+++	++	+	-	-
CMI	+++	++	+	+/-	-
Lepromin test	+++	+	+/-	-	-
Antibodies to lepra bacilli	+/-	+/-	+	++	+++
Phagocytic cells	Mature epitheloid	Immature epitheloid	Immature epitheloid	Macrophage	Macrophage
Type-1 reaction	-	+	+	+	+
Type-2 reaction	-	-	-	+/-	++

Table-4: Ridley & Jopling classification

Features	Paucibacillary	Multibacillary
Pathology		
Leprosy	TT, BT & I-Indian types	LL, BL & BB types
Nerve involvement	1	≥ 2
Skin lesions	1-5	≥ 6
Diagnosis		
Microscopy	-Ve	+Ve
Treatment (Multi drug therapy)		
Indication	To avoid the drug resistance in monotherapy	
Course	6 months	For 1 year or until skin smear becomes -ve.
Drugs	- Rifampicin (highly bactericidal) 600 mg once a month under supervision & - Dapson 100mg daily self administered	- Rifampicin: 600mg once a month, - Dapson 100mg daily and - Clofazimine 50mg daily
Follow-up	Annually at least for 4 years.	Annually at least for 8 years.
Other drugs	- Ethionamide or prothionamide may be added (as substitute of clofazamine). - Quinolones, minocycline, clarithromycin, rifapentine, moxifloxacin are other useful drugs - Under leprosy eradication programme single lesion is managed by rifampicin, ofloxacin & minocycline.	

Table-5: Differences between paucibacillay & multibacillary leprosy

➢ **Complications of leprosy:** Two types like

A. **Structural & functional (anatomical & physiological) deformities:** About 25% of untreated patients develop following complications

1. **Nose:** Epistaxis, collapse of the bony part of nose **called saddle-nose [fig.-5(a)]** or anosmia.
2. **Eyes [fig.-5(b)]:** Uveitis, cataracts, loss of eye brows, glaucoma, corneal ulcer, corneal insensitivity & lagophthalmus.
3. **Extremities [fig.-5(c)]:** Plantar ulceration, foot drop & charcot's joints, claw hand, wrist drop etc.

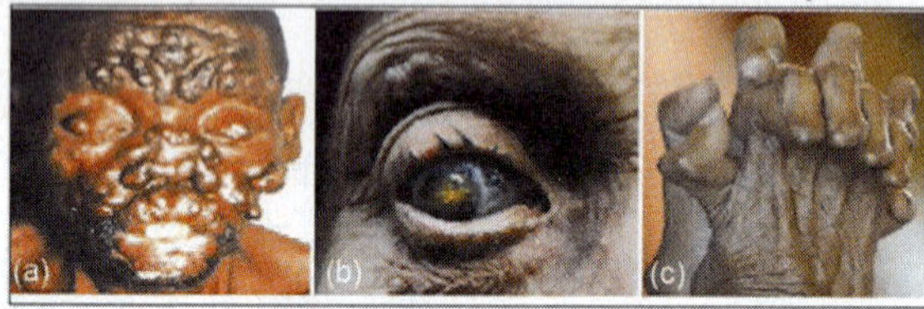

Figure-5: Complications in leprosy

4. **Nerve abscess:** More common in BT. Ulnar nerve is most frequently involved.
5. **Testes:** Orchitis followed by impotence.
6. **Oral lesions:** Small tumour like masses are presents on tongue, lips or hard palate **called lepromas**. They tend to ulcerate. Premaxillary bone recession present frequently with or without tooth loss.

B. **Allergic: Called lepra reaction**

✪ **Definition:** It is an acute exacerbation / allergic response during course of leprosy.

✪ **Types:** Two types of such reaction

a. **Type I** [Reversal reaction or borderline reaction]

- Occurs in initial 6 months.
- Present with macules, papules or plaques.
- No systemic features.
- Examples of type IV hypersensitivity reaction. Predominant response is by T_h1 with increase level of IL-2 & IFN-γ.
- Seen in BT, BB & in BL.
- Treatment is steroids.
- Borderline groups are unstable & they can shift to upgrade or downgrade direction.

1. **Upgrade direction:**
- Present in BL & in treated patients, increased CMI & shift to TT.
- It is a CMI response with influx of lymphocytes in lesions.
- Lesions are swollen and erythematous along with pain and tenderness.

2. **Downgrade direction**
- Present in BT & in untreated or pregnant women, decreased CMI & shift to LL.

- Influx of bacilli in lesion.

b. Type II [ENL, Erythema Nodosum Leprosum]

- Rarely occurs in 1st 6 months.
- Present with painful erythematous papules.
- Systemic features subcutaneous nodule, fever, arthralgia, lymphadenopathy neuritis, uveitis, orchitis & glomerulonephritis are present.
- Example of arthus reaction & main cytokines involved in the reaction is TNF-α. Predominant response is by T_h2 with increase level of IL-6 & IL-8.
- Seen in LL & in BL.
- Develop when patient is under the treatment, because of release of antigen from dead bacilli.
- Characterised by deposition of PMNs, IgG & complement in lesions.
- Treatment is steroids, antipyretics, thalidomide, chloroquine & clofazimine.

✓ **Notes: Lucio phenomenon**

- **Synonym:** Diffuse lepromatosis
- **History:** It is named after Rafael Lucio Nájera (1819 – 1866), a Mexican physician who together with his medical assistant, Alvarado described and observed it in one of his patients in 1852. He himself got infected with this type of Leprosy from which he died in 1886, aged 66 years
- **Geographical distribution:** It seen exclusively in some cases of lepromatous leprosy in Mexico & the Caribbean.
- **Pathogenesis:** It is mediated by immune-complex deposition.
- **Histopathology:** Histopathological changes involving multiple, acute, necrotizing cutaneous vasculitis & thrombosis in the larger vessels of the deeper dermis, ischemic necrosis of the epidermis & superficial dermis, endothelial proliferation & heavy infestation of endothelial cells with AFB.
- **Clinical presentation (fig.-6):**

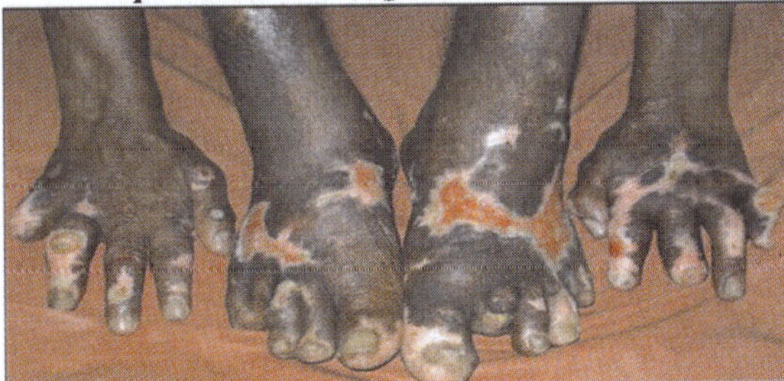

Figure-6: Clinical presentation in Lucio phenomenon

- It is an unusual, non-nodular, diffuse necrotizing skin lesion, especially in untreated cases of lepromatous leprosy.
- It is characterised by recurrent crops of large, sharply demarcated, ulcerative lesions, affecting mainly the lower extremities, but may generalised & become fatal as a result of secondary bacterial infection & sepsis.

- **Treatment:** Treated by anti-leprosy therapy (dapsone, rifampin, & clofazimine), optimal wound care, and treatment for bacteremia, including antibiotics. In severe cases, exchange transfusion is helpful.

❖ Laboratory diagnosis:

➢ **Specimens:**

1. Nasal specimens:

- **Nasal mucosal scraping:**
  - By using blunt scalpel.
  - Erode the nasal septum, remove the piece of mucus membrane & take over the slide.
  - Teased in uniform smear.
  - Not recommended routinely.
- **Nasal secretion:**
  - Early morning sample is advised.
  - Mucus secretion is collected by blowing the nose on a clean cellophane sheet.

2. Skin scraping (slit skin smear):

- Total 5-6 different areas of skin should be sampled like forehead, buttock, chin, cheeks and ear lobules. By using scalpel with blade.
- Edge of the lesion is the preferred site.
- Clean the lesion with spirit & pinched tightly to minimise the bleeding.
- Made a 5 mm long incision to reach up to infiltrated layers.
- Wipe out the blood or secretion; rotate the blade transversely to obtain the tissue pulp below epidermis, over the sterile slide.
- Smear (8 mm size of smear) uniformly over slide.

3. Biopsy: From nodular lesion, thick nerve or from lymph nodes.

➢ **Testing method:**

I. Microscopy: →Follow morphology

II. Culture: → Follow C/Cs

III. Serological tests: Ab detecting tests has some value

1. Tests to detect IgM Ab against PGL-1:

- Latex agglutination test
- ELISA: Sensitivity is 95% in untreated LL & 60% in TT cases. Titre decrease with effective therapy. It also present in non leprosy cases, so rarely useful

2. Tests to detect specific Ab of *M leprae*: Widely used test in this category is fluorescent leprosy antibody absorption (FLA-ABS) test. It is useful to detect the early stage of disease & also to diagnose the subclinical cases. It is 92% sensitive & 100% specific.

IV. Molecular: PCR is in progress.

V. Test to determine the CMI: →Lepromin test

✪ **Principle:** Based on DTH (Delayed Type Hypersensitivity).

- **Ag:** Ag will standardise as per bacilli contents. Three types of antigens.

1. **Lepromin Ag:** Early reaction & contain 40 million bacilli/ml. It is derived from armadillo (Lepromin A), which replaced the human lepromin (Lepromin H).
2. **Mitsuda Ag:** Early & late reaction & contain 160 million bacilli/ml.
3. **Dharmendra Ag:** Early & late reaction & contain 10 million bacilli/ml.

- **Effective factors:**

1. **Age:** It is negative in 1st six months of life & may become positive up to 1 year of age.
2. **BCG vaccine:** It may turn –Ve result to positive (?)

- **Method:** Inject 0.1 ml Ag intradermally on flexor aspect of forearm & examined after 48-72 hours.
- **Result & interpretation:** Two results like early & late as shown in **table-6.**

Early	Late
Fernandez reaction	Mitsuda reaction
Read after 48 hours	Read at 21 days (3 weeks)
Erythema & induration in 24-48 hrs will disappear in 3-5 days.	Nodule formation (by infiltration of lymphocytes, giant cell & epitheloid cells) after 3-4 wks gets ulcerated & disappears in few wks.
Positive if size of erythema & induration is > 10 mm	Positive if size of nodule is > 5 mm
It is the DTH to soluble components of lepra bacilli due to infection or exposure by other ways	It indicates the status of CMI to antigens of lepra bacilli. Positive indicates good CMI & negative indicates poor CMI
Less useful	More useful

Table-6: Result of lepromin test

- **Uses:** It is not used for diagnosis of leprosy. Possible uses are mentioned in **table-7.**

Uses	+Ve result	-Ve result
To classify the leprosy	TT	LL
To assess the prognosis & treatment response	Good	Poor
To assess the host immunity against bacilli	Good	Poor

Table-7: Uses of lepromin test

✓ **Notes: Leprosy centres**

- **Follow chapter → Laboratory diagnosis of bacterial infections**

❖ Prevention:
Early diagnosis & treatment is the best strategies for prevention.

A **General measures:** Isolation of patients.

B **Chemoprophylaxis:** Long term chemoprophylaxis by using dapsone is useful in LL.

C **Immunoprophylaxis:**

- No specific vaccine is available.
- Due to antigenic relationship between lepra bacilli & tubercle bacilli combination of BCG + lepra bacilli (ICRC bacillus) is tried, but without any conclusive evidence.

❖ Treatment:

A. **Chemotherapy:**

- **Monotherapy:** By using dapsone. Due to development of resistance, MDT is recommended.
- **Multi Drug Therapy (MDT): → Follow table-4**

B. **Immunotherapy:**

- **Immunotherapeutic vaccine:** Developed from *Mycobacterium W* by National Institute of Immunology (NII), New Delhi, is able to increase to effect of MDT.

❖ **World leprosy day:** This day was chosen on last Sunday of January in each year in commemoration of the death of Mahatma Gandhi, the leader of India who understood the importance of leprosy.

M. leprae murium

- Produce leprosy in rat characterised by subcutaneous induration, lymphadenopathy, emaciation, ulceration & loss of hair.
- Bacilli are present large numbers in lesions.
- Bacilli resemble to *M. leprae* but distinct from *M. leprae* by DNA studies.

Question bank

Essay/Full question

1) *M. leprae*

Short notes

1) Culture of *M. leprae*
2) Pathogenicity or laboratory diagnosis of *M. leprae*
3) Classification / different types of leprosy
4) Lepromin test
5) Lepra reaction
6) Differences between LL & TT

Short questions for theory/viva questions

1) What is globi?
2) What is morphological & bacteriological index in *M. lepare*?
3) What is lucio phenomenon or diffuse lepromatosis?
4) How lepromin test is useful in management of leprosy.

MCQs for chapter review

M leprae

1) **Which of the following is true regarding globi in a patient with lepromatous leprosy -** (AI 02)
(a) Consist of lipid laden macrophages (b) Consist of macrophages filled with AFB (c) Consist of neutrophils filled with bacteria (d) Consist of activated macrophages
2) **For experimental work lepra bacilli are bets cultured in-** (AI 96)

(a) Armadillos (b) Mouse foot pad (c) Guinea pig (d) Rabbit testes

3) ***Mycobacterium lepra* can be grown in -**
(a) LJ medium (b) Roberson cooked meat medium (c) Foot pad of mice (d) Sabouraud's agar

4) **Lepra bacilli can survive outside the human body up to-**
(a) 7 days (b) 12 days (c) Zero days (d) 5 days

5) **Leprosy affect all of the following except-** (AI 07)
(a) Testes (b) Ovaries (c) Eyes (d) Nerves

6) ***Mycobacterium lepra* is spread by -**
(a) Skin to skin contact (b) Blood transfusion (c) Droplet spread (d) Ingestion

7) **The characteristic finding in a case of leprosy is** (AIIMS, Dec-98, 00)
(a) Culture test is positive in 2-3 months in LJ medium (b) Long contact with tuberculoid leprosy can transmit the disease (c) CMI is seen in Lepromatous leprosy (d) Macule lesion heals spontaneously

8) **Neurological involvement is pronounced in which type of leprosy**
(a) Tuberculoid (b) Lepromatous (c) Borderline (d) Lucio leprosy

9) **Single skin lesion is seen in which type of leprosy-** (AI 93)
(a) LL (b) TT (c) BL (d) BT

10) **Following test is not used for diagnosis of leprosy** (AIIMS- 06)
(a) Lepromin test (b) Slit skin smear (c) Fine needle aspiration cytology (d) Skin biopsy

11) **Mitsuda reaction is read after** (AIIMS- 93)
(a) 3 days (b) 3 hours (c) 3 weeks (d) 3 months

12) **In the management of leprosy, lepromin test is most useful for –** (AI-03)
(a) Herd immunity (b) Prognosis (c) Treatment (d) Epidemiological investigation

13) **Exacerbation of lesions in patients of borderline leprosy is seen in – (PGI, June-01)**
(a) Erythema nodosum leprosum (b) Lepra reaction type-1 (c) Jarisch-Herxheimer reaction (d) Resolving leprosy

14) **Characteristics of type II lepra lepra reaction –** (PGI, Nov-13, 09)
(a) Erythema & oedema (b) ENL (c) Lymphadenopathy (d) Uveitis (e) Trophic ulcer

15) **Main cytokines involved in erythema nodosum leprosum (ENL) reaction is –** (AIIMS-06)
(a) Interleukin -02 (b) Interferon–gamma (c) Tumour necrosis factor- alpha (d) Macrophage colony stimulating factor

16) **ENL is seen in –**
(a) Lepromatous leprosy (b) Tuberculoid type (c) Intermediate leprosy (d) Pure neuritic

17) **Following drug is used for the treatment of type II lepra reaction, except –** (AIIMS-06)
(a) Chloroquine (b) Thalidomide (c) Cyclosporine (d) Corticosteroid

18) **Fastest microbicidal agent against *M. leprae* –** (AI 04)
(a) Clofazimine (b) Dapsone (c) Rifampicin (d) Minocycline

19) **Under leprosy eradication programme, the management of single lesion is -** (AIIMS 02)
(a) Single dose of rifampicin and dapsone (b) Rifampicin and dapsone for 6 months (c) Rifampicin, ofloxacin & minocycline single dose (d) Rifampicin & minocycline for 6 months

20) **True about lepra bacilli is -** (AIIMS May-94)
(a) INH inhibits their growth (b) Anti leprosy vaccine can give lifelong protection (c) *Mycobacterium lepra* can be grown in foot pad of mice (d) Incubation period is 3-4 months

Answers of MCQs & explanation

1) **(b)**
- Follow section, ***M leprae* (morphology)** for explanation

2) **(a)**
3) **(c)**
- Follow section, ***M leprae* (culture characteristics)** for explanation

4) **(b)**
- Follow section, ***M leprae* (resistance)** for explanation

5) **(b)**
- Median nerve & ovaries are never involved in TT
- Other organs involved in the leprosy are explained under the heading of pathogenicity (sites)

6) **(a) & (c)**
- Follow section, ***M leprae* (pathogenicity →mode of transmission)** for explanation

7) **(b) & (d)**
- Culture is not possible in LJ or any other medium. Lepra bacilli can grow only in animals as described in culture characteristics
- Paucibacillary leprosy (TT) contains less numbers of bacilli, so having less risk of transmission & can transmit the infection after longer contact. Multibacillary leprosy (LL) contains large numbers of bacilli & must be considered infectious.
- CMI is absent in lepromatous leprosy
- Macule lesion heals spontaneously in indeterminate type

8) **(a)**
- Neurological involvement occurs early in TT due to external compression by granuloma, more sensory loss (Early hyposthesia or anaesthesia)
- For more explanation follow **table-3 (nerve involvement)**

9) **(b)**
- Lesion is single/few TT & increasing from TT to LL as per spectrum of disease with increasing bacterial load & also loss or absence of CMI

10) **(a)**
- Lepromin test is not used for diagnosis but for other purpose. Uses of lepromin test are explained in **table-6**

11) **(c)**
- Follow section, ***M leprae* (laboratory diagnosis → Lepromin test & table-6)** for explanation

12) **(b)**
- Positive lepromin test indicate good CMI & good prognosis while negative result indicate the poor or absence of CMI & poor prognosis, so turning of negative to positive result following antileprotic drugs, will indicate response to therapy & help in management of leprosy

13) **(b)**
14) **(b)**
15) **(c)**
16) **(a)**
- Follow section, ***M leprae* (pathogenicity →complications →lepra reaction)** for explanation

17) **(c)**
- Lepra reaction can occurs in LL, where CMI is absent or low. Cyclosporin is immunosuppressive agent & can suppress more immunity, if given so not useful

18) **(c)**
- Rifampicin is the only bactericidal drug against *M leprae*

19) **(c)**
- Follow section, ***M leprae* (pathogenicity → therapeutic types & table-5)** for explanation

20) **(c)**
- INH is not the antileprotic drugs
- No any useful anti leprosy vaccine available which can give lifelong protection
- *Mycobacterium lepra* can be grown in foot pad of mice as describe in culture characteristics
- Incubation period is very long from few months to as long as 30 years (2- 5 years).

40 Non Tuberculous mycobacteria (NTM)

Learning heading & subheadings

NTM

- Meaning:
- Synonym:
- Properties:
- Classification:
- Laboratory diagnosis:
- Treatment

Mycobacteria as skin pathogens

NTM

- **Meaning:** Mycobacteria **other than typical tubercle bacilli,** occasionally cause **human disease resembling tuberculosis called NTM.**

- **Synonym:**
  - Anonymous mycobacteria.
  - Unclassified mycobacteria.
  - Atypical mycobacteria.
  - MOTT (Mycobacteria Other Than Tubercle bacilli).

  } Because causing disease other than tuberculosis except *M. kansasi*

  - Environmental mycobacteria: As environment (water, soil etc.) are the common sources.
  - Opportunistic mycobacteria: Because producing infection in person with IDDs
  - Paratubercle bacilli.
  - Tuberculoid bacilli.

- **Properties:**
  - They are saprophytes & natural habitat in water & soil but unlike saprophytic mycobacteria they can infect human / animals & causing opportunistic infection. Infection does not occur in person with normal immunity.
  - They are also present as normal flora in skin, GIT & respiratory tract.
  - Widely present in soil, water and air. Infection with them is quite common due to direct repeated environmental exposure. Such repeated infection will decrease the efficacy of BCG vaccine by cross contamination.
  - They are common where tuberculosis is rare & rare where tuberculosis is endemic.
  - Low virulence compare to *M. tuberculosis.*
  - Overt disease present in immunocompromised & subclinical infection occurs in immunodeficient persons.
  - Person to person infection does not occur.
  - Infection is mainly asymptomatic, which cause weak positive Mantoux reaction.
  - Some species like *M. avium, M. kansasi, M. xenopi* are occurs as laboratory contaminant & mistaken as tubercle bacilli in smear.
  - They are acid as well as alcohol fast.
  - Most NTM are strict aerobes & grow best at acidic pH.
  - They can grow at 25^0C, 37^0C & 45^0C on LJ medium.

- **Classification:** Given by Runyon in 1959 on the basis of pigment production & growth rate.

1. **Group-I: Called photochromogens**
2. **Group-II: Called scotochromogens**
3. **Group-III: Called nonchromogens (nonphotochromogens)**

} Slow grower in 4-12 weeks

4. **Group-IV: Called rapid growers.** Grow in 7 days.

Group-I: Photochromogens

- **Definition:** Produce yellow-orange pigment in dark & in light when young culture is exposed to light for 1 hr in presence of air & re incubated for 24-28 hrs.
- **Species: → Table-1**

Group-II: Scotochromogens

- **Definition:** Produce yellow-orange-red pigment in light & even in dark.
- **Species: → Table-2**

Photochromogens			
Species	Biochemical test	Pathogenic lesion	Other remarks
M kansasii	Nitrate reduction test: +Ve Tween 80 hydrolysis test: + Ve Urease test: + Ve Catalase test: +Ve Pyrazinamide test: -Ve	Chronic Pulmonary disease resembling tuberculosis	Growth at 25 ^{0}C & 37 ^{0}C in LJ medium
M marinum (M. balnei)	Nitrate reduction test: -Ve Urease test: +Ve Pyrazinamide test: +Ve	Skin wart (Swimming pool granuloma or fish tank granuloma), tender nodules (spread in a sporotrichoid pattern) tendonitis	Growth at 25 ^{0}C & variable at 37 ^{0}C
M simiae	Niacin test: +Ve (So, confused with *M. tuberculosis*)	Pulmonary disease	
M. genavense		Infection in HIV patient	
M asiaticum	Niacin test: -Ve	Pulmonary disease & bursitis	
Mnemonic: P- kamasige-as (as per group & order of species in this table, highlighted by under lined)			

Table-1: Species of photochromogens

Scotochromogens			
Features	Biochemical tests	C/Fs	Other features
M. scrofulaceum	Tween 80 hydrolysis: -Ve Urease test: +Ve Pyrazinamide test: -Ve Nicotinamide test: -Ve	Cervical lymphadenitis (scrofula) in children.	Growth at 25 ^{0}C & 37 ^{0}C
M. gordonae	Tween 80 hydrolysis: +Ve Urease test: -Ve Pyrazinamide test: +Ve Nicotinamide test: +Ve	Pulmonary features. Present in tap water.	
M. szulgai	- It is scotochromogen at 37 ^{0}C & photochromogen 25 ^{0}C. - It produces pulmonary infection, lymphadenitis & cutaneous-subcutaneous bursitis.		
M. celatum	It produces pulmonary infection.		
M. flovescens	Intermediate growth rate in 7-10 days at 25^{0}C -37 ^{0}C with butyrous colony & yellow orange pigment. Non pathogenic.		
Mnemonic: S- sgz-ce flo (as per group & order of species in this table highlighted by under lined)			

Table-2: Species of scotochromogens

Group-III: Nonchromogens

Mnemonic:
- **Nonchromogens: No- mai-xup** → Follow text as per group & order of species highlighted by under lined.
- **Rapid growers: R- sp-fca** → Follow text as per group & order of species highlighted by under line.

- **Synonym:** Non photochromogens.
- **Definition:** No pigment production either in light or in dark.
- **Species:**

- ***M malmoense***: It is slow grower & causing pulmonary infection & lymphadenitis.
- ***M. avium***:
  - It causes natural tuberculosis in birds & lymphadenopathy in pigs.
  - It is an opportunistic human pathogen.
- ***M. intracellularae***:
  - Also **called Battey bacilli** because 1st identified in Battey state hospital of tuberculosis, Georgia, USA.
  - It is closely related *M. avium*, so collectively **called MAC (*Mycobacterium* Avium Complex).**
  - MAC is the most common cause of pulmonary disease from atypical category.
  - MAC is the opportunistic pathogen in HIV positive patient when CD4 count is < 50/ cmm. It present with fever, weight loss, abdominal pain, diarrhoea, night sweats & lymphadenopathy. AFB are found in stool, sputum & blood.
- ***M. xenopi***:
  - It is nonchromogen but may form scotochroogenic yellow colonies.
  - It causing pulmonary lesion especially in HIV positive patient & epididymitis.
  - It was originally isolated from toads.
  - It is isolated from hospital water sources & associated with nosocomial outbreak.
  - Differences with MAC: → **Table-3**

Features	MAC	*M. xenopi*
Urease test	-Ve	-Ve
Pyrazinamide test	+Ve	+Ve
Iron uptake	-Ve	-Ve
Catalase test at 68 ^{0}C	-Ve	+Ve
Aryl sulphatase	-Ve	+Ve
Growth at 45 ^{0}C	+Ve	+Ve

Table-3: Differences between MAC & *M. xenopi*

- ***M. ulcerans:*** → **Table-5**
- ***M. paratuberculosis***:
  - Also **called Johne's bacillus.**

- Mainly cattle pathogen. In human cause Crohn's disease but its association is still under question.

- **Other species:** *M. nonchromogenicum, M. gastri, M. terrae, M. shimoidei* etc.

Group-IV: Rapid growers

Features	*M. fortuitum*	*M. chelonae*
- Aryl sulphatase - Growth by 5% NaCl - Iron uptake - Nitrate reduction test	+Ve +Ve +Ve +Ve	+Ve -Ve -Ve -Ve
- Growth on Mac Conkey's agar - Growth at 25 °C & 37 °C	+Ve +Ve	+Ve +Ve
Pathogenic lesion	Pulmonary infection, wound infection, abscess following injection or vaccination.	

Table-4: Species of rapid growers

- **Definition:** Rapid growers are not producing pigment & growth occur within 7 days at 25°C & 37 °C.
- **Species:** → **Table-4**
  - It includes mostly saprophytic bacilli.
  - *M. smegmeatism* & *M. phlei* produce the pigment.
  - *M. fortuitum, M. chelonae & M abscessus* do not produce the pigment. Differences between *M. fortuitum* & *M. chelonae* are given in **table-4.**
  - Other rapid growers are *M. vaccae, M. genevense, M. confluentis* & *M. intermedium.*

❖ Laboratory diagnosis:

- **Specimens:** Sputum, pus / exudates, nodular biopsy etc.
- **Testing methods:**

I. **Microscopy:** By ZN stain.

II. **Culture & biochemical tests:** → **Flow chart-1**

III. **Animal pathogenicity:** Non pathogenic for guinea pig but pathogenic for mouse.

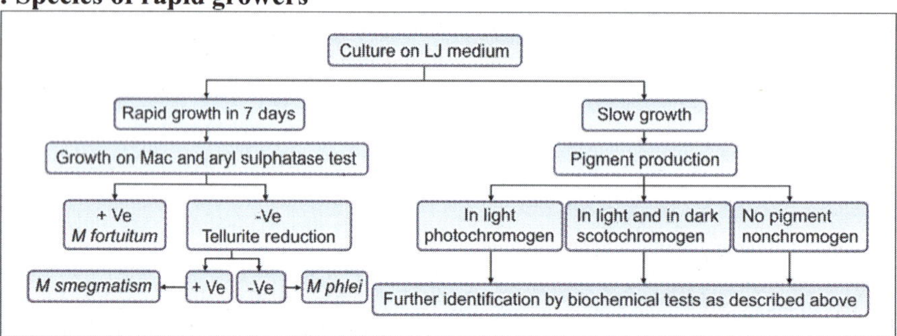

Flow chart-1: Laboratory diagnosis of atypical mycobacteria

Features	*M. marinum (M. balnei)*	*M. ulcerans (M. buruli)*
History & synonym	1st identified in Sweden from swimming pool water **called *M. balnei*** (from **balneum=bath**) later identified from European & American country **called *M. marinum***	1st identified from Australia **called *M. ulcerans*** & than from Buruli district, Uganda with large epidemic **called *M. buruli***
Prevalence	In temperate climate	In tropical climate
Mode of transmission	Swimming pool water	Traumatic injuries
Sites	Prominence like elbows, ankles, nose	Legs or arms
Incubation period	-	Few weeks
Virulence factors	-	Only *Mycobacteria* producing exotoxin **called mycolactone**.
Clinical features	**Swimming pool / fish tank granuloma:** Papular lesion gets ulcerated with spontaneous healing (Self limited)	**Buruli ulcer:** Initially nodule formation gets ulcerated & heals with disfiguring scar (chronic progressive ulcer)
Lab. diagnosis - Samples - ZN stain - LJ medium - Pigment in light - Foot pad of mice inoculation - Guinea pig inoculation	 - Smear from edge of ulcer - Scanty bacilli - Grow in 1-2 weeks at 25-35 °C - Produced - Local inflammation followed by purulent ulcer - Non pathogenic	 - Smear from edge of ulcer - Plenty of bacilli - Grow in 4-8 weeks at 30-33°C - Not produced - Oedema of limb but ulceration is infrequent - Inflammation & necrosis

Table-5: Differences between *M. ulcerans* & *M. balnei*

❖ **Treatment:** Anti tuberculous drugs are useful. Most atypical mycobacteria are resistant to anti tuberculous drugs, so drug are selected after antibiogram.

Mycobacteria as skin pathogens

- ***M. tuberculosis***: Follow chapter → *Mycobacterium tuberculosis* (section → extra pulmonary tuberculosis).
- ***M. leprae*** are able to produce skin infection.
- Some **atypical mycobacteria** are also act as skin pathogens.

1. **Abscesses following injection or vaccination:**
   - *M. fortuitum*
   - *M. chelonei* } **Vide supra**
2. **Swimming pool granuloma / fish tank granulomas:** *M. marinum* / *M. balnei* (**table-5**).
3. **Buruli ulcer:** *M. ulcerans* / *M. buruli* (**table-5**).
4. **Skin lesion:** *M haemophylum*, required haemin for growth & grow at 32 ^{0}C in 2-4 wks.

Question bank

Short notes

1) Atypical mycobacteria.
2) Mycobacteria as skin pathogens.

Short questions for theory/viva questions

1) Name the four pigment producing bacteria.
2) Classify atypical mycobacteria.

MCQs for chapter review

NTM

1) **True about Mycobacterium other than tuberculosis is -** (AIIMS 08)
(a) Causes disseminated infection (b) Occurs in person with normal immunity (c) Causes decreased efficacy of BCG due to cross immunity (d) Person to person transmission seen
2) **Photochrmogenic bacterium is**
(a) *M. kansasii* (b) *M. scrofulaceum* (c) *M. intracellularae* (d) *M. avium*
3) **Which of the following are photochromogens-**
(a) *M. fortuitum* (b) *M. marinum* (c) *M. simiae* (d) *M. kansasi*
4) **Pigment producing atypical mycobacteria-**
(a) *M. fortuitum* & *M. chelonae* (b) *M. xenopi* and MAC (c) *M. gordonae* and *M. szulgai* (d) *M. ulcerans*
5) **Which of the following is not a rapidly growing atypical mycobacteria causing lung infections-** (AIIMS, May 13)
(a) *M. chelonae* (b) *M. fortuitum* (c) *M. abscessus* (d) *M. kansasi*
6) **Battey bacillus is**
(a) Photochromogen (b) Scotochromogen (c) Nonchromogen (d) Rapid grower
7) **A patient with diarrhoea with AFB (+) ve organism in stool. The most likely organism is** (AI-00)
(a) *Mycobacterium avium intracellularae* (b) *Mycobacterium TB* (c) *Mycobacterium leprae* (d) *Mycoplasma*
8) **Scotochromogens are-**
(a) *M. scrofulaceum* (b) *M. avium* (c) *M. szulgai* (d) *M. gordonae*
9) **Scotochromogens produce pigment in**
(a) Light (b) In dark (c) Absence of light (d) Light & dark
10) **Which of the following is slow grower-** (AIIMS, May-13)
(a) *M. kansasii* (b) *M. chelonae* (c) *M. fortuitum* (d) *M. abscessus*

Mycobacteria as skin pathogen

11) **Cutaneous lesion is produced by following bacteria except**
(a) *M. tuberculosis* (b) *M. leprae* (c) *M. marinum* (d) *M. intracellulare*
12) **Fish tank granuloma is seen in**
(a) *M. fortuitum* (b) *M. leprae* (c) *M. marinum* (d) *M. kansasi*

Answers of MCQs & explanation

1) **(c)**
- Follow section, **NTM (properties)** for explanation

2) **(a)**
3) **(b), (c) & (d)** } Follow section, **NTM (Group-I: photochromogens & table-1)** for explanation
4) **(c)**
- Pigment producing atypical mycobacteria are photochrmogens & scotochrmogens.
- *M. fortuitum* & *M. chelonae* are rapid growers & do not produce the pigment.
- M. xenopi, MAC & *M. ulcerans* are nonchromogens & do not produce the pigment.
- *M. gordonae* and *M. szulgai* are scotochrmogens & known to produce the pigment.

5) **(d)**
- *M. chelonae*, *M. fortuitum* & *M. abscessus* are rapid growers while *M. kansasi* is photochrmogen, causing tuberculosis like lesion in lung

6) **(c)**
7) **(a)** } Follow section, **NTM (group-III: nonchromogenes →*M. intracellularae*)** for explanation
8) **(a), (c) & (d)**
- Follow section, **NTM (Group-II: scotochromogens & table-2** for explanation

9) **(d)**
- Photochrmogens produce pigment in light, scotochrmogens produce pigment in light & dark& nonchromogens do not produce pigment

10) **(a)**
- Photochrmogens, scotochrmogens & nonchromogens are the slow growers. *M. kansasii* is the photochromogen
- All other options are belong to rapid growers

11) **(d)**
12) **(c)** } Follow section, **Mycobacteria as skin pathogen & table 5** for explanation

41 Listeria and Erysipelothrix

Learning heading & subheadings

Listeria

Classification:

Listeria monocytogenes

Listeria ivanovi

Erysipelothrix rhusiopathiae

- **Meaning:**
- **Morphology:**
- **Cultural characteristics (C/Cs):**
- **Biochemical reactions (B/Rs):**
- **Pathogenicity:**
- **Laboratory diagnosis:**
- **Prevention:**
- **Treatment:**

Listeria

Classification:

- **Order:** Bacillales
- **Family:** Listeriaceae
- **Genus:** *Listeria*
- **Species:**
  - The genus *Listeria* currently contains 17 species: *L. aquatica, L. booriae, L. cornellensis, L. fleischmannii, L. floridensis, L. grandensis, L. grayi, L. innocua, L. ivanovii, L. marthii, L. monocytogenes, L. newyorkensis, L. riparia, L. rocourtiae, L. seeligeri, L. welshimeri* and *L. weihenstephanensis.*
  - Both *L. ivanovii* & *L. monocytogenes* are pathogenic in mice, but only *L. monocytogenes* is consistently associated with human illness.

Listeria monocytogenes

Meaning & history:

- **Genus name:** *Listeria monocytogenes* was first described by EGD Murray in 1924 based on six cases of sudden death in young rabbits. Murray referred to the organism as *Bacterium monocytogenes* before Harvey Pirie changed the genus name to *Listeria* in 1940 in honour of Joseph Lister (father of antiseptic surgery).
- **Species:** Cause monocytosis after experimental inoculation in rabbits. Monocytosis also occurs in human; hence the species name is *monocytogenes*.

Uses:

1. **Transfection vector:** Because *L. monocytogenes* is an intracellular bacterium, some studies have used this bacterium as a vector to deliver genes *in vitro*. One example of the successful use of *Listeria monocytogenes* in *in vitro* transfer technologies is in the delivery of gene therapies for cystic fibrosis case.
2. **Cancer treatment:** *L. monocytogenes* is being investigated as a cancer immunotherapy for several types of cancer. A live attenuated ADXS11-001 vaccine of *L. monocytogenes* is under development as a possible treatment for cervical carcinoma.

Morphology: →Figure-1(a)

- **Type according to gram stain:** GPB.

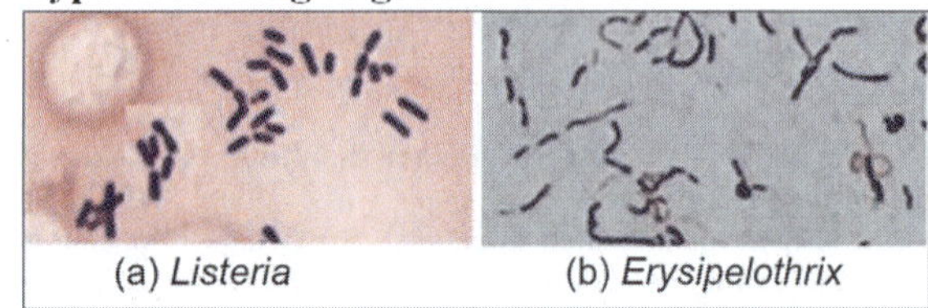

(a) *Listeria* (b) *Erysipelothrix*

Figure-1: GPB under gram stain

- **Size:** 2 -3µm x 0.5 µm.
- **Shape:** Rod shape. Pleomorphic from small to medium coccobacilli. Filamentous forms observed in old culture.
- **Arrangement:** Singly or in pairs or with angle to each other mistaken as diphtheria. Also occurs in short chain.
- **Motility:** Tumbling motility (end over end) with peritrichous flagella at 25^0C (room temperature) but not at 37^0C (body temperature). Motility is due to temperature dependent flagella expression, **called differential motility.**
- **Non sporing & non-capsulated:**

Cultural characteristics (C/Cs):

- **Effective factors:**

- O_2 effect: Facultative anaerobes.
- Co_2 effect: Better growth occurs under 5-10% CO_2 (**Capnophilic bacteria**).
- Optimum temperature: 37^0C (range 1-45^0C).
- pH: Slightly alkaline about 9.6
- Grow on ordinary media. Growth is improved by adding carbohydrates, blood or liver extracts in media.
- It can grow in presence of 0.1% tellurite & 10% salt.

➢ **Culture in media:**

A. Liquid media:

1. Enrichment media:

- Like tryptose phosphate broth & thioglycollate broth
- Samples are collected in enrichment medium like trypticase soy broth & incubated at 4^0C followed by subculture on solid media every week for 1-6 months **called cold enrichment**.

B. Solid media/plating media:

1. **Blood agar:** Produces β-haemolysis may confuse with **β-haemolytic *Streptococci*** (***L. ivanovii*** gives inner zone of β-haemolysis surrounded by α-haemolysis).
2. **Mac Conkey's medium:** Poor growth.
3. **Tryptose phosphate agar:** Colonies are 0.5-1mm, smooth, translucent & easily emulsifiable.

C. Selective media:

1. **Mac Conkey's medium:** Poor growth.
2. **PALCAM agar:** Make the medium selective by adding the Polymyxin, Acriflavine, Lithium chloride, Ceftazidime, Aesculin & Mannitol.

➢ **Culture in animal (Anton test):** Instillation of culture in to the eyes of guinea pig/rabbit produces kerato-conjunctivitis within 24 hours **called Anton test**.

❖ Biochemical reactions (B/Rs):

1. **Sugar fermentation:** Ferments glucose, maltose, rhamnose, salicin & α-methyl D-mannoside with acid production without gas.
2. **I M Vi C test:** - + + -
3. **Catalase test:** +Ve
4. **Oxidase & urease test:** -Ve
5. **H_2S:** -Ve
6. **Aesculin hydrolysis test:** +Ve
7. **CAMP test:** +Ve

❖ **Immunity:** Bacilli are intracellular & antibodies are not protective. CMI is useful.

❖ Pathogenicity:

➢ **Disease name: Called listeriosis.**

➢ **Nature & history of disease:**

- *L. monocytogenes* serotype 4b strains are responsible for 33 to 5% of sporadic human cases worldwide and for all major food borne outbreaks in Europe and North America since the 1980s.
- *L. monocytogenes* was not identified as a cause of food borne illness until 1981, however. An outbreak of listeriosis in Halifax, Nova Scotia, involving 41 cases and 18 deaths, mostly in pregnant women and neonates, was epidemiologically linked to the consumption of coleslaw containing cabbage that had been contaminated with *L. monocytogenes*-contaminated sheep manure. Since then, a number of cases of food borne listeriosis have been reported, and *L. monocytogenes* is now widely recognized as an important hazard in the food industry.
- It is one of the most virulent food borne pathogens, with case-fatality rate is around 20 -30%.
- Responsible for an estimated 1,600 illnesses and 260 deaths in the United States annually, listeriosis ranks third in total number of deaths among food borne bacterial pathogens, with fatality rates exceeding even *Salmonella* (1%) & *Cl. botulinum*.

➢ **Reservoir of infection:**

- Common reservoirs are mammals, fish, birds, animals, ticks & crustacean. Also present as saprophytes in decaying materials, water & soil.
- Study suggests that 10% of human GIT are colonised by *L. monocytogenes*.

➢ **Source of infection:** *Listeria* have tendency to grow at wide range of temperature from (range 1-45^0C, refrigerator to body temperature) hence it present in all hot & cold (refrigerated) items. Common sources are as below.

- Milk of infected animals: Pasteurised or unpasteurised.
- Food: Vegetables like prepared salad, milk products like soft cheese & butter, non vegetable like meat of turkey, undercooked chickens, hot dogs & few others like coleslaw, pate etc.
- Other sources are water, respiratory droplets, contaminated hospital devices etc.

➢ **Mode of transmission:**

A. Direct:

1. **Contact:** *Listeria* is also a common veterinary pathogen, being associated with abortion & encephalitis in sheep and cattle. Occupational **contact** with animal, birds in veterinarian, animal handles & poultry worker is the mode for human entry.
2. **Vertical:** By placenta or by infected birth canal to neonates.

B. Indirect (vehicle borne):

1. **Air borne:** By inhalation of dust.
2. **Food borne:** Unpasteurised (raw) milk of infected animal or cabbage contaminated with sheep manure.
3. **Fomites borne:** To neonates via contaminated hospital equipments or from contaminated hands-fingers of nurse.

➢ **Incubation period:**

- Variable from 3 to 70 days.
- The onset of serious forms of listeriosis is unknown but may range from a few days to three weeks.
- The onset of gastrointestinal symptoms is unknown but probably exceeds 12 hours.

➢ **Portal of entry:** Skin, GIT, respiratory tract etc.

➢ **Sites:** Meninges, brain, spinal cord, blood, uterus & also other organs.

➢ **Precipitating factors (epidemiological determinants):** Three types

I. Agent factors (virulence factors)

A. Antigens:

- Have fourteen O-Ag which are heat stable & four H-Ag which are heat labile.
- Based on agglutination reaction several serovars (1/2a, 1/2b, 1/2c, 3a, 3b, 3c, 4a, 4b, 4ab, 4c, 4d, 4e & 7) are identified.
- 90% of listeriosis is caused by serovar-1/2a, 1/2b & 4b.

B. Toxin:

- Haemolysin-O **called listeriolysin-O**.
- Antigenically similar to streptolysin-O & pneumolysin.

C. Intracellular location: Intracellular nature (ability to survive within mononuclear phagocytes and host epithelial cells) of bacilli helps to evades the host defence like action of complement & antibodies & also the antibiotic effects.

D. Motility: Help in spread of infection from one cell to other cell.

E. Adhesin (organ of adhesion): Two types like

- D-galactose in their teichoic acids help to bound with D-galactose receptors on macrophage's polysaccharides of payer's patches & epithelial cells.
- Other important adhesins are the internalins (A & B are subtypes). To attach with phagocytic cells bacteria required internalin. Internalin A binds to E-cadherin, while internalin B binds to the cell's Met receptors. If both of these receptors have a high enough affinity to *Listeria*'s internalin A and B, then it will be able to invade the cell via an indirect mechanism **called zipper mechanism**.
- Corresponding receptors of adhesions are also found in blood brain barrier & placenta, which provide the channel for manifestation in brain & foetus in uterus.

F. Ability to grow at wide range of temperature: Ability of bacteria to grow at temperatures as low as 0 °C permits exponential multiplication in refrigerated foods. At refrigeration temperature, such as 4 °C, the amount of ferric iron can affect the growth of *L. monocytogenes*.

G. Infective dose: Fewer than 1,000 total organisms may cause disease.

H. Feric iron: Bacteria produce siderophore & are able to obtain the iron from transferring.

I. Endotoxin (LPS): An early study suggested that *L. monocytogenes* is unique among Gram-positive bacteria in that it might possess LPS, which serves as an endotoxin. Later, it was found to not be a true endotoxin. *Listeria* cell walls consistently contain lipoteichoic acids resemble the LPS of Gram-negative bacteria in both structure & function.

II. Host factors

1. **Age:** Neonates & older are at more risk.
2. **Sex:**

- No sex bar but disease is common in pregnancy because the organism has the ability to penetrate the endothelial layer of the placenta.
- Pregnancy encounters 27% of total cases mostly during 3rd trimester.

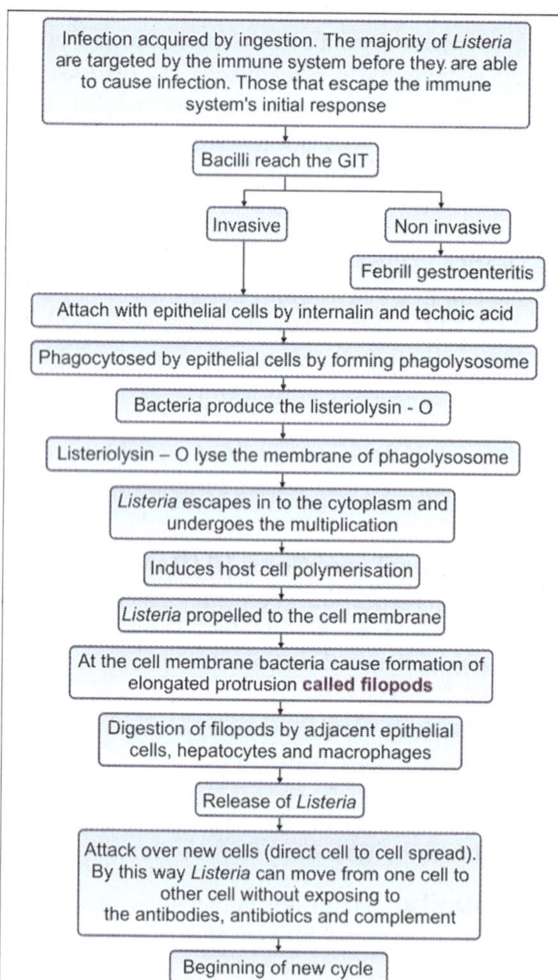

Flow chart-1: Pathogenesis of *L. monocytogenes*

3. **Patients with immunosuppressive condition:** It is an opportunistic pathogen, more in patients with cirrhosis, diabetes, HIV, blood cancer & immunosuppressive therapy otherwise only seven per 1,000,000 healthy people are infected with virulent *Listeria* each year.

III. Environmental factors

1. **Distribution:** Bacilli are distributed mammals, fish, birds, animals, ticks & crustacean. Also present as saprophytes in decaying materials, water & soil.

- **Pathogenesis: →Flow chart-1**
- **Clinical features:** Listeriosis is a food borne illness & defined in two categories.

a. **Noninvasive listeriosis:** Present as febrill gastroenteritis with local GIT features.

b. **Invasive listeriosis:** Following three subtypes.

1. **Pregnancy associated listeriosis:** In pregnant women cause abortion, still birth, premature delivery. Infertility in adult female.
2. **Neonatal listeriosis:** Characterised as neonatal meningitis. It is the 4th (3rd by few authors) most common cause of meningitis in newborns. [*E. coli* (34%) > Group B β-Haemolytic *Streptococci* (*Strept. agalactiae,* 30%) > GNB (8%) > *Listeria monocytogenes* (6%)]. Following two subtypes.

- **Early infection:**
  - Onset in < 5 days (mean age = 1.5 days).
  - Acquired via placenta.
  - Associated with obstetrical complications like pre mature delivery & low birth weight.
  - Common presentation is neonatal sepsis.
  - Common complication is granulomatous infantseptica.
  - Mortality: Very high about > 30 %.
  - Nosocomial outbreak: Absent.
- **Late infection:**
  - Onset in > 5 days (mean age = 14.2 days).
  - Acquired from infected birth canal or from environment or from contaminated hospital equipments or from contaminated hand-finger of nurse.
  - Not associated with obstetrical complications as mentioned earlier.
  - Common presentation is neonatal meningitis.
  - Granulomatous infantseptica is not seen.
  - Mortality: Low about > 30 %
  - Nosocomial outbreak: Present

3. **Listeriosis associated with immunosuppression:**
   - Common in older group.
   - Present with meningitis-meningoencephalitis, conjunctivitis, abscess, urethritis, pneumonia, endocarditis, septicemia etc.

- **Complications:** Surviving neonates of faetomaternal listeriosis may suffer granulomatosis infantiseptica-pyogenic granulomas distributed over the whole body & may suffer from physical retardation.

❖ Laboratory diagnosis:

I. Human samples

- **Specimens:** CSF, blood, sputum, vaginal discharge, placental tissue, lochia, meconium, nasopharyngeal aspirates, gastric aspirates & eye-ear-skin swab.
- **Collection:** Follow **cold enrichment** as mentioned above.
- **Testing methods:**

A. **Microscopy: → Follow morphology**
B. **Culture: → Follow C/Cs**
C. **Biochemical reactions: → Follow B/Rs**

II. Food samples

- **Specimens:** Suspected food materials.
- **Collection:** Follow **cold enrichment** as mentioned above.
- **Testing methods:**

A. **DNA probe:** The methods for analysis of food are complex and time-consuming. The present U.S. FDA method, revised in September 1990, requires 24 and 48 hours of enrichment, followed by a variety of other tests. Total time to identification takes five to seven days, but the announcement of specific non-radio labelled DNA probes should soon allow a simpler and faster confirmation of suspect isolates.

❖ Prevention:

- Early diagnosis & treatment of infection in pregnancy.
- Proper preparation of food by washing of vegetables.
- Use of pasteurised of milk.

❖ Treatment:

- Pregnant patient: Ampicillin or Pn G are effective. Erythromycin is given in patient allergic to Pn.
- Non-pregnant patient: Ampicillin or Pn G are effective. Cotrimoxazole (trimithoprim & sulphamithoxazole) & gentamicin are given in patient allergic to Pn.
- Neonate: Ampicillin.
- Cephalosporin is not effective.

Listeria ivanovii

- *L. ivanovii* gives inner zone of β-haemolysis surrounded by α-haemolysis.
- *L. ivanovii* is a pathogen of mammals, specifically ruminants & has rarely caused listeriosis in humans.

Erysipelothrix rhusiopathiae

❖ Synonym: *Erysipelothrix insidiosa*

❖ **Morphology: →Figure-1(b)**

- **Type according to gram stain:** GPB.
- **Size:** 1-2μm x 0.2-0.4 μm.
- **Shape:** Straight-rod shape, slightly curve or filamentous forms are also observed.
- **Non sporing, non-capsulated & nonmotile:**

❖ **Cultural characteristics (C/Cs):**

- **Effective factors:**
  - O_2 effect: Microaerophilic in primary culture but aerobes & facultative anaerobes on subculture.
  - Optimum temperature: 30-37^{0}C, no growth at 4^{0}C
  - Grow on ordinary media & growth is improved by adding glucose or serum.
  - Shows ***S-R*** forms. **S (Smooth) forms→** forms at 33^{0}C & in alkaline pH, **R (Rough) forms→** forms at 37^{0}C in neutral pH. **R Form** suggests long filamentous form or chain.
- **Media:**

A. **Liquid media:**

1. **Glucose broth:**
2. **Serum broth:**

} **S forms→** uniform turbidity, **R forms→** flocculent or matted growth

B. **Solid media/plating media:**

1. **Nutrient agar:** Growth is improved by adding glucose or serum.
2. **Blood agar:** Shows **S-R** forms. **S form: →** smooth colonies with circular entire edge, 0.5-1mm, low convex, translucent and glistening surrounded by α –haemolysis, forms at 33^{0}C & in alkaline pH. **R→** rough forms at 37^{0}C in neutral pH.

C. **Selective media:**

1. **Liquid selective media:** Liquid media + 0.04% kanamycin & 0.0025% vancomycin.
2. **Solid selective media:** Blood agar + 0.1% sodium azide & 0.001% crystal violet.
3. **Mac Conkey's medium:** No growth.
4. **PT medium:** Black colonies.

❖ **Biochemical reactions (B/Rs):**

1. **Sugar fermentation:** G S L M
   A - A -
   (Other sugars fermented are galactose, fructose with production of acid only.)
2. **Coagulase test:** Tube and/or slide tests are +Ve with rabbit and/or bovine serum.
3. **I M Vi C test:** - - - -
4. **H_2S:** +Ve in TSI
5. **Catalase, oxidase, urease & nitrate tests:** -Ve

❖ **Pathogenicity:**

- **Reservoir of infection:** Animals like fish, pig etc.
- **Mode of transmission:**

1. **Direct contact:** Contact of wounded skin with infected animal tissue or animal products in animal handler. Common in animal handlers.
2. **Rarely by ingestion**

- **Clinical features:**

1. **Animal infection: Erysipelas** in pig, sheep & fish.
2. **Human infection: Erysipeloid** characterized by painful, purplish swelling without pus (pus present in staphylococcal & streptococcal erysipelas). Commonly present on hands & on finger due to direct contact **called seal finger** or **called whale finger.**

- **Complications:**

1. **Local:** Arthritis, Lymphangitis & lymphadenitis.
2. **Systemic:** Septicemia, endocarditis occurs directly by ingestion or due to blood invasion from erysipeloid.

❖ **Laboratory diagnosis:**

- **Specimens:** Tissue or biopsy from local lesion. Blood in systemic infection.
- **Transport:** Samples are collected in liquid selective media, sent to laboratory followed by subculture over plating media.
- **Testing methods:**

I. **Microscopy: → Follow morphology**
II. **Culture: → Follow C/Cs**
III. **Biochemical reactions: → Follow B/Rs**

❖ **Prevention:** Educate the risk group while handling the animals.

❖ **Treatment:** Pn, erythromycin & other antibiotics are effective. It is intrinsically resistant to vancomycin.

Question bank

Case study

1) A 3 weeks old child presented to the paediatrician with the features of meningitis. A presumptive diagnosis of late onset of perinatal infection was made. The CSF culture was positive for gram positive bacilli. Identify the case & answer the following
   a) Name the clinical condition in given case & its causative agent
   b) Describe the morphology & culture characteristics of causative agent
   c) Describe the pathogenicity of causative agent
2) A 30 year old woman with a bad obstetric history presents with fever. The blood culture from the patient grows gram positive small to medium coccobacilli that are pleomorphic, occurring in short chains. Direct wet mount from the culture shows tumbling motility. Identify the case & answer the following
   a) Name the clinical condition in given case & its causative agent
   b) Describe different mode of transmission of causative agent
   c) Describe the laboratory diagnosis of causative agent

Short notes

1) Listeriosis
2) *E. rhusiopathiae*

Short questions

1) What is cold enrichment?
2) What are Anton test & Sereny test?

MCQs for chapter review

L. monocytogenes

1) **All of the following are true about *Listeria* except -** (AI- 04)
(a) Transmitted by contaminated milk (b) Gram negative bacteria (c) Cause abortion in pregnancy (d) Cause meningitis in neonates
2) **True statement about *Listeria*:-**
(a)) Gram negative bacillus (b) Motile by peritrichous flagella (c) Commonest cause of community acquired meningitis (d) Only one serovars known
3) **Listeria culture media -** (AIIMS, May-09)
(a) Baker (b) Korthoff (c) Tinsdale (d) Blood agar
4) **Anton test is used for -**
(a) *Listeria monocytogenes* (b) *Ligionells* (c) *Brucella* (d) *Bordetella*
5) **Major step in pathogenesis of listeriosis is-** (AIIMS, Nov-05)
(a) The formation of antigen-antibody complexes with resultant complement activation and tissues damage (b) The release of hyaluronidase by *L. monocytogenes*, which contributes to its dissemination from local sites (c) The antiphagocytic activity of the *L. monocytogenes* capsule (d) The survival and multiplication of *L. monocytogenes*, within mononuclear phagocytes and host epithelial cells
6) **Most of the cases of *Listeria* are due to-**
(a) 1 (b) 4a (c) 4b (d) 6
7) **In a patient of Listeria meningitis who is allergic to penicillin the treatment of choice is –** (AIIMS 04)
(a) Vancomycin (b) Gentamicin (c) Trimithoprim-sulfamethaxozole (d) Ceftriaxone

E. rhusiopathiae

8) **Route of infection in erysipelod is-**
(a) Ingestion (b) Direct inoculation (c) Inhalation (d) Congenital
9) **Following is the lesion not containing pus-**
(a) Erysipeloid (b) Impetigo (c) boil (d) Erysipelas
10) **Seal finger and whale finger are associated with**
(a) *Listeria* (b) *Erysipelothrix* (c) *Corynebacterium* (d) *Treponema*

Answers of MCQs & explanation

1) **(b)**
- *Listeria* is a gram positive bacterium not gram negative

2) **(b)**
- Gram positive bacillus
- Motile by peritrichous flagella
- Commonest cause of nosocomial meningitis
- Many serovars as mentioned with respective section

3) **(d)** }
4) **(a)** } Follow section ***L. monocytogenes*** **(culture characteristics)** for explanation

5) **(d)**
- Intracellular nature (ability to survive within mononuclear phagocytes and host epithelial cells) of *Listeria* helps to evades the host defence like action of complement & antibodies & also the antibiotic effects.

6) **(c)**
- *L. monocytogenes* serotype 4b strains are responsible for 33 to 5% of sporadic human cases worldwide and for all major food borne outbreaks in Europe and North America since the 1980s.

7) **(b) & (c)**
- Follow section ***L. monocytogenes*** **(treatment)** for explanation.

8) **(b)**
- Follow section ***E. rhusiopathiae*** **(pathogenicity → mode of transmission)** for explanation.

9) **(a)**
- Erysipeloid is caused by *E. rhusiopathiae* not containing pus
- Other lesions are caused by *Streptococci* & *Staphylococci*, are containing pus

10) **(b)**
- Follow section ***E. rhusiopathiae*** **(pathogenicity → clinical features)** for explanation.

42 Actinomycetales

Learning heading & subheadings

- Meaning:
- Uses:
- Classification:
  - *Actinomyces*
  - *Nocardia*
  - Mycetoma
  - Botryomycosis
  - *Tropheryma*

Meaning: **Actino** word derived from **actis** = **rays** like appearance in granules & mycetes from **mykes** = **branching or filamentous** shape like fungi.

Uses: Antibiotics produced from *Streptomyces* spp. are labelled with suffix "mycin" (except rifampicin). Following are the examples

- Streptomycin (1944): From *Streptomyces griseus*
- Kanamycin (1957):From *Streptomyces kanamyceticus*
- Tobramycin (1970): From *Streptomyces tenebrarius*
- Neomycin: From *Streptomyces fradiae*
- Framyctin: From *Streptomyces lavendulae*
- Erythromycin (1952): From *Streptomyces erythreus*
- Rifampicin (Rifampin): From *Streptomyces mediterranei.*

Classification:→ **Flow chart-1**

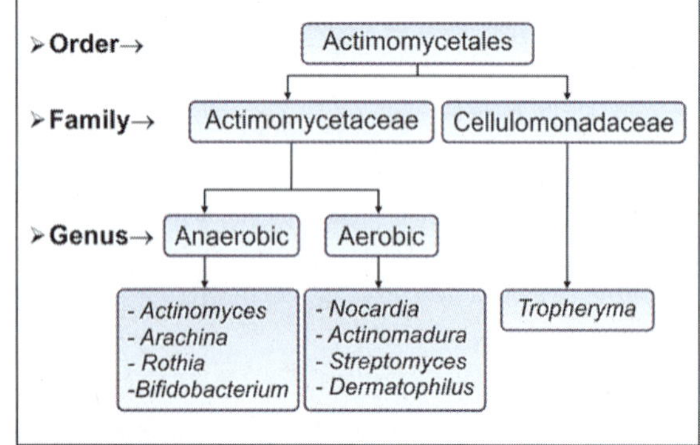

Flow chart-1: Classification of Actimomycetales

Actinomyces

- **Species:** *A. israelii, A. bovis, A. naeslundii, A. viscosus, A. odontolyticum, A. gerencsonei & A. meyeri.*
- **History:** Pathologist Otto Bollinger described the presence of *A. bovis* in cattle in 1877 & shortly afterwards, James Israel discovered *A. israelii* in humans in 1890.
- **Morphology:**
  - **Type according to gram stain:** Gram positive filamentous bacilli / cocco-bacilli as shown in **fig.-1(a)**

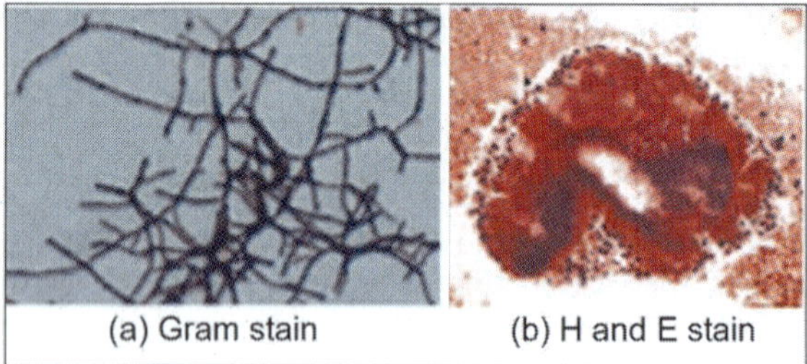

Figure-1: Staining of *Actinomyces* & sulfur granules

  - **Acid fastness:** Non acid fast.
  - **Size:** Variable.
  - **Shape:** Branching (filamentous) like fungi or curved.
  - **Motility:** Non motile.
  - **Spore:** Non-sporing.
  - **Capsule:** Non-capsulated.
- **Cultural characteristics C/Cs):**
  - **Effective factors:**
    - O_2 effect: Strict anaerobe.
    - Temperature: 37°C.
  - **Media:**

A. Liquid Media:

1. **Thioglycollate broth:** *A. israelii* produce fluffy ball like growth. *A. bovis* produce general turbidity.

B. Solid media:

1. **BHIA:** Molar tooth or spidery or bread crumb appearance of colonies after 48-72 hrs.

- **Biochemical reactions (B/Rs):**

1. **Sugar fermentation:** All species ferment the glucose.
2. **Catalase test:** -Ve

- **Pathogenicity:**
  - **Disease name: Called actinomycosis.** It is the chronic granulomatous lesion of connective tissues with multiples sinuses discharging sulfur granules.

- **Reservoir & source of infection:** Normal flora of human mouth, intestine & vagina, so human acts as reservoir & source of infection.
- **Mode of transmission:**
  - **Endogenous infection:** It occurs following disturbances of this flora by trauma, foreign body insertion like Intra Uterine Contraceptive Devices (IUCD), poor oral hygiene etc.
  - **Co- infection:** Actinomycosis is associated with other bacteria like staphylococci, anaerobic streptococci, *Bacteroides, Fusobacter, Bifidobacterium dentium, Haemophilus aphrophilus, Eikenella corrodens* etc.
- **Sites:** Most common sites are cervicofacial (angle of jaw), abdomen, thorax, pelvis, CNS, musculoskeletal, liver, lungs & internal organs.
- **Precipitating factors (epidemiological determinants):**

1. **Age:** Common in young adult from 10-30 years.
2. **Sex:** More in males then females. 60% cases are cervicofacial & 20% cases are abdominal. In female pelvic actinomycosis is common due to use of IUCD.
3. **Occupation:** Common in agriculture workers.
4. **Location:** More in rural areas than urban. In developed countries incidences are declining due to use of antibiotics.
5. **Other factors:** Like poor hygiene.

- **Pathology:**
  - Lesion is characterised by granulomatous swelling with multiples sinuses discharging pus & granules (yellow colour).
  - Granules are < 5mm in size, hard & yellow in colour **called sulfur granules**.
  - Word sulfur indicate the yellow colour of granules, neither the presence of sulfur in granules nor related to any contents.
- **Clinical features:** Most common species causing actimomycosis is *A. israelii* with following features.

A. Lumpy jaw:

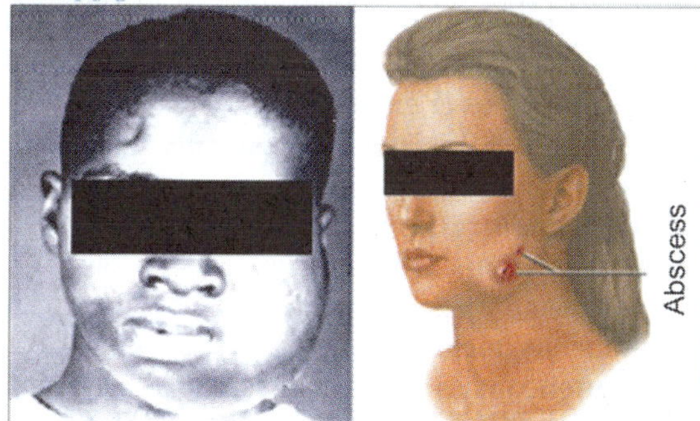

Figure-2: Lumpy jaw in human

- Present on cheeks & submaxillary region.
- It is the most common type & hold about 60% cases of total actinomycosis.
- Most common site is angle of jaw (cervicofacial) & lesion **called lumpy jaw** (**fig.-2**) characterised by painless, hard mass, slow growing, large swelling / abscess that grow on the head and neck. It may be due penetration by oral flora by local trauma during dental treatment, poor oral hygiene, periodontal disease, radiation therapy or accidental injury (broken jaw). It can also affect swine, horses, dogs, sheep & less often wild animals.
- Other cervicofacial lesions are otitis, sinusitis & canaliculitis.

B. Actinomycosis in abdomen: Around caecum.

C. Actinomycosis in thorax: In lungs, pleura & pericardium.

D. Actinomycosis in pelvis: Mostly in IUCD users.

E. Mycetoma: Lesion in subcutaneous tissues.

F. Gingivitis & periodonititis:

❖ Laboratory diagnosis:

- **Specimens:**
  - Pus or discharge from sinus.
  - Tissue biopsy.
  - Sputum.
  - Granules: Collected in test tubes containing sterile saline. Washed several times in sterile saline & slide is prepared by crushing the granules between two slide. Hold the crushed granules by sterile forceps & rubbed over medium for culture.
- **Testing methods:**

I. Microscopy:

1. **Gram stain:**
   - GPB are seen as shown in **fig.-1(a).**
   - Sulfur granules are yellowish in colour. Granules appear centrally as gram positive filaments (due to bacterial colonies) & peripheral as gram negative (due to Ag-Ab complex by host defence mechanism) giving club shape or sun ray appearance.
2. **Haemotoxylin & Eosin stain:** Centrally bacilli & inflammatory cells present peripherally as shown in **fig.-1(b).**
3. **Modified Z N stain:** To differentiate from *Nocardia.*
4. **Fluorescent staining:** Also useful staining method.

II. Culture: →Follow C/Cs

III. Biochemical reactions: → Follow B/Rs

IV. GLC: It detects the products of glucose metabolism.

V. Molecular methods: PCR &RFLP are useful.

❖ Treatment:

- **Antibiotics:** Pn is the drug of choice, will continue for several months. Tetracycline or erythromycin are useful in patients allergic to Pn.
- **Surgery:** If necessary.

Nocardia

❖ **Species:** *N. asteroids, N. brasiliensis, N. caviae (N. otitidiscaviarum)* etc.

❖ **Meaning & history:** The genus was named for Edmond Nocard, a 19th-century veterinarian & biologist.

❖ **Morphology:**

➢ **Type according to gram stain:** Gram positive filamentous bacilli/cocci-bacilli.

➢ **Acid fastness:** Acid fast by 1% sulphuric acid (**fig.-3**) & also weakly acid fast by Kinyoun's staining. Acid fastness is due to presence of intermediate length of glycolipid **called nocardic acid** (as like mycolic acid in *Mycobacteria*).

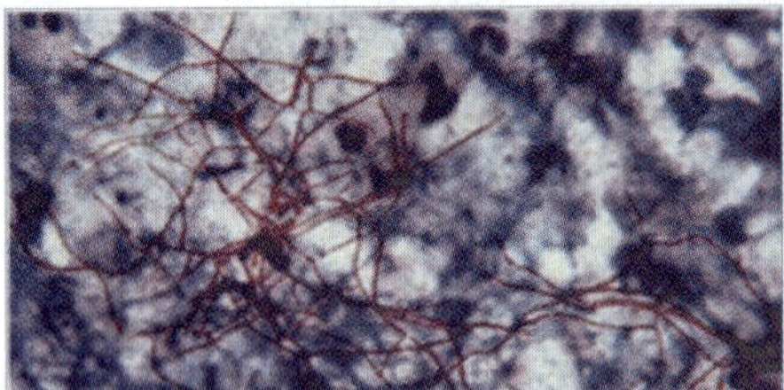

Figure-3: *Nocardia* under ZN stain

➢ **Size:** Variable.

➢ **Shape:** Curved or branching like fungi.

➢ **Motility:** Non motile.

➢ **Spore:** Non-sporing.

➢ **Capsule:** Non-capsulated.

➢ **Other useful staining methods are:** H & E stain

❖ **Cultural characteristics:**

➢ **Effective factors:**

- **O_2 effect:** Strict aerobes.
- **Temperature:** Normal temperature is $37^{o}C$ where growth occurs in 2 days to 2 weeks, but can grow at $45^{0}C$ in 3 days.

➢ **Media:**

A. **Solid media:** Dry, glabrous, wrinkled/folded or may be pigmented (yellow to orange/red colour) & adherent (to the medium) colonies may occurs on following media.

1. **Sabouraud dextrose agar without antibiotics**
2. **Blood agar**
3. **BHIA**

B. **Selective media:**

1. **Sabouraud dextrose agar with chloramphenicol:** chloramphenicol prevents the bacterial contamination by other bacteria.
2. **Buffered yeast extract agar contains polymyxin & vancomycin:** Polymyxin & vancomycin are selective agents.
3. **Medium for paraffin bait technique:** Media contains paraffin (sole source of carbon), are useful to identify the *Nocardia* from soil & clinical samples.
4. **Lowenstein Jensen medium:** Produces moist glabrous colonies.

❖ **Biochemical reactions (B/Rs):**

1. **Sugar fermentation:** Non fermenters but utilise (assimilation) the numbers of sugars oxidatively.
2. **Catalase test:** +Ve
3. **Urease test:** +Ve (By all species).
4. **Hydrolysis of casein, hypoxanthine & tyrosine:** +Ve
5. **Acetamide utilisation test:** +Ve
6. **Growth in lysozyme:** +Ve

❖ **Pathogenicity:**

➢ **Disease name: Called nocardiosis.**

➢ **Nature of disease:**

- Normally found in soil, these organisms cause occasional sporadic disease in humans and animals throughout the world.
- High mortality exceeds 80% especially with brain infection; in other forms, mortality is 50%, even with appropriate therapy.

➢ **Reservoir & source of infection:** Natural habitat in soil & over vegetative materials.

➢ **Mode of transmission:** Exogenous infection from soil via inhalation (pulmonary nocardiosis) or by trauma (skin & subcutaneous nocardiosis).

➢ **Portal of entry:** Skin & respirator system.

➢ **Sites:** Lungs, skin, subcutaneous tissues, brain etc.

➢ **Precipitating factors (epidemiological determinants):** Two types

I. Agent factors (virulence factors)

1. **Cord factor (glycolipid derivative or nocardic acid):** Cell wall of nocardia contains intermediate length of glycolipid **called nocardic acid**. dimycolyltrehalose **called cord factor** which is inhibit the phagocytosis.
2. **Enzymes:** Super oxide dismutase & catalase.

➢ **Pathology:**

- Pulmonary nocardiosis is characterised by granuloma with neutrophilic infiltration, necrosis & abscess.
- Skin & subcutaneous nocardiosis is characterised by granulomatous swelling with multiples sinuses discharging pus & granules.
- Granules are 0.5-2mm in size, soft, lobulated & yellowish-white in colour.

➢ **Clinical features:**

1. **Pulmonary nocardiosis:** Pneumonia, abscess & granulomatous lesion simulating tuberculosis.
2. **Cutaneous nocardiosis:** Abscess, cellulitis etc.
3. **Subcutaneous nocardiosis:** Mycetoma (actinomycetoma).
4. **Systemic nocardiosis:** Brain abscess (most common by *N. asteroides*), keratitis, metastatic complication in kidneys other organs. More in person with IDDs.

II. Host factors

1. **IDDs:** It is an opportunistic pathogen present commonly in person with AIDS, tuberculosis, steroid therapy & organ transplantation.

❖ Laboratory diagnosis:

➢ **Specimens:**
- Pus or discharge from sinus.
- Tissue biopsy.
- Sputum.
- Granules: Collected in test tubes containing sterile saline. Washed several times in sterile saline & slide is prepared by crushing the granules between two slide. Hold the crushed granules by sterile forceps & rubbed over medium for culture.

➢ **Testing methods:**

I. **Microscopy:** →Follow morphology
II. **Biochemical reactions:** → Follow B/Rs
III. **Culture:** →Follow C/Cs

❖ Treatment:

➢ **Antibiotics:**
- Pn is resistant.
- Sulphonamide is the drug of choice.
- Cotrimoxazole (sulphamethoxazole & trimithoprim) or minocycline will continue for several months.
- In immunocompromised persons addition of amikacin & cefotaxime are advisable.

➢ **Surgery:** If necessary.

❖ Differences between *Actinomyces* & *Nocardia*: →Table 1

Features	*Actinomyces*	*Nocardia*
	Staining	
Acid fastness	Non-acid fast	Acid fast
	Culture characteristics	
O_2 effect	Anaerobic	Aerobic
Temperature for growth	37° C	37° C, but can grow at 45°C
Colonies	Non-pigmented	Pigmented
	Biochemical reactions	
Sugar reaction	Fermenter	Assimilation
Catalase	-Ve	+Ve
	Pathology & treatment	
Natural habitat	Mouth, GIT & vagina	Soil
Mode of infection	Endogenous	Exogenous
Infection occurs in	Immunocompetent	Immunodeficient
Granules		
Size	> 5mm	0.5-2 mm
Consistency	Hard	Soft
Colour	Yellow	Yellowish white
Treatment	Pn	Sulphonamide, cotrimoxazole

Table 1: Differences between *Actinomyces* & *Nocardia*

Mycetoma

More details: Follow chapter → Deep mycosis

Botryomycosis

More details: Follow chapter → Micrococcaceae

Tropheryma

❖ **Species:** *Trophyrema whipplei*

❖ **Synonym:** Previously *Trophyrema whippelii* name was given.

❖ **Common name & history:** Disease **called Whipple's disease**, from the name of George Hoyt Whipple who diagnosed the disease 1907. However the causative agent identified later in 2003 in Johns Hopkins hospital **called Whipple's bacilli**.

❖ Morphology:

- It is intracellular pathogen resent in macrophages of lamina propria & mesenteric lymph nodes.
- GPB, however in laboratory it can be stained as GNB or intermediate between GPB & GNB.
- Intracellular location is better stained by Periodic Acid Schiff (PAS) stain.

❖ **Culture characteristics:** Not useful.

❖ Pathogenicity:

➢ **Precipitating factors:**

1. **Age:** Common at 4th-5th decades of life.
2. **Sex:** More in male.

➢ **Clinical features:** Multisystem involvement.
- Endocarditis.
- Intestine: Causing malabsorption syndrome **called whipple's disease** or **called intestinal lipodystrophy** characterised by abdominal pain, diarrhoea, weight loss & mesenteric lymphadenitis.
- Neurological disturbances.
- Polyarthritis.
- Hyperpigmentation of skin.
- Also damage to kidneys, lungs, spleen & liver.

❖ Laboratory diagnosis:

➢ **Specimens:** Intestinal or mesenteric lymph node biopsy.

➢ **Testing methods:**

I. **Microscopy:** PAS stain identifies the intracellular bacilli.
II. **Culture:** Not useful.
III. **Molecular:** PCR targeting 16S ribosomal RNA is useful.
IV. **D-Xylose absorption test:**
- In normal individuals, a 25 g oral dose of D-xylose will be absorbed and excreted in the urine at approximately 4.5 g in 5 hours.

- A decreased urinary excretion of D-xylose is seen in conditions involving the GI mucosa, like small intestinal bacterial overgrowth & Whipple's disease
- In cases of bacterial overgrowth, the values of D-xylose absorption return to normal after treatment with antibiotics. In contrast, if the D-xylose urinary excretion is not normal after a course of antibiotics, then the problem must be due to a non-infectious cause of malabsorption (like celiac disease).

❖ Treatment:

- Pn, ampicillin, tetracycline or cotrimoxazole for 1-2 years.
- Hydroxochloroquine for 12-18 months.
- Chances of relapse of disease are 40%, it treatment taken for less than one year.

Question bank

Case study

1) A 50 year old female patient visited the surgical OPD with history of painless hard soft tissue swelling on left jaw which discharges granules. Macroscopic examination of granules revealed the sulphur granules. Microscopic examination of granules by gram stain suggests gram positive material in centre & gram negative material in periphery. Culture growth occurs under anaerobic incubation. Identify the organism & answer the following
   a) Name the clinical condition & causative agent
   b) Describe the morphology & culture characteristics of causative agent
   c) Write the pathogenicity of causative agent

2) A 40 year old male patient visited the medical OPD with history of fever & coughing. Radiological examination suggests the pneumonia. Sputum examination revealed filamentous GPB that showed acid fastness to 1% H_2SO_4. Culture growth occurs under aerobic incubation. Identify the organism & answer the following
   a) Name the clinical condition & causative agent
   b) Describe the morphology & culture characteristics of causative agent
   c) Write the pathogenicity of causative agent

Short notes

1) Acinomycosis
2) *Nocardia*
3) Whipple's bacilli

Short questions for theory/viva questions

1) Write four differences between *Actinomyces* & *Nocardia.*
2) What is botryomycosis?

MCQs for chapter review

Actinomyces

1) **Most common site for actinomycetes is**
(a)) Cervicofacial (b) Toracis (c) Abdomen (d) Brain
2) **Which of the following is the most predominant constituent of sulfur granules of actinimycosis-** (AIIMS, May- 04)
(a) Organisms (b) Neutrophils and monocytes (c) Monocytes and lymphocytes (d) Eosinophils
3) **Colour of granules of actinomycetes is -**
(a) Black (b) Yellow (c) Red (d) Brown
4) **Sulphur granules are composed of -**
(a) Organisms (b) Leucocytes (c) Erythrocytes (d) Keratinocytes

Nocardia

5) ***Nocardia* can be differentiated from the *Actinomyces* by -**
(a) ZN staining (b) Fontana stain (c) Gram stain (d) O_2 requirement
6) ***Nocardia* resemble *Actinomyces* morphologically but -**
(a) Are anaerobic (b) Are facultative anaerobic (c) Are aerobic (d) Require CO2 for growth
7) **A characteristic infection of *Nocardia asteroides* is-** (AI -12)
(a) Diarrhoea (b) Secondary dissemination to liver (c) Brain abscess (d) Colonic diverticulosis
8) **A clinical specimen was obtained from the wound of a patient diagnosed as nocardiosis. For the selective isolation of *Nocardia* species which of the following would be the best method-** (AIIMS -04)
(a) Paraffin bait technique (b) Castaneda's culture method (c) Craig's culture method (d) Hair bait technique

Answers of MCQs & explanation

1) **(a)**
- Follow section, ***Actimomyces* (pathogenicity → sites)** for explanation.

2) **(a)**
3) **(b)**
} Sulfur granules are yellowish in colour. Granules appear centrally as gram positive filaments (due to bacterial colonies) & peripheral as gram negative (due to Ag-Ab complex by host defence mechanism) giving club shape or sun ray appearance

4) **(b)**
- Follow section, ***Actimomyces* (laboratory diagnosis → microscopy →gram stain)** for explanation

5) **(a) & (d)**
6) **(c)**
} Follow **table-1** for explanation

7) **(c)**
- Follow section, ***Nocardia* (pathogenicity →clinical features)** for explanation

8) **(a)**
- Paraffin is the sole source of carbon & useful for selective isolation of *Nocardia* species
- Castaneda's culture method is the biphasic culture method useful in many bacteria like *S. typhi*, *Brucella* etc.
- Craig's culture method is useful to differentiate motile from non-motile bacteria
- Hair bait technique is useful diagnosis of dermatophytes

43 Enterobactericeae-I

(E. coli, Klebsiella, Proteus etc.)

Learning heading & subheadings

- Definition of Enterobactericeae:
- Classification of Enterobactericeae:
- Colour reaction by Enterobactericeae on different media:

Escherichiae

Klebsielleae

Proteeae

Erwinieae

Yersiniae

New genera of Enterobactericeae

Definition of Enterobactericeae: Any bacterium classified as a member of Enterobactericeae family if it has following criteria.

1. Normal habitat of intestine.
2. Gram-negative bacilli.
3. Non-acid fast.
4. Non-sporing.
5. May be capsulated.
6. May be motile by peritrichate flagella (except *Shigella* & *Klebsiella,* which are nonmotile) not by polar flagella
7. Aerobic and facultative anaerobic.
8. Grow on ordinary media (non fastidious)
9. Ferment glucose with production of A/AG
10. Reduce nitrate to nitrite.
11. Catalase positive (except *Sh. dysenteriae* type 1)
12. Oxidase negative (except *Plesiomonas shigelloides*)

Classification of Enterobactericeae:

A. Based on lactose fermentation in Mac Conkey medium:

1. Lactose Fermenters [LF(s)]:

- Also **called coliform bacilli.**
- Examples: *Escherichia* & *Klebsiella.*
- LF produces pink colonies on Mac Conkey medium.

2. Late Lactose Fermenters [LLF(s)]:

- Also **called paracolon bacilli.**
- Examples: *Shigella sonnei* & *Citrobacter.*
- LLF produces pale colonies earlier & later pink colonies on Mac Conkey's medium.

3. Non Lactose Fermenters [NLF(s)]:

- Examples: *Proteus, Providentia, Morgnella, Salmonella, Shigella* (except *Sh sonnei*) & *Yersinia*
- NLF produces pale/colourless colonies on Mac Conkey's medium.

B. Systemic classification:

- **Bases:** It based on morphological, biochemical, genetical & taxonomical properties.
- **Systems:** Three systems are employed like
1. Bergey's manual (1984).
2. Edward-Ewing classification (1986).
3. Farmer & Kelly classification (1991).
- **Properties of all systems:** All three systems are almost same & classify the family in to tribe / sub-family, genera, species & subspecies / serotypes / biotypes / bacteriophage types / colicin types.
- **Four tribes: →Table 1**

Tribe	Genus
Escherichiae	*Escherichia, Edwardsiella, Salmonella, Shigella & Citrobacter*
Klebsielleae	*Klebsiella, Entrobacter, Hafnia, Serratia, Pantoea , Cedacea*
Proteeae	*Proteus, Morganella, Providencia*
Erwinieae	*Erwinia*
Yersiniae	*Yersinia*
Newer genera: *Plesiomonas, Ewingella, Budvicia, Tatumella , Rahnella & Kluyvera*	

Table-1: Systemic classification of Enterobactericeae family

Colour reaction by Enterobactericeae on different media: →Table 2

Escherichiae

Escherichia coli

- **Meaning & history:** In 1885, the German-Austrian pediatrician Theodor Escherich discovered this organism in the faeces of healthy individuals.
- **Other species of genus:** *E. fergusoni, E. hermanii, E. vulneris, E. blattae* etc.
- **Uses:** *E. coli* is a very versatile host (vector) for the production of heterologous proteins like insulin, enzymes & vaccines by using recombinant technology.

Medium	Sugar	Indicator	Acidic pH	Alkline pH
Sugar media	G,S,L,M,	Andrade's	Pink	colourless
Mac Conkey's	L	Neutral red	Pink	Pale
DCA	L	Neutral red	Pink	Pale
SS agar	L	Neutral red	Pink	Pale
XLD medium	L, S	Phenol red	Yellow	pink
TSI	G, S, L	Phenol red	Yellow	pink
TCBS	S	Bromothymol blue	Yellow	Blue/green
CLED	L	Bromothymol blue	Yellow	Blue/green

Table-2: Colour reaction by Enterobactericeae on different media

❖ Morphology:→ Figure-1(a)

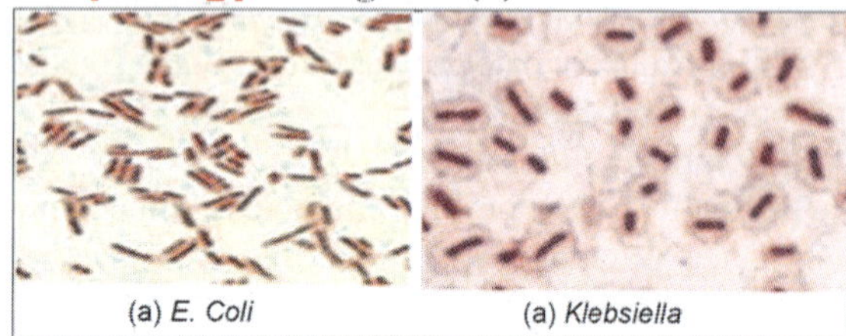

Figure-1: GNB under Gram stain

- **Type according to gram stain:** GNB.
- **Size:** 1–3 µm x 0.4–0.7 µm.
- **Shape:** Straight road.
- **Arrangement:** Singly, in pairs or in small groups.
- **Capsule:** Found in some strain.
- **Motility:** Motile by peritrichate flagella.
- **Spores:** Nonsporing.

❖ Cultural characteristics (C/Cs):

- **Effective factors:**
  - O_2 effect: Aerobe & facultative anaerobes.
  - Temperature: 37^0C.
  - pH: 7.6
- **Culture in media:**

A. Liquid media:

1. **Peptone water:** } Uniform turbidity
2. **Glucose broth:** } & heavy deposit at bottom

B. Semisolid stab agar: 'Fan type' growth outward from stab line.

C. Solid media:

1. **Nutrient agar:** Colonies are large, thick, grayish white, moist, smooth opaque or partially translucent discs. Initially smooth (S) become rough (R) on subculture **called S—R variation**. It is due to loss of cell wall antigens & virulence.
2. **Blood agar:** Produces haemolytic colonies.

D. Selective media:

1. **MacConkey's agar:** Bright pink (**pink spreading**) colony due to lactose fermentation as shown in **fig.-2(a)**.
2. **XLD (Xylose Lysine Deoxycholate) medium:** Yellow colony.
3. **CLED medium (Cysteine Lactose Electrolyte Deficient):** Yellow colony.
4. **DCA (Deoxycholate Citrate Agar):** }
5. **SS (Salmonella-Shigella) agar:** } Growth is
6. **W-B (Wilson-Blair) medium:** } inhibited

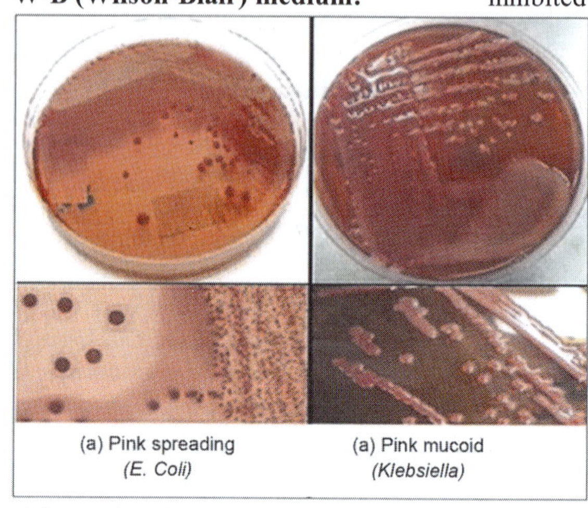

Figure-2: Pink colonies on Mac Conkey's agar

- **Culture in animals:** Uses of animals for cultivation of *E. coli* are described below with diarrheagenic strains of *E. coli.*

❖ Biochemical reaction (B/Rs):

1. **Sugar fermentation [fig.-3(a)]:** *E. coli* ferments maltose & many other sugars with acid & gas.

G	S	L	M
AG	V	AG	AG

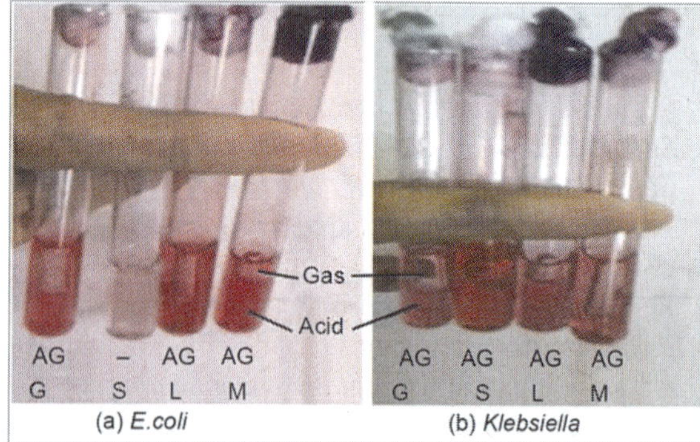

Figure-3: Sugar fermentation tests

2. **I M Vi C tests [fig.-4(a)]:** + + - -
3. **Catalase test:** +Ve
4. **Nitrate reduction test:** + Ve
5. **Oxidase test:** -Ve
6. **H_2S test:** -Ve
7. **Urease test:** -Ve

8. **TSI test [fig.-5(a)]:** AG/A-H_2S (AG = Acid + Gas, A= acid)

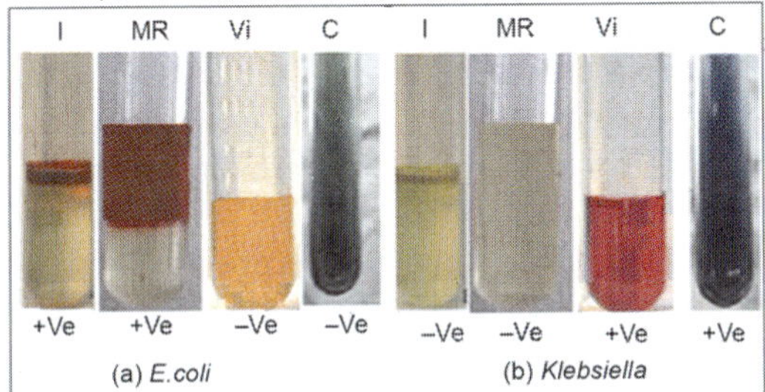

Figure-4: IMViC tests

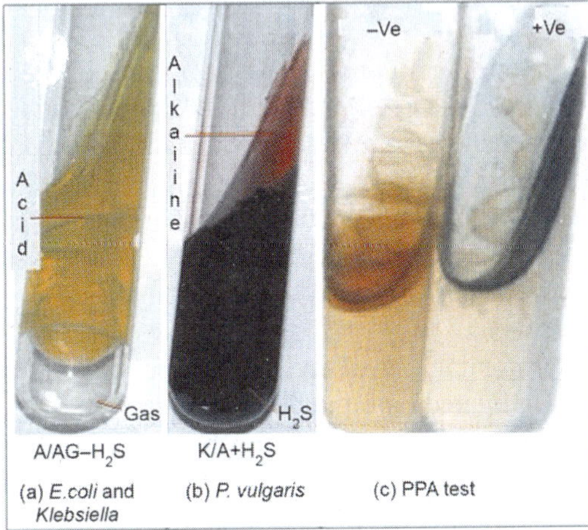

Figure-5: TSI (a & b) & PPA(c) tests

Resistance:

- It survives for several days in water, soil, dust & air & it can be easily killed by moist heat at 60^0C in 30 minutes.
- It also killed by 0.5-1 parts per million (ppm) chlorine in water.

Pathogenicity:

- **Disease name:** It produces following three diseases

I. **Urinary Tract Infection (UTI).**
II. **Diarrhoea**
III. **Other infections**

- **Reservoir of infection:** Human & animals are the reservoirs contain *E coli* as normal flora in the GIT.
- **Source of infection:** Water or food. Bacilli are excreted in faeces & remain viable for some days in the environment; hence detection of bacilli in water, specially a variant **called thermovariant *E. coli*** which survive at 44^0C, is taken as recent contamination from faeces of human or animals.
- **Mode of transmission:** By ingestion of contaminated food & water.
- **Incubation period:** 3 to 5 days, may be short as 1 day & long as 10 days.
- **Portal of entry:** GIT
- **Sites:** Intestinal & extra intestinal.
- **Precipitating factors (Epidemiological determinants):** Following are the factors.

I. **Agent factors (virulence factors)**

A. **Intracellular (cell wall associated) factors:**

i. **Capsular (K) antigen:** (German language **capsule** is termed as **Kapsel**).

- 100 types.
- Polysaccharide in nature inhibits phagocytosis.
- Mask the O-Ag & prevent the agglutination by O antiserum.

ii. **Flagellar (H) antigen:** (H is from **Hauch = mist or film of breath**, Growth on agar resemble like a film of breath on glass).

- 75 types.
- Organ of locomotion.

iii. **Somatic antigen (O Ag or LPS or Endotoxin):** (O is from **Ohne Hauch = without mist/film of breath**, Growth on agar without film).

- 170 types.
- Lipopolysaccharide exhibiting endotoxic activities.
- Also inhibit the phagocytosis & bactericidal effects on complement.

iv. **Fimbrial (Fi) antigen:** Organ of adhesion. Following different types are present in different types of *E. coli.*

1. **Colonisation Factor Antigens:** Present in ETEC & help to adhere with intestinal epithelial cells.
2. **Mannose resistant fimbriae:**
   - So, named because not inhibited by mannose.
   - Different examples are Dr, P, M, S & F1C.
   - P fimbriae help in attachment of *E. coli* with RBCs surface of P blood group **called haemagglutination.**
   - P fimbriae in EHEC, especially in nephritogenic strain & help in attachment with uroepithelial cells.
3. **Fucose (?):** It contains mannose & help in adhesion of human & animal cells.

B. **Extracellular factors:** Exotoxin production.

i. **Haemolysin:** Clinically it is not significant. Produced more by virulent than avirulent strains.

ii. **Enterotoxin:** Following three types.

a. **Heat labile toxin (LT):**

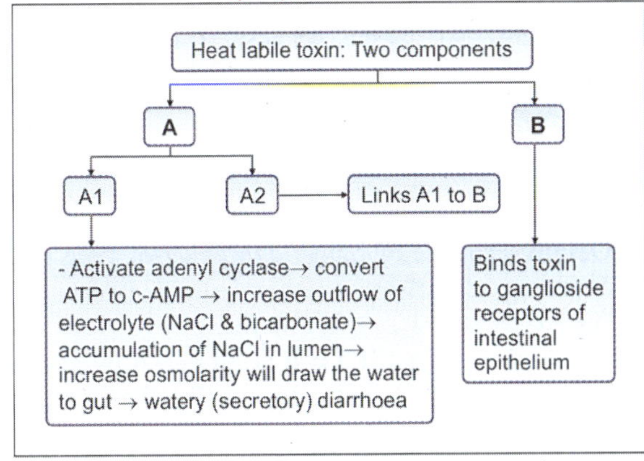

Flow chart-1: Heat labile enterotoxin

Properties:

- It was discovered by De & colleagues from the case of adult diarrhoea.

- Same as cholera toxin but less potent.
- Plasmid encoded.
- **Components/subtypes & action: → Flow chart-1**
- **Diagnostic tests: →Table-3**

Features	LT	ST
In vivo tests		
• **Ligated rabbit ileal loop**		
- Read at 6 hrs	±	±
- Read at 18 hrs	+	-
- Infant rabbit bowel	+	+
- Infant mouse intragastric (4 hrs)	-	+
• **Adult rabbit /guinea pig skin test (Skin blueing test):** To detect the vascular permeability factor (VPF)	+	-
In vitro tests		
Tissue culture test		
- Rounding of Y1 mouse adrenal cells	+	-
- Elongation of chinese hamster ovary cells due to intracellular increase c-AMP	+	-
Serological tests		
ELISA with monoclonal Ab	+	+
Passive agglutination test	+	-
Passive immune haemolysis/Precipitation/Eiken test	+	-
Molecular tests		
DNA probe	+	+

Table-3: Diagnostic tests of LT & ST

b. Heat stable toxin (ST):

- **Properties:** Plasmid encoded.
- **Components/subtypes & action: → Flow chart-2**
- **Diagnostic tests: →Table-3**

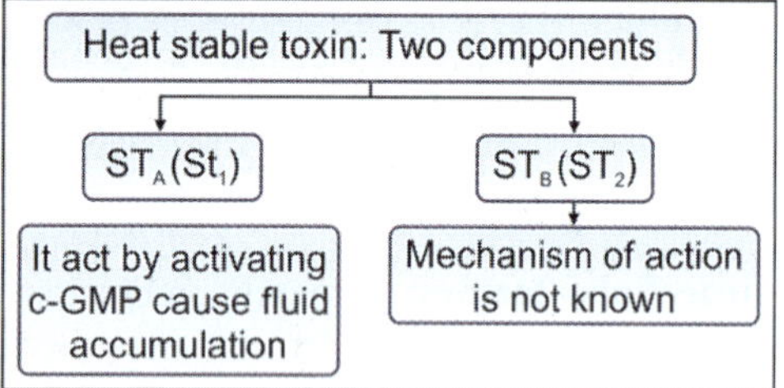

Flow chart-2: Heat stable enterotoxin

c. Verotoxin (VT) / verocytotoxin / Shiga like toxin (SLT):

- **Meaning:** So, called because it is cytotoxic on cultured vero cells, derived from African green monkey kidney cells.
- **Types:** Two main categories according to origin of bacteria.

1. Shiga toxin:

- **Origin:** Produce by *Shigella dysenteriae* type 1.
- **More details:** Follow chapter → Enterobactericeae –III (*Shigella*)

2. Shiga like toxin (SLT): It is produced by bacteria other than *Shigella* but antigenically, biochemically & physically similar to shiga toxin, so **called Shiga-Like Toxin (SLT).**

- **Bacteria producing SLT:** Entero haemorrhagic *E. coli, V. cholerae, Aeromonas hydrophila* & *Campylobacter jejuni.*
- **Properties of SLT:**
  - Gene responsible for production of SLT is bacteriophage coded.
- **Biological action of SLT:** Three types of actions
  - Neurotoxicity:
    - Detected by paralysis & death on injection in to mice or rabbits.
    - It is neurotoxic, but this property is secondary because it not acts directly on CNS but to the blood vessels supplying the nerve.
  - Cytotoxicity:
    - In vitro: Cytopathic changes in cultured Vero or HeLa cells.
    - In vivo: Toxin consists two sub units like binding (B) & active (A). Sub unit A divided in to two fragments like A1 & A2. B helps in adhesion with host cells. A2 links A1 to B. A1 inactivate the host cell 60S ribosome & inhibit the protein synthesis leading to cell death. Cell death resulting discontinuity of mucosa & haemorrhage (blood diarrhoea).
  - Enterotoxicity: It allows the collection of fluid in gut (in ligated rabbit ileal loop).
- **According to neutralisation by shiga antitoxin:** 2 subtypes like VT1 & VT2
  - VT1: Neutralised by shiga antitoxin.
  - VT2: Not neutralised by shiga antitoxin.
- **Diagnostic tests:** Detection of SLT is done by following tests.
  - Culture: Cytopathic changes in cultured Vero or HeLa cells.
  - Serology: Demonstration of VT antibody in sera by latex agglutination test & ELISA.
  - Molecular: DNA probe of VT1 and VT2 gene.

II. Host factors

1. Working around livestock.
2. Consuming unpasteurized dairy product.
3. Eating undercooked meat.
4. Drinking impure water.
5. Age younger and older adults are at a higher risk.
6. Weak immune system.

➢ **Clinical features:** *E coli* causes 3 diseases like UTI, diarrhoea & other infections as defined below.

I. Urinary Tract Infection (UTI)

- **Mode of transmission:**
  - **Ascending:** From faecal contamination of perineum to urethra & kidneys.
  - **Descending:** Spread from distant sites to the kidneys via blood.
- **Serotypes:** O group 1, 2, 4, 6 &7. One serotype can cause UTI at a time but recurrence may be by any serotype.
- **Precipitating factors**

- **Age:** More in children because of faecal contamination.
- **Sex:** More in female than male because of shorter urethra. *E. coli* cause 80-90% of lower UTI (cystitis) in young women.
- **Catheterisation** in 2% cases: *E. coli* is the most common cause of acute UTI (in 80% cases without catheter).
- **Obstruction** by prostatic enlargement, calculi, pregnancy & congenital malformation.

✪ **Types:** Two types as shown in **table-4**

Features	Upper UTI	Lower UTI
Sites	Kidneys & Ureters	Bladder & Urethra
Mode of infection	Ascending & Descending	Ascending
Clinical syndrome	Pyelonephritis	Cystitis & urethritis
C/Fs	Fever, vomiting & loin pain	Dysuria, urgency & frequency
Frequency	Less common	More common
Ags of *E. coli*	K-Ag	Fi-Ag

Table-4: Types of UTI caused by *E. coli*

✪ **Laboratory diagnosis**

♣ **Specimens:** Midstream urine sample.

♣ **Collection:**

a. **Manual:**

1. **In male:** Retract the prepuce, clean the glans with sterile gauze piece, wipe out the initial few drops & collect the mid stream urine in sterile wide open mouth container.
2. **Female:** Separate the labia by fingers, clean the genitals with sterile gauze piece, wipe out the initial few drops & collect the mid stream urine in sterile wide open mouth container.

b. **Catheterisation:** Normally urine is sterile but during voiding may be contaminated by genitals. To avoid such contamination catheterisation is suggested.

c. **Suprapubic aspiration:** In infants.

♣ **Transport:**

- Urine is good medium for growth of bacteria, therefore sent urine immediately to laboratory after collection without delay.
- If delay than store in refrigerator at 4^0C.
- If more delay is expected than add preservatives like 0.1g/10ml boric acid.

♣ **Testing methods:**

a. **Gross examination:**

- Appearance: Turbid.
- pH: pH is acidic in *E coli* infection.

b. **Microscopy:**

- **Wet preparation:** Examine it for the presence of bacteria, pus cells, RBCs, crystals, casts, epithelial cells etc.
- Presence of 3 pus cells per high power field suggests infection.
- **Gram stain: →Follow morphology**

c. **Culture:** Two types

1. **Quantitative:** Pour plate method.

- **Normally urine** is sterile but during voiding may be contaminated by genitals & culture suggests presence of bacteria which is categorised by **Kass concept.**
- **Significant bacteriuria:** $>10^5$ bacteria/ml indicates active infection & require treatment.
- **Doubtful/equivocal:** Between10^4 - 10^5/ml required repeat testing or take proper history.
- **Nonsignificant:** $<10^4$ / ml suggest no significant growth & regarded as a contaminant. However it is significant in patient with antibiotic therapy, diuretic drug & *Staph. aureus* infection.

2. **Semi-quantitative:**

- **Standard loop technique:** Loopful urine (0.004ml or1/250ml) is inoculated on blood agar & Mac Conkey's agar. After overnight incubation at 37 C, colony on blood agar counted and multiplies by 250 to get bacterial count per ml of urine.
- **Dip slide culture:**
- **Dip spoon**
- **Filter paper strip method**

d. **Biochemical reaction: →Follow B/Rs**

e. **Rapid screening tests:**

- **Advantages:** Useful in peripheral setup where culture is not possible.
- **Disadvantage:** Less sensitive & unreliable.
- **Tests:**

1. **Griess nitrate test:** Nitrate is not present in urine & its reduction to nitrite indicates presence of bacteria in urine.
2. **Catalase test:** Bubbles formation indicates Catalase producing bacteria in urine.
3. **Glucose paper test:** Based on utilization of glucose by urinary bacteria.
4. **Triphenyl Tetrazolium Chloride (TTC) test:** Reagent is converted in to pink-red colour indicate the respiratory activity of bacteria.
5. **Microscopic urine examination:** Under the gram stain.
6. **Dip slide culture:** Agar coated slide is exposed to urine sample or urine stream, incubated & observed for growth.

f. **Detection of site of infection:** By antibody coated bacteria test.

- **Principle:** When kidney is infected not bladder, Ab coated bacteria present in urine.
- **Detection:** Immunofluorescent using fluorescent tagged antihuman globulin or by staphylococcal coagglutination.

II. Diarrhoea

Six different types of diarrheagenic strains of *E. coli*

A. Entero Pathogenic *E coli* (EPEC):

- **Clinical features:** Causing watery diarrhoea in infants & children, occur as an institutional outbreaks / sporadic cases.
- **Pathogenesis:**
  - Does not producing the enterotoxin.
  - Bacilli are adhering to the mucosa or cup-like projections ('pedestals') of enterocyte membrane causing disruption of brush border /microvilli.
- **Diagnosis:** (1) Culture on HEP-2 cells (2) Failure to ferment sorbitol (3) Agglutination by specific antiserum.

B. Entero Toxigenic *E coli* (ETEC):

- **Clinical features:** Transmitted by contaminated food & water, not by fomites & no person to person transmission occurs. It causes endemic diarrhoea in infant & children of developing countries. It is the major cause of mortality in developing countries in children < 5 year. Person who visits such country may suffer with disease **called traveller's diarrhoea.**
- **Serotypes:** O6, O8, O15, O25, O27 & O167
- **Pathogenesis**
  - Organ of adhesion: Fimbrial Ag or Colonisation Factor Antigens (CFA-I, II, III & IV).
  - Toxin production (plasmid mediated): LT or ST or both. It is non invasive & effects are due to initial adhesion through CFA followed by toxin production. Toxin alone is not able to give diarrhoea.
- **Diagnosis:** Specimens like feces, food & water.

i. Detection of bacilli: Routine test like microscopy & culture.

ii. Detection of toxins: Tests to detect the LT & ST are given in **table-3.**

C. Entero Invasive *E coli* (EIEC):

- **Clinical features:** Causing mild diarrhoea to dysentery resembling shigellosis, in children & in adults.
- May show antigenic cross reactivity with *Shigella* & initially classified under the **Alkalegenes – Dispar group.**
- **Serotypes:** O28ac, O112ac, O124, O136, O143, O114, O152 & O154.
- **Pathogenesis:** Having VMA (Virulence Marker Antigen) which is plasmid encoded OMP, responsible for invasion & destruction of epithelial cell to elicit dysentery.
- **Diagnosis:**

1. Non-motile.
2. Cell penetration of HeLa or HEP-2 cells in culture.
3. Late or non lactose fermenters with acid without gas.
4. Sereny test: Instillation of suspension of freshly isolate into eyes of guinea pigs or mice leads to mucopurulent conjunctivitis and severe keratitis. It detects the invasive property of bacteria.
5. VMA- ELISA: To detect the VMA.

D. Entero Haemorrhagic *E coli* (EHEC) / Vero Toxigenic *E Coli* (VTEC) / Shiga toxigenic *E. coli* (STEC).

- **Meaning:** Because having haemorrhagic tendency & allow presence of blood in urine & stool.
- **Clinical features:** Causing mild to severe diarrhoea, haemorrhagic colitis (dysentery), HUS (Haemorrhagic/Haemolytic Uremic Syndrome) & food poisoning in children & in elder group in developed countries.
- **Serotypes:** Common by O157:H7 & rare by O26:H1.
- **Pathogenesis:** Produce VT or Shiga Like Toxin (SLT) which target the vascular endothelial cell of intestine and kidney and cause haemorrhagic colitis (dysentery) & HUS.
- **Mode of transmission:** Ingestion of contaminated vegetables (radish/alfalfa) or salad.
- **Diagnosis:** Specimens is feces.

i. Detection of bacilli:

- Sorbitol Mac Conkey's medium (also **called modified Mac Conkey's medium** & contains sorbitol instead of lactose): All *E coli* strains are sorbitol fermenters while O157:H7 is sorbitol non-fermenter. However few studies claimed that few strain of O157:H7 are sorbitol fermenters.
- Cell culture: Demonstration of cytotoxic effect on Vero or Hela cell.

ii. Detection of VT/SLT:

- Serology: Demonstration of VT antibody in sera by latex agglutination test & ELISA.
- Molecular: DNA probe of VT1 and VT2 gene.

E. Entero Aggregative *E coli* (EAEC):

- **Meaning:** Causing aggregation of Hep-2 cells like '**stacked brick formation** ' hence the name.
- **Clinical features:** Causing persistent diarrhoea especially in developing countries & also traveller's diarrhoea.
- **Pathogenesis:** Form low molecular weight heat stable toxin **called EAST (Entero Aggregative heat Stable entero Toxin)** causing shortening of villi, hemorrhagic necrosis and edema.

✓ **Traveller's diarrhoea:** **Follow chapter → Systemic infections**

F. Diffusely Adherent *E coli* (DAEC):

- **Meaning:** Adhere with HEP-2 cells in culture in diffuse pattern hence **called DAEC.**
- **Clinical features:** It causes diarrhoea in children between 2-6 years.
- **Pathogenesis:** Showing diffuse adherence fimbriae contribute to the pathogenesis.

III. Other infections

- **Types:**
- **Peritonitis:** Primary from exogenous entry of bacilli or secondary due to intestinal perforation which allow the distant spread of bacilli.
- **Abscess:** Hepatic abscess or abscess in soft tissue.
- **Wound infections:** Common in diabetic patients.
- **CNS infection:** Especially neonatal meningitis.
- **Nosocomial infection:** Ventilator associated pneumonia.
- **CVS infections:** Endocarditis, shock & SIRS (Systemic Inflammatory Response Syndrome).
- **Bacteremia & septicemia:** Septicemia present with fever, hypotension & DIC usually in debilitated patients with high mortality.
- **Diagnosis:**
  - Specimens: Blood, CSF, pus / swab from wound & sputum.
  - Testing methods: Samples are processed in a routine way.

✓ **Notes:** *E. coli* is the most common cause of acute UTI (in 80% cases without catheter), neonatal meningitis, intra-abdominal abscess & nosocomial infection.

Edwardsiella spp.

- **Species:** Three species as follows.

1. ***Edwardseilla tarda***
   - Tarda from **tardy = weak, because of weak sugar fermentation.**
   - GNB, non-motile & non-capsulated.
   - Ferments only glucose & maltose.
   - Indole, citrate, H_2S, lysine & ornithine decaboxylation tests are positive.
   - Normal intestinal flora in cold-blooded animal like snakes & other.
   - Septic shock, liver abscess & diarrhoea in human
   - Identified from: Pus, blood, urine & CSF.
2. ***Edwardseilla ictaluri*:** Human septicemia.
3. ***Edwardseilla horshinae*:** Human pathogenicity is unknown.

Citrobacter spp.

- **General features:**
  - GNB & motile.
  - Late lactose fermenter.
  - I M Vi C tests: V - + +
  - H_2Sproduction: +Ve
- **Species:** Three species like *Citro. freundii, Citro. Koseri* & *Citro. Amalonaticus.*
  - ***Citro. freundii*:**
    - Formerly **called Ballerup-Bathesda group**.
    - Some strain **(Bhatanagar strain)** share common Ag **(like Vi Ag)** with *S. typhi* & *S. paratyphi C* & confusing the diagnosis.
    - Intestinal flora may produce UTI, gall bladder infection, otitis media & meningitis.

Klebsielleae

Klebsiella spp.

❖ **Meaning:** Genus named after German microbiologist Edwin Kleb (1834-1913).

❖ **Classification:**

A. **Based on capsular (K) antigen:** More than 80 serotypes.

B. **Phage typing:** It is also useful.

C. **Based on biochemical properties:** Many species like *K. pneumoniae, K. granulomatis, K. planticola, K. ornitholytica, K. oxytoca* & *K. terrrigena* .

K. pneumoniae

- **Synonyms:**
  - Friedlander's bacilli: Because 1st discovered by Friedlander.
  - Bacillus mucosus capsulatus.
  - Pneumobacillus.
- **Subspecies:** *K. pneumoniae pneumoniae, K. pneumoniae aerogenes, K. pneumoniae ozaenae* (Abel's bacillus) & *K. pneumoniae rhinoscleromatis* (Frisch's bacillus).
- **Morphology: → Figure 1(b)**
  - **Type according to gram stain:** Gram negative bacilli or cocco-bacilli.
  - **Size:** 1–2µm x 0.5–0.8 µm.
  - **Shape:** Short, plump & straight road.
  - **Arrangement:** Singly, in pairs or in small groups.
  - **Capsule:** Capsulated.
  - **Motility:** Nonmotile.
  - **Spore:** Non-sporing.
- **Cultural characteristics (C/Cs):**
  - **Effective factors:**
    - O_2 effect: Aerobe & facultative anaerobes.
    - Temperature: 37^0C
    - pH: 7.6
  - **Media:**
    1. **Nutrient agar:** Forming large, dome-shaped, mucoid & sticky colonies.
    2. **MacConkey's medium:** Colonies are bright pink-mucoid due to lactose fermentation as shown in **fig.2(b)**.
- **Biochemical reaction (B/Rs):**

1. **Sugar fermentation tests: → Fig.-3(b)**

G	S	L	M
AG	AG	AG	AG

2. **I M Vi C tests [fig.-4(b)]:** - - + +

3. **Catalase test:** +Ve
4. **Nitrate reduction test:** + Ve
5. **Oxidase test:** -Ve
6. **H_2S production:** -Ve
7. **Urease test:** +Ve
8. **TSI test[fig.-5(a)]:** AG/A-H_2S

➢ **Pathogenicity:**

i. ***Klebsiella pneumoniae pneumoniae*:**

✪ **Virulence factors:**

- **Capsule:** Inhibits the phagocytosis.
- **Toxin:** Similar to ST toxin of *E. coli* causing diarrhoea.

✪ **Diseases:**

a. **Pneumonia:**

- **Precipitating factors:**
  - Age: In middle aged or older persons.
  - Diabetes mellitus.
  - Alcoholism.
  - Chronic bronchopulmonary disease.
- **Serotypes:** 1, 2 & 3
- **Clinical features:**
  - Massive mucoid inflammatory exudates of lobar or lobular distribution, involving one or more lobes of lung. Necrosis and abscess formation.
  - Fever & cough are common features.

b. **UTI:**

c. **Diarrhoea:** Due to enterotoxin.

d. **Pyogenic infections:** Abscesses, meningitis & septicemia.

ii. ***Klebsiella pneumoniae aerogenes*:**

a. **Pneumonia**

b. **UTI**

c. **Diarrhoea**

d. **Pyogenic infections:** Like abscesses & septicemia.

e. **Nosocomial infection (NI)**

iii. ***Klebsiella pneumoniae ozaenae*:**

- **Serotypes:** Capsular type 3 to 6.
- **Ozena:** Typical lesion **called ozena** characterised by foul smelling nasal discharge.

iv. ***Klebsiella pneumoniae rhinoscleromatis*:**

- **Serotypes:** Capsular type 3
- **Rhinoscleroma:** Typical lesion **called rhinocleroma** characterised by chronic granulomatous hypertrophy of nose with intracellular bacilli.

➢ **Laboratory diagnosis:**

✪ **Specimens:** Urine, pus, blood, stool, nasal biopsy etc.

✪ **Testing methods:**

1. **Microscopy: →Follow morphology**
2. **Culture : →Follow C/Cs**
3. **Biochemical reaction: →Follow B/Rs**

➢ **Treatment:** Klebsiella are generally resistant to ampicillin, amoxycillin & carbenicillin. They are sensitive to cephalosporin, nitrofurantoin, co-amoxiclav & gentamicin.

K. granulomatis

➢ **Reason of reclassification:** Previously it was not the part of Enterobactariceae family but later it was identified that morphologically & antigenically it is similar to *Klebsiella*, hence reclassified as *K. granulomatis.*

➢ **Synonym:**

1. ***Donovania granulomatis*: Genus name** after **Donovan (1905),** who 1st described the intracellular-bacilli from genital ulcer. **Species name** after **granulomatous forms** of disease
2. ***Calymmatobacterium granulomatis*:**

➢ **Morphology:**

✪ **Type according to gram stain:**

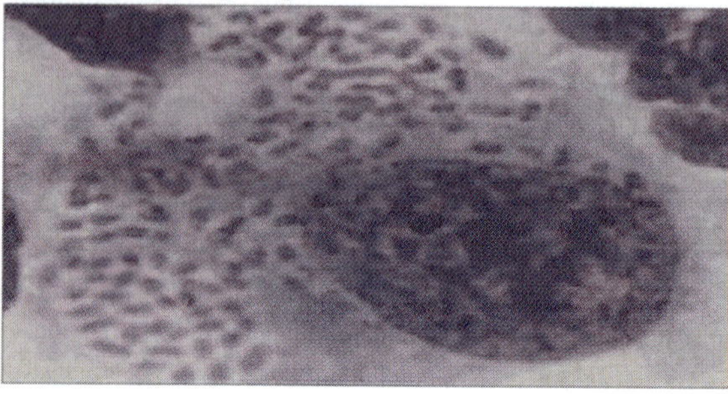

Figure-6: Donovan's bodies under Giemsa stain

- Gram negative cocco-bacilli. Better stained by Wright, Giemsa **(fig.-6)** or Leishman stain as an intracellular bacilli [**called Donovan's intracellular bodies / Donovan's bodies**] **in mononuclear cells** with **bipolar staining** which gives **'safety-pin or telephone handle appearance'** & pinkish capsule.
- Other bacteria with safety pin appearance are *Y. pestis, P. multocida, Francisella tularensis Burkholderia pseudomallei, Haemophilus ducreyi, Brucella abortus, Chromobacter violaceum,* etc.

✪ **Size:** 1–2μm.

✪ **Capsule:** Capsulated.

✪ **Motility:** Nonmotile.

✪ **Spore:** Non-sporing.

➢ **Cultural characteristics (C/Cs):** Grow on

- Modified Levinthal agar.
- Egg yolk medium.
- Egg culture: In yolk-sac off chick embryo.
- Cell culture: HEP-2 cell lines.

➢ **Pathogenicity:**

✪ **Disease name:** Disease **called donovanosis** or **granuloma venereum** or **granuloma inguinale.**

✪ **Mode of transmission:** Sexually intercourse.

✪ **Incubation period:** 1-12 weeks.

✪ **Portal of entry:** Skin/mucosa.

✪ **Sites [fig.-7(a) & (b)]:** Genitals in 90% cases, particularly of labia is common.

✪ **Clinical features:**

- Produce single or multiple, local, subcutaneous nodule that erode through skin to produce granulomatous, sharply defined ulcer **[fig.-7(a) & (b)]** which is painless.
- The granulomatous swelling, may heaped up via subcutaneous tissue to inguinal area which simulates the lymphadenopathy **called pseudo-lymphadenopathy** or **called pseudo-bubo.** In fact absence of true lymphadenopathy is the hall mark of disease.

✪ **Complications:** Pseudo/genital elephantiasis (labial swelling), phimosis & paraphimosis.

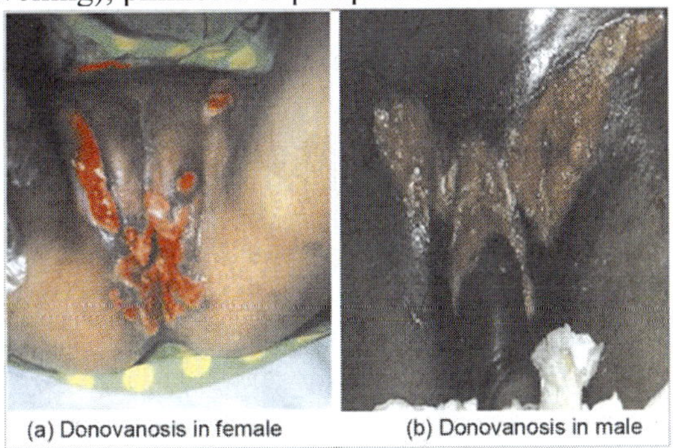

(a) Donovanosis in female (b) Donovanosis in male

Figure-7: Donovanosis in female & male

➢ **Laboratory diagnosis:**

✪ **Specimens:** Clean the ulcer with saline & collect the bits of tissue or biopsy materials.

✪ **Testing methods:**

- Identification of bacilli by microscopy & culture methods as described above.
- Multiplex PCR developed for simultaneous detection of sexually transmitted microbes like *T. pallidum, H. ducreyi, K. granulomatis, C. trachomatis* & HSV.

➢ **Prevention:** Safe sex is the nest way for prevention of disease.

➢ **Treatment:** Azithromycin is the drug of choice. Doxycycline (2nd choice) for 3 weeks is curative. Cotrimoxazole, chloramphenicol, gentamicin, fluoroquinolones & newer macrolides are also effective.

Enterobacter spp.

➢ **General features:**

Test	*E. cloacae*	*E. aerogenes*
Gas from glycerol	-	+
Aesculin hydrolysis	-	+
Lysin edecarboxylase	-	+
Arginine dihydrolase	+	-

Table-5: Species of *Enterobacter*

- Formerly **called *Aerobacter***
- GNB, motile & capsulated
- Lactose fermenter
- I M Vi C test: - - + +

➢ **Species:** Two species as shown **table-5**

➢ **Pathogenicity:** Produce UTI, respiratory infection, wound infection, septicemia, and meningitis.

Hafnia alvei

➢ **General properties:**

- Only one species in this group is *H. alvei.*
- GNB & motile.
- Biochemical reactions are best seen at 30^{0}C.
- Non Lactose Fermenter (NLF).
- I M Vi C tests: - - + + (Best at 22^{0}C).
- Lysin & other decarboxylation tests are positive.

➢ **Pathogenicity:** Opportunistic pathogen & isolated from blood , urine, pus & sputum.

Serratia spp.

➢ **General properties:**

- Gran negative bacilli or cocco-bacilli & motile.
- Strict aerobes.
- Slow lactose fermenter.

➢ **Species:** Three species like *S. marcescens* (*S. prodigiosus*), *S. rubidaea* & *S. liquifaciens.*

- ***S. marcescens* (*S. prodigiosus*):**

1. **Respiratory infection:**
   - Red colour pigment **called prodigiosin.**
   - Best produced at room/ low temp-20^{0}C.
   - Its presence in sputum simulating presence of blood. **called pseudo-haemoptysis**
2. **Nosocomial infection:** Produce by resistant strain
3. **Other infections:** Also causing the meningitis, endocarditis, septicemia, peritonitis etc.

Pantoea spp.

➢ **General properties:**

- *Pantoea* (Greek) means all sources, as it has been isolated from geographical & ecological sources.
- Lactose Fermenter with acid & gas.
- Voges Proskauer test: +Ve.
- Arginine, lysine & ornithine decarboxylation: -Ve

➢ **Species:** Two species like

- *P. agglomerans:* Septicemia & salicin positive.
- *P. dispersa:* Salicin negative.

Proteeae

❖ **Common name:** All the bacteria under the tribe Proteeae are **called *Proteus* bacilli.**

❖ **Meaning:** From Greek god **Proteus who was able to assume any shape**, as bacteria are pleomorphic & can occur variable in size & shape.

❖ **General features:**

1. PPA test:
   - All *Proteus* bacilli produce the enzyme phenyl alanine deaminase which split the phenyl alanine to Phenyl Pyruvic Acid (PPA).

Tribe	Proteeae					
Genus	*Proteus*		*Morgnella*	*Providencia*		
Species	*Pr. vulgaris*	*Pr. mirabilis*	*M. morganii*	*P. alcalifaciens*	*P. stuartii*	*P. rettgeri*
	Features					
Adonitol fermentation	-	-	-	+	+ -	+ -
Trehalose fermentation	+ -	+	+ -	-	+	-
Indole	+	-	+	+	+	+
Methyle red	+	+	+	+	+	+
VP test	-	-	-	-	-	-
Citrate test	+	+	-	+	+	+
PPA test	+	+	+	+	+	+
Urease test	+	+	+	-	+ -	+
H_2S	+	+	-	-	-	-
Ornithin decarboxylation	-	+	+	-	-	-
Swarming	+	+	-	-	-	-
Lesions	Rare human pathogen	UTI & NI	UTI & NI	Diarrhoea	UTI, burns infection	NI

Table-6: Species of Proteeae

- PPA gives acidic pH to medium & detected by PPA test. Positive PPA test indicated by green colour **[fig.-5(c)]** on adding of 10% ferric chloride within 4-5 minutes. Negative will not change the colour of phenyl alanine agar slant.
- This is the single test which distinguishes Proteeae from all other members of Enterobactericeae family.

2. Resistant to KCN.
3. Degrade tyrosine.
4. Lactose, dulcitol & malonate non fermenter.
5. MR test: Positive.
6. VP test: Negative.
7. Arginine or lysine decarboxylation tests: Negative.

❖ **Morphology:** GNB, Pleomorphic bacilli with 1–3 µm x 0.5 µm, non-capsulated, actively motile (non-motile strains are also observed by **Weil-Felix**) by peritrichate flagella.

❖ **Classification:** →**Table-6**

❖ **General scheme to differentiate the Proteus bacilli in laboratory by using routine tests:** →**Flow chart-3**

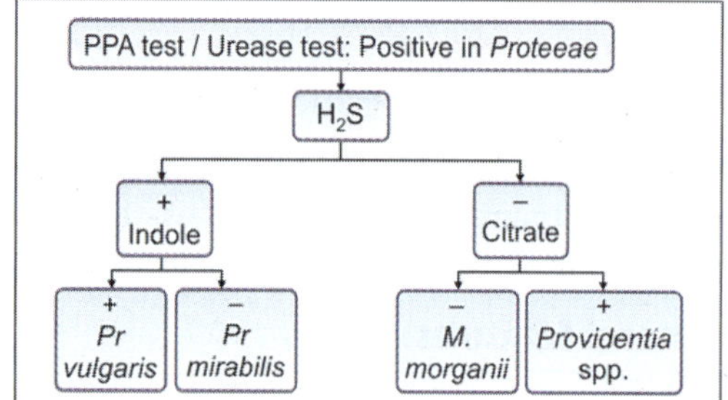

Flow chart-3: Differentiation of *Proteus* bacilli

Proteus spp.

➢ **Cultural characteristics (C/Cs):**

♣ **Effective factors:** Aerobe & facultative anaerobes.

♣ **Media:**

A. **Blood agar:**

✪ **Odour:** Cultures have putrefacient odour described as 'fishy' or 'seminal'.

✪ **Swarming:**

- **Definition**: Rapid (2–10 µm/s) & coordinated translocation of a bacterial population present as thin filmy layer in concentric circles on solid or semi-solid surfaces **called swarming**.
- **History:** Swarming motility was first reported by Jorgen Henrichsen.
- **Mechanism:** Exactly unknown but may be due to multiple, thick & strong flagella which allow the actively motile cells to move away from the site of inoculation in search of nutrients.
- **Types & examples:** Following are the types.

i. **Continuous swarming:** → **Fig.-6 (a)**
- Uniform film of growth on solid media & it is mostly featureless.
- Example: *B. subtilis.*

ii. **Discontinuous swarming:**

1. **Concentric:** → **Fig.- 8(b)**
- Series of concentric circles around site of inoculation. It gives appearance like 'bull's eye'.
- Example: *Pr. mirabilis.*

2. **Dendritic:** → **Fig.-8(c)**
- Branching pattern.
- Example: *P. aeruginosa.*

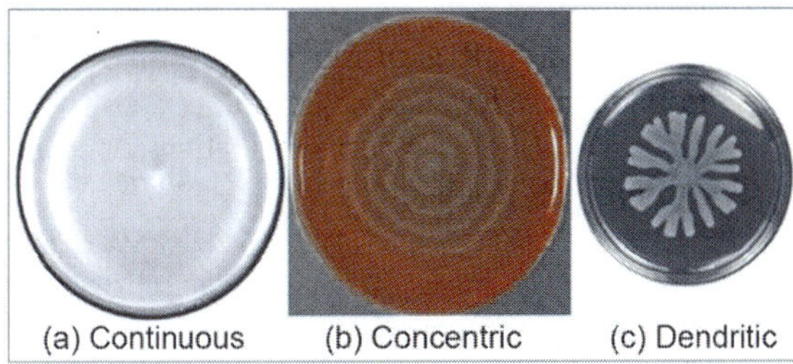

Figure-8: Types of swarming

iii. **Other types & examples:** Also occurs in *Pr. vulgaris*, *Cl. tetani* etc.

- **Disadvantage of swarming growth:** It create problem to isolate the pure growth.
- **Anti swarming methods:**

a. **Physical method:** Agar overlays, poured plates, increasing agar concentration (3-4% or 6%).

b. **Chemical method:** Incorporation of

- Chloral hydrate (1:500)
- Sodium azide (1:500)
- Alcohol (5-6%)
- Sulphonamide
- Neomycin
- Surface active agents
- Boric acid (1:1000)
- p-Nitrophenylglycerol (0.2-0.4 nM in plates requiring 24 hrs incubation & ≤ 1.0 nM in plates requiring 72 hrs incubation).

c. **Other methods:**

1. Incorporation of H-antiserum.
2. Some media also inhibit swarming: Mac Conkey's medium, DCA & XLD are due to bile salt, W & B medium is due to bismuth sulphite & CLED medium due to electrolytes deficiency.

- **Diene's phenomenon: → Fig.-9(a)**

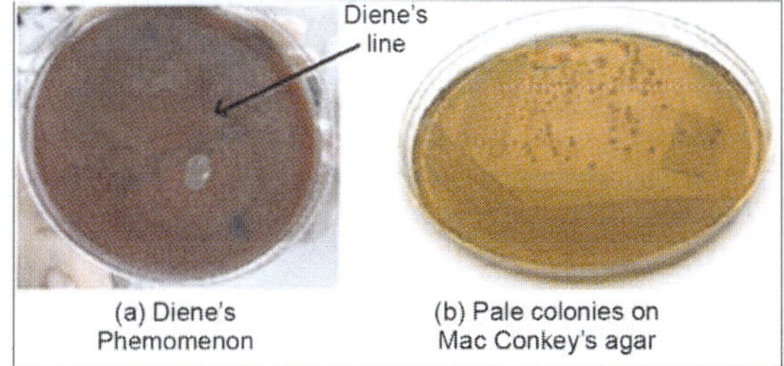

Figure-9: Cultural properties of *Proteus* spp.

o Definition:

- Inoculate **two identical** *Proteus* strains at different point on culture plate without anti swarming agents, resulting swarming growth coalesce without line of demarcation.
- Inoculate **two non-identical** *Proteus* strains at different point on culture plate without anti swarming agents, resulting swarming growth fails to coalesce with line of demarcation. This phenomenon **called Diene's phenomenon** & line of demarcation **called Diene's line.**

o Use: To determine the identical & non-identical *Proteus* strains.

✓ **Note: Diene's stain** →It is useful in identification of *Mycoplasma.*

B. **MacConkey's medium:** No swarming occurs. Smooth, pale (colourless) colonies develop as shown in **fig.-9(b).**

➢ **Antigenic structure:**

- Somatic O Ag.
- Flagellar H Ag.
- Hetreophile antigens:

- Weil and Felix observed that certain nonmotile strains of *Pr. vulgaris*, **called 'X strains',** were agglutinated by sera from typhus fever patients.
- This heterophilic agglutination is due to sharing of common Ag (carbohydrate) between *Proteus* and *Rickettsia.*
- Three nonmotile strains, OX2 & 0X19 of *Proteus vulgaris* & OXK of *Proteus mirabilis* are observed
- They forms basis of Weil-Felix reaction for diagnosis of some Rickettsial infections.

➢ **Typing of *Proteus*:**

1. Bacteriophage typing.
2. Bacteriocin typing.
3. Ribotyping.
4. Diene's phenomenon: Vide supra.

➢ **Pathogenicity:**

✪ **Transmission:**

- **Exogenous:** They are the **saprophytes** available in soil, sewage & animal materials.
- **Endogenous:** Present as **normal flora** in moist areas like skin & intestine in human & animals.

✪ **Clinical features:**

1. **Opportunistic & nosocomial infections:** Likc UTI, wound infection, septicemia & soft tissue infections.
2. **Bladder stone:** Enzyme urease breaks the urea in to ammonia which makes the urine alkaline & damage the renal epithelium. Alkaline urine allows the deposition of phosphate to form the bladder stone (phosphate stone).

➢ **Laboratory diagnosis:**

✪ **Specimens:** Urine, pus & blood.

✪ **Testing methods:**

I. **Microscopy: →Follow morphology**

II. **Culture : →Follow C/Cs**

III. **Biochemical reaction: →Follow table-5**

***Providencia* spp.**

- Three species with all important features are mentioned in **table-6.**
- Motile but not swarm.

Morgnella morganii

- All important features are mentioned in **table-5.**
- Motile but not swarm.
- Found in human & animal faeces.

Erwinieae

Erwinia

➢ **General properties:**
- GNB.
- Motile
- Produce yellow pigment.

➢ **Species:** *E. herbicola* isolated from plant produce UTI & respiratory infection.

Newer genera of Enterobactericeae

➢ ***Plesiomonas:*** Follow chapter → Vibrionaceae, Aeromonadaceae and *Plesiomonas*

➢ **Others genera:** *Ewingella, Budvicia, Tatumella , Rahnella & Kluyvera.*

Question bank

Case study

1) A 20 year male admitted in medical emergency ward with abdominal pain & diarrhoea. Stoll examination revealed pus cells, RBCs & motile bacteria. Gram stain showing GNB & culture reported the lactose fermenting bacteria. Identify the most common pathogen & answer the following
a) Name the two examples of each lactose fermenters (coliform bacilli) & non lactose fermenters (paracolon bacilli)
b) Write the morphology & culture characteristics of causative agent
c) Write the pathogenicity of causative agent

2) A female patient visited the hospital with complain of fever & micturition with pain, frequency & urgency. Mid stream urine sample is collected. Direct microscopy suggests the actively motile GNB. Culture on Mac Conkey's medium gives pink colonies. Identify the most common pathogen & answer the following
a) Write the different mode of transmission of clinical condition
b) Name the other organisms producing similar clinical condition
c) Describe the laboratory diagnosis of clinical condition

3) An adult male visited the hospital with complain of fever & cough. Gram stain of sputum identified capsulated gram negative coccobacilli. Culture on Mac Conkey's medium gives pink mucoid colonies. Identify the most common pathogen & answer the following
a) Define & classify the family to which the causative agent is belong
b) Write the morphology & culture characteristics of causative agent
c) Write the pathogenicity of causative agent

Essay/Full question

1) *E. coli*
2) Proteeae

Short notes

1) Classification of Enterobactericeae
2) Verotoxin / verocytotoxin
3) Diarrheagenic strains of *E. coli*
4) *Klebsiella pneumoniae*
5) *Klebsiella granulomatis* (Donovanosis or Granuloma inguinale)
6) *Proteus*
7) Bacterial swarming

Short questions for theory/viva questions

1) Define: Enterobactericeae.
2) What are coliform bacilli? Write two examples.
3) What are paracolon bacilli? Write two examples.
4) Name four SLT producing bacteria.
5) What is modified Mac Conkey's medium? Write its use.
6) What is Anton test & Sereny test?
7) Write four names of bacteria with safety pin appearance.
8) What is spreading & swarming growth of bacteria?
9) What is Diene's phenomenon & Diene's stain? Write one use of each.
10) Name four VP test positive bacteria.
11) Write four names of media which inhibit the bacterial swarming.

MCQs for chapter review

Definition of Enterobactericeae

1) **Following is not the property of bacterium from Enterobactariceae family**
(a) Catalase positive (b) Oxidase positive (c) Nitrate positive (d) Sugar fermentation

2) **Which is true of Enterobactericeae**
(a)) All are catalase positive except *Shigella dysenteriae* type 1 (b) Nitrate reduction negative (c) Glucose not fermented by all (d) Motility by polar flagellum

Classification of Enterobactericeae

3) **Coliform bacilli are defined as**
(a) Lactose fermenters (b) Non-lactose fermenters (c) Sucrose fermenters (d) a+b

4) ***E. coli* gives pink colour with -** (PGI- 99)
(a) Chocolate agar (b) LJ medium (c) Mac Conkey's medium (d) Saline broth

5) **Enterobactericeae are all except-** (PGI, Dec- 06)
(a) *Pseudomonas* (b) *Klebsiella* (c) *V. cholerae* (d) *Proteus* (d) *E. coli*

E. coli

6) **A 20 year old male had pain in abdomen and mild fever followed by gastroenteritis. The stool examination showed presence of pus cells and RBCs on microscopy. The etiological agent responsible is most likely to be-** (AIIMS, May-13)
(a) Entero Invasive *E coli* (b) Entero Toxigenic *E coli* (c) Entero Pathogenic *E coli* (d) Entero Aggregative *E coli*

7) **Watery diarrhoea in children is caused by-**
(a) EIEC (b) EPEC (c) ETEC (d) EAEC

8) **Which of the following is true about Entero Pathogenic *E coli*** (AI -96)
(a) Cause diarrhoea in infants (b) Acts by invasion of intestinal epithelial cells (c) Adults are mostly affected (d) Affects immunocompromised host

9) **Most common strain of *E. coli* giving rise to traveller's diarrhoea is -**

(a) Entero Invasive *E coli* (EIEC) (b) Entero Pathogenic *E coli* (EPEC) (c) Entero Toxigenic *E coli* (ETEC) (d) Entero Aggegative *E coli* (EAEC)

10) True about Entero Toxigenic *E coli* is - (AIIMS, Nov-10)
(a) Causes epidemic diarrhoea in children in epidemic country (b) Not a cause of traveller's diarrhoea (c) Invasive (d) Spread by contaminated water

11) Regarding ETEC true is- (AIIMS, Nov -10)
(a) Invades submucosa (b) Most common in children of developing countries (c) Fomite borne and person to person (d) Not a common cause of traveller's diarrhoea

12) Most common cause of diarrhoea in children of developing country is -
(a) EIEC (b) EPEC (c) ETEC (d) EAEC

13) All are true about Entero haemorrhagic *E coli* is – (AIIMS, June -99)
(a) Sereny test positive (b) May cause diarrhoea (c) Can cause haemolytic uremic syndrome (d) Verocytotoxin is produced

14) All of the followings are true about HUS except- (AI-12)
(a) Infection may be transmitted by food (b) HUS is caused by Verotoxin producing *Escherichia coli* (c) HUS is more common in children (d) HUS is rarely associated with haemorrhagic colitis.

15) With reference to infection with *E. coli* the following are true except - (AI -05)
(a) Entero Aggegative *E coli* is associated with persistent diarrhoea (b) Entero Haemorrhagic *E coli* can cause haemolytic uremic syndrome (c)) Entero Invasive *E coli* produces a disease similar to salmonellosis (d) Entero Toxigenic *E coli* is a common cause of to traveler's diarrhoea

16) A 20 year old man presented with haemorrhagic colitis. The stool sample grew *Escherichia coli* in pure culture. The following serotype is likely to be the causative agent-(AI-04)
(a) O157:H7 (b) O159:H7 (c) O107:H7 (d) O55:H7

17) Which of these are true of *E. coli* - (PGI, June-02)
(a) The LT (labile toxin) in ETEC acts via c-AMP
(b) In type causing UTI the organism attaches via pilli
(c) The ST (stable toxin) in ETEC is responsible for causing haemolytic uremic syndrome (HUS)
(d) EIEC invasiveness is under plasmid control
(e) In EPEC the toxin helps in invasion by the bacteria

18) Culture media used for diagnosis of EHEC O157:H7 is – (AI-04)
(a) O culture (b) Sorbitol Mac Conkey's medium (c) XLD agar (d) Deoxycholate media

19) In *E. coli* true is -
(a) ETEC is invasive (b EPEC acts via cAMP (c) Pilli present in uropathogenic type (d) ETEC causes HUS

20) Labile toxin of *E. coli* can be detected by following methods except -
(a) Into infant rabbit bowel (b) Into adult rabbit skin
(c) Intragastrically in to infant mouse (d) Into tissue culture of chinese hamster ovary cells (e) Into Y1 mouse adrenal cells

21) Which toxin is not mediated by cAMP - (AIIMS, June -98)
(a) *V cholerae* 01 (b) Heat stable *E. coli* toxin (c) Heat labile *E. coli* toxin (d) *V cholerae* 0137

22) Toxin acting on cGMP -
(a) Heat stable *E. coli* toxin (b) Heat labile *E. coli* toxin (c) Cholera toxin (d) Shiga toxin

23) *E. coli* gets attached to the surface with the help of - (AI-00)
(a) Fucose (b) Concavatin (c) Phyhaemagglutinin (d) Lactin

24) True about *E. coli* is - (AIIMS, May-94)
(a) Sereny test is done to diagnose Entero Toxigenic *E coli* (ETEC) (b) Entero Pathogenic *E coli* (EPEC) is also invasive (c) UTI is caused by single serotype at a time only (d) *E coli* is the most common organism to infect burn wound

25) Most common cause of liver abscess (PGI-00)
(a) *Streptococci* (b) *Staph aureus* (c) *E. coli* (d) *Staph pyogenes*

26) A microbiologist wants to develop the vaccine for prevention of attachment of diarrheagenic *E. coli* to the specific receptors in the gastro intestinal tract. All of the following fimbrial adhesion would be appropriate vaccine candidates except- (AI-04)
(a) CFA-1 (b) Pi-Pilli (c) CS-2 (d) K88

27) Sereny test is useful to detect
(a) Entero Invasive E. coli (b) *V. cholerae* (c) Entero toxigenic E. coli (d) Entero pathogenic E. coli

Klebsiella

28) Friedlander's bacillus is-
(a) *Klebsiella pneumoniae* (b) *Clostridium welchii* (c) *Chlamydiae* (d) *E coli*

29) Which of the following is associated with extremely foul smelling infection-
(a) *Klebsiella rhinoscleromatis* (b) *Klebsiella seeberi* (c) *Klebsiella zygomaticus* (d) *Klebsiella ozaenae*

30) A male patient present with granulomatous penile ulcer. On Wright Giemsa stain tony organism of 2 micron within macrophages are seen. What is the causative organism? (AIIMS, May-04)
(a) LGV (b) *Calymmatobacterium granulomatis* (c) *Neisseria* (d) *Staph aureus*

31) In donovanosis
(a) Pseudolymphadenopathy (b) Penicillin is used for treatment (c) Painful ulcer (d) Suppuative lymphadenopathy

Proteus

32) Diene's phenomenon is seen with - (PGI-02)
(a) *Proteus mirabilis* (b) *Klebsiella* (c) *Proteus vulgaris* (d) *providentia* (e) *Morgnella*

33) *Proteus* antigen cross react with-
(a) *Klebsiella* (b) Rickettsiae (c) *Chlamydiae* (d) *E coli*

Answers of MCQs & explanation

1) (a), **2) (b)** } Follow section, **definition of Enterobactericeae** for explanation
3) (a), **4) (c)** } Follow section **classification of Enterobactericeae** for explanation
5) (a) & (c)
- Because *Pseudomonas* & *V. cholerae* are oxidase positive
- Follow section, **definition & classification of Enterobactericeae** for more explanation

6) (a)
- Because Entero Invasive *E coli* causing dysentery, hence pus cells & RBCs are present in stool
- Even EHEC also causing haemorrhagic diarrhoea (haemorrhagic colitis) but that option is not given

7) (b), **8) (a)** } EPEC Causing watery diarrhea in infants & children, occur as institutional outbreaks / sporadic cases.
9) (c)
- ETEC & EAEC both are known to cause traveller's diarrhoea, but most common by ETEC

10) (d)
- ETEC causing traveller's diarrhoea in children of developing countries
- It is non invasive & effects are due to initial binding by CFA followed by toxin production
- Transmitted by contaminated food & water not person to person

11) (b), **12) (c)** } Follow section, ***Escherichia coli* (diarrhoea →ETEC)** for explanation
13) (a)
- Follow section, ***Escherichia coli* (diarrhoea → EHEC)** for explanation

14) (d)
- HUS is a rare complication following haemorrhagic colitis. Most cases of HUS are associated haemorrhagic colitis but all cases haemorrhagic colitis may not progress to HUS
- Follow section, ***Escherichia coli*** **(diarrhoea → EHEC)** for more explanation

15) (c)
- Entero Invasive *E coli* produces a disease similar to shigellosis not to salmonellosis

16) (a)
- Haemorrhagic colitis is caused by EHEC, where O157:H7 is the most common serotype

17) (a), (b) & (c)
- The ST (stable toxin) in ETEC is act via cGMP
- In EPEC is non-toxigenic

18) (b)
- Follow section, ***Escherichia coli*** **(diarrhoea → EHEC →** detection of bacilli**)** for explanation.

19) (c)
- ETEC is noninvasive
- EPEC does not producing the toxin & no activation of cAMP, which is the property of labile toxin
- HUS is caused by EHEC

20) (c)
- Follow section, ***Escherichia coli*** **[pathogenicity → agent factors (virulence factors) → table-3]** for diagnostic test of LT & ST

21) (b)
- Heat labile *E. coli* toxin & cholera toxin of *V cholerae* 0137 & O1 are structurally & antigenically same, but cholera toxin is hundred times more potent than labile toxin. Both act via cAMP, while Heat stable *E. coli* toxin act via cGMP

22) (a)
- Already explained

23) (a)
- Follow section, ***Escherichia coli*** **[pathogenicity → agent factors (virulence factors) → fimbriae]** for explanation

24) (c)
- Sereny test is done to diagnose EIEC
- EPEC is also non-invasive
- UTI is caused by single serotype at a time only, however recurrence can occur by same or other serotypes
- Most common organism to infect burn wound is *P. aeruginosa* followed by Staph aureus

25) (c)
- *E. coli* is the most common cause of acute UTI (in 80% cases without catheter), neonatal meningitis, intra-abdominal abscess & nosocomial infection

26) (d)
- K is the capsular antigen
- Other three are fimbriae/pilli or types of pilli and known as organs of adhesion
- CFA is found in Entero Toxigenic *E coli.* It has many components. CS-II is the component of CFA

27) (a)
- Follow section, ***Escherichia coli*** **(pathogenicity →diarrhoea → Entero Invasive E coli)** for explanation

28) (a)
- Follow section, ***Klebsiella*** **spp. (*K pneumoniae* →synonyms)** for explanation

29) (d)
- *Klebsiella ozaenae* causing foul smelling nasal discharge

30) (b)
31) (a)
} Follow section, ***Klebsiella*** **spp. (*K granulomatis*)** for explanation

32) (a) & (c)
- Follow section, ***Proteus*** **spp. (cultural characteristics)** for explanation

33) (b)
- Follow section, ***Proteus*** **spp. (antigenic structure)** for explanation

44 Enterobactericeae-II (*Salmonella*)

Learning heading & subheadings

- Synonym & history:
- Nomenclature:
- Morphology:
- Cultural characteristics (C/Cs):
- Biochemical reaction (B/Rs):
- Resistance:
- Antigenic structure:
- Antigenic variation:
- Classification:

Enteric fever / typhoidal group

- Typhoid fever
- Paratyphoid fever

Non-typhoidal group

- *Salmonella* food poisoning
- *Salmonella* septicemia

Synonym & history: *Salmonella typhi* was 1st observed by Eberth in 1880 in the mesenteric nodes & spleen of fatal case and isolated by Gaffky in 1884, so previously **called Eberth-Gaffky bacillus or *Eberthella typhi*.**

Nomenclature:

- **Genus name:** Salmon & Smith described bacilli hence the genus **called *Salmonella*** with removal of earlier genus name *Eberthella*.
- **Species name:** Species name are based on animal source (*S. gallinarium*), name of discoverer (*S. schottmulleri*), name of patients (*S. thompson*) & place of isolation (*S. poona*).

Morphology: → Figure-1

- **Type according to gram stain:** GNB.
- **Size:** 0.5 µm x 1–3 µm.
- **Shape:** Rod shape.
- **Arrangement:** Single, in pair or in small group.
- **Capsule:** Non capsulated.
- **Motility:** Motile with peritrichate flagella (except *S. gallinarum* & *S. pullorum*). It is detected by hanging drop preparation.
- **Spores:** Nonsporing.
- **Fimbriae:** May be present.

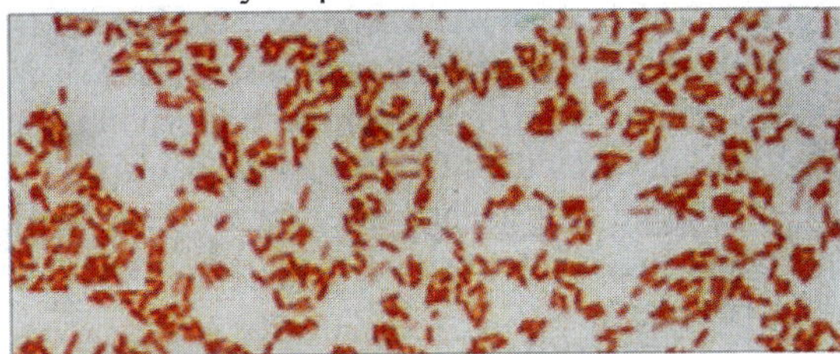

Figure-1: *S. typhi* under gram stain

Cultural characteristics (C/C):

- **Effective factors:**
- O_2 effect: Aerobe and facultative anaerobe.
- Optimum temperature: 37°C (15–41°C).
- pH: 6–8
- *S. typhi* & few other species of *Salmonella* required tryptophan as a growth factor.
- **Culture in media:**

A. Liquid media:

1. **Enrichment media for faeces:** Following media are useful for *Shigella* & *Salmonella* but better for *Salmonella*.
   - Selenite-F broth / selenite broth:
   - *Salmonella Shigella* broth:
   - Tetrathionate broth:
2. **Enrichment media for blood:**
   - Taurocholate broth: Dilution ration is 1:10.
3. **Transport media:**
   - Sach's glycerol buffered saline (Gram negative broth or glycerol saline transport medium): Preserves *Salmonella* & *Shigella* from faecal specimens.
   - Gram negative broth: Transport & selective medium for *Salmonella* & *Shigella* from clinical (faeces, urine, blood etc) & non clinical specimens (water, food etc.). It contains sodium citrate & sodium deoxycholate inhibit the growth of gram positive & coliforms. Collect the specimen; incubate for 6-8 hours followed by subculture on solid media. It is not good for rectal swab.
   - Cary Blair medium: For transportation of EHEC (O157:H7), *Salmonella, Shigella* & *V. cholerae*.

B. Solid media:

1. **Nutrient agar:** Large about 2-3mm, circular, convex & translucent colonies.

C. **Selective media:**

2. **Mac Conkey's agar [fig.-2(a)]:**
3. **DCA:**
4. **S-S agar:**

} Pale colonies due to NLF

5. **W & B medium [fig.-2(b)]:** Jet black colonies due H_2S production by all *Salmonella* species except *S paratyphi A, S. cholerasuis* & few other species that do not form H_2S & produces green colonies.
6. **XLD agar:** Pink colonies with black centre due H_2S production.
7. **Hektoen enteric agar:**

- It is a selective & differential medium, primarily used to recover *Salmonella* & *Shigella* from samples. It contains indicators of lactose fermentation & H_2S production; plus inhibitors to prevent the growth of Gram-positive bacteria.
- Contain bile salts as inhibitory agents & some dyes. Produce green colour colonies with colour fading to the periphery.

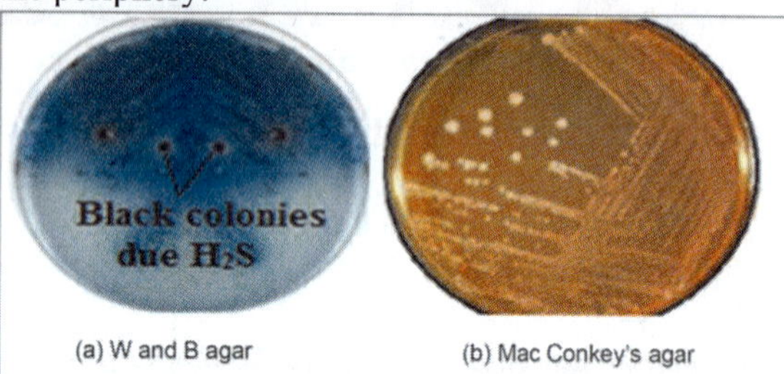

Figure-2: Colonies of *S. typhi*

Biochemical reaction (B/Rs):

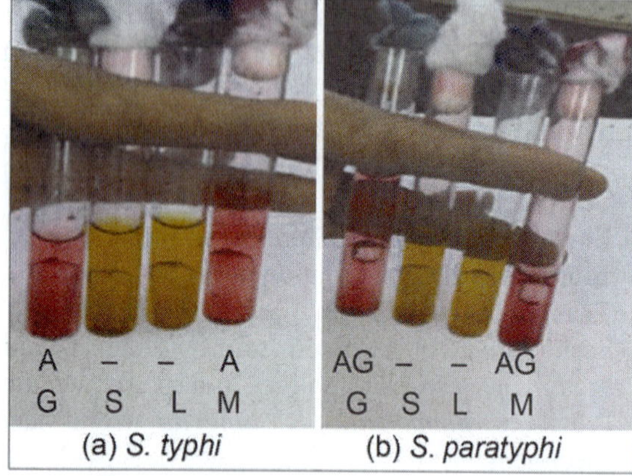

Figure-3: Sugar fermentation tests

1. **Sugar fermentation tests:**

- ***S. typhi*** (anaerogenic = No gas): → **Fig.-3(a)**

G	S	L	M	Maltose	Salicin
A	-	-	A	-	-

- ***S. paratyphi:*** → **Fig.-3(b)**

G	S	L	M
AG	-	-	AG

2. **I M Vi C tests:** - + - V (*S. typhi* & few other *Salmonellae* do not grow on Simmon's citrate medium as they required tryptophan as a growth factor)
3. **Catalase test:** +Ve
4. **Nitrate reduction test:** + Ve
5. **Oxidase test:** -Ve
6. **H_2S production:** +Ve (Except *S paratyphi A & S. cholerae suis*)
7. **Urease test:** -Ve
8. **TSI test:**

- ***S typhi*** = K/A + H_2S
- ***S paratyphi A*** = K/AG-H_2S
- ***S paratyphi B*** = K/AG +H_2S

Resistance: Bacilli are killed by heat at 55^0C in 1 hour / 60^0 C in 15 minutes, boiling, chlorination of water pasteurisation of milk, 5% phenol & mecuric chloride in 5 minutes.

Antigenic structure: Five types of antigens.

i. **Somatic antigen (O Ag or LPS or Endotoxin):**

- **Properties:**
  - Phospholipid-protein-polysaccharide complex forms an integral part of cell wall.
  - Identical with endotoxin & extracted from cell by trichloracetic acid **called Bovine Ag.**
  - Heat stable.
  - Not-destroyed by boiling or by alcohol or by acids.
  - Group specific, so antibody produced is not discriminate between typhoid & paratyphoid fever.
  - Less immunogenic & induces antibody formation slowly & in low titre following infection or immunization.
  - Antibody is not long lasting, so indicates the recent infection.
  - Agglutination takes place more slowly and at higher temperature (50-55 °C).
  - Producing compact, chalky, granular clumps when mixed with O antisera.
- **Biological action:** It is responsible for endotoxic activities.
- **Clinical significance:** Helps to diagnose the typhoid fever by Widal test.

ii. **Flagellar (H) antigen:**

- **Properties:**
  - Protein in nature **called flagellin.**
  - Heat labile.
  - Destroyed by boiling or by treatment with alcohol but not by formaldehyde.
  - Species specific, so antibody produced is discriminate between typhoid & paratyphoid fever
  - Strongly immunogenic & induces antibody formation rapidly & in high titre following infection or immunization.
  - Antibody is long lasting, so indicates the convalescent phase.
  - Agglutinates very rapidly & and at 37°C.

- Producing large, loose & cotton wooly or fluffy clumps, when mixed with H-antisera.
- **Clinical significance:** Helps to diagnose the typhoid fever by Widal test.

iii. Vi antigen:

- **Properties:**
  - Many strains of *S typhi* fail to agglutinate with O antiserum due to presence of surface/envelop antigen which is related with virulence **called Vi Ag.**
  - Felix and Pitt described this antigen (analogous to K Ag of coliforms bacilli).
  - Polysaccharide in nature.
  - Heat labile.
  - Destroyed by boiling or heating at 60 °C for 1 hr or by treatment with N HCl and 0.5 N NaOH but not by alcohol or by 0.2% formalin..
  - Vi Ag prepared by treating suspension with glycerol & alcohol.
  - Vi antigen lost on serial subculture.
  - Bacilli in-agglutinable with O antiserum become agglutinable after loss of Vi Ag.
  - It present in *S typhi, S paratyhi C, S dublin* & in some strain of *Citrobacter freundii* (**Ballerup-Bethesda group**).
  - Less immunogenic & induces antibody formation in low titre following infection or by alcoholised vaccine but no antibody formation following phenolised vaccine.
- **Biological actions:**
  - Inhibit phagocytosis.
  - Resist complement activity.
  - Resist bacterial lysis by alternative pathway & by peroxidase killing.
  - Bacilli with Vi Ag are causing more consistent disease than those are lacking.
- **Clinical significances:**
  - Vi Ag is poorly immunogenic & antibody titre is very low, so not helpful in diagnosis of typhoid fever hence not included in Widal test
  - It is detected by agglutination test. Total absence of Vi antibody indicate poor prognosis (disappear in convalescence phase) and it persistence indicate carrier state.
  - It is used for epidemiological typing of *S. typhi* by using Vi bacteriophage.
  - Also useful for vaccination.

iv. Fimbrial (Fi) Ag: Not important in diagnosis instead causing confusion in diagnosis due to non-specific nature & common sharing with other Enterobacteriaceae.

v. Mucoid (M) antigen:

- **Properties:**
  - Polysaccharide in nature.
  - Responsible for mucoid colony.
  - Present in *S. paratyphi B* & some strain of *E. coli.*
  - Resemble the Vi Ag & prevent agglutination by O antiserum.
  - Heating at 100^0 C for 2.5 hrs makes the strain agglutinable for O antiserum.

Antigenic variations:

a. H – O variation:

- **Principle:** Based on loss of H Ag.
- **Types:** Two types as follows.

1. **Phenotypic variation:** Loss of H Ag by *Salmonella* occurs when they grow on phenol (1:800) agar. It is temporary & H Ag reappears when they grow on media free of phenol.
2. **Genotypic variation:** Loss of H Ag by mutation. It is stable.

- **Use:** Preparation of specific H & O antiserum by following methods.
  - Preparation of O antiserum: By using stable mutant (genotypic variation-No H Ag) like *S. typhi* 901- O strain.
  - Preparation of H antiserum: By obtaining a population of motile cells rich in H Ag with following methods.

1. **Craig's tube :**
2. **U-tube:**

} Follow chapter → Culture methods

b. Phase variation:

- **Properties:**
  - Present in H Ag.
  - Some strain posses both phases **called diphasic** & strain posses only one is **called monophasic**.
- **Types / phases:** Present in H Ag in two phases.

1. **Phase-I:**
   - Species specific.
   - Large numbers of antigens are found in these group & designated as a to z and then z1 to z68.
2. **Phase-II:**
   - Group/genus specific.
   - Antigens are designated by Arabic numerals (1-12).

c. V- W variation:

- Many strains of *S typhi* fails to agglutinate with O antiserum due to presence of surface/envelop antigen & agglutinate with Vi antiserum this **called 'V form'**.
- After several subculture Vi Ag will lost & strain fail to agglutinate with Vi antiserum but agglutinate with O antiserum this **called 'W form'**.
- Intermediate stage when strain agglutinate with both antiserums **called 'VW form'**.

d. S-R variation:

- It indicates the change in the colonies from smooth (S) to rough (R).
- Initially strain producing smooth (S) colony due to presence of O antigen & virulence.
- Strain undergoes mutational changes producing rough (R) & autoagglutinable colony with loss of O Ag & virulence.

- R form common in laboratory due to repeated subculture.
- S-R variation can be prevented by maintaining culture in Dorset egg medium & lyophilisation.

e. **O-Ag variation:** Structural changes in O Ag can be induced by bacteriophage (lysogenisation, which results in new serotypes of *S. anatum* to *S. newington* & later to *S. minneapolis* as shown in **flowchart-1.**

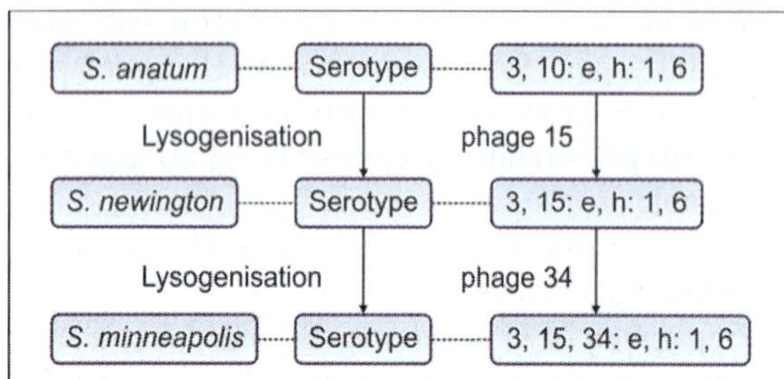

Flowchart-1: O-Ag variation by phage

Classification:

I. Serological (Kauffmann-White) classification:

1. O-Ag (group specific):

- Many serogroups were identified initially & all were labelled as A, B, C.....
- As the numbers increased it labelled as 1, 2, 3.....
- 2 is older group A, 4 is older group B, 9 is older group D & so on.
- Total 67 serogroups are identified by using group specific O-Ag.

2. H-Ag (species specific / serotype specific):

- Around 2300 serotypes are identified by using species specific H-Ag (phase I & phase II).
- Follow **table-1**for some important strains.

Sero-group	Serotype	O Ag	Phase I	Phase II
2-A	*S. paratyphi A*	1, 2, 12	a	-
4-B	*S. paratyphi B*	1, 4, 5, 12	b	1,2
7-C1	*S. paratyphi C*	6, 7 (Vi)	c	1,5
9-D	*S. typhi*	9, 12(Vi)	c	-

Table-1: Kauffmann-White classification

II. Biochemical or Kauffmann classification or biotypes: Four subgenera or subgroups like I, II, III & IV are identified as shown in **table-2.**

Test	I	II	III	IV
Lactose	-	-	+	-
Dulcitol	+	+	-	-
d-Tartrate	+	-	-	-
Malonate	-	+	+	-
Salicin	-	-	-	+
KCN	-	-	-	+

Table-2: Biotypes of *Salmonella*

III. Molecular classification: DNA hybridisation study shows that there are two main species in the genus *Salmonella.* Each species further classified in to subspecies & subspecies in to serotypes or serovars by earlier Kauffmann-White's classification.

i. ***S. enterica*:** Six subspecies as follows. Most of the human infections are caused by subspecies *arizonae* & *enterica.*

1. ***S. enterica*** subsp. *enterica*
2. ***S. enterica*** subsp. *salamae*

3a. ***S. enterica*** subsp. *arizonae*

3b. ***S. enterica*** subsp. *diarizonae*

4. ***S. enterica*** subsp. *houtenae*
6. ***S. enterica*** subsp. *indica*

ii. ***S. bongori*:** Earlier subspecies 5.

IV. Clinical classification: Whole spectrum of disease **called salmonellosis** which includes following clinical conditions as mentioned in **flowchart-2.**

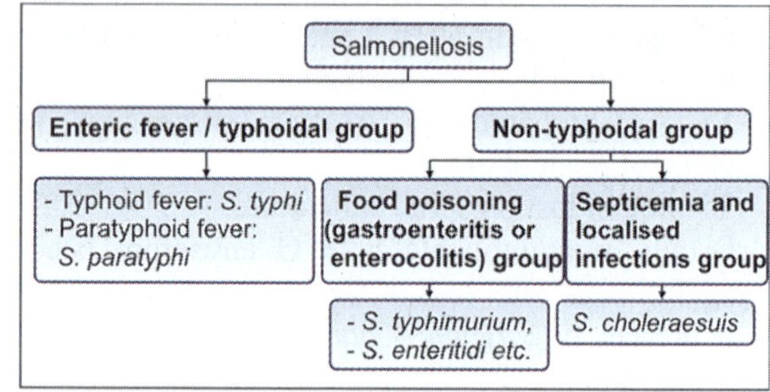

Flowchart-2: Clinical types of salmonellosis

Enteric fever / typhoidal group

❖ **Definition:** Enteric fever / typhoidal group is general terminology which includes typhoid fever caused by *S. typhi* & paratyphoid fever caused by *S. paratyphi* A, B & C.

❖ **Types (pathogenicity):** Two types like typhoid & paratyphoid fever.

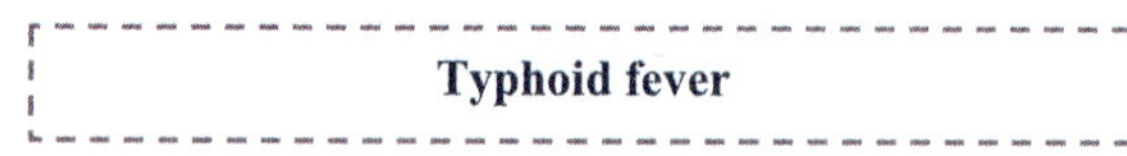

Typhoid fever

➢ **Nature & history of disease:**

- Typhoid fever is distributed worldwide. It may occur as in endemic or epidemic forms.
- About 22 million cases are reported annually with 6,00,000 deaths.

➢ **Reservoir of infection:** *Salmonella typhi* is the obligate pathogen for human. Cases or carriers of *Salmonella* are the reservoir hosts.

➢ **Source of infection:** Water or food.

➢ **Mode of transmission:** Ingestion.

➢ **Incubation period:** 7- 14 days.

➢ **Portal of entry:** GIT.

➢ **Sites:** Intestinal & extra-intestinal (complications).

➢ **Precipitating factors (epidemiological determinants):** Following are the factors.

A. Agent factors (virulence factors)

It includes intracellular (cell wall associated) factors as follows.

i. **Somatic antigen (O Ag or LPS or Endotoxin):**
ii. **Flagellar (H) antigen:**
iii. **Vi antigen:**
iv. **Fimbrial (Fi) Ag:**

} Discussed earlier.

v. **Mucoid (M) antigen:** Discussed earlier.
vi. **Infective dose:** Very high about 10^3-10^6 bacilli can initiate the disease.

B. Host factors

1. **Age:** Common in 5-20 years age.
2. **Local factors:** Following factors can promote the *Salmonella* infection.
   - Low gastric acidity: Bacilli are sensitive to gastric acid. Low acidity due to achlorhydria & use of antacids can enhance the infection.
   - Local disease: *H. pylori* infection, inflammatory bowel disease etc.
   - Gastro intestinal surgery.
   - Suppression of intestinal flora by antibiotics.
3. **Hygiene:** Common in people with poor hygiene.

C. Environmental factors

1. **Urban versus rural:** More common in rural areas than urban. Typhoid fever is eliminated (decreased incidence) from the developed countries due to improved water supply & also in hygiene.

➢ **Pathogenesis: → Flow chart-3**

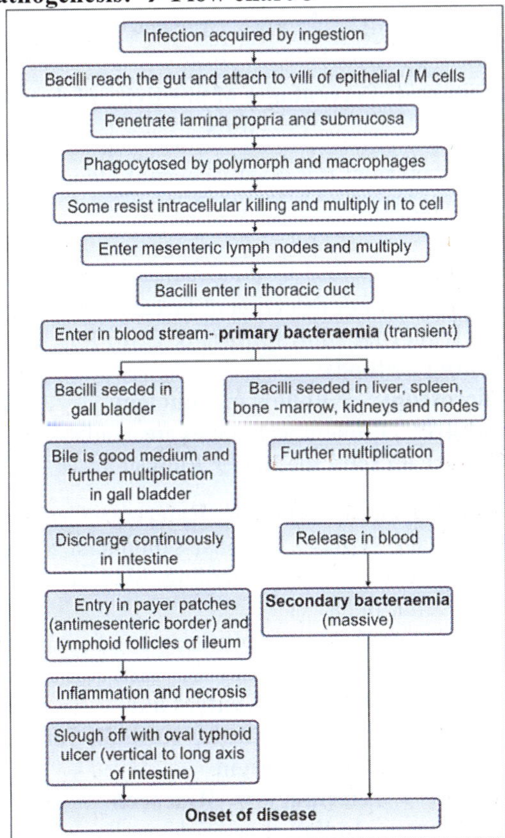

Flow chart-3: Pathogenesis of typhoid fever

✓ **Note:** Intestinal tuberculosis ulcer is horizontal (transverse to long axis of intestine)

➢ **Clinical features:** Very mild to fatal disease.

1. **Local:** Abdominal discomfort with either constipation or diarrhoea. Stool is khakhi-green, slimy **called pea-soop stool**, typically occurs in 3rd week of typhoid fever. At this time patient is in toxic stage & greater risk to develop perforation & haemorrhage. Similar stool occurs in EPEC in infants.
2. **Systemic:**
   - Onset is usually gradual with headache, malaise, anorexia & coated tongue.
   - Undifferentiated continuous fever (**step-ladder pyrexia**) with relative bradycardia & toxemia.
   - Soft & palpable spleen.
   - Hepatomegaly.
   - '**Rose spots** 'on skin during 2nd or 3rd week. Fade on pressure & rarely noticeable in dark-skinned patients.

➢ **Complications:**

1. **Local:** Intestinal perforation & hemorrhage. Stricture is not seen after typhoid but common after tuberculosis.
2. **Systemic:** Case fatality rate is <1%. Circulatory collapse, bronchitis or bronchopneumonia, deafness, cholecystitis, arthritis, abscesses, periosteitis, nephritis, HUS, hemolytic anemia, venous thromboses & neurological like meningitis, peripheral neuritis, cerebellar ataxia, muttering delirium, coma vigil, paranoid psychoses, hysteria, delirium & aggressive behavior.

➢ **Sequel:** Osteomyelitis is rare sequel.

➢ **Relapse:** Slow convalescence & relapse occurs in 5-10 %

➢ **Epidemiological types of typhoid fever:** Two types

i. **Endemic:** Occur throughout the year.
ii. **Epidemic:** Sudden onset by food, water or milk contamination.

Paratyphoid fever

➢ **Nature & history of disease:**

- Paratyphoid fever has variable distribution. *S. paratyphi A* is prevalent in India & other Asian countries, Eastern Europe & South America. *S. paratyphi B* is prevalent in Western Europe & North America. *S. paratyphi C* is prevalent in Eastern Europe & Guyana.
- About 6 million cases are reported annually
- Proportion of typhoid fever to paratyphoid fever A 10:1 with B is rare & C is least.

➢ ***S. paratyphi A & B*** cause paratyphoid fever which resembles to typhoid fever but generally milder.

- *S paratyphi C* causes paratyphoid fever present as septicemia with suppurative complications.

Laboratory diagnosis of enteric fever:

- **Specimens:**

2. **For detection of case:** Blood, bone marrow, bile, pus from suppurative lesion, CSF, sputum & autopsy specimens from liver, spleen mesenteric lymph node etc.
3. **For detection of carrier:** Urine & bile.
4. **For detection of case & carrier:** Stool.

- **Collection:**

1. **Blood for culture:**

- **Collection (amount) of blood:** 5-10ml blood is collected in adult & 2-3ml in paediatric patient by venepuncture
- **Media/containers:** Blood is collected in 50-100ml of taurocholate broth (1:10 dilution) for adult.
- **Processing:** Incubate at 37^{0}C for 24 hrs followed by subculture (S/C) on solid media & selective media which are mentioned above.
- **Advantages:**
  - Rapidly becomes positive with 90% in 1st week, 75% in 2nd week, 60% in 3rd week & 25% after as shown in **figure-4.**
  - Because of cross reactivity by different antigens in Widal test, blood culture is considered as gold standard for diagnosis of enteric fever almost at any time.
- **Disadvantages:**
  - It becomes negative after antibiotic treatment.
  - Blood contains inhibitory or bactericidal substances which are obviated by four fold dilution of blood or by adding liquoid (SPS-Sodium Polyanethol Sulphonate).

2. **Stool for culture:** Bacilli are shed in faeces throughout the course of illness & even in convalescence.

- **Collection:** Collect freshly passed stool
- **Media/containers:** Stool is collected in enrichment broth like selenite-F broth or tetrathionate broth.
- **Processing:** Incubate at 37^{0}C for 24 hrs followed by subculture (S/C) on solid media & selective media.
- **Advantages:**
  - Useful in patient taking antibiotic drug which does not interfere with intestinal bacilli.
  - Detection of case & faecal carrier.
- **Disadvantages:**
  - Bacilli shedding very infrequently in faeces so repeated cultures are required.
  - It will not differentiate between case & carrier.

3. **Urine:**

- **Collection:** Collect the mid-stream urine sample.
- **Media/containers:** Collect it in sterile container
- **Processing:** Centrifuge it. Take sediment in enrichment broth. Incubate at 37^{0}C for 24 hrs followed by subculture (S/C) on solid & selective media.
- **Advantage:** For detection of urinary carrier.
- **Disadvantage:**
  - Bacilli shed infrequently & irregularly in urine, so repeated cultures are required.
  - Positive only during 2nd and 3rd week & than 25% positivity rate.

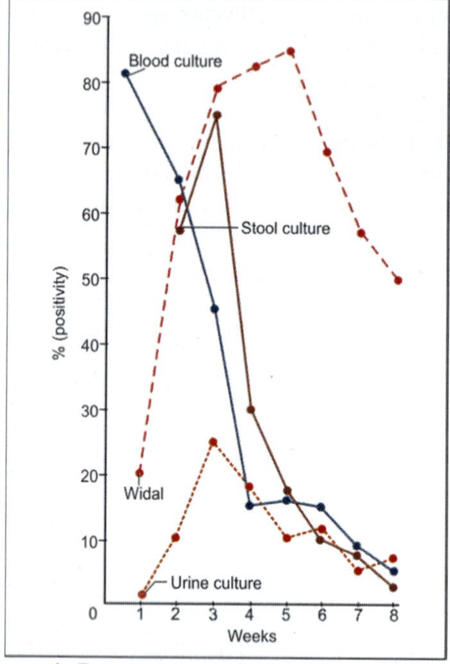

Figure-4: Percentages of positivity of different tests

4. **Bone marrow:** It is positive even if blood culture is negative.
5. **Bile:**

- **Collection:** Collect by duodenal aspiration.
- **Advantage:** For detection of faecal carrier.

6. **Pus from rose spot, sputum & CSF:** Rarely used.

- **Testing methods:**

A. **Microscopy:** → **Follow morphology**

B. **Culture:** Different techniques are available.

i. **Culture on solid media:** → **Flow chart-4**

✓ **Note: National *Salmonella* Reference Centres**

- **For phage typing:** National salmonella Vi phage typing centre →Lady Harding Medical College, New Delhi, India.
- **For Serotyping:** Identification of uncommon serotypes, culture should be sent to **National *Salmonella* Reference Centres like**.

1. **Central Research Institute, Kasauli, India:** For *Salmonella* of human origin.
2. **Indian Veterinary Research Institute, Izzatnagar, India:** For *Salmonella* of animal origin.

ii. **Castaneda culture method / biphasic media (Liquid- broth+ solid - slant phase):** It contains 50-100 ml BHIB & BHIA

- **Advantages:** It avoids the contamination during subculture
- **Culture technique:** Blood or bone marrow is inoculated in broth and incubated in upright position. For subculture bottle is tilted so that broth runs over the slant & then bottle is incubated in upright position.
- **Growth detection:** Next day observed slant for colonies
- **More details of biphasic media:** Follow chapter → Culture methods

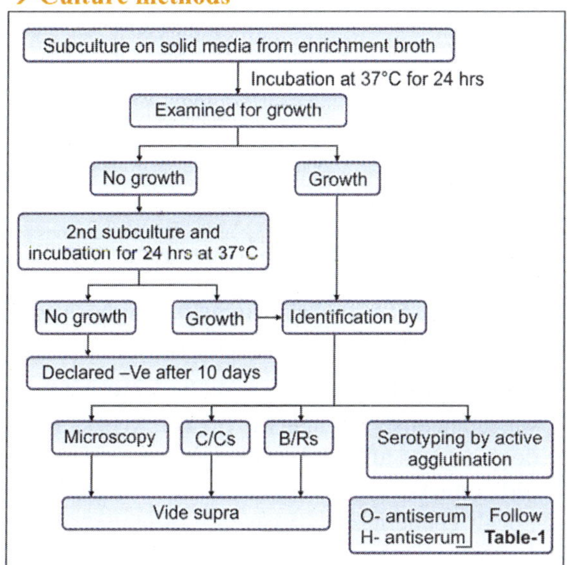

Flow chart-4: Cultivation techniques & identification of growth on solid media

iii. **Clot culture:**

- 5 ml blood in sterile test tube & allowed to clot.
- Separate the serum can be used for Widal test.
- Add streptokinase (100U/ml) to break clot → release bacteria free→ subculture on solid media.
- **Advantage:**
  - It obviates the bactericidal action of serum.
  - Serum is available for serological test.

C. **Serological tests:** Two types

i. **Ab detection tests:** Because of cross reaction by related antibodies, these tests have limited value. Following are useful tests.

1. **Widal test:** Follow chapter → Antigen-antibody (Ag-Ab) reactions.
2. **Typhidot test:** It detects IgG & IgM antibodies to outer membrane proteins antigen.
3. **IDL tubex test:** It detect the IgM antibodies against O9 antigen of *S typhi*
4. **ELISA:** } Both detect the IgM antibodies against LPS-Ag
5. **IgM dip stick test:** } Both detect the IgM antibodies against LPS-Ag
6. **CIE:**
7. **Dot blot assay:** It detects the IgG antibodies against H antigen.
8. **Indirect Haem Agglutination (IHA) Test:**

ii. **Ag detection tests:** By using monoclonal Ab. Samples are blood (early phase) & urine (late phase).

1. **ELISA**
2. **Co-agglutination test:**
   - *Staph. aureus* (Cowan I strain) which contain protein A is fixed with Ab of *S. typhi.*
   - Mixed such sensitised *Staph. aureus* with patient serum containing typhoid Ag (urine also contains typhoid Ag).
   - Typhoid Ag combine with Ab of *S. typhi* & produces clumping of *Staph aureus* **called coagglutination.**
   - Advantage: Test is rapid, sensitive & specific.
   - Disadvantage: Test is positive in 1st week but not after that.

D. **Pathological test:**

i. **Blood picture:** Leucopenia with lymphocytosis.

ii. **Diazo test:**

- **Sample:** Urine
- **Reagent:** Diazo reagent 40 parts of solution A & one part of solution B.
  - Solution A: 0.5g sulphanilic acid, 5ml H_2SO_4 & 100ml distilled water.
  - Solution B: Sodium nitrate 0.5 g/100ml distilled water.
- **Steps:**
  - Mix equal volume of urine & diazo reagent in test tube & add few drops of 30% NaOH.
  - Development of pink/red colour on shaking indicates +Ve test.

E. **Molecular test:** PCR based test are sensitive but costly, so not available widely.

F. **Salmonella typing method:**

i. **Phenotyping methods:**

a. **Bacteriophage typing:** Follow chapter → Laboratory diagnosis of bacterial infections.

b. **Bacteriocin typing:**

c. **Biotyping:**

- For *S. typhi* it described earlier.
- It is also possible in *S typhimurium.*
- Kristensen biotyping by xylose & arabinose fermentation is also useful.
- It also done by production of tetrathionate reductase.

d. **Antibiogram typing:** Not able to differentiate between the other species.

ii. **Genotyping methods:** Useful for the epidemiological purpose & has more discriminating power like

- Pulsed Field Gel Electrophoresis.
- Multi locus enzyme electrophoresis.
- IS-200 profiling.

- Random amplified polymorphic DNA typing.

❖ **Carrier:**

➢ **Definition:** Person who carries the organism without any sign-symptoms of disease **called carrier**. It never presents in normal population & occurs only after infection.

➢ ***S. typhi* carrier:** Two types.

a. **Fecal carrier:** Bacilli persist in gall bladder & shed in feces but for a different period. Antibiotics do not eliminate intestinal bacilli rapidly unlike bacilli blood, so faecal culture is useful after antibiotics course. Faecal carrier is common but less risky.

1. **Convalescent carrier:** Shed bacilli in feces from 3 wk to 3 month after clinical cure.
2. **Temporary carrier:** Shed bacilli in feces > 3 months to < 1 year.
3. **Chronic carrier:** Shed bacilli in feces > 1 year. Example of chronic carrier is Mary Mallon/Typhoid marry **(New York Food handlers or cook)** who over a period of 15 year caused at least seven outbreaks affecting over 200 person.

b. **Urinary carrier:** Bacilli persist in kidneys & shed in urine. Urinary carrier is rare but more dangerous because it is associated with anomalies like calculi or schistosomiasis.

➢ ***S. paratyphi* carrier:** Also occur in paratyphoid bacilli.

➢ **Laboratory diagnosis of carrier:**

- **Faecal carrier:** Repeated bile & stool culture. Collection after purgative gives more chance of isolation. Duodenal aspiration may be useful.
- **Urinary carrier:** Repeated urine culture.
- **Detection of recent carrier:** Detection of Vi antigen for screening purpose.
- **Detection of carrier in cities:**

1. **Sewer swab technique:** Gauze pad left in sewer and drain. Culture and by positive swab one may reach to house harboring carrier.
2. **Filtration technique:** Filtration through millipore membrane followed by culture of membrane.

❖ **General scheme to diagnose case & carrier in enteric fever:** → **Flow chart-5.**

❖ **Prevention:**

A. **General measures:** Improvements in sanitation and provision of protected water.

B. **Immunoprophylaxis:** Following types of vaccine are developed for *Salmonella* spp.

i. **TAB vaccine:**

- **History:** Developed & tested successfully by Almroth Wright in Africa.
- **Preparation:** Heat inactivation of typhoid bacillus at 50-60^{0}C.
- **Preservation:** In 0.5 % phenol.
- **Contain:** *S. typhi*-1000 million & *S paratyphi A* and *B*, 750 million each per ml.

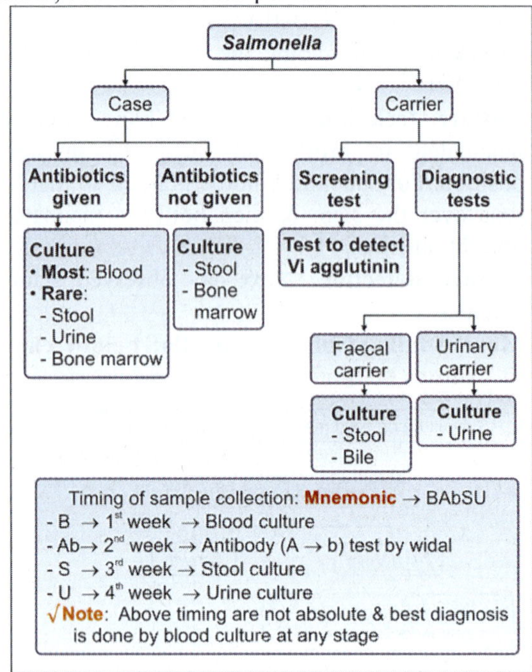

Flowchart-5: General scheme to diagnose case & carrier in enteric fever

- **Administration:** Two doses of 0.5 ml subcutaneously at interval of 4-6 weeks. Booster dose is given after 2-3 years.
- **Side effects:**
  - Local: Tenderness.
  - General: Fever, malaise etc.
  - Reactions are overcome by injecting 0.1 ml intradermally.
- **Uses:**

1. **In non-endemic areas:** For troops, medical & paramedical personnel.
2. **In endemic areas:** For children.

ii. **Typhoral (live typhoid oral) vaccine:**

- **Preparation:** Stable mutant of *S typhi* strain Ty21a, lacking enzyme UDP-galactose-4-epimerase (Gal E mutant). This enzyme is responsible for production of Lipopolysaccharide 'O' Ag which makes the strain virulent.
- **Contain:** Vaccine is enteric coated capsule containing 10^9 viable lyophilised mutant bacilli.
- **Administration:** One capsule orally taken hour before food with a glass of water or milk on Days 1, 3 and 5. No antibiotic should be taken during this period. On ingestion it initiates infection but 'self-destructs' after four or five cell divisions and therefore cannot induce any illness.
- **Side effects:** Diarrhoea, abdominal pain or rashes.
- **Advantages:**
  - Given by oral route & obviate the side effects by injection route.

- Provide local & systemic immunity.
- Safe, long acting & more convenient. It starts protection after 2-3 weeks & immunity will last for 3 years.
- Provide 67-90% protection.
- **Contraindication:** In children with <5 years of age.

iii. Vi vaccine (typhim-Vi):

- **Contain:** Purified Vi polysaccharide antigen (25 ug per dose) from *S typhi* strain Ty2.
- **Administration:** Single subcutaneous or intramuscular injection. Same dose is given to adults & children.
- **Advantage:** Provide protection for 2-3 years thereafter booster dose is recommended.
- **Disadvantages:**
  - Local reaction, but minimal like pain & erythema.
  - It is T-cell independent, hence poorly immunogenic in children < 5 years.
  - Not useful in patient hypersensitive to the vaccine components.
- **Contraindication:**
  - In children with <5 years of age.
  - In allergic patients.

iv. Other types:

a. Monovalent vaccine:

- Heat killed & phenol preserved.
- It contains single antigen or single species.
- As it contains single species it is useful in country like India, where only one species is the major cause of disease.

b. Bivalent vaccine:

- Heat killed & phenol preserved.

c. VirEPA vaccine:

- It is prepared by binding the Vi to the non toxic recombinant protein (identical to *P. aeruginosa* exotoxin A).
- Not marketed yet.
- More immunogenic than typhim-Vi.

❖ Treatment:

a. Treatment of case:

➢ **Earlier (older) sensitive drugs:**

- Chloramphenicol: Initially bacilli were sensitive to chloramphenicol but plasmid mediated resistant strains were identified in 1972 from Mexico & Kerala (India). Resistant strain identified in Calicut, Kerala & later spread in other part of country.
- Ampicillin, amoxicillin, cotrimoxazole & furazolidone: Such strains were sensitive to many drugs like ampicillin, amoxicillin, cotrimoxazole & furazolidone. Resistant develop to these drugs in late 1980 **called multidrug resistant (MDR) *Salmonella*.**

➢ **MDR *salmonella:*** Following drugs are used currently to treat MDR *Salmonella*

- Fluoroquinolones: Ciprofloxacin (drug of choice), ofloxacin or pefloxacin.
- 3rd generation cephalosporins: Ceftriaxone, ceftazidime or cefotaxime
- Azithromycin

➢ **Nalidixic acid resistant *salmonella:*** Resistant also start to develop against ciprofloxacin, which is detected by using nalidixic acid **called nalidixic acid resistant *Salmonella*.** It is either plasmid or chromosome mediated.

➢ **Resistant to ceftriaxone & ampicillin:** Resistant also develop against ceftriaxone, due to production of ESBL & also against ampicillin due to AmpC β-lactamase production.

➢ **Reversal of sensitivity:** *Salmonella* sensitive to newer drugs are now becomes resistant & instead they becomes sensitive to older drugs

b. Treatment of carrier:

1. **Combination of chemotherapy & vaccine:** Ampicillin / amoxicillin can
   - Eliminate the carries state.
   - Prevent the relapse.
2. **Surgical treatment:** Cholecystectomy, pyelolithotomy or nephrectomy.

Non-typhoidal group

Salmonella food poisoning

❖ **Synonym:** It is zoonosis, also **called *Salmonella* gastroenteritis** or ***Salmonella* enterocolitis.**

❖ **Species:** Non typhoidal *Salmonella* like *S. typhimurium* (most common in the world), *S. enteritidis, S. haldar, S. anatum, S. newport, S. seftenberg, S. heidelberg, S. agona, S. virchow, S. Indiana* etc.

❖ Pathogenicity:

➢ **Reservoir of infection:** Human & animals are the reservoir hosts for non typhoidal group, unlike *S. typhi* where only human case/carrier is the reservoir host. However role of human carrier is minimal.

➢ **Source of infection:** Animal product like egg, meat, milk or milk-derivatives.

➢ **Mode of transmission:**

- By ingestion of animal product as mentioned earlier, especially egg & egg products. *Salmonella* can enter through the shell if eggs left on contaminated chicken feed or faeces, and grow inside.
- Also by ingestion of salad / vegetables which are contaminated by manure or poor handling.
- Food contamination by dropping of rat, lizard and other small animal.

- Also occur without food as cross infection in hospital.
- It occurs in developed countries while enteric fever is a problem of developing countries.

➤ **Incubation period:** ≤ 24 hrs

➤ **Portal of entry & sites:** GIT

➤ **Pathogenesis:** It has invasive property & not released any toxin.

➤ **Clinical features:**

- Acute cholerae type diarrhoea: Passage of 1-2 loose stools.
- Acute stage subsides in 2-4 days or progress to dysentery with presence of blood + mucus in stool.
- Abdominal pain & vomiting.
- Typhoid or septicemic kind of fever develops in few days.

❖ **Laboratory diagnosis of food poisoning:** Isolation of bacilli from food or faeces.

❖ **Prevention:** Prevention of food contamination during production, packaging, storage & marketing.

❖ **Treatment:**

- **Non-invasive cases:** Symptoms are subsides in 2-4 days & antibiotics are not necessary.
- **Invasive cases:** Antibiotics are necessary.

✓ **Note: DT 104 strain of *S typhimurium***

- Multidrug resistant strain emerged in early 1990s & associated with an increased risk of blood stream infection & hospitalization. Acquired by raw or partially cooked meat products.

Salmonella septicemia

❖ **Species:** *S. choleraesuis.*

❖ **Clinical features:** Suppurative lesions such as endocarditis, meningitis, pneumonia, deep abscess, osteomyelitis & antecedent gastroenteritis may or may not present.

❖ **Laboratory diagnosis:** Isolation of bacilli from pus, blood or faeces.

Question bank

Case study

1) A paediatric patient visited the hospital with complain of step ladder type of fever since 10 days. Blood is collected for culture & serology. Culture report suggests GNB. Widal test is positive with high titre for H-Ag & O-Ag. Identify the organism & answer the following

a) Name the causative agent & describe the morphology of causative agent

b) Write the pathogenicity of causative agent

c) Describe the laboratory diagnosis of carrier of causative agent

Essay/Full question

1) *S. typhi*

Short notes

1) Biochemical reactions / Pathogenicity / Lab. diagnosis of *S. typhi,*
2) Antigenic structure of *S. typhi.*
3) Antigenic variation of *S. typhi.*
4) Classification of *S. typhi.*
5) *Salmonella* food poisoning.
6) Widat test.
7) Culture techniques for typhoid fever.

Short questions for theory/viva questions

1) What is typhoid merry?
2) Mention the reference centres for *Salmonella* phage typing & Serotyping of human origin.
3) Name the four *Salmonella species* causing food poisoning.

MCQs for chapter review

1) **All of the following *Salmonella* are motile except -**
(a) *S. typhi* (b) *S. enteritidis* (c) *S. gallinarum* (d) *S. typhimurium*

2) **Following are gas producing *Salmonella*** (AI -92)
(a) *S. typhi* (b) *S. enteritidis* (c) *S. cholera* (d) *S. typhimurium*

3) **Growth factor needed for *Salmonella***
(a) Tryptophan (b) Niacin (c) B-12 (d) Citrate

4) **There has been an outbreak of food borne *Salmonella* gastroenteritis in the community and the stool samples have been received in the laboratory. Which is the enrichment medium of choice -** (AIIMS, May-03)
(a) Cary Blair medium (b) V R medium (c) Selenite F medium medium (d) Thioglycolate medium

5) **Agglutination with O antigen of *S typhi* is inhibited by -** (AIIMS-92, AI- 95)
(a) Vi antigen (b) Pilli antigen (c) Flagellar antigen (d) All of the above

6) **True statement about Widal test in typhoid is -** (AI -99)
(a) O-antigen titre remains positive for several months & reaction to it is rapid (b) H-antigen titre remains positive for several months & reaction to it is rapid (c) Both remains positive for several months & reaction to both is rapid (d) None

7) **Most immunogenic in typhoid-**
(a) O antigen (b) H antigen (c) Vi antigen (d) Somatic antigen.

8) **Vi antigen found in –** (PGI, May-13 & June-05)
(a) *S paratyphi A* (b) *S paratyphi C* (c) *S dublin* (d) *Klebsiella pneumoniae* (e) *Citrobacter freundii*

9) **A 24 year old cook in a hostel mess suffered from enteric fever 2 year back. The chronic carrier state in this patient can be diagnosed by -** (AIIMS, Nov-02)
(a) Vi agglutination test (b) Blood culture in brain heart infusion broth (c) Widal test (d) C-reactive protein

10) **Which is true about Widal reaction -** (AI -93)
(a) Antibody to H-Ag appears first and persists (b) Antibody to O-Ag appears first and persists (c) Antibodies to O & H-Ag appears simultaneously and persists (d) None of the above

11) **Pea-soop stool is characteristically seen in**
(a) Cholera (b) Typhoid (c) Botulism (d) Polio in immuno-compromised host

12) **All of the following are true regarding typhoid except -** (AIIMS, June-99)
(a) Urinary carriers are more dangerous (b) Vi Ab is used for detecting carrier (c) Vi is seen in normal population (d) Urine carrier is associated with anomalies

13) **Diagnosis of typhoid in 1st week is done by -**
(a) Widal test (b) Stool culture (c) Blood culture (d) Urine culture

14) In a patient with typhoid, diagnosis after 15 days of onset of fever is best done by- (AI -01,02)
(a) Blood culture (b) Widal (c) Stool culture (d) Urine culture

15) Drug commonly used against enteric fever are all except - (AI-08)
(a) Amikacin (b) Ciprofloxacin (c) Ceftriaxone (d) Azithromycin

16) True about salmonellosi - (PGI-11)
(a) Decreased incidence in developed countries (b) Antacid and prolonged antibiotic administration promote infection (c) Always fatal (d) Food borne to man and animal

17) True about typhoid -
(a) It is caused by food poisoning (b) Water can transmit the disease (c) Ty21a is an oral vaccine (d) Chronic carrier called when transmit up to 6 months (e) Widal test positive in 1st week

18) True about *Salmonella typhi* infection in intestine are- (PGI-01)
(a) Affects payer's patches (b) Common in mesenteric border (c) Erythrophagocytosis is the characteristics (d) Strictures are common (e) Typhoid ulcer always bleed very common

19) True about maximum isolation period of enteric fever- (AIIMS-08)
(a) Till three consecutive negative urine/stool culture samples are obtained from patient (b) After chloramphenicol treatment for 72 hours (c) Disappearance of fever (d) Widal test negative

20) For typhoid endemic country like India, Immunisation of choice is- (AIIMS-02)
(a) TAB vaccine (b) Typhod 21A oral vaccine (c) Monovalent vaccine (d) Any of these

21) About Vi polysaccharide vaccine true is- (AIIMS, Nov-10)
(a) Can be given in patient with yellow fever and hepatitis B (b) Has many contraindications (c) Has many serious systemic side effects (d) Has many serious local side effects

22) All of the following statements about non typhoid *Salmonella* are true except - (AI-09)
(a) Humans are the only reservoirs (b) Transmission is most commonly associated with eggs, poultry & undercooked meat (d) Common in immunocompromised individual (e) Resistance to fluoroquinolones has emerged

23) Typhoid is fever caused by
(a) *S. typhi* (b) *S. para typhi* (c) a+c (d) None of above

24) Food poisoning is produce by
(a) *S. typhi* (b) *S. paratyphi* (c) a+b (d) *S. typhimurium*

25) *Salmonella* gastroenteritis is - (PGI -02)
(a) Mainly diagnosed by serology (b) Blood and mucus present in stool (c) Caused by animal products (d) Symptoms appear by 4-48 hours (e) Features are due to exotoxin released

26) DT 104 strain is belong to which of the following bacteria- (PGI , Nov 11)
(a) *Salmonella gallinarum* (b) *Salmonella typhi* (c) *Salmonella enteritidis* (d) *Salmonella paratyphi A* (e) *Salmonella typhimurium*

27) Microorganisms that can enter freshly laid eggs are
(a) *Salmonella* (b) *Bucella* (c) *Shigella* (d) *Vibrio cholerae*

28) Prolonged *Salmonella* septicemia is caused by- (PGI -95)
(a) *S enteritidis* (b) *S cholera suis* (c) *S typhimurium* (d) *S typhi*

Answers of MCQs & explanation

1) (c)
- All *Salmonella* are motile with peritrichate flagella, except *S. gallinarum & S. pullorum*

2) (a)
- *S. typhi* is anaerogenic, it ferment the sugars with acid only while other can ferment acid with gas

3) (a)
- *S. typhi* & few other *Salmonellae* do not grow on Simmon's citrate medium as they required tryptophan as a growth factor

4) (c)
- Follow section. **culture characteristics (C/Cs)** for explanation

5) (a)
6) (b)
7) (b)
8) (b), (c) & (e)
9) (a)
10) (a)
(5–10) Follow section, **antigenic structure** for explanation

11) (b)
- Follow section, **Enteric fever / typhoidal group (typhoid fever →clinical features)** for explanation

12) (c)
- *Salmonella* carrier never presents in normal population & occurs only after infection.
- Faecal carrier is common but less risky.
- Urinary carrier is rare but more dangerous because it is associated with anomalies like calculi or schistosomiasis.

13) (c)
14) (b)
(13–14) Follow section, **enteric fever / typhoidal group (General scheme to diagnose case & carrier in enteric fever → flow chart-5)** for explanation

15) (a)
- Follow section, **enteric fever / typhoidal group (treatment → treatment of case)** for explanation

16) (a)
- More common in rural areas than urban. Typhoid fever is eliminated (decreased incidence) from the developed countries due to improved water supply & also improvement in hygiene.
- Bacilli are sensitive to gastric acid. Low acidity due to achlorhydria & use of antacids can enhance the infection. Suppression of intestinal flora by antibiotics can promote the infection
- Not always fatal, case fatality rate is <1&
- Transmitted by contaminated food & water to man and animals

17) (a), (b) & (c)
- *S. typhi* is transmitted by contaminated food (food poisoning) & water to man and animals
- Ty21a strain used to prepare the Typhoral (Live Typhoid oral) vaccine of *S typhi*
- Chronic carrier called when transmit the infection for > 1 year
- Widal test positive in 2nd week

18) (a)
- *S. typhi* affects payer's patches which lie along the anti-mesenteric border
- Erythrophagocytosis is not seen it is the characteristics of *E. histolytica*
- Strictures are uncommon, but common in tuberculosis
- Typhoid ulcer bleed very rare

19) (a)
- Maximum isolation period of enteric fever: Till three consecutive negative urine/stool culture samples collected on three separate days

20) (a)
- Typhoid endemic country like India, single species is the species like *S. typhi* is responsible for disease, so Monovalent vaccine is indicated

21) (a)
- Vi polysaccharide vaccine is contraindicated in children < 5 year of age & in allergic patient. No other contraindications, so can be given in patient with yellow fever and hepatitis B

22) (a)
- Human & animals are the reservoir hosts for non typhoidal group, unlike *S. typhi* where only human case/carrier is the reservoir host.

23) (a)
- Enteric fever / typhoidal group include typhoid fever caused by *S. typhi* & paratyphoid fever caused by *S. paratyphi A, B & C*.

24) (c)
25) (c) & (d) } Follow section, **non-typhoidal group (*Salmonella* food poisoning)** for explanation
26) (e)
27) (a)

- Follow section, **non-typhoidal group (*Salmonella* food poisoning → mode of transmission)** for explanation

28) (b)

- Follow section, **non typhoidal group (*Salmonella* septicemia)** for explanation

45 Enterobactericeae-III (*Shigella*)

Learning heading & subheadings

- ❖ Meaning & synonym:
- ❖ Morphology:
- ❖ Cultural characteristics (C/Cs):
- ❖ Biochemical reaction (B/Rs):
- ❖ Resistance:
- ❖ Classification:
- ❖ Antigenic structure:
- ❖ Pathogenicity:
- ❖ Laboratory diagnosis:
- ❖ Prevention:
- ❖ Treatment:

❖ **Meaning & synonym:** 1st identified by **Kiyoshi Shiga** in 1896 from dysentery patient in Japan hence the name. Also **called shiga bacilli** from the name of discoverer.

❖ **Morphology:** → **Fig.-1**

- ➢ **Type according to gram stain:** GNB
- ➢ **Size:** 0.5 µm x 1–3 µm.
- ➢ **Shape:** Short rod.
- ➢ **Arrangement:** Single / pair / small group.
- ➢ **Capsule:** Noncapsulated but few strain has capsular (K) Ag.
- ➢ **Motility:** Nonmotile.
- ➢ **Spores:** Nonsporing.
- ➢ **Fimbriae:** May be present.

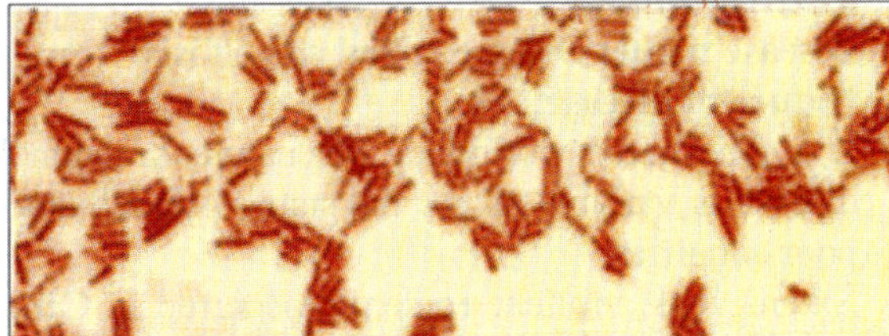

Figure-1: Morphology of *Shigella* under gram stain

❖ **Cultural characteristics (C/Cs):**

➢ **Effective factors:**

- O_2 effect: Aerobes and facultative anaerobes.
- Optimum temperature: 37°C (10–40°C).
- Optimum pH: 7.4

➢ **Culture in media:**

A. **Liquid media:**

1. **Enrichment media for faeces:** Following both enrichment media are useful for *Shigella* & *Salmonella* but better for *Salmonella*
   - Selenite-F broth / selenite broth:
   - *Salmonella Shigella* broth:
2. **Transport media:**
   - Sach's glycerol buffered saline (Gram negative broth or glycerol saline transport medium): Preserves *Salmonella* & *Shigella* from faecal specimens
   - Gram negative broth: Transport & selective medium for *Salmonella* & *Shigella* from clinical (faeces, urine, blood etc) & non clinical specimens (water, food etc.). It contains sodium citrate & sodium deoxycholate inhibit the growth of gram positive & coliforms. Collect the specimen; incubate for 6-8 hours followed by subculture on solid media. It is not good for rectal swab.
   - Cary Blair medium: For transportation of EHEC (O157:H7), *Salmonella Shigella* & *V. cholerae*

B. **Solid media:**

1. **Nutrient agar:** Large about 2-3 mm, circular, convex, smooth, translucent & grey colonies.
2. **Blood agar:** Some strains are haemolytic.

C. **Selective media:**

1. **Mac Conkey's:**
2. **DCA:**
3. **S-S agar:**

} Palc/colourless (**fig.-2**) colonies, except *Sh. sonnei*, which gives pink colonies due to LLF

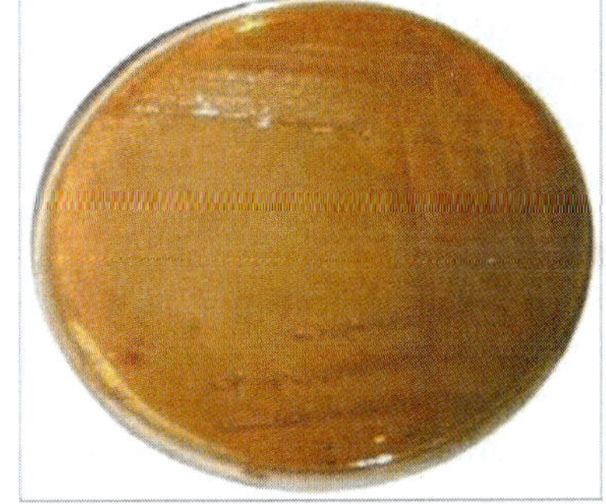

Figure-2: Pale colonies in Mac Conkey's medium by *Shigella*

4. **XLD media:** Pink colonics without black center because of absence of H_2S production.
5. **W & B medium:** Growth is inhibited
6. **Hektoen enteric agar:**
   - It is a selective & differential medium, primarily used to recover *Salmonella* & *Shigella* from patient

specimens. It contains indicators of lactose fermentation & H_2S production; as well as inhibitors to prevent the growth of Gram-positive bacteria.

- Contain bile salts as inhibitory agents & some dyes. Produce green colour colonies with colour fading to the periphery.

➢ **Culture in animal:** → Sereny test

- Instillation of suspension of freshly isolate into eyes of guinea pigs or mice leads to mucopurulent conjunctivitis and severe keratitis.
- Test is non invasive but it detects the invasive property of bacteria.

❖ Biochemical reaction (B/Rs):

1. **Sugar fermentation by *Shigella* spp.:**

- Glucose is fermented by all species with acid without gas production except New Castle & Manchester biotypes of *Sh. flexneri* type 6 & some strain of *Sh. boydii* type 13 & 14 which form gas.
- Mannitol fermentation is useful in classification as shown in **table-1.** *Sh. dysenteriae* does not ferments mannitol while remaining three species can ferment the mannitol with acid without gas production.
- Adonitol, inositol & salicin are not fermented.

Species	G	S	L	M
Sh. dysenteriae	A	-	-	-
Sh. flexneri	A	-	-	A
Sh. boydii	A	-	-	A
Sh. sonnei	A	A (Late fermentation)	A (late fermentation)	A

Table-1: Sugar fermentation by *Shigella* spp.

2. **I M Vi C tests:** V + - -
3. **Catalase test:** All species / serotype are catalase +Ve except *Sh. dysenteriae* type –I.
4. **Nitrate reduction test:** + Ve
5. **Oxidase test:** -Ve
6. **H_2S production:** -Ve
7. **Urease test:** -Ve
8. **TSI test:** K/A – H_2S.

❖ Resistance:

- *Shigella* is killed by heating at 56^0C in one hour & by 5% phenol.
- It can resist gastric acidity also.
- Epidemic strain showed plasmid borne multiple drug resistance.

❖ Classification: 4 species / 4 subgroups, based on biochemical & serological tests.

a. ***Sh. dysenteriae* / subgroup A:** 10 serotypes

- **Type 1 - *Sh. shigae*:**
- Originally described by Shiga.
- Produces shiga toxin.
- Indole & catalase tests are -Ve (only member of Enterobactericeae family with catalase -Ve).
- It is the most virulent, associated with complications (vide infra) & high mortality.
- **Type 2 – *Sh. schmitzi*:**
- Indole & catalase (variable by some strain) tests are +Ve.
- Ferments rhamnose & sorbitol.
- **Type 3 -7:** Large and Sach group.

b. ***Sh. flexneri* (after Flexner) / subgroup B:** It has 6 serotypes with many subtypes & 2 antigenic variants like X & Y which do not possess type specific antigens. Name given from the Flexner, who identified the bacilli by its mannitol fermenting property in Philippines in 1900.

- **Serotype 6 of *Sh. flexneri*:**
- Indole negative.
- Biotype: Three biotypes as follows.

1. Boyd 88: Which ferment glucose & mannitol with acid only.
2. Manchester: Which ferment glucose & mannitol with acid and gas.
3. Newcastle: Ferments glucose with or without production of gas but not mannitol.

c. ***Sh. boydii* (after Boyd) / subgroup C:**

- It has 15 serotypes.
- Name given from the Boyd, who described the bacilli in India in 1931.
- Bacilli resemble to *Sh flexneri* biochemically but not antigenically.
- Less frequent cause of dysentery

d. ***Sh sonnei* (after Sonne) / subgroup D:**

- It has 1 serotype (antigenically homogenous) & classified by colicin typing in to 26 types.
- Name from the Sonne, who described the bacilli in Denmark.
- Indole negative & ferment lactose and sucrose very late (3-8 days) with acid production only.
- Causes mildest form of bacillary dysentery. In many cases it causes diarrhoea.
- Antigenically homogenous but may occur in two forms, phase I & phase II, latter forming large, flatter & irregular colonies.

❖ Pathogenicity:

➢ **Disease name:** Disease **called shigellosis.**

➢ **Nature of disease:**

- It is distributed worldwide but nature & extent of disease is variable as per the status like affluent & poor countries.
- Extensive & virulent epidemic occurred in Central America in 1968. Similar localised outbreak occurred in Bangladesh & in Sri Lanka.
- Several outbreak followed by epidemics occurred in India from 1974.
- Endemic shigellosis is common in poor countries in age group.
- In India, rate of dysentery by different species is variable as mentioned below. *Sh. flexneri* is the

most predominant species while *Sh. boydii* is least frequent.

1. *Sh. dysenteriae*: 8-25%
2. *Sh. flexneri*: 50-85%
3. *Sh. boydii*: 0-8%
4. *Sh. sonnei*: 2-24%

- Epidemics are associated with poverty & poor hygiene. Epidemic is influenced by war & its outcome.

➢ **Reservoir of infection:** Human is the natural host of bacilli. Human case or carrier is the reservoir of infection. Bacilli disappear within few weeks from faeces, so chronic carrier is very rare.

➢ **Source of infection:** Water or food.

➢ **Mode of transmission:**

a. Direct transmission:

1. Contaminated fingers/hands: Hands to mouth.
2. Sexual contact in male homosexual: Skin to skin/mucosa **called gay bowel syndrome.**

b. Indirect transmission (vehicle borne):

1. Food & water borne: *Sh sonnei* especially occurs as food poisoning.
2. Vector borne: Mechanical by flies.
3. Fomites borne: Door handles, lavatory seats etc.

➢ **Incubation period:** 48 hrs (1-7 days).

➢ **Portal of entry:** GIT & skin/mucosa.

➢ **Sites:** Intestinal & extra-intestinal (complications).

➢ **Precipitating factors (epidemiological determinants):** Following are the factors.

I. Agent factors (virulence factors)

A. Intracellular (cell wall associated) factors:

i. Capsular (K) antigen: Present in some strains. It masks the O-Ag & inhibits agglutination by antiserum. It inhibits the phagocytosis.

ii. Somatic antigen (O Ag or LPS or Endotoxin): Present in large number. Causing diarrhoea & ulcer. LPS is responsible for endotoxic activities.

iii. Fimbriae: Organ of adhesion

iv. Invasive property:

- Invasive property is due to a special type of OMP **called VMA (Virulence Marker Antigen)** which is plasmid encoded, responsible for invasion, multiplication of bacilli & destruction of epithelial cells.
- It is detected by VMA ELISA or by culture cells like Hela or Hep-2 cells

v. Cross reactive antigens: There is antigenic sharing between *Shigella, Salmonella* and *E. coli*.

vi. Infective dose: They resist gastric acidity & few bacilli can initiate the disease. Infective dose is very low, about 10-100 bacilli.

B. Intracellular (cell wall associated) factors:

i. Exotoxins/enterotoxins: Two varieties

a. Shiga toxin / verotoxin / verocytotoxin:

- **Bacteria producing shiga toxin:** *Sh. dysenteriae* type-1.
- **Properties of shiga toxin:**

- Less important in pathogenesis, because non-toxigenic strain can invade the mucosa & multiply.
- Earliest exotoxin identified from GNB.
- Chromosome mediated.

- **Biological actions of shiga toxin:** Three types of actions

o Neurotoxicity:

- Detected by paralysis & death on injection in to mice or rabbits.
- It is neurotoxic, but this property is secondary because it not acts directly on CNS but to the blood vessels supplying the nerve.

o Cytotoxicity:

- In vitro: Cytopathic changes in cultured Vero or HeLa cells.
- In vivo: Toxin consists two sub units like binding (B) & active (A). Sub unit A divided in to two fragments like A1 & A2. B helps in adhesion with host cells. A2 links A1 to B. A1 inactivate the host cell 60S ribosome & inhibit the protein synthesis leading to cell death. Cell death resulting discontinuity of mucosa & haemorrhage (bloody diarrhoea → dysentery).

o Enterotoxicity: It allows the collection of fluid in gut (in ligated rabbit ileal loop).

- **Diagnostic tests of shiga toxin:** Detection of shiga toxin is done by following tests.

- Culture: Cytopathic changes in cultured Vero or HeLa cells.
- Serology: Demonstration of antibody in sera by latex agglutination test & ELISA.
- Molecular: DNA probe.

b. *Shigella* enterocytotoxin (ShET):

- **Subtypes:** Two forms

1. *Shigella* enterocytotoxin 1 (ShET 1):

- Secreted from *Sh. flexneri* 2a.
- Structurally similar to cholera toxin.
- Chromosome mediated.

2. *Shigella* enterocytotoxin 2 (ShET 2):

- Secreted from all strain of *Sh. flexneri.*
- Helps in iron uptake.
- Plasmid mediated.

- **Biological action:** Both toxins allow the collection of fluid in gut (in ligated rabbit ileal loop).

II. Host factors

1. **Age:** Common in young children due to poor hygiene, however endemic shigellosis found in all ages.
2. **Immune status:** Bacilli last longer in patient with malnutrition & IDDs like AIDS but disappeared within few weeks from the faeces of normal individual.
3. **Poverty, lack of sanitation & mental status:** Also favours the shigellosis.

- After that 2nd-11th epidemic occurred from AD 558-664 in 8-12 years cycles.
- Finally all known world affected by plague.

2. **The second pandemic:**
- **Called Black Death** because it was present with gangrene of skin-finger-penis.
- Biotypes: *Y. pestis* var *medievalis.*
- Occurred between AD 1347-1351 (14th century) in Europe.
- It began in Black sea & spread to Europe & West Russia.
- It killed 17-28 million people.
- After that epidemic continue from AD 1361 - 1480 in 2-5 years cycles.
- It also affected the all known world.

3. **The third pandemic:**
- **Called modern plague.**
- Biotypes: *Y. pestis* var *orientalis.*
- Occurred between AD 1855-1918 (19th century) in Asia & in other countries.
- It began in Yunnan, a South Western province of China in 1855 & spread to Hong Kong in May 1894, Mumbai 1896, Kolkata 1898, Madagaskar 1898; Egypt, Portugal, Japan, Paraguay & Eastern Africa in 1899; Manila, Glasgow, Sydney & San Francisco in 1900.
- Local epidemics occurred subsequently throughout the world with plenty of victims.
- Finally whole world affected by plague & disease receded by control of rodent & vector.

✪ **In India:**

- **Indian scenario of plague:**

1. **China pandemic (1855-1918):**
- It entered in India in 1896 (Bombay) & spread all over the country with 10 million death by 1918.
- It gradually decline thereafter, however few scattered cases were reported till 1967.

2. **No cases from 1967 to 1994.**
3. **Maharashtra outbreak (1994) of bubonic plague:** It occurred in Beed-Latur district of Maharashtra in August 1994.
4. **Surat epidemic (1994) of pneumonic plague:** It occurred in Surat & adjoining regions of Gujarat & Maharashtra in September in 1994. Around 6000 cases were reported with 60 deaths over a period of 2 months.
5. **Simla outbreak (2002):** It occurred near Rohru of Simla (Himachal Pradesh) in February 2002 with 4 deaths.
6. **Uttaranchal outbreak (2004) of bubonic plague:** It occurred in Dangud village of Uttarkashi district of Uttaranchal in 2004 with 8 cases & four deaths.

- **Indian foci of plague:** Total four foci of plague are known in India.

1. Region near Kolar at the trijunction of Tamil Nadu, Karnataka & Andhra Pradesh.
2. Beed-Latur district of Maharashtra from where Surat epidemic was originated.
3. Rohru in Himachal Pradesh.
4. Dangud village of Uttaranchal.

➢ **Reservoir of infection:** Different types of rodents are the main reservoir as described below.

➢ **Source of infection:** Fleas. Man to man transmission can occur, especially in pneumonic plague.

➢ **Mode of transmission:**

a. **Indirect:**

1. **Flea bite (Vector borne):** Bubonic plague.

- **Mechanisms of introduction of bacilli:** Blocked flea cannot suck the blood because the bacterial masses block the way mechanically, but instead regurgitated the contents of proventriculus (blood mixed bacteria) in to the bite wound thus transmitting the infection.

2. **Air borne:** Pneumonic plague.

b. **Direct contact:** Bubonic or septicemic plague.

- Contact with infected animals (like rodents) during skinning & handling.
- It also acquired by contact of wounded skin (produce by flea bite) with faeces of infected fleas.

➢ **Incubation period:**

a. **Extrinsic incubation period:**

✪ **Definition:** Time taken by vector (flea) to become infective (blocking of proventriculus) after receiving the microorganisms (ingestion of infected blood) **called extrinsic incubation period.**

✪ **Period:** Usually 2 weeks.

b. **Intrinsic incubation period (Incubation period):**

✪ **Definition:** Interval between entry of microorganisms & appearance of 1st clinical features **called incubation period.**

✪ **Period: → Table-2**

➢ **Portal of entry & sites: → Table-2**

Features	Bubonic plague	Pneumonic plague	Septicemic plague
Incubation period	2-7 days	1-3 days	2-7 days
Portal of entry	Skin	Respiratory system	Secondary to other plague
Sites	Femoral & inguinal nodes	Respiratory system	Blood & meninges

Table -2: Differences between varieties of plague

➢ **Precipitating factors (epidemiological determinants):** Following are the five types.

I. Agent factors (virulence factors)

Plague bacilli are antigenically homogeneous, so it is very difficult to discriminate between virulent & avirulent strain & to do serotyping.

i. **Intracellular (cell wall associated) factors:**

a. **pH6 adhesin (ph6 antigen):** Helps in adhesion.

most predominant species while *Sh. boydii* is least frequent.

1. *Sh. dysenteriae*: 8-25%
2. *Sh. flexneri*: 50-85%
3. *Sh. boydii*: 0-8%
4. *Sh. sonnei*: 2-24%

- Epidemics are associated with poverty & poor hygiene. Epidemic is influenced by war & its outcome.

➤ **Reservoir of infection:** Human is the natural host of bacilli. Human case or carrier is the reservoir of infection. Bacilli disappear within few weeks from faeces, so chronic carrier is very rare.

➤ **Source of infection:** Water or food.

➤ **Mode of transmission:**

a. Direct transmission:

1. Contaminated fingers/hands: Hands to mouth.
2. Sexual contact in male homosexual: Skin to skin/mucosa **called gay bowel syndrome.**

b. Indirect transmission (vehicle borne):

1. Food & water borne: *Sh sonnei* especially occurs as food poisoning.
2. Vector borne: Mechanical by flies.
3. Fomites borne: Door handles, lavatory seats etc.

➤ **Incubation period:** 48 hrs (1-7 days).

➤ **Portal of entry:** GIT & skin/mucosa.

➤ **Sites:** Intestinal & extra-intestinal (complications).

➤ **Precipitating factors (epidemiological determinants):** Following are the factors.

I. Agent factors (virulence factors)

A. Intracellular (cell wall associated) factors:

i. Capsular (K) antigen: Present in some strains. It masks the O-Ag & inhibits agglutination by antiserum. It inhibits the phagocytosis.

ii. Somatic antigen (O Ag or LPS or Endotoxin): Present in large number. Causing diarrhoea & ulcer. LPS is responsible for endotoxic activities.

iii. Fimbriae: Organ of adhesion

iv. Invasive property:

- Invasive property is due to a special type of OMP **called VMA (Virulence Marker Antigen)** which is plasmid encoded, responsible for invasion, multiplication of bacilli & destruction of epithelial cells.
- It is detected by VMA ELISA or by culture cells like Hela or Hep-2 cells

v. Cross reactive antigens: There is antigenic sharing between *Shigella, Salmonella* and *E. coli*.

vi. Infective dose: They resist gastric acidity & few bacilli can initiate the disease. Infective dose is very low, about 10-100 bacilli.

B. Intracellular (cell wall associated) factors:

i. Exotoxins/enterotoxins: Two varieties

a. Shiga toxin / verotoxin / verocytotoxin:

- **Bacteria producing shiga toxin:** *Sh. dysenteriae* type-1.
- **Properties of shiga toxin:**
  - Less important in pathogenesis, because non-toxigenic strain can invade the mucosa & multiply.
  - Earliest exotoxin identified from GNB.
  - Chromosome mediated.
- **Biological actions of shiga toxin:** Three types of actions
  - Neurotoxicity:
    - Detected by paralysis & death on injection in to mice or rabbits.
    - It is neurotoxic, but this property is secondary because it not acts directly on CNS but to the blood vessels supplying the nerve.
  - Cytotoxicity:
    - In vitro: Cytopathic changes in cultured Vero or HeLa cells.
    - In vivo: Toxin consists two sub units like binding (B) & active (A). Sub unit A divided in to two fragments like A1 & A2. B helps in adhesion with host cells. A2 links A1 to B. A1 inactivate the host cell 60S ribosome & inhibit the protein synthesis leading to cell death. Cell death resulting discontinuity of mucosa & haemorrhage (bloody diarrhoea → dysentery).
  - Enterotoxicity: It allows the collection of fluid in gut (in ligated rabbit ileal loop).
- **Diagnostic tests of shiga toxin:** Detection of shiga toxin is done by following tests.
  - Culture: Cytopathic changes in cultured Vero or HeLa cells.
  - Serology: Demonstration of antibody in sera by latex agglutination test & ELISA.
  - Molecular: DNA probe.

b. *Shigella* enterocytotoxin (ShET):

- **Subtypes:** Two forms

1. ***Shigella* enterocytotoxin 1 (ShET 1):**
   - Secreted from *Sh. flexneri* 2a.
   - Structurally similar to cholera toxin.
   - Chromosome mediated.
2. ***Shigella* enterocytotoxin 2 (ShET 2):**
   - Secreted from all strain of *Sh. flexneri.*
   - Helps in iron uptake.
   - Plasmid mediated.

- **Biological action:** Both toxins allow the collection of fluid in gut (in ligated rabbit ileal loop).

II. Host factors

1. **Age:** Common in young children due to poor hygiene, however endemic shigellosis found in all ages.
2. **Immune status:** Bacilli last longer in patient with malnutrition & IDDs like AIDS but disappeared within few weeks from the faeces of normal individual.
3. **Poverty, lack of sanitation & mental status:** Also favours the shigellosis.

III. Environmental factors

- Common in developing & poor countries because of poor sanitation.
- It is common in mental hospitals.

➢ **Pathogenesis: → Flow chart-1**

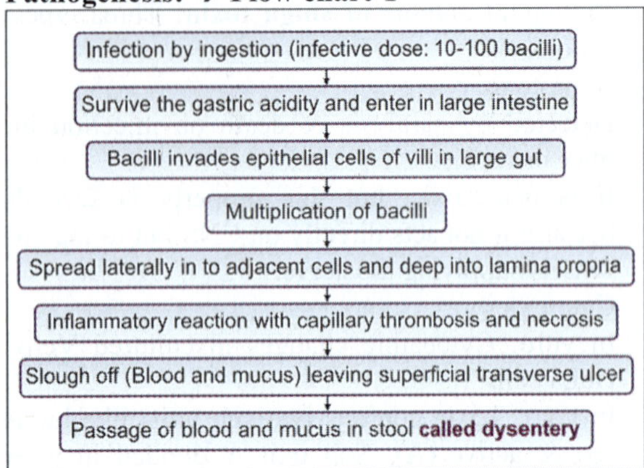

Flow chart-1: Pathogenesis of *Shigella*

➢ **Clinical types:** Whole spectrum of disease **called shigellosis** which includes following clinical conditions.

a. **Bacillary dysentery (invasive diarrhoea/bloody diarrhoea):** Other bacteria causing dysentery are *Cl. difficile* EIEC, EHEC, *Y enterocolitica, C. jejuni, V. parahaemolyticus* & may by few non typhoidal *Salmonella* spp. Following are the clinical features.

1. **Local:** Increase the frequency of stool containing blood & mucus along with abdominal cramps and tenesmus.
2. **General:** Fever & vomiting

b. **Bacteremia:** Bacilli enter in to the blood from the intestinal ulcer & causing bacteremia.

c. **Gay bowel syndrome:** In male homosexual.

➢ **Complications:**

1. **Common complications:** Mostly seen in *Sh. dysentriae* type 1 and includes arthritis, toxic neuritis, conjunctivitis, parotitis & in children intussusception.
2. **Hemolytic uremic syndrome (*Sh. dysentriae* type 1):**
   - Seen in severe cases.
   - Other agents causing hemolytic uremic syndrome are EHEC, *Salmonella* & *C jejuni* & few drugs like cyclosporine, quinine & clopidogrel.
3. **Ekiri syndrome:** It is a toxic encephalopathy cerebral oedema, seizures, altered consciousness & abnormal posture.
4. **Autoimmune reaction (Reiter's syndrome):**
   - Mostly seen by *Sh. flexneri.*
   - Occurs in 3% cases.
   - Develop in patient showing HLA B27.
   - It is the most common organism causing reactive arthritis following diarrhoea.

- More details: Follow chapter → Neisseriae, Moraxellaceae and Mimeae.

❖ Laboratory diagnosis:

➢ **Specimens:** Fresh stool

➢ **Collection & transport:** Collect the sample in transport media as mentioned above & sent to laboratory for testing.

➢ **Testing methods:**

I. **Microscopy: → Follow morphology**
II. **Culture: → Follow C/Cs**
III. **Biochemical reaction: → Follow B/Rs**
IV. **Serological tests:** Agglutination by using polyvalent & monovalent antisera.
V. **Bacteriocin typing:** It is also useful.

❖ Prevention:

- Improving personal & environmental sanitation.
- Chemoprophylaxis & immunoprophylaxis have no role.

❖ Treatment:

- Uncomplicated cases are self-limited but dehydration has to be corrected by ORS (Oral Rehydration Salt) therapy.
- Multiple plasmid mediated drug resistant *Shigella* are widely prevalent.
- Many strains are sensitive to nalidixic acid, norfloxacin & other flouroquinolones.

Question bank

Case study

1) A 10 year old child admitted in hospital with complains of fever, abdominal cramps & diarrhoea, containing blood & mucus. Stool culture identified the NLF bacteria on Mac Conkey's medium. Identify the disease & answer the following
a) Name the causative agent & describe the morphology of causative agent
b) Write the pathogenicity of causative agent
c) Describe the laboratory diagnosis of causative agent

Short notes

1) Shigellosis

Short questions for theory/viva questions

1) Name the species of *Shigella.*
2) Write the sugar fermentation tests in *Shigella* species.
3) Name the four bacteria causing dysentery.
4) What is gay bowel syndrome?

MCQs for chapter review

1) ***Shigella* can be differentiated from *E. coli* by all of the following features except-** (AI -99)
(a)) *Shigella* does not produce gas from glucose (b) *Shigella* does not ferment lactose (c) *Shigella* does not ferment mannitol (d) *Shigella* has no flagella, is non motile
2) ***Shigella* can be divided into subgroup on the basis of ability to ferment-** (AI -97)
(a) Lactose (b) Maltose (c) Fructose (d) Mannitol

3) **Non-lactose fermenters includes all of the following except-**
(a) *Sh. dysenteriae* (b) *Sh. sonnei* (c) *Sh. flexneri* (d) *Sh. boydii*

4) **Most virulent species of *Shigella* is**
(a) *Sh. dysenteriae* (b) *Sh. sonnei* (c) *Sh. flexneri* (d) *Sh. boydii*

5) **All are true about *Shigella* except** (AIIMS, Nov-99)
(a) Large dose is required for infection (b) Associated with haemolytic uremic syndrome (c) Causes bloody diarrhoea with mucus (d) Gut pathology is due to toxin

6) **Which of the following statement regarding *Shigella dysenteriae* types I is true** (AI -99)
(a) It can lead to haemolytic uremic syndrome (b) It produces an invasive enterotoxin (c) It is facultative aerobes (d) It is MR negative

7) **Bacteria causing bacillary dysentery is / are**
(a) *Shigella* spp. (b) *C. jejuni* (c) *V. parahaemolyticu* (d) All of above

8) **Shigellosis is best diagnosed by**
(a) Stool examination (b) Stool culture (c) Sigmoidoscopy (d) Enzyme

9) **All of the following cause haemolytic uremic syndrome** (AIIMS, May-07)
(a) *Shigella* (b) *Campylobacter* (c) EHEC (d) *Vibrio cholerae*

10) **Haemolytic uremic syndrome is caused by** (PGI, May-13, Dec-07)
(a) EIEC (b) *Shigella* (c) *Salmonella* (d) Cholera (e) *Klebsiella*

Answers of MCQs & explanation

1) **(c)**
- Mannitol fermentation is useful in classification of *Shigella* as shown in **Table-1.** *Sh. dysenteriae* does not ferments mannitol while remaining three species can ferment the mannitol with acid without gas production
- *E coli* is motile by peritrichous flagella & ferment glucose & lactose with acid & gas. *Shigella* is non motile & all species can ferment glucose with acid only while lactose is fermented late by *Sh sonnei* with acid only

2) **(d)**
- Mannitol fermentation is useful in classification of *Shigella* as shown in **Table-1.** *Sh. dysenteriae* does not ferments mannitol while remaining three species can ferment the mannitol with acid without gas production

3) **(b)**
- All *Shigella species* are non lactose fermenter except *Sh sonnei* which is late fermenter

4) **(a)**
- *Sh. dysenteriae* is the most virulent, associated with complications (vide infra) & high mortality

5) **(d)**
- Large dose is not required for infection, 10-100 bacilli (**called infective dose**) are enough to elicit the infection
- Associated with haemolytic uremic syndrome & can causes bloody diarrhoea with mucus
- Toxin is not required for gut pathology, even non toxigenic strain can invade & multiply in the enterocytes

6) **(a)**
- *Sh dysenteriae* types I can lead to haemolytic uremic syndrome
- It produces an enterotoxin, which is non invasive
- It is aerobes & facultative aerobes
- It is MR positive

7) **(d)**
- Follow section, **pathogenicity (Clinical types → Bacillary dysentery)** for explanation

8) **(b)**
- Follow section, **culture characteristics** for explanation

9) **(d)**
10) **(b) & (c)**
} Follow section, **pathogenicity (complications)** for explanation

46 Enterobactericeae-IV (*Yersinia*)

Learning heading & subheadings

- Meaning:
- Classification:

Yersinia pestis

Yersinia pseudotuberculosis & Yersinia enterocolitica

Yersinia pseudotuberculosis

Yersinia enterocolitica

Meaning: Genus named from Alexander Yersin who discovered the bacilli along with Kitasato in 1894 from Hong Kong at the beginning of last epidemic, however Yersin bacilli word is not used for all species of genus but only for *Yersinia pestis*

Classification: →Flow chart-1

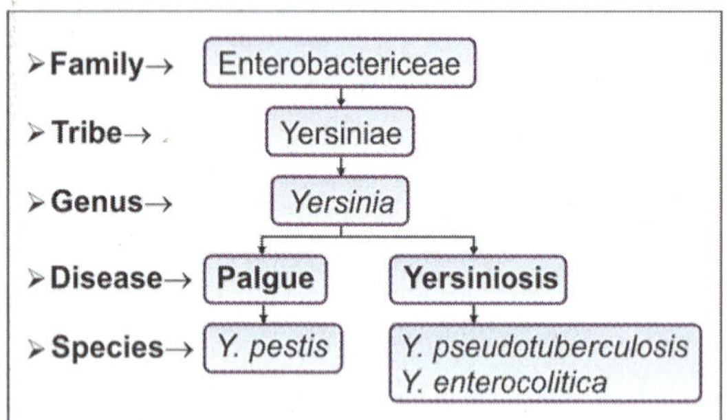

Flow chart-1: Classification of *Yersinia*

Yersinia pestis

❖ **Common name:**

- Plague bacilli, as the disease produced by them.
- Yersin bacilli, from the Alexander Yersin.

❖ **Use:** *Yersinia pestis* is the agent to be used in bioterrorism especially in non endemic regions.

❖ **Morphology:**

➢ **Staining properties: → Fig.-1.**

- **Gram stain:** Gram-negative bacillus or coccobacilli. Also showing bipolar staining (**fig.-1**).
- **Giemsa stain or methylene blue or Wayson stain (fig.-2) or Wright's stain:**
  - It shows bipolar staining **called safety pin** or **telephone handle appearance** with the two ends densely stained and the clear central area.
  - It is more in tissue smear than smear of culture.
  - Other bacteria with safety pin appearance are *P. multocida, Francisella tularensis Burkholderia pseudomallei, Haemophilus ducreyi, Brucella abortus, Chromobacter violaceum, Calymatobacter granulomatis* etc.

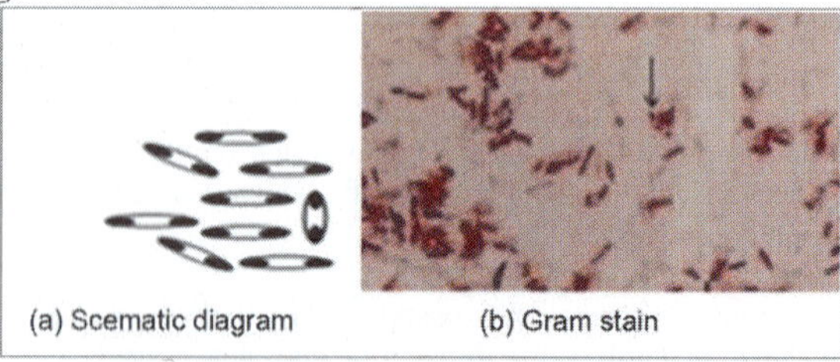

Figure-1: Bipolar staining (safety pin appearance) of *Y. pestis* under gram stain

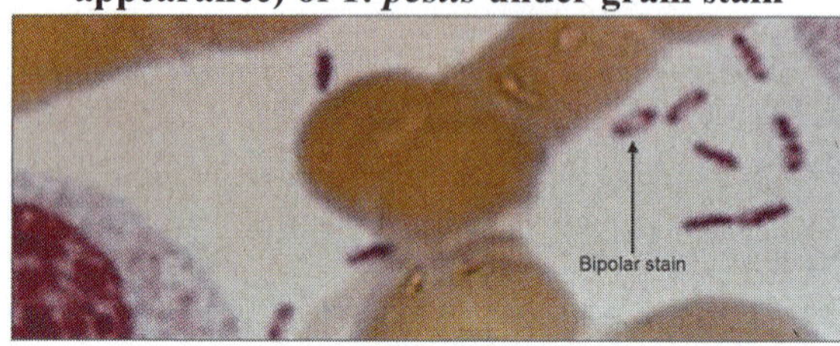

Figure-2: Bipolar staining (safety pin appearance) of *Y. pestis* under Wayson stain

- **Immunofluorescent stain:** Fluorescent antibody technique may be used to identifying the bacilli.

➢ **Size:** 1.5 µm x 0.7 µm.

➢ **Shape:** Short, plump & oval with rounded ends and convex sides.

➢ **Arrangement:** Singly, in small groups & in short chain in liquid medium.

➢ **Motility:** Non-motile.

➢ **Spore:** Non-sporing.

➢ **Slime layer (envelop):** Best develop at 37^0C but rare at its optimum temperature 27^0C.

➢ **Pleomorphism & involution forms**: Ageing culture shows great variation in size & shape like enlarged, elongated, irregular, pear-shaped or globular like yeast cells **called pleomorphism**. It is marked in 3% NaCl **called involution forms** & used for identification of bacilli. It is due to defective cell wall synthesis or autolysis.

❖ Cultural characteristics (C/Cs):

➢ **Effective factors:**

- O_2 effect: Aerobes & facultative anaerobes, but sensitive to O_2 which is overcome by anaerobiosis.
- Temperature: Range is 4 to 45° C, optimum temp. is27^{0}C & slime layer develop at 37^{0}C.
- pH: Range of 5.0 -9.6 & optimum pH is 7.2.

➢ **Culture in media:**

A. Liquid media:

1. **Nutrient broth:** Flocculent growth occurs at the bottom & along the sides of the tube, with little or no turbidity. A delicate pellicle may form later
2. **Oil / ghee broth in flask:** Medium contains oil / ghee at top. A characteristic growth occurs which hangs down into broth from the surface **called 'stalactite growth'** or **called 'stalactites'** as shown in **fig.-3**.

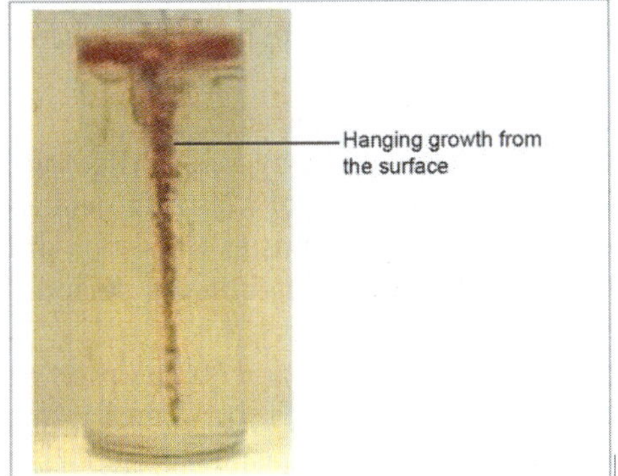

Figure-3: Stalactite growth of *Y. pestis*

B. Solid media:

1. **Nutrient agar:** Colonies are small, delicate, transparent discs, becoming opaque & increase in size on further incubation
2. **Mac Conkey's agar:** Pale/colourless colony due to NLF. It disappear after longer time due to autolysis.
3. **Blood agar:** Nonhaemolytic dark brown coloured colonies due to absorption of haemin.
4. **Haemin containing media:** Absorb the haemin & produces the dark brown pigmented colonies in blood agar & other haemin containing media. Pigment production is essential for biofilm formation & flea blocking.

C. Selective media:

1. **Yersinia specific CIN agar:** It is a selective medium for sputum & contains cefsulodin, irgasan & novobiocin

➢ **Culture in animals:**

- Inoculates exudates from bubo or culture suspension in guinea pig or in white rat.
- Development of oedema, necrosis at injection site & enlargement of regional node, spleen & animal die in 2-5 days.
- Take samples from local sites, nodes, spleen or heart blood & test with microscopy, culture or by B/Rs.

❖ Biochemical reaction [B/Rs):

1. **Sugar fermentation:** G S L M
A - - A
- Also ferments maltose with acid but not rhamnose.
2. **I M Vi C tests: - + - -**
3. **Catalase test:** +Ve
4. **Nitrate reduction test:** + Ve
5. **Aesculin hydrolysis:** +Ve
6. **ONPG (β-galactosidase) test:** +Ve
7. **Oxidase test:** -Ve
8. **H_2S production:** -Ve
9. **Urease test:** -Ve
10. **Gelatin liquefaction test:** -Ve
11. **Ornithine decarboxylation test:** +Ve
12. **Biotyping:**
- Given by **Devignat**
- Three biotypes based on glycerol fermentation & nitrate reduction: → **Table -1**

Biotype	Glycerol fermentation	Nitrate reduction
Y. Pestis var *orientalis*	-	+
Y.Pestis var *antigua*	+	+
Y.Pestis var *medievalis*	+	-

Table -1: Biotypes of *Y. pestis*

❖ Resistance:

- *Y. pestis* is killed by heat (at 55^{0}C), sunlight, drying & 0.5% phenol (in 15 minutes).
- They are susceptible to specific bacteriophages.
- Produce plasmid mediated resistance to many antibiotics.

❖ Pathogenicity:

➢ **Disease name:** It is a zoonosis **called 'plague'.**

➢ **Nature & history of plague:** It can occur as an endemic, localised outbreak, epidemic or in pandemic forms.

✪ **Home land of plague:** Plague is very ancient human disease. Central Asia or Himalaya is **called the home land of human plague**, from where it spread & causing epidemic & pandemic.

✪ **In the World:** Three pandemic reported (600 years interval) in the history with different biotypes.

1. **The first pandemic:**
- **Called Justinian plague**
- Biotypes: *Y. pestis* var *Antigua.*
- Occurred between AD 541-544 (6th century) in Mediterranean countries.
- It began in Egypt & spread to Middle East & Mediterranean Europe.
- It killed 100 million people.

- After that 2nd-11th epidemic occurred from AD 558-664 in 8-12 years cycles.
- Finally all known world affected by plague.

2. The second pandemic:

- **Called Black Death** because it was present with gangrene of skin-finger-penis.
- Biotypes: *Y. pestis* var *medievalis.*
- Occurred between AD 1347-1351 (14th century) in Europe.
- It began in Black sea & spread to Europe & West Russia.
- It killed 17-28 million people.
- After that epidemic continue from AD 1361 - 1480 in 2-5 years cycles.
- It also affected the all known world.

3. The third pandemic:

- **Called modern plague.**
- Biotypes: *Y. pestis* var *orientalis.*
- Occurred between AD 1855-1918 (19th century) in Asia & in other countries.
- It began in Yunnan, a South Western province of China in 1855 & spread to Hong Kong in May 1894, Mumbai 1896, Kolkata 1898, Madagaskar 1898; Egypt, Portugal, Japan, Paraguay & Eastern Africa in 1899; Manila, Glasgow, Sydney & San Francisco in 1900.
- Local epidemics occurred subsequently throughout the world with plenty of victims.
- Finally whole world affected by plague & disease receded by control of rodent & vector.

✪ **In India:**

- **Indian scenario of plague:**

1. **China pandemic (1855-1918):**
   - It entered in India in 1896 (Bombay) & spread all over the country with 10 million death by 1918.
   - It gradually decline thereafter, however few scattered cases were reported till 1967.
2. **No cases from 1967 to 1994.**
3. **Maharashtra outbreak (1994) of bubonic plague:** It occurred in Beed-Latur district of Maharashtra in August 1994.
4. **Surat epidemic (1994) of pneumonic plague:** It occurred in Surat & adjoining regions of Gujarat & Maharashtra in September in 1994. Around 6000 cases were reported with 60 deaths over a period of 2 months.
5. **Simla outbreak (2002):** It occurred near Rohru of Simla (Himachal Pradesh) in February 2002 with 4 deaths.
6. **Uttaranchal outbreak (2004) of bubonic plague:** It occurred in Dangud village of Uttarkashi district of Uttaranchal in 2004 with 8 cases & four deaths.

- **Indian foci of plague:** Total four foci of plague are known in India.

1. Region near Kolar at the trijunction of Tamil Nadu, Karnataka & Andhra Pradesh.
2. Beed-Latur district of Maharashtra from where Surat epidemic was originated.
3. Rohru in Himachal Pradesh.
4. Dangud village of Uttaranchal.

➢ **Reservoir of infection:** Different types of rodents are the main reservoir as described below.

➢ **Source of infection:** Fleas. Man to man transmission can occur, especially in pneumonic plague.

➢ **Mode of transmission:**

a. Indirect:

1. **Flea bite (Vector borne):** Bubonic plague.
   - **Mechanisms of introduction of bacilli:** Blocked flea cannot suck the blood because the bacterial masses block the way mechanically, but instead regurgitated the contents of proventriculus (blood mixed bacteria) in to the bite wound thus transmitting the infection.
2. **Air borne:** Pneumonic plague.

b. Direct contact: Bubonic or septicemic plague.

- Contact with infected animals (like rodents) during skinning & handling.
- It also acquired by contact of wounded skin (produce by flea bite) with faeces of infected fleas.

➢ **Incubation period:**

a. Extrinsic incubation period:

✪ **Definition:** Time taken by vector (flea) to become infective (blocking of proventriculus) after receiving the microorganisms (ingestion of infected blood) **called extrinsic incubation period.**

✪ **Period:** Usually 2 weeks.

b. Intrinsic incubation period (Incubation period):

✪ **Definition:** Interval between entry of microorganisms & appearance of 1st clinical features **called incubation period.**

✪ **Period:** → **Table-2**

➢ **Portal of entry & sites:** → **Table-2**

Features	Bubonic plague	Pneumonic plague	Septicemic plague
Incubation period	2-7 days	1-3 days	2-7 days
Portal of entry	Skin	Respiratory system	Secondary to other plague
Sites	Femoral & inguinal nodes	Respiratory system	Blood & meninges

Table -2: Differences between varieties of plague

➢ **Precipitating factors (epidemiological determinants):** Following are the five types.

I. Agent factors (virulence factors)

Plague bacilli are antigenically homogeneous, so it is very difficult to discriminate between virulent & avirulent strain & to do serotyping.

i. Intracellular (cell wall associated) factors:

a. pH6 adhesin (ph6 antigen): Helps in adhesion.

b. Antigens: Antigenic structure is complex. 20 antigens have been detected by gel diffusion and biochemical analysis.

1. Slime layer / capsular / envelope Ag (fraction 1 or F1 Ag):
- Heat labile.
- Protein in nature.
- Developed at 37°C.
- Plasmid encoded.
- Inhibits phagocytosis.
- Necessary for full virulence.
- Ab to this antigen is protective in mice.
- Necessary for effective vaccine production.

2. Somatic Ag: Two subtypes V & W.
- Always produced together.
- Heat stable.
- Developed at 20 & 37°C.
- Plasmid encoded.
- Inhibit phagocytosis & intracellular killing of bacilli.

c. Unidentified surface component: Absorbs the haemin & aromatic dyes in medium to produce the pigmented colonies which helps in biofilm formation & flea blocking.

d. Purin synthesis: It also contributes in virulence.

ii. Extracellular factors:

a. Bacteriocin: Virulent strains produce a pesticin-I which inhibits the strains of *Y. pseudotuberculosis, Y. enterocolitica* & *E. coli*.

b. Enzymes:

1. Protease:
- Encodes by pla gene.
- It degrades the complement.
- It also activates the mammalian plasminogen.
- They adhere to the extracellular matrix component laminin, thus promoting the dissemination of bacteria.

2. Others: Coagulase & fibrinolysin.

c. Toxins: Called 'plague toxins. Two types.

1. Endotoxin: LPS in nature as like other GNB.

2. Murine toxin:
- So called because active in rat/mice but not in guinea pig or rabbit.
- Protein & heat labile.
- Possessing properties of both exotoxins and endotoxins.
- Toxoided but do not diffuse freely into the medium and released after cell lysis.
- On injection into experimental animals it produces local edema & necrosis with systemic effects on peripheral vascular system and liver.
- Its role in disease in human beings is not known.

d. Siderophore: It helps in acquisition of iron.

iii. Secretory system III: It injects the F1 Ag in to host cells & also the adhesins.

II. Host factors

1. **Age & sex:** No age & sex bar.
2. **Occupational:**
- Risk increased with skinning & handling of animal carcass.
- Laboratory or hospital workers are at high risk.
3. **Movement of people:** In plague foci / region.

III. Environmental factors

1. **Seasonal:** Cool & humid season favours the multiplication of fleas (high flea index).

IV. Rodent factors (reservoir of infection)

✪ **Species:** Following different types of wild rodents are the main reservoirs like
- **Desert rodent (Gerbils):** *Tatera indica*
- **Sewer rodent:** *Rattus novergicus*
- **Field rodent:**
- **Forest rodents (Bandicoot):** *Bandicota indica*
- **Domestic rodent:** *Rattus rattus.* It is responsible only when numbers of other rodents are dwindled.

✪ **Rat fall:** Death of diseased rat **called rat fall**. When diseased rat dies fleas leaves the carcass & in the absence of other rat it bites to human.

V. Vector (flea) factors

✪ **Species:** Following types of flea are responsible.

1. **Rat flea:** *Xenopsylla cheopis* (In North India & more efficient vector), *X. astia* (In South India & less efficient vector) and *Ceratophyllus fasciatus.*
2. **Human flea:** Rare by *Pulex irritants.*

✪ **Blocked flea:**
- Plague bacilli are the natural parasites of rodents. They are infected by bite of rat fleas & fleas acquired the infection from rodents during bite for blood meal (5000 bacilli per 0.5ml blood). In the flea the bacilli multiply in stomach to such an extent that they block the proventriculus, such flea **called blocked flea**.
- Completely blocked flea dies as it cannot obtain the blood meal while partially blocked flea **called enzootic foci** can survive longer up to 4 years inside the burrow. Bacilli continue multiply in flea & can infect the new rodents which may visit such burrow & eventually responsible for re-emergence of plague, hence partially blocked flea is more dangerous.

✪ **Flea index or cheopis index:** Average numbers of flea per rat **called flea index**. Plague outbreak likely occurs in place where flea index in more than 1.

➢ **Natural cycles of plague:** Two cycles as below.

a. Urban cycle or domestic cycle: It is continue between human, rat fleas & domestic rodents.

b. Wild or sylvatic cycle: It occurs in nature between wild rodents & independent to human.

➢ **Clinical types & features of plague:** Three major forms of plague like bubonic, pneumonic and septicemic.

i. Bubonic plague:

✪ **Meaning:**

- Derived from **bubo = groin**, because nodes are involved after the fleas bite.
- It is the common variety of plague.
- Common site is e inguinal lymph nodes.
- Depending upon the site of flea bite any node can be infected like cervical, axillary or submaxillary.
- Cervical or submaxillary nodes are commonly involved in children.
- It is characterised by intense painful swelling. Nodes become enlarged and suppurate as shown in **fig.-4(a).**

ii. Pneumonic plague: Haemorrhagic pneumonia. Cyanosis is very prominent. The bloody mucoid sputum that is coughed out contains bacilli in large numbers. It is highly infectious & in untreated patients, almost invariably fatal (30-100%).

iii. Septicemic plague:

- It occur secondary to bubonic or pneumonic plague or primarily by direct contact from laboratory infection.
- The bacilli enter the bloodstream from the bubo and produce septicemia, cutaneous & mucosal haemorrhage, DIC & gangrene of skin-finger-penis as shown in **fig.-4(b)** (hence the **called black death** to the pandemic of 14th century, killed a quarter of all mankind).
- Meningitis may occur rarely.

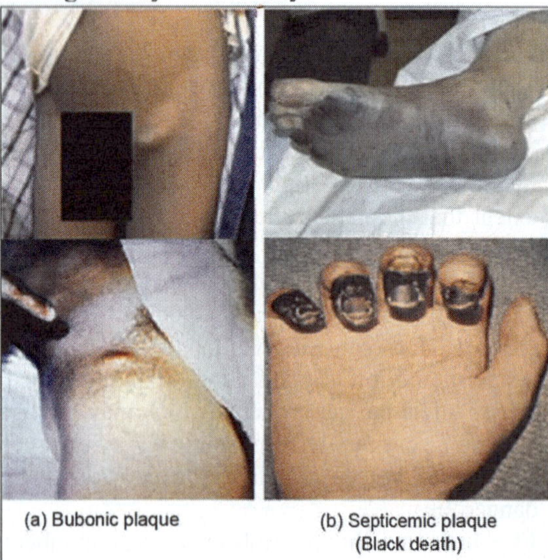

(a) Bubonic plaque (b) Septicemic plaque (Black death)

Figure-4: Features of plague

❖ Laboratory diagnosis:

I. Diagnosis in human:

➢ **Specimens:** Discharge from bubo, sputum or blood (three blood samples are collected over a period of 45minutes).

➢ **Testing methods:**

A. Microscopy: → Follow morphology

B. Culture: → Follow C/Cs

C. Biochemical reaction: → Follow B/Rs

D. Serological tests:

1. **Passive haemagglutination:** Antibody to the F-I antigen may be detected by passive haemagglutination. Rise in titre of antibodies in paired sera or titre of 128 or above in a single serum sample can be considered positive.
2. **ELISA:** Tests developed for IgG and IgM.

E. Molecular tests: PCR is the rapid & sensitive method for accurate diagnosis.

II. Diagnosis in animal:

✪ **Precautions:**

- If rat is died of plague (rat fall) may carry infected fleas & it should be handled with care.
- Apply kerosene to remove ecto-parasite.
- In laboratory carcass should be dipped in 3% Lysol.

✪ **Specimens:** From lymph nodes, spleen, heart blood or bone marrow.

✪ **Testing methods:** Similar to human testing methods.

❖ Prevention:

A. General measures: Control of fleas & rodents.

B. Immunoprophylaxis: Three types of vaccines.

1. **Live vaccine:** Not useful.
2. **Killed vaccine:**

- **Preparation:**
  - Prepared at the Haffkine Institute, Mumbai.
  - It is a whole culture antigen vaccine.
  - A virulent strain of the plague bacillus is grown in casein hydrolysate broth for 2-4 weeks at 32°C and killed by 0.05% formaldehyde.
- **Preservation:** With phenyl mercuric nitrate (Sokhey's modification of Haffkine's vaccine).
- **Administration:**
  - Given subcutaneously.
  - 2 doses at an interval of 1-3 months followed by a third dose 6 months later.
- **Efficacy:**
  - Gives some protection against bubonic plague but not against pneumonic plague.
  - Immunity does not last for more than 6 months. In contrast, an attack of plague provides more lasting immunity.
- **Uses:** Vaccine is recommended to occupationally risky persons, such as plague laboratory or hospital workers.
- **Disadvantages:** It has no value in plague outbreaks & mass vaccination is not advised.

3. **Subunit recombinant F1 (rF1):** Under trial.

C. Chemoprophylaxis: Tetracycline is the drug of choice given for 5 days. Cotrimoxazole is also useful with 5 days course.

❖ **Treatment:**

1. **Chemotherapy:**
- Streptomycin (drug of choice in normal form), doxycycline & chloramphenicol (drugs of choice in pneumonic plague, septicemic plague or meningitis) are effective.
- Patient should be isolated for 24 hours or until pneumonia should be ruled out by effective antibiotic therapy.
- Early treatment with antibiotics has reduced plague mortality from 30-100% to 5-10%.

Yersinia pseudotuberculosis & *Yersinia enterocolitica*

❖ **Yersiniosis:** It is a zoonotic infection with yersiniae other than *Y. pestis* like *Y. pseudotuberculosis* & *Y. enterocolitica*.

I. *Y. pseudotuberculosis*

➢ **Meaning:** Causing tuberculosis like lesion in guinea pig, rabbit & rodent hence the name pseudotuberculosis.

➢ **Synonym:** Formerly **called *Pasteurella pseudotuberculosis.***

➢ **Morphology:**
- **Staining properties:** GNB.
- **Size:** Small.
- **Shape:** Oval.
- **Capsule:** Noncapsulated.
- **Motility:** Motile at 22^0C but not at 37^0C.

➢ **Cultural characteristics (C/Cs):**
- Aerobes & facultative anaerobes.
- Optimum temperature: 29^0C

1. **Nutrient agar:** Colonies are raised / umbonate, granular, 1mm in size & translucent.
2. **Mac Conkey's agar:** Poor growth.
3. **Blood agar:** Nonhaemolytic.

➢ **Biochemical reactions (B/Rs):**

1. **Sugar fermentation:** Rhamnose & melibiose are fermented with acid only.
2. **Urease test:** +Ve
3. **Catalase test:** +Ve
4. **ONPG (β-galactosidase) test:** +Ve
5. **Ornithine decarboxylation test:** -Ve

➢ **Typing:**
- **Thal & Knapp, 1971 serotyping:** Antigenically heterogeneous. 6 serotypes based on heat-stable O-Ag & Heat-labile H-Ag. Most human infection is by type-1.
- Antigenic cross reaction occurs with *Y. pestis.*
- Serotypes 2 & 4 are cross react with Salmonella's Kauffmann-White O group B (Now 4 = *S. parathphi B*) & D (now 9 = *S. typhi*).

➢ **Pathogenicity:**
- **Virulence factor:**
- Adhesin proteins: Inv (invasive) protein, ail (attachment & invasive locus) protein & Yad A (*Yersinia* adhesin A → it binds with collagen & fibronectin to aid the invasion of tissue by organism & also it inactivate the complement).
- Super Ag: Binds with T cells to release cytokines in huge amount.
- **Mode of transmission:**

1. **Contact:** Contact of skin with water.
2. **Ingestion:** By entry of food & vegetables contaminated by animal feces.

- **Clinical features:**

1. **In animals:** Tuberculosis like nodule in liver, spleen, lungs etc.
2. **In human:** Acute mesenteric lymphadenitis simulating acute/subacute appendicitis (**called pseudoappendicular syndrome**) with typhoid like fever, gastroenteritis, hepatosplenomegaly & erythema nodosum.

➢ **Laboratory diagnosis:**
- **Specimens:** Tissue from mesenteric nodes, blood etc.
- **Testing methods:**

A. **Microscopy:** → **Follow morphology**
B. **Culture:** → **Follow C/Cs**
C. **Biochemical reaction:** → **Follow B/Rs**
D. **Serological tests:** Tube agglutination.
E. **Intradermal skin test:** Similar to tuberculin or brucellin test.

II. *Y. enterocolitica*

➢ **Source:** Identified from human, animal & as saprophytes from water-soil, so not a true zoonotic.

➢ **Morphology:**
- **Staining properties:** Gram negative coccobacilli with pleomorphism in old culture.
- **Capsule:** In vivo but not in culture.
- **Motile** By peritrichous flagella at 22^0C but not at 37^0C.

➢ **Cultural characteristics (C/Cs):**
- Aerobes & facultative anaerobes.
- Temperature: Optimum temperature is 22-29^0C. It can grow at 4^0C in refrigerated food may cause food poisoning.

1. **Nutrient agar:** Colonies are smooth & translucent.
2. **Mac Conkey's agar:** Pinpoint pink colonies.
3. **Blood agar:** Nonhaemolytic.
4. **Selective medium:** Schiemann CIN medium is useful to isolate the bacilli from faeces.

➢ **Biochemical reaction (B/Rs):**

1. **Sugar fermentation test:** Sucrose & cellobiose with acid only.
2. **Indole test:** +Ve
3. **VP test:** +Ve

4. **Urease test:** +Ve
5. **Catalase test:** +Ve
6. **ONPG (β-galactosidase) test:** +Ve
7. **Ornithine decarboxylation test:** +Ve

➢ **Typing:**

1. **Biotyping:** Six biotypes. Based on biotypes new species are noticed: *Y. frederikseni*, *Y. intermedia* & *Y. kristenseni.*
2. **Bacteriophage typing:** I-X types.
3. **Serotyping:** Based on O & H Ag. Total 60 serotypes. O3, O8, O9 are responsible for human infection.

➢ **Pathogenicity:**

- **Virulence factor:**
  - Heat stable enterotoxin produced in refrigerated food (<30^0C) causing food poisoning.
  - Adhesin proteins: Different types like MyF Ag, pH6 Ag, inv (invasive) protein, ail (attachment & invasive locus) protein & Yad A (*Yersinia* adhesin A → it binds with collagen & fibronectin to aid the invasion of tissue by organism & also it inactivate the complement).
- **Source of infection:** Identified from human, animal & as saprophytes from water-soil.
- **Mode of transmission:** As like *Y. pseudotuberculosis.*
- **Clinical features:** 3 types of disease in human.

1. **In young children:** Self-limited gastroenteritis with (dysentery) or without blood.
2. **In older children:** Mesenteric lymphadenitis & terminal ileitis mimic appendicitis **called pseudoappendicular syndrome,** but more severe than previous one.
3. **In adults:** Septicemia with high fatality rate.

- **Complications:** Adult type causing polyarthritis, erythema nodosum & Reiter's syndrome.

➢ **Laboratory diagnosis:**

- **Specimens:** Tissue from mesenteric nodes, blood, stool, food water, soil etc.
- **Testing methods:**

A. **Microscopy: → Follow morphology**
B. **Culture: → Follow C/Cs**
C. **Biochemical reaction: → Follow B/Rs**
D. **Serological tests:** Also useful.

Question bank

Case study

1) A 55 years old male is visited the hospital with complains of fever & haemoptysis. Sputum examination with Wayson's stain shows the bacilli with bipolar staining. Identify the case & answer the following
   a) Name the clinical condition & causative agent
   b) Name the four bacteria showing bipolar staining
   c) Describe the morphology & C/Cs of causative agent
   d) Write the pathogenicity causative agent

2) A girl from Manali visit the surgical OPD with complains of fever & painful inguinal swelling. On clinical examination it diagnosed as an inguinal lymphadenopathy. Sample collected from the local lesion & sent for culture. On culture it shows the stalactite growth. Identify the case & answer the following
   a) Name the clinical condition & causative agent
   b) Describe the virulence factors of causative agent
   c) Describe the lab. diagnosis of causative agent

Essay/Full question

1) *Y. pestis*

Short notes

1) Pathogenicity or labortory diagnosis of *Y. pestis*
2) Yersiniosis

Short questions for theory/viva questions

1) Name the four bacteria showing safety pin appearance.
2) What is stalactites?
3) Name the four foci of plague in India.
4) What is blocked flea?
5) Comment: Partially blocked flea is more dangerous than completely blocked flea in plague.
6) What is an enzootic focus of plague?

MCQs for chapter review

Y. pestis

1) **True about *Y. pestis*** (PGI, Dec -03, Dec-06)
   (a) Gram +Ve (b) Gram -Ve (c) Motile (d) Non-motile (e) It is coccobacilli
2) **'Safety pin appearance' is characteristic of**
   (a) *Yersinia pestis* (b) *Anthrax bacilli* (c) *Berkholderia pseudomallei* (d) a+c
3) **All of the following statements about plague are wrong except-** (AIIMS-04)
   (a) Domestic rat is the main reservoir (b) Bubonic is the most common variety (c) The causative agent can survive up to 10 years in the soil of rodent burrows (d) Incubation period for pneumonic plague is one to two weeks
4) **A farmer present to the emergency department with painful inguinal lymphadenopathy and history of fever and flu like symptoms. Clinical examination reveals an ulcer in the leg. Which of the following stain should be used to detect suspected bipolar stained organisms-** (AIIMS, Nov-09, 12 AI-11)
   (a) Albert's stain (b) Wayson's stain (c) Ziehl Neelsen stain (d) Mc Fadyean stain
5) **False statement about plague is -**
   (a) It is gram negative cocco bacillus responding to streptomycin (b) Bubonic plague is the most common form (c) Pneumonic plague develops most rapidly and most frequently fatal (d) The bubo of plague is characterised by intense cellulitis.
6) **True statement about *Y pestis* is/are -** (PGI, June- 04)
   (a) Gram positive (b) Non motile (c) Benzyl penicillin is given in prophylaxis (d) Patients are kept isolated till 48 hours of treatment (e) Repeated blood culture is diagnostic
7) **The drug of choice for chemoprophylaxis in contacts of patient of pneumonic plague-** (AIIMS,Nov-02)
   (a) Penicillin (b) Rifampicin (c) Erythromycine (d) Tetracycline
8) **Which of the following drug(s) is/are used in treatment of plague -** (PGI, Dec-08)
   (a) Streptomycin (b) Tetracycline (c) Ciprofloxacin (d) Chloramphenicol (e) Cotrimoxazole

Y. pseudotuberculosis* & *Y. enterocolitica

9) **True about yersiniosis –**
(a) Zoonosis (b) Caused by *Y pestis* (c) By *Y. enterocolitica* (d) By *Y. pseudotuberculosis*

Answers of MCQs & explanation

1) **(b), (d) & (e)** } Follow section, ***Y. pestis* (morphology)** for explanation
2) **(d)** }
3) **(b)**
- Wild rats are the main reservoir for plague
- Not the *Y. pestis* but partially blocked flea **called enzootic foci** can survive longer up to 4 years inside the burrow.
- Incubation period for different varieties is given in **table-2**

4) **(b)**
- Bipolar stained is done by Wayson's stain from the given options

5) **(d)**
- Options a-c are explained in text with respective sections
- Cellulitis is the features of streptococcal or staphylococcal infection not the features of bubonic plague.

6) **(b), (d) & (e)**
- *Y pestis* is gram negative & tetracycline is given in prophylaxis

7) **(d)**
- Tetracycline is the drug of choice for chemoprophylaxis given for 5 days

8) **(a), (b) & (d)**
- Follow section ***Y. pestis* (treatment)** for explanation

9) **(a), (c) & (d)**
- Follow section, **yersiniosis** for explanation

47 Vibrionaceae, Aeromonadacaeae and *Plesiomonas*

Learning heading & subheadings

Vibrionaceae

- Meaning:
- History:
- Classification:

Non halophilic vibrios

Halophilic vibrios

Aeromonadaceae

Plesiomonas

Vibrionaceae

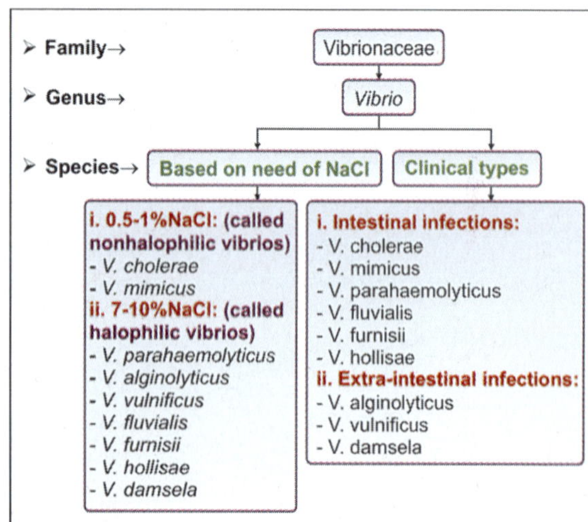

Flow chart-1: Classification of Vibrionaceae

Meaning: *Vibrio* from **vibrare** = **vibrate** because of motile nature of bacteria.

Classification: →**Flow chart-1**

Non halophilic vibrios

Vibrio cholerae

- **Synonym:** ***Vibrio comma*** because of **comma shaped** bacilli.
- **History:** It was 1st isolated by Robert Koch in 1883 in Egypt from cholera patient.
- **Morphology:**

➢ **Type according to gram stain:** GNB [**fig.-1(a)**].

➢ **Size**: 0.2-0.4 μm x 1.5 μm.

➢ **Shape**: Short, curved, cylindrical rod with rounded or pointed ends typically comma shaped.

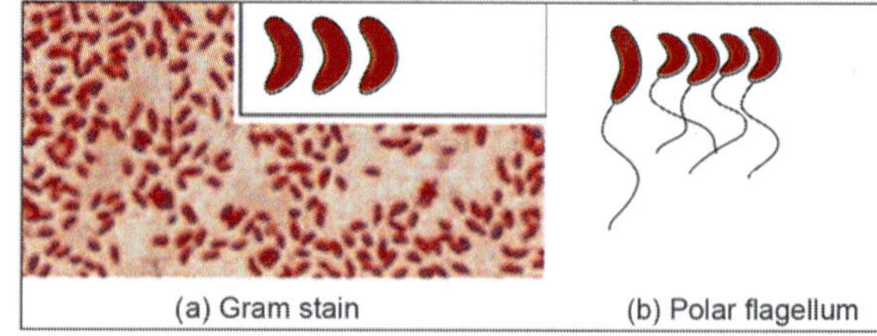

Figure-1: Morphology of *V. cholerae*

➢ **Arrangement:**
- Singly
- In group
- Parallel **called 'fish in stream appearance'** or end to end arrangement giving **S-shape or spiral form** appearance.

➢ **Motility:**
- Actively motile with single sheathed polar flagellum at one pole **called monotrichate flagellum** [**fig.-1(b)**]. It shows darting motility.
- Microscopy from young culture or from acute cholera stool reveals actively motile *Vibrio* suggests **'swarm of gnats'**

➢ **Capsule:** Non-capsulated. Bengal strain (O139) is capsulated.

➢ **Spore:** Non-sporing.

- **Fimbriae:** Special organ for adhesion **called 'Toxin Co-regulated Pilus (TCP)'**. Vibrio colonise throughout the course of infection without damage or invasion to host cell. TCP constantly bind the *Vibrio* with host cell.

❖ Cultural characteristics (C/Cs):

- **Effective factors:**
  - O_2 effect: Strict aerobes also grow anaerobically but growth is slow & scanty.
  - Temperature: Optimum temp. is 37°C (16–40°C).
  - pH: Optimum pH is alkaline pH about 8.2 (6.4–9.6)
  - 0.5-1% NaCl is required for optimal growth. High concentrations of NaCl (>6%) is inhibitory.
- **Culture in media:**

A. Liquid media:

i. Ordinary / basal / simple media:

1. **Peptone water:** Surface pellicle occurs within 6 hrs which breaks on shaking in membranous pieces. Turbidity & powdery deposit develop on continued incubation.

ii. Transport / holding media: Maintain the viability of bacteria during transport but does not allow the no multiplication.

1. **Venkatraman-Ramakrishnan (VR) medium:**
   - pH 8.6-8.8 remains viable for several weeks.
   - Prevent overgrowth of commensals.
2. **Cary- Blair transport medium:**
   - pH-8.4
   - It also useful for *Salmonella, Shigella* & *C. jejuni*
3. **Autoclaved sea water:**

iii. Enrichment medium: Also serve as transport media.

1. **Alkaline Peptone Water (APW):** pH-8.6
2. **Monsur's taurocholate tellurite peptone water:** pH-9.2

B. Semi-solid media:

1. **Gelatin stab culture:** Infundibuliform (funnel-shaped) or napiform (turnip-shaped) colony due to gelatin liquefaction in 3 days at 22 °C.
2. **Semi-solid agar stab culture:** For motility detection.

C. Solid media:

1. **Nutrient agar:** Colonies are moist, translucent, 1-2 mm, round discs with bluish tinge in transmitted light, has distinctive odour.
2. **Blood agar:** Initially α-haemolytic (green zone) later β-haemolytic (clear zone).

D. Selective media:

1. **Alkaline bile salt agar:** pH of medium is 8.2 & colonies are like nutrient agar.
2. **Mac Conkey's agar:** Pale / colourless colony due to NLF **[fig.-2(a)]**.
3. **TCBS (Thiosulphate Citrate Bile salts Sucrose) medium:** Bromothymol blue is the pH indicator gives yellow colony **[fig.-2(b)]** at acidic pH due to sucrose fermentation.

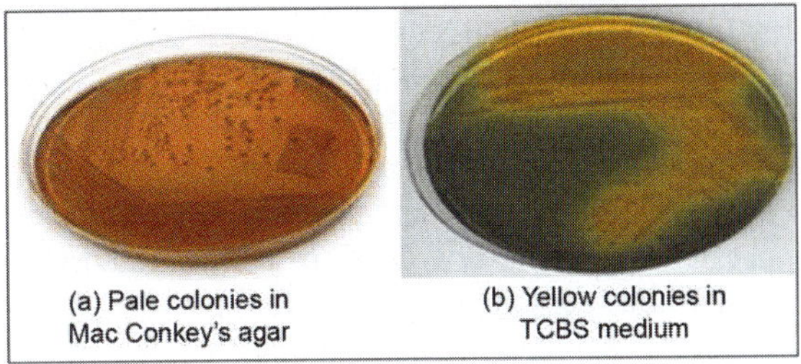

(a) Pale colonies in Mac Conkey's agar (b) Yellow colonies in TCBS medium

Figure-2: C/Cs of *V. cholerae*

4. **Monsur's gelatin taurocholate trypticase tellurite medium:** Small translucent colonies with black centre (black due to tellurite reduction), become large colony after 48 hrs.

- **Culture in animal:** Number of animal models has been used to study the pathogenic mechanisms in cholera. The first of these was the rabbit ileal loop model of De and Chatterjee in 1953. Injection of ligated ileal loop caused fluid accumulation & ballooning.

❖ Biochemical reaction (B/Rs):

1. **Sugar fermentation test:**

G	S	L	M
A	A	-	A

   - Oxidative & fermentative
   - It also ferments maltose & rhamnose with acid only but not inositol or arabinose. It may split lactose very slowly.
2. **I M Vi C tests:** + - V -
3. **Catalase test:** +Ve
4. **Nitrate reduction test:** + Ve
5. **Oxidase test:** +Ve
6. **H_2S production:** -Ve
7. **Urease test:** -Ve
8. **TSI test:** A/A - H_2S
9. **String test:** →**Fig. 3(a)**

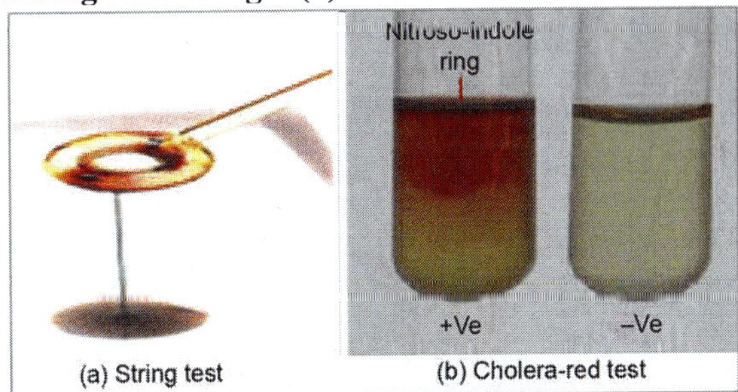

(a) String test (b) Cholera-red test

Figure-3: B/Rs of *V. cholerae*

   - Mix a loopful suspension of *V. cholerae* & a drop of 0.5% sodium deoxycholate in saline on a slide.
   - Suspension loses its turbidity, becomes mucoid and forms **'string'** between loop & mixture when loop is withdrawn slowly away from mixture.
10. **Haemolytic reaction:**
    - Mixed equal volume of broth culture & 1% sheep RBCs.
    - Incubated for 2 hr at 37°C, than kept overnight in refrigerator at 4°C.

- Examine for haemolysis
- Classical Vibrio: Non-haemolytic
- El Tor Vibrio: Haemolytic

11. Cholera red reaction: →Fig. 3(b)

- Indole & nitrates tests are positive by *V. cholerae*.
- Tested by adding few drops of concentrated H_2SO_4 to 24-hour peptone water culture.
- With *V. cholerae* a reddish pink colour **nitroso-indole ring** is formed.

12. Gelatin liquefaction test: +Ve

13. Lysine decarboxylation: +Ve

14. Ornithine decarboxylation: +Ve

15. Arginine decarboxylation: -Ve

16. Tests to differentiate the *V. cholerae* from related genera → Table 1

❖ Resistance:

- *V. cholerae* is killed by heating at 55^0C in 15 minutes, by boiling in few seconds & by drying.
- It grows at low temperature & survives for 2-4 weeks in ice cold water & for 4-6 weeks or longer in ice.
- Its survival in water depends on pH, temperature, salinity & presence of other materials. In clean tape water it survives for 30 days. They can't survive in polluted water of Ganges due to presence of large numbers of vibriophages.
- It can survive for 1-2 days in a food left at room temperature but survives more than 2 weeks in food store in cold temperature.
- It is sensitive to acids but resist high alkalinity. It is killed by normal gastric acidity so required high infective dose & survive for 24 hours in achorhydric patients.
- It is killed by chlorination of water. Chlorination does not kill the spores /sporing bacteria & viruses like polio, hepatitis etc.

❖ Classification of *V. cholerae*:

A. Heiberg classification based on fermentation reaction: →Table 2

Group	Mannose	Sucrose	Arabinose
I	A	A	-
II	-	A	-
III	A	A	A
IV	-	A	A
V	A	-	-
VI	-	-	-
VII	A	-	A
VIII	-	-	A

Table-2: Heiberg classification of *V. cholerae*

B. Gardner and Venkatraman's serological classification: → Flow chart-2 & table-3

Genus	Hugh-Leifson / O-F test		Aminoacid decarboxylation test			String test
	Oxidation (O)	Fermentation (F)	Lysine	Arginine	Ornithine	
Vibrio	+	A	+	-	+	+
Aeromonas	+	A/AG	-	+	-	V
Pseudomonas	+	-	V	V	V	-
Plesiomonas	+	+	+	+	+	-

Table-1: Tests to differentiate the *V. cholerae* from related genera

A: Acid, AG: Acid + gas, V: Variable

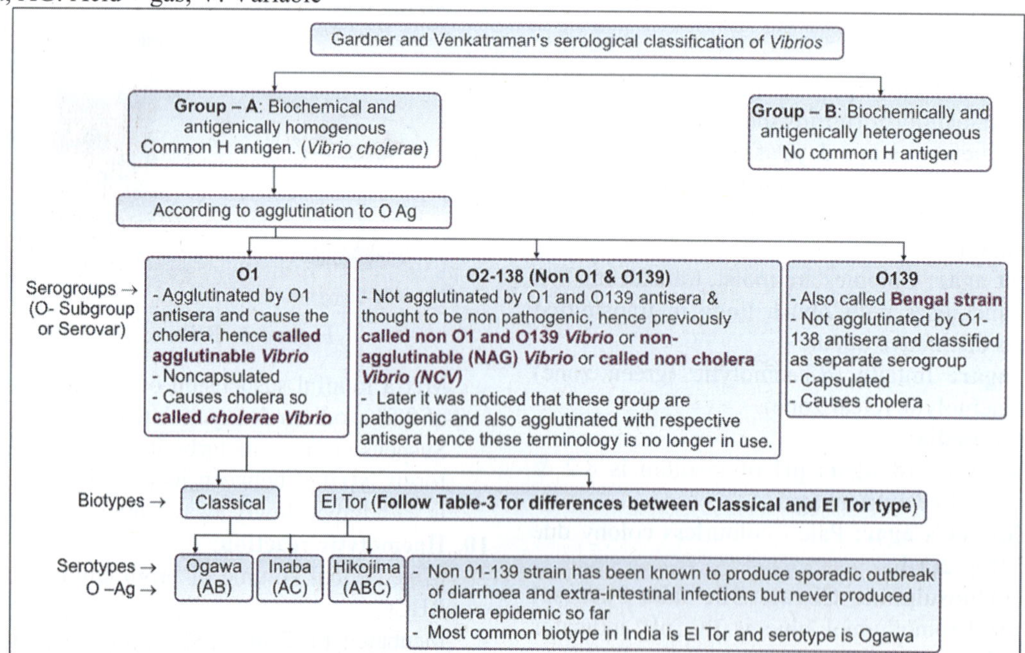

Flow chart-2: Gardner and Venkatraman's serological classification

Test	Classical	El Tor
Haemolysis of Sheep RBCs	-	+
Haemagglutination of Chick RBCs	-	+
Vi test	-	+
Polymixin B sensitivity (50 U)	S	R
Mukharjee phage IV sensitivity	S	R
Sensitivity to El Tor phage V	R	S

Table-3: Differences between Classical & El Tor type

S= Sensitive, R= Resistant

C. Other methods:

1. **Phage typing:** **Follow chapter → Laboratory diagnosis of bacterial infections**
2. **Ribotyping:**

❖ Pathogenicity:

- **Disease name:** Disease **called cholera.**
- **Nature & history of diisease:** It can occur as sporadic, endemic, localised outbreak, epidemic or in pandemic forms.
- **Home land of cholera:** Cholera is very ancient human disease. In Bengal (India), large deltaic area of the river Ganga & Brahmaputra is **called the home land of cholera**, from where it spread & caused many epidemics in different part of country. Till early in the 19th century it was limited to India & many epidemics in the country.
- **Pandemic report:** Total eight pandemic reported in the history mainly by Classical biotypes & rare by El Tor.

a. The first six pandemics:

- Occurred between 1817 to1923.
- All were caused by Classical biotypes.
  Originated from the Bengal to involve most of the world.
- Several thousands of deaths were reported.
- After 6th pandemic it was limited to its home land.

b. 7th pandemic:

- Occurred in 1961.
- Caused by El Tor biotypes.
- Originated from the Sulawesi (Celebes), Indonesia & spread to Hong Kong & Philippines. Entered in India-Pakistan in 1964, in Iran-Iraq in 1965-66, in Russia in 1970-71, in Kenya in 1971, in Portugal-Spain in 1971, in Peru-South America in 1991 & in Central America in 1994, thus encircled the whole world in 30 years.
- 7th pandemic was different form earlier in following ways.

1. Caused by El Tor biotypes.
2. Origin was not India but Indonesia.
3. Low mortality.
4. Less severe with mild to asymptomatic infections. More cases are subclinical.
5. High carrier rate, so remained endemic in many areas & causing periodic epidemics. Secondary attack rate is low, fewer secondary cases in affected families. (**secondary attack rate:** It is defined as the probability that infection occurs among susceptible persons within a reasonable incubation period following known contact with an infectious person or an infectious source).
6. El Tor biotypes is much hardier than the Classical & survive much longer in the environment, thus involved entire world including countries of Central America, South America, Australia & other affluent countries which were never affected before.
7. 7th pandemic which was caused by El Tor biotypes replace the Classical biotypes, thus in India, Classical biotypes was hardly encountered after the El Tor biotypes took root but in Bangladesh Classical biotypes staged comeback in 1982.

c. 8th pandemic (O-139 or Bengal strain):

- Occurred in October 1992 in Madras (Chennai), India & later similar outbreak occurred in other part of India.
- It is not agglutinable by O1-138 & identified as newer strain **called O139.**
- It was limited to coastal areas of Bay of Bengal up to West Bengal, India & adjacent areas of Bangladesh hence **called Bengal strain.**
- It replaced the El Tor *Vibrio* (of 7th pandemic).
- By January 1993, strain produced epidemic in Bangladesh & rapidly spread in almost 11 Asian countries & threatened to cause the next pandemic. But surprisingly in 1994 El Tor *Vibrio* regained its dominance & threat of an O139 strain diminished.
- It causes cholera, similar to O1 El Tor strain. It is differentiated from O1 strain by following ways

1. Capsulated.
2. More invasive & causing bacteremia & some extra intestinal lesions.
3. Distinct LPS.
4. Not protected by O1 vaccine.
5. Contains novel surface antigens.

- Both O1 El Tor & O139 began to co-exist in endemic areas but are now declining.
- Currently O139 still causing minor cases in India & Bangladesh.

- **Reservoir of infection:** Human (no animal) case or carrier. Infected person can shed the bacilli for 10 days or longer.
- **Source of infection:** Contaminated food & water.
- **Mode of transmission:**

- By ingestion of contaminated food & water which are infected by stool or vomitus of case or carrier.
- Person to person transmission is possible in household contact or in close community contact only by supplying the drinking water with contaminated hands **called domestic spread.**

- Vegetables washed with contaminated water can lead epidemic.
- **Incubation period:** < 24 hrs to 5 days.
- **Portal of entry:** GIT.
- **Sites:** Intestine.
- **Precipitating factors (epidemiological determinants):** Following are the types.

I. Agent factors (virulence factors)

i. Intracellular (cell wall associated) factors:

1. **Endotoxin (lipopolysaccharide/LPS):** Endotoxin, no role in pathogenesis in human but intraperitoneal inoculation in mice causes fatal effect.
2. **Flagella:** Organs of locomotion. Help to reach the epithelial cells.
3. **Fimbriae (TCP):** Special organ for adhesion **called 'Toxin Co-regulated Pilus (TCP)'**. Vibrio colonise throughout the course of infection without damage or invasion to host cell. TCP constantly bind the *Vibrio* with host cell.

ii. Extracellular:

a. Exotoxins: Called enterotoxins with following different types.

1. **Heat labile toxin (LT):**

- **Synonym:** Cholera toxin (CT) or cholera enterotoxin (CTX) or choleragen.

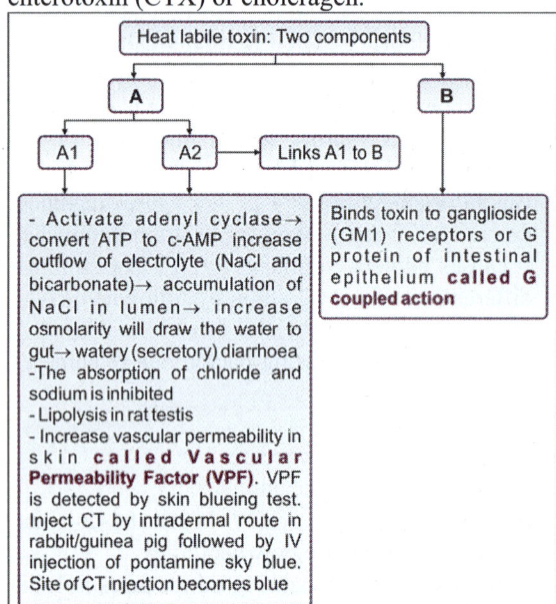

Flow chart-3: Heat labile enterotoxin

- **Properties:**
  - Heat labile *E. coli* toxin (LT) & cholera toxin of *V cholerae* 0137 & O1 are structurally & antigenically same, but cholera toxin is hundred times more potent than labile toxin. Both act via cAMP.
  - Gene for toxin production is bacteriophage coded. It can also replicate as a plasmid which can be transmitted to non toxigenic strain, rendering them toxigenic.
  - Molecular weight (MW): 84, 000
  - It is toxigenic, can induce neutralizing antitoxin.
  - It can be toxoided.
  - It can affect only intestinal epithelial cells, no effect on any other cells.
- **Components & actions: → Flow chart-3**

2. **Vero toxin (VT)** or **vero cyto toxin** or **Shiga Like Toxin (SLT):** Follow chapter → Enterobactericeae-I (*E. coli, Klebsiella* and *Proteus* etc.)
3. **Zona occludens toxin:** Responsible for disruption of tight junction between mucosal cells.

b. Enzymes:

1. **Mucinase:** Help to cross the protective layer of mucin.
2. **Neuraminidase (haemagglutinin protease):**
   - Formerly **called 'cholera lectin'**.
   - It cleaves mucus & fibronectin.
   - It releases the bounded *Vibrio* & favour it's spread to other intestinal part.
3. **Other enzymes:** Like collagenase, elastase, chitinase, nucleotidase, lipase etc. are also helps in spread & virulence of *Vibrio.*

c. Infective dose:

- Bacilli are sensitive to acids (acid prove effective barrier against cholera) but resist high alkalinity.
- They are killed by normal gastric acidity so infective dose is very high about 10^4-10^6 bacilli. It can survive for 24 hours in achorhydric (absence of hydrochloric acid in gastric secretion) patients.
- 10^6 pathogenic *Vibrio* will not cause infection **without food** in normal person but same dose produce infection **with food** in normal person.

d. Siderophore: Required for iron uptake.

✓ **Notes: Regulatory gene**

- **ToxR gene / Tox R protein:** It is a regulatory gene which regulate CT, TCP & other virulence factors of *V cholerae.*

II. Host factors

1. **Age:** No age bar but during epidemic it target more to children.
2. **Immunity:**
   - People with low immunity (HIV infected persons) & lack of preexisting immunity are more prone to disease.
   - Single attack of vibrio can provide 6-9 months immunity, re-infection is possible afterward. Immunity may be local or systemic. Local immunity includes presence of antibodies like IgA, IgG & IgM in faeces **called coproantibodies. (copro = related to dung or faeces)**. Systemic immunity includes vibriocidal antibodies in the serum of patient have been associated with protection against colonisation and disease.

Prevalence of vibrio is measured by measuring the titre of vibriocidal antibodies.

3. **Malnutrition:** Also favours the disease.
4. **Gastric acidity:** Discussed earlier under the heading of infective dose.
5. **Blood group:** Most in O group. Least in AB group. Reason is not known.

III. Environmental factors

1. **Seasons:** Occurs throughout the year but major cases occurs in summer (high temperature), heavy rain fall (flooding).
2. **Habitat:** *V. cholerae* can survive extra-cellularly. Commonly it habitat in brackish estuaries or coastal sew water particularly in small crustacean like crab, copepods or in plankton.
3. **Other factors includes**: Poor sanitation, overcrowding, population mobility (in pilgrimages, marriages, fairs, festivals etc.)

➢ **Pathogenesis: → Flow chart-4**

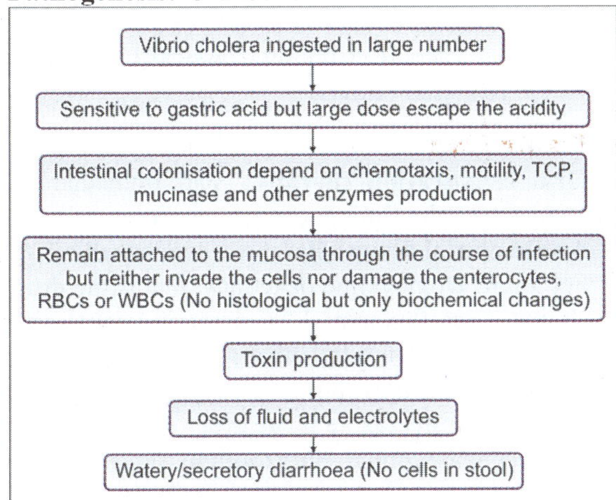

Flow chart-4: Pathogenesis of cholera

➢ **Clinical features:** Clinical severity is variable from asymptomatic case to fatal

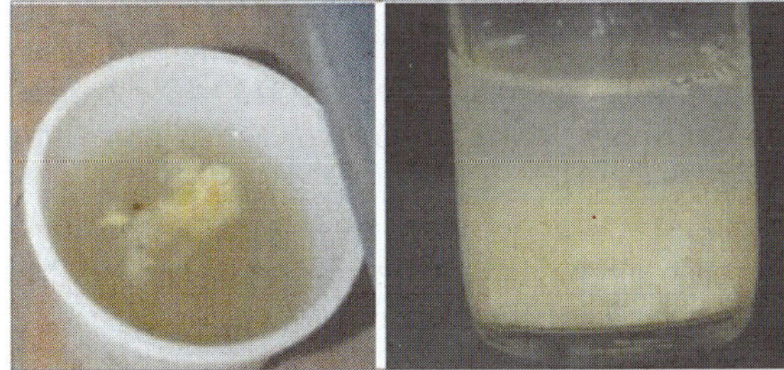

Figure-4: Rice water stool in cholera

- Begins with the sudden onset of painless watery/secretory diarrhoea (no cells in stool) with effortless vomiting.
- Passage of **'rice water stool' (fig.-4)** has fishy, inoffensive sweetish odour may contain mucus flakes but no blood or pus cells.
- Fever is usually absent.
- Hypovolemic shock may cause death in < 24 hrs.

➢ **Complications:** Severe dehydration causes anuria, haemoconcentration, hypovolamic shock, hypokalemia, acidosis, muscular cramps, renal failure, cardiac arrhythmia, pulmonary oedema, paralytic ileus etc.

➢ **Carrier:** Four types of carrier

a. **Incubatory:** Shed the bacilli in faeces for 1-5 days
b. **Convalescent:** Excrete the bacilli for 2-3 weeks
c. **Healthy / contact carrier:** Had subclinical infection & shed the *Vibrio* for 10 days
d. **Chronic carrier:** Shed the bacilli for months or years **(up to 10 years),** more in El Tor than Classical. Persistence gall bladder infection is reason for chronic carrier.

❖ Laboratory diagnosis:

I. Detection of case

A. Detection of case by identifying the bacilli:

➢ **Specimens:** Stool & rectal swab.

➢ **Collection:**

- Stool: Collected before antibiotic, by introducing a catheter in rectum & letting the watery stool flow in sterile screw-capped container.
- Rectal swab: Good quality swab which absorb 0.1-0.2 ml fluid. In convalescence phase dip the swab in enrichment broth & than collect the samples.

➢ **Transport:**

- If specimens can reach to laboratory in few hrs than transfer in enrichment media.
- If long period before reach to laboratory then transfer in transport media.
- If transport media are not available, filter paper strip may be soaked in stool & transfer in plastic envelop.

➢ **Testing methods:**

i. **Macroscopic examination: 'Rice water stool',** inoffensive sweetish odour, may contain mucus flakes.

ii. **Microscopy:**

1. Detection of motility by direct hanging drop preparation.
2. Inhibition of motility by specific antiserum under DGIM or PCM.
3. Detection of whole morphology: By gram stain or by direct immune fluorescence.
4. More details: → Follow morphology

iii. **Culture:** Subculture on solid media from enrichment broth as described in **flow chart-5.**

iv. **Serological test:**

- Not useful in case detection but useful to access prevalence of cholera in area.
- Prevalence of *Vibrio* is measured by measuring the titre of vibriocidal antibodies by agglutination test, IHA & complement based vibriocidal test & antitoxin assay.

v. **Blood picture:**

- Neutrophilia.

- Normal sodium, potassium & chloride level.
- Markedly reduced bicarbonate level.

vi. Typing:

a. Bacteriophage (Vibrio phage) typing: Vide supra

b. Ribo typing:

B. Detection of case by identifying the LT: Follow chapter → Enterobactericeae-I (*E. coli, Klebsiella Proteus* etc.) (section heat labile toxin)

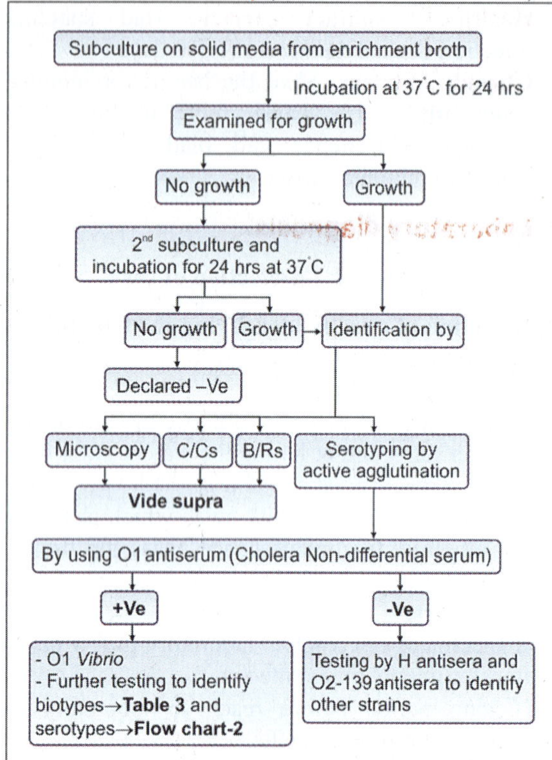

Flow chart-5: Cultivation techniques & identification of growth on solid media

II. Detection of carrier

- **Specimens:** Stool collected by normal defecation or by purgation with mannitol (30g) or with $MgSO_4$ (15-30g) & bile collected by duodenal intubation.
- **Test:** Repeated enrichment & subcultures are required.

III. Detection of source

- **Enrichment technique:** Collect 900ml water → enrichment in 100ml APW (pH-9.2) → incubation for 6-8 hrs at 37°C → subculture on solid media.
- **Filtration technique:** Filtration through millipore membrane → culture the membrane.
- **Sewage** → dilute in saline → filtered through gauze → treated as water.

❖ Prevention:

A. General measures: Chlorination of water & improvement of environmental sanitation.

B. Chemoprophylaxis: Tetracycline is the drug of choice. It is indicated to household contact or close community contact. It is not indicated for total community **called mass prophylaxis**, as it is not able to prevent the spread.

C. Immunoprophylaxis: Ideal vaccine is yet to found. Following are some useful vaccine

a. Injectable killed vaccine:

- **Contain**: Three different types
  1. Vaccine with 8000 million of *V. cholerae* per ml with equal numbers of Ogawa & Inaba serotypes.
  2. Vaccine with equal number of Classical & El Tor *Vibrio*.
  3. Vaccine with O-139 strain.
- **Administration:** By subcutaneous (SC) or by intramuscular (IM) injection.
- **Disadvantages:**
  - Provide only 50-60% immunity.
  - No longer protection. Immunity last for 3-6 months.
  - Does not provide local immunity.

b. Oral vaccine: Two types

1. **Killed oral whole cell vaccine:** With & without inclusion of B subunit of cholera toxin.
2. **Live oral vaccine:** Contain Classical *Vibrio*, El Tor *Vibrio* & O-139 strains.

❖ Treatment:

1. **Oral rehydration therapy:** Start immediately to compensate the fluid & electrolytes loss.
2. **Antibacterial drugs:** Having secondary role.
   - For adult: Doxicycline or tetracycline is the drug of choice. Ciprofloxacin, 3rd generation cephalosporin or erythromycin are the other alternatives.
   - For children: Furazolidine is the drug of choice but in India cotrimoxazole is the drug of choice
   - For pregnant women: Furazolidine (drug of choice).

O2-138 (Non O1&O139)

❖ General features:

- Morphologically & Biochemically similar to O1 & O139 Vibrio, but not agglutinated by O1 & O139 antisera & thought to be non pathogenic, hence previously **called non O1 & O139 *Vibrio*** or **non-agglutinable (NAG) *Vibrio*** or **called non cholera *Vibrio (NCV)***
- Later it was noticed that these group are pathogenic & also agglutinated with respective antisera hence these terminology is no longer in use

❖ Pathogenicity:

- **Mode of transmission:** Ingestion of sea food like raw oyster. In Calcutta found in small pond fish
- **Clinical features:**

1. **Intestinal:** Not causing cholera but gastroenteritis present with abdominal pain, nausea, vomiting, diarrhoea & fever.
2. **Extra-intestinal:** Causing otitis media, wound infection & bacteremia

❖ **Treatment:** Same as like cholera & includes fluid replacement & antibiotics like tetracycline, ciprofloxacin & 3rd generation cephalosporin

Vibrio mimicus

- So, called because biochemically similar to *V. cholerae.*
- Grow at 0.5-1% NaCl & sucrose non-fermenters.
- Causes diarrhoeal disease in Gulf-coast of USA by ingestion of seafood (oyster) similar to *V. parahaemolyticus.*

Halophilic vibrios

❖ **Definition:** Vibrios which grow at high concentration **(7-10%)** of NaCl are **called halophilic vibrios.**

❖ **Classification:**

I. **Causing Gastroenteritis:** *V. parahaemolyticus, V.fluvialis, V. furnisii & V. hollisae.*

II. **Causing extra-intestinal infections:** *V. alginolyticus, V. vulnificus & V. damsel.*

❖ **Differences between *Vibrio comma* & halophilic vibrios:** →**Table-4**

❖ **Species:**

A. ***V. parahaemolyticus***

➢ **History:** Isolated from Japan in 1951 as a causative agent of food poisoning due to ingestion of sea fish.

➢ **Morphology:** Same as like *V. cholerae* except.

- It is pleomorphic when grow on 3% salt agar & in old culture.
- Shows bipolar staining.
- Capsulated.
- Motile with peritrichous flagella in solid & with polar flagella in liquid medium.
- Showing pleomorphism especially when grow on 3% salt agar & in old culture.

➢ **Cultural characteristics (C/Cs):**

- Grow in media with 8% NaCl but not with 10% NaCl. Optimum NaCl is 2-4%.

i. **Liquid media:** Peptone Water with 8% NaCl

ii. **Selective media:**

1. **TCBS medium:** Green colonies with
   - Centre: Opaque & raised.
   - Margin: Translucent & flat.
2. **Wagat-Suma agar (high salt blood agar):**
   - Pathogenic strains from human are β-haemolytic & non-pathogenic strains from environment (water) are nonhaemolytic **called Kanagawa phenomenon.**
   - It is due to heat stable haemolysin.
   - It can swarm on blood agar.

➢ **Biochemical reaction (B/Rs):**

1. **Sugar fermentation tests:** G S L M
   A - - A
   - Also produce acid from maltose, mannose & arabinose. Do not ferment salicin, xylose, adonitol, inositol & sorbitol.
2. **I M Vi C tests:** + - - +
3. **Catalase test:** +Ve
4. **Nitrate reduction:** + Ve
5. **Oxidase test:** +Ve
6. **H_2S production:** -Ve
7. **Urease test:** Some strains are + Ve.
8. **String test:** +Ve

➢ **Resistance:**

- It is killed by heating at 60^0C in 15 minutes.
- It does not grow at 4^0C but can survive refrigerator & freezing.
- Destroyed by drying & putting in distilled water or vinegar.

➢ **Pathogenicity:**

✪ **Virulence factors:**

a. **Antigens:**

1. O-Ag (12 O-groups).
2. K-Ag (59 types).
3. H-Ag.

b. **Toxin:**

1. **Haemolysin:**
   - Produces the heat stable haemolysin.
   - Not significant in virulence but used in laboratory to test for Kanagawa phenomenon & pathogenicity.

Test	*Vibrio comma*	*V. parahaemolyticus*	*V. alginolyticus*	*V. vulnificus*
Indole	+	+	+	+
VP	V	-	+	-
Nitrate	+	+	+	+
Urease	-	Some strain are +	-	-
Lactose	-	-	-	Acid
Sucrose	+	-	+	-
Swarming	-	- / +	+	-
0.5-1% NaCl	+	-	-	-
8% NaCl	-	+	+	+
10% NaCl	-	-	+	<10%

Table -4: Differences between *Vibrio comma* & halophilic vibrios

- Kanagawa phenomenon +Ve: Pathogenic.
- Kanagawa phenomenon –Ve: Non-pathogenic.

2. **Type III secretion system:** It is capable of injecting virulence proteins into host cells to disrupt host cell functions or cause cell death by apoptosis.

- **Mode of transmission:** Ingestion of sea (marine) food like sea-fish, shrimps, crabs or molluscs (oyster). In Calcutta found in small pond fish.
- **Incubation period:** About 24 hours
- **Clinical features:**

1. **Food poisoning:**
- Important cause of food poisoning throughout the world. Not all strains are pathogenic, only Kanagawa phenomenon positive causes food poisoning.
- Present with abdominal pain, nausea, vomiting, diarrhoea & low grade fever.

2. **Dysentery:**
- Less common.
- Occurs in India & Bangladesh.

- **Complications:** Moderate degree of dehydration.
- **Laboratory diagnosis:**
- **Specimens:** Stool
- **Testing methods:**

i. **Macroscopic examination:** Stool with cellular exudates & often blood.

ii. **Microscopy:** → **Follow morphology**

iii. **Culture:** → **Follow C/Cs**

iv. **Biochemical reactions:** → **Follow B/Rs**

B. ***V. alginolyticus***

- Halophilic *Vibrio* is similar to *V. parahaemolyticus* except tolerate 10% NaCl (most salt tolerating species), VP positive & ferments sucrose.
- Found in sea fish & sea-water.
- On exposure produce eye, ear & wound infections in human.

C. ***V. vulnificus***

- Previously **called** L^+ ***Vibrio*** or ***Beneckea vulnifica.***
- Tolerate <10% NaCl, VP –Ve & ferments lactose but not sucrose.
- Infection occurs due to ingestion of oysters.
- Two clinical conditions:

1. Wound infection on exposure to sea water.
2. Ingestion in liver disease patient: Cross the GIT without any GIT symptoms enters in blood & causing septicemia.

Aeromonadaceae

Classification: →Flow chart-6

Morphology:

- **Type according to gram stain:** GNB
- **Motility:** Motile with single polar flagellum. In some strains lateral flagella are found while some non motile strains also found.
- **Capsule:** Capsulated.
- **Spore:** Non-sporing.
- **Fimbriae:** Present.

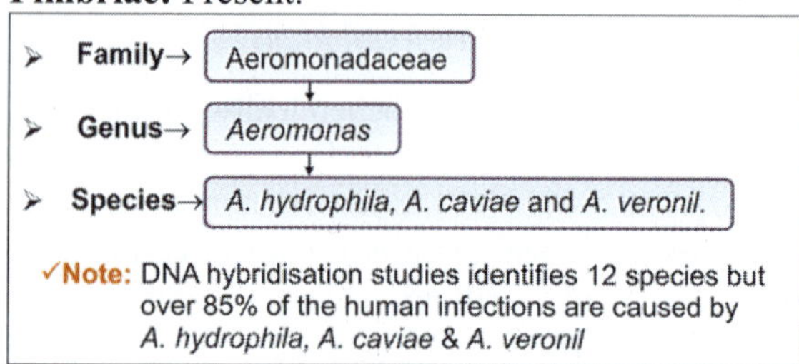

Family→ Aeromonadaceae
Genus→ Aeromonas
Species→ A. hydrophila, A. caviae and A. veronil.
✓Note: DNA hybridisation studies identifies 12 species but over 85% of the human infections are caused by A. hydrophila, A. caviae & A. veronil

Flow chart-6: Classification of Aeromonadaceae

Cultural characteristics (C/Cs):

- **Effective factors:**
  - Temperature: Optimum temperature is 32°C (4–42°C).
  - pH: Range 4.5–9.0
  - Growth is not supported by NaCl.
- **Media:**

1. **Blood agar:** 90% strains produce β-haemolysis while *A. caviae* give non haemolytic colonies.
2. **Mac Conkey's agar:** Pale colonies due to NLF.

Biochemical reactions (B/Rs): → Table-1

Pathogenicity:

- **Virulence factors:**

1. **Fimbriae:** Organ of adhesion.
2. **Capsule:** Inhibit the phagocytosis.
3. **LPS:** Endotoxic actions.
4. **Exotoxins:** Haemolysin, aerolysin, enterotoxin (Shiga Like Toxin/SLT)

- **Reservoir of infection:** Fresh water or brackish water or marine water or polluted water of drained pipes or in sink traps.
- **Source of infection:** Food & water.
- **Mode of transmission:** Ingestion of contaminated food & water.
- **Clinical features:**

a. **Animal disease:** *A. hydrophila* produces the red leg disease in frog & also pathogenic for other cold blooded animals like fish & reptiles.

b. **Human disease:** Following two types.

1. **Intestinal:** Not causing cholera but gastroenteritis present with abdominal pain, nausea, vomiting, watery diarrhoea / dysentery & fever.
2. **Extra-intestinal:**
- Peritonitis.
- Musculoskeletal & wound infection.
- Bacteremia in person with IDDs.
- Respiratory infections: Like pneumonia, pharyngitis & epiglotitis.
- HUS (Haemolytic Uremic Syndrome) due to production of SLT.

Laboratory diagnosis:

- **Specimens:** Stool, vomitus, urine, sputum etc.

- **Testing methods:**
- i. **Microscopy:** → **Follow morphology**
- ii. **Culture:** → **Follow C/Cs**
- iii. **Biochemical reactions:** → **Follow B/Rs**

❖ **Treatment:** Treated by using antibiotics & fluid therapy.

Plesiomonas

❖ **Meaning:**
- **Genus:** ***Plesiomonas*** **(Greek) = Neighbour,** because of close association with *Aeromonas.*
- **Species:** *P. shigelloides,* name given because of antigenically related to *Sh. sonnei.*

❖ **Classification:** →**Flow chart-7**

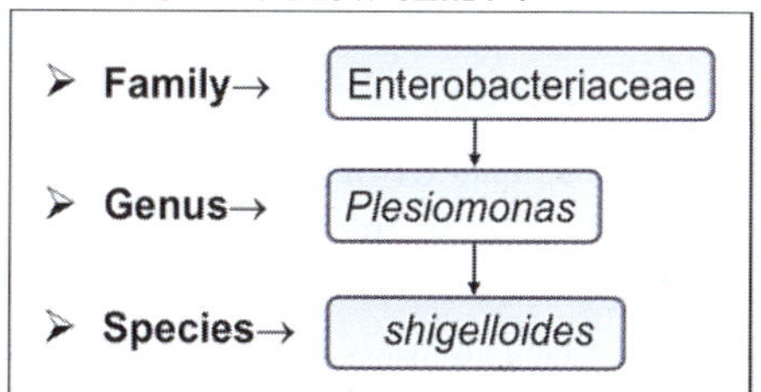

Flow chart-7: Classification of *Plesiomonas*

❖ **General features:**
- Initially listed under Vibrionaceae family but DNA hybridisation study suggests that it is more related to *Proteus* spp., hence shifted to Enterobacteriaceae family.
- It is the only genus in Enterobacteriaceae family which gives oxidase test positive.
- Growth is not stimulated by NaCl.

❖ **Morphology:**
- **Type according to gram stain:** GNB.
- **Motility:** Motile with lophotrichous flagella.

❖ **Cultural characteristics (C/Cs):**
- **Effective factors:**
- Temperature: Optimum temperature is 37°C, but better growth occurs at 30°C.
- Growth is not stimulated by NaCl.
- Differentiated from *Vibrio* & *Aeromonas* by tests mentioned in **table-1** & also by ability to produce resistance to compound O/129.
- **Media:**
1. **Mac Conkey's agar or DCA:** Some strains are LFs give pink colonies while some are NLFs give pale/colourless colonies.

❖ **Biochemical reactions (B/Rs):** → **Table-1**

❖ **Pathogenicity:**
- **Reservoir of infection:** Saprophyte in water and soil. Commensals in animal intestine (like fish) & rare in human intestine.
- **Source of infection:** Food & water.
- **Mode of transmission:** Ingestion of contaminated food & water.
- **Clinical features:**
1. **Intestinal:** Causing gastroenteritis more severe in person with IDDs.
2. **Extra-intestinal:** Arthritis, meningitis, septicemia & cellulitis.

❖ **Laboratory diagnosis:**
- **Specimens:** Stool, blood etc.
- **Testing methods:**
- i. **Microscopy:** → **Follow morphology**
- ii. **Culture:** → **Follow C/Cs**
- iii. **Biochemical reactions:** → **Follow B/Rs**

❖ **Treatment:** Treated by using antibiotics & fluid therapy.

Question bank

Case study

1) A paediatric patient visited the hospital with complains of abdominal pain & diarrhoea. Stool examination revealed rice water appearance & darting type motility under hanging drop preparation. Identify the organism & answer the following
a) Name the clinical condition & causative agent
b) Describe the morphology & culture characteristics of causative agent
c) Write the classification of causative agent
d) Write the pathogenicity of causative agent

Essay/Full question

1) *V. cholerae*

Short notes

1) Classification of Vibrionaceae
2) Morphology or C/Cs or B/Rs or classification of *V. cholerae*
3) Non O1 & non O139 (O2-138) vibrios
4) O139 (Bengal strain) vibrio
5) Halophilic vibrios
6) *Aeromonas*
7) *Plesiomonas*

Short questions for theory/viva questions

1) Name two transport & two enrichment media for *V. cholerae*
2) Write the four differences between Classical & El Tor *Vibrio*
3) Write the two examples of each, nonhalophilic & halophilic *Vibrios*
4) What is Kawagawa phenomenon

MCQs for chapter review

Vibrionaceae

1) **Halophilic *Vibrios* are except-** (PGI, Nov-13, 10)
(a) *V. cholerae* (b) *V. vulnificus* (c) *V. parahaemolyticus* (d) *V. mimicus* (e) *V. alginolyticus*

Vibrio cholerae

2) **True about cholera vibrio is-** (PGI-98)

(a) Can tolerate wide range of alkaline pH (b) Non-motile bacilli (c) Can't be grow in media (d) NaCl stimulates growth

3) **All of the following are true regarding *Vibrio cholerae* except-** (AI-94)
(a) Transported in acidic medium (b) Gram negative (c) Aerobic organism (d) Ferment glucose

4) **The following are true of *Vibrio cholerae* except-** (AI-01)
(a) Produces indole and reduces nitrates (b) Synthesises neuraminidase (c) Dies rapidly at low temperature (d) Vaccine confers long immunity

5) ***Vibrio cholerae* true is -** (PGI-98)
(a) Very resistant to alkaline pH (b) Nutritionally fastidious (c) Best growth at 24^{0}C (d) Rod shaped bacilli

6) **Which of the following statement is true about *Vibrio cholerae* -** (AI-99)
(a) There is no natural reservoir (b) Transported in alkaline peptone water medium (c) Halophilic (d) Oxidase negative

7) **7th pandemic of cholera is caused by -**
(a) El Tor (b) O139 *V. cholerae* (c) Classical *V. cholerae* (d) *V. mimicus*

8) **The characteristic features of EL Tor cholera is all except -** (AI-97)
(a) More of subclinical cases (b) Mortality is less (c) Secondary attack rate is high in family (d) El Tor vibrio is harder and able to survive longer

9) **Strain of *Vibrio cholerae* in Bengal -**
(a) O139 (b) O137 (c) O17 (d) O40

10) **Cholera is caused by -** (PGI, Nov-13, June -09)
(a) *Vibrio cholerae*-01 (b) *Vibrio cholerae*-0139 (c) *Vibrio parahaemolyticus* (d) NAG vibrio

11) **Not true about EL Tor vibrio O1 -** (AI-10)
(a) Animals are the only reservoir (b) Epidemiologically indistinguishable from *V. cholerae*-O139 (c) Human acts as vehicle for spread (d) Efficacy of vaccine against El Tor vibrio is great

12) **True regarding cholera is -** (AIIMS, Dec-95)
(a) Toxin acts on GM1 receptors (b) Toxin action is cAMP mediated (c) Peritrichate flagella (d) Utilise arginine and lysine

13) **Which of the following toxin can stimulate adenylate cyclase with G protein coupled action -**
(a) Shiga toxin (b) Cholera toxin (c) Diphtheria toxin (d) Pseudomonas toxin

14) **Cholera toxin effects are mediated by stimulation of which of the following second messanger -** (AI-12)
(a) cAMP (b) cGMP (c) Ca^{++} - calmodulim (d) IP_3/DAG

15) **Which toxin act by ADP ribosylation -** (PGI -07)
(a) Botulinum toxin (b) Shigella toxin (c) *Vibrio cholerae* (d) Diphtheria toxin (e) Pertusis toxin

16) **Cholera toxin is due to -**
(a) Chromosome (b) Plasmid (c) Phage (d) Transposon

17) ***Vibrio cholerae* is able to stay in GIT because of -** (PGI, May-13, Dec-06)
(a) Acid resistance (b) Bile resistance (c) Motility (d) Binds to specific receptors (e) Anaerobic potential

18) **Which of the following is true of cholera -** (PGI-02)
(a) Recent epidemic was due to classical type (b) Causes secretory diarrhoea (c) Caused by endotoxin (d) Vibriocidal antibodies correspond to susceptibility

19) **True about cholera is-**
(a) Gram negative rod (b) Associated with fever (c) Causes painful watery diarrhoea (d) It is an achlorhydria which renders an individual susceptible to disease

20) **In a patient presenting with diarrhoea due to *Vibrio cholerae*, which of the following will be present-** (PGI, Dec-01)
(a) Abdominal pain (b) Presence of leucocytes in stool (c) Fever (d) Neutrophilia (e) Occurrences of many cases in same locality

21) **Antibiotic treatment of choice for treating cholera in an adult is a single dose of -** (AI-05)
(a) Tetracycline (b) Cotrimoxazole (c) Doxicycline (d) Furazolidone

22) **Drug of choice for treating cholera in pregnant women is -** (AIIMS-05)
(a) Tetracycline (b) Doxicycline (c) Furazolidone (d) Cotrimoxazole

23) **Which of the following is drug of choice for chemoprophylaxis of cholera -** (AIIMS-05)
(a) Tetracycline (b) Doxicycline (c) Furazolidone (d) Cotrimoxazole

24) **True about epidemiology of cholera -** (PGI -03)
(a) Chemoprophylaxis is not effective (b) Boiling cannot destroy the organism (c) Food can transmit the disease (d) Vaccine can give 90% protection

25) **Which is not true about *Vibrio cholera* -** (AI -05)
(a) It is not halophilic (b) Grows on simple media (c) Man is the only natural host (d) Cannot survive in extracellular environment

26) **True about *Vibrio cholera* O139 all except-** (AI -07, 08)
(a) Clinical manifestation are similar to O1 El Tor strain (b) First discovered in Chennai (c) Epidemiologically indistinguishable from O1 El Tor strain (d) Produce O1 polysaccharide

27) **All of the following statement about El Tor Vibrios are true, except -** (AI -10)
(a) Human are the only reservoir (b) Can survive in ice cold after for 2-4 weeks (c) Killed by boiling for 30 seconds (d) Enterotoxin can have direct effects on other tissues besides intestinal epithelial cells

28) **Which of the following about cholera is true -** (AI -90)
(a) Invasive (b) Endotoxin is released (c) Recent infection in India are of classical type (d) Vibriocidal antibodies titre measures prevalence

29) **Which of the following is not associated with *Vibrio cholerae* -**
(a) Haemolytic uremic syndrome (b) Rice water stool (c) Dehydration (d) None

Halophilic *Vibrios*

30) ***V. parahaemolyticus* food poisoning is caused by ingestion of-** (AI-96)
(a) Eggs and poultry products (b) Raw vegetable (c) Catfish, shellfish, sea food (d) Milk products

31) **Which of the following 'vibrios' is most commonly associated with ear infection-** (AI-12)
(a) *V. alginolyticus* (b) *V. parahaemolyticus* (c) *V. vulnificus* (d) *V. fluvialius*

Aeromonanadaceae

32) **Red leg disease is caused by** (PGI-01)
(a) *Pseudomonas* (b) Mouldy sugar cane fibre (c) Conidiosporum (d) *Aeromonas*

Answers of MCQs & explanation

1. **(a) & (d)**
- Follow section, **Vibrionaceae (classification →flow chart-1)** for explanation

2. **(a) & (d)**
- Can tolerate wide range of alkaline pH from 6.4-9.6
- It is motile monotrichous flagellum with darting type of motility
- It can grow in media
- 0.5-1% NaCl stimulates growth

3. **(a)**

- Can tolerate wide range of alkaline pH from 6.4-9.6, so transported in alkaline medium. For more explanation of transport media & their pH, follow section C/Cs (transport media/holding media)
- For explanation of other options follow section morphology, C/Cs & B/Rs

4. (c) & (d)
- Indole & nitrates tests are positive by *V. cholerae.*, tested by cholera red reaction as explained in section B/Rs (Cholera red reaction)
- Option b: Follow section, ***V. cholerae* [pathogenicity → agent factors (virulence factor) → enzymes]** for explanation
- It does not die at low temperature, but it grows at low temperature (16-40^{0}C) & survives for 2-4 weeks in ice cold water & for 4-6 weeks or longer in ice.
- Vaccine confers immunity last for 3-6 months.

5. (a)
- Can tolerate wide range of alkaline pH from 6.4-9.6
- Nutritionally not fastidious, because can grow in simple media
- Best growth at 37^{0}C (optimum temperature)
- Comma shaped bacilli

6. (b)
- Human is the only natural reservoir
- Transported in alkaline peptone water & other media as described in text
- Non-halophilic
- Oxidase positive

7. (a) } Follow section, ***V. cholerae* (pathogenicity →**
8. (c) } **pandemic report → 7th pandemic)** for explanation

9. (a)
- Follow section ***V. cholerae* [pathogenicity → pandemic report →8th pandemic (O-139 or Bengal strain)]** for explanation

10. (a) & (b)
- *Vibrio parahaemolyticus:* Causing food poisoning & dysentery
- NAG vibrio (Non 01-139 strain) has been known to produce sporadic outbreak of diarrhoea & extra-intestinal infections but never produced cholera epidemic so far
- Follow section, ***V. cholerae* (classification of *V. cholerae* →flow chart-2)** for explanation

11. (a), (b) & (d)
- No animals but human beings are the only reservoir
- Epidemiologically El Tor is distinguished from *V. cholerae*-0139 by presence of capsule & also by distinct polysaccharide **called O139 LPS**
- Human acts as vehicle for spread by stool & vomitus
- Efficacy of vaccine against El Tor vibrio is not great

12. (a) & (b)
- It is motile by monotrichate flagella
- It decarboxylase the lysine & ornithine but not arginine
- Follow section, ***V. cholerae* [pathogenicity → agent factors (virulence factors) & flow chart-3]** for more explanation

13. (b) } Follow section ***V. cholerae* [pathogenicity → agent**
14. (a) } **factors (virulence factors) & flow chart-3]**
15. (c) } for explanation

16. (c)
- Follow section, ***V. cholerae* [pathogenicity → agent factors (virulence factors) → exotoxin → heat labile toxin (LT)]** for explanation

17. (c)
- Follow section, ***V. cholerae* (pathogenicity → pathogenesis & flow chart-40** for explanation

18. (b)
- Recent epidemic in 1992 was due to Bengal strain
- Causes watery/secretory diarrhoea
- Endotoxin is not associated with pathogenesis
- Vibriocidal antibodies present in serum are not correspond to susceptibility but provide protection against colonisation & disease

19. (a) & (d)
- Gram negative bacilli with comma shape
- For options b & c follow section, ***V. cholerae* (pathogenicity → clinical features)**
- Bacilli are sensitive gastric acid, so achlorhydria (absence of hydrochloric acid in gastric secretion) which renders an individual susceptible to disease

20. (d) & (e)
- Cholera present with painless watery/secretory diarrhoea (no cells in stool) with effortless vomiting
- Fever is usually absent
- It present as localised outbreak, epidemic or in pandemic forms so many cases will occur at a time in same locality
- Blood picture suggests neutrophilia

21. (c) } Follow section, ***V. cholerae* (treatment)** for explanation
22. (c) }

23. (a)
- Follow section, ***V. cholerae* (prevention → chemoprophylaxis)** for explanation

24. (c)
- Chemoprophylaxis is effective for closed contacts or house hold contact, but not for mass prophylaxis
- For explanation of option b follow section, ***V. cholerae* (resistance)**
- Food & water can transmit the disease
- Vaccine can give 50-60% protection

25. (d)
- *V. cholerae* can survive extra-cellularly in brackish estuaries or coastal sew water particularly in small crustacean like crab, copepods or in plankton

26. (d)
- Options a, b & c: Follow section ***V. cholerae* [pathogenicity → pandemic report →8th pandemic (O-139 or Bengal strain)]** for explanation
- It does not produce O1 LPS but O 139 LPS

27. (d)
- Option d: Follow section, ***V. cholerae* [pathogenicity → agent factors (virulence factors) → exotoxin → heat labile toxin (LT)]** for explanation
- Other options are already explained

28. (b) & (d)
- It can affect only intestinal epithelial cells, no effect on any other cells, so it is non-invasive
- It released endotoxin but not contributing in pathogenesis
- Recent infection in India are of El Tor type
- For explanation of option d, follow section laboratory diagnosis (serological tests)

29. (a)
- Haemolytic uremic syndrome is caused by *Shigella dysenteriae* type 1, EHEC & *C jejuni*
- *V. cholerae* causing diarrhoea with rice water stool appearance & dehydration

30. (c)
- Follow section **halophilic *Vibrios* (*V. parahaemolyticus*)** for explanation

31. (a)
- Follow section, **halophilic *Vibrios* (*V. alginolyticus*)** for explanation

32. (d)
- Follow section **Aeromonadaceae (pathogenicity → Clinical features)** for explanation.

48 Campylobacterales

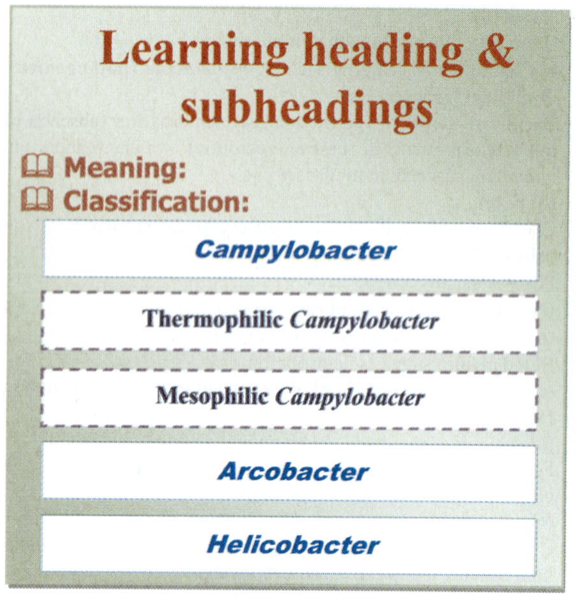

Learning heading & subheadings
Meaning:
Classification:
Campylobacter
Thermophilic Campylobacter
Mesophilic Campylobacter
Arcobacter
Helicobacter

Meaning: **Campylo** from **campylos (Greek)** = **curved** + **Bacter** from **baktron (Greek)** = **rod** because of curve shape of bacillus.

Classification: → **Flow chart-1**

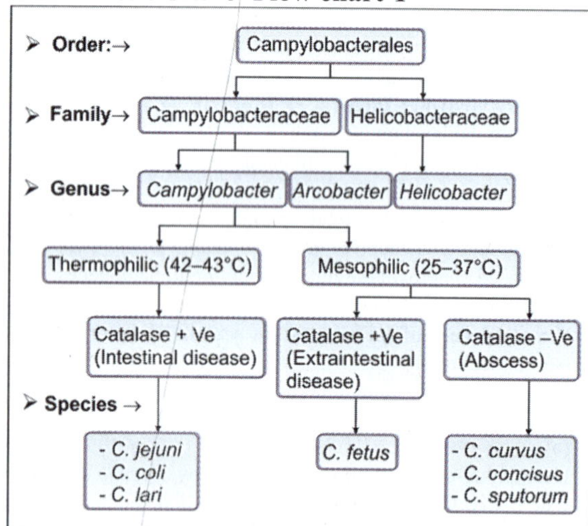

Flow chart-1: Classification of Campylobacterales

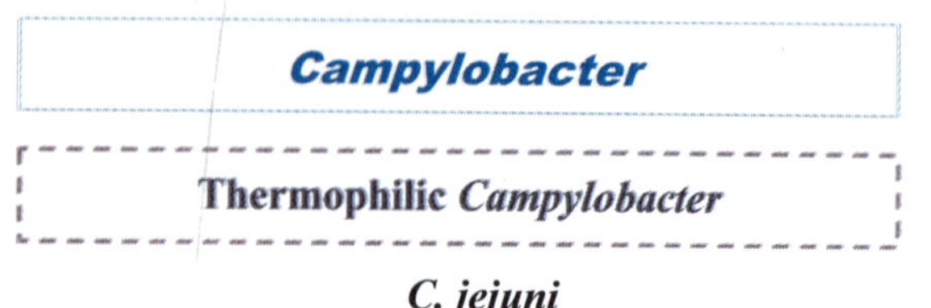

C. jejuni

❖ **History:** In 1886 a pediatrician, Theodor Escherich, observed *Campylobacters* from diarrhoea samples of children. The first isolation of *C. jejuni* was done in Brussels, Belgium, from stool samples of a patient with diarrhoea.

❖ **Morphology:**

- **Type according to gram stain:** GNB (**fig.-1**).
- **Size:** 0.2-0.4 μm x 1.5 -5μm.
- **Shape:** Curved, typically comma shaped, S-shaped or in spiral (gull-wing) forms. Under light microscopy, *C. jejuni* has a characteristic "sea-gull" shape appearance as a consequence of its helical form. When exposed to atmospheric O_2, *C. jejuni* is able to change into a coccal form.

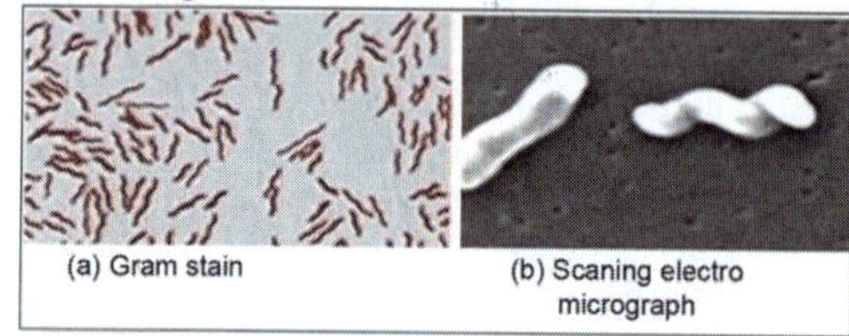

Figure-1: Morphology of *C. jejuni*

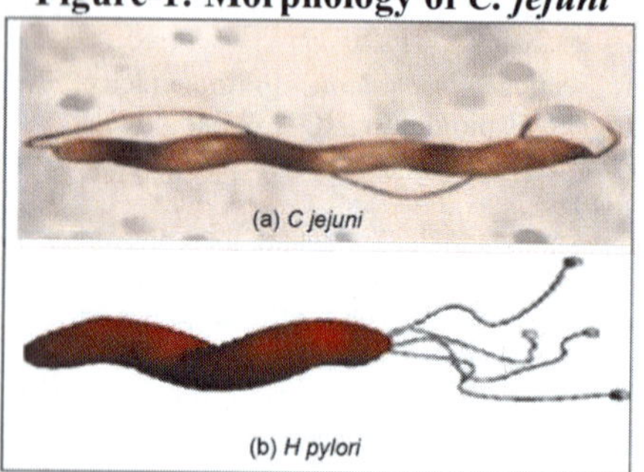

Figure-2: Arrangement of flagella in *C. jejuni* & in *H pylori*

- **Motility: Darting / tumbling motility** with single unsheathed polar flagellum at one end **called monotrichous** or both end **called amphitrichous** [**fig.-2(a)**]. Motility is better examined by DGIM or PCM.
- **Capsule & spores:** Nonsporing & non capsulated.

❖ **Cultural characteristics (C/Cs):**

- **Effective factors:**
  - O_2 effect: Microaerophilic (required O_2 less than environmental O_2 about 5%).
  - Temperature: Thermophilic & can grow at 42-43°C.
  - Growth occurs in incubation under 5% O_2, 10% CO_2, 85% nitrogen.
- **Media:**

A. Liquid media: Cary- Blair transport medium in which bacteria are survive for 1-2 weeks at 4^0C.

B. Solid media:

1. **Nutrient agar:**

2. **Blood agar (*Campylobacter* blood agar):** Non-haemolytic. Blood provides extra nutrition & also inhibits toxic materials forms during growth of bacteria. Charcoal is best substitute for blood.

C. Selective media:

1. Skirrow's medium.
2. Butzler's medium.
3. Campy BAP medium: Lysed bood agar with polymyxin B, amphotericin B, trimithoprim, vancomycin & cephalothin.
4. Modified Charcoal cefoperazone deoxycholate agar (CCDA) medium.
5. CVA medium: Medium contains cefoperazone, vancomycin & amphotericin B.

➢ **Growth properties:** Fresh colonies are flat, moist, translucent, 1-3 mm like water-drops.

❖ Biochemical reaction (B/Rs):

1. **Sugar fermentation test:** Non fermenters
2. **Catalase, oxidase & nitrate reduction test:** + Ve
3. **Hippurate hydrolysis & indoxyl acetate test:** +Ve
4. **H_2S production & urease test:** –Ve
5. **Sensitivity testing:**

- Nalidixic acid: Sensitive
- Cephalothin: Resistant

❖ Pathogenicity:

➢ **Disease name:** Whole spectrum of disease **called campylobacteriasis.** It is zoonosis & most common cause is *C jejuni.*

➢ **Nature & history of disease:** *C. jejuni* infections are extremely common worldwide, although exact figures are not available. New Zealand reported the highest national campylobacteriosis rate.

➢ **Reservoir of infection:** Animals like poultry, cattle, sheep, swine, dog, cat & some birds are the reservoirs. No human reservoir.

➢ **Source of infection:**

- Contaminated food or water which are infected by animal excreta.
- Infected animal products like unpasteurised milk, raw chicken etc.

➢ **Mode of transmission:** It is a zoonosis, human infection acquired by

- Ingestion of raw milk or raw chicken of infected animal.
- Ingestion of food/water contaminated by animal faeces as they are constantly shed in faeces.
- Direct contact with infected animals.
- Oral-anal sex.

➢ **Incubation period:** 1-7 days.

➢ **Portal of entry:** GIT

➢ **Sites:** Mostly intestinal (jejunum, ileum & colon) & extra-intestinal lesion is common in person with IDDs.

➢ **Precipitating factors (epidemiological determinants):**

I. Agent factors (virulence factors)

1. **Enterotoxin:** Same as heat labile toxin of *V. cholerae* enterotoxin
2. **Cytoledal distending toxin / cytotoxin (Shiga Like Toxin?):** No significant role, may be responsible for dysentery.
3. **Infective dose:** *Campylobacter* species are sensitive to the stomach's normal production of hydrochloric acid: as a result, the infectious dose is relatively high, and the bacteria rarely cause illness when a person is exposed to less 10^3 organisms. However for *C jejuni* infective dose is very less about 500 bacilli.
4. **Penetration:** Motility & spiral shape aids in penetration of GI mucosa.

II. Host factors

1. **Age:** *C. jejuni* in children & *C. fetus* in older age.
2. **Sex:** *Campylobacter* organisms are isolated more frequently from males than females. Homosexual men appear to be at increased risk.
3. **Economical status:** In developing countries present as asymptomatic infection except in children < 2 years while in developed countries it is the leading cause of diarrhoea than *Salmonella* & *Shigella.*
4. **Immunity:** Extra-intestinal lesion is common in person with IDDs.

III. Environmental factors

1. **Seasonal:** Peak incidence in summer & early autumn.

➢ **Pathogenesis: → Flow chart-2**

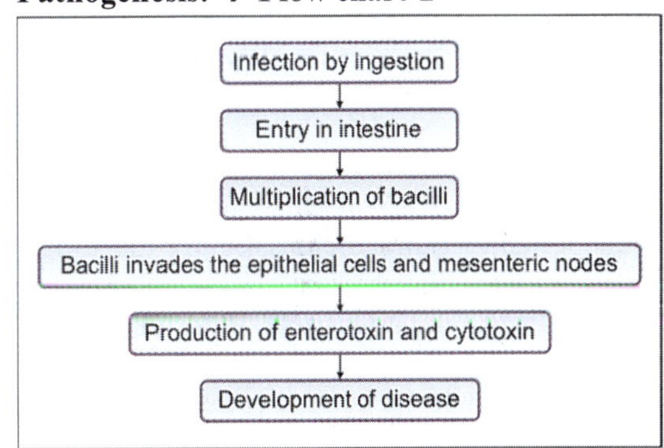

Flow chart-2: Pathogenesis of *C. jejuni*

➢ **Clinical features:**

1. **Intestinal:**

- Illness start with fever, abdominal pain and watery-diarrhoea contains blood (WBC).
- Last for 1-2 weeks & self limiting.

2. **Extra-intestinal:** Very rare but may produce the bacteremia, septicemia, meningitis & vascular infections like endocarditis, aneurysm & thrombophlebitis in immunocompromised hosts.

➢ **Complications:**

Test	C. jejuni	C. coli	C. lari	C. fetus	C. curvus
Growth at 25°C	-	-	-	+	-
Growth at 42°C	+	+	+	-	+/-
Catalase	+	+	+	+	-
H_2S	-	-	-	-	+
Hippurate hydrolysis	+	-	-	-	-
Indoxyl acetate hydrolysis	+	+	-	-	+
Nalidixic acid sensitivity	S	S	R	R	S
Cephalothin sensitivity	R	R	R	S	Not useful

Table-1: Tests to differentiate between *Campylobacter* species

1. **Gastrointestinal perforation**
2. **Haemolytic uremic syndrome**
3. **Thromocytopenic purpura**
4. **GBS (Guillain Barre Syndrome):**
- It is an acute paralytic disease of peripheral nervous system.
- Mainly caused by serotype O19.
- It appears after 1-2 weeks of infection.
- It develops in 0.3 per 1000 infection. 20-40% GBS cases are due to *C. jejuni.*
5. **Septic abortion**
6. **Reactive arthritis**
7. **α-Chain disease:** Lymphoma occurs in MALT.
8. **Periodonitis.**

❖ Laboratory diagnosis:

➢ **Specimens:** Stool or rectal swab.

➢ **Collection & transport:** Collect in Cary-Blair medium & transport immediately to laboratory followed by subculture on solid & selective media.

➢ **Testing methods:**

1. **Microscopy: → Follow morphology**
2. **Culture: → Follow C/Cs**
3. **Biochemical reaction: → Follow B/Rs**
4. **Molecular method:** PCR is useful.
5. **Differentiation of *C. jejuni* from related species: → Table-1**

❖ Prevention:

- Frequent hand washing before & after touching the animal products like chicken.
- Do not drink unpasteurized milk or untreated surface water.
- All poultry should be cooked to reach a minimum internal temperature of 165°F (74°C).

❖ Treatment:

1. **Oral rehydration therapy:** To replace the fluid & electrolytes loss.
2. **Antibiotics:** Erythromycin is the drug of choice.

C. coli & C. lari

➢ ***C. coli:*** Causes the same illness as like *C. jejuni* & differentiated by negative hippurate hydrolysis test

➢ ***C. lari:*** Produces the same illness as like *C. jejuni* & differentiated from *C. jejuni* & *C. coli* by resistance to nalidixic acid.

Mesophilic *Campylobacter*

A. Catalase +Ve group: → *C. fetus*

- **Mode of transmission:** By faeco-oral route.
- **Extra intestinal disease:** Like bacteraemia, septicemia & meningitis in hosts with IDDs.

B. Catalase –Ve group: → *C. curvus, C. concisus, C. sputorum* & *C. mucosalis*

- Dental infection, root canal & abscess in other tissues.

Arcobacter

- Species: *A. cryophilis, A. butzleri* & *A. nitrofigilis.*
- GNB, spiral shape, motile by unsheathed polar flagella.
- Aerotolerant.
- Grow at 15-25°C.
- Catalase & Nitrate : +Ve
- Hippurate hydrolysis: -Ve
- Indoxyl acetate hydrolysis: +Ve
- Nalidixic acid: Sensitive
- Cephalothin: Resistance
- Produce diarrhoeal disease similar to *C. jejuni.*

Helicobacter

H pylori

❖ **Synonyms:** Formerly **called *Campylobacter pylori*** but in 1989, Goodwin *et al.* published sufficient reasons to justify the new genus name *Helicobacter.*

❖ **Meaning: Genus name** (*Helicobacter)* is because of its helical shape & **species name**, because of genitive (close association) to pylorus (pylorus = circular opening of stomach in duodenum).

❖ **History:** It was identified in 1982 by Australian scientists Barry Marshall & Robin Warren, from the person with chronic gastritis and gastric ulcers.

❖ **Uses:** Mucosal colonisation by *H pylori* has protective role & it minimise the occurrence of
- Gastroeosphageal reflux disease.
- Barret's oesophagus.
- Adenocarcinoma of oesophagus.
- Allergic disease like asthma.

❖ **Morphology**

➢ **Type according to gram stain:** GNB under gram stain [**fig.-3(a)**]. Also stained by Giemsa stain or H & E stain, basic fuchsin stain [**fig.-3(b)**], Warthin–Starry silver stain [**fig.-3(c)**], acridine orange stain & phase-contrast microscopy.

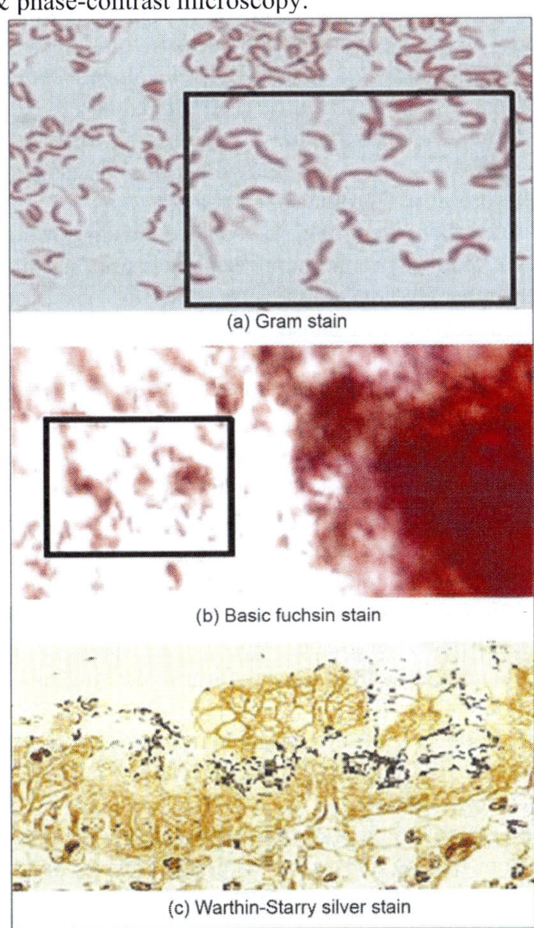

Figure-3: Morphology of *H. pylori*

➢ **Size:** 0.5-0.9 μm x 2.5-3 μm.

➢ **Shape:** Spiral / helical shaped.

➢ **Motility:** Motile with tuft (4-8 in numbers) of sheathed flagella at one pole **called lophotrichous** [**fig.-2(b)**], best seen in liquid medium.

❖ **Cultural characteristics (C/Cs):**

➢ **Effective factors:**
- O_2 effect: Microaerophilic (required O_2 less than environmental O_2 about 5%).
- Optimum temperature: 37°C, some strains can grow at 42-43°C.
- pH: 6.7
- Growth occur in incubation under 5% O_2, 10% CO_2, 85% nitrogen.

➢ **Media:**

A. **Liquid media:**
1. **Peptone water:** Useful for motility detection.
2. ***Brucella* broth:** Contains 1-10% horse or fetal calf serum.

B. **Solid media:** Like
- Blood agar.
- Chocolate agar.
- BHIA with 5% horse blood.
- Tryptose soya agar with 5% sheep blood.
- *Brucella* agar with 5% sheep blood.

C. **Selective media:**
1. Make above solid media selective by adding vancomycin + nalidixic acid + AMB.
2. Campylobacter selective media like Skirrow's medium is also useful.

✪ **Growth properties:** Small colonies develop in 3-7 days.

❖ **Biochemical reaction (B/Rs):**
1. **Sugar fermentation test:** Non fermenters.
2. **Phosphatase, catalase, oxidase test:** + Ve
3. **H_2S Production:** + Ve
4. **Urease test:** Strong positive in a minutes, tested from gastric mucosa.
5. **Nitrate reduction:** -Ve
6. **Nalidixic acid:** Resistance.
7. **Cephalothin:** Sensitive.

❖ **Pathogenicity:**

➢ **Reservoir of infection:** Human is the only reservoir. Only animal infected is monkey.

➢ **Source of infection:** Water contaminated from the faeces of case. Also saliva & gastric mucus.

➢ **Mode of transmission:** It colonise about 50% of human gastric antrum. *H. pylori* are contagious. Exact route is not known, person-to-person transmission by either the oral–oral, oro-gastic (by gastric mucus) or faeco–oral route is most likely. Consistent with these transmission routes, the bacteria have been isolated from faeces, saliva, and dental plaque of some infected people. Transmission occurs mainly within families in developed nations, yet can also be transmitted orally by means of faecal matter through the ingestion of waste-tainted water in developing countries.

➢ **Incubation period:** Few days.

➢ **Portal of entry:** GIT.

➢ **Sites:** It colonises any part of stomach but gastric antrum is the most common site of infection. It colonises the part of oesophagus & duodenum commonly exposed to acid.

➢ **Precipitating factors (epidemiological determinants):**

I. Agent factors (virulence factors)

1. **Motility:** To avoid the acidic environment of the interior of the stomach (lumen), *H. pylori* uses its flagella to burrow into the mucus lining of the stomach to reach the epithelial cells underneath, where it is less acidic.
2. **Adhesin:** Organ of adhesion.
3. **Toxin:** Vacuolating cytotoxin produces the injury to host cells & responsible for ulcer. It is regulated by vacuolating cytotoxin gene.
4. **Urease production:**
- It split urea to ammonia which buffers the gastric acidity & provides protection to the bacilli. It locally raises the pH from about 2 to a more biocompatible range of 6 to 7.
- Enzyme urease is 100 times more active than produced by *Pr vulgaris.*
- Antiurease antibodies are not formed.
5. **Amidase & arginase:** May contribute in production of ammonia.
6. **Molecular mimicry:** Cross reactivity between antigen of gastric mucosa & organism allows the formation of autoantibody responsible for chronic active gastritis.
7. **Cag pathogenicity island:** It is a group of genes (**called cytokine associated genes**) helps in colonisation of bacteria by following mechanisms
- It encode for a specific protein **called Cag A protein.**
- Cag A protein injected by *H pylori* in to the gastric epithelial cells which release the cytokines (IL-1β is the major cytokine) causing cytoskeletal changes & proliferation thereby enabling *H pylori* to colonise the gastric epithelium.
- Cag A gene is highly immunogenic, associated with peptic ulcer disease or gastric adenocarcinoma & patient with peptic ulcer disease or gastric adenocarcinoma have antibodies to Cag A gene.

✓ **Note:** *H pylori* & *H influenzae* are the bacteria whose complete genome has been mapped.

II. Host factors

1. **Age:**
- Common in adult.
- *H pylori* are acquired in childhood but immunity does not develop & prevalence increase with age. Childhood is a risk factor for *H pylori* colonisation.
- People infected in early age are likely to develop more intense inflammation that may be followed by atrophic gastritis with a higher subsequent risk of gastric ulcer, gastric cancer or both. Acquisition at an older age brings different gastric changes more likely to lead to duodenal ulcer.
2. **Smoking:** Increases risk of ulcer & cancer.
3. **Diet:** Preserved food & diet rich in salt increase the risk of cancer while diet rich in vitamin C & antioxidants are protective.
4. **Immunity:** Infection induce the AMI (local & systemic antibodies) & CMI, but not protective.

III. Environmental factors

1. **Economical status:** However, over 80% of individuals infected with the bacterium are asymptomatic, and it may play an important role in the natural stomach ecology. More than 50% of the world's population harbour *H. pylori* in their upper gastrointestinal tract. Infection is more common in developing countries than Western countries. Low prevalence (30% in adult) in developed countries than developing countries (80% in adult).
2. **Other contributory factors are:** Low socioeconomic status, crowding, poor hygiene etc.

➢ **Pathology:** Chronic superficial gastritis.
- Bacteria present over the surface but do not invade the cell. Chronic superficial gastritis is due to primary colonisation not due to re-infection. Reinfection can cause chronic gastritis but rate is very low about 0.5% per year.
- It also **called type B gastritis** (Type A gastritis is due to pernicious anaemia) or **chronic active gastritis.**
- Antral gastritis is linked with duodenal ulcer while pangastritis is linked with gastric ulcer (peptic ulcer) & gastric adenocarcinoma.
- Infection remain lifelong if remain untreated.

➢ **Clinical features:**
- Dyspepsia, stomach (abdominal) pain, nausea, bloating, belching & sometimes vomiting or black stool.
- Pain usually occurs on empty stomach in mid night or in early morning. Pain relieved little after meal.

➢ **Complications:**
1. **Peptic ulcer & duodenal ulcer:** *H pylori* detected from 66% & 77% cases of peptic ulcer & duodenal ulcer respectively.
2. **Chronic atrophic gastritis**
3. **Hypergastrinemia:**
- Gastrin is the hormone released by stomach wall in the blood. It stimulates the secretion of gastric juice.
- Release of gastrin is controlled by somatostatin.
- Antral colonisation of *H pylori*, diminish the somatostatin producing cell, **called D cells** → Decrease release of somatostatin → Loss of inhibitory control over gastrin release → Increase gastrin release **called hypergastrinemia.**
4. **Malignancies:**
- Gastric carcinoma.

- Mucosa Associated Lymphoid Tissue (MALT) lymphoma: Risk is lowered with successful treatment of *H pylori.*

❖ Laboratory diagnosis:

➢ **Specimens:**
- For culture (highly specific but less sensitive because of difficulties in isolation of *H pylori*): Gastric mucosa & vomitus.
- For serology: Stool & blood.
- Molecular: Stool, dental plaque, water & gastric juice.

➢ **Testing methods:** Two types of tests.

a. **Invasive:**

1. **Gastric mucosa collected by endoscopy: → Flow chart-3**

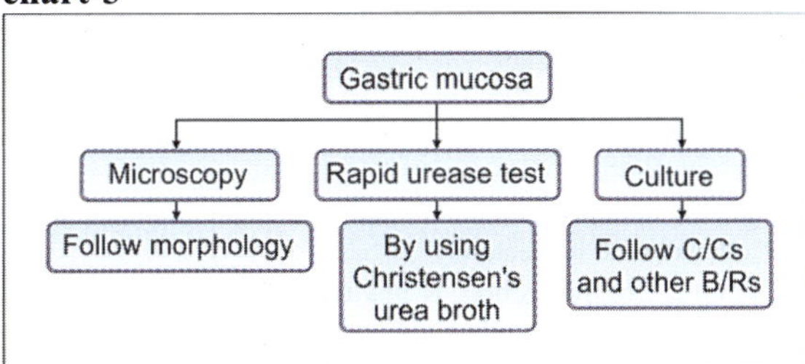

Flow chart-3: Testing of gastric mucosa

b. **Non invasive:**

1. **Urea breath test:**
- **Steps:** Patient drink ^{13}Carbon or ^{14}Carbon - labelled urea solution & then blow in a tube. If urease is present, the urea will be hydrolyses which can be detected in breath film by spectroscopy.
- **Advantages:**
  - Most sensitive (> 90%) & specific (> 90%).
  - Reliable method.
  - Uses to monitor the treatment: It is useful in follow up after treatment & test becomes negative after improvement following antibiotics.
  - Most consistent method.
- **Disadvantage:** It will be positive with massive infection.

2. **Serological tests:**
- **Antigen detection test from stool (coproantigen):**
  - By ELISA.
  - Less accurate than urea breath test.
- **Antibody detection from blood:** Collected by venepuncture → Centrifugation → Separate serum → Detection of IgG by ELISA or by immuno blot assay, but less useful.

3. **Molecular test:** PCR from stool, dental plaque, water & gastric juice.

❖ Prevention:

- Improvement in hygiene.
- Vaccine is under trial to prevent the cancer & other complications.

❖ Treatment:

➢ **Indication:** Neither in asymptomatic person nor as a prophylaxis but in person with
- Duodenal or peptic ulcer.
- Low grade Mucosa Associated Lymphoid Tissue (MALT) lymphoma: Treatment given for *H pylori* can cause regression of gastric lymphoma.

➢ **Therapy: → Flow chart-4**

Other *Helicobacters*

- *H. heilmanii*: Human & animal infection.
- *H. cinnaedi* & *H. fennelliae*: opportunistic pathogen in HIV patient.

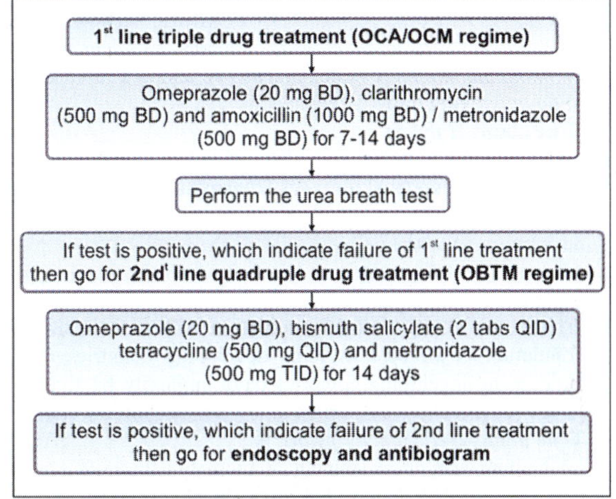

Flow chart-4: Treatment of *H pylori*

Question bank

Case study

1) A 40 year male presented to medical OPD with complain of abdominal pain at mid night which gets relieved on meal. Gram stain of stool revealed helical/spiral shaped GNB. Gastric mucosa collected by endoscopy gives urease test positive. Identify the case & answer the following
a) Name the causative agent of clinical condition
b) Describe the morphology, culture characteristics & biochemical reactions of causative agent
c) Write the pathogenicity of causative agent

Short notes

1) Pathogenicity or Lab. diagnosis of *C. jejuni*
2) Pathogenicity or Lab. diagnosis of *H. pylori*

Short questions for theory/viva questions

1) Name two selective media, each for *C. jejuni* & *H. pylori*

MCQs for chapter review

C. jejuni

1) *Campylobacter* culture media are- (PGI, Dec-08)
(a) Schadlar's agar (b) CVA medium (c) Regan Lowe medium (d) Skirrow's medium (e) *Campylobacter* blood agar

2) All are true statement about *Campylobacter jejuni* except- (AIIMS, Nov-09, May-11)

(a) Human is the only reservoir (b) Can cause GB syndrome (c) Poultry is the source of infection (d) Common cause of campylobacteriasis

H pylori

3) **True about *H pylori*** (AIIMS-97)
(a) Vacuolating cytotoxin (b) Antiurease antibody detection specific for type I (c) Found in jejunum (d) Treatment is A1(OH) 2

4) **True about *H pylori* is all except** (PGI, June -2000)
(a) It split urea & produces ammonia to survive (b) Produces gastric carcinoma (c) Gram -ve curved rods (d) Cag A gene is not associated with risk of duodenal ulcer

5) **Seven sheathed flagella is seen in**
(a) *V cholerae* (b) *H pylori* (c) *Ps aeruginosa* (d) Spirochetes

6) **All are true regarding *H pylori* except** (AIIMS, Sept-96, Feb-97)
(a) Less prevalent in developing countries (b) Ulcer is caused by toxigenic strains (c) Urea breath +ve test is a rapid method of detection (d) Gram –ve organism

7) **True about *H pylori*** (AIIMS-97)
(a) Seen in 85 to 90% cases of gastric ulcer (b) Seen in 20 to 25% cases of duodenal ulcer (c) Transmitted from man to man, faeco-orally & by orogastric route (d) Common in adults of developing countries

8) **All of the following are true about *Helicobacter pylori* except** (AI -98)
(a) About 50% of world population affected (b) 85% of population is affected in some developing countries (c) All children in developing countries have immunity by five years of age (d) Infection is common in low socioeconomic status

9) **True about *Helicobacter pylori* is** (AI -98)
(a) Culture and gram staining of biopsy is the gold standard investigation (b) Controlled urea breath is negative with massive infection (c) Anti urease antibody are produced only by invasive strains (d) Urease activity provides protective environment to the bacilli

10) **Non invasive test for *H pylori*** (PGI, May -13, June 08)
(a) Rapid urease test (b) Urease breath test (c) Stool antigen assay (d) Stomach aspiration culture (e) Biopsy

11) ***H pylori* true about** (PGI, June -2004)
(a) Gram +ve spiral organism (b) It is a protozoa (c) Causes chronic gastritis in adult due to reinfection (d) Treatment causes regression of gastric lymphoma (e) Duodenal mucosa normal

12) **Regarding *H pylori* all are true except** (PGI, June -2002)
(a) Gram -ve bacillus (b) Strongly associated with duodenal ulcer (c) Associated with lymphoma (d) C-14 urea breath test is used in diagnosis (e) It should be eradicated in all cases whenever detected

13) **True about *H pylori*** (PGI, June -2004)
(a) It is flagellated (b) Involved in peptic ulcer disease (c) Hypergastrinemia caused by it (d) Eradication leads to improved life style (e) It is gram –ve organism

14) **True about *H pylori* is all except** (AI-98)
(a) Urea breath test is diagnostic (b) Gram negative flagellate bacilli (c) Risk factor for development of adenocarcinoma (d) It provides lifelong immunity

Answers of MCQs & explanation

1. **(b), (d) & (e)**
- Follow section, ***C. jejuni* [Cultural characteristics (C/Cs)]** of *C jejuni* for explanation

2. **(b)**
- Campylobacteriasis is the zoonosis where animals like poultry, cattle, sheep, swine, dog, cat & some birds are the reservoir & no human reservoir
- Common complication is GB syndrome
- Source is raw milk or raw chicken
- *C jejuni* is the most common cause of campylobacteriasis

3. **(a)**
- Vacuolating cytotoxin produces the injury to host cells & responsible for ulcer
- Antiurease antibody is not formed
- Option c: Follow section, ***H pylori* (pathogenicity →sites)** for explanation
- A1(OH) 2 is not used in treatment

4. **(d)**
- Cag A gene is highly immunogenic, associated with peptic ulcer disease or gastric adenocarcinoma & patient with peptic ulcer disease or gastric adenocarcinoma have antibodies to Cag A gene

5. **(b)**
- *H pylori* is motile by lophotrichous flagella
- *V cholerae* & *Ps aeruginosa* are motile by monotrichous flagella
- Spirochetes have endoflagella

6. **(a)**
- Low prevalence (30% in adult) of *H pylori* in developed countries than developing countries (80% in adult)

7. **(c)**
- *H pylori* detected from 66% & 77% cases of peptic ulcer & duodenal ulcer respectively
- Option c: Follow section, ***H pylori* (pathogenicity → mode of transmission)** for explanation
- Option d: Follow section, ***H pylori* (pathogenicity → host factors)** for explanation

8. **(c)**
- Follow section, ***H pylori* (pathogenicity → precipitating factors → host factors & environmental factors)** for explanation

9. **(d)**
- Culture is highly specific but less sensitive because of difficulties in isolation of *H pylori,* so its not the gold standard
- Controlled urea breath is positive with massive infection
- Anti urease antibody are not produced only by invasive strains
- Urease split urea to ammonia which buffers the gastric acidity & provide protection to the bacilli

10. **(b) & (c)**
- Follow section, ***H pylori* (laboratory diagnosis)** for explanation

11. **(d)**
- It is gram –Ve helical / curved bacteria
- It is not protozoa but bacteria
- Chronic superficial gastritis is due to primary colonisation not due to re-infection. Reinfection can cause chronic gastritis but rate is very low about 0.5% per year
- MALT is caused by *H pylori* & treatment given for *H pylori* can cause regression of gastric lymphoma
- Duodenal mucosa is not normal because *H pylori* can damage duodenal mucosa

12. **(e)**
13. **(a), (b), (c), (d) & (e)**
14. **(d)**

} Follow section, ***H pylori*** for explanation of all options

49 Non-fermenters

Learning heading & subheadings

- Synonym:
- Definition:
- Classification:
  - **Pseudomonas**
    - *Pseudomonas aeruginosa*
    - Other species of *Pseudomonas*
  - **Burkholderia**
    - *Bukholderia cepacia*
    - *Bukholderia mallei*
    - *Bukholderia pseudomallei*
  - ***Alcaligenes faecalis***
  - ***Stenotrophomonas maltophila***
  - ***Flavobacterium meningosepticum***
  - ***Legionella pneumophila***

Synonym: Non-fermenting bacteria

Definition: Non-fermenters are a taxonomically heterogeneous group of bacteria that cannot catabolise glucose & are thus unable to ferment. This does not necessarily exclude that species can catabolise other sugars or have anaerobiosis like fermenting bacteria.

Classification: →**Flow chart-1**

Pseudomonas

Pseudomonas aeruginosa

❖ **Synonym:** *Pseudomonas pyocyanea* or *Bacillus pyocyaneus*

❖ **Morphology:** → **Fig.1**

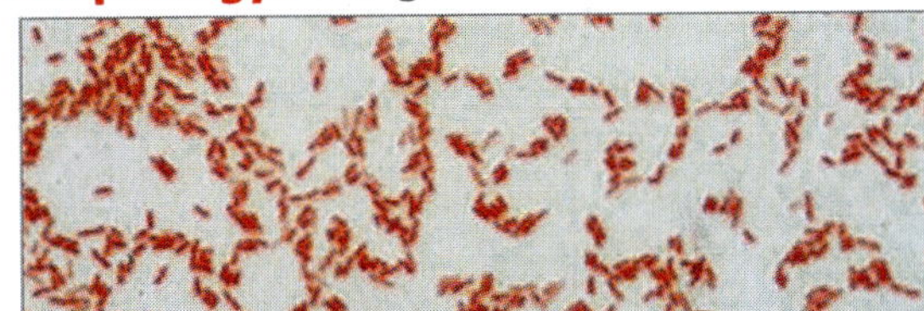

Figure-1: Morphology of *P. aerugoinosa*

- **Type according to gram stain:** GNB.
- **Size:** 0.5μm x 1.5–3μm.
- **Shape:** Short road.
- **Arrangement:** Singly or in pairs or in small group.
- **Motility:** Motile by monotrichous flagellum.
- **Capsule:** Non-capsulated but have slime layer made up by polysaccharide with glycocalyx.
- **Spore:** Non-sporing.
- **Fimbriae:** Present in some clinical isolates.

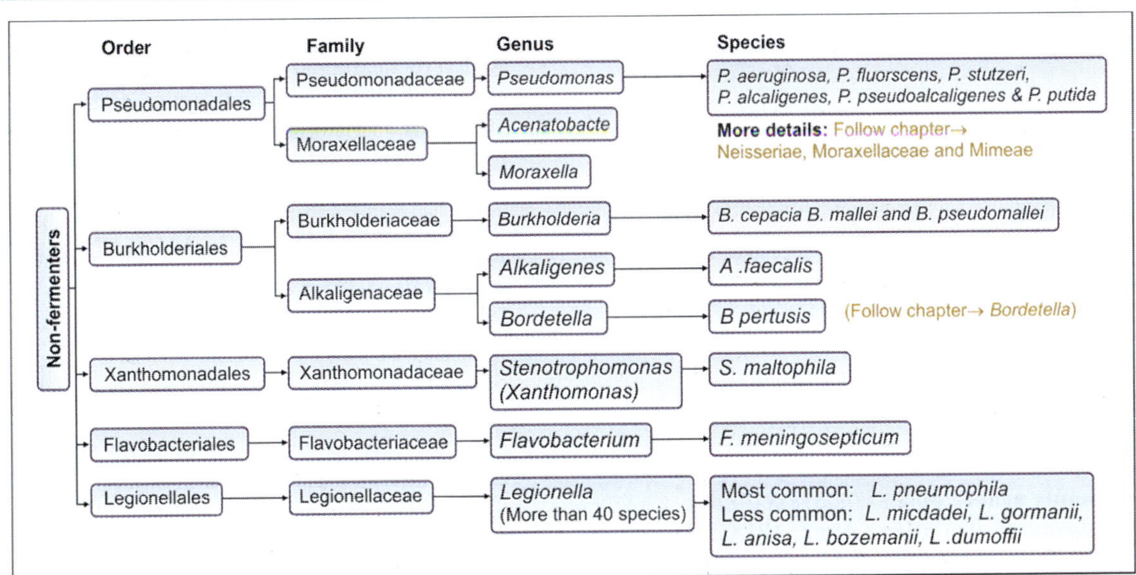

Flow chart-1: Classification of non-fermenters

❖ Cultural characteristics (C/Cs):

➢ **Effective factors:**

- O_2 effect: Strict aerobes can grow anaerobically if nitrate is available.
- Temperature: Optimum temperature is 37°C (6-42°C).
- pH: Neutral pH is required.

➢ **Culture in media:**

A. Liquid media:

1. **Peptone water:** Dense turbidity with surface pellicle.
2. **Enrichment medium:** *Pseudomonas* enrichment broth.

B. Solid media:

i. Nutrient agar plate / slant:

✪ **Growth properties:** Colonies are large, pigmented, opaque & irregular with distinctive musty, mawkish, earthy or sweet grape like odour.

✪ **Pigment production:**

- **Properties of pigments:**

- Diffusible in nature (unlike *Staphylococcus* where pigment is non diffusible) & spread in whole medium from the site of inoculation.
- 10% strains are non-pigmented.

- **Types:** Four types

1. **Pyocyanin: → Fig.2(a)**

- Bluish green phenazine pigment soluble in water and chloroform.
- Produced only by *P. aeruginosa*.
- Inhibits the growth of many other bacteria and makes the organism dominant in mixed infections.

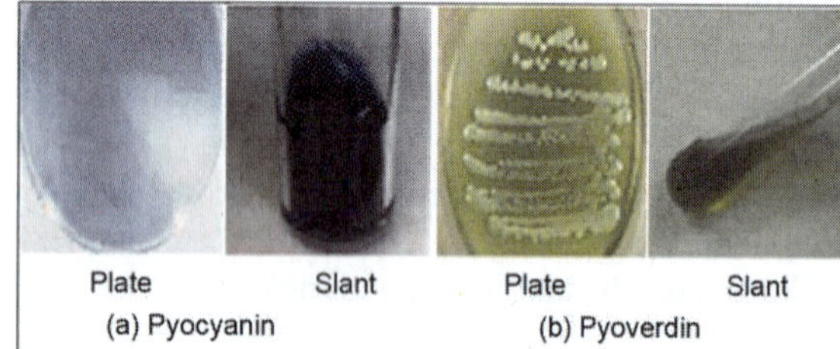

Figure-2: Pigments of *P. aerugoinosa*

2. **Pyoverdin (Fluorescein): → Fig.2(b)**

- Greenish yellow pigment soluble in water but not in chloroform.
- Fluorescein may be produced by other species.
- In old cultures oxidised to yellowish brown pigment.

3. **Pyorubin:** Red in colour.
4. **Pyomelanin:** Brown in colour.

ii. Blood agar: Some strains are haemolytic.

C. Selective media:

1. **Mac Conkey's agar [fig.3(a)]:** } Pale colonies due to NLF
2. **DCA:** }
3. **Cetrimide agar:** Contains 0.03% cetrimide.
4. ***Pseudomonas* Isolation Agar (PIA):** Contains irgasan as selective agent.

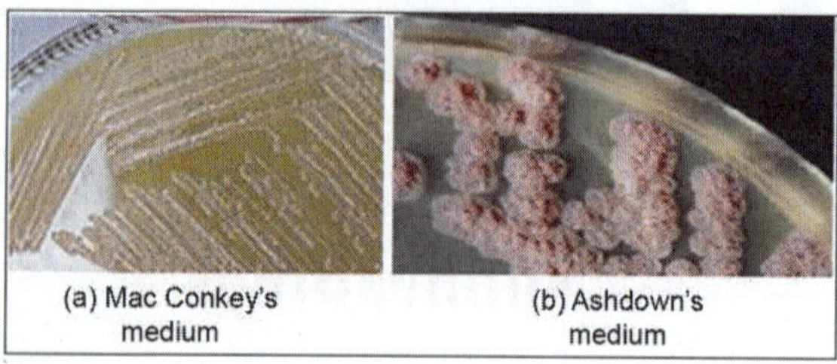

Figure-3: (a) Pale colonies on Mac Conkey's agar by ***P. aeruginosa*** **(b)** Wrinkled purple colonies on Ashdown's medium by ***B. pseudomallei***

D. Media for production & identification of pigments:

1. **Pyocyanin:** Medium P & PIA (selective) are useful for pigment identification.
2. **Pyoverdin (fluorescein):** King's medium B.
3. **Pyorubin:** 1% DL-Glutamate medium.
4. **Pyomelanin:** Furunculosis agar, Davis-Mingioli's mineral salt medium [1% tyrosine].

❖ Biochemical reactions (B/Rs):

1. **Sugar fermentation tests:**

- Non-fermentative but oxidative.
- Oxidised the sugar & produce acid only**.** Sugar is only carbon source
- Peptone water is unsuitable to detect weak acid production, so Hugh & Leifson's (**oxidative-fermentation test**) medium with glucose is useful to detect weak acid production from sugar.

2. **I M Vi C tests: - - - +**
3. **Catalase test:** +Ve
4. **Nitrate reduction test:** + Ve
5. **Oxidase test:** +Ve
6. **H_2S production:** -Ve
7. **Urease test:** -Ve
8. **TSI:** K/Nil or K/K (no change in butt, because non-fermentive & alkaline in slant).
9. **Arginine decarboxylase test:** +Ve

❖ Resistance:

- Killed by heating at 55^0C in 1 hour.
- Resistant to common antiseptics and disinfectants such as quaternary ammonium compounds, chloroxylenol and hexachlorophene. It can grow in bottles of antiseptics like dettol, iodine, cetrimide lotions or soap lotion etc. kept for use in hospitals. Indeed, dettol or cetrimide is incorporated in a media selective for *P aeruginosa*.
- Resistant to many antibiotics **called multidrug resistant or pan drug resistant.**
- Sensitive to acids, beta glutaraldehyde, silver salts and strong phenolic disinfectants.
- Susceptibility to silver: Use of silver sulphonamide compounds as topical cream in burns.

❖ Typing:

Two types of method for typing of bacilli.

A Phenotyping methods:

1. **Serotyping:** 27 serotypes based on O Ag. Less useful because less discriminatory power.
2. **Antibiogram typing:** More useful methods.
3. **Bacteriophage typing:** Less useful because less discriminatory power.
4. **Bacteriocin typing:**
- Bacteriocin **called pyocin** or **called aeruginosin** with three types like R, F & S.
- 105 types are identified based on growth inhibition of indicator strain by pyocin.
- Less useful because less discriminatory power.

B Genotyping methods: Pulsed field gel electrophoresis is best useful because more discriminatory power.

❖ Pathogenicity:

➢ **Reservoir & source of infection:**
- Widely available in hospital environment.
- It can survive & multiply even with minimal nutrients, if moisture is available.
- **Equipments** such as respirators, endoscopes & stitch materials, **articles** such as hospital-bed & cloths, **medicines** such as lotions, creams & eye-ear drops & even **stocks** of distilled water, plants & flowers may be frequently contaminated.

➢ **Mode of transmission:** Direct from environment or contaminated hospital materials.

➢ **Portal of entry:** Skin, respiratory system etc.

➢ **Sites:** Skin, soft tissues, GIT, blood, respiratory system etc.

➢ **Precipitating factors (epidemiological determinants):**

I. Agent factors (virulence factors)

A. Intracellular (cell wall associated):

i. Antigens:
1. Somatic (O) Ag:
2. Flagellar (H) Ag: Organ of locomotion.
3. Slime layer act as capsule: Inhibit phagocytosis.
4. Fimbriae: Organ of adhesion.

ii. Antibiotic resistance: Due to alteration in cell wall & porin channel. Resistance to common antibiotics & antiseptics, establish itself widely in hospitals.

iii. Ability to form biofilms:

B. Extracellular:

i. Pyocyanin pigment:
- Stop ciliary movement of respiratory epithelium & prevent bacteria from host defense.
- Inhibit growth of other bacteria & makes the bacterium dominant in mixed infection.
- Catalyses production of superoxide & H_2O_2.

ii. Toxins:
1. Exotoxin A, S, T, U & Y: A act as NADase. It acts like diphtheria toxin & inhibits the protein synthesis by inhibiting the elongation factor -2 (EF-2).
2. Enterotoxin: Causing collection of fluid in ligated rabbit illeal loop.
3. Haemolysin

✓ **Notes: Toxins act by inhibiting the protein synthesis**
- Diphtheria toxin: } By inactivation of EF-2
- *Pseudomonas* toxin:
- Shiga like toxin (SLT): } By inactivation of 60S ribosome
- Shiga toxin:

iii. Enzymes:
1. Phospholipidase: Breaks down lipids & lecithin facilitating tissue destruction.
2. Elastase: Degrade elastin → damage of lung parenchyma & haemorrhagic lesions
3. Protease: Help to spread in tissues

II. Host factors

1. **Immunity:** It is the common cause of life threatening fever in person with IDDs.
2. **Prolonged hospitalisation:** It favours the infection.

III. Environmental factors

Common in hospital environmental as mentioned earlier.

➢ **Clinical features:** Two types

a. Community acquired infection (outside hospital in community):
1. **Ear infection:** Otitis media. It is the most common agent to cause suppurative otitis media outside the hospital.
2. **Intestinal:** Infantile diarrhoea due to heat labile enterotoxin.
3. **Respiratory tract infection:** Most common cause of respiratory infection in cystic fibrosis patient.
4. **Shanghai fever:** Self limited febrile illness resembling typhoid fever.

b. Hospital acquired (nosocomial) infection: It includes following types
1. **Localised infections (blue pus → fruity odour) of:**
- Traumatic wound.
- Burn wound: Most common agent to cause infection in burns.
- Bed sore.
- Ecthyma gangrenosum & many other skin lesions are occurs in patients with leukemia & malignancy. It occurs singly or in small number on the perineum, buttock & extremities.
- Eye infections.
- Brain abscess.
- Nail bed infection following excessive exposure of hands to detergents & water.
2. **Generalised infections:** Septicemia & endocarditis in debilitated patients.
3. **Iatrogenic infections:**
- Meningitis following lumbar puncture.
- UTI following catheterisation.

i. **Microscopy:** → **Follow morphology**
ii. **Culture:** → **Follow C/Cs**
iii. **Biochemical reactions:** → **Follow B/Rs**
iv. **Serological tests:** Following are useful tests
- Latex agglutination test.
- Indirect Haem Agglutination test (IHA).
- ELISA for IgG & IgM detection.

v. **Molecular test:** PCR.

❖ **Prevention:** Strict aseptic precautions to control the infection.

❖ **Treatment:** Same as *B. mallei.*

Alcaligenes faecalis

❖ **Meaning:**
- **Genus name:** Because **non fermenters & gives alkaline reaction** in litmus milk test.
- **Species name:** Because **identified from faeces.**

❖ **Morphology:**
- **Staining properties:** GNB.
- **Shape:** Short rod.
- **Motility:** Motile by peritrichous flagella.

❖ **Cultural characteristics (C/Cs):**
- **Effective factors:** Strict aerobes.
- **Media:**

1. **Blood agar:** Some strains produce the colonies with greenish discolouration & fruity odour (green apple odour).
2. **Mac Conkey's agar:** Most strains produce the thin & spreading colonies with irregular edge.

❖ **Biochemical reaction (B/Rs):**
1. **Sugar fermentation test:** Non fermentative but oxidative.
2. **Citrate test:** +Ve
3. **Oxidase test:** +Ve
4. **Nitrate reduction:** +Ve
5. **Urease test:** -Ve

❖ **Pathogenicity:**
- **Reservoir & source of infection:** Soil & water saprophytes including IV fluid. Hospital contaminant in respirators, nebulizer etc. Commensals in human & animal intestine.
- **Clinical features:**
  - Causing nosocomial infections like UTI.
  - Common lesions produced are gastroenteritis, typhoid like fever & local sepsis.
  - Also cause opportunistic infections like otitis media, meningitis & pneumonia.

❖ **Laboratory diagnosis:** Faeces, blood, urine, pus etc. are tested by microscopy, culture & by B/Rs as described above.

❖ **Treatment:** Fluoroquinolones & nalidixic acid are the sensitive drugs.

Stenotrophomonas maltophila

❖ **Synonym:** Previously **called** ***Pseudomonas maltophila.***

❖ **Morphology:** GNB, 0.7–1.8 × 0.4–0.7 μm in size & motile due to polar flagella.

❖ **C/Cs:**
- Aerobes.
- Grow well on Mac Conkey's agar producing pigmented colonies.

❖ **B/Rs:**
- Non fermentative but utilise the sugar oxidatively.
- Catalase positive.
- Oxidase test: -Ve (non-oxidative).
- Lysin decarboxylation test: +Ve.

❖ **Pathogenicity:**
- **Reservoir & source of infection:** It is ubiquitous in aqueous environments, soil, and plants. It is a rhizosphere (present in soil surrounding the plant root).
- **Precipitating factors:**

✪ **Virulence factors:**
- Resistant to many broad-spectrum antibiotics by efflux pump mechanism & to carbapenems due to the production of two inducible chromosomal metallo-β-lactamases (designated L1 and L2).
- LPS responsible for endotoxic activities.

✪ **Host factors:**
- It is associated with high morbidity & mortality in severely immunocompromised & debilitated individuals. Risk factors include cystic fibrosis, HIV -AIDS, malignancy, neutropenia, mechanical ventilation, central venous catheters, recent surgery, trauma, prolonged hospitalization, intensive care unit admission and broad-spectrum antibiotic use.
- *S. maltophilia* colonization rates in individuals with cystic fibrosis have been increasing.

- **Clinical features:**
  - **Nosocomial infections like** pneumonia in ventilated patient, UTI, septicemia & wound infections.
  - **Opportunistic infections like** ecthyma gangrenosum in neutropenic patients.

❖ **Laboratory diagnosis:** Bacteria are diagnosed from blood, urine, sputum samples by microscopy, culture & biochemical tests.

❖ **Treatment:** Multi drug resistant & useful antibiotics are tigecycline & polymyxin B. Antibiogram requires nonstandard culture methods (incubation at 30 °C). Testing at the wrong

1. **Serotyping:** 27 serotypes based on O Ag. Less useful because less discriminatory power.
2. **Antibiogram typing:** More useful methods.
3. **Bacteriophage typing:** Less useful because less discriminatory power.
4. **Bacteriocin typing:**
- Bacteriocin **called pyocin** or **called aeruginosin** with three types like R, F & S.
- 105 types are identified based on growth inhibition of indicator strain by pyocin.
- Less useful because less discriminatory power.

B Genotyping methods: Pulsed field gel electrophoresis is best useful because more discriminatory power.

❖ Pathogenicity:

➢ **Reservoir & source of infection:**
- Widely available in hospital environment.
- It can survive & multiply even with minimal nutrients, if moisture is available.
- **Equipments** such as respirators, endoscopes & stitch materials, **articles** such as hospital-bed & cloths, **medicines** such as lotions, creams & eye-ear drops & even **stocks** of distilled water, plants & flowers may be frequently contaminated.

➢ **Mode of transmission:** Direct from environment or contaminated hospital materials.

➢ **Portal of entry:** Skin, respiratory system etc.

➢ **Sites:** Skin, soft tissues, GIT, blood, respiratory system etc.

➢ **Precipitating factors (epidemiological determinants):**

I. Agent factors (virulence factors)

A. Intracellular (cell wall associated):

i. Antigens:
1. Somatic (O) Ag:
2. Flagellar (H) Ag: Organ of locomotion.
3. Slime layer act as capsule: Inhibit phagocytosis.
4. Fimbriae: Organ of adhesion.

ii. Antibiotic resistance: Due to alteration in cell wall & porin channel. Resistance to common antibiotics & antiseptics, establish itself widely in hospitals.

iii. Ability to form biofilms:

B. Extracellular:

i. Pyocyanin pigment:
- Stop ciliary movement of respiratory epithelium & prevent bacteria from host defense.
- Inhibit growth of other bacteria & makes the bacterium dominant in mixed infection.
- Catalyses production of superoxide & H_2O_2.

ii. Toxins:
1. Exotoxin A, S, T, U & Y: A act as NADase. It acts like diphtheria toxin & inhibits the protein synthesis by inhibiting the elongation factor -2 (EF-2).
2. Enterotoxin: Causing collection of fluid in ligated rabbit illeal loop.
3. Haemolysin

✓ **Notes: Toxins act by inhibiting the protein synthesis**
- Diphtheria toxin: } By inactivation of EF-2
- *Pseudomonas* toxin:
- Shiga like toxin (SLT): } By inactivation of 60S ribosome
- Shiga toxin:

iii. Enzymes:
1. Phospholipidase: Breaks down lipids & lecithin facilitating tissue destruction.
2. Elastase: Degrade elastin → damage of lung parenchyma & haemorrhagic lesions
3. Protease: Help to spread in tissues

II. Host factors

1. **Immunity:** It is the common cause of life threatening fever in person with IDDs.
2. **Prolonged hospitalisation:** It favours the infection.

III. Environmental factors

Common in hospital environmental as mentioned earlier.

➢ **Clinical features:** Two types

a. Community acquired infection (outside hospital in community):
1. **Ear infection:** Otitis media. It is the most common agent to cause suppurative otitis media outside the hospital.
2. **Intestinal:** Infantile diarrhoea due to heat labile enterotoxin.
3. **Respiratory tract infection:** Most common cause of respiratory infection in cystic fibrosis patient.
4. **Shanghai fever:** Self limited febrile illness resembling typhoid fever.

b. Hospital acquired (nosocomial) infection: It includes following types
1. **Localised infections (blue pus → fruity odour) of:**
- Traumatic wound.
- Burn wound: Most common agent to cause infection in burns.
- Bed sore.
- Ecthyma gangrenosum & many other skin lesions are occurs in patients with leukemia & malignancy. It occurs singly or in small number on the perineum, buttock & extremities.
- Eye infections.
- Brain abscess.
- Nail bed infection following excessive exposure of hands to detergents & water.
2. **Generalised infections:** Septicemia & endocarditis in debilitated patients.
3. **Iatrogenic infections:**
- Meningitis following lumbar puncture.
- UTI following catheterisation.

- Pulmonary infection following tracheostomy.
- Ventilator associated pneumonia following ventilation.

❖ **Laboratory diagnosis:**

➤ **Specimens:** Urine, pus, blood, sputum, CSF, swab etc.

➤ **Collection:** Collect in enrichment broth & than subculture on solid media

➤ **Testing methods:**

i. **Microscopy: → Follow morphology**
ii. **Culture: → Follow C/Cs**
iii. **Biochemical reactions: → Follow B/Rs**
iv. **Typing: →Vide supra**

❖ **Prevention:** Strict aseptic prequation are required to control the infection.

❖ **Treatment:** *Pseudomonas* is multi drug resistant. Antibiotics are given after antibiogram.

Other species of *Pseudomonas*

Other species like *P. stutzeri, P. fluorscens* & *P. putida* are known to produces the opportunistic infections

Burkholderia

Bukholderia cepacia

❖ **Synonym:** Previously **called** ***Pseudomonas cepacia.***

❖ **Morphology:** GNB which is motile by lophotrichous flagella.

❖ **Cultural characteristics (C/Cs):**

➤ **Effective factors:**

- O_2 effect: Aerobes.
- Temperature: Optimum temperature is 25-35^{0}C.

➤ **Culture in media:**

1. **Nutrient agar:** Growth occurs in 48 hours but on prolonged incubation, colonies become reddish purple.

❖ **B/Rs:**

- Acidifies mannitol, sorbitol and sucrose.
- Oxidase positive.

❖ **Genotyping:** Based on DNA hybridisation method 9 genomovars or groups are identified of which II & III are causing infection in patients of cystic fibrosis.

❖ **Pathogenicity:**

➤ **Virulence factors:**

1. **Pili:** Organ of adhesion.
2. **Elastase:**
3. **LPS:** Endotoxic activities.

➤ **Clinical features:**

1. **Plant pathogen:** Nutritionally very versatile & causing onion rot **[Cepia (Latin) = onion].**
2. **Human pathogen**

- Opportunistic pathogen & causing **fatal necrotising pneumonia** in a patient with cystic fibrosis or chronic granulomatous disease.
- Causes UTI, respiratory & wound infections, peritonitis, endocarditis and septicemia.

❖ **Treatment:**

- Can grow in many disinfectants & even use Pn G as sole source of carbon.
- Inherently multi drug resistant.

Bukholderia mallei

❖ **Synonym:** Previously **called** ***Pseudomonas mallei.***

❖ **History:** Organism was 1st discovered by Loeffler & Schultz in 1882.

❖ **Morphology:**

➤ **Type according to gram stain:** GNB but stains irregularly with beaded form.

➤ **Size:** 0.5µm× 2-5µm.

➤ **Shape:** Slender rod.

➤ **Motility:** Only species of genus which is nonmotile.

❖ **Cultural characteristics (C/Cs):**

➤ **Effective factors:**

- O_2 effect: Aerobes & facultative anaerobes.
- Temperature: Grow at wide range of temperature.

➤ **Culture in media:**

2. **Nutrient agar:** In young culture small & translucent colonies & in aging culture become yellowish & opaque.
3. **Mac Conkey's agar:** No growth.
4. **Medium contains potato:** Produces amber or honey like growth.

➤ **Culture in animal:**

- Intra-peritoneal injection into male guinea pigs: It produces swelling of the testis, inflammation of tunica vaginalis & scrotal skin ulcer **called Straus reaction**. Test is not useful.
- Tunica reaction also caused by *Brucella, Preisz-Nocard bacillus, Actinobacillus* & *P. pseudomallei.*

❖ **Biochemical reactions (B/Rs):**

- Biochemically inactive & attack on glucose only.
- Oxidase –Ve.

❖ **Pathogenicity:**

➤ **Disease name:** Disease **called glanders.**

➤ **Synonym:** In Latin **called malleus.**

- **Reservoir & source of infection:** It is a zoonosis. Common reservoirs are equine animals like horses, mules & asses.
- **Mode of transmission:**
1. **Direct contact:** Transmitted by direct skin contact with infected animals. Common in person who handle the horses.
2. **Inhalation:** Most dangerous bacteria for accidental transmission in laboratory workers.
- **Clinical features:**
a. **Animal infections:** Two forms.
1. **Glanders:** Present with respiratory nodules & profuse nasal discharge.
2. **Farcy:** Skin & subcutaneous lymphatic nodules.
b. **Human infections:** Two forms
1. **Acute:** Febrile illness & nasal discharge.
2. **Chronic:** Skin & respiratory nodules or abscess.

Laboratory diagnosis:
- **Specimens:** Blood, sputum, discharge from lesionetc.
- **Testing methods:**
i. **Microscopy: → Follow morphology**
ii. **Culture: → Follow C/Cs**
iii. **Skin test: Called mallein test** based on DTH, performed by SC, IC or by conjunctival route.

Prevention: Avoid contact with infected animals.

Treatment:
- Bacteria are multi drug resistant. Antibiotics are given after antibiogram.
- Ceftazidime is drug of choice & given with cotrimoxazole, tetracycline, amoxicillin, clavulanate or chloramphenicol.

Burkholderia pseudomallei

Synonym: *Whitmore's bacilli, Actinobacillus whitmori, Malleomyces pseudomallei* or *Loeffrella pseudomallei.*

History:
- Organism was discovered by Whitmore in 1913 hence **called Whitmore's bacilli.**
- Human disease was 1st described by Whitmore & Krishna swami in 1913.

Morphology:
- **Type according to gram stain:**
- Gram stain: GNB.
- Methylene blue stain: Typical '**bipolar safety pin'** appearance.
- **Motility:** Motile by several polar flagella (lophotrichous)
- **Immunofluorescent microscopy:** Also useful.

Cultural characteristics (C/Cs):
- **Effective factors:**
- O_2 effect: Strict aerobes.
- Temperature: Grow at 42^0C.
- **Media:**

A. **Solid media:**
1. **Nutrient agar:**
2. **Blood agar:**
3. **Mac Conkey's agar:**

(1–3: Rough & corrugated colonies)

B. **Selective media:**
1. **Ashdown's medium:** Produces wrinkled purple colonies as shown in **fig.-3(b).**

Biochemical reaction (B/Rs):
1. Forming acid from several sugars.
2. Gelatine liquefaction test: +Ve
3. Arginine decarboxylation test: +Ve
4. Intracellular accumulation of poly-β hydroxyl butyrate.

Pathogenicity:
- **Disease name: Called melioidosis.**
- **Synonym:** Initially limited in Asia & North Australia, later spread to USA military person who return from Vietnam war with exacerbation **called 'Vietnam time bomb'.**
- **Meaning:** Word derived from **melis = disease of asses + eidos = resemblance,** as it resemble to malleus (glander).
- **Reservoir of infection:** Zoonosis (epizootic) particularly in rodents in South East Asia, India & North Australia.
- **Source of infection:** Present as saprophytes in soil & water in endemic area which may act as source of infection.
- **Mode of transmission:** Human infection occurs by
1. **Direct contact:** Contact of abrade skin with contaminated water or soil.
2. **Inhalation:** Dangerous agent used in bioterrorism.
- **Precipitating factors:**
- **Agent factors (virulence factors):** Two heat labile toxins one is lethal & second is necrotising.
- **Host factor:** DM increases the risk.
- **Clinical features:** Four stages
1. **Acute:**
- Acute pulmonary infection: Most common lesion present with extensive necrotising pneumonia may mimics tuberculosis. X-ray shows the upper lobe infiltration.
- Septicemia often fatal (Acute stage has high case fatality).
2. **Subacute:** Typhoid like illness.
3. **Chronic:** Abscess/suppurative foci in skin, subcutaneous tissue, bone & in other organs.
4. **Latent infection:** Survive in RE-system & reactivation can occur.

Laboratory diagnosis:
- **Specimens:** Sputum, pus, blood or urine etc.
- **Testing methods:**

i. **Microscopy:** → **Follow morphology**
ii. **Culture:** → **Follow C/Cs**
iii. **Biochemical reactions:** → **Follow B/Rs**
iv. **Serological tests:** Following are useful tests
- Latex agglutination test.
- Indirect Haem Agglutination test (IHA).
- ELISA for IgG & IgM detection.

v. **Molecular test:** PCR.

❖ **Prevention:** Strict aseptic precautions to control the infection.

❖ **Treatment:** Same as *B. mallei.*

Alcaligenes faecalis

❖ **Meaning:**
- **Genus name:** Because **non fermenters & gives alkaline reaction** in litmus milk test.
- **Species name:** Because **identified from faeces.**

❖ **Morphology:**
- **Staining properties:** GNB.
- **Shape:** Short rod.
- **Motility:** Motile by peritrichous flagella.

❖ **Cultural characteristics (C/Cs):**
- **Effective factors:** Strict aerobes.
- **Media:**

1. **Blood agar:** Some strains produce the colonies with greenish discolouration & fruity odour (green apple odour).
2. **Mac Conkey's agar:** Most strains produce the thin & spreading colonies with irregular edge.

❖ **Biochemical reaction (B/Rs):**
1. **Sugar fermentation test:** Non fermentative but oxidative.
2. **Citrate test:** +Ve
3. **Oxidase test:** +Ve
4. **Nitrate reduction:** +Ve
5. **Urease test:** -Ve

❖ **Pathogenicity:**
- **Reservoir & source of infection:** Soil & water saprophytes including IV fluid. Hospital contaminant in respirators, nebulizer etc. Commensals in human & animal intestine.
- **Clinical features:**
  - Causing nosocomial infections like UTI.
  - Common lesions produced are gastroenteritis, typhoid like fever & local sepsis.
  - Also cause opportunistic infections like otitis media, meningitis & pneumonia.

❖ **Laboratory diagnosis:** Faeces, blood, urine, pus etc. are tested by microscopy, culture & by B/Rs as described above.

❖ **Treatment:** Fluoroquinolones & nalidixic acid are the sensitive drugs.

Stenotrophomonas maltophila

❖ **Synonym:** Previously **called** ***Pseudomonas maltophila.***

❖ **Morphology:** GNB, 0.7–1.8 × 0.4–0.7 μm in size & motile due to polar flagella.

❖ **C/Cs:**
- Aerobes.
- Grow well on Mac Conkey's agar producing pigmented colonies.

❖ **B/Rs:**
- Non fermentative but utilise the sugar oxidatively.
- Catalase positive.
- Oxidase test: -Ve (non-oxidative).
- Lysin decarboxylation test: +Ve.

❖ **Pathogenicity:**
- **Reservoir & source of infection:** It is ubiquitous in aqueous environments, soil, and plants. It is a rhizosphere (present in soil surrounding the plant root).
- **Precipitating factors:**

✪ **Virulence factors:**
- Resistant to many broad-spectrum antibiotics by efflux pump mechanism & to carbapenems due to the production of two inducible chromosomal metallo-β-lactamases (designated L1 and L2).
- LPS responsible for endotoxic activities.

✪ **Host factors:**
- It is associated with high morbidity & mortality in severely immunocompromised & debilitated individuals. Risk factors include cystic fibrosis, HIV -AIDS, malignancy, neutropenia, mechanical ventilation, central venous catheters, recent surgery, trauma, prolonged hospitalization, intensive care unit admission and broad-spectrum antibiotic use.
- *S. maltophilia* colonization rates in individuals with cystic fibrosis have been increasing.

- **Clinical features:**
  - **Nosocomial infections like** pneumonia in ventilated patient, UTI, septicemia & wound infections.
  - **Opportunistic infections like** ecthyma gangrenosum in neutropenic patients.

❖ **Laboratory diagnosis:** Bacteria are diagnosed from blood, urine, sputum samples by microscopy, culture & biochemical tests.

❖ **Treatment:** Multi drug resistant & useful antibiotics are tigecycline & polymyxin B. Antibiogram requires nonstandard culture methods (incubation at 30 °C). Testing at the wrong temperature results in isolates being incorrectly reported as being susceptible when they are, in fact, resistant. Disc diffusion method should not be used, as it is unreliable. Agar dilution should be used.

Flavobacterium meningosepticum

❖ **Meaning:**

- **Genus name:** From **flavus (Latin) = yellow + Bacterium = related to bacteria**, because of yellow colour pigment production by bacteria.
- **Species name:** Associated with meningitis & septicemia produced by it.

❖ **History & synonym:**

- *Flavobacterium meningosepticum*, King, 1959
- *Chryseobacterium meningosepticum*, Vandamme *et al.*, 1994
- *Elizabethkingia meningoseptica*, Kim *et al.*, 2005

❖ **Morphology:**

➢ **Staining properties:** GNB.
➢ **Shape:** Curved rod.
➢ **Motility:** Nonmotile.

❖ **Cultural characteristics (C/Cs):**

➢ **Effective factors:** Required O_2 for growth & grow better at 40^0C.
➢ **Media:**

1. **Blood agar:** Pale yellow colour pigmented colonies produced after 24 hours **[fig.4]** & better at 40^0C.
2. **Chocolate agar:**
3. **Mac Conkey's agar:** Poor growth.

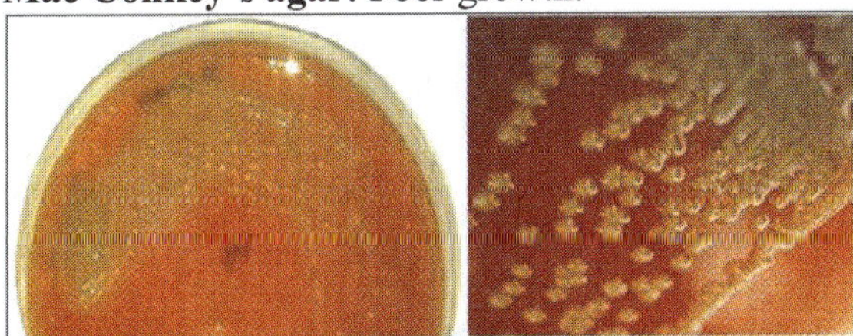

Figure-4: Pigment of *F. meningosepticum* on blood agar

❖ **Biochemical reaction (B/Rs):**

1. **Sugar fermentation test:** Weak fermentative (oxidative) & proteolytic.
2. **Indole test:** +Ve
3. **Catalase test:** +Ve
4. **Oxidase test:** +Ve
5. **Urease test:** -Ve

❖ **Pathogenicity:**

➢ **Reservoir & source of infection:** Ubiquitous saprophytes.
➢ **Clinical features:**

- Nosocomial infections: Neonatal meningitis & septicemia associated with nursery outbreak.
- Also cause opportunistic infections.

❖ **Laboratory diagnosis:** CSF or blood tested by microscopy, culture & by B/Rs as described above.

❖ **Treatment:** Fluoroquinolones & nalidixic acid are the sensitive drugs.

Legionella pneumophila

❖ **Meaning & history:** **Genus named** because 1st identified in member of American **Legion** (Group of soldiers) who attended a convention in Philadelphia in 1976.

❖ **Classification:** →**Flow chart-2**

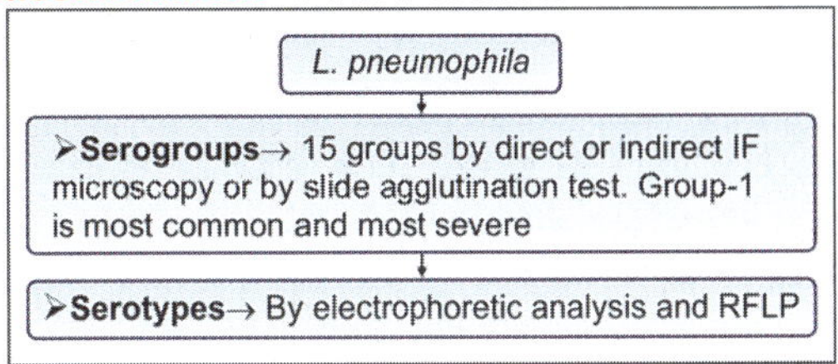

Flow chart-2: Classification of *Legionella* spp.

❖ **Morphology:** → **Fig.-5**

➢ **Staining properties:**

- GNB or gram negative coccobacilli, but difficult to examine under gram stain from sputum. Smear contains numerous leucocytes.
- Better stained by silver impregnation or fluorescent stain.
- Fat globules stain by Sudan black.
- Cell wall of *L. micdadei* is acid fast in nature.

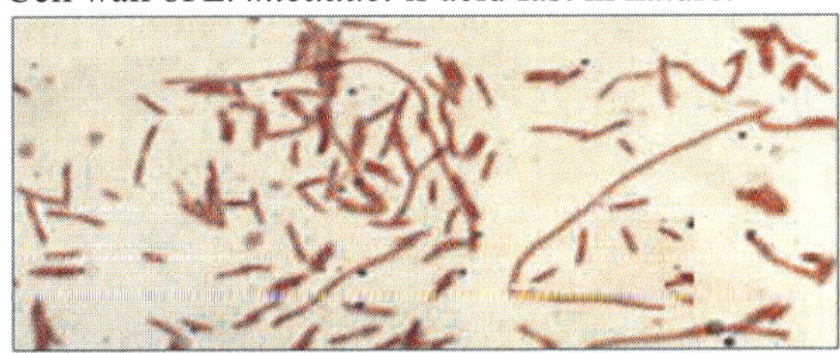

Figure-5: Morphology of *L. pneumophila*

➢ **Size:** 0.2-0.3μm x 1–3μm.
➢ **Shape:** Short rod, coccobacilli with pointed ends & filamentous forms.
➢ **Motility:** Motile by single polar or subpolar flagella at one end.
➢ **Capsule & spore:** Non-capsulated & non-sporing.
➢ **Immunofluorescent microscopy:** Performed by using monoclonal or polyclonal sera.

❖ **Cultural characteristics (C/Cs):** Culture is highly sensitive (80-90%) & specific (100%) for diagnosis.

➢ **Effective factors:**

- O_2 effect: Strict aerobes.
- CO_2 effect: Better growth under 5-10% CO_2 (capnophilic) & high humidity (90%).
- Optimum temperature: 29-40°C.

- pH: 6.9
- Highly fastidious bacteria, better growth occurs in media supplemented with L-cysteine & iron.
- Slow growing colonies may appear after 3-6 days.

➢ **Culture in media:**

A. Liquid media: Enrichment broth prepared from yeast extract, liver extract, L-cysteine & iron. Samples are collected in enrichment broth & after appropriate incubation they are subculture on solid media.

B. Solid/plating media:

1. **BCYE (Buffered Charcoal Yeast Extract) agar with L-cysteine:** It is a complex medium producing opal colonies (opal = stone with milky appearance).
2. **Feeley Gorman (FG) agar:** Diffusible brown pigment is produced which fluoresces dull yellow on UV light exposure. This may be enhanced by addition of tyrosine in medium.
3. **Egg-yolk medium:** Opacity around colonies due to lecithinase production, however not used for diagnostic purpose

C. Selective medium: BCYE agar + vancomycin + cycloheximide + polymyxin-B.

➢ **Culture in animal:** Inoculation in guinea pig by intraperitoneal or by respiratory route. Organism identified from peritoneal exudates, local abscess & spleen materials

➢ **Culture in egg:** Grow in yolk sac of hen's egg.

❖ **Biochemical reaction (B/Rs):** Difficult to perform because of slow growth.

1. **Sugar fermentation test:** Non-fermentative but hydrolyse the starch.
2. **Catalase test:** +Ve
3. **Oxidase test:** Variable
4. **Hippurate hydrolysis test:** +Ve

❖ **Pathogenicity:**

➢ **Disease name:** Disease **called legionellosis** having two forms such as mild influenza like symptoms **called pontiac fever** while bilateral pneumonia **called legionnair's disease**.

➢ **Nature of disease:** Legionnair's disease occurs in epidemic or sporadic form while pontiac fever occurs as localised outbreak with high attack rate.

➢ **Reservoir of infection:**

✪ **Aquatic reservoir:** No carrier or animal reservoir, but aquatic reservoirs like
- Naturally in rivers, mud, stream, lakes etc.
- Artificially in air conditioners or water coolers.

✪ **Protozoa:** Bacteria survive in free living amoeba & in certain protozoa.

➢ **Source of infection:** Aerosols arise from air-conditioner or from shower heads or from infected aquatic reservoirs.

➢ **Mode of transmission:**

- **Inhalation:** Human infection occurs by **inhalation** of aerosols arise from air-conditioner, shower heads, nebulizer, humidifier, device filled with tap water or from infected aquatic reservoir. Aerosolised *Legionella* can survive long & traversed to long distance may lead to epidemic.
- Other modes are like direct instillation in to the lungs or aspiration.
- Human to human transmission does not occur.

➢ **Incubation period:** 24-48 hrs for Pontiac fever & 2-10 days for Legionnaire's disease.

➢ **Portal of entry:** Respiratory system.

➢ **Sites:** Respiratory system & disseminated in other organs by local, blood or lymphatic route

➢ **Precipitating factors (epidemiological determinants):**

I. Agent factors (virulence factors)

1. **Enzyme production:** Produce beta-lactamase responsible for drug resistance.
2. **Intracellular location:** Escape host defence & antibiotic effects. CMI is primary mechanism but not protective.

II. Host factors

1. **Age:** Elderly persons are at greater risk.
2. **Sex:** More in male than female.
3. **Immunity:** Risk increased with pre-existing conditions like alcoholism, smoking, hospitalisation, IDDs etc.

III. Environmental factors

1. **Nutrition to bacteria:** Nutritional requirement is filled by some type of algae in aquatic reservoir.
2. **Economical status:** More in developed countries. In developed countries about 1-3% community acquired & 10-30% hospital acquired pneumonia are due to *Legionella*

➢ **Pathogenesis: → Flow chart-3**

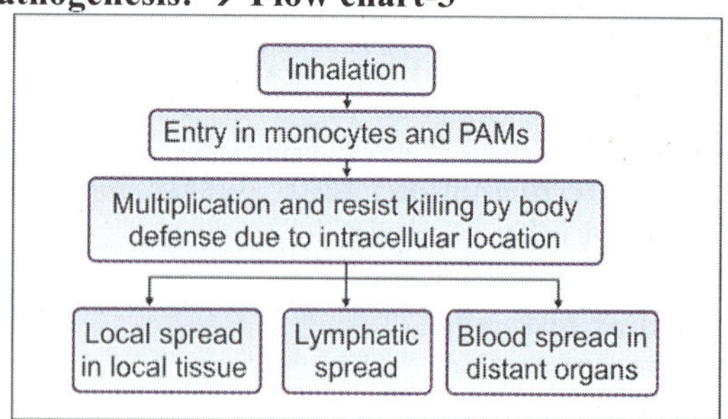

Flow chart-3: Pathogenesis of Legionellosis

➢ **Clinical features:** Two clinical forms.

a. Legionnaire's disease:
- It is a bilateral pneumonia present with fever, non-productive cough & dyspnoea may progress to diarrhoea & encephalopathy (confusion).
- Case fatality is 15-20% due to respiratory failure or shock.

b. Pontiac fever:

- Mild influenza like illness, present with fever, chills, headache & myalgia.
- Self limited.

➢ **Complications:** Mostly in heart like myocarditis, pericarditis & endocarditis.

❖ Laboratory diagnosis:

➢ **Specimens:** Sputum, respiratory aspirates, lung tissue & blood.

➢ **Collection:** In enrichment broth → Transport to lab. → Incubation → Subculture over media.

➢ **Testing methods:** Identification of bacilli by

1. **Microscopy: → Follow morphology**
2. **Culture: → Follow C/Cs**
3. **Biochemical reactions: → Follow B/Rs**
4. **Serological tests:**
   - **Ag detection tests:** From urine by ELISA & latex agglutination test.
   - **Ab detection tests:** From serum by ELISA & IIF test.
5. **Molecular:** PCR.
6. **Chromatography:** High content of fat gives typical profile on GLC.

❖ Prevention: Disinfection of water by silver ionization, commercial copper, super heat & flush methods to remove the biofilms of *L. pneumophila* from water.

❖ Treatment: Quinolones (levofloxacin, ciprofloxacin etc.) & newer macrolides are the drugs of choice. Alternative drugs are tetracycline, rifampicin & cotrimoxazole are useful in severe cases. B-lactam group & aminoglycosides are ineffective.

Question bank

Case study

1) A 40 year male presented to medical OPD with complain of fever & productive cough. Clinically he is diagnosed as cystic fibrosis. Gram stain of sputum revealed gram negative short rod & Culture on Mac Conkey's give NLF colonies. Biochemically it is oxidase & citrate positive. Identify the commonest agent & answer the following
   a) Name the commonest agent causing respiratory infection in cystic fibrosis
   b) Describe the morphology, culture characteristics & biochemical reactions of commonest agent in given case
   c) Write the pathogenicity of commonest agent in given case

Essay/Full question

1) Non-fermenters

Short notes

1) Pathogenicity or laboratory diagnosis of *P. aeruginosa*
2) Glanders
3) Melioidosis
4) Legionellosis

Short questions for theory/viva questions

1) Name the four non-fermentative bacteria.
2) Name the four media useful to detect the pigments of pseudomonas.
3) What is strauss reaction & tunica reaction?
4) What is Vietnam time bomb?
5) Write the etiological agents for glanders & glandular fever (infectious mononucleosis).
6) Write the etiological agents for malleus & melioidosis.

MCQs for chapter review

Pseudomonas

1) **An organism grown on agar shows green coloured colonies; likely organism is -** (AI-01)
(a) *Staphylococccus* (b) *E coli* (c) *Pseudomonas* (d) *Peptostreptococcus*
2) ***Pseudomonas* is which type of bacteria-**
(a) Anaerobic (b) Microaerophilic (c) Strict aerobe (d) Obligate anaerobe
3) **Selective medium to detect the pyoverdin pigment produce by *P. aeruginosa* is**
(a) Mannitol salt agar (b) Furunculosis agar (c) Thayer Martin medium (d) King's medium B
4) **Which bacteria act by inhibiting protein synthesis -** (AI-01, 98)
(a) *Pseudomonas* (b) *Staphylococccus* (c) *Streptococccus* (d) *Klebsiella*
5) **Ecthyma gangrenosum is caused by -**
(a) *Pseudomonas* (b) *Streptococccus* (c) *Staphylococccus* (d) *H influenzae*
6) ***Pseudomonas* infection not cleaned by**
(a) Dettol (b) Hypochlorite (c) Chlorine (d) Betadine

Bukholderia pseudomallei

7) **All of the following causes melioidosis**
(a) *Bukholderia pseudomallei* (b) *Bukholderia mallei* (c) *Bukholderia cepacia* (d) None
8) **The following statement is true regarding melioidosis except -** (AI, 05)
(a) It is caused by *Bukholderia mallei* (b) The agent is gram negative aerobic bacteria (c) Bipolar staining of etiological agent is seen methylene blue stain (d) The most common form of melioidosis is pulmonary infection

Legionella pneumophila

9) **All of the following are correct regarding *Legionella* except** (AIIMS, Nov- 04)
(a) *Legionella* can be grown on complex media (b) *Legionella pneumophila* sero group 1 is the most common serogroup isolated from humans (c) *Legionella* are communicable from infected patients to others (d) *Legionella pneumophila* is not effectively killed by polymorpho nuclear leucocytes
10) **A 60 year old man is diagnosed to be suffering from Legionnaire's disease after the returns home from attending a convention. He could have acquired it -** (AI-03)
(a) From a person suffering from the infection while travelling in the aeroplane (b) From a chronic carrier in the convention centre (c) From the inhalation of the aerosol in the air conditioned room at convention centre (d) By sharing a towel with a fellow delegate at the convention centre
11) **Aerosol spread leading to epidemic is seen in infection with** (AIIMS, Nov- 01)

(a) *Legionella* (b) *Haemophilus* (c) Influenza virus (d) *Mycoplasma*

12) Devi a 28 year female, has diarrhoea, confusion high grade fever with bilateral pneumonitis. The diagnosis is (AI, 2000)
(a) *Legionella* (b) *Neisseria meningitidis* (c) *Streptococus pneumoniae* (d) *H influenzae*

13) Which of the following is a good medium to use for diagnosis of Legionnaire's disease (AIIMS, Nov- 01)
(a) Thayer martin medium (b) BCYE agar (c) Bordet Gengu medium (d) Chocolate agar

14) True about *Legionella* (PGI, Dec-06)
(a) Epidemic (+) (b) Splenomegaly (c) Easily seen in sputum (d) Scanty neutrophils with fed organisms (e) Purulent sputum common

Answers of MCQs & explanation

1. (c)
- *Pseudomonas* is the only organism producing the green colour pigment which gives green colonies over agar.
- *Staphylococccus* also produce pigment but colours are white (*Staph albus*), lemon yellow (*Staph citrus*) or orange (*Staph aureus*)
- *E coli* & *Peptostreptococcus* are non pigmented

2. (c)
- Follow section, ***Pseudomonas* (culture characteristics → effective factors)** for explanation

3. (d)
- Follow section, ***Pseudomonas* (culture characteristics → media for production & identification of pigments)** for explanation

4. (a)
- Toxins act by inhibiting the protein synthesis
- Diphtheria toxin: } By inactivation of EF-2
- *Pseudomonas* toxin: }
- Shiga like toxin (SLT): } By inactivation of 60S ribosome
- Shiga toxin: }

5. (a)
- Follow section, ***Pseudomonas* (pathogenicity → clinical features)** for explanation

6. (a)
- *Pseudomonas* can grow in bottles of antiseptics like dettol, iodine, cetrimide lotions or soap lotion etc. kept for use in hospitals. Indeed, dettol or cetrimide is incorporated in a media selective for *P aeruginosa*.

7. (a)
- *Bukholderia mallei*: Causing glander
- *Bukholderia cepacia:* Causing fatal necrotising pneumonia & infection in other systems

8. (a)
- Melioidosis is caused by *Bukholderia pseudomallei*

9. (c)
- *Legionella* can be grown on complex medium like BCYE agar
- Sero group 1 is the most common & most sever sero group isolated from humans
- *Legionella* are not communicable from infected patients to others (no man to man transmission)
- *Legionella pneumophila* is not effectively killed by polymorpho nuclear leucocytes because of intracellular location, it escape host defence & antibiotic effects

10. (c) } Follow section. ***Legionella pneumophila***
11. (a) } **pathogenicity → mode of transmission)** for explanation

12. (a)
- Bilateral pneumonitis is caused by *Legionella*

13. (b)
- Follow section, ***Legionella pneumophila* (culture characteristic → solid/plating media)** for explanation

14. (a)
- Legionnaire's disease present as epidemic or sporadic, it does not present with splenomegaly
- Option c & d: Follow section, ***Legionella pneumophila* (morphology)** for explanation
- Sputum is non productive

50 Pasteurellales

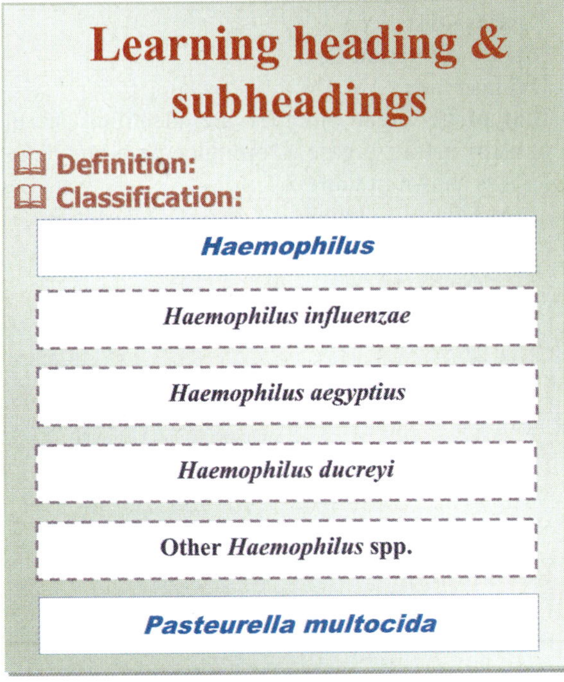

Learning heading & subheadings
Definition:
Classification:
Haemophilus
Haemophilus influenzae
Haemophilus aegyptius
Haemophilus ducreyi
Other Haemophilus spp.
Pasteurella multocida

Definition: Gram negative bacteria that live on mucosal surfaces of birds and mammals, especially in the upper respiratory tract.

Classification: →Flow chart-1

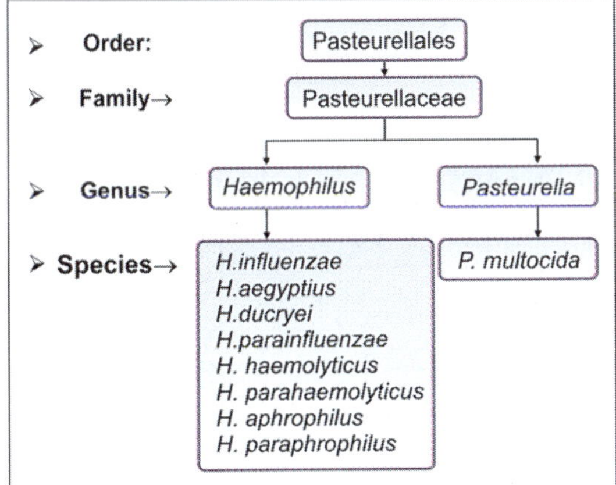

Flow chart-1: Classification of Pasteurellales

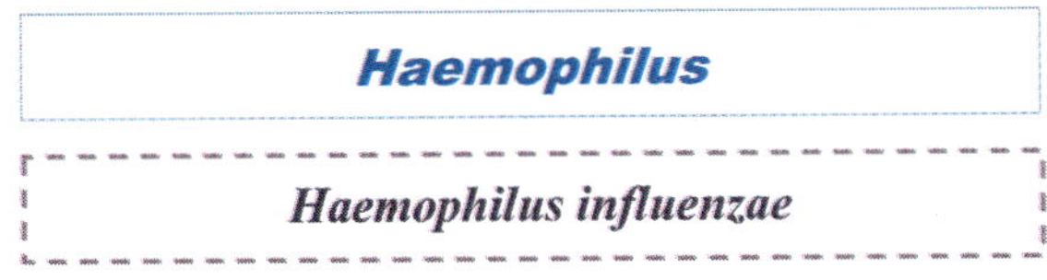

- **Meaning:** *Haemophilus* word includes **Haemo = blood + Philus = friendly** means **blood loving** because bacteria required growth factor X & V (**one/both**)which are present in blood.

- **Synonym:**
  - Influenza bacillus.
  - Pfeiffer's bacillus, because **Pfeiffer** (1892) identified it in sputum of patients of **1889-90 influenza pandemic** as a causative agent of human influenza. But later it proved by Smith, Andrew & Laidlaw in 1933 that human influenza is due to influenza virus hence it remained as *H. influenzae.*

- **Morphology:** → **Fig.-1**

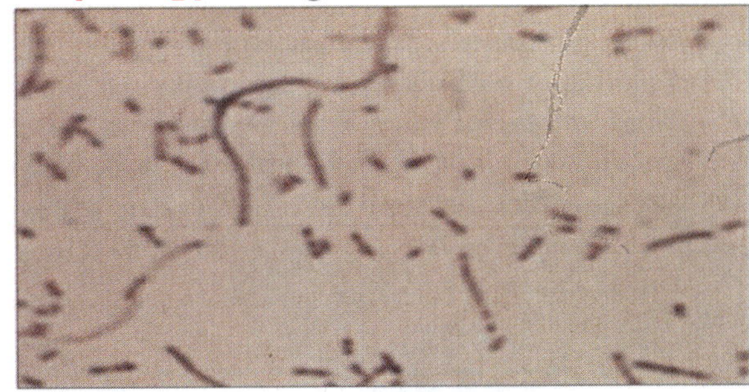

Figure-1: Morphology of *H. influenzae*

- **Type according to gram stain:**
  - Gram negative coccobacilli but better stained by using dilute carbol fuchsin or safranin as counter stain.
  - Better result with Loeffler's methylene blue stain.
- **Size:** 0.3μm x 1μm.
- **Shape:** Pleomorphic. Coccobacilli in sputum & in young culture & filamentous in CSF.
- **Capsule:** Capsulated & it is detected by quelling reaction or by negative staining.
- **Motility & spore:** Nonmotile & non sporing.
- **Fimbriae:** Present.
- **Immunofluorescent microscopy:** Also useful method.

- **Cultural characteristics (C/Cs):**
- **Effective factors:**

Features	X factor	V factor
Heat	Stable	Labile at 120^{0}C in few min.
Act as	Haemin or haematin	Bacterial vitamin or coenzymes-NAD / NADP
Function	For synthesis of haem enzymes - oxidase, catalase & peroxidase	Hydrogen acceptor in cell metabolism

Table-1: Factors required for growth of *H. influenzae*

- O_2 effect: Aerobes but grow anaerobically. (facultative anaerobes)
- CO_2 effect: Mostly require 5-10% CO_2 (capnophilic).
- Temperature: Optimum temp. is 37^0C.
- Fastidious in nature & required X and V factors for growth as mentioned in **table-1.**

➢ **Culture in media:**

A. Liquid media:

1. **Phenol red broth (contains NAD):** For sugar fermentation test.
2. **Filde's peptic digest - blood broth:** Nutrient broth + peptic digest of blood.
3. **Levinthal's medium:** Contains mixture of boiled-filtered blood & nutrient broth.

B. Solid media:

1. **Blood agar:** V factor available inside the unlysed RBCs & it is not available free in medium hence bacteria produce scanty growth or no growth.
2. **Blood agar with *Staph. aureus* streaking:**

- *Staph aureus* produce V factor which favours the growth of *H. influenzae*. Colonies are large near the streaking line because more V factor is available while small colonies away from streaking line **called satellitism** as shown in **fig.-2.**

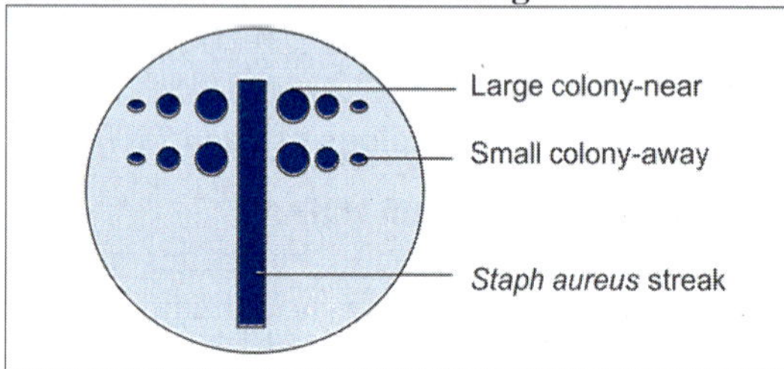

Figure-2: Satellitism

3. **Chocolate agar:** Superior than blood agar because both X and V factors are available freely.
4. **Levinthal's agar:** Translucent colonies with iridescence by capsulated strain.
5. **Filde's peptic digest -blood agar:** Nutrient agar + peptic digest of blood.

C. Selective medium: Blood agar + bacitracin + sucrose + haemin X factor + V factor disc + phenol red.

- Bacitracin: Makes the medium selective for *H. influenzae* & *H. parainfluenzae.*
- Sucrose: Fermented by *H parainfluenzae* gives yellow colonies while not fermented by *H. influenzae* give colourless colonies.
- Haemin X factor: Required as growth factor for *H influenzae.*
- Later add V factor disc: *H influenzae* will identified as satellite growth around disc.
- Phenol red: pH indicator.

❖ Biochemical reaction (B/Rs):

1. **Sugar fermentation test:** Glucose & xylose are fermented with acid production only but not lactose, sucrose & mannitol.
2. **Catalase test:** +Ve
3. **Nitrate reduction test:** + Ve
4. **Oxidase test:** +Ve
5. **Biotyping:** Eight biotypes are identified on the basis of indole, urease & ornithine decarboxylation tests as shown in **table-2.**

Biotypes	Indole	Urease	Ornithine decarboxylase
I	+	+	+
II	+	+	-
III	-	+	-
IV	-	+	+
V	+	-	+
VI	-	-	+
VII	+	-	-
VIII	-	-	-

Table-2: Biotypes of *H. influenzae*

❖ Resistance:

- *H. influenzae* is killed by heat at 55^0C in 30 minutes.
- Culture is maintained for long time by lyophillisation.
- Plasmid born resistance is common to many antibiotics.

❖ Pathogenicity:

➢ **Reservoir of infection:** Human case.

➢ **Source of infection:** Nasopharyngeal or respiratory droplets.

➢ **Mode of transmission:**

- **Endogenous infection:**
  - Organisms are located as normal flora in nasopharynx.
  - Spread: Possibly as per **flow-chart -2.**

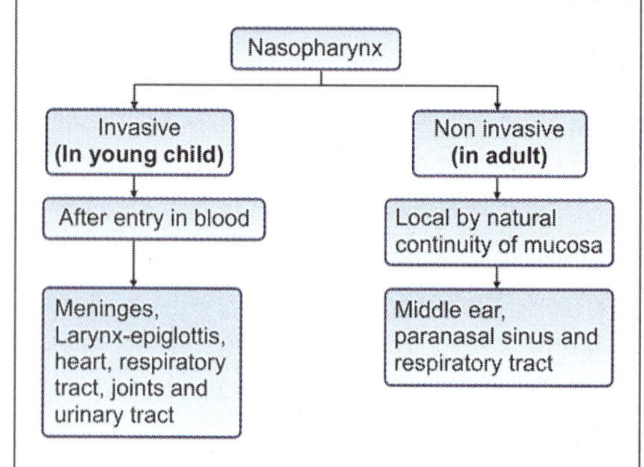

Flow chart-2: Spread of *H. influenzae*

- **Exogenous infection:** By inhalation of nasopharyngeal or respiratory droplets.

➢ **Incubation Period:** Unknown, probably short about 2-4 days.

- **Portal of entry:** Respiratory tract in case of exogenous infection.
- **Sites:** Meninges & respiratory system.
- **Precipitating factors (epidemiological determinants):**

I. Agent factors (virulence factors)

a. **Plasmid:** Encodes for drug resistance.
b. **Fimbriae:** Organ of adhesion.
c. **IgA protease:** Decrease the local immunity.
d. **Antigens:** Three major surface antigens.

1. **Capsular polysaccharide:** It is a major antigenic determinant.
- **Pittman typing:** Six capsular types from a-f where b is the most common **called Hib (*Haemophilus influenzae* type b)** & responsible for 95% of *Haemophilus influenzae* meningitis. It is invasive type.
- Typing is based on agglutination, Quelling reactions, precipitation, coagglutination or ELISA.
- It inhibits the phagocytosis. It does not induce the alternative complement pathway.
- All the types contain hexose & hexosamine sugars while type b contains ribose & ribitol **called PRP (Polyribosyl Ribitol Phosphate)** antigen & produce IgG, IgM & IgA which are bactericidal & protective, hence this PRP-Ag is included in vaccine.
- Non capsular strain can't typed & are **called untypable strains** & produce non-invasive or local disease.

2. **Outer membrane proteins (OMP) Ag:**
- Contribute in adhesion & invasion.
- 13 serotypes of Hib are identified on the bases of OMP Ag.
- Antigens produce the antibodies which are protective.

3. **Lipo oligosaccharide (LOS):**
- OMP & LOS subtyping have an epidemiological value.
- LOS has endotoxic action but differ from LPS of other gram negative bacteria.

II. Host factors

1. **Age:** Common in young children. Young house hold contacts of patients with systemic *H influenzae* infection are at increased risk of infection.
2. **Immunity:** Maternal antibodies against type b can transfer from mother to child & provide protection to the child up to the age of 6 months. Waning of such antibodies titre increase the risk of infants to the type b *H influenzae.*

- **Clinical features:** Two types

a. **Invasive:** 95% infections are caused by type b.

✪ **Meningitis:**
- More in young children (2 month-3 year) with 90% case fatality rate.
- Less in old children because of development of immunity by subclinical infection.
- Enter in meninges by blood from nasopharynx.

✪ **Laryngo epiglottitis (called croup):**
- Causes epiglottitis & uvulitis producing laryngeal or respiratory obstruction.
- > 2 years children are vulnerable.
- Can be fatal in 2 hours & required urgent tracheostomy.

✪ **Respiratory tract infections:**
- **Pneumonia:**
  - Present with meningitis & empyema.
  - Present as lobar pneumonia or bronchopneumonia.
  - Present in older children & adults.
- **Bronchitis:** Acute exacerbation of chronic bronchitis & bronchiectasis.

✪ **UTI:** In children with urinary tract abnormalities.

✪ **Suppurative lesions:** Brain abscess, arthritis, endocarditis, pericarditis & cellulitis in buccal or periorbital part.

b. **Non-invasive:**
- Mostly caused by untypable strains.
- By local spread from nasopharynx to cause acute otitis media (2nd most common cause), sinusitis & exacerbation of chronic bronchitis, bronchiectasis or COPD.

✓ **Note: Order of strain to produce the infection**
- Next to *Haemophilus influenzae* type b, untypable strains are the most relevant in clinical infections.

❖ Laboratory diagnosis:

- **Specimens:** CSF, blood, sputum, throat or nasopharyngeal swab, pus from lesion, urine, aspirates from joint-pleural-pericardial-bronchus etc.
- **Testing methods:**

i. **Microscopy: → Follow morphology**
ii. **Culture: → Follow C/Cs**
iii. **Biochemical reaction: → Follow B/Rs**
iv. **Serological tests:** PRP-Ag detection by passive haemagglutination, CIE, ELISA & *Staph aureus* coagglutination test.
v. **Molecular test:** Are also useful.

❖ Prevention:

A. **General measures:** Isolation of *H. influenzae* patients & avoiding contact with children.
B. **Immunoprophylaxis:** Two types of vaccine.

i. **Hib PRP vaccine:**
- It is poorly immunogenic in children < 2 years.
- Useful for children > 2 year & adults.

ii. **Conjugate vaccine:**
- Hib PRP is more immunogenic in children < 2 years when conjugated with DPT (**triple vaccine**) or meningococcal vaccine.
- Also available as **pentavalent vaccine** which available in different types preparation.

1. **Pentvac** contains Diphtheria, Pertusis, Tetanus, HBV & *H. influenza* type b (Hib).
2. **Pentaxim** contains D, P, T, IPV & Hib.

C. **Chemoprophylaxis:**

- Rifampicin for 4 days prevents secondary infection in contacts & also eradicates the carrier state.

❖ **Treatment:**

1. **Meningitis:** Treated by cefotaxime or ceftazidime.
2. **Respiratory infection:** Treated by ampicicillin & cotrimoxazole.
3. **Resistant to antibiotics:** It is plasmid mediated & treated by amoxycillin + clavulanate or by clarithromycin.

Haemophilus aegyptius

❖ **Synonym:**

- Previously **called *H. aegypticus.***
- Koch - Weeks Bacillus because 1st observed by Koch from the case of conjunctivitis in Egypt (hence the species **called *aegyptius***) in1883 & cultivated by Weeks in New York in 1887,

❖ **Cultural characteristics (C/Cs):**

- Nutritionally exacting.
- Growth is improved by adding factor X & V.
- On heated blood agar grow very slowly & poorly, producing 0.5mm colonies after 48hrs.

❖ **Biochemical reaction(B/Rs):** It is similar to biotype-III of *H. influenzae* & differentiated as

- Failure to ferment **xylose.**
- **Indole** negative.
- Sensitive to **troleandomycin.**
- Strong **haemagglutination** with human or guinea pig RBCs at 4^0C.

❖ **Pathogenicity:**

➢ **Clinical features:** It produces highly contagious conjunctivitis **called pink eye**. Common in tropical & subtropical countries & may occur in epidemic form.

➢ **Complications:** Bacilli enter in blood from the conjunctiva & produce the fulminant septicemia **called Brazilian Purpuric Fever (BPF).**

- So called because 1st noticed in Brazil in 1984 & now endemic in South America.
- Present as fever, purpura, hypotensive shock & death.
- Common in infant & children with high fatality.

❖ **Treatment:** Local sulphonamide or gentamicin.

Haemophilus ducreyi

❖ **Meaning:** Species name came from **Ducreyi** who identified the bacilli from chancroid lesion in 1890 & he noticed that disease is transmitted by inoculation in the skin of forearm.

❖ **Morphology:**

➢ **Type according to gram stain:** GNB but stain like GPB, frequently showing the bipolar staining.

➢ **Size:** 0.6 µm x 1 – 1.5 µm.

➢ **Shape:** Short ovoid bacilli.

➢ **Arrangement:**

1. Small **groups** or **whorls.**
2. Parallel chains of bacilli giving **'school of fish appearance'** or **'rail road track appearance'.**

❖ **Cultural characteristics (C/Cs):**

➢ **Effective factors:**

- Co_2 effect: Growth is improved by incubation under 10% CO_2 & high humidity for 2-8 days.
- Temperature: Optimum temp. is 35^0C.
- Difficult to grow.
- Require factor X only.

➢ **Culture in media:**

A. **Solid media:**

1. **Blood agar:** Grow on fresh clotted/coagulated human or rabbit blood agar.

B. **Selective medium:**

1. **Gibco Chocolate agar:**

- Chocolate agar enriched with fetal calf serum, factor X (1% Isovitale X) & vancomycin.
- After inoculation, incubate the plate at 35-37^0C for 5 days.
- Growth may start after 48 hrs produce pinpoint colonies which become 1-2mm in next 48-72 hrs & smear examination revealed chain of bacilli.
- Bacteria are antigenically homogenous & growth is confirmed by slide agglutination.
- They are biochemically inert.

➢ **Culture in animal:** Intradermal inoculation of culture in rabbit produces a local ulcer.

➢ **Culture in egg:** Grows in Chorio Allontoic Membrane (CAM) of chick embryo.

❖ **Biochemical reaction (B/Rs):** Not significant.

❖ **Pathogenicity:**

➢ **Disease name: Called chancroid** or **soft sore** or **soft chancre.**

➢ **Mode of transmission:** Sexual intercourse (venereal disease).

➢ **Clinical features:** Non-indurated, tender, irregular swelling on external genitalia gets ulcerated (**fig.-3**).

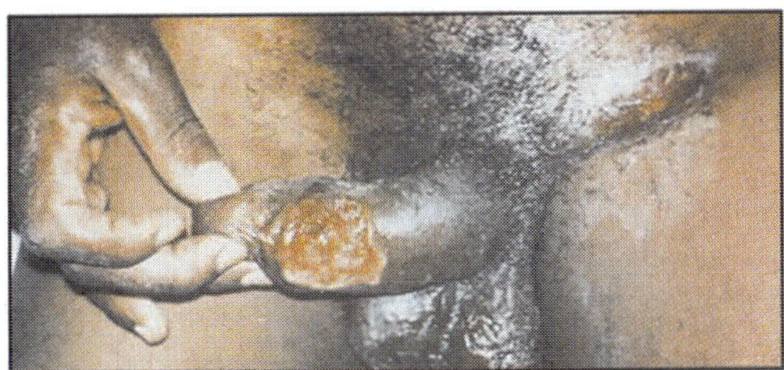

Figure-3: Chancroid

- **Complication:** Infection is localized, spreading to only to regional lymph nodes. Lymph nodes enlarged & painful.
- **Differences between chancroid & chancre:** → Table-3

Laboratory diagnosis:

- **Specimens:** From base & margin of ulcer by using saline-moistened swab.
- **Testing methods:**

i. **Microscopy:** → **Follow morphology**

Chancroid	Chancre
Caused by *H. ducreyi*	Caused by *T. pallidum*
Also **called soft sore** or **soft chancre**	Also **called hard sore** or **hard chancre** or **Hunterian chancre**
Non-indurated swelling	Indurated swelling
Multiple	Single
Painful [**Cry** (from du**c**re**y**i) due to pain]	Painless
Irregular	More circumscribed
Local spread to regional nodes	Spread to regional node by lymph or blood
Regional nodes are painful	Regional nodes are swollen, discrete, rubbery & painless

Table-3: Differences between chancroid & chancre

ii. **Culture:** → **Follow C/Cs**

iii. **Multiplex PCR:** It is developed for simultaneous detection of sexually transmitted microbes like *T. pallidum, H. ducreyi* & HSV.

Prevention: Safe sex.

Treatment:

Single dose of azithromycin is the drug of choice. Sulphonamide or tetracycline is effective. In resistant cases erythromycin, cotrimoxazole, ciprofloxacin or ceftriaxone are useful drugs.

Other *Haemophilus* spp.

↓

Follow table-4

Pasteurella multocida

Meaning:

Species of genus, *P. aviseptica* (**chicken cholera bacilli**) was used by **Pasteur** to produce the 1st attenuated bacterial vaccine, hence the name **Pasteurella.**

Synonym: Formerly **called *P. septica.***

Morphology:

- **Staining properties:** Gram negative coccobacilli & showing bipolar staining under methylene blue.
- **Size:** 0.7 µm x 0.3-0.6µm.
- **Motility:** Nonmotile.
- **Capsule:** Capsulated at 37^0C.

Cultural characteristics (C/Cs):

Aerobic & facultative anaerobes & optimum temperature is 37^0C.

1. **Nutrient agar:** 0.5-1mm circular colonies.
2. **Mac Conkey's agar:** No growth occurs.
3. **Blood agar:** Non haemolytic colonies.
4. **Three different forms of colonies:**

- Smooth colonies: Capsular & virulent strain.
- Rough colonies: Non capsular & avirulent strain.
- Mucoid colonies: Intermediate between capsular & non capsular strain.

Biochemical reaction (B/Rs):

1. **Sugar fermentation test:** Glucose & sucrose are fermented with acid production only.
2. **Indole test:** +Ve
3. **Urease test:** -Ve
4. **Catalase test:** +Ve
5. **Oxidase test:** +Ve
6. **ONPG (β-galactosidase) test:** -Ve
7. **Ornithine decarboxylation test:** +Ve

Classification:

Antigenically homogeneous. Total 15-types are identified based on 4-K Ag & 11-O Ag.

Pathogenicity:

- **Reservoir of infection:** Human & domestic animals like dog, cat etc. are the reservoirs.
- **Source of infection:** Saliva of dog, cat & other domestic animals. Human body carries the bacteria in respiratory tract & in sinuses as commensals.
- **Mode of transmission:**
  - Transmitted by dog bite or cat bite.
  - Contact with infected animals.
  - Also present in human respiratory tract and in nasal sinuses as commensals, which are carry to traumatic site by blood.
- **Clinical features:**

1. **Animals:** Haemorrhagic septicemia.
2. **Human:** Following two types of illness.

- **Local:** Cellulitis, abscess, adenitis & osteomylitis following animal bites.
- **Systemic:** Meningitis following head injury, respiratory infection (like pneumonia, bronchitis or sinusitis), appendicitis & abscess in appendix.

Laboratory diagnosis:

- **Specimens:** Pus, tissue from nodes, blood, CSF & sputum are the useful samples.

Features	H. parainfluenzae	H. haemolyticus	H. parahaemolyticus	H. aphrophilus	H. paraphrophilus
Factors	V	X & V	V	X	V
Flora in	Respiratory tract	Throat	Throat, mouth	Mouth	-
infection	Endocarditis Pharyngitis Urethritis	Oral cavity (**β-haemolysis on blood agar)**	Oral sepsis Endocarditis	Jaw infection, brain abscess & endocarditis	Opportunistic pathogen

Table-4: Differences between *Haemophilus* spp.

- **Testing methods:**

1. **Microscopy: → Follow morphology**
2. **Culture: → Follow C/Cs**
3. **Biochemical reactions: → Follow B/Rs**

- **Treatment:** Tetracycline, streptomycin & penicillin are effective.

Question bank

Case study

1) A 6 year old patient admitted in hospital with complains of fever & seizure. Altered sensorium & neck rigidity are identified on examination. CSF microscopy suggests capsulated pleomorphic GNB. Satellitism is the property of culture test. Identify the organism & answer the following

a) Name the causative agent & describe the morphology of causative agent

b) Write the pathogenicity of causative agent

c) Describe the laboratory diagnosis of causative agent

Essay/Full question

1) *H. influenzae.*

Short notes

1) Pathogenicity or laboratory diagnosis of *H. influenzae.*

2) H. ducreyi

3) P. multocida

Short questions

1) What are satellitism and stalactites?

MCQs for chapter review

MCQs

Haemophilus influenzae

1) **Which of these need both X and V factors-** (PGI-99)
(a) *Haemophilus influenzae* (b) *H. ducryei* (c) *H. paraphrophilus* (d) *H. aegyptius* (e) *H. haemolyticus*

2) **The major antigenic determinant of *H. influenzae* is –** (PGI -99)
(a) 'M' protein (b) Capsular polysaccharide (c) Catalase (d) Coagulase

3) **About *H. influenzae* all true except -** (AIIMS, Nov-09, Nov-10)
(a) Requires factor X and V for growth (b) Rarely present as meningitis in children less than 2 months of age (c) Capsular polypeptide protein is responsible for virulence (d) MC invasive disease of *H. influenzae* is meningitis

4) **Disease caused by *Haemophilus*** (PGI, June-99)
(a) Chancroid (b) Influenza (c) Acute epiglottitis (d) Brain abscess (e) Brazilian pupuric fever

5) **Satellitism is seen in culture of**
(a) *Haemophilus* (b) *Streptococcus* (c) *Klebsiella* (d) *Proteus*

6) **True about *H. influenzae***
(a) Grow on sheep blood agar & CO2 (b) It is not capsulated (c) Invasive strain is most common (d) Gram positive

Haemophilus ducreyi

7) **A 20 year old male patient present to the STD clinic with a genital ulcer. The gram stain of the smear from ulcer shows gram negative coccobacilli. The most appropriate media for culture would be** (AI-04)
(a) Thayer Martin medium (b) Blood agar with X & V factors (c) Chocolate gar with isovitate X (d) Tellurite blood agar

8) **Chancroid is caused by**
(a) *H. ducreyi* (b) *T pallidum* (c) Gonococcus (d) HSV

9) **A patient has multiple necrotic ulcers with tender inguinal lymphadenopathy. The likely diagnosis is** (AIIMS, Dec-94)
(a) *Haemophilus ducreyi* (b) *Chlamydia trachomatis* (c) Herpes simplex (d) *Candida albicans*

Pasteurella multocida

10) **Most common mode of transmission of *Pasteurella multocida* is -** (AI -09)
(a) Animal bites or scratch (b) Aerosols or dust (c) Contaminated tissues (d) Human to human

Answers of MCQs & explanation

1) **(a), (d) & (e)**
- Factor X & V: *H. influenzae*, *H. aegyptius* & *H. haemolyticus*
- Factor X: *H. ducryei* & *H. aphrophilus*
- Factor V: *H. parainfluenzae*, *H. parahaemolyticus* & *H. paraphrophilus*

2) **(b)**
- Follow section, ***Haemophilus influenzae* [pathogenicity → agent factor (virulence factors)]** for explanation

3) **(c)**
- Capsule is polysaccharide not polypeptide which is responsible for virulence

4) **(a), (c). (d) & (e)**
- Chancroid: Caused by *H. ducryei*
- Acute epiglottitis & Brain abscess: Caused by *H. influenzae*
- Brazilian pupuric fever: Caused by *H. aegyptius*

5) **(a)**
- Follow section, ***Haemophilus influenzae* (culture characteristics → solid media)** for explanation

6) **(c)**
- Does not grow on sheep blood agar
- It is capsulated
- Invasive strain is most common than non-invasive
- Gram negative

7) **(a)**
- Genital ulcer shows gram negative coccobacilli, which is probably *Haemophilus ducreyi* which does not grow on blood agar but it can grow on Gibco Chocolate agar enriched with fetal calf serum, factor X (1% Isovitale X) & Vancomycin
- Thayer Martin medium is a selective medium for *N gonorrhea* & *N meningitidis*

- Tellurite blood agar is a selective medium for *C diphtheriae*

8) (a)

- *H. ducryei* causing chancroid
- *T pallidum* causing chancre
- Follow **table-3** for differences between chancroid & chancre

9) (a)

- Features in given case are of *H. ducryei*. Follow **table-3** for explanation.

10) (a)

- Follow section, ***Pasteurella multocida*** **(pathogenicity →mode of transmission)** for more explanation

51 Bordetella

Learning heading & subheadings

- *Bordetella pertusis*
- *Bordetella parapertusis*
- *Bordetella bronchoseptica*
- *Bordetella avium*

Bordetella pertusis

❖ **Meaning & history:**

- **Genus name:** It came after **Jules Bordet** who identified the bacilli along with **Octave Gengou** from the sputum of children suffered with disease in 1900 & successfully cultivated in complex medium in 1906.
- **Species name:** It came from the word **pertussis** = **intense cough** a characteristic feature of disease.

❖ **Synonym:** Bordet – Gengou bacillus from the name of its discoverers.

❖ **Morphology:** →**Fig.-1**

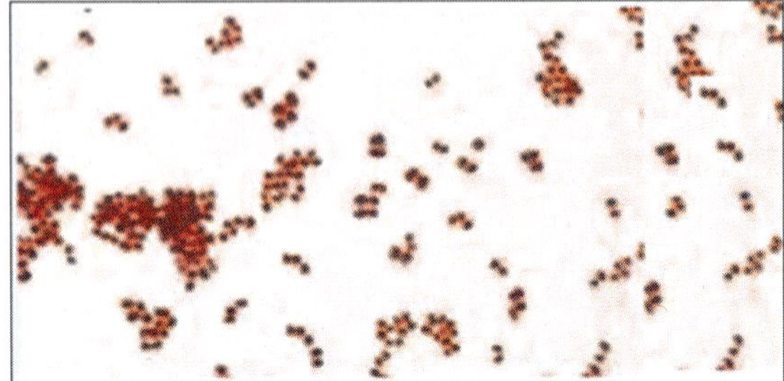

Figure-1: Morphology of *B. pertusis*

➢ **Type according to gram stain:** Gram negative coccobacilli.
➢ **Size:** Small about 0.5 µm.
➢ **Shape:** In primary culture ovoid-coccobacilli but in subculture becomes long-thread like.
➢ **Arrangement:** Culture smear shows loose clumps with space in between **called 'thumb print appearance'.**
➢ **Capsule:** Capsule is present but disappears on repeated cultivation. It is detected with capsular-stain but not by specific antiserum. It does not contribute in pathogenicity.
➢ **Nonmotile & non sporing.**
➢ **Polar bodies (metachromatic granules):** Detected by toludine blue.
➢ **Fimbriae:** Present in freshly isolated strains.
➢ **Immunofluorescent microscopy:** is also useful.

❖ **Cultural characteristics (C/Cs):**

➢ **Effective factors:**
- O_2 effect: Strict aerobes.
- Temperature: Optimum temp. is 35-36^{0}C.
- Fastidious in nature & require special complex media for growth.

➢ **Media:**

A. Solid media:

1. **Nutrient agar:** No growth occurs but achieved by adding charcoal or starch.
2. **Bordet – Gengou (Regan-Lowe) medium:** It is the blood agar contains glycerine & potato. Blood is not to enrich the medium but it neutralise the inhibitory substance produced during culture growth.
3. **Charcoal agar:** It replaces the Bordet – Gengou medium. Charcoal serves as like blood.

B. Selective medium:

1. **Regan-Lowe medium:** Blood agar with glycerine, potato & cephalosporin (selective agent).

➢ **Growth properties:**

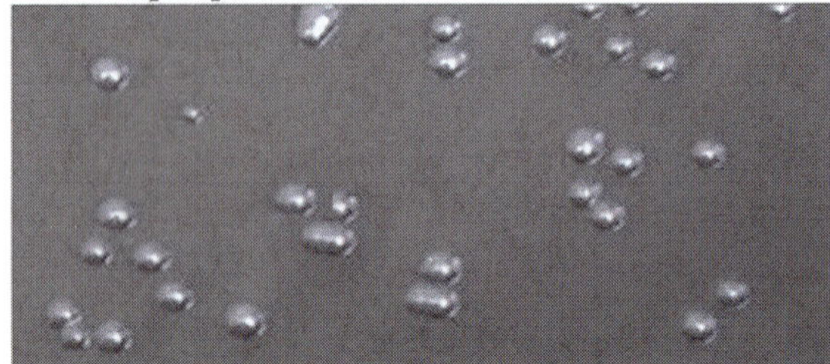

Figure-2: Mercury drop colonies on Regan-Lowe medium

- Growth is slow.
- Small, dome shaped, smooth, opaque, viscid, greyish white & glistening colonies develop after 3-5 day which appear like **'bisected pearls' or 'mercury drops'** as shown in **fig.-2**.
- Confluent growth present as an **'aluminium paint appearance'.**

❖ **Biochemical reaction (B/Rs):**

- Biochemically inactive.
- Non-fermenter.
- Oxidase & catalase are positive.
- Urease, nitrate & citrate negative.

❖ **Resistance:** *B. pertusis* is killed by

- Heating at 55^{0}C in 30 minutes.

- Drying.
- Disinfectant.

❖ Variation:

a. S-R variation: Initially fresh isolates produce smooth (S) colonies labelled as Phase-I, on repeated subculture it lost the surface Ag and pass through Phase- II & III and finally becomes rough (R) labelled as Phase – IV.

- Phase-I: Virulent.
- Phase-IV: Avirulent.

b. Modulation: Change in colour of colonies in Bordet – Gengou medium is **called modulation**. It is due to variation in capsular (K) Ag by nature of medium. Three modes are observed like X, I & C.

1. **X:** From Xanthine means yellow, because of yellow colour colony.
2. **I:** From Intermediate, because intermediate colony between yellow & blue.
3. **C:** From Cyanine means blue, because blue colour colony.

❖ Pathogenicity:

➢ **Disease:** Disease **called pertussis or whooping cough.**

➢ **Meaning:** Pertusis mean intense cough.

➢ **Nature & history of disease:** Distributed worldwide. It may occur in the form of epidemic outbreak. Recent epidemic occurred in Washington in 2012. In India cases are declining due to vaccination.

➢ **Reservoir of infection:** Human case is the only reservoir, no animal reservoir. There is no evidence of chronic carrier or subclinical infection.

➢ **Source of infection:** Respiratory droplets generated during coughing, sneezing or talking.

➢ **Mode of transmission:** Very contagious disease. Whooping cough is the most infectious disease & non-immune seldom escapes the disease. It is transmitted by

- Respiratory droplets generated during coughing, sneezing or talking.
- Fomites borne.
- Direct contact.

➢ **Incubation period:** 1-2 weeks (7-14 days).

➢ **Portal of entry & site:** Respiratory system.

➢ **Precipitating factors (epidemiological determinants):**

I. Agent factors (virulence factors)

1. Pertussis toxin:

- **General properties:**
  - Extracellular.
  - MW: 1, 17,000.
  - Toxoided & produce antibody which is protective, hence included in acellular vaccine.
- **Structure:**
  - Structurally it is similar to LT of *E coli* or cholera toxin of *V cholerae.*
  - It has two subunits like A (active) & B (binding). It binds with G protein of host cell (like respiratory epithelium) by B subunit followed by action by A subunit. It activates the adenyle cyclase which cleaves ATP to cAMP. Increase cAMP is responsible to increase secretion from cells like insulin.
- **Biological actions:** As follows
  - Lymphocytosis Producing Factor (LPF): As name suggest causing lymphocytosis in human & in animals.
  - Histamine Sensitising Factor (HSF): Sensitise only animal not human with histamine.
  - Islet Activating Protein (IAP): It activate the intracellular cAMP in pancreatic islet & increase the insulin secretion in animal not in human.

2. Surface agglutinogens:

- It is genus or species specific.
- It is associated with fimbriae.
- Favours the adhesion of bacilli with respiratory epithelium.
- 14 factors or types are identified by agglutination absorption test. Help in serotyping & epidemiological studies.
- Factors 1-6 are in *B. pertussis.*
- Factor 7 is common in all species.
- Factor 12 is in *B. bronchoseptica.*
- Factor 14 is in *B. parapertussis.*
- Disease is mostly by factors 1, 2 & 3. They also produce protective Ab, hence factors 1, 2 & 3 are included in acellular vaccine.

3. Filamentous Haem Agglutinin (FHA):

- Appear as filamentous structure under electron microscope, hence the name.
- It adhere the *B pertusis* with cilia of respiratory epithelium.
- It also favour adhesion of other bacteria like *H. influenzae* & *Strept pneumoniae* to respiratory epithelium **called piracy of adhesion.**
- Produce protective Ab, hence FHA is included in acellular vaccine.
- It is one of three haemagglutinin produced by *B pertusis* other two are lipid factor & pertusis toxin.

4. Pertactin:

- It is an OMP Ag present in virulent strain of *B. pertusis.*
- It produces protective Ab, hence included in acellular vaccine.

5. Adenylate Cyclase (AC) Toxin: Catalysing the cAMP activity.

6. Tracheal Cyto Toxin (TCT): Causing ciliary damage to tracheal epithelium.

7. Heat-labile toxin: Inactivated at 56^0C after 30 min. Dermonecrotic in nature.

8. **LPS:**
- As like endotoxin of other GNB.
- Heat stable.

Present in the whole cell pertusis vaccine but not considered as protective.

II. Host factors

1. **Age:**
- High mortality & incidence occurs in 1st year of life. It is a disease of children below school age as maternal antibodies are not protective thereafter incidence is decline due to vaccination.
- Atypical form present in adult as **bronchitis**, serve as source of infection in infant & children.

2. **Sex:** More in female at all age.
3. **Immunity:**
- Childhood pertusis is on the decline rate due to immunisation but adult pertusis is on the rise due to waning of immunity.
- Natural infection gives immunity but not long lasting & second attacks have been reported.

III. Environmental factors

- Overcrowding, poverty, poor hygiene, rural areas etc.
- Secondary attack rates are high (about 90%) in unimmunized close house hold contacts.

➢ **Clinical features:**

✪ **Adults:** Atypical form present as **bronchitis**, serve as source of infection in infants & children.

✪ **Children:** Disease **called pertussis or whooping cough.**

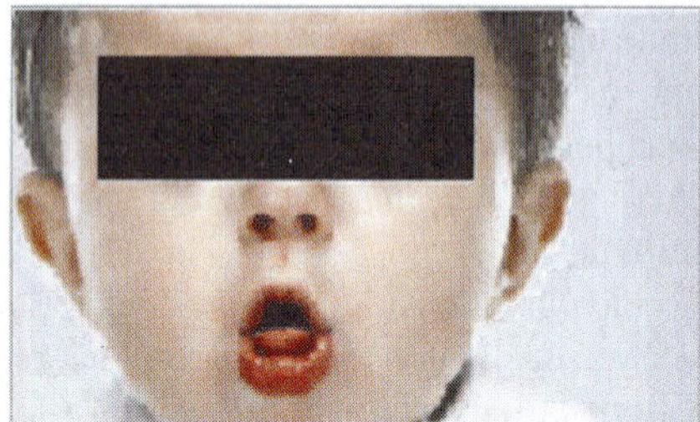

Figure-3: Protrusion of tongue in pertusis

- **Common features:**
- Present in <1 year child.
- Outbreaks first described in the 16th century.
- It is a major cause of childhood fatality prior to vaccination, so vaccination should be started earlier.

- **Species involvement:** 95% by *B. pertussis*, 5% by *B. parapertussis*, rare by *B. bronchoseptica.*
- **3 Stages of disease:** Total duration is 6-8 weeks (each stage will last for 2 weeks).

1. **1st / Catarrhal stage:**
- Insidious onset with fever & dry cough.
- Arrested with early treatment.
- Stage of maximum infectivity for other children.

2. **2nd / Paroxysmal stage:**
- Increase the intensity (with violent spasm) & frequency of cough (become continuous), followed by long inrush of air in almost empty lungs with a characteristic audible sound/whoop (hence the name whooping cough). It is followed by vomiting also (post tussive vomiting).
- Cough is sever & during coughing there may be visible neck vein distension, bulging of eyes, protrusion of tongue (**fig.-3**) & cyanosis may occur.
- Symptoms getting worst at night.
- Stage to develop maximum complications.

3. **3rd / Convalescent stage:** Intensity & frequency of cough gradually decline.

- **Pseudo-whooping cough:** Similar disease produced by other organism like adenovirus and *Mycoplasma pneumoniae.*

➢ **Complications:**

1. **Pressure effect:** Violent coughing produces subconjunctival haemorrhage, subcutaneous emphysema. pneumothorax, abdominal pain, inguinal hernia etc.
2. **Respiratory:** After ciliary damage inflammation extend into lungs producing local diseases like bronchiectasis, diffuse bronchopneumonia & lung collapse (atelactesis).
3. **Neurological:** Convulsion, coma may give permanent sequelae like epilepsy, paralysis, retardation, blindness or deafness.

❖ Laboratory diagnosis:

➢ **Specimens & Collection:** Bacilli are present in respiratory specimen in large amount & easily demonstrated in 1st stage, scanty in 2nd stage & not in 3rd stage. Culture of nasopharyngeal secretion is the gold standard for diagnosis. Following types respiratory or nasopharyngeal specimens are collected.

1. **Cough plate method:** Culture plate is held 10-15cm in front of patient's mouth during coughing, so respiratory droplets directly inoculated in medium.
2. **Pernasal nasopharyngeal swab:** Flexible nichrome wire swab is inserted in nasal cavity till reach to nasopharynx.
3. **Peroral (post nasal) nasopharyngeal swab:** West's post nasal swab is inserted in oral cavity till reach to nasopharynx.

➢ **Transport:** In 0.25- 0.5 ml cas-aminoacid solution (pH, 7.2), modified Stuart's transport medium or in Mischulow's charcoal agar.

➢ **Testing methods:**

a. Blood pictures:

1. Leucocytosis (Total count is - 20, 000-30, 000 per cmm) with relative lymphocytosis (60-80%).
2. ESR increased when secondary infection occur.

b. Microscopy: →**Follow morphology**

c. **Culture:** → **Follow C/Cs**
d. **Biochemical reaction:** → **Follow B/Rs**
e. **Serological tests:**
1. **Ab detection from serum:** Ab appears very late & useful in retrospective diagnosis. Serum will be collected few weeks after the onset of disease. It is detected by agglutination, gel precipitation or by CFT.
2. **Ab detection from nasopharyngeal secretion:** Particularly IgA by ELISA is useful in culture negative cases.

f. **Molecular:** PCR is more sensitive & more reliable.
g. **Typing:**
1. **Serotyping:** As described in surface agglutinogen.
2. **Genotyping:** Done by PFGE or by gene sequencing.

❖ **Prevention:**

A. **General measures:** Isolation of patients & avoiding contact with infected children.
B. **Immunoprophylaxis:** Two types of vaccine.
1. **Whole cell killed vaccine:**
- **Preparation:**
  - **Plain vaccine:** Prepared from smooth phase-I strain. Attenuated by 0.2% merthiolate during several months storage at 4^0C.
  - **Alum absorbed vaccine:** Provide long lasting immunity. Less side effects & more safe.
- **Administration:**
  - It is given with diphtheria & tetanus toxoid as **triple vaccine (DTP or DPT) or penta vaccine** which available in different types preparation: (1) Pentaxim contains D, P, T, IPV & Hib vaccine. (2) Pentavac contains D, P, T, HBV & Hib vaccine.
  - Pertusis components are adjuvant & increase the immunogenicity of diphtheria toxoid & tetanus toxoid.
  - Given by subcutaneous or by intramuscular route.
  - Three (Primary) doses are given at 6th weeks, 10th week & 14th week of age.
  - Booster dose is given after 1year.
  - Booster dose is also given in children < 5 years of age, if they had been previously immunised. It also given after 5 years but whooping cough is rare after 5 years.
- **Efficacy:** Gives 90% protection.
- **Side effects:**
  - **Mild:** Fever & local soreness.
  - **Severe:** Hyperpyrexia, shock, seizure-convulsion & encephalopathy (1 in 5-10 million cases).
- **Contraindications:**
  - Further dose is contraindicated if encephalopathy developed.
  - Allergic patients.
  - After 5-6 years.
  - Children with history of epilepsy.

2. **Acellular vaccine:**
- **Preparation:** From bacillus components like PT, FHA, agglutinogens 1,2,3 (fimbrial antigen 1,2,3) & pertactin (OMP Ag).
- **Advantages:** Less side effects, more safe & given after 5-6 years.

C. **Chemoprophylaxis:** Erythromycin is the drug of choice for contact for 10 days.

❖ **Treatment:** Antibiotics are useful when started in 1st ten days. Macrolides like erythromycin, azithromycin & clarithromycin are drugs of choice. Cotrimoxazole & chloramphenicol are also useful.

Bordetella parapertusis

➢ **History:** It was isolated in 1937 from the mild case of whooping cough.
➢ **Morphology:** Morphologically same as pertusis but antigenically it is different.
➢ **C/Cs:**
1. **Nutrient agar:** It produces the brown diffusible pigments on nutrient agar after 2 days of incubation.
2. **Charcoal blood agar:** Grow very rapidly than pertusis & also agglutinated more strongly than pertusis antiserum.

➢ **Pathogenicity:** Causing whooping cough in 5% cases. Uncommon in most countries. It is very mild may be due to lack of production of pertusis toxin or other virulence factors.
➢ **Prevention:** Pertusis vaccine is not protective for *B parapertusis.*
➢ **Differences between *B. pertussis, B. parapertussis* & *B. bronchoseptica:*** → **Table-1**

Features	*B. pertussis*	*B. parapertussis*	*B. bronchoseptica*
Motility	-	-	+
Nutrient agar	-	+	+
Bordet-Gengou medium	Grow in 3-6 days	Grow in 1-2 days	Grow in 1 day
Urease	-	+	+
Nitrate	-	-	+
Oxidase	+	-	+

Table-1: Differences between *B. pertussis, B. parapertussis* & *B. bronchoseptica*

Bordetella bronchoseptica

➢ **History:** Originally isolated from dog with bronchopneumonia in 1911.
➢ **Morphology:** Motile by peritrichate flagella. Antigenically same as *B. pertusis* & *B. abortus*.
➢ **C/Cs:** Grow on ordinary media without blood.
➢ **B/Rs:** Alkaline reaction in litmus milk test.

- **Pathogenicity:** Naturally present in respiratory tract of many animals. Human infection is acquired from such animals. Causing whooping cough in 0.1% cases.
- **Difference between *B. pertussis, B. parapertussis & B. bronchoseptica:* → Table-1**

Bordetella avium

- **Pathogenicity:** It causes respiratory disease in turkey.

Question bank

Case study

1) A 4 months old child carried to paediatric OPD from the rural area with complain of sever cough since 8-10 days and apnoea during the bouts, followed by vomiting. Nasopharyngeal swab is collected & proceed to culture showing "bisected pearls" colonies. Identify the case & answer the following
a) Name the clinical condition & causative agent.
b) Describe the morphology, culture characteristics & biochemical reactions of causative agent
c) Write the pathogenicity of causative agent

Essay/Full question

1) *Bordetella*

Short notes

1) Pathogenicity or lab. diagnosis or immunoprophylaxis of *B. pertusis.*

Short questions for theory/viva questions

1) What is modulation in *B. pertusis*?
2) What is pseudo-whooping cough?
3) What is piracy of adhesion?
4) Write the four differences between *B. pertusis* & *B. parapertusis*

MCQs for chapter review

Bordetella pertusis

1) **Culture media for pertusis is-** (PGI -94)
(a) LJ medium (b) Chocolate agar (c) Wilson Blair medium (d) Bordet Gengou medium
2) **A 7 month old partially immunised child presented with cough ending in characteristic whoop. Which of the following is considered the best type of specimen to isolate the organism and confirm the diagnosis** (AIIMS, May-11, AI-11)
(a) Nasopharyngeal swab (b) Cough plate method (c) Tracheal aspirate (d) Sputum
3) **Whooping cough is caused by**
(a) *B pertusis* (b) *H influenzae* (c) Pneumococcus (d) Meningococcus
4) **Usual incubation period of pertusis is** (AIIMS-05)
(a) 7-14 days (b) 3-5 days (c) 21-25 days (d) Less than 3 days
5) **What is true about *B. pertusis*** (PGI -95)
(a) Adhere to normal mucosa (b) Destroy cilia (c) Local tissue destruction (d) All of above
6) **Acellular pertusis vaccine contains** (AIIMS, May-11)
(a) Pertactin, flagillary haemagglutinin, cytotoxin, endotoxin (b) Pertactin, flagillary haemagglutinin, fimbriae, endotoxin (c) Pertactin, cytotoxin, fimbriae, pertusis toxin (d) Flagillary haemagglutinin, pertusis toxin, fimbriae
7) **All are true statements regarding pertusis except-** (PGI -12)
(a) Secondary attack rate average 90% in unimmunised contacts (b) Incubation period is around 14 days (c) Erythromycin is the drug of choice (d) Can affect people of any age (e) Main source of infection is chronic carrier

Answers of MCQs & explanation

1. **(d)**
- Follow section, ***Bordetella pertusis* [cultural characteristics (C/Cs)]** for explanation
2. **(a)**
- Culture of nasopharyngeal secretion is the gold standard for diagnosis, so it is the best specimens
3. **(a)**
4. **(a)**
- Follow section, ***Bordetella pertusis* (pathogenicity → incubation period)** for explanation
5. **(d)**
- Adhere to normal mucosa by Filamentous Haem Agglutinin (FHA)
- After adhesion it destroy cilia by tracheal cytotoxin
- After ciliary damage inflammation extend into lungs producing local diseases like bronchiectasis, diffuse bronchopneumonia & lung collapse (atelactesis)
6. **(d)**
- Follow section, ***Bordetella pertusis* (prevention → immunoprophylaxis →acellular vaccine)** for explanation
7. **(e)**
- Human case is the only reservoir, no animal reservoir. There is no evidence of chronic carrier or subclinical infection in pertusis

52 Brucella

Learning heading & subheadings

- Species:
- Morphology:
- Cultural characteristics (C/Cs):
- Biochemical reaction (B/Rs):
- Resistance:
- Antigenic variation:
- Typing:
- Pathogenicity:
- Laboratory diagnosis
- Prevention:
- Treatment:

❖ Species:

A. Human pathogens:

1. ***Brucella melitensis*:**
   - **Genus name** came from army doctor **David Bruce** (1886), who isolated organism from the spleen & **species name** came from the place Melita (Roman name, actual name Malta), from where it was isolated.
   - Natural pathogen for sheep, goat & camel but it can cause infection in human by raw milk.
2. ***B. abortus*:** Causing **abortion in cattle** (cow & buffalo) hence the species name **is abortus.** Identified by Bang in 1897.
3. ***B. suis*: Swine (pig)** pathogen hence the species name is **suis.** Isolated by Traum from pig in USA in 1914.
4. ***B. canis*: Canine (dog)** pathogen hence the species name is **canis.** Isolated from the case of canine abortion. Occasionally causes human disease.

B. Animal pathogens:

1. ***B ovis*:** Causing abortion in sheep.
2. ***B neotomae*:** Identified from desert wood rat.

✓ **Note: Other animal pathogens**

- *Yersinia pestis:* Wild rodent
- *Francisella tularensis:* Rabbit

❖ Morphology:

- **Type according to gram stain:** Gram negative coccobacilli also showing bipolar staining.
- **Size:** Small, 0.5 -1.5μm x 0.5-0.7 μm & mistaken as cocci as was done by Bruce & **called** *Micrococcus melitensis.* Irregular forms observed in culture.
- **Shape:** Short rod like coccobacilli.
- **Arrangement:** Singly or in pairs or in short chains or in clusters.
- **Nonmotile, non sporing & non-capsulated:**
- **Immunofluorescent microscopy:** It is also useful.

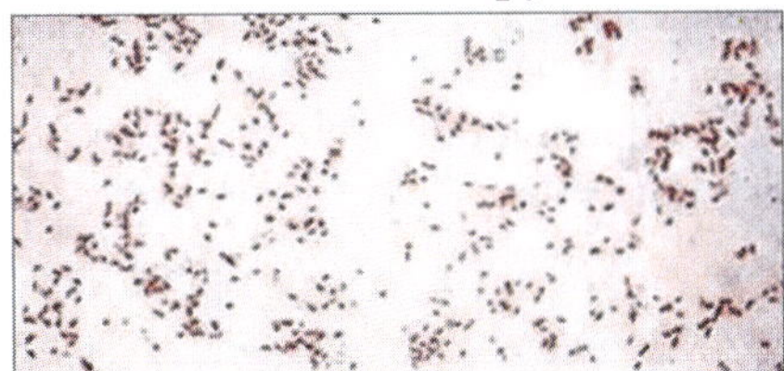

Figure-1: Morphology of *B. abortus*

❖ Cultural characteristics (C/Cs):

- **Effective factors:**
  - O_2 effect: Strict aerobes.
  - Co_2 effect: Better growth occurs under 5-10% CO_2 (capnophilic).
  - Temperature: Optimum temp. is 37^0C.
  - pH: Optimum pH is 6.6-7.4
  - Slow & scanty growth on ordinary media & growth is improved by adding serum or liver extract
- **Culture in media:**

A. Liquid media:

1. **Nutrient broth:**
2. **Liver infusion broth:**
3. **Serum dextrose broth:**
4. **Trypticase soy broth:**

} Uniform growth with powdery or viscous deposit at bottom in old culture

B. Solid media:

1. **Nutrient agar:**
2. **Liver infusion agar:**
3. **Serum dextrose agar:**
4. **Serum potato infusion agar:**
5. **Trypticase soy agar:**
6. **Tryptose agar:**

} Small, moist, translucent & glistening colony.It change to smooth, rough or mucoid forms with antigenic & virulent changes. Culture should not be declared –Ve before 6-8 weeks

C. Selective medium: Bacitracin, polymyxin & cycloheximide are added in above media to make them selective.

D. Castaneda method/biphasic (liquid/broth phase + solid/slant phase) medium:

- Advantages: Avoid the contamination during subculture.
- Culture technique: Blood or bone marrow is inoculated in broth and incubated in upright position. For subculture bottle is tilted, so that broth runs over the slant & then bottle is incubated in upright position.
- Growth detection: Next day observed slant for colonies.

- **Culture in animals:** Guinea pig is the most susceptible laboratory animal.

- Tunica reaction is elicited in male guinea pig after intraperitoneal inoculation.
- Inject the bacilli in thigh of guinea pig. Animal will die after 6-8 weeks. Collect the samples from regional lymph nodes or from spleen and proceed for culture. Blood is collected for Ab detection.

❖ Biochemical reaction (B/Rs):

1. **Glucose fermentation test:** Non-fermenter.
2. **I M Vi C test: - - - -**
3. **Oxidase test: +Ve**
4. **Catalase test: +Ve**
5. **Nitrate reduction test: +Ve**
6. **Urease test: +Ve**

❖ Resistance:

B. abortus is killed by heating at 60^0C in 10 minutes, sunlight, acid, pasteurisation & 1% phenol in 15 minutes.

❖ Antigenic structure:

A Somatic antigen:

- Somatic antigen of *Brucella* contains two epitopes like A & M & present in different species in different amount as follows.

1. ***B melitensis*:** Contains 20 times as much A as M.
2. ***B. abortus*:** Contains 20 times as much M as A.
3. ***B. suis*:** Intermediate antigenic pattern.

- Advantages: Helpful for serotyping & identification of species.
- Disadvantage: Serotyping is not straightforward, because species diagnosed serologically as *B. abortus* may be behave biochemically as *B melitensis* & vice versa.

B Cross reactive antigens: Antigenic cross reaction may occurs with following bacteria.

1. ***V. cholerae*:** Cholera vaccine produces the *Brucella* agglutinin last for 3 years.
2. ***E. coli*:** 0:116 & 0:157.
3. ***S. typhi*:** 0:30 or N antigen of Kauffman & White. Also Vi Ag like L antigen of *Brucella.*
4. ***S. maltophila***
5. ***Y. enterocolitica*:**
6. ***F. tularensis*:**

❖ Typing:

A. Biotyping:

➢ **Based on**: CO_2 requirement, H_2S production, tolerance to bacteriostatic dyes (like basic fuchsin & thionin), agglutination to monospecific sera, phage lysis [Tblisi (Tb) phage] & biochemical test with amino acids & carbohydrates

- ***B melitensis*:** 3 biotypes (1-3)
- ***B. abortus*:** 7 biotypes (1-6 & 9)
- ***B. suis*:** 4 biotypes (1-4)

✓ **Note: Biotypes of *B. suis* on the basis of H_2S production**

- H_2S positive: **Called American strain**
- H_2S negative: **Called Danish strain**

➢ **Reference centre for biotyping:** Central Veterinary Laboratory, New Haw, UK.

B. Bacteriophage typing: **Follow chapter → Laboratory diagnosis of bacterial infections**

❖ Pathogenicity:

➢ **Disease name:** It is a zoonosis **called brucellosis** (also **called Mediterranean fever, Malta fever** or **undulant fever**). Most human infection in India is by *B melitensis* acquired from goats or sheep.

➢ **Nature of disease:** Endemic in areas with availability of large numbers of animals like Mediterranean zone, Eastern Europe, Central Asia, Mexico & South America.

➢ **Reservoir of infection:** Following animals are the reservoirs.

- ***B. melitensis*:** Sheep, goat & camel. Most common & most virulent human pathogen
- ***B. abortus*:** Cattle
- ***B. suis*:** Swine
- ***B. canis*:** Dog

} rare or intermediate human pathogens

➢ **Source of infection:** Animal products like milk, dairy products prepared from infected milk (cheese, ice cream etc.) & meat. Human products like vaginal discharge. Bacteria are also present in excreta of animals like urine or faeces. Most common animals responsible for human infection are sheep & goat.

➢ **Mode of transmission:** No man to man transmission can occurs however possible by sex, breast feeding or via placenta. Common routes are mentioned below.

a. Direct:

1. **Contact:**
   - Contact during sexual intercourse.
   - Occupational contact with infected animals/animal tissues in butcher, veterinarian & animal handlers.
   - Contact of abraded skin with infective materials.
2. **Inoculation:** Accidentally in laboratory in conjunctiva or in mucosa.
3. **Vertical:** By placenta & breast feeding.

b. Indirect (vehicle borne):

1. **Air borne:** By inhalation of dust particles arise from dried animal material like wool.
2. **Water & food borne:** Ingestion of
   - Milk: A Maltese bacteriologist Zammit noticed that *B. melitensis* is transmitted to human by goat's milk.
   - Meat or animal products prepared from infected animals.
   - Contaminated water from animal excreta (urine, faeces) or carcass.
   - Contaminated raw vegetables from animal excreta (urine, faeces) or carcass.
3. **Vector borne:** In animal by blood sucking arthropod (ticks).

➢ **Incubation period:** 10-30 days.

- **Portal of entry:** Skin, GIT, respiratory system etc.
- **Sites:** Blood, RE system, placenta, muscles etc.
- **Precipitating factors (epidemiological determinants):**

I. Agent factors (virulence factors)

1. **Intracellular location:** Helps in survival against antibodies & drugs
2. **LPS:** Having endotoxic actions

II. Host factors

1. **Occupational factors:** Like laboratory workers, veterinary doctors, butchers, forest officers & animal handlers are at most risk.
2. **Presence of erythritol in placenta:** Growth is enhanced due to presence of erythritol.

- **Pathogenesis:** → **Flow chart-1**

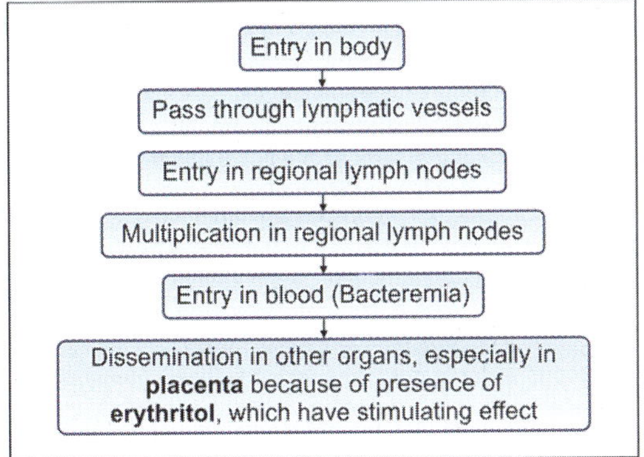

Flow chart-1: Pathogenesis of *Brucella* spp.

- **Clinical features:** Brucellosis is present with non specific sign & symptoms.

1. **Acute/subacute brucellosis:**
   - Associated with prolonged bacteremia.
   - Present as irregular fever (undulating/on-off fever in some cases), chills, joint-muscle pain, asthmatic attack, sweating, exhaustion, anorexia, constipation, nervous irritability etc.
2. **Chronic brucellosis:**
   - Non bacteremic, low grade infection with periodic exacerbation of minor symptoms like sweating, joint pain, lassitude, minimal or no fever.
   - Sage of hypersensitivity with minimal or no fever.
   - Immunity is mostly CMI. Th1 try to eliminate the intracellular-bacilli via releasing of TNF-α, TNF-β, IL-1 & IL-12. Tissue reaction to *Brucella* consist granuloma formation with epithelial cells, giant cell, lymphocytes & plasma cells heals with fibrosis & some time with calcification.
   - Granuloma occurs in RE system like spleen, lymph node (lymphadenopathy), liver (hepatomegaly) etc.
3. **Latent brucellosis:** Survive in RE-system & produce late infection. No symptoms but diagnosed with positive serological tests.

- **Complications:** They are associated with bones, joints, nerve system or with visceral organs.

✓ **Note: Variation in presentation as per species**

1. ***Brucella melitensis*:** Acute & aggressive features.
2. ***B. abortus*:** Chronic & insidious features.
3. ***B. suis*:** Focal abscess.
4. ***B. canis*:** Acute gastrointestinal symptoms.

❖ Laboratory diagnosis:

A. Human brucellosis

- **Specimens:** Blood, bone marrow, urine, aspiration from nodes, sputum, CSF, breast milk, vaginal discharge, seminal fluid etc.
- **Collection:** Collect in trypticase broth , incubates at 37^0C under 5-10% CO_2 & than s/c on solid media
- **Testing methods:**

i. **Microscopy:** → **Follow morphology**
ii. **Culture:** → **Follow C/Cs**
iii. **Biochemical reactions:** → **Follow B/Rs**
iv. **Serological tests:**

✪ **Immunological markers:** Both IgM & IgG are appearing 7-10 days after infection. As the disease progress IgM will decline with same or rising titre of IgG. In chronic stage IgM may often be absent & only IgG can be detected. It detects IgM, so positive in acute stage while negative or weakly positive in chronic stage, hence the result will be read carefully & a negative result may not exclude the brucellosis

✪ **Tests to detect antibodies:**

1. **Tube agglutination test/ Standard Agglutination Test (SAT):**

- **Principle:** Based on tube agglutination.
- **Ag:** LPS Ag of *B abortus.*
- **Ab:** Patient serum.
- **Method:**
  - Mix the equal volume of serial diluted patient's serum with antigen suspension.
  - Incubate at 37^0C for 24 hour or for 50^0C for 18 hours.
- **Significant titre:** It is 1:160. In endemic areas rising titre is confirmed by repeating the test after 2-4 weeks.
- **Blocking antibodies:** It detects IgM, while IgG & IgA are act as blocking Abs or nonagglutinating Abs.
- **False +Ve test:**
  - Due to immunisation.
  - Due to cross reactive antigens from different bacteria as mentioned above.
  - Cholera induced agglutinin may be differentiated by the agglutination absorption test or treatment of serum with 2-mercaptoethanol (2ME).
- **False –Ve test:**
  - Due to prozone phenomenon which is eliminated by dilution method by using 4% saline.
  - Due to effect of blocking antibodies which are eliminated by

- Prior heating of serum at 55^{0}C for 30 minutes.
- Dilution of patient's serum by using 4% saline.
- Detection of blocking antibodies by Coombs test.

2. **CFT:** More useful to detect IgG/chronic stage.
3. **ELISA:**
- Sensitive & specific test.
- It detect IgM & IgG separately, so useful to differentiate between acute & chronic stage.

4. **2-mercaptoethanol (2ME) agglutination test:**
- It destroys the IgM (by breaking the disulphide bond of IgM) from the samples contains both IgG & IgM, so it detects only IgG **called 2ME resistant IgG.**
- It is superior than routine agglutination test.
- 2ME resistant IgG can fall after adequate therapy, so reducing titre of IgG can indicates the adequate therapy & no further progress of disease.

5. **Rose Bengal card test:**
6. **Dip stick test:**

v. **Brucellin test:** Based on DTH, like tuberculin test.

vi. **Molecular test:** Like PCR.

B. Animal brucellosis

- **Specimens:** Milk (cream of the milk).
- **Testing methods:** Same as like human brucellosis.
- **Some rapid test for human & animal brucellosis:**

1. **Rapid plate agglutination test:**
2. **Rose Bengal test.**
3. **Whey agglutination test.**
4. **Milk ring test:**
- Milk is mixed with *Brucella* Ag (prepared from killed *Brucella* & stained with haematoxylin).
- Incubated in water bath at 70^{0}C for 40-50 min. & Read the result.
- +Ve: Blue ring at top, leaving milk unstained if milk contains Ab.
- -Ve: No ring at top, leaving milk in blue colour if no Ab in milk.

❖ Prevention:

A. General measures:

- Prevention of consumption of milk & other product of infected animals.
- Milk borne infection is controlled by pasteurization.
- Identification & slaughtering of infected animals & development of certified *Brucella* free herds.

B. Immunoprophylaxis: Two types of vaccine.

1. **Animal vaccine:** Prepared from strain 19 & protective in cattle.
2. **Human vaccine:** Live attenuated vaccine is prepared but not suitable for human use.

C. Chemoprophylaxis: Doxycycline plus rifampicin is given after exposure.

❖ Treatment: By using antibiotics.

- **For children & pregnant women:** Cotrimoxazole with rifampicin or Gentamicin are effective.
- **For adult:**
  - Gold standard: Doxycycline daily for 45 days (6 weeks) with streptomycin by IM injection for 2 weeks.
  - WHO regime: Rifampicin for 6 weeks plus doxycycline daily for 6 weeks. Relapse or treatment failure can occur in 5-10% cases.
- **For CNS involvement:** Cotrimoxazole is added to the regime with continuation for 6 months.

Question bank

Case study

1) A farmer rearing sheep, presented in hospital with complain of fever. Clinical examination ruled out the lymphadenopathy & hepatomegaly. Liver biopsy revealed non caseating granuloma while standard agglutination test from serum measured 1: 1280 titre. Identify the case & answer the following
a) Name the clinical condition & causative agent.
b) Describe the morphology, culture characteristics & biochemical reactions of causative agent
c) Write the pathogenicity of causative agent
d) Describe the serological tests of causative agent

Essay/Full question

1) *Brucella*

Short notes

1) Pathogenicity or laboratory diagnosis of *Brucella melitensis*

Short questions for theory/viva questions

1) What is milk ring test?
2) Write the different mode of transmission of brucellosis.

MCQs for chapter review

1) ***Brucella melitensis* is commonly found in (animal) -** (PGI, Nov -13, May-11)
(a) Pig (b) Camel (c) Sheep (d) Goat (e) Reinder

2) **A farmer presented with fever off and on for the past 4 years was diagnosed to be suffering from chronic brucellosis. All of the following serological tests would be helpful in the diagnosis at this state except -** (AI-11)
(a) Standard Agglutination Test (b) 2 mecaptoethanol test (c) Complement fixation test (d) Coomb's test

3) **All are true about *Brucella* except-** (AIIMS, May -11)
(a) *Brucella abortus* is capnophilic (b) Transmission by aerosol route can occur occasionally (c) Pasteurisation destroy it (d) 2ME is used to detect IgA

4) **Treatment of brucellosis-** (PGI, June-08)
(a) Doxycycline (b) Streptomycin (c) Erythromycin (d) Pencillin (e) Rifampin

Answers of MCQs & explanation

1. **(b), (c) & (d)**
- Follow section, **species** for explanation

2. **(a)**
- SAT is useful to diagnose the acute stage (IgM)

3. **(d)**
- 2ME is used to detect IgG

4. **(a), (b) & (e)**
- Follow section, **treatment** for explanation

53 Miscellaneous GNB

Learning heading & subheadings

- *Francisella tularensis*
- *Chromobacterium violaceum*
- *Gardnerella vaginalis*
- Rat bite fever (RBF)
- HACEK group
- *Capnocytophaga* spp.

Francisella tularensis

❖ **Classification:** →Flow chart-1

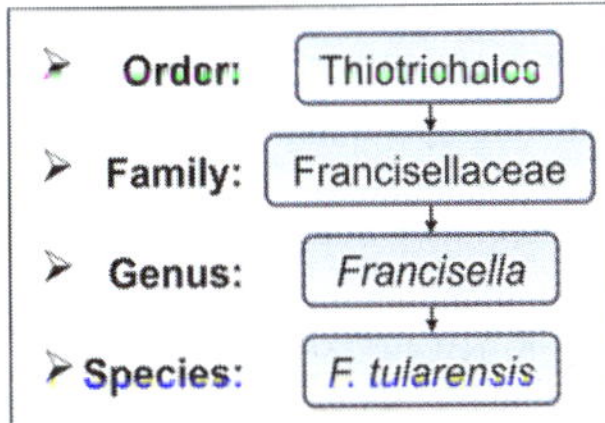

Flow chart-1: Classification of *F. tularensis*

❖ **Meaning:**

- **Genus name:** Named after Francis for pioneering studies on tularemia a disease of rabbits & other rodents.
- **Species name:** 1st described in Tulare country, California, hence **disease** is tularemia & **species** is tularensis.

❖ **Synonym:** Formerly **called *Pastuerella tularensis*** or **called *Brucella tularensis.***

❖ **Morphology:**

➢ **Staining properties:** Gram negative coccobacilli with 10% carbol fuchsin 7 showing bipolar staining.

➢ **Size:** 0.3-0.7 µm x 0.2µm.

➢ **Shape:** Pleomorphic with bacillary or filamentous forms.

➢ **Motility:** Nonmotile.

➢ **Capsule:** Capsulated & resemble to ***Mycoplasma*** being filterable, multiply by budding & filamentous formation besides binary fission.

❖ **Cultural characteristics (C/Cs):**

➢ **Effective factors:**

- Strict aerobes.
- Optimum temperature: 37^{0}C.
- Fastidious in growth requirements.

➢ **Culture in media:**

A **Liquid media:** Contain casein hydrosylate, thiamine & cystine.

B **Solid media:**

1. **Francis' blood dextrose cystine agar:** Minute droplet like transparent colonies appears after 3-5 days.

❖ **Biochemical reaction (B/Rs):**

1. **Sugar fermentation test:** Glucose & maltose are fermented with acid production only
2. **Indole test:** -Ve
3. **Urease test:** -Ve
4. **Catalase test:** Variable
5. **Ornithine decarboxylation test:** -Ve

❖ **Biotypes:** Based on virulence & epidemiological nature. Highly virulent in N. America & low virulent in Europe & in Asia.

❖ **Pathogenicity:** Disease **called tularemia** (plague like disease).

➢ **Mode of transmission & clinical features:**

1. **Direct contact:** Infection occurs by direct contact with animal tissue in butchers.
2. **Tick bite:** Local ulcer & adenitis.
3. **Deer fly bite:** There is evidence that deer flies in the western U.S. are involved in the transmission of tularemia, so also **called deer fly fever** or **rabbit fever**. Compared to ticks, deer flies are minor vectors of tularemia. Bite produces pain, swelling & itching.
4. **Accidental transmission in laboratory:** Ocular & other symptoms.

5. **Ingestion of meat or water contaminated by animal excreta:** Typhoid like fever. (Also **called Lemming fever** in Norway because of water contamination by excreta of lemmings = water rats)
6. **Inhalation:** Influenza like symptoms.

❖ **Laboratory diagnosis:**
➢ **Specimens:** Material from local lesion or blood.
➢ **Tested methods:**
1. **Microscopy: → Follow morphology**
2. **Culture: → Follow C/Cs**
3. **Biochemical reactions: → Follow B/Rs**
4. **Serological test:** Agglutination, CFT, Coombs test & haemagglutination test.

❖ **Prevention** An attenuated vaccine is available which can be administered by scarification to persons who are subject to high risk of infection.

❖ **Treatment:** Drug of choice is streptomycin. Other drugs like tetracycline, gentamicin & fluoroquinolones are also effective.

Chromobacterium violaceum

❖ **Morphology:**
➢ **Staining properties:** GNB & also showing bipolar staining.
➢ **Size:** 0.6–0.9 µm x 1.5–3-4 µm.
➢ **Shape:** Long road in shape.
➢ **Motility:** Motile by single flagella at one end (monotrichous) or at both ends (amphitrichous).
➢ **Spore & capsule:** Nonsporing & non capsulated.

❖ **Cultural characteristics (C/Cs):**

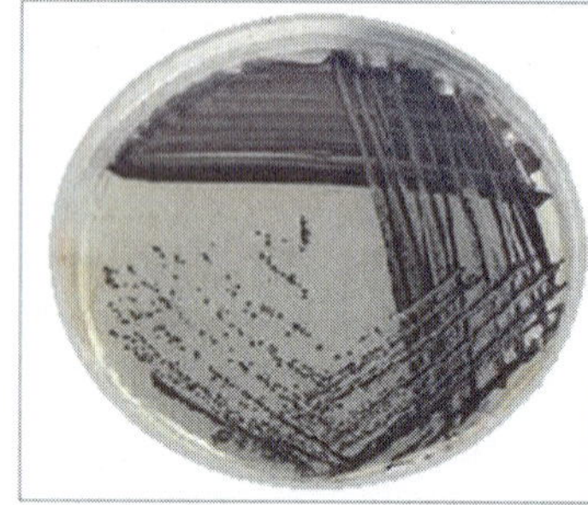

Figure-1: Pigment of *C. violaceum* on nutrient agar

➢ **Effective factors:**
- O_2 effect: Aerobes & facultative anaerobes.
- Temperature: Grow at 35-37^{0}C.

➢ **Media:**
1. **Nutrient agar:**
- Produce violet pigment **called violacein (hence the word *violaceum*)** as shown in **fig.-1.**
- It is soluble in ethanol & insoluble in water and in chloroform.
2. **Mac Conkey's agar:** Pale colonies due to NLF.

❖ **Biochemical reaction (B/Rs):**
1. **Sugar fermentation test:** Ferment glucose with acid production only.
2. **Urease test:** -Ve
3. **Catalase test:** +Ve
4. **Oxidase test:** +Ve

❖ **Pathogenicity:**
➢ **Reservoir of infection:** Soil & water saprophytes.
➢ **Source of infection:** Water.
➢ **Mode of transmission:** Gain entry via contact with wound or by ingestion of contaminated water.
➢ **Clinical features:** Skin lesion, local abscess or septicemia in immunosuppressed persons.

❖ **Laboratory diagnosis:** Pus swab or blood tested by microscopy & culture as described above.

Gardnerella vaginalis

❖ **Meaning:** **Genus name** is given in honour of **HL Gardner & Dukes (1955),** who described the bacilli. **Species name** is given as bacteria are habitat in vagina.

❖ **Synonym:**
- **Formerly called *Corynebacterium vaginalis*** because under gram stain they appear gram positive like *Corynebacterium* but catalase –Ve hence excluded from the group.
- **Formerly called *Haemophilus vaginalis* because** 1st identified over blood agar, but doesn't required factors X & V hence excluded from the *Haemophilus* group.

❖ **Morphology:**
➢ **Staining properties:** GNB to gram variable.
➢ **Shape:** Rod shape to pleomorphic.
➢ **Motility, capsule & spore:** Non-motile, non capsulated & non-sporing.
➢ **Metachromatic granules:** Are also present.

❖ **Cultural characteristics (C/Cs):**
➢ **Effective factors:**
- O_2 effect: Anaerobes.
- CO_2 effect: Better growth occurs under 5-10% CO_2 (capnophilic).

➢ **Media:**
1. **Blood agar:** Produce β-haemolysis on human or rabbit (but not sheep) blood agar.
2. **Two layer plate:** Base with Columbia agar & top with Columbia agar containing 5% old blood gives better result.
3. **Peptone Starch Dextrose agar (PSD):** To identify mix bacteria with colony morphology, but required skill & experience.
4. **Selective media:** Blood agar + colistin (or gentamicin) + nalidixic acid + AMB.

❖ **Biochemical reaction (B/Rs):**

1. **Sugar fermentation:** Ferments glucose, mannose, dextrin, fructose, galactose & ribose with acid production while variable result with lactose, xylose & sucrose.
2. **Catalase:** -Ve
3. **Hippurate hydrolysis:** +Ve

❖ Classification:

1. **Biotypes:** Eight biotypes based on β-galactosidase, lipase & hippurate hydrolysis tests.
2. **Serotyping:** Also developed by using mono & polyclonal sera.

❖ Pathogenicity:

➢ **Disease name:** Disease **called bacterial vaginosis** (not vaginitis, because no sign of inflammation). It is actual not an infection but an alteration of vaginal flora.

➢ **Mode of transmission:** It present in vagina of 40% healthy women causing endogenous infection along with other bacteria.

➢ **Precipitating factors (epidemiological determinants):**

1. **Age:** Infection is most common in sexually active girls in child bearing age.
2. **Co-infections:** Presence of local genital infections (like gonorrhea) or systemic disease (like HIV).
3. **Unprotected intercourse.**
4. **Vaginal douching.**
5. **Use of antibiotics:** *Lactobacilli* present in adult vagina (specially **called Doderlein's bacilli**) convert glycogen in to lactic acid & provide local protection by acidic pH. Use of antibiotics reduced the *Lactobacilli* & vagina is dominated by other anaerobes like *G vaginalis*, *Bacteroides*, *Mobiluncus* & rare by *Mycoplasma hominis* & *Prevotella* etc.

➢ **Clinical features:** Discharge is not from cervix but from vagina with foul/fishy odour & better identified under speculum examination.

➢ **Complications:** Preterm labour, post-cesarean endometritis etc.

❖ Laboratory diagnosis:

➢ **Amsel's criteria:** Based on **clinical background** (gold standard) as follows.

1. Vaginal discharge which adhere to vaginal wall on clinical examination.

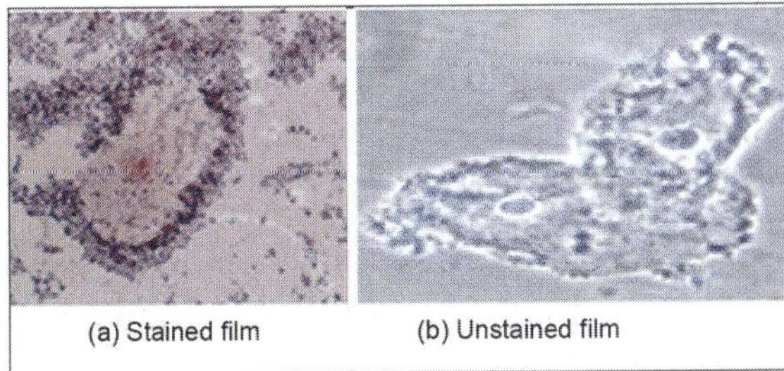

(a) Stained film (b) Unstained film

Figure-2: Clue cells

2. Foul smelling detected by **Whiff test:** A drop of 10% KOH was put on vaginal secretions taken on a glass slide and presence of ammonical odour.
3. Increased vaginal pH ≥5.0 measured by pH meter.
4. Clue cells **(**epithelial cell with surface covered by bacilli**)** are seen in stained/unstained films **(fig.-2).**

If three/four of the above criteria are found, indicates bacterial vaginosis.

➢ **Laboratory method:**

- **Specimens:** Vaginal swab or vaginal discharge.
- **Testing methods:**

a. Microscopy:

1. **Wet film:** Performed bed side after collection. The wet film was examined for the presence of clue cells (>20%) which are vaginal epithelial cells with granular surface and blurred margins because of attached bacteria. Leucocytes also decrease in secretion.
2. **Gram stained smears:** These smears were examined for presence of altered vaginal flora in form of gram negative cocco-bacilli studding vaginal epithelial cells instead of normally predominant gram positive *Lactobacilli*. Gram stain diagnosis was based on a criteria score described by **Nugent et al** as shown in **table-1**. Nugent criteria score vaginal flora as normal (0-3), intermediate (4-6) and bacterial vaginosis (7-10).

Score	Organism morphotype Per High Power Field		
	Lacto-bacillus (parallel-sided, GPB)	***Gardnerella / Bacte-roides*** (tiny, gram variable coccobacilli and rounded, pleomorphic, GNB with vacuoles)	***Mobi-luncus*** (curved, GNB)
0	>30	0	0
1	5-30	<1	1-5
2	1-4	1-4	>5
3	<1	5-30	
4	0	>30	

Table-1: Nugent's Scoring System

b. Culture: → **Follow C/Cs**

c. Biochemical reaction: → **Follow B/Rs**

❖ Treatment: Metronidazole (drug of choice) given 500mg twice daily for 7 days. It endogenous infection may not required treatment also.

Rat bite fever (RBF)

❖ Definition: Triad of relapsing fever, rash & arthralgia occurring days or weeks after rat bite.

❖ Etiological agents: Two types

I. ***Streptobacillus moniliformis*: Called haverhill fever** or **erythema arthriticum epidemicum** or **streptobacillary RBF.**

II. ***Spirillum minus*****:** **Called sodoku** or **spirillary RBF.**

I. *Streptobacillus moniliformis*

❖ **Meaning:**

- **Genus name:** *Strepto* came from **streptos (Greek) = curved /twisted+ bacillus from baculus (Latin) = rod**, indicating straight rod shaped bacteria with curve.
- **Species name:** Word *moniliformis* = necklace.

❖ **Morphology: → Fig.-3(a)**

➢ **Staining properties:** Highly pleomorphic GNB.

➢ **Size:** Variable in size from 0.1 to 0.5 μm x 2.0 to 5.0 μm, and can potentially grow up to 10 to 15 μm, with long, curved segments from 100 to 150 μm.

➢ **Shape:** Short rod to pleomorphic.

➢ **Arrangement:** In culture it appears in chain with variable length **[fig.-3(a)]**, beaded forms or axial fusiform swelling.

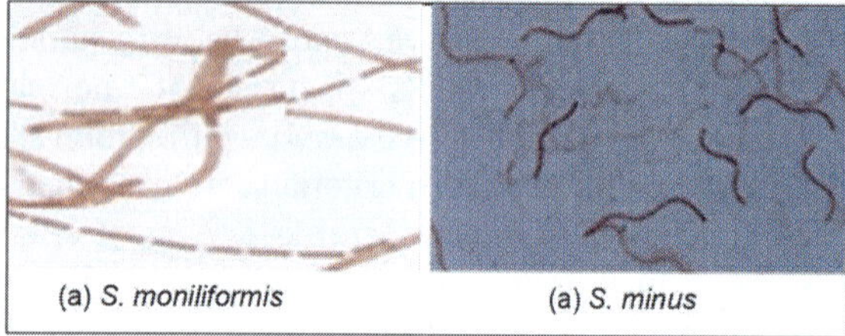

Figure-3: Morphology of agents causing RBF

➢ **Motility:** Non-motile.

➢ **Capsule & spore:** Non- capsulated & non-sporing.

➢ **L-forms:** Are also present.

❖ **Cultural characteristics (C/Cs):**

➢ **Effective factors:**

- Aerobes & facultative anaerobes or microaerophilic.
- Incubation required at 37°C in humid atmosphere for 3-days.
- Growth is improved by adding blood or 20% serum in medium.

➢ **Culture in media:**

A. Liquid media:

1. **20% Serum nutrient broth:** Bacteria produce **'fluffy ball colonies'.**

B. Solid media:

1. **20% Serum nutrient agar (moist plate not dry):**
2. **Loeffler's serum (moist slope):**

- **Growth properties:** Incubation required at 37°C in humid atmosphere. Colonies develops after for 3-days which are raised, smooth, 1-2mm, grey in colour, granular & short life will dies in 3-4 days.
- Smear examination shows chain of bacilli with variable length, beaded forms, axial fusiform swelling or L-forms.

➢ **Culture in animal:** Inoculation in mice produce generalised infection with swelling of legs or feet.

❖ **Biochemical reaction (B/Rs):**

1. **Sugar fermentation:** Ferments glucose & few other sugars with acid production only.
2. **Catalase, oxidase, urease & indole test:** -Ve

❖ **Pathogenicity:**

➢ **Disease name & meaning:** **Called haverhill fever,** because 1st human case was observed in **Haverhill, USA.**

➢ **Synonym:**

- **Streptobacillary RBF**
- Also **called erythema arthriticum epidemicum** because involvement of joint & epidemic outbreak.

➢ **Nature of disease:** Epidemic outbreak can occur.

➢ **Reservoir of infection:** Rat.

➢ **Source of infection:** Rat or water-milk-food contaminated by rat products.

➢ **Mode of transmission:** Rat bite or by ingestion of water-milk-food contaminated by rat products.

➢ **Incubation period:** 2-10 days.

➢ **Portal of entry:** Skin or GIT.

➢ **Sites:** Joints & other body parts.

➢ **Clinical features:**

1. **Animal like rat/mice:** Multiple arthritis with swelling of legs or feet.
2. **Human:** Characterized by sudden onset of fever, headache, myalgia, petechial rash & arthritis. Relapse in untreated cases.

❖ **Laboratory diagnosis:**

➢ **Specimens:** Blood or joint fluid.

➢ **Testing methods:**

1. **Microscopy: → Follow morphology**
2. **Culture: → Follow C/Cs**
3. **Biochemical reactions: → Follow B/Rs**
4. **Serological test:** Agglutination, CFT etc.
5. **Animal inoculation:** In mice generalised infection with swelling of legs or feet can occur.

❖ **Prevention:** Rat control & use of sterile water-milk-food.

❖ **Treatment:** Respond to tetracycline, erythromycin & penicillin.

II. *Spirillum minus*

❖ **History:** It was 1st observed in rat by Carter in 1888 in India & diagnosed as causative agent of RBF by Japanese workers.

❖ **Morphology: → Fig.-3(b)**

➢ **Staining properties:** GNB but better stained by Giemsa, Leishman's stain or by Fontana stain.

➢ **Size:** 0.2-0.5 μm × 2-5-10 μm.

➢ **Shape:** Rigid spiral in shape with tight coils at regular interval of 1μm as shown in **fig.-3(b).**

➢ **Motility:** Darting motility by single flagella at both ends (amphitrichous) or by tufts (2-7) of flagella at both ends (amphilophotrichous) examined by DGIM.

❖ Cultural characteristics (C/Cs):

- Microaerophilic.
- Can't grow on artificially prepared nutritional media.
- Animal culture: Identification done by animal culture in mouse or guinea pig. In mouse, no sign of illness but after 5-14 days bacilli identified in blood or peritoneal fluid.

❖ Pathogenicity:

- **Disease name:** **Called sodoku.**
- **Synonym:** Also **called spirillary RBF.**
- **Reservoir & source of infection:** Present in rat & also present in stagnant fresh water.
- **Mode of transmission:** Transmitted by rat bite.
- **Incubation period:** 1-4 weeks.
- **Clinical features:**

1. **Animal:** Slow progressive septicemia & die in few weeks.
2. **Human:** Inflammation at the site of rat bite, enlargement of regional lymph nodes with fever & skin rash.

- **Complication:** 10% mortality due to endocarditis.

❖ Laboratory diagnosis:

- **Specimens:** Exudates from local lesion, lymph node aspirates or blood.
- **Testing methods:** Identification of bacilli by **microscopy & animal culture** as described above.

❖ **Prevention:** Rat control & use of doxycycline or oral penicillin after rat bite is effective.

❖ **Treatment:** Respond to tetracycline, erythromycin & penicillin.

HACEK group

❖ **Meaning:** Name is given by using initial of following genera

- ***H**aemophilus* (*parainfluenzae, aphrophilus, paraphrophilus*)
- ***A**ctinobacillus* *actinomycetemcomitans*
- ***C**ardiobacterium* *hominis*
- ***E**ikenella* *corrodens* and
- ***K**ingella* *kingae*

a. ***Haemophilus* spp.:** Follow chapter → Pasteurellales

b. ***Actinobacillus actinomycetemcomitans*:**

- **Morphology:** GNB / GN coccobacilli & nonmotile.
- **C/Cs:**
  - ✪ **Effective factors:** Microaerophilic & best growth under 5-10% CO_2.
  - ✪ **Media:** Nutrient agar, blood agar, chocolate agar → star shaped colonies.
- **B/Rs:** Ferment Glucose with acid production only. Catalase & oxidase are positive.
- **Pathogenicity:**
  - **Dental pathogen:** Normal flora of mouth causes **periodontal infection.**
  - **Mycetoma:** In 30% cases of mycetoma, it is associated with *A. israelii*.
  - **Other infections:** Endocarditis, pericarditis, meningitis, pneumonia, UTI, abscess, empyema etc.

c. ***Cardiobacterium hominis*:**

- **Meaning:** Produces disease in person with pre-existing heart disease, hence the name.
- **Morphology:** GNB. Pleomorphic & nonmotile.
- **C/Cs:**
  - ✪ **Effective factors:** Facultative anaerobes. Best growth under 3-5% CO_2 & high humidity.
  - ✪ **Media:** Nutrient agar, blood agar & yeast extract agar.
- **B/Rs:**
  - Ferment plenty of sugars.
  - Indole & oxidase tests: Positive
  - Catalase & nitrate: Negative
- **Pathogenicity:** Normal flora of nose & throat, may cause endocarditis specially in pre-existing cardiovascular disease.
- **Treatment:** Respond to many antibiotics. Streptomycin & penicillin are the drugs of choice.

d. ***Eikenella corrodens*:**

- **Meaning:** Jerking motility helps bacilli to spread & to produce corrosive effect (corroding appearance) over blood agar hence the species **called corrodens.**
- **Morphology:** GNB, shows unusual jerking or twitching motility not due flagella but by contractile-fimbriae like filamentous appendages. Jerking motility helps bacilli to spread & to produce corrosive effect (corroding appearance) over blood agar.
- **C/Cs:**
  - Aerobes & facultative anaerobes.
  - Good growth under humid atmosphere & 5-10% CO_2.
  - Require haemin for growth.
  - Growth occurs on nutrient agar.
  - Blood agar: Fimbriate strain produce **'corroding appearance'** & non-fimbriate strain produce **'non-corroding appearance'.**
  - Selective medium: Nutrient agar + haemin + clindamycin + KNO_3.
- **B/Rs:**
  - Not-ferments sugar.
  - Indole & catalase test: Negative.
  - Oxidase test: Positive.
- **Pathogenicity:** Norma flora of mouth, respiratory tract & GIT. They produce opportunistic infection like endocarditis & mixed infection with other bacteria like-periodontal disease, wound infection,

subcutaneous-brain-liver-skin abscess, meningitis, osteomyelitis, pneumonia etc.

- **Treatment:** Respond to tetracycline & penicillin.

e. ***Kingella kingae*:**

- **Morphology:** GN bacilli or coccobacilli & sometimes gram negative diplococcus like *Neisseria.*
- **C/Cs:** Grow on Thayer-Martin medium.
- **B/Rs:** Catalase is negative & oxidase is positive.
- **Pathogenicity:** Normal flora of mouth responsible for endocarditis & bone-joint-tendon infections.

Capnocytophaga spp.

❖ **Meaning:** Genus name came from **"Capno" for its dependence on CO_2 + "cytophaga" for its flexibility and mobility shift** (gliding motility).

❖ **Species:** This genus includes 8 different species.

A. **Isolated oral cavity of humans:**

- *Capnocytophaga ochracea,*
- *C. gingivalis*
- *C. granulosa*
- *C. haemolytica*
- *C. sputigena*
- *C. leadbetteri*

B. **Isolated oral cavity of animals like dog & cat :**

- *C. canimorsus*
- *C. cynodegmi*

C. canimorsus

- **Meaning:** Species name came from **canine = dog,** because transmitted by dog bite.
- **History:** First observed in 1976 by Bobo & Newton from the case with meningitis & septicemia bitten by 2 different dogs on 2 consecutive days.
- **Morphology: → Fig.-4**

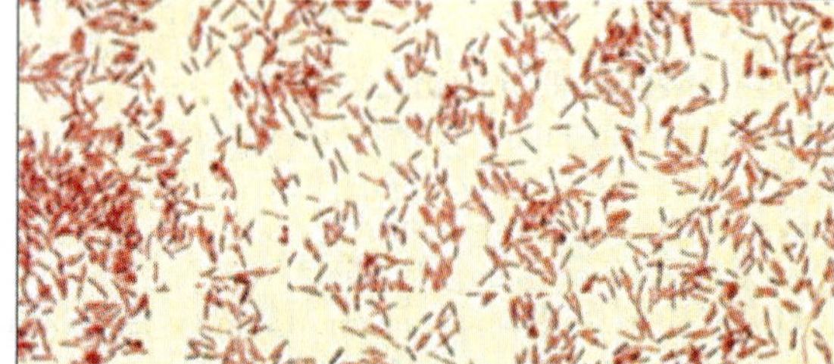

Figure-4: Morphology of *C. canimorsus*

✪ **Staining properties:** GNB.
✪ **Size:** 1-3 μm in length.
✪ **Shape:** Rod shape. After growth on agar plates, longer rods with curved shape.
✪ **Motility:** Non flagellates but showing gliding motion, although this can be difficult to see.

- **Cultural characteristics (C/Cs):**

✪ **Effective factors:**

- O_2 effect: Anaerobes.
- CO_2 effect: Better growth occurs under 5-10% CO_2 (capnophilic).
- Fastidious can grow on media enriched with blood.
- Slow growing colonies may appear after 18-24 hours or longer (48-72 hrs).

✪ **Media:**

1. **Blood agar:** With 5% sheep or rabbit blood.
2. **BHIA:**
3. **Chocolate agar:**

✪ **Growth properties:** At 18 hours, colonies are usually less than 0.5 mm. in diameter spotty & convex. At 24 hours, colonies may be up to 1 mm. in diameter. After 48 hours, colonies are narrow, flat & smooth with spreading edges. At this time purple, pink, orange or yellow colour pigmented colonies may appear, but once they are scraped from the agar plate they are always yellow.

- **Biochemical reactions (B/Rs):** Difficult to perform because of slow growth.

1. **Sugar fermentation test:** Ferments maltose & lactose.
2. **Catalase test:** +Ve
3. **Oxidase test:** +Ve
4. **Arginine dihydrolase test:** +Ve
5. **Nitrate reduction, urease test & H_2S production:** -Ve

- **Pathogenicity:**

✪ **Reservoir & source of infection:** It is a zoonosis. Bacteria present as a normal oral flora in canine and feline species & in human also.
✪ **Incubation period:** Symptoms appear after 2-3 days of exposure or after 1weeks.
✪ **Mode of transmission:**

- **Endogenous infection:** Periodontal infection due to activation of oral flora in individual with IDDs.
- **Exogenous infection:** Transmission may occur from animals through bites, licks or even close proximity with animals.

✪ **Precipitating factors (epidemiological determinants):**

I. Agent factors (virulence factors)

1. **Enzymes:** Produce beta-lactamase responsible for drug resistance.

II. Host factors

1. **Age:** Middle-aged and elderly persons are at greater risk. More than 60% of sufferers are fifty years of age or older.
2. **Distribution:** Worldwide. Cases have been reported in the USA, Canada, Europe, Australia & South Africa.
3. **Immunity:** *C. canimorsus* generally has low virulence in healthy individuals, but cause severe illness in persons with pre-existing conditions like

- Splenectomy.
- Alcoholism.
- Immuno-suppression due to the use of steroids (glucocorticoids) in SLE patients.
- Beta thalassemia.
- Smoking.

4. **Occupational:** Individuals who spend a greater portion of their time with canines & felines are at high risk like veterinarians, breeders, pet owners, and animal keepers.
5. **Type of animal bite:** Chance of infection after dog bites are 3-20% while after cat bite, it may be as high as 50%.

✪ **Clinical features:**

- **Periodontal infections:** Due to activation of oral flora in individual with IDDs.
- **Mild flu like symptoms:** It includes fever, vomiting, diarrhoea, malaise, abdominal pain, myalgia, confusion, dyspnoea, headaches and skin rashes such as exanthema.
- **More severe case:** Fulminant septicemia, endocarditis, DIC & meningitis. Prior treatment with methylprednisolone has been shown to prolong bacteremia in these infections, which enables the progression of endocarditis.

➢ **Laboratory diagnosis:** Because of slow growth of bacteria difficult to diagnose by laboratory methods. Clinical history of dog or cat bite helps in diagnosis. Such history enable microbiologist for longer incubation of culture in suspected cases.

✪ **Specimens:** Blood or CSF.

✪ **Testing methods:** Identification of bacilli by

1. **Microscopy: → Follow morphology**
2. **Culture: → Follow C/Cs**
3. **Biochemical reactions: → Follow B/Rs**
4. **Molecular:** PCR

➢ **Treatment:** Pn G is the drug of choice, but bacteria are able to produce beta-lactamase, so imipenem / cilastatin, clindamycin or combinations having beta-lactamase inhibitor are indicated.

Question bank

Short notes

1) Tularemia
2) *Chromobacter violaceum*
3) Hever hill fever
4) Sodoku
5) HACEK group
6) *Capnocytophaga canimorsus*

Short questions for theory/viva questions

1) Name the causative agent for following disease
Sanghai fever, Sodoku, Haverhill fever & Pontiac fever

MCQs for chapter review

Gardnerella vaginalis

1) **A-40-year-old woman presented to the gynecologist with complain of profuse vaginal discharge. There was no discharge from the cervical os on the speculum examination. The diagnosis of bacterial vaginosis was made based upon all of the following findings on microscopy except** (AI-06)
(a) Abudance of gram variable coccobacilli (b) Absence of *Lactobacilli* (c) Abundance of polymorph (d) Presence of clue cells

Rat bite fever

2) **Rat bite fever may be caused by** (PGI-85)
(a) *Leptospira canicola* (b) *Streptobacillus moniliformis* (c) *Borrelia recurrentis* (d) *Spirillum minus*

HACEK group

3) **HACEK group includes all except-**(AIIMS, Nov-07,May-08)
(a) *Haemophilus aphrophilus* (b) *Acinetobacter baumanni* (c) *E. corrodens* (d) *Cardiobacterium hominis*
4) **True about HACEK group of bacteria is?**
(a) Anaerobes (b) Includes *Coxiella burnetii* (c) Gram positive (d) Required CO_2 for growth

Answers of MCQs & explanation

1) **(c)**
- Follow section ***Gardnerella vaginalis*** for explanation

2) **(b) & (d)**
- Follow section **rat bite fever** for explanation

3) **(b)**
- Follow section **HACEK group (meaning)** for explanation

4) **(d)**
- HACEK group bacteria are not anaerobes but microaerophilic
- It does not includes *Coxiella burnetii*
- All are gram negative
- Required 5-10% CO_2 for growth

54 Non sporing anaerobes

Learning heading & subheadings

- ❖ Definition:
- ❖ Clinical significances:
- ❖ Classification:
- ❖ Important features of anaerobes:
- ❖ Pathogenicity:
- ❖ Laboratory diagnosis
- ❖ Treatment:

❖ **Definition:** Bacteria which do not have spores & survive in absence of oxygen are **called non sporing anaerobes.**

❖ **Clinical significances:**
- Present as normal flora in intestine & produces the vitamins.
- *Lactobacillus acidophilus* present in adult vagina (specially **called Doderlein's bacilli**) convert glycogen in to lactic acid. Such acidic pH of vagina provides local protection.
- Produces toxin (toxaemia) & other metabolites to elicit the local plus systemic disease.

❖ **Classifications:** **Follow → Table 1**

❖ **Important features of anaerobes:**

➢ ***S. ventricularis***: GPC arranged in group of eight.

➢ ***P. niger***:
- Family: Peptococcaceae.
- GPC arranged singly, in pair or in cluster but never in chain.
- It produces the black colony on blood agar.
- Produces the H_2S.

➢ ***Peptostreptococcus* spp.:**
- Family: Peptostreptococcaceae.
- GPC arranged in pair or in chain.

➢ ***V. parvula***:
- Family: Veilonellaceae.
- GNC arranged in pair or in short chain.

➢ ***Eubacterium* spp.:** GPB present as dental pathogen (periodonitis).

➢ ***Propionibacterium* spp.:**
- GPB present as normal flora of skin.
- Anaerobes & aerotolerant.
- *P acne:* Isolated from acne lesion.
- *P avidum* & *P granulosum:* Pathogenic role is unknown.

➢ ***Lactobacillus* spp.:**
- GPB.
- Showing bipolar staining.
- They ferment the materials like milk or cheese with production of acid.
- They are acidophilic & grow best at pH < 5.

➢ ***Mobilincus* spp.:**
- Gram variable bacilli.
- Curved in shape.
- Motile in nature

➢ ***Bifidobacterium* spp.:**
- Branching pattern like Y-shape hence the name.
- Non motile & pleomorphic in nature.

➢ ***Bacteroides fragilis***:

✪ **Morphology:**
- **Type according to gram stain:** Gram negative bacilli or coccobacilli.
- **Size:** 0.4-0.8 μm×1-4 μm.
- **Shape:** Rod shape.
- **Arrangement:**
- **Motility:** Non motile.
- **Capsule:** Capsulated.
- **Spore:** Non-sporing.
- **Other species of genus *Bacteroides*:** *B. ovatus, B. distasonis, B. vulgates, B. thetaiotaomicron* etc.

✪ **Culture characteristics (C/Cs):**
- **Effective factors:**
  - O_2/ Co_2 effect: Strict anaerobe & grow best under 10% Co_2.
  - Temperature: 37^0C
- **Blood agar:** Under 10% Co_2 & in anaerobic condition it produces smooth, circular, convex, 0.2-0.5mm, translucent or opaque, light gray colonies. Colonies are non haemolytic in 24 hours, but becomes β-haemolytic after longer incubation.

✪ **Biochemical reactions (B/Rs):**
1. **Sugar assimilation:** Strongly saccharolytic.
2. **Sugar fermentation:** Ferments plenty of sugars.
3. **Aesculin hydrolysis test:** +Ve

✪ **Resistance:** It produces the β-lactamase (penicillinase) which is responsible for drug resistance among β-lactam group.

- **Pathogenicity:**
- **Reservoir & source of infection:** Most common anaerobes isolated from the bowel & other samples. Normal stool contains 10^{11} *Bacteroides* / gram than 10^{8} facultative anaerobes / gram.
- **Mode of transmission:** Endogenous infection due to disturbances of this flora.
- **Sites:** GIT, lungs, brain & soft tissues.
- **Precipitating factors (epidemiological determinants):**

a. **Agent (virulence) factors:** It produces the lesions by following virulence factors.

1. **Polysaccharide capsule:** It releases the IL-7, IL-8 & TNF responsible for intra-abdominal abscess.
2. **Endotoxin (LPS):** Causing endotoxic activities. Structurally & functionally it is different from other endotoxin of aerobic GNB by it's low toxicity for fever & shock which is actually from inflammation following infection rather than direct infection & low frequency for DIC & purpura.
3. **Aggresins:** It includes the enzymatic activities like protease, neuraminidase, DNAase, heparinise etc.

b. **Host factors:** All favours the bacterial invasion from respective surfaces like trauma, tissue necrosis, diabetes mellitus, IDDs, chronic steroid therapy, antibiotic therapy, presence of foreign body, malnutrition, cancer etc.

- **Clinical features:** Brain & lung abscess, pneumonia, wound infection, peritonitis, hepatic abscess & other abdominal infection occurs mostly following surgery.

- **Laboratory diagnosis:** As like other anaerobes described below.

- **Treatment:** Metronidazole is effective, resistance is rare but reported.

- ***Porphyromonas* spp.:** Differ from *B. fragilis* by ability to produce the pigment & asaccharolytic property.
- ***Prevotella melaninigenica*:**
  - Initially called *Bacteroides melaninogenica.*
  - It produces the haemin derived black or brown pigment.
  - Moderately saccharolytic.
  - Colonies produces the brick-red fluorescence when exposed to UV light.
  - Other species of like *P. deticola* & *P. buccalis* are non pigmented.
- ***Fusobacterium* spp.:** Long thin spindle shaped GNB.

Pathogenicity:

- **Mode of transmission:**
- **Endogenous infection:**
  - **Normal flora:** Non sporing anaerobes are normal flora of human body as shown in **table-1.**
  - **Precipitating factors:** All favours the bacterial invasion from respective surfaces like trauma, tissue necrosis, diabetes mellitus, IDDs, chronic steroid therapy, antibiotic therapy, presence of foreign body, malnutrition, cancer etc.
- **Poly-microbial** Anaerobic infections are generally poly-microbial.
- **Co-infection:** Anaerobic infections are present with aerobic bacteria.
- **Agent factors (virulence factors):**
  - **Capsule:** It inhibits phagocytosis e.g. *Bacteroides fragilis*
  - **Enzyme production:** Helps in spread of infection.
  - **Toxin production:** E.g. *Fusobacterium necrophorum*
- **Pathogenesis:** Exact mechanism are unknown but may be due to reduced blood supply → reduction in Eh potential→ anoxic damage to tissues.
- **Clinical feature favours the anaerobic infection:**
  - Foul & nauseating odour.
  - Gas production gives crepitation on clinical examination.
  - Black pus.
  - Prolonged cellulitis, ulcer & abscess which are refractory to treatment.

Laboratory diagnosis:

- **Specimens collection & transport:**
  - Anaerobes are normal flora of human body, collect the sample in such a way to avoid mixture of resident flora & their presence will not prove casual role.
  - Anaerobes are very sensitive to O_2, care is required for minimum air exposure.
  - Airtight container or anaerobic media (RCMM, Thioglycollate broth etc.) are preferable.
  - Also transport in **PRAS (Pre Reduced Anaerobic Sterilised) medium:** Tube contains nitrogen fitted tightly with butyl stopper.
  - Stuart's transport medium is also useful.
  - Swabs are generally not ideal, but if collected then sent in to Stuart's medium.
  - Sputum is not ideal. Lung abscess or tracheo bronchial aspiration is recommended.
  - Type of sample & method depends on site of infection.
  - Some accepted methods are thoracocentesis, aspiration by needle- syringe, surgical excision etc.
  - Abscess/discharge-aspiration by needle-syringe & inject in airtight bottle.
  - Blood in BHIA or in anaerobic media.
- **Testing methods:**

A. **Microscopy:** Gram stain.

B. **Culture:** Selective medium (Blood agar + neomycin + yeast extract + haemin + Vitamin K)

- **Incubation:** At 37^0C with 5-10% CO_2 in anaerobic (gas pack) jar.

Group	Anaerobes	Normal flora in				Pathogenic lesions
		Skin	mouth	GIT	Vagina	
GPC	***Sarcina*** *S. ventricularis*					Non-pathogenic
	Peptococcus *P. niger*	-	+	+	-	Abscess formation in soft tissues
	Peptostreptococcus *Pst.anaerobius* *Pst. asaccharolytic* *Pst. tetradius* *Pst. prevoti*	-	+	+	+	Puerperal sepsis, wound infection, gangrenous appendicitis, UTI, abscess in brain & in other internal organs, Osteomyelitis
GNC	*Veillonella parvula*	-	+	+	+	Pathogenic role is uncertain
GPB	***Eubacterium*** *E brachy* *E timidum* *E nodatum*	-	+	+	-	Periodonitis
	Propionibacterium *P acne*	+	-	-	-	Acne, endocarditis
	P avidum *P granulosum*					Pathogenic role is uncertain
	Lactobacilli					
	L salivarius,	-	+	+	-	Pathogenic role is uncertain
	L acidophilus	-	-	+	+	
	L casei	-	+	-	-	
	L odontolyticum	-	+	-	-	
	L catenaforme					Causing bronchopneumonia
	Mobilincus					
	M mulieris	-	-	-	+	Bacterial vaginosis. **Clue cells** (epithelial cell with surface covered by bacilli) are seen in stained/unstained films
	M curtisii	-	-	-	+	
	Bifidobacterium dentium	-	+	+	-	Dental caries
	Actinomyces	-	+	+	+	More details →Follow chapter: Actinomycetales
GNB	***Bacteroides*** *B fragilis*	-	-	+	+	Brain & lung abscess, pneumonia, wound infection, peritonitis, hepatic abscess & other abdominal infection
	Porphyromonas					
	P gingivalis	-	+	-	-	Periodontal disease
	P endodontalis	-	+	-	-	Dental root canal infection
	Prevotella *P melaninogenica*	-	+	+	+	Liver abscess, lung abscess, brain abscess, mastoiditis, abdominal, gum & oral infections
	Fusobacterium					Oral & pleuropulmonary infections
	F nucleatum	-	+	-	-	Liver & abdominal infection, thrombo-phlabitis called Lemierre's syndrome
	F necrophorum	-	-	+	-	
	Leptotrichia *L buccalis*	-	+	-	-	Initially called *F. fusiforme*, causing Vincent angina (More details: Follow chapter →Spirochetales)
Spirochaetes	***T. pallidum*** ***B. vincenti***	More details →Follow chapter: Spirochetales				

Table-1: Types, sites as normal flora & pathogenic lesions of non-sporing anaerobes

- **Extra plate:** Aerobic incubation, as control & to identify co-infection by aerobes.

C. **Biochemical reaction:**

D. **Serological test:**

E. **Rapid methods:**

i. **GLC (Gas Liquid Chromatography):**

ii. **Sensitivity testing:** By using gentamicin & metronidazole disc.

iii. **Ultraviolet light (Wood's lamp) exposure:** E.g. exposure of culture or even wound dressing gives bright red fluorescence in ***P. melaninogenica.***

❖ Treatment:

- **Selection of antibiotics:** Drug resistance is a common problem in anaerobic infections. Drug selection depends on
  - Site of infections.
  - Type of anaerobes.
  - Sensitivity pattern of anaerobes.
- **Antibiotics:**
  - Commonly useful antibiotics are penicillin, 2nd generation cephalosporin, chloramphenicol, fucidin, trimithoprim, clindamycin, tetracycline, imipenam, & aztreonam.
  - Bacteroides are sensitive to metronidazole.

Question bank

Essay/Full question

1) Non sporing anaerobes.

Short notes

1) *Bacteroides fragilis*
2) Laboratory diagnosis of non sporing anaerobes.

Short questions for theory/viva questions

1) Write the two clinical significances of non sporing anaerobes.
2) What are Doderlein's bacilli?

MCQs for chapter review

Clinical significances

1) **Doderlein's bacilli word is associated with**
(a) *Clostridium* (b) *Lactobacilli* (c) *Treponema* (d) *Borrelia*

2) **True about anaerobic infection**
(a) Causes toxemia (b) Causes systemic infections (c) Both (d) None

Classifications & important features of anaerobes

GPC

3) **One of the following infection is caused by anaerobic gram positive cocci** (AI -95)
(a) Puerperal infection (b) Food poisoning (c) Endocarditis (d) Septicemia

4) **All are used for anaerobic streptococci except-** (AIIMS, Dec-97)
(a) Penicillin (b) Carbenicillin (c) Clindamycin (d) Vancomycin

Bacteroides

5) **With reference to *Bacteroides fragilis* following statements are true except:** (AI-07, AIIMS, Nov-12,11, May-06, Nov-06, May-03)
(a) *Bacteroides fragilis* is the same frequent anaerobes isolated from clinical samples (b) *Bacteroides fragilis* is not uniformly sensitive to Metronidazole (c) The lipopolysaccharide formed by *Bacteroides fragilis* is structurally & functionally different from the other conventional endotoxin (d) Shock and disseminated intravascular coagulation are common in *Bacteroides* bacteremia

Prevotella

6) **A patient is present with frontal abscess. Foul smelling pus is aspirated. Pus shows red fluorescence on ultraviolet examination. The most likely organism causing frontal abscess is-** (AIIMS, May-02)
a) *Bacteroides* (b) *Peptostreptococcus* (c) *Pseudomonas* (d) *Acanthamoeba*

Answers of MCQs & explanation

1) **(b)** } Follow section, **clinical significances** for explanation
2) **(c)** }
3) **(a)**
   - Lesions produced by anaerobic gram positive cocci are listed in **table-1,** common lesion by anaerobic gram positive cocci from the given options is puerperal infection
4) **(b)**
5) **(d)**
   - *Bacteroides fragilis* is the most common anaerobes isolated from the bowel & other samples.
   - Metronidazole is the drug of choice but resistant strain has been reported
   - Option C & D: Follow section, **important features of anaerobes (*Bacteroides fragilis*)** for explanation
6) **(a)**
   - All organisms are able to produce the brain abscess, but with red fluorescence is *P. melaninigenica* which was initially classified as a species of *Bacteroides*
   - Other microbes which get fluorescence under UV light are
     - **Bright green:** *Microscporum audounii, M. ferruginium, M. canis* & *Pseudomonas* in burns wound
     - **Dull green:** *Trichophyton schoenleinii*
     - **Dull yellow:** *Microscporum gypseum*
     - **Golden yellow:** *Malassazia furfur*
     - **Coral-red:** *Corynebacterium minutissimum* (Erythrasma)
     - **Brick-red:** *Prevotella melaninogenica*

55 Spirochetales

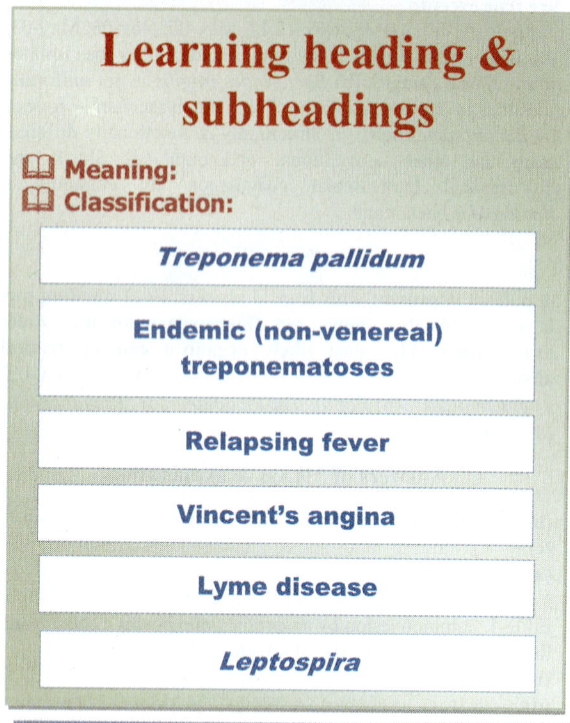

Meaning: From **speira = coil + chaita = hair** indicating flexuous spiral forms.

Classification: → **Flow chart-1**

Treponema pallidum

❖ **Meaning:** Word derived from **trepos = turn + nema = thread + pallidum = pale staining.**

❖ **History:**

- *Treponema pallidum* was first identified by Fritz Schaudinn and Erich Hoffmann in 1905.
- The first effective treatment (Salvarsan) was developed in 1910 by Sahachirō Hata in the laboratory of Paul Ehrlich which was followed by the introduction of penicillin in 1943.

❖ **Morphology:**

➢ **Staining properties:** GNB, but better stained by following methods.

A. **Vital stain:** It is a wet mount & maintains the viability of bacteria & useful for motility detection.

✪ **Types of motility:** 3 types of motility.

1. **Flexion & extension:** During movement secondary curve appear which disappear after sometime, but primary coils remain unchanged.
2. **Translatory motility:** Whole organism move in one direction.
3. **Cork screw motility:** Movement around long axis

✪ **Endoflagella:** Having endoflagella but not useful for motility and remain in periplasmic space between peptidoglycan and outer membrane.

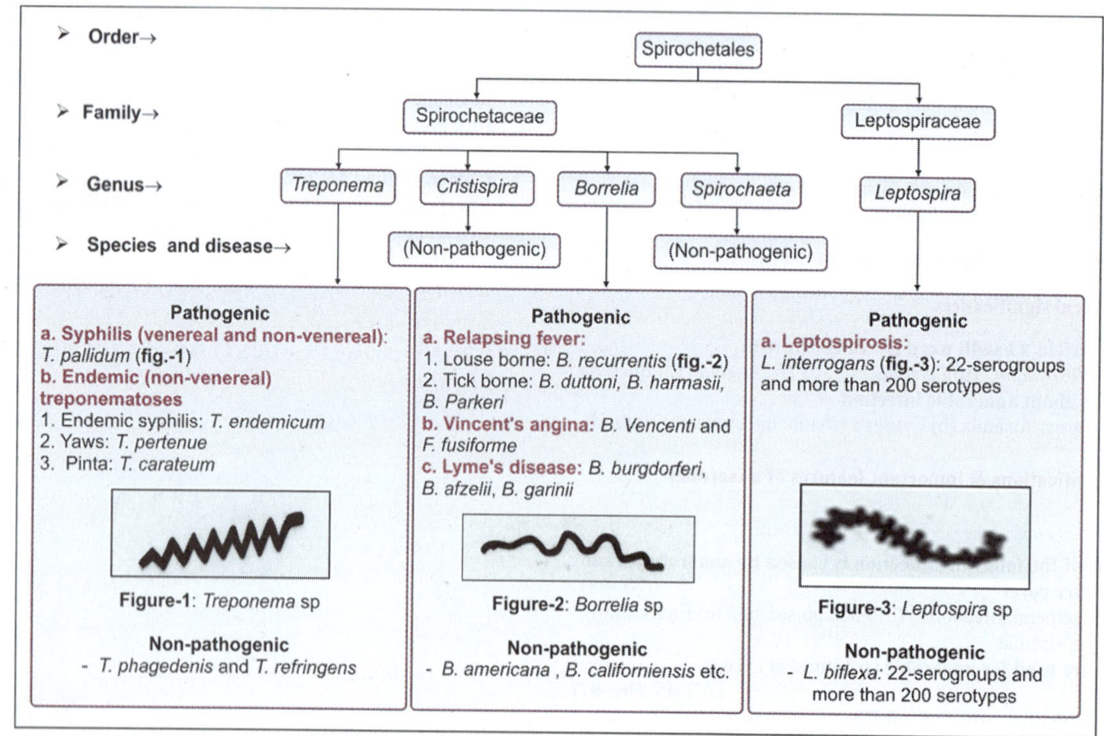

Flow chart-1: Classification of Spirochetales

✪ **Detection of motility:** By following two microscopic techniques.

i. **Dark Ground Illumination Microscopy (DGIM):**
- Prepare the wet films from exudates, apply thin cover slips & examine under the DGIM **(fig.- 4).**
- **Disadvantages:** Low sensitivity, so required 10^4 /ml *Treponema* for test to be +Ve.

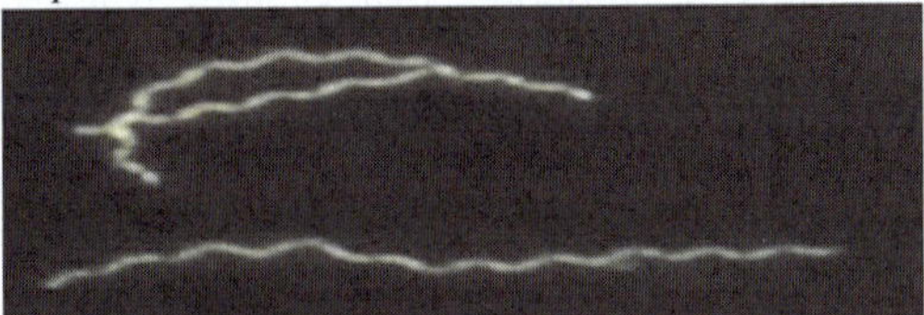

Figure-4: ***T. pallidum*** **under DGIM**

ii. **Phase Contrast Microscopy (PCM):**

B. **Supra vital stain:** Following are useful stains.

i. **Silver impregnation stains:** Like
- Fontana stain **(fig.-5)** from culture.
- Levaditi's stain from tissue section.

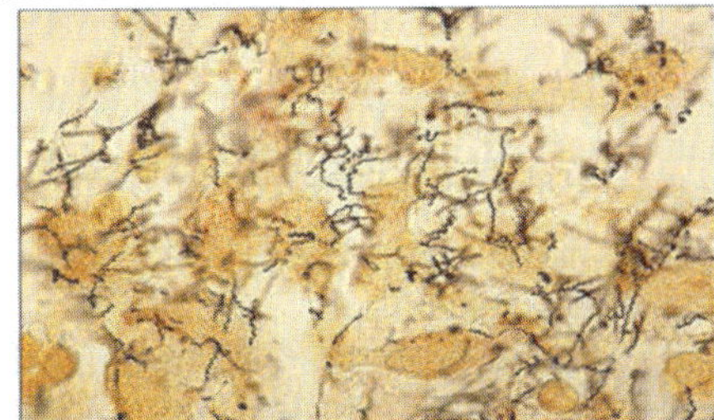

Figure-5: ***T. pallidum*** **under Fontana's stain**

ii. **Histopathological stain:** Like Giemsa stain.

iii. **Negative stains:** Like Nigrosin / Indian ink.

iv. **Direct fluorescent antibody test for *T pallidum* (DFA-TP):**
- Prepare the smear from exudates & fixed with acetone.
- Stain with reagent containing fluorescent tagged anti-*T pallidum* antiserum (specific monoclonal Ab) & examine under the fluorescent microscope.
- **Advantage:** Safe & more reliable.

➢ **Size:** 10 μm long ×0.2 μm.

➢ **Shape:** Regular spiral in shape with 10 coils at interval of 1 μm and sharp end.

➢ **Non-sporing.**

➢ **Non-capsulated.**

❖ **Cultural characteristics (C/Cs):**

➢ **Effective factors:**
- O_2 effect: Strict anaerobes & killed by 0_2 exposures.
- Generation time: 30-33 hours.

➢ **Media & cultivation techniques:**

A. **Pathogenic *Treponema*:**
- Do not grow in artificial culture media.
- It maintained for many decades by serial testicular passage in rabbits e.g. Nichol's strain of *T pallidum*
- Nichol's strain is useful to prepare the antigen for species specific treponemal tests.

B. **Non-pathogenic *Treponema*:**
- Grow in artificial culture media.
- *T. phagedenis* (Reiter's strain, Kazan's strain) and *T. refringens* (Noguchi's strain) can grown in **thioglycollate medium containing serum.**
- Reiter's strain is useful to prepare the antigen for group specific treponemal tests.

❖ **Resistance:** Organisms are killed by
- Heating at 41-42^{0}C in 1 hr.
- Refrigerating at 0-4^{0}C in 1-3 days.
- Drying.
- 0_2 exposures.
- Distilled water.
- Antibiotics.
- Disinfectants like soap, arsenic, mercury & bismuth.

❖ **Antigenic properties:** Two types of antigens.

A. **Non-treponemal / non-specific / cardiolipin / cholelecithin antigen:**
- It released not from *Treponema* itself, but from infected host cell like bullock heart, so **called non-treponemal / non-specific** or **cardiolipin (cardia = heart & lipin = for lipid contain) antigen** & is biochemically a diphosphatidyl glycerol.
- Among the lipid portion it contains cholesterol & lecithin hence also **called cholelecithin antigen.**
- Antibody produced by this antigen is **called reagin antibody** which is IgG or rarely IgM in nature.
- Antigen was standardised by Pangborn in 1945.
- Reagin antibody reacts in standard or nonspecific or non treponemal tests for syphilis, such as Wassermann, Kahn, VDRL etc.

✓ **Note: Reagin antibody**

▪ **IgE antibody of type-I hypersensitivity:** It also **called reagin antibody**; however there is no correlation between two antibodies.

B. **Treponemal / specific antigen:** Two subtypes

i. **Group specific antigen:**
- Biochemically lipopolysaccharide-protein in nature.
- Found in pathogenic and in nonpathogenic treponemes.
- Antibody to this antigen is detected by preparing the antigen from nonpathogenic strain like **Reiter's strain.**

ii. **Species specific antigen:**
- Polysaccharide in nature.
- Found in pathogenic treponemes & it is species specific.
- Antibody to this antigen is detected by preparing the antigen from pathogenic strain like **Nichol's strain.**

❖ **Immunity in syphilis:**

- **Humoral immunity** is not effective.
- **Cell mediated immunity** is more relevant.
- **Phagocytosis** is predominant in early syphilis.
- Primary infection provides some immunity to re-infection.
- **Premunition (concomitant infection, infection immunity)**
- Re-infections do not appear in person already having active infection **called premonition.**
- It occurs in some parasitic infections also.
- Patient becomes susceptible to re-infection only when his original infection is cured.
- **Syphilis & AIDS**
  - Transmission: Abraded skin of syphilis patient allows the more chances of transmission of HIV.
  - Clinical features: Syphilis progress more rapidly in AIDS patients. Concurrent infection may leads to early development of late syphilis & neurosyphilis even after treatment of primary or secondary stage.
  - Diagnosis:
- Poor serological response due to absence of immunity & high titre in STS perhaps due to B cell activation which may not fall even after treatment.
- Negative treponemal tests with advancement of disease due to immune paralysis in end stage.

❖ Pathogenicity, laboratory diagnosis, prevention & treatment:

➢ **Disease name:** Whole spectrum of disease caused by genus *Treponema* **called treponematoses.** Disease caused by *Treponema pallidum* **called syphilis.**

✓ **Note: Treponematoses**

- **Definition:** Whole spectrum of disease caused by genus *Treponema* **called treponematoses.**
- **Classification:** Two categories

1. **Venereal treponematoses**: Like venereal syphilis.
2. **Non-venereal (endemic) treponematoses:** Following four conditions.

- **Non-venereal syphilis:** By *T pallidum* **(flow chart-1).**
- **Endemic syphilis / non-venereal syphilis / bejele:** By *T endemicum* **(flow chart-1).**
- **Yaws:** Follow **table-2.**
- **Pinta:** Follow **table-2.**

➢ **Meaning of syphilis:** Syphilis word derived from the person name **syphilus** who died due to disease.

➢ **Nature & history of syphilis:**

- It is distributed worldwide.
- There are two hypotheses know for the origin of syphilis. 1st proposes that syphilis was carried to Europe from the Americas by the crew of Christopher Columbus as a by product of the Columbian exchange **called Columbian theory**, while the other proposes that syphilis previously existed in Europe but went unrecognized **called pre-Columbian theory**. The 1st written records of an outbreak of syphilis in Europe occurred in 1494 / 1495 in Naples, Italy, during a French invasion.
- Because it was spread by returning French troops, the disease was " **called French disease**", and it was not until 1530 than the term "syphilis" was first applied by the Italian physician & poet Girolamo Fracastoro
- With the discovery of penicillin & also no any extra human reservoir it is expected to eradicate the disease.
- Incidences have been increase with advancing life style, customs & habits.

➢ **Classification of syphilis: → Flow chart-2**

I. Venereal syphilis

✪ **Reservoir of infection:** Only human.

✪ **Source of infection:** Human body fluid like exudates from the lesion.

✪ **Mode of transmission:** Approximately 30% persons are infected after unprotected sexual intercourse with infected person. Spirochetes enter through minor abrasion in skin & mucosa.

✪ **Incubation period:** 10-90 days.

✪ **Infective dose:**

- Infectivity is maximal in first two year of disease (primary, secondary & tertiary). After 5 years the risk is minimal.

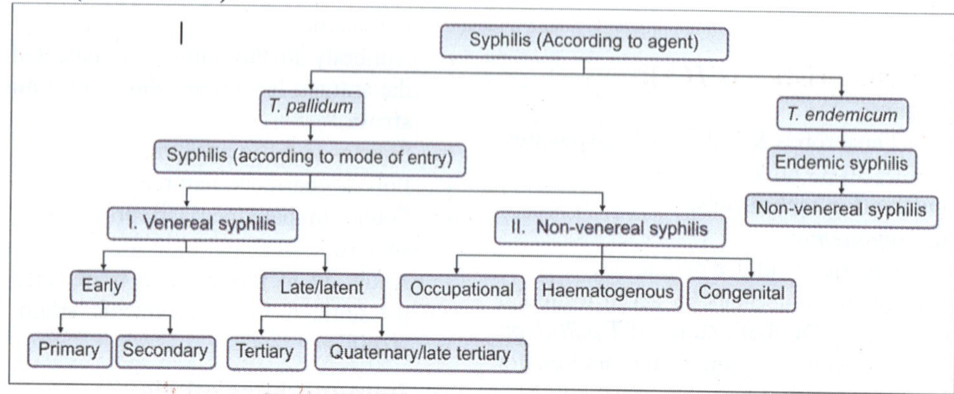

Flow chart-2: Classification of syphilis

- Infective dose is small about 60 treponemes are capable of infecting 50 human volunteers.
- **Portal of entry:** Skin/ mucosa.
- **Sites:** Skin, genital organs, liver, bones, brain, CVS, CNS etc.
- **Pathogenesis, stage of disease & clinical features of venereal syphilis: → Flow chart-3 & fig.-6-8**

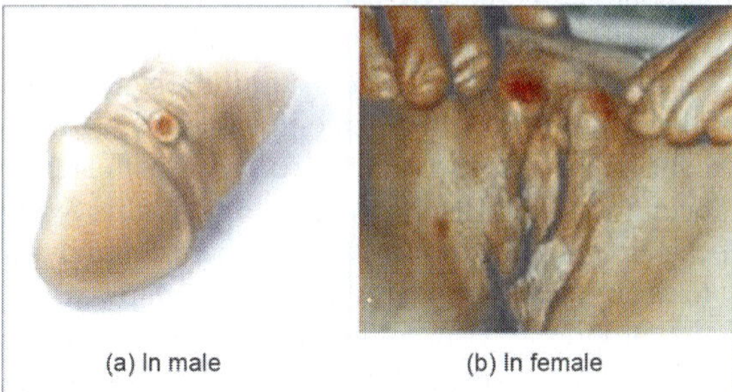

(a) In male (b) In female

Figure-6: Chancre in primary syphilis

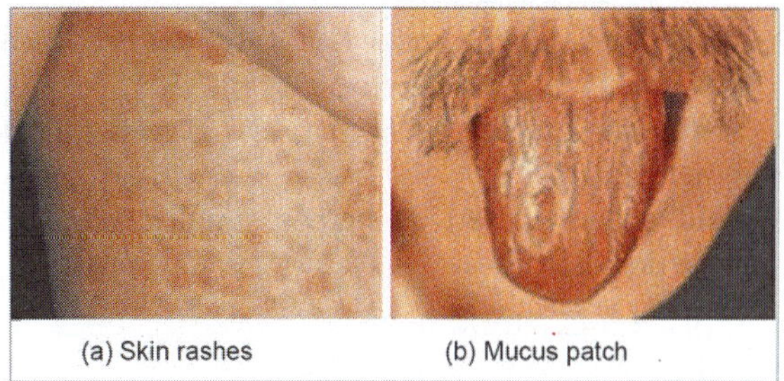

(a) Skin rashes (b) Mucus patch

Figure-7: Skin rashes & mucus patch in secondary syphilis

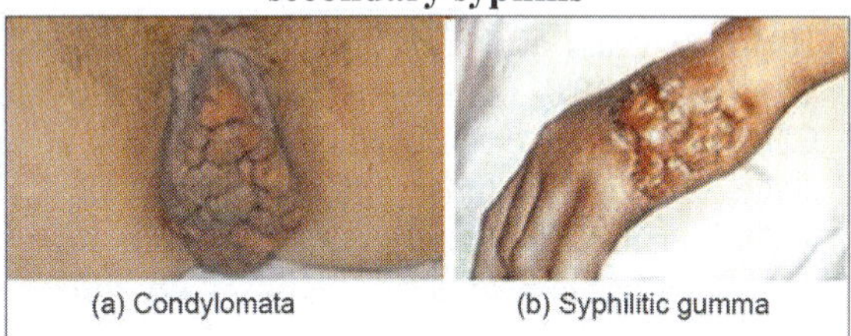

(a) Condylomata (b) Syphilitic gumma

Figure-8: Condylomata in secondary syphilis & syphilitic gumma in tertiary syphilis

Pathogenesis | **Stage of disease** | **Clinical features**

Organism enter by sexual contact

↓

Local multiplication in skin → **Primary syphilis** →

- **Chancre/ Hard chancre**: Also **called Hunterian chancre** from the name of John Hunter, who produced experimental lesion on himself and described the disease. It begins with single, painless, avascular, ulcerated, indurated swelling with exudative discharges. Present mostly on genitals (**fig.-6**) and rarely on mouth and nipples. Chancre is covered by thick glairy exudates rich in spirochetes. Sometimes bacilli may enter in blood and lymph before the appearance of chancre and patient may be infectious in late incubation period. Chancre heals without treatment in 10-40 days with thin scar or may persist in an individual with IDDs
- **Lymphadenopathy**: Mostly inguinal nodes are involved. It could be bilateral and nodes are swollen, rubbery, discrete and non-tender.

Local multiplication in skin branches to:

- In 75% cases chancre completely disappear in 10-40 days without treatment.
- In some cases → Bacilli multiply and disseminated via blood → **Secondary syphilis**: Begin after 6 months of healing of primary syphilis. →

- **Asymptomatic**: Patient is asymptomatic in initial 1-3 months. Bacilli are abundant in secondary lesions, so more infective than primary stage and lesions are variable in distribution, intensity and duration..
- **Papule**: Skin rashes over back or front [**fig.-7 (a)**], palms and soles
- **Mucus patches**: In mucosa of oro-pharynx [**fig.-7 (b)**]
-**Condylomata lata**: It is benign growth or warty lesion, present at muco-cutaneous junctions like perianal region [**fig.-8 (a)**], vulva and scrotum. Most infective (Condylomata > skin rash > primary stage).
- **Other features**: May involve the eyes, bone and meninges.

Bacilli multiply and disseminated via blood branches to:

- Secondary syphilis completely disappear spontaneously or in 3-4 years & serum test are -Ve
- Secondary syphilis completely disappear but serological test are +Ve **called quiescence period** → **Late syphilis/ latent syphilis** →

Tertiary syphilis: Lesion contains few bacilli, so less infective. It may represent the allergic manifestation. Following are the main features
- Aortic aneurysm
-Syphilitic gumma/Gumatous syphilis [**fig.-8 (b)**]: Granulomatous lesion in any organs but mostly in bone and skin
- CNC: Meningitis or meningovascular syphilis

Late tertiary/quaternary syphilis: Following features several decades after the infection
-Tabes dorsalis (degeneration of posterior route of spinal cord)
-GPI (Generalised Paralysis of Insane)

✓ **Note: Chancre redux** or **chancre monoredive**

- **Definition and cause**: It's a relapse or re-appearance of chancre due to insufficient treatment of early syphilis and accompanied by enlarged lymph node. It does not contain spirochetes and reaction may be allergic type.

Flow chart-3: Pathogenesis, stage of disease & clinical features of venereal syphilis

✓ **Notes: Soft sore / chancroid / soft chancre & cold sore / fever blister / herpes labialis**

- **Soft sore:** Caused by *H. ducreyi* & pain full (for more details, **follow chapter → Pasteurellales**).
- **Cold sore:** Caused by herpes simplex virus (for more details, **follow chapter → Herpesviridae**).

✓ **Note: Neurosyphilis**

- **Cause:** Caused by *T. pallidum.*
- **Clinical features**: It usually occurs in people who have had chronic, untreated syphilis, usually about 10 to 20 years after first infection & develops in about 25%–40% of persons who are not treated. CDC advises that neurosyphilis can occur at any stage of a syphilis infection. It may be asymptomatic. Commonly nerve system is infected in tertiary & late tertiary syphilis with following features.

o Tertiary syphilis: Meningitis or meningovascular syphilis.

o Late tertiary syphilis: Following features several decades after the infection.

- Tabes dorsalis (Degeneration of posterior route of spinal cord).
- GPI (Generalised Paralysis of Insane).

- **Diagnosis:** Tests available for syphilis are not giving 100% accuracy in diagnosis of neurosyphilis. It based on clinical findings, CSF picture & non treponemal tests.

o Specimens: CSF

o Tests:

1. CSF picture: Lymphocytic pleocytosis, Normal glucose but high (moderate) protein.
2. Non treponemal tests:
   - VDRL-CSF: Invasion of bacilli stimulates the production of non treponemal (non-specific) antibodies in CSF, so it is the standard test for diagnosis of neurosyphilis. However, VDRL has 90% specificity & 30% sensitivity in neurosyphilis. It becomes negative after 1 year of treatment so, useful to monitor the neurosyphilis.
   - RPR: It is not done from CSF. It showing only 50% of sero-conversion after treatment, so not useful to monitor the treatment.
3. Other tests: Like FTA-ABS, TPHA & TPPA are less useful because the treponemal (specific) antibodies have tendency to cross the CSF, so enough antibodies are already present in CSF before the development of neurosyphilis. Such tests are positive from CSF even in absence of neurosyphilis.

- **Treatment & monitoring:** Penicillin is used to treat neurosyphilis; however, early diagnosis and treatment is critical. Two examples of penicillin therapies include
  - Aqueous penicillin G 3–4 million units every four hours for 10 to 14 days.
  - One daily intramuscular injection & oral probenecid four times daily, both for 10 to 14 days.
  - Follow-up blood tests are generally performed at 3, 6, 12, 24, and 36 months to make sure the infection is gone. CSF analysis is generally performed every 6 months.
- **Effect of HIV on neurosyphilis:** Neurosyphilis remain unheard after penicillin therapy. However, concurrent infection of *T. pallidum* with HIV has been found to affect the course of syphilis. Syphilis can lie dormant for 10-20 years before progressing to neurosyphilis, but HIV may accelerate the rate of the progress. Also, infection with HIV has been found to cause penicillin therapy to fail more often. Therefore, neurosyphilis has once again been prevalent in societies with high HIV rates & limited access to penicillin.

✪ **Laboratory diagnosis of venereal syphilis:**

A Microscopy:

♣ **Specimens:**

- **Blood:** By vene puncture
- **Lymph node tissue:** By aspiration method
- **Exudates from lesions:** Clean the lesion with a gauze piece soaked in warm saline and margins gently scraped so that superficial epithelium is abraded. Apply gentle pressure at base of lesion. Collect the exudates without mixing the blood.
- **Biopsy/tissue materials:** Collected from chancre, condylomata, syphilitic gumma etc. Condylomata lata is most infectious.

♣ **Indications:** Applicable in primary, secondary & congenital syphilis with superficial lesions.

♣ **Microscopical findings: →Follow Morphology**

B Culture: →Follow C/Cs

C Serological tests:

♣ **Specimens:** Serum, plasma & CSF.

♣ **Tests:** Two main types of tests as below

i. Non-treponemal tests (non-specific tests, reagin antibody dependent tests, STS-Standard Tests for Syphilis):

- **Based on** detection of reagin antibody of cardiolipin antigen.
- **It creates confusion** with IgE antibody in atopy, though there is no connection between two.
- **Clinical application & sensitivity of non-treponemal tests**
  - Tests are reactive 3-5 weeks after acquiring the primary infection or 7-10 days after appearance of chancre.
  - Sensitivity is 60- 70% in primary syphilis and titre is low about 1:8.

- Sensitivity is 100% in secondary syphilis and titre is 16-128 or more.
- Sensitivity is 60- 70% in latent/late syphilis.
- High titre & higher positivity rate also noticed in congenital syphilis.
- Also useful to detect neurosyphilis especially VDRL test.
- Quantitative tests are useful to monitor patient's response against treatment, to indicate stage of disease, to detect re-infection and to eliminate the effect of prozone phenomenon. Reagin tests are preferred to monitor the efficacy of antibacterial therapy because they usually become negative or decreasing in titre following treatment.
- If treatment started in early syphilis reagin antibody test become negative within 6-18 months, but if treatment is started late it remain positive in low titre.
- All serological tests are false positive in endemic treponematoses like yaws, pinta & endemic syphilis & can't differentiate the endemic treponematoses.

• **Tests:**

a. **Wasserman compliment fixation test:** Not used now.
b. **Kahn test:** Tube flocculation test, not used now.
c. **VDRL test:** } Follow chapter →Antigen-antibody (Ag-Ab) reactions
d. **RPR test:**
e. **Automated RPR** } Large scale testing.
f. **VDRL-ELISA**
g. **Unheated Serum Reagin Test (USRT):** It is similar to VDRL test except for
- EDTA is used as an Ag stabiliser & daily preparation of antigen is not required.
- Preheating of serum does not required as choline chloride is used to remove the inhibitors.

h. **TRUST:**
- Full name: Toludine Red Unheated Serum Test.
- Ag is more stable, so can be stored at room temperature 26-31° C.
- TRUST is performed by using unheated serum.
- It is same as like RPR test but Ag is coated with toludine red instead of carbon particle & resulting clumps are in red colour.

ii. **Treponemal (specific) tests:** Two types like group specific & species specific.

a. **Group specific test:**

• **Antigen prepared by** using non-pathogenic *Treponema* like Reiter strain.

• **Clinical application & sensitivity**
- It avoids Biological False Positive (BFP).
- It's sensitivity & specificity are lower than species specific test.

• **Test:** Only one test in this category like **Reiter Protein Complement Fixation Test (RPCFT).**

b. **Species specific test:**

• **Antigen prepared by** using pathogenic *Treponema* like Nichol's strain.

• **Clinical application & sensitivity**
- Distinguish positive STS from BFP.
- It's sensitivity & specificity are higher in late/latent syphilis.

• **Tests:** Three subtypes of tests in species specific category.

* **By using live strain:**

1. **TPI (*Treponema Pallidum* Immobilisation) test:**
- Test serum is incubated with complement and *T. pallidum* maintained in complex medium anaerobically.
- Motility examined under dark ground illumination.
- If antibodies are present in test serum, treponemes are immobilized.
- Positive test: ≥50% of treponemes are immobilized
- Negative test: ≤ 20% of treponemes are immobilized.
- Intermediate/inconclusive: If in between 20%-50%.
- Test is considered as gold standard, but because of its complexity it is available in highly equipped laboratory.

* **By using killed strain:**

1. ***Treponema Pallidum* Agglutination (TPA) test:**
- Killed suspension of *Treponema* is mixed with test serum & incubated.
- Examine the clumps under DGIM.
- Gives false positive results, so not in use.

2. ***Treponema Pallidum* Immune Adherence (TPIA) test:**
- Killed suspension of *Treponema* is mixed with test serum, complement, RBCs & incubated.
- In presence of antibody *Treponema* adhere on RBCs.
- Gives false positive results, so not in use.

3. **Fluorescent Treponemal Antibody (FTA) test:**
- Indirect immune fluorescence test.
- It's modified test is useful.

4. **Fluorescent Treponema Antibody- ABSorption (FTA-ABS) test:**

o Steps:
- It is a modification of FTA test.
- The patient serum is 1st diluted with non pathogenic Reiter's strain to remove group specific treponemal antibodies.
- Patient serum is layered on a slide previously coated with killed *T pallidum.* Treponemal antibodies present in patient serum are bound with *T pallidum.*
- Add the fluorescent labelled anti human Ig & examine the slide under the microscope.

o Advantages:
- Most sensitive & specific test in all stage of syphilis.

- It is the 1st serological test to be positive following infection.
- It is useful to detect the neurosyphilis from CSF.
- It is useful to detect the congenital syphilis by detecting the IgM from foetal serum **called IgM FTA-ABS test.**

o Disadvantages:
- Available in well equipped laboratory.
- False positive result may occur in Lyme disease which is corrected by VDRL test with negative result.

* **By using treponemal extracts:**

1. ***T. pallidum* Haem-Agglutination (TPHA) test:**

o Steps:
- Treponemal antigen is coated with RBCs.
- Mix such antigen with test sera containing antibody.
- Haem agglutination (clumping of RBCs) occurs.
- Test is employed as an automated micro-haemagglutination test (MHA-TP).

o Advantages:
- Highly specific & sensitive as like FTA-ABS test except in primary stage (65-85%).
- It is simple, economical, no special equipment required & commercially available. **These advantages** make TPHA a standard confirmatory test.

2. **Latex agglutination test or *Treponema pallidum* Particle Agglutination (TPPA) test:**
- *T. pallidum* antigens are coated with latex/gelatin particles.
- As specific as TPHA, and most sensitive in all stages of syphilis.

3. **Enzyme Immuno Assays (EIA):** *T. pallidum* antigens are coated in micro-titre well & detection of IgG & IgM separately.
4. **Western blot (WB) assay:** Highly sensitive & specific for detection of IgG & IgM antibodies separately.

♣ **Sensitivity & specificity of serological tests in different stages of syphilis: →Table-1**

Stage	Primary	Secondary	Late	Specificity
VDRL	78%	100%	71%	98%
RPR	86%	100%	73%	98%
FTA-ABST	84%	100%	96%	97%
TPHA	76%	100%	94%	99%
TPPA	88%	100%	*	98%
EIA	90%	100%	*	99%
WB	90%	100%	*	98%

Table-1: Sensitivity & specificity of serological tests in different stages of syphilis

* Sensitivity not known

♣ **Key points to be remember about serological tests:**

- Tests are reactive 3-5 weeks after acquiring the primary infection or 7-10 days after appearance of chancre.
- Most sensitive serological test in all stages of syphilis: TPPA test.
- 1st serological test to be positive following infection: FTA-ABS test.
- Test of choice for rapid diagnosis from clinical samples: RPR test.
- Test for monitoring the therapy: VDRL test or RPR test.
- Screening test for large numbers of samples: VDRL test or RPR test.
- Confirmatory test: FTA-ABS test or TPPA test, EIA or TPHA test because having high specificity.
- Neurosyphilis best diagnosed by non treponemal tests while IgM in congenital syphilis is best diagnosed by treponemal tests.

D **Molecular tests:** PCR based techniques are useful.

✪ **Prevention of venereal syphilis:**

A. **General measures:**
- Avoiding sexual contact with infected person.
- Use of physical barrier like condoms.
- Use of antiseptics like potassium permanganate.
- Transfusion syphilis is prevented by refrigerating the blood at 0-4^{0}C for1-3 days before transfusion

B. **Chemoprophylaxis:** Penicillin is useful

C. **Immunoprophylaxis:** No effective vaccine is available.

✪ **Treatment & monitoring of venereal syphilis:**

- **Treatment:**

a. **Patient not allergic to penicillin G (Pn G):**

1. **Early syphilis:**
- Single injection of 2.4 million units.
- Adverse reaction: **Called Jarisch-Herxheimer reaction** is frequent but harmless. It is due to hypersensitivity or due to liberation of toxic products like tumour necrosis factors form killed treponemes.

2. **Late syphilis:**
- Inject the 2.4 million units every week for 3 weeks.
- Adverse reaction: **Called Jarisch-Herxheimer reaction** is rare but dangerous.

b. **Penicillin G (Pn G) allergic patients:** Doxycycline/ tetracycline is effective.

- **Monitoring:**
- **Treponemal tests:** Antibodies titre by treponemal tests like FTA-ABS test or TPPA test or TPHA test, remain high even after clinical improvement, so treponemal tests have little or no value in management of syphilis.
- **Non-treponemal tests:** Antibodies titre by non-treponemal tests like VDRL test & RPR test, start to decline or become negative after treatment, so it is better to use non-treponemal tests for

management of syphilis following treatment. VDRL should be done at 3 months interval for at least 1 year. Sometimes patient have low antibodies titre to non-treponemal tests in spite of successful treatment **called serofast reaction** which may be due to treatment failure

a. **For early syphilis:** Following successful treatment there should be at least fourfold decline in the titre at the end of 3rd or 4th month & eightfold decline in the titre at the end of 6th or 8th month.

b. **For late/latent syphilis:** Titre decline gradually following successful treatment & low titre may persist for a years.

1. Non-venereal syphilis

A Occupational syphilis:

- Present in doctors & nurses.
- Primary chancre occurs on hands/fingers.

B Haematogenous syphilis:

- Transmitted by blood transfusion.
- Primary chancre does not occur.

C Congenital syphilis:

✪ **Mode of transmission of congenital syphilis:**

- Transmission can take place through placenta (and at birth from infected mother's genital?) at any stage of pregnancy but foetal lesions develop after 4 months of gestation when foetal immune system starts to develop.
- A woman with early syphilis can infects foetus in 75-90% cases.
- A woman with late or 2 yr old syphilis can infects foetus in 35% cases.

✪ **Clinical features of congenital syphilis:**

- **Maternal features:** Increase risk to pregnancy. It causes abortion, live birth, stillbirth & stigmata of syphilis.
- **Features in new born:** Three types

○ Early congenital syphilis: Features develop in 0-2 years.

- May be asymptomatic.
- Symptomatic newborns, if not stillborn, are born premature, with an enlarged lymph nodes, liver & spleen, skeletal abnormalities (like osteochondritis, periosteitis & osteitis), pneumonia, anaemia, seizure, thrombocytopenia, leucocytosis, jaundice & a bullous skin disease **called pemphigus syphiliticus.**
- Newborns will typically not develop a primary syphilitic chancre, but may present with signs of secondary syphilis (which involve skin & mucosa) like generalized skin rashes, syphilitic rhinitis / snuffles" **[fig.-9 (a)]**, the mucus from which is laden with the *T. pallidum* bacterium, and therefore highly infectious. Rarely, the symptoms of syphilis go unseen in infants so that they develop the symptoms of late congenital syphilis.

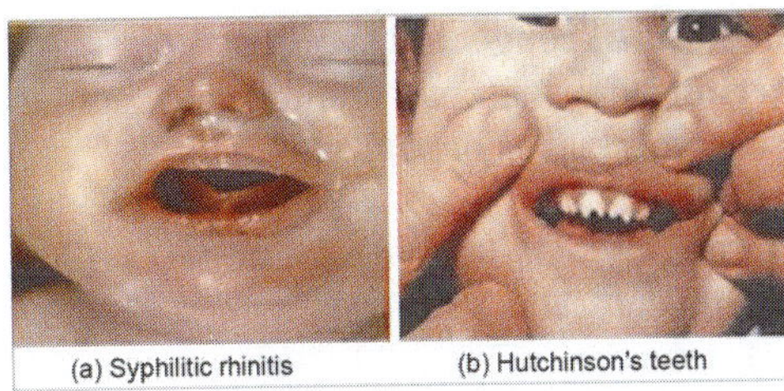

(a) Syphilitic rhinitis (b) Hutchinson's teeth

Figure-9: Congenital syphilis

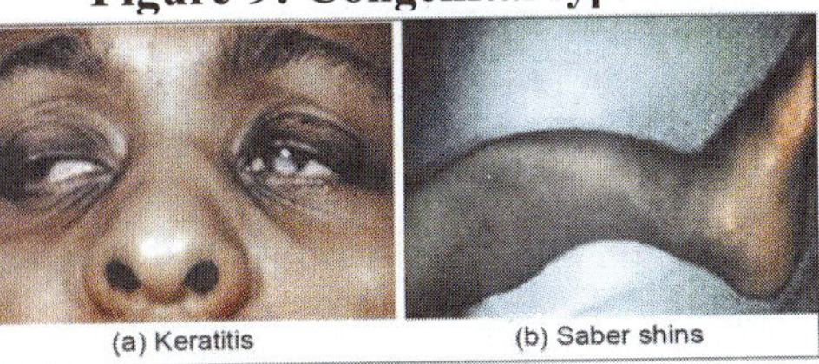

(a) Keratitis (b) Saber shins

Figure-10: Congenital syphilis

○ Late congenital syphilis: Features develop ≥ 2 years.

- Subclinical infection in 60% cases.
- Interstitial keratitis.
- Deafness from auditory nerve disease.
- Clutton's joints: Bilateral swollen knees or knee effusion.
- Gummatous periosteitis.
- Destruction / perforation of bony & cartilage part of nasal septum.

○ Residual stigmata: With damage to bones, teeth, eyes, ears & brain.

- **Hutchinson's triad** consisting of deafness (due to auditory nerve disease), Hutchinson's teeth [centrally notched or blunted, widely spaced peg-shaped upper central incisors as shown in **fig.-9 (b)**], and interstitial keratitis [an inflammation of the cornea as shown in **fig.-10(a)**, which can lead to corneal scarring and potentially blindness].
- Mulberry molars: Permanent first molars with multiple poorly developed cusps.
- Frontal bossing: Prominence of the brow ridge.
- Saddle nose: Collapse of the bony part of nose.
- Hard palate defect.
- Swollen knees.
- Du Bois sign: Narrowing of the little finger.
- Poorly developed maxillae.
- Protruding mandible.
- Petechiae.
- Saber shins: Malformation of tibia with sharp anterior bowing **[fig.-10(b)].**
- Lymph node enlargement.
- Jaundice.
- Pseudo-paralysis.
- Rhagades: Linear scars at the angles of the mouth & nose due to bacterial infection of skin lesions.
- Higoumenakis sign, enlargement of the sternal end of clavicle in late congenital syphilis.
- Death from congenital syphilis is usually due to bleeding into the lungs.

✪ **Diagnosis of congenital syphilis:**

- **Specimens:** Placenta, umbilical cord, nasal discharge, skin lesions etc.
- **Tests:**

A **Microscopy:** DGIM to demonstrate *T pallidum.*

B **Serological tests:**

1. **IgM detection**
   - 1st Ab appears after infection is IgM which detected after 2nd week of infection.
   - IgM doesn't cross the placenta, its presence in neonatal serum **called syphalotoxemia** which indicates congenital syphilis. It helps to differentiate it from passively transferred maternal antibodies.
   - IgM detected by treponemal test like IgM FTA-ABST test, TPHA test & EIA (syphilis capita M test). IgM also detected by VDRL test from whole sera. Commercially available tests are not recommended for IgM detection.
2. **Parallel testing of maternal & neonatal sera:** When above tests are not available parallel testing of maternal & neonatal sera is done in which neonatal sera shows the high titre than maternal sera.
3. **Serial testing of neonatal sera:** It is done to detect the presence of passively transferred maternal antibodies in neonatal serum by using VDRL test. Such titre decrease rapidly & VDRL test become negative by 3 months.

C **Molecular:** PCR base technique.

D **Radiological:** Abnormal x-rays.

✪ **Prevention of congenital syphilis:** It is prevented if pregnant mother is identified & treated before 4 months /16 weeks. High risk to foetus in untreated women like greatest risk in the early stages of infection, but the disease can be passed at any point during pregnancy, even during delivery (if the child had not already contracted it). A woman in the secondary stage of syphilis decreases her foetus's risk if she receives treatment before the last month of pregnancy.

✪ **Treatment of congenital syphilis:**

- An afflicted child can be treated by using antibiotics like an adult; however, any developmental symptoms are likely to be permanent.
- Kassowitz's law is an empirical observation used in context of congenital syphilis stating that the greater the duration between the infection of the mother and conception, the better is the outcome for the infant. Features of a better outcome include less chance of stillbirth and of developing congenital syphilis.
- The CDC recommends treating symptomatic or babies born to infected mother with unknown treatment status with procaine penicillin G, 50,000 U/kg dose IM a day in a single dose for 10 days. Treatment for these babies can vary on a case by case basis. Treatment cannot reverse any deformities, brain or permanent tissue damage that has already occurred.

Endemic (non-venereal) treponematoses

↓

Table-2

Relapsing fever

❖ **Meaning:**

- It occurs with 5-10 relapses, hence the name relapsing fever.
- Relapsing fever has been known since the time of Hippocrates & has occurred in epidemic, endemic & sporadic forms.

Features	Endemic syphilis	Yaws	Pinta
Synonym	Bejel, siti, dichuchwa, njovera, skerljevo etc.	Pian, framboesia, bouba etc.	Mal del pinto, carate, azul, purupuru etc.
Agent	*T. endemicum*	*T. pertenue*	*T. carateum*
Transmission	In young children via person to person contact by use of contaminated utensils for drinking & eating purpose	- Direct contact - Some times flies may act as mechanical vector	Direct contact
Age	Early childhood	Early childhood	Late childhood
Primary syphilis	Not seen but present on nipples of mother infected by their children (oral lesion)	Extra genital papules (limbs) which break down to form ulcerative granuloma	Extra genital papules (limbs, face) without ulcer but develops in lichenoid / psoriatic patch
Secondary / tertiary syphilis	Same as syphilis	Same as syphilis but CVS (heart) & CNS (nerve) features are rare	Secondary lesion are characterised by hypo or hyperpigmentation
Lab. diagnosis	Same as syphilis		
Treatment	All endemic treponematoses are treated by benzathine penicillin		
Relapse	Unknown	Common	None

Table-2: Types of endemic (non-venereal) treponematoses

Types	Louse borne	Tick borne
Etiological agent	*Borrelia recurrentis*	*B. duttonii, B. harmasii, B. parkeri*
Nature	Epidemic	Endemic or sporadic **called place disease**
Distribution	East Africa (Sudan & Ethiopia)	North America, Central Asia & Africa
Vector	*Pediculus humanus corporis*	*Ornithodorus lahorensis, O. tholozoni, O. Crossi* & fowl tick like *Aargus persicus*
Reservoir	Human. Louse is not the reservoir because transova-rial transmission does not occurs in louse	Human, rodents & tick because transovarial transmission occurs in ticks.
Source	Head louse	Tick & their excreta
Mode of transmission	*Borrelia* are present in blood not in saliva or excreta of vector, so transmitted by rubbing the vector against the abraded akin but not by bite or by rubbing the excreta	*Borrelia* are present in all parts of vector & transmitted by bite or by rubbing the excreta/vector against abraded akin
Severity	More & highly fatal	Less sever & less fatal
Jaundice & haemorrhage	More common	Less common
Relapse	Less	More

Table-3: Types of relapsing fever

❖ **Etiological agents:** Two types **(table-3)**

❖ **Morphology: →Figure -11(a)**

➢ **Staining properties:** GNB, but better stained by Giemsa, Leishman or dilute carbol fuchsin.

➢ **Size:** 8-20μm × 0.2-0.5μm.

➢ **Shape:** Irregular spiral shape with 3-5 wide open coils & pointed ends.

➢ **Motility:** Lashing motility examined by wet mount under DGIM or under PCM.

❖ **Cultural characteristics (C/Cs):**

➢ **Effective factors:**

- O_2 effect: Microaerophilic.
- Temperature: 33°C.

➢ **Culture in media:** Grow with difficulties in Noguchi's medium.

➢ **Culture in animal:**

- Inoculate intraperitoneally 1-2ml of patient's blood in white mice.
- Bacteria multiply in animal & appear in large number in peripheral blood within two days.
- Prepare smear from tail vein of animal after 2 days & examined daily for 2 weeks.

➢ **Culture in egg:** Growth occurs in Chorio Allantoic Membrane **(CAM)** of chick embryo.

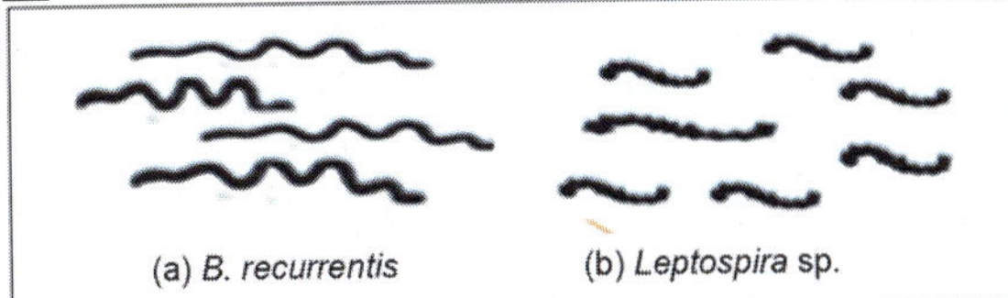

Figure-11: Morphology or *B recurrentis* & *Leptospira* spp.

❖ **Antigenic structure:**

- One of the reasons behind occurrence of relapse in relapsing fever is due to antigenic variation in "vmp gene" of *Borrellia*. Vmp gene is located in linear plasmid which shows the DNA rearrangement.
- Due to antigenic variation newer strain is not protected by antibodies of earlier strain. Ultimate protection to the disease occurs after multiple attacks due to development of immunity to all strains.

❖ **Pathogenicity:**

➢ **Reservoir & source of infection: → Table-3**

➢ **Mode of transmission:**

- **Louse borne: → Table-3**
- **Tick borne: → Table-3**
- **Congenital:** By placenta
- **Occupational:** By accidental contact to laboratory workers.

➢ **Incubation period:** 1-10 days.

➢ **Portal of entry:** Abraded skin.

➢ **Sites:** Bacteria present in blood during febrile period & in brain during afebrile period.

➢ **Clinical features: → Table-3**

- Sudden onset of fever (bacteria are in blood) which last for 3-5 days followed by afebrile period (bacteria are in brain).
- After afebrile period of 3-5 days another bouts of fever.
- Fever subsides after 5-10 relapses.

❖ **Laboratory diagnosis:**

➢ **Specimens:** Blood.

➢ **Testing methods:**

A **Microscopy: → Follow Morphology**

B **Culture: →Follow C/Cs**

C **Serological tests:**

- Weil-Felix reaction is developed.
- Rarely useful because giving false + Ve reaction.

- Borrelia antibody produces agglutinin with Proteus OX-K Ag.

D **Molecular test:** Multiplex PCR to target the various *Borrelia spp.* causing relapsing fever.

❖ **Prevention:** Identification & eradication of vectors. No vaccine is available.

❖ **Treatment:** Tetracycline, chloramphenicol, penicillin & erythromycin are effective.

Vincent's angina

❖ **Synonyms:** Fusospirochetosis.

❖ **Etiological agents:** It is a symbiotic infection, caused by *Borrelia vincenti* & *Fusobacter fusiforme.*

❖ **Morphology:** →**Table-4 & fig.-12.**

Features	*B. vincenti*	*F. fusiforme*
Synonym	*Treponema vincenti*	*Fusiform bacilli*
Micro-scopy	Gram –Ve but better stained by Giemsa/ dilute carbol fuchsin	Gran –Ve bacilli & stained by Gram stain
Size	5-20μm × 0.2-0.6μm	3-10 μm × 1μm
Shape	Irregular spiral with 3-5 wide open coils & pointed end	Spindle with pointed end
Motility	Motile	Non-motile
Cultural characte-ristics	Heartly's broth enrich with ascitic fluid (Strict anaerobes)	In blood agar contains vanco-mycin + neomycin, it produces grey colour non-haemolytic colony
Biochemi-cal test	Not useful	Indole test→ +Ve

Table-4: Differences between *B. vincenti* & *F. fusiforme*

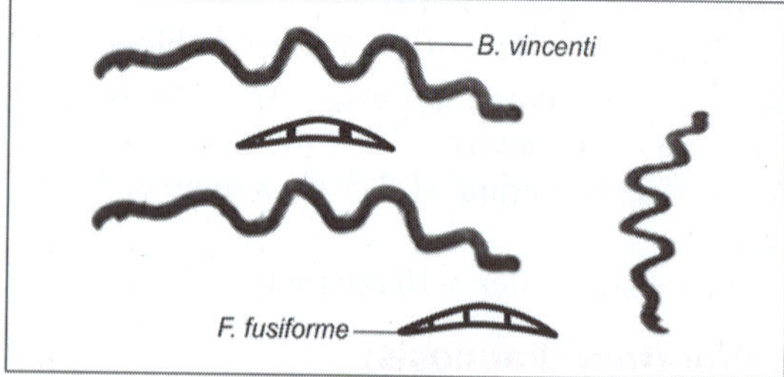

Figure-12: Morphology of *B. vincenti* & *F. fusiforme*

❖ **Pathogenicity:**

➢ **Reservoir& source of infection:** Both are normal flora of oral cavity in man.

➢ **Mode of transmission:** Both are normal flora of oral cavity. Endogenous infection occurs by activation of flora in malnutrition & viral infections.

➢ **Clinical features:**

- It is ulcerative gingivostomatitis or oropharyngitis.
- It also identified from other clinical conditions like lung abscess, phagedenous skin, ulcer, gangrenous balanitis, choleric diarrhoea, dysentery etc. but significance is not known.

❖ **Laboratory diagnosis:**

➢ **Specimens:** Exudates from lesion of oral cavity.

➢ **Testing methods:**

A **Microscopy:**
B **Culture:**
C **Biochemical reaction:**
} → Follow **table-4**

❖ **Treatment:** Penicillin & metronidazole are the effective drugs.

Lyme disease

❖ **Meaning:** New spirochetal infection identified in 1975 while studying a cluster of juvenile arthritis in **Lyme**, Connicticut, USA hence **called Lyme disease**. However later it was identified from other part of world.

❖ **Synonym:** Lyme arthritis & Lyme borreliosis.

❖ **Etiological agent:**

- Causative agent of Lyme disease was identified in1985 by Bergdorfer in USA hence **called *B. bergdorferi***. *B mayonii* is also a causative agent of Lyme disease in USA.
- In Europe & Asia, *B afzelii* & *B garinii* are the causative agents of Lyme disease.

❖ **Morphology:**

➢ **Type according to gram stain:** GNB.

➢ **Size:** 4-30μm ×0.2 μm in size.

➢ **Motility:** Motile in nature.

❖ **Cultural characteristics (C/Cs):**

➢ **Effective factors:**

- O_2 effect: Microaerophilic
- Temperature: 33°C

➢ **Medium:** They are fastidious bacteria grow on BSK (Barbour-Stoenner- Kelly) medium (best **called Kelly's medium**) after an incubation period of ≥ 2 weeks.

❖ **Pathogenicity:**

➢ **Reservoir of infection:** Rodents, deers & other mammals.

➢ **Source of infection:** Vector like tick.

➢ **Mode of transmission:** By bites of *Ixodid* ticks

- **USA:** *Ixodid dammini.*
- **Europe:** *Ixodid raciness.*

- **Incubation period:** 1-2 weeks, but can be much shorter (days) or much longer (months to years).
- **Portal of entry:** Skin.
- **Site:** Skin, eyes, muscle, bone, joints, hearts, CNS etc.
- **Precipitating factors (epidemiological determinants):**

I. Agent factors (virulence factors)

1. **Antigenic variation:** It present in cell surface lipoprotein **called VlsE surface protein**. Due to antigenic variation newer strain is not protected by antibodies of earlier strain.
2. **Change in shape & shedding of cell wall:** In the tick & mice, bacteria have thick cell wall & spiral shape, if it maintains such thick cell wall & spiral shape immune system can control the infection. However in the human body it can shed its cell wall & assume the different shape so it is not recognised by immune system & protect itself.

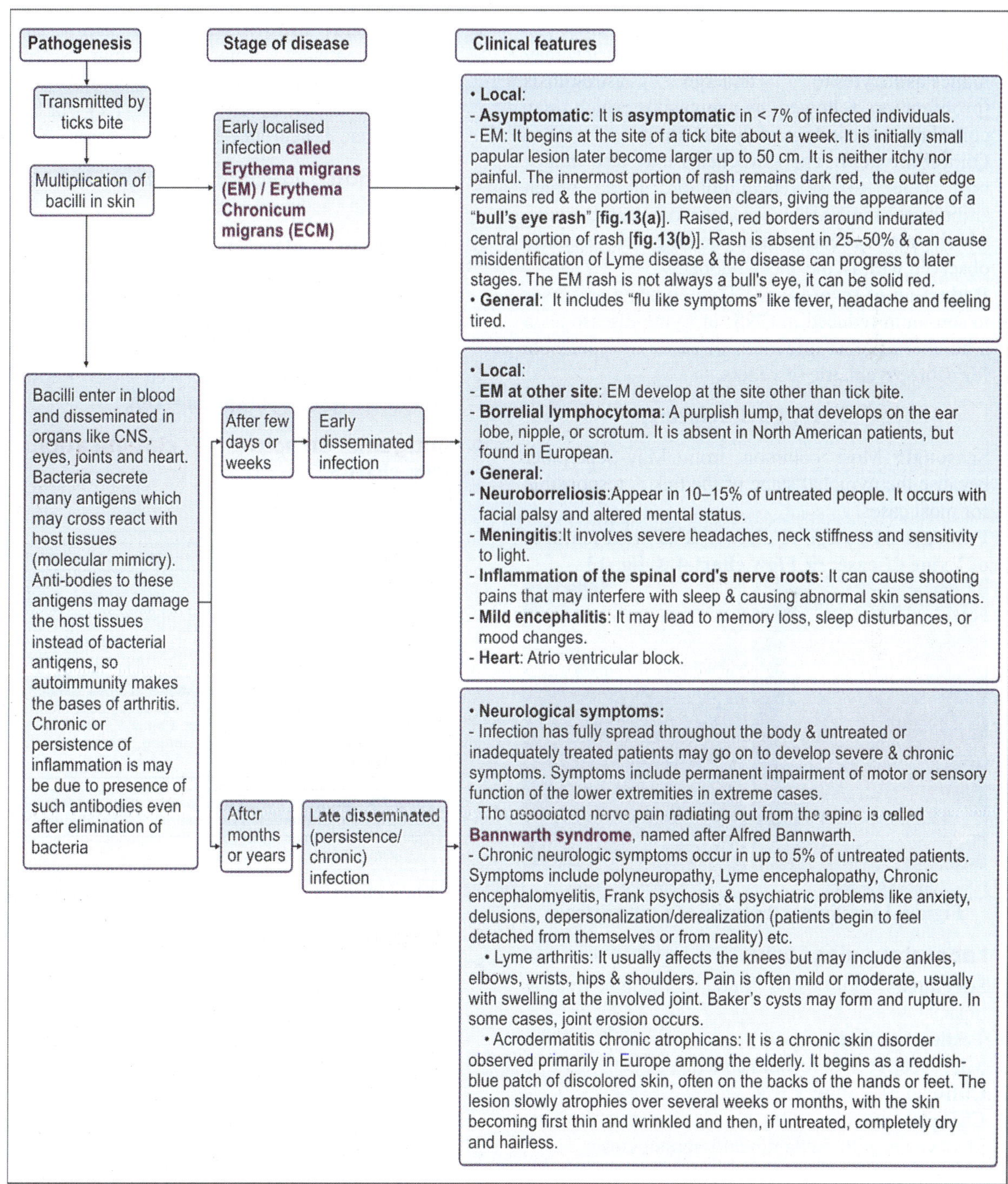

Flow chart-4: Pathogenesis, stage of disease & clinical features of Lyme disease

II. Vector factors

1. **Tick saliva:** It accompanies the spirochete into the skin during the feeding process, contains substances that disrupt the immune response at the site of the bite & provides a protective environment where the spirochete can establish infection.

III. Host factors

1. **Age:** Common in elderly people.
2. **Host protease:** The spread of *B. burgdorferi* is aided by the attachment of the host protease plasmin to the surface of the spirochete.
3. **Astrogliosis:** In the brain, *B. burgdorferi* may induce astrocytes to undergo astrogliosis (proliferation followed by apoptosis), which may contribute to neurological dysfunctions.
4. **Quinolinic acid:** The spirochetes may also induce host cells to secrete quinolinic acid, which stimulates the NMDA receptor on nerve cells, which may account for the fatigue & malaise observed with Lyme encephalopathy.
5. **Reduction of tryptophan:** Tryptophan, a precursor to serotonin reduced in CNS in Lyme disease & in a number of other infectious diseases is responsible for neuropsychiatric disorders.

IV. Environmental

1. **Seasonal:** Most common from May-September because the nymphal stage of the tick is responsible for most cases.

➢ **Pathogenesis, stage of disease & clinical features of Lyme disease: → Flow chart-4 & fig.-13**

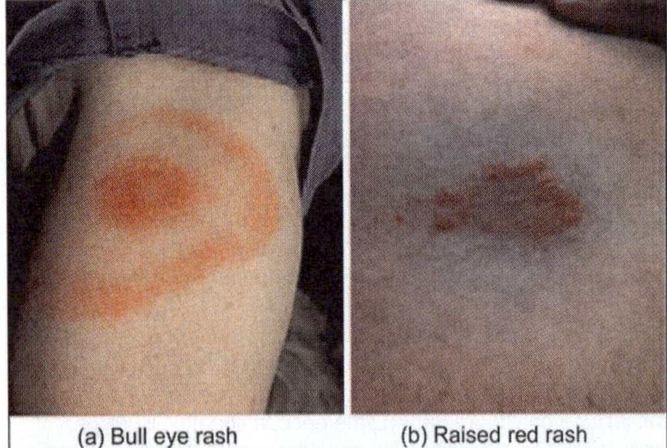

Figure-13: Clinical features of Lyme disease

❖ **Laboratory diagnosis:**

➢ **Specimens:** Skin lesion, blood, CSF, joint fluid & ticks.

➢ **Testing methods**

A. **Microscopy:** Not recommended

B. **Culture: → Follow C/Cs**

C. **CSF picture:**
- Pleocytosis with predominant lymphocytosis.
- Increased protein.
- Normal glucose.
- Presence of IgM, IgG & IgA in CSF indicate the intrathecal synthesis of antibodies.

D. **Serology:**
- Most useful.
- Antibodies develop after 1-2 months.
- Initial IgM response followed by IgG.
- Detected by ELISA, IF and immunoblotting test.
- False positive test may be seen with FTA-ABS test.

E. **Molecular test:** PCR is most sensitive from joint fluid but sensitivity is poor from blood, urine & CSF samples.

❖ **Differential diagnosis:** Lyme disease should be differentiated from multiple sclerosis, rheumatoid arthritis, fibromyalgia, chronic fatigue syndrome, lupus, Crohn's disease, HIV or other autoimmune & neurodegenerative diseases.

❖ **Prevention:** Identification & eradication of vectors. No vaccine is available.

❖ **Treatment:** Doxycycline, amoxicillin & cefuroxime are effective.

Leptospira

❖ **Meaning:** Lepto word derived from **Leptos = thin/fine** + **spira** from **speira = coil.**

❖ **Antigenic structure & classification:** → **Flow chart-5**

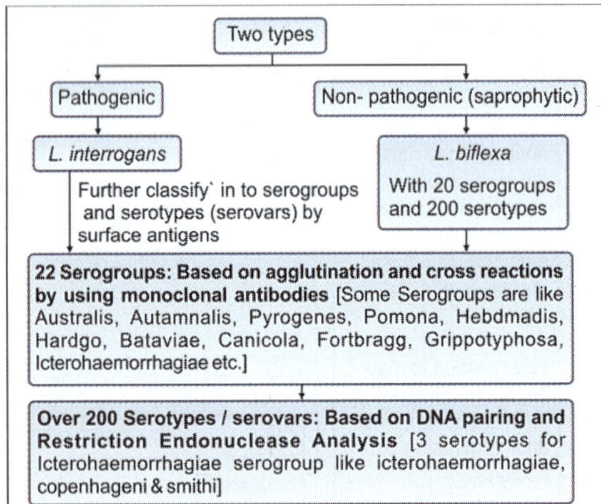

Flow chart-5: Classification of *Leptospira* spp.

❖ **Morphology:** →**Fig.-11(b)**

➢ **Staining properties:**
- GNB but better stained by Giemsa & aniline dyes.
- Very thin so better result obtained by silver impregnation stain.
- Immunofluorescent staining & microscopy is also useful technique.

➢ **Size:** 6-20μm × 0.1μm.

➢ **Shape:** Both ends are like hooks of umbrella or like interrogation mark with several coils together which are distinguished under DGIM in living state or under electronic microscopy.

➢ **Motility:**

- Actively motility with spinning or translation type of motility.
- Motility examined by wet mount under DGIM.

❖ Cultural characteristics (C/Cs):

➢ **Effective factors:**

- Aerobic and microaerophilic.
- Optimum temp: 25-30° C.
- Optimum pH: 7.2-7.5
- Generation time: In media it is 12-16 hours & 4-8 hours in animals.

➢ **Culture in laboratory media:**

✪ **Media:**

i. Liquid media:

1. **By using serum:** Korthof's medium & Stuart's medium.
2. **By using serum derivatives like albumin:** EMJH (Ellinghausen McCullough Johnson Harris) medium.

ii. Semisolid media (0.5% agar): Fletcher's medium, growth occurs few mm below surface in ring form **called Dinger's ring,**

iii. Solid media: Liquid media + 2% agar,

iv. Selective media: By adding 5-fluouracil in above mentioned media.

✪ **Technique: → Flow chart-6**

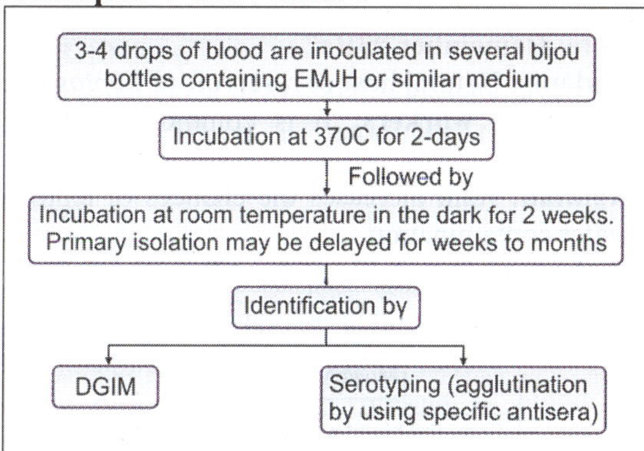

Flow chart-6: Cultivation technique in media

➢ **Culture in animal: → Flow chart-7**

➢ **Culture in egg:**

- Grow in CAM of chick embryo
- *Leptospira* may be demonstrated in the blood of allantoic vessels 4-5 days after inoculation.

➢ **Points to be remember for isolation & identification:**

- **Blood:**
  - It is less sensitive for microscopy.
  - Chances of isolation are increased by culturing the blood every day in the early stage of disease.
- **Urine:** Direct culture of urine is less useful due to presence of contaminant but isolation is possible after animal culture.
- **CSF:** Leptospira are also isolated from CSF.
- **Reference centre for serotyping:**
  - Identification of serotype & serovars is generally a complicated procedure in *Leptospira* due to presence of plenty of antigens & also cross reactivity between the antigens. In such cases sample will be referred to WHO/FAO reference laboratory.

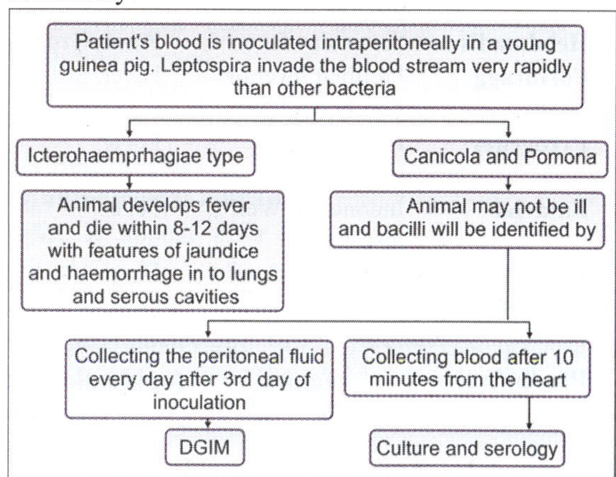

Flow chart-7: Animal cultivation technique

❖ Pathogenicity:

➢ **Disease name:** It is a zoonosis & whole spectrum of disease **called leptospirosis** but different names are given as per causative serovar as mentioned in **table -5.**

➢ **History & distribution:**

- Present in all countries except Antarctica.
- In India, it is common in Tamil Nadu, Kerala & Andaman (**called Andaman haemorrhagic fever**).

➢ **Reservoir of infection:** Rat for Weil's disease & for other types reservoir are mentioned in **table -5**

➢ **Source of infection:** Water or mud contaminated from excreta (like urine) of animals.

➢ **Mode of transmission:**

- Direct contact of abraded skin with contaminated water or mud from **urine** of infected animals.
- It also transmitted by intact mucosa of mouth, nose & conjunctiva.
- Bacteria are also present in **milk** of infected animals, but die very rapidly so human infection is not possible by such milk.
- Not sheds in **saliva**, so animal bite is not significant.
- Man is the dead end or aberrant host. No evidences of human to human transmission are found.

➢ **Incubation period:** 7-10 days (range 2-26 days).

➢ **Portal of entry:** Abraded skin or intact mucosa.

➢ **Sites:** Blood, liver, kidneys, meninges etc.

- **Tests:**

1. Cross Agglutination and Absorption Test (CAAT):

- Identification of serotype & serovars is generally a complicated procedure in *Leptospira* due to presence of plenty of antigen & also cross reactivity between the antigens. In such cases sample will be referred to WHO/FAO reference laboratory.
- Cross reactivity is eliminated by using the agglutination absorption test which gives more accurate diagnosis.

E. Molecular: PCR, DNA pairing, RFLP, PFGE are useful techniques.

➢ **Faine's criteria:**

- It is a WHO approved guideline used for the diagnosis of leptospirosis.
- It based on clinical, epidemiological & laboratory findings.

II. Diagnosis of animal leptospirosis

Leptospirosis in rodents & in other animal is diagnosed by

A. Culture methods: From piece of kidney.

B. Serological tests: As like human tests.

III. Diagnosis of *Leptospira* from water

Leptospira are present in water are diagnosed by

A. Animal culture methods: If a shaved & scarified area of the skin of young guinea pig immersed in infected water for an hour, infection develops through the abrasions.

❖ **Prevention:**

A. General measures: Like

- Rodent control
- Use of protective cloths during working in water loaded agricultural area
- Disinfection of water.

B. Immunoprophylaxis: No effective vaccine is available. Vaccine has been developed with some success for animals. In human vaccine is tried for risky persons.

C. Chemoprophylaxis: 200 mg doxycycline by oral route, once in a week is the drug of choice.

❖ **Treatment:**

- Mild case: 100 mg doxycycline by oral route, twice in day for 7 days. Amoxicillin is also effective.
- Severe case: 1-2 million units of Pn is given by IV injection 6 hourly for 7 days. A mild Jarisch-Herxheimer reaction may occur. Alternative drug is ceftriaxone or cefotaxime.

Question bank

Case study

1) A male patient who is occupationally a truck driver has visited the STD clinic with complain of painless, indurated genital lesion with superficial ulcer & non-tender, discrete, swollen regional lymph nodes persisting for 3 weeks. Laboratory report suggests the reactive VDRL test with 1:32 titre. Identify the organism & answer the following
a) Name the causative agent & describe the morphology of causative agent
b) Write the pathogenicity of causative agent
c) Describe the lab. diagnosis of causative agent

2) A female patient working in water flooded rice field farm with bare foot & abraded skin is admitted in medical OPD. She is giving history of fever since 15 days. History ruled out the presence of jaundice features since 7days. Motile bacteria examined under DGIM & with umbrella handle like appearance. Identify the organism & answer the following
a) Name the causative agent & describe the morphology of causative agent
b) Write the pathogenicity of causative agent
c) Describe the lab. diagnosis of causative agent

Essay/Full question

1) *T. pallidum*

Short notes

1) Classification of spirochetales.
2) Pathogenicity or laboratory diagnosis of *T. pallidum.*
3) Neurosyphilis
4) STS
5) VDRL test
6) RPR test
7) Congenital syphilis
8) Endemic treponematosis
9) Relapsing fever
10) Vincent's angina or Fusospirochetosis
11) Lyme disease or Lyme arthritis
12) Leptospirosis
13) Weil's disease

Short questions for theory/viva questions

1) Write the one use of each Nichol's strain & Reiter's strain of *T pallidum.*
2) Mention the different types of syphilis.
3) Mention the different types of treponematoses.
4) Write four examplesof STS.
5) What is syphalotoxemia?
6) What is serofast reaction in syphilis?
7) What is chancre redux?
8) What is Hutchinson's triad?
9) What is Dinger's ring?
10) Write the role of hook of *Leptospira* in virulence.

MCQs for chapter review

Classification

1) Spirochetes among following are- (PGI, Dec -10)
(a) Syphilis (b) *Leptospira* (c) *Mycoplasma* (d) *Brucella* (e) *Borrelia*

Treponema pallidum

2) *Treponema pallidum* was first identified by-
(a) Fraenkel (b) Fritz Schaudinn and Erich Hoffmann (c) Nicolaicu (d) Ogston

3) Stain for *Treponema*
(a) Fontana's stain (b) Acid fast stain (c) Methenamine silver stain (d) PAS

4) **Following is true about *T. pallidum,* except-** (PGI-98)
(a) Can be transmitted in rabbit testis (b) Motile by peritrichate flagella (c) To visualise, dark ground microscope is used (d) TPI test is very useful

5) **Refrigerated blood stored up to 48 hours before transfusion can destroy which of the following**
(a) HIV (b) Hepatitis B (c) *Treponema pallidum* (d) *P vivax*

6) **All are true about secondary syphilis except-** (PGI, May-10, 13)
(a) Gumma formation (b) Condylomata lata (c) Palmar erythema (d) Chancre may occur (e) Mucosal patch

7) **"Chancre redux" is a clinical features of** (AIIMS, Nov-06)
(a) Early relapsing syphilis (b) Late syphilis (c) Chancroid (d) Recurrent herpes simplex infection

8) **In a syphilis patient site which does not help in isolation of organism--**
(a) Gumma (b) Primary chancre (c) Mucosal patch (d) Maculopapular rash

9) **Primary lesion of *Treponema pallidum* is known as**
(a) Chancre (b) Hard chancre (c) Soft sore (d) Cold sore

10) **True about primary chancre –** (PGI, Dec-08)
(a) Painless ulcer (b) Painless lymphadenopathy (c) Covered with exudate (d) Indurated lesion (e) Organism can be cultured from exudative fluid

11) **True about primary chancre –** (PGI, Dec-04)
(a) Multiple ulcers (b) Painless solitary ulcer (c) Most infective state (d) Heals automatically in few months without treatment (e) Penicillin is the drug of choice

12) **Investigation of choice for detection of syphilis in a patient after 2 course of complete therapy-** (AI-02)
(a) FTA-ABS (b) VDRL (c) TPI (d) Dark ground microscopy

13) **Most sensitive test for *Treponema-*** (AIIMS, May-10)
(a) VDRL (b) RPR (c) FTA-ABS (d) Kahn

14) **Confirmatory test for syphilis-**
(a) VDRL (b) FTA-ABS (c) RPR (d) None

15) **Regarding syphilis all are true except -** (AIIMS, Nov-93)
(a) VDRL titre decease or even absent after treatment (b) VDRL becomes positive after 10-14days of infection (c) Earliest serological test to become positive in untreated primary syphilis is TPHA (d) Yaws and pinta can't be differentiated by serological tests

16) **All are true about FTA-ABS in syphilis except-** (AI -00)
(a) FTA-ABS becomes negative after treatment (b) Present in secondary syphilis (c) It is specific test (d) May be positive in Lyme disease

17) **Dark ground microscopy is used for –** (PGI-98)
(a) TPI (b) FTA-ABS (c) Kahn test (d) VDRL

18) **Nichol's treponemes are used in –**
(a) Wasserman reaction (b) VDRL (c) RPR test (d) TPI test

19) **RPR test is belong to**
(a) Treponemal test category (b) Non-treponemal test category (c) Standard Test for Syphilis category (d) b+c

Neurosyphilis

20) **Diagnostic test of choice for neurosyphilis is –** (PGI, May-13, 10)
(a) VDRL (b) FTA-ABS (c) TPI (d) RPR

21) **25 year old labourer 3 years back presented with penile ulcer not treated. Later he got neurological treatment for which he got treated. Test to monitor response to treatment is -** (AIIMS, Nov-09)
(a) VDRL (b) FTA-ABS (c) TPI (d) RPR

Congenital syphilis

22) **Features of congenital syphilis are –** (PGI, May-10)
(a) Snuffles is late manifestation (b) Perforation in cartilagenous part of nose (c) Mulberry molar (d) Saddle nose deformity

23) **Congenital syphilis can be best diagnosed by -** (AI -01)
(a) IgM FTA-ABS (b) IgG FTA-ABS (c) VDRL (d) TPI

24) **Hutchinson's triad consisting of**
(a) Keratitis (b) Urethritis (c) Arthritis (d) Deafness (e) Notched or blunted upper central incisors

Endemic (non-venereal) treponematoses

25) **Non-venereal treponematoses is/are-** (PGI, May -10)
(a) *T. pertenue* (b) *T. carateum* (c) *T. pallidum* (d) *T. cuniculi*

26) **Regarding yaws all are true except –** (AI-08)
(a) Caused by *T. pertenue* (b) Sexually transmitted (c) Cross reactive antibodies with, syphilis (d) Drug of choice is the penicillin

27) **All of the following about "yaws" are true except –** (AI -11)
(a) Caused by *Treponema pertenue* (b) Transmitted non venereally (c) Secondary yaws can involve bone (d) Late stage of yaws involve heart and nerves

28) **Bejel is caused by-** (PGI, May -10)
(a) *T. pallidum* (b) *T. endemicun* (c) *T. pertenue* (d) *T. carateum*

Relapsing fever

29) **Which of the following microorganisms uses antigenic variation as a major means of evading host defenses –** (AIIMS, Nov -04)
(a) *Streptococcus pneumoniae* (b) *Borrelia recurrentis* (c) *Mycobacterium tuberculosis* (d) *Listeria monocytogenes*

30) **Antigenic variation is/are seen in** (PGI, Nov -10, 13)
(a) *Treponema pallidum* (b) *Neisseria* (c) *Corynebacterium* (d) *Borrelia recurrentis*

31) ***Borrelia* undergoes antigenic variation due to –**
(a) Plasmid (b) Transposon (c) Intrinsic mutation (d) All of above

32) **Louse borne relapsing fever is caused by –**
(a) *B. duttonii* (b) *B. recurrentis* (c) *B. parkeri* (d) *B. burgdorferi*

33) **Tick borne relapsing fever is/are caused by –**
(a) *Borrelia recurrentis* (b) *Borrelia duttonii* (c) *Borrelia burgdorferi* (d) *Borrelia hermsii* (e) None of above

34) **True about *Borrelia recurrentis* –**
(a) Causes leptospirosis (b) Water borne disease (c) Vector borne disease (d) Transmitted by tick

Vincent's angina

35) **Vincent's angina is caused by –**
(a) *B. vincenti* (b) *F. fusiforme* (c) *B. recurrentis* (d) *B. burgdorferi-*

Lyme disease

36) **The following are true regarding Lyme disease except-** (AI-03)
(a) It is transmitted by *Ixodid tick* (b) Erythema chronicum migrans may be a clinical features (c) *Borrelia recurrentis* is an aetiological agent (d) Rodent act as natural host

37) **Which of the following are not the manifestations of *Borrelia burgdorferi* –** (PGI, May-10 & 13)
(a) Erythema chronicum migrans (b) Acrodermatitis chronica atrophicans (c) Lymphogranuloma venereum (d) Granuloma fasiale (e) Lichen panus

38) **Lyme disease is**
(a) A mite borne illness caused by *Borrelia burgdorferi* (b) A tick borne illness caused by *Borrelia burgdorferi* (c) A louse borne illness caused by *Borrelia burgdorferi* (d) Non vector borne illness caused by *Borrelia burgdorferi*

39) **Kelly's medium is used in the isolation of -** (PGI-81)
(a) *Leptospira* (b) *Borrelia* (c) *Bartonella* (d) *Brucella*

40) **Lyme disease, all are true except-** (AIIMS, May-11, 10)
(a) *Borrelia burgdorferi* replicate locally and invades locally (b) Infection progress in spite of good humoral immunity (c)

Polymorphonuclear lymphocytosis suggest meningial involvement (d) IgA intrathecally confirms meningitis

41) **"Erythema chronicum migrans" is caused by –**
(a) *B. burgdorferi* (b) *Toxoplasma gondii* (c) *Toxocara canis* (d) *Strongyloides stercoralis*

Leptospirosis

42) **A bacterial disease that has been associated with 3 "Rs" i.e. rats, rice fields and rain fall is –** (AI -05)
(a) Leptospirosis (b) Plague (c) Melioidosis (d) Rodent - bite fever

43) **Reservoir of Leptospira –** (AI -05)
(a) Cat (b) Dog (c) Rat (d) Monkey

44) **Not used in leptospirosis –** (AIIMS, May-10)
(a) Microscopic agglutination test Widal test (b) Dark field illumination (c) Macroscopic agglutination test (d) Weil Felix reaction

45) **Culture media of leptospirosis –** (AIIMS, May-09)
(a) Kortof (b) Perkin (c) Tinsdale (d) Baker's

46) **The following about leptospirosis is true except–** (PGI-02)
(a) High fever with chills (b) Seen in sewage workers (c) Jaundice is present (d) Acute renal failure may occur (e) Tetracycline is the drug of choice

47) **All of the following statements about leptospirosis are true except–** (AI-09)
(a) Infection acquired by direct contact with infected urine (b) Mortality is 5-15% in severe cases (c) Antibodies are usually detectable in the first week (d) IV penicillin is recommended for treatment of severe cases

48) **Which of the following statements about leptospirosis is true –** (AI-11)
(a) Rats are primary reservoirs (b) Fluoroquinolones are the drug of choice (c) Person to person transmission is common (d) Hepato renal syndrome may occur in up to 50% of patients

49) **A sewage workers presents to the emergency department with fever and jaundice. Laboratory findings reveal an elevated BUN and serum creatinine suggestive of renal failure. Which of following antibiotics is recommended?** (AI-11)
(a) Cotrimoxazole (b) Erythromycin (c) Ciprofloxacin (d) Penicillin G

50) **Which of the following is transmitted by rat urine-**
(a) *Leptospira* (b) *Listeria* (c) *Legionella* (d) *Mycoplasma*

51) **Which human infection spread through urine** (PGI-06)
(a) *Leptospira* (b) *Legionella* (c) Plague (d) Diphtheria

52) **Weil's disease is caused by-**
(a) *Leptospira* (b) *Listeria* (c) *Mycoplasma* (d) *Legionella*

53) ***Leptospira* canicola infection usually present as-**
(a) Aseptic meningitis (b) Jaundice (c) Diarrhoea and vomiting (d) Lobar pneumonia

Answers of MCQs & explanation

1) **(a), (b) & (e)**
- Follow section, **classification (flow chart-1)** for explanation

2) **(b)**
- Follow section, ***Treponema pallidum* (history)** for explanation

3) **(a)**
- Follow section, ***Treponema pallidum* (morphology)** for explanation

4) **(b)**
- *Treponema pallidum* have endoflagella & it is motile, but endoflagella have no role in motility.
- For explanation of 'option a' follow C/Cs, 'option c' follow morphology & 'option d' follow serological tests of written under the section *Treponema pallidum*

5) **(c)**
- Option a, b & d: Not killed by refrigeration
- Option c: Follow section, ***Treponema pallidum* (resistance)** for explanation

6) **(a), (c) & (d)**
7) **(a)**
} Follow section. ***Treponema pallidum* (pathogenicity → flow chart -3)** for explanation

8) **(a)**
- Gumma is a tertiary syphilis with few bacilli, so less useful in isolation while secondary lesion condylomata lata, palmar erythema & mucosal patch & primary lesion like chancre have more bacilli & helpful for diagnosis

9) **(d)**
- Primary lesion of *Treponema pallidum* is known as chancre / hard chancre / Hunterian chancre while soft sore is caused by *Haemophilus ducreyi* & cold sore is due to herpes simplex virus.

10) **(a), (b), (c) & (d)**
- Pathogenic *T pallidum* are more in exudative fluid but difficult to culture

11) **(b), (d) & (e)**
- Primary chancre present with solitary ulcer. Condylomata lata is the most infectious stage.

12) **(b)**
- VDRL test is useful to monitor the therapy. Follow section *Treponema pallidum* (treatment & monitoring of venereal syphilis) for more explanation.

13) **(c)**
14) **(b)**
} Follow section, ***Treponema pallidum* (serological tests → FTA-ABS test)** for explanation

15) **(b) & (c)**
- VDRL becomes positive 3-5 weeks after acquiring the primary infection or 7-10 days after appearance of chancre
- Earliest serological test to become positive in untreated primary syphilis is FTA-ABST

16) **(a)**
- FTA-ABS is species specific test, remain positive after treatment, highly positive in all stage of syphilis & false positive in Lyme disease

17) **(a)**
- Treponema is immobilised by specific antiserum in presence of complement. Such immobilisation is examined under DGIM **called TPI (*Treponema Pallidum* Immobilisation) test.**

18) **(d)**
- Nichol's strain is useful to prepare the antigen for species specific treponemal tests. From the given options treponemal test is TPI

19) **(d)**
- Follow section, ***Treponema pallidum* (venereal syphilis → laboratory diagnosis of venereal syphilis)** for explanation

20) **(a)**
- Follow section, ***Treponema pallidum* (neurosyphilis → diagnosis)** for explanation

21) **(a)**
- Given case is neurosyphilis where best diagnostic test is VDRL. Follow section neurosyphilis (**diagnosis**) for more explanation about other options.

22) **(b), (c) & (d)**
- Snuffles is early manifestation in congenital syphilis

23) **(a)**
- Follow section, ***Treponema pallidum* (diagnosis of congenital syphilis → serological tests →IgM detection)** for explanation

24) **(a), (d) & (e)**
- Follow section, ***Treponema pallidum* (clinical features of congenital syphilis →late congenital syphilis)** for explanation

25) **(a) & (b)**
- Follow section, **endemic (non-venereal) treponematoses (classification & table-2)** for explanation

26) **(b)**
27) **(d)**
28) **(b)**
} Follow **table-2** for explanation

29) (b) } *Borrelia recurrentis* causing relapsing fever is under
30) (d) } goes the antigenic variation & escape the host defence
31) (a)
- *Borrelia recurrentis* showing antigenic variation in Vmp gene which is located in linear plasmid

32) (b) } Follow section, **relapsing fever** (**table-3**)
33) (b) & (d) } for explanation
34) (c)
- *Borrelia recurrentis* causing relapsing fever which is transmitted by vector (louse). Follow section relapsing fever for more explanation

35) (a) & (b)
- It is a symbiotic infection caused by *Borrelia vincenti* & *Fusobacter fusiforme.*

36) (c)
- *Borrelia recurrentis* causing relapsing fever while Lyme disease is caused by *Borrelia burgdorferi*

37) (c), (d) & (e) } Follow section, **Lyme disease** (**flow chart-4**)
38) (b) } for explanation
39) (b)
- Kelly's medium is used in the isolation of *Borrelia burgdorferi* which is the causative agent of Lyme disease

40) (c)
- Meningial involvement in Lyme disease suggests mononuclear lymphocytosis not the polymorphonuclear lymphocytosis. Follow section Lyme disease for explanation of other options.

41) (b)
- Erythema chronicum migrans" is is a feature of Lyme disease which is caused by *Borrelia bergdorferi*

42) (a)
- Follow section, **leptospirosis (note → "3Rs"**) for explanation

43) (c)
- Rat is the reservoir for Weil's disease. For other types & respective reservoir, follow section, **leptospirosis (classification & table-5**).

44) (d)
- Weil Felix reaction is useful for *Rickettsia*

45) (a)
- Follow section, **leptospirosis** (**culture characteristics**) for explanation

46) (e)
- Tetracycline is not the drug of choice. Follow section, **leptospirosis** (**treatment**) selection of drug of leptospirosis.

47) (c)
- Antibodies (IgM) appear after 1st week, detectable titre present in 2nd week, reaches peak level in 3rd- 4th (1:10,000 titre) week, then decline slowly & becomes undetectable in a six months

48) (a)
- Rat is the reservoir for Weil's disease. For other types & respective reservoir, follow section classification (**table-5**).
- Pn / doxicycline is the drug of choice as per severity
- Person to person transmission does not occur
- Hepato renal syndrome may occur in up to 10% of patients

49) (d)
- Given case is of leptospirosis, where drug of choice is Penicillin G from the given options.

50) (a)
- Leptospira: It is a zoonosis transmitted by direct contact of abraded skin with contaminated water or mud from urine of infected animals like rat
- Listeria: It is a zoonosis transmitted directly by contact or vertical route & indirectly by air borne, water borne, food borne & fomite borne
- Legionella: Transmitted by inhalation of aerosols arise from air-conditioner, shower heads, nebulizer, humidifier, device filled with tap water or from infected aquatic reservoir
- Mycoplasma: Transmitted by inhalation route & person to person transmission is possible by close contact

51) (a)
- Option a: Follow section **leptospirosis (pathogenicity → mode of transmission)** for explanation
- Follow **respective chapters** for explanation of other options.

52) (a)
- Weil's disease is a one type of leptospirosis caused by Ictero haemorrhagiae serovars of *Leptospira*

53) (a)
- *Leptospira* canicoal present as an influenza like illness or aseptic meningitis

56 Mycoplasmatales

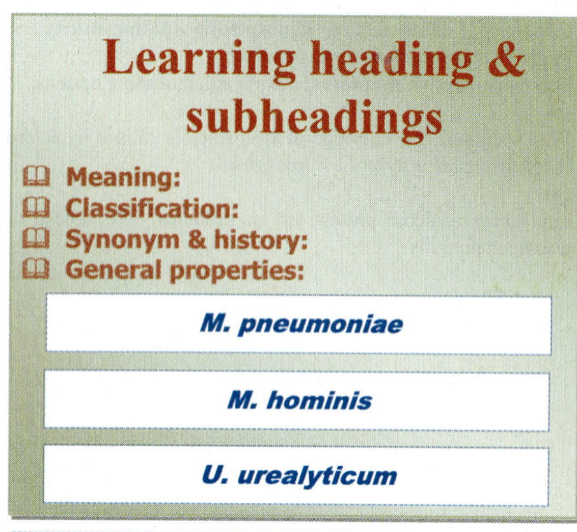

Learning heading & subheadings
Meaning:
Classification:
Synonym & history:
General properties:
M. pneumoniae
M. hominis
U. urealyticum

Meaning:

Myco from **Mykes (Greek) = branching / filamentous form + Plasma = plasticity of nature**

Classification:

→ **Flow chart-1 & table-1**

Synonym & history:

a. Pleuro Pneumonia Like Organism (PPLO):

- As it cause bovine pleuropneumonia in animals.
- The first member of this group *Mycoplasma mycoides* subsp. *mycoides* was isolated by Roux & Nocard in 1898 from cattle with pleuropneumonia.

b. Eaton agent or Eaton's agent:

- Eaton 1st isolated the bacteria in hamster & cotton rat.
- He also transmits the infection in chick embryo by amniotic inoculation.
- Because it is smaller in size & can pass through filter as like virus, initially it **called Eaton agent** & grouped as virus but later grouped as bacteria because multiply by binary fission, sensitive to antibiotics, having both DNA & RNA & can grow on artificially prepared media.

General properties:

- **Cell wall deficient:** The inability to synthesize a peptidoglycan cell wall is due to the absence of genes encoding its formation.
- **Growth:** It can grow in cell free media / artificially prepared nutritional media.
- **Habitat:** Free living in the environment but in human can habitat in respiratory system or in the genital organs.
- **Species:** Around 16 human pathogens are known few are mentioned in **flow chart-1** & **table-1.**
- **Pleomorphism:** Cell wall deficient & no fixed size or shape. Smallest prokaryotes.
- **Cell culture contaminants:**
  - *Mycoplasma* species are the common contaminants in viral cell culture & interfering not in cytopathic effect but in growth of viruses.
  - They also interfere with reading of serological testing.
  - It originated from the workers or from animals sera or from trypsin used in cell culture.
  - It's very difficult to eliminate the *Mycoplasma* as contaminant & change of cell line is required.
- **Drug resistance:** They are cell wall deficient & completely resistant to cell wall dependent drugs like β-lactam which include penicillin & cephalosporin.

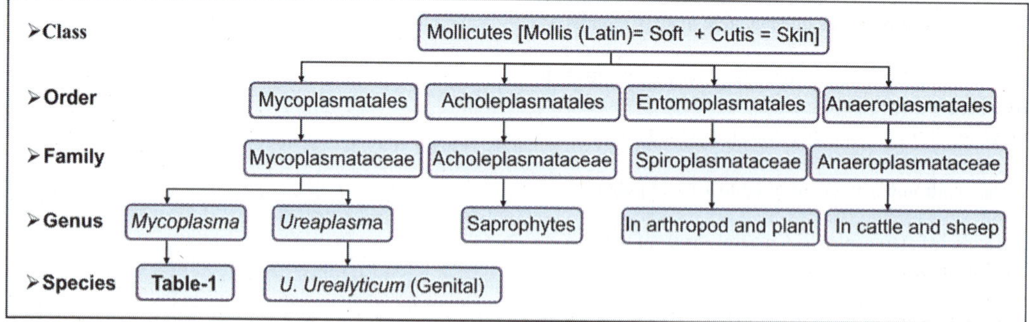

Flow chart-1: Classification of Mollicutes

Pathological status	Habitat	Mycoplasma spp.
Established pathogen	Respiratory system	*M. pneumoniae*
Presumed pathogen	Genital	*M. hominis,*
Non pathogen	Mouth	*M. orale, M. buccale, M. salivarium & M. faucium*
	Genital	*M. fermentans, M. genitalium, M. penetrans, M. spermatophilum & M. primatum*

Table-1: *Mycoplasma* spp.

Features	*Mycoplasma*	L-forms
Type	Stable (natural) type cell wall deficiency	Stable or unstable type cell wall deficiency
Filterable	Yes	No
Cell wall	Peptidoglycan precursor are absent	Peptidoglycan precursor are may present
Cell membrane	Sterol present	Sterol absent
Disease	Can cause disease	Cant's cause disease but may cause persistence of infection

Table-2: Differences between *Mycoplasma* & L-forms

➤ **Persistence of infection:** The persistence of *M. pneumoniae* infections even after treatment is associated with its ability to mimic host cell surface composition.

➤ ***Mycoplasma* & L-forms:**
- *Mycoplasma* showing stable type of L – forms but genetic, biochemical & antigenic evidences are against the possibilities.
- *Mycoplasma* species are the common contaminants in viral cell culture & interfering not in cytopathic effect but in growth of viruses.
- Differences between *Mycoplasma* & L-forms are shown in **table-2.**
- For more details of L forms **follow chapter → Morphology of bacteria.**

➤ **Opportunistic pathogen:**
- *Mycoplasma* can causes more sever & prolonged infection in HIV & in immunodeficient persons.
- AIDS associated *Mycoplasma* are *M. incognitus*, *M. fermentans* (**urine**) *M. penetrans* (**urine**) *M. pirum* (**blood**) etc.

M. pneumoniae

❖ Morphology:

➤ **Staining properties:**
- Gram negative but better stained by Giemsa stain.
- Colony on solid media is stained by Diene's stain.
- Fluorescent staining is also useful.

➤ **Size:**
- Smallest free living microorganisms.
- Highly pleomorphic & no fixed size.
- About 125-250nm in size.
- Because of smaller size & plasticity it can pass through bacterial filters [**other bacteria which can pass through filter are *F. tularensis, Coxiella burnetii* & *Chlamydiae*** (PLT agent / PLT virus)**]**.

➤ **Shape:**
- Highly pleomorphic & no fixed shape.
- Present in different forms like coccoid, balloon, disc, ring or star or granules or filamentous forms as shown in **fig.-1 (a) (helical→ *Spiroplasma*).**

➤ **Motility:** No flagella but showing gliding motility.

➤ **Cell wall:**
- Devoid of cell wall, bounded by a single trilaminar unit membrane containing sterols.
- Sterol present in membrane maintains the rigidity of bacterial cell.
- *M. pneumoniae* are the only bacterial cells that possess cholesterol in their cell membrane (obtained from the host) and possess more genes that encode for membrane lipoprotein variations than other *Mycoplasma.*

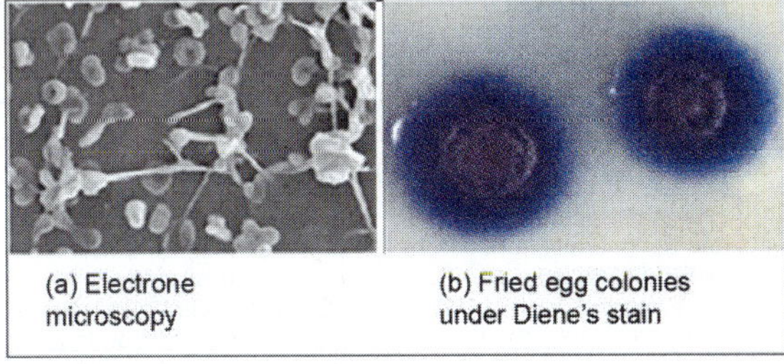

(a) Electrone microscopy
(b) Fried egg colonies under Diene's stain

Figure-1: Morphology & C/Cs of *M. pneumoniae*

➤ **Multiplication:** By binary fission, budding or beaded forms are also noticed.

➤ **Organ for adhesion:** No fimbriae but shows bulbous enlargement with which they attach to neuraminic acid receptor holding host cells & also on RBCs **called haemadsorption.**

➤ **L-forms:** Present & stable type.

➤ **Other features:** Nonsporing, non flagellated & non fimbriated.

❖ Cultural characteristics (C/Cs):

➤ **Effective factors:**

O_2 effect: Aerobes & facultative anaerobes.
- Temperature: Optimum growth at 35-37°C.
- pH: 7.8
- Growth factors: Require sterol and cholesterol for growth. Media are enriched with 20% horse/human serum (source of cholesterol) & yeast extract. 30% human ascetic fluid is also useful instead of serum for enrichment.

➤ **Culture in media:**

A. Liquid medium (enrichment medium):

i. *Mycoplasma* / PPLO broth: BHIB + peptone water + yeast extract+ horse/human serum + phenol red + glucose. It also useful as transport medium.

B. Solid media:

i. *Mycoplasma* glucose agar: Mycoplasma broth + agar.

ii. SP4 agar: Contains phenol red as an indicator & give yellow colour colony.

C. Biphasic media: It contains liquid & solid phase.

D. Selective media:

i. Liquid selective media: *Mycoplasma* broth + Penicillin (Pn) + polymyxin B + AMB.

ii. Solid selective media:

- *Mycoplasma* glucose agar + Pn +Polymyxin B + AMB.
- Thallous acetate is inhibitory for *U. urealyticum* & *M. genitalium,* so rarely useful as selective agent.

➢ **Cultivation techniques: → Flow chart-2**

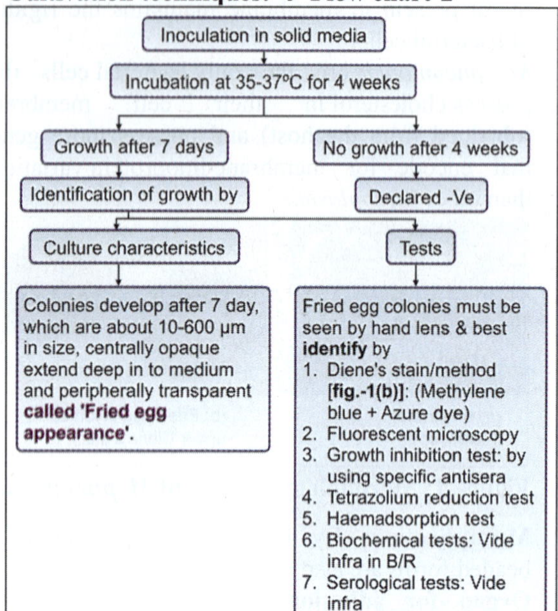

Flow chart-2: Cultivation techniques of *M. pneumoniae*

✓ **Note: Diene's phenomenon** → It is useful to identify the identical & non-identical *Proteus* strains (swarming).

➢ **Culture in egg:** It can grow in chicken embryo.

❖ Biochemical reaction (B/Rs):

1. **Glucose fermentation:**
   - Ferments glucose with acid production only.
   - Tested by using Mycoplasma broth.
2. **Urease test & arginine hydrolysis:** Negative

❖ Resistance:

- Destroyed by heat at 45^{0}C in 15 minutes.
- Resistant to penicillin & other β-lactam due to absence of cell wall.
- They are sensitive to surface active agents like taurocholate, digitonin & some antibiotics like tetracycline & erythromycin.
- *M. pneumoniae* can grow in presence of 0.0002% methylene blue, while other species are inhibited.

❖ Pathogenicity:

➢ **Disease name: Called primary atypical pneumonia.** *M. pneumoniae* is the most common cause.

➢ **Meaning:**

✪ **Called primary** because it develops independently of other diseases.

✪ **Called atypical** because of following reasons

- **Etiological agents:** Typical pneumonia always signals bacterial causes but it is caused by atypical microbes (other than bacteria *Strept. pneumoniae*, *H. influenzae* & *Moraxella catarrhalis*). These atypical organisms include special bacteria, viruses, fungi & protozoa as follows
  - Bacteria: *M. pneumoniae* (most common cause), *Chlamydiae psittaci*, *Chlamydiae pneumoniae*, *Coxiella burnetii*, *Legionell pneumophilla* & *Francisella tularensis*
  - Viruses: Adeno virus, Respiratory Syncitial Virus (RSV), influenza virus, para-influenza virus, *Coxsackievirus*, human corona virus etc.
  - Fungi: *Pneumocystic jiroveci*, *Histoplasma capsulatum*, *Coccidioided immitis* etc.
  - Protozoa: *Toxoplasma gondii*
- **Pathology & clinical presentation:** In addition, this form of pneumonia is atypical in presentation (less pulmonary & more systemic symptoms) with moderate amounts of sputum, no consolidation, only small increases in white cell counts & no alveolar exudate.

➢ **Synonym:**

- Affected person not too sick, so **called "walking pneumonia"**.
- Patchy inflammatory changes are present in alveolar septa & in interstitial space, so **called interstitial pneumonia.**

➢ **Nature of disease:** Distributed worldwide. Reinfection & epidemic cycling is thought to be a result of P1 adhesin subtype variation. About 40% of community-acquired pneumonia is due to *M. pneumoniae* infections.

➢ **Reservoir of infection:** Human.

➢ **Source of infection:** Respiratory droplets.

➢ **Mode of transmission:**

1. **Inhalation:** Transmitted by inhalation of respiratory or nasopharyngeal droplets.
2. **Contact:** Person to person transmission by close contact is also possible, typically in military persons.

➢ **Incubation period:** 1-3 weeks.

➢ **Portal of entry:** Respiratory system.

➢ **Sites:** Pulmonary & extra pulmonary sites.

➢ **Precipitating factors (epidemiological determinants):**

I. Agent factors (virulence factors)

a. Nuclease enzymes: Degrades the host cell nucleic acid to generate the precursor for synthesis of their own nucleic acid.

b. Antigens:

1. **Protein Ag:**

- **Called P_1** or **cytadhesin** which helps in adhesion to respiratory epithelium & block the ciliary movement **called ciliostasis.**
- It is detected by ELISA.

2. **Glycolipid Ag:**
- For adhesion with RBCs & responsible for haemolytic anaemia.
- Forms the basis for detection of heterophile antibodies by cold agglutination test.
- Identified by CFT.

3. **Hydrogen peroxide:** It can injure the host cell by reducing glutathione, damaging lipid membranes & causing protein denaturation.
4. **Cytotoxin:** It has ADP ribosylating & vacuolating properties as like pertusis toxin.
5. **Lipoproteins:** Present in cell membrane & appear to induce inflammation.

II. Host factors

1. **Age:** More in children & elder group.
2. **Other risk groups:** Outbreaks of *M. pneumoniae* infections tend to occur within groups of people in close & prolonged proximity, including schools, institutions, military bases & households.

III. Environmental factors

1. **Seasonal:** The incidence of disease does not appear be related to season or geography; however, infection tends to occur more frequently during the summer and fall months when other respiratory pathogens are less prevalent.

➢ **Pathology:**

- **Macroscopic:** Patchy inflammatory changes in the interstitial areas.
- **Microscopic:**
- No signs and symptoms of lobar consolidation, meaning that the infection is restricted to small areas, rather than involving a whole lobe. As the disease progresses, however, the look can tend to lobar pneumonia.
- Alveolar septa are widened & oedematous infiltrated by lymphocytes, macrophages & occasionally by plasma cells.
- Absence of leucocytosis.
- Lack of alveolar exudates, so moderate amount of sputum or no sputum at all (non-productive).

➢ **Clinical features:**

- It present in interstitial space but not in alveoli so, respiratory symptoms like sputum production is minimal or not at all and manifested with some atypical features fever, malaise, headache, sweating, myalgia, sore throat etc.
- Dry irritating cough followed later by a productive cough with radiographs showing consolidation.
- It also causes pharyngitis, tracheo-bronchitis & sinusitis.
- Clear without antibiotic therapy.
- Consolidation in lower lobe can be observed by X-ray.

➢ **Complications:** Otitis, myringitis, rashes, meningitis, encephalitis, haemolytic anaemia etc.

❖ Laboratory diagnosis:

➢ **Specimens:** Throat swab, sputum, respiratory secretions etc.

➢ **Testing methods:**

I. Microscopy: → Follow morphology

II. Culture: → Follow cultural characteristics

III. Biochemical reaction: →Vide supra

IV. Blood picture: No leucocytosis but raised ESR in 50% of patients

V. Serological tests:

A Antigen detection tests: Antigen can be detected in respiratory specimens by

1. Immunofluorescence test
2. CIE
3. ELISA
4. Immuno Blot test

B Antibody detection tests:

i. Specific tests: So called because performed by using antigen from *Mycoplasma.*

a. More sensitive tests:

1. Immunofluorescence test
2. Haemagglutination inhibition test
3. Metabolic inhibition test

b. Less sensitive tests:

1. IHA test
2. CFT

ii. Nonspecific tests: So called because performed by using antigen from other cells.

1. ***Streptococcus* MG test:**
- Do the serial dilution of patient serum.
- Add the heat killed suspension of *Streptococcus* MG.
- Observe for the agglutination after overnight incubation at 37°C.
- 1:20 is significant titre.

2. **Cold agglutination test:**
- In patient with primary atypical pneumonia high proportion of antibodies are produced that agglutinate human O cell at low temperature.
- Do the serial dilution of patient serum.
- Add the 0.2 % human O group cells.
- Do the overnight incubation at 4°C & observed for the clumps..
- Clumps will dissociate at 37°C.
- 1: 32 or above is significant titre.

3. **Indirect Coombs test:** Is also useful in some cases.

VI. Molecular: DNA probe, PCR etc.

❖ Treatment:

- Macrolides like azithromycin (500 mg orally on 1st day followed by 250 mg/day for 5 days),

erythromycin & clarithromycin are the drugs of choice.
- Other alternatives are tetracycline / doxycycline or fluoroquinolones like levofloxacin, moxifloxacin & gemifloxacin (no levofloxacin) are effective.

M. hominis

❖ **Morphology:** Similar to *M. pneumoniae.*

❖ **Cultural characteristics (C/Cs):** All media of *M. pneumoniae* are supplemented with arginine instead of glucose **called H-broth & H-agar** produce large fried egg colonies identify by Diene's stain.

❖ **Biochemical reaction (B/Rs):** Do not ferment glucose but arginine hydrolysis test is +Ve.

❖ **Resistance:** Resistant to penicillins & rifampicin, so difficult to eliminate from the cell culture, animal host & human host.

❖ **Pathogenicity:**

➢ **Mode of transmission:**

1. **Contact:**
- Vaginal intercourse.
- Oral-to-genital contact.
2. **Vertical/Congenital:**
- Vertically from mother to her infant in utero.
- From infected birth canal.
3. **Tissues transplantation:** Acquisition through transplanted tissues.

➢ **Precipitating factors:**

1. **Age:** These are inhabitant of genitourinary tract particularly in the sexually active adults. Neonates specially girls are colonised during birth from infected birth canal, but this colonisation does not persist & becomes only about 10% up to age of pre-puberty. After puberty colonisation increase about 15% in men & women due to sexual activity.
2. **Immunodeficiency disease:** It also favours the infection.
3. **Race:** It is more common in African Americans than in Caucasians.

➢ **Clinical features:**

✪ **Uro-genital:**
- NGU: Non-Gonococcal Urethritis
- PID: Pelvic Inflammatory Disease
- Cervicitis
- Urethritis
- Cystitis
- Endometritis
- Chorioamnionitis

✪ **Extra-genital:**
- Pyelonephritis
- Infectious arthritis
- Surgical and nonsurgical wound infections
- Bacteremia
- Pneumonia
- Meningitis
- Salpingitis
- Septic arthritis

❖ **Laboratory diagnosis:** Same as *M. pneumoniae* but differentiated by growth on **H-broth** & **H-agar** & ability to hydrolyse arginine.

❖ **Treatment:** Tetracyclines, macrolides, erythromycin, macrolides, ketolides & quinolones are used to treat infections.

U. urealyticum

❖ **Morphology:** Similar to *M. pneumoniae.*

❖ **Cultural characteristics (C/Cs):** All media of *M. pneumoniae* are supplemented with urea instead of glucose **called U-broth & U-agar** produce very tiny colony hence **called T strain** or **T forms of *Mycoplasma.***

❖ **Biochemical reaction (B/R):** Glucose fermentation & arginine hydrolysis are negative but urease test is positive.

❖ **Pathogenicity:**

➢ **Mode of transmission:**

1. **Contact:**
- Vaginal intercourse
- Oral-to-genital contact
2. **Vertical / congenital:**
- Vertically from mother to her infant in utero or
- From infected birth canal.

➢ **Precipitating factors:**

1. **Age:** These are inhabitant of genitourinary tract particularly in the sexually active adults. Neonates specially girls are colonised during birth from infected birth canal, but this colonisation does not persist & becomes only about 10% up to age of pre-puberty. After puberty colonisation increase about 45-75% in men & women due to sexual activity.

➢ **Clinical features:**

a. **In men:**
- Non Gonococcal Urethritis (NGU) / Non specific urethritis
- Epididymitis
- Proctitis
- Reiter's syndrome (urethritis, conjunctivitis & arthritis)

b. **In women:**
- Acute urethral syndrome
- Bartholinitis
- Endometritis
- Salpingitis

- Pelvic Inflammatory Disease (PID)
- Reiter's syndrome (cervictis / urethritis, conjunctivitis & arthritis)
- Fitz – Hugh Curtis syndrome (peritonitis & perihepatic inflammation)

➢ **Complications:** Infertility, abortion, ectopic pregnancy, premature delivery, antenatal morbidity, puerperal sepsis, post partum fever, Low Birth Weight (LBW) of infant & chorioamnionitis.

❖ **Laboratory diagnosis:** Diagnosed from genital discharges by same methods as like *M. pneumoniae* but differentiated by growth on **U-broth** & **U-agar** & urease positive.

❖ **Treatment:**

- Doxycycline is the drug of choice but azithromycin is also used as a five-day course instead of a single dose that would be used to treat *Chlamydia* infection.
- Streptomycin is an alternative, but less popular because it must be injected.

Question bank

Essay/Full question

1) *M. pneumoniae*

Short notes

1) Classification of *Mollicutes*
2) Morphology/ pathogenicity / laboratory diagnosis of *M. pneumoniae*
3) Primary atypical pneumonia (interstitial pneumonia).
4) Genital *Mycoplasma.*

Short questions for theory/viva questions

1) What is Eaton agent?
2) Write the four differences between *Mycoplasma* & L-forms
3) Name four bacteria causing primary atypical pneumonia
4) What is T-strain or tiny strain of *Mycoplasma*?
5) What is Diene's stain / method & Diene's phenomenon?

MCQs for chapter review

General properties

1) **The following statements are true with references to *Mycoplasma* except-** (AIIMS, Nov-05)
(a) They are the smallest prokaryotic organisms that can grow in cell free culture media (b) They are obligate intracellular organisms (c) They lack a cell wall (d) They are resistant to Beta-lactam drugs

M. pneumoniae

2) **Which of the following needs cholesterol and other lipids for growth**
(a) *Y pestis* (b) *Pseudomonas* (c) *Proteus* (d) *Mycoplasma*
3) **Diene's method is used for –** (PGI -99)
(a) *Mycoplasma* (b) *Chlamydiae* (c) Plague (d) Diphtheria
4) **Fried egg colony is seen in culture of -**
(a) *Mycoplasma* (b) *Legionella* (c) *Trachoma* (d) *Haemophilus*
5) **In references to *Mycoplasmas,* the following are true except** (AIIMS, May-05)
(a) They are inhibited by penicillin (b) They can reproduce in cell free media (c) They have an affinity for mammalian cell membrane (d) They can pass through filters of 450 nm pore size
6) **True about *Mycoplasma,* are all except-** (AIIMS, May-08)
(a) They are L forms (b) Sterol enhance growth (c) Can grow in cell free media (d) When grow in liquid medium do not produces turbidity.
7) **True about *Mycoplasma* is-** (AIIMS, Dec-95)
(a) Causes lung infection (b) Penicillin is drug of choice (c) Thick cell wall (d) Thallium acetate inhibits the growth
8) ***Mycoplasma pneumoniae* is characterised by all except-** (AIIMS, June-98)
(a) Diagnosed by serum cold antibody (b) Treatment is erythromycin (c) Cannot be culture from sputum (d) Raised ESR
9) **Atypical pneumonia can be caused by the following microbial agents except-** (AI -05)
(a) *Mycoplasma* (b) *Legionell pneumophilla* (c) Human corona virus (d) *Klebsiella pneumoniae*

U urealytocum

10) **Ureaplasma naturally resistant to**
(a) Erythromycin (b) Tetracycline (c) Chloramphenicol (d) Cephalosporin

Answers of MCQs & explanation

1) **(b)**
- Option b: *Mycoplasma* are not the obligate intracellular organisms because it can grow in cell free media & it also living free in the environment
- Option a, c & d: Follow section, **general properties** for explanation

2) **(d)**
- Follow section, ***M. pneumoniae* (culture characteristics → effective factors)** for explanation

3) **(a)** } Follow section, ***M. pneumoniae* (culture characteristics**
4) **(a)** } **→ cultivation technique & flow chart-2** for explanation
5) **(a)**
- *Mycoplasma* are cell wall deficient & completely resistant to cell wall dependent drugs like β-lactam which include penicillin & cephalosporin
- *Mycoplasma* can grow in cell free media like PPLO broth etc.
- Option c & d: Follow section, **synonym & history (Eaton agent)** for explanation

6) **(a)**
- *Mycoplasmas* are naturally deficient to cell wall which is stable while L form is cell wall deficiency due to effect of penicillin which is induced artificially & it may be stable or unstable.
- Sterol & cholesterol are required for growth of bacteria
- *Mycoplasma* can grow in cell free media like PPLO broth etc.
- Not produces turbidity in liquid medium

7) **(a)**
- Causes lung infection **Called primary atypical pneumonia**
- Penicillin is not effective because no cell wall
- Thallium acetate does not inhibits the growth

8) **(c)**
- Antigens from *Mycoplasma* are producing the antibodies that agglutinate human O cell at 4°C
- It can be culture from sputum & ESR raised in 50% of patients

9) **(d)**
- Follow section, ***M. pneumoniae* (pathogenicity → etiological agents)** for explanation

10) **(d)**
- *Ureaplasma* are cell wall deficient & completely resistant to cell wall dependent drugs like β-lactam which include penicillin & cephalosporin

57 Chlamydiales

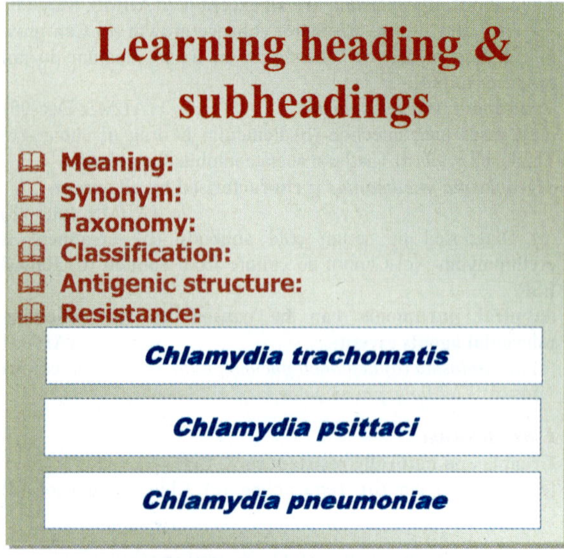

Meaning:

Word Chlamydiae derived from **chlamys = helmet (mentle)**, because inclusion body encloses within the cells.

Synonyms:

1. *Chlamydophila*
2. **PLT agent / PLT virus:** It causes psittacosis-lymphogranuloma–trachoma in human, so **called PLT agent / PLT virus.**
3. **Energy parasite:** Lack enzyme of electron transport channel (ETC) & dependent on the host cells for energy & nutrition, so **called energy parasite.**
4. **Bedsonia:** Because of pioneering work by **Sir Samuel Bedson** on organism causing psittacosis, this group also **called Bedsonia.**
5. **Basophilic viruses:** *Chlamydia* produces intracytoplasmic inclusion body which is basophilic in nature hence sometimes **called basophilic viruses.** Viruses are produced eosinophilic type of inclusion body.

Taxonomy:

➢ **Was considered as virus:** Because many features are similar to viruses like

1. Obligate intracellular organism in human, animal or bird's cells with tropism for squamous epithelial cells & macrophages of GIT & respiratory system
2. Pass through filter.
3. Failure to grow in cell free media.
4. Producing the inclusion body.

➢ **Now accepted as bacterium:** Because many features are similar to bacteria like

1. Have both DNA & RNA.
2. Have a cell wall but lack of peptidoglycan.
3. Have ribosomes.
4. Replicate by binary fission without an "eclipse phase".
5. Sensitive to antibiotics.

Classification:

Based on antigenic properties as shown **flowchart-1.**

Antigenic structure:

Three types of antigen as shown in **table-1**

Resistance:

- Heat sensitive & killed by heat at 56^0c in a minute.
- Also killed by disinfectants like phenol, formalin, ethanol & ether.
- Infectivity is maintained for several days at 4^0C.
- It can be preserved by lyophillisation or at -70^0C.

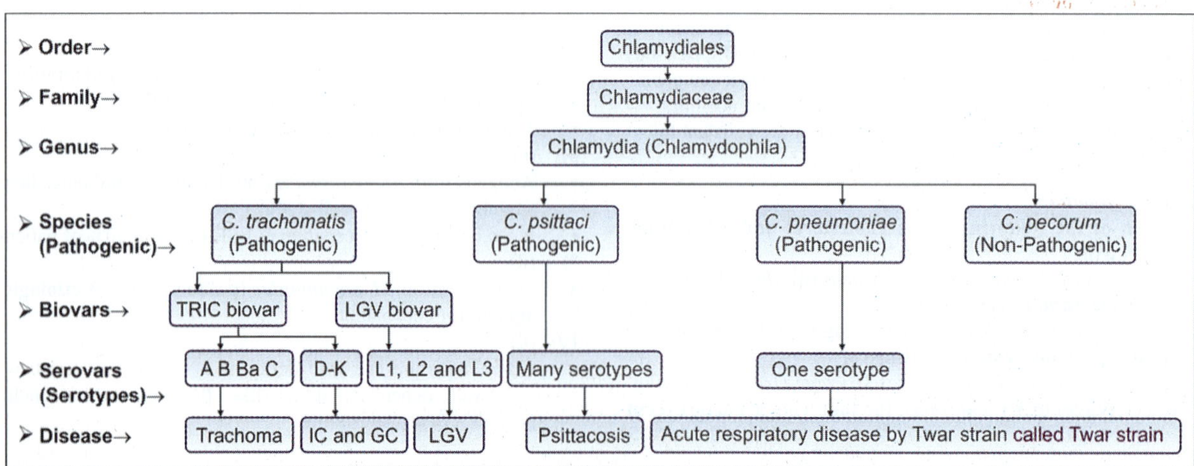

Flowchart-1: Classification of Chlamydiales

No.	Type of antigen	Bio-chemistry	Properties	Identification
1	Genus/Group specific	Lipopolysaccharide	Like LPS of GNB	CFT
2	Species specific	Protein (for classification in to species)	Present at envelop surface.	----
3	Serotype/ intra species specific	Protein (for serotying of *Chlamydia* spp.)	MOMP (Major Outer Membrane Protein)	Micro-IF

Table-1: Antigenic properties of Chlamydiales

Chlamydia trachomatis

❖ **History:** Characteristic inclusion body **called Halberstaedter - Prowazek body**, because it was detected by Halberstaedter –Prowazek in 1907 from conjunctival smear from orangutans.

❖ **Biovars & serovars:** → **Flow chart-1**

❖ **Life cycle:** → **Fig.-1 & flow chart-2**

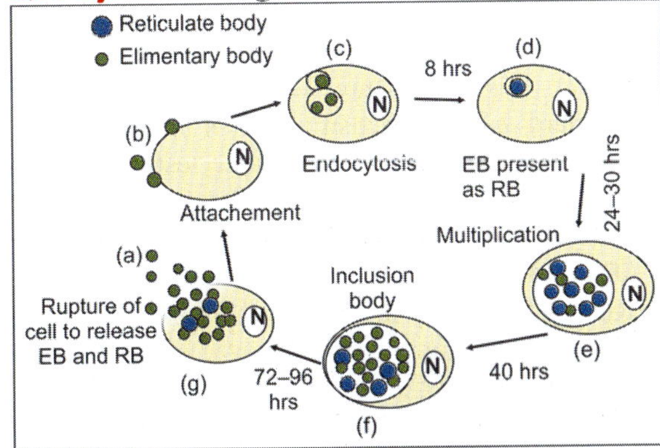

Figure-1: Life cycle of *Chlamydia* spp.

Free EB **[fig.1(a)]**

↓

EB attach to the host cell **[fig.1(b)]**. Molecules responsible for attachment is may be MOMP.

↓

EB enter in the host cell by endocytosis **[fig.1(c)]**. It is separated from host cell cytoplasm by endosomal membrane around it **called phagocytic vacuole**.

↓

Exact mechanisms to escape the intracellular killing are unknown but may be due to secretion of antigens by *Chlamydia*, which are settled on endosomal membrane and prevent the fusion of **phagocytic vacuole** with lysosome to form phagosome/phagolysosome.

↓

After 8 hrs EB identified as RB **[fig.1(d)]**.

↓

In 24-30 hrs RB undergoes multiplication by budding method, which is continuing for 40 hrs to form multiple EB and RB **[fig.1(e)]**. All EB and RB are collected within a membrane inside the host cells **called inclusion body [fig.1(f)] [called HP body** in *C trachomatis* and **called LCL body** in *C psittaci* as shown in **table 3)]**

↓

After 72-96 hrs cell get rupture **[fig.1(g)]** to release the EB and RB in *C trachomatis* **(cycle completed in 48 hrs in *C. psittaci*)**

↓

EB infect the other cell to continue the life cycle

Flow chart-2: Life cycle of *Chlamydia* spp.

❖ **Morphology:**

➢ **Cell wall & staining properties:**

- **Structure:**
  - Outer cell wall of *C. trachomatis* resemble to gram negative bacteria.
  - It has high lipid contents but devoid of peptidoglycan & N acetyle muramic acid. Perhaps it contains tetrapeptide linked matrix.
- **Staining & microscopy:**

A. Light microscopy:

- It identifies both the inclusion (HP) body & EB.
- EB also **called Miyagawa's granulocorpuscles.**
- *Chlamydia* are gram negative but better stained by

1. **Lugol's iodine:** Inclusion body of *C trachomatis* contains glycogen matrix, so stained with iodine & sensitive to sulphadiazine & cyclosporine. Inclusion body of *C psittaci* does not contain glycogen matrix, so not stained with iodine.
2. **Giemsa stain**
3. **Castaneda stain**
4. **Machiavello stain**
5. **Giminea stain**

B. Direct immuno fluorescent microscopy:

- By using monoclonal Ab
- Identify both inclusion body & EB in conjunctival / cervical / urethral specimens.
- More sensitive and specific.

➢ **Phases:** It is biphasic with two morphological forms as explained in **table-2.**

Features	Elementary Body (EB)	Reticulate Body (RB)
Synonym	Miyagawa granulocorpuscle	Initial body
Location	Extracellular	Intracellular
Size	200-300 nm	500-1000 nm
Shape	Spherical shape	Pleomorphic
Projection	Few	More
Function	Infective	Reproductive by binary fission
Metabolic activity	Inactive	Active
RNA:DNA ratio	1:1	3:1
Cell wall	Trilaminar & rigid cell wall like GNB	Fragile & pliable
Trypsin digestion	Resistant	Sensitive

Table-2: Morphological forms of Chlamydiales

➢ **Inclusion body: →Table-3**

Features	HP body	LCL Body
Full form	Halberstaedter - Prowazek body	Levinthal Cole Lillie body
Agent	*C. trachomatis*	*C. psittaci*
Nature	Compact	Vacuolated
Contain	Glycogen matrix	No glycogen matrix
Iodine stain	Yes	No
Sensitive	To sulphadiazine & cyclosporine	Only to cyclosporine
Habitat	Eye, genital organs	Respiratory system
Maturity time	In 72-96 hrs	In 48 hrs
Released from host cell	Released with scaring of host cell	Released with lysis of host cell

Table-3: Differences between HP & LCL body

❖ **Cultural characteristics (C/Cs):** Not grow in artificially prepared nutritional media or cell free media. Cultivation is done by using following methods.

➢ **Culture in animal:**

- **Animal used is:** Mouse
- **Growth:**
  - Only LGV biovar (L1, L2 & L3) infect the mouse by intracerebral route not the TRIC biovar.
  - TRIC biovar can kill the animal if introduced by intravenous route due to toxic effects.
  - Growth is detected by detecting the elementary body.
- **Disadvantages:**
  - Only historical value, no longer in use.
  - Reactions are variable by different species.

➢ **Culture in eggs:**

- **History:** This technique was developed by Tang & colleagues in 1957.
- **Pre-treatment of egg:**
  - It is required to avoid the contamination.
  - It is done with pre-treatment of egg culture with streptomycin or with polymyxin B.
- **Growth:**
  - It grows in yolk sac of 6-8 days old chick embryo.
  - Egg is incubated at 35^{0}C in a humid atmosphere. Blind passage may be necessary for isolation.
  - Growth is detected by identifying the group specific complement fixing antigen, elementary & inclusion bodies.
- **Disadvantage:** Less sensitive, time consuming & cumbersome.

➢ **Culture in cells/tissues:**

- **Cells used are:** McCoy cells, Hela cells, BHK-21 & Afrcian green monkey kidney cells (Vero cells). Cells are non-replicating (stationary phase).
- **Pre-treatment of cell culture:**
  - It is required to enhance the chlamydial replication & to increase the detection of inclusion bodies.
  - It is done with pre-treatment of cell culture with irradiation or cycloheximide or 5-iodo-2-deoxyuridine or with diethyaminoethanol (DEAE) dextran.
- **Incubation:** Culture is incubated under 10% CO2 for 48-72 hours. Shorter for *C. trachomatis* & longer for others.
- **Growth:**
  - LGV biovar is more infective than TRIC biovar.
  - Growth is enhanced by centrifugation of cells after inoculation which promotes the contact between the cell monolayer & chlamydial particles.
  - Growth is identified by detecting the inclusion bodies.
- **Advantage:** Highly specific but less sensitive (90%). Tissue culture was considered as gold standard but less sensitive (than molecular tests) which is replaced by molecular tests (vide infra) which are highly sensitive & specific & now considered as gold standard.
- **Disadvantages:**
  - Risk of laboratory infection/contamination.
  - Time consuming.
  - Labour intensive.
  - Required expertise & technically demanding.

❖ **Pathogenicity, diagnosis, prevention & treatment:**

➢ **Precipitating factors (epidemiological determinants):**

I. Agent factors (virulence factors)

a. **LPS:** During intracellular multiplication LPS accumulate on host cell surface induce inflammatory & immunological response which is responsible for production of disease.
b. **Host cell destruction:** When inclusion body gets mature, host cell is not able to hold the weight & finally gets rupture to release the EB.
c. **Intracellular location:** Escape the host defence & effects of antibiotics.
d. **MOMP:** It may help in attachment with host cells.

II. Host factors

a. Poor hygiene & lack of education about transmission of infection.

➢ **Diseases name:** *Chlamydia* produce following diseases.

I. **Trachoma**
II. **Inclusion conjunctivitis (IC)**
III. **Genital Chlamydiasis (GC)** } **Genital Infections (GI)**
IV. **Lympho Granuloma Venereum (LGV)** } **Genital Infections (GI)**

I. Trachoma

- **Meaning:** Name is given from **trakhus (Greek) = rough,** because of roughness of conjunctiva in disease.
- **Definition:** It is a chronic kerato-conjunctivitis characterized by
  - Follicular hypertrophy.
  - Papillary hyperplasia.
  - Pannus formation.
  - Cicatrisation.
- **Synonym:** Also **called Egyptian ophthamia** or **blinding trachoma** or **endemic blinding trachoma** or **endemic trachoma** or **granular conjunctivitis.**
- **Cause:** By serovars/serotypes A, B, Ba & C of *C. trachomatis.*
- **Distribution:** Distributed worldwide & 500 million people estimated to be affected. Endemic in Middle East, Africa, India & the Far East.
- **Reservoir of infection:** Human case.
- **Source of infection:** Conjunctival discharge is the main source of infection; therefore the secondary bacterial infection which increases the discharge is helpful for its transmission.
- **Mode of transmission:** Infection transmitted from eye-to-eye by

1. **Direct contact:** Direct contact with dust (air borne) or infected water.
2. **Fingers/fomites borne:**
   - Contact with contaminated fingers of patients, doctors, nurses etc.
   - Contact with infected tonometer.
   - Contact with common towel, handkerchief, bedding & surma-rods.
3. **Vector borne:** Mechanical transmission by flies.

- **Incubation period:** Variable about 5-12 days & influenced by the dose of infection.
- **Portal of entry:** Conjunctiva.
- **Sites:** Conjunctiva & cornea.
- **Predisposing factors:**

1. **Age:** Common in infant & in early childhood otherwise no age bar.
2. **Sex:** More in female in numbers & in severity.
3. **Race:** No race bar but common in Jews & less in Negros.
4. **Climate:** Common in dry & dusty weather.
5. **Occupation:** Dust, smoke & sunlight are increasing the risk therefore it is common in outdoor workers.
6. **Socioeconomic status:** Common in developing countries due to
   - Poor hygiene.
   - Overcrowding.
   - Abundantly flies population.
   - Common sharing of towel, handkerchief, bedding & surma-rods.
   - Lacks of education especially about spread of disease.

- **Pathology:** Following two phases

A. **Active trachoma:** Insidious (subacute / gradual but with harmful effect) onset.

i. **Conjunctival pathology:** → **Fig.-2**

a. **Congestion:**

b. **Follicles:**

- **Macroscopic:**
  - Looks like boiled sago grains.
  - Present on upper palpebral (tarsal) conjunctiva but may be present on upper & lower fornix. Sometimes also in bulbar (ocular) conjunctiva.
- **Microscopic:**
  - Centrally: Contains mononuclear histiocytes, multinucleated cells **called Leber cells** & few lymphocytes.
  - Peripherally: Contains lymphocytes & blood vessels.

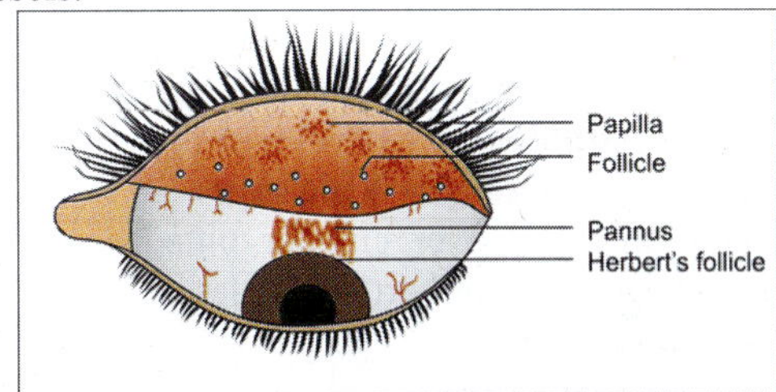

Figure-2: Pathology of trachoma

c. **Necrosis:**
- Present in later stage.
- Necrosis & Leber cells help to differentiate the trachoma from other forms of follicular conjunctivitis.

d. **Papillary hyperplasia:**
- It contains blood vessels centrally surrounded by lymphocytes.
- It is a raised area which gives red appearance to conjunctiva.

ii. **Corneal pathology:** → **Fig.-3**

a. **Superficial keratitis**

b. **Herbert's follicles:** Histologically similar to conjunctival follicles.

c. **Pannus formation:**

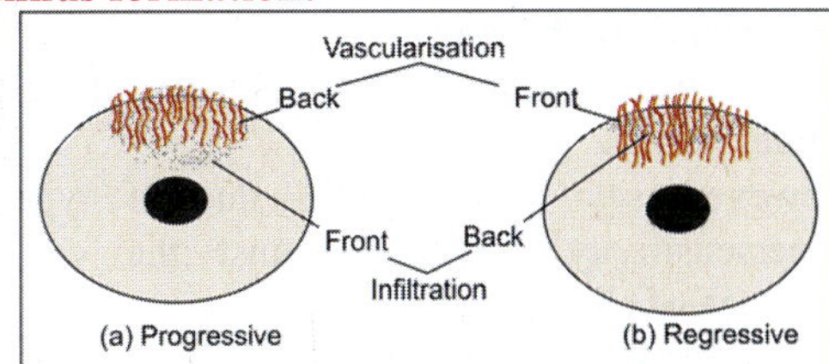

Figure-3: Pannus formation

- **Definition:** Central blood vessels surrounded by lymphocytes **called pannus formation.**
- **Types:** It has two types like progressive & regressive.

1. **Progressive:** → **Fig.3(a)**

- Cellular infiltration is ahead to vascularisation.
- Present in active trachoma.

2. **Regressive: → Fig.3(b)**

- Vascularisation is ahead to cellular infiltration.
- Present in cicatricial trachoma.

d. **Corneal ulcer:**

- Present at the advancing edge of pannus.
- It is chronic in nature which may become chronic or indolent.

B. **Cicatricial trachoma:**

i. **Conjunctival pathology:**

a. **Scaring:**

- Shape: Irregular, star shaped or linear.
- Site: Linear scar present in the sulcus subtarsalis **called Arlt's line.**

b. **Concretion:**

- Mechanisms of formation: It is not a calcification but formed due to accumulation of dead epithelial cells with mucus deposition **called gland of Henle.**
- Size: Pin point to 2mm.

c. **Others:** It includes pseudocyst & symblepharon.

ii. **Corneal pathology:**

a. **Regressive pannus: → Vide supra**

b. **Herbal pits:** Oval or circular pitted scar formed due to healing of Herbert's follicles.

c. **Corneal opacity:**

d. **Total corneal pannus:**

iii. **Lid pathology:** It includes

- Trichiasis: Rubbing of eyeball by eyelashes.
- Tylosis: Thickening of lid margin.
- Ptosis: Droping of eye lid.
- Madarosis: Loss of eyelashes.
- Ankyloblepharon: Fusion of part or all the margin of eyelids.
- Entropion: Inward folding of eyelids usually lower lids.

iv. **Lacrimal apparatus pathology:** It includes

- Chronic dacryocystitis.
- Chronic dacryoadenitis.

✪ **Pathogenesis:**

A **Active trachoma:** Subacute inflammatory response with congestion, follicles, hyperplasia & pannus formation.

B **Cicatricial trachoma:**

- Scar formation is due to continued mild chronic inflammation.
- However, scar formation is due to type –IV hypersensitivity reaction against the continued presence of chlamydial antigen.

✪ **Clinical features of trachoma:**

A. **Active trachoma:** Symptoms depend on presence or absence of secondary bacterial infections.

i. **Without secondary infection:** It includes

- Mild foreign body sensation.
- Lacrimation.
- Slight stickiness of lids.
- Scanty mucoid discharge.
- Redness of eye.

ii. **With secondary infection:** It includes

- High mucopurulent discharge.
- Stickiness of eye lids.

B. **Cicatricial trachoma:**

- Conjunctival & corneal xerosis.
- Blindness (blinding trachoma).

✪ **Grading of trachoma:**

A. **McCallan classification:** McCallan classify the trachoma in following four stages in 1908.

i. **Stage-1 (Infiltration or incipient trachoma:** Hyperaemia of conjunctiva, immature follicle & highest infectivity is present.

ii. **Stage-2 (Florid infiltration or established trachoma):** Mature follicle, papillae & progressive corneal pannus.

iii. **Stage-3 (Scaring or cicatrising trachoma):** Scar formation in palpebral conjunctiva.

iv. **Stage-4 (Stage of sequelae or healed trachoma):** Features due to cicatrisation. This stage is non-infectious.

B. **WHO classification:** WHO classify the trachoma in following five stages in 1987.

i. **TF (Trachomatous inflammation - follicular):** Follicles are present& minimum 5 follicles are required to diagnose this stage with size of ≥ 0.5 mm.

ii. **TI: (Trachomatous inflammation - intense):** Inflammatory thickening of upper tarsal conjunctiva which obscures more than half of the normal deep tarsal vessels.

iii. **TS: (Trachomatous scaring):** White scar formation in palpebral (tarsal) conjunctiva.

iv. **TT: (Trachomatous trichiasis):** At least one eye lash rubbing the eyeball

v. **CO: (Corneal Opacity):** Easily visible opacity present over pupil & cause significant visual loss (less than 6/18).

✪ **Diagnosis of trachoma:** Conjunctival scraping / swab is the sample tested by microscopy & culture methods as described earlier in the section of morphology & C/C s respectively.

✪ **Prevention of trachoma:**

- Improvement in hand hygiene & health education about transmission of trachoma.
- Control of flies.

✪ **Treatment of trachoma:** Local & oral administration of antibiotics is advised for trachoma.

- Doxycycline is the drug of choice.
- Erythromycin is the drug of choice for pregnant women.
- Single dose of azithromycin can gives good effect.

II. Inclusion conjunctivitis (IC)

- **Cause:** By serovars/serotypes D, E, F, G, H, I, J & K.
- **Sub-Types:** Two subtypes as follows.

a. In new born: Called inclusion blenorrhoea.

- **Synonym:** Ophthalmia neonatorum.
- **Mode of transmission:** From the infected birth canal to the new born.
- **Incubation period:** 5-12 days after birth.
- **Clinical features:**
  - Benign & self limited.
  - Micro-pannus.
  - Conjunctival scar.
  - Chances of recurrences.
- **Complication:** Infantile pneumonia at 4-16 weeks of age & present with cough, wheezing & fever.
- **Diagnosis:** Same as trachoma.
- **Prevention:** Control of mother's infection.
- **Treatment:** Azithromycin is effective.

b. In adult: Called swimming pool conjunctivitis.

- **Synonym:** Adult inclusion conjunctivitis.
- **Mode of transmission:** By contact with contaminated swimming pool water from genital secretion of others/self.
- **Clinical features:** Follicular hypertrophy & muco-purulent discharge.
- **Diagnosis:** Same as trachoma.
- **Prevention:** Avoiding contact with contaminated swimming pool water.
- **Treatment:** Tetracycline or azithromycin may be given orally.

III. Genital Chlamydiasis (GC)

- **Cause:** By serovars/serotypes D, E, F, G, H, I, J & K.
- **Mode of transmission:** Sexual intercourse.
- **Clinical features:** Mostly asymptomatic but may manifest as follows.

o <u>In Women</u>:
- Acute urethral syndrome
- Bartholinitis
- Endometritis
- Salpingitis
- Pelvic Inflammatory Disease (PID)
- Reiter's syndrome (cervictis, conjunctivitis, arthritis)
- Fitz –Hugh Curtis syndrome (Peritonitis & Perihepatic inflammation)

o <u>In Men</u>:
- Non Gonococcal Urethritis (NGU)/ Non specific urethritis
- Epididymitis
- Proctitis
  Reiter's syndrome (urethritis, conjunctivitis, arthritis)

- **Complications:**
  - Infertility,
    Abortion
  - Ectopic pregnancy
  - Premature delivery
  - Antenatal morbidity
  - Puerperal sepsis
  - Post partum fever
  - Low birth weight of infant
  - Chorioamnionitis
- **Diagnosis:**

o <u>Specimens:</u>
- Urethral mucosa scraping / swab
- Cervical mucosa scraping / swab
- Vaginal mucosa scraping / swab
- Anal mucosa scraping / swab
- Urine

o <u>Testing methods:</u>

A Microscopy: → Follow morphology

B Culture: → Follow C/Cs

C Serological tests:

- **Methods:**

i. Detection of antigens:

1. Micro IF
2. ELISA

ii. Detection of antibodies:

1. CFT (group specific)
2. Micro IF (type specific)
3. ELISA also useful

- **Disadvantages of serological methods**: Not useful in non-invasive condition like trachoma & IC.

D Molecular methods:

- **Indications:**
  - To diagnose the case.
  - To diagnose the asymptomatic carrier.
  - To separate the biovar & serovars.
- **Advantages:**
  - Highly sensitive & specific method, replace the gold standard method like cell culture.
  - It is rapid tes.
- **Disadvantages:**
  - Expensive.
  - Required expertise & technically demanding.
- **Tests:**

1. DNA probe
2. PCR
3. LCR
4. Transcription mediated amplification
5. Strand displacement assay

- **Prevention:** Safe sex.
- **Treatment:** Tetracycline is effective.

IV. Lympho Granuloma Venereum (LGV)

- **Synonyms:** Lympho granuloma inguinale, poradenitis, climatic bubo & tropical bubo.
- **Cause:** By serovars/serotypes L1, L2 & L3.

- **Mode of transmission:** Sexual intercourse.
- **Incubation period:** 3 days -5 weeks.
- **Clinical features:** Three stage of disease.

1. **Primary stage:** Painless papulo-vesicular (ulcerative) lesion on extra-genital sites.
2. **Secondary stage:**
   - Suppurative enlargement of inguinal lymph nodes in male & intrapelvic-pararectal lymph nodes in female. Secondary stage (lymphadenopathy) lesion is bilateral & tender while primary stage (papulo-vesicular) lesion is painless.
   - It breakdown to form pus discharging sinus.
3. **Tertiary stage:**
   - Scaring due to healing of sinus.
   - Lymphatic blockage.

- **Complications:**
  - Infection spread to eyes, joints & meninges.
  - In female it leads to rectal stricture. It also causes the elephantiasis of vulva **called genital eliphantiasis** or **esthiomene.**

✓ **Note: Other cause of genital eliphantiasis**

- Filariasis [*W bancrofti* (more) & *B malayi* (less)]
- Donovanosis (*K granulomatis*): Actually causing pseudoeliphantiasis (labial swelling)

- **Diagnosis:**

A **Microscopy:** → **Follow morphology**
B **Culture:** → **Follow C/Cs**
C **Serological tests:** Same as GC.
D **Molecular methods:** Same as GC.
E **Allergic test:** → **Frei's test:**

- **Principle:** Based on delayed type of hypersensitivity.
- **Indication:** For LGV.
- **Antigen:** Originally prepared from bubo pus & later from mouse brain or yolk sac culture **called lygranum.**
- **Method:**
  - Antigen introduced intradermally in one forearm & other arm as control.
  - Observe for the reaction.
- **Result:** Induration of ≥ 7 mm in 2-5 days indicates +Ve reaction.
- **Disadvantages:**
  - Not useful in non-invasive conditions like trachoma & IC.
  - False +Ve results are very frequent.

- **Prevention:** Safe sex.
- **Treatment:** Tetracycline for three weeks.

Chlamydia psittaci

❖ **Meaning:** Psittaci word derived from **psittcos = parrot**, because disease transmitted from parrot to human.

❖ **Synonyms:** Ornothosis (**ornithos = birds**) when acquired by non-psittacine (non-parrot) bird.

❖ **Serovars:** → **Flow chart-1**

❖ **Morphology:**

- Produce the inclusion body **called LCL body** in 24 hours.
- More details: Follow **table-2, figure-1, flow chart-2 & table-3**.

❖ **Cultural characteristics (C/Cs):** Not grow in artificially prepared nutritional media/cell free media. Cultivation is done by using following methods

A. **Animal inoculation:**
- **Animal used is:** Mouse.
- **Growth:** It infects the animal by intracerebral, intranasal, intraperitoneal & subcutaneous routes.

B. **Eggs inoculation:** It grows in yolk sac of old chick embryo.

C. **Tissue culture:** Grow well in cell culture media but because of risk of laboratory infection cell culture should not be attempted.

❖ **Pathogenicity:**

- **Disease name:** Disease **called psittacosis** if acquired from parrot or **called ornithosis** if acquired from non-psittacine bird (bird other than parrot)
- **Reservoir of infection:** Bird like parrot.
- **Source of infection:** Bird excreta & droppings or nasal discharge & aerosols from human case.
- **Mode of transmission:**
  - Inhalation of particle from bird excreta.
  - Parrot (bird) bites.
  - Case to case transmission may occur as *Chlamydia* may sheds in nasal discharge, droppings & aerosols from the patients.
- **Incubation period:** 10 days.
- **Portal of entry:** Respiratory tract.
- **Sites:** Respiratory system, GIT etc.
- **Precipitating factors:**

a. **Occupational:**
1. **Laboratory workers:** High frequency in laboratory workers.
2. **Other workers:** It is common in poultry workers, pigeon farmers, pet shop owner, bird fanciers, veterinarians etc.

b. **Overcrowding**
c. **Caging:**
d. **Type of strain:** Strains from the parrots & turkeys are more virulent than other sources.

- **Clinical features:** Mild influenza like symptoms including diarrhoea, mucopurulent discharge & emaciation to fatal pneumonia.
- **Complications:**
  - Septicemia.
  - Meningoencephalitis.

- Endocarditis.
- Pericarditis.
- Arthritis.
- Typhoid like syndrome.

❖ Laboratory diagnosis:

➢ **Specimens:**
- Blood.
- Sputum.
- Lung tissues cells like PAMs (Pulmonary Alveolar Macrophages).

➢ **Testing methods:**

I. Microscopy:

A. Light microscopy:
- Useful to detect the LCL body.
- Chlamydia are gram negative but better stained by

1. Giemsa
2. Castancda
3. Machiavello
4. Giminea stains
5. Lugol's iodine: LCL body is devoid of glycogen matrix so not stained with **Lugol's iodine** & only sensitive to cyclosporine but not to sulphadiazine.

B. Immuno Flourescent microscopy: Is also useful.

II. Culture: → **Follow C/Cs**

III. Serological tests: Like CFT (group specific) & micro IF (type specific).

Chlamydia pneumoniae

❖ **History:** It was 1st reported by Grayston et al. in 1986 from the adult patient with acute respiratory disease in Taiwan & **called TWAR strain** (from Taiwan) of *C psittaci* due to sharing of common group specific antigen but later identified as separate species by
- Species specific antigen.
- DNA hybridisation.
- REA.
- Ability to grow in cell culture.
- Only human source availability without availability of animal or avian sources.

❖ **Cultural characteristics (C/Cs):** Grow very poorly in cell culture. Can be isolated by using HEP-2 or human fibroblast cell lines.

❖ Pathogenicity:

➢ **Mode of transmission:** Human to human infection by inhalation.

➢ **Incubation period:** 1-3 weeks.

➢ **Portal of entry:** Respiratory tract.

➢ **Sites:** Respiratory system, sinuses etc.

➢ **Precipitating factors:**

1. **Overcrowding**
2. **Age:** Common in young children.

➢ **Clinical features:**

1. **Respiratory system:**
   - Primary atypical pneumonia (walking pneumonia) like *M. pneumonia.*
   - Sinusitis.
   - Pharyngitis & bronchitis.
   - Adult onset of asthma.
2. **CVS system:** Associated with atherosclerosis of coronary, carotid & cerebral arteries.

❖ Laboratory diagnosis:

➢ **Specimens:**
- Blood.
- Sputum.

➢ **Testing methods:**

I. Cultural: Grow very poorly, so not useful.

II. Serological test:
1. CFT.
2. ELISA.
3. Micro IF.

III. Molecular:
1. DNA hybridization.
2. Restriction endonuclease analysis.

❖ **Treatment:** Azithromycin or clarithromycin are the effective drugs.

Question bank

Case study

1) A 5 year children visited the eye clinic with mucopurulent discharge & redness of eye. Clinical examination of eye shows the follicle in conjunctive. Conjunctival scraping revealed inclusion body stained with iodine. Identify the organism & answer the following
   a) Name the causative agent & describe the morphology & life cycle of causative agent
   b) Write the pathogenicity causative agent
   c) Write the laboratory diagnosis of causative agent

2) A 25 year old man present in STD clinic with painless ulcer on extra-genitals. On physical examination bilateral tender inguinal lymphadenopathy was noticed.. Identify the organism & answer the following
   a) Name the clinical disease & causative agent
   b) Describe the morphology & life cycle of causative agent
   c) Write the pathogenicity causative agent
   d) Write the laboratory diagnosis of causative agent

Essay/Full question

1) *C. trachomatis*

Short notes

1) Classification of Chlamydiales
2) Morphology & life cycle of *C. trachomatis*
3) Trachoma
4) Lympho Granuloma Venereum
5) Psitacosis
6) *C. pneumonuae*

Short questions for theory/viva questions

1) Write the differences between elementary body & reticulate body of *C. trachomatis.*

2) Write the differences between HP & LCL body.
3) Write the importance of Lugol's iodine in identification of *C. trachomatis & C. psittaci.*

MCQs for chapter review

Taxonomy

1) **Taxonomically Chlamydia is a -**
(a) Bacteria (b) Virus (c) Fungus (d) Nematode

Classification

2) **Which of the following has one serotype -**
(a) *C. psittaci* (b) *C. pneumoniae* (c) *C. trachomatis* (d) None

C. trachomatis

3) **The following statements are true regarding *Chlamydiae* except –** (AIIMS, May-05)
(a) Erythromycin is effective for therapy of chlamydial infections (b) Their cell wall lack a peptidoglycan layer (c) They can grow in cell free culture media (d) They are obligate intracellular bacteria
4) ***Chlamydiae trachomatis,* false is -** (AIIMS, Nov-06, AI-11)
(a) Elementary body is metabolically active (b) It is biphasic (c) Reticulate body divides by binary fission (d) Inside the host cell it evade phagolysosome
5) **All of the following are true about *Chlamydiae* except –**
(a) Gram positive (b) Causes trachoma (c) Causative organism of psittacosis (d) Are also called basophilic viruses
6) ***Chlamydiae trachomatis,* serovars D-K causes -** (AI-98)
(a) Arteriosclerosis (b) Trachoma (c) Lympho granuloma venereum (d) Urethritis
7) ***Chlamydiae* causes all the following disease except -** (AI-95)
(a) Non Gonococcal urethritis (b) Pneumonia (c) Trachoma (d) Parotitis
8) ***Chlamydiae trachomatis* is associated with the following except -** (AI-05)
(a) Endemic trachoma (b) Inclusion conjunctivitis (c) Lympho granuloma venereum (d) Community acquired pneumonia
9) ***Chlamydiae* causes-** (PGI, Dec-00)
(a) Infertility (b) Pneumothorax (c) Pelvic inflammatory disease (d) Congenital malformation in fetus
10) **The following is not a method of isolation of *Chlamydia* from clinical specimens-** (AIIMS, Nov-05)
(a) Yolk sac inoculation (b) Enzyme immune assay (c) Tissue culture using irradiated McCoy cells (d) Tissue culture using irradiated BHK cells
11) ***Chlamydiae* in asymptomatic carrier, the most sensitive test is -** (AIIMS, Nov-09)
(a) Tissue culture (b) Nucleic acid amplification test (c) Serology (d) Serum electrophoresis
12) **The most sensitive method for detecting cervical *Chlamydiae trachomatis* infection is-** (AI -04)
(a) Direct fluorescent antibody test (b) Enzyme immunoassay (c) Polymerase chain reaction (d) Culture on irradiated McCoy cells
13) **All of the following statements about *Chlamydiae trachomatis* are true except –** (AI-09)
(a) Genital chlamydial infection are often asymptomatic (b) Can be cultured (c) Inclusion conjunctivitis is caused by *Chlamydiae trachomatis,* serotypes D-K (d) Penicillin is the treatment of choice
14) **Frei's test is useful for diagnosis of-**
(a) *Mycoplasma* (b) *Rickettsia* (c) Sarcoidosis (d) *Chlamydia*
15) **Genital eliphantiasis is seen in –**
(a) *Rickettsia* (b) Chancroid (c) Lymph granuloma venereum (d) Syphilis
16) **Genital eliphantiasis is seen in –** (PGI-06)
(a) Donovanosis (b) Lymph granuloma venereum (c) Congenital syphilis (d) Herpes simplex

C psittaci

17) **Chlamydiae psittacosis, all are true except -** (AI-07)
(a) Acquired from bird's droppings (b) Causes urethritis (c) Causes pneumonia (d) Treatment is tetracycline
18) **Levinthal Cole Lillie bodies are seen in -** (AI-07)
(a) LGV (b) Psittacosis (c) Kala azar (d) Chicken pox

C pneumoniae

19) **Which of the following statement is true regarding *Chlamydiae pneumoniae* –** (AI -05)
(a) Fifteen serovars have been identified as human pathogen (b) Mode of transmission is by bird excreta (c) The cytoplasmic inclusion present in the sputum specimen are rich in glycogen (d) Group specific antigen is responsible for the production of complement fixing antibodies

Answers of MCQs & explanation

1) **(a)**
- Follow section, **taxonomy** for explanation

2) **(b)**
- Follow section, **classification** for explanation

3) **(c)**
- *Chlamydiae* can't grow in cell free culture media/artificially prepared nutritional media.
- For explanation of option a follow section **treatment**, for option b follow section **morphology** (cell wall) & for option d follow section **taxonomy**.

4) **(a)**
- For explanation of option a, b & c follow **morphology (phases & table-2)** & for option d follow section **life cycle**.

5) **(a)**
- *Chlamydiae* is gram negative, causes trachoma & psittacosis
- Option d: Follow section **synonyms** for explanation

6) **(d)**
- Serovar D-K causes genital chlamydiasis which is present with urethritis & with other manifestation as described earlier in text in the section pathogenicity
- Arteriosclerosis is caused by *C pneumoniae*
- Trachoma is caused by serovars A, B, Ba & C while Lympho granuloma venereum caused by serovars L1, L2 & L3 of *C trachomatis*

7) **(d)**
8) **(d)**
9) **(a) & (c)**

} Follow section, **pathogenicity of *C trachomatis, C psittaci & C pneumoniae*** for explanation

10) **(b)**
- Enzyme immune assay is the serological method used for detection of Ag or Ab not for isolation of bacteria

11) **(b)**
12) **(c)**

} Tissue culture was considered as gold standard but less sensitive (90%) which is replaced by molecular tests like nucleic acid amplification test, PCR, LCR etc. which are highly sensitive & specific & now considered as gold standard.

13) **(d)**
- Penicillin is not the treatment of choice & useful drugs for *Chlamydiae* are from tetracycline group or from macrolide group

14) **(d)**
- Frei's test is the allergic test done to diagnose the LGV caused by *Chlamydiae trachomatis* serovars L1, L2 & L3

15) **(c)**
16) **(a) & (b)**

} Follow section ***C trachomatis* [pathogenicity → Lympho Granuloma Venereum (LGV)]** for explanation

17) **(b)**
- Follow section ***C pneumoniae*** for explanation

18) **(b)**
- Follow **table-3** for explanation

19) **(d)**
- Follow **table-1** for explanation.

58 Rickettsiales, *Coxiella* and *Bartonella*

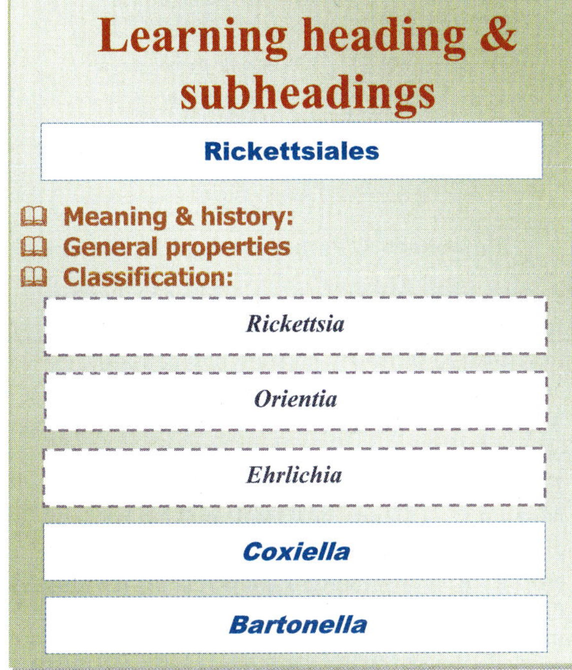

Learning heading & subheadings

Rickettsiales

- Meaning & history:
- General properties
- Classification:

Rickettsia

Orientia

Ehrlichia

Coxiella

Bartonella

Rickettsiales

Meaning & history:

- Order, family & genus named after **Howard Taylor Ricketts**, who discovered the spotted fever rickettsia in 1911 & died due to illness (typhus fever) acquired during his studies.
- Species *R. prowazekii* is named by Da Rocha Lima in honour of Von Prowazek.
- Charles Nicolle notices the role of lice in transmission of epidemic typhus.

General properties:

Obligate intracellular bacilli/coccobacilli, gram negative in nature, transmitted by arthropod.

Taxonomy:

- **Was considered as virus:** Because many features are similar to viruses like
1. Obligate intracellular.
2. Failure to grow in cell free media.
- **Now accepted as bacterium:** Because many features are similar to bacteria like
1. Both DNA & RNA.
2. Have a cell wall poorly stain with gram stain & mostly gram negative bacilli/coccobacilli in nature
3. Contains ribosomes.
4. Replicate by binary fission.
5. Sensitive to antibiotics.

Classification: →Flow chart-1

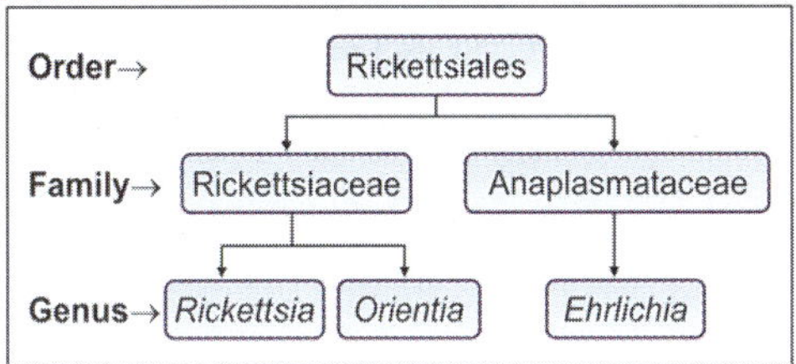

Flow chart-1: Classification of Rickettsiales

✓ **Note: Reasons for exclusion of *Coxiella* & *Bartonella* from Rickettsiales**

- ***Coxiella***: It is excluded from order Rickettsiales because not the arthropod borne.
- ***Bartonella***: It is excluded from order Rickettsiales because not the obligate intracellular, can grow in cell free media & differ in genetic properties.

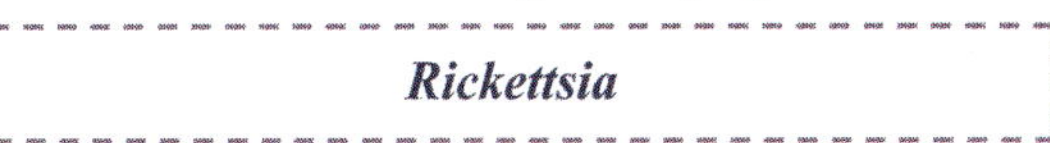

Rickettsia

Morphology:

- **Staining properties:** It is Gram negative. Stains bluish purple with Giemsa & Castaneda stains & red with Gimenez & Machiavello stains.
- **Size:** 0.3-0.6 µm x 0.8-2 µm in size.
- **Shape:** Pleomorphic coccobacilli.
- **Motility:** Nonmotile.
- **Capsule:** Non capsulated.
- **Layers:** Under electron microscope three layers are seen like outer slime layer, cell wall & inner plasma membrane.

Cultural characteristics (C/Cs):

➢ **Effective factors:**
- No growth in cell-free media (obligate intracellular).
- Optimum temperature: 32-35^{0}C.
- Growth occurs in the cytoplasm (typhus group) of infected cells, in nucleus & cytoplasm (spotted fever group) or in cytoplasmic vacuole (*Coxiella*).

➢ **Culture in animals:**
- Guinea pigs & mice are useful animal.
- When male guinea pigs are inoculated intraperitoneally with *R. typhi*, it develop fever, scrotal enlargement, inflammatory adhesions between the layers of the tunica vaginalis & testis cannot be pushed back into the abdomen **called tunica reaction or Neill-Mooser reaction.**

➢ **Culture in eggs:**
- Grow in the yolk sac of chick embryos.
- This technique was discovered by Cox.

➢ **Culture in cells:**
- Rickettsia can grow in detroit 6, HeLa, HEP-2, mouse fibroblast & other continuous cell lines.
- Not a satisfactory method.

❖ Resistance:
- Destroyed by heat at 56^{0}C & at room temperature.
- It is preserved in skimmed milk or in SPG (Sucrose Potassium Phosphate & Glutamate) medium.

❖ Antigenic structure:

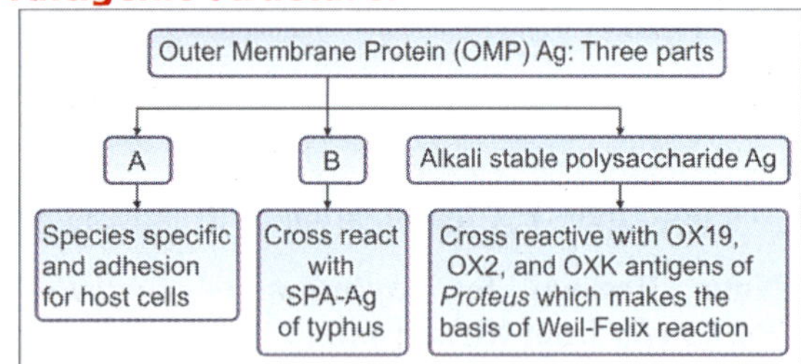

Flow chart-2: Antigens of spotted fever group

1. **Typhus fever group:**
- It contains Surface Protein Antigen (SPA)
- It is species specific & cross react with B-antigen of spotted fever group.

2. **Spotted fever group:** OMP-Ag as shown in **flow chart-2.**

❖ Pathogenicity:
➢ **Pathogenesis: → Flow chart-3**

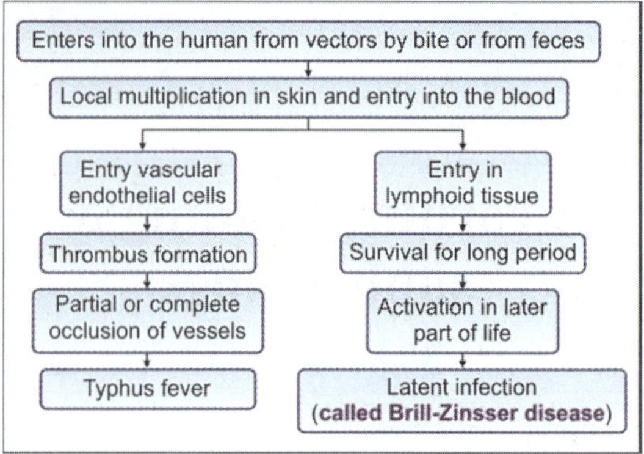

Flow chart-3: Pathogenesis of *Rickettsia*

➢ **Pathological types:** Two types like **(A) Typhus fever group** & **(B) Spotted fever group** are described in **table-1** with subtypes, causative agents, vector & reservoir.

A. **Typhus fever group:** Bacteria present in cytoplasm with following subtypes.

i. **Epidemic typhus:**

➢ **Meaning:** Typhus = cloud/smoke, because of cloudy state of consciousness.

➢ **Synonym:** Louse-borne typhus, classical typhus & Gaol fever.

✪ **Etiological agent:** *R. prowazekii*

✪ **Mode of transmission:**
1. By bite of head louse *Pediculus humanus corporis.*
2. By rubbing the faeces of louse against abraded skin produced during scratching.
3. Inhalation of aerosol from dried louse faeces.
4. Instillation in conjunctiva.

Diseases	Species of *Rickettsia*	Insect vector	Reservoir
A. Typhus fever group: In cytoplasm			
Epidemic typhus (Mnemonic: pp)	*R. prowazekii*	Head louse	Human
Recrudescent / latent typhus (Brill Zinsser disease)	*R. prowazekii*	Head louse	Human
Endemic typhus (murine typhus/flea borne typhus)	*R. typhi (R. mooseri)*	Rat flea	Rodents
	R. felis (feline rickettsiae)	Cat flea	Cat
B. Spotted fever group: In nucleus & in cytoplasm			
Indian / South African / Kenyan - tick typhus **Mediterranean / Israeli / Astrakhan -spotted fever** **Boutonneuse fever**	*R. conorii*	Tick	Rodent
Rocky mountain spotted fever	*R. rickettsii*	Tick	Rodents, Dogs
Siberian tick typhus	*R. siberica*	Tick	Cattle
Sub Saharan African tick typhus	*R. africae*	Tick	?
Queensland tick typhus	*R. australis*	Tick	Bush rodent
Oriental spotted fever	*R. japonica*	Tick	?
Rickettsial pox	*R. akari*	Mite	Mice

Table-1: Pathological types of *Rickettsia*

✪ **Incubation period:** 5-15 days

✪ **Clinical features:** Disease start with chills & fever. Rash appears on the 4th -5th day on the trunk and spreading over the limbs but sparing face, palms and soles. Patient progress to stupurous & delirium.

➢ **Complication:** Death in 40% cases

ii. **Brill Zinsser disease:**

➢ **Meaning: Brill** identified typhus like disease in New York, in Jewish immigrants from Europe. **Zinsser** identified the bacilli from such case & proved that it was a recrudescences of infection acquired before many years

➢ **Synonym:** Latent typhus, Recrudescent typhus

➢ **Etiological agent:** *R. prowazekii*

➢ **Clinical feature:**

- In patient who recover from epidemic typhus , bacteria remain latent in lymphatic tissue or organs for years
- Such latent bacteria become reactivated and lead to recrudescent typhus
- Milder disease, duration of disease is shorter, case fatality is lower.

iii. **Endemic typhus:**

✪ **Synonym:** Flea borne typhus or murine typhus

✪ **Etiological agents:**

- *R. typhi* (*R. mooseri*): Transmitted by the rat flea *xenopsylla cheopis*
- *R. felis:* Transmitted by the cat flea *Ctenocephalus felis*

✪ **Mode of transmission:**

1. By bite of rat/cat flea
2. By rubbing the faeces of flea against abraded skin, produced during scratching
3. Inhalation of aerosol from dried faeces of flea
4. Ingestion of food contaminated by excreta of rat or cat flea

B. **Spotted fever group:** Bacteria present in nucleus & in cytoplasm with following subtypes

i. **Indian / South African / Kenyan - tick typhus or Mediterranean / Israeli / Astrakhan - spotted fever or Boutonneuse fever:** *R.conori*

ii. **Rocky Mountain spotted fever:** *R. rickettsii.* Lungs are infected in 7-16% cases.

iii. **Siberian tick typhus:** *R. siberica*

iv. **Sub Saharan African tick typhus:** *R. africae*

v. **Queensland tick typhus:** *R. australis*

vi. **Oriental spotted fever:** *R. japonica*

✪ **Mode of transmission:** All above diseases are transmitted by tick bite like *dermacentor andersoni* & by some other ticks like *Rhipicephalus sanguinens, Haemaphysalis leachi, Amblyoma* & *Hyalomma.* Transovarial transmission of *Rickettsia* is present in ticks & mites but not in louse & fleas.

vii. **Rickettsial pox:**

✪ **Meaning:** Because resembles to chickenpox

✪ **Synonym:** Vesicular or varicelliform rickettsiosis

✪ **Etiological agent:** The causative agent is *R. akari* (from akari meaning mite).

✪ **Mode of transmission:** By bite of mite *Liponyssoides sanguineus*

✪ **Clinical features:** Self limited-neonatal-vesicular exanthema like chickenpox

❖ **Laboratory diagnosis of *Rickettsia*:** Very dangerous pathogen to work in laboratory.

➢ **Specimens:** Blood.

➢ **Testing methods: → Flow chart-4**

a. **Culture: Follow culture characteristics**

b. **Molecular:** PCR

c. **Serological tests:**

1. Weil-Felix reaction: More details, **Follow chapter → Antigen-Antibody (Ag-Ab) reactions**
2. Others tests are CFT, agglutination of rickcttsial suspensions, passive haemagglutination test, toxin neutralization test, immunofluorescence, radioisotope precipitation & radio immuno assay.

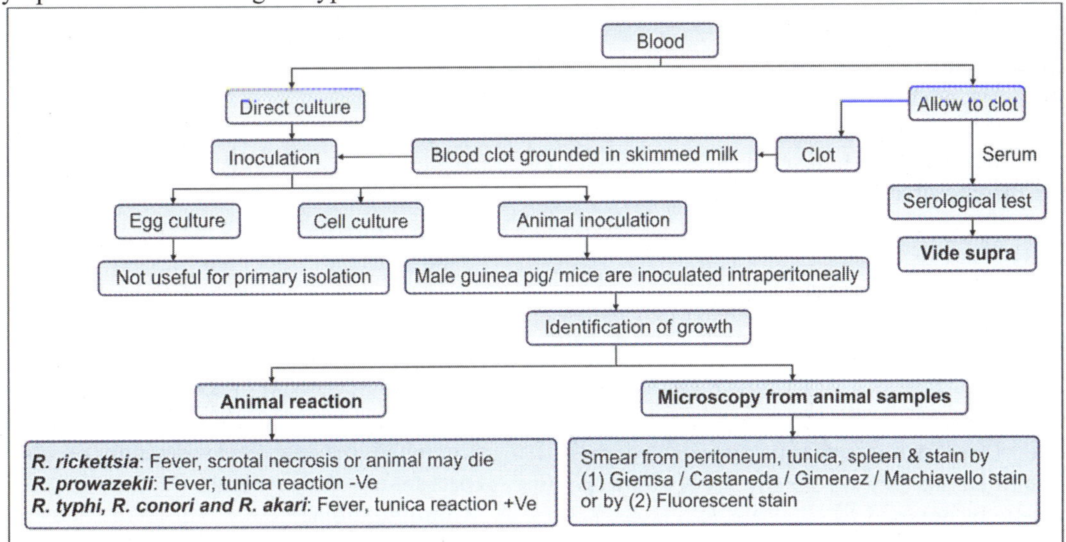

Flow chart-4: Laboratory diagnosis of *Rickettsia*

❖ **Prevention of *Rickettsia*:**

A. **General measures:**

- Control of vectors & animal reservoirs.
- Sterilisation of contaminated cloths, beds, pillows of infected persons.
- Wearing of protective cloths before entering in endemic area.

B. **Immunoprophylaxis:** Different type killed & live vaccines are developed for epidemic typhus, but none of them is satisfactory.

i. **Killed vaccines:**

1. **Weigl's vaccine:** Inactivated by phenol & prepared from intestinal contents of lice infected per rectum by *R. prowazekii*. Mass production is a problem with this vaccine.
2. **Mouse lung vaccine:** Formalin inactivated & produced by Castaneda.
3. **Yolk sac vaccine:** Developed by Cox & effective.

ii. **Live vaccines:**

- Prepared from the attenuated strain.
- Highly immunogenic.
- Also prepared against Rocky Mountain spotted fever.
- Develop mild disease after administration.

❖ **Treatment:** Tetracycline, chloramphenicol or ciprofloxacin are the drug of choice.

Orientia

❖ **Species:** *Orientia tsutsugamushi*

❖ **Meaning:** Tsutsuga = dangerous & Mushi = insect or mite borne.

❖ **Synonym:** Formerly it was know with names like *R. tsutsugamushi* or *R. orientalis* .

❖ **History:** It was 1st observed in Japan, where it was found to be transmitted by mites.

❖ **Morphology:**

- ➢ **Staining properties:** Gram negative but better stained with Gimenez stain.
- ➢ **Size:** 0.6μm x 1.2-3.0 μm in size.
- ➢ **Shape:** Pleomorphic coccobacilli.
- ➢ **Motility:** Nonmotile.
- ➢ **Capsule:** Non capsulated.

❖ **Cultural characteristics (C/Cs):** Unable to grow in cell-free media & can grow only in cell monolayers.

❖ **Classification:** *Orientia* are antigenically variable. Three major antigenic types (serotypes) are identified as follows. Many more serotypes continue to be reported.

1. **Karp:** It accounts 50% of all infections.
2. **Gilliam:** It accounts 25% of all infections.
3. **Kato:** It accounts less than10% of all infections.
4. **Kawasaki:**

❖ **Pathogenicity:**

➢ **Disease name:** Disease **called scrub typhus** because originally it found in scrub jungle.

➢ **Synonym:**

- Also **called chigger borne typhus** as transmitted by Mite's larva **called chigger** (only stage fed on the host). Chiggers feed on serum of warm blooded animals while adult mites fed on plants.
- Also **called Japanese river disease.**

➢ **Nature & history of disease:** It occurs all along East Asia, from Korea to Indonesia & in the pacific Islands including Australia.

➢ **Reservoir of infection:** Rodents & birds.

➢ **Source of infection:** Mites. It transmitted transovarially in mites.

➢ **Mode of transmission:**

- **Vector:**
  - It is transmitted by bite of trombiculoid mite's larvae **called chigger** (hence disease **called chigger borne typhus**).
  - Mite inhabits in sharply demarcated area in soil **called mite islands.**
  - When human visit such **mite islands** it enters by the bite of mite's larva.
- **Species:**
  - In India: *Leptotrombidium deliensis.*
  - In Japan: *Leptotrombidium akamushi.*

➢ **Incubation period:** 1-3 weeks.

➢ **Portal of entry:** Skin.

✪ **Sites:** Skin, lymph nodes, lungs, meninges etc.

✪ **Precipitating factors (epidemiological determinants):**

1. **Zoonotic tetrad:** Four factors are essential for development of disease like *Orientia tsutsugamushi*, chiggers, rats & secondary or transitional form of vegetation **called zoonotic tetrad.**
2. **Occupation:** It is a serious problem in military persons especially during jungle warfare. It was recognised in Indo-Burmese theatre in the 2nd World war.
3. **Environmental:** It is common in scrub jungle, sandy beaches, mountain deserts & equatorial rain forests where plenty of moisture & scrub vegetations are available.

➢ **Clinical features:** Eschar (present in < 50% of western) at the site of vector's bite, maculopapular rash, regional lymphadenopathy, fever, headache, conjunctivitis etc. Rash develop on 4-6 days & present in < 40% patients.

➢ **Complications:**

- Pneumonia & encephalitis.

- Case fatality rate is 7% in untreated cases.

❖ **Laboratory diagnosis:** Weil-Felix positive with OX-K antigen.

❖ **Prevention:**

A. **General measures:** Organism is highly virulent & should be handled in laboratory with bio safety level-3.

B. **Immunoprophylaxis:** Because of constant antigenic variation it is very difficult to develop the protective vaccine & vaccine developed for one locality may not be effective for other locality.

❖ **Treatment:**

- B-Lactam is not effective because of lack of peptidoglycan in cell wall.
- Aminoglycosides are not effective because of intracellular location of bacteria where amino-glycosides do not penetrate.
- Doxycycline, rifampicin & azithromycin are effective.

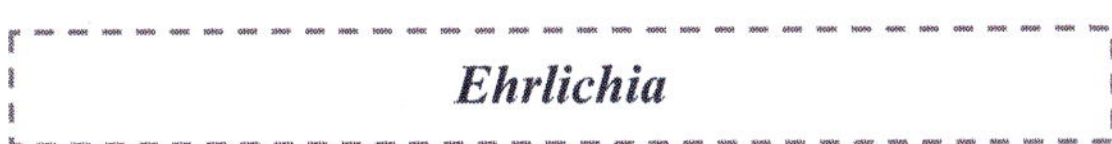

Ehrlichia

❖ **Morphology:**

➢ **Staining properties:** Gram negative but better stained by Giemsa or Wright stain or IF-stain.

➢ **Size:** Small in size.

➢ **Arrangement:** Obligatory intracellular bacteria having an affinity towards blood cells-neutrophils, lymphocytes & monocytes. In the cytoplasm of infected phagocytic cells they grow within phagosomes in a clusters as like mulberry **called morula** (**morula = mulberry**). Morula stain by Giemsa stain.

❖ **Cultural characteristics (C/Cs):** Relative successful method by culturing over DH82 cell line [derived from canine (dog) histiocytoma].

❖ **Pathogenicity:**

➢ **Disease name: Called ehrlichiosis.**

➢ **Types & other details:** Three types of disease as mentioned in **table-2.**

Features	Glandular fever	Human Monocytic Ehrlichiosis (HME)	Human Granulocytic Ehrlichiosis (HGE)
Species	*E. sennetsu*	*E. chaffensis*	*E. equi (E. phagocytophila)*
M/T	Ingestion of fish	Tick bite → *Amblyoma*	Bite of *Ixodid tick*
C/F	Lymphoid hyperplasia, atypical lympho-cytosis	Leucopenia, multisystem involvement, thrombo-cytopenia	Leucopenia, thrombo-cytopenia

Table-2: Types of ehrlichiosis

❖ **Laboratory diagnosis:**

➢ **Specimens:** Blood, CSF etc.

➢ **Testing methods:**

1. **Microscopy:** Prepare smear from blood & CSF → Stain by Giemsa / Wright stain or by IF-stain → examined by microscope → positive test indicates the presence of morula in blood & CSF monocytes.
2. **Culture: → Follow C/Cs**
3. **Molecular:** Nested PCR.

❖ **Prevention:** Vector control is effective.

❖ **Treatment:** Doxycycline & tetracycline are the effective drugs.

Coxiella

❖ **Species:** *Coxiella burnetii*

❖ **Synonym & Meaning:**

- Earlier the etiological agent of the disease was unknown hence it was **called 'Query' or Q fever**.
- In Australia, Burnet identified the causative agent as a rickettsia, it was **named *R. burnetii.***
- Same time same agent was identified from ticks in USA, by Cox **called *R. diaporica* (Diapor = ability to pass through pores of filter)**.

❖ **Taxonomy:** As the Q fever agent is not truly an arthropod borne & differed from other Rickettsiales member in many features, it has been excluded from Rickettsiales & renamed as *Coxiella burnetii.*

❖ **Morphology:**

➢ **Staining properties:** Pleomorphic, small Gram-negative rods better stained by Giminez & other rickettsial stains.

➢ **Size:** 0.2-0.4 µm x 0.4-1µm.

➢ **Shape:** Sometimes spherical with 0.5 – 0.3 µm size.

➢ Able to pass through filter.

❖ **Cultural characteristics (C/Cs):**

A. **Animal inoculation:** Guinea pig, hamster & mouse are useful animals.

B. **Egg culture:** It grows well in yolk sac of chick embryo.

C. **Cell culture:** It grows in human embryo lung fibroblast cell culture.

❖ **Resistance:**

- In dried faeces it survives for a year or more at 4^0C & in meat at least for 1 month.
- Not completely inactivated by 1% phenol in 1 hour & at 60^0C in 1 hour (heat resistant).
- In milk *Coxiella burnetii,* may survive pasteurisation by Holder method but killed by Flash method.

❖ **Antigenic or phase variation:**

- *Coxiella* are not showing antigenic cross reaction with *Proteus* or other *Rickettsia.*
- Two types of phase variations.

1. **Phase-I:**
- Fresh isolates present in guinea pig.
- Autoagglutinable.
- Phagocytosed in absence of antibody.
- Strong immunogenic elicits good antibody response against both phases.

2. **Phase –II:** Phase-I will convert in to Phase –II on repeated passage in yolk sac. Phase-II antibody is more suitable for CFT.

❖ **Pathogenicity:**

➢ **Disease name:** Disease is zoonosis **called 'Query' or 'Q fever'.**

➢ **Nature & history of disease:**
- Derrick investigated an outbreak of typhoid like fever in abattoir workers in Brisbane, Australia in 1935 by inoculating the blood from the patient to know the causative agent.
- It is distributed worldwide.

➢ **Reservoir of infection:** Tick like *Ixodid ticks.*

➢ **Source of infection:** Animal or animal products.

➢ **Modes of transmission:**

a. **Animal transmission:** Transmitted to cattle, sheep and poultry by *Ixodid ticks.* Transovarial transmission occurs in ticks but tick is not responsible for human transmission.

b. **Human transmission:** Person to person transmission is very rare. Ticks are less for human transmission which is possible by following routes

1. **Contact:**
- Occupationally through handling wool or hides, meat or other animal products contaminated with the organism especially in abattoir workers.
- Direct contact with abraded skin will favour the infection.

2. **Ingestion:** Ingestion of milk from infected animals
3. **Inhalation:** Inhalation of aerosols arises from dried tick faeces.

➢ **Incubation period:** 3-30 days.

➢ **Portal of entry:** Skin, GIT & respiratory system.

✪ **Sites:** Lungs, liver, brain, meninges, endocardium etc.

✪ **Precipitating factors (epidemiological determinants):**

I. Agent factors (virulence factors)

1. **Intracellular nature:** It is an obligate intracellular pathogen in monocytes-macrophages & evades the host defence. It share many features of *Rickettsia* like intracellular parasitism, cell wall composed of peptidoglycan, presence of DNA plus RNA & susceptibility to antibacterial agents but differs by heat resistant nature & no arthropod borne transmission.
2. **Dismutase:** Resistant to the acidic environment of phagolysosome by producing superoxide dismutase

II. Host factors

1. **Occupation:** Common in abattoir workers who are handling the products of infected animals like meat, wools or hides.
2. **Poor hygiene:** Also common in person drinking the raw milk of infected animals.

III. Environmental factors

1. **Environmental contamination:** Environment is regularly contaminated by bacteria, as they are abundantly present in tick's faeces & products of conception. They survive in dried faeces for long period.

➢ **Pathogenesis:** It induces the autoantibodies particular to cardiac & smooth muscles.

➢ **Clinical features:** Clinical picture is variable & sometimes present as asymptomatic infection. It present as acute & chronic form as follow

1. **Acute Q fever:** Characterized by primary atypical pneumonia/interstitial pneumonia.
2. **Chronic Q fever:** Bacteria spread throughout the body & causing hepatitis, meningo-encephalitis or endocarditis. Spontaneous recovery is usual.

➢ **Complications:**
- **Post Q fever fatigue syndrome:** Present with fever, headache, myalgia, sweating, arthralgia & muscle fasciculation. Spontaneous recovery may occur.
- **Latent infection:** Coxiella may remain latent in the tissues of patients for 2-3 years.

❖ **Laboratory diagnosis:**

➢ **Specimens:** Sputum, blood, milk/tissue of infected animals etc.

➢ **Testing methods:**

I. **Microscopy:→ Follow morphology**
II. **Culture: → Follow C/Cs**
III. **Serological tests:** Complement fixation test or indirect immunofluorescence assay are useful.
IV. **Molecular method:** PCR.

❖ **Prevention:**
- In milk *C burnetii*, may survive pasteurisation by Holder method but killed by Flash method.
- Vaccines are developed like formalin killed whole cell vaccine & trichloracetic acid extract vaccine, but not useful.

❖ **Treatment:** Tetracycline, erythromycin, clarithromycin, rifampicin or ciprofloxacin are effective drugs.

Bartonella

❖ **Properties:**
- It is not obligate intracellular (also extracellular) parasite hence excluded from Rickettsiaceae family.
- Transmitted by arthropods.

- Invades blood cells & endothelial cells.

❖ Morphology:

- **Staining properties:** GNB better stain by Wharthin -Starry technique.
- **Size:** 0.5 µm x 1–3 µmin size.
- **Shape:** Pleomorphic & rod shape.
- **Motility:** Motile with tuft of polar flagella.
- **Immunofluorescent microscopy**: It is also useful for identification.

❖ Cultural characteristics (C/Cs):

- **Effective factors:**
  - Can grow in cell free media.
  - Temperature: 35-37^{0}C.
  - O_2 or CO_2 effect: Better growth under 5% CO_2.
- **Culture in media:**

A. Liquid media:

- BHIB supplemented with 10% haemin is a useful medium.
- Growth occurs at 35-37^{0}C after 12-15 days.
- BHIB is useful for biochemical reactions.

B. Solid media:

1. BHIA
2. Trypticase soy agar
3. Rabbit, sheep, human blood agar

} Produces agar adherent colonies

- **Culture in cells:** Vero cells are useful for cultivation.

❖ Biochemical reactions (B/Rs): Tests are performed by using BHIB

1. Oxidise ribose.
2. Gelatin liquefaction test: +Ve
3. Hippurate hydrolysis: +Ve
4. Aesculin hydrolysis: +Ve

❖ Pathogenicity: Three different species & disease as shown in **table-3.**

❖ Laboratory diagnosis:

- **Specimens:** Blood, lymph node biopsy etc.
- **Testing methods:**

I. Microscopy: **:→ Follow morphology**

II. Culture: → Follow C/Cs

III. Biochemical tests: → Follow B/Rs

IV. Serological tests: Are also useful.

V. Physiological methods: GLC to identify fatty acids component.

VI. Molecular methods: Further classification based on protein profile by Sodium Dodycile Sulphate-Poly Acramide Gel Electrophoresis (SDS-PAGE), RFLP & PCR.

Species	*B. bacilliformis*	*B. (Rochalimaea) quintana*	*B. henselae*
Reservoir	Human only	Human only	Cats & other feline
Mode of trans-mission	By sandfly bite (*Lutzomyia*)	By human head louse (*Pediculus humanus corporis*). No vertical transmission occurs in lice. Faeces become infectious after 5-10 days & lice remains infectious for life. Auto inoculated due to scratching.	- By cat scratch or cat bite - Also by cat flea (*Ctenocephalides felis*)
Clinical features	**1. Oroya fever (Carrion's disease):** - Fever & progressive anemia due to bacterial invasion of RBC. - High mortality in untreated cases. **2. Verruga peruana:** - A late sequel. - Nodular ulcerating skin lesion. - Bacilli seen inside RBC & in the skin lesions	**1. Trench fever / five-day fever / Quintana fever:** - Fever last for 5 days (hence the name), followed by remission & recurrence after 5 days with about 12 recurrences. - Non fatal disease - Slow course & prolonged convalescence leads to loss of manpower. **2. Chronic infection (latent infection) :** Recrudescence may occur after 20 years	1. Cat scratch disease: - Also caused by *Afipia felis* - Present with fever & lympha-denopathy. Lymph node contains granulomatous lesion with central star shaped necrosis (called stellate necrosis) surrounded by histiocytes, B cells & giant cells called stellate abscess 2. Lesions in patients with HIV / IDDs: - Bacillary angiomatosis: Vascular nodules or tumours appear on the skin, mucosa and other locations - Bacillary peliosis: In liver and spleen 3. Bacteremia &endocarditis:
Other key points	Above two conditions were noticed in 1885 by the Peruvian medical students Daniel Carrion. He inoculated himself with material from verruga & developed Oroya fever, hence also called **Carrion's disease**	- Disease named trench fever as it was occurred in soldiers fighting in the trench in Europe - The word quintana means fifth, referring to five day fever	

Table-3: Pathogenicity of *Bartonella* spp.

Mnemonic: A/t mode of transmission (Vector & disease name followed by agent's name)

- **LET – pq** → Louse borne, Epidemic typhus & Trench fever - *R. prowazekii* & *B. quintana*
- **FEn –tf** → Flea borne & Endemic typhus - *R. typhi (R. mooseri)* & *R. felis*
- **TSE – cce**→ Tick borne, Spotted fever group & Ehrlichiosis - *R. conorii* (& others except *R. akari*) *E. chaffensis* & *E. equi*
- **MRS –at** → Mite borne, Rickettsial pox & Scrub typhus - *R. akari* & *O tsutsugamushi*
- **IGQ –sb** → Ingestion/Inhalation , Glandular fever & Q fever - *E. sennetsu* & *C. burnetti*
- **SO-b** → Sand fly & Oroya fever - *B. bacilliformis*

Question bank

Essay/ Full question

1) Q –fever (*Coxiella burnetii*)

Short notes

1) *Rickettsia*
2) *Orientia*
3) *Ehrlichia*
4) Cat scratch disease

Short questions for theory/viva questions

1) What is tunica reaction or Neil-Mooser reaction?
2) Name the causative agent for following disease.
Q-Fever, Oroya fever, Trench fever & cat scratch disease

MCQs for chapter review

Rickettsiales

Rickettsia

1) ***Rickettsiae* -** **(AIIMS -94)**
(a) Multiply only within living cell (b) Produce typhus fever of epidemic type only (c) Transmitted by arthropod vectors (d) Respond to tetracycline therapy
2) **All are true about *Rickettsia* except -** **(AIIMS, June -99)**
(a) Obligate intracellular (b) Gram +ve bacill (c) Arthropods are vectors (d) Weil-Felix test is diagnostic
3) **Neil – Mooser reaction is used to diagnose** **(PGI -99)**
(a) *Rickettsiae* (b) *Chlamydiae* (c) *Mycoplasma* (d) Herpes
4) **A man present with fever, chills 2 weeks after a louse bite. There was a maculopapular rash on the trunk which spread peripherally. The cause of this infection can be -** **(AIIMS -03)**
(a) Scrub typhus (b) Endemic typhus (c) Rickettsial pox (d) Epidemic typhus
5) **Brill-Zinsser disease is**
(a) Epidemic louse borne typhus (b) Endemic louse borne typhus (c) Q fever (d) Rocky mounted spotted fever
6) **It is true regarding endemic typhus that -** **(AIIMS -06)**
(a) Man is the only reservoir of infection (b) Flea is a vector for the disease (c) Rash developing in to eschar is the characteristic presentation (d) Culture of the etiological agent in tissue culture is the diagnostic
7) **Which of the following statement is true about endemic typhus -** **(AI -03)**
(a) It is caused by *R rickettsii* (b) It is transmitted by bite of fleas (c) Has no mammalian reservoir (d) Can be culture in chemical defined media
8) **Following is the etiological agent of Rocky mounted spotted fever -** **(AIIMS, May-05)**
(a) *Rickettsia rickettsii* (b) *Rochalima quintana* (c) *Rickettsia tsutsugamushi* (d) *Coxiella burnetii*
9) **Vascular endothelial infection is caused by**
(a) *Rickettsiae* (b) *Mycoplasma* (c) *Chlamydiae* (d) None
10) **Primary site of multiplication of rickettsial organisms is in the-**
(a) Parenchymal cells of the liver (b) Endothelial cells of small vessels (c) Media of arteries (d) Advantitia of all blood vessels
11) **Which of the following used for *Rickettsia* -**
(a) Weil-Felix reaction (b) Rose Waller test (c) Paul- Bunnel test (d) VDRL

Orientia

12) **Disease caused by *Rickettsia* & *Orientia* is transmitted by -** **(PGI -11)**
(a) Rat flea (b) Tick (c) Louse (d) Tromiculid mite (e) Gamaxid mite
13) **Mite is a vector for -** **(PGI, May-13, June -08)**
(a) *R. typhi* (b) *R. prowazekii* (c) *R. rickettsii* (d) *R tsutsugamushi* (e) *R. conorii*
14) **Transovarial transmission is a features of** **(PGI -98)**
(a) Scrub fever (b) Epidemic typhus (c) Endemic typhus (d) Trench fever
15) **True about scrub typhus is?**
(a) Transmitted by larvae of tromiculid mite (b) Incubation period is 3-4 days (c) Eschar is diagnostic (d) Caused by *Rickettsia typhi*
16) **All are true regarding scrub typhus except?**
(a) Caused by *R tsutsugamushi* (b) Spread by mites (c) Caused by bite of adult mite on vertebrate host (d) Tetracycline is effective
17) **Which is not transmitted by arthropod -** (AIIMS, Feb -97)
(a) *Rickettsia prowazekii* (b) *Coxiella burnetii* (c) *Rickettsia akari* (d) *Rickettsia rickettsii*

Ehrlichia

18) ***E. chaffensis* is causative agent of**
(a) HME (b) HGE (c) Glandular fever (d) None

Coxiella

19) **All of the following statement are true regarding Q fever except -** **(AI -03)**
(a) It is a zoonotic disease (b) Human disease is characterised by an interstitial pneumonia (c) No rash is seen (d) Weil –Felix reaction is very useful for diagnosis
20) **Mode of transmission of Q fever -** **(AIIMS -04)**
(a) Bite of infected louse (b) Bite of infected tick (c) Inhalation of aerosol (d) Bite of infected mice

Bartonella

21) **All are true about *B quintana* except -**
(a) Causes trench fever (b) Not detected by Weil – Felix reaction (c) Recurrence is common (d) Tick is the vector
22) ***B henselae* causes all except -**
(a) Oroya fever (b) Cat scratch disease (c) Bacillary angiomatosis (d) SABE
23) **Most common cause of bacillary angiomatosis is**
(a) *B quintana* (b) *B bacilliformis* (c) *B henselae* (d) *B elizabethi*
24) **Cat scratch disease is-** **(PGI-98)**
(a) Associated with positive Frei's skin test (b) Caused by DNA virus (c) Associated with a pathognomic histological

picture (d) Associated with regional lymphadenopathy (e) Associated with Hanger-rose test

Answers of MCQs & explanation

1) (a), (c) & (d)

- *Rickettsia* can multiply only within living cell (obligate intracellular) *in vivo* (like nucleus of vascular endothelial cells) & *in vitro* (like detroit 6, HeLa, HEP-2, mouse fibroblast & other continuous cell lines)
- Produce typhus fever of epidemic & endemic type
- Transmitted by bite or faeces of insect as mentioned in **table-1**
- Respond to tetracycline therapy

2) (b)

- *Rickettsia* is gram negative. Follow section ***Rickettsia*** for explanation of other options.

3) (a)

- Follow section, ***Rickettsia*** **(culture characteristics)** for explanation.

4) (d)

- From the given option louse borne infection is epidemic typhus
- Scrub typhus & Rickettsial pox are mite borne
- Endemic typhus is flea borne

5) (a)

- Follow section, *Rickettsia* **(pathogenicity → pathological types → Brill-Zinsser disease)** for explanation.

6) (b)

- Rodent & cat are the only reservoir as mentioned in **table-1**
- Flea is a vector & no eschar formation in disease
- Tissue culture is available but not satisfactory, so diagnostic methods are molecular (PCR) & serological

7) (b)

- Endemic typhus is caused by *R typhi*. Other options are already explained

8) (a)

- Follow section, ***Rickettsia*** **(pathogenicity → pathological & table-1** for explanation.

9) (a)
10) (b)
} Follow section, ***Rickettsia*** **(pathogenicity → pathogenesis & flow chart-3**) for explanation.

11) (a)

- Rose Waller test is used for RF or RA factor, Paul- Bunnel test for infectious mononucleosis & VDRL for syphilis detection

12) (d)
13) (d)
} *R. akari* & *O tsutsugamushi* are the mite borne pathogens. *O tsutsugamushi* was previously known as *R tsutsugamushi*

14) (a)

- Transovarial transmission to offspring is present in ticks & mites but not in louse & fleas. Scrub fever is mite borne, epidemic typhus & trench fever are louse borne while endemic typhus is flea borne

15) (a)

- Scrub typhus is caused by *O tsutsugamushi* & transmitted by larvae (**called chigger**) of trombiculide mite but not by adult stage. Incubation period is 6-21 days. Eschar is not diagnostic because it absent in < 50% of Westerners.

16) (c)

- Scrub typhus is transmitted by larvae (**called chigger**) of trombiculide mite but not by adult stage.

17) (b)

- Follow section, **table-1 &** ***Coxiella*** for explanation.

18) (a)

- Follow section, ***Ehrlichia*** **(pathogenicity → types & other details & table-2)** for explanation.

19) (d)

- The test is not diagnostic (negative) in Rickettsial pox, trench fever & Q fever

20) (c)

- Follow section, ***Coxiella*** **(pathogenicity → mode of transmission)** for explanation.

21) (d)
22) (a)
23) (c)
} Follow section, ***Bartonella*** **(table-3)** for explanation.

24) (c) & (d)

- Frei's skin test is useful for Lympha granuloma venereum caused by *Chlamydia trachomatis*
- Cat scratch disease is
  - Caused by bacteria not by virus
  - Associated with a pathognomic histological picture like stellate abscess
  - Associated with regional lymphadenopathy
  - Not associated with Hanger-rose test

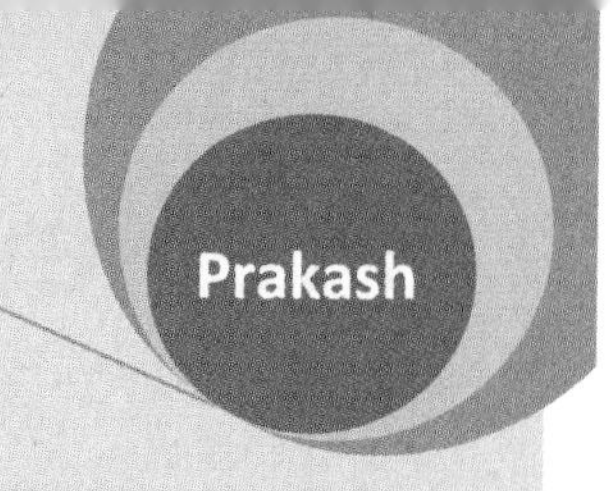

Section IV
Virology

Preview of Virology

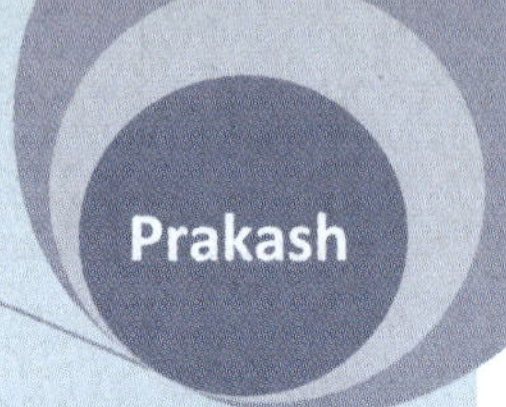

Almost all the viruses are written with following headings & subheadings

- **Meaning / Common name / Synonym:**
- **History:**
- **Geographical distribution & genotypes:**
- **Classification:**
- **Morphology:** With appropriate figures
  - **Shape:**
  - **Size:**
  - **Genome & capsid:**
  - **Envelope:**
  - **Others:** Like viral proteins, inclusion body etc.
- **Culture characteristics (C/Cs):**
  - i. **Egg culture:**
  - ii. **Animal culture:**
  - iii. **Tissue / cell culture:**
- **Resistance:**
- **Antigenic structure & serotypes:**
- **Immunity:**
- **Pathogenicity:**
  - **Disease name:**
  - **Synonym:**
  - **Nature or history of disease:**
  - **Reservoir of infection:**
  - **Source of infection:**
  - **Mode of transmission:**
  - **Incubation period:**
  - **Portal of entry:**
  - **Sites:**
  - **Precipitating factors (epidemiological determinants):**
  - **Pathogenesis:**
  - **Clinical features:**
  - **Complications:**
- **Laboratory diagnosis:**
  - **Specimens:**
  - **Testing methods:**
    - A. **Microscopy:**
    - B. **Culture:**
    - C. **Serological tests:**
    - D. **Molecular methods:**
- **Prevention:**
  - **General measures:**
  - **Chemoprophylaxis:**
  - **Immunoprophylaxis:**
- **Treatment:**

59 General properties of viruses

Learning heading & subheadings

Introduction

➢ **Meaning:** Virus is a **Greek word means poison.** Term virus was coined by Edward Jenner in 1798.

➢ **Definitions:**

✪ **Virion:** Extracellular infectious virus particle **called virion.**

✪ **Viroids:** Virus particle without extracellular phase **called viroids. (Vide infra)**

➢ **Differences between bacteria & viruses: →Table-1**

Bacteria	Viruses
Prokaryotes category	Neither prokaryotes nor eukaryotes
Larger, measured in µm	Smaller, measured in nm
Both DNA & RNA	One type of nucleic acid (NA), either DNA or RNA, but never both.
Nucleic acid surrounded by plasma membrane	Nucleic acid surrounded by a protein coat.
Thick cell wall contains peptidoglycan and LPS	Some viruses have additional outer lipoprotein envelope.
Contain organelles like mitochondria, golgi apparatus, ribosomes etc.	No cellular organelles
Extra-cellular except *M tuberculosis, Chlamydiae* spp. etc.	Intra-cellular
Contains the enzymes necessary for reproduction	Lack the enzymes necessary for reproduction
Multiply by binary fission	Multiply by replication of NA & synthesis of the viral protein.
Growth occurs on artificially prepared (cell free) media.	No growth on artificially prepared media.
Not pass through filter except few like *M pneumoniae, F. tularensis, C. burnetii, Chlamydiae* spp.	Pass through filter
Sensitive to antibiotics	Not sensitive to antibiotics
Few bacteria are motile	Motility absent

Table-1: Differences between bacteria & viruses

Morphology

❖ **Size: →Fig.-1**

- Viruses are very smaller than bacteria.
- Size is measured in nm.
- As they are very small, can pass through filter so **called filterable viruses**.
- Determined by electron microscopy.
- Some larger viruses can be examined by light microscope like pox virus.
- Variable in size: Like

1. Smallest (also smallest DNA) virus: *Parvovirus* [Parvo (Latin) = small] about 20 nm in size. It is as small as largest protein particle like haemocyanin.

2. Largest (also largest DNA) virus: Pox virus about 300 nm in size. It is as large as smallest bacteria like *Mycoplasma.*
3. Smallest RNA virus: Picornaviridae about 27-30 nm in size.
4. Largest RNA virus: Paramyxoviridae about 100-300 nm in size.

❖ **Shape:** →**Fig.-1**

- Viruses are very variable in shape.
- Most are spherical (like *Parvovirus*, picorna virus etc.) some are irregular.
- Rabies virus: Bullet shape.
- Ebola virus: Filamentous in shape.
- Pox virus: Brick shape.
- Tobacco Mosaic Virus (TMV): Rod shape.
- Bacteriophage virus: Tad pole in shape.

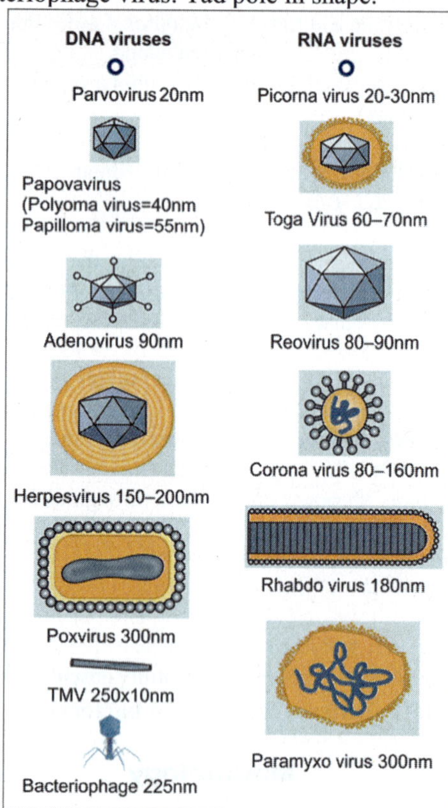

Figure-1: size & shape of different viruses

❖ **Structure:** Structure of virus consists following components from inner to outer **(fig.-2).**

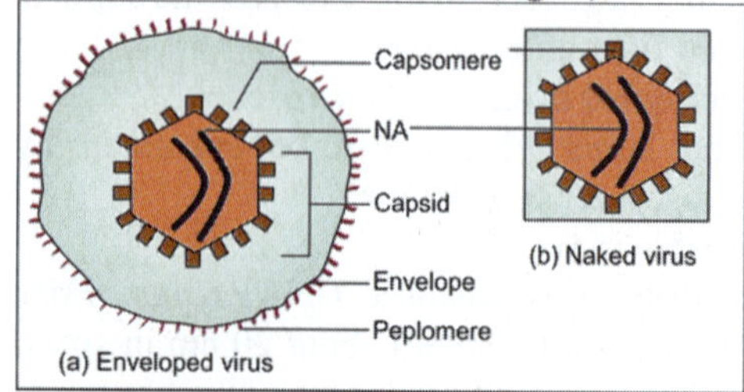

Figure-2: Structure of virus

A. Nucleic Acid (NA) / genome / core:

➢ **Types:** It may be either DNA or RNA (never both).

➢ **Properties:**
- Fully developed viral particles composed of nucleic acid in centre.
- Protein ranges from about 1% - 50%.
- It is extracted by treatment with detergent or phenol red.
- In some viruses like picorna virus, papova virus extracted NA is able to initiate the infection.

➢ **Organisation of NA:**

✪ **Strands:** It may be single stranded (ss) or double stranded (ds).

✪ **Pattern:** It may be circular or linear (non-segmented or segmented.

i. Circular genome: Circular like coil without ends.
1. Papovaviridae
2. Poxviridae

ii. Linear genome:

a. Non segemented: Only single piece.
1. Togaviridae
2. Rhabdoviridae
3. Some bacteriophages

b. Segmented genome: With multiple pieces.

1. Retroviridae:
- Two segments of ss-RNA (+)
- *Lentivirus* (Visna virus, SIV & HIV)

2. Orthomyxoviridae:
- Eight segments of ss-RNA (-)
- *Influenzavirus*

3. Bunyaviridae:
- Three segments of ss-RNA (-)
- *Hantavirus, Nairovirus, Phlebovirus & Ukuvirus*

4. Reoviridae:
- 10-12 segments of ds-RNA (+/-)
- *Reovirus, Orbivirus & Rotavirus*

5. Arenaviridae:
- Two segments of ss-RNA (-)
- *Mammarenavirus* (LCM virus, Junin virus & Machupo virus)

Mneumonic → ROBRA

B. Capsid or shell:

➢ **Definition:** NA surrounded by a protein coat **called capsid**.

➢ **Biochemistry:** Structural unit of capsid **called capsomere** which is made up by protein.

➢ **Functions of capsid:**
- It protects the NA from deleterious agents like nuclease or other environmental agents.
- It introduces the NA in to host cell by adsorbing to cell surfaces.
- Provides antigenic property to virus.

➢ **Three types (symmetry) of capsid:**

a. Icosahedral (cubical) symmetry: → **Fig.-3**
- NA is surrounded by equilateral triangle of capsomere (like soccer ball).
- Examples: Herpes viruses, adeno viruses etc.

- Composed of 12 vertices/corners & 20 facets/sides.
- Each facet has an equilateral triangle.
- Two types of capsomere in this type of capsid.
1. Pentons: Present at vertices, always 12 in numbers
2. Hexons: Present at facets, in variable numbers.

b. Helical (spiral tube) symmetry: →Fig.-4

- NA surrounded by capsomeres which are arranged together in tube shape structure.
- Examples: The helix can be either rigid in TMV or flexible in influenza viruses.

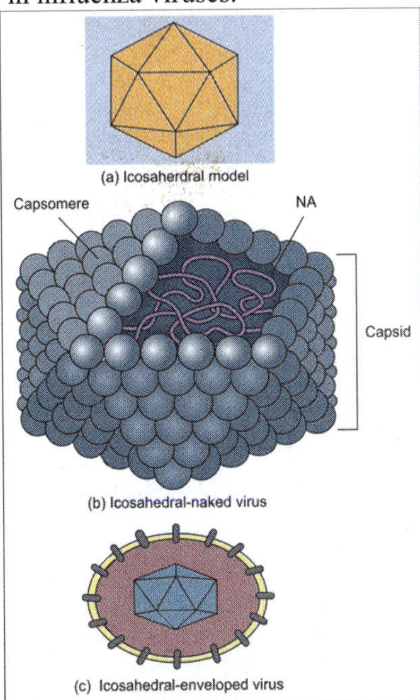

Figure-3: Icosahedral symmetry of capsid

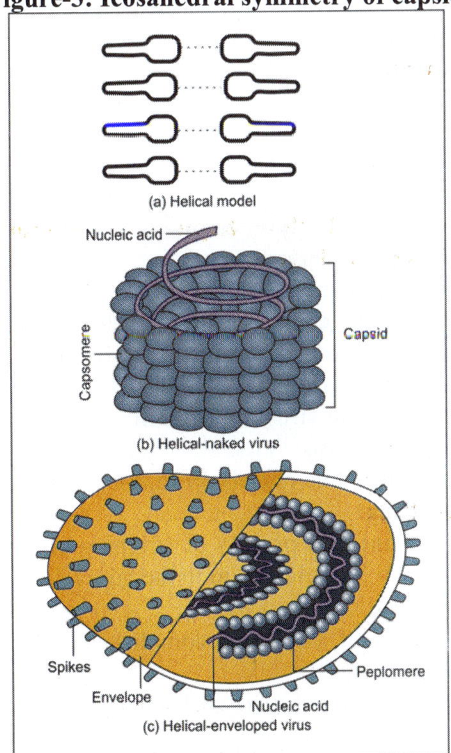

Figure-4: Helical symmetry of capsid

c. Complex symmetry: →Fig.-5

- These viruses possess a capsid that is neither purely helical nor purely icosahedral, and that may possess extra structures such as protein tails or a complex outer wall.
- Examples:

1. **Pox viruses:**

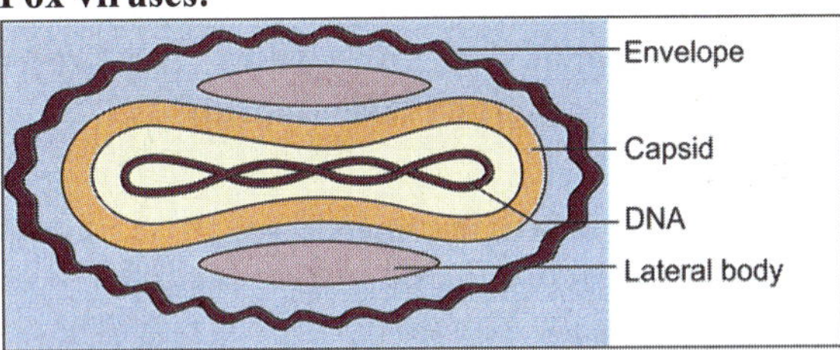

Figure-5: Complex symmetry of capsid (pox virus)

- Largest virus & complex viruses that have an unusual morphology.
- The viral genome is associated with proteins within a central disk structure **called nucleoid**. The nucleoid is surrounded by a membrane and two lateral bodies of unknown function. The virus has an outer envelope with a thick layer of protein studded over its surface **(fig.-5).**

2. **Enterobacterio phage T4:** It has a complex structure consisting of an icosahedral head bound to a helical tail, which may have a hexagonal base plate with protruding protein tail fibres. This tail structure acts like a molecular syringe, attaching to the bacterial host and then injecting the viral genome into the cell.
3. **Arenaviridae:**

C. Envelope & peplomeres: →Fig.-2

➢ **Definitions:**

- Some viruses have an outer lipoprotein layer **called envelope**.
- Some envelopes have spikes like projections **called peplomeres**, from peplos meaning envelop.
- Viruses with envelop are **called envelop viruses** while some viruses without envelop are **called naked viruses**.

➢ **Biochemistry:**

- Envelope is made up by lipoprotein where lipid derived from the host cell plasma membrane by budding & proteins are viral encoded.
- Peplomeres are glycoproteins.

➢ **Types of peplomeres with example:** Influenza virus has two kinds of peplomeres.

1. **H (haemagglutinin):** It allows the virus to attach to host cells (and red blood cells).
2. **N (neuraminidase):** It is an enzyme that allows the mature viral particles to escape from the host cell.

➢ **Functions:** It confers properties on viruses like

1. **Chemical:** Enveloped viruses are susceptible to lipid solvents like ether, chloroform & bile salts.

2. **Antigenic:** Viral neutralisation by specific antibodies to envelop or peplomere antigens.
3. **Biological:** Follow H & N **(vide supra)** peplomeres of influenza viruses.

✓ **Note:**

- **Enveloped viruses [fig.2-(a)] =NA + capsid + envelope**
- **Non-enveloped (naked) viruses [fig.2-(b)] = nucleic acid + capsid (nucleocapsid)**

D. Fibrils:

- Additional features in some viruses.
- It protrudes from vertices.
- Example: Adenoviruses.

E. Enzymes: Most viruses do not possess any enzymes for biosynthesis or energy production. They remain dependant on host cells; except influenza virus has neuraminidase & retrovirus has reverse transcriptase which transcribes RNA to DNA.

Resistance

1. **Heat and cold:**

- Viruses are heat labile & generally destroyed by heating at 50-60^0 C for 30 minute or at 4^{0}C in a day.
- They are stable at low temperature.
- Viruses can be preserved at -70^{0}C or for long storage it is preserved by lyophilisation (freeze drying).

2. **pH:**

- Viruses can be preserved at neutral pH (7.3).
- All viruses are killed at alkaline pH.
- Entero viruses are resistance to acidic pH, while rhinoviruses are susceptible to acidic pH.

3. **Disinfectants:**

- Viruses are most resistant to disinfectants.
- Most common virucidal agents are $KMNO_4$, H_2O_2, hypochlorite, iodine & chlorine (but affected by organic matter present in water).
- Formaldehyde & BPL (Beta Propio Lactone) are virucidal & used to prepare the killed vaccine.
- Enveloped viruses are susceptible to lipid solvents like ether, chloroform & bile salts. Susceptibility can be used to distinguish envelope viruses from non- envelope.
- Naked viruses are most resistant to disinfectants.
- Salts: Many viruses can be stabilized by salt in concentrations of 1 mol/L. e.g. $MgCl_2$, $MgSO_4$ & Na_2SO_4.

4. **Radiation:** Ultraviolet, X-ray and high-energy particles inactivate viruses.
5. **Antibiotics:** Antibacterial agents have no effect on viruses.

Viral multiplication

❖ **Total six steps:** →**Fig.-6**

i. Attachment or adsorption:

➢ **Definition:** Specific binding between virus & specific receptors on the host cellular surface **called adsorption**.

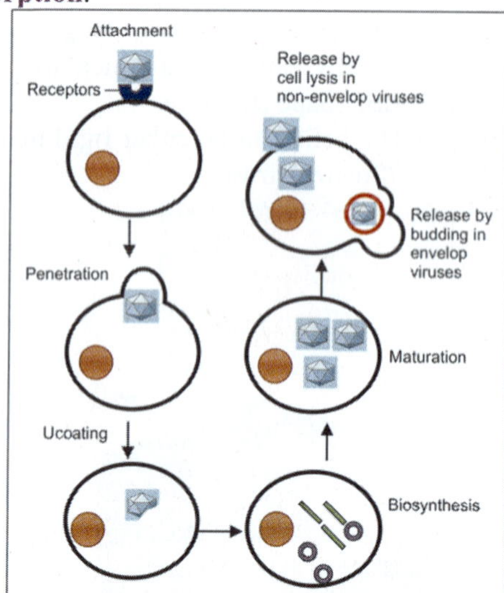

Figure-6: Viral multiplication

➢ **Examples:**

- HIV infects CD4 cells by specific receptors for gp120.
- Influenza virus attach to glycoprotein receptors on respiratory epithelium by haemagglutinin (H).
- Polio virus can attach to lipoprotein receptors present on primate, not on rodent cell.
- However some viruses like picorna virus can directly inject the NA in to the host cells, which are resistant to infection by whole virus.

ii. Penetration

➢ **Bacterial virus:**

- Bacterial virus **called bacteriophage**. It can enter in to bacteria by complex mechanisms due to tough bacterial cell wall.
- More details: **Follow chapters → Bacteriophages & Genetics of bacteria.**

➢ **Human virus:**

- Human virus can enter in host cell by mechanisms resembling phagocytosis **called 'viropexis.'**
- Naked virus: Human host cells do not have tough wall, so whole virus can enter in cell.
- Enveloped virus: Viral envelop fuse with plasma membrane while nucleocapsid can enter in to cell.

iii. Uncoating:

➢ **Definition:** It is process of stripping of envelop & capsid, so NA released in to the host cell.

➢ **Features:**

- Uncoating of virus is accomplished by lysosomal enzymes.
- Bacteriophage don't require uncoating because their nucleic acid is injected into the host cell.
- In Poxvirus uncoating is two step process.

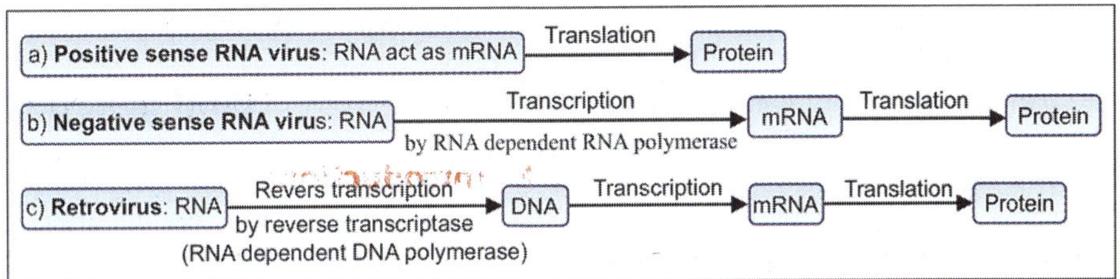

Flow chart -1: Mechanisms of translation in RNA viruses

- 1st step: Stripping of envelop by lysosomal enzymes.
- 2nd step: Stripping of capsid by specific viral uncoating enzymes.

iv. Biosynthesis:

➢ **It includes the synthesis of**
- NA.
- Capsid.
- Enzymes (regulatory protein): Helps in biosynthesis by inhibiting the host cell metabolism.

➢ **Sites of biosynthesis:** Depend on type of particles to be synthesised & type's of virus.

✪ **Biosynthesis of NA:**
- DNA viruses: In nucleus except poxvirus in which NA synthesised in cytoplasm.
- RNA viruses: In cytoplasm except orthomyxovirus, paramyxovirus & retrovirus in which NA synthesised in nucleus.

✪ **Biosynthesis of viral proteins:** Take place only in cytoplasm.

➢ **Steps of biosynthesis:**

a. Transcription:

✪ **Definition:** Process of synthesis of mRNA from viral NA.

✪ **Classes:** Six classes are described by Baltimore in 1970.

- **Class-1:**
  - ds-DNA virus: Like adeno, herpes, papova virus, where DNA enters in host cell nucleus & use host cell enzymes for transcription.
  - Partially ds-DNA virus: Like hepadna virus where duplex is formed by DNA polymerase in cytoplasm, than mature NA enters in to host cell nucleus & uses host cell enzymes for transcription.
- **Class-2:** ss-DNA virus like parvovirus. DNA enters in host cell nucleus, converted in to duplex & than uses host cell enzymes for transcription.
- **Class-3:** ds-RNA virus like reo virus. ds-RNA transcribed to mRNA by viral polymerase.
- **Class-4:** Plus (positive) strand ss-RNA viruses like picorna virus & toga virus. RNA itself acts as mRNA & translated to viral proteins as shown in **flow chart-1(a).**
- **Class-5:** Minus (negative) strand ss-RNA virus like rhabdo virus, orthomyxo virus & paramyxo virus. Virus possesses their own RNA polymerase (RNA dependent RNA polymerase) which transcribed RNA to mRNA which translates to protein as shown in **flow chart-1(b).**
- **Class-6:** Like retro viruses. Conversions of ss-RNA to ds-DNA by enzyme reverse transcriptase (RNA-dependent DNA polymerase, DNA polymerase), DNA transcribed to mRNA which translate to protein as shown in **flow chart-1(c)**.

b. Translation:

✪ **Definition:** Process of synthesis of early or non-structural proteins from mRNA.

✪ **Features:** These are enzymes which induce & maintain the synthesis of viral components by inhibiting the host cell metabolism.

c. Replication: It includes the replication of viral NA.

d. Synthesis of late or structural proteins: Like capsid.

v. Maturation & assembly:
- After synthesis of viral particles, they undergoes to maturation & assembly to produce the complete virus.
- In adeno virus & herpes virus it takes place in nucleus.
- In picorna virus & pox virus it takes place in cytoplasm.
- At this stage non-enveloped virus are complete, while in enveloped virus only nucleocapsid is synthesised followed by envelope synthesis from host cell membrane by budding method.
- This envelop undergoes modification to introduce virus specific Ags like haemagglutinin (H) in influenza virus.

vi. Release: Release of daughter virus is possible by following mechanisms.

➢ **Host cell lysis:** Viruses can be released from the host cell by lysis, a process that kills the host cell by bursting its membrane and cell wall if present. This is a feature of many viruses like bacteriophage and some animal viruses like poliovirus.

➢ **Budding:** Enveloped viruses (e.g. HIV) typically are released from the host cell by budding. During this process the virus acquires its envelope, which is a modified piece of the host's plasma or other internal membrane.

➢ **Some viruses undergo a lysogenic cycle:**
- No release of progeny virus, but viral genome is incorporated by genetic recombination into the host's chromosome.

- Such viral genome "**called provirus**" or in the case of bacteriophage "called **prophage**".
- "Provirus" or "prophage" is behaves like host genome & multiply simultaneously with host cell's genome & confers certain new properties in host cell **called lysogenic conversion**.
- Examples of lysogenic conversion:

a. **Malignant transformation by oncogenic virus:** Normal cells changed to malignant cells.

b. **Conversion of nontoxigenic strain of bacteria in to toxin producing strain:** Like

1. *C. diphtheriae:* Diphtheria toxin.
2. *V. cholerae:* Cholera toxin.
3. *EHEC:* Verotoxin.
4. *Cl. botulinum:* Toxin C & D.
5. *S. pyogenes:* Exotoxin A & C.

❖ **Eclipse phase:**

- From the stage of entry to synthesis of daughter virions, virus remained underground or disappeared & can't be demonstrated in host cells **called eclipse phase**.
- It is about 15-30 minutes in bacteriophage & 15-30 hrs in human virus.

❖ **Burst size:**

- Release of progeny of virus per infected cell **called burst size**.
- It is estimated in bacteriophage & difficult to measure in human virus.

❖ **Abnormal replicative cycle:**

✪ **Incomplete viruses:** Due to defective assembly, progeny virions released may not be infective **called incomplete viruses**.

✪ **von Magnus phenomenon:** Such incomplete viruses are seen when cell infected with high dose of influenza virus, where progeny released have high haemagglutinin titre but low infectivity **called von Magnus phenomenon**. It is due to formation of incomplete virus particles lacking NA.

✪ **Abortive infection:** Due to defect in release virus infection in some cells does not lead to production of progeny virion **called abortive infection**.

✪ **Defective virus:**

- Some virus when infect the cells are not able to give rise fully formed progeny **called defective viruses**.
- Defective viruses can give rise fully formed progeny, only when they are co- infected by helper virus like

- Rouse Sarcoma Virus (RSV) is not able to synthesise the envelope by self. When it co-infected by helper virus like Avian Leukosis Virus (ALV), resulting progeny are with envelop. The envelope Ags of progeny RSV is therefore determined by the type of helper virus.
- HDV (defective virus) & HBV (helper virus).
- Adeno associated satellite virus (defective virus) & adeno virus (helper virus).

Viral genetics

❖ **Introduction:** Two main mechanisms for genetic inheritance of virus like mutation & recombination. Additionally virus also exhibits non-heritable mechanisms due to interaction between viral products.

Mutation

➢ More details: Follow chapter → Genetics of bacteria

➢ **Some important points are highlighted at here.**

- **Frequency of mutation:** It is same as bacteria: 10^{-4}-10^{-8}
- **Change in antigenic properties:** It confers certain new properties in virus like virulence, host range, antigenicity (**antigenic drift & antigenic shift in Influenza virus)**, pock or plaque morphology & drug resistance.
- **Conditional lethal mutation:**

- A mutation may affect an organism in such a way that the mutant can survive only in certain environmental condition **called conditional lethal mutation**.
- Example: A temperature sensitive mutant (ts mutant) can survive at permissive temperature of 35°C but not at restrictive temperature of 39°C.
- Uses in study of viral genetics & vaccine production (influenza vaccine).

Recombination

➢ **Definition:** Transfer of genetic materials or genetic information from one cell to other cell in viruses (viruses are different but related) **called genetic recombination.**

➢ **It occurs between:**

- Two active (infectious) viruses.
- One active & one inactive virus.
- Two inactive (non-infectious) viruses.

➢ **Methods of viral gene transfer:** Following types.

i. **Intramolecular recombination:**

- Occurs when two closely related viruses are infect the host cell.
- Two viruses exchange the NA & form the hybrid that harbours the genes from both species.
- It occurs in ds-DNA & in some RNA viruses.

ii. **Reassortment:**

- Occurs when different strains of same virus are growing together with different antigens.
- Like one human strain, one avian strain & two pigs (swine) strains of influenza virus (total four strains) growing together in pig with different H & N Ags.

- A hybrid may obtain H-Ag from one parent & N-Ag from other, resulting a novel virus is formed like **swine origin influenza virus (S-OIV) or H1N1 2009 pandemic strain**.

iii. **Cross reactivation /marker rescue/ reactivation:**

- Occurs when active strain & related inactive strain infect the host cell together.
- A progeny virus may possess gene from active strain & one or more genes from inactive strain.
- Example:
  - Epidemic strain of influenza virus (A_2) which grows very poorly in eggs.
  - When such active strain (A_2) grown in eggs along with standard strain (A_1) -activated by radiation, resulting progeny contains growth properties of A_1 & antigenic properties of A_2.
  - Useful in preparation of influenza vaccine.

iv. **Multiplicity reactivation:**

- When cell is infected by larger dose of single virus (high MOI-Multiplicity Of Infection), inactivated by UV radiation, it produce changes in host cell gene & produces the live virus **called multiplicity reactivation.**
- Disadvantage: Vaccine inactivated by UV radiation is not safe.

v. **Lysogenic conversion : vide supra**

vi. **Pseudovirion:**

- Normally viral NA is enclosed by viral capsid, but sometimes host NA is enclosed by viral capsid **called pseudovirion**.
- Example: Papova virus.

vii. **Transduction:**

- Transfer of host NA from one cell to other cell by bacteriophage **called transduction**.
- Used to correct the inborn errors of metabolism.

❖ Interaction between viral products (Non-heritable mechanisms)

i. **Phenotyping mixing:**

- **Transcapsidation:**
  - When two different viruses are infecting the host cell, NA of one virus is surrounded by capsid of other virus **called transcapsidation**.
  - It is not a stable change; on subsequent passage original capsid will form.

ii. **Genotyping mixing:**

- **Heterozygosis:**
  - Incorporation of more than one complete genome in to virus.
  - On subsequent passage, two types of viral progeny will form.

iii. **Complementation:**

- **Definition:**
  - Functional interaction between two viruses, in which one or both may be defective.
  - One virus provides gene product to other virus which is defective & resulting other virus will replicate & progeny virus are like parent virus.
- **Example:**
  - When rabbit is infected with heat inactivated virulent myxoma virus & active avirulent fibroma virus, it develops fatal myxomatosis.
  - Heat inactivated myxomavirus is not able to produce infection due to deficiency of DNA dependent RNA polymerase.
  - When co-infected by fibroma virus, it provides the required enzyme to produce infection.

iv. **Interference:**

- **Definition:** Presence of one virus will interfere the function of other virus.
- **Mechanism:** Interference is produced by
  - Interferon production.
  - Destruction of receptors required for attachment.
  - Auto-interference: High MOI (Multiplicity Of Infection) inhibit the production of own progeny virus.
- **Clinical significance:** Useful in controlling polio outbreak by administration of live attenuated polio virus vaccine (OPV), which interfere with wild polio virus. On other hand presence of pre-existing virus will interfere the vaccine virus.

v. **Enhancement:** Presence of one virus will increase the effect of (CPE) other virus **called enhancement.**

Viral taxonomy

❖ **Definition:** It is the description, identification, nomenclature & orderial classification of organisms according to their presumed natural relationships.

❖ Nomenclature::

➢ **Order:** Labelled by adding the suffix **'virales'.**

➢ **Family:**
- Family is classified on the basis of morphology, genome structure and strategies of replication.
- Virus family: Labelled by adding the suffix **'viridae'.**
- Virus subfamily: Labelled by adding the suffix **'virinae'.**

➢ **Genus:**
- Genus is classified on the basis of physicochemical / serological differences.
- Genus name give by adding the suffix ***'virus'*** & it is written in Italic pattern.

➢ **Species:** No exact system for species nomenclature.

❖ Classification:

➢ **Properties:**
- All microbes are grouped either in prokaryotes or in eukaryotes. Viruses are not classified in any group.

- Viral classification system is proposed by an International Committee on Taxonomy of Viruses in 2000.

➢ **Bases for classification:**

✪ **Two main types based on NA**

- DNA viruses: Deoxyrebo viruses
- RNA viruses: Rebo viruses

✪ **Further types based on**

- **Morphology:** Size, shape, type of symmetry, presence or absence of envelope.
- **Genome:** Size of genome, strandedness (ss or ds), linear or circular, positive (+) or negative (-) sense.
- **Physico-chemical or serological properties.**

✪ **Classification:**

I. DNA viruses: Deoxyrebo viruses
II. RNA viruses: Rebo viruses
} **Follow Table-2**

Naked or enveloped	Virus family	Genus/species	Capsid symmetry	Nucleic acid type
DNA viruses				
Enveloped	Poxviridae	Smallpox virus, cow pox virus, sheep pox virus, orf virus, monkey pox virus & vaccinia virus	Complex	ds
	Herpesviridae	Herpes simplex virus, varicella-zoster virus, cyto megalo virus, Epstein–Barr virus etc.	Icosahedral	ds
	Hepadnaviridae	Hepatitis B virus	Icosahedral	Circular, partially ds
Naked	Adenoviridae	Adeno virus	Icosahedral	ds
	Papovaviridae	HPV, SV-40 virus, JC virus & BK virus	Icosahedral	ds circular
	Parvoviridae	Parvovirus B19	Icosahedral	ss
RNA viruses				
Enveloped	Togaviridae	*Rubivirus* (Rubella virus), *Pestivirus, Alphavirus*	Icosahedral	ss (+)
	Flaviviridae	Dengue virus, HCV, Yellow fever virus	Icosahedral	ss (+)
	Arenaviridae	*Mammarenavirus* (LCV, Junin virus, Machupo virus)	Complex	ss (-)
	Orthomyxoviridae	*Influenzavirus*	Helical	ss(-)
	Paramyxoviridae	*Rubulavirus* (Mumps virus), *Pneumovirus* (RSV), *Morbilivirus* (Measles virus), *Henipavirus* (Nipah virus)	Helical	ss(-)
	Bunyaviridae	*Hantavirus, Nairovirus, Phlebovirus, Ukuvirus*	Helical	ss(-)
	Rhabdoviridae	*Vesicullovirus* (Vesicular stomatitis virus, Chandipura virus), *Lyssavirus* (Rabies virus)	Helical	ss(-)
	Filoviridae	Ebola virus, Marburg virus	Helical	ss(-)
	Coronaviridae	Human Corona virus	Helical	ss (+)
	Retroviridae	*Lentivirus* (Visna virus, SIV & HIV)	Icosahedral	ss(+)
Naked	Reoviridae	*Rotavirus, Orbivirus , Coltivirus, Orthoreovirus*	Icosahedral (two capsid)	ds (+/-)
	Picornaviridae	*Enterovirus, Rhinovirus, Hepatovirus /Heparnavirus* (HAV)	Icosahedral	ss (+)
	Caliciviridae	*Norwalk virus, Hepevirus* (HEV)	Icosahedral	ss (+)
	Astroviridae	*Astrovirus*	Icosahedral	ss

Table-2: Classification of viruses

Mnemonics:

- **DNA viruses:**
- **Enveloped DNA viruses: PH2→** Poxviridae, Herpesviridae, Hepadnaviridae
- **Naked BNA viruses: AP2→** Adenoviridae, Papovaviridae, Parvoviridae
- **DNA virus = icosahedral capsid:** All the DNA viruses whether enveloped or naked have, icosahedral type of capsid except Poxviridae having complex variety of capsid
- **DNA virus = no helical capsid:** DNA viruses have no helical type of capsid
- **DNA virus = ds NA:** All the DNA viruses have, ds NA except Parvoviridae has ss NA
- **RNA viruses:**
- **Enveloped RNA viruses: FABRic FOT-PCR→** Flaviviridae, Arenaviridae, Bunyaviridae, Rhabdoviridae, Filoviridae, Orthomyxoviridae, Togaviridae, Paramyxoviridae , Coronaviridae , Retroviridae
- **Naked RNA viruses: Astro-PCR→**Astroviridae, Picornaviridae, Caliciviridae, Reoviridae
- **RNA virus = icosahedral & helical capsid:** RNA viruses have icosahedral or helical type of capsid except Arenaviridae having complex variety of capsid
- **RNA virus = ss NA:** All the RNA viruses have ss NA except Reoviridae has ds NA
- **Icosahedral capsid = Naked virus :** Naked viruses whether DNA or RNA have icosahedral type of capsid
- **Icosahedral capsid = DNA virus + naked RNA:** All the DNA viruses (except Poxviridae) & naked RNA viruses have icosahedral type of capsid

Subviral agents

❖ Viroids:

➤ **Definition:** Virus particle without extracellular phase **called viroids**.

➤ **History:** 1st introduced by Diener in 1971.

➤ **Morphology:**

- Genome: Contains ss-RNA, which is smaller than normal virus. HDV may resemble to viroid.
- Capsid & envelope: Absent.
- Contains enzyme RNA polymerase II which instead of synthesising RNA from DNA, uses the rolling cycle to synthesise RNA by using viroid's RNA as template.

➤ **Resistant:**

- Resistant to heat.
- Sensitive to nuclease.

➤ **Pathogenicity:**

- Potato spindle tuber viroid: First viroid to be identified. It is a plant pathogen causing potato spindle tuber disease.
- Also cause human & animal diseases.

❖ Prions:

➤ **Definition:** Proteinaceous infectious virus like-particles without nucleic acid (NA) **called prions**.

➤ **History:** Prion was identified by Stanley B Prusiner, awarded with Nobel Prize in 1997.

➤ **Morphology:**

- Contains protein without NA.
- MW of protein is50, 000 & size is 4-6nm.

➤ **Resistant:**

- Sensitive to protease.
- Resistant to nuclease, heat (90^{0}C for 3min.) & UV-rays.
- Routine methods like autoclaving (120^{0}C for 20 min.), boiling, radiation etc. are not effective.
- Prions are killed by autoclaving at 134^{0}C for 5 hours with prior treatment with acidic detergent or by treatment with 2N NaOH for several hours or by 0.5% sodium hypochlorite for 2 hours.

➤ **Pathogenicity:**

✪ **Disease name:** Disease **called prion disease.**

✪ **Incubation period:** Long incubation period may be up to 30 years, but once the disease sets in, progress is fast.

✪ **Sites:** CNS.

✪ **Pathogenesis:** Many theories are proposed for the pathogenesis of prion disease as follows.

- **Stanley B Prusiner theory:** It is mentioned in **flow chart-2**. Because of his great work he was awarded with Noble Prize in 1997.
- **Abnormal protein folding:** α helix structure of PrP^c change to β structure PrP^{sc} **called misfoled or unfold protein.** This unfolded protein is dangerous because it unfold many other folded prion protein. Unfold protein undergoes replication & spread throughout tissues without using DNA or RNA to produce the disease.

✪ **Pathology:**

- Progressive vacuolation in the dendritic & axonal process of the neurons.
- Extensive astroglial hypertrophy & proliferation.
- Spogiform encephalopathy & neuro-degeneration in the grey matter.
- Amyloid plaques present in brain.
- Gliosis.
- No inflammation.
- Absence of immune response (non-immunogenic).

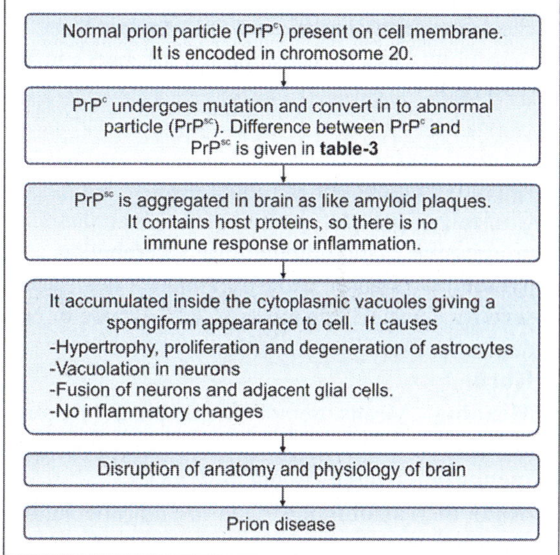

Flow chart-2: Pathogenesis of prion particle

Features	PrP^c	PrP^{sc}
Full form	Prion particle cellular	Prion particle scrapie
Forms	Normal form	Active or pathogenic form
Structure	Elongated polypeptide with more α helix & less β structure	Globular polypeptide with less α helix & more β structure
Location	Cell membrane	Cytoplasm
Protease	Sensitive	Resistant

Table-3: Differences between PrP^c & PrP^{sc}

✪ **Clinical types::** Two types of prion diseases.

a. Prion diseases in animals:

1. **Mink encephalopathy:** Spread to mink when they fed on scrapie infected sheep's meat.
2. **Scrapie:** Transmitted vertically from ewe to lamb.
3. **Bovine spongiform encephalopathy (BSE, Mad cow disease):** Spread to cattle when they fed on scrapie infected sheep's meat. Enzootic occurred in 1986 in Britain.

b. Prion diseases in human:

1. **CJD (Creutzfeldt-Jacob Disease):**
- **Nature or history of disease:**
- A variety of CJD (vCJD) was occurs in persons < 45 years in Britain in 1996, due to consumption of beef, infected with BSE & many cattle were slaughtered before anxiety was allayed.
- It occurs in sporadic due to mutation in prion.
- It also occurs in inherited (familiar) forms.
- **Mode of transmission:**
- Iatrogenic: Due to
- Corneal transplantation.
- Dura mater graft implantation (>160 cases have been reported).
- Injection of pituitary growth hormone from infected person (>180 cases have been reported).
- Electro encephalogram electrode implantation.
- Ingestion: Due to consumption of beef, infected with BSE.
- Hereditary
- **Clinical features:**
- Defective higher cortical functions.
- Clinically present with senile encephalopathy, progressive inco-ordination, cerebellar gait, pyramidal signs, extra-pyramidal dysfunctions, seizures, visual impairment, 90% myoclonus, & dementia. Death occurs within a year.

2. **Kuru:**
- **Meaning:** Means tremor characteristic feature of disease.
- **Incubation period:** About 5-10 years.
- **Mode of transmission:** Due to anthropophagy or Cannibalism.
- It is the act or practice of humans, eating the flesh or internal organs of other human beings.
- Word came from Caníbales, the Spanish name for the Caribs, a West Indies (New Guinea) tribe that formerly practiced cannibalism after the death of relatives due to customs.
- Was identified in New Guinea & disease was stopped after stopping the cannibalism
- **Clinical features:** Cerebellar ataxia, tremor & death.
- **Nobel Prize:** Given to Carlton Gajdusek in 1976 for his contribution in disease.

3. **GSSS (Gerstmann Straussler Scheinker Syndrome):**
4. **Fatal familial insomnia:**

- **Laboratory diagnosis:**
- **Specimens:** Brain biopsy & CSF.
- **Testing methods::**

1. **Light microscopy:** Histopathological changes like
   - Hypertrophy, proliferation & degeneration of astrocytes.
   - Vacuolation in neurons.
   - Fusion of neurons & adjacent glial cells.
   - No inflammatory changes.
2. **Conformation dependent assay:** It is specific diagnosis for measurement of PrP^{sc}.
3. **Stress protein 14-3-3:** Elevated in CSF.
4. **Sequencing the gene:** It is important to detect the mutation to identify the familiar CJD.
5. **Abnormal EEG:** In late stage of disease, high voltage, tri-phasic sharp discharges are observed.
6. **MRI:** Greater than 90% cases showing the increased intensity in the basal ganglia & cortical ribboning.

- **Prevention:** No effective measures are available.
- **Treatment:** Several measures using drugs like quinacrine & anti-PrP antibodies eliminate the prion particles from the cultured cells but failed to do so *in vivo*.

Important terminology

- Equine: Horse
- Feline: Cat
- Bovine: Cattle (cow/buffalo)
- Canine: Dog
- Murine: Rat/mice
- Simian: Monkey
- Swine (Porcine): Pig
- Avian: Birds
- Caprine: Sheep/goat

Question bank

Essay/Full question

1) Morphology of viruses.

Short notes

1) Structure of viruses.
2) Viral capsid.
3) Viral multiplication.
4) Mutation.
5) Viral recombination.
6) Classification of viruses or viral taxonomy.
7) Prion particle

Short questions for theory/viva questions

1) Write the four differences between viruses & bacteria.
2) What is capsid? Write its two functions.
3) What is peplomere? Write its two functions.
4) What is eclipse phase?
5) What is von Magnus phenomenon?
6) Define: Burst size, incomplete virus, von Magnus phenomenon & abortive viral infection.
7) What is defective virus? Write two examples.
8) Define: Provirus & prophage.
9) Write four examples of bacteria producing toxin after phage conversion.
10) Define: Virion & viroid.

MCQs for chapter review

Introduction

1) **False about viruses is**
(a) Ribosome absent (b) Mitochondria absent (c) Motility absent (d) Nucleic acid absent
2) **Following is not the property of virus**
(a) Contains both DNA & RNA (b) Neither prokaryotes nor eukaryotes (c) No growth on media (d) Pass through filter
3) **Which of the following does not possess both DNA & RNA**
(a) Bacteria (b) Fungi (c) Viruses (d) Spirochetes
4) **All of the following are general properties of viruses except** (AI-94)
(a) May contain both DNA and RNA (b) Form extracellular infectious particles (c) Heat labile (d) Not affected by antibiotics

Morphology

5) **Brick shaped virus is**
(a) Chicken pox (b) Small pox (c) CMV (d) EBV
6) **Rabies virus is in**
(a) Bullet shape (b) Spherical shape (c) Brick shape (d) Rod shape
7) **Smallest DNA virus is**
(a) Herpes virus (b) Adenovirus (c) Parvovirus (d) Poxvirus
8) **The virus with smallest genome**
(a) Reovirus (b) Parvovirus (c) Picornavirus (d) HIV
9) **Segmented genome is found in all except**
(a) Influenzavirus (b) Reovirus (c) Bunyavirus (d) Rhabdovirus
10) **Segmented genome is found in** (AIIMS, June-98)
(a) Retrovirus (b) Rotavirus (c) Poliovirus (d) Rhabdovirus
11) **Segmented RNA is found in**
(a) Influenza virus (b) Rabies virus (c) Herpes virus (d) Molluscum contagiosum virus
12) **Segmented double stranded RNA virus is seen in** (PGI-97)
(a) Reo virus (b) Myxovirus (c) Rabies (d) Parvovirus
13) **DNA covering material in a virus is called as** (PGI -96)
(a) Capsomere (b) Capsid (c) Nucleocapsid (d) Envelope
14) **Symmetric protein shell which encase the nucleic acid core of virus**
(a) Capsomere (b) Capsid (c) *Basidiomycetes* (d) Fungi imperfecti

Viral multiplication

15) **von Magnus phenomenon** (PGI-97)
(a) Is a normal replicative cycle (b) Virus yield has low haemagglutination (c) Virus has high infectivity (d) Virus yield has high haemagglutination titre but low infectivity

Viral genetics

16) **One virus particle prevents multiplication of second virus. This phenomenon is** (PGI-96)
(a) Viral interference (b) Mutation (c) Supervision (d) Permutation

Viral taxonomy

17) **Adeno virus**
(a) ds-DNA (b) Enveloped (c) Complex symmetry of capsid (d) None
18) **Human papilloma virus contains**
(a) ds-DNA (b) ss-DNA (c) ds-RNA (d) ss-RNA
19) **Lipid envelope is found in which virus** (PGI-98)
(a) Reo (b) Herpes (c) Picorna (d) All of the above
20) **In which of the following has genome double stranded nucleic acid** (PGI, Nov-13, May-10)
(a) Orthomyxoviruses (b) Poxviruses (c) Papovaviruses (d) Reoviruses
21) **Which of the following DNA viruses possesses a capsid with icosahedral symmetry and no lipid envelope** (PGI-87)
(a) Herpesvirus (b) Adenovirus (c) Poxvirus (d) Papovavirus
22) **Which is not a DNA virus**
(a) Parvovirus (b) Papovavirus (c) Poxvirus (d) Rhabdovirus
23) **Which of the following is not a RNA virus** (AIIMS, Nov-08)
(a) Ebola (b) Simian-40 (c) Rabies (d) Vesicular stomatitis virus
24) **Which is enveloped virus**
(a) Dengue virus (b) Nor walk virus (c) Hepatitis A virus (d) Adeno virus
25) **Non enveloped ss RNA virus is**
(a) Picorna virus (b) Pox virus (c) *Retrovirus* (d) *Bunyavirus*
26) **Which of the following virus has negative sense RNA** (AI -98)
(a) Rabies (b) Reovirus (c) Corona virus (d) Calci
27) **Negative sense nucleic acid genome is found in** (PGI, May-10)
(a) Polio virus (b) Rabies (c) Measles (d) Picorna virus (e) Influenza

Subviral agents

28) **Which of the following infectious agent lacks RNA**
(a) Virus (b) *Staphylococci* (c) Prions (d) *Cryptococcus*
29) **True about viroid is**
(a) Causes tumour in animals (b) Lack envelope like covering (c) Have only genetic material (d) Visible on light microscope
30) **True about prion protein disease is all except,** (AIIMS, Nov-01)
(a) Myoclonus is seen in 10% if the patients (b) Caused by infectious protein (c) Brain biopsy is diagnostic (d) Commonly manifest as dementia
31) **Prions are best killed by**
(a) Autoclaving 121^{0}C (b) 5% formalin (c) Sodium hydroxide (d) Sodium hypochlorite
32) **Which of the following is correct about prions** (AIIMS, Nov-12)
(a) Long incubation period (b) Destroyed by autoclaving 121^{0}C (c) Nucleic acid present (d) Immunogenic
33) **Prions are** (AI -08)
(a) Made up of bacterial and viral particles (b) Immunogenic (c) Infectious (d) RNA particles
34) **Prions consist of** (AIIMS, Nov-07)
(a) DNA and RNA (b) DNA, RNA and protein (c) RNA and protein (d) Only proteins
35) **Regarding prion protein which of the following statement is true** (AIIMS, Nov-08)
(a) It is a protein product coded in viral DNA (b) It catalyse abnormal folding of other proteins (c) It protects disulfide bond from oxidation (d) It cleaves normal proteins
36) **True about prion is** (AI -11)
(a) Encoded by viral genome (b) Associated with misfolding of protein (c) Non infectious (d) Immunogenic
37) **Which of the following is not a prion associated disease**
(a) Scrapie (b) Kuru (c) Creutzfeldt-Jacob disease (d) Alzheimer disease
38) **Which of the following is not a prion disease**
(a) Bovine spongiform encephalopathy (b) Transmissible mink encephalopathy (c) Scrapie (d) Progressive multifocal leucoencephalopathy
39) **Mad cow disease (Bovine spongiform encephalopathy) is similar to man in** (AI -11)
(a) Alzheimer disease (b) Creutzfeldt-Jacob disease (c) Hutington's chorea (d) Picks disease
40) **Mad cow disease (spongiform encephalopathy) occurs due to** (AIIMS, Dec -97)
(a) CJ virus (b) Arena virus (c) Kuru virus (d) Parvo virus
41) **Mad cow disease is due to**
(a) Slow virus (b) *Mycoplasma* (c) Bacteria (d) Fungi
42) **Human cannabilism is associated with**
(a) Q fever (b) Sleeping sickness (c) Trachoma (d) Kuru

43) **Fatal familial insomnia is associated with** (AI -99)
(a) Prion disease (b) Degeneration disease (c) Neoplastic disease (d) Vascular disease

Answers of MCQs & explanation

1) **(d)**
2) **(a)**
3) **(c)**

Follow **table-1** for explanation

4) **(a)**

- Follow section, **introduction, table-1 & resistance (heat and cold)** for explanation

5) **(b)**
6) **(a)**
7) **(c)**
8) **(b)**

Follow section, **morphology (size & shape)** for explanation

9) **(d)**
10) **(a) & (b)**
11) **(a)**
12) **(a)**

Follow section, **morphology [structure → nucleic acid (NA) / genome / core]** for explanation

13) **(b)**
14) **(b)**

Follow section, **morphology (structure → capsid or shell)** for explanation

15) **(d)**

- Follow section, **viral multiplication (Abnormal replicative cycle → von Magnus phenomenon)** for explanation

16) **(a)**

- Follow section, **viral genetics (recombination → viral interference)** for explanation

17) **(a)**
18) **(a)**
19) **(b)**
20) **(b) & (d)**
21) **(b) & (d)**
22) **(d)**
23) **(b)**
24) **(a)**
25) **(a)**
26) **(a)**
27) **(b), (c) & (e)**

Follow section, **viral taxonomy (table-2)** for explanation

28) **(b) & (c)**

- Follow section, **subviral agents (viroids)** for explanation

29) **(c)**
30) **(a)**
31) **(c) & (d)**
32) **(a)**
33) **(c)**
34) **(d)**
35) **(b)**
36) **(b)**
37) **(d)**
38) **(d)**
39) **(b)**
40) **All options are wrong**
41) **(a)**
42) **(d)**
43) **(a)**

Follow section, **subviral agents (prion)** for explanation

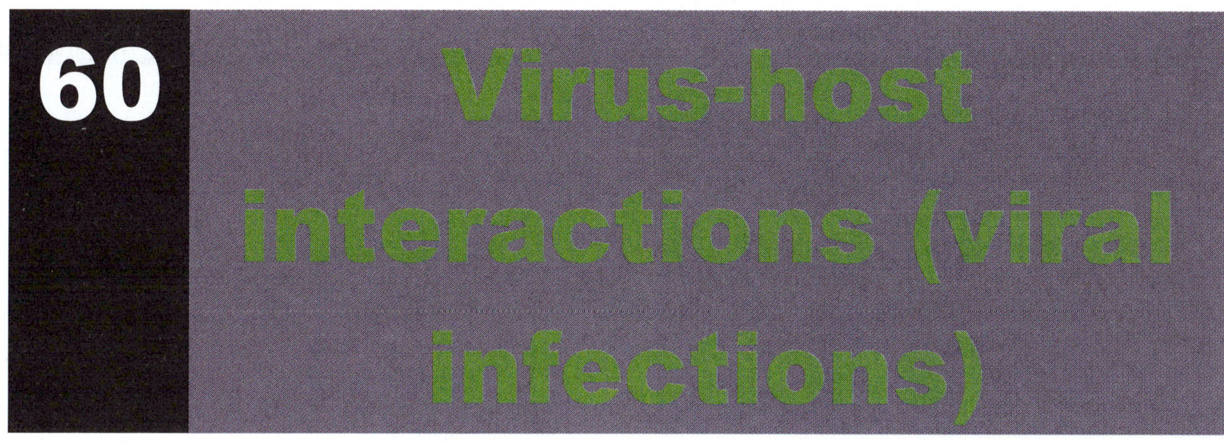

60 Virus-host interactions (viral infections)

Learning heading & subheadings

Introduction

Immune response (Ir) to viral infections

Introduction

❖ **Effects on cell by virus:** Sometimes virus causes no damage **called steady state infection** or causing following types of damage.

➢ **Types of cellular damage:**

- Cytocidal: Cell death like in polio virus (virus causing cell degeneration leading of cell death.
- Cytolysis: Cell lysis like in bacteriophage virus (virus multiply in cell to produce daughter viruses, so cell is not able to hold the weight & finally die).
- Cell proliferation: E.g. MCV.
- Malignant transformation: E.g. oncogenic virus.
- Cyto Pathic Effect (CPE): In tissue / cell culture.
- Morphological changes: E.g. inclusion body formation by rabies virus, ballooning of cells in herpes virus.
- Fusion of adjacent infected cell leading to polykaryocytosis or syncytium formation.
- Damage to chromosomes by measles, mumps, adenovirus, CMV etc.
- Antigenic changes on surfaces:

1. Haemagglutinin on surface of influenza infected cell: Causing haemadsorption of RBCs.
2. Tumour Ags on surface of cell infected by oncogenic virus.

➢ **Mechanisms of cellular damage:**

- Shutting down of protein or DNA synthesis.
- Accumulation of toxic viral molecules causing distortion of cellular architecture.
- Alteration of plasma membrane permeability, which release the lysosomal enzymes causing autolysis.

❖ **Mode of transmission:** Two categories as below

a. **Direct modes:** Not required mediator/vehicle.

1. **Droplet nuclei:**

Time	Infections
Antenatal / before birth / congenital / transplacental / teratogenic	- Rubella (congenital rubella syndrome) - CMV (congenital cytomegalovirus infection) - Herpes viruses (HSV causing congenital herpes simplex while VZV causing foetal varicella syndrome & congenital / neonatal varicella) - HBV - HIV-AIDS - Zika virus - Parvovirus B19 - Chikungunya virus
Intranatal / during birth (transcervical)	- CMV - HSV - HPV
Postnatal / after birth by breast feeding	- CMV - HIV

Table-1: Vertical viral infections

- Droplet nuclei/particles of saliva or nasopharyngeal secretion arise during coughing, sneezing, speaking, talking or invasive procedure (bronchoscopy) enter in to other host directly who is in close contact.
- Such particles are ≥ 5 μm in diameter & spread to short distance (< 3 feet) & directly enter in other host. However such larger particle can be filtered by nose.
- Particles ≤ 5 μm in diameter are traverse to long distance & produces the air borne (indirect) infection described later in this chapter.
- Infection by droplet nuclei is increased in close contact, overcrowding & lack of ventilation.
- **Viruses** transmitted by droplet nuclei are influenza virus, mumps virus, rubella virus, adeno virus & parvo virus B19

2. **Inoculation / injection under skin or mucosa:** By contaminated needle / syringe like HIV, HBV, HCV etc.
3. **Contact with skin/mucosa:**
- Sexually Transmitted Diseases / Infections (STD or STI): **Follow chapter → Systemic infections**
- Direct skin-to-skin contact: Like HHV-1 & 2 (HSV-1 & 2 respectively), HHV-3 (VZV), pox virus, MCV etc.
4. **Vertical: → Table-1**

b. Indirect modes: Required mediator/vehicle.

1. **Inhalation (air borne):**
- Particles arise during coughing, sneezing, talking or invasive procedure from patients which are ≤ 5 µm in diameter are traverse to long distance & produces the air borne infection.
- Some droplet nuclei settle over different objects & become part of dust & cause air borne infection.
- **Viruses** transmitted by air borne route are influenza virus, measles virus, VZV and haemorrhagic fever viruses causing pneumonia.
2. **Ingestion (food & water borne):** Polio virus, *Rotavirus*, HAV, HEV, adeno virus, reo virus etc.
3. **Blood borne:** By transfusion of blood or blood products like HHV-4 (EBV), HHV-5 (CMV), HHV-8 (KSHV), HBV, HCV, HDV, HTLV-I, HTLV-II, HTLV-III (HIV), parvovirus B19, zika virus etc.
4. **Saliva borne:**
- From human saliva like HHV-4 (EBV), HHV-6 (HBLV), HHV-7 (RK virus), ECHO virus, mumps virus etc.
- From monkey bite like Herpes virus simiae or B virus.
- From dog's saliva like rabies virus.
5. **Vector borne:**
- **Mosquitoes borne:**
- *Aedes*: Chikungunya virus, yellow fever virus, dengue virus, zika virus, Rift Valley fever virus (also by *Culex*), orungo virus etc.
- *Anopheles*: O'nyong-nyong virus.
- *Culex*: JEV, St. Louis encephalitis virus, Ilheus virus, West Nile virus, Murray Valley encephalitis virus, Oropouche virus, Rift Valley fever virus & African horse sickness virus.
- **Ticks borne:**
- Russian Spring Summer Encephalitis (RSSE) virus.
- Central European encephalitis virus.
- Western Siberian encephalitis virus.
- Powassan encephalitis virus.
- Louping ill virus.
- Kyasanur forest disease virus.
- Omsk haemorrhagic fever virus.
- Nairobi sheep disease virus.
- Crimean Congo Haemorrhagic Fever (CCHF) virus.
- Kolarado tick fever virus.
- **Sandfly borne:**
- *Phlebotomus*: Sandfly fever virus or three day fever virus, chandipura virus (also by *Sergentomyia*).
- *Lutzomyia shannoni*: Vesicular stomatitis virus.
- *Sergentomyia:* Chandipura virus.
6. **Fomites borne:** Contamination of fomites like towel, handkerchief, pen, pencils, clothes, cups, spoon, keys etc may transmit the infection like HAV, swine flu etc.
7. **Unclean hands & fingers:** Swine flu, SARS-CoV, MERS-CoV etc.

❖ Pathogenesis of virus or spread of virus in the body:

➢ **History:** Spread of viral infection was 1st studied by Fenner in 1948 by using the mousepox as the experimental model.

➢ **Pathogenesis: →Flow chart-1**

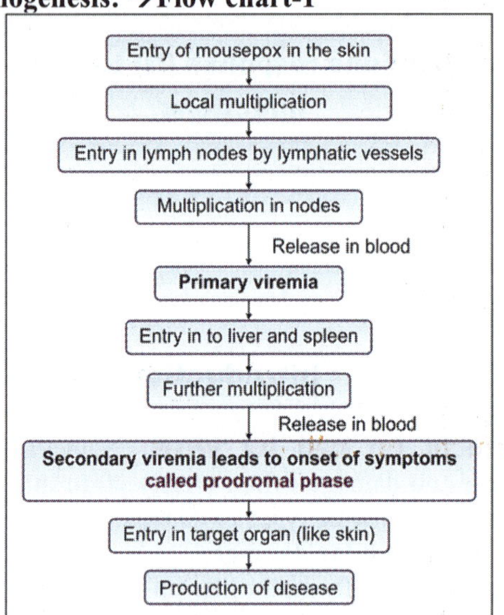

Flow chart-1: Pathogenesis of viral infections

➢ **Incubation period (IP):**

✪ **Definition:** It is an interval between entry of virus & development of clinical sign-symptoms.

✪ **Effective factors:** Duration depends on

- **Sites of entry, multiplication & lesion:**
  - Sites of entry & sites of lesion are same:
    - Short IP.
    - About 1-3days.
    - Like GIT virus: *Rotavirus*.
  - Sites of entry& sites of lesion are distant:
    - Long IP.
    - About 10-20days.
    - Like poliovirus: Enters by GIT & lesion in CNS.
- **Direct deposition of virus in blood:**
  - Short IP.
  - About 5-6 days.
  - Like dengue virus or yellow fever virus.
- **Nature of multiplication:** Long IP if virus multiply slowly
  - About months or years.

- Like in HBV IP is 2-6 months & in HIV after primary infection AIDS will start approximately after 10 years.

Immune response (Ir) to viral infections

❖ **Types of Ir:** Two main types.

A. **Specific (immunological):** Two subtypes.

i. **AMI (HI):**

- Different classes of antibodies are formed.
- IgM & IgG play major role in blood & tissue immunity.
- IgA: It provides local or mucosal immunity.
- Antibodies neutralise the virus by following mechanisms.
  - Prevent adsorption to cell.
  - Increase viral degradation.
  - Prevent release of viral progeny.
  - Along with complement causing surface damage to viral envelops & cytolysis of viral infected cell.
- Not all antibodies neutralise the virus but enhance the viral infectivity & contribute to viral pathogenesis by
  - Activation of complement system followed by lysis of infected cell.
  - Immune complex type of injury.

ii. **CMI:**

- Cytotoxic T cells (Tc) directly kills the viral infected cells.
- Sensitised T cells release the cytokines which enhance phagocytosis.
- Release of interferon (IFN) from T cells, which inhibits the viral multiplication & limit the infection.
- CMI also take part in DTH following viral vaccination.

B. **Non-specific:**

i. **Phagocytosis:**

- **Microphages**: No role in viral clearing.
- **Macrophage:** Phagocytose the virus and important in clearing virus from bloodstream.

ii. **Body temperature:**

- **Protection:** Fever act as a natural defence against viral disease as most viruses are inhibited by temperature above 39□^{0}C.
- **Damage:** However few exception are
  - Herpes simplex: Reactivated by fever and produce 'fever blisters'.
  - Herpes fibrilis: Accompany with fever & other bacteria like *Strept pneumoniae*, *Strept pyogenes*, *Haemophilus influenza* & parasite like malaria.

iii. **Age:** most viral infections are commoner and more dangerous at the two extremes of age.

iv. **Hormones:**

- **Corticosteroid:** Administration enhances most viral infection. Because of depression of immune response and inhibition of IFN synthesis.
- **Examples:**
  - Coxasackie B1 not cause disease in adult mice but induce fatal infection in mice treated with cortisone.
  - Varicella & vaccinia are lethal in patients on cortisone.

v. **Malnutrition:** Some viral infections, such as measles, produce a much higher incidence of complications and a higher case fatality rate in malnourished children than in well fed patients.

vi. **Interferon (IFN):**

➢ **History:** IFN was discovered in 1975 by Issacs and Lindemann, who showed that when chick CAM is treated with live or inactivated influenza virus produce antiviral substances which rendered the cell resistant to viral infection.

➢ **Definition:** It is a protein produce by vertebrate cell due to viral or non-viral stimulation.

➢ **Mechanism of action:**

- It has no direct action on virus but acts on other cells of same species, rendering them refractory to viral infection.
- It inhibit the viral transcription in infected cell.
- On exposure cell produce TIP (Translation Inhibiting Protein), which inhibit the viral translation without affecting the cell.
- TIP is actually a combination of three enzymes like protein kinase, oligonucleotide synthetase & RNAase.

➢ **Properties:**

- **Synthesis:**
  - IFN synthesis begins within about an hour of induction and reaches in high levels in 6-12 hrs.
  - It synthesised vary rapidly than Ab, hence play primary role in defence.
  - It is produced from host cells, not from virus so it a host protein.
  - Increased production: It increased by increasing the temperature up to 40^{0}C.
  - Decreased production: It decreased by increasing the O_2 tension & by steroid therapy.
- **Species specific:** IFN produce by one species can protect the same or related species. So IFN produce by human cell can protect human cell or related species like monkey but not other species like mouse or chick.
- **Cell's factors:** Cellular transcription and protein synthesis necessary for IFN production.
- **Virus's factors:**
  - IFN is not virus specific because IFN induce by one virus can protect against any viral infection.
  - Viruses are varying in their susceptibility to IFN.
  - Virus are vary in their capacity to induce IFN production like

61 Laboratory diagnosis of viral infections

Learning heading & subheadings

Diagnosis

📖 **Steps:**

- Sample collection
- Transportation & storage
- Sample rejection criteria
- Testing methods

Viral assay

Diagnosis

📖 **Steps:** Following are the different steps employed for diagnosis of bacterial infections.

◇ **Sample collection:**
◇ **Transportation & storage:**
◇ **Sample rejection criteria:**
◇ **Testing methods:**

Sample collection

❖ **Precautions:** Following precautions are to be taken before collecting the sample.

- Take all the aseptic precautions.
- Wearing the PPEs (Personal Protective Equipments) like disposable gloves, eye shields, apron, cap, mask & shoes cover.
- Selection of proper site.
- Use disposable needle & syringe.
- Container should be sterile, leak proof & securely fastened.
- Paired serum samples for serological tests one in acute stage & second 7-14 days later.
- Use appropriate transport medium whenever necessary.
- Filling the request form with complete data.
- If spillage of sample then wipe it with 10% sodium hypochlorite.
- Proper waste disposal of hazardous material.

❖ **Collection:**

- Collect the samples in Viral Transport Media (VTM).
- Collections of different samples according to system infected are shown in **table-1.**

System	Specimens
CNS	CSF
GIT	Gastric aspirate, gastric biopsy, rectal swab & stool
Genital tract	Discharge
Respiratory system	Sputum, throat or nasopharyngeal materials
Urinary system	Urine
Ear/eye	Ear / conjunctiva / corneal discharge or scrapings
Skin	Macular, popular or ulcer scraping or fluid
Common for HIV, HBV, HCV, HDV	Blood (serum)

Table-1: Samples according to system infected

Transportation & storage

❖ **Transportation:**

- Transport the samples with triple layer packing & biohazard symbol.
- More details about triple layer packing & biohazard symbol: Follow chapter → Laboratory diagnosis of bacterial infections.

❖ **Storage:** If there is delay in transport of sample then it should be stored in refrigerator.

Sample rejection criteria

- More details: **Follow chapter → Laboratory diagnosis of bacterial infections.**

Testing methods

Following are the different testing methods.

I. Microscopy

A. Light (simple) microscopy: It is useful to detect the following things.

➢ **Viruses:** Viruses are very small in size & difficult to see under the light microscope, however some virus **like poxvirus** can be examined under light microscope.

➢ **Viral antigens:**
- It is detected by **immunoperoxidase staining.**
- Tissue section or cells coated with viral antigens are stained by antibodies fixed with horse redish peroxidise enzyme, followed by adding of hydrogene peroxide & coloured reagent (benzidine derivative).
- Coloured complex formed can be viewed under light microscope.

➢ **Inclusion body:** It visible under light microscope.

✪ **Definition:** It is an intracellular aggregate of viral proteins or antigens.

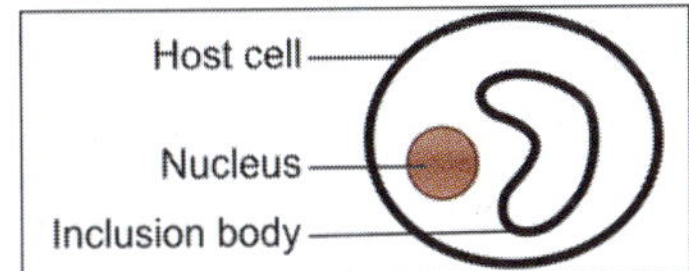

Figure-1: Intra-cytoplasmic inclusion body

✪ **Properties:**
- **Morphology:** Variable in size & shape.
- **Structure:** It includes protein from microbes & rarely from host cells.
- **Location:** It may be intranuclear, intra-cytoplasmic or mixed.
- **Staining properties:** Variable in staining reaction.
  - Acidophilic: Stain pink with Giemsa or eosin methylene blue. E.g. All the viral inclusion bodies are acidophilic like Cowdry type A, polio etc. except adenovirus inclusion body & "Owl eyes" in cytomegalovirus.
  - Basophilic: E.g. Adeno virus & "Owl eyes" in cytomegalovirus.

✪ **Mechanism of formation:** When genes from one organism are expressed in another the resulting protein sometimes forms inclusion bodies.

✪ **Etiological classification:** Two main types.

i. Infectious origin:

a. Bacterial (basophilic):
- H.P. (Halberstaedter Prowazeki) body: *C. trachomatis*
- LCL (Levinthal-Cole-Lillie) body: *C. psittaci*

b. Parasitic: *Babesia* spp. & malaria.

c. Viral: Three subtypes as per location in cell.

1. Intracytoplasmic (acidophilic): → Fig.-1
- **Poxviridae family**
  - Paschen body in variola virus infection (smallpox).
  - Guarnieri body in vaccinia virus infection.
  - Bollinger body in fowlpox virus.
  - Henderson-Peterson body or molluscum body (larger size 20-30μm) in molluscum contagiosum virus (MCV) infection.
- **Rhabdoviridae family:** Negri body in infected brain cell by rabies virus.

2. Intranuclear: Also **called Cowdry type inclusion body.** Two subtypes as follows.
- **Cowdry type A** (acidophilic)**:** Variable in size & with granular appearance.
  - Lipschutz body: In herpes simplex virus, varicella zoster virus.
  - Torres body in yellow fever virus.
- **Cowdry type B:** More circumscribed & often multiple.
  - Polio virus (acidophilic).
  - Adeno virus (basophilic).
  - "Owl eye" in cytomegalovirus (basophilic).

3. Both intranuclear & intracytoplasmic: Warthin-Finkeldey body in measles.

ii. Non-infectious origin: Inclusion body in RBCs is present in many non-infective conditions like as Hb precipitate, lead poisoning, anaemia etc.

✓ **Note: Pseudo-inclusions body**
- It is the invaginations of the cytoplasm into the cell nuclei, which may give the appearance of intranuclear inclusions body. It may appear in papillary thyroid carcinoma.

✪ **Clinical significance:** Easily examined under light microscope & helps in diagnosis of viral infection.

B. Electron microscopy:
- Viruses are very small, so simple microscopy is not useful & examined by electron microscopy.
- In some viruses it is the only method like viruses causing diarrhoea.

C. Immuno electron microscopy: Specific Ab is added to react with viral Ag & then examined under electron microscopy.

D. Immunofluorescent (IF) microscopy: Both direct & indirect are useful.

II. Viral culture

Virus can't grow over artificially prepared nutritional (chemically defined or cell free) media. Three techniques are employed for viral cultivation.

A. Animal culture:

➢ **History:** Human volunteer was used by Reed & colleagues in 1900 to work on yellow fever.

➢ **Commonly used animals:**

- **Infant suckling mice:**
  - Used for coxsackie & arbo virus.
  - Virus is inoculated by intraperitoneal, subcutaneous, intracerebral or by intranasal route.
- **Other animals are:** Guinea pigs, rabbits, ferrets etc.

➢ **Indication for growth detection in animals:** By death, disease or visible lesion production in animals.

➢ **Disadvantages:** Animal immunity & latent microbes in animal are interfere with viral growth

➢ **Uses:** To study the
- Immune response (Ir) or virus-host interaction.
- Pathogenesis.
- Epidemiology.
- Oncogenesis.

B. Embryonated egg culture:

➢ **History:** Developed by Good pasture in 1931.

➢ **Different parts to be inoculated: →Fig.-2**

i. Inoculation in Chorio Allantoic Membrane (CAM): →Pock assay
- Used for vaccinia or variola virus, HSV, pox virus & Rous sarcoma virus cultivation.
- Visible lesion **called pock** with different morphology by different virus.
- Number of pock will estimate the number of particle in suspension.

ii. Allantoic cavity: Used for orthomyxovirus (influenza) or paramyxovirus (mumps virus) cultivation.

iii. Amniotic cavity: Used for influenza virus, mumps virus, avian adenovirus, new castle disease virus etc.

iv. Yolk sac: Used for some viruses (may like herpes virus), *Chlamydiae* spp. & *Rickettsia* spp.

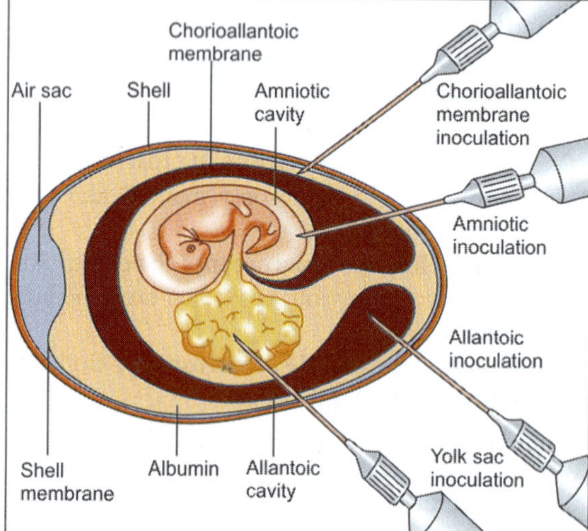

Figure-2: Different parts of hen's egg

➢ **Disadvantages:**
- It does not allow the study of virus-host interaction
- Many viruses are fail to grow, so primary isolation of such virus is not possible

➢ **Uses:**
- **Hen's eggs:** To prepare the vaccine of
  - Influenza virus: Influenza virus vaccine is prepared by allantoic cavity inoculation.
  - Yellow fever virus: 17D strain vaccine.
  - Rabies virus (Flury strain): Live attenuated chick embryo vaccine (non-neural vaccine).
- **Duck's eggs:** To prepare the inactivated duck egg (non-neural) vaccine for rabies virus.

C. Cell / tissue culture:

➢ **History:**
- Steinhardt was the first to use tissue culture in virology in 1913. He maintained the vaccinia virus in fragments of rabbit cornea.
- Enders, Robbins & Weller were made the method most useful for virus cultivation since 1949 by cultivating neurotropic virus like poliovirus in non-neural tissue.

➢ **Advantages:** Cheaper and easier.

➢ **Disadvantages:** Bacterial contamination in tissue culture can be overcome by using the antibiotics.

➢ **Types:** Three types of tissue culture.

i. Organ culture:
- Done by using bits of organs with preservation of normal anatomy & physiology.
- Useful for viruses which are special pathogens for certain organs.
- Example: Tracheal ring for coronavirus.

ii. Explant culture:
- Done by mincing the tissue **called explants culture.**
- Example: Mincing of adenoid tissue for adenovirus.

iii. Cell culture:

✪ **Preparation of cell culture media (monolayer):**
- **Pre-treatment:** Done by dissociating the tissue in to cells by using proteolytic enzymes (trypsin) or by mechanical shaking.
- **Preparation of media:** Such cells are washed, counted & suspended in containers like bottles, petri dish or test tubes or flask to prepare the cell culture media.
- **Adding of different ingredients in media:**
  - Media are enriched by adding vitamins, amino acids, salts, glucose, 5-10% foetal-calf serum.
  - Antibiotics to prevent the bacterial contamination.
  - Set the appropriate pH about 7.2-7.4
  - pH indicator (phenol red) to notice the pH change.
  - Buffer system contains bicarbonate in equilibrium with atmospheric CO_2 (5%).
- **Incubation of media:**
  - Tissue culture flask or bottle is incubated horizontally in presence of CO_2 (5%), either as a stationary culture or roller drum culture. Rolling in roller drum provides better aeration, which is useful for some fastidious bacteria like *Rotavirus.*

- On incubation cell adhere to glass or plastic surface & divide to form the cell monolayer in a week.

✪ **Subtypes of cell culture media:** Three types based on origin, chromosomal character & numbers of generation through which they can be maintained.

a. Primary cell culture:

- **Properties:** Prepared from normal cells, freshly taken from organs.
- **Disadvantages:**
  - High cost.
  - Short life: Limited numbers of divisions about 5-10.
  - Can't be maintained in serial culture.
  - Presence of latent virus in animal cell.
- **Examples:**
  1. Rhesus monkey kidney cell culture: For isolation of *Enterovirus,* myxo viruses & adeno viruses.
  2. Human amnion cell culture.
  3. Chick embryo fibroblast cell culture.
- **Uses:**
  - Primary isolation of virus.
  - For vaccine preparation.

b. Secondary or diploid cell strains:

- **Properties:**
  - Prepared from normal host cells.
  - Cells that retains the original diploid chromosome number & karyotype during serial sub-cultivation.
  - Undergoes around 50 divisions before goes to death.
- **Advantages:** Susceptible to wide range of human virus.
- **Examples:**
  1. Human diploid (secondary) fibroblast cell culture: For isolation of
     - Herpesviridae: HSV, VZV, EBV & CMV
     - Picornaviridae: *Enterovirus* (polio virus, coxsackie virus A 7, 9 & 16, ECHO virus etc.), *Rhinovirus* & *Hepatovirus* (*Heparnavirus*).
     - Paramyxoviridae: *Parainfluenzavirus.*
  2. HL-8 cell: Rhesus embryo cell strain.
  3. WI-38 cell: Human embryonic lung cell strain.
  4. MRC-5 cell.
- **Uses:**
  - Primary isolation of some fastidious virus.
  - For preparation of viral vaccine like HAV, chickenpox, rabies & MMR etc.

c. Continuous cell lines:

- **Properties:**
  - Cells that prepared from cancer cells which pass through indefinite divisions.
  - Maintained by serial subculture or stirred at -70^{0}C for future use.
- **Examples:**
  1. HeLa cell: Human carcinoma of cervix cell line.
  2. HEP-2 cell: Human epithelioma of larynx cell line.
  3. KB cell: Human carcinoma of nasopharynx cell line.
  4. McCoy cell: Human carcinoma of synovial cell line.
  5. Detroit-6 cell: Sternal marrow cell line.
  6. Chang C/I/L/K cell: Human Conjunctiva (C), Intestine (I), Liver (L) & Kidney (K) cell line.
  7. Vero cell: African green (vervet) monkey kidney cell line.
  8. BHK-21 cell: Baby Hamster Kidney cell line.
- **Uses:**
  - Primary isolation of virus.
  - Vaccine preparation like vero cells for rabies vaccine.

✪ **Methods for detection of viral growth in cell culture:**

a. Cytopathic effects (CPE):

- **Definitions:**
  - CPE: Many viruses are causing morphological changes in the cell culture **called CPE**.
  - Cytopathogenic virus: Virus causing CPE **called cytopathogenic virus**.
- **Properties:**
  - CPE can be examined under microscope.
  - Different virus produces specific CPE & helps in presumptive viral diagnosis.
  - CPE can appear early or late in the course of the viral infection.
- **Two types of CPE:**

1. **Cytocidal (cell death) or cell degeneration:** herpes virus, *Enterovirus* etc.
2. **Non-cytocidal:** Like
   - Inclusion body formation: E.g. in rabies & other viruses.
   - Transformation: E.g. in oncogenic viruses.
   - Infected cells are round up & piled up on top of each other: E.g. vesicular stomatitis virus.
   - Syncytium formation by cell fusion: E.g. in measles virus.
   - Clumping of cells looks like grapes: E.g. in adeno virus.
   - Discrete focal degeneration. E.g. in herpes virus.
   - Rapid CPE with crenation of cells & degeneration of entire cell sheet. E.g. in entero viruses.
   - Prominent cytoplasmic vacuolation: E.g. SV-40 virus.

b. Metabolic Inhibition (MI):

- When virus grow in culture produces acid due to metabolism.
- Addition of specific inhibitors will inhibit the metabolism & no acidic production, which is detected by pH indicator like phenol red.

c. Interference: Growth of non-cytopathogenic virus can be inhibited by growing it with cytopathogenic virus.

d. **Transformation:** Tumour formation by oncogenic virus in cell culture.

e. **Haemadsorption:**

- **Definition:** When haemagglutinating virus grows in guinea pigs RBCs containing culture, it adsorbs the RBCs on surfaces **called haemadsorption.**
- **Examples:**

- Orthomyxoviridae: Influenza virus.
- Paramyxoviridae: Mumps virus, parainfluenza virus & measles virus.
- Picornaviridae: *Enterovirus* (polio virus, coxsackie virus ECHO virus etc.), *Rhinovirus* & *Hepatovirus* (*Heparna virus*).
- Reoviridae: *Rotavirus, Orbivirus, Coltivirus* & *Orthoreovirus.*
- Rhabdoviridae: Lyssa virus 1 (rabies virus).

f. **Immunofuorescent microscopy:**

- Viral antigen from cell culture is detected by staining the culture growth with fluorescent labelled antibody & examining under the microscope.
- Highly sensitive & most useful method.

g. **Electron microscopy (EM):** Virus growth in cell culture is detected by examining the culture under electron microscope.

h. **Detection of enzymes:** Virus growth in cell culture is detected by detecting enzyme like reverse transcriptase in culture fluid.

i. **Gene detection:** By PCR or nucleic acid probe.

j. **Immunoperoxidase staining:** As described above under the heading of light microscopy.

✪ **Uses:**

1. **For cultivation of following microbes:**

- Bacteria: *Rickettsia* spp. *Orientia tsutsugamushi, Chlymydiae* spp. & *Ehrlichia* spp.
- Viruses: Almost all viruses are growing in cell free media. Other useful viral cultivation techniques for viruses are egg culture & animal culture.
- Fungi: *Pneumocystis jiroveci.*
- Few protozoa: *T gondii.*

2. **For preparation of vaccine:**

✪ **Limitations:** Organisms mentioned in **table-2** are not growing in tissue/cell culture media.

Parafungal agents	
Rhinosporidium seeberi	
Viruses	
Molluscum contagiosum virus (Also not growing in egg & animal culture)	All hepatitis viruses except HAV
Parvovirus B19	Rota viruses except type A
Parasites	
Metazoa	

Table-2: Microbes can't grow in cell culture media

III. Serological tests

- **Paired sera:** Examination of single serum is meaningless except for IgM specific test. For serological examination testing of paired sera are advisable as follows

- Acute sample: In early infection.
- Convalescent sample: 10-14 days after.

- **Different tests:** Antigens or antibodies are detected by ELISA, precipitation, RIA, CFT, agglutination, haemagglutination, flow through assay etc.

IV. Molecular methods

- **Advantages:** High sensitivity & specificity.
- **Disadvantages:** High cost & not available in peripheral centres.
- **Methods are**

- Hybridisation.
- PCR: For DNA viruses.
- RT- PCR: For RNA viruses.
- Real time PCR.

Viral assay

❖ **Definition:** It is an assay to measure or to quantitate the viral content of a specimen.

❖ **Methods:** Two types of assay.

A. **Measurement of total virus particle:**

i. **Direct count:**

- By simple negative staining the viral particles are directly counted by electron microscope.
- A known concentration of latex particles can be mixed with viral suspension.
- Ratio between latex particles & viral particles can gives idea about virus count.

ii. **Haemagglutination titre:**

✪ **Advantage:** Simple method.

✪ **Disadvantage:**

- At least 10^7 virus (like influenza) are required in specimens.
- Low sensitivity.

B. **Measurement of infectious virus particle:**

i. **Quantitative assay:**

✪ **Features:**

- It measures the actual number of infectious particles in specimen.
- It is like estimation of bacterial viable count.

✪ **Types:**

a. **Plaque assay:**

- **History:** It was introduced by Dulbecco in 1952.
- **Steps:**

- Viral suspension is added to monolayer of cell culture, allow for absorption & medium is covered by agar gel to spread of virus.
- Viral progeny spread to immediate vicinity of infected cell.
- In this situation each virus produce lesion **called plaques**, which is examined by unaided eye.
- Each plaque is assumed to come from a single viral particle.

b. Pock assay: →Follow embryonated egg culture

ii. Quantal assay:

✪ **Features:**

- It measures the presence or absence of particle in specimens.
- It can be done in animal, tissue culture or in eggs.

✪ **Steps:**

- Dilutions of virus are prepared.
- Constant volume of each dilution is injected into a number of test animals.
- At each dilution the proportion of infected individuals is scored (death or disease, cytopathic effect, recognition of progeny).
- Highest dilution that shows the effect in 50% of animals **called 50% infectious dose (ID_{50}).**
- ID_{50} is calculated by statistical method developed by Reed & Muench.

Question bank

Essay/Full question

1) Lab. diagnosis of viral infections.

Short notes

1) Inclusion body.
2) Viral culture.
3) Viral assay.

Short questions for theory/viva questions

1) Write four examples of intracytoplasmic or intranuclear inclusion bodies.
2) Name the inclusion body of following viruses. Variola virus, Vaccinia virus, fowpox virus & MCV
3) Define: Inclusion body & pseudo- inclusion body.
4) Write four methods to detect the viral growth in tissue culture.
5) Write four name of viruses which can be cultivated on human diploid (secondary) fibroblast cell culture.
6) Name four viral vaccines prepared by using embryonated egg culture technique.
7) Define: Pock & plaque
8) What is CPE?
9) Name four bacteria growing in cell culture media.
10) Name four viruses not growing in cell culture media.

MCQs for chapter review

Diagnosis

1) **Inclusion body is seen in -**
(a) *Rickettsiae* (b) *Chlamydiae* (c) *Mycoplasma* (d) *H pylori*
2) **Both intranuclear and intracytoplasmic inclusion is seen in**
(a) Pox virus (b) Herpes virus (c) Measles virus (d) Mumps virus
3) **Bollinger bodies are seen in**
(a) Chickenpox (b) Cowpox (c) Fowlpox (d) Smallpox
4) **Appearance of Cowdry type A inclusion bodies**
(a) Granular (b) Circumscribed (c) In polio (d) None
5) **Inclusion body present in rabies is**
(a) Negri body (b) Bollinger body (c) Lipschutz body (d) Torres body
6) **Inclusion bodies of vaccinia is known as** (PGI-86)
(a) Guanieri bodies (b) Negri bodies (c) Asteroid bodies (d) Schuffner bodies
7) **Owl's eye intranuclear inclusion body is seen in**
(a) Herpes zoster (b) Herpes simplex (c) CMV (d) EBV
8) **Influenza virus culture is done in**
(a) Chorio allantoic membrane (b) Allantoic cavity (c) Yolk sac (d) All
9) **Which of the following produces pocks on chorio allantoic membrane of chick embryo** (AIIMS, Dec-94)
(a) Myxo virus (b) Varicella (c) Herpes simplex (d) Cytomegalo virus
10) **Pocks on chick embryo are formed by all except** (PGI-97)
(a) Variola (b) Vaccinia (c) Chickenpox (d) Cowpox
11) **Viruses can be isolated from clinical samples by cultivation in the following except** (AI-05)
(a) Tissue culture (b) Embryonated eggs (c) Animals (d) Chemically defined media
12) **Which of the following is primary cell line (culture)**
(a) Chick embryo fibroblast (b) Hela cells (c) Vero cells (d) WI-38
13) **Human fibroblast cell line is used for cultivation of**
(a) Adenovirus (b) Poliovirus (c) HIV (d) Measles
14) **Hep-2 cells are types of**
(a) Primary cell culture (b) Diploid cell strain (c) Continuous cell line (d) Explant culture
15) **Which is not a cytopathic effect of virus**
(a) Syncytium formation (b) Budding (c) Ballooning and floating (d) Focal degeneration
16) **Susceptible cultured cells infected with which of the following viruses would exhibit haemadsorption with the appropriate erythrocyte** (AIIMS, 84, 93)
(a) Sindbis virus (b) Rabies virus (c) Measles virus (d) Respiratory syncytial virus
17) **Which of the following grow in cell culture media**
(a) *Chlamydia* (b) *Ureaplasma urealyticum* (c) *Pseudomonas* (d) *Trophyremma whippeli*
18) **One of the following virus is not a cultivable virus** (AI-97)
(a) Papova (b) Parvovirus B-19 (c) Herpes (d) Adenovirus
19) **Laboratory diagnosis of viral respiratory tract infection can be established by all of the following tests except** (AI-04)
(a) Detection of virus specific IgM antibodies in single serum specimen (b) Demonstration of viral antigens by indirect immunofluorescence assay in nasopharyngeal washing (c) Isolation of viruses using centrifugation enhanced culture (d) Detection of viral haemagglutination inhibiting (HAI) antibodies in a single serum specimen

Viral assay

20) **Viral plaques is made in lab for** (AIIMS, Dec-94)
(a) Quantitative assay of infectivity of virus (b) Diagnosis of virus (c) Qualitative assay of infectivity of virus (d) Type of virus
21) **Plaque formation in virus is done for** (AI-98)
(a) Isolation and typing of viruses (b) Cloning separation of specific viruses (c) Determining infectivity of viruses (d) Assessing of multiplication of viruses
22) **Virus quantification is done by**
(a) Egg inoculation (b) Haemadsorption (c) Plaque assay (d) Electron microscopy

Answers of MCQs & explanation

1) **(b)**

- *Rickettsiae*, *Mycoplasma* & *H pylori* are not producing any type of inclusion body

2) (c)
3) (c)
4) (a)
5) (a)
6) (a)
7) (c)

Follow section, **diagnosis [testing methods → microscopy → Light (Simple) microscopy → inclusion body)** for explanation

8) (b)
9) (c)
10) (c)

Follow section, **diagnosis [testing methods → culture → embryonated egg culture)** for explanation

11) (d)
12) (a)
13) (b)
14) (c)

Follow section, **diagnosis [testing methods → culture → cell / tissue culture)** for explanation

15) (b)
- Budding is the reproductive method of fungi & few bacteria like *Mycoplasma pneumoniae & Francisella tularensis*

16) (b) & (c)
- Follow section, **diagnosis [testing methods → culture → cell / tissue culture → methods for detection of viral growth in tissue culture → haemadsorption)** for explanation

17) (a)
- Follow section, **diagnosis [testing methods → culture → cell / tissue culture → uses)** for explanation

18) (b)
- Follow section, **diagnosis [testing methods → culture → cell / tissue culture → limitations & table-2)** for explanation

19) (a) & (d)
- For serological testing paired sera are advisable
- Follow section, **diagnosis (testing methods → serological tests)** for explanation

20) (a)
21) (c)
22) (c)

Follow section, **viral assay [methods → quantitative assay)** for explanation

62 Poxviridae

Learning heading & subheadings

- Classification:
- Antigenic structure:

Human diseases

- Variola virus
- Vaccinia virus
- Monkeypox virus
- Cowpox virus
- Buffalopox virus
- Orfpox virus
- Paravaccinia (pseudocowpox) virus
- Molluscum Contagiosum Virus
- Yabapox virus
- Tanapox virus

Classification:

- **Family:** Poxviridae.
- **Two subfamily:**

A. Subfamily: Chordopoxvirinae.

- **Genus:** Following are the genera.

a. *Orthopoxvirus*:

- Poxvirus infecting mammalian are **called** *Orthopoxvirus*.
- Following are the species.
  - Variola virus (natural virus causing smallpox in human).
  - Vaccinia virus (artificial virus).
  - Cowpox virus.
  - Buffalopox virus.
  - Monkeypox virus.
  - Cantagalo & Arcatuba virus.

b. *Avipoxvirus*:

- Poxvirus infecting birds are **called** ***Avipoxvirus***.
- Following are the species.
  - Turkypox virus.
  - Canarypox virus.
  - Fowlpox virus (Inclusion body **called Bollinger body**).
  - Pigeonpox virus.

c. *Capripoxvirus*:

- Poxvirus infecting goat & sheep are **called** *Capripoxvirus*.
- Following are the species.
  - Sheeppox virus.
  - Goatpox virus.
  - Lumpy skin disease virus.

d. *Leporipoxvirus*:

- Poxvirus infecting leporids like rabbits, squirrel or hares are **called *Leporipoxvirus***.
- Following are the species.
  - Myxomavirus.
  - Fibroma virus.

e. *Parapoxvirus*:

- Poxvirus infecting ungulates are **called** *Parapoxvirus*.
- Following are the species.
  - Human orf virus.
  - Paravaccinia (pseudocowpox) virus.
  - Bovine papular stomatitis virus.
  - Deerpox virus.
  - Sealpox virus.

f. *Suipoxvirus*:

- Poxvirus infecting swine (pig) are **called** *Suipoxvirus*.
- Following is the species.
  - Swinepox virus.

g. *Molluscipoxvirus*: Following is the species.

- Molluscum contagiosum virus (MCV).

h. *Yatapoxvirus*: Following are the species.

- Yabapox virus (Yaba monkey tumour virus).
- Tanapox virus.

B. Subfamily: Entomopoxvirinae.

- Do not infect the mammalian.

Antigenic structure:

- All pox share common nucleoprotein (NP) antigen.
- Antigenic cross reactivity is present in between th different pox viruses.
- Twenty different antigens like heat labile L, heat stable S, LS (complex of L & S), agglutinogen and haemagglutinin present in different pox virus.

Species	Reservoir	Distribution	Human disease
Orthopoxvirus			
Variola virus	Human	Eradicated	Smallpox
Vaccinia virus	Human	-	Local skin lesion (Artificial virus) & used for vaccination
Monkeypox virus	Rodents & monkeys	Africa	Rare, skin or systemic lesions
Cowpox virus	Cows	Europe	Rare, skin or systemic lesions
Buffalopox virus	Water buffalo	Indian subcontinent	Rare, skin lesions
Cantagalo & Arcatuba virus	Cattle	South America	Rare, skin or systemic lesions
Parapoxvirus			
Orf virus	Sheep & goats	Worldwide	Rare, local skin lesions **called contagious pustular dermatitis**
Paravaccinia (pseudocowpox) virus	Cattle	Worldwide	Rare, local skin lesions **called milker's nodule (node)**
Bovine papular stomatitis virus	Cattle	Worldwide	Rare, local skin lesions
Deerpox virus	Deer	Deer herds	Local pox skin lesions
Sealpox virus	Seal	Seal colonies	Local pox skin lesions
Molluscipoxvirus			
Molluscum Contagiosum Virus (MCV)	Human	Worldwide	Benign skin nodules **called molluscum contagiosum**
Yatapoxvirus			
Yabapox virus	Monkeys	Unknown	Local skin tumour
Tanapox virus	Monkeys	Africa (Zaire)	Rare, local skin lesions

Table-1: Poxvirus causing human disease

Human diseases

Four genera of *Poxviridae* with respective species causing human disease are listed in **table-1.**

Variola virus

❖ **History:** Microscopically identified by Buist in1887.

❖ **Use:** Useful as biological weapon.

❖ **Morphology:** → **Fig.-1**

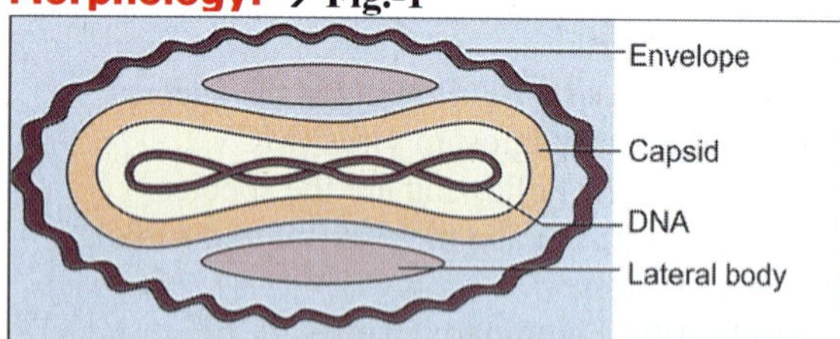

Figure-1: Morphology of variola virus (complex symmetry)

- **Shape:** Brick shaped.
- **Size:** 300 x200x100nm, largest of all animal viruses & only virus visible under the light microscope.
- **Genome & capsid:** ds-DNA surrounded by double layer capsid (complex variety of capsid).
- **Envelope:** Lipoprotein in nature.
- **Lateral body:** On either side of capsid (between capsid & envelop) a lens-shaped body is present **called lateral body**. Function is unknown.
- **Inclusion body**
  - **Called Paschen body.**
  - Intracytoplasmic.
  - Identified by Paschen in 1906 from smallpox lesion
  - Detected under light microscopy.
- **Multiplication:** Virus replicates in **cytoplasm** of infected cells.
- **Electron microscopy:** For rapid diagnosis.

❖ **Culture characteristics (C/Cs):**

i. **Egg culture:**

- Grow on CAM of 11-13 days old hen's egg and form 'pocks' in 48-72 hrs.
- Highest temperature above which pocks are not produced **called ceiling temperature.**
- **Variola:**
  - Pocks are small, shiny, white, convex, non- necrotic & non-haemorrhagic.
  - Ceiling temperature: For variola major is 38^0C & for variola minor is 37.5^0C.
- **Vaccinia:**
  - Pocks are large, irregular, greyish, flat, necrotic & haemorrhagic.
  - Ceiling temperature: 41^0C.

ii. **Tissue culture:**

- Commonly used cells are: Hela cells, Vero cells & chick embryo cell.
- Guarnieri bodies (eosinophilic inclusion bodies): Identified in stained smear.
- Vaccinia, not variola produce plaque in chick embryo cell culture.

iii. **Animal culture:** Monkey, rabbit, calves & sheep are useful.

❖ Resistance:

- Susceptible to UV light, formalin & oxidising disinfectants.
- Resistant to 50% glycerol and 1% phenol.
- Enveloped, even though not inactivated by ether.

❖ Pathogenicity:

➢ **Disease name:** Human pox caused by variola virus is **called smallpox.**

➢ **Nature & history of disease:**

- **Ancient scourge:** Killed many millions.
- **Last variola major:** It was detected in Saiban Bibi, a Bangldeshi woman at Karimganj Railway station, Assam in 24th may 1975.
- **Last variola minor:** It was detected in Merca, Somalia in October, 1977.
- **Last outbreak:** Natural small pox ceased in 1977, but small outbreak was occurred in August 1978 in Birmingham in medical school following accidental spread from laboratory. It was promptly identified & controlled but incident gave message regarding hazards of keeping stock. After that all stock were destroyed by direction from WHO.
- **Stock of virus & vaccine:** Large stock was maintained at CDC, Atlanta, USA and at Centre for Research on Virology & Bio-technology Koltsova, Russia but they were destroyed in June 30 1999. Large stock of small pox vaccine is maintained by WHO for rapid deployment in case of bioterrorism or re-emerging of disease.
- **Global eradication:**

- Globally eradicated on 8th may, 1980.
- Factors contributed in eradication were

1. Use of freeze dried vaccine.
2. Multiple puncture technique of vaccination by using bifurcated needle, which was simple, effective & economical.

➢ **Reservoir of infection:** No animal /vector reservoir but only human reservoir.

➢ **Source of infection:** Respiratory droplets.

➢ **Mode of transmission:**

- Via droplets/aerosol in early phase of disease.
- Via close contact.

➢ **Portal of entry:** Respiratory tract.

➢ **Sites:** Skin.

➢ **Incubation period:** 12 days.

➢ **Pathogenesis:** → **Flow chart-1**

➢ **Clinical features:**

✪ **Clinically two types of smallpox:**

1. Variola major: High mortality & classical smallpox.
2. Variola minor: Low mortality & alastrim.

✪ **Features:**

- **Prodromal phase:** Non specific febrile & prostrating flu-like illness last for 3-5 days.
- **Eruptive phase:** Characteristic rash – single crop of centrifugal exanthems passed through macular, vesicular & pustular stages (**fig.-2**) before scabbing and heal by scar formation in 2-4 wks.

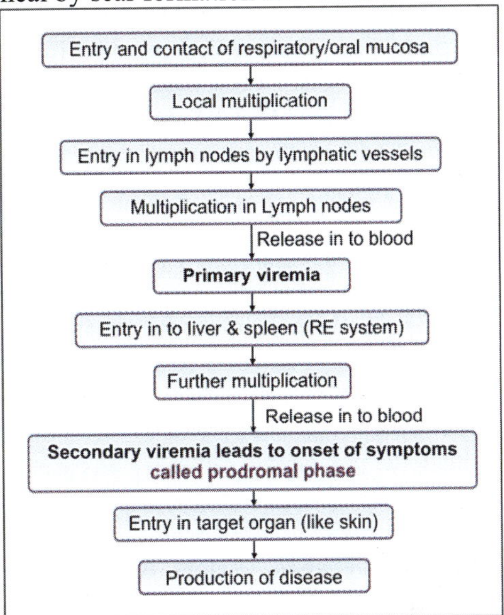

Flow chart-1: Pathogenesis of pox (variola) virus

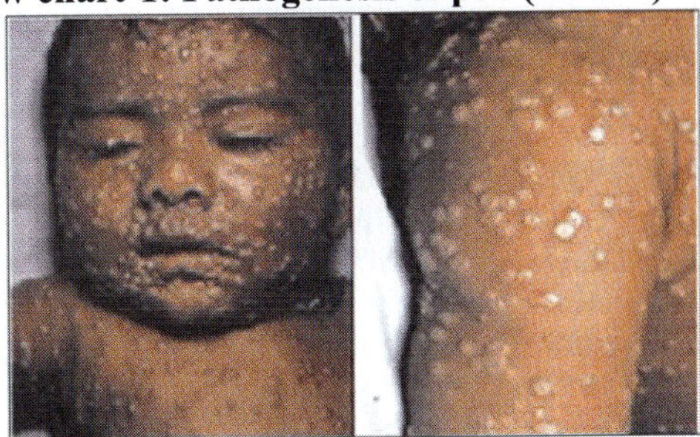

Figure-2: Small pox lesions

❖ Laboratory diagnosis:

➢ **Specimens:**

- **Prodromal phase:** Blood.
- **Eruptive phase:** Fluid, scraping or scab from lesion.

➢ **Testing methods:**

A. **Microscopy:** → **Follow morphology**

B. **Culture:** → **Follow C/Cs**

C. **Serological & molecular methods are also useful**

❖ Prevention:

- It is eradicated from the world & routine vaccination is now stopped.
- 1st vaccine of small pox was developed from cowpox lesion by Edward Jenner.
- Freeze dried vaccine was used for control. It is injected by multiple puncture with bifurcated needle in upper arm.

Vaccinia virus

- It is similar to variola virus & both can be considered together.
- Initial cowpox vaccine virus was maintained by serial arm-arm passage in human, it underwent some permanent changes & become different from cowpox & smallpox **called vaccinia virus.**
- As it not occurs in nature, so **called artificial virus**.
- Inclusion body produced by vaccinia virus **called Guarnieri body.**
- **Uses:**
- For preparation of smallpox vaccine.
- As a vector to prepare recombinant vaccine like HBV, HIV & rabies.
- To prepare pharmacological product like neuropeptide.
- **Disadvantage:** Not suitable as a vector for human use due to its pathogenic effect.
- **Pathogenicity:** Non-pathogenic but may cause local skin lesions.
- **Differences between variola & vaccinia virus: →Table-2**

Features	Variola	Vaccinia
Type of virus	Natural	Artificial
Ceiling temp.	$37.5^0/38^0c$	41^0c
Pock morphology	Small, shiny, white, convex, non- necrotic & non haemorrhagic	Large, irregular greyish, flat, necrotic & haemorrhagic
Plaque on chick embryo tissue culture	NO	Yes
Inclusion body	Paschen body	Guarnieri body
Pathogenicity	Small pox	Local skin lesion
Use for vaccine preparation	No	Yes

Table-2: Differences between variola & vaccinia virus

Monkeypox virus

- Clinically same as smallpox.
- Rodents are the primary reservoir followed by monkeys.
- Transmitted by direct contact with animals. Person-to-person transmission occurs rarely.
- Distributed in Africa.
- First outbreak was reported in USA in 2003 with more than 70 cases. It was transmitted from pet prairie dog that got infection from rodents.
- It produces local lesion like small pox but mild in nature & systemic illness like fever & lymphadenopathy.

Cowpox virus

- Rodents or cats are the primary reservoirs followed by cow.
- Cow lesions are present on udder or teats & enter in human during milking.
- Distributed in Britain & Europe.
- Fatal outbreak was reported in wild animals like cheetahs & elephants.
- Human lesions appear on hands or fingers & with rare systemic illness like fever.
- Distinguished from variola & vaccinia virus by haemorrhagic lesion in CAM & in rabbit skin & also by restriction endonuclease analysis.

Buffalopox virus

- It was identified from cattle in India in 1934.
- Lesions appear on hands of persons in contact of infected animal.
- Epizootic was occurred in buffaloes.
- Clinically as like smallpox & distinguished by laboratory methods.

Orfpox virus

- Disease of sheep and goats.
- Transmitted to human by animal contact.
- Single papulo-vesicular lesion with central ulcer on hand, forearm or face **called contagious pustular dermatitis** or **infectious labial dermatitis** or **ecthyma contagiosum** or **thistle disease** or **scabby mouth.**
- Virus is different from variola & vaccinia virus & morphologically similar to paravaccinia virus.

Paravaccinia (pseudocowpox) virus

- Morphologically similar to orf virus.
- Cow lesions are enter in human during milking.
- Human lesion is ulcerative nodule on skin **called Milker's nodule.**
- Different from cowpox as not grow in eggs, but grow in bovine kidney culture.

Molluscum Contagiosum Virus (MCV)

❖ **History:** MCV was first described & later it was named by Bateman in the early nineteenth century.

❖ **Geographical distribution & types:**
- Distributed worldwide.
- Four types of virus from MCV-1 to MCV-4.
- MCV-1 is the most common & most prevalent (75-90%) & MCV-2 is common in adults.

❖ **Morphology:** Same as other pox virus as described above under variola virus.

❖ **Culture characteristics (C/Cs):** Virus cannot be cultivated in egg, animal or tissue culture.

❖ **Pathogenicity:**

➢ **Disease name:** Disease **called molluscum contagiosum.**

➢ **Synonym:** Water wart.

➢ **Nature or history of disease:**

- Incidence has been increased globally since 1966.
- Approximately 122 million people were affected worldwide by MCV as of 2010 (1.8% of the population).

➢ **Reservoir & source of infection:** Human.

➢ **Mode of transmission:**

- Direct contact to infected skin or contaminated clothes or toys (Common use of towels by barbers or swimming pools).
- Sexual intercourse.
- Autoinfection by scratching the lesion or by contact of normal skin with infected skin.

➢ **Portal of entry:** Skin.

➢ **Sites:**

- Lesions are most commonly found on the face, arms, legs, torso & armpits in children (Except palm & sole).
- Adults typically have molluscum lesions in the genital region and this is considered to be a sexually transmitted infection; however, if genital lesions are found on a child, sexual abuse should be suspected.

➢ **Precipitating factors:**

1. **Age:** Common in children between 4-11 years & sexually active adults.
2. **IDDs:** Common in AIDS patients.
3. **Sexual activity:**

➢ **Clinical features:**

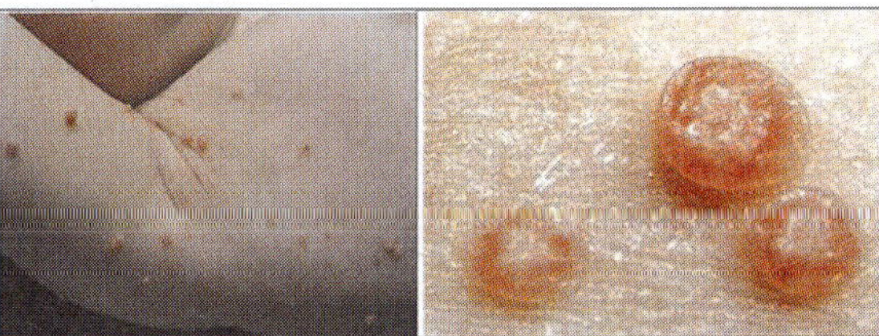

Figure-3: Lesions of MCV

- Lesions are flesh/pink-coloured, dome-shaped, pearly in appearance, 1–5 mm in diameter & with a dimpled centre **called umbilicated nodule** as shown in **fig.-3.**
- Lesions are generally not painful, but they may itch or become irritated.
- Self limited condition & disappear in 6 months to 5 years without treatment but last longer in person with IDDs.

➢ **Complications:** Picking or scratching the bumps may lead to

- Spread of the viral infection.
- Bacterial infection.
- Scarring.
- Eczema in 10% cases.

❖ **Laboratory diagnosis:**

➢ **Specimens:** Skin scraping or excision biopsy.

➢ **Testing methods:**

1. **Light microscopy:**
   - By using H & E stain.
   - Very large (20-30μm), hyaline, intracytoplasmic & eosinophilic inclusion bodies detected in in epithelial cells **called molluscum bodies** or **called Henderson-Petterson bodies.**
2. **Electron microscopy:** For virus detection.
3. **Culture: → Follow C/Cs**
4. **Molecular:** PCR.

❖ **Treatment:**

A. Medications:

- For mild cases, over-the-counter wart medicines, such as salicylic acid may shorten infection duration.
- Daily topical application of tretinoin cream.
- Cantharidin to be an effective and safe treatment for removing the lesions.
- Oral cimetidine has been used as alternative treatment for pediatric population as it is more difficult to use more invasive and discomforting application.
- Placebo-controlled trials have demonstrated the efficacy of a combination of essential oils & iodine in the treatment of molluscum in children.

B. Imiquimod: A form of immunotherapy.

C. Surgery:

- Cryosurgery: Liquid nitrogen is used to freeze and destroy lesions.
- Scraping them off with a curette.

D. Laser: Pulsed dye laser therapy is a safe and effective treatment for molluscum contagiosum and is generally well-tolerated by children.

Yabapox virus

- Monkey tumour virus related to poxvirus.

Tanapox virus

- Identified from the epidemic of febrile illness along the Tana river, Kenya in hence the name.
- Patient had single pock like lesion on the upper part of body.
- Antigenically unrelated to other poxvirus & can grow in human & monkey tissue culture but not in eggs.

- Monkeys are the susceptible animals.
- It is active in Zaire.

Question bank

Essay/Full question

1) Poxviridae.

Short notes

1) Classify Poxviridae.
2) Human pox virus.
3) Variola virus.
4) MCV.

Short questions for theory/viva questions

1) Who discovered the small pox vaccine? What was the source?
2) Name the four species of poxviridae causing human disease.
3) Name the inclusion body of following viruses: Variola virus, Vaccinia virus, fowpox virus & MCV.
4) Write the four differences between variola & vaccinia virus.

MCQs for chapter review

Classification

1) **Small pox belong to which genus of poxviruses**
(a) *Parapoxvirus* (b) *Capripoxvirus* (c) *Laporipoxvirus* (d) *Orthopoxvirus*
2) **Which of the following is not a pox virus** (AIIMS-92)
(a) Cow pox (b) Molluscum contagiosum (c) Small pox (d) Chicken pox
3) **Following virus is of pox virus**
(a) Variola (b) Coxsackie (c) ECHO (d) HSV

Antigenic structure

4) **The protection against small pox by previous infection with cowpox represent** (AIIMS.May-04)
(a) Antigenic cross reactivity (b) Antigenic specificity (c) Passive immunity (d) Innate immunity

Human diseases

5) **Vaccine preparation requires which virus as vector** (PGI, May-13)
(a) *Rhinovirus* (b) Vaccinia (c) Adeno virus (d) Ebola (e) Hepatitis B
6) **Which virus cannot be cultivated**
(a) Vaccinia (b) Variola (c) Molluscum contagiosum (d) Cowpox
7) **Which virus would not grow in egg, animal cells**
(a) Cowpox (b) Vaccinia (c) Variola (d) Molluscum
8) **Most common molluscum virus**
(a) 1 (b) 2 (c) 3 (d) 4
9) **Umbilicated nodules are produced by**
(a) Pox virus (b) *Enterovirus* (c) *Rhinovirus* (d) Myxo virus

Answers of MCQs & explanation

1) (d)
2) (d)
3) (a)
} Follow section, **classification** for explanation

4) (a)
- Small pox & cowpox viruses are belong to same family & protection is due to antigenic cross reactivity
- Follow section, **antigenic structure** for more explanation

5) (b)
- Follow section, **human diseases (vaccinia virus → uses)** for explanation

6) (c)
7) (d)
8) (a)
9) (a)
} Follow section, **human diseases (molluscum contagiosum virus)** for explanation

63 Herpesviridae

Learning heading & subheadings

Meaning: The word herpes is taken from the **herpein (Greek) = To creep or crawl**. This refers the spreading nature of skin lesion.

Classification: → **Table-1**

Morphology: →**Fig.-1(a)**

- **Shape:** Spherical or oval shaped.
- **Size:**
  - Enveloped virus: 300 nm.
  - Naked virus: 100nm.
- **Genome & capsid:** Virus contains ds-DNA surrounded by icosahedral variety of capsid.
- **Envelope:** Present with spikes about 8nm long.
- **Teguments:** Space between capsid & envelope is taken up by amorphous protein material **called teguments.**
- **Multiplication:** Virus replicates in **nucleus** of infected cells.
- **Inclusion body**
  - **Called Lipschutz body.**
  - Intranuclear Cowdry type-A.
  - Detected under light microscopy by Giemsa stain.
- **Tzanck test:**
  - **History:** Arnault Tzanck, 1947.
  - **Tzanck cells:** Multinucleated giant cells **called Tzanck cells**, are formed due to fusion of acanthoytic keratinocytes in pemphigus vulgaris, herpes simplex, herpes zoster & chicken pox.

Order: Herpesvirales, Family: Herpesviridae						
Sub family	**Genus**	**Species**	**Common name**	**Target cell type**	**Latency**	**Transmission**
α-herpesvirinae	*Simplexvirus*	HHV-1	Herpes Simplex Virus-1 (HSV-1)	Mucoepithelial	Neuron	Contact, aerosols
α-herpesvirinae		HHV-2	Herpes Simplex Virus -2 (HSV-2)	Mucoepithelial	Neuron	Close contact usually sexual
α-herpesvirinae	*Varicillovirus*	HHV-3	Varicella Zoster Virus (VZV)	Mucoepithelial	Neuron	Contact or respiratory route
γ-herpesvirinae	*Lymphocrypto-virus*	HHV-4	Epstein-Barr Virus (EBV)	B-cell, epithelial	B-cell	Kissing, transfusions transplantation,
β-herpesvirinae	*Cytomegalo-virus*	HHV-5	Cyto Megalo Virus (CMV)	Epithelia, monocytes, lymphocytes	Monocytes, lymphocytes and possibly others	Contact, blood transfusions, transplantation, congenital
β-herpesvirinae	*Roseolovirus*	HHV-6	Human B-cell Lymphotropic Virus (HBLV)	T lymphocytes and others	T -lymphocytes and others	Contact, respiratory route
β-herpesvirinae		HHV-7	R K virus	T lymphocytes and others	T -lymphocytes and others	Unknown
γ-herpesvirinae	*Rhadinovirus*	HHV-8	Kaposi's Sarcoma associated Herpes Virus (KSHV)	Endothelial cells	Unknown	Exchange of body fluids?

Table-1: Classification of Herpesviridae

scar. It present mostly on cheeks, chin, around mouth & on the forehead.

- **Other cutaneous variety of herpes:**
- **Napkin rash:** Occurs in infant on the buttock.
- **Fever blister or herpes labialis [fig.-2(a)] or cold sore:** Fever by any cause reactivates the virus & blister formation **called fever blister** or **herpes labialis.**

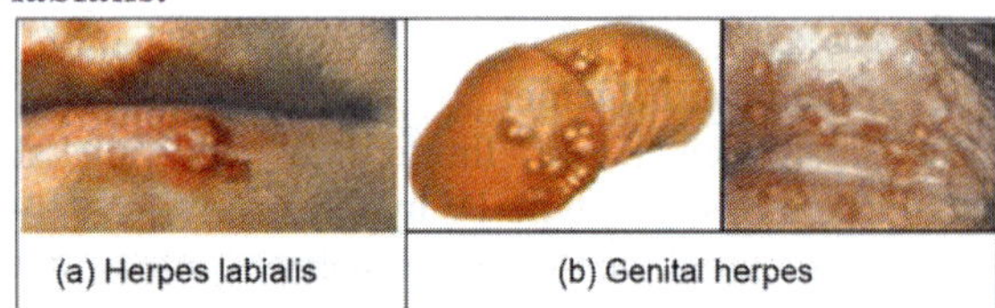

(a) Herpes labialis (b) Genital herpes

Figure-2: Herpes lesions

- **Eczema herpeticum:** Generalised eruption in children with eczema by herpes.
- **Herpetic whitlow:** Occupational herpes on fingers or hands in doctors or nurses characterised by vesicle with ulcer.
- **Herpes gladiotorum:** Mucocutaneous lesions present on the body of wrestlers.
- **Kaposi's varicelliform eruption:** Vaccinia virus also produce similar lesion, which clinically indistinguishable from herpes. Both are collectively **called Kaposi's varicelliform eruption**.

b. **Oral cavity:**

- **Primary infection:**
- Common in buccal mucosa.
- Acute gingivostomatitis & pharyngitis are the most common **primary infection**.
- Tonsilitis or ulcerative stomatitis are also the rare **primary infections.**
- **Recurrent infection:** Herpes labialis occurs as **recurrent infection** & present with painful vesicles near lips.
- **Complication:** Vesicle gets ulcerated & can predispose to **secondary bacterial infection**.

c. **GIT:**

- **Oesophagitis:** Present with dysphagia, substernal pain & weight loss.
- **Hepatitis:** It is the inflammation of liver.
- **Rectal & perianal lesions:** Occurs in homosexual.

d. **Respiratory system:** Pharyngitis, tracheobronchitis & pneumonitis.

e. **Ocular herpes:** More by HSV-1.

- **Conjunctiva:** Follicular conjunctivitis with vesicle of lid.
- **Cornea:** Acute keratoconjunctivitis & dendritic ulcer which may heal with scar or with corneal blindness.
- **Retina:** Choreoretinitis & acute necrotising retinitis.

f. **CNS infection:**

- **Encephalitis:**
- Acute onset with fever & neurological symptoms.
- Occurs in 10-20% cases with 95% chances are in HSV-1 than HSV-2.
- It acquired by olfactory bulb in children & in adult it occurs due to reactivation from trigeminal nerve.
- Involve the temporal lobe at most.
- In neonates sometimes HSV-2 may cause encephalitis without any skin lesions.
- **Meningitis:** Self limiting disease & healed in weeks without sequelae. Recurrent condition **called Mollaret's meningitis.**
- **Complications:** Also causes
- Sacral region (Autonomous nerve system involvement).
- Transverse myelitis.
- Guillian –Barre syndrome.
- Bell's palsy (Peripheral nerve system involvement)

g. **Visceral:** Disseminated infections in patients with IDDs, malnutrition & burns.

h. **Genital:**

- **Primary infection [Fig.-2(b)]:** It is more severe & present with fever & severe painful vesiculo-ulcerative lesion on external genitalia, while latent infection is mild.

i. **Neonatal (congenital) herpes:**

- Transmitted in utero, during birth or after birth.
- Risk is more with HSV-2 (75% of total cases) than HSV-1 & with primary infection than recurrent infection in mother.
- **Localised lesion:** Occurs over skin, eyes or mouth.
- **Generalised lesion:** In multiple organs including encephalitis with high mortality & survival with neurological impairment.

j. **Oncogenic (not proved):** HSV-1 associated with carcinoma of lips & HSV-2 associated with carcinoma of cervix.

❖ Laboratory diagnosis:

➢ **Specimens:** Vesicle fluid, scraping from lesion, saliva, corneal scraping, CSF or brain biopsy at autopsy.

➢ **Testing methods:**

A. **Microscopy: → Follow morphology**

B. **Culture: → Follow C/Cs**

C. **Serological tests:**

- Primary infection: High Ab titre
- Latent infection: Low Ab titre
- Tests are: CFT, ELISA or neutralisation based test.

D. **Molecular methods:** PCR or DNA hybridisations are the useful methods for diagnosis & for differentiation between HSV-1 & 2.

❖ **Prevention:** No effective vaccine is developed. It is controlled by avoiding contact with infected person & also by safe sex.

❖ Treatment:

- Idoxuridine: Used topically for eye infection.

- Acyclovir & vidarabin: Drug of choice for deep & systemic infection.
- Early treatment with intravenous acyclovir improves the outcome of encephalitis.
- Valacyclovir and famciclovir are effective orally.
- When resistance develop to these drugs, foscarnet may be useful.

HHV-3

❖ **Common name:** Varicella Zoster Virus (VZV).

❖ **History:**
- Weller & Stoddard isolated the virus from both, chickenpox & zoster lesions, but they were not cleared that both lesions were due to same virus.
- This confusion was cleared by Von Bokay in 1888 & he noticed that both lesions were due to same virus.
- Differences between two lesions were defined by Heberden in late 18th century.

❖ **Geographical distribution & genotype (clade):** Worldwide distribution. There are five clades of VZV as follows.
- Clade1 & 3: European/North American strain.
- Clade 2: Asian strain, especially from Japan.
- Clade 4: Strain from Europe but its geographic origins need further clarification.
- Clade 5: Appears in India.

❖ **Morphology:** Same as like HSV.

❖ **Culture characteristics (C/Cs):**

i. **Egg culture:** } No growth
ii. **Animal culture:** }
iii. **Tissue culture:** Commonly used cells are: Hela cells, Vero cells, human embryonic cell culture, human amnion & human fibroblasts.

❖ **Antigenic structure:** Only 1antigenic type & can be differentiated from HSV-1 & 2 by specific antisera.

❖ **Immunity:** Single attack confers long lasting immunity.

❖ **Clinical type:** It produces two types of disease (Suggested by Von Bokay in 1889) like **varicella** (chickenpox → Primary infection) & **zoster** (herpes zoster or zona or shingles → Latent infection), hence **called varicella- zoster virus (VZV)**.

Varicella (Chickenpox)

➢ **Pathogenicity:**

✪ **Nature of disease:** In children it is common but mild while in adults it is rare but severe.

✪ **Reservoir of infection:** Human.

✪ **Source of infection:** Skin, buccal mucosa lesion, vesicular fluid & aerosols. Infectivity is maximum in early stage, decrease with advancing of lesion & scabs are generally non-infectious.

✪ **Mode of transmission:**
- Via droplets/aerosols.
- Via close contact.
- Vertical from mother to child.

✪ **Incubation period:** 14-21 days.

✪ **Portal of entry:** Skin or mucosa (conjunctiva) or respiratory tract.

✪ **Sites:** Mainly on trunk & spread to face, arms & legs.

✪ **Precipitating factors (epidemiological determinants):**

1. **Age:** Usually mild form in childhood but more severe in adults & during pregnancy.
2. **Pregnancy:** More severe infection.
3. **IDDs:** More common in person with IDDs like AIDS.

✪ **Pathogenesis:** → **Flow chart-2**

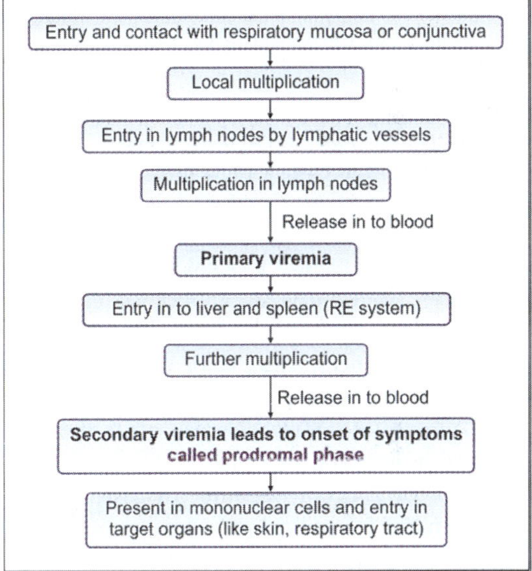

Flow chart-2: Pathogenesis of chickenpox

✪ **Clinical features:**

i. **In children:**

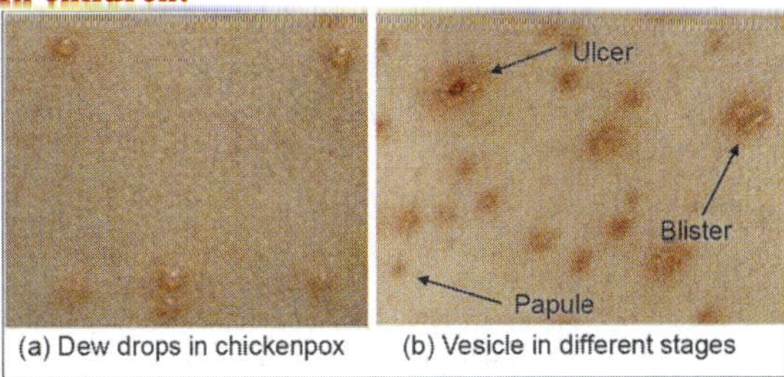

Figure-3: Chickenpox

- **Prodromal (pre eruptive) phase:** Mild illness like fever, back pain & malaise.
- **Eruptive:** Characteristic rash developed with following features.

- Centripetal, mainly on trunk & look like a "**dew drop**" lying on skin as shown in **fig.-3(a).**
- It spread less common to arms & legs.
- It passes through the stage of macule, papule, vesicle, pustule & may be ulcer **[fig.-3(b)]** & scab.
- Oral lesions: Vesicle form of rash sometimes also develops in oral mucosa, gingival, tongue, palate & pharynx. Vesicle gets rupture to form painless ulcer.

ii. In adults: Entire disease is more severe than children and rash is very profuse.

iii. Varicella in pregnancy: Primary infection during pregnancy is more severe and complicated to pneumonia. Chances of infection to foetus depend on period of gestation.

a. Infection in 1st half (early) of pregnancy: Usually foetus is asymptomatic and 3% chance of foetal transmission **called foetal varicella syndrome**, which is characterised by

- Scarring of skin.
- Hypoplasia of limbs.
- CNS defects.
- Eye defect like choreoretinitis.
- Infant's death.

b. Infection near the time of delivery (late half of pregnancy): The condition **called congenital (neonatal) varicella.** Chickenpox is more severe for new born if it developed to mother in late pregnancy. However severity is variable as follows.

1. **Mother rash occur a weeks or more before delivery:** Both virus & antibodies can enter in foetus & foetus can escape the disease.
2. **Mother rash occur less than a weeks or in two days of delivery.**

- Only viruses, no antibodies can cross the placenta & develop neonatal varicella.
- It may vary from a mild disease to a fatal disseminated infection.

✪ **Complications:**

- Secondary bacterial infection of the vesicles by *Staphylococcus* or *Streptococcus.*
- Encephalitis/encephalopathy: Most common extracutaneous site is CNS (or most common complication) following chickenpox.
- Viral pneumonia: Most serious complication following chickenpox.
- Haemorrhagic chickenpox.
- Acute cerebral ataxia.
- Reye's syndrome: Characterised by acute encephalopathy with fatty degeneration of liver. Aspirin should be avoided as it increases the risk of Reye's syndrome.

➢ **Laboratory diagnosis:** Diagnosed more by it's clinical presentations & laboratory help is rarely required. Laboratory diagnosis is required only for atypical presentations, particularly in the immunocompromised patient.

✪ **Specimens:** Vesicle fluid & scraping from lesions.

✪ **Testing methods:**

A. Microscopy:

- **Direct detection:** By Tzanck test.
- **Electron microscopy (EM):** May be used for vesicle fluids but cannot distinguish between HSV and VZV.
- **Immunofluorescent (IF) microscopy:** From skin scrapings can distinguish between HSV and VZV.

B. Culture: → Follow C/Cs.

C. Serological tests: ELISA for IgM (recent infection) & IgG (past infection) & Counter Immuno Electrophoresis (CIE).

D. Molecular methods: PCR.

➢ **Prophylaxis:** Two methods.

a. Active immunisation:

- **Types of vaccine:**

1. **Live attenuated vaccine:**

- It was developed by serial passage of virus in tissue culture in 1974 by Takahashi in Japan from a **patient named Oka**, hence **called Oka strain**.
- Heat labile & stored frozen.

2. **Modified lyophilised form of the vaccine:**

- It is now available.
- Stored between 2-8^{0}C.

- **Dose & route:**

- For children < 12 years: Single SC dose.
- For children > 12 years: Two SC dose, at 6-10 weeks apart.

- **Reaction:** Local vesicle develops, but heals quickly.
- **Contraindication:** Pregnancy.

b. Passive immunisation: By Varicella Zoster Immunoglobulin (VZIg).

- **Indication:** For immunodeficient patients.
- **Dose & route:** 1.25-5ml by IM route within 72 hours of infection.
- **Disadvantage:** Not useful for treatment.

➢ **Treatment:**

- **Indication:** For immunodeficient, elders and complicated varicella.
- **Drugs:**

- Steroids are contraindicated, as it enhances the risk of pneumonia and disseminated disease.
- Chicken pox in children: Symptomatic treatment is given & no antiviral drugs.
- Chicken pox in adults: Acyclovir.
- Zoster: Famciclovir or valcyclovir are effective.
- Post herpetic neuralgia: Gabapentin, analgesics & anti viral drugs.

Zoster (herpes zoster or zona or shingles)

- **Meaning:** Herpes from **herpein = to creep + Zoster from zoster = girdle.**
- **Pathogenicity:** It is due to viral reactivation.

Precipitating factors:

1. **Age:** Usually in old age around 50 years.
2. **IDDs:** More common in person with HIV infection & other IDDs.
3. **Malignancy:** Hodgkin's disease.

Pathogenesis:

- After primary infection, virus remains latent in trigeminal (semilunar/Gasserian or Gasser's) ganglion for several years & reactivated in old age around 50 years when immunity waned (due to disease like AIDS, age factor etc.) or by other stimuli.
- Virus tracks down the area supplied by spinal cord segment D3-L2 & ophthalmic branch of trigeminal nerve & rarely by facial nerve.
- The reactivation is associated with nerve.
- Inflammations with pain precede to skin lesion.
- Virus produce zoster lesion in skin or mucosa.

Clinical features:

- **Nerve:**
  - Intensive pain which may last for months (**post-herpetic neuralgia**).
  - Pain & paresthesia may persist for weeks / months.
- **Skin:** The rash is identical in nature but limited distribution & heals in 2 weeks.
- **Eyes:**
  - Herpes zoster ophthalmicus is common & problematic.
  - Two or more ocular features are keratitis, conjunctivitis, episcleritis, iridocyclitis & glaucoma.
- **Ears:** Ramsay hunt syndrome characterised by eruption in external auditory canal.

Complications:

- Lower motor neuron paralysis.
- Meningoencephalitis.
- Generalised herpes by haematogenous spread.

- **Diagnosis:** Same as chickenpox.
- **Treatment:** Follow chickenpox.

HHV-4

Common name: Epstein - Barr Virus (EBV).

History: Virus was observed in culture lymphoma cells by Epstein, Barr & Achong in 1964.

Geographical distribution & genotypes:

- Distributed worldwide.
- Two genotypes like EBV type 1 & EBV type 2 based on digestion of genome by restriction enzyme and comparing the resulting digestion patterns by gel electrophoresis.
- Both types are equally prevalent in Africa but type 1 is dominant in rest of the world.
- Two subtypes have different EBV nuclear antigens. Both are differ in their transforming capabilities & reactivation ability.

Morphology: Same as like other HSV but antigenically different.

Culture characteristics (C/Cs): Not useful.

Resistance: Enveloped, inactivated by fat solvent like ether, chloroform, bile salts & alcohol.

Antigenic structure: Three classes of antigens.

1. Early antigens: These are non-structural antigens help in viral replication.
2. Late antigens: These are structural antigens of viral capsid & envelop.
3. Latent phase antigens: These are synthesized during latent infection like
   - EBV nuclear antigen: It has six subtypes.
   - EBV latent membrane antigen: It has two subtypes.

Immunity: Antibodies are formed but not protective.

Pathogenicity:

- **Disease name:** EBV produces
  1. Oral hairy leukoplakia.
  2. Infectious mononucleosis.
  3. Malignancies: Like
     - Nasopharyngeal carcinoma.
     - Burkit's lymphoma.
     - Lymphoma (Hodgkin's & Non-Hodgkin's lymphoma).
- **Nature of disease:** EBV is ubiquitous. Virus can produce the periodic reactivation, latent infection & lifelong persistence.
- **Reservoir of infection:** Human.
- **Source of infection:** Human saliva, blood or blood products.
- **Mode of transmission:**
  a. **Direct:** Oral contact during kissing, so **called kissing disease.**
  b. **Indirect:** By transfusion of blood/blood products & bone marrow transplantation.
- **Incubation period:** 4-8 weeks.
- **Portal of entry:** Oral mucosa or skin (skin in case of blood transfusion).
- **Sites:** B lymphocytes.
- **Precipitating factors (epidemiological determinants):**

1. **Age:**
   - EBV is common in infant & children of developing countries & usually asymptomatic.
   - EBV is common in adolescence & early adulthood patient of affluent countries & develops IM.
2. **IDDs**: Like AIDS or malaria or organ transplant.

3. **Genetic factors:** EBV infection is associated with X-linked lymphoproliferative (XLP or Duncan syndrome) disease.
4. **Environmental & racial factor:**
   - Nasopharyngeal carcinoma is common in men of **Chinese** origin.
   - Hyperendemic malaria prevalent in **Africa** is impairing the immune system of children & co-infection with EBV produces Burkit's lymphoma.
5. **Co-infection**: EBV infection is also associated with CMV infection.

➢ **Pathogenesis & clinical features: → Flow chart-3 & fig.-4.**

➢ **Complications:**
- **Most common:** Neurological like meningitis / meningoencephalitis.
- **Others:** Splenic rupture, cardiac, pulmonary & haematological (autoimmune haemolytic anaemia may be due to formation of cold agglutinin) complications.

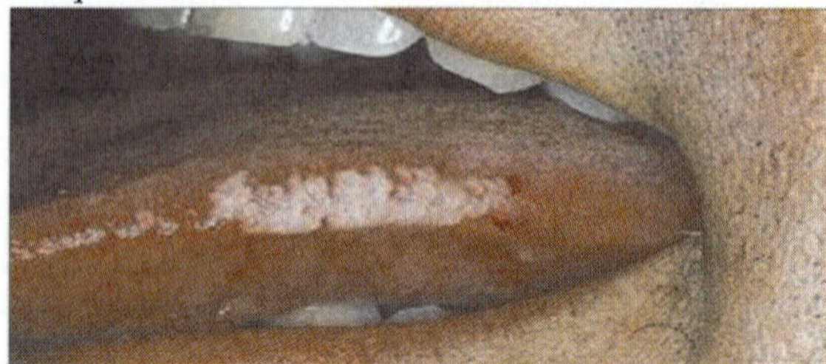

Figure-4: Oral hairy leukoplakia

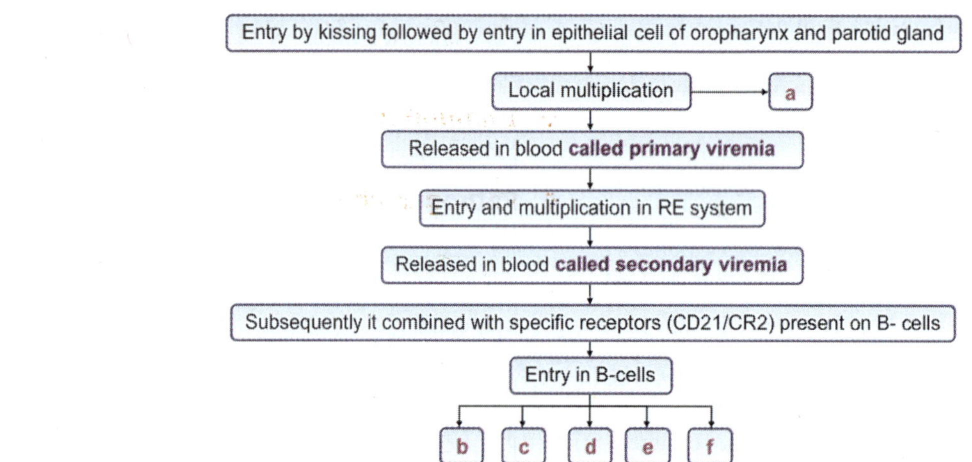

a. **Shedding and malignancies:** Shedding in saliva for months or long time and produce nasopharyngeal carcinoma.
b. **Cell lysis:** Lysis of B-cell and release of progeny virus
c. **Long time survival in B-cell:** It transformed (immortalised) the B –cell.
d. **Reactivation:**
1. **In immunocompetent person:** Checked by T-cell and no reactivation
2. **In immunodeficient person:** Following types of malignant lesions are produced
- **In patient with malaria:**
  - Hyperendemic malaria prevalent in Africa is impairing the immune system of children and co-infection with EBV produces the Burkit's lymphoma. Memory B cells are the reservoir of EBV and Burkit's lymphoma is the tumour of B cells.
  - Immunosuppressive effect of malarial parasite allows the virus proliferation and interference with immune mechanisms to neoplastic cells
- In patient with AIDS:
  - Reactivation of virus in person with AIDS and produce the lymphoma (Hodgkin's and Non-Hodgkin's lymphoma).
  - EBV-DNA regularly found in tumour cell.
- **In patient with AIDS and organ transplantation:** Oral hairy leukoplakia characterised by white patch on the side of the tongue (**fig.-4**) with a corrugated or hairy appearance. This white lesion cannot be scraped off; it is benign and does not require any treatment, although its appearance may have diagnostic and prognostic implications for the underlying condition like AIDS. The white appearance is created by hyperkeratosis (overproduction of Kertain) and epithelial hyperplasia.

e. **Polyclonal activation of B-cell (autoimmunisation):** To produce heterophile-Ab, detected by **Paul-Bunnel test**
f. **Infectious mononucleosis / glandular fever / kissing disease:**
- Formation of Ag (neoantigen) on B-cell surface, which induce blast-transformation in T-cell.
- Multiple atypical (blast) T-cell are examined in peripheral smear **called infectious mononucleosis**.
- **Characterised by:**
  - Usually a self-limited disease and resolved in 2-4 weeks
  - It consists of fever, sore throat (most common symptom), lymphadenopathy (most common sign), splenomegaly and mild transient rash
  - Jaundice may be seen due to hepatitis.
  - Presence of > 20% atypical lymphocytes (lymphocytosis not monocytosis) in the blood. Atypical lymphocytes are characterised by round or irregular nuclei with abundant flowing cytoplasm taking dark staining at periphery.
- Other causes of infectious mononucleosis:
  - **Infectious:** CMV, *Toxoplasma gondii* and HHV-6 (variant - B).
  - **Non-infectious:** Non-specific stimuli.

Flow chart-3: Pathogenesis & clinical features of EBV

Features	Paul Bunnell test (performed 1st)	Differential absorption test		
		Serum treated with guinea pig kidney cells	Serum treated with ox RBCs	Paul Bunnell test (Repeat)
Infectious mononucleosis	+Ve	No absorption	Absorption	+Ve= Pre-treatment with guinea pig kidney cells -Ve= Pre-treatment with ox RBCs
Serum therapy	+Ve	Absorption	No Absorption	-Ve for both sera
Normal serum	+Ve	Absorption	No absorption	+Ve= Pre-treatment with ox RBCs -Ve= Pre-treatment with guinea pig kidney cells

Table-3: Differential absorption test

❖ Laboratory diagnosis:

➢ **Specimens:** Blood, saliva etc.

➢ **Testing methods:**

A. Microscopy:

- Indirect IF microscopy is useful.
- Other details: Follow morphology.

B. Blood picture:

- Initially leucopenia due to reduction in polymorph count but later leucocytosis due to appearance of abnormal mononuclear cell (atypical lymphocytes / blast T cells). > 20% lymphocytes are atypical in peripheral blood.
- Atypical lymphocytes in peripheral smear.

C. Cell culture: Time consuming, so rarely useful.

D. Serological tests: Best method.

i. Tests for detection of antigens: Like viral capsid-Ag.

- ELISA, CFT, gel diffusion techniques are useful.

ii. Tests for detection of antibodies: Two types of antibody.

a. Tests for detection of heterophile (non-specific) Abs:

1. Paul-Bunnell test:

♣ **History:** It was developed by John R Paul (American physician, 1893-1971) & Walls W. Bunnell (American physician, 1902-1966).

♣ **Principle:** Based on detection of heterophile antibodies by agglutination reaction. Heterophile antibodies have the ability to agglutinate red blood cells of different animal species like sheep, horse & cow/ox. The Paul-Bunnell test uses sheep RBCs.

♣ **Antibody:**

- Patient serum contains heterophile antibodies.
- In infectious mononucleosis, IgM heterophile antibodies appear early in 1st week in 40% cases & in 3rd week in 80-90% cases & remain detectable for the first 3 months of infection & then disappear.
- Heterophile antibodies are also present in normal individual or after serum therapy (injection of serum) & makes the confusion in diagnosis of infectious mononucleosis, which are differentiated by absorption test in which heterophile antibodies are absorbed by ox red blood cells but not by guinea-pig kidney cells.

♣ **Antigen used:** Sheep RBCs.

♣ **Method:**

- Inactivate the patient serum by heating at 56°C for 30 minutes.
- Do the serial dilution of patient serum in tube & mix the equal volume of 1% sheep RBCs.
- Incubate the tube at 37°C for 4 hours.

♣ **Results:**

- +Ve: Agglutination of RBCs.
- –Ve: No agglutination.

♣ **Interpretation:**

✪ **Positive:** It is positive infectious mononucleosis in children & young adults. Agglutination titre of >256 is considered as significant.

✪ **Negative:** Test is negative in children < 5 year, elderly & in patient without symptoms of infectious mononucleosis.

✪ **False positive:** Due to presence of heterophile antibodies in normal individual or after serum therapy, which are differentiated by differential absorption test as follows.

Differential absorption test

- **Principle (table-3):** Differential absorption test based on absorption of heterophile antibodies of infectious mononucleosis by ox red blood cells but not by guinea-pig kidney cells while heterophile antibodies of normal individual & due to serum therapy are absorbed by guinea-pig kidney cells but not by ox red blood cells.
- **Result (table-3):**

♣ **Use:** For diagnosis of heterophile antibodies.

2. Monospot or mononuclear spot test:

- It is rapid test which based on detection of heterophile Ab by slide agglutination reaction. It uses the horse RBCs.
- Test serum is initially treated with guinea-pig kidney cells & ox red blood cells.
- Advantages: It is rapid test, simple to perform, high sensitivity about 75% & specificity (90%) & it replaced differential absorption test.
- Disadvantages: False positive result is seen in connective tissue disease, lymphoma, viral hepatitis & malaria.

b. Tests for detection of specific EBV antibodies: Following different types of antibodies are detected by ELISA against different antigen of EBV.

1. **Ab to viral capsid-Ag:**
- IgM detection: Indicates the recent infection.
- IgG detection: Indicates the past infection.
2. **Ab to nuclear-Ag:** It suggest past infection but four fold rise in titre suggest the current infection.
3. **Ab to early-Ag (called EA-D Ab):** Ab to early Ag is elevated in acute infection & Burkit's lymphoma & it is distributed in nucleus & cytoplasm of infected cells.
4. **Ab to early-Ag (called EA-D Ab):** Ab to early Ag is elevated in nasopharyngeal carcinoma & it is restricted to the cytoplasm of infected cells.

E. Molecular methods:
- PCR.
- Hybridisation: Most sensitive method.
- Real time PCR (Quantitative PCR / qPCR).

❖ **Prevention:** No specific vaccine is available.

❖ **Treatment:** There is no specific treatment. Acyclovir is effective.

HHV-5

❖ **Common name:** Cyto Megalo Virus (CMV) or previously **called salivary gland virus.**

❖ **Meaning:** Name is given by Weller and co-workers in 1960, because infected cell [Cyto (Greek) = cell] is enlarging [Megalic (Greek) = large].

❖ **History:**
- Inclusion bodies & inclusion-bearing cells were first shown by Ribbert in 1881.
- Goodpasture and Talbert in 1921 were the first to suggest the "cytomegalic " nature of infected cells
- The introduction of exfoliative cytology methods allowed identification of characteristic cells in the urine of infected infants. Smith in 1956, Rowe and co-workers in 1956, and Weller et al in 1957 independently isolated human CMV strains.
- In 1960, Weller and co-workers proposed the term "cytomegalovirus" and subsequently isolated CMV from the urine of infants with generalized disease.

❖ **Geographical distribution:** In USA & also in some developing countries. Up to 80% asymptomatic persons containing the antibodies showing the high prevalence.

❖ **Morphology:**
- ➢ Largest among the all herpes viruses about 150-200nm.
- ➢ Showing prominent intranuclear Cowdry type-B inclusion body **called "owl's eye" (fig.-5).**
- ➢ Other morphology is same as like HSV & VZV.

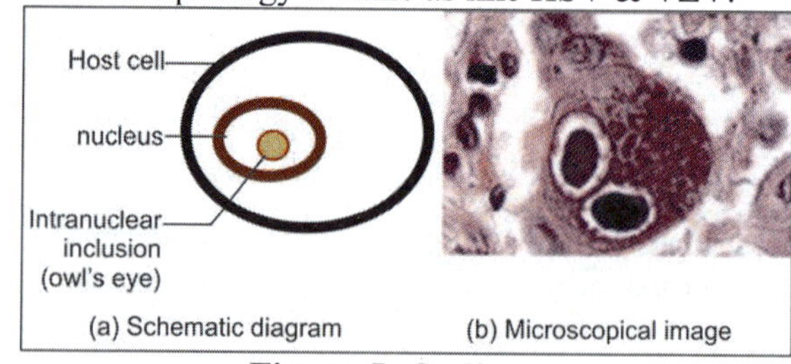

Figure-5: Owl's eye

❖ **Culture characteristics (C/Cs):**
- CPE developed in human fibroblasts after 50 days.
- Growth is identified by IF microscopy.

❖ **Resistance:** Enveloped, inactivated by fat solvent like ether, chloroform, bile salts & alcohol.

❖ **Antigenic structure:** Human CMV is unrelated antigenically to animal CMV except simian CMV with which it shows the minor antigenic cross reactivity. Human isolates may carry minor genetic & antigenic differences but clinically not significant.

❖ **Immunity:** Antibodies are formed but not protective.

❖ **Pathogenicity:**
- ➢ **Nature of disease:** Virus can produce the periodic reactivation, latent infection & lifelong persistence.
- ➢ **Reservoir of infection:** Human.
- ➢ **Source of infection:** Saliva, blood, urine, milk, semen & cervical secretion. Congenitally infected child had high viruria for 4-5 years & they are highly infectious in early infancy.
- ➢ **Mode of transmission:**

a. Direct:
1. **Close contact:** By body fluid & during coitus.
2. **Vertical:** From mother to child.
- Antenatal: By placenta.
- Intranatal: Contact with maternal body fluid during delivery.
- Postnatal: By breast feeding.

b. Indirect:
1. **Vehicle borne:** By blood, blood products **(post-transfusion mononucleosis)** & organ transplantation.

- ➢ **Portal of entry:** Skin or mucosa.
- ➢ **Sites:** Respiratory system & foetal organs.
- ➢ **Precipitating factors (epidemiological determinants):**

1. **Age & IDDs:** Disseminated lesion in neonate & person with IDDs, while asymptomatic in normal children & immunocompetent person. Most common pathogen causing infection following organ transplantation.
2. **Poor hygiene:**

3. **Socio-economical status:**
- More in person with low socio-economical status.
- 90% patients are sero-positive in developing countries while 40-70% people are sero-positive in developed countries.

➢ **Pathogenesis:**
- Glycoprotein receptors (spikes or peplomere) present on viral surface are combines with Fc piece of irrelevant Ig, resulting masking of virus & prevent access to specific anti-CMV Ab.
- Once infected, the person carries the virus for life, which may be activated from time to time.
- It may multiply in epithelium of respiratory system, salivary glands, kidneys & cervix and sheds in the urine, saliva, tears, semen, breast milk & cervical secretion.

➢ **Clinical features:**

a. **Primary infection:**
- Asymptomatic in older children & adult with prolonged latency & occasional reactivation.
- Reactivation can also lead to vertical transmission.
- It is common following transfusion **called post-transfusion mononucleosis**.
- Primary infection sometimes present with **infectious mononucleosis like syndrome** & characterised by malaise, myalgia, fever, liver function abnormalities, lymphocytosis **without heterophile Ab** in serum.
- Primary infection in person with IDDs is more severe and present with pneumonia, hepatitis or generalised disease or even fatal infection.

b. **Vertical infection:**
1. **Antenatal (congenital):** Transmission by placenta **called cytomegalic inclusion disease**. It is the most common virus causing intrauterine infection. It is associated with
- Hepatosplenomegaly (most features).
- Jaundice.
- Thrombocytopenic purpura.
- Haemolytic anaemia.
- Microcephaly.
- Choreoretinitis & cerebral calcification resembling toxoplasmosis.
- Often death.
- Survival shows mental retardation.
2. **Intranatal infection:** Usually asymptomatic.
3. **Postnatal infection:** Usually asymptomatic.

c. **Oncogenic:** Carcinoma of prostate & Kaposi's sarcoma.

d. **Infection following organ transplantation:** CMV is the most common pathogen causing infection following organ transplantation & present with fever, leucopenia, hepatitis, pneumonitis, oesophagitis, gastritis, colitis, retinitis & meningo-encephalitis.

❖ **Laboratory diagnosis:**

➢ **Specimens:** Urine, saliva, tears, semen, breast milk & cervical secretion & blood (buffy coat).

➢ **Testing methods:**

A. **Microscopy:** → **Follow morphology**

B. **Cell culture:** → **Follow C/Cs**

C. **Serological tests:** Little value
- ELISA, IHA, CFT are useful.
- IgM detection for diagnosis of congenital infection.

D. **Molecular methods:** Most useful method of diagnosis. Available test is PCR.

❖ **Prevention:**

➢ **General measures:**
- Screening and matching the CMV status of the donor and recipient.
- Use of CMV negative blood for transfusions.

➢ **Chemoprophylaxis:** Acyclovir & ganciclovir are used for prophylaxis.

➢ **Immunoprophylaxis:**
- **Active immunisation:**
  - Live attenuated vaccine (Towne 125 & AD 169 strain) & purified CMV polypeptide vaccine are developed.
  - Effective vaccine is not available.
- **Passive immunisation:** Administration of CMV immunoglobulin to sero negative recipients prior to transplant.

❖ **Treatment:** Ganciclovir & foscarnet are effective in persons with IDDs.

HHV-6

❖ **Common name:** Human B-Cell Lymphotropic Virus (HBLV).

❖ **History:** 1st isolated in 1986 from blood of patient with lymphoproliferative disease.

❖ **Subtype:** Two variant (A & B) has been identified.

❖ **Pathogenicity:** Disease produced by Variant-B.

➢ **Mode of transmission:** Ubiquitous & spread by saliva.

➢ **Clinical features:**
- **In children:** Paediatric disease **called sixth disease** or **roseola infantum** or **exanthema subitum** & characterised by high grade fever & skin rashes.
- **In adults:** Infectious mononucleosis like syndrome & focal encephalitis.
- **In person with IDDs:** Pneumonia & disseminated diseases.

HHV-7

❖ **Common name:** R K virus but this name is no longer in use.

❖ **DNA homology:** It shares 30-50% DNA homology with HHV-6.

❖ **History:** 1st isolated in 1990 from CD4 cells of healthy person.

❖ **Pathogenicity:**

➢ **Disease name:** Disease **called exanthema subitum.**

➢ **Mode of transmission:** Spread by saliva.

➢ **Clinical features:**

- Disease mainly present in children.
- Combine with specific receptors present on CD4 cells & causes further depletion of CD4 cells in HIV patient.
- Present with fever, seizure, ptyriasis rosea, respiratory symptoms & GIT symptoms.

HHV-8

❖ **Official name:** Kaposi's Sarcoma- associated Herpes Virus (KSHV).

❖ **History:**

- 1st isolated in 1994 from tissue of Kaposi's sarcoma from HIV patient, however its causal relationship with Kaposi's sarcoma is still to prove hence **called Kaposi's sarcoma associated Herpes Virus (KSHV)**
- Also identified from Kaposi's sarcoma without HIV.

❖ **Pathogenicity:**

➢ **Distribution & transmission:**

1. **Oral secretion:** Highly prevalent in Africa (endemic) with transmission by oral secretion.
2. **Homosexual practise:**
   - Low prevalence in Asia, North Europe & North America.
   - Rate is higher in male homosexual.
3. **Blood borne:** Also transmitted by blood, blood products, contaminated needle & syringe in drug abuse & by organ transplantation.

➢ **Clinical features:**

- **In immunocompetent:** Present fever & rash.
- **In immunodeficient like HIV / AIDS and following organ transplantation:** It causes

1. Kaposi's sarcoma:
   - Most common cancer occurs in AIDS patient.
   - It is a cancer of lymphatic endothelium & forms vascular channels that fill with blood cells, giving the tumour its characteristic bruise-like appearance.
   - The most typical feature of Kaposi sarcoma is the presence of spindle cells forming slits containing RBCs. The tumour is highly vascular, containing abnormally dense & irregular blood vessels, which leak RBCs into the surrounding tissue & gives dark colour to tumour. Inflammation around the tumour may produce swelling and pain.
   - The spindle cells of Kaposi sarcoma differentiate toward endothelial cells, probably of lymph vessel rather than blood vessel nature.
2. Primary effusion lymphoma (body cavity lymphomas).
3. Castleman's disease (lymphoproliferative disease of B cells).

❖ **Diagnosis:**

➢ **Specimens:** Saliva, blood, lymphoid tissues etc.

➢ **Testing methods:**

A. **Serological tests:** ELISA, indirect immunofluorescent test & Western blot test are useful.

B. **Molecular methods:** PCR for DNA detection.

✓ **Notes: Exanthema (exanthem) versus enanthema (exanthem)**

▪ **Exanthema (exanthem):**

- **Definition:** Skin eruption or skin rash is **called exanthema.** Sometimes it is considered as exanthematous fever also.
- **Causative agents:**
  - **Old list of causative agents:** Total six organisms were classified as under this list like
    1. First disease: Measles (rubeola) caused by measles virus.
    2. Second disease: Scarlet fever caused by *Strept pyogenes.*
    3. Third disease: German measles (rubella) caused by rubella virus.
    4. Fourth disease: Caused by *Staph aureus*. It was described in 1900 but it's existence is not widely accepted today.
    5. Fifth disease: Erythema infectiosum or slapped cheek disease caused by parvo virus B19.
    6. Sixth disease: HHV-6 (roseola infantum or exanthema subitum) & HHV-7 (exanthema subitum).
  - **Other organisms:** In addition to above mentioned diseases many other viral diseases are considered as exanthem like
    1. Varicella zoster (chickenpox & zona): Caused by varicella zoster virus.
    2. Mumps: Caused by mumps virus.
    3. Disease caused by *Rhinovirus*.
    4. Rocky mounted spotted fever: Caused by *R. rickettsia*
    5. Tick borne diseases.
    6. Viral haemorrhagic fever.

▪ **Enanthema (enanthem):**

- **Definition:** Mucosal eruption is **called enanthema.**
- **Causative agents:** It occurs with viral exanthema. Following are the common enanthematous conditions.

1. Small pox: Caused by variola virus
2. Measles (rubeola): Caused by measles virus.
3. Chickenpox: Caused by varicella zoster virus.
4. Roseola infantum: Caused by HHV-6.
5. Hypersensitivity:

Ceropethacine herpes virus-1

- **Common name:** Herpes virus simiae or B Virus.
- **Meaning:** From initial B of the name of patient virus **called B virus.**
- **History:** 1st isolated in 1934 by Sabin & Wright from brain of laboratory worker who developed fatal ascending myelitis after being bitten by healthy monkey.
- **Pathogenicity:**

➢ **Mode of transmission**

- Monkey bite.
- Contact of monkey tissue infected with virus.

➢ **Clinical features:**

- Vesicle in buccal mucosa which gets ulcerated & shed the virus to infect the contact.
- Disease is fatal (60% mortality) & survival shows the neurological sequelae.

- **Prevention:**

- Antigenically same as like HHV but HHV-Ab does not neutralise the B virus.
- Formolised vaccine is tried for laboratory worker who are at risk.

Question bank

Case study

1) A 8 year old child is brought to the hospital with history of fever & vesicle on the lips. Mother had given the history of similar illness to 2-3 colleagues of his school. Scraping is done from the vesicular lesion for Tzanck test. Tzanck cells are identified under microscopy. Identify the clinical conditions & answer the following
   a) Name the clinical condition & causative agent.
   b) Write pathogenicity of clinical condition
   c) Write the diagnosis of clinical condition

2) A 25 year old male is brought to the hospital with history of fever & sever painful vesicle on the external genitalia. Later he developed the neck rigidity. CSF is collected & it's testing reported the presence of predominant lymphocytes with normal glucose & elevated level of protein. Scraping is done from the vesicular lesion for Tzanck test. Tzanck cells are identified under microscopy. Identify the clinical conditions & answer the following
   a) Name the clinical condition & causative agent.
   b) Write pathogenicity of clinical condition
   c) Write the diagnosis of clinical condition

3) A 50 year old HIV +Ve male visited the medical OPD with history of severely painful vesicular lesion on the right side of the spine on the lumbar region. He reported the similar lesion on the trunk before many years, but with very low severity which was healed with formation of scab & at that time he was HIV –Ve. Identify the clinical conditions & answer the following
   a) Name the clinical condition & causative agent.
   b) Name the exanthematous clinical conditions with causative agents.
   c) Write pathogenicity of clinical condition
   d) Write the diagnosis of clinical condition

4) A 20 year old male visited the medical OPD with history of fever & sore throat since 5 days. Blood is collected for cell count which reported the lymphocytosis with atypical lymphocytes in peripheral blood. Identify the clinical conditions & answer the following
   a) Name the clinical condition & causative agent.
   b) Write pathogenicity of clinical condition
   c) Write the diagnosis of clinical condition

5) A 40 year old man with kidney transplantation before 2 months visited the medical OPD with history of fever & features suggestive of bilateral diffuse interstitial pneumonia. The laboratory report suggested the ds-DNA virus with owl's eye inclusion body. Identify the clinical conditions & answer the following
   a) Name the most common agent in given condition.
   b) Write pathogenicity of clinical condition
   c) Write the diagnosis of clinical condition

Essay/Full question

1) Herpesviridae

Short notes

1) Classification of Herpesviridae.
2) HSV-1 & 2.
3) VZV.
4) EBV.
5) CMV.
6) Chicken pox.
7) Infectious mononucleosis.
8) Paul Bunnell test.
9) Exanthema versus enanthema.

Short questions for theory/viva questions

1) Write four differences between HSV-1 & HSV-2.
2) What is Tzanck test?
3) Name the four virus transmitted by saliva.
4) Name the four cancer causing herpes viruses with cancer produced by them.
5) What are exanthema & enanthema?
6) Write four examples of viral exanthematous fever.
7) Write 1 pathogenic disease produced by each RK & BK virus.

MCQs for chapter review

Classification

1) **Varicella are classified under** (AI-96)
(a) *Enterovirus* (b) Retro virus (c) Pox virus (d) Herpes virus

Morphology

2) **Herpes simplex virus is** (AI-91)
(a) Single stranded DNA (b) Double stranded DNA (c) Single stranded RNA (d) Double stranded RNA

HHV-1 & 2

3) **Herpes simplex virus causes all except**
(a) Encephalitis (b) Pharyngitis (c) IMN (infectious mononucleosis) (d) Whitlow

4) **Encephalitis is caused by**
(a) HSV-1 (b) EBV (c) Infectious mononucleosis (d) CMV

5) **A neonate develop encephalitis without any skin lesion, most probable causative organism is** (AIIMS-02)
(a) HSV-1 (b) HSV-II (c) Meningococci (d) *Streptococci*

6) **Regarding HSV-2 infection** (PGI, June-02)
(a) Primary infection is usually wide spread (b) Recurrent attacks are due to reactivation of latent infection (c) Encephalitis can be caused by HSV-2 (d) New born may acquire infection via the birth canal at the time of labour (e) Treatment is with acyclovir

7) **Following is true for HSV-1**
(a) Small pock (b) Poor replication in chick embryo fibroblast culture (c) Above belt infection (d) a+b+c

8) **True about herpes virus** (PGI, May-13, Dec-03)
(a) HSV encephalopathy is treated with acyclovir (b) Oropharyngeal involvement is common in HSV-1 (c) Recurrent genital involvement is common in HSV-1 (d) Recurrence is rare in HSV-1

HHV-3

9) **Herpes zoster is caused by** (AI-99)
(a) Herpes simplex type I (b) Herpes simplex type II (c) Epstein Barr virus (d) Varicella

10) **Infectivity of chicken pox last for** (AI-02)
(a) Till the last scab falls off (b) 6 days after onset of rash (c) 3 days after onset of rash (d) Till the fever subsides

11) **Rash pattern in chickenpox is**
(a) Centripetal (b) Centrifugal (c) Localised (d) All

12) **Most common extra skin manifestation of varicella is involvement of**
(a) CNS (b) Lungs (c) Kidneys (d) CVS

13) **Hypoplasia of limb and scarring is caused by**
(a) Varicella (b) Herpes simplex (c) Rubella (d) *Toxoplasma*

14) **Tests for chicken pox**
(a) Fluorescent Ab test (b) ELISA (c) Widal (d) PCR

15) **Chickenpox** (PGI-85)
(a) Is commonly seen in a congenital form (b) May be severe in a new born child infected by the mother in late pregnancy (c) Affects limbs more that the trunk (d) May cause pneumonitis (e) Should be treated with intravenous vidarabine when there is evidence of hepatitis.

16) **Shingles are seen in**
(a) IMN (b) Herpes zoster (c) Chickenpox (d) Small pox

17) **Zoster recurrence occur after infection with** (AI-99)
(a) HSV 1 (b) H SV 2 (c) Varicella (d) Small pox

18) **Varicella zoster remains latent in** (AI-10)
(a) Lymphocytes (b) Monocytes (c) Trigeminal ganglion (d) Plasma cells

19) **Which virus reactivates & involves the eye** (AI-98)
(a) Herpes zoster (b) CMV (c) EB virus (d) Enterovirus 70

20) **Zoster ophthalmicus is due to**
(a) Primary herpes infection of eye (b) Herpes reactivation in optic nerve (c) Herpes reactivation in Gasserion gaglion (d) Herpes infection of eye in immunocompromised patient

21) **Treatment of herpes zoster**
(a) Zidovudin (b) Valacyclovir (c) Ribavarin (d) Nevirapine

HHV-4

22) **Oral hairy leukoplakia caused by**
(a) Epstein Barr Virus (b) CMV (c) HIV (d) HZV

23) **African Butkitt's lymphoma is caused by**
(a) Epstein Barr Virus (b) CMV (c) HIV (d) HZV

24) **Epstein Barr Virus causes autoimmunity by** (AI -12)
(a) Molecular mimicry (b) Inducing inappropriate expression of class II MHC (c) Release of sequestere antigens (d) Polyclonal activation of B cells

25) **All are associated with EBV except**
(a) Infectious mononucleosis (b) Nasopharyngeal carcinoma (c) Oral hairy leukoplakia (d) Epidermodysplasia

26) **EB virus causes all except** (AIIMS, Nov-99)
(a) Infectious mononucleosis (b) Nasopharyngeal carcinoma (c) Burkit's lymphoma (d) Carcinoma of cervix

27) **EB virus has been implicated in the following malignancies except** (AI -04)
(a) Hodgkin's disease (b) Non-Hodgkin's disease (c) Nasopharyngeal carcinoma (d) Multiple myeloma

28) **True about infectious mononucleosis is** (PGI, June-08, May-13)
(a) Associated with heterophile antibodies (b) Monocytosis (c) Associated with cold agglutinin (d) Associated with CMV infection (e) Self limited disease

29) **A patient with sore throat has positive Paul Bunnell test. The causative organism is**
(a) EBV (b) Herpes virus (c) Adenovirus (d) CMV

30) **Paul Bunnell antibodies are reactive in all except**
(a) Ox (b) Sheep (c) Dog (d) Horse

31) **Most sensitive test for diagnosis of infectious mononucleosis**
(a) Monospot test (b) Paul Bunnell test (c) Lymphocytosis in peripheral smear (d) Culture of the virus

32) **Lymphocytosis with atypical lymphocytes are seen in infection with**
(a) HSV (b) HBV (c) EBV (d) RSV

33) **Burkit's virus is**
(a) EBV (b) HPV (c) HIV (d) HAV

34) **IMN true is all except**
(a) Caused by EBV (b) Also called kissing disease (c) Diagnosed by Paul Bunnel test (d) RNA virus

HHV-5

35) **The most common presentation of congenital CMV infection is** (PGI-94)
(a) Hepatosplenomegaly (b) Microcephaly (c) Cerebral calcification (d) Chorioretinitis

36) **Which of the following does not establish a diagnosis of congenital CMV infection in a neonate** (AI-95)
(a) Urine culture of CMV (b) IgG CMV antibodies in blood (c) Intranuclear inclusion bodies in hepatocytes (d) CMV viral DNA in blood by polymerase chain reaction

37) **The most sensitive and rapid test for diagnosis of CMV retinitis is** (AIIMS, May-13)
(a) Viral isolation from the intraocular fluid (b) Nucleic acid detection from the intraocular fluid (c) Viral antigen detection in vitreous (d) Viral antibody detection in the blood by ELISA

38) **Immunocompromised patient due to transplantation is suffering from pyrexia and neutropenia. Most likely cause is** (PGI-97)
(a) HSV (b) CMV (c) Gram (-) ve organism (d) Gram (+) ve organism

39) **All are true regarding cytomegalo virus except**
(a) It is a DNA virus (b) Most commonly infected in last trimester (c) Diagnosed by increased IgA in foetal blood (d) Most common cause of congenital viral infection

HHV-6

40) **HHV-6b causes**
(a) Carcinoma of cervix (b) Carcinoma of endometrium (c) Clear cell carcinoma (d) Focal encephalitis

HHV-8

41) **Kaposi sarcoma is caused by**
(a) Human herpes virus-2 (b) Human herpes virus-4 (c) Human herpes virus-6 (d) Human herpes virus-8

42) **HHV-8 causes**
(a) Burkit's lymphoma (b) Nasopharyngeal carcinoma (c) Kaposi sarcoma (d) Hepatic carcinoma

43) **The tissue of origin of Kaposi sarcoma is** (AIIMS, May-05)
(a) Lymphoid (b) Vascular (c) Neural (d) Muscular

44) **Multifocal tumour of vascular origin in a patient of AIDS** (AI-00)
(a) Kaposi sarcoma (b) Astrocytoma (c) Gastric carcinoma (d) Primary CNS lymphoma

Common MCQs of herpes group

45) **All of the following are true about herpes group virus except** (AI -98)
(a) Ether sensitive (b) May cause malignancy (c) HSV-II involves below diaphragm (d) Burkit's lymphoma involves T cells

46) **True about virus is**
(a) HSV-1 causes encephalitis (b) EBV affects T lymphocytes (c) CMV is always symptomatic (d) Herpes zoster is not reactivated

Answers of MCQs & explanation

1) **(d)**
- Varicella is actually a varicella zoster virus belong to family Herpesviridae
- Follow section, **classification** for more explanation

2) **(b)**
- Follow section, **morphology (genome & capsid)** for more explanation

3) **(c)**
- Follow section, flow chart -3 for causes of IMN (infectious mononucleosis)
- Follow section, **HHV-1 & 2 (pathogenicity → clinical features)** for pathogenic lesions caused by herpes simplex virus

4) **(a)**
5) **(b)**
6) **(a), (b), (c), (d) & (e)**
7) **(d)**
8) **(d)**

} Follow section, **HHV-1 & 2 (pathogenicity →clinical features) & table-2** for explanation

- Follow section, **HHV-1 & 2 (pathogenicity treatment) & table-2** for more explanation

9) **(d)**
10) **(b)**
11) **(a)**
12) **(a)**
13) **(a)**
14) **(a), (b) & (c)**
15) **(b) & (d)**
16) **(b)**
17) **(c)**
18) **(c)**
19) **(a)**
20) **(c)**
21) **(b)**

} Follow section, **HHV-3** for more explanation

22) **(a)**
23) **(a)**
24) **(d)**
25) **(d)**
26) **(d)**
27) **(d)**
28) **(a), (c), (d) & (e)**
29) **(a)**
30) **(c)**
31) **(a)**
32) **(c)**
33) **(a)**
34) **(d)**

} Follow section, **HHV-4 & flow chart-3** for more explanation

35) **(a)**
36) **(b)**
37) **(b)**
38) **(b)**
39) **(c)**

} Follow section, **HHV-5** for more explanation

40) **(d)**
- Follow section, **HHV-6** for more explanation.

41) **(d)**
42) **(c)**
43) **(b)**
44) **(a)**

} Follow section, **HHV-8** for more explanation

45) **(c) & (d)**
- Herpes viruses are envelop virus, which is made up by lipoprotein. This envelope is sensitive lipid solvents like ether, chloroform etc.
- Herpes viruses like HHV-1, 2, 4, 5 & 8 are causes malignancy
- HSV-II involves below the west not below the diaphragm
- Burkit's lymphoma involves B cells not the T cells

46) **(a)**
- EBV affects B lymphocytes
- CMV is asymptomatic in older children & adult with prolonged latency & occasional reactivation
- Herpes zoster is reactivated from trigeminal gaglion

64 Other DNA viruses

(Hepadnaviridae, Adenoviridae, Papovaviridae and Parvoviridae)

Hepadnaviridae

- Viruses are responsible for hepatitis in human & it is better to discuss it with other hepatitis viruses.
- More details: Follow chapter → Hepatitis viruses.

Adenoviridae

❖ **Meaning:** Name is given because; it was grown & identified from the adenoid tissues.

❖ **Use:** Carry inserted DNA up to 7kb & act as vector in gene therapy.

❖ **History:** 1st identified by Rowe & colleagues in 1953 by growing the surgically removed adenoid tissue on plasma clot culture.

❖ **Geographical distribution:** Worldwide.

❖ **Classification & antigenic structure:**

➢ **Family:** Adenoviridae.

➢ **Genus:** All adenoviruses share common complement fixing antigens.

✪ **Two genera:**

1. ***Mastadenovirus***: Infect the mammals.
2. ***Aviadenovirus***: Infect the birds.

- **Subgenus or subgroup: →Table-1**
  - Human adeno viruses are divided into six subgroups (A to F) based on certain properties like haemagglutination, fibre length, DNA analysis & oncogenic potential as shown in **table-1.**
  - Group specific Ag present on **hexons** and can be detected by ELISA or by IF test.
- **Serotype: →Table-1**
  - Each group is divided in many serotypes by type specific Ag.
  - More than 50 serotypes are identified as shown in **table-1.**
  - Type specific Ag is present on **pentons & fibres.** It is detected by neutralisation test.

Sub-genus	Serotype	Haemagglutination	
		Red cells	Pattern
A	12,18,31	Rat	Partial
B	3, 7, 11, 14, 16, 21, 34, 35	Monkey	Complete
C	1, 2, 5, 6	Rat	Partial
D	8, 9, 10, 13, 15, 17, 19, 20, 22-30, 32, 33, 36-39, 42 - 47	Rat	Complete
E	4	Rat	Partial
F	40,41	Rat	Partial

Table-1: Subgroup & serotypes of human adeno viruses

❖ **Morphology: →Fig.-1**

➢ **Shape:** Appear like space vehicle (satellite).

➢ **Size:** Non-enveloped (naked virus) about 70-75 nm in size.

➢ **Genome & capsid:** ds-DNA surrounded by icosahedral variety of capsid.

➢ **Capsomeres:**

- Total 252 in numbers, arranged with 20 triangular facets & 12 vertices.

- 240 capsomeres have six neighbour **called hexons** while 12 capsomeres have five neighbour **called pentons.**
- Penton consist penton base anchored in capsid & rod like projection or fibre with knob at distal end.

➢ **Envelope:** Non enveloped (naked) virus.

➢ **Electron microscopy (EM):** For diagnosis of virus present in faeces.

➢ **IF microscopy:** For eye or nasopharynx samples.

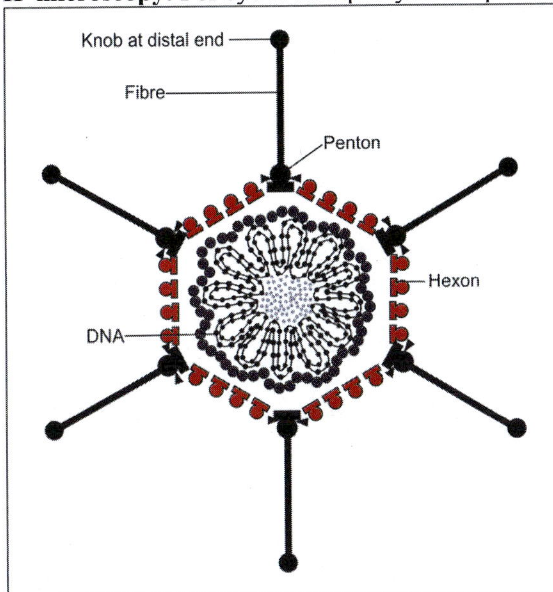

Figure-1: Morphology of adeno virus

❖ Culture characteristics (C/Cs):

i. Tissue culture:

- Grow only in human cells like: Hela cells, HEP-2 & human embryonic kidney cell.
- Growth is identified by intranuclear inclusion bodies, rounding of cell or aggregation in grape like cluster.
- Viral antigen from culture is identified by CFT, neutralisation test or by Haemagglutination test.

ii. Animal culture: Animals are not susceptible.

❖ Resistance:

- Inactivated at 50^{0}C.
- Non-enveloped resist by ether & bile salts.

❖ Pathogenicity:

➢ **Nature of disease:** One serotype can produce many diseases & same disease can be produced by many serotypes. Different serotypes are producing endemic, epidemic or outbreak.

➢ **Reservoir of infection:** Human.

➢ **Source of infection:** Respiratory droplets, faeces, eye discharge, urine etc.

➢ **Mode of transmission:**

- Via droplets/aerosol in early phase of disease.
- Via close contact.
- Faeco-oral route.

➢ **Portal of entry:** Respiratory tract, GIT, conjunctiva etc.

➢ **Sites:** Respiratory tract, eyes, bladder, intestine etc.

➢ **Clinical features: →Table-2**

Features	Serotypes
Respiratory	
Pharyngitis	1-7
Pneumonia	3,7
Acute Respiratory Distress (ARD) in military person	4,7
Pharyngo-conjunctival fever	3,7,14
Eye	
Epidemic kerato-conjunctivitis (shipyard eye)	8,19, 37
Acute follicular (swimming pool) conjunctivitis	3,4,7, 11
GIT	
Diarrhoea (in children)	40,41
Others	
Acute haemorrhagic cystitis	11,21
Generalised exanthema, Mesenteric adenitis & intussusception & oncogenic (not for human)	
Tumour production (noticed by Huebner in 1962)	
Sarcoma in baby hamster	12, 18
Tumours in animals	12, 18 & 31
Transformation of cell culture	All types
Human cancer	Not produced

Table-2: Clinical features of adeno viruses

❖ Laboratory diagnosis:

➢ **Specimens:** Serum, nasopharyngeal or throat samples, eye sample like conjunctival scraping, stool & urine.

➢ **Testing methods:**

A. Microscopy: → Follow morphology

B. Culture: → Follow C/Cs

C. Serological test: ELISA

D. Molecular methods: PCR

❖ Treatment:

No specific antiviral drugs are available, only symptomatic treatment is given.

❖ Prevention:

A General measures:

- Hand washing.
- Use of paper towels than cloths towel, which easily gets dry.
- Chlorination of water to prevent the water related transmission.
- Strict aseptic techniques during eye examination.

B Immunoprophylaxis:

- **Aim:** To prevent the epidemic in communities & in military person.
- **Vaccination:**
  - Killed & live vaccine for prevention of ARD.
  - No vaccine is available for general use.

- Live vaccine available as gelatin coated capsule, contains type 4 & 7, used orally in military persons. It was highly effective but due to manufacturer issues it is not in use since 1999.

Papovaviridae

❖ **Meaning:** From initial of its genera *Papillomavirus* + *Polyomavirus*.

❖ **Classification:** →Flow chart-1

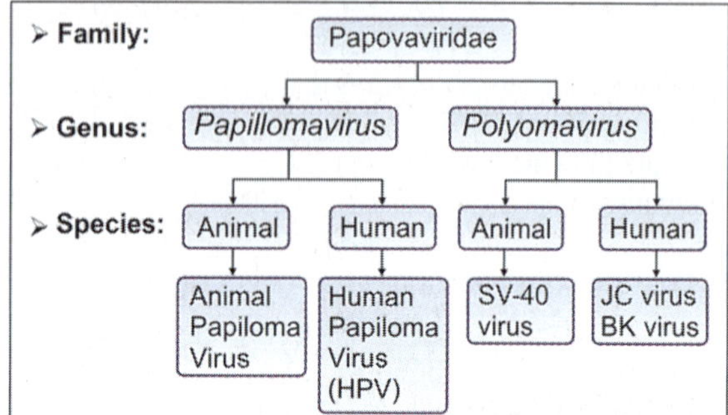

Flow chart-1: Classification of Papovaviridae

✓ Note: SV-40 (Simian Vacuolating-40) virus.
- It causing the polyoma (malignant tumour) in mice.

❖ **Morphology:**
➢ **Size:** Small.
➢ **Genome & capsid:** ds-DNA surrounded by icosahedral variety of capsid.
➢ **Envelope:** Non enveloped (naked) virus.

HPV

✪ **History:** Virus nature was identified in 1907.
✪ **Geographical distribution:** Worldwide.
✪ **Morphology:**
- **General morphological features:** → Vide supra.
- **Genomic structure:** Two types of genes.

a. **Early region genes:**
- Codes for non structural proteins.
- Like E1-E7.
- Products of these genes are codes with oncogenic potential.

b. **Late region genes:**
- Codes for structural proteins like capsid. Two types like L1 (for major capsid protein) & L2 (for minor capsid protein).

✪ **Culture characteristics (C/Cs):** HeLa (Human carcinoma of cervix) cells used for culture are containing HPV-18 DNA.
✪ **Resistance:**
- The virus is relatively hardy and immune to many common disinfectants.
- Exposure to 90% ethanol for at least 1 minute, 2% glutaraldehyde, 30% savlon, and/or 1% sodium hypochlorite can disinfect the pathogen.
- The virus is resistant to drying and heat, but killed by 100 °C (212 °F) and UV radiation.

✪ **Types:** Over 170 types are identified based on DNA sequences of L1 gene. They are labelled as 1, 2, 3 etc. & disease produced by particular types is described in pathogenicity.
✪ **Immunity:** Some HPV types like 16, 18, 31 & 45 are not controlled by immune system resulting lifelong infection & development of cancer.
✪ **Pathogenicity:**
- **Disease name:** It produces two types of lesions in human like
  - Precancerous lesions **called warts** or **verucca** or **human papilloma** or **human papillomatosis.** It is a cauliflower like growth raising beyond the surface.
  - Cancer: Squamous cell carcinoma.
- **Reservoir & source of infection:** Human.
- **Mode of transmission:**
  - Direct skin-to-skin contact.
  - Vaginal and anal sex.
  - Occasionally it can spread from a mother to her baby during pregnancy.
  - Not spread via common items like toilet seats.
- **Portal of entry:** Skin or mucosa.
- **Sites:**
  - Skin of arms, face, forehead or feet.
  - Sole.
  - Finger nail region.
  - Genitals like cervix, vulva, vagina, penis & anus
  - Larynx & mouth.
- **Precipitating factors:**

1. **Age:** Common in children & adults.
2. **IDDs:** Epidermodysplasia verruciformis occurs in immunocompromised individuals.

- **Clinical features:** → **Fig.-2 & table-3**

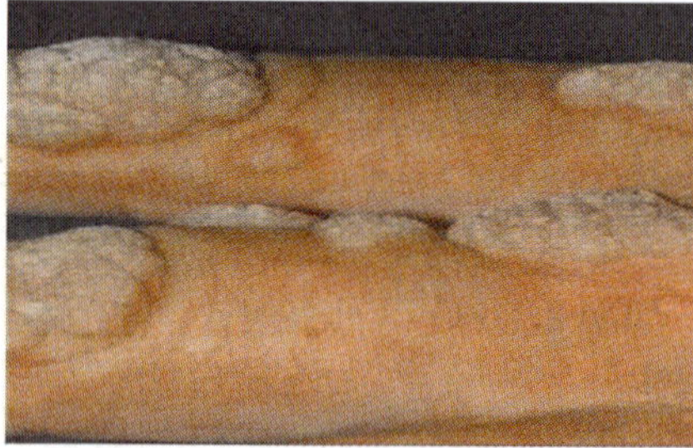

Figure-2: Skin wart (Verruca vulgaris) caused by HPV

- **Complication:** Recurrence is the common problem after treatment.

✪ **Diagnosis:**
- **Specimens:** Biopsy from warts.
- **Testing methods:**

A. **Naked eye:** Most lesions are visible naked eye. 5% acetic acid can be applied to improve the visibility.
B. **Microscopy:** → **Follow morphology**

Disease	HPV type
Warts (verucca or papilloma or papillomatosis)	
Common warts (Verruca vulgaris): Most common type of wart. Seen commonly on hands, feet & rarely on knees or elbows in young children.	2, 7, 22
Plantar warts (Verruca plantaris): Found on the soles; grow inward, generally causing pain when walking. Seen in adolescent & young adult.	1, 2, 4, 63
Flat warts (Verruca plana): Found on the arms, face or forehead. Seen in young children and teens	3, 10, 8
Anogenital warts (Conduloma acuminate) Seen on ano-genital parts & most common in sexually disease active adults.	6, 11, 42, 44 and others
Anal dysplasia (lesions)	6, 16, 18, 31, 53, 58
Epidermodysplasia verruciformis: Occurs in person with IDDs & tendency to change to SCC particularly in sun exposed areas.	more than 15 types (5, 8)
Focal epithelial hyperplasia (mouth)	13, 32
Mouth papillomas	6, 7, 11, 16, 32
Verrucous cyst	60
Laryngeal papillomatosis	6, 11
Cancer	
Oropharyngeal cancer	16
Laryngeal or oesophageal carcinoma	16 & 18
Genital cancers: Seen in cervix, vulva, vagina, penis & anus	Highest risk: 16, 18, 31, 45 Other high-risk: 33, 35, 39, 51, 52, 56, 58, 59 Probably high-risk: 26, 53, 66, 68, 73, 82

Table-3: Clinical features of HPV

C. Culture: → Follow C/Cs.

D. Serological test: Ab detection is not much useful.

E. Molecular methods: PCR or hybrid capture assay used to detect the DNA & specific type.

F. Cytological study:

- Papanicolaou smears (Better **called pap smears**) prepared from cervical or anal scraping.
- Histopathological staining of biopsies.

✪ **Prevention:**

A. General measures: Use of barrier method like condom.

B. Immunoprophylaxis:

- **Preparation:** Vaccine is prepared from major capsid protein like L1.
- **Types:** Two types of vaccine.

1. Quadrivalent:
   - Contain type 6, 11, 16 & 18.
   - Licensed in USA & recommended by CDC for administration to girls & young women from 9-26 years of age.
   - Three doses by IM route: After the 1st dose, 2nd dose should be given 2 months later & 3rd dose should be given 6 months after the 1st dose.
   - Among contains of vaccine, types 16 & 18 are the most common types for cervical cancer worldwide with prevalence rate is >70%. Vaccine offered the protection against HPV 16 & 18 & prevents the cervical cancer.
2. Bivalent: Contains high risk type 16 & 18.

- **Efficacy:** Recombinant vaccine is available which is highly effective & reduces the rate of all infection including cervical cancer. Efficacy is >90%.
- **Contraindication:** Pregnancy.

✪ **Treatment:** HPV lesions generally heal spontaneously.

A. Medications: Topical application of podophyllum.

B. Imiquimod: It is a form of immunotherapy.

C. Surgery: Like cryosurgery & electrodessication. Recurrence & scaring is common following surgical excision of wart, so not recommended.

D. Laser: Also useful.

E. Immunotherapy: Prepared from two main oncogenes like E6 & E7, especially in treatment of cancer but still under trial.

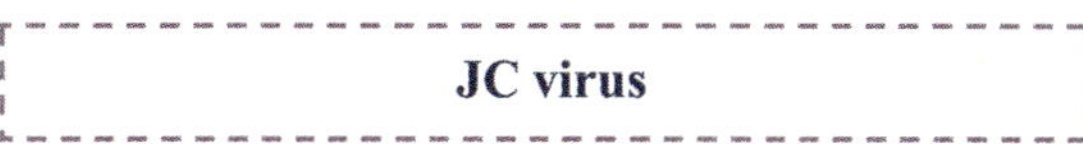

JC virus

✪ **Meaning & history:**

- John Cunningham virus, from the initial of patient's name. Patient was suffered with Progressive Multifocal Leucoencephalopathy (PML) & virus was identified from the brain of this patient in 1965 by ZuRhein, Chou, Silverman & Rubinstan by EM.
- Later it was isolated in culture.

✪ **Geographical distribution & genotypes:** It infects 70-90% of people. Antibodies are identified from human serum. Different typing systems are given according to its distribution.

i. Genotype: Following 8 types are found.

- **Type 1 & 4:**
  - Bothe types are closely related.

- Found in Europe & Northern Japan, North-East Siberia & Northern Canada.
- **Type 2:** Several variants like
- 2A: Found in Japanese population & Native Americans.
- 2B: Found in Eurasians.
- 2D: Found in Indians.
- 2E: Found in Australians & Western Pacific populations.
- **Type 3 & 6:**
- Bothe types are found in Sub-Saharan Africa.
- Type 3 present in Ethiopia, Tanzania & South Africa.
- Type 6 found in Ghana.
- **Type 5:** No more detail is known.
- **Type 7:** Several variants like
- 7A: Found in Southern China & South East Asia & Native Americans.
- 7B: Found in Northern China, Japan & Mongolia.
- 7C: Found in Northern & Southern China.
- **Type 8:** Distributed in Papua New Guinea & Pacific Island.

ii. **Other subtypes:**

a. **European type:** Like a, b & c.

b. **African types:**

1. **Minor: Called Af1** distributed in Central & West Africa.
2. **Major: Called Af2** distributed throughout the Africa & also in West & South Asia.

c. **Asian types:** Like B1-a, B1-b, B1-d, B2, CY, MY & SC.

- **Morphology:** → Vide supra
- **Culture characteristics (C/Cs):** Grow in human foetal glial cell culture.
- **Pathogenicity:**
- **Reservoir of infection:** Human.
- **Source of infection:** Contaminated sewage water from urine of patients.
- **Mode of transmission:** Mostly by ingestion of contaminated water.
- **Portal of entry:** GIT.
- **Sites:** Brain & colon/rectum.
- **Precipitating factors:**

1. **Age:** Infection acquired in childhood & also by adolescent.
2. **IDDs:** It produces the PML & other lesions only in immunodeficient persons due to
   - AIDS.
   - Immunosuppressive drug like rituximab etc.
   - Organ transplantation.

- **Pathogenesis:** Probably as shown in **flow chart-2.**
- **Clinical features:** Two types of latent form in immunocompromised patients.

1. **Progressive Multifocal Leucoencephalopathy (PML):**
   - Subacute demyelinating (degenerative) disease of older person whose immunity is suppressed by malignancy or by other IDDs.
   - Deterioration of motor function, speech & vision.
   - Death in 3-4 months.
2. **Malignancy:**
   - Virus is malignant & produces malignant gliomas following intracerebral inoculation in new born hamsters.
   - JC virus is found from the human colorectal cancer in immunodeficient subjects but still it is controversial to accept it as causative agent.

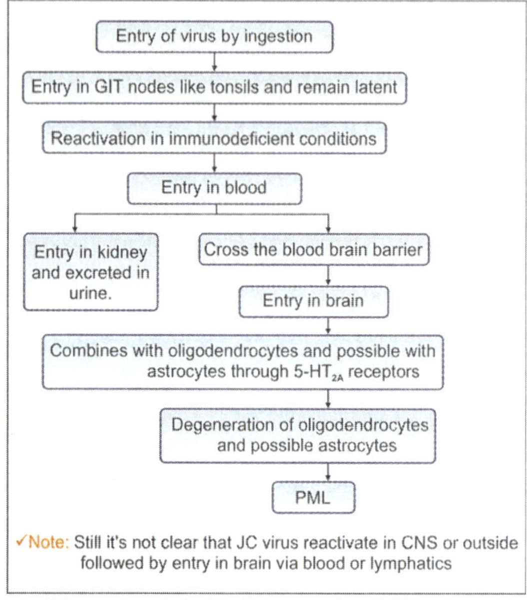
Entry of virus by ingestion
Entry in GIT nodes like tonsils and remain latent
Reactivation in immunodeficient conditions
Entry in blood
Entry in kidney and excreted in urine.
Cross the blood brain barrier
Entry in brain
Combines with oligodendrocytes and possible with astrocytes through 5-HT_{2A} receptors
Degeneration of oligodendrocytes and possible astrocytes
PML
✓Note: Still it's not clear that JC virus reactivate in CNS or outside followed by entry in brain via blood or lymphatics

Flow chart-2: Pathogenesis of JC virus

- **Diagnosis:**
- **Specimens:** Brain biopsy & serum.
- **Testing methods:**

1. **Microscopy:** EM is useful.
2. **Culture:** Grow in human foetal glial cell culture.
3. **Serological tests:** Ab is detected from serum.
4. **Molecular method:** PCR for identification & to differentiate JC virus from BK virus.

- **Prevention:** Avoidance of immunosuppressive drug like rituximab.

BK virus

- **Meaning & history:** Isolated in 1971 from the urine of renal transplant patient. Name is given from the initial of patient
- **Geographical distribution:** It is distributed in 80% of population in asymptomatic form.
- **Morphology:**
- It is similar to JC virus , since their genomes share 75% sequence similarity.
- Both of these viruses can be identified and differentiated from each other by carrying out

serological tests using specific antibodies or by using a PCR based genotyping approach.
- EM is also useful.

✪ **Culture characteristics (C/Cs):**
- Grow in primary & continuous cell cultures.
- Both JC & BK viruses agglutinate guinea pig & chicken RBCs.

✪ **Pathogenicity:**
- **Reservoir & source of infection:** Human. Excreted in respiratory droplets or in urine.
- **Mode of transmission:** Exactly not known but person to person transmission is possible from urine or respiratory droplets.
- **Portal of entry:** May be respiratory system.
- **Site:** Kidneys.
- **Precipitating factors:** Latent infection occurs in patient with immunocompromised conditions like
  - Renal or organs or bone marrow transplant.
  - Immunosuppressive therapy like tacrolimus and mycophenolate mofetil.
- **Pathogenesis:** Virus remain in latent form in kidney for very long time & reactivated in Immunocompromised patients due to renal or organ transplant to produce renal dysfunction.
- **Clinical features:**
  - Asymptomatic infection: Present in 80% population.
  - Primary infection:
    - Present in immunocompetent patients.
    - Mild infection, present with fever or respiratory symptoms.
  - Latent infection:
    - Present immunocompromised patients.
    - Virus reactivated in patient with renal or organ transplant leading to renal dysfunction, seen by a progressive rise in serum creatinine and an abnormal urinalysis revealing renal tubular cells and inflammatory cells.
    - It is also associated with ureteral stenosis and interstitial nephritis.
    - In bone marrow transplant recipients it is notable as a cause for hemorrhagic cystitis.

✪ **Diagnosis:**
- **Specimens:** Kidney biopsy & serum.
- **Testing methods:**
1. **Microscopy: → Follow morphology.**
2. **Culture: → Follow C/Cs.**
3. **Serological tests:** Ab is detected from serum.
4. **Molecular method:** PCR for identification & to differentiate JC virus from BK virus.

✪ **Prevention:** Switch tacrolimus to cyclosporine.

✪ **Treatment:** Therapeutic option includes.
- Leflunomide: A pyrimidine synthesis inhibitor is now generally accepted as the second treatment option behind reduction of immunosuppression.
- Cidofovir.
- Intravenous immunoglobulin.
- Fluoroquinolones: Ciprofloxacin lower viral loads but no data on survival and graft loss exist.

Parvoviridae

❖ **Meaning:** Family name given from word **parvo (Latin) = small**, because it is the smallest virus about 20 nm in size. As small as largest protein molecules like haemocyanin.

❖ **Classification:** →**Flow chart-3**

❖ **Morphology:**
- **Size:** 20 nm (smallest virus).
- **Non enveloped (naked) virus.**
- **Genome & capsid:** Only DNA type virus with ss-DNA. It is surrounded by icosahedral variety of capsid.
- **EM:** Detection of parvovirus from blood by EM.

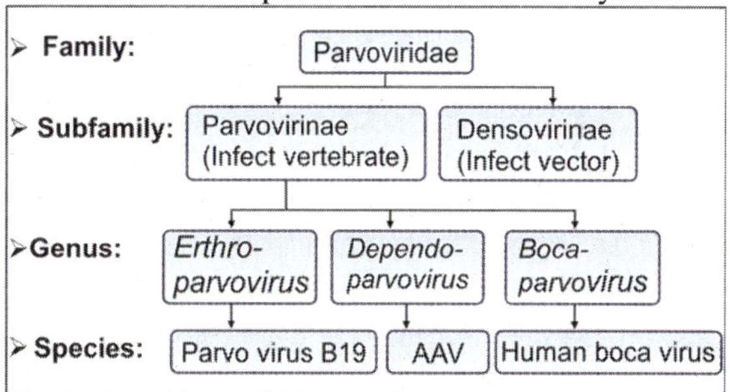

Flow chart-3: Classification of Parvoviridae

Parvo virus B19

✪ **Synonym:** B19 virus or erythro virus B19.

✪ **Meaning:**
- **Family name:** From **parvo (Latin) = small**, because of smallest virus.
- **Genus name:** Having capability to invade the precursors of RBCs in bone marrow, hence the genus **called erythroparvovirus.**
- **Species name:** It was identified in the well number B-19 of larger size microtitre plate, hence the species **called B19.**

✪ **History:** It was discovered by Australian virologist Yvonne Cossart in 1975.

✪ **Geographical distribution & genotypes:**
- Worldwide distribution.
- Genotypes: Three genotypes are identified.

✪ **Morphology:**
- **General morphological features:** → Vide supra
- **Genomic structure:** Two types of genes like VP1 & VP2. Both are encode for structure protein, where VP2 is the major capsid coding gene.

- **Culture characteristics (C/Cs):** Difficult to grow in culture.
- **Immunity:** Past infection provide protection in half populations.
- **Pathogenicity:**
- **Disease name:** In children it produces the disease **called erythema infectiosum** or **slapped cheek disease** or **5th disease.**
- **Nature of disease:** May produces the epidemic. Last epidemic year was occurred in1998. Outbreaks can arise especially in nurseries and schools.
- **Reservoir & source of infection:** Human. Cat and dog parvo viruses do not infect the human.
- **Mode of transmission:** By
  - Respiratory route: Primary mode of transmission.
  - Blood.
  - Placenta: ≥ 30% chances of transplacental transmission.
- **Incubation period:** Symptoms appear after 6 days. (Average 16-17 days).
- **Portal of entry:** May be respiratory system.
- **Sites:** Skin & blood cells.
- **Precipitating factors (epidemiological determinants):**

1. **Age:** In children of 5-10 years.
2. **Immuno deficiency disease (IDD):** Also favours the disease.

- **Pathogenesis:**
  - Virus having capability to invade the precursors of RBCs in bone marrow.
  - It combines with specific receptors present on RBCs surface **called P antigen** (also **called globoside**).
  - It enters in RBCs & lyses the cell causing **erythema infectiosum (slapped cheek disease or 5th disease).**
  - Sometimes it is associated with aplastic anaemia due to destruction of RBCs precursors.
- **Clinical features:**

a. In immunocompetent host:

1. **Respiratory infection:** It present with macula-papular rash & arthralgia.
2. **Erythema infectiosum or slapped cheek disease:**
   - Common in children of 5-10 years.
   - Starts with erythema of cheeks (**fig.3**) & spread to trunk & limbs, followed by lymphadenopathy & arthralgia.
   - Also **called 5th disease**, as it is 5th in the list of old six exanthematous diseases.
   - A usual brief viral prodromal phase with fever, headache, nausea & diarrhoea.
   - As the fever breaks, a red rash forms on the cheeks, with relative pallor around the mouth ("slapped cheek rash"), sparing the nasolabial folds, forehead, and mouth.
   - "Lace-like, (reticular)" red rash on trunk or extremities then follows the facial rash. Infection in adults usually only involves the reticular rash, with multiple joint pain (arthralgia) predominating.
   - Exacerbation of rash by sunlight, heat, stress.
   - Teenagers or young adults may develop the so-**called "papular purpuric gloves and socks syndrome"**.

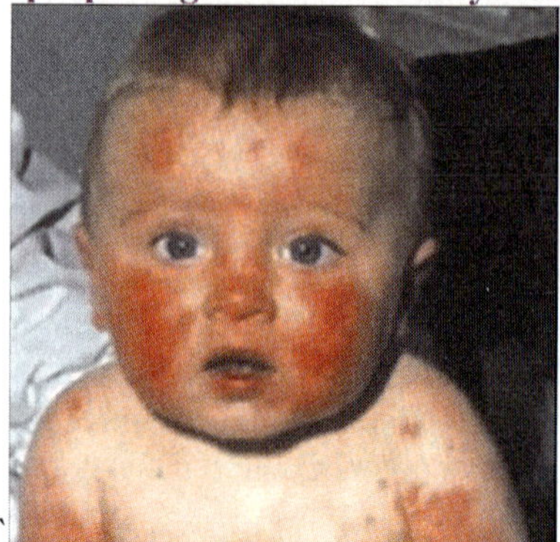

Figure-3: Slapped cheek disease

3. **Acute arthropathy:**
   - Commonly present in adult with arthralgia & arthritis.
   - It involves the peripheral joints like wrists & knees.
   - It is non destructive & resolves by three weeks.
   - Sometimes associated with rash.
4. **Aplastic crisis:**
   - "**Aplastic crisis**" means rapid & severe anaemia due to temporary cessation of RBCs production (erythropoiesis).
   - It also **called reticulocytopenia** or **marrow failure**
   - It is most dangerous in children with pre-existing bone marrow stress, like haemolytic anaemia, sickle cell disease or hereditary spherocytosis
   - Viruses enter in the reticulocytes (immature RBCs or erythroid progenitors) & destroy them, so reticulocyte count is decrease in blood (reticulocytopenia) followed by temporary cessation of RBCs production.
   - Due to reduce RBCs, there is rapid & severe anaemia (aplastic crisis) which is treated with blood transfusion.
5. **Haemophagocytic syndrome:**
   - It is a haematological disorder characterised by uncontrolled proliferation of lymphocytes & macrophages (histiocytes).
   - It also **called haemophagocytic lymphohistiocyto-sis.**
   - Rarely caused by parvovirus B19.
   - It seen more in children than adults.

b. In immunocompromised host: Persistent anaemia.

c. In pregnancy: Infection in 2nd & 3rd trimester causes non-immune foetal hydrops and foetal loss (abortion).

- **Laboratory diagnosis:**
- **Specimens:** Blood/serum, tissues or respiratory specimens.

- **Testing methods:**

A. **Microscopy: → Follow morphology**

B. **Culture: → Follow C/Cs**

C. **Serological tests:**

- IgM Ab is diagnosed in early stage. It indicates the recent infection & remains elevated for 2-3 months.
- IgG Ab is diagnosed in later stage. It indicates the late infection & persists for years.
- Ag is detected by immunohistochemistry method from bone marrow or foetal tissues.

D. **Molecular tests:** Real time PCR, which is most sensitive & detects the viral load. In acute infection viral load is 10^{12}DNA copies / ml

- **Prevention:** No effective vaccine is available.
- **Treatment:**
  - No specific antiviral is available.
  - Symptomatic treatment is given.
  - Neutralising immunoglobulins are given.

AAV

- **Full name:** Adeno Associated Virus **(AAV).**
- **Synonym:** Adeno satellite virus.
- **Meaning:**
- **Genus name:** *Dependoparvovirus*, as dependent on adenovirus (helper virus) for multiplication.
- **Species name:** So **called**, because it is a defective virus & required adeno virus (helper virus) for multiplication. It can multiply only in cells co-infected with adenovirus.
- **Morphology: → Vide supra**
- **Typing:** Following serotypes are identified by EM, IF test & CFT.
- **Human origin:** 1, 2 & 3.
- **Simian origin:** 4
- **Pathogenicity:** Exactly not known.

Human boca virus

New parvo virus identified from children with acute respiratory disease & gastroenteritis, but its pathogenic role is not clear.

Question bank

Case study

1) A 6 year old male child is brought to the hospital with history of fever & diarrhoea followed by redness over the cheeks sparing the other parts of face. Different laboratory tests from blood identify the ss-DNA virus. Identify the clinical conditions & answer the following

a) Name the clinical disease with causative agent.

b) Write pathogenicity of clinical condition

c) Write the diagnosis of clinical condition

Essay/Full question

1) Papovaviridae

Short notes

1) Adenoviruses
2) HPV
3) JC virus
4) BK virus
5) Parvovirus B19

Short questions for theory/viva questions

1) What is 5th disease?
2) What is aplastic crisis? Name the one virus responsible for it.
3) Write the one pathogenic disease produced by each RK virus & BK virus.

MCQs for chapter review

Adenoviridae

1) **Virus causing haemorrhagic cystitis, diarrhoea & conjunctivitis is** (AI-01)
(a) RSV (b) *Rhinovirus* (c) Adeno virus (d) Rota virus

2) **Pharyngoconjunctival fever is caused hy**
(a) Adenovirus 3 and 7 (b) Adenovirus 11, 21 (c) Adenovirus 40, 41 (d) Adenovirus 8, 19

3) **Adenovirus causes all except**
(a) Haemorrhagic cystitis (b) Diarrhoea (c) Respiratory tract infection (d) IMN

Papovaviridae

4) **Most common tumour caused by HPV is** (AIIMS-97)
(a) Warts (b) Carcinoma of cervix (c) Nasopharyngeal carcinoma (d) Lymphoma

5) **Condyloma accuminata is caused by**
(a) HSV (b) HPV (c) HIV (d) VZV

6) **Condyloma accuminata is caused by HPV types of**
(a) 18, 31 (b) 17, 12 (c) 6, 11 (d) 16, 18

7) **Human papillomatsis is caused by**
(a) HSV (b) HPV (c) HIV (d) HBV

8) **Most common type of HPV associated with cervical cancer**
(a) 6, 11 (b) 5, 8 (c) 16, 18 (d) 6, 8

9) **HPV vaccine is** (AIIMS, Nov-09)
(a) Monovalent (b) Bivalent (c) Quadrivalent (d) Both bivalent and quadrivalent

10) **True about HPV vaccination** (PGI, Nnov-09)
(a) Given in women age group 20-40 years (b) Primary dose consists of 2 doses (c) Efficacy >70% for cervical cancer (d) Two types are available in market (e) Protect against HPV 16 & 18

11) **Which of the following statement is correct** (PGI-05)
(a) Viral warts usually resolve spontaneously (b) Plantar warts should not be excised (c) Callosity is formed occupationally (d) Corns are viral in etiology (e) Plantar warts are painless

12) **All of the following are true about the papovavirus except** (AI-95)
(a) They are non-enveloped icosahedral viruses (b) Produce papilloma (c) RNA virus (d) SV-40 oncogenic

13) **Post transplant nephropathy after 1 month is most likely be due to?** (AIIMS, May-14)
(a) Hepatitis C (b) HHV-6 (c) BK virus (d) Herpes simplex virus

14) **PML is caused by** (PGI-00)
(a) CMV (b) Papova virus (c) HIV (d) Polio virus

Parvoviridae

15) **The virus which causes aplastic anaemia in chronic haemolytic disease is** (PGI-96)
(a) Adenovirus (b) Hepatitis virus (c) EB Virus (d) Parvovirus

16) **Infection with which of the following agents is particularly dangerous for anaemic patients**
(a) Adeno virus (b) Cytomegalovirus (c) Herpes simplex virus (d) Parvo virus

17) **In parvovirus infection what is common in adult** (PGI, June-97)
(a) Bone marrow aplasia (b) PRCA (c) Erythema infectiosum (d) Arthropathy

18) **Parvovirus infection is associated with** (PGI, June-08)
(a) Hydrops foetalis (b) Aplastic anaemia (c) Abortion (d) Sixth disease (e) Haemophagocytic syndrome

19) **All of the following statements about parvovirus B-19 are true except** (AI-09)
(a) DNA virus (b) Crosses placenta in < 10 % cases (c) Can cause severe anaemia (d) Can cause aplastic crisis

20) **All of the following statements about parvovirus B-19 are true except** (AI-11)
(a) < 10 % spread by transplacental route (b) Respiratory route is the primary mode of transmission (c) It is a DNA virus (d) Affects erythroid progenitors

21) **False regarding erythema infectiosum is**
(a) Caused by HHV6 (b) Marked erythema of the cheeks or slapped cheek appearance often with relative circum oral pallor (c) Infection during pregnancy can result in hydrops foetalis due to foetal anaemia (d) Arthritis is a complication

22) **Slapped cheek sign is seen in**
(a) Parvo virus B19 (b) JC virus (c) *Rotavirus* (d) Mumps

Answers of MCQs & explanation

1) (c)
2) (a)
3) (a), (b) & (c)
} Follow **table-2** for explanation

4) (a)
5) (b)
6) (c)
7) (b)
8) (c)
} Follow section, **Papovaviridae & table-3** for explanation

9) (d)
10) (d) & (e)
} Follow section, **Papovaviridae (immunoprophylaxis)** for explanation

11) (a), (b) & (c)
- Viral warts are mostly caused by HPV. which usually resolve spontaneously
- Recurrence & scaring is common following surgical excision of wart (plantar warts), so not recommended.
- Callosity is formed occupationally which is characterised by superficial circumscribed yellowish white flat thickened patch of hyperkerotic material.
- Corn is the hyperkeratosis of skin at pressure points usually on sole, foot & toes. It is painful
- Plantar warts causing pain on walking

12) (c)
- Papovavirus is ds -DNA virus
- SV-40 causing the polyoma (malignant tumour) in mice

13) (c)
- Neuropathy following renal or organ transplantation is common by BK virus

14) (b)
- Follow section, **Papovaviridae (JC virus → pathogenicity → clinical features)** for explanation

15) (d)
16) (d)
17) (d)
18) (a), (b), (c) & (e)
19) (b)
20) (a)
21) (a)
22) (a)
} Follow section, **Parvoviridae (parvo virus B19)** for explanation

65 Picornaviridae

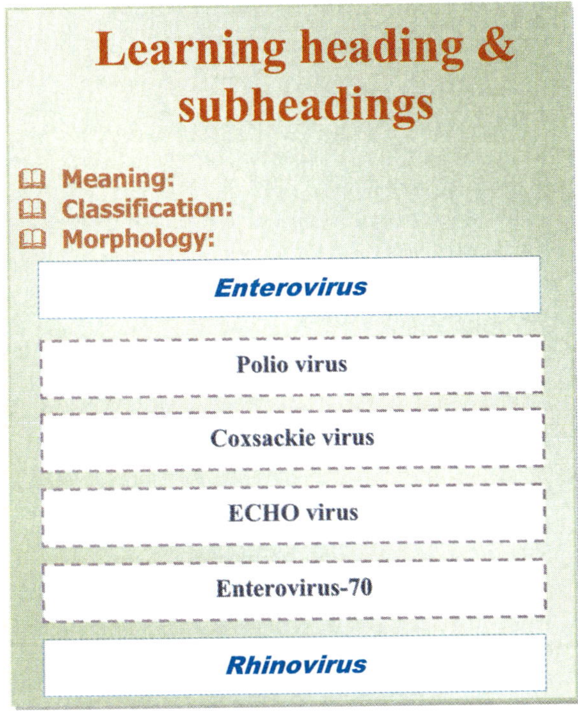

Meaning: Picorna word derived from pico + RNA where **pico = small size about** 27-30nm & **RNA = type of genome in virus.**

Classification:

- **Family:** Picornaviridae.
- **Genus:** Two groups like human & animal pathogens.

A. Human pathogens: Following four genera.

a. ***Enterovirus* (EV):** Affect the enteric tract.

1. **Polio virus:** 1 – 3.
2. **Coxsackie virus:**
   - Coxsackie virus A: 1-24.
   - Coxsackie virus B: 1 – 6.
3. **ECHO virus:** 1–34.
4. **Other entero viruses (EV):** 68 – 72.
   - EV-68: Pneumonia & bronchitis.
   - EV-69: No human disease.
   - EV-70: Acute haemorrhagic conjunctivitis (AHC).
   - EV-71: HFMD, meningitis & encephalitis.
   - EV-72: Reclassified as *Hepatovirus* (HAV).

b. ***Rhinovirus*:** Affect the nasal mucosa.

- >100 serotypes.
- Tissue culture type: H, M & O.

c. ***Hepatovirus (Heparnavirus* = Hepa (liver) + rna (RNA genome):**

- HAV (Hepatitis A virus) which infects the liver.
- Previously it was classified as EV 72.
- More details: Follow chapter → Hepatitis viruses.

d. ***Parechovirus*:**

B. Animal pathogens: Following two genera.

a. ***Aphthovirus*:** Foot & mouth disease in cattle.

b. ***Cardiovirus*:** Encephalo-myocarditis in mice.

Morphology: →**Fig.-1**

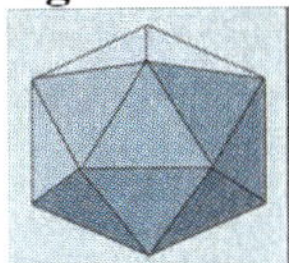

Figure-1: Morphology of Picronaviridae (polio virus)

- **Shape:** Spherical.
- **Size:** 27 nm having 60 subunits, each consist four viral proteins (VP-1 to VP-4).
- **Genome & capsid:** ss-RNA (+) surrounded by icosahedral variety of capsid.
- **Non enveloped (naked virus)**
- Eosinophilic intranuclear Cowdry type-B inclusion bodies may be seen in stained preparation.

Enterovirus

Polio virus

History:

- It was first isolated in 1909 by Karl Landsteiner & Erwin Popper by inoculation of spinal cord & faecal extract in to monkey from the fatal case of polio.
- Virus infecting nerve system, but its non neural cultivation technique over human embryonic cell was developed by Nobel Laureate, Enders, Wellers & Robbins in 1949 with development of CPE.

Geographical distribution:

- **World scenario:** It was present in many countries, but almost eradicated from many countries by successful vaccination except Pakistan, Afghanistan & Nigeria (abbreviated as PAN countries) where scattered cases are present.
- **Indian scenario:** Polio is eradicated from the India & WHO declared it as polio free in 2014.

Use: Polio virus is one of the most well-characterized viruses & has become a useful model for understanding the biology of RNA viruses.

Morphology: → Vide supra

Culture characteristics (C/Cs):

i. **Egg culture:** Old strain can grow, not the fresh isolates.

ii. **Animal culture:** Animals are susceptible.

- Monkey is infected by intraspinal/intracerebral mode.
- Chimpanzees or cynomolgus monkey may be infected orally.

iii. Tissue culture:

- Grow only in human & monkey cells.
- Human: Human diploid (secondary) fibroblast cell line.
- Monkey: Primary monkey kidney culture is useful. Growth is indicated by typical CPE in 2-3 days.
- Infected cells round up, pyknotic or refractile.
- Eosinophilic **intranuclear Cowdry type-B inclusion bodies** may be seen in stained preparation.
- Viral antigen from culture is identified by neutralisation test.
- Cell monolayer produce plaques with agar overlay.

❖ Resistance:

- Inactivated at 55^0C for 30 minutes.
- Non-enveloped resist to lipid solvent like ether, chloroform & bile salts.
- Also resist to proteolytic enzyme.
- Destroyed by formaldehyde, oxidising agents & chlorination.

❖ Antigenic structure & serotypes:

➢ **By neutralisation test:**

- **Types:** 3 types of strain.

1. **Type 1 (Brunhilde & Mahoney):**
   - Most commonly associated with paralysis.
   - Mostly causes epidemic.
   - Poor vaccine response, so difficult to eradicate.
2. **Type 2 (Lencing & Mefi):**
   - Causes endemic infections.
   - In India paralysis by type-2 is common.
   - Most effective antigen.
3. **Type 3 (Leon & Sauket):**
   - Causes epidemic.
   - Most common Vaccine Associated Polio (VAP) virus.

- **Cross reaction:** Immunity is type specific & cross reaction is common between 1 & 2, 2 & 3 but little or none between 1& 3.

➢ **By CFT, ELISA or precipitation test:** Two Ags.

1. **C (Capsid) Ag:**
   - C antigen **also called heated (H) antigen** - associated with empty or noninfectious virus.
   - It is less specific & reacts with heterotypic sera.
   - Anti-C- Ab is not protective.
2. **D (Dense) Ag:**
   - D antigen **also called Native (N) antigen** - associated with whole virion and is type specific.
   - Anti-D-Ab is protective, so potency of the injectable polio vaccine measured in terms of D-antigen units.

❖ Immunity:

a. Humoral immunity: It is protective but type specific.

✪ **Circulating antibodies (IgM & IgG):**

- IgM: Appear within a week & last for about six months.
- IgG: It persist for life.
- Both protect to the systemic infection but not to local (intestinal/mucosal) infection, so virus continuously shed in faeces.
- They protect against the virus of same serotype.

✪ **Secretory antibody (IgA):**

- It is synthesised locally by intestinal mucosa & provide local immunity.
- It is present in mother's milk & protects the child from infection.

b. Cell mediated immunity: Virus also induces the CMI but its role is uncertain.

❖ Pathogenicity:

➢ **Disease name: Called polio.**

➢ **Synonym:** Also **called poliomyelitis.**

➢ **Nature of disease:** It is endemic & epidemic in nature.

➢ **Reservoir of infection:**

- Human is the only natural reservoir of infection due to shedding of virus in **faeces** for 3-4 months. There is no chronic carrier, but person with IDDs can shed it for longer time.
- It may be patient (case) or symptomless carrier.
- For every one case about 1000 subclinical cases in children & 100 in adults are present; which are act as reservoirs.

➢ **Source of infection:**

- Food & water contaminated from human faeces.
- In early stage it also sheds in **throat secretion** & possible source of infection to contact.

➢ **Mode of transmission:**

- Faeco-oral route: Ingestion of food & water contaminated from human faeces.
- Inhalation.
- Entry through conjunctiva from droplets of respiratory secretions -possible mode of entry in close contacts of patients in early stages of the disease.
- Direct neural transmission in case of tonsillectomy.

➢ **Incubation period:** 7-14 days on average (range is 4 days - 4 weeks).

➢ **Portal of entry:** GIT.

➢ **Sites:** Brain & spinal cord.

➢ **Precipitating factors (epidemiological determinants):** Two types.

a. Agent factors:

- Dose of infection.
- Virulent or avirulent strain.
- Types of strain (**vide supra**): Type 1 & 3 are causing epidemic disease while type 2 causes endemic disease.

b. Host factors:

1. **Age:** Adults are more susceptible than children.
2. **Sex:** It has been noted as 3 males to one female.
3. **Pregnancy:** More risk due to hormonal changes.
4. **IDDs:** It is more severe & virus shedding is more prolonged in person with IDDs.
5. **Tonsillectomy:** During the incubation period may predispose the bulbar poliomyelitis. It also precipitates the direct neural transmission.
6. **Heavy exercise:** Heavy exercise & increase muscular activities are increases the risk of paralysis.
7. **Vaccination:**
- Injection of alum precipitated triple vaccine (DPT) may precipitate the paralysis in inoculated limbs.
- Mechanisms are uncertain.
8. **Trauma:** It may leads the viral entry in to local nerve fibres or segment of spinal cord corresponding to the site may be more susceptible to viral damage due to reactive hyperaemia.

c. Environmental factors:

1. **Rainy season:** In India most cases were reported in rainy season during June –September.
2. **Cold environment:** Polio virus survives for long time in cold environment.
3. **Overcrowding & poor sanitation:** Also provide the opportunities for exposure.

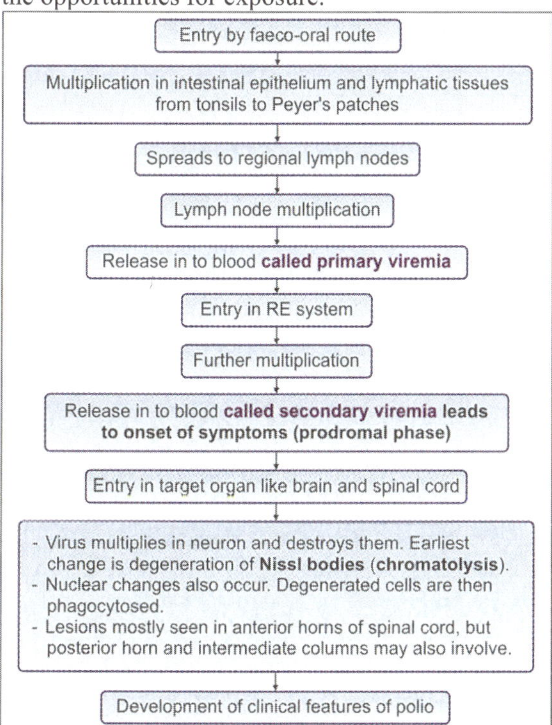

Flow chart-1: Pathogenesis of polio

- **Pathogenesis:** Virus is spread by haematogenous & neural routes.

1. **Haematogenous route: → Flow chart-1**
2. **Neural route:** Neural transmission occurs following tonsillectomy.

- **Clinical features: → Fig.-2**

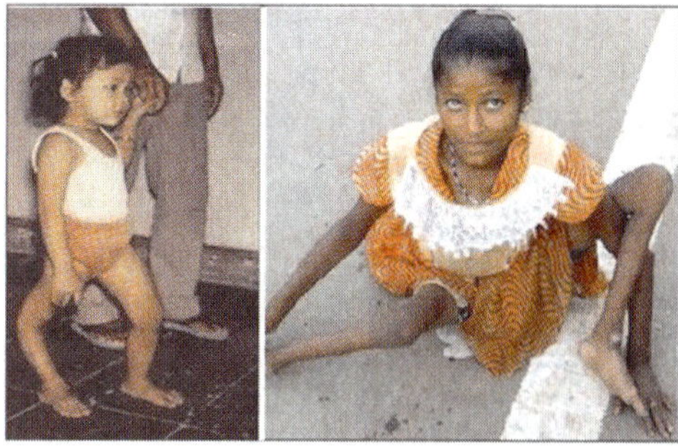

Figure-2: Cases of polio

- **Stages of paralysis:**

a. Inapparent infection:
- About 90-95 % cases are asymptomatic.
- Only 5-10% produces the clinical illness.

b. Minor illness or abortive polio:
- Occurs in 4-8 % of the infections.
- Associated with primary viremia & production of minor symptoms like fever, headache, sore throat and malaise lasting for 1-5 days.
- It **called the minor illness** and in many cases this is only manifestation.

c. Non-paralytic polio:
- Sometimes the infection will not progress beyond the stage of aseptic meningitis & there is no paralysis.
- Features of aseptic meningitis (stage of CNS invasion by virus) like fever (biphasic fever), headache, neck stiffness & rigidity are present.
- Aseptic meningitis occurs in 1 % cases.

d. Major illness or paralytic polio: It present with flaccid paralysis with following features.

- **Duration:** If the infection progresses, minor illness followed 3-4 days later by major illness.
- **Frequency:** Occurs in <1 % of the infections.
- **Sites of paralysis:**
  - Paralysis may be bulbar, spinal & bulbospinal.
  - It affects the proximal muscles 1st followed by distal muscles.
  - Quadriceps is the most common muscle affected in leg, while in hand most common affected muscle is oppenens pollicis. Tibialis anterior is the most common muscle undergoes to complete paralysis.
- **Tripod sign:**
  - Synonym: Also **called "Amoss's sign"** & first described by the American pathologist Harold Lindsay Amoss (1886-1956).
  - Paralysis start from the hip & proceeds towards extremities which leads to typical '**tripod sign**'.
  - In tripod sign patient sit with flexed hip & both arms extended towards the back for support as shown in **fig.-3(a)**.
  - Tripod sign is a useful sign of meningeal irritation. It is used for diagnosing conditions like meningitis, subarachnoid haemorrhage, and poliomyelitis.
- **Other important points:**

- It is characterised by descending, asymmetric, acute flaccid paralysis.
- Cranial nerves are involved but no sensory loss
- No autonomic disturbance.
- Non progressive.
- Lower motor neuron (LMN) type.
- Exaggerated tendon reflexes are absent
- **Recovery:** Recovery of paralysed muscle takes place in next 4-8 weeks & usually complete after 6 months, leaving behind the residual paralysis with variable degree.
- **Mortality:** Mortality is 5-10% due to respiratory failure.
- **Biphasic course:** Some time disease progression occurs in two phase. In 1st phase aseptic meningitis occurs with full recovery. In 2nd phase return of fever with paralysis in 1-2 days.
- **Post polio atrophy syndrome:** A recrudescence of paralysis and muscle wasting has been observed in individual, usually decades (20-40 years) after the episode of paralytic polio.

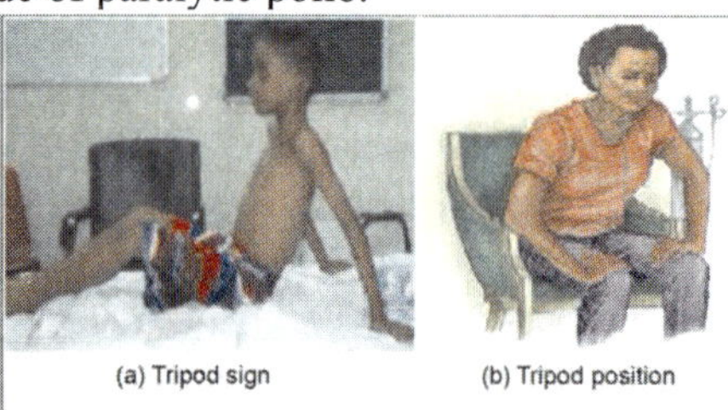
(a) Tripod sign (b) Tripod position

Figure-3: Tripod sign & tripod position

✓ **Note: Tripod position**

- **Features:** In tripod position, one sits or stands leaning forward and supporting the upper body with hands on the knees or on another surface as shown in **fig.-3(b)**.
- **Causes:** It mostly occurs when patient feel respiratory distress like in chronic obstructive pulmonary disease.

➢ **Complications:**

1. **Mortality:** In 5-10% cases due to respiratory failure
2. **Post polio muscle atrophy syndrome:** Recrudescence of paralysis & muscle wasting has been occurred in individual, usually 20-40 years after the episode of paralytic polio.

❖ Laboratory diagnosis:

➢ **Specimens:** Blood, throat swab, stool & CSF.

➢ **Testing methods:**

A. Microscopy: → Follow morphology.

B. Culture: → Follow C/Cs.

C. Serological tests:

- Less useful method.
- Antibodies are developed after paralysis.
- Antibodies are detected by CFT or by neutralisation test.

D. Molecular methods:

- **RT- PCR:**
- **Sequencing:**
- Three types of polio strain are in circulation in environment like wild strain, OPV strain & vaccine derived polio viruses (VDPVs).
- All three can be differentiated by sequencing.

❖ Prevention:

➢ **Aim:** To eradicated the polio.

➢ **Types of immunisation:**

A. Active immunisation: By using vaccines.

✪ **Types of vaccines:** Two types of vaccines (both are effective).

i. Killed vaccine:

- **Synonym:** Injectable polio vaccine or inactivated polio vaccine (IPV) or Salk vaccine.
- **History:** Developed by Salk & his team, in 1957 at the University of Pittsburgh.
- **Preparation:**
- Prepared by using all three types of polio viruses.
- Type 1 (40 units), 2 (8 units) & 3 (32 units) are grown in a monkey kidney tissue culture (Vero cell line), which are then inactivated with formalin.
- **Dose:**
- **Route:** By IM or SC route.
- **Schedule (according to national immunisation schedule):** First three doses are given at 6th, 10th & 14th week & fourth dose at 6-12 months & fifth dose at school entry age. Five doses should be completed before school age. Then additional dose every 5 year up to age of 18 year.
- **Protection by IPV:** The injected Salk vaccine confers IgM, IgG & serum IgA (systemic) mediated immunity in the bloodstream, which prevents polio infection from progressing to viremia and protects the motor neurons, thus eliminating the risk of bulbar polio and post-polio syndrome.
- **Mixed or combination:**
- In some states pentavalent vaccine (**Pentvac**) contains Diphtheria, Pertusis, Tetanus, HBV, H influenza type b (Hib) is given at 6th weeks, 10th weeks & 14th weeks with OPV.
- Other same preparation is **Pentaxim** contains D, P, T, IPV & Hib given with OPV & HBV.
- **Advantages:**
- More stable & safe than live vaccines because the dead microbes can't mutate back to their disease-producing state.
- No disease to contact.
- Don't require refrigeration, can be easily stored and transported at ambient temperature.
- Given in combination with polyvalent vaccine.
- Useful for person with immunodeficiency disease & on steroid therapy.
- Useful in pregnancy also.

- **Disadvantages:**
- Weaker immune response than live vaccines. So it would likely take several additional doses or booster doses to maintain a person's immunity.
- Short lived immunity.
- Provides only systemic, but not local immunity.
- Local reaction at the site of injection.

ii. **Live vaccine:**

- **Synonym:** Oral polio vaccine (OPV) or Sabin vaccine.
- **History:** Developed by Coprowsky, Cox & Sabin. All three were used initially, now Sabin vaccine (1957) is in routine use.
- **Preparation:**
- Prepared by using all three types of polio viruses.
- Vaccine contains **(1)** 3, 00, 000 TCID 50 of Type 1 virus, **(2)** 1, 00, 000 TCID 50 of Type 2 virus & **(3)** 3, 00, 000 TCID 50 of Type 3 virus.
- Vaccine is temperature sensitive. It makes thermostable by adding some salts like $MgCL_2$ & Na_2 SO_4. These salts act as pH < 7. The pH of vaccine is maintained by keeping the vial airtight.
- Viruses are grown in a primary monkey kidney or in human diploid cell culture.
- **Dose:**
- **Route:** Two drops by oral route; repeat if child spit out.
- **Schedule (according to national immunisation schedule):** Initial dose given immediately after birth **callled zero dose polio**. First three doses are given at 6th, 10th & 14th week & fourth dose at 6-12 months & fifth dose at school entry age. Five doses should be completed before school age. Then additional dose every 5 year up to age of 18 year.
- **Reason for requirement of three doses:** Single dose is enough to provide sufficient immunity, but in practise three doses are required to ensure multiplication by all three viruses after overcoming interference by themselves.
- **Advantages:**
- OPV produces secretory IgA & provides immunity in the intestine (local), the primary site of wild poliovirus entry, which helps to prevent infection with wild virus in areas where the virus is endemic.
- Also provide systemic immunity (IgG).
- The live virus used in the vaccine is shed in the stool & can be spread to others within a community & provides herd or community immunity.
- Confer strong & long lasting immunity.
- More economical than IPV.
- Given by oral route, so highly trained person is not required.
- **Disadvantages:**

a. **Temperature sensitive:** Heat labile & inactivated, if temperature is not maintained during storage & transportation.

b. **Vaccine originated polio:** Two types.

1. **Vaccine Associated Polio virus (VAP):**

- Vaccine virus causing polio **called vaccine associated paralytic polio**.
- Virus shows the < 1% genetic divergence from the parental strain **called OPV-like isolate.**
- It is ubiquitous at the place where OPV is given spread by faeco-oral route to close contact.
- It occurs in 1 case out of 2.5 million doses of OPV
- It is more common in person with IDDs (increase risk by 3000 fold) & following 1st dose than subsequent dose.
- Most common in Sabin serotype 3 (60%) followed by Sabin type 2.

Features	IPV	OPV
Synonym	Killed or Salk vaccine	Live or Sabin vaccine
Attenuation	By formalin	Live attenuated
Route	IM or SC	Oral
Contraindication	Not in IDD	Yes in IDD
Cost	Virus contains are 10,000 times higher than OPV, hence costlier	Cheap
Role	Prevent paralysis not reinfection	Prevent paralysis & reinfection
Immunity	Short lived	Long lived
Protection	Less	More
Ig produced	IgG, IgM	IgA & IgG
Local immunity	No	Yes
CMI	Poor/no	Yes
Reversion to virulence	No	Yes
Excretion of vaccine microbes & transmission to non-immune contacts	No	Yes
Interference by other virus in host	No	Yes
Heat stability	No	Yes
Temp. maintenance during storage & transport	No	Yes

Table-1: Differences between IPV & OPV

2. **Vaccine Derived Polio virus (VDP):**

- Virus shows the > 1% genetic divergence from the parental strain (if it shows < 1% then **called OPV-like isolate**).
- Most common in Sabin serotype 2 (90%) followed by Sabin type 1. It is more common in types 2 of vaccine because wild strain of type 2 is eradicated & not circulating in the community since 1999 (type 2 is eradicated in 1999).
- Since 2000 VDP outbreaks have occured in 18 countries with majority of type 2 (87.1%). In 2013 over 700 strains have been isolated worldwide. Around 50% of such strains were from India & Nigeria.

- To avoid chances of VDP by type 2 it is eradicated from trivalent vaccine. Such trivalent vaccine is replaced by bivalent vaccine contains type 1 & 3.
- Another reason (probably) for removal of type 2 is probably due to acquirement of cross protection between types 1 & 2, and types 2 & 3 but little or no between 1 & 3.

✪ **Differences between IPV & OPV: →Table-1**

✪ **Contraindications:**

- IDDs (for OPV)
- Pregnancy: vaccination will be delayed unless immediate protection is required.
- Diarrhoea: It's not the contraindication, but the dose given to child with diarrhoea is not counted & repetition of dose is required.

✪ **Effective factors on vaccine failure:**

a. **Breast-milk:**

- Colostrum contains high level of IgA. Ingestion of OPV three days after the child birth may interfere with OPV.
- Breast milk after 4th day contain low level of IgA, may not interfere with OPV.

b. **Pre-existing viral disease:**

- ***Enterovirus*** may prevent the colonisation by vaccine virus & effect over immunity.
- **Coxsackie B** may interfere while **coxsackie A** may be synergistic.

c. **Improper cold-chain maintenance:** The shelf life of the vaccine is 4 months at 4-8^{0}C & 2 years at -20^{0}C. Improper storage & cold chain failure may be partly responsible for apparent OPV failure.

d. **pH:** OPV best act at pH below 7. pH is maintained by keeping the vaccine air tight.

✪ **Criteria for attenuation of strain:**

- Should not be neurovirulent as tested by intraspinal inoculation in monkey.
- Should be stable & should not acquire neuro-virulence after serial enteric passage.
- Should be able to induce intestinal infection & immune response following feeding.
- Should possess genetic characteristics (marker) by which they can be differentiated from wild virulent properties.

✪ **Marker to differentiate wild from attenuated strain:**

a. **D marker:** Wild strain will grows at low level of bicarbonate but the avirulent strain will not.

b. **ret 40:** Wild strain will grows well at 40^{0}C but not the avirulent strain.

c. **MS:** Wild strain will grows in a stable cell line of monkey kidney, but the avirulent strain grows poorly.

d. **Mc Bride's intratypic antigenic marker:** Shown by rate of inactivation by specific antiserum.

e. **Other methods:** Above markers are not sufficient. Other methods used are

1. Molecular epidemiology: By using monoclonal-Ab.
2. Oligonucleotide finger printing.
3. Nucleic acid sequencing.

✪ **Eradication of poliomyelitis:**

- **Strategies for eradication:**
  - Conduct PPI.
  - High level of routine immunisation.
  - Monitoring of vaccination.
  - Diagnosis of all cases of acute flaccid paralysis by polio or non-polio.
  - Early diagnosis from stool.
  - Outbreak control of cases to stop transmission.
- **Goal & drawback:** in 1988, WHO had proposed the global eradication of poliomyelitis by the year 2000, by global immunisation with OPV. Poor progress in immunisation in many countries has been the setback to this objective.

✪ **Pulse Polio Immunisation (PPI):** term pulse indicates mass immunisation by OPV on a single day to all children between 0-5 years in the community regardless of previous or routine immunisation.

✪ **Mopping up:** Door-to door immunisation in high risk district where wild virus is known or suspected to circulate.

✪ **Endgame strategic plan (2013-18):**

- **Aim:** To eradicate the polio from the entire world by 2018.
- **Strategies:**
  - Third dose of OPV will be replaced by IPV by the end of 2015.
  - Trivalent OPV will be replaced by bivalent OPV (type 1 &3) six months after starting the IPV up to mid 2016.
  - Complete replacement of OPV by IPV by 2019
- **Certification:** Implementation of containment programme & to certify the world as polio free by end of 2018.
- **Future planning:** Utilisation of infrastructure, fund, manpower, knowledge & experience for other health programme that has been created to eradicate the polio.

B. **Passive immunisation:**

- Done by using Ig.
- OPV & IPV eliminate the use of passive immunisation
- 0.25-0.3 ml/kg/body weight is protective.

❖ **World polio day:** It was fixed on 24th Oct of every year by Rotary International over a decade ago to commemorate the birth of Jonas Salk, who led the first team to develop a vaccine against poliomyelitis.

Coxsackie virus

❖ **Meaning:** 1st patients came from the Coxsackie village of New York, hence the genus name.

❖ **History:**
- It was first isolated in 1948 by Dalldorf & Sickles by inoculation of faecal extract in to suckling mice from the paediatric case of paralytic polio, from which polio1 was isolated.
- It caused paralysis in inoculated mice.

❖ **Geographical distribution:** Different serotypes of coxsackie A & coxsackie B are distributed in different regions.

❖ **Morphology:** → Vide supra

❖ **Culture characteristics (C/Cs):**

i. Animal culture:
- Infect the suckling mice but not the adult mice,
- Inoculation done by subcutaneous, intraperitoneal or intracerebral route.
- Identification done by histopathology & by neutralisation test.
- Coxsackie A: Produces generalised myositis, flaccid paralysis & death in a week.
- Coxsackie B: Produce patchy focal myositis, spastic paralysis, necrosis of brown fat, pancreatitis, hepatitis, myocarditis & encephalitis.

ii. Tissue culture:
- A7, A9 & all coxcackie B can grow in monkey kidney tissue culture.
- A7 & A9 can grow in human diploid (secondary) fibroblast cell line.
- A21 grow in Hela cells.

❖ **Resistance:** Non-enveloped resist to lipid solvent like ether, chloroform & bile salts.

❖ **Antigenic structure & serotypes:** Two groups like A & B, are identified by neutralisation test & pathological changes in suckling mice.

I. **Coxsackie A:** 1-24 serotypes (type 23 is same as echovirus-9 & type 24 is as echovirus-34).

II. **Coxsackie B:** 1-6 serotypes (all type share common complement fixing Ag).

❖ **Immunity:** Immunity is type specific.

❖ **Pathogenicity:**
➢ **Nature of disease:** Coxsackie B produces the epidemic every 2-3 years.
➢ **Reservoir of infection:** Human.
➢ **Source of infection:** Food & water contaminated from human faeces.
➢ **Mode of transmission:** By faeco-oral route.
➢ **Portal of entry:** GIT.
➢ **Sites:** → **Table-2**
➢ **Precipitating factors:**
1. **Age:** Young infants are commonly infected.
➢ **Clinical features:**

I. Coxsackie A

1. **Herpangina (vesicular pharyngitis):**
- Occurs in children.
- Local features: Small vesicle on fauces & posterior pharyngeal wall which break down to form ulcer.
- Systemic features: Fever, headache, vomiting & abdominal pain.
2. **Aseptic meningitis:**
- Mostly A7 & A9.
- Maculopapular rash may be present.
- Type-7 produced outbreak of paralysis in Scotland, Russia & elsewhere.
- Erroneously referred as type-4 polio virus.
3. **Produced by A9, A16 & B1-3:**
- Exanthematous disease occurs in young children.
- Papulovesicular lesion present on skin & oral mucosa.
- Resolved in 1-2 weeks.
- Occur as sporadic cases & as an outbreak.
4. **Conjunctivitis:** Rarely by A24.
5. **Produced by entero virus 71:**
- Occurred as extensive epidemic in 1970 in East Asia from Taiwan to Singapore.
- Present with pulmonary haemorrhage, aseptic meningitis, encephalitis, flaccid paralysis with many fatalities.
6. **Hand foot and mouth disease (HFMD): → Fig.-4**
7. **Minor respiratory infection:** Like common cold caused by A10, A21 & A24.

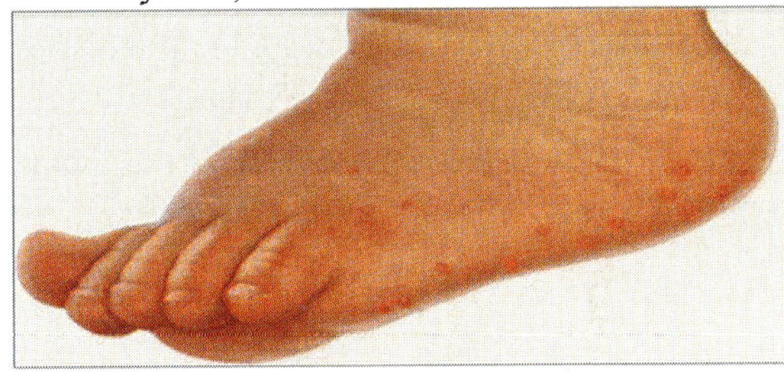

Figure-4: Foot disease

II. Coxsackie B

1. **Aseptic meningitis:** Caused by all group B viruses
2. **Hand foot and mouth disease (HFMD):** Caused by B 1-3 viruses.
3. **Epidemic pleurodynia or Bornholm disease:**
- So called because 1st described in **Danish Island of Bornholm.**
- Occur as sporadic cases & as epidemic.
- Present with fever, chest paint & abdominal pain.
4. **Myocarditis and pericarditis:** Occurs in newborn, older children & adult with high fatality.
5. **Juvenile diabetes:** Associated with B4, but causal role is still to prove.
6. **Orchitis:**
7. **Minor respiratory infection:** Like common cold caused by B3.
8. **Transplacental & neonatal transmission:** Serious disseminated disease in newborn which may

include meningitis, encephalitis, hepatitis & adreno-cortical involvement.

9. **Post-viral fatigue syndrome:** Associated with group B, but causal role is still to prove.

❖ **Differences between Coxsackie A & B:** → **Table-2**

❖ **Laboratory diagnosis:**

➢ **Specimens:** Stool & sample from lesion

➢ **Testing methods:**

A. **Microscopy:** → **Follow morphology**

B. **Culture:** → **Follow C/Cs**

C. **Serological test:** Not useful because of many serotypes

D. **Molecular method:** PCR is more useful as it is sensitive & serotype specific.

Features	Coxsackie A	Coxsackie B
Intracerebral inoculation in mice	Flaccid paralysis & systemic myositis	Spastic paralysis & focal myositis
Sites	More in skin & mucosa	More in heart, pancreas, pleura & liver
Clinical features	Follow text	Follow text
Serotypes	1-26	1-6
Receptors	Intercellular adhesion molecules	Coxsackie virus & adenovirus receptors

Table-2: Differences between coxsackie A & B

❖ **Prevention:** Vaccination is not useful because of several serotypes & immunity is type specific.

❖ **Treatment:** Self limited disease & symptomatic treatment is required.

ECHO virus

❖ **Full name:** **E**ntero **C**ytopathogenic **H**uman **O**rphan Viruses.

❖ **Meaning:** Not associated with any particular disease at the time of discovery hence **called orphan viruses**. However later it identified as a causative agent of many disease but the original name is still persist.

❖ **History:** The first isolation of echoviruses occurred from the faeces of asymptomatic children early in the 1950, just after cell culturing had been developed.

❖ **Geographical distribution:** Worldwide.

❖ **Morphology:** → Vide supra

❖ **Culture characteristics (C/Cs):**

i. **Animal culture:**

- Animals are less susceptible.
- Monkey & new born mice produce paresis on inoculation.

ii. **Tissue culture:** Grow only in human or monkey cells.

- Human cells: Human diploid (secondary) fibroblast cell line.
- Monkey cells: Primary monkey kidney culture is also useful. Growth is indicated by typical cytopathic effects.
- Viral antigen from culture is identified by neutralisation or haemagglutination test.

❖ **Resistance:**

- Echoviruses are infective & stable over a wide range of pH (3-10).
- Non-enveloped resist to lipid solvent like ether, chloroform, bile salts & alcohol.

❖ **Antigenic structure & serotypes:** By neutralization tests, classified into 34 serotypes. But type 10 & 28 removed from the group & classified as Reovirus-1 & Rhinovirus-1 respectively.

❖ **Pathogenicity:**

➢ **Nature & history of disease:**

- Epidemics have been reported in Panama, Mexico, Switzerland, Cuba, the United States, and Turkey. Asian-Pacific countries have reported major enteroviral epidemics with significant morbidity and mortality. A Thai hospital reported the first nosocomial outbreak of hand-foot-and-mouth disease due to echovirus type 11.
- Epidemic of fever & aseptic meningitis is common by serotypes, 4, 6, 9, 16, 20, 28 & 30.

➢ **Reservoir of infection:** Human

➢ **Source of infection:** Mostly contaminated food & water. Rarely it presents in saliva & swimming pool water.

➢ **Mode of transmission:**

- By faeco-oral route.
- Respiration of oral secretions such as saliva.
- Fomites (inanimate objects) borne.
- Contaminated swimming and wading pools can also transmit the virus.
- Also, there are well-documented reports of transmission via the contaminated hands of hospital personnel.

➢ **Incubation period:** 4-6 days after the infection.

➢ **Portal of entry:** GIT.

➢ **Sites:** Meninges, GIT liver, spleen, bone marrow, heart and lungs.

➢ **Pathogenesis:** → **Flow chart-2**

➢ **Precipitating factors:**

1. **Age:** Common in children younger than 15 years.
2. **Sex:** More in male child.
3. **Seasonal:** Epidemic is common in summer.
4. **Overcrowding & poor sanitation:** Also increase the exposure risk.
5. **IDDs:** Opportunistic pathogen in immuno-compromised individual.

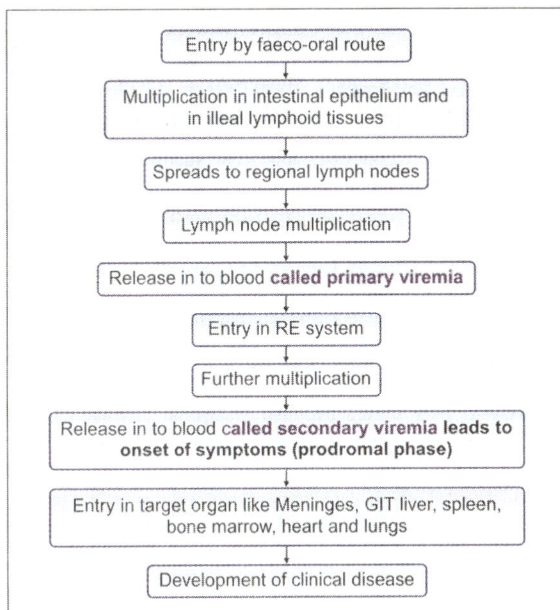

Flow chart-2: Pathogenesis of ECHO virus

- **Clinical features:**
- More than 90% infections are asymptomatic.
- Aseptic meningitis: Epidemic present with fever with rash & aseptic meningitis. Produced by serotypes like 4, 6, 9, 16, 20, 28 & 30.
- Respiratory infections: Common by 1, 11, 19, 20 & 22.
- Gastroenteritis: By 18.
- **Complications:** Occasional cases of paralysis & hepatic necrosis have been reported.

Laboratory diagnosis:

- **Specimens:** Throat swab, stool & CSF.
- **Testing methods:**

A. **Microscopy: → Follow morphology**
B. **Culture: → Follow C/Cs**
C. **Serological tests:**

- Not used routinely.
- Useful in epidemic to identify causative serotype.

Prevention: Vaccination has not attempted.

Treatment:

- No specific drug is available.
- Symptomatic treatment is given.
- The anti-viral drug pleconaril interferes with the binding of the echovirus particle to the cell membrane & the drug also hinders the uncoating of virions by attaching itself to the viral protein capsid.

Entero virus-70

Synonym: Also **called Acute Haemorrhagic Conjunctivitis Virus (AHCV).**

Geographical distribution: Distributed in tropical countries.

Morphology: → **Vide supra**

Culture characteristics (C/Cs): By tissue culture

- Grow in human embryonic kidney or Hela cells.
- Can grow in monkey kidney cells.

Resistance:

- Entero virus 70 is sensitive to a solution of 500 ppm sodium hypochlorite with a contact time of 2 minutes.
- It is resistant to phenyl mercuric borate and isopropyl alcohol.
- It can be inactivated by extreme heat (>56°C), ultraviolet light & drying.
- It can survive at least 24 hours on inanimate surfaces under high humidity conditions.
- It is stable in liquid environments and can survive for many weeks in water, body fluids and sewage.

Immunity: Not specific.

Pathogenicity:

- **Disease name:** Disease **called acute hemorrhagic conjunctivitis (AHC).**
- **Nature or history of disease:**
- It occurs in epidemic or pandemic forms.
- The first pandemic of acute hemorrhagic conjunctivitis, affecting hundreds of millions of people, occurred in 1969 in Africa. It spread to several parts of Africa, Middle East, India, South East Asia, Japan, England & Europe.
- Since then the virus has been associated with large outbreaks, mainly in tropical areas.
- **Reservoir of infection:** Human.
- **Source of infection:** Eye secretion.
- **Mode of transmission:** Direct or indirect contact (introduction of the virus into the eye through infected hands and fomites) with eye secretions. No vector borne transmission occurs.
- **Incubation period:** 24 -48 hrs.
- **Portal of entry:** Eye.
- **Sites:** Ophthalmic & non ophthalmic sites.
- **Precipitating factors:** Health workers are at more risk.
- **Clinical features:**

1. **Acute hemorrhagic conjunctivitis:**

- It present with eye pain, photophobia, swelling of eye lid and varying redness of the conjunctiva (from subconjunctival petechiae to haemorrhage).
- Disease resolved in 10 days.
- Transient corneal involvement may occur in some cases.
- Other virus produce same lesion: Also caused by Coxsackie type A-24. Both viruses show intratypic antigenic difference.

2. **Non-ophthalmic symptoms:** Such as

- Neurologic dysfunction.

17) Common antibody produced by IPV & OPV is
(a) IgA (b) IgM (c) IgG (d) a+c

18) Which viral disease transmitted by oro-faecal route
(a) Dengue (b) Polio virus (c) Hepatitis B (d) Influenza virus

19) Virus which spread by haematogenous and neural route is
(a) Rabies virus (b) Varicella zoster virus (c) Polio virus (d) EB virus

Coxsackie virus

20) Suckling mice is used for isolation of
(a) Coxsackie virus (b) Pox virus (c) Herpes virus (d) Adenovirus

21) Following virus can be grown in suckling mice
(a) Coxsackie virus (b) Rhino virus (c) ECHO virus (d) Polio virus

22) *Enterovirus* causes all except (AIIMS, Nov-01, AI-09)
(a) Haemorrhagic fever (b) Pleurodynia (c) Herpengina (d) Aseptic meningitis

23) Mode of spread of *Enterovirus*
(a) Vector mediated (b) Droplet infection (c) Faeco-oral route (d) Skin contact

24) Coxsackie A virus does not causes
(a) Herpengina (b) Hand foot and mouth disease (HFMD) (c) Laryngotracheobronchitis (d) Aseptic meningitis

25) Coxsackie group A commonly causes
(a) Conjunctivitis (b) Aseptic meningitis (c) Hepatitis (d) Myocarditis

26) Herpengina is caused by
(a) Adenovirus (b) Enterovirus-72 (c) Coxsackie virus A (d) Coxsackie virus B

27) Herpengina is caused by
(a) *Enterovirus* (b) *Rhinovirus* (c) Myxo virus (d) Rabies virus

28) Coxsackie B virus causes all except
(a) Aseptic meningitis (b) Herpangina (c) Myocarditis (d) Bornholm disease

Entero virus - 70

29) Acute haemorrhagic conjunctivitis is caused by (AI-97)
(a) Entero virus 70 (b) Adeno virus (c) Polio virus (d) Hepadna virus

30) Acute haemorrhagic conjunctivitis is caused by (AI-97)
(a) Entero virus 70 (b) Adeno virus (c) Coxsackie A2-4 (d) Hepadna virus

31) Epidemic haemorrhagic conjunctivitis is caused by
(a) HSV (b) VZV (c) HIV (d) Picorna virus

32) Which of the following does not conjunctivitis
(a) Adeno virus (b) *Enterovirus* (c) Coxsackie virus (d) Herpes virus

33) Entero viruses causes
(a) Acute haemorrhagic conjunctivitis (b) Acute follicular conjunctivitis (c) Posterior follicular conjunctivitis (d) Epidemic kerato conjunctivitis

Mixed MCQs

34) All are included in picorna group of viruses except
(a) Encephalo myocarditis (b) HEV (c) Foot and mouth virus (d) Polio virus

35) All of the following clinical features are associated with entero viruses except (AI-04)
(a) Myocarditis (b) Pleurodynia (c) Herpengina (d) Haemorrhagic fever

36) True statements about entero viruses (PGI, May-13)
(a) Composed of segmented genome (b) Stable at pH 4 (c) Causes pleurodynia (d) Causes encephalitis (e) Causes meningitis

Answers of MCQs & explanation

1) (a)
2) (c)
3) (a)
} Follow section **classification** for explanation

4) (a)
5) (c)
6) (c)
7) (a)
8) (b)
9) (b)
10) (c)
11) (c)
12) (d)
13) (a)
14) (d)
15) (b)
16) (b)
17) (d)
} Follow section ***Enterovirus* (polio virus)** for explanation

18) (b)
- Dengue is transmitted by bite of *Aedes aegypti*, hepatitis B by blood & influenza virus by inhalation route.

19) (c)
- Rabies virus spread by neural route
- Varicella zoster virus & EB virus spread through blood route
- Polio virus spread by blood **(flow chart-1)** & also by neural route following tonsilectomy

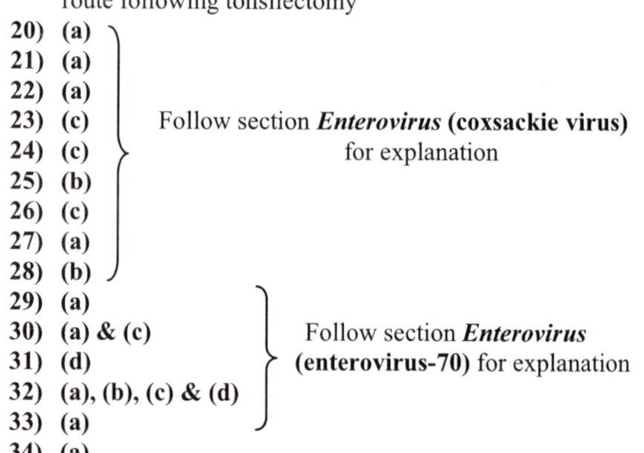

20) (a)
21) (a)
22) (a)
23) (c)
24) (c)
25) (b)
26) (c)
27) (a)
28) (b)
} Follow section ***Enterovirus* (coxsackie virus)** for explanation

29) (a)
30) (a) & (c)
31) (d)
32) (a), (b), (c) & (d)
33) (a)
} Follow section ***Enterovirus* (enterovirus-70)** for explanation

34) (a)
- Viruses from Picornaviridae cause encephalo myocarditis [encephalitis (polio virus) & myocarditis (coxsackie virus B)] & HFMD (coxsackie virus A & B).
- It includes HAV (EV-72, *Hepatovirus*) not HEV (*Hepeviridae*)

35) (a)
- Myocarditis & pleurodynia are caused by Coxsackie B (*Enterovirus*) while herpengina is caused by Coxsackie A (*Enterovirus*)
- Haemorrhagic fever:
  - Nor caused by *Enterovirus*
  - More details: **Follow chapter → Other group of viruses** (section → Haemorrhagic fever viruses)

36) (b), (c), (d) & (e)
- Composed of non-segmented genome
- Stable at wide range of pH from 3-10
- Pleurodynia, encephalitis & meningitis are caused by coxsackie viruses (*Enterovirus*)

66 Orthomyxoviridae

Learning heading & subheadings

- Myxoviruses:
- Meaning:
- Classification:

Influenzavirus

Swine origin influenza virus (S-OIV) or H1N1 2009 pandemic

Strains of influenza virus causing bird flu (avian flu)

Myxoviruses:

- **Called myxoviruses** because virus have affinity for mucus (**myxa = mucus**) & include the two families like Orthomyxoviridae & Paramyxoviridae.
- Orthomyxoviridae is described here & for Paramyxoviridae follow separate chapter.

Meaning: **Orthos (Greek) = straight** related to infection in vertebrate animal + **myxa (Greek) = mucus,** related to affinity of virus for mucin.

Classification:

- **Family:** Orthomyxoviridae.
- **Genus:** Following are the genera.

1. *Influenzavirus A*: Influenza A virus.
2. *Influenzavirus B*: Influenza B virus.
3. *Influenzavirus C*: Influenza C virus.
4. *Isavirus*.
5. *Thogoto virus*.
6. *Quaranja virus*.

✓ **Note: Species or types of influenza virus**

- There are three genera of influenza virus: *Influenza virus A, Influenza virus B & Influenza virus C*. Each genus includes only one species or type like influenza A virus, influenza B virus and influenza C virus respectively.

Influenzavirus

❖ **History:** Virus was 1st isolated in 1933 by Smith, Andrews & Laidlaw.

❖ **Geographical distribution:** Worldwide.

❖ **Morphology:** →**Fig.-1**

- **Shape:** Spherical, filaments in fresh isolates with several μm in length & visible under **DGI microscope**.

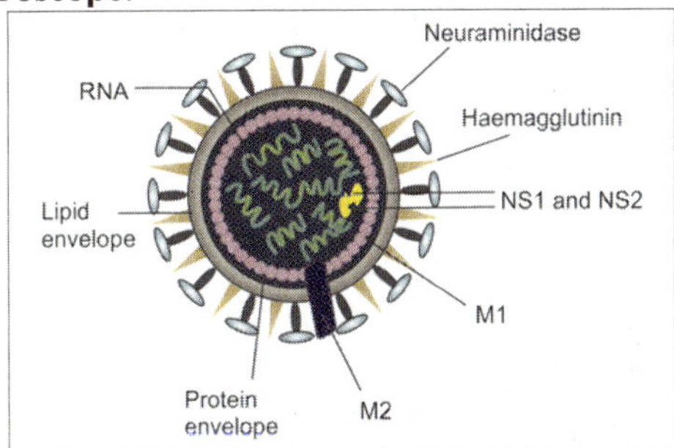

Figure-1: Morphology of Influenza virus

- **Size:** 80-120 nm, pleomorphism is common.
- **Genome:** ss-RNA (-) with 8 pieces. It present with RNA dependent RNA polymerase.
- **Capsid:** NA is surrounded by helical variety of capsid.
- **Envelope:**
  - Nucleocapsid is surrounded by bilayer envelope which consist inner protein & outer lipid layer.
  - Protein is virus coded & lipid is derived from host cell membrane by budding method.
  - Membrane protein also **called matrix** or **M protein**.
  - Two components of M protein like M1 & M2.
- **Peplomeres:**
  - Envelop consist projecting spikes **called peplomeres.**
  - Types: Two types like H & N. Both are strain specific.

a. **Haemagglutinin (H):**

- Triangular in cross section.
- Total 15 Subtypes from H1- H15.

b. **Neuraminidase (N):**

- Mushroom like.
- Destroying the haemagglutinin (H) receptors on host cells hence **called Receptor Destroying Enzyme (RDE)** & causes reversal of haemagglutination & releases the bounded virus to infect the other cells **called elution.**
- Glycoprotein enzyme destroys the cell receptors by splitting of N-acetyl neuraminic acid from it
- Total 9 subtypes from N1-N9.

- **Synthesis:** In nucleus.
- **Viral proteins:**
  - **Structural:**
    - Like PBF1, PBF2, PB2, PA, RNP, H, N & M proteins.
    - PBF1, PBF2& PB2 are responsible for viral transcription & replication.

- **Non-structural:** Like NS1 & NS2.

❖ Culture characteristics (C/Cs):

i. Egg culture:

- Grow well in amniotic cavity of chick embryo.
- After a few egg passages, virus grows well in the allantoic cavity also, except type C.
- It does not damage the chick embryo, which may hatch out normally.
- Virus growth is detected from allantoic & amniotic fluids.
- When passage serially in eggs, using undiluted infected allantoic fluid as inocula, the progeny virus will show high haemagglutinin titre, but low infectivity **called von Magnus phenomenon** & it is due to formation of incomplete virus particles lacking nucleic acid (NA).

ii. Animal culture:

- **Ferrets:** Intranasal instillation produces acute respiratory disease.
- **Mice:**
  - Intranasal instillation produces fatal respiratory disease.
  - Intracerebral inoculation produces fatal encephalitis.

iii. Tissue culture:

- Grow only in primary monkey kidney cells & some continuous cell lines.
- Growth is identified by CPE, haemadsorption & demonstration of haemagglutinin in culture fluid.

❖ Resistance:

- Inactivated at 50^0C for 30 minutes.
- Enveloped virus inactivated by lipid solvents like ether, chloroform & bile salts.
- Also destroyed by formalin, phenol & iodine.

❖ Antigenic structure: Two types of antigen.

A. Internal Ag or Ribonucleoprotein (RNP) Ag or Soluble (S) Ag:

- Occurs in supernatant in virus containing fluid when centrifuged.
- Also **called S-Ag.**
- Detected by CFT & precipitation test.
- Three serotypes (A, B & C→ **vide infra**) based on RNP-Ag.
- Not showing antigenic variation.
- Anti-RNP Ab develops after infection but not after killed vaccine.

B. Surface Ag or formerly called viral (V) Ag:

- ➢ Ab to V-Ag is identifying by CFT.
- ➢ **Two types:**

a. Haemagglutinin (H):

- ✪ **Biochemical nature:** Glycoprotein & composed of two polypeptide chain HA1 & HA2.
- ✪ **Function:** It is responsible for adhesion of virus with mucoprotein receptors on respiratory epithelium **(adsorption)** & on RBCs **(haemadsoption)** and causing haemagglutination of erythrocytes.
- ✪ **Subtypes:** Total 15 subtype from H1- H15, only four have been found in human isolates so far.
- ✪ **Anti-H-Ab**: Develops after infection & immunisation, which prevent haemadsoption or adsorption.
- ✪ **Haemagglutination:**
- **Definition:** When viral suspension is mixed with fowl RBCs, it produces clumping of RBCs **called haemagglutination**.
- **Method:**
  - It is performed in test tube or in plastic tray.
  - Add the red cells with serially diluted viral suspension & examine for haemagglutination.
  - Highest dilution of viral suspension which produces haemagglutination **called haemagglutination titre**.
- **Result:** RBCs which are not agglutinated settle at bottom in form of 'button' while agglutinated cells produces shield-like pattern.
- **Uses:**
  - Haemagglutination provide convenient method for **detection & titration** of the influenza virus in the egg & culture fluid.
  - Haemagglutinin is more resistant to physical & chemical agents than infectivity & can be used for **inactivated virus** like in the standardisation of killed influenza virus vaccine.
  - Haemagglutination & elution are helps in **purifying & concentrating** the virus.
- **Features of haemagglutination:**
  - It is followed by elution.
  - Viral particle released by elution are capable to haemagglutinate the other cells and the released red cells will not haemagglutinate by the same strain but haemagglutinate by other myxovirus.
  - Receptor gradient: Arrange myxo virus in the series & on treatment of red cell with particular virus will remove receptors for preceding virus but not for virus later in the series **called receptor gradient**.
  - Receptor gradient for myxo virus is mumps, New Castle Disease (NCD) & influenza.
  - It takes place at wide temperature range (0-37^0C).
  - Virus is varying in their ability to agglutinate the red cell of different species. Type A & B agglutinate the fowl, human, guinea pigs & other species. Type C agglutinates the fowl RBCs at 4^0C.
- **Haemagglutination inhibition (HAI): → vide infra**

b. Neuraminidase (N):

- ✪ **Biochemical nature:** Glycoprotein in nature.
- ✪ **Function:** Elution (vide supra).
- ✪ **Subtypes:** Nine subtype from N1-N9.
- ✪ **Anti-N-Ab:**
  - It formed following infection & immunisation.
  - It is not protective as like anti- haemagglutinin-Ab.

Old classification	Newer classification by WHO (1971)	Modified classification by WHO	Nomenclature of strain
Asw/ A swine	Hsw N1	H1N1	A swine/Wisconsin/15/30 (H1N1)
A0	H0 N1		A/PR/8/34 (H1N1)
A1	H1N1		A/FM/1/47 (H1N1)
A2 (Asia)	H2 N2	H2 N2	A/Singapore/1/57 (H2N2)
A2 (Hong Kong)	H3N2	H3N2	A/Hong Kong/1/68 (H3N2)

Table-1: Classification & nomenclature of strains of Influenza virus A

- It prevents the release of progeny virus & thus prevents the spread of infection.

✪ **Properties:**

- It is a strain specific antigen.
- Showing variation in antigenic structure, temperature optima & heat stability.

Also present in some bacteria like *V. cholerae* (red cell pre-treated with *V. cholerae* culture suspension will resist haemagglutination by influenza virus due to destruction of receptors by RDE of *V. cholerae*).

❖ **Antigenic classification:** Three species or types like influenza A virus, influenza B virus & influenza C virus are identified based on antigenic nature of the internal or ribonucleo protein & M protein.

A. Type A or Influenza A virus: → **Table-1**

➢ **Properties:**

- Moderate to severe illness.
- Highest antigenic variability.
- Infect the humans, animals & birds.
- It cause pandemics.

➢ **Subtypes:** Based on variation on surface antigens.

i. Older classification: Based only on H-Ag. Within each subtypes strains shows the gradual antigenic drift.

- In 1930, earliest strain isolated from swine (pig) **called Asw (A swine)**.
- In 1934, earliest strain isolated from human **called A0**.
- In 1946, haemagglutinin undergoes changes & new strain identified **called A1 or A/ or A prime**.
- In 1957, new pandemic strain identified in Asia **called A2 (Asia)**. Isolated from Singapore.
- In 1968, new strain emerged in Hong Kong **called A2 (Hong Kong)**.

ii. Newer classification by WHO-1971: Based on antigenic variation of both H & N Ags.

- Based on H-Ag, earlier Asw, A0, A1, A2 (Asia) & A2 (Hong Kong) were designated as Hsw, H0, H1, H2 & H3 respectively.
- Based on N-Ag, earlier A0, A1 were classified in N1 category while A2 (Asia) & A2 (Hong Kong) were categorised as N2.

iii. Modified classification by WHO: Earlier classification of WHO-1971 was again modified.

- Based on grouping together Hsw, H0 & H1under the heading H1.

B. Type B or Influenza B virus:

➢ **Properties:**

- Changes less rapidly than type A.
- It is the exclusive human pathogen except susceptibility to seals.
- It cause epidemic & sporadic.

➢ **Subtypes:** Not showing marked changes for further sub typing.

C. Type C or Influenza C virus:

➢ **Properties:**

- Milder epidemics in humans only.
- It is endemic throughout the world.

➢ **Subtypes:** Significant antigenic variation is not demonstrated in type C for further sub typing.

❖ **Nomenclature of strain:** Complete designation of strain will include the type, place of origin, serial number & year of isolation followed by antigenic subtypes of H & N in brackets, for example A/Hong Kong/1/68 (H3N2) as shown in **table-1.**

❖ **Antigenic variation:**

- It is highest in type A, less in type B & not demonstrated in type C.
- Internal RNP Ag & M protein Ag are stable, but H & N antigens undergo antigenic variation.

A. Variation in H & N antigens: Two types of antigenic variation as described below.

i. Antigenic drift:

- Minor, gradual, sequential change in antigenic structure & production of new Ag which is related with previous Ag **called antigenic drift.**
- New antigen is related with previous Ag & neutralised by antiserum of previous Ag.
- Caused by point mutations in gene due to selection pressure by immunity in the host population.
- Occurs in type A & B.
- May result in epidemic & minor outbreak.
- Occurs at frequent interval about 2-3 years in type A & 4-7 years in type B.

ii. Antigenic shift:

- Major, sudden & drastic change in antigenic structure & production of new Ag which is unrelated with previous Ag **called antigenic shift.**

- New antigen is unrelated with previous Ag & not neutralised by antiserum of previous Ag.
- Caused by exchange of gene segments (genetic re-assortment).
- Occurs in type A only.
- May result in major epidemic & pandemic.
- Occurs less frequently at 10-12 year interval.

B. P-Q-R variation:

- **History:** It is identified by Van der Veen & Mulder
- **Definition:** Influenza strains with same subtype, even strains isolated from outbreak –may behave differently in neutralisation tests with antisera **called P-Q-R variation**.
- **Principle:** It is due to rearrangement of antigenic determinant on the surface of the virion. P-Q-R phases are inconvertible by passaging the virus in the presence of appropriate antiserum.
- **Phases:**
- **P-Phase:** Strains in P -phase were neutralised by homologous antiserum in high titre & heterologous antiserum in low titre. In P-phase the dominant Ag is on the surface which reacts with specific Ab with high avidity.
- **Q-Phase:** Strains in Q- phase were poorly neutralised by homologous & heterologous antiserum. In Q-phase the dominant Ag is buried under the surface & hence inaccessible to the Ab.
- **R-Phase:** Strains in R- phase were neutralised by both homologous & heterologous antiserum in high titre.

C. O-D variation:

- **History:** It is observed by Burnet & Bull in 1943.
- **Definition:** Influenza virus type A underwent certain changes when serially passed in eggs **called O-D variation**.
- **Principle:** O-D variation is result of mutation.
- **Phases:**
- **O (original)-phase:**
- Initial or fresh isolate.
- Grow well in amniotic cavity of chick embryo but poorly or not at all in the allantoic cavity.
- It produces agglutination of mammalian RBCs (guinea pig & human) in high titre & week or no agglutination of fowl RBCs.
- Filamentous forms were common.
- Infectious to human.
- **D (Derived) -phase:**
- Isolates after eggs passage.
- Grow equally in the amniotic & allantoic cavities
- It produces equal or better agglutination of fowl RBCs than mammalian RBCs (guinea pig & human).
- No filamentous forms.
- Relatively non-infectious to human.

❖ Immunity:

a. Humoral immunity:

- Single attack produces the effective antibodies provide protection for 1-2 years, however problem is frequent antigenic variation by virus.
- IgA is synthesised locally by respiratory mucosa & provide local immunity.
- When individual repeatedly attack by different strain of influenza virus type A, antibodies are formed to earlier & also to newer strains, but the dominant antibodies are formed by earliest strain than the latest strain **called the doctrine of original antigenic sin**.

b. Cell mediated immunity: Virus also induces the CMI, but its role is uncertain.

❖ Pathogenicity:

- ➢ **Disease name:** Disease **called influenza.**
- ➢ **History of influenza A pandemic:**

Years	Antigenic type	Nature	Common name
1918-33	H1N1 (former HswN1 / Asw)	Pandemic	Spanish flu
1933-46	H1N1 (former H0N1 / A0)	Epidemic	-
1946-57	H1N1 (former A1)	Epidemic	-
1957-68	H2N2 [former A2 (Asia)]	Pandemic	Asian flu
1968-69	H3N2 [former A2 (Hong Kong)]	Pandemic	Hong Kong flu
1977-78	H1N1 (former A1)	Pandemic	Russian or red flu
2009 to present	H1N1	Pandemic	Swine flu

Table-2: Calendar of influenza pandemic

- **Seroarcheology:** Outbreak data before the isolation of virus (1933) are based on serological survey of individuals alive during those years.
- **Influenza pandemic: → Table-2**
- **WHO role:** It occurs at irregular interval since 1173 & it is as very challenging disease, hence worldwide surveillance is maintained by WHO.
- **Spanish flu (pandemic)**
- Most sever pandemic was reported in 1918-33 **called Spanish flu** with 200 million case & 20 million death. India suffered with 10 million death.
- The antigenic type detected was H1N1 (former HswN1/Asw).
- **Epidemic:**
- After the discovery of influenza virus epidemic was reported by H1N1 (former H0N1/ A0) strain from 1933-46.
- Next epidemic was reported by H1N1 (former A1) strain from 1946-57.
- **Asian flu (pandemic)**
- Next pandemic was originated from China & spread to world in 1957-68 **called Asian flu.**
- The antigenic type detected was H2N2 [former A2 (Asia)] with low mortality but with high morbidity.
- **Hong Kong flu (pandemic)**

- Hong Kong pandemic was originated in 1968-69 **called Hong Kong flu.**
- The antigenic type detected was H3N2 [former A2 (Hong Kong)] with less severity.
- **Russian flu or red flu (pandemic)**
- Re-emergency of previous A1 strain again occurred in China & then spread to Russia in 1977-78 **called red flu** facetiously.
- The antigenic type detected was H1N1 (former A1 strain) with low mortality.
- **Swine flu (pandemic): →Vide infra**
- **Reservoir of infection:** Human, birds, animals etc.
- **Source of infection:** Respiratory secretion.
- **Mode of transmission:**
- Via droplets/aerosol in early phase of disease.
- Rarely via contacts.
- **Incubation period:** 1-3 days.
- **Portal of entry:** Respiratory system.
- **Sites:** Pulmonary & extra-pulmonary.
- **Precipitating factors (epidemiological determinants):**

a. **Agent factors:** Virus factors like antigenic shift, antigenic drift, availability of reservoir or source are important in production of disease.

b. **Host factors:**

1. **Age:** More in children & adolescent due less pre-existing immunity.
2. **Pregnancy:**
3. **Migration:** Host migration will increase the spread.
4. **Immunity:**

- Less in person with pre-existing immunity like adult.
- More in person with low immunity due to presence of other disease like cardiovascular disease, chronic respiratory disease, AIDS, diabetes, cancer etc.

c. **Environmental factors:**

1. **Climate:** In temperate climate epidemic is common in winter while in tropical countries epidemic may occurs in monsoon.
2. **Overcrowding:** Attack is high in close communication in school, institution, camp, fair, marriage etc.

- **Pathogenesis:**
- Neuraminidase reduces the viscosity of the mucus film lining the respiratory epithelium & exposes the cell surface to adhere with haemagglutinin spikes of virus.
- Ciliated cells of respiratory epithelium are damaged & more vulnerable to bacterial infection.
- Viral pneumonia is occur in more severe cases and associated with hyperaemia, thickening of alveolar walls, capillary thrombosis & inflammatory cell infiltration.
- In late stage there is infiltration by macrophages which engulf & remove desquamated alveolar cells.
- **Clinical features:**
- It present with mild coryza to fulminating pneumonia.
- Common symptoms like fever, headache, myalgia, cough, rhinitis, ocular symptoms, abdominal pain & vomiting may occur.
- **Complications:**

1. **Pulmonary:**

- Croup (young children).
- Primary influenza virus pneumonia.
- Secondary bacterial infection: Secondary bacterial pneumonia is more common than primary influenza virus pneumonia. Secondary bacterial infection is caused by
  - *Streptococcus pneumoniae.*
  - *Staphylococcus aureus.*
  - *Haemophilus influenzae.*

2. **Extra-pulmonary:**

- Congestive failure, myocarditis & encephalitis.
- With type B:
  - Reye's syndrome: Degenerative changes in liver, brain & kidney especially in young children.
  - GIT symptoms like gastric flu.

❖ Laboratory diagnosis:

- **Specimens:** Nasal, nasopharyngeal or throat samples.
- **Testing methods:**

A. **Microscopy: → Follow morphology**

B. **Culture: → Follow C/Cs**

C. **Serological test:**

i. **CFT:**

- Detection of Ab against RNP-Ag of type A, B & C.
- Detection of Ab against V-Ag.

ii. **Radial immunodiffusion:**

- Detection of Ab against RNP-Ag, haemagglutinin & neuraminidase.
- Used for screening, not for diagnosis.

iii. **Haemagglutination Inhibition (HAI):**

- **Full name:** Haemagglutination inhibition test.
- **Principle:** It based on detection of Ab against haemagglutinin-Ag.
- **Disadvantages:**

1. **Non-specific inhibitors:**

- Interference by presence of non-specific inhibitory substances like α (Francis), β (Chu) & γ (Shimojo)
- They are mostly glycoprotein.
- They are inactivated by treatment of sera with RDE, trypsin, potassium periodate, kaolin & CO_2.
- Single technique is not effective to inactivate the inhibitors.

2. **Subtype specific:** Ab against haemagglutinin-Ag is subtype specific, so it is necessary to use the antigen of strain currently causing infection.

- **Advantages:** Convenient & most sensitive method.
- **Method:**
- Paired sera are used.

- Remove the inhibitors & do the serial dilution of sera.
- Add the influenza virus.
- Then add the fowl RBCs.
- Highest dilution of serum which inhibits the haemagglutination **called haemagglutination inhibition titre**.

D. Molecular methods:

1. RT-PCR:
- It is the most sensitive, specific & rapid method.
- It also detects the type like A, B, C & strain (subtype) like H or N.

2. Real time RT-PCR (qRT –PCR):
- It is a quantitative method to quantitate the viral load in sample.
- Specific qRT –PCR has been designed to diagnose the swine flu & avian flu.

❖ Prevention:

- **General measures:** Frequent hand washing, avoiding contact with patients, wearing face makes are useful protective measure.
- **Chemoprophylaxis:** Rimantadine & amantidine are useful which block theM2 protein, which acts as ion channel.
- **Immunoprophylaxis:** By using following types of vaccine.

i. Live attenuated vaccine: Vaccines contain a living microbe that has been weakened (attenuated) in the laboratory, so it can't cause disease.

1. **Vaccine prepared from natural virus by serial egg passage:** Cause disease in children after intranasal instillation, so rarely useful.
2. **Vaccine prepared from ts mutant:** Grow at 32-34^{0}C but not at 37^{0}C.
3. **Recombinant vaccine:** Obtained by hybridisation between ts mutant of established strain & new strain.

ii. Killed/ inactivated vaccines:
- Viruses are grow in the allantoic cavity of chick embryo & inactivated by treatment with formalin.
- Allergic reaction in persons who are allergic to egg.
- Administered by subcutaneous route.
- Causes local reaction.

iii. Subunit vaccine: Virus is disrupted by treatment with detergent, so vaccine contains H & N subunits.

❖ Treatment:

- Rimantadine & amantadine are useful, but resistance may occur.
- Zanamivir & oseltamivir are also useful prevention & treatment.

Swine origin influenza virus (S-OIV) or H1N1 2009 pandemic

❖ Classification:

- **Family:** Orthomyxoviridae.
- **Genus:** *Influenzavirus.*
- **Strain:**
  - Strain emerged due to genetic reassortment **(fig.-2)** between four strains of type A in pig. Two are endemic in pig (swine), one is endemic in human & one is endemic in birds (avian), resulting novel virus **called swine origin influenza virus (S-OIV) or H1N1 2009 pandemic strain**, however it's not fair to use the word swine flu.
  - Pig possesses the receptors that can bind to swine, human & avian influenza viruses, such viruses co-infect & combine to form the novel virus.
  - It is less virulent compare to avian flu because it lacks the PB1F2 protein required for NA transcription & replication.
  - It produces low mortality but high morbidity.

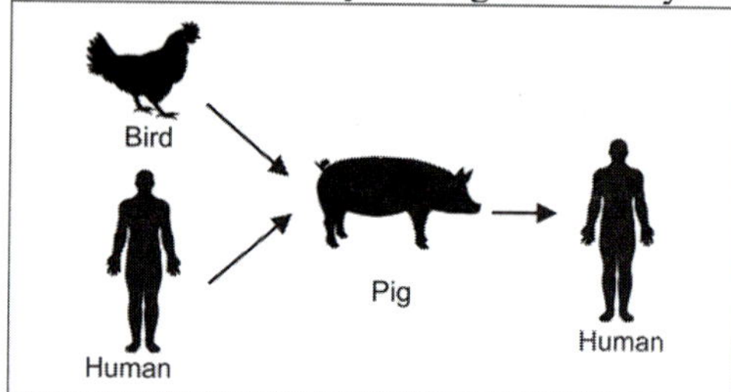

Figure-2: Genetic reassortment of H1N1

❖ Morphology: Same as *Influenzavirus*.

❖ Culture characteristics (C/Cs): Same as *Influenzavirus*.

❖ Resistance: Same as *Influenzavirus*.

❖ Pathogenicity:

- **Disease name: Called swine flu** (It came from swine (pig), hence **called swine flu.**), or **called A/H1N1/2009 pandemic** however it's not fair to use this word.
- **History of swine flu pandemic:**
  - It emerged in California in March 2009 & spread in entire world including India (pandemic) with plenty of death. WHO declared the pandemic in 11th June 2009.
  - In India Since 2009, 53,943 cases are reported with 3315 deaths.
- **Reservoir of infection:** Pig & human.
- **Source of infection:** Respiratory droplets.
- **Mode of transmission:** It can spread from person to person account its rapid spread. Following are the possible modes for entry in human.
  - Via droplets/aerosol.
  - Fomites borne.
  - Via contaminated hands.
- **Incubation period:** 1-3 days.
- **Portal of entry:** Respiratory system.
- **Sites:** Pulmonary & extra-pulmonary.
- **Precipitating factors:** Follow categor -B(ii).

- **Clinical features:** Total three categories.

A. **Category A:**
- Patients with mild fever plus cough/sore throat with or without body ache, headache, diarrhoea & vomiting.
- No testing of the patient for H1N1 is required.
- They do not require oseltamivir (temiflu) and required symptomatic treatment.
- The patients should be monitored for their progress and reassessed at 24 to 48 hours by the doctor.
- Patients should confine themselves at home & avoid mixing up with public & high risk members in the family.

B. **Category B:** Two sub categories.

i. **Category-B (i):** Following sign-symptoms in addition to all category-A.
- High grade fever and severe sore throat.
- No testing of the patient for H1N1 is required.
- Require oseltamivir.
- Require home isolation.

ii. **Category-B (ii):** In addition to all the signs and symptoms mentioned under Category-A, patient having one or more of the following high risk.
- Children less than 5 years old.
- Pregnant women.
- Age: 65 years or older.
- Patients with lung diseases, heart disease, liver disease, kidney disease, blood disorders, diabetes, neurological disorders, cancer and HIV/AIDS.
- Patients on long term cortisone therapy.
- No test for H1N1 is required.
- Treated with oseltamivir.
- All patients of Category-B (i) and (ii) should confine themselves at home and avoid mixing with public and members in the family.

C. **Category C:** Following sign-symptoms in addition to category-A & B.
- Breathlessness, chest pain, drowsiness, fall in blood pressure, sputum mixed with blood & bluish discolouration of nails.
- Irritability among small children, refusal of feed.
- Worsening of underlying chronic conditions.
- Require testing for H1N1.
- Immediate hospitalization and treatment.

Laboratory diagnosis:

- **Indication of testing:** Category-C.
- **Specimens:**
- **Respiratory specimens:** Any two of the following.
  - Nasal swab or throat swab or nasopharyngeal swab
  - Can be collected into the same VTM (Viral Transport Medium) or normal saline.
- **Serological specimens:** Paired serum samples are most useful.
  - Acute sample: Within 7 days after symptom onset.
  - Convalescent sample: More than 21 days after symptom onset at (an interval of 14 days).
- **Storage of specimens:**
- **For specimens in VTM:**
  - Transport to laboratory as soon as possible.
  - Store specimens at 4°C before and during transportation within 48 hours.
  - Store specimens at -70°C beyond 48 hours.
  - Avoid freeze-thaw cycles.
- **For serological specimens:**
  - Store specimen at 4°C within 48 hours.
  - Store specimens at -20°C beyond 48 hours.
  - Avoid repeated freeze-thaw cycles.
- **Transport of specimens:** In triple layer packing.
- **Testing:**

1. **Confirmatory test:** Real time RT-PCR (qRT-PCR).
2. **Other tests:** Virus isolation by cell culture, neutralisation test & genomic sequencing are useful.

Prevention:

- **General measures:**
  - Early diagnosis, treatment & isolation of case.
  - Implementation of standard infection control practices like droplet precautions, contact precautions & air borne precautions.
  - Use of appropriate Personal Protective Equipments (PPE) cap, mask (N95 mask for health care workers), gloves, apron, shoe cover, goggles etc. and standard work precautions, proper disinfection and waste disposal.
  - Restricting entry in swine flu ward.
  - Education of the staff, patients and their visitors.
  - Minimize close contact (less than 3 feet) with the case as far as possible, asks the patient to use face mask/ handkerchief / tissue paper while coughing.
  - Avoid use of articles touched by the patient.
- **Chemoprophylaxis:** Oseltamivir (temiflu) is given for prophylactic purpose.
- **Immunoprophylaxis:** Both live (nasal spray) & killed (injectable) vaccines are available.

Treatment: Oseltamivir (temiflu) & zanamivir (relenza) are useful drug.

Strains of influenza virus causing bird flu (avian flu)

Geographical distribution: Worldwide.

Classification:

- **Family:** Orthomyxoviridae.
- **Genus:** *Influenzavirus.*
- **Strains:**
  - The majority of human cases are from A/H5N1 & A/H7N9. A/H5N1 is associated with higher rate (>50%) of pneumonia & extra-pulmonary manifestation like diarrhoea & CNS involvement.

- Other avian strains can cause human infection are A/H7N7 (Netherland) & A/H9N2 (Hong Kong).
- A/H7N9 stain caused outbreak in China in 2013. It formed due to genetic reassorment of eight bird's virus like H from domestic duck, N from wild bird & remaining six from domestic poultry contains H9N2 (**fig.-3**).
- Strain is most virulent as it posses the PB1F2 proteins.
- It has high mortality (>60%) & low morbidity.

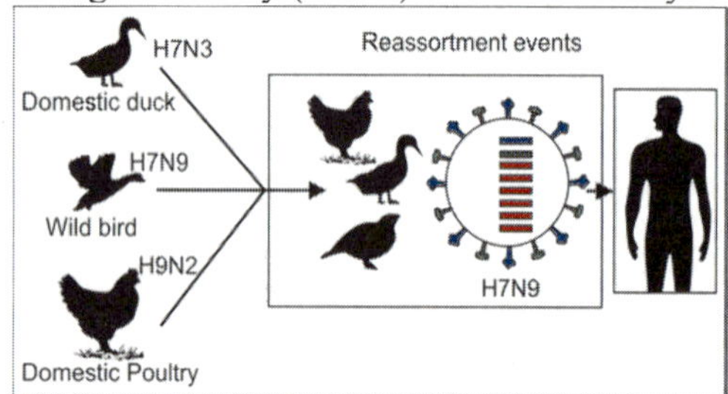

Figure-3: Genetic reassortment of H7N9

❖ **Morphology:** Same as influenza virus.

❖ **Culture characteristics (C/Cs):** Same as influenza virus.

❖ **Resistance:** Same as influenza virus.

❖ **Pathogenicity:**

➢ **Disease name: Called avian flu.**

➢ **Meaning:** From **Avian (Latin) = bird**, because it is an infectious viral disease of birds.

➢ **Synonym:** Also **called bird flu**.

➢ **History of bird flu epidemic:**

- There is no human to human transmission of bird flu, only 500 cases were reported from 1977-2010 from Asia & Middle East.
- Epidemic was occurred in Hong Kong (A/H9N2) in 1997 with 18 reported cases & six deaths. All the human cases were infected from poultry without human to human transmission & immediate slaughtering of 1.6 million hens was done to prevent the further spread, pandemic threat & before the strain became virulent to start human to human spread.
- Next epidemic was occured in China (A/H7N9) in 2013.

➢ **Reservoir of infection:** Birds like duck, poultry & other domestic & wild birds.

➢ **Source of infection:** Bird excreta like faeces & discharge from nose, mouth & eyes.

➢ **Mode of transmission:**

- **Bird to bird transmission:** Virus present in bird's faeces which contaminate the water of ponds or lakes. Aquatic birds like duck may get infection from such contaminated water by ingestion. Virus multiplies in the intestine of bird & excreted in faeces to continue the cycle. Duck is the major link to carry the virus, from wild & domestic birds to human, pig, other animals or other birds.
- **Bird to human transmission:**
  - Inhalation: Inhalation of dust particles arised from infected bird's excreta.
  - Direct contact with birds or excreta present on their body during slaughtering or plucking.
  - It's not transmitted by ingestion of poultry food (chicken).

➢ **Incubation period:** 2-3 days.

➢ **Portal of entry:** Respiratory system.

➢ **Sites:** Pulmonary & extra-pulmonary.

➢ **Precipitating factors:** Poultry workers are at most risk.

➢ **Pathogenesis:** The strain is more virulent due to presence of PBF2 protein, which target host mitochondria & induces apoptosis.

➢ **Clinical features:**

- **In birds:**
  - Ruffled (disarrange) feathers.
  - Drop in egg production.
  - High mortality.
- **In human:**
  - Conjunctivitis.
  - Flu-like illness: Fever, cough, sore throat & muscle aches.
  - Pulmonary: Pneumonia.
  - Extra-pulmonary: Nausea, abdominal pain, diarrhoea, vomiting and sometimes neurologic changes like altered mental status, seizures etc.

➢ **Complications:** Multi organs disease & death. Less morbidity due to no human to human transmission but mortality rate is >60%.

❖ **Laboratory diagnosis:**

➢ **Specimens:** Nasal swab or throat swab collected in VTM (Viral Transport Medium) or normal saline.

➢ **Transport of specimens:** In triple layer packing.

➢ **Testing:**

1. **Confirmatory test:** Real time reverse transcriptase (qRT-PCR).
2. **Other test:** Virus isolation by cell culture.

❖ **Prevention:**

➢ **General measures:**

- Early diagnosis, treatment & isolation of case.
- Avoid exposure to poultry.
- Slaughtering of infected birds.
- Other general measures are same as like swine flu.

➢ **Chemoprophylaxis:** Oseltamivir (temiflu) 70-90% protection.

➢ **Immunoprophylaxis:**

- Effective vaccine is developed to H5N1 avian influenza.
- Vaccine against emerged avian strain is developed & given to the person at risk.

❖ **Treatment:** Oseltamivir, peramivir or zanamivir are the effective drugs.

❖ **Differences between swine flu & bird flu:** → Table-3

Features	Swine flu	Bird flu
Common strains	H1N1	H5N1 & H7N9
Person to person transmission	Yes	No
Nature	Pandemic	Epidemic
PB1F2 protein	Absent	Present
Virulent	Less virulent with low mortality & high morbidity	More with high mortality (>60%) & low morbidity
Reservoir	Pigs & Humans	Birds

Table-3: Differences between swine flu & bird flu

Question bank

Case study

1) A 65 year old male is brought to the hospital with history of mild fever & sore throat before 3 days. Later he developed high grade fever & mixture of blood in sputum. Throat swab was collected & sent to the reference laboratory to rule out the etiological agent. Lab report revealed ss-RNA with negative polarity. Identify the clinical conditions & answer the following
a) Name the clinical condition & its etiological agent.
b) Write pathogenicity of clinical condition.
c) Write diagnosis of clinical condition.

Essay/Full question

1) *Influenzavirus*

Short notes

1) Pathogenicity / laboratory diagnosis of *Influenzavirus*.
2) H1N1 2009 pandemic or swine flu.
3) Bird flu.

Short questions for theory/viva questions

1) What is antigenic shift & antigenic drift in *Influenza virus*?
2) Write four differences between antigenic shift & antigenic drift in *Influenza virus*.
3) What is elution?
4) Write the functions of H & N spikes of *Influenza virus*.
5) Write the four differences between swine flu & bird flu.

MCQs for chapter review

Classification

1) Myxo virusis include (PGI, Dec-08)
(a) Orthomyxovirus (b) Influenza (c) Measles (d) Polio (e) HSV

2) Influenza virus belongs to which family
(a) Paramyxoviridae (b) Orthomyxoviridae (c) Bunyaviridae (c) Togaviridae

Morphology

3) Influenza virus, has
(a) 5 segments of ss RNA (b) 8 segments of ds DNA (c) 8 segments of ss DNA (d) 8 segments of ss RNA

4) Receptor destroying enzyme is
(a) Haemagglutinin peplomere (b) Neuraminidase peplomere (c) Matrix protein (d) Reverse transcriptase

Influenzavirus

5) True statement about influenza A is (AI-99)
(a) It has double stranded segmented RNA (b) Pandemic are caused by antigenic drift (c) Nucleocapsid antibody is not specific (d) Haemagglutinin and neuraminidase is strain specific

6) Antigenic variation seen in which of the following (PGI, Dec-08)
(a) Influenza virus (c) Hepatitis virus (d) Yellow fever virus (e) Leptospira

7) False about antigenic drift (AIIMS-94)
(a) Occur under pressure for immunity (b) Responsible for epidemic of influenza (c) Occurs only in influenza A (d) Occur every 10-12 year

8) False about antigenic drift
(a) Causes pandemic (b) Occurs due to mutation (c) Occurs more frequently (d) Affected by previous antibody

9) Antigenic shift
(a) Occurs every 2-3 weeks (b) Gradual change over time (c) Result from genetic recombination (d) Occur in all influenza virus

10) Not true regarding influenza virus is (AIIMS-99)
(a) All types exhibit antigenic shift (b) Only A type shows antigenic drift (c) Drift is accumulation of point mutations (d) None of above

11) Which of the following is true regarding influenza
(a) It is caused by enveloped DNA virus (b) Laboratory studies may show neutropenia early in the course of disease (c) Primary infectious pneumonia is less common than secondary bacterial pneumonia (d) Antiviral agents given early prevents complications

12) Reye's syndrome following influenza is most commonly associated with (AIIMS-93)
(a) Type A (b) Type B (c) Type C (d) Non of above

13) Influenza vaccine is administered
(a) Subcutaneously (b) Intradermal (c) Nasal drops (d) Iintrathecal

A/H1N1/2009 pandemic or swine flu

14) H1 N1 is a type of
(a) SARS virus (b) Influenza type A virus (c) Influenza type B virus (d) Influenza type C virus

15) Swine flu is caused by
(a) H1N1 (b) H5N1 (c) C3N1 (d) H3N3

Avian flu

16) H5 N1 is a strain of (AI-08)
(a) Avian flu (b) New vaccine against AIDS (c) Agent for japanese encephalitis (d) Causes chikungunya fever

Answers of MCQs & explanation

1)	(a)	Follow section, **classification** for explanation
2)	(b)	
3)	(d)	Follow section, **morphology** for explanation
4)	(b)	
5)	(d)	Follow section, ***Influenzavirus*** for explanation
6)	(a)	
7)	(c) & (d)	
8)	(a)	
9)	(c)	
10)	(a) & (b)	
11)	(c)	
12)	(b)	
13)	(a) & (c)	

14) (b) } Follow section, **A/H1N1/2009 pandemic or swine flu**
15) (a) } for explanation
16) (a)

- Follow section, **avian flu** for explanation

67 Paramyxoviridae

Learning heading & subheadings

- Myxoviruses:
- Morphology:
- Antigenic structure:
- Classification of Paramyxoviridae:

Rubulavirus
- Mumps virus

Parainfluenzavirus
- Parainfluenza viruses

Pneumovirus
- RSV

Morbilivirus
- Measles virus

Avulavirus
- Avian avula virus 1

Henipavirus
- Nipah henipa virus
- Hendra henipa virus

Metapneumovirus
- Human metapneumo virus

Myxo viruses:

- These are **called myxoviruses** because virus have affinity for mucus (**myxa = mucus**) & include the two families like Orthomyxoviridae & Paramyxoviridae.
- For Orthomyxoviridae follow separate chapter & Paramyxoviridae is described here
- Differences between Orthomyxoviridae & Paramyxoviridae: → **Table-1**

Features	Orthomyxoviridae	Paramyxoviridae
Size	80-120nm	100-300nm
Shape	Round & fresh isolates are filamentous	Pleomorphic
Genome	8-Pieces	Single / non-segmented & linear
Size of nucleocapsid	9nm	18nm
Synthesis of RNA	Nucleus	Cytoplasm
Genetic reassortment	Common	Absent
Dependent RNA synthesis	Required for multiplication	Not required
Effect of Actinomycin D`	Inhibits the multiplication	Does not inhibits the multiplication
Antigenic stability	Variable	Stable
Haemolysis	Absent	Present

Table-1: Differences between Orthomyxoviridae & Paramyxoviridae

✓ **Note: In few paramyxovirus RNA synthesis take place in nucleus also**

Morphology: →Fig.-1

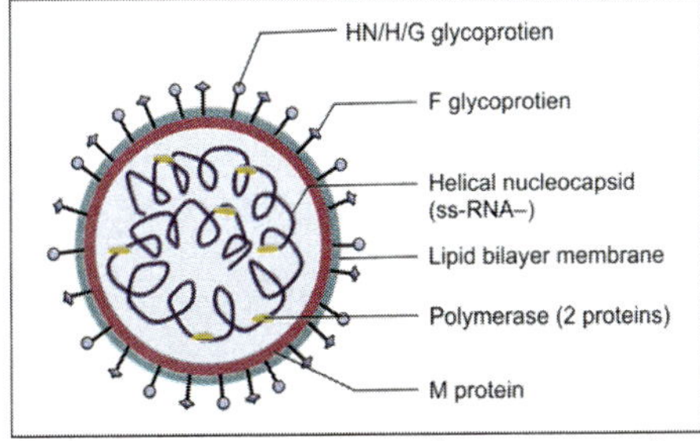

Figure-1: Morphology of paramyxovirus

- Resemble to orthomyxovirridae.
- **Shape:** Round or rarely long filamentous shape.
- **Size:** Larger than orthomyxovirridae about, 100-300 nm. Pleomorphism is common & some time up to 800nm.
- **Genome:** ss-RNA (-).
- **Capsid:** NA is surrounded by helical variety of capsid.
- **Envelopes:** Nucleocapsid is surrounded by bilayer envelop which consists inner protein (M protein) & outer lipid layer.
- **Peplomeres:**
  - Envelop consist projecting spikes **called peplomeres.**

Features	*Rubulavirus*	*Parainfluenza virus*	*Pneumovirus*	*Morbilivirus*	*Henipavirus*	*Metapneumo virus*
Nucleocapsid's size (nm)	18	18	13	18	Not identified	13nm
F-protein	+	+	+	+	+	+
Haemolysin	+	+	-	+	Not identified	-
Haemagglutinin	+	+	-	+	-	-
Neuraminidase	+	+	-	-	-	-
Inclusion body in cytoplasm (C) or nucleus (N)	C	C	C	N & C	Not identified	Not identified

Table-2: Differences between common species of Paramyxoviridae

- They are glycoprotein in nature.
- Two types: H/HN and F.

1. **Haemagglutinin (H or HN):**
- Longer spikes.
- Help in adsorption.
- May also possess neuraminidase activity, hence **called H or HN protein.**

2. **Fusion (F) protein:**
- Help in fusion of viral envelop with plasma membrane, which is the essential step in viral infection.
- Mediates the haemolytic activity.
- Responsible for cell-to-cell fusion, which leads to giant cell or syncytium formation.

Antigenic structure: Do not undergoes the genetic recombination or antigenic variation, hence all paramyxovirus are antigenically stable.

Classification of Paramyxoviridae:

- **Family:** Paramyxoviridae.
- **Genus & species:** Contains six genera mentioned below with human species. Differences between all genera are shown in **table-2.**

1. ***Rubulavirus*:** Mumps virus.
2. ***Parainfluenzavirus*:** Parainfluenzae virus type1-4.
3. ***Pneumovirus*:** Respiratory Syncytial Virus (RSV).
4. ***Morbillivirus*:** Measles virus.
5. ***Avulavirus:*** Avian avula virus 1 (New castle disease virus or ranikhet virus).
6. ***Henipavirus:***
- Nipah henipa virus (nipah virus).
- Hendra henipa virus (hendra virus).
- Cedar henipa virus (cedar virus).
- Ghanaian bat henipa virus (kumasi virus).
- Mojiang henipa virus (mòjiāng virus).
7. ***Metapneumovirus:*** Human metapneumo virus.

Rubulavirus

Mumps virus

❖ **History:**
- It cause non-suppurative enlargement of parotid gland in children.
- As epidemic parotitis, it had been described by Hippocrates in the 5th century BC.
- Viral origin of mumps virus was demonstrated by Johnson & Goodpasture in 1934 by its experimental transmission in monkey.
- Embryonated eggs cultivation was done by Habel in 1945.
- Tissue culture was done by Henle & Deinhardt.

❖ **Geographical distribution:** It is endemic worldwide, but less in developed countries due to vaccination.

❖ **Morphology:** →Vide supra.

❖ **Culture characteristics (C/Cs):** Inoculate immediately after collection as the virus is labile.

i. **Egg culture:**
- Grow well in amniotic cavity of 6-8 days old **chick embryo.**
- Growth is detected after 5-6 days by haemagglutination, haemagglutination inhibition or by indirect IF test.

ii. **Tissue culture:**
- Grow in Vero, Hela or in human amnion cells.
- CPE is not reliable.
- Growth is identified by haemadsorption or haemadsorption inhibition by specific antiserum after 1-2 weeks.
- More rapid result is obtained by IF test within 2-3 days after inoculation.

❖ **Resistance:**
- Inactivated at room temperature & by ether, UV light, formalin etc.
- Stored at -70°C or by lyophilisation.

❖ **Antigenic structure & serotypes:**
- **Two complement fixing Ag:**
  - Soluble (S) or internal-Ag.
  - Viral (V) or surface-Ag.
- **Serotype:** Antigenically stable & only 1 serotype.

❖ **Immunity:**

a. **Humoral immunity:**

- **Antibodies to Soluble (S) or internal-Ag:**
  - It produced after 3-7 days of onset of symptoms but disappear in 6 months.
  - It indicates current or recent infection.
- **Antibodies to Viral (V) or surface-Ag:**
  - It produced after 1 month of onset of symptoms but persist for a year.
  - It indicates late infection.
- **Antibodies to Haemagglutinin (H or HN)-Ag:**
  - It **called Haemagglutination Inhibition (HI) Ab**
  - It provides the effective immunity even produced after subclinical infection.
- **Lasting immunity:**
  - Single attack provides the long lasting immunity, so no chances of second attack.
  - All antibodies are widely present in community.
  - Antibodies also transfer from mother to child to elicit the passive immunity; hence mumps is less before the 6 months of age.

b. **Cell mediated immunity:** Virus also induces the CMI, but its role is uncertain.

c. **Interferon:** It also appears early in mumps infection.

❖ Pathogenicity:

➢ **Disease name:** Disease **called mumps.**

➢ **Nature of disease:** It occurs as epidemic in school children between 5-15 years of age & also in overcrowded community like army camps.

➢ **Reservoir of infection:** Human like patients in the late incubation or in early stage of disease. No any known animal reservoir exist.

➢ **Source of infection:**
- Respiratory droplets, saliva & urine from patients are the main sources.
- Period of infectivity (communicability): Virus present in saliva 1 week before & 1-2 weeks after the onset of parotitis, however peak infectivity is occurs 1 or 2 day before the parotitis & subsides very rapidly. Most contagious period is 1-2 days before the onset of symptoms.
- It also present in urine for 1-2 weeks after the onset of symptoms, but its role in transmission of infection is uncertain.
- Secondary attack rate: It is high about 86%.

➢ **Mode of transmission:**
- Via inhalation.
- Via conjunctiva.
- Direct contact.
- Fomites contaminated by saliva & also by urine of patient.

➢ **Incubation period:** 12-25 days.

➢ **Portal of entry:** Respiratory system.

➢ **Sites:** Parotid glands.

➢ **Precipitating factors:**

1. **Age:**
   - Epidemic occurs in children & young adults (5-15 years).
   - All antibodies are wide in community.
   - Antibodies are also transfer from mother to child to elicit the passive immunity; hence mumps is less before the 6 months of age.
2. **Close contact & overcrowding:** Spread is common in house hold persons & people living in overcrowding areas like army camp, school etc. due to close contact.
3. **Seasonal:** Peak incidence in winter & spring.
4. **Immunity:** Single attack by vaccine or infection, provide the long lasting immunity, so no chances of second attack.

➢ **Pathogenesis: →Flow chart-1**

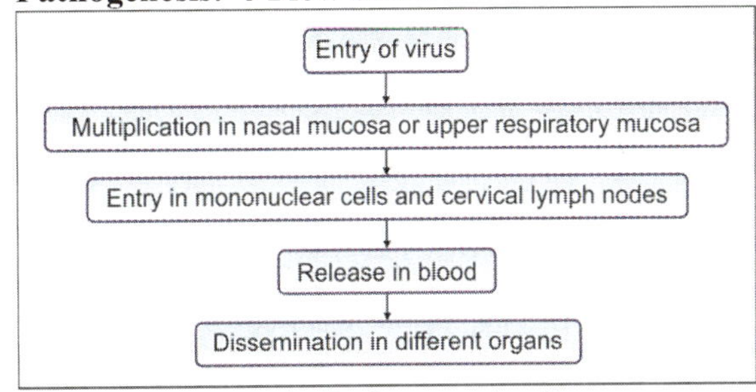

Flow chart-1: Pathogenesis of mumps

➢ **Clinical features:**

- **Prodromal phase:** Present with fever, malaise, headache, nausea & loss of appetite.
- **Disease phase:**
  - Non-suppurative enlargement of parotid gland (parotitis → **fig.-2**) present in 70-90% cases, which may be unilateral or bilateral & present with local pain, tenderness & fever.

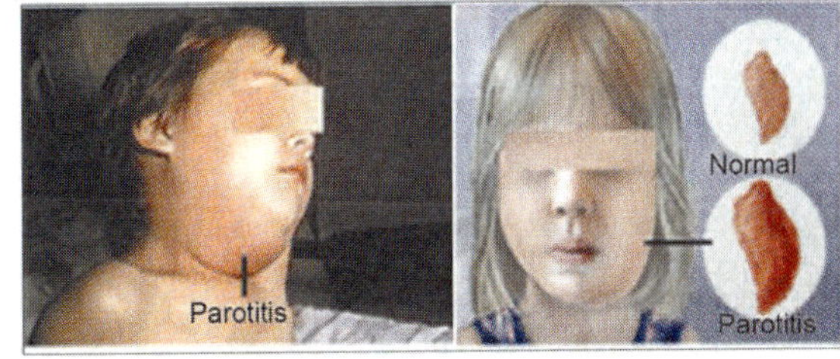

Figure-2: Parotitis in mumps

- Patients complain earache on affected side prior to the parotitis.
- Pain & stiffness on opening the mouth.
- Pain subsides over 1-2weeks.
- Skin over parotid gland is not warm or erythematous.
- Involvement of sublingual & submanidibular glands may occur sometimes.

➢ **Complications:**

1. **Orchitis:**
   - It is the most common complication of mumps among post-pubertal males.
   - Occurs in 25-40% cases.

- Common in adult & occur 7-10 days after the parotitis.
- It presents with fever, chills & pain.
- Unilateral in 75% cases.
- Bilateral is very rare, but when present result in atrophy, low sperm count & role in sterility is not found.

2. **Pancreatitis:**
- Present with upper abdominal pain, nausea & vomiting.
- Occurs in children in 4% cases.

3. **Oophoritis:**
- Present with lower abdominal pain, nausea & vomiting.
- Occurs in post pubertal women in 5% cases.
- Usually unilateral.

4. **Diabetes:**
- Occurs in children in few cases.
- Exact mechanisms are unknown.

5. **Meningo-encephalitis:**
- CNS involvement occurs in 60% cases indicated by pleocytosis in the CSF, but only 10% shows the symptoms of meningitis (aseptic meningitis).
- Aseptic meningitis may develop before, during, after or in absence of parotitis.
- Mumps meningitis or mumps meningo-encephalitis usually resolve without sequelae, but sensory-neural deafness may sometimes result in 5 per 1, 00, 000 cases.
- Atypical mumps: Mumps without parotitis with aseptic meningitis **called atypical mumps.** It occurs in children in 10% cases.

6. **Abortion:**
- Spontaneous abortion in 25% cases, if occur in 1st trimester.
- Congenital malformation may not occur.

7. **Other rare complications:** Thyroiditis, neuritis, hepatitis, myocarditis, transverse myelitis, facial palsy, hydrocephalus, cerebellar ataxia etc.

❖ Laboratory diagnosis:

➢ **Typical case:** Diagnosis based on clinical parameters.

➢ **Atypical case:** Required laboratory help.

✪ **Specimens:** Virus may be isolated from
- Saliva in 4-5 days.
- Urine up to 2 weeks.
- CSF in 8-9 days after onset of illness.

✪ **Testing methods:**

A. **Microscopy:** →**Follow morphology**

B. **Culture:** →**Follow C/Cs**

C. **Serological tests:**

i. **CFT:**
- Detection Ab against S-Ag in acute phase serum is presumptive evidence of current infection.
- Cross reacting antibodies (IgG type) with parainfluenzae viruses cause problem.

ii. **IgM ELISA:** Cross reacting antibodies will not interfere, because they are IgG type.

iii. **HAI:** Cross reacting antibodies (IgG type) with parainfluenzae viruses cause problem.

D. **Molecular methods:** RT-PCR is more rapid & sensitive.

❖ Prevention:

➢ **General measures:**
- Avoid contact with patients in early stage.
- Patient can usually return to work or school about one week after diagnosis of mumps. By this point, patient is no longer contagious.
- Mumps return to normal after ten days of illness.

➢ **Immunoprophylaxis:**

i. **Active immunisation:** By using following type of live attenuated vaccine.

✪ **Preparation:** Vaccines contain **Jeryl-Lynn strain** that has been attenuated by egg passage & grow in chick embryo fibroblast cell culture.

✪ **Administration:**
- **Route:** IM.
- **Dose:** 0.5ml alone or in combination with MMR vaccine after 1 yr. 2nd dose is given at 4-6 years (pre-school time).

✪ **Complication:** Post vaccine aseptic meningitis or local reaction at the site of injection.

✪ **Advantage:** Provide effective protection for at least 10 years.

✪ **Disadvantage:** It may not prevent the disease if given after exposure.

✪ **Contraindications:**
- Patient allergic to egg protein or to neomycin.
- Pregnancy.
- Before 1 year, as maternal Ab does not allow the vaccine virus to multiply before 1 year.
- IDDs.

ii. **Passive immunisation:** By using specific Ig, but protective role is doubtful.

❖ Treatment:

Antibiotics are not effective, symptomatic treatment t is given as follows.
- Bed rest during weakness or tiredness.
- Analgesic & antipyretic such as acetaminophen & ibuprofen, to bring down pain & fever.
- Soothe swollen glands like parotid or testis by applying intermittent ice packs on them.
- Drink plenty of fluids to avoid dehydration due to fever.
- Eat a soft diet of soup, yogurt and other foods that aren't hard to chew (chewing may be painful when your glands are swollen).
- Avoid acidic foods and beverages that may cause more pain in your salivary glands.

Parainfluenzavirus

Parainfluenza viruses

❖ **History, C/Cs, antigenic structure & serotypes :** Four types from 1-4 based on antigenicity including CPE & pathogenicity.

A. Parainfluenza virus-1
- It includes **Sendai virus (HA-1)** & **HA-2.**
- **Sendai virus (HA-1)** was discovered in 1952 in Japan.
- It is natural parasite in mice.
- Antigenically similar virus was identified in 1958 from children with acute respiratory infection by haemadsorption (HA) in cell culture named **HA-2.**
- HA-1 is mice variety & HA-2 is human variety.
- Sendai virus grow in eggs, with infected fluid showing high titre of haemagglutinin, resembling the influenza virus so **called haemagglutinating virus of Japan or influenza virus type-D.**

B. Parainfluenza virus-2
- Was discovered in 1955 from children with croup (acute laryngotracheobronchitis), so **called Croup Associated virus (CA virus).**
- Grow in monkey kidney cell culture with syncytium formation.
- Antigenically similar viruses like simian viruses 5 & 41 cause natural infection in monkeys.

C. Parainfluenza virus-3
- It was discovered in 1958 from children with acute respiratory infection by haemadsorption (HA) in cell culture. Previously named **HA-1.**
- Antigenically similar virus **called Shipping Fever (SF-4)** cause respiratory illness in cattle.

D. Parainfluenza virus-4
- Was discovered in 1960 in Japan from children with mild respiratory infection.
- Two subtypes like A & B.

❖ **Geographical distribution:** Worldwide.

❖ **Morphology:** → Vide supra

❖ **Culture characteristics (C/Cs):** Parainfluenza virus can grow on human diploid (secondary) fibroblast cell line.

❖ **Immunity:** Initial infection minimise the chances of reinfection.

❖ **Pathogenicity:**
➢ **Nature of disease:** Type 3 is more endemic while 2 & 3 cause epidemic disease.
➢ **Reservoir of infection:** Human.
➢ **Source of infection:** Virus present in respiratory secretions for about two weeks.
➢ **Mode of transmission:** By inhalation or by finger.
➢ **Portal of entry:** Respiratory system.
➢ **Site:** Respiratory system.
➢ **Precipitating factors:** Type-3 cause infection before 1 year while 2 &3 cause infection at pre-school age.
➢ **Clinical features:** Cause respiratory disease without viremia. Initial infection is very serious in type 1-3 but mild in type 4.
- **Type-1 & 2:** Croup (acute laryngotracheo-bronchitis).
- **Type-3:** Lower respiratory infection like bronchitis, bronchiolitis & pneumonia.
- **Type-4:** Minor respiratory illness like sore throat & hoarseness of voice.

❖ **Laboratory diagnosis:**
➢ **Specimens:** Nasal or throat swabs.
➢ **Testing methods:**

A. Morphology: →**Follow morphology**

B. Cell Culture:
- Grow in primary monkey kidney cell culture or continuous monkey cell lines.
- Growth is identified by CPE (only in type-2), haemadsorption, haemadsorption inhibition, haemagglutination inhibition or by IF test.

C. Serological test:
- Interference by cross reacting sera is major drawback.
- Paired sera are tested by ELISA, neutralisation, HI, CFT.

D. Molecular methods: RT-PCR is more rapid & sensitive.

❖ **Prevention:** No effective vaccine is available.

❖ **Treatment:** Antibiotics are not effective, symptomatic treatment is given.

Pneumovirus

RSV

❖ **History & synonym:** RSV was 1st isolated from chimpanzee with coryza, so **called chimpanzee coryza agent.**

❖ **Meaning:** So called because it causes respiratory disease in children with cell fusion & syncytium formation.

❖ **Geographical distribution:** Worldwide.

❖ **Morphology:** Same as other paramyxo viruses with following differences.
➢ **Shape:** Pleomorphic.
➢ **Size:** 150-300 nm.
➢ **Nucleocapsid:** 13 nm.
➢ **Envelopes:** Nucleocapsid is covered by envelop.
➢ **Peplomeres:**
- **Properties:**
- They are present as projecting spike over envelop

- They are glycoprotein in nature.
- They do not possess haemolytic, haemagglutinin & neuraminidase properties.

• **Two types:** G and F.

1. **G protein:** Helps in adsorption with host cells.
2. **Fusion (F) protein:**

- Helps in fusion of viral envelop with plasma membrane, which is the essential step in viral infection.
- Responsible for cell-to-cell fusion, which leads to syncytium formation.

❖ Culture characteristics (C/Cs):

- No growth in eggs.
- Grow in Hela or HEP-2 cells.
- Growth is identified by syncytium formation.
- CPE (only in type-2) seen after 10 days.
- Rapid diagnosis is done by IF test.

❖ Resistance:

- Inactivated at room temperature.
- Stored by lyophilisation.

❖ Antigenic structure & serotypes:

- Antigenically stable.
- Only one serotype.
- However by using monoclonal-Ab two subtypes are observed like A & B.

❖ Immunity:

a. **Humoral immunity:**

- Antibodies are produced but their role is not clear, however reinfection is mild compare to primary infection.
- IgA is more protective than IgG.
- Antibodies also transfer from mother to child to elicit the passive immunity, hence newborns are protected.

b. **Cell mediated immunity:** It is more important than CMI in recovery of infection.

c. **Interferon:** It also appears but not in high level.

❖ Pathogenicity:

➢ **Nature of disease:**

- It causes annual epidemic in the temperate regions during winter & in the tropics during the rainy season.
- Outbreaks are common in paediatric ward, nurseries & day care centres.

➢ **Reservoir of infection:** Human.

➢ **Source of infection:** Virus present in respiratory droplets aroused during coughing or sneezing for 1-3 weeks & for a month in person with defective CMI.

➢ **Mode of transmission:**

- Via inhalation.
- By contaminated fingers.
- Fomites borne.

➢ **Incubation period:** 4-6 days.

➢ **Portal of entry:** Respiratory system.

➢ **Site:** Respiratory system.

➢ **Precipitating factors:**

1. **Age:** Common between 6 weeks-6 months with peak at 2-3 months. Almost 70% of children affected by the age of 1 year & almost all by 2 year of age.
2. **Diseases:** Infection is sever in premature infants, underlying congenital cardiac disease, bronchopulmonary dysplasia, nephritic syndrome, organ transplantation & other immunity lowering conditions.
3. **Seasonal factors:** Epidemic in the temperate region during winter & in the tropic during the rainy season.
4. **Environmental factors:** Infection is more common in children wards, nurseries, day care centres & over crowded communities like military persons.
5. **Immunity:**

- Antibodies also transfer from mother to child to elicit the passive immunity, hence newborns are protected.
- More common & virus sheds in respiratory secretion very longer in person with defective CMI.

➢ **Pathogenesis:** Large numbers of lymphocytes are migrate to the sites of infection & producing

- Peribronchiolar infiltration of inflammatory cells.
- Submucosal oedema.
- Necrosis of bronchiolar epithelium.
- Formation of plugs consisting of mucus, cellular debris and fibrin which occlude the smaller bronchioles.

➢ **Clinical features:**

• **Infants & young children:**

- Lower respiratory tract infections: It out rank the other pathogens & most common cause of lower respiratory tract infections like bronchitis, bronchiolitis & pneumonia in infant (< 1 year child) & young children. It occurs in 25-40% of infected infants. Chest X-ray shows peri-bronchial thickening, diffuse interstitial infiltration & rarely lobar consolidation.
- Otitis media.
- Sudden death syndrome.

• **Older children & adult:** Influenza like upper respiratory tract infection like common cold, running nose, sore throat & cough.

➢ **Complications:**

- Secondary bacterial infection.
- Exacerbation of asthma & COPD.
- Recurrent infection is common in children & adults but mild in nature.

✓ **Note: Most common viral agents**

- For lower respiratory tract infections like bronchitis, bronchiolitis & pneumonia in infants (< 1 year child) & young children: RSV

- For croup (acute laryngotracheobronchitis): Parainfluenza virus-2

❖ **Laboratory diagnosis:**
➢ **Specimens:** Nasal or nasopharyngeal swab.
➢ **Testing methods:**
A. **Microscopy: →Follow morphology.**
B. **Cell Culture: →Follow C/Cs.**
C. **Serological tests:** Paired sera are tested by ELISA, neutralisation or CFT,
D. **Molecular methods:** RT-PCR is more rapid & sensitive.

❖ **Prevention:**
- No effective vaccine is available.
- Attempt had been made with formalinised vaccines, but it developed more serious illness than control group on subsequent exposure of infection.

❖ **Treatment:**
- Ribovirin is effective in aerosol form in hospitalised patient & it reduces the virus shedding
- Symptomatic treatment t is given.

Morbilivirus

Measles viruses

❖ **History:** Virus was isolated by Enders & Peebles in 1954 in monkey & human kidney cells.

❖ **Geographical distribution & genotypes (clades):**
- Distributed worldwide.
- 8 clades of measles, which are further grouped in to 23 recognised genotypes by WHO.
- Genotype B3 is most common worldwide while in India D8 is common.

❖ **Morphology:** Same as other paramyxoviruses with following differences.
➢ **Shape:** Spherical & often pleomorphic.
➢ **Size:** 150-250 nm.
➢ **Genome:** ss-RNA (+).
➢ **Capsid:** NA is surrounded by helical type of capsid.
➢ **Envelope:** Nucleocapsid is surrounded by bilayer envelop which consists inner protein (M protein) & outer lipid layer.
➢ **Peplomeres:**
• **Properties:**
- They are present as projecting spike over envelop.
- They are glycoprotein in nature.
• **Two types:** G and F.
1. **Haemagglutinin (H):** Helps in adsorption but no neuraminidase activity.
2. **Fusion (F) protein:**
- Helps in fusion of viral envelop with plasma membrane, which is the essential step in viral infection.
- Mediates the haemolytic activity.

➢ **Inclusion body:** Numerous acidophilic nuclear & cytoplasmic inclusions.
➢ **Giant cells:** Multinucleated giant cells **called Warthin-Finkeldey cells** are found in lymphoid tissues. Theyare examined by Giemsa stain.
➢ **IF microscopy:** It is also a useful technique.

❖ **Culture characteristics (C/Cs):** Inoculate the specimen very immediately after collection as the virus is labile.
i. **Egg culture:** Grow in amniotic cavity of hen's egg.
ii. **Tissue culture:**
- Grow in Vero, Hela or in human amnion cells.
- CPE after weeks.
- Growth is identified by syncytium formation, acidophilic nuclear & cytoplasmic inclusion & giant cell (**Warthin-Finkeldey**) formation.
- More rapid result is obtained by IF test.

❖ **Resistance:** Inactivated by heat, ether, UV light & formalin.

❖ **Antigenic structure:** Antigenically stable (only one strain/type is exist), share antigen with the viruses of canine distemper & bovine rinderpest.

❖ **Immunity:**
- It not occurs in 1st 6 months of life due to passive protection by maternal antibodies.
- One attack confers solid immunity.
- In non immune person, infection always results in disease.

❖ **Pathogenicity:**
➢ **Disease name:** Disease **called measles.**
➢ **Synonym:** Also **called rubeola.**
➢ **Meaning:** Rubeola = red spot, which indicates the characteristic of disease.
➢ **Nature & history of disease:**
- Measles is very ancient disease & initially it was confused with other exanthematous diseases like smallpox. After 1629 it considered as separate entity.
- Basic knowledge of measles was given by Peter Panum (Danish medical students), from the epidemic occurred in Faroe Island in 1846 with involvement of 75% cases. It spared the olders who were alive during previous epidemic.
- Viral origin of measles was established by Goldberger & Anderson in 1911 by inoculation of blood & nasopharyngeal filtrates in monkeys from the case of measles.
- Next was occurred in 1951 in Greenland which affected almost all indigenous population.

- It is endemic throughout the world & produces epidemic every 2-3 years.
- Epidemics are usually seen in late winter & early spring, with peak in April.

➢ **Reservoir of infection:** Human only. No animal reservoir exists.

➢ **Source of infection:**

- Period of infectivity (communicability): Virus present in respiratory droplets aroused during coughing or sneezing, 3 days before the onset of symptoms until the disappearance of rash. Infectivity is maximum in prodromal phase & declined with onset of rash.
- It also present in blood, washed leucocytes & in tears during prodromal phase (last for 2-4 days).
- IT can be recovered from the urine up to 4 days after the appearance of rash.
- Infectivity from blood, urine & tears is unclear.
- Secondary attack rate: High.

➢ **Mode of transmission:**

- Via inhalation of aerosols & respiratory secretion aroused during coughing or sneering.
- Enter via conjunctiva.

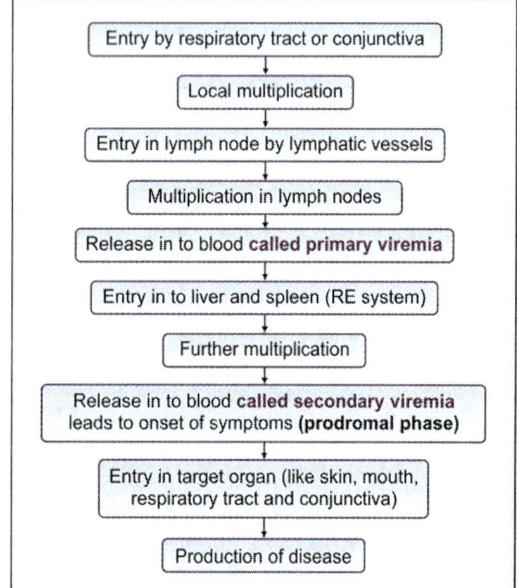

Flow chart-2: Pathogenesis of measles

➢ **Incubation period:** 10-14 days. It may be shorter up to infants & longer up to 3 weeks in adult. Fever occurs after 10 day & rash occur after 14 day.

➢ **Precipitating factors:**

1. **Age:**
   - It not occurs in 1st 6 months of life due to passive protection by maternal antibodies.
   - Common between 6 months to3 years of age in developing country & after 5 years in developed country.
2. **Seasonal:** Epidemic usually seen in late winter & early spring, with peak in April.
3. **Malnutrition:** Common in malnourished child with mortality 400 times higher than well nourished child.
4. **Immuno deficiency disease (IDD):** No protection and infection is almost resulting in clinical disease in immunocompromised host.

➢ **Pathogenesis: →Flow chart-2.**

➢ **Clinical features:**

- **Prodromal phase:**
  - It (fever) begins on 10th day after infection & last up to 14th day (last for 2-4 days).
  - It consist malaise, fever, conjunctival injection (redness of the eyes), cough & nasal discharge.
  - Koplik's spot: It is a small bluish white ulceration on buccal mucosa opposite the 1st & 2nd lower molars, appears 1-2 day after fever & 1-2 days before rash begins. Its presence is pathognomonic of measles.
- **Eruptive phase:**

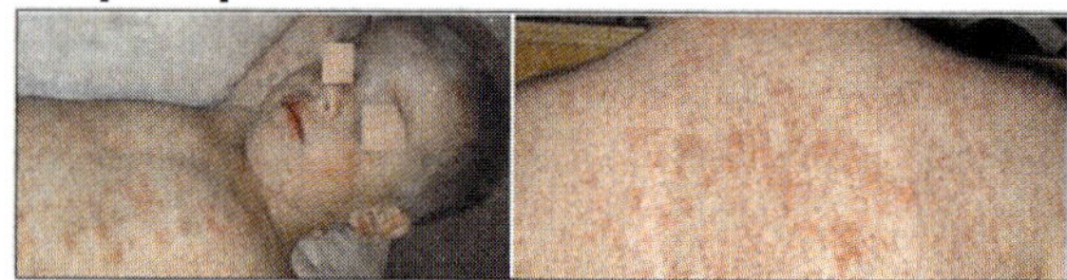

Figure-3: Rashes of measles

- Rash (**fig.-3**) appear 3-4 day after prodromal illness.
- Red maculopapular rash typically appear on forehead at first & then extend down to involve the lower extremities in 2-3 days.
- It disappears in same order in 3-6 days, leaving behind brownish discolouration & finely granular desquamation.
- Generally: Fever (10th day) → Koplik's spot (12th day) → rash (14th day).

➢ **Complications:**

✪ **General:** Weight loss, growth retardation & child remains week for number of days.

✪ **Secondary infection:** Increased susceptibility to bacterial (pneumonia, otitis media), fungal (candidosis) & viral (bronchitis, croup) infection.

✪ **GIT:** Diarrhoea may leads to malnutrition & vitamin A deficiency.

✪ **Respiratory:**

- By virus itself like Hecht's pneumonia (Giant cell pneumonia) & acute laryngo tracheo bronchitis (croup).
- Reactivation of pulmonary tuberculosis.

✪ **CNS:** Encephalitis & transverse myelitis.

✪ **Haematological:** Thrombocytopenia leading to purpura & bleeding from mouth, intestines & genitourinary tract.

✪ **Immune depression:** Suppression of CMI (delayed type of hypersensitivity). Allergic tests like Mantoux and other skin tests are negative.

✪ **In pregnant women:** Spontaneous abortion & premature delivery.

➤ **Sequelae: Called SSPE.**

✪ **Full form:** Subacute Sclerosing Pan Encephalitis.

✪ **Causes:**

- Very rare & delayed sequelae of measles infection occur several years after the primary infection.
- Also rarely by rubella infection.

✪ **Clinical presentation:**

- Occurs very late after initial infection of measles.
- Deterioration of mental & motor functions.
- Death 1-3 years after onset of symptoms.

✪ **Diagnosis:**

- **Samples:** Brain cells, CSF & blood.
- **Tests:**
  - **Microscopy** of brain cells shows the evidence of measles infection.
  - **Culture:** Virus is isolated by co-cultivation of infected brain cells & cells of non-neural origin.
  - **Serological tests** from blood & CSF reveals the measles antibodies.
  - CMI is absent in SSPE.

❖ Laboratory diagnosis:

➤ **Typical case:** Diagnosis is based on clinical ground.

➤ **Atypical case & differentiation from rubella:** It required laboratory help.

✪ **Specimens:** Virus may be isolated from

- Nasal secretion, throat swab & conjunctival swab.
- Blood.
- CSF in SSPE.

✪ **Testing methods:**

A. **Microscopy: → Follow morphology**

B. **Culture: →Follow C/Cs**

C. **Serological tests:**

- CFT, HAI & neutralisation test.
- Detection of measles specific IgM-Ab in single specimen between one & two weeks after the onset of rash is confirmatory.
- Detection of Ab in CSF is diagnostic of SSPE.

E. **Molecular method:** RT-PCR is more rapid & sensitive.

❖ Prevention:

➤ **General measures:**

- Avoid the contact with patient.
- Staying away from school or work and avoiding social activities.

➤ **Immunoprophylaxis:**

i. **Active immunisation:** By using following types of live attenuated vaccines.

a. **Given by injection route:**

✪ **Types:** Three types of preparations.

1. **Edmonston strain:**
   - Original vaccine developed by multiple passages through human kidney, amnion & chick embryo culture.
   - Due to risk of febrile rash (vaccination measles) further attenuation is necessary.
2. **Schwartz & Moraten strain:** Safe but effective only in children older than 15 months.
3. **Edmonston & Zagreb strain:**
   - Effective in infant of 4-6 months.
   - Attenuated by passage in human diploid cells.

✪ **Administration:**

- Given single or in combination like MR or MMR or MMRV (Measles, Mumps, Rubella & Varicella).
- **Route:** By SC route & also effective IM route.
- **Dose:** 0.5ml at 9 months of age according to National immunisation schedule with vitamin A.

✪ **Complication:**

- Mild measles illness (fever & rash).
- Toxic Shock Syndrome (TSS) due to contaminated vial or due to use of same vial for more than one session or next day. Vial should not be used after 4 hours of its opening.

✪ **Advantage:** Single injection start protection in 12 days & last for 20 years.

✪ **Contraindications:**

- Patient allergic to neomycin or other components of vaccine.
- Pregnancy.
- IDDs.

✪ **Measles eradication:**

- **Objectives:** As single dose of measles vaccine provide long lasting immunity, it is possible to eradicate the measles with following objectives.
  - Achieving 96% vaccination in less than 1 year children.
  - Cumulating in the immunity gap be prevented.
- **Progress:** Considerable progress has been achieved in USA & some other countries.

b. **Given by intranasal route:** Live attenuated vaccine given by intranasal route to young babies gives good protection irrespective of effect of maternal Ab.

ii. **Passive immunisation:** Specific Ig is given in dose of 0.25 ml/kg of body weight, 3-4 day after exposure.

❖ Treatment:

Antibiotics are not effective, symptomatic treatment is given as follows.

- Acetaminophen to relieve fever and muscle aches.
- Rest to help to boost up the immune system.
- Plenty of fluids (six to eight glasses of water a day).
- Humidifier to ease a cough and sore throat.
- Vitamin A supplements.

Avulavirus

Avian avula virus 1

- **Synonyms:**
  - It is an avian paramyxovirus type-1.

- In India it **called ranikhet virus.**
- It also **called newcastle disease virus,** as it was first identified in Java, Indonesia, in 1926, and in 1927, in Newcastle-upon-Tyne, England (whence it got its name).

- **Bird infection:** It is a natural pathogen of bird causing explosive outbreak of pneumoencephalitis or influenza with high mortality.
- **Human infection:** Self-limited conjunctivitis in poultry worker & other in contact with infected birds.
- **Prevention:** By vaccine & by slaughtering the infected birds.

Henipavirus

* **Genus:** *Henipavirus*, this new genus was identified in 1990 in an outbreak in Malaysia & Australia.
* **Human species:** Nipah & hendra virus.

- These are zoonotic paramyxo viruses.
- Fruit bats are the natural host.
- Mortality is very high & classified as bio-safety level-4 agents.

Nipah henipa virus

❖ **Common name / synonym & history:** Commonly **called nipah virus**, because it was first identified in 1999 during an outbreak among pig farmers with respiratory & neurological features in **Kampung Sungai Nipah**, Malaysia.

❖ **Geographical distribution & genotypes (clades):** Malaysia, Bangladesh, India, Cambodia, Thailand, Indonesia, Madagascar, Ghana & the Philippines as shown in **fig.-5.** The most likely origin of this virus was in 1947 (95% credible interval: 1888–1988). There are 2 clades of virus —one with its origin in 1995 (95% credible interval: 1985–2002) and a second with its origin in 1985 (95% credible interval: 1971–1996).

❖ **Morphology:** →Vide supra

❖ **Culture characteristics (C/Cs):** It is identifiable under cell culture.

❖ **Resistance:** Nipah virus is killed by heat, drying and cleaning with detergents.

❖ **Pathogenicity:**

➢ **Disease name:** It is a zoonosis (from pig and/or fruits bat) **called nipah virus infection.**

➢ **Nature or history of disease:**

- April,1999, Malaysia & Singapore: Nipah virus was identified in April 1999, when it caused an outbreak of neurological & respiratory disease on pig farms in **Kampung Sungai Nipah**, Malaysia (Peninsular), resulting in 257 human cases, with 105 deaths & the culling of one million pigs. In Singapore, 11 cases, including one death, occurred in abattoir workers exposed to pigs imported from the affected Malaysian farms. No new outbreaks have been reported in Malaysia and Singapore since 1999.
- January 31–23 February, 2001, Siliguri, India: 66 cases with 74% deaths. 75% of patients were either hospital staff or had visited one of the other patients in hospital, indicating human-to-human transmission.
- April – May, 2001, Meherpur, Bangladesh: 13 cases with 9 (69%) deaths.
- January, 2003, Naogaon district, Bangladesh: 12 cases with 8 (67%) deaths.
- January – February, 2004, Manikganj & Rajbari districts, Bangladesh: 42 cases with 14 (33%) deaths.
- 19 February – 16 April, 2004, Faridpur, district, Bangladesh: 36 cases with 27 (75%) deaths.
- January, 2005, Tangail district, Bangladesh: 12 cases with 11 (92%) deaths. The virus was probably contracted from drinking date palm juice, contaminated by fruit bat's droppings or saliva.
- January and February, 2007, Thakurgaon, Bangladesh: 7 cases with 3 deaths.
- February – May, 2007, Nadia district, India: 50 suspected cases with 3–5 fatalities.
- March and April, 2007, Kushtia district, Bangladesh: 8 cases with 5 deaths.
- February – March, 2008, Manikganj & Rajbari districts, Bangladesh: 9 cases with 8 deaths.
- January, 2010, Bhanga subdistrict, Faridpur, Bangladesh: 8 cases with 7 deaths.
- March, 2010, one physician of Faridpur Medical College Hospital caring for confirmed nipah cases was died.
- February, 2011: Hatibandha, Lalmonirhat, Bangladesh. The deaths of 21 school children.
- May, 2018, Perambra near Calicut, Kerala, India: Deaths of 13 people (Till date of this book written).

➢ **Reservoir of infection:**

- Fruit bats are the natural host of the nipah virus. Based on seroprevalence data & virus isolations, the primary reservoir / natural host for nipah virus was pteropid fruit bats, including *Pteropus vampyrus* (large flying fox), & *Pteropus hypomelanus* (small flying fox), both of which occur in Malaysia.
- In Bangladesh and neighboring parts of India, the reservoir is *Pteropus giganteus.*
- Nipah virus has been isolated from Lyle's flying fox (*Pteropus lylei)* in Cambodia, & viral RNA found in urine & saliva from *P. lylei* and Horsfield's round leaf bat (*Hipposideros larvatus*) in Thailand.
- Antibodies to nipah viruses have also been found in fruit bats in Madagascar (*Pteropus rufus, Eidolon*

dupreanum & Ghana (*Eidolon helvum*) indicating a wide geographic distribution of the viruses. No infection of humans or other species have been observed in Cambodia, Thailand or Africa thus far.

- **Source of infection:** Pig is the intermediate host & act as source for human infection. However, human infection can also occur from bats, which also serve as source for human infection.
- **Mode of transmission: → Fig.-4**

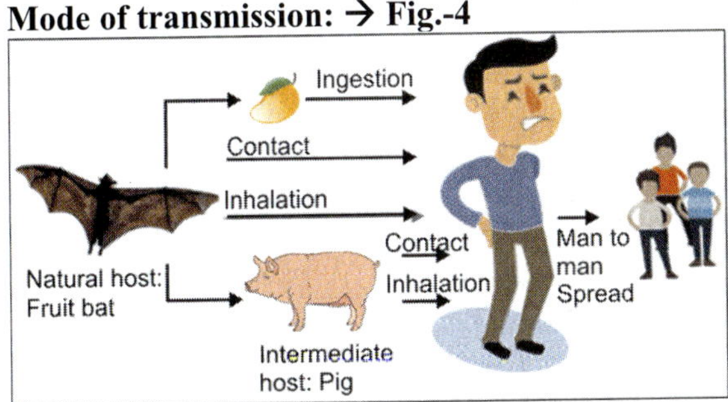

Figure-4: Transmission of nipah virus

- **Transmission to pig:** Fruit bats are the natural host of nipah virus shedding virus in urine, faeces & saliva. Contacts with such bat's products allow the transmission in pig.
- **Transmission to human:** Human infection occurs by following ways.

1. **Fruits bat to human:**
   - Ingestion: Consumption of partially eaten fruits by bats or palm juices contaminated by bat's saliva or droppings.
   - Contact: Transmission possible directly from bats to human via contact.
   - Inhalation: Transmission also possible directly from bats to human via inhalation.
2. **Pig to human:**
   - Contact: Contact with tissues or nasopharyngeal / throat secretions of infected pig.
   - Inhalation: Inhalation of respiratory droplets arise from pigs.
3. **Human to human transmission:** It occurs by close contact or by respiratory droplets of infected patients especially in hospital staff (nosocomial infection) or in family members. In Siliguri, India, 2001 & from 2001 to 2008, in Bangladesh, around half of reported cases were due to human-to-human transmission through providing care to infected patients.

- **Incubation period:** 4-14 days.
- **Portal of entry:** Respiratory system or GIT.
- **Sites:** Respiratory system & brain.
- **Precipitating factors (epidemiological determinants):**

1. **Occupational:** Common in forest workers or pig farmers.

- **Pathogenesis:** Ephrine B2 has been identified as the main receptor for the *Henipavirus*.
- **Clinical features:**

- **In human:**
  - Respiratory features: Flu like symptom including fever, headache, cough, abdominal pain, nausea, vomiting & weakness. Problems with swallowing & blurred vision are relatively common.
  - CNS features: Encephalitis present with drowsiness, disorientation, confusion etc. About a quarter of the patients have seizures & about 60% become comatose & might need mechanical ventilation. In patients with severe disease, their conscious state may deteriorate & they may develop severe hypertension, fast heart rate, and very high temperature.
- **In pig:** It causes a porcine respiratory & neurologic syndrome (Asymptomatic to acute fever, laboured breathing, trembling, twitching & muscle spasms), locally **called "barking pig syndrome" or "one mile cough."**

- **Complications:**
  - Nipah virus is also known to cause relapse encephalitis. In the initial Malaysian outbreak, a patient presented with relapse encephalitis some 53 months after his initial infection.
  - High mortality.

❖ Laboratory diagnosis:

- **Specimens & testing methods:**

A. **Culture:** Cell culture.
B. **Serological tests:** ELISA from serum.
C. **Molecular methods:** RT-PCR from body fluids.

❖ Prevention:

- **General measures:**
  - Avoid the consumption of uncooked fruits and fruit products. Such foods, contaminated with urine or saliva from infected fruit bats, are the most likely source of this outbreak.
  - Stop toddy tapping in the area as toddy can become contaminated with saliva or bat urine.
- **Chemoprophylaxis:** No specific drug is available
- **Immunoprophylaxis:** While no vaccine currently exists, a 2012 study of a trial vaccine developed using the outer proteins of hendra virus was shown to induce protection against nipah in African green monkeys.

❖ **Treatment:** There is no definitive treatment for nipah encephalitis, apart from supportive measures, such as mechanical ventilation & prevention of secondary infection. Ribavirin an antiviral drug, was tested in the Malaysian outbreak, and the results were encouraging, though further studies are still needed.

Hendra henipa virus

❖ Common name / synonym & history:

- Originally it **called "equine morbillivirus"**

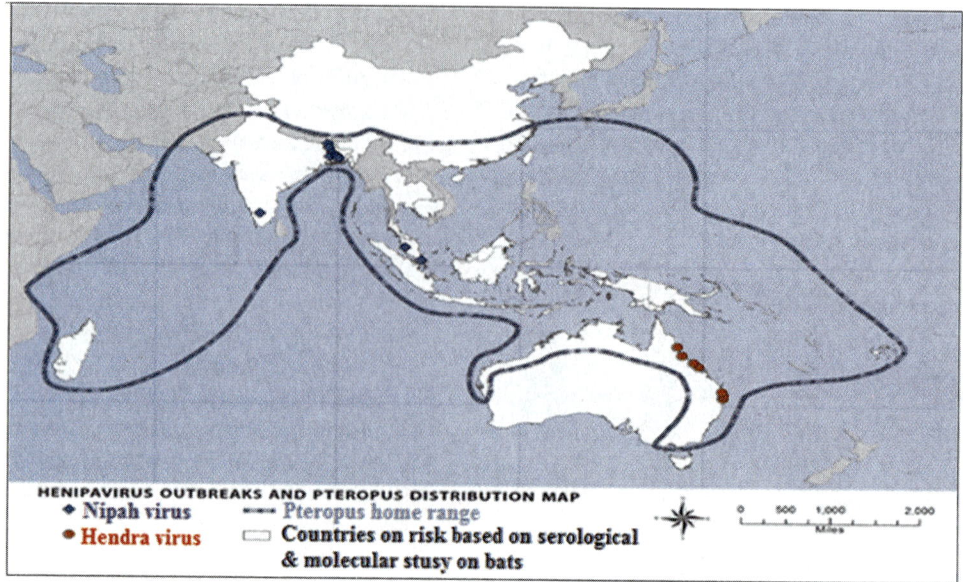

Figure-5: Geographical distribution of nipah virus, hendra virus, bats & countries on risk

- Also **called hendra virus**, as it was discovered in September 1994 when it caused the deaths of 13 horses, & a trainer at a training complex at 10 Williams Avenue, **Hendra**, a suburb of Brisbane in Queensland, Australia.

❖ **Geographical distribution:** Australia. These virus have all been on the east coast of Australia with the most northern event at Cairns, Queensland & the event furthest south at Kempsey, New South Wales as shown in **fig.-5.**

❖ **Morphology:** →Vide supra.

❖ **Culture characteristics (C/Cs):** Virus isolation is done from the CSF or throat swabs.

❖ **Resistance:** Hendra virus is killed by heat, drying and cleaning with detergents.

❖ **Pathogenicity:**

➢ **Disease name:** It is a zoonosis (from horse) **called hendra virus infection.**

➢ **Nature or history of disease:**

- 1st outbreak occurred in September 1994 when it caused the deaths of 13 horses, & a trainer at a training complex at 10 Williams Avenue, **Hendra**, a suburb of Brisbane in Queensland, Australia. Trainer was died due to respiratory & renal failure. Two days later total 19 horses were ill & of them 13 were died & 6 were euthanised to prevent the further transmission
- 2nd outbreak occurred in August 1994 (chronologically preceding the first outbreak) in Mackay 1,000 km north of Brisbane resulting in the deaths of two horses and their owner. Owner developed meningitis, recovered fully but died 14 months later with neurological sign. This outbreak was diagnosed retrospectively by the presence of hendra virus in the brain of the patient.
- On 26 July 2011 a dog living on the Mt Alford property was reported to have hendra virus antibodies, the first time an animal other than a flying fox, horse, or human has tested positive outside an experimental situation.
- Since 1994 to 2013, hendra infections in humans remain rare; only 7 cases have been noticed.
- As of June 2014, a total of 50 outbreaks of hendra virus have occurred in Australia, all involving infection of horses. As a result of these events, 83 horses have died or been euthanised. A further 4 died or were euthanised (total 87) as a result of possible hendra infection. Four of these outbreaks have spread to humans as a result of direct contact with infected horses.

➢ **Reservoir of infection:** Fruit bat (flying fox) is the main reservoir. A seroprevalence of 47% is found in the flying foxes, suggesting an endemic infection of the bat population throughout Australia. Flying fox experimentally infected with the hendra virus develop a viremia (no illness) then excrete the virus in their urine, faeces and saliva for approximately one week. Following types of species are observed.
- Little red flying fox *(Pteropus scapulatus).*
- Black flying fox *(Pteropus alecto).*
- Grey-headed flying fox *(Pteropus poliocephalus).*
- Spectacled flying fox *(Pteropus conspicillatus).*

➢ **Source of infection:** Horse is source of human infection (mentioned as intermediate host by few authors).

➢ **Mode of transmission:**

- **Bats to horses:** Actual mode of transmission between bats & horses has not been determined; however horses may be infected with hendra after exposure to bodily fluid from an infected flying fox. This often happens in the form of urine, feces, or masticated fruit covered in the flying fox's saliva when horses are allowed to graze below roosting sites. The 7 human cases have all been infected only after contact with sick horses. As a result, veterinarians are particularly at risk for contracting the disease.
- **Horse to human:**
- Exact mode is unknown but transmission of hendra virus to humans can occur after direct contact to body fluids & tissues or excretions of horses infected with hendra virus.
- There is no evidence that the virus can be passed directly from flying foxes to humans, dogs to humans, environment to humans, or, from humans to horses.
- There is no evidence of airborne spread (where tiny particles remain suspended in the air).
- Till date, no human-to-human transmission has been documented.

➢ **Incubation period:** 9-16 days.

➢ **Portal of entry:** Exactly not known.

➢ **Sites:** Lungs & CNS.

➢ **Precipitating factors (epidemiological determinants):**

1. **Occupational:** Common in forest worker or dealing with horse business (recreational exposure).

➢ **Pathogenesis:** Ephrine B2 has been identified as the main receptor for the *Henipavirus.*

➢ **Clinical features:**

- **In human:**
- Respiratory features: Severe flu-like illness (fever, cough, sore throat, headache and tiredness), haemorrhage & oedema of lungs.
- CNS features: Meningitis or encephalitis.
- **In horse:** Pulmonary oedema, congestion and/or or neurological signs.

➢ **Complication:** Case fatality rate in humans is 60% and in horses 75%, hence hendra virus has been classified as a bio safety level- 4 agent.

❖ **Laboratory diagnosis:**

➢ **Specimens & testing methods:**

A. **Culture:** →**Follow C/Cs**

B. **Serological tests:** Detection of antibody by ELISA (IgG and IgM) from serum & CSF.

C. **Molecular methods:** Viral RNA detection by real time polymerase chain reaction (RT-PCR) from serum, CSF, or throat swabs.

❖ **Prevention:**

➢ **General measures:**

- Combined efforts: It is a zoonosis; one must understand the social, ecological, and biological contributions that may be facilitating this spillover.
- Deforestation: It is other measure of prevention.
- Avoiding contact: Avoiding contact with ill horses especially in occupational persons.
- Health education: Knowledge regarding seasonal trend of hendra virus in fruit bats is help to contain the disease.
- Notification: Suspected cases of Hendra virus infection in horses should be notified.
- Improvement in hygiene: It is important to pay attention to standard hygiene practices when interacting with any horse like washing hands etc.

➢ **Chemoprophylaxis:** No specific drug is useful.

➢ **Immunoprophylaxis:**

i. **Vaccine for horse:**

- Subunit vaccine is prepared from G (surface) protein of virus, which is effective in ferret.
- Local swelling in horse is the side effect & useful for pregnant mares.

ii. **Vaccine for human:** National Institute of Allergy and Infectious Diseases (NIAID) developed subunit vaccine for nipah virus & hendra virus from G (surface) protein formulated with adjuvant. Both vaccines produced neutralising antibodies in laboratory animals & trial began in 2015 to develop monoclonal antibodies as a complimentary treatment for humans, who exposed to hendra virus infected horses.

❖ **Treatment:** The drug ribavirin has been shown to be effective against the viruses in vitro, but the clinical usefulness of this drug is uncertain.

Metapneumovirus

Human metapneumo virus

- **History:** Resemble to RSV & identified in 2001 by molecular methods.
- **Disease:**
- Children: Respiratory illness.
- Adults: Leukemia & lymphoma.
- Olders: Are also infected by virus.

Question bank

Case study

1) A 15 year old male child is brought to the hospital with fever & painful swelling on right side of cheek. On clinical examination it seems parotitis. 10 days after he developed scrotal swelling, this was ruled out as an orchitis on clinical background. Urine is collected & sent to the referral laboratory which reported ss-

RNA virus with negative polarity. Identify the clinical conditions & answer the following.

a) Name the clinical condition & its etiological agent.
b) Write pathogenicity & diagnosis of clinical condition.
c) How you can prevent this clinical condition?

2) A 11 year old male child is brought to the hospital with history of fever, conjunctivitis, cough & nasal discharge since 10 days. His mother was not able to give complete immunisation history. On mouth examination bluish white ulceration on buccal mucosa against lower molars was identified. Later he developed red maculopapular rash on forehead at first which extend down to involve the lower extremities in 2-3 days. Identify the clinical conditions & answer the following

a) Name the clinical condition & its etiological agent.
b) Write pathogenicity & diagnosis of clinical condition.
c) How you can prevent this clinical condition?

Essay/Full question

1) Mumps virus.
2) Paramyxoviridae.

Short notes

1) Classification of Paramyxoviridae.
2) Mumps virus.
3) Parainfluenzae virus type1-4.
4) RSV.
5) Measles virus.
6) Measles vaccine.
7) Nipah virus.

Short questions for theory/viva questions

1) Write the scientific name for following viruses:
   - Haemagglutinating virus of Japan
   - Croup Associated virus
   - Chimpanzee coryza agent
   - Ranikhet virus
2) What is atypical mumps?
3) Name the two viral strains useful to prepare the vaccine for measles.

MCQs for chapter review

Classification

1) Paramyxo viruses include
(a) Retro virus (b) Polio virus (c) Parainfluenza (d) Rabies

2) Measles virus is (PGI-97)
(a) Paramyxovirus (b) Polio virus (c) Parainfluenza (d) Picorna virus

3) Which of the following statement is / are true of all paramyxo viruses include
(a) They contain single stranded RNA genome of negative polarity (b) Envelope is derived from the host cells plasma membrane (c) They have a cytoplasmic site of replication (d) They enter the body by the respiratory route

Mumps virus

4) With reference to mumps which of the following is true (AI-06)
(a) Meningoencephalitis can precede parotitis (b) Salivary gland involvement is limited to the parotid (c) Patient is not infectious prior to clinical parotid enlargement (d) Mumps orchitis frequently leads to infertility

5) Commonest complication of mumps is (AI-00)
(a) Orchitis and oophoritis (b) Encephalitis (c) Pneumonia (d) Myocarditis

6) Regarding mumps, which is true? (AIIMS, Nov-07)
(a) Causes SSPE (b) Mumps causes aseptic meningitis in children (c) Sublingual gland is involved (d) All

RSV

7) Virus lacking haemagglutinin and neuraminidase but having membrane fusion protein is
(a) RSV (b) CMV (c) HSV (d) EBV

8) The most common etiological agent for acute bronchiolitis in infancy is (AI-06)
(a) *Influenzavirus* (b) *Parainfluenzavirus* (c) *Rhinovirus* (d) Respiratory syncytial virus

Measles virus

9) Which of the following statement is the 'least common' complication of measles? (AIIMS-06)
(a) Diarrhoea (b) Pneumonia (c) Otitis media (d) SSPE

10) Subacute sclerosing pan encephalitis is the delayed manifestation of
(a) Influenzae (b) Measles (c) Mumps (d) Polio

11) Giant cell (Hecht's) pneumonia is due (PGI, Dec-98)
(a) CMV (b) Measles (c) Malaria (d) *P carinii*

12) Which of the following is not true about measles? (AI-08)
(a) High secondary attack (b) Only one strain cause infection (c) Not infectious in prodromal period (d) Infections confer lifelong immunity

Answers of MCQs & explanation

1) (c)
2) (a) } Follow section, **classification** for explanation

3) (a), (b), (c) & (d)

- Option (b) & (c) are partially correct because
  - Envelope is made up by lipoprotein where, lipid derived from the host cell plasma membrane by budding & proteins are viral encoded
  - Paramyxoviruses replicate in cytoplasm but in few paramyxovirus RNA synthesis take place in nucleus also.

4) (a)
5) (a)
6) (b) } Follow section, **mumps virus** for explanation

7) (a)
8) (d) } Follow section, **RSV** for explanation

9) (d)
10) (b)
11) (b)
12) (c) } Follow section, **measles virus** for explanation

68 Arboviruses and Roboviruses

Learning heading & subheadings

Arboviruses

Meaning: Arboviruses means **Ar**thropod (vector) **bo**rne **viruses**, as they are transmitted by arthropod or vector or insect.

Definition: Diverse group of RNA viruses that are transmitted by blood sucking arthropod.

Geographical distribution: Worldwide distribution. More numerous in the tropical than in the temperate zone.

General properties:

- Taxonomically all the viruses are RNA type but belong to different families.
- Over 500 viruses have been listed, out of which about 100 can infect human.
- In India more than 40 viruses have been identified, of which more than 10 can infect human.
- Viruses are multiply inside the insects & establish a lifelong harmless infection in them; hence viruses transmitted mechanically by vectors are not included in this group.

Classification:

- It includes RNA viruses which are dissimilar in properties.
- Classification based on ecological & epidemiological, physical & chemical consideration
- Families & respective genera are mentioned in **table-1.**
- Species of each family & genus are further classified on the bases of clinical syndrome like

1. Fever and/or rash, and/or arthralgia group.
2. Encephalitis group.
3. Haemorrhagic fever group.
4. Multiple syndrome like dengue virus.

Resistance:

- Inactivated at room temperature & also by ether, chloroform & bile salts.
- Infectivity can be retained at -70^{0}C or by lyophilisation.

Antigenic structure:

- Three antigens are important in serological studies like
  - Haemagglutinin Ag.
  - Complement fixing Ag.
  - Neutralising Ag.
- Antigenic cross reaction occurs between arboviruses.
- Plaque reduction neutralisation test (PRNT) shows the greatest specificity for the identification of the arboviruses.

Arboviruses found in India:

➤ **Common:** Chikungunya virus, Dengue virus & Japanese encephalitis (JE) virus.

- **Rare:** Kyasanur Forest disease (KFD) virus, West Nile virus, Sindbis virus, Crimean Congo Haemorrhagic Fever (CCHF) virus, Ganjam virus, Vellore virus, Chandipura virus, Bhanja virus, Umbre virus, Sathuperi virus, Chittor virus, Minnal virus, Venkatapuram virus, Dhori virus, Kaisodi virus & Sandfly fever virus, Zika virus (3 cases found in Gujarat in May-2017).

Family	Genus	Arbovirus species	
Togaviridae	*Rubivirus*	Rubella virus (Not an arbovirus)	
	Alphavirus	**i. Encephalitis causing viruses:** **a. Eastern Equine Encephalitis (EEE) virus** **b. Western Equine Encephalitis (WEE) virus** **c. Venezuelan Equine Encephalitis (VEE) virus**	**ii. Febrile illness & arthritis causing viruses** **a. Chikungunya virus** **b. O'nyog-nyog virus** **c. Semliki Forest Virus** **d. Sindbis virus** **e. Others:** Mayaro virus & Ross River virus
Flaviridae	*Hepacivirus*	HCV (not an arbovirus)	
	Pegivirus	GB (G Barker) virus C (not an arbovirus)	
	Pestivirus	Bovine viral diarrhoea 1 (not an arbovirus)	
	Flavivirus	**Mosquito borne species** **A. Encephalitis group** **i. Japanese encephalitis (JE) virus** **ii. St. Louis encephalitis virus** **iii. Ilheus virus** **iv. West Nile virus** **v. Murray Valley encephalitis virus** **B. Fever /haemorrhagic fever group** **i. Yellow fever virus** **ii. Dengue virus** **iii. Zika virus**	**Tick borne species** **A. Encephalitis viruses group** **i. Russian Spring Summer Encephalitis (RSSE) virus** **ii. Central European encephalitis virus** **iii. Western Siberian encephalitis virus** **iv. Powassan encephalitis virus** **v. Louping ill virus** **B. Haemorrhagic fever viruses group** **i. Kyasanur forest disease (KFD) virus** **ii. Omsk haemorrhagic fever virus**
Bunya-viridae	*Bunyavirus*	**i. California encephalitis virus** **ii. Oropouche virus**	
	Phlebovirus	**i. Sand fly or *Phlebotomus* fever or *Pappataci* fever or three day fever virus** **ii. Rift Valley fever virus (haemorrhagic fever virus)**	
	Nairovirus	**i. Nairobi sheep disease virus** **ii. Crimean Congo Haemorrhagic Fever (CCHF) virus** **iii. Hazara virus** **iv. Ganjamvirus**	
	Hantavirus	It is a robovirus **(table-2)**, not an arbovirus	
Reoviridae	*Rotavirus*	Not an arbovirus	
	Orbivirus	**i. African horse sickness virus** **ii. Orungo virus** **iii. Kemerovo virus**	**iv. Palyam virus** **v. Kasba virus** **vi. Vellore virus**
	Coltivirus	**i. Kolarado tick fever virus**	
	Orthoreovirus	Not an arbovirus	
Rhabdo-viridae	*Lyssavirus*	Not an arbovirus	
	Vesiculovirus	**i. Vesicular stomatitis virus** **ii. Chandipura virus**	

Table-1: Classification of arboviruses

Family	Genus	Robovirus species	
Bunya-viridae	*Hantavirus*	**i. Hantaan virus** **ii. Seoul virus** **iii. Puumala virus**	**iv. Prospect Hill virus** **v. Sin Nombre virus**
Arena-viridae	*Mammarenavirus*	**A. Old world viruses** **i. Lymphocytic Chorio Meninigitis (LCM) virus** **ii. Lassa fever virus (haemorrhagic fever virus)**	**B. New world viruses (haemorrhagic fever viruses)** **i. Junin virus** **ii. Machupo virus** **iii. Guanarito virus** **iv. Sabia virus** **v. White water arroyo virus** **vi. Lujo virus**
	Reptarenavirus	Infecting snakes (not a human pathogen)	

Table-2: Classification of roboviruses

Togaviridae

❖ **Meaning:** Word derived from '**toga**' = **Roman mantle or cloak**, which refer to viral envelope.

❖ **Classification:**
➢ **Family:** Togaviridae.
➢ **Genus:** Two genera like *Rubivirus* & *Alphavirus*

I. *Rubivirus*

♣ **Properties:** It is not the arthropod borne & different from other arboviruses.
♣ **Species:** Rubella virus.
- Causing rubella.
- More details: Follow chapter → Other RNA viruses (Rubella virus and Coronaviridae).

II. *Alphavirus*

♣ **Properties:**
- About 32 species are identified under this genus, of which 13 are known to infect the human.
- All are mosquitoes borne viruses.
- Cross reaction occurs in haemagglutination and complement fixation test.
- Neutralisation test is more specific.

♣ **Species:** Two categories.

i. Encephalitis causing viruses:
- Causing encephalitis in horse and in human.
- Transmitted by *Culex* & *Anopheles* mosquitoes.

a. Eastern Equine Encephalitis (EEE) virus:
- Causing epidemic & sporadic cases of encephalitis in eastern Canada, USA & Caribbean.
- Formalin inactivated vaccine is developed.

b. Western Equine Encephalitis (WEE) virus:
- Causing epidemic in America.
- Formalin inactivated vaccine is developed.

c. Venezuelan Equine Encephalitis (VEE) virus:
- Causing influenza like illness & encephalitis in Central & South America.
- Live attenuated vaccine has been developed.

ii. Febrile illness & arthritis causing viruses:

a. Chikungunya virus:

✪ **History:** Virus was 1st isolated from human case & mosquito in Tanzania in 1952.

✪ **Geographical distribution & typing:**
- Virus is present in Africa South East Asia regions including India & also in Europe & America.
- Genotyping: Three genotypes are seen according to its distribution like
1. West African genotype.
2. East/Central/South African genotype.
3. Asian genotype.

✪ **Morphology:** → **Fig.-1**
- **Shape:** Spherical in shape.
- **Size:** 50-70 nm.
- **Genome:** ss-RNA (+).
- **Capsid:** Icosahedral capsid.
- **Envelope:** Nucleocapsid is surrounded by envelop contains peplomeres like E1 & E2.
- **Replication:** Replicate in host cell cytoplasm & released by budding.

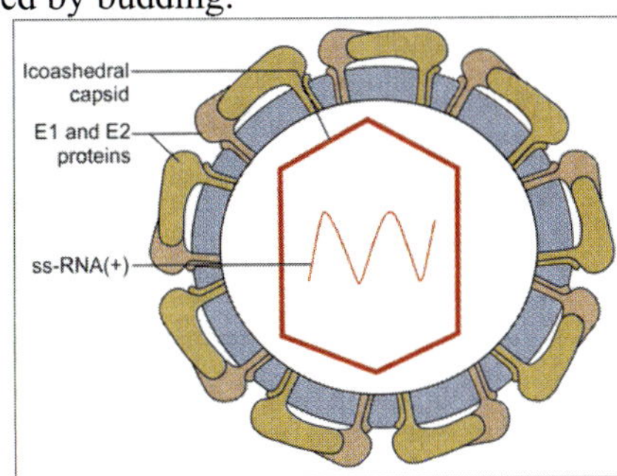

Figure-1: Chikungunya virus

- **Viral proteins:** Two types.
  - Structural proteins:
    - Protein for capsid.
    - Envelope glycoproteins: Two in numbers
1. **E2:** E2 binds to host cell receptors. Virus enters in the host cell through endocytosis.
2. **E1:** It is fusion peptide which, when exposed to the acidity of the endosome in eukaryotic cells, dissociates from E2 & initiates membrane fusion that allows the release of nucleocapsids into the host cells.
  - Non-structural proteins: Three in number like NS1, NS2 & NS3.

✪ **Culture characteristics (C/Cs):** Virus is isolated in monkey cell lines.

✪ **Resistance:** Virus contains lipoprotein envelope & sensitive to lipid solvents like ether & chloroform.

✪ **Antigenic structure & serotypes:** Structural & non structural antigens are seen & no serotypes.

✪ **Immunity:**
- IgM develops after 4 days of infection & last for 3 months.
- IgG develops after 2 weeks & last for years.
- Antibodies are diagnostically useful, so detection of IgM or four fold rise in IgG titre is more significant.

✪ **Pathogenicity:**
- **Disease name:** Called chikungunya.
- **Meaning:** Chikungunya is derived from native word **Kungunyala** (Kimakonde language) = **Bending or folding**, as the patient develop **stooped or doubled up or contort** posture in disease due to severe joint pain.
- **Nature & history of disease:**
  - World scenario: It was detected 1st in Tanzania in 1952 then up to 1960 it produced small outbreaks in Africa & Asia. After inactivity for many decades, it re-emerges since 2005 with millions of cases in Africa, South East Asia, Europe & America. Most

recent epidemic was occurred in Colombia in 2014-15 with 82,977 cases.

- o Indian scenario:
- Emerging (Initial) infection: First outbreak reported in 1963 in Kolkata followed by outbreak in 1964 in Pondicherry, Chennai-Vellore region & then in 1973 in Barsi, Maharashtra.
- Quiescent period: Virus remained silent from 1973-2005.
- Re-emerging infection (Re-union outbreak): Chikungunya re-emerged in 2005-06 from the Southern India (Andhra Pradesh, Tamil Nadu, Kerala, Karnataka) with 2,58, 000 cases from entire country. Later it spread to other parts of India, Asia, Africa, Europe & America. This novel virus is due following reasons.

1. Mutation: Where alanine in 226 position of E1 glycoprotein is replaced by valine.
2. New vector: Mutant virus is 100 times more infective to *Aedes albopticus* than *Aedes aegypticus.*

- **Reservoir of infection:** Human is the reservoir during epidemic or acute infection (urban cycle) because virus is available in high amount in blood during this stage. From human the virus has been taken up by mosquito & spread to other human. During other time (sylvatic cycle) monkeys, birds & other vertebrates are the reservoir.
- **Source of infection:** Mosquito.
- **Mode of transmission:**
- By mosquito bite: Two types of cycle.

1. Urban cycle: Maintained between human & *Aedes aegypti* (original virus & novel virus) or *Aedes albopticus* (novel virus).
2. Sylvatic cycle: Occurs in African forests. Cycle has been maintained between monkeys & forest mosquitoes like *A. furcifer, A. taylori, A. africanus & A. luteocephalus.*

- Rarely shows the congenital transmission.
- By blood transfusion.
- **Incubation period:** About 5 days (3-7 days).
- **Portal of entry:** Skin.
- **Sites:** Skin, conjunctiva, joints, lymph nodes & haemopoietic system.
- **Precipitating factors (epidemiological determinants):** Almost similar to other mosquito borne diseases as follows.

1. **Agent (virulence) factors:** Like novel virus which is 100 times more infective to *Aedes albopticus* than *Aedes aegypticus.*
2. **Vector factors:** Like density, life span, choice of host, resting habit, breeding habit, time of biting & resistance to insecticides.
3. **Host factors:**

- **Age:** Chronic chikungunya virus-induced arthralgia is common in old age group.
- **Sex:** More in male than female because of outdoor visit & better covering of clothes in female.
- **Arthritis:** Joints with arthritis are more likely affected with more severe pain. It also favours the development of chronic chikungunya virus-induced arthralgia.
- **Human habit:** Sleeping outside & not using mosquito repellents like net, cream etc.
- **Migration:** Migration to endemic areas increases the spread.

4. **Environmental factors:** Mostly after rainy season in July-November.

- **Pathogenesis:** It's not clearly understood, but after entry it can multiply in epithelial cells, endothelial cells, fibroblasts, monocytes, skeletal muscle progenitor cells and in myofibers.
- **Clinical features:**
- o Chikungunya fever:
- Present with maculopapular rash (**fig.-2**), sudden onset of fever, crippling joint pain, joint stiffness (predominantly in ankles & wrists), immobility, tenosynovitis, lymphadenopathy & conjunctivitis.
- Biphasic fever with remission after 1-6 days.

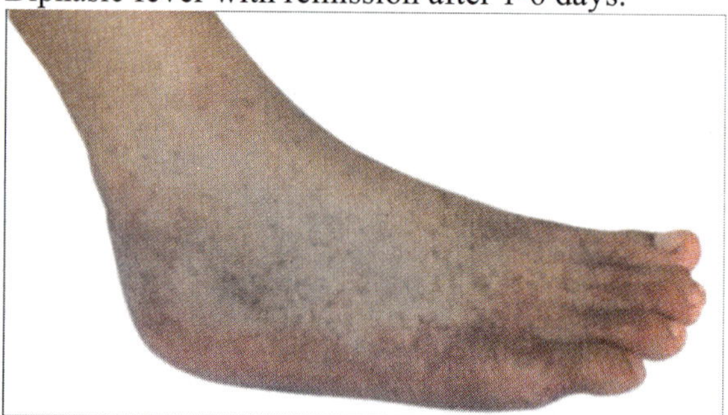

Figure-2: Rashes of chikungunya on right feet

- o Chikungunya haemorrhagic fever: Haemorrhagic tendency was present in epidemic of 1963.
- **Complications:**

1. **Chronic chikungunya virus-induced arthralgia:**

- More common in older age group & persons with arthritis.
- Arthralgia last for many years.
- Exact reason for this is not know but may be due to chronic persistence infection by virus.
- Virus or viral antigen can be detected from the synovial fluid.

2. **Neurological disorders:** Reported very rarely like

- Guillain–Barré syndrome.
- Palsies.
- Meningoencephalitis.
- Flaccid paralysis.
- Neuropathy.

✪ **Diagnosis:**

- **Specimens:** Blood/serum or synovial fluid.
- **Testing methods:**

1. **Microscopy: → Follow morphology.**

2. **Culture:** → **Follow C/Cs.**
3. **Serological tests:** IgM or IgG ELISA used from paired serum samples.
4. **Molecular test:** Real time RT-PCR.

✓ **Note: Following institutes in India are supplying ELISA kits of chikungunya to different laboratories.**
- National Institute of Virology (NIV), Pune, India.
- National Institute of Communicable Disease (NICD), Delhi, India.

✪ **Prevention:**
- **General measures:** Mosquitoes controlling measures like
  - Removal of water reservoir.
  - Use of anti-adults & anti-larval measures like insecticides & biological agents.
  - Using full sleeves shirts & pants.
  - Garments can be treated with pyrethroids, a class of insecticides that often has repellent properties.
  - As infected mosquitoes often feed and rest inside homes, securing screens on windows and doors will help to keep mosquitoes out of the house.
  - Use of bed nets for sleeping infants & young children in day time to avoid day bite.
  - Use of mosquito repellents creams, coil, mats or liquid.
- **Immunoprophylaxis:**
  - Currently no approved vaccine exists.
  - Vaccine under trial: Live measles vaccine virus (**Schwartz strain**) is used as a vector, in to the genome of which five structural genes from chikungunya virus have been incorporated.

✪ **Treatment:** No specific antiviral drug is available, symptomatic treatment is given as follows.
- Bed rest.
- Plenty of fluids to prevent dehydration.
- Take medicine such as paracetamol to reduce fever and pain.
- Do not take aspirin and other non-steroidal anti-inflammatory drugs (NSAIDS until dengue can be ruled out to reduce the risk of bleeding).

b. O'nyog-nyog virus:
- Antigenically related to chikungunya & cause similar disease.
- Virus was 1st isolated in Uganda & confirmed to Africa.
- Transmitted by *Anopheles.*

c. Semliki forest virus:
- Virus was 1st isolated in Uganda in 1942 from Aedes mosquitoes.
- Not associated with human illness though neutralising antibodies have been seen in Africa.

d. Sindbis virus:
- Virus was 1st isolated in the Sindbis district of Egypt in 1952 from *Culex* mosquitoes.
- Also isolated from other country.
- Not associated with human illness though neutralising antibodies have been seen in India.

e. Others:
- Mayaro virus.
- Ross River virus.

Flaviviridae

❖ **Meaning:** Flavi word derived from '**flavus**' **(Latin)** = **yellow,** refer to the species, yellow fever virus of this family.

❖ **Classification:**
- **Family:** Flaviviridae.
- **Genus:** Four genera like *Hepacivirus, Pegivirus, Pestivirus* & *Flavivirus.*

I. *Hepacivirus*

- **Properties:** It is not an arthropod borne & different from other arboviruses.
- **Species:** Hepatitis C virus (HCV).
  - Causing hepatitis.
  - More details: **Follow chapter → Hepatitis viruses.**

II. *Pegivirus*

- **Properties:** It is not an arbovirus.
- **Species:** GB (G Barker) virus C.
- **History:** Discovered in 1995 by G Barker.
- **Synonym:**
  - Formerly **called Hepatitis G virus (HGV)**, but wrongly it was interpreted as HGV because neither it is hepatotropic nor causing hepatitis. In fact it multiplies in bone marrow & spleen & not known to cause any human disease **called orphan virus**.
- **Distribution & genotypes:** It has six genotypes & each has its own geographical distribution.
- **Pathogenicity:**
  - It is transmitted by blood/blood products & by sexual intercourse.
  - It's RNA has been found from the patient of hepatitis, haemodialysis, IV drug addicts & blood donor, but it's role in hepatitis is still to be decided.
  - It's genome resembles to HCV genome except, it lacks protein corresponding to the core protein of HCV that forms the nucleocapsid. HGV infection occurs independently & it does not required HCV. However its prevalence is higher in patient with HCV & HIV.
  - It shows the 35% prevalence in HIV infected persons, but surprisingly this dual infection protect against HIV & patients survive longer.
- **Diagnosis:**

- HGV RNA can be detected by RT-PCR from the blood.
- It produces the Ab, which is protective but not useful in diagnosis.

III. *Pestivirus*

- **Properties:** It is not an arbovirus.
- **Species:** It includes animal species like bovine viral diarrhoea virus 1.

IV. *Flavivirus*

- **Properties:**
  - Many species are identified under this genus, of which few are known to infect the human.
  - Species are mosquitoes borne or tick borne.
- **Species:** Two categories like mosquito borne species & tick borne species.

Mosquito borne species

Two groups like encephalitis group & fever / haemorrhagic fever group as follows.

A. Encephalitis group: Five species

i. Japanese encephalitis (JE) virus:

- **Meaning:** So called because virus was 1st isolated from Japan and causing inflammation of brain [encephalitis from **encephalon (Greek) = brain**].
- **History:** Virus was 1st isolated from Japan during an epidemic in 1935.
- **Geographical distribution & genotypes:**
  - **Most prevalent:** In Korea & Japan in the North & in India & Malaysia in the South.
  - **Genotypes:** Five genotypes are identified on the bases of envelop gene.
    - The Muar strain is the prototype strain of genotype V & isolated from a patient in Malaya in 1952.
    - Genotype IV appears to be the ancestral strain & distributed in the Indonesian–Malayasian region.
- **Morphology:** → Fig.-3

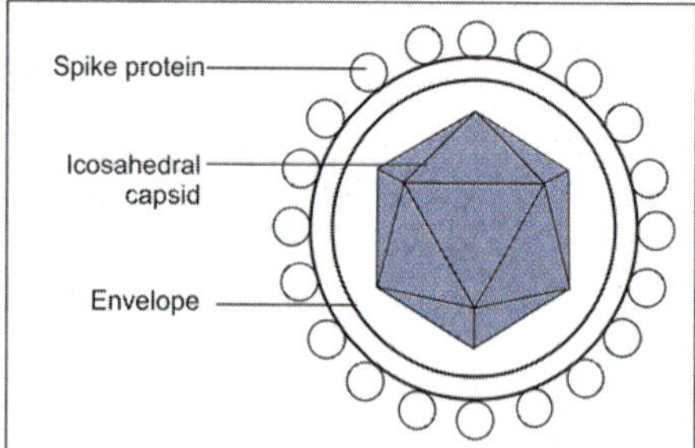

Figure-3: Morphology JEV

- **Shape:** Spherical.
- **Size:** 40 -50 nm.
- **Genome:** ss-RNA (+).
- **Capsid:** Icosahedral capsid.
- **Envelope:** Nucleocapsid is surrounded by envelop.
- **Viral proteins:**
  - Structural proteins: Like capsid, matrix protein & envelop protein.
  - Non-structural proteins: Like NS1 & NS2a, NS2b, NS3, N4a, NS4b & NS5
- **Culture characteristics (C/Cs):**
  - It is a dangerous pathogen to deal in a laboratory (BSL-3).
  - Cultivation is done on Vero cells using serum free medium from CSF or brain tissues collected at autopsy.
- **Resistance:** Enveloped virus sensitive to lipid solvents.
- **Antigenic structure**: Virus contains structure antigens such as capsid antigen & envelope antigen & several non-structural antigens like NS1, NS2a, NS2b, NS3, N4a, NS4b & NS5.
- **Immunity:** Primary infection provides lifelong protection.
- **Pathogenicity:**
  - **Disease name:** Disease **called japanese encephalitis.**
  - **Synonym:** Formerly **called japanese encephalitis B** to distinguish it from encephalitis A (**encephalitis lethargica, Von Econom's disease**), which was prevalent then after.
  - **Nature & history of disease:**
    - In the world:
      - It was 1st isolated from Japan during an epidemic in 1935.
      - Several outbreaks occur thereafter.
      - It has seasonal trend (Summer-Autumn) in the temperate zone, but not evident in tropical areas.
      - *Culex tritaeniorhynchus* is the principal vector in this region.
    - In India:
      - Tamil Nadu outbreak: In India virus was 1st isolated in 1955 from mosquitoes of *Culex vishnui complex* from Vellore during an outbreak of encephalitis in Tamil Nadu. Virus was continued active in Tamil Nadu & Andhra Pradesh in subsequent years in paediatric populations & shown the endemic nature. Most of the cases were occurred between October – November.
      - West Bengal outbreak: It was limited up to Southern part till 1973 and then large outbreak of encephalitis occurred in West Bengal in adult populations with 50% mortality. Cases were reported between June – October.
      - Periodic outbreak in other part of country after 1976: After 1976 virus spread in other part of country with occurrence of periodic outbreak or sporadic cases in Dibrugarh (Assam), Gorakhpur (Uttar Pradesh), Haryana, Maharashtra, Goa, Kolar (Karnataka), Andhra Pradesh, Tirunelveli plus South Arcot (Tamil Nadu), Puducherry & finally in Kerala.

- **Reservoir of infection:** *Ardeid* birds (herons & egrets) are the reservoir host while pigs are the amplifier hosts.
- **Source of infection:** Vector is the source for human infection.
- **Mode of transmission:**
- By mosquitoes bite: *Culex tritaeniorhynchus* is the worldwide vector including India while in India it also transmitted by *Culex vishnui complex.*
- Natural cycle has been worked out in Japan as shown in **fig.-4**.
- Human to human transmission does not occur, so human is not the reservoir & also the dead end host.
- Bird to bird (common like herons & egrets & rare like pigeon, ducks & sparrows) spread has been take place.
- Animal (cattle besides pigs) to animals spread has been take place; however animal may not develop viremia & may not contribute in spread of infection. *Culex tritaeniorhynchus* has predilection for cattle which minimise the exposure to human. Another reason for low human infection is high cattle-pig ration in India.
- Mosquitoes to mosquitoes spread are possible by transovarial route.

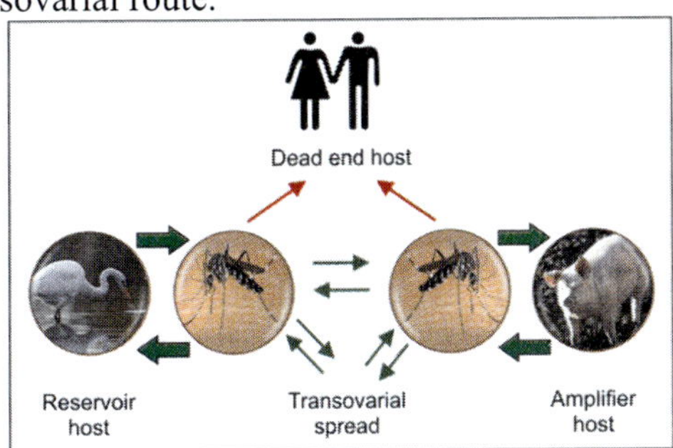

Figure-4: Natural cycle of JEV

- **Incubation period:** 2-15 days.
- **Portal of entry:** Skin.
- **Sites:** Brain.
- **Precipitating factors (epidemiological determinants):**

1. **Agent factors:** Not specific.
2. **Host (human, animal & birds) factors:**
   - All individual infected by virus may not produces the clinical infection; ratio of overt infection is 1:300 to 1:1000.
   - Cattle-pig ratio: More numbers of cattle minimise the chances of human infection.
3. **Vector factors:** Same as described in chikungunya virus.
4. **Seasonal:** Common in summer- autumn season in temperate region.

- **Pathogenesis:** After entering in brain virus activate the microglial cells to release the interleukin-1 (IL-1) and tumour necrosis factor alpha (TNF-α), which can cause toxic effects in the brain. Additionally, other soluble factors such as neurotoxins, excitatory neurotransmitters, prostaglandin, reactive oxygen & nitrogen are secreted by activated microglia.
- **Clinical features:**
  - <u>Prodromal phase:</u>
    - Large majority of cases are asymptomatic.
    - Present with sudden onset of fever, nausea & vomiting. Fever is high & continuous.
  - <u>Encephalitis phase:</u>
    - Start after 1-6 days.
    - Present with neck rigidity, convulsion, altered sensorium & coma.
- **Complications:**
  - Mortality in 50% cases.
  - Neurological damage in 50% of survival.

✪ **Diagnosis:**

- **Specimens:** Blood/serum, CSF or brain tissue collected at autopsy.
- **Testing methods:**

1. **Microscopy: → Follow morphology**
2. **Culture: → Follow C/Cs**
3. **Serological tests:**
   - Immunological markers of JEV are shown in **fig.-5.**
   - IgM detected by capture ELISA but less sensitive due to cross reactivity by other flavi viruses. IgM antibodies are usually detectable 3-8 days after onset of illness and persist for 30-90 days, but longer persistence has been documented. Therefore, positive IgM antibodies occasionally may reflect a past infection or vaccination. Serum collected within 10 days of illness onset may not have detectable IgM and the test should be repeated on a convalescent sample.
   - PRNT is best useful, confirmatory test & based on detection of neutralising antibodies.
   - IgG ELISA also a useful test

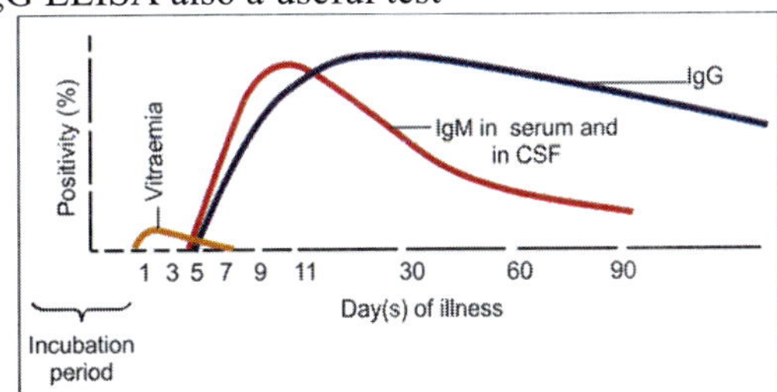

Figure-5: Immunological markers of JEV

4. **Molecular test:** RT-PCR.
5. **Other test:** Histopathological study with immuno-histochemistry.

✪ **Prevention:**

- **General measures:**
  - Slaughtering of pigs. A million pigs were slaughtered in Malaysia in 1999 to stop the epidemic of encephalitis.
  - Mosquitoes control measure as described in chikungunya virus.
- **Vaccination:**

a. **Vaccination of human:**

1. **Killed vaccine:** Following two types.

o Nakayama strain vaccine:

- **Preparation:** Formalin inactivated mouse brain vaccine prepared by using Nakayama strain (genotype-III) in Japan in 1930. In India it is prepared at Central Research Institute, Kasauli.
- **Dose:** Two doses of 1 ml each (0.5ml for child < 3 years) by subcutaneous route at two weeks interval followed by booster after 6-12 months (at least before 1 year) in order to achieve full immunity.
- **Revaccination:** The neutralizing antibody persists in the circulation for at least two to three years and perhaps longer. The total duration of protection is unknown, but because there is no firm evidence for protection beyond three years, boosters are recommended every three years for people who remain at risk.
- **Advantage:** Successfully used in Japan & in India.
- **Disadvantage:** Short lived immunity, high cost & side effects like redness, pain, utricaria & neurological autoimmune reaction in human due to cross reactivity mouse brain.

o Beijing strain vaccine:

- Formalin inactivated mouse brain vaccine prepared by using Beijing strain.
- In India it is prepared at Central Research Institute, Kasauli.

o Beijing P3 strain vaccine:

- It is cell line derived vaccine.

2. **Live attenuated vaccine:**

- **Preparation:** Vaccine prepared in China (licensed in India) by using JE strain SA 14-14-2 passed through weanling mice. It is produced in baby hamster kidney cells.
- **Dose:** Two doses at one year interval by subcutaneous route.
- **Advantage:** Effective to prevent clinical illness.
- **Inclusion in Universal Immunisation Programme in India:** Under this programmes it is given to 5-15 years children in 83 endemic districts of four states like Uttar Pradesh, West Bengal, Karnataka & Assam.

b. **Vaccination of pigs:** It has been proposed

✪ **Treatment:** There is no specific antiviral treatment for JEV is available. Treatment is supportive to relieve symptoms and to stabilize the patient.

ii. **St. Louis encephalitis virus:**

- Transmitted by *Culex tarsalis.*
- Wild birds are the reservoir.
- Most prevalent in North & Central America.
- Cause large epidemic in recent years.
- Cause mild febrile illness to frank encephalitis.
- Case fatality is 2-20%.

iii. **Ilheus virus:**

- Most prevalent in South & Central America.
- Cause mild febrile illness and encephalitis is rare.
- Maintained in cycle by mosquitoes (may be *Culex* or other genera), wild birds & monkeys.

iv. **West Nile virus:**

- Virus was 1st isolated from West Nile province of Uganda.
- Maintained in cycle by *Culex* mosquitoes & wild birds.
- In India it has been isolated from Culex mosquitoes and patients of febrile illness & encephalitis from Rajasthan to Karnataka.

v. **Murray Valley encephalitis virus:**

- Virus was 1st isolated during an epidemic of encephalitis from Murray River Valley in 1951.
- It is confirmed to Australia & New Guinea.
- Maintained in cycle by *Culex annulirostris* & wild birds and break out in epidemic.

B. **Fever / haemorrhagic fever group:** Three species.

i. **Yellow fever virus:**

✪ **History:**

- Virus was 1st identified in early 17th century.
- Later it was identified from certain part of Africa and South and Central America in 20th century.
- Virus was isolated by Theiler in after intracerebral inoculation in mice.

✪ **Geographical distribution & genotypes:**

- It is endemic in West Africa & South plus Central America. It is not present in rest of the world including India.
- India is considered as receptive area because of availability of vector (*Aedes aegypti*) & non-immune human.
- Genotypes: Seven genotypes are identified based on genomic sequence, five of that are endemic in Africa and two in South America.

✪ **Morphology:** Almost same as JEV.

- **Shape:** Spherical.
- **Size:** 40 -50 nm.
- **Genome:** ss-RNA (+).
- **Capsid:** Icosahedral capsid.
- **Envelope:** Nucleocapsid is surrounded by envelop & also contains membrane protein & spike's protein.
- **Viral proteins:**

o Structural proteins: Like capsid, matrix protein & envelop protein.

o Non-structural proteins: Like NS1 & NS2a, NS2b, NS3, N4a, NS4b & NS5.

- **Inclusion body:** Presence of intra nuclear **Cowdry type-A** (acidophilic) inclusion body **called Torres body** in yellow fever. Examined under light microscopy.

- **Histological findings:** All the necrosed cells of liver are coalesces to form multinucleated cell **called Councilman body.**
- **IF microscopy:** Yellow fever antigen may be demonstrated in formalin fixed tissues of liver, kidney, and heart by immunocytochemical staining.

✪ **Culture characteristics (C/Cs):** Virus is cultivated on Vero cells using serum free medium.

✪ **Resistance:** Enveloped virus sensitive to lipid solvents.

✪ **Antigenic structure:** Antigenically homogenous & only one serotype is known to exist.

✪ **Immunity:**

- Indian population is non-immune to yellow fever.
- Single infection confers lifelong immunity & second attack is uncommon.
- Infant born of immune mother have passive immunity for 6 months.
- India is endemic for dengue & presence of dengue antibodies may provide little protection to yellow fever, however yellow fever vaccine is not providing any amount of protection to dengue.

✪ **Pathogenicity:**

- **Disease name:** Disease **called yellow fever.**
- **Meaning:** The name "**yellow fever**" originated from its propensity to cause jaundice (Present with yellowish discolouration of sclera) in victims.
- **Synonym:** Yellow Jack (familiar to the pirates of yellow jack).
- **Nature or history of disease:**
  - It is endemic in West Africa & South plus Central America. It is not present in rest of the world including India.
  - 1st epidemic was reported in Kenya in 1992.
  - Outbreak was reported in Peru in 1995 with 440 cases in 1st six months of year.
  - WHO estimated about 200,000 infections and 30,000 deaths every year due to yellow fever with nearly 90% are from only Africa.
- **Reservoir of infection:** Human is the reservoir for urban infection while wild monkey is the reservoir for wild infection.
- **Source of infection:** Vector is the source for human infection.
- **Mode of transmission:**
  - By mosquitoes bite with following two types of cycle.
    - Urban cycle: Cycle is maintained between human & *Aedes aegypti.*
    - Wild cycle: Cycle is maintained between wild monkey mosquitoes like *Haemagogus spegazzinii* in South America & *A. africanus* & *A. simpsoni* in Africa.
  - Mosquito to mosquito spread is possible by transovarial route. Once it infected remains so for life.
- **Incubation period:** 3-6 days.
- **Portal of entry:** Skin.
- **Site:** Liver.
- **Precipitating factors (epidemiological determinants):**

a. **Agent factors:** Virus remains in mosquito throughout the life once infected.

b. **Host factors:**

1. **Age:** Less in below 6 months due to passive protection by maternal antibodies.
2. **Sex:** More in male due to outdoor visit.
3. **Occupation:** Like forest workers are at high risk.
4. **Migration of population:** From endemic to receptive areas increase the risk.

c. **Vector factors:** Same as described in chikungunya virus.

d. **Environmental factors:**

1. **Temperature & humidity:** Temperature >24^{0}C & humidity > 60% favours the multiplication of virus.
2. **Urbanisation:** It bring population closer to the wild cycle

- **Pathogenesis:**
  - After transmission from a mosquito, the viruses replicate in the lymph nodes & infect dendritic cells in particular. From there, they reach the liver and infect hepatocytes, which lead to eosinophilic degradation of these cells and to the release of cytokines.
  - Apoptotic masses **called councilman bodies** appear in the cytoplasm of hepatocytes.
  - Fatality may occur when cytokine storm, shock, and multiple organ failure follow.
- **Clinical features:**
  - Prodromal phase:
    - Present with sudden onset of high grade fever with chills, headache, nausea & vomiting.
    - Pulse is slow despite high temperature.
  - Jaundice phase:
    - Present with jaundice, albuminuria & haemorrhagic manifestation.
- **Complication:** Death due to renal or hepatic failure

✪ **Diagnosis:** Primary diagnosis is based on clinical parameters like signs, symptoms, travel history, activities etc.

- **Specimens:** Blood, tissues like liver, kidney & heart, body fluids etc.
- **Testing methods:**

1. **Blood picture:**
   - Low white blood cell count (leucopenia).
   - Low platelet count (thrombocytopenia).
   - Elevations in liver function tests.
   - Abnormally prolonged blood clotting times.
   - Abnormal electrolyte.
2. **Urine picture:**
   - Abnormal kidney function tests.

- Urine tests may demonstrate elevated levels of urinary protein and urobilinogen.

3. **Microscopy: → Follow morphology.**
4. **Culture: → Follow C/Cs.**
5. **Serology:**

o Type of sera used: Paired acute and convalescent sera should be tested & rising antibody titre provides confirmation of the diagnosis.

o Serologic diagnosis is achieved by:

- IgM antibody-capture ELISA.
- Haemagglutination inhibition (HAI) test.
- CFT.
- Neutralisation test.

o Immune response:

- IgM, haemagglutination inhibition and neutralising antibodies appear within 5-7 days while complement antibodies formed within 7-14 days after onset.
- Cross-reacting antibodies to other species (like dengue virus) of *Flavivirus* often complicate the diagnosis. Because IgM and complement antibodies persist for relatively short periods of time, they provide a marker of recent infection. IgM antibodies wane or disappear after weeks or months and complement antibodies wane after 1-2 months to low levels by about a year after recovery from infection.
- A retrospective diagnosis may be achieved_by demonstrating a fall in IgM or complement antibody titres in appropriately timed serum specimens.

o Significant titre:

- ≥320 by haemagglutination inhibition.
- ≥160 by neutralisation.
- ≥32 by complement fixation.
- ≥256 by immunofluorescence assay or
- A positive result by IgM-capture ELISA.

o Disadvantages:

- Cross-reactive serologic reactions to other species of *Flavivirus* must be excluded.
- False positive result in a patient with history of yellow fever vaccination.

6. **Molecular:** Identification of viral RNA by RT – PCR.

✪ **Prevention:**

• **General measures:**

- Mosquito control measures as described in chikungunya virus.
- It does not exist in India & India is considered as '**receptive area**' because of large numbers of availability & non-immune human.
- Various reasons for absence of yellow fever in India like measures in airport & vaccination.

a. Measures in airport:

1. **Quarantine:** Quarantine of travellers for 6 days coming from endemic areas.
2. **Strict vaccination:** Strict vigilance for vaccination for persons travel to or from endemic areas.
3. **International certificate of vaccination:** It is mandatory for persons travel to or from endemic areas. Certificate is issued 10 days after the date of vaccination & validate for 10 years. Validity is extends for 10 years more from the date of vaccination following revaccination. Vaccine is contraindicated in infants (<1 year) & even vaccine also induce yellow fever in < 1 year, so decision about requirement of certificate for infant is rest on individual country. In this regard, India requires vaccination/certificate too.
4. **Breteau index or *Aedes aegypti* index:** It is defined as numbers of containers showing breeding of *Aedes aegypti* larvae / numbers of house surveyed × 1000. It should be < 1, surrounding 400 meter of air port.

b. Cross reactive immunity: India is endemic for dengue & presence of dengue antibodies may provide little protection to yellow fever, however yellow fever vaccine is not providing any amount of protection to dengue.

• **Vaccination:** It's not occurs in India though vaccination is mandatory for travel to or from endemic areas. Vaccine starts protection after 10 days & continues for 10 years.

a. Killed / neurotropic vaccine / Dakar vaccine:

- **Preparation:** Vaccine prepared from infected mouse brain was used in French West Africa.
- **Disadvantage:** Produce encephalitis so not useful.

b. Live attenuated / non- neurotropic vaccine / 17D vaccine:

- **Preparation:** It is a live attenuated vaccine prepared by Theiler in 1937 in allantoic cavity of chick embryo from **Asibi strain**. In India it is prepared in Central Research Institute, Kasauli.
- **Storage:** It should be transported at temperature range from -30^{0}C to + 5^{0}C.
- **Dosage & administration:** It is available in lyophilised form & reconstituted before use with sterile saline. It should be used within 30 minutes following reconstitution. Single dose is given by subcutaneous injection.
- **Advantages:** Vaccine is safe, effective & provides protection for 35 years.
- **Contraindications:**

1. Children < 9 months (< 6 months in endemic areas).
2. Pregnancy except during outbreak.
3. IDDs like AIDS.
4. People allergic to eggs proteins.
5. Cholera & yellow fever vaccine interact with each other, hence should not be given together. 3 weeks gap should be maintained between two vaccines.

✪ **Treatment:** There is no specific antiviral treatment for yellow fever is available. Treatment is supportive to relieve symptoms and to stabilize the patient.

ii. Dengue virus:

✪ **History:** DEN 1 was isolated in Hawaii in 1944, DEN 2 from New Guinea in 1944, DEN 3 & 4 from Philippines in 1956. Recently DEN 5 is identified in 2013 from Malaysia. Initial 4 types are present in India, but there is no indication of the presence of DENV-5 in India.

✪ **Geographical distribution & genotypes:**
- Widely distributed throughout the tropics & subtropics.
- Virus is confirmed to east coat of India.
- Five genotypes or serotypes of dengue virus are identified as described in history.
- All types are available in India.

✪ **Morphology: →Fig.-6**
- **Shape:** Spherical.
- **Size:** 40-50 nm.
- **Genome:** ss-RNA (+).
- **Capsid:** NA is surrounded by icosahedral capsid.
- **Envelope:** Nucleocapsid is surrounded by bilayer envelop which consist inner protein (M protein) & outer lipid layer.
- **Peplomeres:** Envelop consist haemagglutinin spikes.
- **Viral proteins:** Two types of proteins

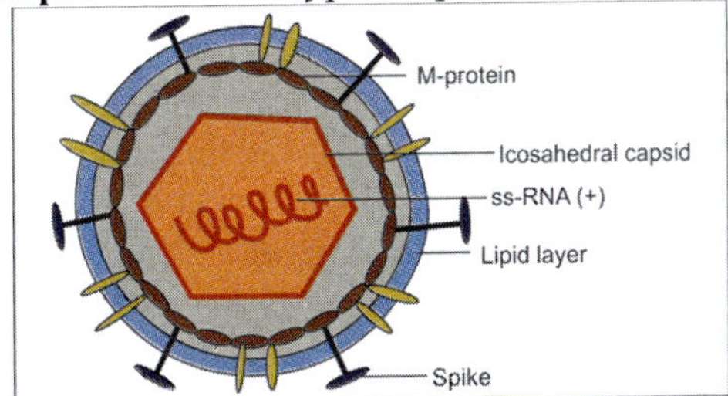

Figure-6: Morphology of dengue virus

a. Structural-proteins:
- C (capsid)-protein.
- M-protein).
- Spikes protein: It is viral haemagglutinin which is a group and type-specific determinants.

b. Non-structural (NS)-Ag: Includes NS1, NS2a, NS2b, NS3, NS4a, NS4b & NS5.

✪ **Culture characteristics (C/Cs):** Virus isolation is best useful in initial 5 days by following culture methods.

1. **Animal culture:** Inoculation in suckling mice, but less sensitive.
2. **Tissue culture:** Grow in Vero or BHK-cells.

✪ **Resistance:** Enveloped virus sensitive to lipid solvents.

✪ **Antigenic structure:** Include the structural & non-structural antigens as described in morphology & with five serotypes/genotypes as described in history.

✪ **Immunity:** Two types of antibodies are produced.

a. Neutralising antibodies:
- It includes the antibodies against both infecting & non infecting serotypes.
- These are protective in nature & shows the 60-80% cross reactivity with other serotypes of dengue virus.
- Antibodies induces long-life protection against the infecting serotype, but they gives short time cross protection against the other types.

b. Non-neutralising antibodies:
- Non-neutralising antibodies are heterotypic (because antibodies produce against non infecting serotypes but not against the infecting serotype) & last lifelong.
- The first (primary) dengue infection causes mostly minor disease, but secondary dengue infection has been reported to cause severe disease (DHF or DSS) in both children and adults. This phenomenon is **called antibody-dependent enhancement**.
- Mechanisms of antibody-dependent enhancement: Antibodies formed following 1st serotype are bound to 2nd serotype, but instead of neutralising 2nd serotype it protect the 2nd serotype against the action of host B-cells resulting more sever disease during secondary infection.
- Antibody-dependent enhancement occurs most when serotype 1 infection is followed by serotype 2.

✪ **Pathogenicity:**
- **Disease name:** Disease **called dengue** or **dengue fever.**
- **Synonym:**
  - Term '**break-borne fever**' was coined during the Philadelphia epidemic in 1780.
  - '**Dandy fever**' in West Indies. Word related with posture & gait in dengue fever in West Indies.
- **Meaning:** Term dengue derived from the **'Ki denga pepo (Swahili language)' = sudden seizure by a demon.**
- **Nature & history of disease:** It occurs in both epidemic & endemic forms. Epidemic starts in rainy season & usually explosive.

○ Global scenario:
- Countries at risk: More than 200.
- New infections annually: 50 million.
- Deaths: 24,000 annually.
- People at risk: 2.5-3 billion.
- Hospitalized cases: 5 00 000/year.
- Disease burden: 4,65,000

○ Indian scenario:
- Dengue is confirmed to east coat of India & cause epidemic in Calcutta & Madras in 1963 along with chikungunya.

- Then major epidemic in West & later in North part in Surat & Delhi 1990 with death due to DHF & DSS.
- All five types are present in country & more than one type has been isolated from same patients.
- **Reservoir of infection:** Human. No animal reservoir is known.
- **Source of infection:** Vector is the source for human infection
- **Mode of transmission:** By bite of *Aedes aegypti* mosquitoes. Extrinsic incubation period is 8-10 days.
- **Incubation period:** 3-14 days.
- **Portal of entry:** Skin.
- **Sites:** Blood, lymph nodes etc.
- **Precipitating factors (epidemiological determinants):**

a. **Agent factors:** Secondary infection by virus is more severe than primary infection due to antibody-dependent enhancement.

b. **Host factors:**

1. **Age:** Common at all ages. Children < 12 years are more prone to develop DHF & DSS.
2. **Sex:** More in males due to outdoor visit.
3. **Immunity:** Secondary infection is less in person having antibodies but more sever if occurs.

c. **Vector factors:** Same as described in chikungunya virus,

d. **Environmental factors:** Widely distributed throughout the tropics & subtropics. Epidemic starts in rainy season & usually explosive.

- **Pathogenesis:** Viremia progress to fever, haemorrhage & shock.
- Initial dengue infection by any serotype **called primary dengue infection**. Subsequent dengue infection, months or year after the primary infection by other serotype, which is more severe, **called secondary dengue infection**.
- There is a hypersensitive or enhancement response due to infection by more than one dengue virus serotype (double infection) as described earlier.
- Subsequent infection may be important: Serotype 1 followed by serotype 2 is more dangerous (it progress to DHF & DSS) than serotype 4 followed by serotype 2.
- Serotype 2 is considered as most virulent.
- **Clinical features:** Traditional (1997) WHO classification divide the dengue in to following three categories (**flow chart-1**).

a. **Dengue fever:**

- Sudden onset of fever which is biphasic (**saddle back**). It present with chills & between 39^0-40^0C temperature & subside in 5-7days. It rise again after 5-8 days hence **called biphasic** or **saddle back fever.**
- Headache.
- Retro-orbital pain.
- Conjunctival injection.
- Pain in back & limbs (**break bone fever**).
- Lymphadenopathy.
- Maculopapular rash appear in 80% cases during remission or during 2nd febrile phase. It last for 2 hrs – several days.

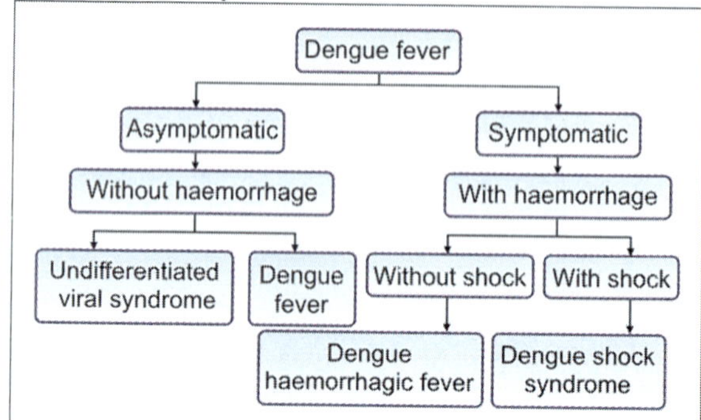

Flow chart-1: Clinical features of dengue

b. **Dengue haemorrhagic fever (DHF):** With haemorrhagic manifestation

- High grade continuous fever.
- Hepatomegaly.
- Thrombocytopenia: Count is ≤ 1, 00, 000/cmm.
- Haematocrit: Increased by 20% or more of base line
- Evidence of haemorrhage which is detected by positive tourniquet test (>20 petechial spots per square inch area in cubital fossa) & spontaneous bleeding from skin, nose, mouth & gums.

c. **Dengue shock syndrome (DSS):** Following feature in addition to all above features.

- Shock: Circulatory failure with rapid & weak pulse, narrowing pulse pressure (20mmHg or less) or hypotension with cold clammy skin & restlessness.

- **Grading of severity of dengue**
- **Grade-I:** Fever with non-specific symptoms and positive tourniquet test.
- **Grade-II:** Grade-I & patients with spontaneous bleeding in skin and/or in other parts like petechiae, pupura, ecchymosis, epistaxis, gum bleeding, haematemesis and/or melaena.
- **Grade-III:** Circulatory failure with rapid & weak pulse, narrowing pulse pressure (20mmHg or less) or hypotension with cold clammy skin & restlessness.
- **Grade-IV:** Shock with undetectable pulse & pressure.
- **2009 WHO classification:** It divide the dengue in to following two categories based on the severity
- Dengue with or without warning sign.
- Severe dengue.

✪ **Laboratory diagnosis:** Diagnosis is usually made clinically on the bases of fever characteristics, blood picture (vide infra), bleeding tendency, pulse, pressure etc.

- **Specimens:**

- Whole blood / plasma / serum / CSF.
- Autopsy materials like liver, spleen, lymph node, thymus, intestine, lungs, skin rashes materials, brain, kidney are collected for virus isolation
- Collect the blood from the heart in autopsy patients.
- Virus also isolated from insect vectors or from animal/bird reservoir.

- **Testing methods:**

a. **Blood picture:**
- Platelet count: ≤ 1, 00, 000/cmm (thrombocytopenia).
- Haematocrit: Increased by 20% or more of base line.

b. **Urine picture:** Proteinuria, haematuria etc.

c. **Microscopy:** → **Follow morphology.**

d. **Culture:** → **Follow C/Cs.**

e. **Serological tests:**

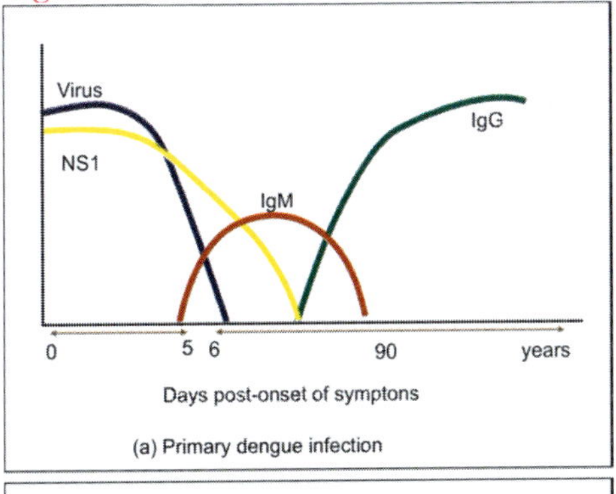

(a) Primary dengue infection

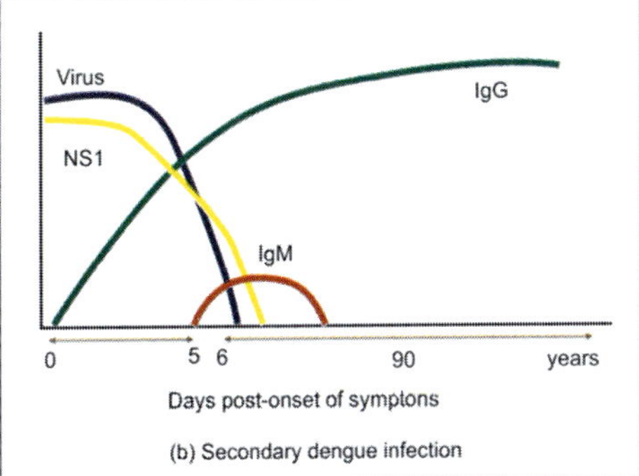

(b) Secondary dengue infection

Figure-7: Immunological reactions in dengue

o Immunological reactions: →**Fig.-7**
- Dengue infection consist the production of IgM & IgG antibodies directed against the spike proteins.
- Immune response varies depending on whether the individual has a primary (1st dengue or other Flavivirus) v/s a secondary (had dengue or other Flavivirus infection in past) dengue infection.
- Primary infection detected by virus isolation or by identifying NS1Ag or by IgM detection followed by IgG detection.
- Secondary infection is detected by IgG detection.
- NS1 appeared in serum from day 1, after the onset of fever & remains positive for 18 days. It's diagnosis differentiate between flavi viruses & also between different serotypes of dengue.
- IgM is produced after 4-5 days & persist for 90 days.
- IgG develops 6-15 days following illness & continue for long time.

o Tests:
- Plaque Reduction Neutralisation Test (PRNT): Most sensitive & specific test but expensive, labour intensive & expensive so routinely not used.
- HAI: It is sensitive but less specific. The haemagglutinin antibodies last for longer, so useful for epidemiological study.
- CFT: Complement fixing antibodies appear later than HI antibodies & last for short period. Can be useful for current infection. Difficult to perform & not useful for epidemiological study
- ICT (Rapid test provides result in few minutes).
- NS1Ag: Detected by ELISA & immunochromatographic test.
- IgM ELISA (MAC-ELISA): Useful for recent infection. Sensitivity is 90% & specificity is 98%.
- IgG ELISA.

f. **Molecular methods:**
- Real time RT-PCR (qRT-PCR) is more rapid & sensitive.
- Genomic sequencing.

✪ **Prevention:**

- **General measures:**
- *Aedes aegypti* breed in stagnant water (e.g. coconut shell, water tank). Cleaning, proper covering or removal of all such water reservoir.
- Other mosquitoes control measures are same as described in chikungunya virus.

- **Immunoprophylaxis:**
- No specific vaccine is available.
- Live attenuated tetravalent vaccine based on chimeric yellow fever dengue virus (CYD-TDV) has been developed by Sanofi Pasteur Company. It is found safe for human use & effective in Phase III clinical trial don in Latin America.

✪ **Treatment:** There is no specific antiviral treatment for dengue is available. Supportive treatment like replacement of fluid & electrolytes loss, platelets transfusion etc. is given.

iii. **Zika virus:**

✪ **Meaning:** So called because virus was 1st isolated from Zika Forest of Uganda in 1947.

✪ **History:**
- Zika virus was first identified in rhesus monkeys in zika forest, Uganda in 1947 through a monitoring network of sylvatic yellow fever. It was identified from the serum of monkey developed fever.
- It was subsequently identified in humans in 1952 in Uganda and the United Republic of Tanzania.

✪ **Geographical distribution & genotypes (lineages):**

- Since the 1950s, virus was limited from Africa to Asia but from 2007 to 2016, it spread eastward, across the Pacific Ocean to the Americas, leading to the 2015 - 16 zika virus epidemic.
- Genotypes (lineages): There are two zika lineages like the African lineage and the Asian lineage. Phylogenetic studies indicate that the virus spreading in the Americas is 89% identical to African genotypes & also closely related to the Asian strain that circulated in French Polynesia during the 2013–2014 outbreaks.

✪ **Morphology: →Fig.-8**

- Morphologically zika virus is related to the japanese encephalitis, west nile, yellow fever and dengue viruses.
- It is spherical & enveloped virus with icosahedral capsid & ss-RNA (+) genome.
- Viral proteins: RNA genome encodes for seven non-structural proteins & three structural proteins.
- Flavi viruses generally replicate in cytoplasm but zika multiply in nucleus of host cells.

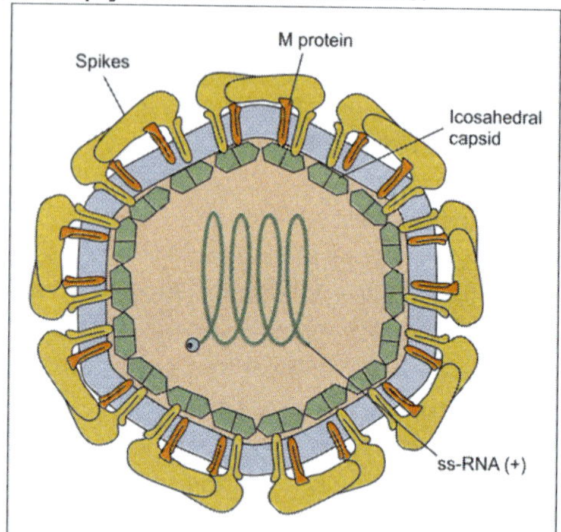

Figure-8: Morphology of zika virus

✪ **Culture characteristics (C/Cs):** Zika has been successfully cultivated on Vero cells.

✪ **Resistance:** Enveloped virus sensitive to lipid solvents.

✪ **Antigenic structure & serotypes:** Include the three structural & seven non-structural antigens as described in morphology.

✪ **Immunity:** Cross reactive immunity may occur due to infection by related flavi viruse like japanese encephalitis, West Nile, yellow fever and dengue viruses.

✪ **Pathogenicity:**

- **Disease name:** Called zika fever.
- **Synonym:** Also called zika virus disease.
- **Nature or history of disease:**

- **Endemic in Africa & South East Asia:** From its discovery to 2007, there were only 14 confirmed human cases of zika infection identified from Africa (Central African Republic, Egypt, Gabon, Sierra Leone, Tanzania, and Uganda) and Southeast Asia (India, Indonesia, Malaysia, the Philippines, Thailand, Vietnam and Pakistan).
- **2007 Zika virus outbreak in Yap Islands:** In April 2007, the first outbreak occurred outside of Africa & Asia on the island of Yap in the Federated States of Micronesia.
- **2013–2014 Zika virus epidemic in Oceania:** Between 2013-14, further epidemics occurred in Oceania (French Polynesia, Easter Island, the Cook Islands & New Caledonia).
- **2015–16 Zika virus epidemic in America:** In early 2016 epidemic occurred in America, actually it began in April 2015 in Brazil and later spread to other countries in South America, Central America, North America and the Caribbean. The zika virus reached Singapore and Malaysia in Aug 2016. In this regards WHO has declared zika virus disease to be "A Public Health Emergency of International Concern (PHEIC)" on 1st February, 2016.
- **Retrospective study:** On 22nd March 2016 Reuters reported that zika was isolated from a 2014 blood sample of an elderly man in Chittagong in Bangladesh as part of a retrospective study.

- **Reservoir of infection:** It is epizootic & monkeys are the reservoir host. Human is the accidental host.
- **Source of infection:** Vector is the source for human infection.
- **Mode of transmission:**

○ Mosquito borne:

- By mosquitoes bite specially *Aedes aegypti* which is active mostly in the daytime.
- Extrinsic incubation period in mosquitoes: About 10 days.
- Virus also documented in other species like *A. africanus*, *A. apicoargenteus*, *A. furcifer*, *A. hensilli*, *A. luteocephalus*, *A. vittatus*, *Anopheles coustani*, *Mansonia uniformis* and *Culex perfuscus*, but their role in transmission is unclear.
- Cycle is maintained between wild monkey & mosquitoes with occasional transmission to human.

○ Other routes: Also transmitted through

- Sexual route.
- Blood transfusion.
- Transplacental with microcephaly in foetus.

- **Incubation period:** Not clear but may be few days.
- **Portal of entry:** Skin.
- **Sites:** Muscles, joints, lymph nodes, brain etc.
- **Precipitating factors (epidemiological determinants):**

a. **Agent factors:** In addition to mosquito bite, virus also spread by sexual route, blood transfusion & through placenta, which increase the risk of infection.

b. **Host factors:**

1. **Age:** No age bar.

2. **Sex:** More in males due to outdoor visit.
3. **Occupation:** Like forest workers are at high risk.
4. **Migration of population:** Migration in to endemic areas increases the risk.
5. **Pregnancy:** At most risk & development of microcephaly to foetus of infected mother.

c. **Vector factors:** Same as described in chikungunya virus.

d. **Environmental factors:**

1. **Urbanisation:** It brings population closer to the wild cycle.

- **Pathogenesis:**
- After the mosquito bite it enters in epidermal keratinocytes, fibroblasts and the Langerhans cells in the skin.
- Further progress is done through lymph nodes & blood stream to produces the viraemia & other features.
- It multiplies in the nucleus of host cell unlike other flavi viruses.
- **Clinical features:** No symptoms or mild symptoms like fever, skin rash, conjunctivitis, muscle and joint pain, malaise or headache. These symptoms normally last for 2-7 days. Feature simulating the dengue fever.
- **Complications:**
- **Foetal damages:** Zika can also spread from a pregnant woman to her foetus. This can results in microcephaly, severe brain malformations, and other birth defects.
- **In adults:** Rarely Guillain–Barré syndrome.

✪ **Laboratory diagnosis:**

- **Specimens:** Blood, urine, semen, CSF or saliva.
- **Testing methods:**

1. **Microscopy: → Follow morphology.**
2. **Culture: → Follow C/Cs.**
3. **Serological tests:**

- PRNT to detect the neutralising antibodies. It is the confirmatory test but available at referral centre like Centres for Disease Control and Prevention (CDC).
- MAC-ELISA: For IgM antibody detection, which appear after 1st week & remain rise up to 12 weeks. It is detected from CSF or serum. Cross reactivity may occur with other flavi viruse, which is cleared by PRNT.

4. **Molecular test:** RT-PCR.

✪ **Prevention:**

- **General measures:**
- Mosquito control measures: Same as described in chikungunya virus.
- Abstinence from sex with infected partners.
- Men who have travelled to an area with zika should use condoms or not have sex for at least six months after their return, even if they never develop symptoms, because the virus is transmissible in semen.
- No pregnancy planning by women living in affected areas & pregnant women not travel to these areas.
- Screening blood donors.
- **Immunoprophylaxis:** There is no effective vaccine

✪ **Treatment:** There is no specific antiviral treatment for zika virus is available. Supportive treatment like replacement of fluid & electrolytes loss, rest & antipyretic like paracetamol is useful.

Tick borne species

Two groups like encephalitis group & haemorrhagic fever group as follows.

A **Encephalitis viruses group:** Following are the members.

i. **Russian Spring Summer Encephalitis (RSSE) virus:**

✪ **History:**

- It causes encephalitis from Scotland to Siberia.
- Its name is given according to variation in clinical features, location & seasonal pattern.

✪ **Pathogenicity:**

- **Disease name:** **Called Russian Spring Summer Encephalitis (RSSE).**
- **Reservoir of infection:**
- Virus transmitted transovarially in ticks which acts as reservoir.
- Wild rodents & migrating birds are other reservoir.
- **Source of infection:** Ticks & milk of infected animals.
- **Mode of transmission:**
- By tick bite: *Ixodid persulcatus.*
- By drinking the milk of infected goats.
- **Clinical features:**
- Encephalitis with high fatality & permanent paralytic sequelae.
- Biphasic meningo-encephalitis may occur.

✪ **Prevention:**

- **General measures:** Avoiding ticks bite.
- **Immunoprophylaxis:** Formalin inactivated vaccine is effective.

ii. **Central European encephalitis virus:** Transmitted by tick bite like *Ixodid ricinus.*

iii. **Western Siberian encephalitis virus:** Transmitted by tick bite like *Ixodid persulcatus.*

iv. **Powassan encephalitis virus:**

- Transmitted by tick bite like *Ixodid cookie.*
- Present in Eastern Canada & USA, where it has been identified from 20 human cases.

v. **Louping ill virus:**

- Transmitted by tick bite like *Ixodid ricinus.*
- Causing acute viral encephalitis in sheep.

- Name given, because infected sheep 'loup' (old Scottish word) or spring in the air.
- Human cases have been reported from Europe.

B Haemorrhagic fever viruses group: Two members.

i. Kyasanur forest disease (KFD) virus:

✪ **History & Meaning:**
- Virus was 1st isolated in Kyasanur forest, Shimoga district of Karnataka, India in 1957.
- It was isolated by National Institute of Virology (NIV), Pune, India from human & dead monkeys.

✪ **Geographical distribution & genotypes:** Virus is distributed in adjoining regions of Shimoga district, Karnataka, India.

✪ **Morphology:** Virus is belongs to the Russian spring summer encephalitis virus group. It is a spherical, enveloped virus of 45 nm in diameter and has a single-stranded, positive-sense RNA genome.

✪ **Culture characteristics (C/Cs):**
- Produces the cytopathic effect on cell culture.
- Mice inoculation: Research using mice models found that virus primarily replicated in the brain. Other research had identified the neurological changes in experimental mice like gliosis, inflammation & cell death in the brain.

✪ **Resistance:** Enveloped virus sensitive to lipid solvents.

✪ **Antigenic properties:** Antigenically related to RSSE virus.

✪ **Pathogenicity:**
- **Disease name:** It is a zoonosis. Transmission cycle involves monkeys & ticks.
  - **Animal:** Called monkey disease or monkey fever, so called (locally) because it first manifested in monkeys as epizootic in 1957 with plenty of deaths.
  - **Human:** Called kyasanur forest disease.
- **Nature & history of disease:**
  - **Animal:** The disease was first manifested as an epizotic outbreak among monkeys killing several of them in the year 1957.
  - **Human:** After its discovery, virus was limited to adjoining talukas of Kyasanur forest like Sagar, Sorab & Shikharpur of Shimoga district. From 1972-75 small foci were found from adjacent areas of North Kanara. In 1982 epidemic (1142 cases & 104 deaths) & epizootic were found in South Kanara. Trend declined after the discovery of vaccine in 1999. From 2003-2012 total 3263 suspected cases were found of which 823 were positive with 28 deaths. From December 2012 to March 2013 total 215 suspected cases were found of which 61 were positive.
- **Reservoir of infection:**
  - Monkeys, porcupines, rats, squirrels, mice, shrews & birds are the reservoir.
  - Virus transmitted transovarially in ticks which acts as reservoir.
  - Wild monkeys are the amplifier host.
  - Man is the accidental & dead end. No human to human transmission can occur.
- **Source of infection:** Vector is the source for human infection.
- **Mode of transmission:** By ticks bite (*Ixodid* or hard tick) like *Haemaphysalis spinigera, H. turtura* etc.
- **Incubation period:** 3-8 days.
- **Portal of entry:** Skin.
- **Sites:** Blood, conjunctiva, muscles etc.
- **Precipitating factors (epidemiological determinants):**

a. **Agent factors:** Causing prolonged viraemia about 8 -10 days.

b. **Host factors:**
1. **Age:** No age bar.
2. **Sex:** More in male due to outdoor visit.
3. **Occupation:** Like forest workers are at high risk.

c. **Vector factors:** About 15 different species of ticks are responsible like *H. spinigera, H. turtura* etc.

d. **Environmental factors:**
1. **Urbanisation:** Dry season from January-June favours the human & monkeys infection because of peak activity by nymph.

- **Pathogenesis:** Not clearly understood.
- **Clinical features:** Two phases.
- **Acute (prodromal) phase:**
  - Sudden onset of fever.
  - Headache.
  - Conjunctivitis.
  - Myalgia.
  - Severe prostration.
- **Haemorrhage phase:** Haemorrhage in skin, mucosa & inner viscera.

✪ **Complication:** The disease has a fatality rate of 3-10%.

✪ **Laboratory diagnosis:**
- **Specimens:** Blood/serum.
- **Testing methods:**
1. **Microscopy: → Follow morphology.**
2. **Culture: → Follow C/Cs.**
3. **Serological tests:**
   - Haemagglutination inhibition test.
   - CFT.
   - Neutralization test.
   - ELISA
4. **Molecular test:** Nested RT-PCR, TaqMan-based real-time RT-PCR.

✪ **Prevention:**
- **General measures:**
  - Vector control measures.
  - Adequate clothing.
  - Vector repellents like dimethylphthalate & DEET.

- Avoid sleeping on ground.
- **Immunoprophylaxis:**
- **Preparation:** A killed (formalin-inactivated) chick embryo kyasanur forest disease virus vaccine is effective & provides some degree of protection. It is developed in the Haffkine institute, Mumbai.
- **Dose:** Two doses at interval of 2 months followed by booster dose at 6-9 months & then every 5 years.
- **Efficacy:** The vaccine has a 62.4% effectiveness rate for individuals who receive two doses & 82.9% for those who receive an additional dose.
- **Target area:** It is recommended in villages, within 5 km range of endemic areas in Karnataka.

✪ **Treatment:** There is no specific antiviral treatment is available. Supportive treatment is given.

ii. Omsk haemorrhagic fever virus:
- Clinically similar to kyasanur forest disease virus.
- Occurs in Russia & Romania.
- Transmitted by *Dermacentor* ticks.

Bunyaviridae

❖ Morphology:
- **Shape:** Spherical.
- **Size:** 100 nm.
- **Genome:** Complex structure with triple segmented ss-RNA (-).
- **Capsid:** NA is surrounded by helical capsid.
- **Envelope:** Nucleocapsid is surrounded by envelop.

❖ Classification:
- **Family:** Bunyaviridae.
- **Genus:** Four genera as described below.

I. *Bunyavirus*

♣ **Properties:** It is a mosquito borne virus.

♣ **Species:** More than 150 species & only few can cause human disease. Some are as follow.

i. California Encephalitis virus:
- Endemic in USA.
- Causing encephalitis, aseptic meningitis & fever.

ii. Oropouche virus:
- Produced large epidemic in Brazil.
- Causing aseptic meningitis & fever.
- Transmitted by midges bite like *Culicoides paraensia.*

II. *Phlebovirus*

♣ **Properties:** It is transmitted by sand flies.

♣ **Species:** Two main members.

i. Sand fly fever or *Phlebotomus* fever or *Pappataci* fever or three day fever virus:
- Transmitted by sand fly like *Phlebotomus pappataci* and fever last for three days hence above mentioned names are given.
- Endemic in Mediterranean coast & Central Asia and extended to East Pakistan to North West India.
- Cases are also reported from Central & South America.
- Twenty antigenic types of which five can cause human disease like Chagres, Candiru, Naples, Silician & Punta Toro.
- Virus transmitted transovarially in sand fly which acts as reservoir.
- Causing self limited febrile illness.

ii. Rift Valley fever virus:

✪ **Meaning:** Named after Rift Valley, Kenya where it was 1st recognised.

✪ **Pathogenicity:**
- **Mode of transmission:**
- By mosquitoes bite: *Culex tritaeniorhynchus* & *Aedes vexans.*
- Also by direct contact with tissues of infected animals.
- **History and clinical features:**
  - Animal infection: Produced large epizootic of hepatitis in sheep & other domestic animals in Africa.
  - Human infection:
- Produce **disease resembling influenza.**
- In 1977-80 it produce extensive epidemic of **fever** in Egypt with many deaths.
- In 1997-98 caused outbreak of **haemorrhagic fever** in Kenya.
- After 2000, it spread outside the Africa & entered in Yemen & Saudi Arabia with hundreds of deaths.

III. *Nairovirus*

♣ **Properties:** Genus is named after one of it's species.

♣ **Species:**

i. Nairobi sheep disease virus:

✪ **Pathogenicity:**
- **Mode of transmission:** By tick bite like *Rhipicephalus.*
- **Clinical features:**
  - Animal infection:
- Produced disease in sheep & goats **called Nairobi sheep disease.**
- Characterised by acute, haemorrhagic gestro-enteritis.
  - Human infection: Produce mild febrile illness.

ii. Crimean Congo Haemorrhagic Fever (CCHF) virus:

✪ **Synonym:** Congo virus has been used in many reports.

✪ **History:** Virus was first identified in Crimea in 1945 & it was identical to the Congo fever virus identified in 1956 in Congo (Zaire), hence the name CCHF virus.

- **Geographical distribution & genotypes:**
- **In the world:** CCHF is found in Eastern Europe, in North-Western China, Central Asia, southern Europe, Africa and the Middle East.
- **In India:** 1st identified in 2011, since then it is wide spread in India.
- **Genotypes:** Based on the genomic sequence data seven genotypes have been recognised like
- Africa 1: Senegal.
- Africa 2: Democratic Republic of the Congo & South Africa.
- Africa 3: Southern and western Africa.
- Europe 1: Albania, Bulgaria, Kosovo, Russia & Turkey.
- Europe 2: Greece.
- Asia 1: Middle East, Iran and Pakistan.
- Asia 2: China, Kazakistan, Tajikistan & Uzbekistan.
- **Morphology: → Fig.-9**
- **Shape:** Pleomorphic.
- **Size:** 80-120 nm.
- **Genome:** ss-RNA (-). Three segments like Small (S), Medium (M) & Large (L). L segment encodes for RNA polymerase, M segment encodes for envelope proteins (Gc and Gn) and the S segment encodes for nucleocapsid.

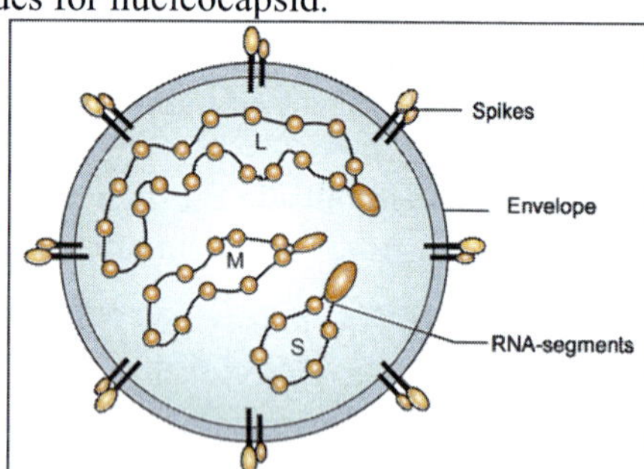

Figure-9: Morphology of CCHF virus

- **Capsid:** NA is surrounded by helical capsid.
- **Envelope:** Nucleocapsid is surrounded envelop.
- **Peplomere:** Envelop consist 5-10nm long spikes.
- **Culture characteristics (C/Cs):** Virus isolation is best useful in initial 5 days.
- **Animal culture:** Inoculation in suckling mice is more sensitive.
- **Tissue culture:** Cell lines used are SW-13, Vero cells, LLC-MK2 & BHK-21 cells. It is most effective in first 5 days.
- **Resistance:** Virus can be inactivated by
- 1% hypochlorite solution.
- 2% glutaraldehyde solution.
- Boiling at 56^{0}C.
- **Pathogenicity:**
- **Disease name:** It is a zoonosis, **called Crimean Congo Haemorrhagic Fever (CCHF)**
- **Nature & history of disease:**
- World scenario:
- CCHF is also endemic in Kosovo.
- On July 28, 2005 total 41 cases of CCHF found in Turkey with one death.
- In September-2010 total 100 cases reported from Pakistan with 10% case fatality.
- As of May 2012, 71 people are reported to have contracted the disease in Iran, with 8 deaths.
- A man died of CCHF in Spain on 25th August, 2016 and infected a nurse. In August 2016 a number of news cases raised the concerns regarding the disease.
- Indian scenario:
- Recently identified in Gujarat. On 19th January, 2011-first case was reported from Sanand, Gujarat, India with 4 deaths including patient along with doctor and nurse.
- In July 2013, the seven persons died due to CCHF in Kariyana village in Babra Taluka, Amreli district, Gujarat, India.
- In December 2014, one person died due to disease that belongs to Madhapar village near Bhuj city, Kutch district of Gujarat, India.
- CCHF has become widespread in India, with the first human case was found in 2011.
- **Reservoir of infection:** Domestic animals like cattle, sheep, goats & others are the reservoir.
- **Source of infection:** Vector is the source for human infection.
- **Mode of transmission:**
- By *Ixodid ticks* (hard ticks) bite **(fig.-10)** like *Hyalomma marginatum* or *H. anatolicum*.
- Other ticks from which virus is identified are *Argas reflexus*, *H. detritum* & *Rhipicephalus sanguineus*.
- Direct contact with blood or infected tissue.
- Aerosols.
- Crushing of an infected tick with bare hands.
- Drinking un-pasteurised milk from infected animals.
- Possible vertical transmission has been reported from mother to child.
- Fomites borne.

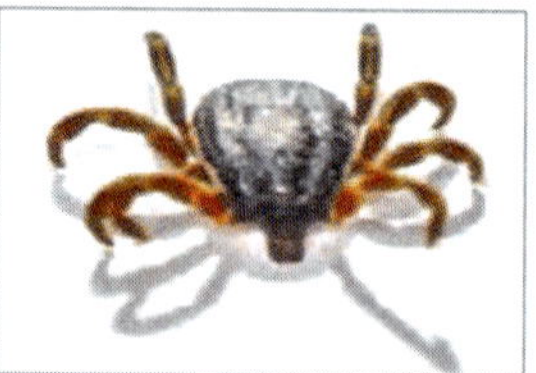

Figure-10: Hard ticks

- **Incubation period:**
- Depends on the mode of acquisition of the virus.
- Following tick bite, the incubation period is usually 1-3 days, with a maximum of nine days.
- Following contact with infected blood or tissues is usually 5-6 days, with a documented maximum of 13 days.
- **Portal of entry:** Skin.

- **Sites:** Symptoms occurs in many systems.
- **Precipitating factors:**

1. **Occupation:**

- Agricultural workers, slaughterhouse workers and veterinarians.
- Health care workers attending on suspect/ probable/ confirmed CCHF cases and not following contact precautions are at high risk of getting infection.

2. **Hospital acquired infection:** Nosocomial outbreak has been reported in many countries.

- **Pathogenesis:** Not clearly understood.
- **Clinical features:**

o Prodromal (pre haemorrhagic) phase:

- Sudden onset of fever [39–41°C, on an average, fever persists for 4–5 days] with chills, severe headache, photophobia, neck pain, dizziness, abdominal pain, diarrhoea, vomiting, myalgia, hypotension, neuropsychiatric changes (early-mood swings, confusion, aggression. Later-sleepiness, depression & lassitude), tachycardia, lymphadenopathy etc.

o Hemorrhagic phase:

- Short & last for 2-3 days.
- Begins on 3rd to 5th day. petechiae, ecchymosis, haematemesis, epistaxis, malaena, leucopenia, thrombocytopenia, haematuria.

o Convalescence phase: Improvement starts by 9-10 days. Pronounced generalized weakness, weak pulse, sometimes complete loss of hair seen.

- **Complications:**
  - Hepato-renal failure, pulmonary failure & DIC.
  - Mortality highest in 2nd week ranging from 5-50%
- **Sequelae:** Polyneuritis, headache, nausea, poor vision, hearing loss, memory loss. Rarely these changes may be permanent. But they may persist for a year or more.

✪ **Differential diagnosis:** The following diseases should be differentiated from CCHF:

- Malaria.
- Leptospirosis.
- Rickettsial diseases.
- Meningococcemia.
- Dengue hemorrhagic fever.
- Haemolytic Uremic Syndrome (HUS).
- Thrombocytopenic purpura.

✪ **Laboratory Diagnosis**

- **Specimens:**
  - Serum or plasma.
  - Tissue samples like liver, spleen, bone marrow, kidney, Lung and brain.
  - Handling of samples required bio-safety level 4 precautions.
- **Testing methods:**

a. **Blood picture:**

- CBC: Leucopenia & thrombocytopenia.
- SGOT, SGPT: Increased level.
- Raised levels of lactate dehydrogenase and creatinine phosphokinase.
- Coagulation tests such as prothrombin time and activated partial thromboplastin time are prolonged.
- Level of fibrinogen might be decreased, and fibrin degradation products could be increased.
- Blood picture returns to normal levels within approximately 5–9 days among surviving patients.

b. **Urine picture:** Haematuria.

c. **Microscopy:** → **Follow morphology.**

d. **Culture:** → **Follow C/Cs.**

e. **Serological tests:**

- **Ab detection:**
  - IgM ELISA: IgM detectable after 6th day of illness & remains detectable for up to four months.
  - IgG ELISA: IgG levels decline but remains detectable for up to five years.
  - Patients with fatal disease do not usually develop a measurable antibody response and in these individuals, as well as in patients in the first few days of illness, diagnosis is achieved by virus detection in blood or tissue samples.
- **Ag detection:** Viral antigens may sometimes be shown in tissue samples using immunofluorescence or ELISA.

f. **Molecular methods:** RT-PCR (rapid & sensitive).

✪ **Prevention:**

- **General measures:**
  - Intensive tick control measures have to be taken by spraying **acericide** drug on all animals in affected and neighbourhood villages.
  - All animals should be covered under effective supervision of animal husbandry department.
  - Insecticide have to be sprayed intensively in all breaks on floor and walls in cattle shades
  - Treatment and spraying with drug has to be repeated after one month.
  - To contain the infection, the admission of the patients should be, in identified hospitals only.
  - Health care staff in the hospitals should be educated with emphasis on protective measures.
  - Surveillance among hospital contacts should be strengthened at hospital setting.
  - Biomedical waste management at the hospitals should be strengthened.
  - Strengthening of health education about causation, transmission and prevention of disease.
  - State wide sero-surveillance in animals to identify prevalence of disease.
  - Insect repellants containing DEET.
  - Wearing protective clothes.
  - Health care workers who had contact with tissue or blood from patients with suspected or confirmed CCHF should be followed up with daily temperature and symptom monitoring for at least 14 days after the putative exposure.

- **Chemoprophylaxis:** Ribavirin is useful.
- **Immunoprophylaxis:** No specific safe & effective vaccine is available. An inactivated mouse brain derived vaccine against CCHF virus has been developed and used on a small scale.

✪ **Treatment:**

- **General supportive therapy:** Intensive monitoring to guide blood and volume component replacement is required.
- **Antiviral drugs:** The antiviral ribavirin has been used in treatment of established CCHF infection with apparent benefits. Both oral & IV formulations seems to be effective.

○ Treatment protocol for adults:

- 2 gm loading dose of ribavirin followed by.
- 4 gm/ day in 4 divided doses (6 hourly)for 4 days.
- 2gm/day in 4 divided doses for 6 days.

○ Treatment protocol for adults: → **Table-3**

Route	Dose	Day 1-4	Day 5-10
IV	17 mg/kg	17 mg/kg 6hr	8 mg/kg 8hr
oral	30 mg/kg	15 mg/kg 6hr	7 mg/kg 6hr

Table-3: Protocol of ribavirin for adult

✪ **Passive immunotherapy:**

- Hyperimmune serum has been tested in few cases.
- A new specific Ig CCHF-venin, has been prepared using the plasma pool of boosted donors. It contains Ab to CCHF virus in a titre of 8.

iii. Hazara virus:

- Virus related to CCHF virus & isolated from Pakistan.
- It also widespread in UAE, Iraq & Iran.

iv. Ganjam virus:

- Virus related to Nairobi sheep disease virus & isolated from ticks collected from sheep & goats in Orissa, India.
- It also isolated from human.
- Accidental transmission in laboratory cause mild febrile illness.

IV. *Hantavirus*

It is not an arbovirus but robovirus and discussed below, under separate heading of **Roboviruses.**

Reoviridae

❖ **Meaning:** It means Respiratory Enteric Orphan Virus because it isolated from respiratory & enteric tract & orphan means without causing any disease.

❖ **Morphology:** → **Fig.-11**

➢ **Shape:** Spherical.

➢ **Size:** 55-57 nm.

➢ **Genome:** ds-RNA (+/-) with 10-12 pieces (11 pieces in *Rotavirus*). It has three segments like large (L), Medium (M) & small (S).

➢ **Capsid:**

- Icosahedral type of capsid with two layers (3 layers in *Rotavirus*).
- Outer layer is fuzzy & indistinct.
- Inner layer has 32 ring shaped capsomere.

➢ **Non-envelope:** Also **called naked virus.**

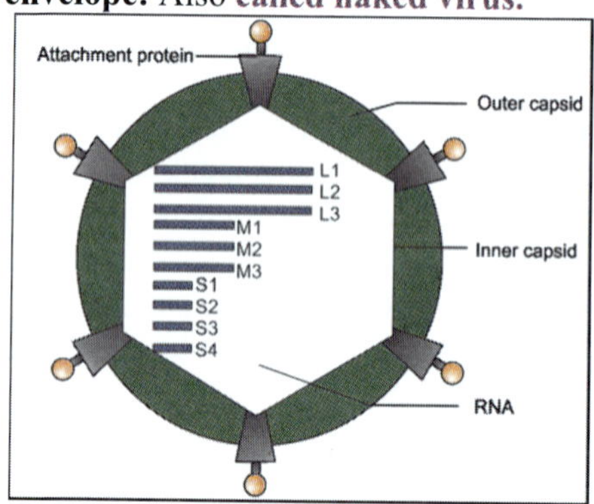

Figure-11: Morphology of Reoviridae

❖ **Resistance:** Virus is naked & resistant to lipid solvents.

❖ **Classification:** →**Flow chart-2**

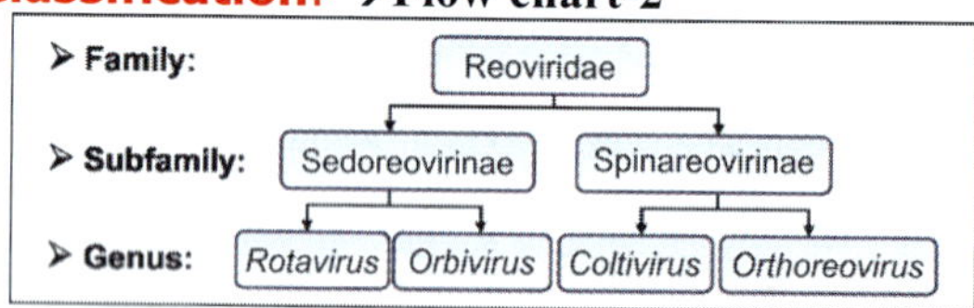

Flow chart-2: Classification of Reoviridae

I. *Rotavirus*

- Rotavirus is not an arbovirus.
- More details: Follow chapter → Other group of viruses

II. *Orbivirus*

✪ **Meaning: Orbi** word derived **orbi (Latin) = ring,** because having 32 ring shaped structure in inner layer of icosahedral capsid. It is considered as an arbovirus.

✪ **Species:** Following are the species.

i. African horse sickness virus:

- Non human pathogens.
- It is a veterinary pathogen & produce epizootic in Iran, Pakistan, Afghanistan & India.
- Transmitted by mosquitoes bite like *Culex*.
- Natural pathogen of horses and mules in India.

ii. Orungo virus:

- Endemic in sub-Saharan Africa.
- It is either subclinical or cause acute febrile illness.
- Transmitted by mosquitoes bite like *Aedes*.

iii. Kemerovo virus:

- Cases have been reported from Russia.
- Causing febrile illness with involvement of meninges.
- Transmitted by tick like *Ixodes persulcatus*.

iv. **Palyam virus:** } All are veterinary pathogens
v. **Kasba virus:**
vi. **Vellore virus:**

III. *Coltivirus*

i. **Kolarado tick fever virus:**
- Only human pathogens in Orbivirus group.
- Distributed in Western USA.
- Transmitted by wood tick *Dermacentor andersoni*, which acts as vector & reservoir.
- Natural pathogen of rodents and in human produce self-limited mild fever without rash.

IV. *Orthoreovirus*

✪ **Serotypes:** Not an arbovirus. Three serotypes: 1, 2 & 3.
✪ **Pathogenicity:** Isolated from respiratory & enteric tract without causing any disease. Transmitted by faeco-oral route or by inhalation.

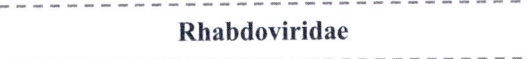

Rhabdoviridae

❖ **Meaning:** Word is derived from **Rhabdos = rod shape**, because of its **shape like rod (bullet).**

❖ **Classification:**
➢ **Family:** Rhabdoviridae.
➢ **Genus:** Two genera like *Lyssavirus* & *Vesiculovirus.*

I. *Lyssavirus*

- It is not an arbovirus.
- More details: Follow chapter → Rhabdoviridae.

II. *Vesiculovirus*

i. **Vesicular stomatitis virus:**
- Virus cause oral mucosal vesicles & ulcers in cattle, horse & pigs as like hand foot mouth disease virus.
- Human infection is rare or present with flu like illness.
- It is a zoonosis, transmitted by sand fly: *Lutzomyia shannoni.*
- Uses:

1. **Oncolytic therapy:** It has been used for oncolytic therapy to reduce the tumour size. Virus spread in melanoma, lung cancer, colon cancer and certain brain tumours in laboratory models of cancer.
2. **Anti-HIV therapy:** Virus can attack HIV infected T-cells. The modified virus was **called a trojan horse virus.**
3. **Vaccine preparation:** Recombinant vesicular stomatitis virus has undergone phase 1 trials as a vaccine for Ebola virus.
4. **Viral model:** To study the properties of viruses in the family Rhabdoviridae, as well as to study viral evolution.
5. **Biomedical research:**
6. **Cytological studies:**

ii. **Chandipura virus:** Arbovirus described below.

✪ **History:**
- Virus was 1st detected by NIV, Pune, India from the serum sample of two adult patients with febrile illness, collected during an outbreak of fever in Chandipur village, Nagpur area, Maharashtra, India in 1967.
- It was discovered by Bhatt & Rodrigues.

✪ **Geographical distribution:** Since its discovery, virus is limited in adjoining regions of Maharashtra, Central India.

✪ **Morphology: →Fig.-12**
- **Shape:** Bullet shaped.
- **Size:** 150-165 nm in length & 50-60 nm wide.
- **Genome:** Linear, ss RNA (-) with RNA dependent RNA polymerase /transcriptase.
- **Capsid:** Helical type.
- **Envelop:** Bilayered contain inner protein (M) & outer lipid layer. Distinct surface projection (spikes) 9-11 nm & glycoprotein in nature.
- **Replication:** In cytoplasm.

✪ **Culture characteristics (C/Cs):** Virus isolation is best useful in initial 5 days.
- **Animal culture:** Inoculation in infant mice is useful.
- **Tissue culture:** Over Vero & BHK-21 cells.

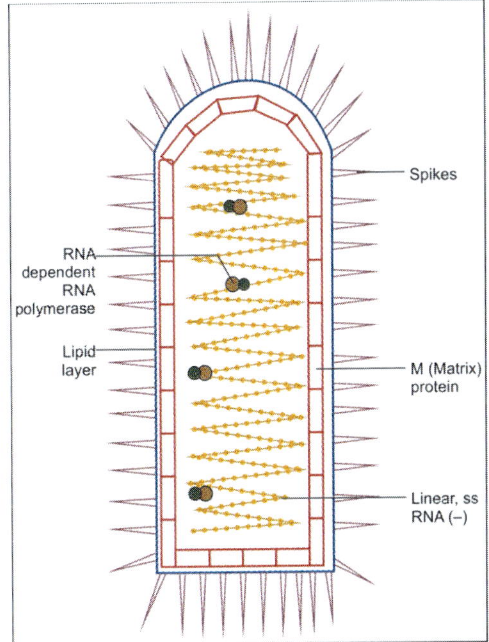

Figure-12: Morphology of Chandipura virus

✪ **Pathogenicity:**
- **Nature & history of disease:**
- It is an emerging virus.
- Since its discovery numbers of unexplained outbreaks of encephalitis occurred in Central India.
- Outbreak occurred in Andhra Pradesh and Maharashtra in June–August 2003 with 329 children affected and 183 deaths.

- Further sporadic cases and deaths in children were observed in Gujarat state in 2004.
- Recent outbreak occured in three districts, Kheda, Vadodara & Panchmahal of Gujarat, India killed 17 people in 2010.
- **Reservoir of infection:** Human.
- **Source of infection:** Vector is the source for human infection.
- **Mode of transmission:** Sand flies species of *Phlebotomus* & *Sergentomyia* are the major vectors for the transmission of virus.
- **Incubation period**: 2-6 days.
- **Portal of entry:** Skin.
- **Sites:** Brain.
- **Precipitating factors:**

1. **Age:** Between 9 months to 14 years.
2. **Sex:** Male : Female ratio is 1:0.77
3. **Seasonality:** Late summer & early monsoon (July-September).
4. **Rural Areas:** Mud, damp soil, other vegetative material (high moisture areas).
5. **Socio-economic class:** Common in lower class.

- **Pathogenesis:** Not clearly understood.
- **Clinical features:** Full clinical picture is still unclear. Preliminary data suggests the range to be from sub-clinical infection / mild to high grade fever to acute encephalitis.
- High grade fever of short duration.
- Vomiting.
- Altered sensorium.
- Generalized convulsions.
- Decerebrate posture.
- Acute encephalitis/ encephalopathy.

✪ **Complication:** Death within few hrs to 48 hrs of hospitalization.

✪ **Differential Diagnosis:** It differentiated from JE virus, paramyxo virus, West Nile Virus & other virus causing encephalitis.

✪ **Laboratory diagnosis:**

- **Specimens:** Blood / serum, throat swab, CSF & urine.
- **Testing methods:**

a. **Microscopy:** → **Follow morphology.**

b. **Culture:** → **Follow C/Cs.**

c. **Serological tests:**

- **Ab detection:**
- IgM ELISA.
- IgG ELISA.
- Neutralisation test.
- CFT.
- Haemagglutination Inhibition test.
- **Antigen Detection:** Viral antigens may sometimes be detected from tissues using immunofluorescence test or by ELISA.

d. **Molecular methods:** RT-PCR is more rapid & sensitive.

e. **Vector diagnosis:**

- Sand flies are collected from houses and around the house of the cases.
- They are transported in plastic jars, identified, pooled, stored at -70^{0}C until processed and tested by RT-PCR.

✪ **Prevention:**

- **General measures:**
- There are no known efficient methods of controlling biting sand flies, but personal protection will help in reducing exposure to their bites.
- Avoid localities, especially at dawn and dusk that are known to be frequented by biting sand flies.
- Wear protective clothing (long sleeves/pants).
- Apply a repellent to exposed skin.
- **Immunoprophylaxis:** No specific vaccine is available.

✪ **Treatment:**

- There is no specific antiviral treatment is available.
- Only intensive supportive & symptomatic treatment is given.
- Close and continuous monitoring is required.

Roboviruses

Meaning: It means **Ro**dent **Bo**rne **Viruses.** However transmission by mites have been reported but not confirmed and in absence of proved arthropod borne transmission it considered as **Robovirus**.

Classification: →**Table-2**

Bunyaviridae

❖ **Classification:**

➢ **Family:** Bunyaviridae.

➢ **Genus:** *Hantavirus.*

➢ **Species:** Five members as follows.

i. **Hantaan virus:**

✪ **Meaning:** Virus is named for the Hantaan River which flows through the endemic region in Korea.

✪ **History:** It came in picture in early 1950s when large numbers of US soldiers serving in Korea got the infection. The cause remained unknown until 1976 when Karl M. Johnson an American tropical virologist and his colleagues, including Korean virologist, Lee Ho Wang (Ho Wang Lee), isolated Hantaan virus from the lungs of striped field mice.

✪ **Geographical distribution:** It is prevalent in Scandinavia, Far East, North Asia, Western Russia, China, South & Central America.

✪ **Morphology:** Same as like other virus of Bunyaviridae family which includes

- Enveloped.
- Single-stranded, negative-sense RNA virus.

- Three genomic segments like large, medium, and small. Segment reassortment within a species appears common.
- Three structural proteins: G1 (glycoproteins), G2 & N (nucleoprotein).

✪ **Pathogenicity:**

- **Disease name:** Disease **called haemorrhagic fever renal syndrome**. Clinically resemble to typhoid, leptospirosis & scrub typhus.
- **Synonyms:**
  - Korean haemorrhagic fever.
  - Epidemic nephrosonephritis.
  - Endemic nephrosonephritis.
  - Manchurian epidemic haemorrhagic fever.
  - Nephropathia epidemica.
  - Rodent borne nephropathy.
- **Reservoir of infection:** Field mouse (*Apodemus agrarius*) is the natural host.
- **Source of infection:** Aerosols from the excreta of rodents like urine, faeces & saliva.
- **Mode of transmission:** By aerosols arise from excreta of rodents like urine, faeces & saliva.
- **Incubation period:** 2-4 weeks.
- **Portal of entry:** Respiratory system.
- **Sites:** Kidneys.
- **Precipitating factors:**
  - There are two seasonal peaks for almost all outbreaks of *Hantavirus* diseases: a small one in spring and a large one in fall. It is due to increase the activities in farms by farmers & exposed to rodents in the fields during planting and harvest periods. Unusually high rainfall in dry parts of the country result in increased food sources for rodents and subsequently increased rodent populations.
  - Fall/winter outbreaks, such as those in Greece, correspond to the movement of rodents from the fields into man-made structures.
- **Pathogenesis:** Exact mechanisms to produce the renal damage are unknown.
- **Clinical features:** Present in two forms.

1. Mild epidemic nephritis: Common in Scandinavia
2. Serious epidemic hemorrhagic fever.

- **Complication:** Death occurs in 10-12% cases.

✪ **Diagnosis:**

- **Specimens:** Blood/serum & urine.
- **Testing methods:**

a. Blood picture:

- Increased levels of serum creatinine (a muscle enzyme), which indicates kidney damage.
- Atypical or elevated white blood-cell count.
- Thrombocytopenia.

b. Microscopy: → **Follow morphology**

c. Serological tests:

- IgM ELISA.
- IgG ELISA.
- Haemagglutination test in paired sera.
- Antigen detection methods are unsuccessful.

d. Molecular methods: RT-PCR (rapid & sensitive).

✪ **Prevention:**

- **General measures:** Rodent control measures.
- **Immunoprophylaxis:**
  - Animal research has shown that immunization with recombinant glycoproteins can partially prevent the infection.
  - Vaccines based on two glycoproteins (G1 and G2) were more effective.

✪ **Treatment:**

- There is no specific antiviral treatment is available
- Symptomatic treatment is given to manage the fluid & electrolyte balance.
- Close and continuous monitoring is required.

ii. Seoul virus:

- Mild type of disease.
- Probably present world-wide.
- Transmitted by rats (*Rattus rattus* & *R. norvegicus*)
- An experimental vaccine for the Seoul virus has been developed.

iii. Puumala virus:

- Responsible for nephropathia epidemica in northern & eastern Europe.
- Transmitted by rats (*Rattus rattus* & *R. norvegicus*).

iv. Prospect Hill virus:

- Isolated from voles in the USA.
- Not associated with human illness.
- Transmitted by rats (*Rattus rattus* & *R. norvegicus*).

v. Sin Nombre virus:

✪ **Meaning:** Meaning name less because newly identified and name is not given.

✪ **History:**

- It was identified in South Western USA in 1993.
- Related virus produces same illness in many parts of South America.

✪ **Pathogenicity:** Disease **called hantavirus pulmonary syndrome.**

- **Mode of transmission:** By inhalation of aerosols arise from excreta of deer mouse & other rodents of Sigmoidontine family.
- **Clinical features:**
  - <u>Prodromal phase</u>:
    - Sudden onset of fever, malaise, myalgia & gastrointestinal symptoms.
    - Last for 3-4 days.
  - <u>Pulmonary phase</u>:
    - Pulmonary oedema identify under radiological picture.
    - In severe cases development of hypotension, tachycardia & tachypnoea leading to death.

Arenaviridae

❖ **Meaning:** Word is came from **arena (Latin)** = **land**, resemble to grains of sand.

❖ **Morphology:** → **Fig.-13**

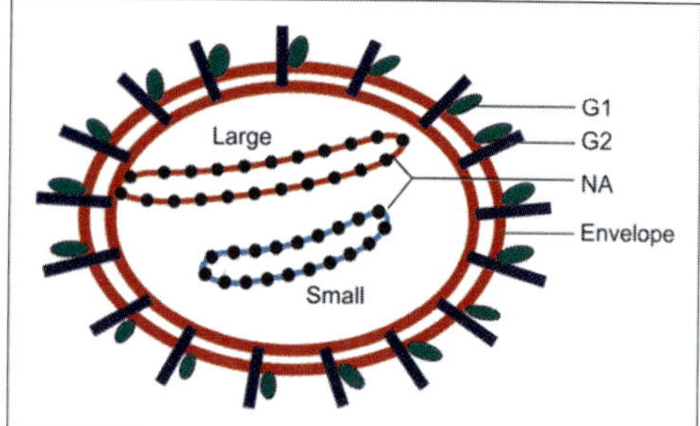

Figure-13: Morphology of Arenaviridae

➢ **Shape:** Spherical or pleomorphic particles. Viral particles are actually ribosomes picked up by virus from host cells during maturation & resembling like sand under EM.
➢ **Size:** 80-300nm.
➢ **Genome & capsid:** ss-RNA (-) in two segment with complex symmetry of capsid.
➢ **Envelope:** Present.

❖ **Classification:**
➢ **Family:** Arenaviridae.
➢ **Genera:** Two genera like *Mammarenavirus* (infecting mammalian hosts) & *Reptarenavirus* (infecting snakes, not a human pathogen).

I. *Mammarenavirus*

Two groups (serogroups?) like old world viruses & new world viruses based on geographical & genetical properties.

A Old world viruses:
✪ **Definition:** Found in the Eastern Hemisphere in places such as Europe, Asia, and Africa.
✪ **Species:** Following two are the old world viruses.

✓ **Note:** LCM virus is the only *Mammarenavirus* to exist in both areas but is classified as an old world virus.

i. Lymphocytic Chorio Meningitis (LCM) virus:
- **Pathogenicity of LCM virus:**
  - Source of infection: Natural parasite of rodents, which excrete the virus in urine & faeces, acts as source for infection.
  - Mode of transmission: From excreta of rodents.
  - Clinical features:
    - Asymptomatic.
    - Influenza like illness.
    - Meningitis.
    - Death due to deposition of immune complex in CNS or Kidney (glomerulonephritis).
- **Diagnosis of LCM virus:**
  - Specimens: Brain/meninges biopsy.
  - Tests:
    - **EM:** Electron dense particles resembling like sand.
    - **Animal inoculation**: In mouse.

ii. Lassa fever virus:
- **Meaning:** 1st noticed in 1969 in American Mission station in Lassa, Nigeria, hence the name.
- **Pathogenicity:**
  - Source of infection: Natural parasite of rodents, which excrete the virus in urine & faeces, acts as source for infection.
  - Mode of transmission:
    - From excreta of rodents.
    - Inhalation.
    - Nosocomial infection.
  - Incubation period: 3-16 days.
  - Clinical features:
    - Causing haemorrhagic fever **called lassa fever**.
    - Case fatality: 35-70%.
- **Diagnosis:** Virus is diagnosed from throat swab, blood & urine of patients.
- **Treatment:** Ribavirin is effective.

B New world viruses

✪ **Definition:** Found in the Western Hemisphere, in places such as Argentina, Bolivia, Venezuela, Brazil, and the United States.
✪ **Species:** Following six are the new world viruses.

i. Junin virus:
- Causing Argentinian haemorrhagic fever.
- Transmitted from rodent's excreta.

ii. Machupo virus:
- Causing Bolivian haemorrhagic fever.
- Transmitted from rodent's excreta.

iii. Guanarito virus: Causing haemorrhagic fever in Venezuala.

iv. Sabia virus: Causing haemorrhagic fever in Brazil.

v. White water arroyo virus: Causing haemorrhagic fever in South Western USA.

vi. Lujo virus: Name is given by using first two letters of the cities involved in the 2008 outbreak of the human viral haemorrhagic fever in, Lusaka (Zambia) & Johannesburg (Republic of South Africa).

Question bank

Case study

1) A 50 year old male is brought to the hospital with stiffness in ankle since 6 months. He was suffered with fever before 6 months & from that time the neck stiffness is continue. Fluid is taken out from the joint & sent to the referral laboratory which suggested the virus induced disease. Identify the clinical conditions & answer the following
a) Name the clinical condition & its etiological agent.
b) Write the morphology of etiological agent.
c) Write pathogenicity & diagnosis of clinical condition.

2) A 25 year old male is brought to the hospital with high fever & headache & retro-orbital pain. On clinical examination petechial rashes, hepatomegaly & positive tourniquet test were ruled out. Blood picture reported the thrombocytopenia with 30,000/cmm count. All lab report suggested it could be virus induced condition. Identify the clinical conditions & answer the following

a) Name the clinical condition & its etiological agent.
b) Write the morphology of etiological agent.
c) Write pathogenicity & diagnosis of clinical condition.

Essay/Full question

1) Arboviruses.
2) Arboboviruses prevalent in India.
3) Flaviviridae.
4) Roboviruses.

Short notes

1) Chikungunya virus.
2) Japanese encephalitis virus.
3) Yellow fever virus.
4) Dengue virus.
5) Zika virus.
6) Kyasanur Forest Disease (KFD) virus.
7) CCHF virus.
8) Chandipura virus.
9) Arboviruses.
10) Hantaan virus.
11) Mammarenavirus.

Short questions for theory/viva questions

1) Name four arboboviruses prevalent in India.
2) Name four mosquito borne viruses.
3) Name four flaviviruses.
4) Name four roboviruses.
5) What is primary & secondary dengue infection?
6) What is antibody-dependent enhancement in dengue? Write its clinical significance.
7) Comment: Secondary dengue infection is more severe than primary dengue infection.

MCQs for chapter review

Arboviruses

Classification

1) **Following are arboviral diseases** (PGI, June-03)
(a) KFD (b) West Nile fever (c) Ganjam virus (d) RSV (e) Puumala virus

2) **Which of the following is/are arboviral diseases** (PGI, June-09)
(a) Japanese encephalitis (b) Dengue (c) Yellow fever (d) Hand foot mouth disease (e) Rocky mountain spotted fever

3) **Group B (flavi viruses) arboviruses is/are** (PGI, Dec-06)
(a) Dengue fever (b) Rift valley fever (c) Chikungunya (d) JE (e) Yellow fever

4) **Virus causing haemorrhagic fever are** (PGI, June-03)
(a) Lassa fever virus (b) Yellow fever virus (c) West Nile virus (d) Crimean Congo virus (e) Ross river virus

5) **Fever & haemorrhagic rashes are seen in all except** (PGI, June-03)
(a) Dengue fever (b) Lassa fever (c) Rift valley fever (d) Sand fly fever (e) Yellow fever

6) **Haemorrhagic fever is not caused by**
(a) Yellow fever (b) KFD (c) Japanese encephalitis (d) Dengue fever

7) **Hepatitis C virus resembles which of the following virus group**
(a) Picorna viruses (b) Herpes viruses (c) Hepadna viruses (d) Flavi viruses

8) **Which of the following viral infection is transmitted by tick?** (AI-05)
(a) Japanese encephalitis (b) Dengue fever (c) Kyasanur Forest Disease (KFD) (d) Yellow fever

Arboviruses found in India

9) **Which of the following is not common in India**
(a) Japanese B encephalitis (b) Lassa fever (c) KFD (d) Dengue

Togaviridae

10) **Chikungunya virus is transmitted by**
(a) *Aedes aegypti* (b) *Culex visnoi-complex* (c) *Aedes albopticus* (d) *Mansonia indiana*

Flaviridae

11) **Choose the false statement regarding hepatitis G virus**
(a) Also called GB virus (b) Blood borne RNA virus (c) Mostly infected with HCV (d) Respond to lamivudine

12) **Following is true kyasanur forest disease except** (AI-04)
(a) Transmitted by soft ticks (b) Caused by retrovirus (c) Incubation period is 3-8 days (d) Killed vaccine available

13) **Which of the followings are true regarding KFD** (PGI-97)
(a) It is zoonosis (b) Affects monkeys (c) Caused by bacteria (d) Caused by *Rickettsia*

14) **KFD is transmitted by** (AI-91)
(a) Fleas (b) Mite (c) Tick (d) Mosquito

15) **Vector of Japanese B encephalitis virus is**
(a) *Anopheles* mosquito (b) *Culex* mosquito (c) *Aedes* mosquito (d) All of the above

16) **In Japanese encephalitis pig acts as** (PGI-00)
(a) Amplifier host (b) Definitive host (c) Intermediate host (d) Any of the above

17) **JE virus life cycle in nature run between?**
(a) Pigs-mosquitoes (b) Cattle-birds (c) Pigs-humans (d) Birds-pigs

18) **Amplifier host is**
(a) Pigs in JE (b) Dog in rabies (c) Man in JE (d) Cattle in JE

19) **True about dengue fever** (PGI, May-13)
(a) Caused by 4 serotypes (b) Effective vaccine available (c) Presents with fever and joint pain (d) Virus belongs to *Flavivirus* genus (e) Contains segmented RNA

20) **Dengue is transmitted by**
(a) *Mansonia annulifera* (b) *Culex fatigans* (c) *Anopheles punctulatus* (d) *Aedes aegypti*

21) **Dengue haemorrhagic fever is caused by** (AI-09)
(a) Type I dengue virus (b) Reinfection with the same serotype of dengue virus (c) Reinfection with the different serotype of dengue virus (d) Infection is in the immunocompromised host

22) **Most virulent dengue fever strain is**
(a) 1 (b) 2 (c) 3 (d) 4

23) **In India, human infections has been reported with dengue virus type**
(a) Type 1 & 2 (b) Type 3 & 4 (c) Type 1 & 5 (d) Type 2 & 5

24) **Most sensitive diagnostic test for dengue is** (AIIMS, Nov-08)
(a) IgM ELISA (b) Complement fixation test (c) Neutralisation test (d) Electron microscopy

25) **Most specific for dengue diagnosis**
(a) IgM ELISA (b) Tissue culture (c) CFT (d) Electron microscopy

26) **Which of the following statement is true regarding arboviruses** (AI-04)
(a) Yellow fever is endemic in India (b) Dengue has only one serotype (c) Kyasanur Forest disease (KFD) is transmitted by

ticks (d) Mosquito of *Culex visnoi-complex* is the vector of dengue

Bunyaviridae

27) CCHF (Crimean Congo Haemorrhagic Fever) virus is belong to
(a) Flaviviridae family (b) Arenaviridae family (c) Togaviridae family (d) Bunyaviridae family

28) True about CCHF
(a) Zoonosis (b) Develop petechial rashes (c) Transmitted by mites (d) Recently disease has been reported in Gujarat (e) It has high fatality

Reoviridae

29) Which of the following viruses composed of two distinct capsids enclosing the double stranded RNA
(a) Adeno virus (b) Reo virus (c) Herpes virus (d) Myxo virus

Roboviruses

Hantavirus

30) All are true regarding *Hantavirus* except (AIIMS, Sept-96)
(a) DNA virus (b) Carried by rodents (c) Cause recurrent respiratory infection (d) Haemorrhagic manifestation may occur

31) True about *Hantavirus* (PGI-02)
(a) *Hantavirus* pulmonary syndrome (b) Transmitted by arthropod (c) Transmitted by rodents (d) Haemorrhagic fever with renal failure (e) *Hantavirus* pulmonary syndrome acquired from person to person

32) Hantaan virus (PGI-96)
(a) Is a DNA virus (b) Causes haemorrhagic fever with renal involvement (c) Belong to Retroviridae family (d) Person to person transmission

Answers of MCQs & explanation

1) (a), (b) & (c)
- Follow section, **arboviruses (classification & table-1)** for explanation
- RSV is paramyxovirus
- Puumala virus is robovirus **(table-2)**

2) (a), (b), (c)
- Follow section, **arboviruses (classification & table-1)** for explanation
- Hand foot mouth disease is caused by coxsackie virus
- Rocky mountain spotted fever is caused by *Rickettsia rickettsii*

3) (a), (d) & (e)
4) (a), (b) & (d)
5) (d)
6) (c)
7) (d)
8) (c)
} Follow section, **arboviruses (classification & table-1) & table-2** for explanation

9) (b)
- Follow section, **arboviruses (arboviruses found in India)** for explanation
- Lassa fever is robovirus & found in the Eastern Hemisphere in places such as Europe, Asia, and Africa

10) (a) & (d)
- Follow section, **arboviruses (Togaviridae → Chikungunya virus)** for explanation

11) (c) & (d)
- Option a, b & c: Follow section, **arboviruses (Flaviviridae → *Pegivirus*)** for explanation
- Lamivudine is reverse transcriptase inhibitor & useful in HBV & HIV.

12) (a) & (b)
13) (a) & (b)
14) (c)
} Follow section, **arboviruses [Flaviridae → Kyasanur Forest Disease (KFD) virus]** for explanation

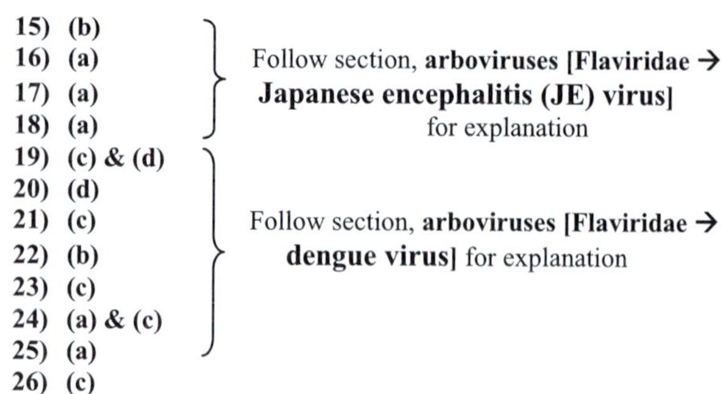

15) (b)
16) (a)
17) (a)
18) (a)
} Follow section, **arboviruses [Flaviridae → Japanese encephalitis (JE) virus]** for explanation

19) (c) & (d)
20) (d)
21) (c)
22) (b)
23) (c)
24) (a) & (c)
25) (a)
} Follow section, **arboviruses [Flaviridae → dengue virus]** for explanation

26) (c)
- Follow section, **arboviruses [Flaviviridae → Yellow fever virus, Dengue virus & Kyasanur Forest disease (KFD) virus]** for explanation

27) (d)
28) (a), (b) (d) & (e)
} Follow section, **arboviruses [Bunyaviridae → *Nairovirus* → Crimean Congo Haemorrhagic Fever (CCHF) virus]** for explanation.

29) (b)
- Follow section, **arboviruses (Reoviridae → morphology)** for explanation

30) (a)
31) (a), (c) & (d)
32) (b)
} Follow section, **roboviruses (Bunyaviridae → hantaan virus & sin Nombre virus)** for explanation

69 Rhabdoviridae

Learning heading & subheadings

- Meaning:
- Classification:

Lyssavirus

- Lyssa virus -1
- Lyssa virus -2
- Lyssa virus -3
- Lyssa virus -4
- Lyssa virus -5 & 6
- Lyssa virus -7

Meaning: Word derived from **rhabdos (Greek)** = **rod**, because of its **shape like rod (bullet).**

Classification:
- **Family:** Rhabdoviridae.
- **Genus:** Two genera.

A. *Lyssavirus*:
- Name derived from word **Lyssa (Greek)** = **rage** (violent / anger).
- Seven species or serotypes as shown in **table-1.**

Species	Common name	Isolated from
Lyssa virus-1	Rabies virus	Warm blood animals
Lyssa virus-2	Lagos bat or Natal bat virus	Bat/cat
Lyssa virus-3	Mokola virus	Cat/dog/human
Lyssa virus-4	Duvenhage virus	Human/bat
Lyssa virus-5	European bat-I virus	Bat/human
Lyssa virus-6	European bat-II virus	Bat/human
Lyssa virus-7	Australian bat virus	Bat/human

Table-1: Species or serotypes of *Lyssavirus*

B. *Vesiculovirus*: Follow chapter → Arboviruses and Roboviruses

Lyssavirus

Lyssa virus-1

- **Common name:** Rabies virus.
- **Meaning:** Rabies word came from **rabidus (Latin)** = **mad** (In Sanskrit **Rabhas**), indicating the features of disease produced by virus.
- **History:** All extant rabies viruses appear to have evolved within the last 1500 years.
- **Geographical distribution & genotypes:**
  - Mostly present in all countries but few countries are rabies free (no case in animal or human for 2 years) like Australia, Antarctica, Britain, Iceland, Ireland, China, Taiwan, Japan, Malta & New Zealand.
  - In India Andaman – Nicobar Islands & Lakshadweep are considered as rabies free.
  - There are 7 genotypes of rabies virus based on genomic sequence. Genotype 1 is present in Asia, Africa & Americas as a result of European exploration and colonization. In Eurasia cases, are due to three of these—genotype 1 & to a lesser extent genotypes 5 and 6.
- **Use:** Rabies virus is used in research for viral neuronal tracing to establish synaptic connections and directionality of synaptic transmission.
- **Morphology:** →**Fig.-1 & 2**

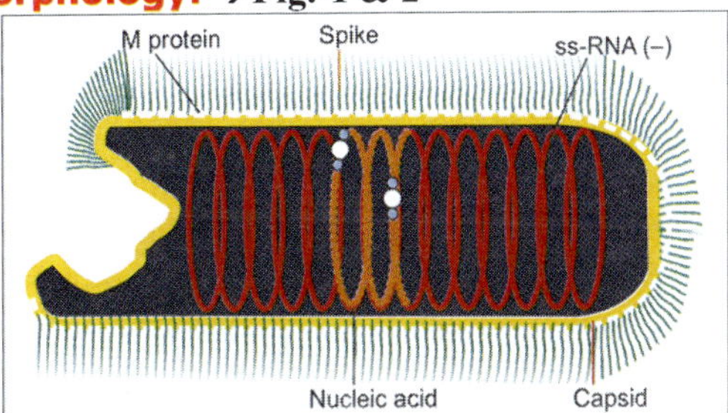

Figure-1: Schematic diagram of rabies virus

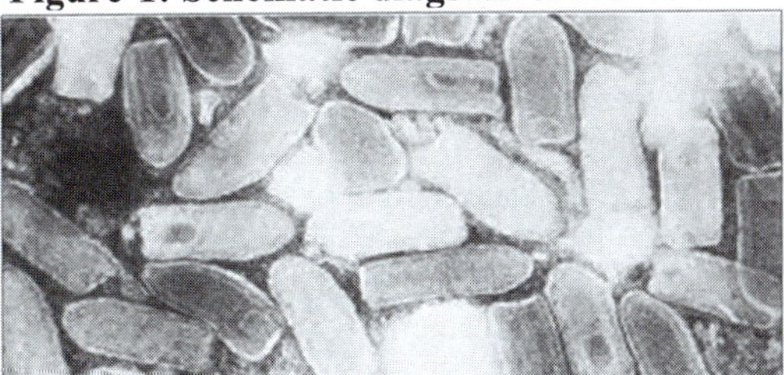

Figure-2: Microscopical image of rabies virus

- **Shape:** Bullet with one round or conical end & other end is concave or planar.
- **Size:** 100 nm in length & 70-75 nm in breadth.

- **Genome & capsid:**
- Single, linear ss-RNA (-) surrounded by helical capsid.
- Also presence of RNA dependent RNA polymerase.
- **Envelope:**
- Nucleocapsid is surrounded by bilayer envelop which consist inner protein **called matrix (M protein)** & outer lipid layer.
- M protein invaginated & also forms bleb at planar end.
- Envelop shows projecting glycoprotein spikes, which are absent at planar end.
- **Multiplication:** In cytoplasm.
- **Inclusion body:**

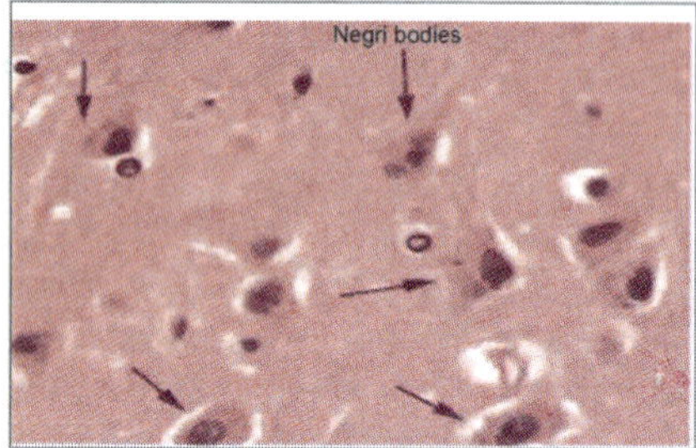

Figure-3: Negri bodies

- Detection of intracytoplasmic **Negri bodies** in brain tissues (cerebellum & hippocampus) & neurons. It present in Purkinje cells of cerebellum & pyramidal neurons of hippocampus & rare in cortical & brain stem neurons. Brain tissue is collected at post-mortem.
- Absent in 20% cases.
- Impression smear is stained with **Seller's technique** (basic fuchsin & methylene blue) & detection of intracytoplasmic inclusion bodies **called Negri bodies (fig.-3)** under light microscopy. Negri bodies are pathognomic of rabies.
- Name is given from the name of Adelchi Negri.
- Negri bodies are differentiated from other bodies like canine distemper virus inclusion bodies.
- It also stained by **Giemsa or Mann's method.**
- Negri bodies are composed of matrix protein & virus particles/antigens.
- Shape: Oval or spherical.
- Size: 3-27 μm.
- Purplish pink with basophilic granules.
- **Immuno fluorescent microscopy:** Useful as ante-mortem methods for diagnosis of rabies antigen from specimens like corneal scarping, saliva or skin biopsy from face or neck.

❖ Culture characteristics (C/Cs):

i. Egg culture:

- Grow in yolk sac of chick embryo.
- Serial passage attenuate the strain & used for vaccine production (**Flury & Kelev**).

ii. Animal culture:

- Experimental infection can be produced in all laboratory animals but mice are most useful.
- Produce fatal encephalitis in 5-30 days after intracerebral inoculation.
- Two types of viruses are demonstrated as shown in **table-2.**

Street virus	Fixed virus
Virus isolated from naturally infected human or animal **(natural rabies virus) called street virus**	After several serial intracerebral inoculation in rabbits, virus undergoes changes & such modified virus **(artificial rabies virus) called fixed virus**
Produce fatal encephalitis after long & variable incubation period of 1-12 weeks	Produce fatal encephalitis after short & fixed incubation period of 6-7 days
Affect the salivary gland	Do not affect the salivary gland
Less neurotropic	More neurotropic
More infectivity by any route	Less infectivity by route other than intracerebral (More neurotropic)
Forms the Negri body	Does not forms the Negri body
Not used for vaccine production	Used for vaccine production

Table-2: Differences between street virus & fixed virus

iii. Tissue culture:

- Grow in cells like Vero cells, WI-38, BHKP-21 & CER.
- Growth is identified by CPE, IF test (2-4 after inoculation) & neutralisation test.

❖ Resistance:

- **Inactivation:**
- Inactivated by heating at 50^0C in 1 hr & 60^0C in 5 minutes. It dies at room temperature but survive for weeks when stabilised by 50% glycerol. It survives at 4^0C for weeks.
- It also inactivated by phenol, formalin, Beta Propio Lactone (BPL), sunlight & UV radiation.
- **Sensitivity:**
- Enveloped virus sensitive to lipid solvents like ether, chloroform & acetone.
- It also sensitive to ethanol, iodine, quaternary ammonium compound, soap & detergents.
- **Preservation:**
- Preserved at -70^0C or by lyophilisation.
- For storage in dry ice, the virus has to be sealed in vials, as it is inactivated to CO_2 exposure.

❖ Antigenic structure: Lyssa virus -1 (rabies virus) is a single species & it has no any serotype or strain.

- **Spikes (glycoprotein) Ag:**

- It mediates the binding of virus with Ach (Acetylcholine) receptors in neural tissue.
- Induce the synthesis of haemagglutination inhibition (HAI) Ab.
- Induces protective virus neutralizing antibody.
- Stimulates cytotoxic T- cell immunity.
- It is serotype (species) specific-Ag.
- Used to prepare the subunit vaccine.

➢ **Nucleic acid Ag:**
- Induce complement fixing Ab.
- Ab is not protective.
- It is group specific-Ag.
- Antibody is used for immuno fluorescent test.

➢ **Other Ags:** Includes two membrane proteins, glycolipid & RNA dependent RNA polymerase.

❖ **Immunity:** Antibodies to spike antigens are protective while to nucleic acid antigens are not protective.

❖ **Pathogenicity:**

I. In animal:

➢ **Disease name: Called rabies.**

➢ **Incubation period:** 3-6 weeks (range from 10 days to a year).

➢ **Clinical features:**

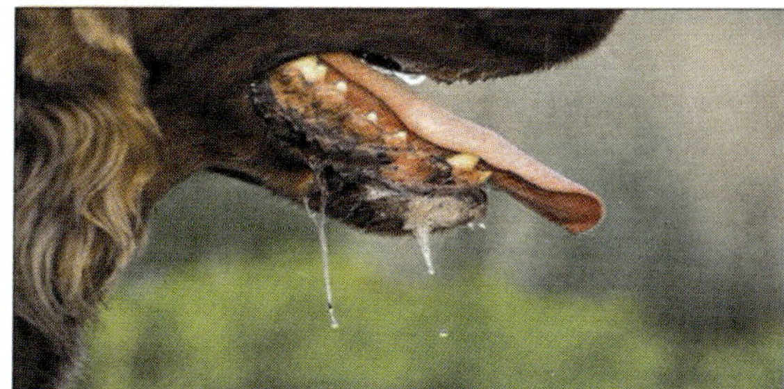

Figure-4: Rabies in dog (dribbling of saliva from mouth)

- **Prodromal phase:**
- Animal become restlessness.
- Snapping at imaginary object.
- Licking or gnawing at the site of bite.
- **Disease phase:** Develop in furious rabies or dumb rabies.

o Furious rabies (mad dog syndrome):
- Dog runs amok, biting without provocation & indiscriminately.
- Dropping of lower jaw & dribbling of saliva from mouth as shown in **fig.-4.**
- Paralysis & convulsion.

o Dumb rabies (paralytic rabies):
- It is the paralytic form in which the animal lies huddled, unable to feed.
- Dog may not bite, but attempt to feed are dangerous.
- It is infectious.
- In 60% cases virus shed in saliva.
- Animal die in 3-5 day.

II. In human:

➢ **Disease name: Called hydrophobia** word came from two words **hydro = water + phobia = fear**, as patients feels inability/fear to drink water. In animal there is no feature of hydrophobia.

➢ **Nature or history of disease:**
- It is enzootic & epizootic in wild & domestic animals.
- It is endemic in >150 countries.
- 55,000 deaths occurs per year in rural areas of Asia & Africa.
- In India it accounts 20,000 deaths per year.

➢ **Reservoir of infection:** Two types of animal reservoirs like
- **Domestic animals:** Dogs, cats & cattle.
- **Wild animals:** Jackals, wolves, foxes, bats, mongooses & skunks.

➢ **Source of infection:** Virus is present in saliva of dog. Dog become infective 3-4 days before the onset of symptoms in to it.

➢ **Mode of transmission:**
- **By bite:**
- Urban area: By bite of infected animal like dog or cats.
- Sylvatic (wild) area: By bite of wild animal like jackals wolves, foxes, mongoose, shunks & bats.
- **Non-biting exposure:**
- Airborne transmission from aerosols generated from infected bats.
- Corneal transplants: Human to human transmission is not possible or rare. A case has been reported due to corneal transplantation from unknown case of rabies virus infection. A case of child biting to parents also on record.
- It is present in human saliva but not infectious to human, so no danger to deal with patient.
- Lick on abrasion of skin or mucosa.
- **Natural cycle:** Following two cycles.

1. **Cycle in mustelids & viverrids:** From mustelids & viverrids, it transfer to wild animals like wolves, jackals, wolves & later shift to domestic animals like dog, cat etc.
2. **Cycle in bat:**
- Present in vampire bats (asymptomatic), insectivorous bats (symptomatic) & furgivorous bats (asymptomatic).
- It remains in respiratory system (pneumotropic) & transmitted to human (neurotropic) or animals (neurotropic) by aerosols from bats.
- Human infection is mostly by visiting the caves colonised by infected bats.

➢ **Incubation period:**
- 1-3 months; however it is short up to weeks or long up to year depending on the site of bite, numbers of wounds, species of biting animal, severity of bite,

amount of virus injected, protection provided by clothing & treatment taken.

- Incubation period is short: When bite is
  - On head, face or upper extremities, less distance from brain.
  - By wild animal.
  - Severe.
  - In children.
- Incubation period is long.
  - When bite is on legs.
  - In adults.

➢ **Portal of entry:** Skin or mucosa.

➢ **Site:** Brain (cerebellum & hippocampus), spinal cord & neurons. Enter very rapidly (centrifugal spread) along the sensory & autonomic nerves to various part including salivary glands, kidneys, heart & retina without the stage of viraemia.

➢ **Precipitating factors (epidemiological determinants):**

1. **Age:** Occurs at any age but patients with 5-15 years of age are at more risk.
2. **Occupations:** Laboratory workers, veterinarians, dog handlers, hunters & field / forest workers are at high risk.
3. **Locations:** Rabies is mostly by bite of domestic animals, however in USA it is due to bite by wild animals.

➢ **Pathogenesis: → Flow chart-1**

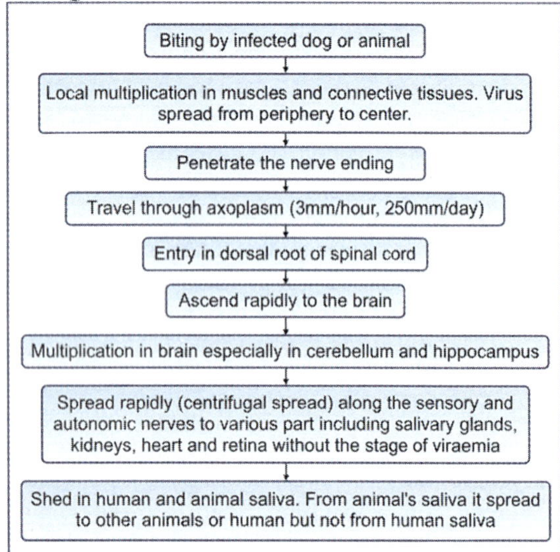

Flow chart-1: Pathogenesis of rabies virus

➢ **Clinical features:**

- **Prodromal phase:** Last for 2-4 days & present with following features.
  - Fever, malaise, headache, fatigue & anorexia.
  - Pain or paresthesia & fasciculation at the site of virus entry.
  - Apprehension, anxiety, agitation, irritability, nervousness, insomnia & depression.
  - Excessive libido, priapism & spontaneous ejaculation.
- **Acute encephalitis phase:**
  - Bizarre behavior (hyperactivity), agitation or seizures between normal periods. It is spontaneous or precipitated by external stimuli.
  - Hydrophobia in spite of intense thirst.
  - Attempt of drinking brings painful spasm of larynx or pharynx producing choking or gagging.
  - Generalised convulsion.
  - Encephalitis is very severe which may involve rhombecephalon (brain stem-mid brain & floor of the fourth ventricle in the medulla), basal ganglia, spinal cord & dorsal root ganglia.
  - Intracytoplasmic **Negri bodies** present in neurons & brain tissues (cerebellum & hippocampus).
- **Coma:**
- **Death:** Death occurs within 1-6 days due to respiratory failure. However, death is almost certain (100% mortality) & recovery with survival is almost rare.

❖ Laboratory diagnosis:

I. In animal:

➢ **Indications:**

- To assess the risk of infection.
- To decide the post exposure prophylaxis.

➢ **Specimens:**

- Animal carcass like salivary glands.
- Severed head.
- Brain (including cerebellum & hippocampus for Negri bodies) in two portion.

1. In 50% glycerol saline.
2. Zenker's fixative.

➢ **Testing methods:**

A. **Microscopy: → Follow morphology.**
B. **Culture: → Follow C/Cs.**
C. **Serology:** Ag detection by immunofluorescent test.

II. In human:

➢ **Indication:** Rabies diagnosis in human is based on clinical ground & laboratory help is required to differentiate from other cause of encephalitis.

➢ **Specimens:**

- **Ante-mortem specimens:** Corneal scraping, saliva, CSF or skin biopsy from face or neck.
- **Post-mortem specimens:** Brain biopsy (cerebellum & hippocampus).

➢ **Testing methods:**

A. **Microscopy: → Follow morphology.**
B. **Culture: → Follow C/Cs.**
C. **Serological test:**

- **Ab detection tests:** Ab detection from CSF is more useful than serum. It developed early in CSF following infection but not by immunisation. It developed late in serum following infection & immunisation.

- Antibody is diagnosed by ELISA, indirect fluorescent antibody test, rapid fluorescent focus inhibition test, CFT, HAI & neutralisation test.
- **Ag detection tests:** Ag is detected by immunofluorescent microscopy from corneal scarping, saliva or skin biopsy from face or neck.

D. Molecular methods: RT- PCR from saliva or brain tissue is rapid & more sensitive method.

❖ Prevention:

I. In animal:

- Post exposure prophylaxis & neural vaccine are not generally useful.
- Single dose of cell culture vaccine is given by IM route at 12 weeks of age provide protection for 3 years.
- Repeat the dose at an interval of every 3 year.

II. In human:

➢ **Pre-exposure prophylaxis:** Vaccine is ideally given before exposure.

✪ **Indications:** In persons who are at risk like

- Veterinarians.
- Dog handlers.
- Rabies research laboratory workers.

✪ **Vaccine:** Human diploid cell culture vaccine is safe & effective.

✪ **Vaccination schedule:**

- Three doses are given on days 0, 7 & 21/28 or 0, 28 & 56 by IM or by ID route.
- Antibody titre should be checked every 6 months for 2 year & there after every 2 year. Booster dose is given if titre falls < 0.5IU/ml (or after 1 year & then every 5 year).

➢ **Post exposure prophylaxis:** It is considered as anti-rabies treatment.

✪ **Indications:**

- In persons bitten or scratched or licked by an animal which is rabid (shows sign of rabies) or cannot be identified/traced.
- Animal dies within 10 days of observation.
- All bites by wild animals, as wild animals are difficult to trace.
- Unprovoked bites.
- All laboratory test of animal are positive for rabies.

✪ **Steps:** It includes local treatment, animal observation & immunisation.

Local treatment

- **Advantage:** It reduces the 80% chances of development of rabies.
- **Treatment:**

- Prompt cauterisation destroys the virus.
- Wash bite area with soap &water.
- Disinfection of wound with quaternary ammonium (cetavlon) compound, 0.1% benzalkonium chloride, iodine or by 70% ethanol.
- Rabies antiserum around skin of bite area.
- Vaccinate with human diploid cell culture vaccine immediately.
- Tetanus antiserum.
- Antibiotics.
- Post-pone the wound suturing: Suturing should not be done immediately, as it allows the virus spread in deeper tissues. If necessary, it should be done 24-48 hours later, applying minimum possible stitches & under cover of anti-rabies serum locally.

Animal observation

Observe the animal for 10 days. If animal survive then discontinue the vaccine.

Immunisation

It includes the active immunisation & passive immunisation as follows.

A. Active immunisation:

☑ **Types of vaccines:** Two types of vaccines.

i. Neural vaccines:

♣ **Disadvantages:** Serious risk with neurological complication, so no longer in use. Originally it was developed by Louis Pasteur & modified later.

♣ **Types of neural vaccine:**

a. Semple vaccine (sheep brain vaccine):

- **History:** Developed by Semple in 1911 at Central Research Institute, Kasauli, India. It was widely used over half a century.
- **Preparation:** It is inactivated vaccine prepared from 5% suspension of sheep brain infected with fixed virus & inactivated with phenol at 37^0C.

b. Beta Propio Lactone (BPL) vaccine:

- **History:** It is a modified Semple vaccine.
- **Preparation:** It is inactivated by BPL instead of phenol.
- **Advantages:**

- More antigenic.
- Small dose is effective.

c. Suckling (infant) mouse brain vaccine:

- **Preparation:**

- Encephalitogenic factor is absent or less in non-myelinated neural tissue of new born animals. It is the basis for this vaccine.
- Vaccine is prepared from brain of infant mouse, rabbit or rat.

- **Disadvantages:**

- Occasionally produce neurological reaction.
- Not used in India, because required large quantities.

ii. Non-neural vaccines:

♣ **Advantages:** No neurological complication.

♣ **Types of non-neural vaccines:** Three types like egg derived vaccines, tissue (cell) culture vaccine & subunit (recombinant) vaccine.

a. **Egg derived vaccines:** Vaccines are prepared following allantoic cavity inoculation. Two subtypes as follows

1. **Inactivated (purified) duck egg vaccine:**

- **Preparation:** Prepared from fixed virus grown in duck egg & inactivated by BPL. Duck egg is larger & provides more yield than hens's egg.
- **Disadvantages:** Less immunogenic & required multiple doses about 16-25 to obtain desired antibody response hence no longer in use.

2. **Live attenuated chick embryo (hen's egg) vaccine:**

- **Preparation:** Two types of preparation by using **Flury strain.**
  - Low egg passage: At 40-45 egg passage for dogs.
  - High egg passage: At 180 egg passage for cats & cattle.

✓ **Notes: Egg culture vaccines**

- **Live attenuated / non- neurotropic vaccine / 17D vaccine of yellow fever virus:** It is prepared by Theiler in 1937 in allantoic cavity of chick embryo from **Asibi strain**. In India it is prepared in Central Research Institute, Kasauli.
- **Live attenuated vaccine of influenza virus:** It is prepared from natural virus by serial egg passage.
- **Live attenuated vaccine of mumps virus:** Vaccines contain **Jeryl-Lynn strain** that has been attenuated by egg passage & grow in chick embryo fibroblast cell culture.
- **Egg derived vaccines of rabies virus:** Above two vaccines.

b. **Tissue (cell) culture vaccines:** Three subtypes as follows. These vaccines are most potent, required less number of doses, low cost & few side effects hence most recommended & also currently used in India.

1. **Human diploid cell culture vaccine (HDCV):**

- **History:** Developed by Koprowsky, Wiktor & Plotkin.
- **Preparation:** Prepared from fixed virus (**Pitman Moore strain**) grown on human diploid cells (WI 38 or MRC 5) & inactivated (killed) by BPL or by tri-n-butyl phosphate.
- **Advantages:**
  - Highly immunogenic & effective.
  - Free from side effect (safe).
- **Disadvantages:** High cost.

2. **Purified chick embryo cell culture (fibroblast) vaccine:**

- **Preparation:** Prepared by growing the virus on chick embryo fibroblast cell culture.
- **Advantages:**
  - Highly immunogenic & effective.
  - Free from side effect (safe).
  - Low cost.
  - Recommended by WHO.

3. **Purified Vero cell vaccine:**

- **Preparation:** Prepared by growing the virus on Vero cell culture.
- **Advantages:**
  - Highly immunogenic & effective.
  - Free from side effect (safe).
  - Low cost.

c. **Subunit (recombinant) vaccine:**

- **Preparation:**
  - Prepared from recombinant glycoprotein-Ag present on surface, which is protective.
  - It is given orally. It is used successfully in animals but still under trial for human use.

☑ **WHO guidelines for post-exposure prophylaxis:** → **Table-3**

Category of risk	Type of exposure	Severity	Prophylaxis
I (No risk)	Touching, feeding or licks on intact skin	None	Not required
II (Minor risk)	Licks on broken skin, scratches or abrasions without bleeding	Minor	- Wound treatment - Vaccine - Observe the animal for 10 days
III (Major risk)	- Transdermal bites or scratches, licks on broken skin - Bites by wild animal	Severe	- Wound treatment - Ig - Vaccine, discontinue if animal survive after 10 days

Table-3: WHO guidelines for post-exposure prophylaxis

✓ **Notes: Best practise**

- It is now well established that irrespective of class of wound, the combined administration of single dose of anti-rabies serum, full course of vaccine & local treatment of the wound is considered as the best post exposure prophylaxis of rabies.
- In India, post exposure prophylaxis is indicated following exposure to any animal bite except rat.

☑ **Vaccination schedule (of tissue / cell culture vaccine):** Two regimes like IM & ID abbreviated in **flow chart-2.**

- **Essen or IM regime** (1-1-1-1-1)**:** By intramuscular (IM) route.
  - 0.5-1ml.
  - Five-six doses are given on days 0, 3, 7, 14, 30 & 90 (last dose is optional in patient receiving Ig). 0 indicate the date of 1st dose not the date of animal bite.
  - Same dose for children & adults.
- **ID regime (Thai Red Cross Schedule):** By intradermal (ID) route.
  - 0.1ml

Notes:

- To abbreviate the regime remember the days, as 0,3,7,14,28/30 and 90
- No = No injection

Days	0	3	7	14	28/30	90	Regime
Sites	1	1	1	1	1	optional	1-1-1-1-1(IM)
2-Sites	2	2	2	No	2	No	2-2-2-0-2(ID)
8-Sites	8	No	4	No	1	1	8-0-4-0-1-1(ID)

Flow chart-2: Regimes of rabies vaccine

- 2 sites ID schedule: Two injections (two different sites) of reconstituted vaccine on days 0, 3, 7 & 28 **called 2-2-2-0-2** or **2-2-2-2 regime** or **two sites ID schedule.**
- 8 sites ID schedule: Vaccine is given at 8 sites on day 0 followed by injection at 4 sites on day 7 & single injection on days 28 & 90 **called 8-0-4-0-1-1** or **eight sites ID schedule.**

☑ **Sites:** Directly in muscle by IM route & intradermally over the muscle by ID route.

- In deltoid region.
- Anterolateral aspect of the thigh: In infants or young children.
- Avoid the gluteal region, as it is less immunogenic due to presence of gluteal fat which delayed the presentation of vaccine's antigens to Antigen Presenting Cells (APCs).

☑ **Vaccine failure:**

- Occur in spite of full course of vaccination.
- It is common with neural vaccine.
- Rare with local treatment of wound followed by full course of vaccination by human diploid cell culture vaccine along with Ig.
- Due to safety of human diploid cell culture vaccine it is advisable to use it.

☑ **Post exposure prophylaxis in immunised person:** Vaccine provides protection for five year. Re-vaccination depends on the severity of wound bite & antibody titre.

- Severe bite & titre unknown: Three doses on 0, 3 & 7 days.
- Less severe bite & titre > 0.5IU/ml: Two doses on 0 & 3 days.

B. Passive immunisation:

☑ **Two types of Ig:**

a. Equine rabies Ig:

- **Preparation:**
- Prepared from hyperimmune horse.
- Two types of preparation.

1. **Crude preparation:** Risk of anaphylaxis.
2. **Purified preparation:** Low risk.

b. Human rabies Ig:

- **Disadvantages:**
- Less availability.
- High cost.
- **Advantage:** Free from risk.
- **Administration:**
- Ig is given before or along with vaccine.
- 20 IU/kg of body weight.
- Half dose is given at wound site & half in gluteal region.

❖ **Treatment:**

- No specific anti-rabies treatment is available except sedation.
- It was reported that complete recovery occurred from established case of rabies after supportive measure & treatment of complication.

❖ **World rabies day:** It is celebrated on 28th Sept of every year which is the anniversary of the death of Louis Pasteur who with his colleagues developed the 1st effective rabies vaccine.

Lyssa virus-2

❖ **Common name:** Lagos bat virus or Natal bat virus.

❖ **History:** Was isolated from the pooled brain of frugivovorus bats from Lagos Island, Nigeria in 1956.

❖ **Pathogenicity:** Produce rabies like illness after intracerebral inoculation & produce Negri bodies in brain of monkey but not mice or dogs.

Lyssa virus-3

❖ **Common name:** Mokola virus.

❖ **History:**

- Virus was isolated from shrews capture near Ibadan, Nigeria in 1968.
- Also found in wild & domestic animals in Africa in later part.
- Also recovered from two children, one of them is died.
- Antibody identified from a case acquired laboratory infection.

Lyssa virus-4

❖ **Common name:** Duvenhage virus.

❖ **History:** Virus was isolated from the brain of man died due to clinical rabies in Africa after being bitten by bat.

Lyssa virus-5 & 6

❖ **Common name:** European bat virus-I & European bat virus –II respectively.

❖ **History:**
- Virus was isolated from European bat hence the name.
- Can infect the human.

Lyssa virus-7

❖ **Common name:** Australian bat virus.

❖ **History:**
- Australia was free from rabies or related viruses till 1996, but then after virus was isolated from Australian bat hence the name.
- Can infect the human who are in contact with bats.

Question bank

Case study

1) A 35 year old male is brought to the hospital with fever & anorexia since 4 days. Relative informed that person is occupationally forest workers & before 3 months he was bitten by wild animal. At that time he took only treatment of local wound & no any vaccine was taken. On clinical examination it was ruled out that patient is feeling difficulty in drinking the liquid. Later he developed convulsion. Convulsion becomes generalised & patient died. Brain biopsy is collected during post-mortem & sent to referral laboratory for histo-pathological study, which reported the Negri bodies in brain tissue. Identify the clinical conditions & answer the following

a) Name the clinical condition & its etiological agent.
b) What is the cause of death in given clinical condition?
c) Write the morphology of etiological agent
d) Write pathogenicity of clinical condition
e) How you can treat the disease, if any patient came immediately to hospital following animal bite.

Essay/Full question

1) Rhabdoviridae
2) Rabies virus

Short notes

1) Pathogenicity by rabies virus in human
2) Rabies vaccine

Short questions for theory/viva questions

1) Name the four factors effective over the incubation period in rabies
2) Mention the common sites for presence of Negri body in rabies
3) Name two artificial viruses
4) Write the two examples of each, neural & non-neural vaccine of rabies virus.
5) Write the taxonomical & genomic differences between lassa fever virus & lyssa virus
6) Name the four viruses in which vaccines are prepared by using eggs or egg culture.
7) Comment: Immediate suturing of wound in rabies, following animal bite is not advised.

MCQs for chapter review

Lyssa virus-1

1) **Which of the following statement is true about rabies virus** (AI,-03)
(a) It is double stranded RNA virus (b) Contains a DNA - dependent - RNA – polymerase (c) RNA has a negative polarity (d) Affects motor neurons
2) **Following statements are true about Negri bodies except**
(a) They are pathognomic of rabies (b) They are found in brain (c) They are cytoplasmic inclusion bodies (d) They do not contain rabies virus antigen
3) **Staining useful for ante-mortem diagnosis of rabies is**
(a) Seller (b) Macchiacillo (c) Giemsa (d) Fluorescent
4) **Negri bodies are found in** (AI-96)
(a) Hypothalamus (b) Hippocampus (c) Mid brain (d) Medulla
5) **Antirabies vaccine is prepared by**
(a) Street virus (b) Fixed virus (c) Line virus (d) Wild virus
6) **About rabies true is** (PGI, Dec-06)
(a) Vaccine causes lifelong immunity (b) Multiple strain are found (c) CNS infection occurs through viraemia (d) Bullet shaped non-enveloped, double stranded RNA virus
7) **True about rabies virus is** (AIIMS, May-94, AI-97)
(a) Rabies is diagnosed by immunofluorescence (b) Rabies causes lifelong immunity (c) Rabies has various strains of viruses (d) Rabies vaccine is always live attenuated
8) **Rabies virus is inactivated by** (PGI-97)
(a) Phenol (b) UV radiation (c) BPL (d) All
9) **Speed of rabies virus in axon is?**
(a) 1 mm per hour (b) 3 mm per hour (c) 5 mm per hour (d) 7 mm per hour
10) **Street rabies virus causes**
(a) Natural rabies (b) Laboratory passage in rabbit (c) Fatal encephalitis in 6 days (d) Negri bodies not seen
11) **Regarding rabies, true is** (AI-00)
(a) Incubation period depends on the site of bite (b) Diagnosis is by eosinophilic intranuclear inclusion (c) It is a RNA virus (d) Caused only by dogs
12) **In rabies the characteristic pathological manifestation is** (AI-97)
(a) Ventriculitis (b) Brain stem encephalitis (c) Basal ganglia affection (d) Meningitis
13) **A 15 year old girl was admitted to the infectious disease hospital with a provisional diagnosis of rabies, The most suitable clinical specimen that can confirm the antemortem diagnosis is** (AIIMS, Nov-04)
(a) Serum for anti-rabies IgG antibody (b) Corneal impression smear for immunofluorescence (c) CSF sample for viral culture (d) Giemsa stain on smear
14) **Rabies virus**
(a) Can be isolated from the blood of infected patients (b) Has multiple antigenic types (c) Can be transmitted by dog 4 weeks before the dog becomes noticeably ill (d) Produce infection that is almost fatal to humans
15) **Neurological complication following rabies vaccine is common with**
(a) HDCV (b) Chick embryo vaccine (c) Semple vaccine (d) Duck egg vaccine
16) **All of the following rabies vaccines are commercially available except** (AI-99)
(a) Killed sheep brain vaccine (b) Human diploid cell vaccine (c) Vero continuous cell vaccine (d) Recombinant glycoprotein
17) **For the treatment of case of class–II dog bite, all of the following are correct except**
(a) Give Ig for passive vaccine (b) Give ARV (c) Immediate stitch wound under antibiotic cover (d) Immediately wash wound with soap and water
18) **All are true of rabies except** (AIIMS-92)
(a) 100% mortality (b) Spreads from periphery (c) Infects only the brain (d) Prophylactic immunisation of people at risk
19) **For the treatment of case of class–III dog bite, all of the following are correct except** (AI-05)

(a) Give Ig for passive vaccine (b) Give ARV (c) Immediate stitch wound under antibiotic cover (d) Immediately wash wound with soap and water

20) **Vaccines prepared by embryonated hen's eggs are** (PGI-04)
(a) Measles (b) Rabies (c) Rubella (d) Varicella

21) **All vaccines developed from embryonated eggs except** (PGI, May-13)
(a) Influenza (b) Hepatitis A (c) Yellow fever (d) Rabies (e) CMV

22) **Numbers of doses of HDCV required for pre-exposure prophylaxis** (AI-97)
(a) 7 (b) 5 (c) 3 (d) 1

23) **Type of vaccine available commercially for rabies are all except**
(a) Inactivated sheep brain vaccine (b) Genetically engineered glycoprotein vaccine (c) Duck embryo vaccine (d) HDCV

24) **Recommended vaccine for rabies**
(a) Semple (b) Duck embryo vaccine (c) Suckling mouse brain vaccine (d) HDCV

25) **Which anti-rabies vaccine has been recommended by WHO**
(a) Duck cell vaccine (b) Chick fibroblast vaccine (c) HDCV (d) Sheep brain vaccine

26) **The schedule of HDCV in rabies is** (AI-96)
(a) 0, 3, 7, 14 & 28 (b) 0, 3, 10 & 30 (c) 3, 7, 14, 16 & 18 (d) 0, 7, 14, 16 & 18

27) **In rabies, human diploid cell culture vaccine for post exposure vaccination is given on the following days.** (AI-98)
(a) 0, 7, 28 then booster dose in 90 days (b) 0, 7, 28 then booster dose in 2 years (c) 0, 3, 7, 14, 28 then booster dose in 90 days (d) 0, 3, 7 and booster dose in 90 days

28) **Schedule of intradermal rabies vaccine is**
(a) 2-2-0-1-0-1 (b) 8-0-4-0-1-1 (c) 8-4-4-1-0-1 (d) 2-0-2-0-1-1

29) **What is the correct recommended schedule (on days) for post-exposure treatment of person who has been vaccinated for rabies previously with HDC**
(a) 0, 3 and 7 (b) 0, 3, 7 and 14 (c) 0, 3, 7, 14 and 28 (d) 0 and 3

30) **Sites for injection of cell culture rabies vaccine**
(a) Gluteus (b) Subcutaneous (c) Deltoid (d) Anterior abdominal wall

Answers of MCQs & explanation

1) (c)
2) (d)
3) (d)
4) (b)

} Follow section, **Lyssa virus -1 (morphology)** for explanation

5) **(b)**
- Follow section, **Lyssa virus -1 [culture characteristics (C/Cs) → table-2]** for explanation.

6) **(d) Partially correct**
7) **(a)**

} **Explained below** ↓

- Vaccine provide immunity for 5 years
- Only species no any strain/serotype or subspecies found in rabies virus
- CNS infection occurs without viraemia
- Bullet shaped, enveloped, ss RNA (-) virus
- Rabies is diagnosed by Ag detection from cornea, saliva or skin biopsy from face or neck by immunofluorescence

8) **(d)**
- Follow section, **Lyssa virus -1 (resistance)** for explanation

9) **(b)**
- Follow section, **Lyssa virus -1** (pathogenicity **→pathogenesis → flow chart-1)** for explanation

10) **(a)**
- Follow section, **Lyssa virus -1 [culture characteristics (C/Cs) → animal culture & table-2]** for explanation

11) **(a) & (c)**
- Follow section, **Lyssa virus -1 [pathogenicity → incubation period]** for explanation of option a & morphology for explanation of option c
- Diagnosis is by eosinophilic intracytoplasmic not intranuclear inclusion
- Caused by dog & also by bite of other animal

12) **(b) & (c)**
- Follow section, **Lyssa virus -1 (pathogenicity → clinical features → acute encephalitis phase)** for explanation

13) **(b)**
- Follow section, **Lyssa virus -1 (laboratory diagnosis)** for explanation

14) **(d)**
- Rabies virus
  - Spread via nerves, so can't be isolated from the blood of infected patients
  - Has only one type
  - Can be transmitted by dog 3-4 days before the dog becomes noticeably ill
  - Produce infection that is almost fatal to humans

15) **(c)**
- Neurological complications are common following neural type (like Semple vaccine) of rabies vaccine. Follow section, **Lyssa virus -1 (prevention → in human → immunisation)** for explanation.

16) **(d)**
- Recombinant glycoprotein is still under trial for human use. Follow section, **Lyssa virus -1 (prevention → in human → immunisation)** for explanation.

17) **(a) & (c)**
- Follow section, **Lyssa virus -1 (prevention → table-3)** for explanation.

18) **(c)**
- For options a, b & c follow section, **Lyssa virus-1 (pathogenicity)** & for options d follow section, **Lyssa virus-1 prevention → in human → Pre-exposure prophylaxis → indications)** for explanation.

19) **(c)**
20) **(b)**
21) **(b) & (c)**
22) **(c)**
23) **(b)**
24) **(d)**
25) **(b)**
26) **(a)**
27) **(c)**
28) **(b)**
29) **(a)**
30) **(c)**

} Tissue /cell culture vaccine are most recommended for use. Follow section, **Lyssa virus -1 (prevention → in human → immunisation)** for explanation.

70 Retroviridae

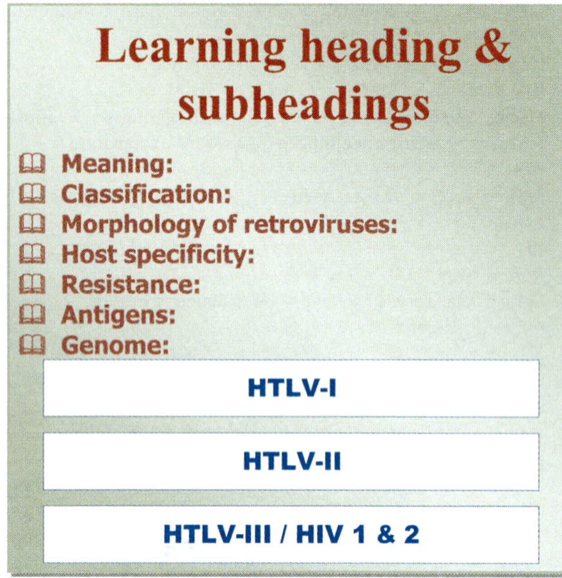

Learning heading & subheadings
Meaning:
Classification:
Morphology of retroviruses:
Host specificity:
Resistance:
Antigens:
Genome:
HTLV-I
HTLV-II
HTLV-III / HIV 1 & 2

Meaning: Retro word derived from **retro = reverse** because having enzyme reverse transcriptase (**RNA dependent DNA polymerase**).

Classification:

- **Family:** Retroviridae.
- **Subfamily:** Two subfamilies.

I. **Spumaretrovirinae:**

- **Meaning:** Spuma = foam.
- **Contains:** 'Foamy viruses' causing asymptomatic infection in animals.
- **Genus & species:**

A. **Spumavirus:** Simian foamy virus& human foamy virus.

II. **Orthoretrovirinae:** Following are the genera & respective species.

A *Alpharetrovirus*: Avian leukosis virus & Rous sarcoma virus.

B *Betaretrovirus*: Mouse mammary tumour virus. (**Bittner's milk factor**)

C *Gammaretrovirus*: Murine leukemia virus & feline leukemia virus.

D *Deltaretrovirus*:

i. **Animal species:** Bovine leukemia virus.

ii. **Human species:**

1. Human T-cell Lymphotropic Virus-I (HTLV-I):
   - Causing T cell leukemia, tropical spastic paresis & demyelinating disease.
2. Human T-cell Lymphotropic Virus-II (HTLV-II):
   - Causing T cell leukemia

E *Epsilonretrovirus*: Walleye dermal sarcoma virus.

F *Lentivirus*:

- **Meaning:** Lenti = Slow because causing slow virus diseases.
- **Species:**

i. **Species causing slow viral diseases in animals:**

a. **Visna virus or visna-maedi virus or maedi-visna virus or ovine lenti virus:**

- **Disease name:** Two types of disease in sheep.

1. **Visna:**
   - **Called visna** when infecting the brain in sheep. Demyelinating disease of sheep was identified in 1935 & eradicated in 1951 by slaughtering the all animals.
   - **Incubation period:** About 2 years.
   - **C/Fs:** Paresis & paralysis followed by death.
2. **Maedi:**
   - **Called maedi** when infecting the lungs in sheep.
   - **Incubation period:** About 2-3 years.
   - **C/Fs:** Fatal haemorrhagic pneumonia in sheep.

b. **Caprine arthritis encephalitis virus:** Arthritis.

c. **Equine infectious anaemia virus:** Anaemia.

ii. **Species causing Immuno deficiency Disease (IDD):**

a. **In primates:**

1. **Animal:**

- **Simian Immunodeficiency Virus (SIV):** Causing Simian-AIDS (S-AIDS).
  - Types of SIV: Isolated from
  - Chimpanzee **called SIV-CPZ** (like HIV-1).
  - Sooty-Mangabeys **called SIV-SM** (like HIV-2).
  - Rhesus-Macaque **called SIV-MAC** (like HIV-2).

2. **Human:**

- **Human immunodeficiency virus (HIV):** Causing Human-AIDS (H-AIDS).

Features	HIV-1	HIV-2
Origin	1st indication in 1981, USA	In 1986, West Africa
Distribution	World-wide & in India	West Africa & few report from western & southern India
Origin for human infection	Chimpanzees (*Pan troglodytes troglodytes*)	Sooty Mangabey monkeys (*Cercocebus atys*)
Virulence	More	Less
Spread	Rapid	Slow
Resembles to SIV	Less	More
vpu gene	Present	Absent
vpx gene	Absent	present
Envelope Ags	gp120 & gp41	gp36

Table-1: Differences between HIV-1 & HIV-2

- o <u>Types of HIV</u>: Two main types based on molecular & antigenic variation like
- HIV-1.
- HIV-2.
- o <u>Similarities between HIV-1 & HIV-2</u>:
- Envelope Ags of both types are different (**follow table-1**), but cross-reactivity occurs between nucleocapsid-Ags.
- HIV-2 has 40% genetic identity with HIV-1.

<u>Differences between HIV-1 & HIV-2</u>: →**Table-1**

b. In non-primates:

1. **Animal:** Feline T-cell Lymphotropic Virus (FTLV) which cause Feline-AIDS (F-AIDS).

Morphology of retroviruses:

- **Shape:** Spherical.
- **Size:** 100nm.
- **Genome & capsid:**
  - Two identical ss-RNA (+) with enzyme reverse transcriptase (**RNA dependent DNA polymerase**).
  - Genome surrounded by double shell, icosahedral variety of capsid.
  - Inner shell is cone shape & contains genome.
- **Envelope:** It contains lipoproteins envelope.

Host specificity:

Three categories of retroviruses depending on their nature to infect host cells.

1. **Ectotropic:** Multiplying in the cells of native host species.
2. **Amphotropic:** Multiplying in the cells of native & foreign species.
3. **Xenotropic:** Multiplying in the cells foreign species but not in the native species.

Resistance:

- **Inactivated by**
  - Heating 56^{0}C in 30 min.
  - Mild acids.
  - Ether.
  - Formalin.
- **Stable:** At -30^{0}C.

Antigens:

Two types.

1. **Type specific:** Present on envelop.
2. **Group specific:** Present on nucleocapsid.

Genome:

Three genomes.

1. **gag:** Encodes for nucleocapsid proteins (antigens).
2. **pol:** Encodes for enzyme RNA dependent DNA polymerase (reverse transcriptase) proteins (antigens).
3. **env:** Encodes for envelop glycoproteins (antigens).
4. **Other genes:** In addition to above genes, some extra genes are present in retroviruses like px gene (in HTLV-I), tat / tex & LTRs etc.

HTLV-I

- **Full form:** Human T cell lymphotropic virus-I.
- **Synonym:** Also **called human T-cell leukemia-lymphoma virus** because known to cause adult T-cell leukemia / lymphoma.
- **History:** HTLV-I was discovered by Robert Gallo and colleagues in 1980 from the cell culture of adult patient with cutaneous T cell lymphoma (mycosis fungoides) & leukemia (Sezwary syndrome) in the USA.
- **Geographical distribution & genotypes:**
  - **Distribution:** Distributed worldwide, but disease present only in endemic areas like Japan & Caribbean.
  - **Genotypes:** Six genotypes from A to F. The great majority of infections are caused by the cosmopolitan subtype A.
- **Morphology:** Same as other retroviruses as described earlier.
- **Culture Characteristics (C/Cs):** It is done by co-cultivation of normal lymphocytes with infected lymphocytes. Virus growth is detected in normal cells by identifying the antigen of HTLV-I.
- **Resistance:** Same as other retroviruses as described earlier.
- **Immunity:** The virus displays relatively low antibody production variability. Natural immunity does occur in humans.
- **Pathogenicity:**
  - **Nature or history of disease:**
    - In USA, HTLV-I/II seroprevalence rate among volunteer blood donors is 0.016%.
    - Sero-prevalence rate of HTLV-I in Japan is 10%.
    - HTLV-1 and HTLV-2 are both involved in actively spreading epidemics, affecting 15-20 million people worldwide. HTLV-1 is the more clinically significant of the two, as it has been proven to be the etiologic agent of multiple disorders. At least 500,000 of the individuals infected with HTLV-I eventually develop rapidly fatal leukemia, while others will develop a debilitative myelopathy, uveitis, infectious dermatitis or another inflammatory disorder.
  - **Reservoir of infection:** Human.
  - **Source of infection:** Blood or breast milk.
  - **Mode of transmission:** HTLV-I and HTLV-II can be transmitted by
    - Sexual intercourse.
    - Blood to blood contact (e.g. by blood transfusion or sharing needles when using drugs).

- Breast feeding.
- **Portal of entry:** Skin or mucosa.
- **Sites:** T cells (both CD4 & CD8), B cells, CNS, skin etc.
- **Precipitating factors (epidemiological determinants):**

1. **Age:** Common in adult.
2. **Risk group:** Person required multiple blood transfusion or taking IV drugs are at great risk.

- **Pathogenesis:**
  - It acts by inserting its genome in host cell DNA **called provirus** which continuously spread from cell to cell.
  - Unlike HIV there are no free virions of HTLV-I free in blood.
  - It has a tax (tex) gene which have oncogenic potential.
- **Clinical features:**
  - Adult T cell leukemia/lymphoma: Rapid onset & fatal in nature.
  - Tropical spastic paraparesis.
  - Debilitative myelopathy or demyelinating disease.
  - Uveitis.
  - Infectious dermatitis / cutaneous T cell lymphoma.
  - Inflammatory disorder.
  - Arthropathy.
- **Complication:** Death & autoimmune disease.

Laboratory diagnosis:

- **Specimens:** Blood/serum.
- **Testing methods:**

A **Microscopy: → Follow morphology.**
B **Culture: → Follow C/Cs.**
C **Serological tests:** ELISA, Western blot, immunofluorescence assay (IFA) etc.
D **Molecular tests:** RT-PCR.

Prevention:

- **General measures:**
  - Screening of blood, organs & tissue of donors.
  - Safe sex.
  - High-risk behavior modification like drug abuse.
  - Avoid direct contact with blood and body fluid.
  - Use of disposable & sterile medical devices.
- **Vaccine:** Experimental vaccination using envelope antigens has been shown to be successful in animal models.

Treatment:

- Prosultiamine: Vitamin B-1 derivative, which has been shown to reduce viral load & symptoms.
- Azacytidine: Anti-metabolite, which has been credited with the cure of a patient in Greece.
- Tenofovir disoproxil (TDF): Reverse-transcriptase inhibitor used for HIV.
- Cepharanthine: An alkaloid from stephania cepharantha hayata& phosphonated carbocyclic 2'-oxa-3'aza nucleosides (PCOANs).
- A newer formulation of TDF, **called tenofovir alafenamide (TAF)**, also has promise as a treatment with less toxicity.

HTLV-II

Full form: Human T cell lymphotropic virus-II.

History: It is closely related to HTLV-I & also discovered by Robert Gallo and colleagues from patient with adult T cell leukemia in Japan & Caribbean.

Geographical distribution: Distributed in certain Native Americans tribes & Africa.

Pathogenicity:

- Transmission, replication & pathogenesis are similar to HTLV-I/
- HTLV-II is associated with T cell malignancies, mild neurologic diseases& chronic lung infections.

HTLV-III / HIV 1 & 2

Full form: Human T cell lymphotropic virus-III or Human immunodeficiency virus.

History & synonym:

- 1st indication was came in 1981, when there were outbreak of two unknown diseases like Kapsosi's sarcoma & *Pneumocystis jirovecii* pneumonia in young adult in Los Angeles & New York, USA who were homosexual & addicted to injected narcotics. They appeared to lose immune system rendering them vulnerable to secondary infections especially avirulent organisms & malignancies. This condition was **called AIDS (Acquired Immuno Deficiency Syndrome).**
- In 1983, virus was isolated by Luc Montagnier & colleagues at Pasteur Institute, Paris from African patient of lymphadenopathy hence **called Lymphadenopathy associated virus (LAV).**
- In 1984 it was isolated by Robert Gallo & colleagues at National Institute of Health (NIH), USA from AIDS patients & **called Human T cell lymphotropic virus-III (HTLV-III),** as HTLV-I & II were already described to cause human leukemia.
- Later, many similar isolates were identified from AIDS patient & in 1986 all such isolates were **called HIV** by International Committee on Virus Nomenclature.
- HIV was diagnosed on clinical background but antibodies detection method like ELISA was established in 1986.
- HIV-2 discovered in 1986, antigenically distinct virus endemic in West Africa.

- **In India** 1st case of HIV infection has been found in female sex workers in Chennai in 1986 & 1st case of AIDS was found in Bombay in 1986.

❖ Geographical distribution & genotypes:

- **Distribution:→Table-1**
- **Genotypes / clades:** Following three genotypes based on sequence analysis of gag and env genes.
  - M (M = Major) group:
    - It causes worldwide infection of HIV-1.
    - This group contains total 10 subtypes from A-J.
    - A: Most prevalent & found worldwide.
    - B: In USA & Europe, commonly spread by homosexual & blood route.
    - C: It is most common in **India & China.** Commonly spread by heterosexual route.
    - E: Common in Thailand. This types is no considered as separate type but recombinant type of A & E **called AE type** or **called CRFs (circulating recombinant forms).**
    - Common types in Africa: A, C & D.
    - Common types in Asia: B, C & E.
  - O (O = Outlier) : A few HIV-1 strains isolated from West Africa (Cameroon & Gabon) do not fall in group M and designated Group O (for outlier).
  - N (N = New) group: Later isolates of HIV-1 from Cameroon are different from M & O **called N group**.
- **Significance of genotyping:**

1. **Diagnostic:** Almost all diagnostic kits contains antigens of M types which missed the prevalence of O types, so it is advisable to includes the antigens of genotype prevalent in country.
2. **Transmission (transmissibility of subtypes):** American type (B genotype) is mostly transmitted by homosexual practise or by blood while Asian & African types (A & C) are transmitted by heterosexual practise.

- **Other typing methods:**

1. **Typing according to growth characters:** Isolates identified from carrier are slow growing & infects only to peripheral blood lymphocytes while from case of AIDS are fast growing & infecting lymphocytes plus monocytes in cell culture.
2. **Transmissibility of subtypes: → Vide supra**

❖ Morphology:→Fig.-1

- **Shape:** Spherical.
- **Size:** 90-100nm.
- **Genome& capsid:**
  - Two identical ss-RNA (+) with enzyme reverse transcriptase (**RNA dependent DNA polymerase**).
  - Conversions of ss-RNA in to ss-DNA & then in to ds-DNA by enzyme reverse transcriptase (RNA-dependent DNA polymerase, DNA polymerase). DNA transcribed to mRNA which translate to protein. ds-DNA may integrated in to host cell chromosome after infection **called provirus.**
  - Provirus remains in host cell for long time, influences the viral function & also initiates the viral replication.
  - Genome surrounded by double shell & icosahedral variety of capsid. Inner shell is cone shape & contains genome.
- **Envelope:**
  - It contains lipoproteins envelope.
  - Lipid derived from the host cell plasma membrane by budding & proteins (glycoprotein-gp) are viral encoded.
  - Protein present as trans-membrane pedicle (gp41) & projecting spike (gp120).
  - gp120 helps in adsorption of virus with specific receptorspresent on CD4 cell surface, while gp41 helps in cell fusion.

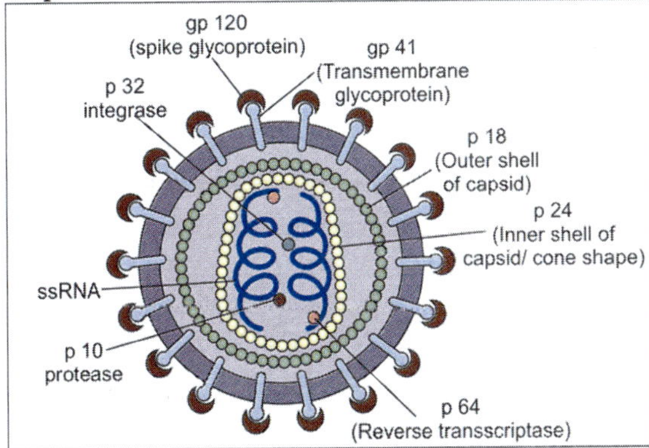

Figure-1: Morphology of HIV

❖ Culture characteristics (C/Cs): Two types of methods.

1. **Direct culture method:** In vitro cultivation of patient cells in presence of phytohaemagglutinin.
2. **Co-cultivation method:**

- **Method:** Co-cultivation between patient's lymphocytes & normal lymphocytes in presence of interleukin-2.
- **Result:** Virus growth is detected by demonstrating Ags or reverse transcriptase enzyme in normal cells.
- **Disadvantages:**
  - Risk of HIV infection.
  - Available at higher centre with adequate infection containment facilities.

❖ Resistance:

- **Sterilisation (physical methods):** It is heat labile (thermo labile). It is inactivated by
  - Autoclaving at 121^0C (15 lbs pressure) for 20 min.
  - Dry heat 170^0 C for 1hours.
  - Boiling for 20 minutes.
- **Disinfection (chemical methods):** Minimum 30 minutes' contact time required to kill HIV with following agents.

- Extreme of pH: 1.0 or 13.0
- Sodium hypochlorite (0.5-1%).
- Ethanol (70%) or isopropanol (35%).
- Lysol (0.5%) for 10 minutes.
- Providone iodine.
- Hydrogen peroxide (0.3%) for 10 minutes.
- Formalin (3-4%).
- Glutaraldehyde (2% **called cidex**).
- House hold bleaching powder (10%) for 10 minutes, for infected needles or syringes.

❖ Viral genome & gene products (antigens):

➢ **Genes:** Two types of genes as follows.

A. Structural genes: Following three types.

i. gag gene:

- Encodes for nucleocapsid (NA/genome/core + capsid/shell) antigens of virus.
- Expressed as a precursor protein p18 (p17 by some authors) which is cleaved into 3 proteins like p15, p18 and p24.

ii. env gene:

- Encodes for envelope glycoprotein of virus.
- Precursor glycoprotein gp160, which is cleaved into 2 proteins gp120 (forms the surface spikes) & gp41 (trans-membrane anchoring protein).

iii. pol gene:

- Encodes for reverse transcriptase & other viral enzymes like integrase (p32), protease (p10) & endonuclease.
- Reverse transcriptase is expressed as a precursor protein cleaved into p31, p51 & p66.

B. Non-structural genes: Following are types.

i. tat gene (trans activating gene): Enhance the expression of all viral genes.

ii. nef gene (negative factor gene): Down regulate the viral replication.

iii. rev gene (regulator of virus gene): Enhance the expression of structural proteins.

iv. vif (viral infectivity factor gene): Influence the infectivity of viral particles.

v. vpu (in HIV-1) and vpx (in HIV-2): Enhancing maturation & release of progeny virus from cells. Helps to differentiate between HIV-1 & HIV-2

vi. vpr: Stimulate the promoter region of virus.

vii. LTRs (Long terminal repeat sequences): One at either end, containing sequences giving promoter, enhancer and integration signals.

➢ **Antigenic structure:** It includes different products of gens (antigens) as follows.

✪ **Major antigens (products of gene) of HIV:**

a. Envelope-Ags:

1. Projecting spikes glycoprotein: gp120 (principle envelopes Ag).
2. Trans-membrane pedicle glycoprotein: gp41.
3. gp36 for HIV-2.

b. Nucleocapsid-Ags:

1. Principle nucleocapsid Ag (inner shell): p24.
2. Other nucleocapsid Ags (outer shell): p15, p18 & p55.

c. Enzyme-Ags:

1. Reverse transcriptase: p31, p51 & p66.
2. Integrase: p32
3. Protease: p10

✓ **Note: Way of numbering/naming the antigens**

- Number indicates the molecular weight of antigen in kilodaltons.

✪ **Diversity of HIV:**

- **HIV shows frequent diversity (variation) in**
  - Antigens: most common in envelope-Ags & rare in other Ags.
  - Nucleotide sequences.
  - Cell tropism.
  - Growth characteristics.
  - Cytopathology.
  - Place (place to place variation).
  - Person (person to person variation).
  - Different site of same person.
- **Reason for variation:** It is due to error prone nature of reverse transcription.

❖ Immunity:

a. Cell mediated immunity (CMI):

- After entry virus binds by gp120 Ag to CD4 receptors presents on $CD4^+$ (helper or inducer T cells) cells & resulting breakdown of cells with leucopenia & reversal of CD4:CD8 ratio.
- Decreasing $CD4^+$cells is an indirect indicator for decreasing CMI which is responsible for development of malignancies, opportunistic infections & inability to mount the DTH.

b. Humoral immunity (HI):

- As the CMI decreasing HI is increased for the compensatory mechanisms resulting increasing the production of antibodies like IgA, IgM & IgG, but these are not protective (useless antibodies).
- IgM synthesised at 4-6 weeks followed by IgG.
- IgM disappear in 8-10 weeks while IgG persist throughout **(fig.-2).**
- Decrease response to Ag & also production of type-III hypersensitivity & autoimmunity by useless antibodies.
- In end stage (AIDS) complete paralysis of immune system & decreasing antibodies like anti-p24.

❖ Pathogenicity:

➢ **Disease name:** Called AIDS.

➢ **Synonym:** Also, called slim disease, because patient becomes very slim due to weight loss.

➢ **Nature or history of disease:**

- **Global scenario:**
  - 1st outbreak was occurred in USA in 1981.
  - It had been originated from Africa probably from SIV & spread to USA via Haiti.

- Since the time of discovery of AIDS epidemic, it claimed about 78 million people with 38 million deaths.
- By the end of 2013 about 35 million people are living with HIV with global prevalence of 0.8% in adults.
- Sub–Saharan Africa is the worst affected region in the world with one adult harbouring HIV in every 20 adults & showing 71% prevalence out of total world HIV patients.

- **Indian scenario:**
- In India 1st case was detected in 1986.
- By the end 2011 total 20.8 lakh adults & 1.4 lakh children are living with HIV-AIDS.
- As far as people living with HIV-AIDS are concerned, Andhra Pradesh (undivided) is worst affected state followed by Maharashtra & Karnataka.
- As far as prevalence (numbers of cases per 100 populations) is concerned Nagaland is the worst affected state followed by Mizoram & Manipur.
- Nagaland has higher prevalence (0.88%) than the global prevalence by the end 2012-13.

➢ **Reservoir of infection:** Both human carrier & case. Actual origin for HIV is shown in **table-1.**

➢ **Source of infection:**
- Body fluid: Like blood, semen, milk & vaginal secretions are infectious. It present in saliva, but no confirmed case of salivary transmission has been reported. It is inactivated by inhibitory substances like secretory leucocyte protease, fibronectin & glycoproteins, which prevent transmission of HIV.
- It also presents in urine, CSF & tears but not able to transmit the disease.
- Cells/tissues.

➢ **Mode of transmission:** Following are the different mode for transmission of HIV. Percentage in brackets indicates the chances of infection per exposure.

a. Direct:

1. **Direct contact**
   - Direct contact (splash) of infected body fluid (blood) with abraded skin/mucosa (in eyes, mouth & nose in hospital worker): Chances of risk are **0.09%**.
   - During sexual intercourse (**0.1-1%**):
   - Oral.
   - Vaginal (heterosexual): Male to female transmission is approximately 8 times higher than female to male transmission. Heterosexual mode is the most common mode of transmission of HIV, especially in developing countries.
   - Anal: More risk than vaginal intercourse.
   - Digital sex.
2. **Inoculation under skin/mucosa:** By contaminated needles or syringe in IV drug users or in hospital staff or surgical wound (**0.5-1%**). Percutaneous injury transmits HBV (**30%**) > HCV (**3%**) > HIV (**0.5-1%**). Lower Segment Cesarean Section (LSCS) decreasing the HIV transmission.
3. **Vertical or mother to baby (30%):** Risk is maximum when mother is recently infected or already developed AIDS. Range of vertical transmission is 15-25% in developed countries & 25-35% in developing countries.
   - **Antenatal (23-30%):** By placenta.
   - **Intranatal (50-65%):** Contact of infected mother's blood to abraded skin/mucosa of baby. Maximum risk than antenatal & postnatal transmission.
   - **Post-natal (12-20%):** By breast milk.

b. Indirect:

1. **Vehicle borne transmission:** By body fluid or by tissues.
   - Transfusion of blood or blood products (>**90%**).
   - Organ or semen transplantation (**50-90%**).
   - Virus load is maximum in blood, genital secretions and CSF. Variable in breast milk & saliva. Zero to minimal in other body fluids.

✓ **Note:** Retroviruses are also classified as exogenous & endogenous retroviruses, as below.

- **Exogenous retroviruses:** It includes the horizontal transmission from one host to another as mentioned earlier.
- **Endogenous retroviruses:** It includes the hereditary (vertical) transmission from parents to offspring, where virus is integrated in to host cell genome, **called provirus**. Provirus behaves like host cell gene, regulate by host cell gene & spread to offspring. However, provirus is usually silent, non-pathogenic & do not cause any disease or malignancies.

➢ **Not transmitted by:**
- **Vector:** By Mosquitoes or by any other arthropods
- **Activities:** Like shaking hands, hugging (body to body contact), dry kissing, putting cheeks together or by eating in same dishes.
- **Sharing common things:** Like cloths, towels or bed sheets.
- **Non living objects:** Like air, food & water.

➢ **Incubation period (IP):**
- Uncertain & from months to year or 10 years or more.
- Long incubation period, because of latent infection by provirus & time to time release of progeny virus.

➢ **Portal of entry:** Skin/mucosa.

➢ **Sites:** Almost all body organs/tissues/cells are susceptible to HIV infection

➢ **Precipitating factors (epidemiological determinants):**

1. **Age:**
   - More in sexually active young adults.

- Children are infected in <3% cases.

2. **Sex:**
- In America, Australia & Europe: More in men.
- In Africa ratio is equal.

3. **Occupation:**
- Health workers are at increased risk.
- More in prostitutes.

4. **No use of condoms:** Sexual intercourse with infected partners without using condoms or suitable devices increased risk.
5. **Iatrogenic:** Use of unsterile needle, syringes or surgical instruments by hospital staff may precipitate the infection.
6. **High risk groups:**
- Drug addicts.
- Patients required multiple blood transfusions like hemophiliacs.

7. **Mode of entry:** Infection is result from entry of HIV-infected cells than the cell free virus.

➢ **Pathogenesis:**

a. **Viral multiplication:→Flow chart-1**

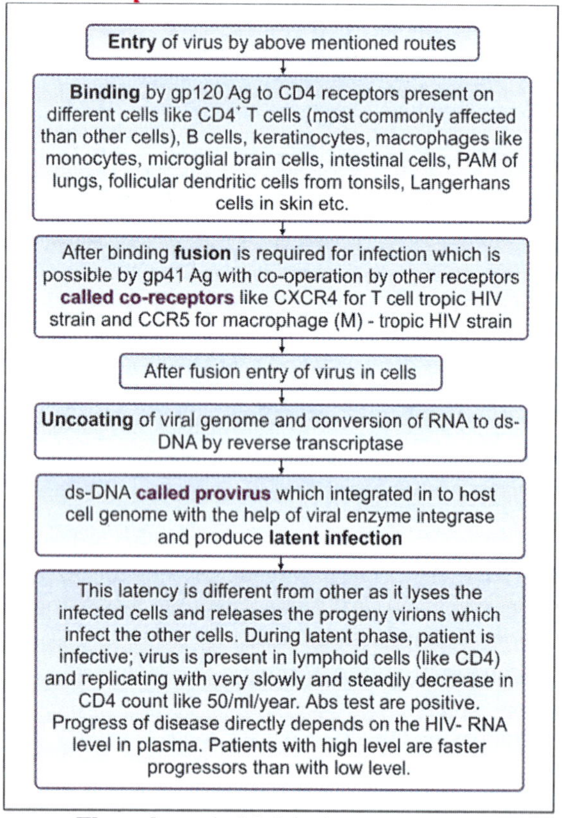

Entry of virus by above mentioned routes

↓

Binding by gp120 Ag to CD4 receptors present on different cells like $CD4^{+}$ T cells (most commonly affected than other cells), B cells, keratinocytes, macrophages like monocytes, microglial brain cells, intestinal cells, PAM of lungs, follicular dendritic cells from tonsils, Langerhans cells in skin etc.

↓

After binding **fusion** is required for infection which is possible by gp41 Ag with co-operation by other receptors **called co-receptors** like CXCR4 for T cell tropic HIV strain and CCR5 for macrophage (M) - tropic HIV strain

↓

After fusion entry of virus in cells

↓

Uncoating of viral genome and conversion of RNA to ds-DNA by reverse transcriptase

↓

ds-DNA **called provirus** which integrated in to host cell genome with the help of viral enzyme integrase and produce **latent infection**

↓

This latency is different from other as it lyses the infected cells and releases the progeny virions which infect the other cells. During latent phase, patient is infective; virus is present in lymphoid cells (like CD4) and replicating with very slowly and steadily decrease in CD4 count like 50/ml/year. Abs test are positive. Progress of disease directly depends on the HIV- RNA level in plasma. Patients with high level are faster progressors than with low level.

Flow chart-1: Multiplication of HIV

b. **Disease progression:**

- **HIV infects & destroys the CD4 cells resulting**
- Decrease T4 numbers (Selective T-cell deficiency)
- Reversal of T4:T8 ration.
- Reduce lymphocytes in lymph node biopsy & also in peripheral blood (Lymphopenia).
- Decrease release of IL-2, γ-IFN & other interleukins which reduces the CMI.
- Decrease the DTH which gives false negative skin tests.
- **When CMI decrease, body increase AMI by compensatory mechanisms resulting**
- Hypergammaglobulinemia (mostly useless antibodies) particularly raised IgA, IgG & in children raised IgM level.
- Immune complex diseases (type-III hypersensitivity) due to presence of useless antibodies.
- Autoimmunity due to presence of autoantibodies.
- Decrease response to Ag due to presence of useless Ab.
- **HIV infects & destroys other cells like**
- Platelets: It produces thrombocytopenia.
- Monocytes & microphage: Resulting decrease cytotoxic activity, chemotaxis, intracellular killing & antigen presentation.
- Cells of CNS: Producing dementia (**called pre senile dementia**) & degenerative neurological lesions. HIV can cross the blood brain barrier & neurological changes are due to direct HIV effects or by opportunistic infection or by malignancies.
- **Clinical manifestations in HIV infection are not due to virus but due to immunodeficiency resulting**
- Secondary (opportunistic) infection by other microbes.
- Malignancies.

➢ **Clinical features:** Disease passes through following different stages.

I. **Acute HIV infection or acute HIV syndrome or acute retroviral syndrome or sero-conversion illness:**
- Minor flu like or acute infectious mononucleosis (glandular fever) like symptoms may occur. It includes fever, rash, headache, fatigue, malaise, lymphadenopathy etc. Symptoms occur 6 to 12 weeks after infection.
- Only Ags (p24) are present while Abs are absent but develops after **window period** (4 weeks after infection) or in later part hence **called sero-conversion illness.**
- These symptoms are due to effect by viral multiplication & by immune complex.
- There is significant decrease in CD4 count in this stage.

II. **Asymptomatic or latent infection:**
- Virus remains latent in infected cells for very long time without any clinical sign-symptoms.
- Abs test are positive.
- Progress of disease directly depends on the HIV-RNA level in plasma. Patients with high level are faster progressors than with low level.

III. **Persistent generalised lymphadenopathy (PGL):**

- It is defined as enlarged lymph node with > 1 cm size in two or more non-contagious sites that last for at least 3 months.
- It is differentiated from other causes of lymphoma.

IV. AIDS Related Complex (ARC): Patients present with considerable immunodeficiency with major & minor features.

i. Major sign:
- Fever > 1 month.
- Diarrhoea > 1 month.
- >10% of weight loss.

ii. Minor sign:
- Cough> 1 month.
- Herpes-zoster infection (shingles).
- Oral candidiasis (thrush).
- Hairy cell leukoplakia.
- Kaposi's sarcoma (KS).
- Salmonellosis.
- Tuberculosis.
- Splenomegaly.

V. AIDS:

✪ **Development of AIDS:**
- It is the end stage of HIV infection.
- After clinical infection, AIDS has been developing approximately in 10 years, however about 5-10% patients escape the development of AIDS for long time around 15 years or more **called long term survival** or **chronic non-progressors**.

✪ **Clinical definition of AIDS:** Irreversible damage of immune defence (CD4 count is < 200) with opportunistic infection and/or malignancy.

✓ **Note: Exclusion of tests from the clinical definition of AIDS**
- Serological & molecular tests are excluded from the definition of clinical AIDS, because they also become positive in other stages of HIV infection like acute HIV syndrome & PGL.

✪ **Opportunistic infections (with agents) & malignancies:**

i. Bacterial:
- Mycobacteria: *M. tuberculosis* & Non-Tuberculous Mycobacteria (NTM) like *M. avium intracellulare* (MAC) are the common agents. Tuberculosis is the most common opportunistic infection in AIDS patient. In developing/tropical countries like India, *M. tuberculosis* is the most important pathogen with multidrug resistant strains. *M. avium intracellulare* is most common when $CD4^{+}$ count fall <50/cmm.
- Salmonellosis: *Salmonella* spp.
- Campylobacter: *Campylobacter* spp.
- Nocardia: *Nocardia* spp.
- Actinomycetes: *Actinomycets* spp.
- Legionellosis: : *Legionella* spp.

ii. Viral:
- Varicella Zoster virus (herpes zoster).
- Herpes simplex viruses: Common pathogen causing genital lesions in AIDS patient. Genital lesions in AIDS patient are also common by *H ducreyi.*
- Cyto megalo virus (CMV): Most common ocular complication by CMV in AIDS patient is retinitis when $CD4^{+}$ count fall <50/cmm. It is usually bilateral & present with retinal exudates & perivascular haemorrhage.
- EBV: Oral hairy leukoplakia.
- JC virus: It produces the PML (Progressive Multifocal Leuco-encephalopathy) & other lesions only in immunodeficient persons due to AIDS, immunosuppressive drug like rituximab or organ transplantation.

iii. Fungal:
- Candidiasis: Caused by *Candida* spp.
- Pneumocystosis: Caused by *Pneumocystis carinii.* Now species name changed to *Pneumocystis jiroveci.* It is the most common in USA & other Western countries. Pneumonia occurs in patient when $CD4^{+}$ count fall <200/cmm& required prophylaxis.
- Cryptococcosis: Caused by *Cryptococcus* spp. It is the most common cause of acute meningitis in AIDS patient. It causing infection when CD4 count fall < 100/cmm. Other opportunistic microbes affecting CNS in AIDS patient are *Toxoplasma gondii*, *M. tuberculosis* & herpes (herpetic encephalitis).
- Aspergillosis: Caused by *Aspergillus* spp.
- Histoplasmosis: Caused by *Histoplasma capsulatum.*
- Penicilliosis: Caused by *Penicillium marneffei.*

iv. Parasitic:
- **Protozoa:**
  - Toxoplasmosis: Occurs when $CD4^{+}$ count fall <200/cmm. Most common cause of seizure in AIDS patient. Toxoplasmosis may present with other features like hemiparesis, vomiting & headache.
  - Diarrhoeal parasites: Mostly causes persistent diarrhoea. Most common type of diarrhoea is cryptosporidiosis.
- Isosporiasis: Caused by *Isospora belli.*
- Cryptosporidiosis: Caused by *Cryptosporidium* spp.
- Microsporidiasis: Caused by *Microspora* spp.
- **Metazoa (helminths/worms):** Strongyloidiasis is the most common helminthic infection in AIDS patient caused by *Stroglyloide stercoralis.*

v. Malignancies:
- Kaposi's Sarcoma (KS): Most common tumour in AIDS patient.
- Lymphoma: Hodgkins & non-Hodgkin's type. Most common lymphoma is immuno blastic lymphoma

while among the brain tumour the most common lymphoma is primary CNS lymphoma.
- Cervical cancer

vi. Others:
- HIV encephalopathy.
- HIV associated nephopathy or cardiomyopathy.

✪ **End stage:**
- Patient present with sign-symptoms of respiratory system, GIT system, skin, CNS (dementia) & malignancies.
- Illness progress inexorably & death of patients in months or years.

➢ **Clinical classification:** CDC, USA classified HIV infection in to following different stages in 1993, based on clinical presentation & CD4 count as mentioned below. This classification was revised by WHO in 2007.

✪ **Group –I:** Acute HIV syndrome.
✪ **Group –II:** Asymptomatic infection.
✪ **Group–III:** Persistent generalised lymphadenopathy.
✪ **Group–IV:** Other diseases with following subgroups.

- **Subgroup A:** ARC.
- **Subgroup B:** Neurological diseases.
- **Subgroup C:** Secondary infectious diseases with following two subgroups.
  - C1: CMV or other herpes diseases, pneumocystosis, cryptococcosis, cryptosporidiosis, toxoplasmosis or strongyloidiasis.
  - C2: Oral hairy leukoplakia, salmonellosis, nocardiosis, tuberculosis, bacteremia or thrush.
- **Subgroup D:** Secondary cancer like Kaposi's sarcoma, lymphoma.
- **Subgroup E:** Other conditions.

✓ **Note: Correlation between CD4 count & opportunistic infections**

- **400-200/cmm:** *M. tuberculosis*, Varicella Zoster virus, Herpes simplex, candidiasis, oral hairy leukoplakia, Kaposi's Sarcoma (KS)
- **<200/cmm:** Pneumocystosis, cryptococcosis, toxoplasmosis
- **<50/cmm:** *M. avium intracellulare* & CMV retinitis.

❖ Paediatric AIDS:

➢ **Rate:** It occurs in 30% cases from infected mothers.

➢ **Mode of transmission:** Vide supra.

➢ **Clinical features:**
- Early deficiency of AMI leads recurrent bacterial infections.
- Failure to thrive.
- Persistent oral candidiasis.
- Tuberculosis.
- Lymphadenopathy.
- Recurrent diarrhea.
- Abnormal neurological findings.
- Lymphocytic interstitial pneumonia.
- Kaposi's sarcoma, Cryptococcosis& Toxoplasmosis are rare compared to adults.

❖ Laboratory diagnosis:

➢ **Policy:**
- In India, it is decided by National Aids Control Organisation (NACO), Delhi.
- NACO provides guidelines for serological testing & interpretation of results.
- It also maintains the uniformity & quality in reporting the incidence & prevalence of disease.

➢ **Indications:**
- To diagnose, to treat & to prevent the HIV-AIDS
- To screen the blood before transfusion.
- Antenatal screening of mother for **P**revention of **P**arent **T**o **C**hild / vertical **T**ransmission (PPTCT) transmission of HIV.
- Promoting voluntary counseling and confidential testing.
- Screening of all those who are at high risk.
- Post exposure management.

➢ **Steps:**
1. Suspect HIV infection (from history).
2. Pretest counseling at ICTC/PPTCT.
3. Informed consent.
4. Sample collection.
5. Sample transport.
6. HIV testing & interpretation of result.
7. Confidential reporting.
8. Posttest counseling.
9. Refer HIV positive to ART (Anti-Retroviral Therapy) Centre to assess clinical & immune status (CD4 count) & for ART.
10. Follow up counseling as required.

➢ **Specimens:** Best sample is blood/serum, but can use CSF, saliva, cervical secretions, semen, tears or materials from organ biopsy.

➢ **Testing methods:** It includes following three types.

I. Non-specific tests or tests to detect immune status or immunological tests:
- TLC: Leucopenia (<2000cmm).
- CD4 count: <200cmm. CD4 count is very low in full blown AIDS (end stage) as suggested in **fig.-2.**
- CD4:CD8 ratio: Reversed.
- Platelets: Thrombocytopenia.
- Antibodies status: Raised IgG & IgA.
- Diminished CMI: All skin tests are negative or false negative.
- Abnormal lymph node biopsy.

II. Specific tests or tests to detect HIV-AIDS:

A. Microscopy: → **Follow morphology.**

B. Culture: → **Follow C/Cs.**

C. Serological tests:

✪ **Types:** Two types like Ag & Ab detection tests.

i. Ag detection tests:

- **Ag synthesis:** P24 is the earliest Ag seen in blood after 2 weeks **(fig.-2)**. However, if the infecting dose is small like needle prick injury, appearance may be delayed.
- **Clinical Significance:**

a. Diagnosis:

- Earliest marker appears in blood & useful for diagnosis of HIV infection in **window period.**
- Time required for synthesis of Ab after entry of virus is **called window period**. It is about 4-6 weeks.
- Newborns& children, where immune system is immature & Abs are not synthesised & disease will have diagnosed by p24.
- Also, detected from CSF.

b. Infectivity: Virus & p24 Ag titre is high in acute phase, decline/absent in latent (asymptomatic) phase due to Ab formation (**sero-conversion illness mostly after 4 weeks**) & again high in the end, which shows maximum infectivity in initial part & end part while less in latent phase **(fig.-2).** However sometimes p24 Ag which is already bound to Ab, gets dissociated from Ag-Ab complex & can be detected by capture ELISA in 30-50% cases.

c. Prognosis: Helps to monitor the disease progress.

- **Test:** P24 Ag is detected by ELISA.

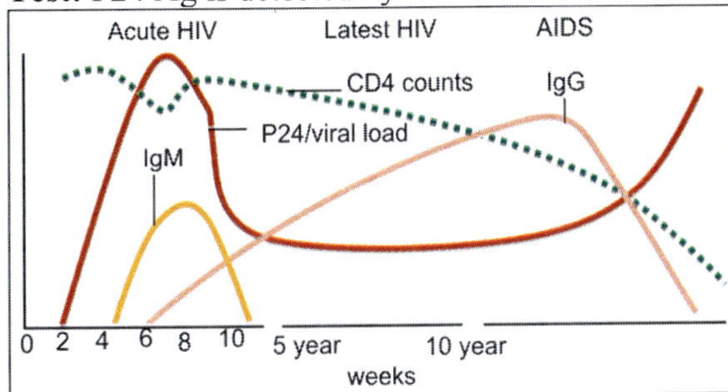

Figure-2: HIV markers in different stage of HIV infection

ii. Ab detection tests:

- **Ab synthesis:**
- IgM synthesised at 4-6 weeks followed by IgG.
- IgM disappear in 8-10 weeks while IgG persist throughout **(fig.-2).**
- When clinical AIDS established with severe immunodeficiency some Ab components may disappear like anti-p24.
- **Clinical Significance:**

a. Screening:

- Aim: To prevent the transmission.
- Definition: Application of HIV testing whether voluntary or mandatory in entire population or target group.
- Not possible in entire population.
- Possible in target group like blood/organ/semen donors, IV drug abuser, antenatal women etc.
- Best useful: Screening is best useful when done for P24 Ag detection.

b. Diagnosis: Most useful for diagnosis of HIV.

c. Sero-epidemiology: Ab survey is most useful in identifying the geographical extent of HIV infection & other epidemiological studies like spread of HIV infection from identified sources.

d. Prognosis:

- Loss of anti-p24 Ab from serum indicates end stage of disease & irreversible breakage of immunity.
- End stage also associated with high antigenic titre of p24 & high viral load in circulation.
- **Disadvantages:** Not useful.
- In **window period** as antibodies are not synthesised
- In **end stage** of disease because of total immunodeficiency.
- When **infection occurs by other virus** like HIV-2 testing is done by using HIV-1 antigens alone.
- **Subtypes of Ab detection tests:** Two types of Ab detection tests as shown in **table-2** with name & differences.

Screening tests	Confirmatory tests
High sensitivity	High specificity
False +Ve	Few or no false +Ve
Low cost	High cost
Easy to perform	Requires special instruments & expert person

Table-2: Differences between antibody detection tests

a. Screening tests:

1. HIV-ELISA:

- Most sensitive about 99.5%.
- More details: Follow chapter → Antigen - antibody (Ag-Ab) reactions.

2. Rapid tests:

- Particle agglutination (latex, RBCs & gelatin).
- Immunoconcentration test (flow through / vertical / dot blot assays).
- ICT (lateral flow assay).
- ELISA based rapid tests (immuno-comb HIV-1 & 2 bi-spot method).

b. Confirmatory tests:

1. Western Blot (WB) test:

- **Advantage:** More specific test than screening tests.
- **Disadvantage:** Less sensitive than screening tests.
- **Detection of antibodies:** It detects the individual antibodies from serum against various antigens of HIV like
- gag gene: p15, p18 and p24.
- pol gene: p31, p51 & p66.
- env gene:gp160, gp120 & gp41.
- **Interpretation of results:**
- WHO criteria: Presence of at least two env bands out ofgp160, gp120 & gp41 with or without gag or pol bands.

- CDC criteria: Presence of any two bands out ofp24, gp160, gp120 & gp41.
- **More details:** Follow chapter → Genetics of bacteria.

2. **Line Immuno Assay.**
3. **Immunoflourescent test.**

✪ **Strategies for HIV testing by using serological tests:**

- **Introduction:**
- It includes three strategies (I, II, III) by using screening test like ELISA or rapid tests.
- In case of discordant/indeterminate result WB test/RT-PCR is used for confirmation.
- A1, A2, A3 represent test-1, test-2 & test-3 respectively.
- Serologically HIV-AIDS is declared positive when three tests are reactive with two different principles or antigens. Same kit should not be used again.
- **Strategies:** Three strategies.

a. **Strategy –I:**

- Indication: For transfusion or transplantation.
- Tests: It is a single test strategy as shown in **flow chart-2.**

b. **Strategy –II:** Following two categories.

1. **Strategy –IIA:**
   - Indication: For sentinel surveillance.
   - Tests: It is a two tests strategy as shown in **flow chart-3.**
2. **Strategy –IIB:**
   - Indication: For diagnosis of an individual with AIDS indicator disease system.
   - Tests: Three tests strategy as shown in **flow chart-4.**

c. **Strategy –III:**

- Indication: For diagnosis of HIV infection in asymptomatic individual.
- Test: It is a three tests strategy as shown in **flow chart-5.**

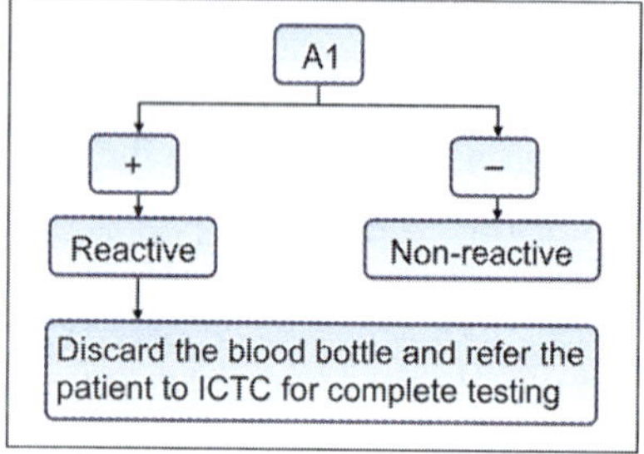

Flow chart-2: Strategy-I of HIV testing

D. Molecular methods:

✪ **List of tests:**

1. RT-PCR or Real Time RT-PCR (qRT-PCR).
2. Branched DNA assay.
3. NASBA.

✪ **Uses:**

1. Highly sensitive & specific test, considered as gold standard for diagnosis & confirmation of HIV. RT-PCR can detect as less as 40copies / ml of HIVRNA, where DNA assay & NASBA detect when concentration is > 50 copies / ml & > 80 copies / ml respectively, hence RT-PCR is considered as most sensitive than other molecular methods.
2. Most sensitive methods can detect very few copies of RNA from clinical samples.
3. For diagnosis of HIV in window period within 12 days of exposure before the availability of p24 Ag in blood.
4. For monitoring the HIV infection: → Vide infra.
5. To detect the drug resistance.
6. To differentiate between HIV -1 & 2.

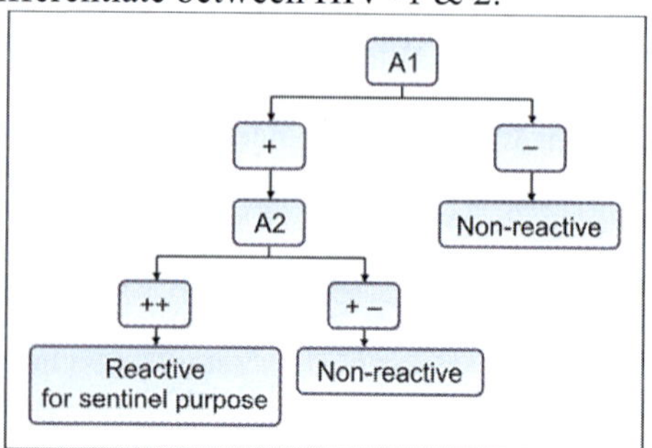

Flow chart-3: Strategy-IIA of HIV testing

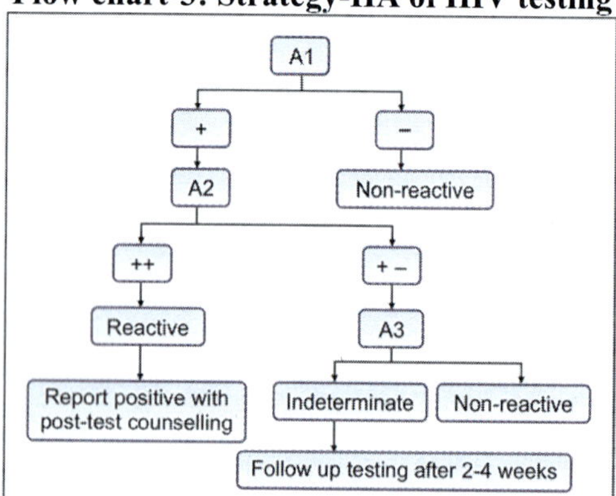

Flow chart-4: Strategy-IIB of HIV testing

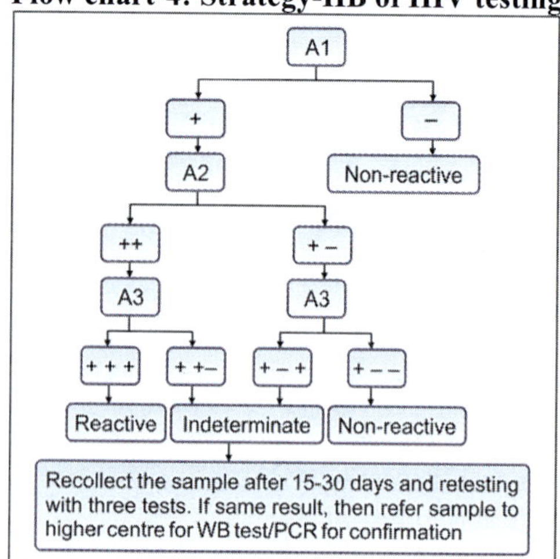

Flow chart-5: Strategy-III of HIV testing

III. **Other tests to diagnose the opportunistic infection:** Routine microbiological methods are enough like microscopy & culture.

✓ **Note: Suggested test of HIV as per time after exposure**

- **Nucleic acid detection:** In 12 days } **window period**
- **p24 detection:**After 2 weeks
- **Ab detection:** After 4 weeks

➢ **Laboratory monitoring of HIV infection:** Some tests are important in monitoring the course of HIV infection.

a. **CD4 count:**
- CD4 count indicates the immune status of patients.
- Count <200 indicates requirement of ART.
- Count <50 indicates serious risk.
- CD4 count is low in full blown AIDS (end stage) as suggested in **fig.-2.**

b. **Viral load test:**
- It is the amount of HIV-RNA in one ml of blood.
- It is measured by two methods like RT-PCR & branched DNA assay (bDNA).
- It indicates response to ART, progress of disease & clinical outcome.
- Viral load is high in full blown AIDS (end stage) as suggested in **fig.-2.**

c. **B-2-microglobulin & neopterin:**
- Both the substances are measured in serum or urine.
- Both substances are low in asymptomatic phase & high in end stage.

➢ **HIV-marker in different stages: →Table-3 & fig.-2**

Stage	P24	IgM	IgG	Western Blot pattern
Acute	+	-/+	-	Partial p24 and/orgp120
Latent	-	+	-	Full pattern
ARC	-	-	+	Loss of p24
AIDS	+	-	-	Loss of p24

Table-3: HIV-marker in different stages

➢ **Testing in children below 18 months:**

✪ **Serological tests:** Not useful because child has immature immune system, so antibodies are not formed & also there is interference by maternal antibodies.

✪ **Detection of virus / viral product** as follows
- P24 Ag detection by ELISA.
- Viral nucleic acid by RT-PCR: Most useful method
- Viral culture method: Labour intensive, so less useful.

❖ Prevention:

➢ **General measures:**
- Improvement in health education.
- Screening of blood, organs & tissues of donor.
- Safe sex.
- High-risk behavior modification like drug abuse.
- Avoid direct contact with blood and body fluid.
- Use of disposable & sterile medical devices.

➢ **Immunoprophylaxis:**

- **It's difficult to develop effective HIV vaccine:** Due to following reasons.
- High mutation in virus: It is due to error prone nature of enzyme reverse transcriptase. Mutation can occur in any gene but most common in *env* gene even though there is formation of antibodies against *env* antigens. Due to high mutation, it shows extensive genetic diversity & evades the host's defence & creates problems in development of effective HIV vaccine.
- Long latent period between exposure & appearance of symptoms.
- Lack of ideal animal model.
- Difficult to get human volunteers for vaccine trials
- Viral genome get incorporated in to host cell genome (**called provirus**) very soon after exposure, hence it provides very short time to control the infection.

- **Types of vaccine:** Following type of vaccine are developed but still under trial.

1. **Modified whole virus vaccine**
2. **Subunit vaccine:** Prepared from envelope gp 120
3. **Vector vaccine:** Most of the vaccine trials are based on this principle. It is done by inserting the immunogen of HIV in non-pathogenic bacteria or viruses like
   - Canarypox virus: Insertion of gp 120 gene.
   - Adenovirus type 5.
   - AAV.
   - Modified Vaccinia Ankara virus: Virus was used by International AIDS Vaccine Initiative in collaboration with NACO, India.
4. **Target cell protection** by Anti-CD4-antibody or by genetically engineered CD4 cells.

➢ **Post-exposure prophylaxis (PEP):**

✪ **Definition:** It is a short-term ART to avoid the HIV infection after occupation exposure like
- Skin injury by needle/sharp items.
- Splash of PIMs over non-intact skin.
- Splash of PIMs over intact skin for prolonged duration.
- Splash of PIMs over mucosa (intact or abraded).

✪ **Guidelines for PEP:**
- It should be initiated within 2 hours but not > 72 hours. If it started very soon it reduces the risk of HIV transmission up to 80%.
- Do not wait for the result of HIV testing to start the PEP.
- Risk of transmission following needle prick injury: HIV is 0.5-1%, HCV is 3-10% & HBV is 6-30%
- Risk of transmission following splash of blood to mucosa of eyes, mouth & nose: HIV is 0.09%.
- Base line HIV tests should be done at the time of exposure & if found negative then it should be repeated at 6 week, 3 months, 6 months & 1 year after exposure.

✪ **PEP regimens:**

i. **To prevent the neonatal transmission:**
- Start the zidovudine treatment to HIV infected mother from the beginning of 2nd trimetser to the

delivery & to baby for 6 weeks following birth. It decreases the HIV transmission from22.6% to <5%.

- Single dose of nevirapine is administered to the mother at the onset of labour & to the baby within 72 hours after birth. It decreased the transmission by 50%. It is the preferred regime in developing countries.

i. **To prevent the transmission following occupation exposure:** It reduces the occupational transmission rate of HIV up to 79%. Following two regimens are useful.

1. **Basic regimen:** Two drugs for 4 weeks.
- Zidovudine: 300mg twice a day.
- Lamivudine: 300mg twice a day.
2. **Expanded regimen:** Three drugs for 4 weeks which includes basic regimen plus
- Indinavir: 800mg thrice a day or
- Nelfinavir: 750mg thrice a day.

✪ **Selection of PEP:**

- **Depends on:**
- Severity of exposure.
- Type of exposure.
- HIV status of the source: Source includes the potentially infectious materials (PIMs) like blood, body fluid, CSF, synovial fluid, pus etc. or instruments contaminated by these PIMs.
- **HIV Exposure Code (EC): →Flow chart-6**

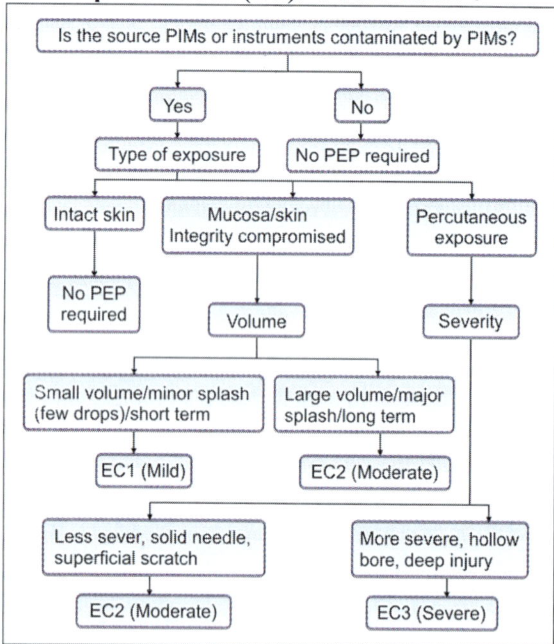

Flow chart-6: HIV Exposure Code (EC)

- **HIV Status Code (SC): →Flow chart-7**
- **Selection of regimens: → Table-4**

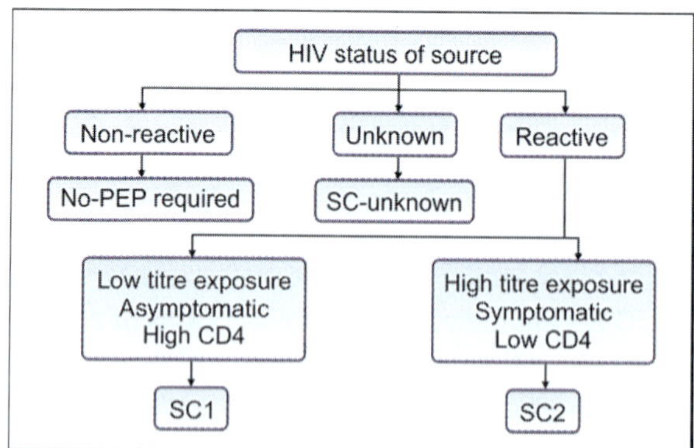

Flow chart-7: HIV Status Code (SC)

EC	SC	PEP
1	1	Nor required
1	2	Basic
2	1	Basic
2	2	Expanded
3	½	Expanded
2/3	unknown	Basic

Table-4: Selection of PEP regimens

❖ Treatment:

i. **General measures:** Understanding & cooperation by hospital staff & relative.

ii. **Specific treatment for tumours & opportunistic infections:** Early diagnosis & treatment of such conditions are required.

iii. **Immuno restorative therapy:** It includes administration of IL, thymic factor, leucocyte transfusion & bone marrow transplantation, but not helpful.

iv. **ART:**

➢ **Role of ART:** It not kill the virus or clear the disease but having following roles to improve & to prolong the life of patients
- Arrest the progress of disease.
- Reduction in viral load as long as possible.
- Immune restoration both quantitative & qualitative.
- Reduction of HIV transmission.

➢ **Classification of ART agents:**

1. **Nucleoside reverse transcriptase inhibitors:** AZT (Azidothymidine, Zidovudine), didanosine, zacitabine, abacavir, emtricitabine & lamivudine.
2. **Non-nucleoside reverse transcriptase inhibitors:** Nevirapine, efavirenz & delavirdine.
3. **Protease inhibitors:** Ritonavir, nelfinavir, saquinavir, amprenavir, lopinavir, fosamprenavir, atazanavir & tipranavir.
4. **Fusion inhibitor:** Enfuvirtide.
5. **Integrase inhibitor:** Raltegravir.
6. **CCR5 receptor inhibitor:** Maraviroc.

➢ **Indications to start ART:**
- Stage I & II: Start ART if CD4 count falls < 350 cells/cmm/
- Stage III & IV: Start ART irrespective of CD4 count.
- HIV with tuberculosis.
- HIV in pregnant women.
- HIV with HBV/HCV infection.

➢ **Selection of ART:**

- Mono therapy is contraindicated.
- Combination therapy which includes minimum three drugs like lamivudine + another drug from same group (e.g. zidovudine) + one drug from Non-nucleoside reverse transcriptase inhibitors group (nevirapine/efavirenz).
- Regimens recommended by NACO:

1. **Preferred regimens:** Lamivudine + zidovudine + Nnevirapine.
2. **Alternate regimens:** Lamivudine + zidovudine + efavirenz or lamivudine + stavudine + efavirenz or lamivudine + stavudine + nevirapine.

➢ **Problems with ART:**

- High cost.
- Side effects like lipid abnormalities & drug interactions.
- Drug resistance.
- Immune reconstructive inflammatory syndrome: It is an overwhelming inflammatory response syndrome due to reduction in viral load & recovery in immune system by drug. Such recovered immune system gives exaggerated immune response to previously acquired opportunistic infections makes the symptoms of infection worse.

❖ **World HIV-AIDS day:** Since 1988, 1st December of every year is celebrated as an AIDS day to raise the awareness of AIDS pandemic caused by HIV by Josh Lowe & mourning those who have died of the disease.

Question bank

Case study

1) A 30-year-old male with history of multiple sex is admitted in hospital with complains of diarrhoea, significant weight loss & fever for the last 1 months. On clinical examination, enlarged lymph nodes were found at multiple sites. Identify the clinical conditions& answer the following

a) Name the clinical condition & its etiological agent.
b) Write the morphology of etiological agent.
c) Write pathogenicity of clinical condition.
d) Write laboratory diagnosis of clinical condition.

2) A lady with labour pain admitted in hospital. A resident doctor got needle prick injury during the management of patient. A blood is collected for different lab investigation from this lady. Laboratory report of lady was found HIV positive. Answer the followings.

a) How you prevent the HIV transmission to baby?
b) Which mode of delivery allow the less transmission of HIV to baby?
c) How you diagnose HIV in new born baby?
d) What are the chances of HIV transmission by needle prick injury & through placenta?
e) Which ART (regime) you prescribed to the resident doctor?
f) How you diagnose HIV in resident doctor in first 2 weeks?
g) Describes different measures for prevention of HIV -AIDS?

Essay/Full question

1) Retroviridae.
2) HIV.

Short notes

1) Classification of Retroviridae.
2) HTLV-I.
3) Pathogenicity / laboratory diagnosis of HIV.
4) HIV genome or genotyping.
5) Genetical & antigenic structure of HIV.
6) Post-exposure prophylaxis of HIV.
7) ART.

Short questions for theory/viva questions

1) Write four differences between HIV-1 & HIV-2.
2) How you can cultivate the HIV?
3) Mention two examples of each, sterilisation & disinfection methods for HIV.
4) Mentions the different types of HIV antigens.
5) Write the clinical classification of HIV infection given by CDC, USA in 1993.
6) What is window period in HIV? Write its clinical significance.
7) Define window period & incubation period. Mention the window period & incubation period in HIV-AIDS.
8) Write two screening & two confirmatory tests for diagnosis of HIV-AIDS.
9) Name the most sensitive & specific test for diagnosis of HIV-AIDS.
10) Write four advantages of HIV-AIDS diagnosis by molecular methods.
11) Name the laboratory diagnostic tests for HIV in window period & after window period.
12) How you can declare any patient, clinically & serologically as a HIV-AIDS patient?
13) Comment: Human saliva does not allow the transmission of HIV.
14) Comment: RT-PCR considered as most sensitive method for diagnosis of HIV among the all molecular methods.
15) Comment: Development of HIV vaccine is difficult.
16) Comment: Use of ART in HIV-AIDS patient may sometime causes inflammatory syndrome.

MCQs for chapter review

Classification

1) **HIV is a which type of virus**
(a) Picorna virus (b) Pox virus (c) Retro virus (d) Herpes virus

Genome

2) **HTLV extra gene is**
(a) Gag (b) Pol (c) Env (d) px

HTLV-I

3) **HTLV-I causes which of the following?**
(a) Tropical spastic paraparesis (b) Familial medeterranian fever (c) Cutaneous T cell lymphoma (d) Burkit's lymphoma

HTLV-III or HIV-1 & 2

4) **HIV virus was discovered in** (AIIMS, May-14)
(a) 1976 (b) 1983 (c) 1996 (d) 1988
5) **Subtype of HIV most common in India**
(a) A (b) B (c) C (d) D
6) **Reverse transcriptase of HIV is**
(a) DNA polymerase (b) DNA dependent RNA polymerase (c) RNA dependent DNA polymerase (d) None
7) **HIV virus contains** (AI-02)
(a) Single stranded DNA (b) Single stranded RNA (c) Double stranded DNA (d) Double stranded RNA

8) **What is the sequence which a retrovirus follows on entering a host cell** (AI-00)
(a) RNA-DNA-RNA (b) RNA-DNA (c) DNA-RNA (d) DNA-RNA-DNA

9) **The HIV can be destroyed in vitro by which of the following**
(a) Boiling (b) Ethanol (c) Cidex (d) All of above

10) **HIV gene is/are** (PGI, June-01)
(a) gp73 (b) p24 (c) gp120 (d) gp5 (e) None

11) **Nef gene in HIV is for use**
(a) Enhancing the expression of genes (b) Enhancing viral replication (c) Decreasing viral replication (d) Maturation

12) **Which of the following is not a structural gene of HIV**
(a) Gag (b) Pol (c) Env (d) Tat

13) **Which of the following genes are present in HIV genome** (PGI-06)
(a) Gag (b) Tat (c) p500 (d) Kinase (e) p24

14) **Gene coding for core of HIV is**
(a) Gag (b) Pol (c) Env (d) Tat

15) **Which of the following gene is associated with encoding of reverse transcriptase**
(a) Gag (b) Pol (c) Env (d) Ltr

16) **Gag gene encodes for**
(a) Reverse transcriptase (b) Core antigen (c) Envelope (d) gene activation

17) **A HIV mother delivers a baby. All are true except** (AIIMS, Nov-99)
(a) Risk of HIV in the baby is up to 90% (b) HIV infection cannot be diagnosed in the baby with available methods (c) AIDS can be transmitted from mother to child during delivery (d) Breast feeding can transmit AIDS

18) **In the heterosexual transmission of HIV**
(a) There is a greater risk of transmission from man to woman (b) There is a greater risk of transmission from woman to man (c) Risk is equal in either ways (d) HIV infection is not transmitted by heterosexual act.

19) **True about HIV** (PGI-00)
(a) Not transmitted through semen (b) More chances of transmission during LSCS than normal labour (c) More infectious than hepatitis B (d) Male to female transmitted > female to male

20) **Mother to child transmission of HIV**
(a) 25% (b) 50% (c) 60% (d) 75%

21) **The chances that a health worker gets HIV from an accidental needle prick is** (PGI, June-99)
(a) 1% (b) 10% (c) 95% (d) 100%

22) **Most common mode of transmission of HIV worldwide is**
(a) Heterosexual (b) Homosexual (c) IV drug abuse (d) Contaminated blood products

23) **HIV is transmitted by following route except**
(a) Blood transfusion (b) Sexual intercourse (c) Saliva (d) Organ transplantation

24) **Percentages of HIV infection by sexual intercourse are**
(a) 0.1-1% (b) 30% (c) 50-90% (d) More than 90%

25) **HIV is not transmitted by**
(a) Sexual contact (b) Percutaneous transmission (c) Transplacental transmission (d) Body to body contact

26) **HIV can** (PGI, June-08)
(a) Cross blood brain barrier (b) RNA virus (c) Inhibited by 0.3% H_2O_2 (d) Thermostable

27) **Regarding HIV infection, not true is** (AI-01)
(a) p24 is used for early diagnosis (b) Lysis of infected CD4 cells is seen (c) Dendritic cells do not support replication. (d) Macrophage is a reservoir for the virus

28) **Regarding HIV which of the following is not true** (AI-02)
(a) It is a DNA retrovirus (b) Contains reverse transcriptase (c) May infect host CD4 cells other than T lymphocytes (d) Causes a reduction in host CD4 cells at late stage of disease.

29) **HIV affects** (AIIMS-98)
(a) Only T helper cells (b) T helper and macrophages (c) NK cells (d) B lymphocytes

30) **HIV infects most commonly** (AIIMS, June-00, AI-09)
(a) CD4+ helper cells (b) CD8+ cells (c) Macrophage (d) Neutrophil

31) **AIDS involves** (AI-98)
(a) T-helper cells (b) T-suppressor cells (c) T-cytotoxic (d) B-cells

32) **HIV can infect all except**
(a) Circulating dendritic cells (b) CD4 T lymphocytes (c) Macrophages (d) Cytotoxic T cells

33) **Receptors for HIV** (AI-09)
(a) CD4 (b) CC3 (c) CD5 (d) CD56

34) **The receptor through which M tropic HIV strains bind**
(a) CCR5 (b) CXR4 (c) CXCR5 (d) Any of the above

35) **Latent phase of HIV** (PGI, Dec-06)
(a) Viral replication (b) Sequestered in lymphoid tissue (c) Infective (d) Non-infective (e) Rapid decline of CD4 is common

36) **HIV infection is associated with** (PGI, June-02)
(a) A glandular fever like illness (b) Generalised lymphadenopathy (c) Gonococcal septicaemia (d) Sinus disease (e) pre-senile dementia

37) **In diagnosis of AIDS, criteria include the following except** (PGI, Dec-01)
(a) CD4<200 (b) CD4<500 (c) CD4:CD8 = 1 (d) Presence of any of the opportunistic infections like tuberculosis, pneumocytosis, cytomegalovirus infection (e) Western Blot positive

38) **Sero-conversion in HIV infection takes place in**
(a) 2 weeks (b) 4 weeks (c) 9 weeks (d) 12 weeks

39) **Most common opportunistic in AIDS in India**
(a) Toxoplasmosis (b) Cryptococcosis (c) Cryptosporidium (d) TB

40) **Most common agent causing tuberculosis in AIDS patient in tropical countries is -** (AI-97)
(a) *Mycobacterium tuberculosis* (b) *Mycobacterium intracellulare* (c) *Mycobacterium parvum* (d) *Mycobacterium* atypical

41) **In India, most common cause of TB in HIV-** (PGI-00)
(a) *M. tuberculosis* (b) *M. avium intracellulare* (c) *M. bovis* (d) *M. scrofulaceum*

42) **CMV retinitis in HIV occurs when CD4 counts falls below** (AI-02)
(a) 50 (b) 100 (c) 200 (d) 150

43) **An HIV patient complains of visual disturbances. Fundal examination shows bilateral retinal exudates and perivascular haemorrhage. Which of the following viruses are most likely to be responsible for this retinitis.** (AI-04)
(a) Herpes simplex (b) Varicella zoster (c) Cytomegalo virus (d) EBV

44) **The most common organism amongst of the following that causes acute meningitis in AIDS patient is -** (AI-05)
(a) *Streptococcus pneumoniae* (b) *Streptococcus agalactiae* (c) *Cryptococcus neoformans* (d) *Listeria monocytogenes*

45) **Common CNS lesion in HIV is caused by** (PGI, June-09)
(a) *Cryptococcus* (b) *Toxoplasma* (c) Neurocysticercosis (d) Mucormycosis (e) Lymphoma

46) **Important features of AIDS are** (PGI, June-01)
(a) Follicular tonsillitis (b) Lichen panus (c) Oral candidiasis (d) Hairy leukoplakia (e) Mitotic division of oral cavity

47) **Which of the following lesion is associated with HIV infection** (AIIMS, May-04)
(a) Hairy leukoplakia (b) Erythroplakia (c) Oral lichen panus (d) Bullous pemphigoid

48) **In a patient having HIV infection, oral ulcer is most commonly due to** (PGI-00)
(a) *Candida* (b) Cryptococcosis (c) *Histoplasma* (d) *Trychophyton*

49) Persistent diarrhoea in AIDS is caused by A/E (PGI-01)
(a) *Microspora* (b) *Cryptococcus* (c) *Cryptosporidia* (d) *Isospora belli* (e) *Giardia lamblia*

50) Most common causative agent of diarrhoea in AIDS
(a) Toxoplasmosis (b) Cryptococcosis (c) *Cryptosporidium* (d) *Mycobacteria*

51) Most common genital lesion in HIV patients is (AI-10)
(a) *Chlamydia* (b) Herpes (c) Syphilis (d) *Candida*

52) Fungal infections associated with AIDS patient are (PGI-03)
(a) *Pneumocystis carinii* (b) *Penicillium marneffei* (c) *Candida* (d) *Cryptococcus* (e) *Cryptosporidium*

53) Commonest helminthic infection in AIDS is (AI-99)
(a) *Trichuris trichuria* (b) *Strongyloides stercoralis* (c) *Enterobius vermicularis* (d) *Necator americanus*

54) Which of the following lesion is not seen in HIV patient with CD4 count less than 100 per micro litre, who has non productive cough? (AIIMS, June-99)
(a) *Mycobacterium tuberculosis* (b) *Pneumocytis carinii* (c) *Mycoplasma pneumoniae* (d) Cryptococcal infection

55) True about HIV all except
(a) PML caused by JC virus (b) CNS lymphoma is the most common CNS tumour (c) CMV is the most common cause of retinitis (d) Most common cause of seizure is *Candida*

56) A person with AIDS related complex is suffering from
(a) Opportunistic infection (b) Cancer related to AIDS (c) Generalised lymphadenopathy (d) Herpes zoster

57) In HIV patient hemiparesis, headache, vomiting occur due to infection of which organism.
(a) Gonococcal infection (b) Toxoplasmosis (c) Streptococcal infection (d) None

58) All are true about AIDS except
(a) Seen in heterosexual only (b) Caused by retro virus (c) Candidiasis is also common feature (d) Retro virus is thermo labile

59) In HIV window period indicates (AIIMS, Nov-07)
(a) Time period between infection and onset of first symptoms. (b) Time period between infection and detection of antibodies against HIV (c) Time period between infection and minimum multiplication of the organism (d) Time period between infection and maximum multiplication of the organism

60) HIV can be detected and confirmed by (AI-05)
(a) Polymerase chain reaction (PCR) (b) Reverse Transcriptase-PCR (c) Real Time -PCR (d) Mimic PCR

61) When compared to Western Blot technique, ELISA test is (AI-93, 96)
(a) Less sensitive, less specific (b) More sensitive, more specific (c) Less sensitive, more specific (d) More sensitive, less specific

62) More sensitive test for HIV infection
(a) Western Blot (b) ELISA (c) Agglutination test (d) CFT

63) Screening test for AIDS
(a) ELISA (b) PCR (c) Western Blot (d) CD4 count

64) More specific test for HIV infection
(a) Western Blot (b) ELISA (c) Agglutination test (d) CFT

65) Confirmatory test for AIDS
(a) ELISA (b) Rapid tests (c) Western Blot (d) CD4 count

66) Following is the marker of HIV infection in blood (AIIMS-94)
(a) Reverse transcriptase (b) DNA polymerase (c) RNA polymerase (d) None

67) All of the following methods are used for the diagnosis of HIV infection in a 2 month old child, except- (AIIMS, May-03)
(a) DNA-PCR (b) Viral culture (c) HIV ELISA (d) p24 antigen assay

68) A patient comes to hospital with history of sore throat, diarrhoea and sexual contact 2 weeks before. The best investigation to rule out HIV is (AI-00)
(a) p24 antigen assay (b) ELISA (c) Western Blot (d) Lymph node biopsy

69) False about p24 is
(a) Seen after 3 weeks of infection (b) Cant be seen in first week (c) Cant be detected after sero-conversion (d) Detected by ELISA

70) Antenatal maternal HIV diagnosis is of importance in
(a) To prevent vertical transmission (b) To terminate (c) To discharge (d) To isolate the patient

71) Which of the following is the most sensitive for diagnosis of HIV?
(a) RT-PCR (b) bDNA assay (c) NASBA (d) p24 detection

72) Full blown immuno deficiency syndrome is
(a) High viral titres with low CD4 count (b) Low viral titres with low CD4 count (c) Low viral titres with high CD4 count (d) High viral titres with high CD4 count

73) Maternal to child transmission of HIV is prevented by (AIIMS, Nov-11)
(a) Nevirapine (b) Lamivudine (c) Didanosine (d) Abacavir

74) A resident doctor sustained a needle stick injury while sampling blood of a patient who is HIV positive, A decision is taken to offer him post exposure prophylaxis. Which one of the following would be the best recommendation? (AIIMS, Nov-03)
(a) Zidovudine + Lamivudine for 4 weeks (b) Zidovudine + Lamivudine + Nevirapine for 4 weeks (c) Zidovudine + Lamivudine + Indinavir for 4 weeks (d) Zidovudine + stavudine + Nevirapine for 4 weeks

75) Which of the following is true regarding HIV infection (AI-04)
(a) Following needle stick injury infectivity is reduced by administration of nucleoside analogues (b) CD4 counts are the best predictors of disease progression (c) Infected T cells survive for a month in infected patients (d) In latent phase HIV has minimal replication

Answers of MCQs & explanation

1) **(c)**
- HIV is a retro virus , belongs to Retroviridae family

2) **(d)**
- Follow section, **genome** for explanation

3) **(a) & (c)**
- Follow section, **HTLV-I (pathogenicity → clinical features)** for explanation

4) **(b)**
- Follow section, **HTLV-III / HIV-1 & 2 (history & synonym)** for explanation

5) **(c)**
- Follow section, **HTLV-III / HIV-1 & 2 (Geographical distribution & genotypes → genotypes / clades)** for explanation

6) **(c)**
7) **(b)**
8) **(a)**

} Follow section, **HTLV-III / HIV-1 & 2 (morphology)** for explanation

9) **(d)**
- Follow section, **HTLV-III / HIV-1 & 2 (resistance)** for explanation

10) **(e)**
11) **(c)**
12) **(d)**
13) **(a) & (b)**
14) **(a)**
15) **(b)**
16) **(b)**

} Follow section, **HTLV-III / HIV-1 & 2 [viral genome & gene products (antigens)]** for explanation

17) **(a) & (b)**

- Risk of HIV transmission from mother to baby is 15-25% in developed countries & 25-35% in developing countries
- HIV infection can be diagnosed in the baby by
- P24 Ag detection by ELISA
- Viral nucleic acid by RT-PCR
- AIDS can be transmitted from mother to child during delivery (intranatal) & by breast feeding (postnatal).

18) **(a)**
19) **(d)**
20) **(a)**
21) **(a)**
22) **(a)**
23) **(c)**
24) **(a)**
25) **(d)**

(18–25) Follow section, **HTLV-III / HIV-1 & 2 (pathogenicity → mode of transmission)** for explanation

26) **(a), (b) & (c)**
- Option a: Follow section, **HTLV-III / HIV-1 & 2 (pathogenicity → pathogenesis → HIV infects & destroys other cells like)** for explanation
- Option b: Follow section, **HTLV-III / HIV-1 & 2 (morphology)** for explanation
- Option c & d: Follow section, **HTLV-III / HIV-1 & 2 (resistance)** for explanation

27) **(c)**
- Option a: Follow section, **HTLV-III / HIV-1 & 2 (laboratory diagnosis → p24 Ag detection)** for explanation
- Option b, c & d: Follow section, **HTLV-III/HIV-1 & 2 [pathogenicity → pathogenesis (flow chart-1)]** for explanation

28) **(a)**
- Option a & b: Follow section, **HTLV-III/HIV-1 & 2 (morphology)** for explanation
- Option c & d: Follow section, **HTLV-III/HIV-1 & 2 [pathogenicity → pathogenesis (flow chart-1)]** for explanation

29) **(b) & (d)**
30) **(a)**
31) **(a) & (d)**
32) **(d)**
33) **(a)**
34) **(a)**

(29–34) Follow section, **HTLV-III/HIV-1 & 2 [pathogenicity → pathogenesis (flow chart-1)]** for explanation

35) **(a), (b), (c) & (e)**
36) **(a), (b) (e)**

(35–36) Follow section, **HTLV-III/HIV-1 & 2 [pathogenicity → pathogenesis (flow chart-1) & clinical features]** for explanation

37) **(b), (c) & (e)**
- Follow section, **HTLV-III / HIV-1 & 2 (pathogenicity → clinical features → AIDS → clinical definition of AIDS)** for explanation

38) **(b)**
- Follow section, **HTLV-III / HIV-1 & 2 (pathogenicity → clinical features → acute HIV infection)** for explanation

39) **(d)**
40) **(a)**
41) **(a)**
42) **(a)**
43) **(c)**
44) **(c)**
45) **(a) & (b)**
46) **(c) & (d)**
47) **(a)**
48) **(a)**
49) **(b) & (e)**
50) **(c)**
51) **(b)**
52) **(a), (b), (c) & (d)**
53) **(b)**
54) **(c)**
55) **(d)**
56) **(a)**

(39–56) Follow section, **HTLV-III / HIV-1 & 2 (pathogenicity → clinical features → AIDS →opportunistic infections & malignancies)** for explanation

57) **(b)**
58) **(a)**
- AIDS is seen in both heterosexual & homosexual persons

59) **(b)**
60) **(b)**
61) **(d)**
62) **(b)**
63) **(a)**
64) **(a)**
65) **(c)**
66) **(a)**
67) **(a) & (c)**
68) **(a)**
69) **(a)**
70) **(a)**
71) **(a)**
72) **(a)**

(59–72) Follow section, **HTLV-III / HIV-1 & 2 (laboratory diagnosis)** for explanation

73) **(a)**
74) **(c)**

(73–74) Follow section, **HTLV-III / HIV-1 & 2 (prevention → post exposure prophylaxis)** for explanation

75) **(a)**
- HIV progress is assessed by viral load (HIV-RNA) not by CD4 count.

71 Other RNA viruses

(Rubella virus and Coronaviridae)

Learning heading & subheadings

- Rubella virus
- Coronaviridae
  - Severe Acute Respiratory Syndrome-related Corona Virus
  - Middle-East Respiratory Syndrome-related Corona Virus

Rubella virus

❖ Classification:

➢ **Family:** Togaviridae.

➢ **Genus:** Following two genera.

A. ***Rubivirus:***

✪ **Species:** Rubella virus → Described below.

B. ***Alphavirus:*** Follow chapter → Arboviruses and Roboviruses.

❖ History:

- Teratogenic complication was diagnosed by Australian ophthalmologist Norman Gregg in 1941, with sudden increase of cataract in infant with rubella.
- Research from different countries shows that rubella produce triad of congenital malformation of cataract, deafness & cardiac defect.
- Rubella virus was isolated in 1962 by tissue culture method.

❖ Geographical distribution & genotypes:

- **Distribution:** Distributed worldwide. Over 100 000 babies are born with congenital rubella syndrome every year.
- **Genotypes:** On the basis of differences in the sequence of the E1 protein, two genotypes have been described which differ by 8 - 10%. These have been subdivided into 13 recognised genotypes – 1A, 1B, 1C, 1D, 1E, 1F, 1G, 1H, 1I, 1J, 2A, 2B & 2C. For typing, WHO recommends a minimum window that includes nucleotides 8731 to 9469. Following is the distribution pattern
  - 1A, 1E, 1F, 2A & 2B: Found in China.
  - 1C: Found in Central & South America.
  - 1E: Found in Africa, Americas, Asia & Europe.
  - 1G: Found in Belarus, Cote d'Ivoire and Uganda.
  - 1J: Found in Japan & Philippines.
  - 2B: Found in South Africa.
  - 2C: Found in Russia.

❖ Morphology: →Fig.-1

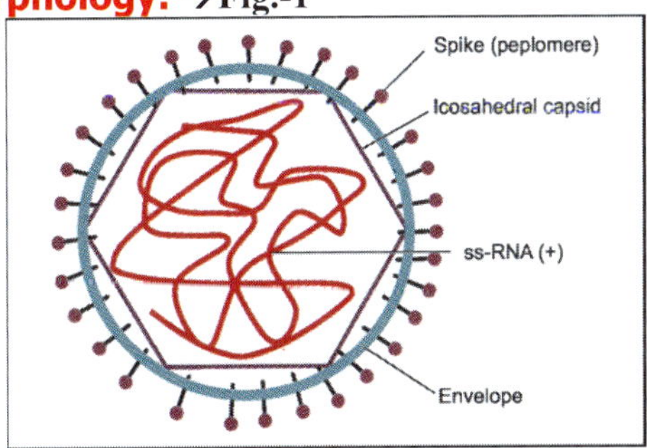

Figure-1: Morphology of rubella virus

➢ **Shape:** Spherical.

➢ **Size:** 50-70 nm.

➢ **Genome:** ss-RNA (+) with icosahedral capsid.

➢ **Enveloped:** Lipoprotein envelope contains haemagglutinating spikes. They agglutinate the goose, pigeon, one-day-old chick & human RBCs at 4^0C.

➢ **Viral proteins:**

- **Structural:** Like capsid (C) & envelope (E1 & E2) proteins.
- **Non-structural:** Like p150 & p90.

❖ Culture characteristics (C/Cs):

i. Animal culture:

- Experimental infection can be produced in monkeys.
- Pregnant rabbit can be used as laboratory model to study the congenital malformation.

ii. Cell culture:

- Can grow in primary cell culture.
- Also grow in continuous cell lines like
  - RK (Rabbit Kidney) -13 cells: Growth is identified by CPE.
  - BHK-21 & Vero cells: No CPE, but growth is identified by interference or by using challenger virus like ECHO-11.

❖ **Resistance:** Inactivated by heat (56^0C), ether, chloroform, formaldehyde, BPL & desoxycholate.

❖ **Antigenic structure & serotypes:** No antigenic variation, only one sero types is known.

❖ Immunity:

- Single attack provides the lifelong immunity & secondary attack is rare.
- Passive immunity is occurs in infants of immune mother for 4-6 months following birth due to presence of passively transferred IgG.

❖ Pathogenicity:

- **Disease name:** Disease **called rubella.**
- **Synonym:** Also **called german measles.**
- **Nature or history of disease:**
  - Disease occurs worldwide throughout the year with peak in spring.
  - Epidemic occurs every 6-8 years & major pandemic every 20-25 years.
  - Last post natal global epidemic was occurred in 1962-65.
  - However due to use of effective vaccine epidemics are less encountered now a days.
- **Reservoir of infection:** Human only case. Carrier stage does not exist.
- **Source of infection:**
  - It present in nasopharyngeal / throat secretion, blood, CSF & urine.
  - Period of infectivity (communicability): It starts a week before the onset of symptoms to about a week after rash appear.
- **Mode of transmission:**
  - By inhalation.
  - By placenta.
- **Incubation period (IP):** 2-3weeks.
- **Portal of entry:** Respiratory system.
- **Sites:** Skin CNS, bones, joints, foetal organs etc.
- **Precipitating factors (epidemiological determinants):**

a. **Agent factors:** Rubella virus is less communicable than measles virus because of absence of coughing. Infectivity is highest before & after a week of appearance of rash.

b. **Host factors:**

1. **Age:**
   - Infants of immune mother are protected up to 4-6 months.
   - Common in children between 3-10 years.
   - 10-40% people can reach to adulthood without experiencing the rubella in the absence of immunisation.
2. **Pregnancy:**
   - About 10-40% people can reach to adulthood without experiencing the rubella in the absence of immunisation, thus child bearing age remains rubella susceptible.
   - In India, 40% female are infected with rubella during child bearing age.
   - Foetal damage by rubella is related to stage of pregnancy.
   - 1st trimester is the most dangerous because, organs are developing. It cause chromosomal breakages & inhibition of mitoses in infected embryonic cells.
   - If infection occurs in 1st trimester resulting foetal death & spontaneous abortion.
   - If occurs late resulting congenital malformation.
   - Percentages of foetal damage at different stage of pregnancy are mentioned in **table-1.**

c. **Environmental factors:**

1. **Climate:** It occurs throughout the years, with peak in the spring.

Weeks of pregnancy	Foetal infection (%)	Foetal damage (%)	Overall foetal risk
< 11	90	100	90
11-16	55	37	20
17-26	33	0	0
>27	53	0	0

Table-1: Percentages of foetal risk at different stage of pregnancy

- **Pathogenesis:** After the entry virus replicates locally in the nasopharynx & then spread to the lymph nodes. Viremia develops after 7-9 days & last until 14th day by which time both antibodies & rashes appear simultaneously suggesting an immunological basis for the appearance of rash.
- **Clinical features:**
  - **Prodromal phase:** It consist coryza, low-grade-fever & sore throat.
  - **Lymphadenopathy:** Post-auricular & posterior cervical lymph nodes are enlarged; however rubella cases without lymphadenopathy are also documented.
  - **Rash:** Pinkish, minute, discrete, macular rash typically appear on face & then extend to neck, trunk & extremities sparing the palms & soles.

✪ **Complications:**

- Arthralgia & arthritis.
- Subacute Sclerosing Pan Encephalitis (SSPE): It is very rare.
- Thrombocytopenic purpura.
- Pregnancy: It produces following effects.
  - 1st trimester (before 12 weeks): Foetal death & spontaneous abortion.
  - Later stage: Congenital malformation **called congenital rubella syndrome**. Two types.

a. **Classical congenital rubella syndrome:** Triad of cataract, deafness & congenital cardiac defect in babies.

b. **Expanded congenital rubella syndrome:** Babies are present with extra features like

- Hepato-splenomegaly.
- Thrombocytopenic purpura.
- Myocarditis.
- Bone lesions.

- Glaucoma.
- Retinopathy.
- Mental, motor & growth retardation.

❖ **Laboratory diagnosis:**

I. **In pregnancy or a case except congenital malformation**

➢ **Specimens:** Throat swab, blood, serum etc.

➢ **Testing methods:**

A. **Microscopy: → Follow morphology.**

B. **Culture: → Follow C/Cs.**

C. **Serological test:**

- ELISA to detect IgM & IgG.
- As IgM is not transported by placenta & synthesised after 20 weeks of gestational age, its presence in the before this time, indicates intrauterine infection & its detection is useful in diagnosis of congenital rubella infection.
- IgG can cross the placenta & it can survive in infants for a period of 6 months. Persistent beyond 1 year in an unvaccinated child suggest the diagnosis of congenital rubella.

D. **Molecular methods:** RT-PCR is rapid & more sensitive method.

II. **In congenital malformation**

➢ **Specimens:** Virus is present in all parts of infected infants. Commonly used specimens are urine, CSF, throat swab, blood etc.

➢ **Testing methods:**

A. **Microscopy: → Follow morphology.**

B. **Culture: → Follow C/Cs.**

C. **Serological test:** ELISA to detect IgM & IgG.

- IgM cant cross the placenta & its presence in infant's blood indicates uterine infection.
- Normal IgG can cross the placenta & remain in infant's blood for 6 months & then disappear. Lasting for more than 6 months indicates uterine infection.

D. **Molecular methods:** PCR is rapid & more sensitive method.

❖ **Prevention:** It is important to acquire protection before child bearing age.

➢ **Active immunisation:** By using live attenuated vaccine.

- **History:** Vaccine was developed in 1979.
- **Preparation:** Prepared by serial passage of virus (**RA 27/3 strain**) in human diploid cell culture.
- **Administration:**
  - Given alone or in combination with MMR or MMRV (MMR + varicella) vaccine to all women with child bearing age & also to children of 1-14 years.
  - **Dose:** 0.5ml.
  - **Route:** SC injection.
- **Advantages:**
  - Well tolerated.
  - Provide protection for 14-16 years or life-long.
- **Disadvantages:** Some side effects like
  - Local reactions.
  - Fever, rash, arthralgia & lymphadenopathy.
- **Contraindications:**
  - Immune deficient persons like leukemia, AIDS etc.
  - Pregnancy is contraindicated after vaccination at least for 3 months.
  - Infants < 1 year, to avoid possible interference to maternal antibody.

❖ **Treatment:** Rubella is mild, self limited condition & no specific treatment is available.

Coronaviridae

❖ **Meaning:** Name is given from the word **corona** = **solar**, because spherical shape & projecting spikes gives solar like appearance.

❖ **Classification:**

➢ **Family:** Coronaviridae.

➢ **Subfamilies:** Two subfamilies like Coronavirinae & Torovirinae.

I. **Coronavirinae:**

➢ **Genera & species:** Following four genera with human species.

A. ***Alphacoronavirus***:

i. **Human corona virus 229E.**

ii. **Human Corona virus NL63 (New heaven corona virus).**

B. ***Betacoronavirus***:

i. **Human corona virus OC43.**

ii. **Severe Acute Respiratory Syndrome-related Corona Virus (SARS-CoV).**

iii. **Human corona virus HKU1.**

iv. **MERS-CoV [Middle-East Respiratory Syndrome related Corona Virus,** previously **called Novel coronavirus 2012** or **called Human Corona Virus-Erasmus Medical Centre (HCoV-EMC)].**

✓ **Note: Order of discovery of above human corona viruses.**

- For many years, scientists knew about only two human corona viruses (HCoV-229E & HCoV-OC43).
- The discovery of SARS-CoV in 2002-03 added a third human coronavirus.
- By the end of 2004, three independent research labs reported the fourth human coronavirus, NL63 or New Haven coronavirus.
- Early in 2005, a research team at the University of Hong Kong reported a fifth human coronavirus in two patients with pneumonia, named it Human coronavirus HKU1.

- In September 2012, a sixth new type of coronavirus, Novel Coronavirus 2012 was identified and now officially labelled as Middle East respiratory syndrome coronavirus (MERS-CoV).

C. ***Gammacoronavirus*:** It includes avian pathogens.

D. ***Deltacoronavirus*:** It includes bulbul & other pathogens.

II. Torovirinae:

➢ **Genera & species:** Following two genera. Both includes animal/avian pathogens.

A ***Torovirus*:** Includes the species causing gastroenteritis in human, cattle, pigs & horses.

B ***Bafinivirus*:** It is a white bream pathogen.

❖ **History:** Corona viruses were first described in the 1960s from the nasal cavities of patients with the common cold. These viruses were subsequently named human coronavirus 229E and human coronavirus OC43.

❖ **Morphology:** → **Fig.-2**

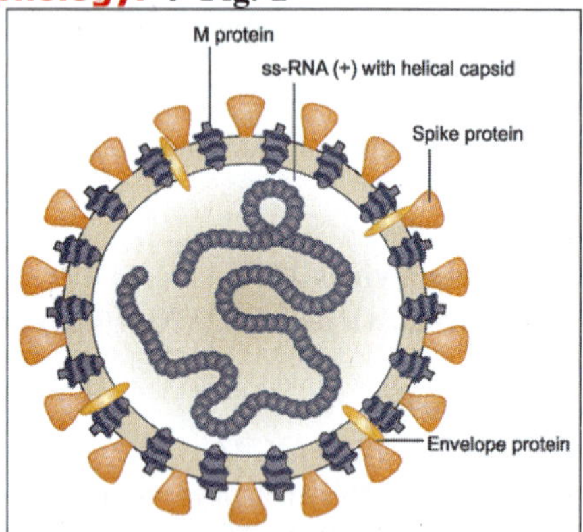

Figure-2: Morphology of Coronaviridae

➢ **Shape:** Spherical or pleomorphic.

➢ **Size:** 100nm.

➢ **Genome & capsid:** ss-RNA (+) with helical variety of capsid.

➢ **Enveloped:** Carrying club or petal shape spikes (peplomeres) on surface, giving solar like appearance.

➢ **Viral proteins:** Two types like

- **Structural proteins:** Four structural proteins like nucleocapsid, spike, membrane (M) and envelope.
- **Accessory proteins:** It also encodes for eight unique proteins, **called accessory proteins.**

❖ **Culture characteristics (C/Cs):**

i. Organ/cell culture:

a. Organ culture:

- Done by inoculating human embryonic trachea with nasopharyngeal secretion (tracheal ring culture).
- Inhibition of ciliary movement indicates the virus growth.
- No longer in use.

b. Cell culture: Vero cells & human diploid embryonic fibroblast cells are useful. SARS-CoV was isolated by using the Vero cells.

ii. Animal culture: Also useful.

Severe Acute Respiratory Syndrome-related Corona Virus

✪ **Abbreviation:** SARS-CoV.

✪ **History:** Virus was isolated in February 2003 on Vero cells. SARS-CoV is thought to be an animal virus, uncertain animal reservoir, perhaps bats, that spread to other animals (civet cats) and first infected humans in the Guangdong province of southern China in 2002.

✪ **Geographical distribution:**

- The distribution is based on the 2002–2003 epidemic. The disease appeared in November 2002 in the Guangdong province of southern China. This area is considered as a potential zone of re-emergence of SARS-CoV.
- Other countries/areas in which chains of human-to-human transmission occurred after early importation of cases were Toronto in Canada, Hong Kong Special Administrative Region of China, Chinese Taipei, Singapore, and Hanoi in Viet Nam.

✪ **Morphology:** → **Vide supra.**

✪ **Culture characteristics (C/Cs):** → **Vide supra.**

✪ **Resistance:** It is an envelope virus susceptible to lipid solvents. There are two groups of corona viruses like

1. **Acid –stable corona virus:** Causing gastroenteritis in human & animals.
2. **Acid –labile corona virus:** Causing common-cold like illness.

✪ **Immunity:** Human corona virus has many serotypes, resulting immunity is poor & reinfection can occur with same serotypes.

✪ **Pathogenicity:**

- **Disease name:** Disease **called Severe Acute Respiratory Syndrome (SARS).**
- **Nature or history of disease:**

- **2002-03, epidemic:** Epidemic started in late 2002 in Guangdong province of southern China. It spread in to almost 26 countries of North America, South America, Europe, and Asia before the SARS global outbreak of 2003 was contained. It reported 8098 cases with 774 deaths. Epidemic was identified by Dr Carlo Urbani from Guangdong who visited the Hong Kong, fell ill & died due to it after infecting 12 persons who had stayed in the same hotel.
- **Current scenario:** Currently, no areas of the world are reporting transmission of SARS. Since the end of the global epidemic in July 2003, SARS has

reappeared four times – three times from laboratory accidents (Singapore and Chinese Taipei), and once in southern China where the source of infection remains undetermined although there is circumstantial evidence of animal-to-human transmission.

- **Indian scenario:** India escaped the 2002-03 epidemics of SARS; however few suspected cases were detected & quarantined.

- **Reservoir of infection:** Human & some animal like monkeys, Himalayan pal, civets, racoon, dogs, cats & rodents are the reservoir.
- **Source of infection:** Virus is excreted in respiratory secretion & stool from the patient, which carry the risk for transmission. Infectivity is more in 2nd week of illness.
- **Mode of transmission:**
  - Inhalations of aerosols arise during coughing or sneezing. Such droplets carry the risk up to 3 feet. Virus deposited on mucosa of nose, mouth & eyes.
  - Contact: The virus also can spread when a person touches a surface or object contaminated with infectious droplets and then touches his or her mouth, nose, or eye(s).
  - In addition, it is possible that the SARS virus might spread more broadly through the air (airborne spread) or by other ways that are not now known.
- **Incubation period:** 2-10 days.
- **Portal of entry:** Respiratory system.
- **Sites:** Respiratory system & GIT.
- **Precipitating factors (epidemiological determinants):**

1. **Close contact with the patients:** Close contact means having cared for or lived with someone with SARS or having direct contact with respiratory secretions or body fluids of a patient with SARS. Examples of close contact include kissing or hugging, sharing eating or drinking utensils, talking to someone within 3 feet, and touching someone directly. Close contact does not include activities like walking by a person or briefly sitting across a waiting room or office.
2. **Age:** The mortality rate was much higher for those over 50 years old in 2003 outbreak.
3. **Occupation:** Laboratory workers are at risk.

- **Pathogenesis:** Virus settle on mucosa of nose, eyes & mouth, later spread to other organs.
- **Clinical features:**
  - **Initially in few days:** Flu-like symptoms which include fever, malaise, myalgia, headache, diarrhoea & shivering (rigors).
  - **In 1st/2nd week:** Cough (initially dry), shortness of breath & diarrhoea are present.
- **Complications:**
  - Secondary bacterial infections.
  - Lymphopenia (low lymphocytes).
  - Liver or heart failure.
  - Respiratory distress/failure leading to death.

✪ **Diagnosis:**

- **Specimens:** Respiratory specimens like sputum, nasopharyngeal secretion & serum.
- **Testing methods:**

1. **Microscopy: → Follow morphology.**
2. **Culture: → Follow C/Cs.**
3. **Serological tests:**
   - IgM antibody is produced. This peaks during the acute or early convalescent phase (week 3) and declines by week 12.
   - IgG Ab is produced later and peaks at 12th week.
   - Antibodies are detected by HAI test or by ELISA.
4. **Molecular test:** RT-PCR is useful for rapid diagnosis.
5. **Chest x-ray:** It is ordered to confirm the pneumonia.

✪ **Prevention:**

- Isolation of patients & avoid contact with relatives.
- Hand washing before and after touching animals, and should avoid contact with sick animals.
- Surface disinfection.
- No specific vaccine is available.

✪ **Treatment:** No specific antiviral drugs are available, supportive measures are given. Antibiotics are prescribed to prevent the secondary bacterial infections.

Middle-East Respiratory Syndrome-related Corona Virus

✪ **Abbreviation:** MERS-CoV.

✪ **Synonym:** Previously **called Novel corona virus 2012** or **called Human Corona Virus-Erasmus Medical Centre 2012 (HCoV-EMC 2012).**

✪ **Common name:** SARS like virus, Novel coronavirus.

✪ **History:**

- Virus was isolated by Dr. Ali Mohamed Zaki in 2012 from the sputum samples of a person who fell ill in a 2012 outbreak in Saudi Arabia. Initially it was **called SARS like virus** & disease **called Saudi SARS**.
- As it diagnosed in 2012 & newer in the list of coronavirus so **called Novel coronavirus 2012.**
- After the Dutch Erasmus Medical Centre sequenced the virus in 2012, the virus **called Human Corona Virus-Erasmus Medical Centre 2012 (HCoV-EMC 2012)**.
- The official name for the virus is Middle East Respiratory Syndrome Corona Virus (MERS-CoV).

✪ **Geographical distribution:**

- The virus started the epidemic in Saudi Arabia & as of July 2015, MERS-CoV spread in over 21 countries, including Saudi Arabia, Jordan, Qatar,

Egypt, the United Arab Emirates, Kuwait, Turkey, Oman, Algeria, Bangladesh, Indonesia (none were confirmed), Austria, the United Kingdom, South Korea, the United States, Mainland China, Thailand, and the Philippines.

- **Genotypes (clades):** Two clades like A and B were reported. The earliest cases of MERS-CoV were of clade A (EMC/2012 and Jordan-N3/2012) & newer cases were different from A were from clade B.

✪ **Morphology: → Vide supra**

✪ **Culture characteristics (C/Cs):** Over culture cells (like Vero cells) it produces the CPE, ballooning & syncytium formation.

✪ **Resistance:**

- It is sterilised by autoclave at 1210C for 15 minutes.
- It is susceptible to 70% alcohol or 0.5% sodium hypochlorite.

✪ **Pathogenicity:**

- **Disease name:** Initial disease **called Saudi SARS.** Actually it **called Middle East Respiratory Syndrome (MERS).**
- **Nature or history of disease:**
  - **2012 epidemic in Saudi Arabia:** It started in Saudi Arabia & later spread to other countries as mentioned earlier. By October 30, 2013, there were 124 cases and 52 deaths in Saudi Arabia.
  - **2015 outbreak in Republic of Korea:** In May 2015, an outbreak of MERS-CoV occurred in the Republic of Korea, when a man who had travelled to the Middle East, visited 4 different hospitals in the Seoul area to treat his illness. This caused one of the largest outbreaks of MERS-CoV outside of the Middle East.
  - **Indian scenario:** It is not reporter from India yet.
- **Reservoir of infection:** Unknown but may be acquired from camels or bats.
- **Source of infection:** Exactly not known but may be the respiratory droplets arise during sneezing & coughing from patient. Raw camel meat or milk may be the source for animal to human spread.
- **Mode of transmission:**
  - Animal to human transmission: The route of transmission from animals (camels) to humans is not fully understood.
  - Human-to-human transmission: Not even human to human transmission occurs until there is as close contact with the patient, especially in health care workers.
- **Incubation period:** 2-14 days.
- **Portal of entry:** May be respiratory tract.
- **Sites:** Respiratory system, GIT & kidneys also.
- **Precipitating factors (epidemiological determinants):**

1. **Virus (agent) factor:** The risk of sustained person-to-person transmission appears to be very low until there is as close contact with the patient. The cells MERS-CoV infects in the lungs only account for 20% of respiratory epithelial cells, so a large number of virions are likely needed to be inhaled to cause infection.
2. **Occupation:** Laboratory workers are at risk.

- **Pathogenesis:** After entering in the body it target the human bronchial epithelium and kidneys.
- **Clinical features:** No symptoms or mild symptoms like fever, cough, shortness of breath, diarrhoea & nausea / vomiting.
- **Complications:** Kidney failure or even death.

✪ **Diagnosis:**

- **Specimens:** Respiratory specimens like sputum, nasopharyngeal secretion & serum.
- **Testing methods:**

1. **Microscopy: → Follow morphology.**
2. **Culture: → Follow C/Cs.**
3. **Serological test:** ELISA, immunofluorescent assay or micro-neutralisation test are useful.
4. **Molecular test:** RT-PCR is useful for rapid diagnosis.
5. **Chest x-ray:** It is ordered to confirm the pneumonia.

✪ **Prevention:**

- Isolation of patients & avoid contact with relatives.
- Avoid to visit the place where camels or their products like meat, milk etc. are available.
- Hand washing before and after touching animals, and should avoid contact with sick animals.
- Surface disinfection.
- No specific vaccine is available.

✪ **Treatment:** No specific antiviral drugs are available, supportive measures are given.

Question bank

Case study

1) A 30-year-old female visited the obstetric OPD with 2 months (8 weeks) amenorrhoea with complain of fever. On clinical examination, rashes on face & post-auricular enlarged lymph nodes were found. Ultra-sonography was advised as a part of routine check-up, which reported the dead foetus & female went for termination of pregnancy. Identify the clinical conditions & answer the following

a) Name the clinical condition & its most common etiological agent.
b) Write the morphology of etiological agent.
c) Write pathogenicity of clinical condition.
d) Write laboratory diagnosis of clinical condition.

Essay/Full question

1) Coronaviridae.

Short notes

1) Rubella virus.
2) Human coronaviruses.
3) SARS-CoV.
4) MERS-CoV.

Short questions for theory/viva questions

1) Write the common manifestation (complications) caused by Rubella virus in pregnant women.
2) Name any four species of human corona virus.

MCQs for chapter review

Rubella virus

1) **Incubation period of rubella is** (AI-93)
(a) 18-72 hours (b) 2-3 weeks (c) 1-3 months (d) > 1year
2) **All of the following statements are true about congenital rubella except** (AI-05)
(a) It is diagnosed when the infants has IgM antibodies at birth (b) It is diagnosed when IgG antibodies persist for more than 6 months (c) Most common congenital defects are deafness, cardiac malformations and cataract (d) Infection after 16 weeks of gestation results in major congenital defects
3) **Risk of the damage to foetus by maternal rubella is maximum if mother gets infected in** (AIIMS-05)
(a) 6-12 weeks of pregnancy (b) 20-24 weeks of pregnancy (c) 24-28 weeks of pregnancy (d) 32-36 weeks of pregnancy
4) **Classical triad of congenital rubella includes all except**
(a) Cataract (b) Deafness (c) Retinitis (d) CHD (Congenital Heart Disease)
5) **The congenital rubella syndrome**
(a) May be prevented by vaccination in early pregnancy (b) Causes IUGR (c) Causes cataract (d) Causes deafness only if acquired before 16 weeks of gestation
6) **Rubella vaccine is contraindicated in all except**
(a) Patient on immunosuppressant (b) Girls with leukemia (c) Girls between 11-14 years (d) Pregnancy

Coronaviridae

7) **Following is/are the human corona virus (es)**
(a) 229E (b) NL63 (c) OC43 (d) SV40
8) **SARS true are** (PGI, June-06)
(a) Severe acute respiratory syndrome (b) Documented respiratory route spread (c) Effective vaccine available (d) Group corona virus
9) **Causative agent of SARS**
(a) H1N1 (b) Corona virus (c) *Rotavirus* (d) RSV

Answers of MCQs & explanation

1) **(b)**
2) **(d)**
3) **(a)**
4) **(c)**
5) **(b) & (c)**
6) **(c)**

(Answers 1–6: Follow section, **rubella virus** for explanation)

7) **(a), (b) & (c)**
- Options a, b & c: Follow section, **Coronaviridae (classification)** for explanation
- SV40 virus is belongs to Papovaviridae family. It is not a human pathogen. It causing the polyoma (malignant tumour) in mice.

8) **(a), (b) (d) & (e)**
9) **(b)**

(Answers 8–9: Follow section, **Coronaviridae (severe acute respiratory syndrome related corona virus)** for explanation)

72 Bacteriophages

Learning heading & subheadings

- ❖ **Meaning:**
- ❖ **Definitions:**
- ❖ **History:**
- ❖ **Classification:**
- ❖ **Morphology:**
- ❖ **Life cycle:**
- ❖ **Uses:**
- ❖ **Phage assay:**

❖ **Meaning:** Bacteriophage word derived from two words like **bacteria + phagein (Greek) = to devour or to eat bacteria**, means virus which eats the bacterium.

❖ **Definition:** Taxonomically unrelated (either DNA or RNA) viruses which eat the bacteria are **called bacteriophages**. Commonly abbreviated as **phages**.

❖ **History:** In 1917 Twort & d'Herelle observed the lysis of dysentery bacillus broth culture from stool filtrate of dysentery patients & gave the name as bacteriophage to such lytic agent.

❖ **Classification:** Bacteriophage group contains either DNA or RNA viruses as shown in **table-1**.

❖ **Morphology:** *E. coli* T-even phages **(fig.-1)** like T2, T4, T6 etc. served as model to describe the properties of bacteriophage.

➢ **Shape:**

- **T-even phage:** Tad pole shape.
- **Some phages are filamentous / spherical in shape**

➢ **Parts:**

✪ **Head:**

- **Size:** 28-100 nm.
- **Shape:** Hexagonal.
- **NA (Genome):** Some phage contains DNA while some contains RNA but never both. NA is surrounded by capsid. It may be ss or ds.

✪ **Tail:** Hollow core surrounded by contractile sheath.

✪ **Base plate with prong & tail fibers:** Helps in adsorption to host cell.

Naked or enveloped	Virus family	Genus/species	Nucleic acid type	Capsid & morphology
		DNA type bacteriophages		
Enveloped	Lipothrixviridae	Acidianus filamentous virus 1	Linear dsDNA	Rod-shaped
	Ampullaviridae		Linear dsDNA	Bottle-shaped
	Globuloviridae		Linear dsDNA	Isometric
	Plasmaviridae	MV-L2 phage	Circular dsDNA	Pleomorphic
Naked	Myoviridae	*E .coli* phage/coli phage (T even phage like T2, T4, T6 phage), Mu, PBSX, P1Puna-like, P2, I3, Bcep 1, Bcep 43, Bcep 78	Linear dsDNA	Icosahedral, contractile tail
	Sipho(stylo) viridae	*E .coli* phage (like T1, T5), λ phage, phi, C2, L5, HK97, N15	Linear dsDNA	Icosahedral, noncontractile tail (long)
	Podo(pedo)-viridae	*E .coli* phage/coli phage (like T3, T7 phage), P22, P37	Linear dsDNA	Icosahedral, noncontractile tail (short)
	Rudiviridae	Sulfolobus islandicus virus 1	Linear dsDNA	Rod-shaped
	Tectiviridae	PRD1 phage	Linear dsDNA	Icosahedral, isometric
	Bicaudaviridae		Circular dsDNA	Lemon-shaped
	Clavaviridae		Circular dsDNA	Rod-shaped
	Corticoviridae	*Pseudomonas* phage MP2	Circular dsDNA	Icosahedral, isometric
	Fuselloviridae		Circular dsDNA	Lemon-shaped
	Guttaviridae		Circular dsDNA	Ovoid
	Inoviridae	M13, MV-L1, *E .coli* phage fd	Circular ssDNA	Helical capsid, filamentous
	Microviridae	*E .coli* phage (X174 phage)	Circular ssDNA	Icosahedral, isometric
		RNA type bacteriophages		
Enveloped	Cystoviridae	Phage ϕ6	Segmented dsRNA	Icosahedral, spherical
Naked	Leviviridae	Phage MS2, Qβ	Linear ssRNA	Icosahedral, isometric

Table-1: Classification of bacteriophages

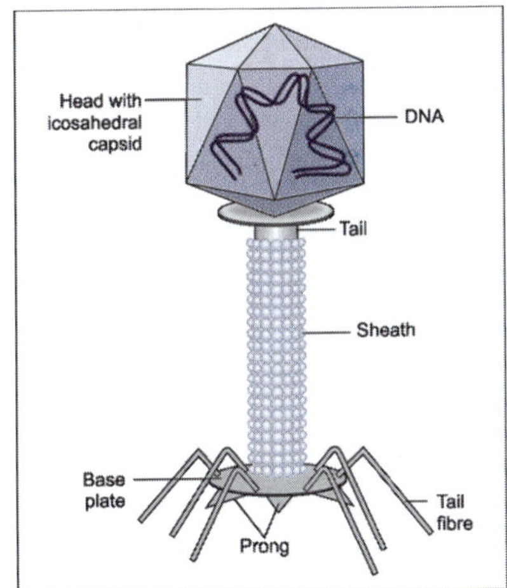

Figure-1: *E. coli* phage (T-even phage)

❖ **Life cycle:** Follow chapter → Genetics of bacteria.

❖ **Uses:**

a. **Therapeutic:** Initially it was used in treatment of bacterial infection, but not satisfactory.

b. **Transduction:**

- To transfer the genetic information between two cells. It transduced not only the chromosome but plasmid, episome & transposon are also tranduced.
- More details: Follow chapter → Genetics of bacteria.

c. **Model:** To study the virus-host interaction.

d. **Cloning vector:** In genetic manipulation.

e. **Control of bacterial population:** Presences of 10^8 phages per ml of water suggest that they have a role in control of bacterial population.

f. **Diagnosis of bacteria & bacteriophage typing:**

- For identification & epidemiological typing of bacteria which are difficult to distinguish by biochemical & serological methods.
- More details: Follow chapter → Laboratory diagnosis of bacterial infections.

g. **Phage conversion:**

- Presence of phage over bacteria confers certain new properties in bacteria **called phage conversion**.
- Following non-toxigenic strain of bacteria becomes toxigenic after infection by phage & producing the toxin.

1. *C. diphtheriae:* Diphtheria toxin.
2. *V. cholerae:* Cholera toxin.
3. *EHEC:* Verotoxin.
4. *Cl. botulinum:* Toxin C & D.
5. *S. pyogenes:* Streptococcal Pyrogenic Exotoxin (SPE) A & C.

h. **Alteration of antigenic properties of *Salmonella*:**

- Structural changes in O Ag of *Salmonella* can be induced by bacteriophage (lysogenisation), which results in new serotypes of *S. anatum* to *S. newington* & later to *S. minneapolis*.
- More details: Follow chapter → Enterobactericeae-II (*Salmonella*).

❖ **Phage assay:**

➢ **Definition:**

- It is one type of plaque assay, but when virus is bacteriophage **called phage assay**.
- When phage is apples to bacterial culture, it produce lytic zone **called plaque**.

➢ **Uses:**

- Give idea about numbers of phages in suspension.
- For purification of phages.
- Size, shape & nature of plaque give idea about type of phage.

Question bank

Essay/Full question

1) Bacteriophage.

Short notes

1) Life cycle of bacteriophage.
2) Uses of bacteriophage.

Short questions for theory/viva questions

1) Write four uses of bacteriophage.
2) Define: Transduction & lysohenic conversion.
3) Draw the morphological labelled diagram of bacteriophage.
4) Define: provirus & prophage.
5) Write four examples of bacteria producing toxin after phage conversion.

MCQs for chapter review

History

1) **Bacteriophage was discovered by**
(a) Edward Jenner (b) Twort & d' herelle (c) Smith, Andrew & Laidlaw (d) Johnson & Goodpasture

Uses

2) **Bacteriophages are mostly needed for** (AIIMS-97)
(a) Bacterial identification (b) Epidemiologically (c) As antibacterial agent (d) Conversion property in bacteria

3) **All of the following statements are true about bacteriophages except** (AIIMS, Nov-98)
(a) It is a virus that infect the bacteria (b) It helps in transduction of bacteria (c) It imparts toxigenicity to bacteria (d) It transfer only chromosomal gene.

4) **Which of the following statement is true about bacteriophages** (AIIMS, May-11)
(a) It is a bacterium (b) It helps in transformation (c) It imparts toxigenicity to bacteria (d) It transfer only chromosomal gene.

Answers of MCQs & explanation

1) **(b)**
- Follow section, **history** for explanation

2) **(a), (b) & (d)**
3) **(d)**
4) **(c)**

} Follow section, **uses** for explanation

73 Hepatitis viruses

Learning heading & subheadings

- Meaning:
- Definition:
- List of viruses causing hepatitis:
- Classification:
- World hepatitis day:

DNA virus

Hepadnaviridae - HBV

RNA viruses

Picornaviridae - HAV

Flaviridae - HCV

Deltavirus - HDV

Hepeviridae - HEV

Differences between hepatitis viruses

Meaning: From **hepa (Greek) = liver + itis = inflammation**, because infecting & causing inflammation of liver.

Definition: Group of heterogenous or taxonomical unrelated viruses (HBV is DNA type & others are RNA type) causing inflammation of liver.

List of viruses causing hepatitis:

A. Hepatitis viruses group:

- Hepatitis A Virus (HAV).
- Hepatitis B Virus (HBV).
- Hepatitis C Virus (HCV).
- Hepatitis D Virus (HDV).
- Hepatitis E Virus (HEV).
- Hepatitis G Virus (HGV).

B. Others: They are not from hepatitis group but causing inflammation of liver (hepatitis).

- Yellow fever virus.
- Lassa fever virus.
- Marburg virus.
- Cytomegalo virus (CMV).
- Herpes simplex virus (HSV).
- Varicella-Zoster Virus (VZV).
- Rubella virus.
- Measles virus.
- Coxsackie virus.

Classification: Two ways to classify the hepatitis viruses as follows.

I. Systemic / taxonomical classification. → Flow chart-1

II. Based on mode of transmission:

A Parenteral transmission: By route other than oral.

- Hepatitis B Virus (HBV).
- Hepatitis C Virus (HCV).
- Hepatitis D Virus (HDV).
- Hepatitis G Virus (HGV).

B Non-parenteral (faeco-oral) transmission: By oral route.

- Hepatitis A Virus (HAV).
- Hepatitis E Virus (HEV).

III. Epidemiological & clinical types:

A. Infectious / infective / type A hepatitis:

- Occur sporadically or epidemic.
- Affect young adult or children.
- Transmitted by faeco-oral route.
- Example: HAV.

B. Transfusion / serum/ type B hepatitis / homologous serum jaundice:

- Transmitted by transfusion of blood or blood products.
- Example: HBV.
- As it is transmitted by homologous serum used for prevention or treatment, so **called homologous serum jaundice.**

C. Non- A non-B hepatitis (NANB): Includes all viruses causing hepatitis but not diagnosed as HAV or HBV like

i. **HCV:** Transmitted by transfusion of blood or blood products.

ii. **HDV:** Defective virus depends on helper virus like HBV & also **called Delta virus.** Transmitted by transfusion of blood or blood products.

iii. **HEV:** Transmitted by faeco-oral route.

iv. **HGV:** Follow chapter → Arboviruses and roboviruses (section → Flaviviridae).

World hepatitis day: It is celebrated on 28th July of every year with aims to raise global awareness & to encourage the prevention, diagnosis & treatment of hepatitis A, B, C, D & E.

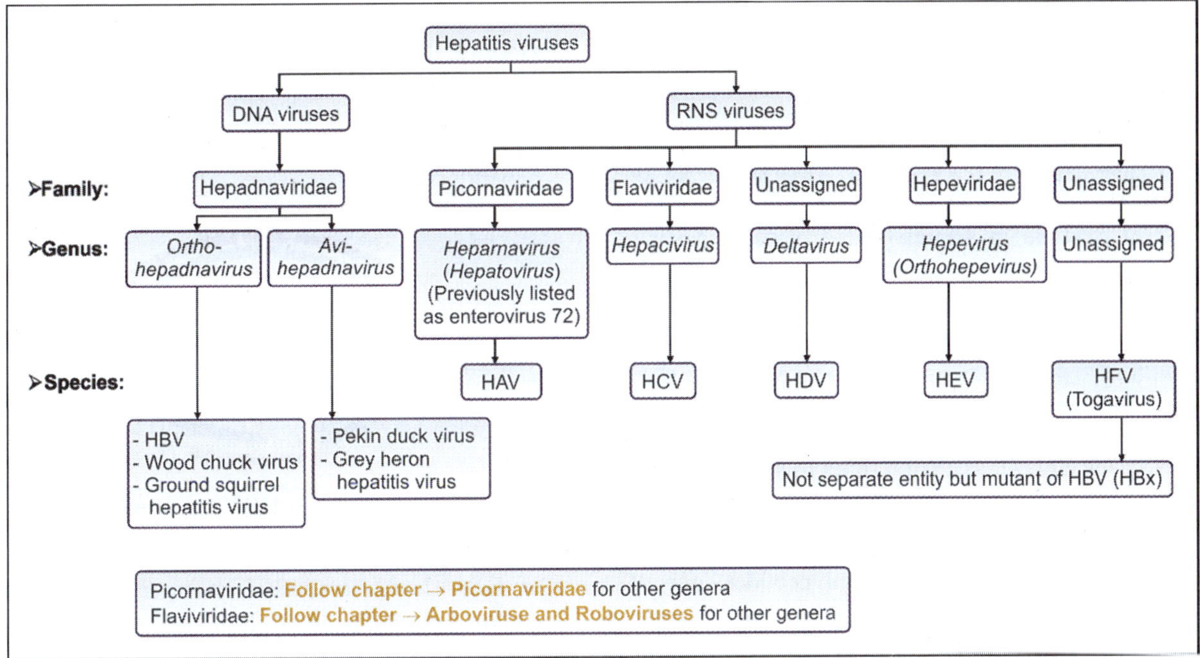

Flow chart-1: Hepatitis viruses group

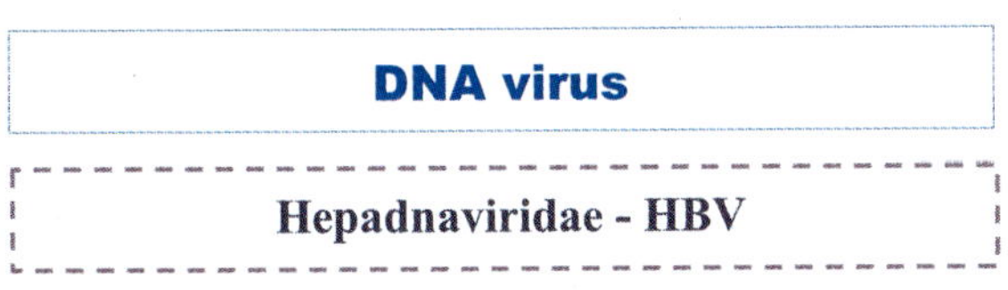

DNA virus

Hepadnaviridae - HBV

❖ **Synonym:** Complete virus particle **called Dane particle.**

❖ **History:**

- In 1965, it was identified by Baruch Blumberg in serum of Australian aboriginal person, who received multiple transfusion & in 1968 it **called surface Ag of HBV (HBsAg) or Australian Ag.**
- David Dane and others discovered the virus particle in 1970 by electron microscopy **called Dane particle.**
- By the early 1980s the genome of the virus had been sequenced.

❖ **Geographical distribution & genotypes:**

- **Distribution:** Distributed worldwide & more than 1/3 of world's population is infected by HBV.
- **Genotypes:**
- Eight major genotypes (A–H). The genotypes have a distinct geographical distribution and are used in tracing the evolution and transmission of the virus.
- Differences between genotypes affect the disease severity, course, a complications, response to treatment and possibly vaccination.
- There are two other genotypes I and J but they are not universally accepted as of 2015.
- Genotypes differ by at least 8% of their sequence and were first reported in 1988 when six were initially described (A–F). Two further types have since been described (G and H).
- Most genotypes are now divided into sub-genotypes with distinct properties.
- ¼ of them becomes carrier & develops chronic liver diseases like chronic hepatitis, cirrhosis & Hepato Cellular carcinoma (HCC).

❖ **Morphology:** →**Fig.-1**

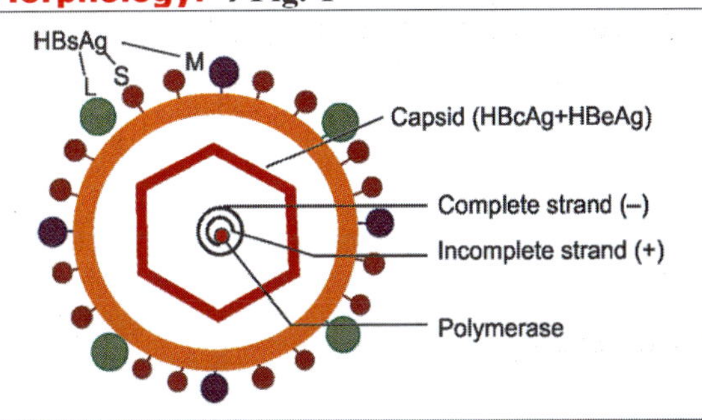

Figure-1: Morphology of HBV

➤ **Shape:** Spherical.

➤ **Size:** 42 nm.

➤ **Genome:**

- HBV contains ds-DNA with one complete strand & other incomplete strand.
- Incomplete strand contains DNA polymerase (DNA dependent DNA polymerase), so **called plus (+) stand** & complete strand **called minus (-) strand.**
- DNA polymerase has two functions **(1)** DNA dependent DNA polymerase **(2)** RNA dependent reverse transcriptase. It repairs the gap in plus strand & makes the genome fully-ds.

- **Capsid:** DNA surrounded by icosahedral variety of capsid contains two antigens like HBcAg & HBeAg.
- **Nucleocapsid (nucleic acid + capsid):** 27nm in diameter.
- **Envelope:** HBV is enveloped virus & contains surface (envelope) Ag **called Australian Ag** or **HBsAg.**
- **Viral particle in serum:** Three types of particle are observed in serum under EM as shown in **fig.-2.**

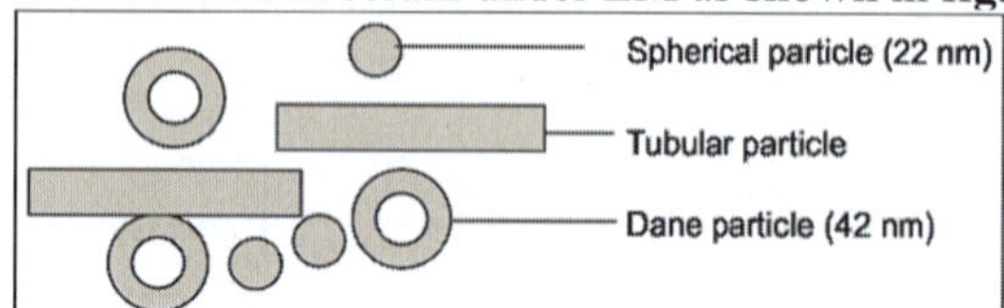

Figure-2: HBV particles in serum

1. **Spherical particles:** Single wall & 22nm in size. It is the surface components of HBV (HBsAg). HBsAg contains two major polypeptides, one of which is glycosylated.
2. **Tubular particles:** These are identical to spherical particles of HBV (HBsAg). Similar in breadth to spherical particles about 22nm but elongated with variable length.
3. **Dane particles:** Complete virus with 42 nm in size. These particles were identified by Dane in 1970, so **called Dane particle.** These particles are made up of

- Outer layer: **Called envelope** & it contains HBsAg.
- Inner layer: **Called nucleocapsid** & it contains HBcAg, HBeAg & partially ds-DNA (core Ag).

❖ Culture characteristics (C/Cs):

i. **Animal culture:** Chimpanzee is infective experimentally & can be used as laboratory model.

ii. **Cell culture:**

- Non-cultivable *in vitro.*
- DNA of HBV can be cloned in yeast & bacteria for vaccine preparation.

❖ Resistance:

- Resistant to heat.
- Inactivated by 2% glutaraldehyde (cidex) & sodium hypochlorite (10,000 ppm chlorine).

❖ Genetic organisation: Different antigens of HBV are encodes by following genes **(fig.-3)**.

a. **S-gene:** Three regions.

- **Pre-S1:** Encodes for large (L) proteins, not found free in circulation.
- **Pre-S2:** Encodes for middle (M) protein.
- **S-region:** Encodes for major (S) protein. M & S proteins are free in circulation as HBsAg particles.

b. **P-gene:** It is the largest (longest) gene & encodes for enzyme DNA polymerase.

c. **C-gene:** Two-regions.

- **Pre-C region:** Encodes for HBeAg.
- **C-region:** Encodes for HBcAg.

d. **X-gene:** Encodes for non-particular protein **called HBxAg**. It has trans-activating effect on viral & some cellular genes. It leads to replication of HBV & some other virus like HIV. HBxAg & its antibody are present in patient with severe chronic hepatitis & HCC.

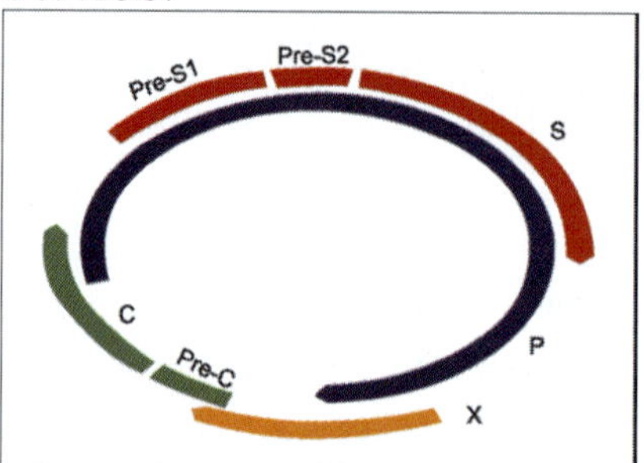

Figure-3: HBV genome

❖ Mutation in genes of HBV: Mutation in genes of HBV leads to clinical emergency of mutant strain. Following three types of mutations are identified in genes of HBV.

a. **Pre-C region mutation:**

- Mutation in pre-C region results in absence of HBeAg.
- It is due to nonsense mutation in the pre-c region leading to formation of stop codons.
- It is distributed in Mediterranean countries & Europe.
- Patients infected with HBV carrying such mutant are diagnosed late & rapidly progress to chronic stage & cirrhosis.
- Diagnostically HBeAg is absent while other markers are as usual.

b. **S-gene mutation (in 'a' components of HBs Ag):**

- Such mutant **called escape mutants.**
- It present in 'a' components of HBsAg in S-gene. It is due to substitution of single amino acid from glycine to arginine at position 145.
- It observed in following cases.

1. Infants born to HBe Ag positive mothers.
2. Liver transplant recipient, who underwent the procedure for hepatitis B & who were treated with a high potency human monoclonal anti-HBs preparation.
3. In patients who were actively & passively immunised for HBV. In such cases antibody pressure may favour the evolutionary changes in 'a' component.

- Presence of S-gene mutant may create the problems in diagnosis & immunisation of HBV.

c. **P-gene mutation:**

- It present in YMDD locus of P-gene of HBV reverse transcriptase.
- It results in development of resistant to lamivudine.

❖ Antigenic structure::

- **Major antigens (products of gene) of HBV:**

a. **Envelope-Ag:** HBsAg.
b. **Capsid-Ags:** HBcAg & HBeAg.

➢ **Antigenic diversity of HBsAg:**

✪ **Components:** It contains group specific & type specific components as follows.

- **Group specific:** Group specific component is 'a'.
- **Type specific:** Type specific components are d-y' & 'w-r'. In addition to all these few other components like x, f, t, j, n, & g are also reported, but not been adequately studied.

✪ **Antigenic types:** Virus is divided into four major serotypes like adr, adw, ayr & ayw based on epitopes present on its envelope (HBsAg). These types are not important in immunity, because each types showing the dominant a variant. Each type shows the distinct geographical importance as follows.

- adr: Common in South & East India & far East.
- adw: Common in Europe, Australia & America.
- ayr: Very rare prevalent.
- ayw: Common from West Asia through the Middle East, to West & Northern India.

❖ Immunity:

a. **AMI:** Antibodies forms after onset of jaundice within week or two weeks. Order is 1st HBcAg then HBeAg & later HBsAg antibodies. Development of HBsAg antibodies indicates the recovery.

b. **CMI:**

- Development of CMI to HBsAg also noticed.
- Hepatocytes carries the antigens are subject to kill by ADCC or by other cytotoxic T-cells
- Absence of immune response may not cause hepatitis but may produce carrier stage, hence infants & immune-deficient persons are become carrier than case.

❖ Pathogenicity:

➢ **Disease name:** Disease **called hepatitis B.**

➢ **Synonym:** Also **called transfusion / serum / homologous serum jaundice.**

➢ **Nature or history of disease:** Disease is usually sporadic & no seasonal outbreak occurs, though occasional outbreak occurs in hospitals, orphanages & asylum.

➢ **Reservoir of infection:** Only human & no animal reservoirs.

➢ **Source of infection:**

- Blood/blood products & body fluids are the main sources.
- Percutaneous injury by infected needle or syringe is transmits HBV (**30%**) > HCV (**3%**) > HIV (**0.5-1%**).
- Period of infectivity (communicability): Virus present in blood/blood products & body fluid during incubation period & acute phase of disease. People infected with HBV remain carrier as long as they carry HBsAg in blood. Individual become non-infectious once HBsAg is replaced by anti-HBsAg Ab. Infectivity is determined by HBeAg. It is maximum when HBeAg is elevated.

➢ **Mode of transmission:** Two modes.

a. **Direct:**

1. **Direct contact:** Contact of contaminated devices like scalpel, scissor, endoscope etc. with abraded skin.
2. **Inoculation** under skin or mucosa by contaminated needles, syringes or by tattooing. Chances of infection are very high about 30%, compared to HCV & HIV with 3% & 0.5-1% respectively.
3. **Sexual intercourse:** More in male homosexual. It present in semen, so screening before donation of semen is obligatory.
4. **Perinatal (vertical):** Mother to infant. Infectivity is more if mother is HBeAg positive. Among the all hepatitis, HBV has maximum perinatal transmission. Risk includes HBV (+) > HCV & HDV (±) > HAV & HEV (-).

- **Antenatal (trans-placental):** Low rate (20%) but higher than HCV (6%).
- **Intranatal:** More common during birth by contact of maternal blood with skin or mucosa of foetus.
- **Post-natal:** Infection by breast milk is possible but efficiency is very low. However, it is advisable to stop feeding if mother is infective & baby is ensured by other sources.

b. **Indirect:**

1. **Vehicle (fluid) borne:**

- By transfusion of contaminated blood or blood products or cryoprecipitate.
- It present in other body fluids like semen, saliva, urine, bile, faeces & breast milk, but of these only semen & saliva can transmit the infection.

- As it survive in mosquitoes for 2 weeks, after blood meal but not able to multiply so **no vector borne** transmission.

➢ **Incubation period (IP):** 1-6 months.

➢ **Portal of entry:** Skin or mucosa.

➢ **Sites:** Liver.

➢ **Precipitating factors (epidemiological determinants):**

1. **Age:** In children due to perinatal transmission (babies of mothers with chronic HBV infection).
2. **Occupation:**

- Health workers are at high risk.
- Sex workers and homosexuals are particular at risk.
- Barbers.

3. **High risk groups are:** Drug addicts, person required blood transfusion or organ transplantation.
4. **HIV & HBV:** About 10% of population infected with HIV is co-infected with HBV. HBV does not alter the progress of HIV, but co-infection with HIV will increase the chances of development of

chronic hepatitis, cirrhosis & Hepato Cellular Carcinoma (HCC) by HBV.

➢ **Pathogenesis:**
- It based on immune response.
- Hepatocytes carries the antigens are subject to kill by ADCC or by other cytotoxic T-cells.
- Absence of immune response may not cause hepatitis but may produce carrier stage, hence infants & immune-deficient persons are become carrier than case.
- Mechanism: → **Flow chart-2**

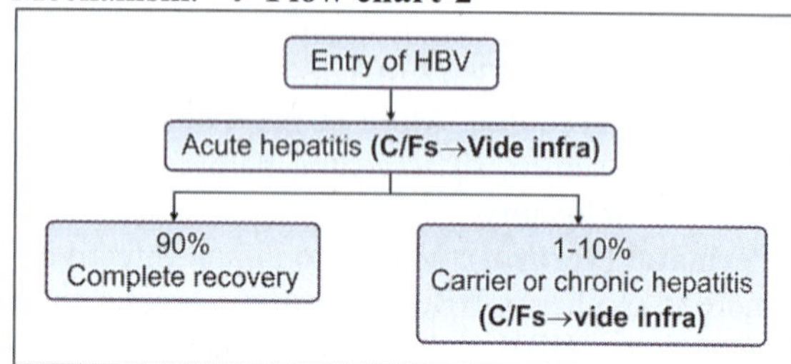

Flow chart-2: Pathogenesis of hepatitis B

➢ **Clinical features (C/Fs):** In 90% patients it present as acute hepatitis with following features.
- Insidious onset with minimal fever.
- Extra-hepatic features are more like arthralgia, utricaria, glomerulonephritis.
- Complete recovery occurs in 90% cases in 1-2 months & virus eliminated from circulation in 6 months & patient remains immune thereafter.
- Simultaneous **HDV infection** leads to fatal fulminant hepatitis (poorest the prognosis).
- 1-10% (poor prognosis) cases develop carrier or chronic hepatitis.

➢ **Complications:** In 1-10% patients it moves to chronic stage with following manifestations.
- Fulminant hepatitis: Instead of insidious onset, acute hepatitis sometimes present with severe & sudden onset **called fulminant hepatitis.**
- Chronic hepatitis.
- Cirrhosis.
- Hepato Cellular Carcinoma (HCC).
- Extra-hepatic: It includes glomerulonephritis, popular acrodermatitis of child hood (Gianotti-crosti syndrome), poly arteritis nodosa, arthritis, angio-oedema etc. These are may be due to immune complex (type-III hypersensitivity) deposition.

➢ **Carrier:**
- **Definition:** Person carries HBsAg in blood for more than six months without any sign-symptoms.
- **Types:** Two types.

a. Super carrier:
- High titre of HBsAg with HBeAg, DNA polymerase & HBV in circulation.
- High infectivity.
- Generally raised transaminase.
- A quarter of carriers are HBeAg positive.

b. Simple carrier:
- Low titre of HBsAg with negative HBeAg, DNA polymerase & HBV.
- Low infectivity.
- Many super carriers become simple carrier in time.

- **Other important aspects about carrier stage:**
- Carrier rate is different in different countries depending on the living standard.
- India falls in intermediate group with high rate (2-7%) in South part while low in North part.
- Following infection 90% neonates, 30% children & 5-10% adults are carrier.
- There are 350 million carrier worldwide, of them 45 million are in India next to China.

❖ Laboratory diagnosis:

➢ **Specimens:** Blood/serum.

➢ **Testing methods:**

A. **Microscopy:** → **Follow morphology.**

B. **Culture:** → **Follow C/Cs.**

C. **Serological tests:**

✪ **Following are the serological markers detectable from serum of patient.**
- **Antigens (Ags):** HBsAg & HBeAg (HBcAg is enclosed in capsid & not released in circulation, hence not detectable; however its antibody is detectable).
- **Antibodies (Abs):** Anti-HBc, anti- HBs & anti-HBe.

✪ **Immunological reactions in HBV infection: →Fig.-4**

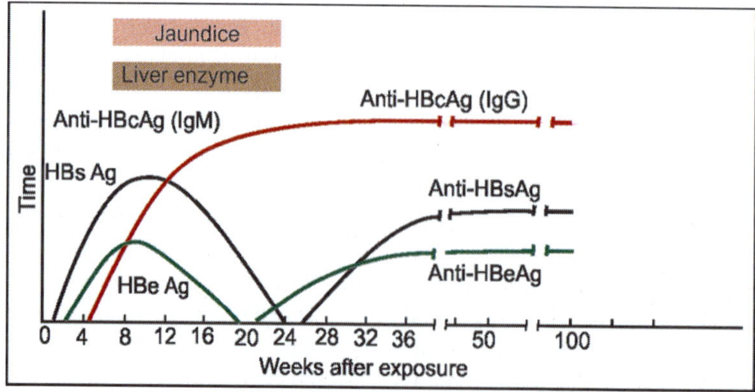

Figure-4: Serological markers of HBV

- **HBsAg & anti-HBs:**
- HBsAg is the 1st marker detectable after infection, even before elevation of liver enzymes (transaminase). It reaches peak at 8th-12th weeks & disappears at 24th weeks (6 months). If last for more than 6 months **indicates carrier or chronic stage**. When it disappears, its antibody, anti- HBs start to appear & remain for very long time.
- Anti-HBs is protective & provide resistance (immunity) to HBV. It's presence without any serological markers (protective antibody) indicate immunisation or recovery from infection.
- **HBcAg & Anti-HBc:**
- HBcAg is enclosed in capsid & not releases in circulation, hence not detectable freely in blood. It remains in hepatocytes, from where it can be detected by immunohistochemical staining. Intra hepatic HBcAg indicate active viral replication.
- Anti-HBc, is detectable after 1st week. It is the earliest Ab seen in blood than other. It remains life-long & serves as useful indicators for HBV infection even in absence of others. It is IgM in nature in initial 6 months & indicates **recent infection** then after becomes IgG which indicates **remote infection** & used as **epidemiological markers**. Anti-HBc distinguishes between recent & remote infection.
- **Acute stage markers:** HBsAg is the earliest marker. For diagnosis of acute stage HBbsAg, HBV DNA & HBe Ag are also useful, but IgM anti-HBcAg is most significant.
- **HBeAg & anti-HBe:**
- HBeAg develops almost same time or little later with HBsAg. Its presence indicates intrahepatic viral replication & DNA polymerase in blood reflecting **high infectivity**.
- Disappearance of HBeAg is followed by anti-HBe.

✪ **Test commonly used are:**
- ELISA.
- Some rapid test like ICT & latex particle agglutination test are also useful.

✪ **Serological pattern in HBV infection: →Table-1**

Stage	HBs Ag	HBe Ag	DNA	Anti-HBc	Anti-HBs	Anti-HBe
Acute	+	+	+	IgM	-	-
Chronic	+	+	+	IgG	IgG	-
Carrier	+	-	-	IgG	-	+/-
Immu-nity	-	-	-	-	+	-

Table-1: Serological pattern in HBV infection

D. Molecular methods:
- Hybridisation & PCR are rapid & more sensitive methods.
- HBV-DNA: Like HBeAg it indicates viral replication in liver & viral infectivity. Both these two present every time, so they can't differentiate between acute & chronic stage. They help to assess the progress of infection to chronic stage. They are the quantitative marker for HBV replication. In a carrier HBV is actively multiplying & is highly infectious **called super carrier**.
- Level of HBV-DNA is correlates with the degree of liver damage indicated by raised ALT & AST.
- **Markers for active viral replication:** HBV-DNA, DNA polymerase, HBeAg, Intra-hepatic HBcAg & liver enzymes.

E. Other supportive test:
- Alanine aminotransferase (ALT).
- AST.
- Bilirubin.

❖ Prevention:

➢ **General measures:**
- Improvement in health education.
- Screening of blood, organs & tissues before donation.
- Safe sex like use of condom.
- High-risk behavior modification like drug abuse.
- Avoid direct contact with blood and body fluid.
- Use of disposable & sterile medical devices.

➢ **Immunoprophylaxis:**

A. Active immunisation: Three types of vaccine.

i. Plasma derived vaccine:
- **History:** Introduced in 1982 & was used in past.
- **Preparation:**
- Prepared from pooled plasma of human carrier contains HBsAg, inactivated by formalin & formulated in alum.
- 1.0 ml contains 20 microgram of HBsAg.
- **Advantages:** Highly immunogenic.
- **Disadvantages:**
- Limited availability, because human source.
- Not free from possible risk of pathogens.

ii. Cloned (recombinant or genetic engineered) vaccine:
- **History:** It was prepared in 1986 & gradually replaced the plasma derived vaccine.
- **Preparation:** Prepared by cloning the S-gene of HBV in **Baker's yeast.** It contains non-glycosylated particles alone. Two types of formulations are available.

1. **Single:**
2. **Combined (pentavac):** Contains Diphtheria, Pertusis, Tetanus, HBV, H influenza type b (Hib).

- **Advantages:**
- Highly immunogenic & sero-conversion occurs in 90% cases.
- Safe & effective.
- **Disadvantage:** High cost.
- **Administration:**
  - Route: By IM route.

- Site:
  - In deltoid region or antero-lateral aspect of the thigh in infants.
  - Avoid the gluteal region, as it is less immunogenic because less numbers of APCs in gluteal fat delaying the presentation to T or B cells.
- Doses:
  - 10-20 microgram in adult & half in children <10 years.
  - Three doses are given on 0, 1 & 6 months with alum adjuvant.
  - Birth dose is given with BCG vaccine but at different site.
- Inclusion in national immunisation schedule:
  - It also included in national immunisation schedule & given alone or in combination with Diphtheria, Pertusis, Tetanus, HBV, Hib (**pentavac**) at 6th, 10th & 14th week.
- **Interruption of vaccine schedule:**
  - It does not require restarting of schedule.
  - If primary series is missed after 1st dose then give 2nd dose immediately followed by 3rd dose after 4 weeks.
  - If 3rd dose is interrupted, then give it immediately.
- **Efficacy:** Long lasting immunity up to 15 years, however some research witnessed with lifelong immunity.
- **Testing:** Effect of vaccine is tested by detecting anti-HBs.
- **Contraindications:**
  - Persons allergic to vaccine components.
  - Neither pregnancy nor lactation is a contraindication.
  - HIV-AIDS, chronic liver disease, renal failure & diabetes shows the low immunogenicity.

iii. Synthetic peptide vaccine:

- **Preparation:** Contains all antigenic components of HBsAg (Pre-S1, Pre-S2 & S).
- **Advantages:** High sero-conversion & long lasting immunity.

B. Passive immunisation: By using pooled normal human Ig.

- **Preparation:** Hyperimmune hepatitis B immunoglobulin is prepared from human volunteers with high anti-HBs titre.
- **Administration:**
  - 0.05-0.07ml/kg by IM route exposed within 48 hours of exposure.
  - It may not prevent the infection, but protect against illness & carrier state.

C. Combined immunisation:

- **Indication:**
  - Non-immune person.
  - Babies born to carrier mother.
- **Administration:**
  - 0.05-0.07ml/kg Ig of HBV is given immediately within 24 hrs by IM route followed by full course of HBV vaccine.
  - When Ig of HBV is not available, vaccine alone provides full protection. HBV Ig does not interfere with Ab response to HBV vaccine.

❖ Treatment:

- No specific anti-HBV treatment is available.
- Interferon-α alone or in combination with lamivudine (inhibit the reverse transcriptase & also used for HIV) & famcyclovir is effective in chronic hepatitis.

RNA viruses

Picornaviridae - HAV

❖ History: It was demonstrated by Feinstone & colleagues in 1973 from the faeces of experimentally infected human volunteers by Immuno Electron Microscopy (IEM).

❖ Geographical distribution & genotypes:

- **Distribution:** Distributed worldwide.
- **Genotypes:** Seven genotypes including four humans and three simian have been described.
  - Human genotypes: They are numbered as I-III & VII. Two subtypes have been described for genotypes I-III like IA, IB, IIA, IIB, IIIA & IIIB. Genotype III has been isolated from both humans and owl monkeys. Commonest human isolate is IA.
  - Simian genotypes: They are numbered as IV-VI.

❖ Morphology: →Fig.-5

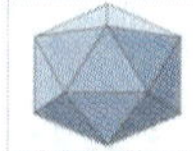

Figure-5: Morphology of HAV

- **Shape:** Spherical.
- **Size:** 27 nm.
- **Non enveloped:** **Called naked virus.**
- **Genome & capsid:** ss-RNA (+) surrounded by icosahedral variety of capsid.

❖ Culture characteristics (C/Cs):

- HAV is the only hepatitis virus which can be cultivated in cell culture (in vitro).
- It can grow in human & simian cell culture.
- Chimpanzees & marmosets can be infected experimentally.
- It has also been clones.

❖ Resistance:

- Resistant to heat at 60^0C for 1 hr & pH at 3.
- Also resistant to ether, chloroform & bile salts.
- Inactivated by formalin (1:4000), chlorine (1ppm for 30 min.) & boiling for 1 minute.
- Preserved at 4^0C temperature or below.

❖ **Antigenic structure:** Only one serotype is known.

❖ **Immunity:**
- Primary infection produces the lifelong immunity, however about 10-15% can get secondary infection.
- Antibodies are formed in 90% of population due to repeated exposure up to age of 10 years & incidences are decline after 10 years & in adult.

❖ **Pathogenicity:**
➢ **Disease name:** Disease **called hepatitis A.**
➢ **Synonym:** Also **called infectious hepatitis / infective hepatitis / type A hepatitis.**
➢ **Nature or history of disease:**
- Hepatitis A occurs sporadically or in form of outbreak.
- Shellfish have been known to be responsible for outbreak.
- Outbreaks are common in military camps, neonatal ICUs, day care centres, summer camp, families & institutes.

➢ **Reservoir of infection:** Human is the only known reservoir, however chimpanzees can acquire the infection from human & can transmit it to human.
➢ **Source of infection:**
- Contaminated food, water or milk.
- It excreted in human faeces before & after 2 weeks of jaundice.
- It also present in saliva & urine but clinically it is not significant.
- Virus present in blood for a very short time (short viremia) before 2 weeks of jaundice & after 1 week of jaundice, so no or very rare blood/serum transmission.
- Period of infectivity (communicability): Virus shed in faeces during incubation period (before 2 weeks of jaundice) & in prodromal phase (after 2 week of jaundice), but not in icteric phase.
- Secondary attack rate: Transmission from patient to case is 10-20%.

➢ **Mode of transmission:**
- By faeco-oral route (infected food handlers, raw shellfish).
- Vertical transmission is not possible.

➢ **Incubation period (IP):** 2-6 weeks.
➢ **Portal of entry:** GIT.
➢ **Sites:** Liver.
➢ **Precipitating factors (epidemiological determinants):**

a. **Agent factors (virulence factors):**
- It produces the very brief viremia hence parenteral transmission is absent or very rarc. Chronic viremia does not occur.
- Virus persists in nature continuously & cases may occur throughout the year.

b. **Host factors:**
1. **Age:**
- Most common infection occurs in children & adolescent between 5-14 years, but illness is mild like mild anicteric gastroenteritis or subclinical.
- More icteric in adults & causes acute icteric febrile illness.
- Anicteric to icteric ratio in children is 12:1 while in adults is 1:3.
- Antibodies are developed after the age of 10 years in 90% of population due to repeated exposure, so remain protected.

2. **Sex:** Both are equally affected.

c. **Environmental factors:**
1. **Overcrowding & poor sanitation:** Common in developing countries & persons with poor sanitation. Incidence is decline in persons with improved personal hygiene.
2. **Seasonal factor:** In India it is common in rainy season. In temperate regions, the disease shows the autumn-winter predilection, but in the tropics no seasonal distribution is evident.

➢ **Pathogenesis: →Flow chart-3**

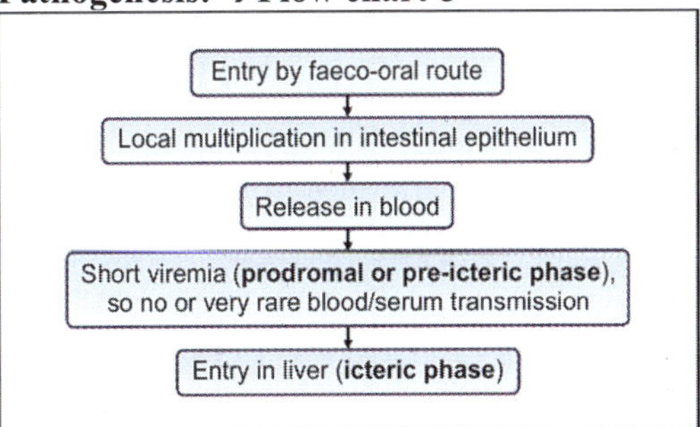

Flow chart-3: Pathogenesis of hepatitis A

➢ **Clinical features:** Large numbers of cases are asymptomatic. Overt illness (acute hepatitis) occurs in 5% cases with following features.
- **Prodromal or pre-icteric phase:**
  - Acute onset with fever, malaise, anorexia, nausea, vomiting & liver tenderness is seen in 5% of cases
  - Symptoms are subsides with onset of jaundice.
- **Icteric (jaundice) phase:** Jaundice which recovered in 99% cases over a period of 4-6 weeks.

➢ **Complications:** HAV & HEV are not showing carrier stage. Carrier stage present in HBV, HCV & HDV. HAV is also not responsible for chronic stage like cirrhosis, chronic hepatitis & HCC. Following are main complications of HAV.
- Fulminant hepatitis.
- Mortality in 0.1-1% cases.

❖ **Laboratory diagnosis:**
➢ **Specimens:** Faeces & serum.
➢ **Testing methods:**

A. **Microscopy: → Follow morphology.**
B. **Culture: → Follow C/Cs.**
C. **Serological tests:**

✪ **Serological markers:** Two types of antibodies (IgM & IgG) are developed.

✪ **Immunological reaction: →Fig.-6**

- **IgM:**
  - It indicates the recent or early infection.
  - It appears in acute phase, reaches peak at 2nd week & disappears at 12th week.
- **IgG:**
  - It indicates the remote or late infection.
  - It appears a week after IgM, reaches peak at 7th-8th week & persists for long time or may be for life.

✪ **Methods:** IgM & IgG Abs are diagnosed by ELISA.

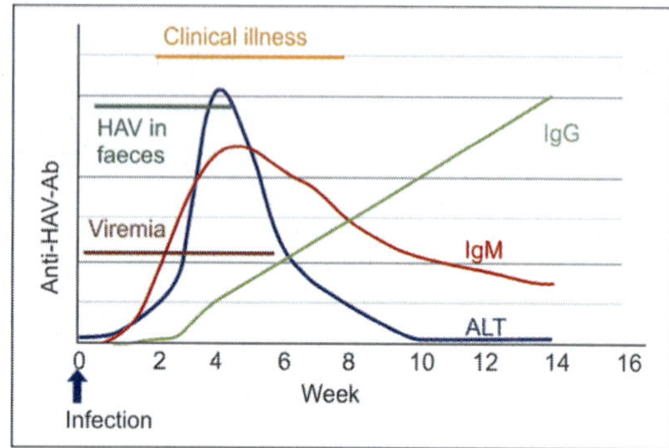

Figure-6: Markers of HAV

D. Molecular methods: RT- PCR is rapid & more sensitive method, performed from faeces.

E. Other supportive test:
- Alanine aminotransferase (ALT).
- Bilirubin.

❖ Prevention:

➢ **General measures:**
- Improvement in hygiene.
- Prevention of faecal contamination of food & water.

➢ **Immunoprophylaxis:**

A. Active immunisation: Two types of vaccine.

i. By using human diploid cell culture vaccine:

- **Preparation:** Alum conjugated vaccine prepared by growing HAV on human diploid cell culture & inactivated by formalin.
- **Advantages:**
  - Effective.
  - Free from side effect (safe).
- **Administration:** Two IM injection start protection after 4 weeks & lasting for 10-12 years.

ii. By using human foetal lung fibroblast vaccine:

- **Preparation:** Vaccine is prepared human foetal lung fibroblast such as MRC-5 & WI-38.
- **Advantages:** Provide 94% protection.
- **Administration:** Single IM injection followed by booster after 6-12 months.

B. Passive immunisation: By using pooled normal human Ig.

- **Administration:**
  - 0.2-0.12ml/kg of body weight by IM route before exposure or in early incubation period.

❖ Treatment:

- No specific anti-HAV treatment is available.
- Supportive measures are given.

Flaviviridae - HCV

❖ History & synonym:

Virus was identified in 1889 & **called parenterally transmitted NANB hepatitis virus.** Major cause (about 80%) of parenterally transmitted NANB- hepatitis.

❖ Geographical distribution & genotypes:

- **Distribution:**
  - It is estimated that 150–200 million people or approximately 3% of the world's population are living with chronic hepatitis C. About 3–4 million people are infected per year and more than 3, 50, 000 people die HCV disease.
  - World-wide prevalence of HCV is 0.2-2% in blood donors & 80% in IV drug users.
  - In India seroprevalence of HCV is 0.3-11.3%.
- **Genotypes:** There are seven major genotypes of HCV from 1-7. They are varying in distribution & also in drug susceptibility.
  - The genotypes are divided into several subtypes like 1a &1b for genotype 1.
  - In the United States about 70% of cases are caused by genotype 1, 20% by genotype 2 and about 1% by each of the other genotypes.
  - Genotype 1: World wide.
  - Genotype 4: Egypt.
  - Genotype 5: South Africa.
  - Genotype 6: Hong Kong.
  - Genotype 1 & 3: India.
  - Genotype 1b responds poorly to therapy than other types.

❖ Morphology: →Fig.-7

➢ **Shape:** Spherical.

➢ **Size:** 50-60 nm.

➢ **Genome & capsid:** Linear, ss-RNA (+) surrounded by icosahedral variety of capsid.

➢ **Envelope:** Envelope present & carrying glycoprotein spikes like E1 & E2.

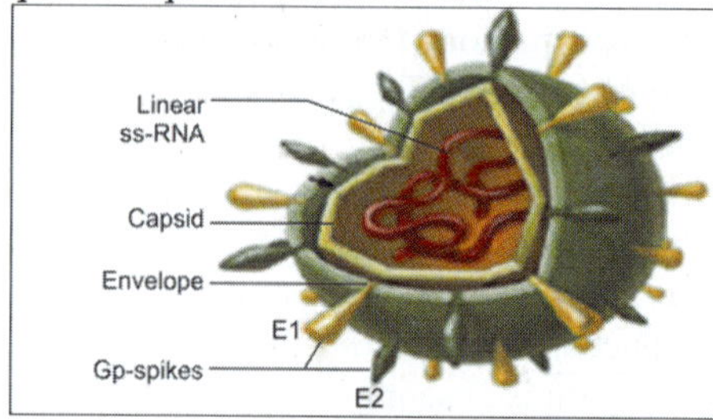

Figure-7: Morphology of HCV

❖ Culture characteristics (C/Cs):

i. Animal culture: Chimpanzee is infective *in vitro.*

ii. Cell culture:

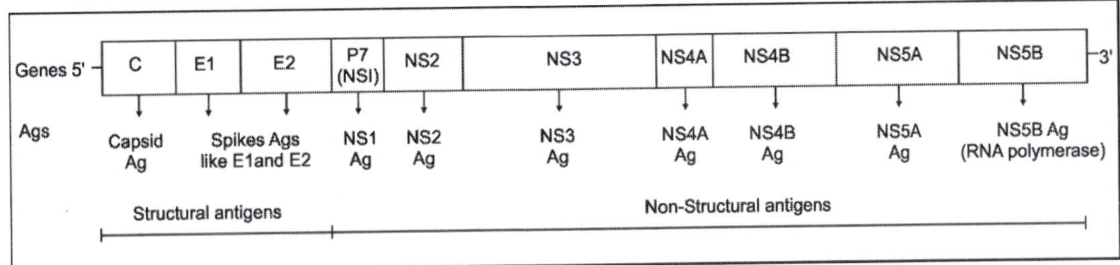

Figure-8: Genetic organisation & antigenic structure of HCV

- Non-cultivable *in vitro.*
- HCV can be cloned in *E. coli.*

❖ **Resistance:** Enveloped virus sensitive to lipid solvents.

❖ **Genetic organisation & antigenic structure:** Genes present in HCV encodes for structural & non structural antigens as shown in **fig.-8**. In HCV genes & antigens have almost same name.

a. **Structural antigens:** It includes
- Capsid antigens (encodes by C gene): C22, C33, C100.
- Spikes (encodes by E1 & E2 genes): Glycoprotein antigens like E1 & E2.

b. **Non- structural antigens:** Encodes by NS genes & antigens are like NS1 (p7 function as ion channel), NS2, NS3, NS4A, NS4B, NS5A & NS5B (function as RNA polymerase).

❖ **Mutation in genes of HCV:** The most variable gene in HCV is E2 gene followed by NS genes; hence they are more prone to undergoes mutations. Mutation in E2 gene enables the emergency of mutant strain, which results in
- Establishment of chronic infection.
- Failure of development of effective vaccine.

❖ **Immunity:** Because of genetic variation, there is less homologous or heterologous post-infection immunity. Protective (neutralising) antibodies are produced against E2 antigens.

❖ **Pathogenicity:**
➢ **Disease name:** Disease **called hepatitis C.**
➢ **Synonym:** Also **called parenterally transmitted NANB hepatitis.**
➢ **Nature or history of disease:** About 3% of people of the world population are infected with HCV. High prevalence has been documented from Africa (10%), South America & Asia. In India prevalence is 1%.
➢ **Reservoir of infection:** Only human & no animal reservoir.
➢ **Source of infection:** Blood/blood products & body fluid.
➢ **Mode of transmission:** Two modes like

a. **Direct:**
1. **Direct contact:** Contaminated devices like scalpel scissors, endoscope etc. with abraded skin or during medical procedure.
2. **Inoculation** under skin or mucosa by contaminated needles, syringes in drug abusers or by tattooing.
3. **Sexual intercourse:** But less important.
4. **Perinatal (vertical):** From mother to foetus is possible but at lower rate (6%) than HBV (20%). It depends on degree of viraemia which is detected by HCV RNA. It is not transmitted by breast feeding.

b. **Indirect:**
1. **Vehicle (fluid) borne:** By transfusion of contaminated blood or blood products or by organ transplantation.

➢ **Incubation period (IP):** 15-160 days.
➢ **Portal of entry:** Skin or mucosa.
➢ **Sites:** Liver.
➢ **Precipitating factors (epidemiological determinants):**
1. **Age:** In adults due to drug abuse or promiscus sexual behaviour.
2. **Occupation:**
- Health workers are at increased risk.
- Sex workers and homosexuals are particular at risk.
- Barbers.
3. **High risk groups are:** Drug addicts, person required blood transfusion or organ transplantation.
4. **Immunodeficient persons:** Are at high risk.

➢ **Clinical features (C/Fs):** In 20% patients it present as acute hepatitis with following features.
- Asymptomatic or anicteric.
- Symptoms are generally mild & vague includes decreased appetite, fatigue, nausea, muscle /joint pains & weight loss.
- Overt jaundice seen in 5% cases.

➢ **Complications:** It is the most common virus among the hepatitis group which moves to chronic stage in 50-80% cases (hence **called notorious virus**) with following complications.
- Chronic hepatitis (60-70%).
- Cirrhosis (5-20%): HCV is most common indicator for liver transplantation following cirrhosis.
- Hepato Cellular Carcinoma (HCC): Occurs in 1-5% cases & it accounts about 25% of total liver patients. It is next to HBV to produce HCC. Co-

infection of HCV with HBV increases the risk for cirrhosis & HCC.

- Extra hepatic: It includes glomerulonephritis, arthritis, joint pain, mixed cryoglobulinemia etc. These are may be due to immune complex (type-III hypersensitivity) deposition.

➢ **Carrier:** In India carrier rate is 1-20%.

❖ Laboratory diagnosis:

➢ **Specimens:** Blood/serum.

➢ **Testing methods:**

A. **Microscopy: → Follow morphology.**

B. **Culture: → Follow C/Cs.**

C. **Serological test:**

- **Antigen detection:** ELISA to detect structural (capsid) or NS3, NS4 & NS5 antigens.
- **Antibody detection:**

- Anti-HCV antibodies develop after 2-3 months of exposure **(fig.-9)**, so not useful in acute stage.
- Different types of antibodies are detected by ELISA like anti-NS5 (3rd generation assay), anti-C22/C33 (2nd generation assay) & anti-C100 (1st generation assay).
- In acute infection, antibody present variably in 50-70% cases & in chronic it present in 95% cases.

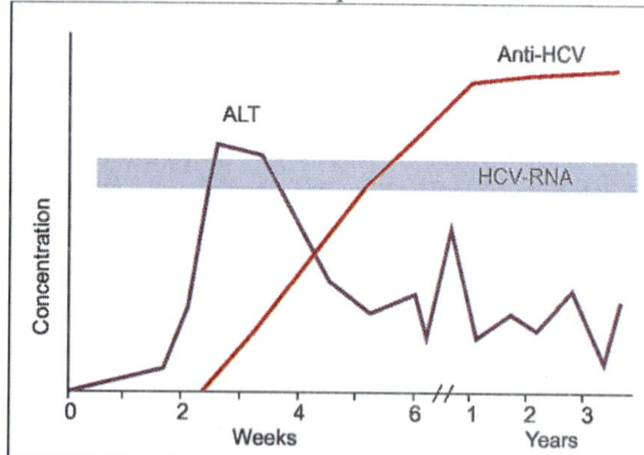

Figure-9: Markers of HCV

D. **Molecular methods:** HCV RNA can be detected within few days after exposure, even before Ab production & elevation of enzymes. Molecular methods are not reliable to know the disease progression or prognosis, but help in predicting the drug response. It is considered as a gold standard. Different methods are

- Branch DNA assay: Less sensitive (detection limit 10^3IU/ml).
- RT-PCR: More sensitive (detection limit 10-10^2IU/ml).
- Transcription mediated amplification (TMA).
- Real time RT-PCR (q RT-PCR): It is the quantitative method & most sensitive test among all.

❖ Prevention:

➢ **General measures:**

- Improvement in health education.
- Screening of blood, organ & tissues of donor.
- Safe sex.
- High-risk behavior modification like drug abuse.
- Avoid direct contact with blood and body fluid.
- Use of disposable & sterile medical devices.
- Those with chronic hepatitis C are advised to avoid alcohol & medications toxic to the liver.
- Cases should be vaccinated for hepatitis A and hepatitis B.
- Ultrasound surveillance for HCC is recommended in those with accompanying cirrhosis.

➢ **Immunoprophylaxis:** No specific active or passive prophylaxes are available.

❖ Treatment:

HCV induces chronic infection in 50–80% of infected persons. In rare cases, infection can clear without treatment. Approximately 40–80% of cases required treatment.

1. **Medications:**

- **Selection & duration of drugs:** Depend on genotypes.

- HCV genotype 1a: 12 weeks of ledipasvir & sofosbuvir or 12-24 weeks of paritaprevir, ombitasvir, dasabuvir, and ribavirin.
- HCV genotype 1b: 12 weeks of ledipasvir & sofosbuvir or 12 weeks of paritaprevir, ombitasvir and dasabuvir.
- HCV genotype 2: 12-16 weeks of sofosbuvir & ribavirin.
- HCV genotype 3: 12 weeks of sofosbuvir, ribavirin & pegylated interferon.
- HCV genotype 4: 12 weeks of ledipasvir and sofosbuvir or paritaprevir, ritonavir, ombitasvir & ribavirin or 24 weeks of sofosbuvir & ribavirin.
- HCV genotype 5 or 6: sofosbuvir & ledipasvir.
- Sofosbuvir with ribavirin and interferon appears to be around 90% effective in those with genotype 1, 4, 5, or 6 diseases.
- Sofosbuvir with just ribavirin appears to be 70 to 95% effective in type 2 and 3 disease but has a higher rate of adverse effects.

- **Success rate:**

- Treatments that contain ledipasvir and sofosbuvir for genotype 1 have success rates of around 93 to 99% but are very expensive.
- In genotype 6 infection, pegylated interferon and ribavirin is effective in 60 to 90% of cases. There is some tentative data for simeprevir use in type 6 disease as well.
- Prior to 2011, treatments consisted of a combination of pegylated interferon alpha and ribavirin for a period of 24 or 48 weeks, depending on HCV genotype. This produces cure rates of between 70 and 80% for genotype 2 and 3, respectively, and 45 to 70% for genotypes 1 and 4.

Adverse effects with these treatments were common, with half of people getting flu like symptoms and a third experiencing emotional problems. Treatment during the first six months is more effective than once hepatitis C has become chronic.

2. **Surgery:** Liver transplantation in cirrhosis due to hepatitis C Treatment with pegylated interferon and ribavirin post transplant decreases the risk of recurrence to 70%.
3. **Alternative therapies:** Like milk thistle, ginseng & colloidal silver. However, no alternative therapy has been shown to improve outcomes in hepatitis C and no evidence exists that alternative therapies have any effect on the virus at all.

Deltavirus - HDV

❖ Introduction:

- The delta agent is a defective virus & always required helper virus like HBV. It has no independent existence.
- It shows similarities with plants viruses like viroids or satellite viruses.

❖ History:

- Virus was identified in Italy in 1977 by Rizzetto & colleagues as nuclear-antigen in nuclei of liver cell of patients infected with HBV.
- This nuclear antigen initially considered as HBV antigen and was **called the delta antigen**.
- Subsequent experiments in chimpanzees showed that the delta antigen was a structural part of a pathogen that required HBV infection to replicate. The entire genome was cloned and sequenced in 1986. It was subsequently placed in its own genus *Deltavirus*.

❖ Geographical distribution & genotypes:

✪ **Distribution:**

- Distributed worldwide & about 5% of HBsAg positive people are co-infected with HDV.
- High-prevalence areas: It includes the Mediterranean, Middle East, Pakistan, Central and Northern Asia, Japan, Taiwan, Greenland and parts of Africa (mainly the horn of Africa and West Africa), the Amazon Basin and certain areas of the Pacific.
- High-prevalence areas: It includes North America, Northern Europe, South Africa and Eastern Asia.
- It is not prevalent in India in spite of maximum HBV carrier.

✪ **Genotypes:**

- **Older typing:** Initially 3 genotypes were identified from I-III with subtypes.
  - Genotype I: Found in Europe, North America, Africa and some parts of Asia.
  - Genotype II: Found in Japan, Taiwan & Yakutia (Russia).
  - Genotype III: Found exclusively in South America (Peru, Colombia, and Venezuela).
  - Some genomes from Taiwan and the Okinawa islands have been difficult to type but have been placed in genotype II.
- **Newer typing:** At least 8 genotypes of this virus from 1-8. Phylogenetic studies suggest an African origin for this pathogen.
  - Genotypes 1:,Restricted to certain geographical areas.
  - Genotypes -2: It is (Previous type -IIa) found in Japan, Taiwan and Yakoutia & Russia.
  - Genotypes -4: It is (previous type -IIb) found Japan and Taiwan.
  - Genotypes -3: Found in the Amazonian regions.
  - Genotypes -5, 6, 7 &8: Found in Africa. Genotype 8 usually found only in Africa but also found in South America and may have been imported into South America during the slave trade.

❖ Morphology: →Fig.-10

- **Shape:** Spherical.
- **Size:** 36 nm.
- **Genome & envelope:** Linear, ss-RNA (-) surrounded by HBsAg (envelope protein) of HBV, hence **called dependent virus.**
- **IF microscopy:** Ag of HDV is detected from nuclei of liver cells by IF test.

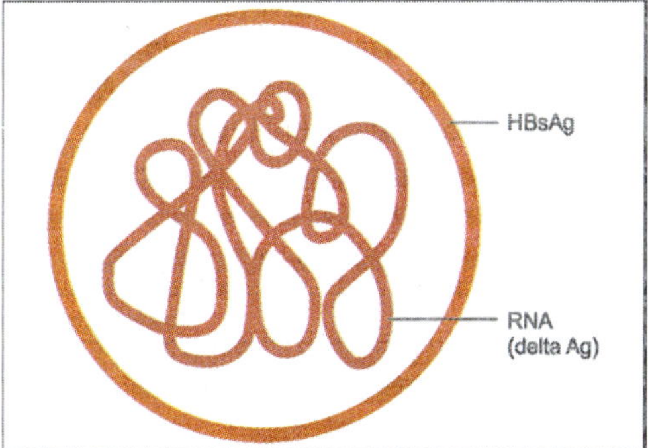

Figure-10: Morphology of HDV

❖ Culture characteristics (C/Cs):

Woodchuck (animal) is an ideal model for study of HDV infection.

❖ Pathogenicity:

- **Disease name:** Disease **called hepatitis D.**
- **Synonym:** Also **called hepatitis delta.**
- **Nature or history of disease:** Globally 5% of HBV patients are infected with HDV.
  - It is endemic in Mediterranean countries where it is transmitted by close personal contact.
  - In non-endemic areas like North Europe or North America it is transmitted by blood/blood products.
  - It may cause outbreak in person infected with HBV with high mortality.

- **Reservoir of infection:** Only human & no animal reservoir.
- **Source of infection:** Blood/blood products & body fluid.
- **Mode of transmission:**

1. **Per-cutaneous exposures:** Injecting drug abuse, blood or by blood products.
2. **Per-mucosal exposures:** Sex contact.
3. **Vertical:** From mother to child.

- **Incubation period (IP):** 1-6 months.
- **Portal of entry:** Skin or mucosa.
- **Sites:** Liver.
- **Precipitating factors (epidemiological determinants):**

1. **Age:** Any age.
2. **High risk groups:**

- Patients required multiple blood transfusions like hemophiliacs.
- In drug addicts.

- **Clinical features:** Two types of infection according to transmission as mentioned in **table-2.**

Features	Co-infection	Superinfection
Definition	HDV & HBV transmitted simultaneously	Infection by HDV in a person already infected with HBV or carrier
Status	Healthy	Infected or carrier
Risk of development of		
- Fulminant disease - Chronic hepatitis - Cirrhosis	- > HBV alone - Rare - Rare	- > co-infection - High - More
HCC	Rare	More
Mortality	Rare	More
Diagnosis		
Ags	HBsAg	HBsAg & HBeAg
Abs	Anti-HBc (IgM) & Anti-HDV (IgM)	Anti-HBc (IgG) & Anti-HDV (IgM, IgG)
Nucleic acid	HDV RNA	

Table-2: Differences between co-infection & superinfection of HDV

- **Co-infection**
  - HDV & HBV transmitted simultaneously.
  - Transient & self limited.
  - Clinically indistinguishable from hepatitis B.
  - Rarely progress to chronic stage at a rate similar to HBV alone.
  - HBV vaccine is effective to prevent against HDV.
- **Superinfection**
  - Infection by HDV in a person already infected with HBV or carrier.
  - Usually develop more serious & chronic infection.
  - It deteriorates the underlying HBV infection. Following stage

1. **Acute stage:** HDV replicates actively with high transaminase levels with suppression of HBV.
2. **Chronic stage:** HDV replication decrease, fluctuating transaminase levels with high HBV. Disease progress to chronic hepatitis, cirrhosis & HCC in 5-20% cases. Mortality is >20%.

❖ Laboratory diagnosis:

- **Specimens:** Blood/serum & liver biopsy.
- **Testing methods:**

A. **Microscopy:** → **Follow morphology.**

B. **Animal culture:** → **Follow C/Cs.**

C. **Serological tests:**

- **Co-infection**
  - Anti-HBc (IgM) & anti-HDV (IgM) are elevated but anti-HDV (IgM) appears late & frequently short lived.
  - Anti-HDV (IgM) develops, 2-3 weeks after infection, immediately replaced by IgG. However IgM also present in chronic infection.
  - IgM detected by ELISA.
  - Co-infection: Anti-HBc (IgM) & anti-HDV (IgM).
- **Superinfection**
  - HBV is already present so, HBV markers already available are HBsAg, HBeAg & Anti-HBc (IgG).
  - HDV markers are Anti-HDV IgM & anti-HDV IgG.
  - Superinfection: Anti-HBc (IgG), Anti-HDV (IgM) & anti-HDV (IgG).

D. **Molecular methods:** RNA sequencing & DNA probe are rapid & sensitive methods.

❖ Prevention:

- **General measures:**
  - Screening of blood, organs or tissues for HBV is automatically minimise the risk of HDV, as HDV does not exist without HBV.
  - Safe sex.
  - High-risk behavior modification like drug abuse.
  - Avoid direct contact with blood and body fluid.
  - Use of disposable & sterile medical devices.
- **Immunoprophylaxis:** No specific active or passive prophylaxis are available for HDV, but immunisation by HBV is effective as HDV cant infect the person immunised to HBV.

❖ Treatment:

- Pegylated interferon alpha: It is the only drug effective against HDV & to reduce the viral load. More than 1 year of therapy may be necessary.
- Liver transplantation may be considered for cases of fulminant hepatitis and end-stage liver disease.
- New therapeutic agents: Such as prenylation inhibitor or myrcludex are useful to inhibit the virus entry in hepatocytes. Myrcludex is under trial as of October 2015.

Hepeviridae - HEV

❖ Synonym:

- Enterically transmitted NANB hepatitis virus.
- E-NANB hepatitis virus.

- Epidemic-NANB hepatitis virus (because causing epidemic).

❖ **History:** Infection with this virus was first documented in 1955 during an outbreak in New Delhi, India. Virus was discovered in 1990 (?).

❖ **Geographical distribution & genotypes:**

Features	Areas with poor water supply	Areas with safe water supply
Reservoir of infection	Human	Animals like monkey, cat, dog, pig, deer etc.
Source of infection	Water/food	Animal tissues (like pork in UK)
Mode of transmission	By ingestion of water/food	By ingestion of raw tissues of animal (liver)
Genotype	1 & 2	3
Nature of disease	Sporadic /epidemic	Sporadic
Countries	Developed	Developing

Table-3: Pattern of HEV

- **Distribution:** Virus is distributed worldwide. Two patterns are observed as shown in **table-3.**
- **Genotypes:** Four genotypes are identified based on the nucleotide sequences of the genome. Genotypes 1 & 2 are restricted to humans & often associated with large outbreaks & epidemics in developing countries with poor sanitation. Genotypes 3 & 4 infect humans, pigs and other animal species & have been responsible for sporadic cases of HEV in both developing & industrialized countries.

1. **Genotype 1:**
- Five subtypes.
- Common in 15-35 years & mortality is about 1%.
- Isolated from tropical & several subtropical countries in Asia & Africa.

2. **Genotype 2:**
- Two subtypes.
- Isolated from Mexico, Nigeria & Chad.

3. **Genotypes 3:**
- Ten subtypes.
- Common Japan.
- Common in people older than 60 years and the mortality is between 5 and 10%.
- Isolated almost worldwide including Asia, Europe, Oceania, North & South America.

4. **Genotypes 4:**
- Seven subtypes.
- Common Japan.
- Common in people older than 60 years & the mortality is between 5 and 10%.
- Limited distribution.

❖ **Morphology:** →**Fig.-11**

➢ **Shape:** Spherical. Virus have 32 cup shape depressions on surface, hence it was initially classified under the genus *Calcivirus* of family Calciviridae. **Calci** derived from **calyx** = **cup**. Now it is classified under the genus *Hepevirus* of family Hepeviridae.

➢ **Size:** 32-34 nm.

➢ **Genome & capsid:** ss-RNA (+) surrounded by icosahedral variety of capsid.

➢ **Envelope:** It is non enveloped virus.

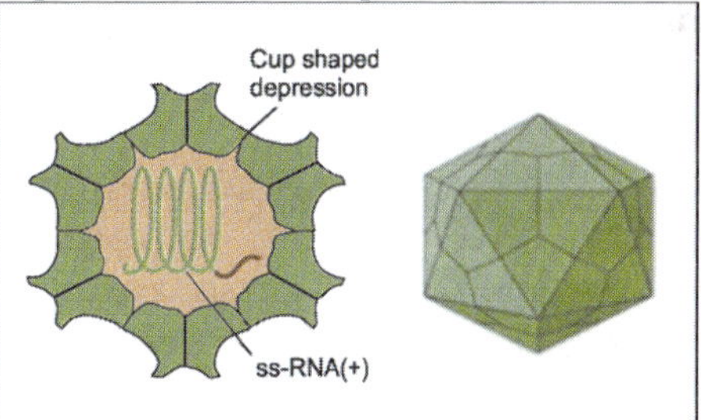

Figure-11: Morphology of HEV

❖ **Culture characteristics (C/Cs):**
- Prevalent in animal reservoir like pigs.
- Experimentally can be transmitted in primates.
- In vitro cultivation has not been successful so far.
- Virus genome has been cloned.

❖ **Resistance:** Non-enveloped virus resistant to lipid solvents.

❖ **Antigenic structure:** RNA antigen **called HEV-Ag.** Only one serotype.

❖ **Immunity:** Secondary attack rate is very low in house hold contact about 2-3% compare to 10-20% in HAV.

❖ **Pathogenicity:**

➢ **Disease name:** Disease is zoonotic **called hepatitis E.**

➢ **Synonym:** Also **called enterically transmitted NANB hepatitis** or **E-NANB hepatitis** or **Epidemic-NANB hepatitis virus.**

➢ **Nature or history of disease:** HEV is the most common cause of viral hepatitis in India, Africa, & Central America. In India, Maximum cases about 30-60% are sporadic type. In other countries it is uncommon & occurs due to travellers from endemic areas. It also causes epidemic. Major epidemic reported in the world are
- 1955–1956, outbreak in New Delhi, India: 30,000 cases within six weeks.
- 1976–1977, outbreak in Burma: 20,000 cases.
- 1978, outbreak in Kashmir, India: 52,000 cases.
- 1991, outbreak in Kanpur, India: 79,000 cases.
- Between 1986 -88, epidemic in China: 100,000 cases.
- 2004, outbreak in Sub –Saharan areas: Two outbreaks one is in Chad & second in Sudan with high fatalities.
- 2005, outbreak in England & Wales: Zoonotic from deer & swine with 329 cases.

Features	A	B	C	D	E
Size	27nm	42nm	50-60nm	36nm	32-34nm
Type	RNA	DNA	RNA	RNA	RNA
Family	Picornaviridae	Hepadnaviridae	Flaviviridae	?	Hepeviridae
Genus	*Heparna virus (Hepatovirus)*	*Orthohepadnavirus*	*Hepacivirus*	*Deltavirus*	*Hepevirus*
Mode of Transmission	Faeco-oral	Percutaneous Permucosal	Percutaneous Permucosal	Percutaneous Permucosal	Faeco-oral
Incubation period	2-6 weeks	1-6 months	15-160 days	1-6 months	15-60 days
Chronic Infection	No	Yes	Yes	Yes	No
Malignancy	No	Yes	Yes	No	No
Carrier	nil	Yes	Yes	No	No

Table-4: Differences between hepatitis viruses

- October 2007, largest epidemic in Kitgum District of northern Uganda: No previous epidemics had been documented here. By June 2009 the epidemic had caused illness in 10,196 persons and 160 deaths.
- 2011, a minor outbreak: It was reported in Tangail, a neighbourhood of Dhaka, Bangladesh.
- July 2012, outbreak in South Sudanese refugee camps in Maban County near the Sudan border: It claimed 400 cases and 16 deaths as of September 13, 2012.
- 2nd February 2013, epidemic in Sans Frontieres: About 4,000 patients & 88 deaths have been reported by "Medical charity Medecins Sans Frontieres.
- April 2014, outbreak in Biratnagar Municipality, Nepal: Over 6,000 locals were infected with 9 deaths.

➢ **Reservoir of infection: → Table-3.**

➢ **Source of infection: → Table-3.**

- Secondary attack rate: Transmission from patient to case is 1-2%.

➢ **Mode of transmission: → Table-3.**

➢ **Incubation period (IP):** 15-60 days.

➢ **Portal of entry:** GIT.

➢ **Sites:** Liver.

➢ **Precipitating factors (epidemiological determinants):**

1. **Age:** Young adults (15-40 years) unlike HAV common in children.
2. **Pregnancy:** More sever (fulminant hepatitis) & high fatality rate of 20-40% in pregnancy especially in 3rd trimester.
3. **Immunocompromised host:** It develop chronic hepatitis with high mortality in person due to organ transplantation & immunosuppressive therapy.
4. **Seasonal factor:** Outbreaks most commonly occur after heavy rainfall & monsoons because of their disruption of water supplies.
5. **Poor hygiene & poor sanitation:** These are the most favouring factors.
6. **Economical status:** Common in developing countries but zoonotic infection is common in developed countries.

➢ **Clinical features:** Clinically resemble to HAV. Both have acute onset with mild & self limited illness with low case fatality of 1%.

➢ **Complication:** Fulminant hepatitis occurs in 1-2% cases, but risk increase up to 20% in pregnancy especially in 3rd trimester. There is no chronic or carrier stage in hepatitis E infection.

❖ Laboratory diagnosis:

➢ **Specimens:** Faeces, bile & serum.

➢ **Testing methods:**

A. **Microscopy: → Follow morphology.**

B. **Culture: → Follow C/Cs.**

C. **Serological test: → Fig.-12**

- IgM & IgG Abs are diagnosed by ELISA.
- IgM appear early with ALT & indicates the acute infection.
- IgG replace IgM after 2-4 weeks & last for years indicates the past infection.

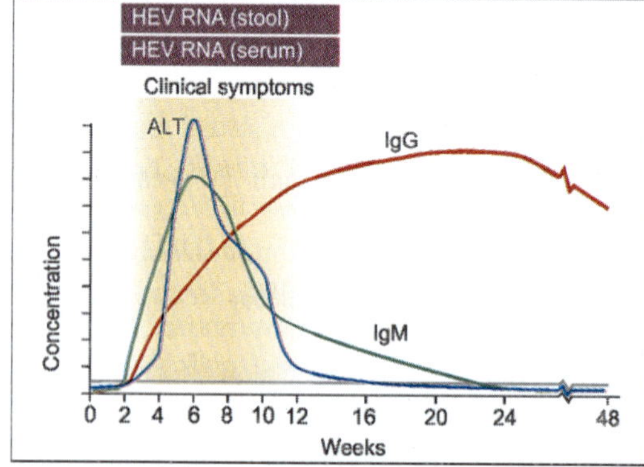

Figure-12: Markers of HEV

❖ Prevention:
Transmission of HEV can be reduced by

- Maintaining quality standards for public water supplies.
- Establishing proper disposal systems for human faeces.

- HEV 239: China prepared the recombinant vaccine by using this strain but not available globally.

❖ Treatment:

- It is self-limiting disease, hospitalization & treatment is generally not required.
- Ribavirin is given to people with fulminant hepatitis, symptomatic pregnant women & immunosuppressed people.
- In some specific situations, interferon has also been used successfully.

Differences between hepatitis viruses

↓

Table-4

Question bank

Case study

1) A 35-year-old male, who received multiple transfusion of blood admitted in hospital with nausea, vomiting, loss of appetite, abdominal pain & passing yellowish dark coloured urine. On clinical examination yellowish sclera was noticed. Blood is collected & sent for serological testing. Laboratory reported positive test for HBsAg & IgM anti-HBcAg with negative reports for HCV, HAV & HEV. Identify the clinical conditions & answer the following

a) Name the disease with clinical stage & its etiological agent.
b) Write the morphology & genetic structure of etiological agent.
c) Write pathogenicity & diagnosis of clinical condition.
d) How you can prevent this clinical condition?

Essay/Full question

1) Hepatitis viruses.
2) HBV.

Short notes

1) Classification of hepatitis viruses.
2) Genomic organisation & mutation in the genes of HBV & HCV.
3) Pathogenicity/lab. diagnosis of HBV (Australian antigen)
4) HBV vaccine.
5) HAV.
6) HCV.
7) HDV.
8) HEV.

Short questions for theory/viva questions

1) Mention the immunological markers of HBV present in serum
2) Write different antigenic types of HBV.
3) Write different modes of entry of HBV.
4) Comment: HAV have no or very rare blood/serum transmission.
5) Comment: HCV called notorious virus among the all hepatitis group.

MCQs for chapter review

Classification

1) **Non-parenteral hepatitis is** (AIIMS-96, AI-00)
(a) Hepatitis A (b) Hepatitis B (c) Hepatitis C (d) Hepatitis D
2) **Which of the following hepatitis virus is a DNA virus** (AIIMS, May-03, PGI, Dec-04)
(a) Hepatitis C virus (b) Hepatitis B virus (c) Delta agent (d) Hepatitis E virus
3) **Hepatitis B is caused by**
(a) RNA virus (b) DNA virus (c) Retrovirus (d) Prion
4) **Which hepatitis virus had been called as enterovirus**
(a) HAV (b) HBV (c) HCV (d) HEV

Hepadnaviridae - HBV

5) **All of the following are components of Dane particle except-** (AIIMS-98)
(a) Surface antigen (b) Core antigen (c) C-antigen (d) Delta antigen
6) **Which of the following is not present in Dane particle?**
(a) Core antigen (b) Surface antigen (c) p53 (d) None of above
7) **Australian antigen is associated with**
(a) HBsAg (b) HBcAg (c) HBeAg (d) None of above
8) **HBV present in India is**
(a) adw (b) ayw (c) adr (d) ayr
9) **Reverse transcriptase of HBV is coded on following gene-** (AI-00)
(a) C gene (b) S gene (c) P gene (d) X gene
10) **Which is longest DNA of hepatitis B virus**
(a) P gene (b) X gene (c) S gene (d) C gene
11) **Hepatitis B is not transmitted by**
(a) Blood transfusion (b) Pasteurised albumin (c) Cryoprecipitate (d) Sexual contact
12) **Which of the following hepatitis virus have significant perinatal transmission** (AI-03)
(a) HEV (b) HCV (c) HBV (d) HAV
13) **Which is not true about hepatitis B virus**
(a) DNA virus (b) Transmitted by faeco-oral route (c) Can be transmitted from mother to child (d) Contains reverse transcriptase
14) **HBV, all are true except**
(a) DNA virus (b) Spread by blood transfusion (c) HBsAg marker of infection (d) Least chances of chronicity
15) **Presence of HBeAg in patients with hepatitis indicates-** (AIIMS-92)
(a) Simple carrier (b) Late convalescence (c) High infectivity (d) Carrier status
16) **HBV is associated with all of the following except**
(a) Hepatic cancer (b) Chronic hepatitis (c) Hepatic adenoma (d) Cirrhosis
17) **Which of the following hepatitis has a poor prognosis**
(a) Hepatitis A (b) Hepatitis B (c) Non A non B type (d) Hepatitis C
18) **Incubation period of HBV is** (AI-00)
(a) 45 to180 days (b) 6 to 60 days (c) 10 days (d) 10 hrs
19) **Hepatitis B virus is not secreted in**
(a) Saliva (b) Semen (c) Stool (d) All of above
20) **Hepatitis B vaccination is given to a patient. His serum will reveal.** (AIIMS, May-02)
(a) HBsAg (b) Anti- HBsAg (c) IgM anti-HBcAg and HBsAg (d) IgM and IgG anti-HBcAg
21) **Which of the following antigen is found within the nuclei of infected hepatocytes and not usually in the peripheral circulation in hepatitis B infection** (AI-00)
(a) HBeAg (b) HBcAg (c) anti-HBc (d) HBsAg
22) **Serological testing of patients shows HBsAg, anti- HBc and HBeAg positive. The patient has**
(a) Chronic hepatitis B with low infectivity (b) Acute hepatitis B with high infectivity (c) Chronic hepatitis B with high infectivity (d) Acute on chronic hepatitis
23) **Acute hepatitis B can be earliest diagnosed by** (AIIMS, Nov-01)

(a) IgM anti-HBc Ab (b) HBsAg (c) IgG anti-HBc Ab (d) anti-HBsAg Ab

24) In a patient of active chronic hepatitis B all are seen except (AIIMS -07)
(a) HBsAg (b) IgM anti-HBc Ab (c) HBe Ag (d) anti-HBsAg

25) Anti HBsAg Ab (AIIMS-93)
(a) Resistance to hepatitis B (b) Acute infection (c) Good prognosis (d) Hepato cellular carcinoma

26) In a patient only anti HBsAg is positive in serum, all other markers are negative. This indicates (AIIMS-00)
(a) Acute hepatitis (b) Chronic active hepatitis (c) Persistent carrier (d) Hepatitis B vaccination

27) First antibody to appear in HBV
(a) IgM anti-HBe (b) IgG anti-HBe (c) IgM anti-HBc (d) IgM anti-HBs

28) The best diagnostic test for recent hepatitis B is (AIIMS-03, PGI -97, 99)
(a) HBsAg (b) IgM anti-HBc (c) anti-HBe (d) anti-HBs

29) Best epidemiological tool for investigation of hepatitis B is (AIIMS-00, AI -97)
(a) Anti-HBsAg (b) anti-HBcAg (c) anti-HBeAg (d) HBcAg

30) Active replication in hepatitis B infection is indicated by?
(a) HBeAg (b) HBsAg (c) HBcAg (d) Anti-HBsAg

31) Infectivity of HBsAg is best/commonly diagnosed by
(a) HBeAg (b) HBsAg (c) HBV DNA (d) Anti-HBsAg

32) Which of this is not a marker of active replicative phase of chronic hepatitis B? (AIIMS-08)
(a) HBV DNA (b) HBV DNA polymerase (c) Anti HBc (d) AST and ALT

33) Best means of giving hepatitis B vaccine is
(a) Subcutaneous (b) Intradermal (c) Intramuscular deltoid (d) Intramuscular gluteal

34) A blood donor is not considered for safe transfusion, if he has (AI-00)
(a) Anti HBsAg +ve (b) Anti HBsAg and HBcAg +ve (c) HBsAg +ve and IgM anti HBcAg +ve (d) Anti-HBc+ve

35) Hepatitis B virus vaccine contains
(a) HBsAg (b) HBc (c) HBe (d) All of above

36) A mother is HBsAg is positive at 32 weeks of pregnancy. What should be given to newborn to prevent the neonatal infection. (AIIMS-02)
(a) Hepatitis B vaccine + immunoglobulin (b) Immunoglobulin only (c) Hepatitis B vaccine only (d) Immunoglobulin followed by vaccine 1 month later.

Picornaviridae - HAV

37) Cultivable (in vitro) hepatitis is (AIIMS, May-07)
(a) Hepatitis A (b Hepatitis B (c) Hepatitis C (d) Hepatitis D

38) Transmission of hepatitis A virus occur (PGI-99)
(a) One week before and one week after onset of symptoms (b) 2 week before onset of symptoms (c) 2 week after onset of symptoms (d) 1 week after onset of symptoms

39) Hepatitis A is transmitted by (AI-93)
(a) Blood route (b) Inhalation (c) Faeco-oral route (d) All

40) Age group affected by hepatitis A virus (PGI-99)
(a) Children (b) Adult (c) Old age (d) Any age

41) About hepatitis A true is (PGI, Dec-08)
(a) Causes mild illness in children (b) 3% incidence of carrier state (c) 10% transmission to HCC (d) Vertical transmission never seen

42) Carrier state does not exist for
(a) Hepatitis B virus (b Hepatitis A virus (c) Non A Non B hepatitis (d) Delta agent

43) True about hepatitis A virus
(a) Causes cirrhosis (b) Helps HDV replication (c) Common cause of hepatitis in children (d) Causes chronic hepatitis

44) Hepatitis A virus is best diagnosed by (AI-01)
(a) IgM antibodies in serum (b) Isolation from stool (c) Culture from blood (d) Isolation from bile

45) Potent (prophylactic) vaccine is available for
(a) Hepatitis C (b) Hepatitis A (c) Hepatitis D (d) Hepatitis E (e) Hepatitis B

Flaviviridae - HCV

46) HCV is (PGI, Dec-05, June -08)
(a) Enveloped RNA (b) Non-enveloped RNA (c) Non-enveloped positive strand RNA (d) DNA virus

47) Maximum hepatitis C virus transmission to foetus in pregnancy depends on (PGI-00)
(a) Duration of illness (b) Time of infection (c) Route of delivery (d) HIV infection (e) High level of HCV infection

48) Hepatitis C virus, true finding is (AIIMS, Dec-98)
(a) Spreads along faeco-oral route (b) Antibody to HCV may not be seen in acute stage (c) Does not cause chronic hepatitis (d) It cannot be cultured

49) Commonest hepatotropic virus causing increased chronic carrier state is
(a) HEV (b) HAV (c) HBV (d) HCV

50) Next to HBV, virus implicated in hepato cellular Ca is (PGI-98)
(a) HCV (b) Herpes (c) HAV (d) HEV

51) Which of the following statement about hepatitis C is true (AI-09)
(a) DNA virus (b) Most common indication for liver transplant (c) Does not causes liver cancer (d) Does not cause co-infection with hepatitis B

52) Which hepatitis virus is notorious for causing chronic hepatitis evolving to cirrhosis
(a) HEV (b) HAV (c) HBV (d) HCV

53) True about HCV includes all except
(a) Highest rate of chronicity among all hepatitis viruses (b) Can be cultured (c) Diagnosed by detection of HCV RNA (d) Transmitted through transfusion of infected food

54) HCV is associated with (AI-00)
(a) Anti-LKM-1 antibody (b) Scleroderma (c) Cryoglobulinemia (d) Polyartritis nodosa

55) Chronic liver disease is caused by
(a) Hepatitis B (b Hepatitis A (c) Hepatitis C (d) Hepatitis E

Deltavirus - HDV

56) Which of the following is a defective virus (AI-01)
(a) HAV (c) HBV (c) HCV (d) HDV

57) Dependent virus is
(a) HAV (c) HBV (c) HDV (d) HCV

58) HBV and HDV false is
(a) Bothe can infect simultaneously (b) HDV causes more serious infection due to superinfection (c) HDV cannot infect in absence of HBV (d) DNA viruses

59) HDV is
(a) ss-RNA virus (b) ss-DNA virus (c) ds-RNA virus (d) ds-DNA virus

60) Chronic hepatitis is seen in
(a) Hepatitis C (b Hepatitis D (c) Hepatitis A (d) Hepatitis E

61) Which of the following does not go in to chronic hepatitis stage
(a) HEV (b) HDV (c) HBV (d) HCV

Hepeviridae - HEV

62) Which of the following is calcivirus (AIIMS, Nov-01)
(a) Hepatitis E (b Hepatitis B (c) Hepatitis C (d) Hepatitis A

63) Which is ss-RNA un-enveloped virus
(a) HBV (b) HEV (c) HCV (d) None

64) Most common route of spread of Hepatitis E is
(a) Sex (b) Faeco-oral route (c) Blood transfusion (d) IV injections

65) With which of the following viral hepatitis infection in pregnancy, the maternal mortality is highest (AIIMS-06)

(a) Hepatitis A (b Hepatitis B (c) Hepatitis C (d) Hepatitis E

66) **A young pregnant woman present with fulminant hepatic failure. The most likely aetiological agent is-** (AI-04)
(a) Hepatitis B virus (b Hepatitis C virus (c) Hepatitis E virus
(d) Hepatitis A virus

67) **During epidemic of Hepatitis E fatality is maximum in**
(a) Pregnant woman (b) Infants (c) Malnourished male (d) Adolscent

68) **Regarding hepatitis E true is-** (AIIMS-98)
(a) Occurs with hepatitis B (b Single stranded DNA virus (c) Occurs along with HIV (d) Mortality increased in pregnancy

69) **Hepatitis E clinically resembles-**
(a) Hepatitis A (b Hepatitis B (c) Hepatitis C (d) Hepatitis D

Mixed MCQs for all hepatitis viruses

70) **The commonest cause of viral hepatitis in India**
(a) Hepatitis A virus (b Enterically transmitted NANB hepatitis
(c) Hepatitis C virus (d) Hepatitis B virus

71) **All the statements are correct about hepatitis viruses except**
(a) Maximum chances of chronic infection is HCV (b Pregnant woman with HEV has 10-20% chances of mortality (c) Vaccine is available only against HBV (d) HBV and HCV has oncogenic potential

72) **All of the following hepatitis virus can be transmitted through blood except**
(a) Hepatitis B (b) Hepatitis C (c) Hepatitis D (d) Hepatitis E

73) **Which of the following is not matched correctly**
(a) Hepatitis D – Defective virus (b) Hepatitis C – Parenteral transmission (c) Hepatitis B – RNA virus (d) Hepatitis E – Faeco-oral transmission

Answers of MCQs & explanation

1) (a)
2) (b)
3) (b)
4) (a)
Follow section, **classification & flow chart-1** for explanation

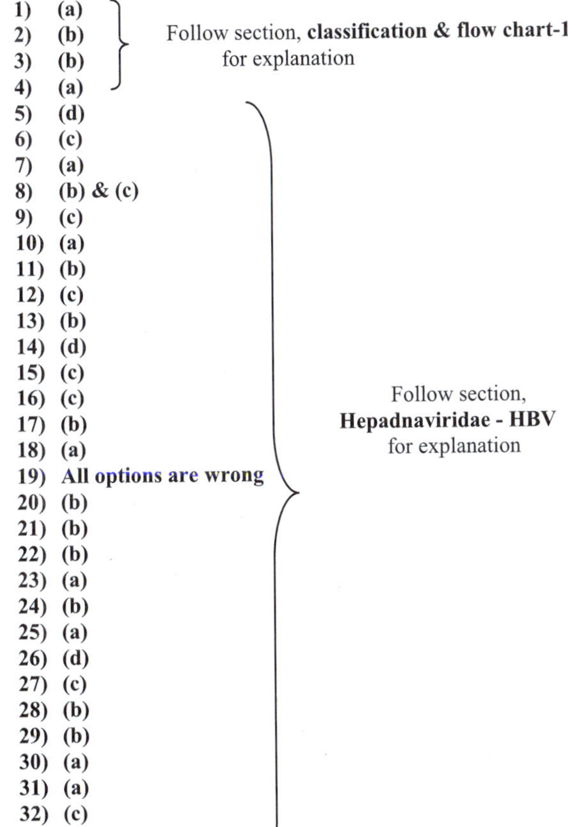

5) (d)
6) (c)
7) (a)
8) (b) & (c)
9) (c)
10) (a)
11) (b)
12) (c)
13) (b)
14) (d)
15) (c)
16) (c)
17) (b)
18) (a)
19) All options are wrong
20) (b)
21) (b)
22) (b)
23) (a)
24) (b)
25) (a)
26) (d)
27) (c)
28) (b)
29) (b)
30) (a)
31) (a)
32) (c)
33) (c)
34) (c)
35) (a)
Follow section, **Hepadnaviridae - HBV** for explanation

36) (a)
- Combined immunisation is better effective in given case.

37) (a)
38) (b) & (c)
39) (c)
40) (a)
41) (a) & (d)
42) (b)
43) (c)
44) (a)
Follow section, **Picornaviridae - HAV** for explanation

45) (b) & (e)
- Among the hepatitis viruses potent vaccine available for HAV & HBV

46) (a)
47) (e)
48) (b) & (d)
49) (d)
50) (a)
51) (b)
52) (d)
53) (b) & (d)
Follow section, **Flaviviridae - HCV** for explanation

54) (a) & (c)
- Anti-LKM Ab is anti-kidney liver microsomal Ab. It is developed due homology between viral particles & host tissues (cytochrome P450 system). Following three types
- Anti-LKM Ab: HCV
- Anti-LKM Ab: Drug (tienilic acid) induced hepatitis
- Anti-LKM Ab: HDV & autoimmune poly endocrine syndrome.

55) (a) & (b)
- Chronicity of hepatitis viruses: HCV (50-80%, most notorious) > HDV (5-20%) > HBV (1-10%) > HAV= HEV (Almost none)

56) (d)
57) (c)
58) (d)
59) (a)
Follow section, ***Deltavirus* - HDV** for explanation

60) (a) & (b)
61) (a)
Among the hepatitis viruses, type B, C & D are causing chronic hepatitis while A & E are causing chronic hepatitis.

62) All options are wrong
- HEV have 32 cup shape depressions on surface, hence it was initially classified under the genus *Calcivirus* of family *Calciviridae*. **Calci** derived from **calyx** = **cup**. So as per older classification option 'a' is right but now it is classified under the genus *Hepevirus* of family *Hepeviridae*, so all options are wrong.

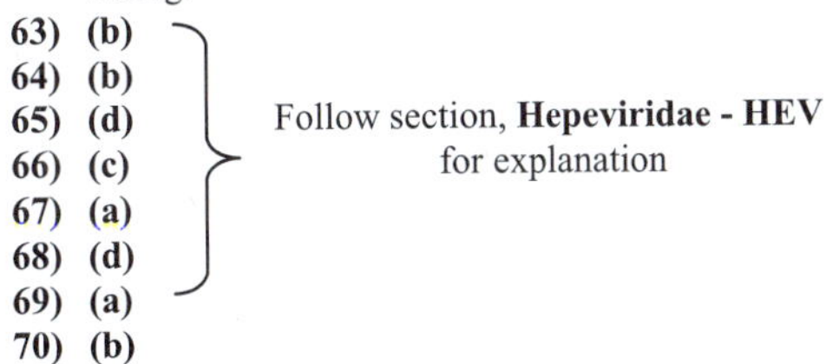

63) (b)
64) (b)
65) (d)
66) (c)
67) (a)
68) (d)
Follow section, **Hepeviridae - HEV** for explanation

69) (a)
70) (b)
- HEV is the most common cause of viral hepatitis in India, Africa, & Central America.

71) (c)
- Potent vaccine is available against HBV & HAV.

72) (d)
- HEV transmitted by faeco-oral route.

73) (c)
- HBV is DNA virus.

74 Other group of viruses

(Haemorrhagic fever viruses, diarrhoeal viruses, slow disease viruses, encephalitis viruses, glomerulonephritis viruses and oncogenic viruses)

Haemorrhagic fever viruses

Classification:

I. Systemic / taxonomical classification

A DNA viruses:

i. **Poxviridae:** Pox viruses causing humna lesion like variola virus.

ii. **Herpesviridae:** Like VZV

B RNA viruses:

i. **Paramyxoviridae:** Measles virus.

ii. **Togaviridae:** Chikungunya virus.

iii. **Flaviridae:** Two groups like mosquito borne & tick borne as follows.

➢ **Mosquito borne species**

1. Yellow fever virus.
2. Dengue virus.
3. Zika virus.

➢ **Tick borne species**

1. Kyasanur forest disease (KFD) virus.
2. Omsk haemorrhagic fever virus.

iv. **Bunyaviridae:**

- ***Nairovirus:*** Crimean Congo Haemorrhagic Fever (CCHF) virus.
- ***Phlebovirus:*** Rift Valley fever virus.
- ***Hantavirus:*** Hantaan virus & puumala virus.

v. **Arenaviridae:** Lassa fever virus & all new world viruses are haemorrhagic viruses.

vi. **Filoviridae:** → **Vide infra**

II. Clinical classification: It based on many features like clinical presentation, mode of transmission etc.

A. **Exanthematous viruses with hemorrhagic property:** Small pox, chicken pox, measles (All are described in respective chapters).

B. **Arboviruses:**

- **Mosquitoes borne:** Yellow fever virus, dengue virus & chikungunya virus.
- **Tick borne:** KFD virus, Omsk haemorrhagic fever virus & CCHF virus.

C. **Roboviruses:**

- **Haemorrhagic fever renal syndrome:** Hantaan virus.
- **Haemorrhagic fever:**
- Lassa fever virus & all new world viruses are the haemorrhagic species.

D. **Other like:** Like Filoviridae.

Filoviridae

❖ **Classification:** →**Flow chart-1**

❖ **Meaning:**

- **Name of family:** It is given from the word **filum** = **thread**, because thread like shape of virus.
- **Name of genera:**

- *Ebolavirus*: Genus name is came from the Ebola River, because the 1st case was identified from the village Yambuku near to Ebola river in Zaire (now the Democratic Republic of the Congo) in 1976.
- *Marburgvirus*: Genus name is came from the Marburg, Germany, at where the 1st infection was occurred in laboratory workers, who were working with tissue of African green monkeys (*Chlorocebus aethiops*).

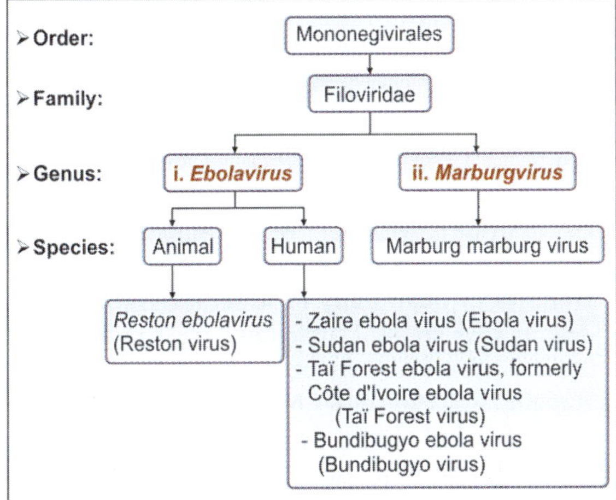

Flow chart-1: Classification of Filoviridae

Morphology: →Fig:-1

- **Shape:** Elongated like as thread.
- **Size:** 80nm in breath & 800-1000 (sometimes up to 14, 000) nm in length.
- **Genome & capsid:** ss-RNA (-) with helical variety of capsid.
- **Envelope:** Present.

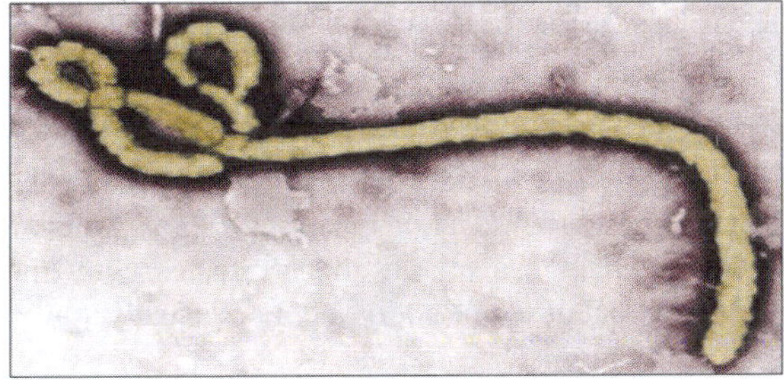

Figure-1: Morphology of Filoviridae (*Ebolavirus*)

i. *Ebolavirus*

Zaire ebola virus

- **Common name:** Ebola virus.
- **Abbreviation:** ZEBOV or EBOV.
- **History:** It was 1st isolated in 1976 from Yambuku, Zaire (now the Democratic Republic of the Congo).
- **Geographical distribution:** Sub-Saharan regions.
- **Morphology:**
- **General morphological features:** → Vide supra
- **Genomic structure:** This viral genome codes for seven structural proteins & one non-structural protein as shown in **fig.-2.**

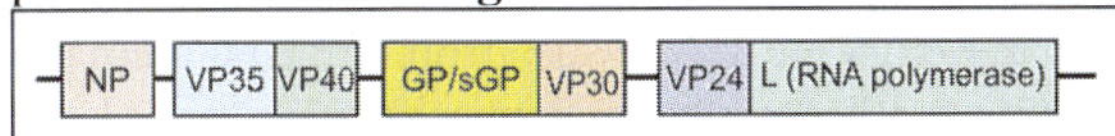

Figure-2: Genomic structure of Ebola virus

- **Culture characteristics (C/Cs):** It is cultivated on Vero cells but culture method is not able to differentiate between the members Filoviridae & also great risk of laboratory transmission (BSL-4).
- **Resistance:**
  - The virus is able to survive on objects for a few hours in a dried state.
  - It can survive for a few days within body fluids outside of a person.
  - The Ebola virus may be able to persist for more than 3 months or up to years in the semen after recovery, which could lead to infections via sexual intercourse.
  - It is an envelope virus susceptible to lipid solvents.
- **Immunity:** Recovery from Ebola depends on good supportive clinical care and the patient's immune response. People with ebola infection develop antibodies that last at least for 10 years.
- **Pathogenicity:**
- **Disease name:** Disease **called ebola virus disease.**
- **Synonym:** Also **called ebola hemorrhagic fever** or simply **called ebola.**
- **Nature or history of disease:**
  - The disease (also virus) was first identified in 1976 in two simultaneous outbreaks, one in Nzara village in Sudan & other in Yambuku village near the Ebola River in Zaire (from which the disease/virus takes its name).
  - Ebola outbreaks occur intermittently in tropical regions of sub-Saharan Africa.
  - Between 1976 and 2013, the World Health Organization reports a total of 24 outbreaks involving 1,716 cases.
  - The largest outbreak to date was the epidemic in West Africa, which occurred from December 2013 to January 2016 with 28,616 cases and 11,310 deaths.
  - On 8 August 2014, the WHO declared the epidemic to be an international public health emergency. It was declared no longer an emergency on 29 March 2016.
  - Measures taken in India to prevent the spread of 2013-16 outbreaks: Persons with acute fever & who has been in Guinea, Liberia, Sierra Leone or Mali in past 21 days were kept in quarantine in the airport until tested negative for Ebola virus.
- **Reservoir of infection:** Fruit bats ((*Hypsignathus monstrosus*, *Epomops franqueti* & *Myonycteris*

torquata) are the main reservoir hosts. End hosts are humans and great apes.

- **Source of infection:** Body fluid (like blood, semen breast milk etc.) & tissues from infected animals or human. Contaminated objects & water are also the source of infection.
- **Mode of transmission:** Following are the possible cycle as shown in **fig.-3.**

o Fruit bats to fruit bats:

o Fruit bats to animals: Bats drop partially eaten fruits and pulp, then land mammals such as gorillas, monkeys & duikers feed on these fallen fruits. This chain makes possible indirect transmission from the natural host to animal populations.

o Animals to animals: From one animal to other animal.

o Fruit bats to human: Exact route is unclear.

o Animals to human: Direct contact of abraded skin/mucosa with infected animals such as a gorillas or monkeys or their body fluid.

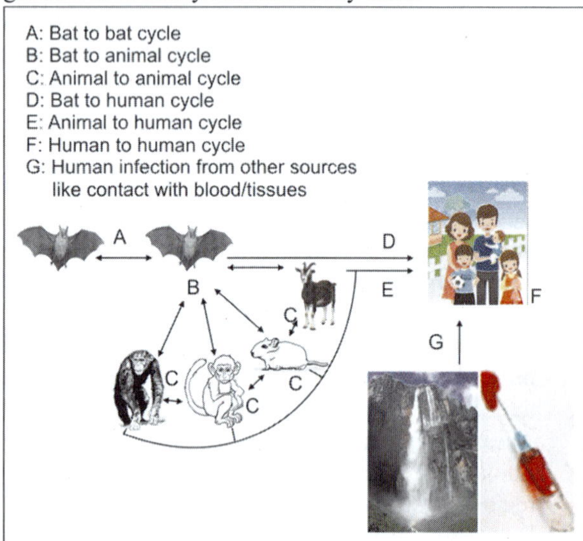

Figure-3: Cycle of Ebola virus

o Human to human:

- Direct contact of abraded skin/mucosa with blood & bodily fluids (including urine, saliva, faeces, vomit, breast milk and semen) from infected persons. It has not been reported to be transmitted through sweat.
- Sexual transmission: Virus sheds in semen for several months after recovery from illness.
- Breast milk may be infectious in survivors for few months.

o Human infection from other sources:

- Contact with contaminated water.
- Objects like clothes, bedding, needles, syringes/sharps or medical equipments that have been contaminated with the virus.
- Airborne transmission has not been documented due to low levels of the virus in the lungs and other parts of the respiratory system in primates.

- **Incubation period:** 2-21 days (average 8-10 days).
- **Portal of entry:** Skin or mucosa.
- **Sites:** Endothelial cells (cells lining the inside of blood vessels), liver cells, immune cells such as macrophages, monocytes etc. and dendritic cells.
- **Precipitating factors (epidemiological determinants):**

a. **Agent factors:** Even after a person recovers from the acute phase of the disease, Ebola virus survives for months in certain organs such as the eyes and testes.

b. **Host factors:**

1. **Occupation:** Medical & paramedical workers, forest workers & veterinarian are at high risk.
2. **Handler of dead body or animal tissues:** Because dead bodies are still infectious, the handling of the bodies of Ebola victims (during cremation or embalming) can only be done while observing proper barrier/ separation procedures.

c. **Environmental factors:**

1. **Climate:** Ebola virus outbreaks tend to occur when temperatures are lower and humidity is higher than the usual for Africa.

- **Pathogenesis:** Following entry in body, virus enters in endothelial cells (cells lining the inside of blood vessels), liver cells, immune cells such as macrophages, monocytes etc., and dendritic cells. Immune cells carry the virus to nearby lymph nodes where further reproduction of the virus takes place. From there, the virus can enter the bloodstream and lymphatic system and spread throughout the body. Macrophages & lymphocytes undergo programmed cell death leading to an abnormally low concentration of lymphocytes in the blood. This contributes to the weakened immune response seen in those infected with Ebola virus. Breakdown of endothelial cells leads multiple bleeding points.
- **Clinical features:** Causing haemorrhagic fever.
  - Fever, severe headache, muscle pain, weakness, fatigue, diarrhoea, vomiting, abdominal (stomach) pain.
  - Unexplained haemorrhage (bleeding or bruising) outside or inside the body like oozing from the gums, blood in the stools.
- **Complications:** High case fatality rate about 90%.

✪ **Diagnosis**

- **Specimens:** Virus is diagnosed from blood & other body fluids of patients.
- **Testing methods:**

1. **Microscopy: → Follow morphology**

2. **Culture:** → Follow C/Cs
3. **Serological test:** ELISA (capture) to detect antigens & antibodies like IgM & IgG.
4. **Molecular methods:** RT-PCR is rapid & more sensitive method.

✪ **Prevention:**

- **General measures:**
- Avoid contact with infected person.
- Avoid sharing objects used by patients.
- Avoid funeral or burial rituals that require handling the body of someone who has died from Ebola.
- Avoid contact with bats and nonhuman primates or blood, fluids, and raw meat prepared from these animals.
- Wearing personal protective equipments like boots, gowns, gloves, masks and goggles in health set up.
- Sterilizing equipment and surfaces.
- Surveillance.
- Isolation of patients & avoid contact with relatives.
- **Immunoprophylaxis:** No specific vaccine is available.

✪ **Treatment:** No specific treatment is available. Supportive care like

- Rehydration with oral or intravenous fluids.
- Symptomatic treatment includes blood products, immune therapies and drug therapies.

Sudan ebola virus

- **Common name:** Sudan virus.
- **Abbreviation:** SUDV or SEBOV.
- **History:** It was discovered from the Sudan country in 1976 hence the name.
- **Distribution:** It is endemic in Sudan and / or Uganda
- **Morphology:**
- Same as other Ebola viruses as described earlier.
- Genome: It has a genome with three gene overlaps (VP35/VP40, GP/VP30, VP24/L). It has a genomic sequence different from Ebola virus by ≥30%.
- It also shows the genetic, biochemical and immunologic differences with Zaire ebola virus.
- **Culture:**
- Difficult to isolate compare to Zaire strain in cell culture.
- Less lethal for suckling mice: 10 particles of Zaire ebola virus can kill the animal while 10, 000 of Sudan ebola virus can't do the same.
- **Pathogenicity:**
- It causes disease similar to Zaire bola virus in human and non-human primates.
- First outbreak occurred in Southern Sudan in June 1976.
- The most recent outbreak occurred in June-August, 2012 in Uganda with 24 confirmed cases and 17 deaths.
- The case fatality rate is 55-65%.

Tai forest ebola virus

- **Common name:** Tai forest virus.
- **Synonym:** Formerly **called Côte d' Ivoire ebolavirus.**
- **Abbreviation:** CIEBOV or TAFV.
- **History:** It was discovered from the Tai National park in Côte d' Ivoire in 1995 from the dead chimpanzee, hence the name.
- **Distribution:** It is endemic in Côte d' Ivoire.
- **Morphology:**
- Same as other Ebola viruses as described earlier.
- It has a genome with three gene overlaps (VP35/VP40, GP/VP30, VP24/L).
- It has a genomic sequence different from Ebola virus by ≥30%.
- **Pathogenicity:** It causes disease similar to Zaire bola virus.

Bundibugyo ebola virus

- **Common name:** Bundibugyo virus.
- **Abbreviation:** BEBOV or BDBV.
- **History:** It was discovered from the cases of viral hemorrhagic fever outbreak began in the Bundibugyo & Kikyo townships of Bundibugyo District in western Uganda on August 1 of 2007, hence the name.
- **Distribution:** It is endemic in Uganda.
- **Morphology:**
- Same as other Ebola viruses as described earlier
- It has a genome with three gene overlaps (VP35/VP40, GP/VP30, VP24/L).
- It has a genomic sequence different from Ebola virus by ≥30%.
- **Pathogenicity:**
- It causes disease similar to Zaire bola virus.
- 1st outbreak occurred in 2007–2008 in Bundibugyo district, Uganda with 149 cases and 37 deaths. Case fatality was 25%.
- 2nd outbreak occurred in 2012 in Province Orientale, Democratic Republic of the Congo with 57 cases and 29 deaths. Case fatality was 51%.

ii. *Marburgvirus*

Marburg marburg virus

✪ **Meaning:** →Vide supra.

✪ **Morphology:** Same as other filoviruses.

✪ **Pathogenicity:**

- **Disease name:** Disease **called marburg virus disease.**

- **Nature or history of disease:**
- 1st outbreak occurred in 1967 in two cities, Marburg and Frankfurt of Germany & also in capital, Belgrade of Yugoslavia.
- Many outbreaks were reported between 1967-2012.
- Recent outbreak occurred in 2014 in Uganda with 1 case and 1 death.
- **Mode of transmission:**
- Person to person transmission.
- Sexual transmission.
- Laboratory acquires infection.
- **Clinical features:**
- Causing haemorrhagic fever.
- Case fatality: 35%.
- **Diagnosis:** Virus is diagnosed from tissue, blood, semen & anterior chamber of eye of patients by microscopical, culture, serological & molecular methods.

Diarrhoeal viruses

Synonym: Gastroenteritis viruses.

Taxonomical classification: Following viruses are causing diarrhoea.

I. DNA viruses:

A. Adenoviridae:
- Produce diarrhoea in children in summer seasons.
- Common serotypes responsible are: 40 & 41.

II. RNA viruses:

A. Reoviridae: *Rotavirus* (rota virus A to rota virus H).

B. Calciviridae: *Norovirus* (norwalk virus) *Sapovirus* (sapporo virus).

C. Astroviridae: *Astrovirus* (human astro virus).

D. Coronaviridae: SARS-CoV, MERS-CoV & *Torovirus* are known to produces the diarrhoea.

E. Orthomyxoviridae: Influenza A/H5NA & Influenza A/H1N1 are also known to produces the diarrhoea.

F. Picornaviridae: *Enterovirus* like polio virus, coxsackie virus & ECHO virus.

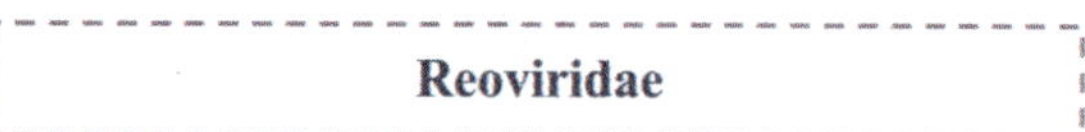

Reoviridae

Classification: →Flow chart-2

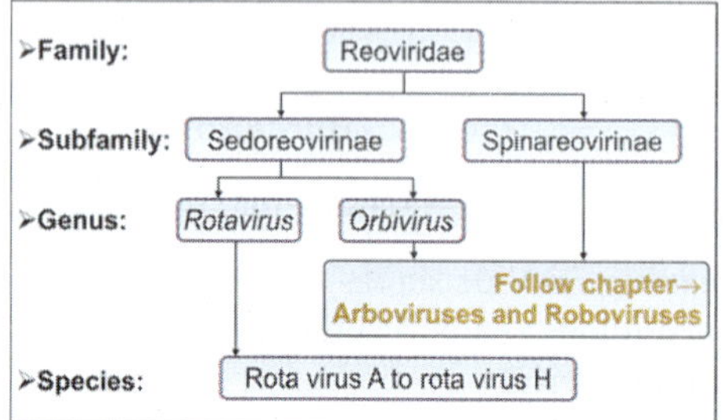

Flow chart-2: Classification of *Rotavirus*

Rotavirus

- **Meaning:** Word derived from **rota (Latin) = wheel**, because outer shell shows radiating spikes giving appearance like wheel.
- **History:** Virus was identified by Ruth Bishop & colleagues in 1973, in Melbourne, Australia from ultrathin section of biopsy under EM by using negative staining.
- **Geographical distribution & genotypes:**
- **Distribution:** Distributed worldwide.
- **Genotypes: → Vide infra**
- Total 8 species of *Rotavirus* (may be based on common group Ag present in inner shell) from rota virus A to rota virus H.
- Most common human species is A (about 90% of human infections are by species A) & other rare are B and C.
- A–E species cause disease in other animals.
- E and H in pigs.
- D, F and G in birds.
- **Morphology: → Fig.-4**
- **Shape:** Spherical.
- **Size:** 60-80 nm.
- **Genome:** ds-RNA (+/-) with 11 pieces in *Rotavirus* (10-12 pieces in other species of Reoviridae).
- **Capsid:** Icosahedral type of capsid with three layers in *Rotavirus* (2 layers in other species of Reoviridae).
- **Non-envelope:** Also called naked virus.

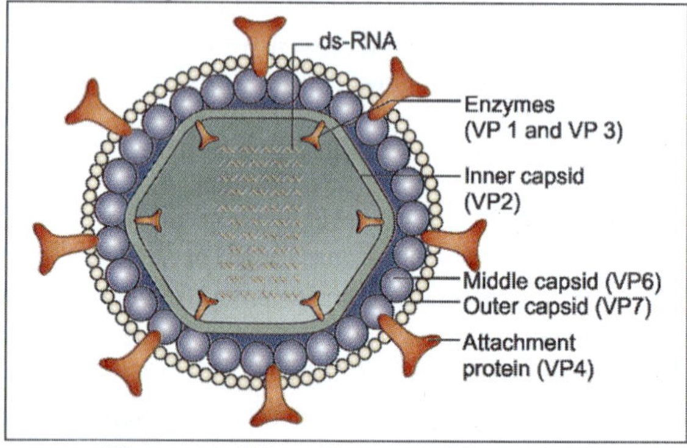

Figure-4: Morphology of *Rotavirus*

- **Immune Electron Microscopy (IEM):** It is expensive & required 10^6 particles/ml of stool for better result.
- **Viral proteins (VP):** Two types.
- Structural: VP1 (RNA polymerase), VP2 (inner capsid), VP3 (guanylyl transferase), VP4 (attachment protein), VP6 (middle capsid) & VP7 (outer capsid)
- Non-structural proteins: NSP1, NSP2, NSP3, NSP4, NSP5 & NSP6

✓ **Note: Three types of viral particles in *Rotavirus***

1. **Complete or double shelled virus:** 70nm & smooth surface & radiating spikes giving wheel like appearance.
2. **In-complete or single shelled virus:** 60nm, no outer shell & rough surface.
3. **Empty particle:** Without RNA core.

➢ **Culture characteristics (C/Cs):**

- Human rota viruses are not growing on cell culture media except rota virus A. Growth of rota virus A is facilitated by adding the trypsin & rolling the tissue culture.
- Calf & simian rota virus can grow very easily over cell culture & useful to prepare the antigens for serological studies.

➢ **Resistance:** Virus is naked & resistant to lipid solvents. Virus is stable in environment for long period.

➢ **Antigenic structure, serotypes & genotypes:**

- Within rota virus A there are different strains, **called serotypes**.
- As with influenza virus, a dual classification system is used which based on two proteins on the surface of the virus. The glycoprotein VP7 defines the G serotypes and the protease-sensitive protein VP4 defines P serotypes.
- G serotypes is further classified as G1, G2, G3 ... G19, while typing of P serotypes is challenging. However genotyping of P is possible & labelled as P[1], P[2] P[3] .... P[28].
- Most widely used system for expressing typing of rotavirus is G serotype & P genotype.
- Most common type present in India & in world is G1P[8], which account about 70% of total isolates.
- Because the two genes that determine G-types and P-types can be passed separately to progeny viruses different combinations (genetic reassortment) are found.

➢ **Immunity:**

- Children below six months are protected by maternal Ab.
- Initial attack (clinical or subclinical infections) in child age provides immunity, so less in older children & adults. However some strain produce diarrhoea in older children & adults **called Adult Diarrhoea Rota Virus (ADRV).**

➢ **Pathogenicity:**

✪ **Disease name:** Disease **called rota virus diarrhoea.**

✪ **Nature or history of disease:**

- Produces the epidemic mostly in winter season.
- Outbreak of rota virus B diarrhoea in older children & adults was reported from different part of China, so **called Adult Diarrhoea Rota Virus (ADRV).**
- Group A: Causes endemic diarrhoea in infants & young children.
- Group B: Causes outbreak of diarrhoea in adults & children.
- Group C: Causes sporadic & occasionally outbreak of diarrhoea in children.

✪ **Reservoir of infection:** Human.

✪ **Source of infection:** The faeces of an infected person can contain more than 10^{10} infectious particles per gram; fewer than 100 of these are required to transmit infection to another person. Large numbers of viral particles makes the diagnosis very easy.

✪ **Mode of transmission:**

- Faeco-oral route: By ingestion of contaminated food & water.
- Fomites borne.
- Contaminated hands or contact with infectious surface.
- Respiratory route is also possible.

✪ **Incubation period:** 2-3 days.

✪ **Portal of entry:** GIT. Entry also possible by respiratory tract.

✪ **Sites:** GIT.

✪ **Precipitating factors (epidemiological determinants):**

a. **Agent factors:**

- Virus is stable in environment for long period.
- Fewer than 100 particles are required in faeces to transmit infection to another person.
- It is estimated that about half the children hospitalised for diarrhoea treatment are from rotavirus origin.
- NSP4 (considered as enterotoxin) increase the vascular permeability & increase the secretion.

b. **Host factors:**

1. **Age:**

- Common in infant & young children between 6-24 months.
- Children below six months are protected by maternal Ab.
- Nearly every child in the world is infected with rotavirus at least once by the age of five.

2. **Poor hygiene & Low socio-economical status:** Precipitate the infection.
3. **IDDs:** Usually viruses are excreted for 2-12 days but in HIV or malnourished person it prolonged.

c. **Environmental factors:**

1. **Season:** *Rotavirus* & other viral diarrhoea are common in winter while of bacterial origin are common in summer.

2. **Climate:** In tropical countries *Rotavirus* occurs throughput the years but peak in cool seasons.

✪ **Pathogenesis:**
- After entry, virus damages the enterocytes (villous epithelium) in small intestine, resulting secretory diarrhoea.
- It damage the small intestinal mucosa & sparing the gastric & colonic mucosa.
- NSP4 (act as enterotoxin) increase the vascular permeability & increase the secretion.

✪ **Clinical features:**
- Acute watery diarrhoea, abdominal pain, vomiting with or without fever.
- Green colour or pale (yellow) stool without blood or mucus.
- Self limited & recovery occurs in 5-10 days.
- Low mortality.

➢ **Diagnosis:**

✪ **Specimens:** Stool, mucosal biopsy & serum.

✪ **Testing methods:**

i. **Microscopy: → Follow morphology**

ii. **Culture: → Follow C/Cs**

iii. **Serological tests:**
- **Ag detection:** From the stool by ELISA, latex particle agglutination & immunofluorescent microscopy.
- **Ab detection:** IgM & IgG are detected from serum by ELISA.

iv. **Molecular methods:** RT-PCR is rapid & more sensitive method.

➢ **Prevention:**

✪ **General measures:** Sanitation & health education.

✪ **Immunoprophylaxis:** By using vaccine.

- **Types of vaccine:** Vaccine is developed but not in wide use. Following two types of live attenuated vaccines are developed.

a. **Monovalent human rotavirus vaccine (Rotarix):**

o Preparation: It is live attenuated vaccine prepared by using the serotypes G1, G2, G3, G4 & G9.

o Dose:
- Two doses are given orally between 2-4 months.
- 1st dose at 6 weeks & 2nd dose at 10 weeks, not beyond 12 weeks.
- Interval between two doses should be at least 2 weeks.
- Two doses are completed by the age of 16 weeks, not after 24 weeks.

b. **Pentavalent bovine-human reassortment vaccine (Rota Teq):**

o Dose:
- Three doses are given orally, at 2,4 & 6 months.
- 1st dose at 6 -12 weeks & subsequent dose after 4-10weeks.
- Should not be initiated after 12 weeks & all three doses should be completed before 32 weeks.

- **Advantages:** Both vaccines are safe & effective.
- **Disadvantage:** Intussusception when given to infants >12 weeks.

➢ **Treatment:** Rehydration therapy to overcome the fluid & electrolyte loss. No specific antiviral treatment is available.

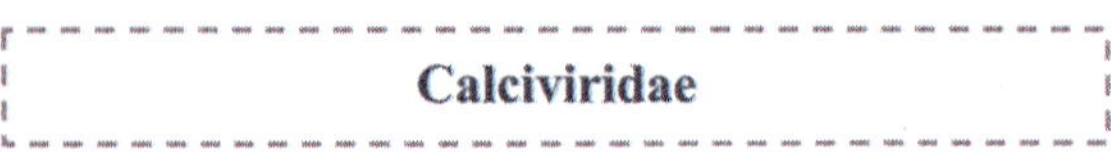

❖ **Classification: →Flow chart-3**

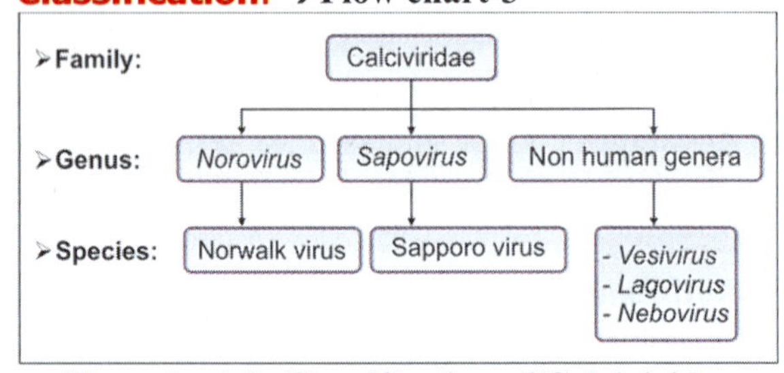

Flow chart-3: Classification of Calciviridae

❖ **Morphology:**

➢ **Shape:** Spherical.

➢ **Size:** 23-40 nm.

➢ **Genome:** ss-RNA (+) which is linear (non segmented).

➢ **Capsid:** Icosahedral type of capsid.

➢ **Non-envelope:** Also **called naked virus.**

Norwalk virus

✪ **Meaning & History:** Name given from Norwalk, Ohio, USA where epidemic of acute gastroenteritis was occurred in children & teachers at Bronson Elementary school.

✪ **Common name:** Winter vomiting virus.

✪ **Pathogenicity:**
- **Mode of transmission:** Faeco-oral route by consumption of raw oyster.
- **Clinical features:** Diarrhoea in adults & children.

✪ **Laboratory diagnosis:**
- **Specimens:** Faeces.
- **Testing methods:**

i. **Microscopy: → Follow morphology**

ii. **Culture:** Not cultivated.

iii. **Serological test:** Antibodies are diagnosed by ELISA & some other test.

Sapporo virus

- It causes sporadic & occasional outbreaks of diarrhoea in infants, children & adults.

Astroviridae

❖ **Meaning:** Astro meaning star shape.

❖ **Classification:**
➢ **Family:** Astroviridae.
➢ **Genus:** *Astrovirus*.
➢ **Species:** Human astro virus.

❖ **Morphology:**
➢ **Shape:** Star shape (**fig.-5**).
➢ **Size:** 28 nm.
➢ **Genome & capsid:** ss-RNA (+) type, icosahedral types of capsid.

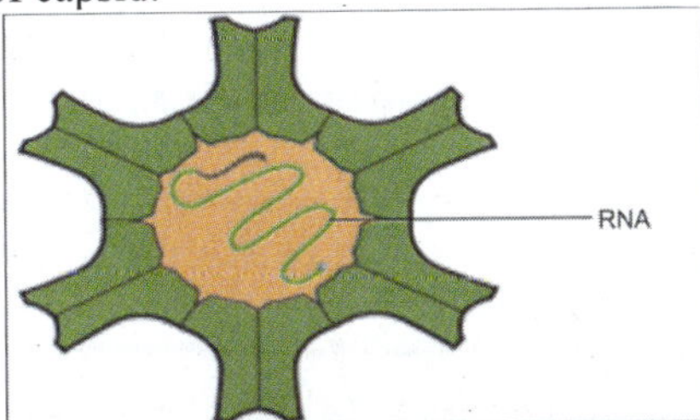

Figure-5: Morphology of *Astrovirus*

Human astro virus

✪ **Serotypes:** Seven serotypes of which type is most common to cause diarrhoea.
✪ **Pathogenicity:** It causes sporadic & occasional outbreaks of diarrhoea in infants, children & adults.

Slow disease viruses

❖ **History:**
- Concept of slow virus disease was given by Sigurdsson in 1954, a veterinary pathologist.
- He examined slow progressing infection in sheep like scrapie, visna & maedi.

❖ **Definition:** Slow virus diseases are defined with following criteria.
- Long incubation period from months to years.
- Long course of illness with remission & exacerbation.
- Fatal termination.
- Common in CNS.
- Genetic predisposition.
- Absence of immune response or immune response may contribute to disease. No interferon production.
- No inflammation.
- On cytopathogenic effect in vitro.

❖ **Types:** Following three types.

A. Group A (*Lentivirus*):
➢ **Viruses & diseases:**
i. **Visna virus or visna-maedi virus or maedi-visna virus or ovine lenti virus:** Visna & maedi.
ii. **Caprine arthritis encephalitis virus:** Arhtritis.
iii. **Equine infectious anaemia virus:** Anaemia.
➢ **More details:** Follow chapter → Retroviridae

B. Group B (Prion diseases):
➢ **Virus & disease:** Caused by subviral agent **called prion** & disease **called prion disease** with following types.

i. **Prion disease in animals:**
1. Mink encephalopathy.
2. Scrapie.
3. Bovine spongiform encephalopathy (BSE, Mad cow disease).

ii. **Prion disease in human:**
1. CJD (Creutzfeldt-Jacob Disease).
2. Kuru.
3. GSSS (Gerstmann Straussler Scheinker Syndrome).
4. Fatal familial insomnia.

➢ **More details:** Follow chapter → General properties of viruses.

C. Group C:
➢ **Viruses & diseases:**
i. **Measles virus:**
- **SSPE.**
- **More details:** Follow chapter → Paramyxoviridae.

ii. **JC virus:**
- **PML.**
- **More details:** Follow chapter → Other DNA viruses.

Encephalitis viruses

❖ **Systemic / taxonomical classification:**

A. DNA viruses:
i. **Poxviridae:** Pox viruses causing humna lesion like variola virus.
ii. **Herpesviridae:**
- Like HSV-1, HSV-2, VZV, EBV & CMV.
- These viruses causes sporadic encephalitis.
- CMV causes meningo-encephalitis in patient with organ transplantation.

B. RNA viruses:
i. **Picronaviridae:** These viruses cause sporadic encephalitis.
1. **Polio virus:** 1 – 3.
2. **Coxsackie virus:**
- Coxsackie virus A: 9.
- Coxsackie virus B: 3, 4, 5 & 6.
3. **ECHO virus:** 6, 9, 17 & 19.
4. **Other entero viruses (EV):** EV-71.

ii. **Orthomyxoviridae**: *Influenzavirus*.
iii. **Paramyxoviridae:**
1. ***Rubulavirus*:** Mumps virus (sporadic encephalitis).

2. ***Morbillivirus***: Measles virus.
3. ***Henipavirus:*** Nipah virus (epidemic encephalitis).

iv. **Togaviridae *(Alphavirus):*** Causes epidemic of encephalitis. Mosquito borne viruses like
1. Eastern Equine Encephalitis (EEE) virus.
2. Western Equine Encephalitis (WEE) virus.
3. Venezuelan Equine Encephalitis (VEE) virus.

v. **Flaviridae *(Flavivirus):*** Causes epidemic of encephalitis. Two groups like mosquito borne & tick borne as follows.

➢ **Mosquito borne species**
1. Japanese encephalitis (JE) virus.
2. St. Louis encephalitis virus.
3. Ilheus virus.
4. West Nile virus.
5. Murray Valley encephalitis virus.

➢ **Tick borne species**
1. Russian Spring Summer Encephalitis (RSSE) virus.
2. Central European encephalitis virus.
3. Western Siberian encephalitis virus.
4. Powassan encephalitis virus.
5. Louping ill virus.

vi. **Bunyaviridae *(Bunyavirus):*** California encephalitis virus Causes epidemic of encephalitis.

vii. **Rhabdoviridae:** Rabies virus causes sporadic encephalitis.

viii. **Retroviridae:** HIV.

❖ **Pathogenicity, laboratory diagnosis, prevention & treatment:** Follow → Respective chapters.

Glomerulonephritis viruses

❖ **Classification:**

I. Systemic / taxonomical classification

A. DNA viruses:

i. **Herpesviridae:** Like EBV & CMV.
ii. **Hepadnaviridae:** HBV.
iii. **Papovaviridae:** BK virus.
iv. **Parvoviridae:** Parvo virus.

B. RNA viruses:

i. **Paramyxoviridae:** Measles virus & mumps virus.
ii. **Picornaaviridae:** Coxsackie virus.
iii. **Flaviridae:**

➢ ***Hepacivirus***: HCV.

➢ ***Flavirus***: Dengue virus.

iv. **Bunyaviridae:**

➢ ***Hantavirus***: Hantaan virus & puumala virus.

v. **Retroviridae:** HIV.

II. Clinical classification:

A. **Focal segmetal glomerulosclerosi:** HIV, HBV, parvo virus & coxsackie virus.

B. **Membrane proloferative glomerulonephritis:** HIV, HBV, HCV, CMV & EBV.

C. **Diffuse proloferative glomerulonephritis:** Coxsackie virus.

D. **Membranous nephropathy:** HBV & HCV.

E. **Endocapillary proloferative glomerulonephritis:** Measles virus & dengue virus.

F. **Mesangio proloferative glomerulonephritis:** Mumps virus & parvo virus.

G. **Haemorrhagic fever renal syndrome:** Hantaan virus & puumala virus.

H. **Renal dysfunction, ureteral stenosis and interstitial nephritis:** BK virus.

❖ **Pathogenicity, laboratory diagnosis, prevention & treatment:** Follow → Respective chapters.

Oncogenic viruses

More details: Follow chapter → Oncogenic microbes

Question bank

Essay/Full question

1) Haemorrhagic fever viruses.
2) Diarrhoeal viruses.
3) Encephalitis viruses.
4) Slow disease viruses.
5) Glomerulonephritis viruses.

Short notes

1) Arenaviruses.
2) Zaire ebolavirus.
3) *Rotavirus.*

Short questions for theory/viva questions

1) Name four viruses of Filoviridae family causing human infection.
2) Name four viruses causing diarrhoea.

MCQs for chapter review

Haemorrhagic fever viruses

1) **Haemorrhagic fever is caused by** (PGI, June-03)
(a) West Nile fever (b) Sand fly fever (c) Ebola virus (d) All of above

2) **Ebola virus is a** (PGI, June-03)
(a) Reo virus (b) Filo virus (c) Herpes virus (d) *Rotavirus*

Diarrhoeal viruses

3) **The viruses causing gastroenteritis are** (PGI, Dec-08)
(a) *Rotavirus* (b) Nor walk virus (c) Adeno virus (d) Hepadna virus (e) *Enterovirus*

4) **Which virus does not cause diarrhoea**
(a) *Rotavirus* (b) *Reovirus* (c) Adeno virus (d) Pox virus

5) **Diarrhoea is not a feature of**
(a) *Rotavirus* (b) *Calcivirus* (c) *Enterovirus* (d) Rhabdo virus

6) **All are cultivable virus except** (AIIMS, Dec-97)
(a) *Rotavirus* (b) *Enterovirus* (c) ECHO virus (d) Coxsackie virus
7) **Viral enterotoxin is detected as possible mechanism of pathogenesis in** (AI-98, PGI-02)
(a) Adenovirus (b) *Rotavirus* (c) *Calcivirus* (d) *Astrovirus*
8) ***Rotavirus* causes**
(a) Acute non-bacterial gastroenteritis in adult (b) Infantile diarrhoea (c) Teratogenic effects (d) Respiratory infection in immunocompromised
9) **All are true about *Rotavirus* except** (AIIMS-97)
(a) Causes diarrhoea in man and children (b) Rota B can be grown in culture (c) Rota C can cause diarrhoea in children (d) Culture cannot be done
10) **Which of the following is true about *Rotavirus*** (AI-94)
(a) Commonly affects children (b) Double stranded DNA (c) Can be grown easily on cell culture (d) Egg shell appear under electron microscope
11) **The following is true of *Rotavirus***
(a) Easily grow in cell culture (b) Double stranded DNA (c) Terminal ileum will destroyed (d) Adult and old people account for 60% infection
12) ***Rotavirus* is diagnosed by** (AIIMS, Dec-99)
(a) IgM specific antibody in stool (b) ELISA demonstrate antibody in stool (c) Immunofluorescence antigen in stool (d) Culture of *Rotavirus*
13) ***Rotavirus* infection is diagnosed by the presence of** (AI -00)
(a) Antigen in stool by ELISA (b) Virus in stool (c) Antigen in blood (d) Antibody in stool
14) **Best vaccine for *Rotavirus* infection is** (AI-98)
(a) Asymptomatic neonatal vaccine (b) DNA vaccine (c) Genetic reassortment (d) Capsular component vaccine
15) **Genetic reassortment is seen with** (AIIMS, Nov-10)
(a) *Astrovirus* (b) Herpes virus (c) *Rotavirus* (d) *Hepadnavirus*
16) **Vaccination causing intussusception** (PGI, Nov-13, Dec-07)
(a) *Rotavirus* (b) Parvo virus (c) Inactivated polio (d) BCG (e) Measles

Slow disease viruses

17) **Which of the following is not considered to be a slow virus disease**
(a) Kuru (b) Scrapie (c) Creutzfeldt-Jacob disease (d) Maedi (e) Sarcoidosis
18) **All of the following human diseases are caused by prion except**
(a) SSPE (b) Visna (c) CJD (d) Kuru
19) **Creutzfeldt-Jacob Disease is caused by** (PGI -96)
(a) Prion (b) JC virus (c) Genetic factors (d) Nutritional deficiency

Encephalitis viruses

20) **Encephalitis is caused by** (AIIMS-98)
(a) HSV-1 (b) EBV (c) Infectious mononucleosis (d) CMV
21) **Most common cause of sporadic viral encephalitis is** (AIIMS-04)
(a) Japanese encephalitis (b) Herpes simplex encephalitis (c) HIV encephalitis (d) Rubeola encephalitis
22) **Not a cause of epidemic encephalitis** (PGI, May-14)
(a) Herpes simplex virus (b) Rabies (c) West Nile virus (d) Nipah virus (e) Japanese encephalitis virus

Glomerulonephritis viruses

23) **Renal involvement is seen in which of the following infections?** (PGI-03)
(a) Cytomegalovirus (b) Polyoma virus (c) Human pailloma virus (d) HIV (e) HBV

Answers of MCQs & explanation

1) **(c)**
- Follow section, **haemorrhagic fever viruses (classification)** for explanation.

2) **(c)**
- Follow section, **haemorrhagic fever viruses (classification) & Filoviridae** for explanation

3) **(c)**
4) **(d)**
5) **(d)**
}- Follow section, **diarrhoeal viruses (classification)** for explanation

6) **(a)**
7) **(b)**
8) **(b)**
9) **(b)**
10) **(a)**
11) **(c)**
12) **(c)**
13) **(a) & (b)**
14) **(c)**
15) **(c)**
16) **(a)**
}- Follow section, **diarrhoeal viruses (*Rotavirus*)** for explanation

17) **(e)**
18) **(a) &(b)**
19) **(a)**
}- Follow section, **slow disease viruses** for explanation

20) **(a), (b), (c) & (d)**
21) **(b)**
22) **(a) & (b)**
}- Follow section, **encephalitis viruses (classification)**for more explanation

23) **(a), (d) & (e)**
- Follow section, **glomerulonephritis viruses (classification)** for explanation

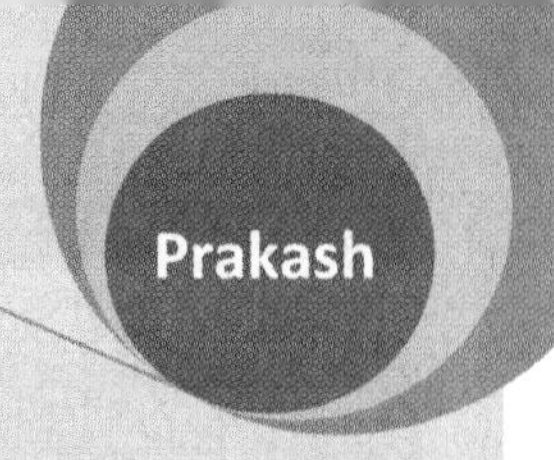

Section V
Mycology

Preview of Mycology

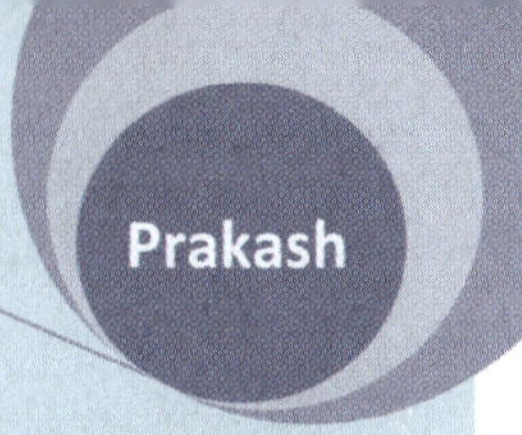

Definition:

Classification:

All fungal infections within each group are written with following headings & subheadings

- **Meaning / synonym:**
- **Definition:**
- **Etiological agent:**
- **Pathogenicity:**
- **Reservoir of infection:**
- **Source of infection:**
- **Mode of transmission:**
- **Incubation period:**
- **Portal of entry:**
- **Sites:**
- **Precipitating factors (epidemiological determinants):**
- **Pathogenesis:**
- **Clinical features:**
- **Complications:**
- **Laboratory diagnosis: (with appropriate figures)**
- **Specimens:**
- **Testing:**

A. Microscopy:

i. Wet mount preparation:

a. Direct 10% KOH :

i. Differential stains:

a. Microbiological stains:

b. Histopathological stains:

B. Culture:

- **Routine media:**
- **Cultivation technique:**
- **C/Cs:**
- **LCB/PHOL stain:**
- **Selective media:**
- **Spores producing media:** For some fungus

C. Biochemical reactions (B/Rs): For some fungus

i. Sugar fermentation & assimilation test:

ii. Urease test:

D. Serological tests:

E. Molecular method:

F. Skin test:

G. Animal inoculation:

H. Gag Liquid Chromatography:

I. Special tests:

- **Prevention:**
- **Treatment:**

75 General properties of fungus

Learning heading & subheadings

Introduction

❖ **Meaning:** **Fungus** (**Latin**) & **Mykes** (**Greek**) both have same meaning as **mushroom (types of edible fungi),** because it has mushroom like appearance.

❖ **Definition:**

- Microorganism with mushroom like appearance **called fungus** (plural; **fungi**).
- Branch of medical science related with study of fungus and disease produce by it is **called Mycology**.

❖ **History:** **Raynold Jacques Sabouraud** (1964-1936) is **called the father of Mycology**.

❖ **Properties:**

➢ **Taxonomy:** Eukaryotes **(Eu = true + karyotes = nucleus),** because contains mature nucleus. Actually fungi are branching filamentous in nature & **prefix Myco** is used for some bacteria like *Mycobacteria* & *Mycoplasma* because they have branching-filamentous form as like fungi.

➢ **Morphology:**

✪ **Capsule:**

- *Cryptococcus neoformans* is the only capsulated fungus.
- Capsule aid in virulence & also help in diagnosis of fungus.

✪ **Cell wall:** Present & contains polysaccharides like chitin, glucans, mannans, chitosan, cellulose etc. mixed with polypeptide.

✪ **Plasmalemma (cytoplasmic membrane):** Present inner to cell wall & contains glycoproteins, lipid & ergosterol.

✪ **Cytosol (cytoplasm):**

- Fungus is eukaryotic microbes & contains nucleus, nuclear membrane, mitochondria, golgi apparatus, endoplasmic reticulum, ribosomes etc.
- It contains both DNA & RNA.

✪ **Reproduction:** By

- **Asexual methods:** Hyphal extension, budding or fission.
- **Sexual methods:**
  - Meiosis.
  - Mitosis.
  - Unknown: In many fungi sexual methods of reproductions are unknown. Such fungi **called fungi imperfecti.**

✪ **Chlorophyll:** It is absent, so not able to do photosynthesis & remain dependent on host cell for nutrition.

✪ **Differences between bacteria & fungi: Table-1.**

Features	Bacteria	Fungi
Taxonomy	Prokaryotes	Eukaryotes
Cell	Unicellular	Uni / multicellular
Cell wall / envelope	Thick & contains peptidoglycan and LPS	It contains chitin, manna & other polysaccharides
Sterol in plasma membrane	Absent (Except in *Mycoplasma* & *Ureaplasma*)	Present (like cholesterol, ergosterol etc.)

Table-1: Differences between bacteria & fungi

❖ **Useful properties of fungi:**

A. Food industries:

1. **Mushroom of basidiomycetes:** Used to prepare the food.
2. To alter the **texture, flavour, digestibility & palatability** of natural & processed food.
3. ***Candida fukuyamaensis***: To prepare the Russian manchurian tea, used as medicine in many disease.
4. ***Endomyces***: To prepare the fat.
5. ***Torulopsis***: To prepare the protein.
6. ***Saccharomyces***: To prepare the alcohol.

B. Drugs preparation:

1. ***Penicillium notatum***: Penicillin was discovered from this fungus by Alexander Fleming in 1928.

2. ***Penicillium chrysogyneum***: Also useful to prepare the penicillin.
3. ***Penicillium griseofulvum***: For gresiofulvin.
4. ***Acremonium (Cephalosporium) chrysogyneum:*** To prepare cephalosporin.
5. ***Aspergillus tereus***: To prepare simvastatin (cholesterol lowering agent).
6. ***Claviceps purpura***: To prepare ergot alkaloids like ergometrine or ergotamine.
7. ***Tolypocladium inflatum:*** Cyclosporine an Immunosuppressive drug derived from these fungi.

C. **Vaccine preparation:** Certain fungi like *Saccharomyces cerevisiae*, *Hansenula polymorpha* & *Pichia* spp. are used for as a cloning vector to prepare recombinant vaccine of HBV.

D. **Research model:** *Neurospora crasa* acts as an ideal model to study host-pathogen relationship.

E. **Vector control:**
1. ***Culicinomyces clavosporus***: Used in malaria eradication.
2. ***Coelomomyces***: It is able to kill the larva of mosquitoes.

F. **Agriculture:**
1. ***Beavaria bassiana***: Used to control the banana root borer, sugar cane borer, Sweet potato weevil & rice water weevil.
2. ***Vertcilium lecani***: Used to control the Sweet potato white fly, most damaging pest in Cuba.
3. ***Trichoderma***: Used to control the soil-borne disease that attacks the tobacco, tomatoes & peppers.

❖ Harmful properties of fungi:

A. **Diseases in human:**

i. **Mycosis (mycoses):**
- Disease produced by fungus invasion in body **called mycosis** (Plural; **mycoses**).
- All the diseases are described in respective chapters.

ii. **Allergic reactions:**
- **Types:** Two types like "id' reaction & systemic disease.
- **More details:** Follow chapter → Miscellaneous topics in Mycology

B. **Fungal food poisoning:**
- **Types:** Two types like mycetism (mycetismus, muscarinism) & mycotoxicoses.
- **More details:** Follow chapter → Miscellaneous topics in Mycology

C. **Spoiling of stored food:**
- It spoils the stores grains, fruits, vegetables & foodstuff.
- It present as **bread molds** in stored food.
- About 10% of world's foods are spoiled by fungal contamination.

D. **Decaying of materials:** Fungi causing decaying of leather, timber, fabrics, electric devices etc.

E. **Fungal growth on plasticize products:**
- It grows on plastic items like computer disks, videotapes, audiotapes etc.
- Commonly encountered fungi are *Alternaria, Aspergillus, Epicossum, Paecilomyces, Penicillium & Trichoderma.*

F. **Biological warfare:**
1. **Yellow rain:**
- Yellow rain was the subject of a 1981 political incident in which the US Secretary of State Alexander Haig accused the Soviet Union of supplying T-2 mycotoxin to the Communist states in Vietnam, Laos and Cambodia for use in counterinsurgency warfare. Refugees described many different forms of attacks, including a sticky yellow liquid falling from planes or helicopters, which was **called yellow rain**. Those exposed claimed neurological & physical symptoms including seizures, blindness and bleeding with over ten thousand deaths.
- Sample analysis from the victims reported the presence of *Trichothecene* mycotoxins, including T-2 toxin, diacetoxyscirpenol (DAS) & deoxynivalenol (DON), however presence of mycotoxin in yellow rain was challenged by later studies.

2. ***Coccidioides immitis***: It transmitted by inhalation & dangerous to work with it in laboratory enables it use in war.

Classification

I. **Morphological classification:** Four types.

A. **Yeast: →Fig.-1(a)**
- Unicellular & spherical. Cells are without budding **called yeast cells** or in budding forms **called budding yeast cells**.
- Developed by asexual (budding) method.
- No hyphae or filamentous form.
- **Colony:** Creamy or pasty.
- **Examples:** *Cryptococcus neoformans, Saccharomyces cerevesiae, Rhodotorulla* (?) etc.

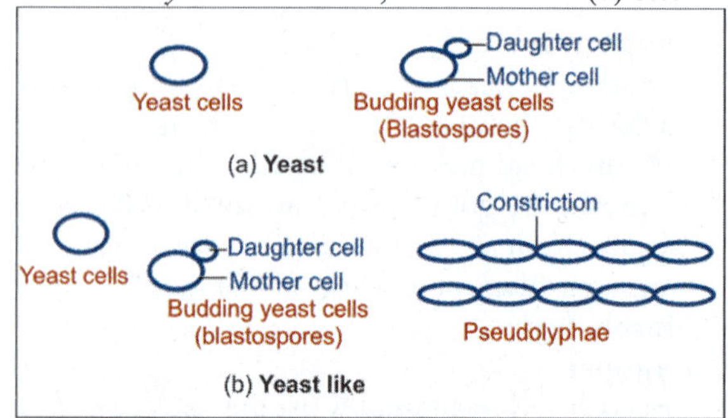

Figure-1: Yeast, budding yeast cell & pseudohyphae

B. **Yeast like: →Fig.-1(b)**

- Unicellular & spherical or oval. Cells are without budding **called yeast cells** or in budding forms **called budding yeast cells**. During budding process in budding yeast cells, daughter cell incompletely gets separated from mother cell & produces a chain of elongated budding yeast cells **called pseudohyphae**.
- Developed by asexual (budding or binary fission) methods.
- **Colony:** Creamy or pasty.
- **Example:** *Candida* spp.

C. Mold / filamentous:

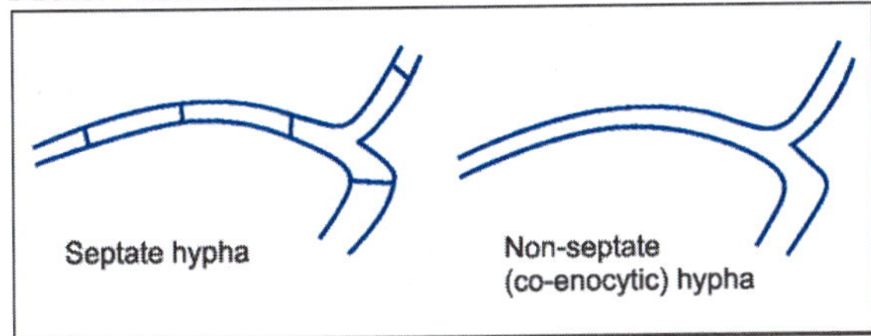

Figure-2: Types of hyphae

- Multicellular.
- Developed by asexual (budding / binary fission) or by sexual methods.
- Filamentous hyphae **(fig.-2)** which may be septate or non-septate (co-enocytic).
- **Colony:** Cottony, woolly, velvety, granular & pigmented.
- **Examples:**
  - Dermatophytes.
  - *Geotrichum candidum.*
  - *Coccidioides immitis.*
  - *Aspergillus* spp.
  - Zygomycetes like *Mucor, Rhizopus* etc.

D. Dimorphic fungi:

- Grow at two different temperatures hence **called dimorphic fungi.**
- **37^0C:** Yeast or parasitic phase.
- **22^0C:** Mold or mycelial phase.
- **Examples:** Following six genera authentically designated as dimorphic fungi.
  - All systemic fungi like *Histoplasma capsulatum, Coccidioides immitis, Blastomyces dermatitidis* & *Paracoccidioides brasiliensis.*
  - *Sporothrix schenckii.*
  - *Penicillium marneffei* (other species are not dimorphic & can grow at 25^0C as mold).

II. Systemic (taxonomical) classification: It includes naming & typing of fungus.

➢ **Five kingdom system of classification:**

- All organisms can be placed in five kingdoms like monera, protista, fungi, plantae & animalia by R. H. Whittaker in 1969, **called five kingdom system of classification.**
- Fungi were initially classified with the plants, but in 1969 it is classified in a separate kingdom as **"fungi"** under the superkingdom **"eukaryotes".**
- General scheme of classification includes Superkingdom → Kingdom → Phylum (Division was used initially now replaced by phylum) →Class → Order → Family (Tribe) → Genus → Species (Specific Epithet) →Subspecies (subsp.) / Variety (var.) / Forma (f.) / Forma specials (f. sp.) as mentioned in **table-2.**
- The name of phylum, class, order & family ends by adding suffix **"mycota", "mycetes", "ales"** & **"aceae"** respectively as shown in **table-2.**

Superkingdom →Eukaryotes			
Kingdom → Fungi			
Taxon	**Suffix**	**Teleomorph (sexual)**	**Anamorph (asexual)**
Plylum	***mycota***	Ascomycota	Deuteromycetes
Class	***mycetes***	Ascomycetes	Hyphomycetes
Order	***ales***	Onygenales	Moniliales
Family	***aceae***	Onygenaceae	Moniliaceae
Genus	-	*Ajellomyces*	*Histoplasma*
Species	-	*capsulatus*	*capsulatus*
Variety	-	*capsulatus*	*capsulatus*

Table-2: General scheme of classification of fungi

➢ **Binomial nomenclature:**

- Binomial nomenclature (scientific name) system was proposed by Swedish botanist in 1758 which include genus name at 1st followed by species/epithet name in Italic pattern.
- In case of male scientist species name ends with suffix **"ii"** and In case of female scientist species name ends with suffix **"eae".**
- Both singular & plural are written same but in abbreviation sp. & spp. are used for singular & plural respectively.
- Genus name: Latin noun & start with capital letter with Italic pattern.
- Species / epithet name: Start with small letter with Italic pattern irrespective of person or place name. It based on different properties of unit like *albicans* from white colony, *brisiliensis* from place of origin, *marneffei* from scientists etc.
- Example: *Histoplasma capsulatum.*

➢ **Trinomial nomenclature:**

- The word in the name (second epithet) might by subspecies (subsp.) / variety (var.) / forma (f.) / forma specials (f. sp.) and also italicized or underlined.
- Example: *Histoplasma capsulatum* var. *capsulatum, Histoplasma capsulatum* var. *duboisii* & *Histoplasma capsulatum* var. *farciminosum.*

➢ **Classification:** It based on spore formation methods as mentioned below. This classification also used other supportive features like fatty acids analysis, zymogram pattern, DNA hybridisation, RFLP etc.

A. Asexual spores: Developed by budding, binary fission or by apical elongation.

i. **Blastospores: →Fig.-1**
- Developed by budding method.
- Budding part of yeast cells **called blastospores.**
- Example: *Cryptococcus neoformans.*

ii. **Chlamydospores:**
- Developed by apical elongation method.
- Pre-existing hyphal cells becomes thick, double wall & circular **called chlamydospores.**
- **Examples:** *Candida* spp., *Paracoccidioides brasiliensis.*
- **Chlamydospores producing media:** Rice starch agar & cornmeal agar incubate at 20^0C.

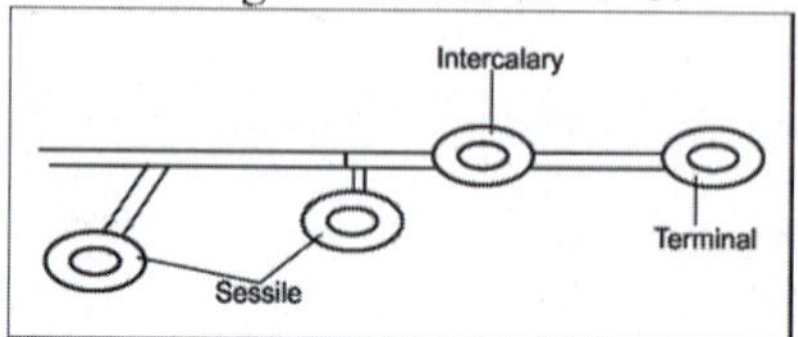

Figure-3: Subtypes of Chlamydospores

- **Subtypes:** Three subtypes as shown in **fig.-3.**
1. Terminal
2. Sessile
3. Intercalary

iii. **Arthrospores: →Fig.-4**
- Developed by apical elongation method.
- Pre-existing hyphal cells becomes thick, double wall & cuboidal or rectangular or barrel shaped **called arthrospores.**

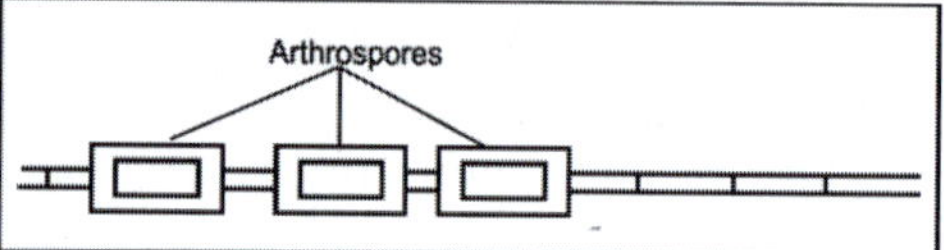

Figure-4: Arthrospores

- Detached after fracture of supporting cell.
- **Examples:**
- Dermatophytes.
- *Geotrichum candidum.*
- *Coccidioides immitis.*
- *Hortae werneckii.*
- *Trichosporon beigelii.*

iv. **Sporangiospores: →Fig.-5**

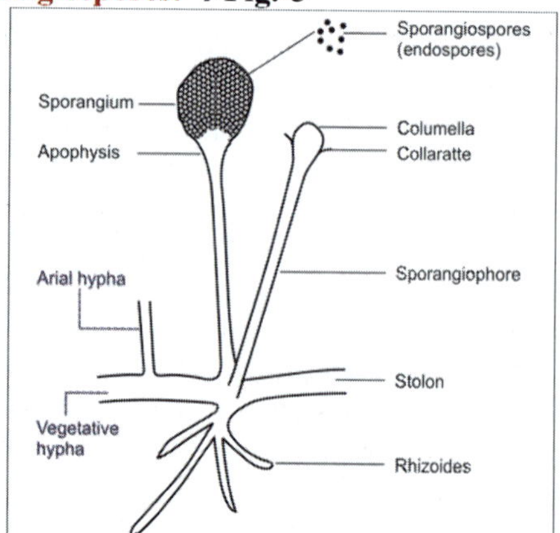

Figure-5: Sporangiospores

- Developed by mitosis.
- Endogenous spores formation.
- Spores are enclosed in a sac like structure **called sporangium** & spores **called sporangiospores.**
- **Example:** Zygomycetes.

v. **Conidiospores (conidia): →Fig.-6**
- Developed by mitosis.
- Exogenous spores formation.
- Spores are arranged in a chain like structure & arise from a wase like structure **called phialides (conodia producing cell).**
- **Example:** *Aspergillus* spp.
- **Subtypes of conidia:**

a. **Microconidia:** Further divided as
1. **Basipetal:**
- Youngest conidium at base.
- **Examples:** *Penicillium, Aspergillus, Scopulariopsis brevicaulis.*
2. **Acropetal:**
- Youngest conidium at top.
- **Examples:** *Alternaria & Cladosporium.*

b. **Macroconidia:**
1. **Dictyoconidia:**
- Macroconidia with transverse & longitudinal septa.
- **Examples:** *Alternaria & Bipolaris.*
2. **Phragmoconidia:**
- Macroconidia with only transverse septa.
- **Example:** *Curvularia.*

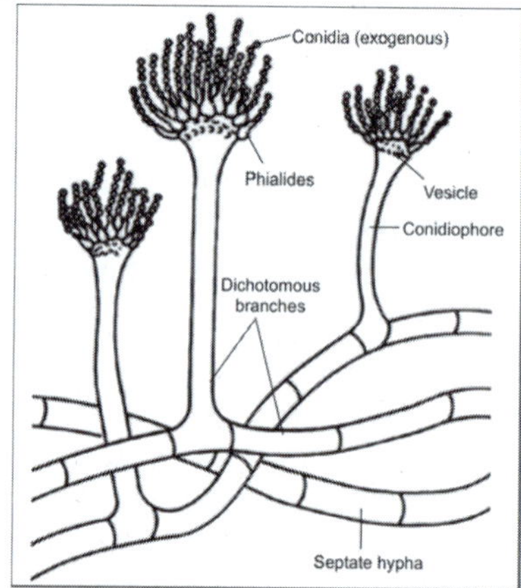

Figure-6: Conidiospores

vi. **Aleurospores: →Fig.-7**
- Macroconidia arranged the side of hyphae by a supporting cell **called aleurospores.**
- Released after detachment from cell.
- **Examples:** *Epidermophyton & Microsporum canis.*

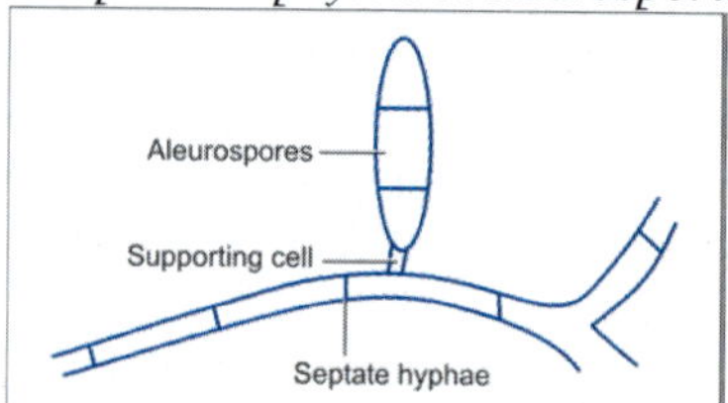

Figure-7: Aleurospores

Spores	Phylum	Class	Order	Family	Genus	Species
Kingdom: Fungi						
Non-Septate (aseptate / co-enocytic) hyphae						
Zygospores	Zygo-mycota	Zygomycetes (Phycomycetes)	Mucorales	Mucoraceae	*Mucor*	*M. racemosus*
					Rhizomucor	*R. pusillus*
					Rhizopus	*R. arrhizus*
						R. microspores
					Absidia	*A. corymbifera*
					Apophysomyces	*A. elegans*
				Cunninghamellaceae	*Cunninghamella*	*C. bertholletiae*
				Saksenaeaceae	*Saksenaea*	*S. vasiformis*
				Thamnidaceae	*Cokeromyces*	*C. recurvatus*
				Syncephalastraceae	*Syncephalastrum*	*S. recemosum*
			Entomophorales	Ancylistaceae	*Conidiobolus*	*C. coronatus*
				Basidiobolaceae	*Basidiobolus*	*B. ranarum*
Septate hyphae						
Ascospores	Asco-mycota	Ascomycetes	Pneumocystidales	Pneumocystidaceae	*Pneumocystis**	*P. jirovecii*
		Pyrenomycetes (Unitunicate)	Microascales	Microascaceae	*Pseudoallescheria*	*P.boydii*
					Scopulariopsis	*S. brevicaulis*
			Ophistomatales	Ophistomataceae	*Sporothrix*	*S shenckii*
			Sordariales	Sordariaceae	*Neurospora*	*N crasa*
			Hypocreales	Nectriaceae	*Fusarium*	*F graminiarum*
				Hypocreaceae	*Acremonium*	*A falciforme*
		Pyrenomycetes (Bitunicate)	Dothideales	Dothideaceae	*Hortaea*	*H werneckii*
				Piedraiaceae	*Piedraia*	*P hortae*
		Plectomycetes	Eurotiales	Trichocomaceae	*Aspergillus*	*A flavus, A niger*
					Penicillium	*P marneffei*
			Onygenales	Onygenaceae	*Chrysosporium*	*C parvum*
					Ajellomyces	*A capsulatus*
Basidio-spores	Basidio-mycota	Basidiomycetes	Tremellales	Cryptococcaceae	*Trichosporon*	*T beigelii*
		Pucciniomycetes	Sporidiales	Sporidiobolaceae	*Rhodotorula*	*R glutinis*

Table-3: Sexual spores with taxonomical types of fungi

Spores	Phylum	Class	Order	Family	Genus	Species
Non-Septate (aseptate / co-enocytic) hyphae & sexual spores						
Oospores	Oomycota	Oomycetes	Pythiales	Pythiaceae	*Pythium*	*P insidiosum*
No hyphal structure, Asexual spores						
Spores	-	Mesomycetozoea	Dermocytida	-	*Rhinosporidium*	*R. seeberi*
Sporangio-spores	Chloro-phyta	Trebouxiophyceae	Chlorellales	Chlorellaceae	*Prototheca*	*P. wickerhamii* *P. zopfii*

Table-4: Parafungal agents

✓ **Notes:**

- **Pneumocystis* has no hyphae but taxonomically classified as fungus as Ascomycetes, however still is controversial to classify it as fungus & better to classify as atypical fungus under the new phylum **called Protomycota.**
- Tables do not include all fungi but only fungus important at undergraduate level.

> **Mnemonic:**
> - **Asexual spores:** ABC – CAS → Above explanation
> - **Sexual spores:** ZABO → **Table- 3**

B. Sexual spores: Developed by miosis & mitosis, present as dimorphic fungi. Sexual spores with taxonomical types are shown in **table -3 & fig.-8.**

C. Un-known method (sexual spores): Exact method of sexual reproduction is unknown and such fungi are **called Miosporic fungi** or **Mitosporic fungi** or **Deuteromycetes** or **Deuteromycota** or **Hyphomyctets** or **Fungi imperfecti.**

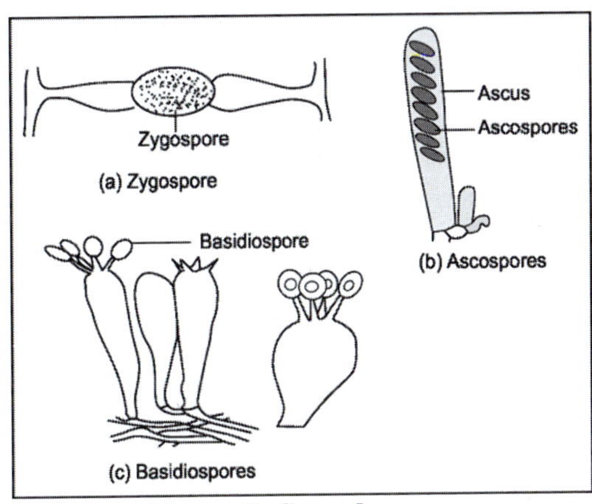

Figure-8: Sexual spores

➢ **Parafungal agents:**
- Few pathogens like *Pythium insidiosum, Rhinosporidium seeberi* & *Prototheca* are producing disease similar to mycosis **called parafungal agent.**
- Sexual spores: Produced by *Pythium insidiosum.*
- Asexual spores: Produced by *Rhinosporidium seeberi* & *Prototheca.* In *Prototheca spores* are produced by internal septation & cleavage.
- They are studied in mycology but not classified in the kingdom fungi. Their classification is given **table-4.**

III. Clinical classification:

➢ **Nomenclature:**
- Fungal disease **called mycosis (singular) / mycoses (plural).**
- Name of fungal disease are given by adding the suffix **"sis"** or **"mycosis"** to genus name, however it is not satisfactory because same fungus causing many diseases & same disease is caused by many fungi.
- Some names of the fungal diseases are given by adding the suffix **"i"** to genus & species name, like Histoplasmosis capsulati/duboisii/farciminosi.

➢ **Types:** Two types.

A. Superficial mycoses: Follow chapter → Superficial mycoses

B. Deep mycoses: Follow chapter → Deep mycoses

IV. Ecological classification: **→Flow chart-1**

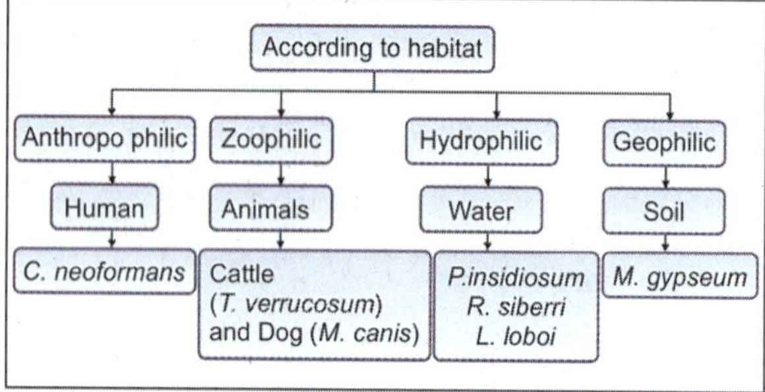

Flow chart-1: Ecological types of fungus

Hyphae, Pseudohyphae & Mycelium

❖ Hypha (Plural; Hyphae):

➢ **Meaning:** Hypha derived from **huphe (Greek) = Web.**

➢ **Definition:** It is an elongated, tubular & branching structure of fungus.

➢ **Types of hypha:**

A. According to presence or absence of septa: →Fig. 2

i. Septate hyphae

ii. Non-septate hyphae (co-enocytic):

B. According to projection: →Fig.-5

i. Arial hyphae:
- Hyphae projected in air & containing spores **called arial hyphae.**
- Concerned with developmental function.

ii. Vegetative hyphae:
- Hyphae submerged with surface or media **called vegetative hyphae.**
- Concerned with nutritional function.

C. According to colour:

i. Dark (brown-black) hyphae:
- Brown-black pigmented hyphae occurs in some fungi & such fungi **called phaeoid fungi or demateceous fungi or black fungi.**

ii. Hyaline hyphae:
- Colourless hyphae occur in some fungi & such fungi **called hyaline fungi.**

D. According to morphology: →Fig.-9

i. Racquet hyphae:
- Enlargement of hyphal cell in-between length of hyphae with one broad end & other pointed end **called racquet hyphae.**
- **Example:** *T. mentagrophytes & E. flocossum*

ii. Nodular hyphae or knot organ:
- In-between length of hyphae presence of swelling, like knot **called nodular hyphae.**
- **Examples:** *T. mentagrophytes, M. canis* etc.

iii. Spiral hyphae:
- Hyphae present spiral shape.
- **Example:** *T. mentagrophytes.*

iv. Favic chanderlier:
- At the end of hyphae presence of multiple small projections like horn of reinder or chanderlier **called favic chanderlier.**
- **Examples:** *T. violaceum & T. schoenleinii.*

v. Pectinate body:
- One surface of hyphae is uniform while other shows some projections like broken comb **called pectinate body.**
- **Example:** *M. audounii.*

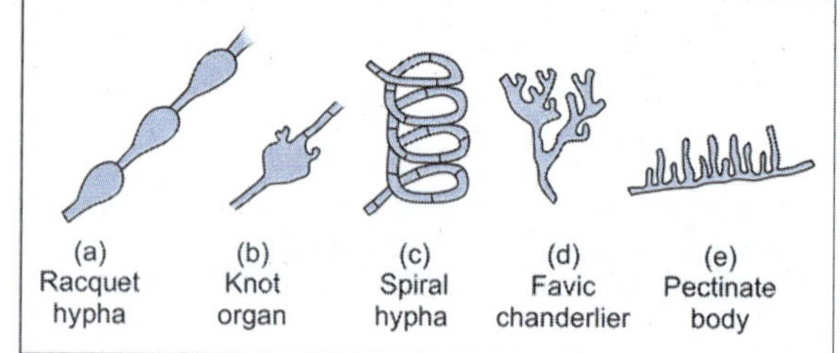

Figure-9: Morphological types of hyphae

❖ Pseudohyphae:

➢ **Definition:** →Vide supra

➢ **Differences between hyphae & pseudohyphae: →Table-5**

❖ Mycelium:

➢ **Definition:** It is an entangled mass of hyphae.

➢ **Morphology: →Fig.-10**

Features	Hyphae	Pseudohyphae
Reproduction	By apical elongation	By budding
Morphology	Fig.-2	Fig.-1
Hyphal cell	Cuboidal / rectangular	oval
Constriction in between two cells	Absent	Present
Cell wall	Uniform due to absence of constriction	Not uniform due to presence constriction
Dividing septum	Straight	Oblique/curved

Table-5: Differences between hyphae & pseudohyphae

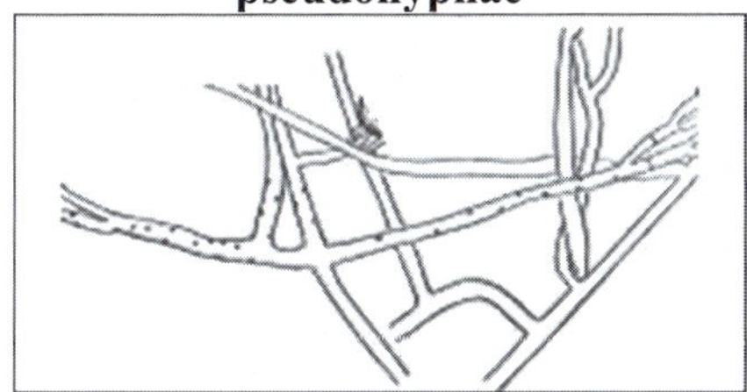

Figure-10: Mycelium

Pathogenicity or virulence of fungi

- **Precipitating factors (epidemiological determinants):** Virulence of fungi is affected by following three factors **called precipitating factors** or **epidemiological determinants.**

I. **Agent factors (virulence factors or determinants of virulence):**
II. **Host factors:**
III. **Environmental factors:**

I. Agent factors (virulence factors or determinants of virulence)

♣ **Factors:** Following are the different types.

A. **Intracellular or cell associated:**

i. **Adhesion:** Cell wall glycoprotein helps in attachment with host cell **called adhesin.**

ii. **Cell wall components:**

a. **Polysaccharide & polypeptide complex in cell wall:**
- Provide rigidity & structural integrity to cell.
- It acts as a barrier against the effect of deleterious agents on fungi.
- Glucans is antiphagocytic.

b. **Endotoxin:**
- It is a glycoprotein present in cell wall of *Candida, A flavus* & *A fumigates.*
- It is responsible for tissue necrosis, pyogenic & anaphylactic reaction.

iii. **Other components related to bacterial cell:**

a. **Capsular (K) Ag:** Capsular (K) antigen present in different *Cryptococcus* which inhibit the phagocytosis.

B. **Extracellular:**

i. **Enzymes:** → Table-6

Enzyme	Sources	Actions
Elastase	*A flavus, A fumigatus* & dermato-phytes	Enhances the fungal invasion in elastin containing tissues like lungs, skin, blood vessels etc. by degrading the elastin & scleroprotein
Alkaline protease	*A flavus, A fumigatus* & *Rhizopus* spp.	Enhances the fungal invasion in tissues like lungs, by degrading the elastin & collagen
Keratinase Collagenase	Dermato-phytes	Enhances the fungal invasion in tissues like skin by degrading the scleroprotein
Acid protease	*A fumigatus* & *candida* spp.	Cleavage of IgA to reduce the local immunity
Urease	*C. neoformans*	Convert urea in to ammonia which act as nitrogen source

Table-6: Enzymes, sources & actions in fungi

ii. **Toxins:** Follow chapter → Miscellaneous topics in Mycology (section →fungal food poisoning)

iii. **Antigens:** Produce allergic reaction **called id reaction** (candidid in *Candida* & dermatophytid in dermatophytes).

iv. **Pigment:** Melanin pigment produce by *Cryptococcus neoformans*, which protect fungus against the UV radiation & effects of immune cells.

v. **Mannitol production:** It produced by*Cryptococcus neoformans* & protects the fungus from intracellular killing by phagocytes.

C. **Others:**

i. **Fungal dimorphism:** All the dimorphic fungi (mentioned above) have two forms like mycelium & yeast phase, possess different antigenic & surface features, and require different host mechanisms to contain them.

ii. **Thermotolerance:**
- Ability of fungus to survive at 37^0C makes it a potent human pathogen.
- *Cryptococcus neoformans* can survive at higher temperature about 41-43^0C.

iii. **Resistance to antimicrobial products released by host cells:** Like yeast, spherules etc. are showing resistant to antimicrobial products like H_2O_2 released by host cells to evade the host defence.

iv. **Phenotypic switching:** *C albicans* has ability to adapt the different changing condition of host, which helps to evade the host defence mechanism & survival of fungus.

v. **Survival in acidic pH:** Fungus grows best at acidic ph & it may tolerate the gastric acidity.

II. Host factors

1. **Trauma:** Local trauma may precipitate the fungal infection.
2. **Immunosuppressive disease or conditions:** Following conditions favour the fungal infections
- Long term steroid therapy.
- Antibiotic therapy.
- DM.
- Immunosuppressive therapy.
- Renal transplantation.
- Malignancy.
- AIDS.
3. **Occupation:** Common in wooden workers like carpenters, farmers etc.
4. **Sex:** Common in female due to wet work.
5. **Wet areas:** Moisture may precipitate the fungal infection in areas like inguinal, axilla, foot due to constant wearing of shoes etc.

III. Environmental factors

1. **Economical status:** Common in developing countries.

Question bank

Essay/Full question

1) Classification of fungi

Short notes

1) Useful & harmful properties of fungi
2) Taxonomical (systemic) classification of fungi
3) Fungal spores
4) Fungal hyphae
5) Virulence factors of fungi

Short questions for theory/viva questions

1) Write four differences between bacteria & fungi.
2) Comment: Fungus is not able to do photosynthesis.
3) Write four differences between hyphae & pseudohyphae.
4) Write four examples of asexual spores of fungus.
5) Write four examples of sexual spores of fungus.
6) Define: Vegetative hyphae & aerial hyphae.
7) What is pectinate body & favic chanderlier?
8) What is mycelium (in fungus)?

MCQs for chapter review

Introduction

1) **Fungus useful for penicillin preparation is**
(a) *Penicillium notatum* (b) *Aspergillus tereus* (c) *Candida fukuyamaensis* (d) *Penicillium marneffei*

Classification

2) **Which of the following is only yeast**
(a) *Candida* (b) *Mucor* (c) *Rhizopus* (d) *Cryptococcus*
3) **Fungi that posses capsule is** (PGI-99)
(a) *Blastomyces dermatitidis* (b) *Histoplasma* (c) *Cryptococcus* (d) *Coccidioides immitis*
4) **Which of the following is false regarding dimorphic fungi**
(a) Occurs in two growth forms (b) Can cause systemic infection (c) *Cryptococcus* is an example (d) *Coccidioides* is an example
5) **Dimorphic fungi behave like yeast at**
(a) <10^0C (b) Body temperature (c) >40^0C (d) In vitro
6) **Dimorphic fungus** (PGI, Dec-02)
(a) *Candida* (b) *Cryptococcus* (c) *Blastomycosis* (d) *Coccidioidomycosis* (e) *Sporothrichosis*
7) **All are dimorphic fungi except** (AIIMS-09)
(a) *Blastomyces dermatitidis* (b) *Histoplasma* (c) *Penicillium marneffei* (d) *Phialophora*
8) **Dimorphic fungus**
(a) *Candida* (b) *Histoplasma* (c) *Rhizopus* (d) *Mucor*
9) **The following fungi are thermally dimorphic except** (AIIMS, Nov-03, AI-97)
(a) *Sporothrix schenckii* (b) *Cryptococcus neoformans* (c) *Blastomyces dermatitidis* (d) *Histoplasma capsulatum*
10) **Budding reproduction in tissue is seen in**
(a) *Cryptococcus, Candida* (b) *Candida, Rhizopus* (c) *Rhizopus, Mucor* (d) *Histoplasma, Candida*
11) **The fungi which do not have sexual phase belong to which of the following groups** (PGI-94, 96, 97)
(a) Phycomycetes (b) Fungi imperfecti (c) Basidiomycetes (d) Ascomycetes
12) **Barrel shaped spores (arthrospores) are seen with**
(a) *Blastomyces* (b) *Histoplasma* (c) *Coccidioides* (d) *Candida*
13) **A sporangium contains** (AIIMS-02)
(a) Spherules (b) Sporangiospores (c) Chlamydospores (d) Conidia
14) **Following is the asexual spore**
(a) Oospore (b) Zygospore (c) Ascospore (d) Blastospore
15) **Aseptate hyphae are seen in**
(a) Phycomycetes (b) Ascomycetes (c) Basidiomycetes (d) Deuteromycetes
16) **Ascospore is**
(a) Asexual spore (b) Sexual spore (c) Conidia (d) None of above
17) **Which of the following is produced sexually** (AIIMS-81)
(a) Ascospore (b) Conidium (c) Odium (d) Yeast bud
18) **Fungal spores may be produced** (AIIMS-02)
(a) Singly (b) In chains (c) In sporangium (d) All of above
19) **Human fungal infection is known as**
(a) Mycosis (b) Mycoses (c) a+b (d) Fungosis

Answers of MCQs & explanation

1) **(a)**
- Penicillin was discovered from *Penicillium notatum* by Alexander Fleming in 1928

2) **(d)**
- *Candida* is yeast like
- *Mucor & Rhizopus* are mold (filamentous) type

3) **(c)**
- In *Histoplasma capsulatum*, species name indicating the capsulated property of fungus but it in non capsulated
- *Cryptococcus neoformans* is the only capsulated fungus

4) **(c)**
5) **(b)**
6) **(c), (d) & (e)**
7) **(d)**
8) **(b)**
9) **(b)**
10) **(a)**

(Answers 4–10: Follow section, **classification (morphological classification)** for explanation)

11) **(b)**

- Phycomycetes, Basidiomycetes & Ascomycetes are showing sexual method of reproduction while in Fungi imperfecti method of reproduction is unknown

12) (c)

- Follow section, **classification [systemic (taxonomical) classification → asexual spores → arthrospores]** & **figure-4** for explanation

13) (b)

- Follow section, **classification [systemic (taxonomical) classification → asexual spores → sporangiospores]** & **figure-5** for explanation

14) (d)

- Oospore, zygospore & ascospore are the sexual spores

15) (a)
16) (b)
17) (a)

} Follow **table-3** for explanation

18) (d)

- Follow section, **classification [systemic (taxonomical) classification]** to know about all types of fungal spores, method of production & for other details.

19) (c)

- Mycosis is singular form for fungal infection while mycoses are the plural form for fungal infection.

- **Principle:** Haematoxylin is oxidised to haematin on air or light exposure (or by adding oxidising agents in stain) which stains nuclei in blue with mordant effect by metal while eosin, stains cytoplasm & tissue fibres in pink colour.
- **Uses:** It is used in many diagnostic settings.

2. **PAS (Periodic Acid Schiff) stain:**

- **Ingredients:** Stain contains periodic acid & Schiff's reagent (basic fuchsin, distilled water, potassium/sodium metabisulphite, HCL & decolouring charcoal).
- **Principle:** It based on the principle of **Feulgen reaction** where oxidisation of polysaccharide of fungi & bacteria by periodic acid releases aldehydes that yield red colour compound with basic fuchsin of Schiff's reagent. Nuclei stain blue, fungi magenta/red & background as light green. Protein & nucleic acids remain unstained.
- **Uses:** Stain is used for diagnosing fungi in tissues that are stained darker than surrounding tissues.
- **Disadvantages:**
  - It also stains the tissue contains carbohydrate making fungus demonstration more difficult.
  - Few microbes like *Actinomycetes* (*Nocardia*) are not stained by PAS stain.
  - It stains only live not the dead fungi.

3. **Gridley's fungal stain:** Almost parallel to PAS stain.

- **Ingredients:** Stain contains chromic acid & Schiff's reagent (aldehyde fuchsin, distilled water, sodium metabisulphite, HCL & tartrazine).
- **Principle:** Oxidisation of polysaccharide of fungi & bacteria by chromic acid releases aldehyde that yield purple colour compound with aldehyde fuchsin of Schiff's reagent. Fungi (mycelia & yeast cells), elastic tissues & mucin stains in purple & background in yellow colour.
- **Uses:** Stain is used for diagnosing fungi in tissues with purple colour & background in yellow colour.
- **Disadvantages:** It stains the mucin & elastic fibres present in tissue in purple colour, making fungus demonstration more difficult.

4. **GGMS (Grocott Gomori's Methenamine Silver) stain:**

- **Ingredients:** Stain contains chromic acid, methenamine silver nitrate, sodium metabisulphite, sodium thiosulphate etc.
- **Principle:** Oxidisation of polysaccharide of fungi & bacteria by chromic acid releases aldehyde which reduces methenamine silver nitrate to metallic silver. Metallic silver deposited al the place where aldehydes is available yielding brown-black colour to the fungal cell wall & bacteria, tissue pale green, cytoplasma old rose & mucopolysaccharide dark grey.
- **Uses:**
  - It also stains the *Actinomycetes* (like *Nocardia, Actinomyces, Actinomadura* & *Streptomyces*) which are not stained by PAS stain.
  - It stains both live & dead fungi compared to PAS stain which stain only live fungi.
  - For *Pneumocystis jirovecii,* stains the cyst wall in black colour.

5. **Mayer's mucicarmine stain:**

- **Ingredients:** Stain contains carmine (red colour) dye, aluminium hydroxide & aluminium chloride. Aluminium hydroxide & aluminium chloride has mordant effect.
- **Principle:** It based on carminophilic property of microbe. Carminophilic means ability of microbes to eat carmine (red colour) dye, especially due to presence of mucin (glycoprotein) in cell wall or due to polysaccharide capsule. Here mucin part of cell (like cancer cells & *R. seeberi*) stains in red, capsule in deep rose colour while nuclei in blue colour.
- **Uses:**
  - *R. seeberi* (mucin in cell wall): Sporangium & endospores stain in red colour while nuclei in blue colour.
  - *C. neoformans* : Capsule stains deep rose in colour
  - Cancer cells: Because malignant cells contain mucin.

6. **Masson Fontana Silver (MFS) stain:**

- **Ingredients:** Stain contains silver nitrate (of Fontans's silver stain used for *T pallidum*).
- **Principle:** Melanin produced by fungi stains black in colour by silver nitrate.
- **Uses:** For melanin producing fungi like *C. neoformans* & black (phaeoid) fungi. Fungi stain black & nuclei in red.

7. **Giemsa stain:** For trophozoites & sporozoites (internal nuclei) of cyst of *Pneumocystis jirovecii,* where nuclei are stain in pink colour & cytoplasm in blue colour.
8. **Alcian blue stain:** For capsulated fungus like *C. neoformans.*

iii. Fluorescent Microscopy (FM) & staining:

a. Fluorochrome staining:

- By using dye like Calco Flour White (CFW) stain
- It directly binds with fungal cell wall present in samples & enhances the fungal visualisation.

b. Immunofluorescent staining: Detection of antigen or antibody by using a dye like FITC (Fluorescin Iso Thio Cyanate).

II. Culture

- **Culture media**

i. Routine fungal culture media:

- It includes **Sabouraud Dextrose Agar (SDA)** with antibiotics like cycloheximide which prevent the contamination by saprophytic fungi & gentamicin plus chloramphenicol prevent the bacterial growth & makes the medium selective for fungus.

- **Two sets** of media are used
- 1st set is incubated at room temperature (20-25°C) for mycelial phase.
- 2nd set is incubated at 37°C for yeast phase.

ii. Nutritionally deficient (spore producing) media:

- Deficiency of nutrition allows the spore production.
- **Chlamydospores producing media** are
- Cornmeal or cornmeal tween agar.
- Rice starch agar.

iii. Selective media:

a. *Candida* selective media: Used to differentiate *Candida* spp.

- Tetrazolium reduction medium.
- Chrom agar.

b. *Cryptococcus* selective media:

- Bird seed (niger seed) agar: } Brown colour colony
- Sunflower seed agar: }

c. Dermatophyte selective media:

- Dermatophyte test medium: Red colony.
- Dermatophyte identification medium: Purple colony.

d. *Aspergillus* selective medium:

- Czapek-Dox agar: To differentiate the *Aspergillus* spp.

e. *Malassezia* selective medium: PYG (Peptone Yeast extract Glucose) agar.

➢ **Culture technique & identification of growth: →Flow chart-1**

III. Biochemical reactions (B/Rs)

i. Sugar fermentation & assimilation test: To differentiate the *Candida* species & other yeast or yeast like fungi

ii. Urease test: Positive in fungus like *Cryptococcus neoformans, Trichosporon beigelii, Trichophyton mentagrophytes* & *Rhodotorula mucinaginosa.*

IV. Serological tests

Like ELISA, precipitation based tests, RIA, CFT, agglutination tests etc. are useful to detect the fungal infections.

V. Molecular tests

- **Advantages:** High sensitivity & specificity
- **Disadvantages:** high cost & not available in peripheral centre
- **Methods:** DNA probe, hybridisation, PCR etc.

VI. Other tests

A. Skin test: Based on DTH.

B. Animal inoculation: Laboratory animals like rabbits, guinea pig etc. are useful.

C. Gag Liquid Chromatography: To detect the fungal metabolites like D-arabinitol, D-mannose.

D. Wood's lamp examination:

➢ **Synonym:** Black light lamp or UV-A light lamp or ultraviolet light lamp.

➢ **History:** It was devised by Robert Williams Wood in 1903 using "Wood's glass".

➢ **Principle:**

- Made up with barium silicate & nickel oxide.
- It transmits the UV light (at a wavelength of approximately 365 nanometers) which produce different fluorescence on exposure to skin.

➢ **Uses:**

i. Infectious conditions:

1. **Bright green:** *Microscporum audounii, M. canis, M. ferruginium* & *Pseudomonas* in burns wound.
2. **Dull green:** *Trichophyton schoenleinii.*
3. **Dull yellow:** *Microscporum gypseum.*
4. **Golden yellow:** *Malassazia furfur* (causing ptyriasis versicolor).
5. **Coral-red:** *Corynebacterium minutissimum* (causing erythrasma).

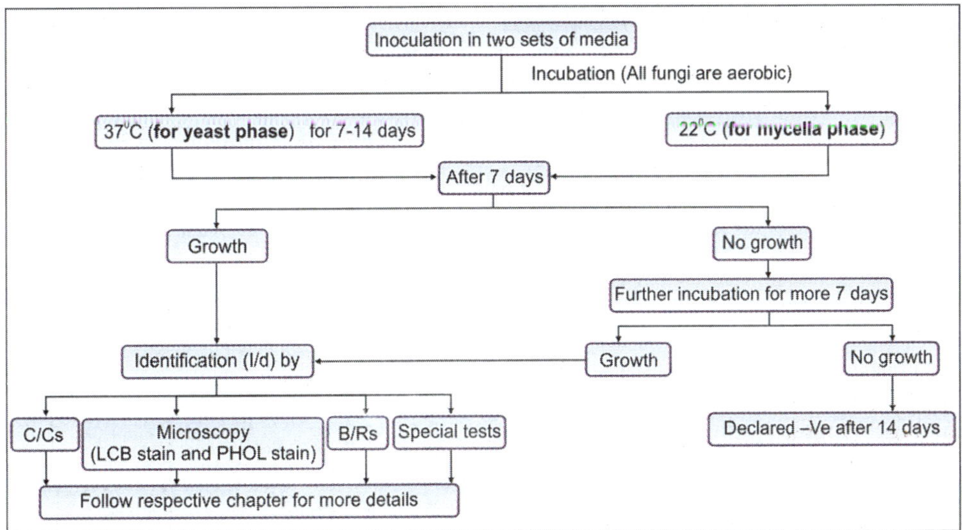

Flow chart-1: Fungal culture technique & identification of growth

6. **Brick-red:** *Prevotella melaninogenica.*
7. *Propionibacterium acnes*: It's causing acne & exhibits an orange glow.

ii. Non-Infectious conditions:

1. **Ethylene glycol poisoning:** Manufacturers of ethylene glycol-containing antifreezes commonly add fluorescein, which causes the patient's urine to fluoresce under Wood's lamp.
2. **Vitiligo:** Wood's lamps have also been used to differentiate hypopigmentation from depigmentation such as with vitiligo. A vitiligo patient's skin will appear yellow-green or blue under the Wood's lamp.
3. **Porphyria cutanea tarda:** In this condition urine turns pink upon illumination with Wood's lamp.
4. **Tuberous sclerosis:**
5. **Melanoma:**
6. **Freckles:**
7. **Phototherapy:** Bili light. A type of phototheraphy that uses blue light with a range of 420-470 nm, used to treat neonatal jaundice.

E. Special tests:

i. Teased mount: Teased out the beats of colony over glass slide, put LCB stain & examine under microscope. It does not give 'In situ' appearance but separate the fungus from mass & makes the easy examination.

ii. Slide culture: → **Fig.-2**

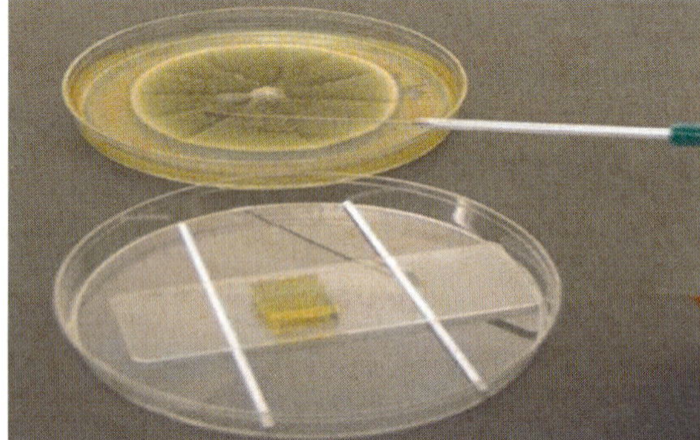

Figure-2: Slide culture

- Preserve the in situ (undisturbed) fungal growth under microscope.
- Place a sterile slide in petri-dish.
- Place a 1cm SDA block on slide.
- Inoculate the test species at four sides of agar block.
- Cover the agar block with cover slip.
- Incubate at 25^0c for 48 hrs.
- Take new slide & add a drop of LCB stain.
- Transfer the cover slip from petri-dish slide to new slide & examine under the microscope.

iii. Cellophane tape mount: Cellophane touch to the colony in media & fix on slide with LCB stain. Examine the in situ appearance under microscope.

iv. Exo-antigens tests: Free antigen of fungus produce during growth in culture broth.

v. Germ tube test:

➢ **Synonym & history:** Also **called Reynold-Braude phenomenon**, because it was first reported by Reynolds and Braude in 1956.

➢ **Indications:** For rapid identification of *Candida* species like

1. ***Candida albicans* (+):**
   - Half rate of positivity than *Candida dubliniensis*
   - Approximately 95–97% of *C. albicans* isolates develop germ tubes when incubated in a proteinaceous media
2. ***Candida dubliniensis* (++):**
   - Double rate of positivity than *Candida albicans*

➢ **Principle:** Formation of germ tube is associated with increased synthesis of protein and ribonucleic acid. Germ tube solutions contain serum, essential nutrients for protein synthesis. It is lyophilized for stability.

➢ **Material required:**

- Culture: Suspected *Candida* culture plate.
- Reagent: Serum (human, sheep, foetal bovine) or other commercially produced media.
- Others: Test tubes, loop or wooden applicator, Pasteur pipettes, slides, cover slips & microscope.

➢ **Method:**

✪ **Steps:**

- Mix fungal culture with sheep or human serum or foetal bovine serum & incubate at 37^0C for 2-4 hrs.
- Take one drop over slide, put cover slip (wet mount) & examined under microscope.
- Wet mount can also be prepared by using the KOH.

✪ **Control:**

- **Positive control:** *C. albicans* (ATCC 10231).
- **Negative control:** *C. tropicalis* (ATCC 13803) or *C. glabrata* (ATCC 2001).

✪ **Results:**

- **Positive test:**
  - A short hyphal (filamentous) extension arising laterally from a yeast cell, with no constriction at the point of origin (**fig.-3**).
  - Examples: *Candida albicans* & *C. dubliniensis.*
- **Negative test:**
  - No hyphal (filamentous) extension arising from a yeast cell or a short hyphal extension constricted at the point of origin.
  - Examples: *C. tropicalis*, *C. glabrata* & other yeasts.

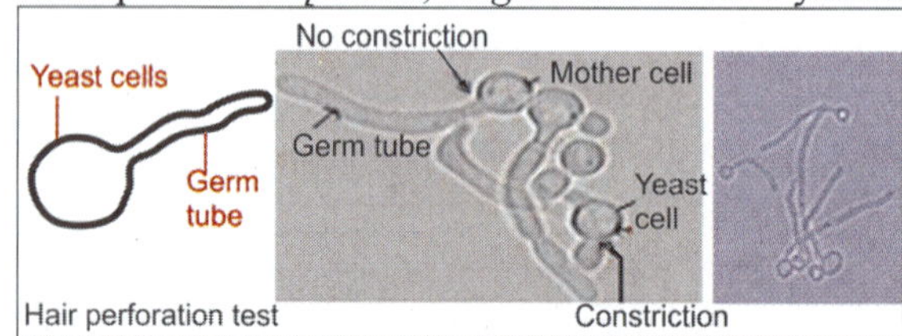

Figure-3: Germ tube

➢ **Features of germ tube:**

- Germ tube is half the width and 3 -4 times the length of the yeast cell.
- There is no presence of nucleus.
- Non-septate.
- No presence of constriction at the point of origin.

➢ **Advantages:**
- Rapid test for diagnosis & differentiation of *Candida albican*s from other *Candida* isolates. It can be performed in less than three hours.
- Easy to perform.

➢ **Disadvantages (limitations):**
- Germ tube is not confused with pseudohyphae or buds, as there is no constriction at the site of origin of germ tube from yeast cells.
- *Candida tropicalis* may produce pseudo-germ tubes after 3 hrs of incubation but they show constriction at the point of origin.
- Too heavy inoculum will inhibit germ tube formation.
- This test is only part of the overall scheme for identification of yeasts. Further testing is required for definite identification.

➢ **Other methods to detect the germ tube:** By using
- Milk medium.
- Amino acid synthetic medium.
- Muller Hinton agar also used for germ tube formation in both this media.

➢ **Clinical significance of germ tube:** Germ tube is one of the virulence factors of *Candida albican*s.

vi. Dalmau plate culture:

➢ **Indication:** For in situ identification of chlamydospores.

➢ **Method:** To set up a yeast morphology plate, dip a flamed sterilized straight wire into a light inoculum (sterile distilled water suspension) and then lightly scratch the wire into the surface of a cornmeal/tween 80, rice/tween 80 or yeast morphology agar plate, then place a flamed cover slip onto the agar surface covering the scratches. Dalmau morphology plates are examined in situ using the lower power microscope for the presence of spores.

vii. Hair baits technique:

➢ **Indication:** For identification of keratinophilic fungi from soil.

➢ **Principle:** Based on utilisation of keratin by fungus.

➢ **Method:**
- Place soil samples in sterile petri dish.
- Place the around 30 pieces of sterile (by autoclave) horse's hairs on top of soil.
- Wet the soil surface by using sterile distilled water (don't flood it).
- Add more water & incubate at 30^0C.
- When white to brown fungal growth appear around the hairs, transfer them with fungal growth on SDA plate in scattered manner. Bury one end of hair under agar surface.
- Take hair with fungal growth for microscopic observation under LCB mount.
- When fungal colonies appear on SDA plate, make the LCB mount for identification of fungus under microscope.
- Fungi which grow on SDA plate should be transferred to other plate for further confirmation.

viii. Hair perforation technique:
- Place filter paper strip in sterile petri dish & cover the strip by using sterile distilled water.
- Add small portion of sterilised pre-pubertal or infant's hair in to water.
- Add 5-6 drops of 10% yeast extract to speed up the reaction.
- Inoculate the colony directly on hair & incubate at 25^0C for 4 weeks.
- Take the hair on slide, prepare the LCB mount & examine under microscope for perforation of hair shaft as shown in **fig.-4.**
- Test is positive in *T. mentagrophytes* & *M. canis* & negative in *T. rubrum* & *M. equinum.*

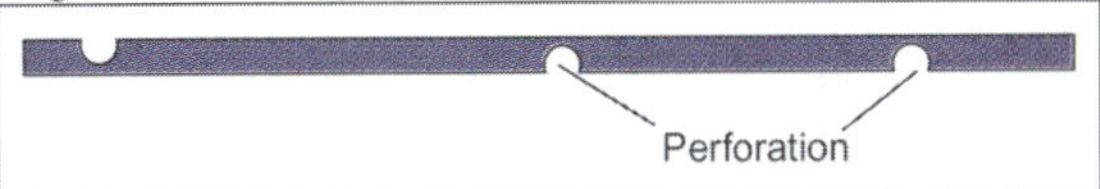

Figure-4: Hair perforation test

F. Antifungal sensitivity test: Report the result with antifungal sensitivity pattern.

Laboratory fungal contaminants

❖ **Introduction:**
- Mycology laboratory encounter more contaminant than actual pathogens.
- They always create the confusion in the diagnosis of actual pathogen.
- It's very difficult to draw a line between contaminants & actual pathogens, however contaminants can be differentiated by

1. Repeated growth in all clinical specimens.
2. Presence of growth in un-inoculated areas (pathogens can grow only at the inoculated site but not anywhere).
3. May be absent in direct smear examination.

❖ **Classification:** Almost many are described in respective chapters. All they are summarised in following five groups.

A Zygomycets:
- *Absidia* species.
- *Mucor* species.
- *Rhizopus* species.
- *Syncephalustrum* species.
- *Cunninghamella* species.

B Hyaline hyphomycetes

- *Acremonium* species.
- *Aspergillus* species.
- *Chrysosporium* species.
- *Fusarium* species.
- *Penicillium* species.
- *Paecilomyces* species.
- *Scopulariopsis* species.
- *Sepedonium* species.
- *Trichoderma* species.
- *Trichothecium* species.
- *Verticillium* species.

C Phaeoid fungi

- *Alternaria* species.
- *Aureobasidium* species.
- *Bipolaris* species.
- *Chaetomium* species.
- *Cladosporium* species.
- *Curvularia* species.
- *Helminthosporium* species.
- *Nigrospora* species.
- *Phoma* species.

D Yeast & yeast like

- *Geotrichum* species.
- *Rhodotorula* species.
- *Saccharomyces* species.
- *Trichosporon* species.
- *Ustilago* species.

E Look alike fungi

- *Sepedonium* species.
- *Malbranchia* species.
- *Chrysosporium* species.
- *Acrodonium* species.

Question bank

Essay/Full question

1) Laboratory diagnosis of fungal infections.

Short notes

1) Fungal stains.
2) Fungal culture.
3) Germ tube test.
4) Fungal laboratory contaminants.

Short questions for theory/viva questions

1) Comment: Thick tissue or skin scraping sample is treated with 10% KOH.
2) Name two selective culture media for each, *Candida* spp. & *C. neoformans.*
3) Name four fungus giving urease test positive.
4) What is fungal slide culture?
5) What is germ tube test?
6) What is hair bait technique & hair perforation technique?
7) Mention the four laboratory fungal contaminants.

MCQs for chapter review

Testing methods

1) **KOH wet mount can be prepared for**
   (a) Bacteria (b) Virus (c) Fungus (d) Parasite
2) **Culture medium for fungus is** (PGI-94)
   (a) Tellurite medium (b) NNN medium (c) Chocolate medium (d) Sabouraud's medium
3) **Which dye is most suitable for fungus demonstration in biopsy-** (AIIMS, Nov- 09)
   (a) Alizarin red (b) Veirhoff dye (c) Manson's trichome (d) PAS
4) **Correctly matched stain** (PGI, May-13, June-06)
   (a) Mucicarmine- *Cryptococcus* (b) Giemsa- *Candida* (c) Methanamine silver – *Histoplasma* (d) Gram's – *Pneumocystis carinii*
5) **Stain used for staining fungal elements-** (AIIMS, Nov- 09)
   (a) Acid fast stain (b) Mucicarmine (c) Methenamine silver (d) Gram stain
6) **Common stain for fungal hyphae** (AIIMS, May-13)
   (a) Methylene blue (b) Gomori methenamine silver (c) Congo red (d) Oil red O
7) **Fungal staining is done by**
   (a) Calcofluor white (b) Leishman stain (c) ZN stain (d) None
8) **Wood lamp can be used for evaluation of -** (PGI, June-02)
   (a) Tinea capitis (b) Freckles (c) Vitiligo (d) Tuberous sclerosis
9) **Reynold-Braude phenomenon, is seen in**
   (a) *Candida albicans* (b) *Candida psitasi* (c) *Histoplasma* (d) *Cryptococcus*
10) **Germ tube test is used in diagnosis for**
   (a) *Candida albicans* (b) *Cryptococcus* (c) *Histoplasma* (d) Coccidioidomycosis
11) **Hair perforation test is positive in infection with** (PGI-97)
   (a) *Trichohyton* (b) *Microsporum* (c) *Epidermophyton* (d) All of above

Answers of MCQs & explanation

1) **(c)**
- KOH will liquefy the keratin or thick tissue present in samples & makes the clear fungal examination. It could be done by slide or tube method.

2) **(d)**
- Tellurite medium: It is useful for *C. diphtheriae*, *Staph. aureus, E. faecalis, E. rhusiopathiae*
- NNN medium: It is useful for parasite like *Leishmania* spp. & *T. cruzi*
- Chocolate medium: It is useful for growth of fastidious bacteria, like *H. influenzae, Staphylococcus* spp., *Neisseria* spp., *Streptococcus* spp. & *Pneumococcus*
- Sabouraud's medium: Acidic pH favour the growth of fungus

3) **(d)**
- Follow section, **testing methods (microscopy & staining → differential stains → histopathological stains)** for more details

4) **(a)**
- Giemsa- *Pneumocystis carinii*
- Methanamine silver – *Pneumocystis carinii & Actinomycetes*
- Gram's – *Candida & all fungi stain gram positive*
- Follow section, **testing methods (microscopy & staining → differential stains → histopathological stains)** for more details

5) **(b), (c) & (d)**
- Acid fast stain is for acid fast bacteria & parasites
- Follow section, **testing methods (microscopy & staining → differential stains → histopathological stains)** for more details

6) **(b)**
- From the given options only fungal stain is Gomori methenamine silver. Follow section, **testing methods (microscopy & staining)** for more details

7) **(a)**
- From the given options Leishman stain is for parasites & ZN stain is for acid fast bacteria plus parasites. Follow section, **testing methods (microscopy & staining)** for more details

8) (a), (b), (c) & (d)
- Tinea capitis is caused by *Microscporum* spp. or *Trichophyton* spp. (dermatophyte category), which fluoresce in different colour under UV light.
- Follow section, **testing methods (other tests → Wood's lamp examination →uses)** for explanation of other options

9) (a) } Follow section, **testing methods (other methods →**
10) (a) } **germ tube test)** for explanation.

11) (a)
- Follow section, **testing methods (other tests → hair perforation technique)** for explanation

77 Superficial mycoses

Learning heading & subheadings

- Definition
- Classification:
  - Surface mycoses
  - Cutaneous mycoses

Definition: Fungal infections present in the skin & its appendages (like hair & nail) **called superficial mycoses.**

Classification: Two subtypes like surface mycosis & cutaneous mycosis.

Surface mycoses

❖ **Definition:** Fungi affecting the outer most layer (dead layer or stratum corneum) of skin & its appendages like hairs & nails **called surface mycoses.**

❖ **Properties:** It does not produce the inflammatory reaction but only produces the cosmetic effects.

❖ **Examples:** Following four are examples.

I. **Malassezia infections**
II. **Tinea nigra**
III. **Piedra**
IV. **Onychomycoses**

I. Malassezia infections

➢ **Etiological agent:** *Malassezia furfur.*

➢ **Synonym:** Agent was previously **called *M. ovalis*** or ***Pityrosporum ovale.***

➢ **Pathogenicity:**

✪ **Reservoir & source of infection:** It is the resident flora of human & animals.

✪ **Mode of transmission:** It is a normal flora of skin & infection is endogenous.

✪ **Portal of entry:** Endogenous infection.

✪ **Sites:**

- Occurs in area rich in sebaceous glands (excessive sweating).
- Lesions are found in neck, trunk, face, scalp, upper limbs & shoulders.

✪ **Precipitating factors (epidemiological determinants):**

1. **Age:** Common in teenager.
2. **Sex:** Equal infection in both sexes.
3. **Other factors:** Hormonal factors, excessive sweating & immunosuppressive status are responsible for recurrence.

✪ **Pathogenesis:** It is a lipophilic fungus. It interferes with melanin production resulting hypo or hyper pigmented patches on skin.

✪ **Clinical features:**

A. **Pityriasis (tinea) versicolor [fig.-1(a)]:** Fungus interferes with melanin production resulting hypo or hyper pigmented patches on skin & non-inflammatory macular lesion with fine scales.

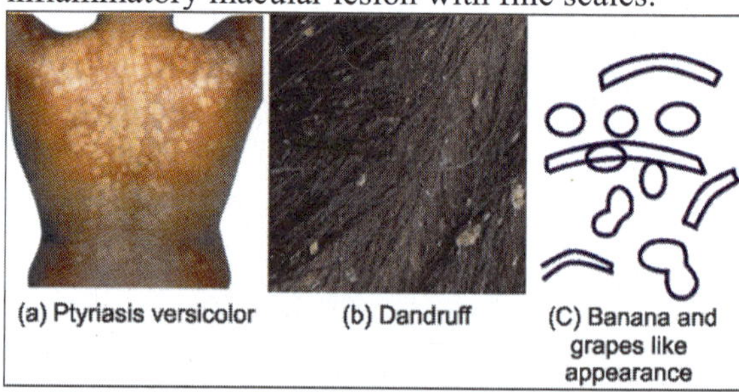

Figure-1: Images of *M. furfur*

B. **Seborrheic dermatitis [dandruff or pityriasis capitis, fig.-1(b)]:**

- **Meaning: Sebo** from **Sebum (Latin)** = **Grease** and **rrhoea** from **rhoea (Greek)** = **discharge/flow.**
- Whitish, dry & loose flakes on scalp.

✪ **Complications:** Recurrence is common due to hormonal factors, excessive sweating & immunosuppressive status.

➢ **Laboratory diagnosis:**

✪ **Wood's lamp examination:**

- Made up with barium silicate & nickel oxide.
- It transmits the UV light which produces golden yellow fluorescence.

✪ **Specimens:**

- Epidermal scales picked up by forceps or by using cellophane tap.
- Skin scraping.
- All the samples are collected in black envelope.

✪ **Testing:**

A. **10% KOH:** Cluster of round yeast cells with 2-7μm size & short, curved hypha gives appearance **called banana & grapes like** or **Spaghetti & meatballs like appearance [fig.-1(c)].**

B. **Culture:**

- **Medium:** SDA + antibiotics + tween-80 + olive oil. lipophilic fungus grow with difficulties on medium after adding the olive oil.
- **C/Cs on SDA:** Small, creamy & yellow colony.
- **LCB/PHOL stain:** Spherical yeast cells & short curved hyphae.

➢ **Prevention:** Removal of precipitating factors to prevent the recurrence.

➢ **Treatment:** Two types of treatment.

A. **Local:**

- 25% sodium thiosulphate.
- 10% surfur ointment.
- Whitefield ointment.
- 1-2% imidazole cream.
- Selenium sulphide shampoo for dandruff.
- Shampoo for dandruff which includes 2% ketoconazole & 1% zinc pyrithone.
- Lotion for ptyriasis versicolor which includes clotrimazole plus selenium sulphide (Candid TV).
- Topical terbinafine is useful for both ptyriasis versicolor & dandruff.

B. **Systemic:** It includes

- Pulse therapy of fluconazole 150 mg once or twice a week for 2-3 months.
- Others orally used drugs are itraconazole, ketoconazole etc.

II. Tinea nigra

➢ **Meaning: Tinea = fungal infection & nigra = black**

➢ **Definition:**

- Superficial fungal infection of palm or sole by black fungi **called tinea nigra.**
- It also **called superficial phaeohyphomycosis,** because caused by black fungi.

➢ **Etiological agent:** *Exophiala werneckii.*

➢ **Synonym:** Agent also **called *Hortae werneckii*** or ***Cladosporium werneckii*** or ***Phaeoannellomyces werneckii.***

➢ **Pathogenicity:**

✪ **Reservoir and source of infection:** It present in soil, sewage, decaying vegetation, wooden stick, salted fish & sea water. It is halophilic fungus & optimally can grow at 3-6% NaCl of sea water, but can tolerate up to 10% NaCl.

✪ **Mode of transmission:** Infection commonly acquired from sea water during bathing.

✪ **Incubation period:** 2-7 weeks.

✪ **Portal of entry:** Skin.

✪ **Sites:** Palm & soles with excessive sweating which precipitate the infection due to halophilic (required high salt for growth) nature of fungus.

✪ **Precipitating factors (epidemiological determinants):**

1. **Age:** Teenager or < 20 years.
2. **Sex:** Females are infected 3-5 times more than males.
3. **Hyperhydrosis:** Common in patient with excessive sweating.

✪ **Pathogenesis & clinical features:**

- Fungus increases the melanin production.
- Presence of brown-black pigmented macular lesion on palm **called tinea nigra palmaris [fig.-2(a)]** or sole **called tinea nigra plantaris [fig.-2(b)].**

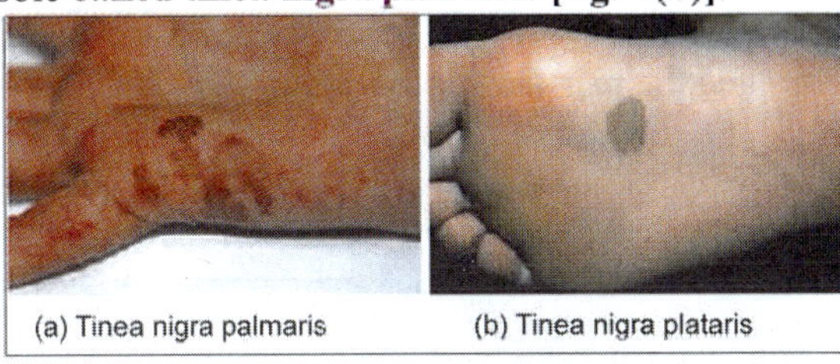
(a) Tinea nigra palmaris (b) Tinea nigra plataris

Figure-2: Types of tinea nigra

➢ **Laboratory diagnosis:**

✪ **Specimens:** Skin scraping collected in black envelope.

✪ **Testing:**

A. **10% KOH:** Cluster of round budding yeast cells with 2-8μm size & brown-septate-branched hyphae.

B. **Culture:**

- **Media:** SDA + antibiotics.
- **C/Cs on SDA:** Brown-black colony.
- **LCB/PHOL stain:** Cluster of round budding yeast cells with 2-8μm size & brown-septate-branched hyphae.

➢ **Prevention:** No standard guidelines for prevention.

➢ **Treatment:** Two types of treatment.

A. **Local:** Application of keratolytic agents like

- Whitefield ointment.
- 10% salicylic acid ointment.

B. **Systemic:** Orally used drugs are itraconazole (200 mg daily for three week), griseofulvin etc.

III. Piedra

* **Meaning:** From **piedra (Spanish) = stone**, because of nodule like formation within the hair shaft.

* **Definition:** It is a fungal infection of hair characterised by nodule formation along the hair shaft.

* **Types:** Following two types.

A. **White piedra:**

➢ **Synonym:** Also **called trichomycosis nodularis** or **trichosporonis nodosa.**

➢ **Etiological agent:** *Trichosporon beigelii.*

➢ **Pathogenicity:**

- **Reservoir of infection:** It present in soil & stagnant water.
- **Source of infection:** Stagnant water.
- **Mode of transmission:**
  - Exactly not known but may be due to contact with stagnant water of swimming pool.
  - Pubic white piedra may be transmitted by sexual intercourse.
- **Portal of entry:** Direct contact to hair with contaminated swimming pool stagnant water.
- **Sites:** Axillary, pubic, moustache & beard area.
- **Precipitating factors (epidemiological determinants):**

1. **Age & sex:** Variable from country to country.
2. **Race:** It is common in person with black complex.

- **Clinical features:** Greyish-white soft nodule around the hair shaft as shown in **[fig.-3(a)].**

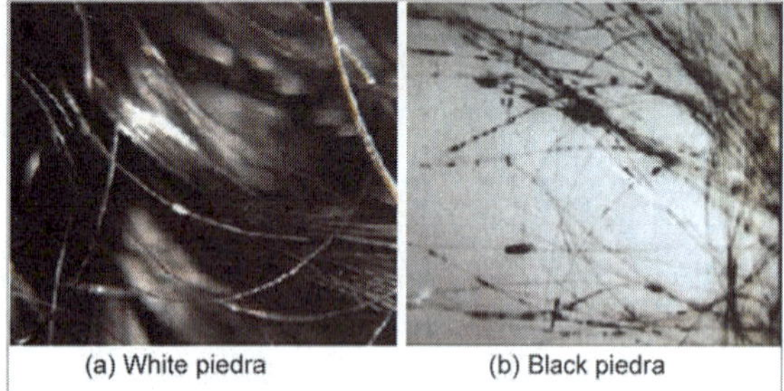
(a) White piedra (b) Black piedra

Figure-3: Types of piedra

- **Complications:** Scalp colonisation may lead persistent infection & recurrence.

➤ **Laboratory diagnosis:**

- **Specimen:** Hair pieces.
- **Testing:**

i. **10% KOH:** Hyaline septate hypha with arthrospores.

ii. **Culture:**

- **Media:** SDA + antibiotics.
- **C/Cs on SDA:** White creamy colony.
- **LCB/PHOL stain:** Hyaline septate hyphae.

➤ **Prevention:** Good personal hygiene helps to prevent the infections.

➤ **Treatment:**

i. **Removal of hair:** It is the best treatment for both piedra, however in female due to habit of keeping long hair it is not possible to cut the hairs.

ii. **Local:**
  - Coating of hairs with azole derivatives.
  - Antifungal shampoo or topical lotion.

iii. **Systemic:** White piedra is difficult to treat due to scalp colonisation by fungi, however azoles or AMB are effective.

B. Black piedra:

➤ **Synonym:** Disease also **called tinea nodosa.**

➤ **Etiological agent:** *Piedraia hortae.*

➤ **Pathogenicity:**

- **Reservoir of infection:** It present in soil & infect monkey as well as man.
- **Source of infection:** Contaminated combs, pillows & bed sheets.
- **Mode of transmission:** Common sharing or contact with infected items like combs, pillows & bed sheets.
- **Portal of entry:** Direct contact to hair during combing or sharing infected pillow.
- **Site:** Hair of scalp, moustache & beard area.
- **Precipitating factors (epidemiological determinants):**

1. **Age:** 16-29 years.
2. **Sex:** More in girls than boys.
3. **Life style (occupation):** Common in hostels girls due to sharing common combs, pillows & bed sheets.

- **Clinical features:** Presence of hard, black nodules along the hair shaft **[fig.-3(a)],** produce metallic sound during combing of hair.

➤ **Laboratory diagnosis:**

- **Specimen:** Hair pieces.
- **Testing:**

i. **10% KOH:** Dark septate hyphae around hair shaft with asci containing ascospores.

ii. **Culture:**

- **Media:** SDA + antibiotics.
- **C/Cs on SDA:** Brown-black colony.
- **LCB/PHOL stain:** Dark septate hyphae.

➤ **Treatment:**

i. **Removal of hair:** } Same as white piedra.
ii. **Local:** }

iii. **Systemic:** Terbinafine in a dose of 250 mg for 6 weeks is effective for black piedra.

IV. Onychomycoses

➤ **Meaning: Onycho** from **Onyx (Greek) = nail & Mycosis = fungal disease**

➤ **Definitions:**
  - Fungal infections of nail **called onychomycoses [fig. 4(a)].**
  - Fungal infections of nail by dermatophytes are **called tinea unguium.**

➤ **Etiological agents:**

A. Dermatophytes: Called tinea unguium.
  - *T. mentagrophytes.*
  - *T. rubrum.*
  - *E. flocossum.*

B. Non-dermatophytes:
  - *Scopulariopsis brevicaulis.*
  - *Scytalidium dimidiatum.*
  - *Scytalidium hyalinum.*
  - *Aspergillus flavus.*
  - *Aspergillus fumigates.*
  - *Acremonium* species.
  - *Fusarium oxysporum.*

- *Onychocola Canadensis.*
- *Geotrichum candidum.*
- Yeast like: *C. albicans.*

➢ **More details about etiological agents:** Follow respective chapters.

➢ **Prevention:** Improvement in hygiene.

➢ **Treatment:**

a. **Treatment of dermatophytes:**
- Treated by using pulse therapy of itraconazole & terbinafine for 6-12 months.
- Clinical cure of onychomycoses is define as disappearance of almost all lesion & residual lesions are not >10%.
- Mycological cure is defined as negative microscopy & culture.

b. **Treatment of non-dermatophytes:** Itraconazole is effective for *S. brevicaulis*, *Aspergillus* spp. & *Fusarium oxysporum*.

Cutaneous mycoses

❖ **Definition:** Fungal infections of skin layer beneath the dead layer **called cutaneous mycoses.**

❖ **Properties:** Produces the inflammatory & allergic reactions.

❖ **Examples:** Following two are examples.

I. **Candidiasis**
II. **Dermatophytoses**

I. Candidiasis

➢ **Synonym:**

✪ **Moniliasis:** Because previously the genus was **called *Monilia*** or **called *Odium*** (species was referred as *Monilia albicans* or *Odium albicans*).

✪ **Candidosis:** Both candidisis & candidosis are correct terminology for the disease. 'Osis' used as suffix in European countries while 'asis' in USA & rest of the world.

➢ **Definition:** It is an infection of skin, its appendages, subcutaneous tissue & internal organs by *Candida* species.

➢ **Etiological agents:** Caused by *Candida* species like
- *Candida albicans* (*Monilia albicans*).
- *C. krusei.*
- *C. kefyr* (*C. pseudotropicalis*).
- *C. glabrata.*
- *C. guilliermondi.*
- *C. tropicalis.*
- *C. parapsilosis.*
- *C. lusitaniae.*
- *C. dubliniensis.*
- *C. visvanathii.*
- *C. pelliculosa (Pichia anomala).*

➢ **Pathogenicity:**

✪ **Reservoir & source of infection:** It is a normal flora of skin-mucosa & infection is endogenous.

✪ **Mode of transmission & portal of entry:** Endogenous transmission.

✪ **Sites:** Many sites like skin, mucosa, meninges, GIT etc.

✪ **Precipitating factors (epidemiological determinants):**

a. **Agent factors (virulence factors):**
1. **Adhesin:** Adhesin present on cell wall helps to bind with host cells.
2. **Toxin:** It is glycoprotein like bacterial endotoxin & produce pyogenic & anaphylactic reaction.
3. **Enzymes:**
   - There are more than 14 hydrolytic enzymes are produce by *Candida* like protease, proteinase, lipase, phospholipase, esterase, phosphatase etc.
   - They help in fungal invasion.
4. **Phenotyping switching:** It is an ability of fungus to adapt the different changing condition of host, which helps to evade the host defence mechanism & survival of fungus.
5. **Antigens:** Produce allergic reaction **called id reaction** or **candidid.**

b. **Host factors:**
1. **Age:** Old age.
2. **Trauma:** Local trauma or 3rd degree burn may precipitate the infection.
3. **Immunosuppressive disease or conditions:** It causes infection in immunocompetent & also in individual with immunosuppressive disease or conditions like

- **Drugs:**
  - Long term steroid therapy.
  - Antibiotic therapy: Kills the bacteria & reduce the nutritional competition with *Candida* spp.
  - Contraceptive pills.
  - Intravenous drug abuse.
- **Metabolic disease:** Like diabetes mellitus.
- **Infectious disease:** Like AIDS.
- **IDDs**
  - CMI deficiency disease: Like neutropenia, leukemia, Di George syndrome, chronic mucocutaneous candidiasis etc.
  - Combined immunodeficiency of AMI & CMI: Like SCID (Severe Combined Immuno Deficiency).
- **Malnutrition:** Malnutrition due to deficiency of vitamins like B_6, folic acid & minerals like zinc or iron etc.

c. **Environmental factors:** Common in developing countries.

✪ **Clinical features:** Two types of disease.

i. **Infectious disease:** Following groups

a. **Cutaneous (skin + appendages):**
1. Generalised skin infection.
2. Intertriginous: Skin folds infection.

3. Paronychia: Nail folds infection.
4. Onychomycosis **[fig.-4(a)]**: Nail infection.
5. Diaper dermatitis [diaper rash or napkin candidiasis, **[fig.-4(b)]**: Macula-papular skin rash in infant by using wet diaper which may form vesicles or pustules.
6. Candidal granuloma: Chronic granulomatous lesion with giant cells over face, trunk, scalp or legs.

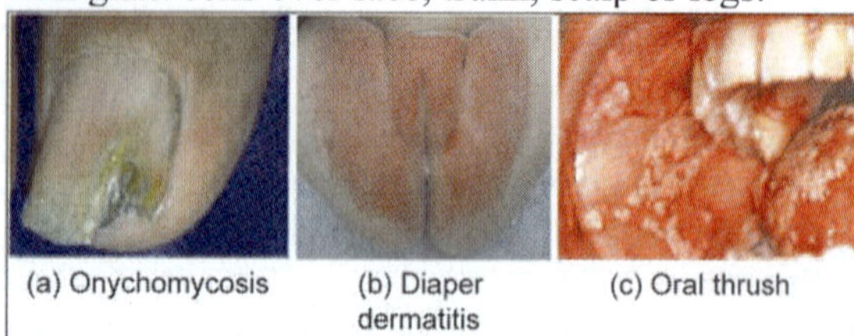

(a) Onychomycosis (b) Diaper dermatitis (c) Oral thrush

Figure-4: Types of candidiasis

b. Mucosal:
1. Oral: Thrush **[fig.-4(c)]**, glossitis, cheilitis & stomatitis.
2. GIT: Oesophagitis & gastritis.
3. Genital: Balanitis, balanoposthitis & vulvovaginitis.
4. Respiratory mucosa: Tracheitis & bronchitis.

c. Systemic:
1. CNS: Meningitis & encephalitis.
2. Respiratory: Pneumonia.
3. Urinary tract: Urethritis.
4. CVS: Endocarditis, candidemia (*Candida* infection of blood).
5. Bone & Joint: Arthritis & osteomyelitis.
6. Eye: Keratitis & endophtalmitis.
7. Ear: Otomycocsis.
8. Nosocomial infection also occurs.

ii. Allergic diseases:
- **Called 'id' reaction** or **candidids.**
- Present with eczema, utricaria, asthma, gastritis or irritable bowel syndrome.

➢ **Laboratory diagnosis:**

✪ **Specimens:** Urine, CSF, blood, discharges, mucosal biopsy etc.

✪ **Testing:**

A. Microscopy:

i. Wet mount preparation:

a. Direct 10% KOH:
- **Morphology:** Round or oval budding yeast cells with pseudohyphae as shown in **fig.-5.**

ii. Differential stains:

a. Microbiological stains:
- **Gram stain:** Looks gram positive in nature, round or oval budding yeast cells with pseudohyphae **(fig.-6).**

B. Culture:
- **Routine media:** SDA with antibiotics.
- **Selective media:** Used to differentiate *Candida* spp.
- Tetrazolium reduction medium.
- Chrom agar.
- **Chlamydospores producing media:** Deficiency of nutrition allows the spore production. They are produced at 20^{0}C. Chlamydospores producing media are
- Cornmeal or cornmeal tween agar.
- Rice starch agar.
- **Cultivation technique:** Follow chapter → Laboratory diagnosis of fungal infections (section →flow chart-1)
- **C/Cs on SDA:** Creamy-white colonies on SDA **(fig.-7).**
- **Identification of culture growth by LCB/PHOL stain:** Round or oval budding yeast cells with pseudohyphae are noticed.

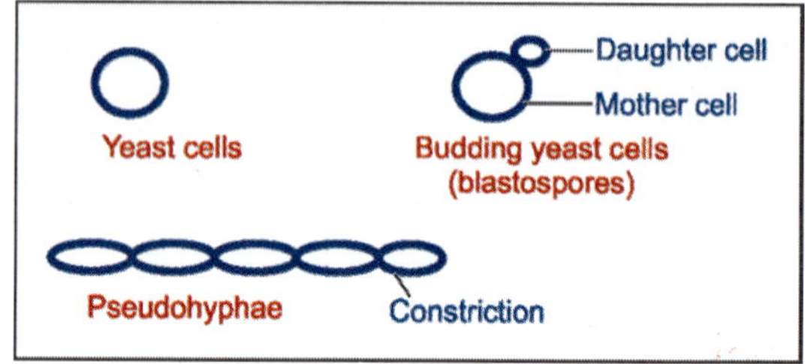

Figure-5: Morphology of Candida

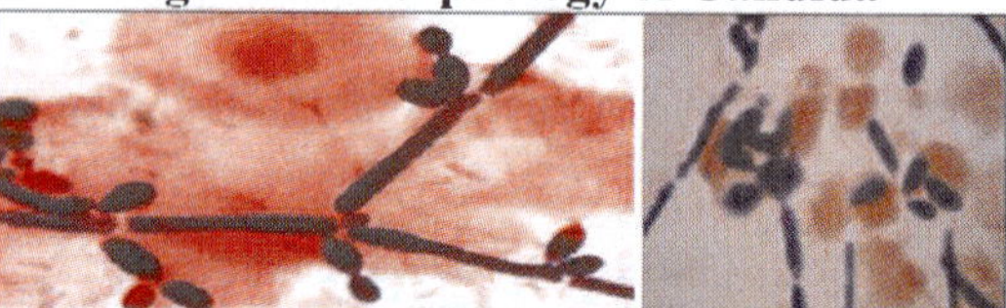

Figure-6: *Candida* under gram stain

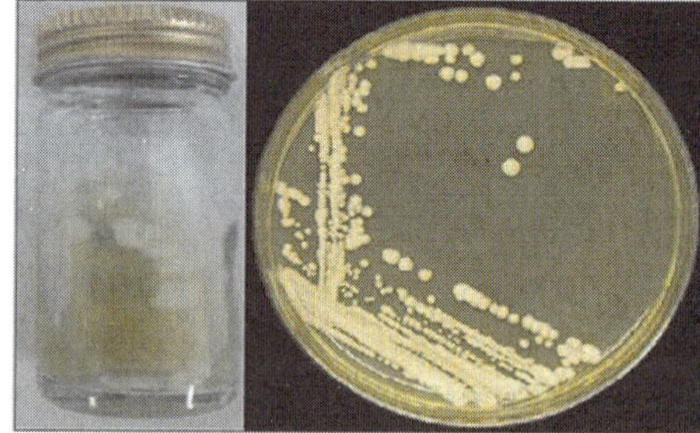

Figure-7: *Candida* on SDA in bottle & petri dish

C. Biochemical reactions (B/Rs):

i. Sugar fermentation & assimilation test: To differentiate the *Candida* species & other yeast or yeast like fungi.

D. Serological test: Like ELISA, precipitation, RIA, CFT, agglutination etc.

E. Molecular method:
- **Advantages:** High sensitivity & specificity.
- **Disadvantages:** High cost & not available in peripheral centre.
- **Methods:** DNA probe, hybridisation & PCR.

F. Skin test: Based on DTH.

G. Animal inoculation: Laboratory animals like rabbits, guinea pig etc. are useful.

H. Gag Liquid Chromatography: To detect the fungal metabolites like D-arabinitol & D-mannose.

I. Special tests:

i. **Teased mount:**
ii. **Slide culture:**
iii. **Cellophane tape mount:**
iv. **Germ tube test:**
v. **Dalmau plate culture:**

} **Follow chapter → Laboratory diagnosis of fungal infections**

J. **Antifungal sensitivity test:** Report the result with antifungal sensitivity pattern.

➢ **Prevention:**
- Removal of precipitating factors mentioned earlier.
- Appropriate antifungal drugs to prevent the deep seated infections.

➢ **Treatment:** Three types of treatment.

A. **Local chemotherapy:** Local oral or mucocutaneous lesions are treated by applying
- 1% gentian violet.
- Nystatin.
- Azole cream.

B. **Systemic chemotherapy:** Intravenous AMB with flucytosine for systemic candidiasis. Oesophageal & vulvovaginal candidisis is treated by oral fluconazole.

C. **Immunotherapy:**
- Candidiasis in blood is common in patient with neutropenia.
- Immunotherapy by using cytokines like G-CSF & GM-CSF is useful, which activate the neutrophils against *Candida* species.

II. Dermatophytoses

➢ **Synonym:**
- Tinea
- Ring worm

➢ **Definitions:**

✪ **Dematophytoses:** Superficial fungal infections of skin, hairs & nails caused by dermatophytes **called dermatophytoses.**

✪ **Dematomycoses:** Infections of skin due to different fungi like *Candida* & by cutaneous manifestation of deep mycoses **called dermatomycoses.**

➢ **Etiological agents:** Caused by dermatophytes which are classified in different groups.

A. **Systemic classification:** Three different genera & around 42 species. →**Table-1 & fig.-5.**

B. **Ecological types:** Based on habitat **(flow chart-1)**

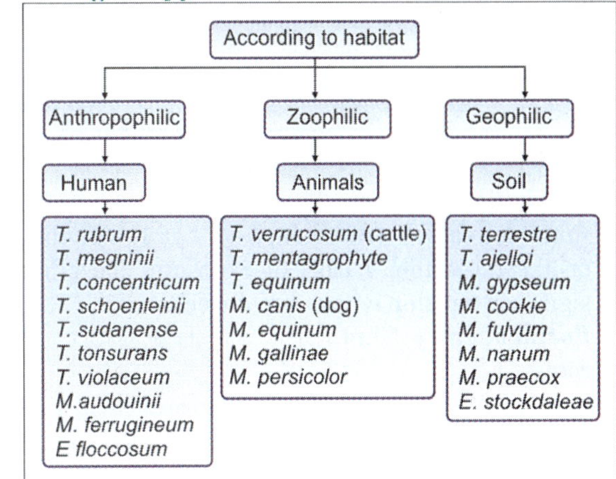

Flow chart-1: Ecological types of dermatophytes

➢ **Pathogenicity:**

✪ **Reservoir & source of infection:** It present on all living (human, animal) & non-living objects (soil, water, materials available at barber's shop etc.) or fomites. All such objects are the sources of infection.

✪ **Mode of transmission:**
- It present on all living & non-living objects or fomites. Transmitted by direct contact with such objects or fomites. Hyphae then penetrate the stratum corneum.
- Zoonotic infection by zoophilic fungi due to direct contact with animals.
- *T. capitis* transferred from barbershop by sharing the common materials like scissors, razor, blade & headrest. Headrest of vehicle also transmits the *T. capitis.*

Genus	***Trichophyton*** **[fig. 8 (a) & (d)]**	***Microsporum*** **[fig. 8(b) & (e)]**	***Epidermophyton*** **[fig. 8(c)]**
Species	*T. mentagrophytes* *T. violaceum, T. schoenleinii* *T, verrucosum, T. rubrum*	*M. gypseum,* *M. canis* *M. audounii, M.nanum*	*E. floccosum* *E. stockdaleae*
Habitat	Skin, hair & nail	Skin & hair (no nail)	Skin & nail (no hair)
C/Cs on SDA	Powdery, velvety or waxy with pigmentation	Cottony, powdery or velvety with white-brown pigments	Powdery & greenish yellow
Macroconidia	Rare, thin-smooth wall & blunt pencil end in shape	Numerous, thick-rough wall, pointed end & boat shape	Numerous, smooth wall & club shape
Microconidia	Abudant & grapes like arrangement	Scanty	Absent

Table-1: Systemic classification & differences between genera of dermatophytes

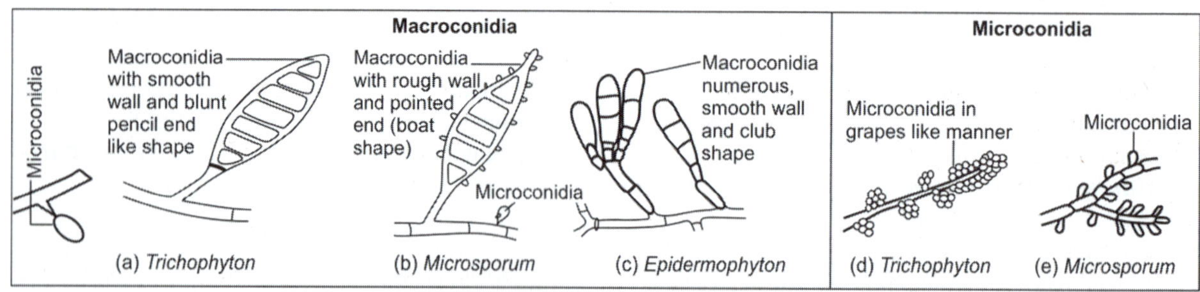

Figure-8: Macroconidia & microconidia in dermatophytes

- **Incubation period:** Fluorescence produced by some dermatophytes, such as *M. canis*, can appear on the fur within 7 days of exposure, and clinical signs can develop within 2 to 4 weeks.
- **Portal of entry:** Skin.
- **Sites:**
  - Skin of scalp, moustache area, beard area, chest, shoulder, neck, groin, perineum & plantar aspect of foot, toes, interdigital web space.
  - Nail.
  - Hair.
- **Precipitating factors (epidemiological determinants):**

a. Agent factors (virulence factors):

1. **Keratophilic:** Grow only in dead keratinised tissues.
2. **Enzymes:** Keratinases, elastase & collagenase helps in fungal invasion.
3. **Fungal metabolites:** Produces erythema, vesicles & pustules. When hyphae becomes old, they breakdown to release the arthrospores which clears the central ringworm lesions.
4. **Antigens:** Produce allergic reaction **called id reaction** or **dermatophytid.**

b. Host factors:

1. Excessive Sweating.
2. Tight fitting garments like socks & underwear.
3. Poor hygiene.
4. Trauma.

c. Environmental factors: As per differences in the environmental condition species of dermatophytes shows the different geographical distribution as follows.

- **South Pacific, Couth & Central America:** *T. tonsurans* & *T. concentricum.*
- **Other Western countries:** *T. rubrum* & *M. canis*
- **Central & West Africa:** *T. sudanense, T .gourvilii* & *T. yaoundei.*
- **European countries:** *M. canis* & *T. mentagrophytes.*
- **Japan:** *M. ferrugineum.*
- **New Zealand & Australia:** *T. rubrum* & *M. distortum.*
- **India:** *T. rubrum, T. mentagrophytes* & *E. floccosum.*

- **Pathogenesis:** Fungus grows only in dead keratinised tissues & releases fungal metabolites which help in invasion & also for allergic reactions.
- **Clinical features:** Two types of disease.

i. Infectious diseases: Following groups

a. Tinea capitis: Scalp infection with following variants (**fig.-9**).

1. Kerion:

- **Kerion** (**Greek**) means **honeycomb.**
- Inflammatory boggy mass on scalp with multiple sinuses sometimes may discharge the mycetoma like grains.
- Mostly caused by *T. mentagrophytes* & *T. verrucosum.*

2. Favus (tinea favosa):

- **Favus** (**Latin**) means **honeycomb**
- Honeycomb like fungal growth within hair follicles of scalp may produces cup like crusts (scutula), alopecia & scarring.
- Mostly caused by *T. schoenleinii* & rarely by *T. violaceum* & *M. gypseum.*

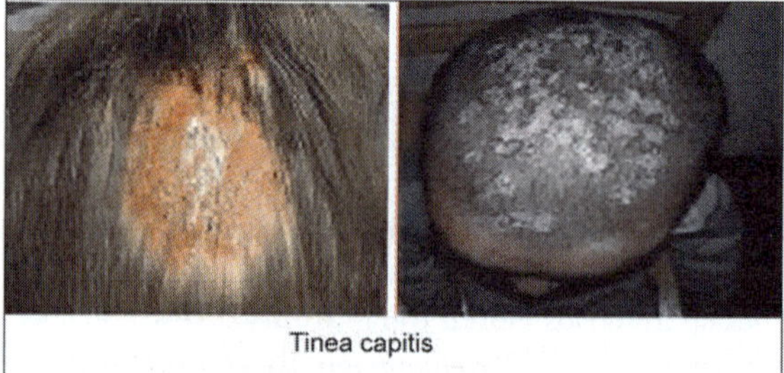

Tinea capitis

Figure-9: Tinea capitis

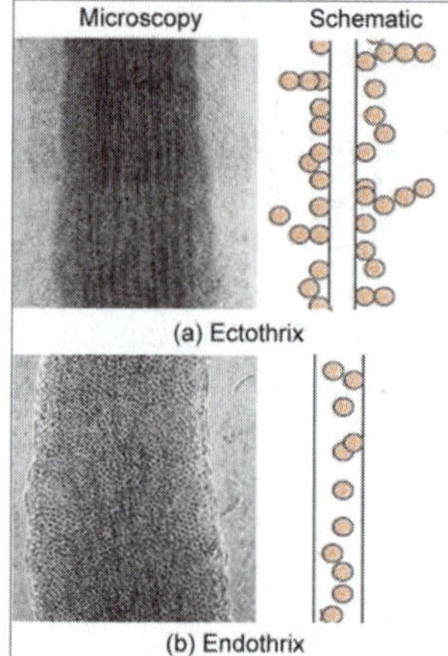

Figure-10: Ectothrix & Endothrix hair infection

3. Black dot:
- Endothrix type of invasion of fungus in hair shaft with abundant sporulation.
- It produces breakage of hair from scalp surfaces & black dot formation over the surface.
- Mostly caused by *T. tonsurans* & *T. violaceum*.

4. Ectothrix hair infection: →Fig.-10 (a)
- Presence of arthrospores appears as mosaic or in chain outer to the hair shaft.
- Mostly caused by *T. mentagrophytes, T, verrucosum, M. gypseum, M. canis* & *M. audouinii.*

5. Endothrix hair infection: →Fig.-10(b)
- Presence of arthrospores inside the hair shaft.
- Mostly caused by *T. schoenleinii, T. violaceum* & *T. tonsurans.*

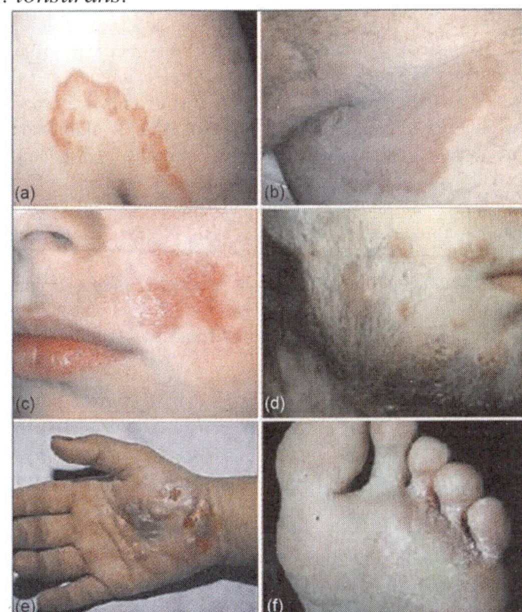

Figure-11: (a) Tinea corporis (b) Tinea cruris (c) Tinea faciei (d) Tinea barbae (e) Tinea mannum (f) Tinea pedis

b. Tinea corporis (tinea glabrosa): Infection in non-hairy skin like trunk & limbs [**fig.-11(a)**] caused by *T. rubrum.*

c. Tinea cruris (jock itch):
- Infection of groin & perineum area [**fig.-11(b)**]. Itching is predominant feature.
- Caused by *T. rubrum* & *E. floccosum*

d. Tinea faciei: Infection of facial skin excluding beard area [**fig.-11(c)**].

e. Tinea barbe (barber's itch): Infection of beard & moustache area [**fig.-11(d)**] of skin. Mostly by *T. verrucosum*, *T. mentagrophytes* & rare by *M. canis* & *T. rubrum.*

f. Tinea mannum: Infection of palm [**fig.-11(e)**] caused by *T. rubrum, T. mentagrophytes* & *E. floccosum.*

g. Tinea pedis (athlet's foot):
- Infection of plantar aspect of foot, toes & interdigital web space [**fig.-11(f)**].
- It mostly occurs in athletes (like football player) & person wearing shoes for long time.
- It is precipitated by warmth & moisture produce by shoes.
- Caused by *T. rubrum, T. mentagrophytes* & *E. floccosum.*

h. Tinea imbricata:
- Concentric rings of papulo squamous scales produce intense pruritus which may leads to lechnification.
- Caused by *T. concentricum.*

i. Tinea gladiatorum:
- Occurs in wrestlers on areas like chest, shoulder & neck directly comes in contact with infected wrestler.
- Caused by *T. tonsurans.*

j. Tinea incognito: Occurs due to steroid therapy.

k. Tinea unguium: Infection of nail.

ii. Allergic diseases:
- **Called 'id' reaction** or **dermatophytid.**
- Present in two forms.

1. Lichen scrofulosorum-like.
2. Pompholyx-like.

➢ **Differential diagnosis:**

1. Leprosy.
2. Secondary syphilis.
3. Psoriasis.
4. Eczema.
5. Lichen planus.
6. Alopecia.
7. Contact dermatitis.

➢ **Laboratory diagnosis:**

✪ **Wood's lamp examination:**
- Made up with barium silicate & nickel oxide.
- It transmits the UV light which produces fluorescence by some fungi & by some bacteria.

1. **Bright green:** *M. audounii, M. ferruginium, M. canis* & *Pseudomonas* in burns wound.
2. **Dull green:** *T. schoenleinii.*
3. **Dull yellow:** *M. gypseum.*

✪ **Specimens:** Skin, hair & nail.

✪ **Testing:**

A. Microscopy:

i. Wet mount preparation:

a. Direct 10% KOH:
- **Subtypes:**

1. **Slide method:** Useful for thin samples like epidermal scales, skin scraping, hair etc
2. **Tube method:** Useful for thick samples like nail,

- **Morphology:** Hyaline septate hyphae with arthrospores **(fig.-12).**

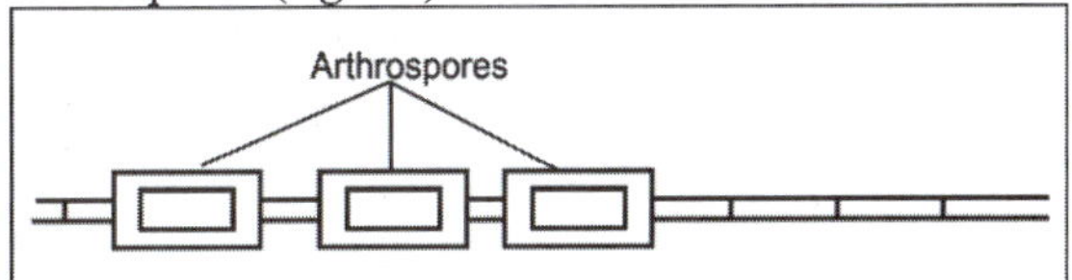

Figure-12: Arthrospores

ii. **Differential stains:**
a. **Microbiological stains:** Rarely useful.
b. **Histopathological stains:** For nail.
- PAS stain.
- GGMS stain.

iii. **Fluorescent Microscopy (FM) & staining:**

B. **Culture:**
- **Routine media:** SDA with antibiotics.
- **Selective media:**
  - Dermatophyte test medium: Red colony.
  - Dermatophyte identification medium: Purple colony.
- **Cultivation technique:** **Follow chapter → Laboratory diagnosis of fungal infections** (section →flow chart-1)
- **C/Cs on SDA: → Table-1**
- **Identification of culture growth by LCB/PHOL stain:**
  - Macroconidia & microconidia are identified as described in **table-1.**
  - Also there is presence of racquet hypha, knot organ, spiral hypha, fevic chanderlier & pectinate body **as described in chapter → General properties of fungus.**

C. **Biochemical reaction (B/Rs):**
i. **Urease test:** To differentiate the *T. mentagrophytes* (+Ve) from *T. Rubrum* (-Ve).

D. **Serological tests:** Like immunodiffusion test.

E. **Molecular method:**
- **Advantages:** High sensitivity & specificity.
- **Disadvantages:** High cost & not available in peripheral centre.
- **Methods:** DNA probe, hybridisation & PCR.

F. **Skin test:** Based on DTH.

G. **Animal inoculation:** Guinea pig is useful.

H. **Special tests:**
i. **Teased mount:**
ii. **Slide culture:**
iii. **Cellophane tape mount:**
iv. **Hair bait technique:**
v. **Hair perforation test:**

} **Follow chapter → Laboratory diagnosis of fungal infections**

➢ **Prevention:**
- Improvement of hygiene.
- Live spore vaccine, killed hyphal vaccine cell wall vaccine & soluble cytoplasmic extract vaccine of *T. mentagrophytes* var. *erinacei* had been studies in guinea pig. Out of this live spore vaccine produces the immunity as like natural infection.

➢ **Treatment:** Two types of treatment.

A. **Local:**
- Whitefield ointment.
- Tolnaftate.
- Azole creame.

B. **Systemic:** 500 mg oral griseiofulvin is given two divided doses for 3-6 months. A single dose of 2g is given in tinea capitis. Ketoconazole is also useful.

Question bank

Case study

1) In HIV-AIDS patient, gram stain of lung aspirate shows the yeast like morphology. Identify the organism & answer the following
a) Name the most common causative agent & draw the diagram of morphology of causative agent in given case.
b) Describe the virulence factors of causative agent.
c) Write the clinical manifestation of causative agent.
d) Write the laboratory diagnosis of causative agent.

2) A 50 year HIV +Ve female visit the medical OPD with complain of ulcer on oral cavity. Oral examination rule out white patches over tongue & other part of oral mucosa. Tissue taken from ulcer & proceed by gram stain & culture on corn meal agar. Gram stain revealed budding yeast cell with pseudohyphae & corn meal agar produces the chlamydospores. Identify the organism & answer the following
a) Name clinical infection (disease) & the most common causative agent of it.
b) Write two selective & two spore producing media of causative agent.
c) Write the clinical classification of fungi with examples in each category.
d) Write in details about pathogenicity of causative agent in given case.

3) A 25 year football player visit the surgical OPD with complains of ulcer on plantar aspect of foot. It is suspected as dermatophyte type lesion on clinical examination. Tissue taken from ulcer & proceed with culture on sabouraud's agar, which revealed smooth wall pencil shaped macroconidia & plenty of microconidia. Identify the organism & answer the following
a) Name clinical infection (disease) & the most common causative agent of it.
b) Name four fungi causing infection in to toe nail.
c) Write the differences between different genera of dermatophytes.
d) Write in details about pathogenicity of causative agent.
e) Write the laboratory diagnosis of causative agent.

Essay/Full question

1) Superficial mycoses.

Short notes

1) Malassezia infections.
2) Tinea nigra.
3) Piedra.
4) Onychomycosis.
5) Candidiasis.
6) Dermatophytoses.

Short questions for theory/viva questions

1) Write four examples of surface mycoses.
2) What is onychomycoses? Name two etiological agents.
3) Define: Dermatophytoses & dermatomycoses.
4) What is chlamydospore? Name two chlamydospores producing media.

5) Write four differences between *Trichophyton & Microsporum / Trichophyton & Epidermophyton / Epidermophyton & Microsporum*
6) What is clinical cure & mycological cure of onychomycoses?
7) Name the one example of each lipophilic, halophilic, keratophilic & hydrophilic fungus.

MCQs for chapter review

Surface mycoses

1) Ptyriasis versicolor is caused by
(a) *E. flocossum* (b) *M. gypseum* (c) *M. furfur* (d) *T. tonsurans*

2) Which of the following are difficult to isolates from culture
(a) *Candida* (b) Dermatophytes (c) *Cryptococcus* (d) *Malassezia furfur* (e) Coccidioidomycosis

3) Selenium sulphide is indicated for
(a) Tinea versicolor (b) Tinea corporis (c) Mixed mycotic infections (d) Candidiasis only

4) Black piedra is produced by
(a) *Piedra hortae* (b) *Trichsporon beigelii* (c) *Hortae werneckii* (d) *Malassezia furfur*

5) White piedra is produced by
(a) *Piedra hortae* (b) *Pityrosporum orbicularae* (c) *Hortae werneckii* (d) *Trichsporon beigelii*

Cutaneous mycoses

6) True about *Candida albicans* is (AIIMS, May-94)
(a) *Candida* is pathogenic to mice (b) Its growth is inhibited by Griseofulvin (c) *Candida* shows mycelia and chlamydospores on corn meal agar (d) *Candida* is present in normal faeces

7) The following is not true of *Candida albicans* is (AI-92)
(a) Yeast like fungus (b) Forms chlamydospores (c) Blastomere is seen in isolates (d) Causes meningitis in immunocompromised

8) *Candida albicans* causes all of the following except (AI 95)
(a) Endocarditis (b) Mycetoma (c) Meningitis (d) oral thrush

9) Which fungal infection is common in neutropenia (AIIMS -99)
(a) *Candida* (b) *Histoplasma* (c) *Aspergillus niger* (d) *Aspergillus fumigates*

10) Most common fungal infection in febrile neutropenia is (AI -01)
(a) *Aspergillus niger* (b) *Candida* (c) Mucormycosis (d) *Aspergillus fumigates*

11) *Candida albicans* infection is predisposed by all except (AIIMS, Sept-96)
(a) Menstruation (b) Diabetes (c) Minipill users (d) Combined pill users

12) Candidiasis is associated with all except
(a) Oral contraceptive pill (OCP) (b) IUCD user (c) Diabetes (d) Pregnancy

13) *Candida* has predilection for all except
(a) Diabetes (b) Extreme of age (c) Athletes (d) Pregnant female

14) *Candida* is most implicated in causation
(a) Conjunctivitis (b) Tinea capitis (c) Desert rheumatism (d) Thrush

15) Which of the following disease is endogenous in origin (PGI-80)
(a) Aspergillosis (b) Candidiasis (c) Phycomycosis (d) All of the above

16) Which of the following fungus does not infect hair
(a) *Trichohyton* (b) *Microsporum* (c) *Epidermophyton* (d) *Trichosporon*

17) Dermatophytes not infecting nail is
(a) *Trichohyton* (b) *Microsporum* (c) *Epidermophyton* (d) *Trichosporon*

18) Dermatophytes infecting
(a) Subcutaneous tissue (b) Systemic organs (c) Nails, hair and skin (d) Superficial skin and deeper tissue

19) Which of the following infecting hair, akin and nail
(a) *Trichohyton* (b) *Microsporum* (c) *Epidermophyton* (d) None of above

20) Trichohyton species which is zoophilic
(a) *T. tonsurans* (b) *T. violaceum* (c) *T. mentagrophytes* (d) *T. schoenleinii,*

21) Which of the following is spread from animals to man (AI -92)
(a) *T. rubrum* (b) *T. tonsurans* (c) *E. flocossum* (d) *T verrucosum*

22) Which of the following does not produces dermatophytosis in India (PGI, Nov-13, Dec-04)
(a) *T. rubrum* (b) *T. mentagrophytes* (c) *Microsporum distortum* (d) *Epidermophyton flocossum*

23) Most common cause of tinea capitis
(a) *M canis* (b) *Epidermophyton flocossum* (c) *T tonsurans* (d) *M distortum*

24) Kerion is caused by (PGI-98)
(a) *Candida* (b) *Streptococcus* (c) Dermatophytes (d) Herpes

25) Black dot ring worm is caused by
(a) *Microsporum* (b) *Trichohyton* (c) *Epidermophyton* (d) *Candida*

26) T capitis (endothrix) is caused by (PGI, Dec-00)
(a) *Epidermophyton* (b) *T. tonsurans* (c) *T. violaceum* (d) *Microsporum* (e) *T. rubrum*

27) Tinea cruris is caused by (PGI-97)
(a) Epidermophyton (b) Trichohyton (c) Microsporum (d) *Candida*

28) Dermatophytids are
(a) Fungal hyphae in skin (b) Vegetative fungal cells in keratinised tissue (c) Cutaneous lesions secondary to hypersensitivity to fungal antigens (d) Dead fungal tissue

Answers of MCQs & explanation

1) (c)
- Ptyriasis versicolor is a type of surface mycosis caused by *M. furfur* while *E. flocossum*, *M. gypseum* & *T. tonsurans* are the dermatophytes causing cutaneous mycosis.

2) (d), **3) (a)** — Follow section, **surface mycosis (*Malassezia* infections)** for explanation

4) (a), **5) (d)** — Follow section, **surface mycosis** for the explanation of all options & disease produced by all given fungus.

6) (c) & (d)
- *Candida* is human pathogen with endogenous origin
- Systemic chemotherapy of candidiasis includes intravenous AMB with flucytosine for systemic candidiasis. Eosophageal & vulvovaginal candidisis is treated by oral fluconazole.

7) (c)
- Blastomere is the segmented embryo present in the egg of hook worm parasites like *Ancyclostoma duodenale* & *Nectar americanus*

8) (b), **9) (a)**, **10) (b)**, **11) (a)**, **12) (b)**, **13) (c)**, **14) (d)**, **15) (b)** — Follow section, **cutaneous mycosis (candidiasis)**

16) (c), **17) (b)**, **18) (c)**, **19) (a)** — Follow section, **table-1** for explanation

20) (c), **21) (d)** — Follow **flow chart-1** for explanation

22) (c)

- Follow section, **cutaneous mycosis (dermatophytosis → pathogenicity → precipitating factors → environmental factors)** for explanation

23) (c)
24) (c)
25) (b)
26) (b) &(c)

Follow section, **cutaneous mycosis (dermatophytosis → pathogenicity → clinical features → tinea capitis)** for explanation

27) (a) & (b)

- Follow section, **cutaneous mycosis (dermatophytosis → pathogenicity → clinical features → tinea cruris)** for explanation

28) (c)

- Follow section, **cutaneous mycosis (dermatophytosis → pathogenicity → clinical features → allergic diseases)** for explanation

78 Deep mycoses

Learning heading & subheadings

- Definition
- Classification:
  - Subcutaneous mycoses
  - Systemic mycoses
  - Opportunistic mycoses

Definition: Fungal infections present in the tissues below the skin & in different systems **called deep mycoses.**

Classification: Three subtypes like subcutaneous mycoses, systemic mycoses & opportunistic mycoses.

Subcutaneous mycoses

❖ **Definition:** These are the fungal infections of subcutaneous tissues.

❖ **Properties:** Mostly transmitted by trauma.

❖ **Examples:**

I. **Mycetoma**
II. **Sporotrichosis**
III. **Chromomycosis**
IV. **Rhinosporidiosis & Oculosporidiosis**
V. **Lobomycosis**
VI. **Subcutaneous zygomycosis**

I. Mycetoma

➢ **Synonym:**

✪ **Madurella mycosis**

✪ **Maduramycosis:** As it was 1st diagnosed in Madura district of Tamil Nadu, India by Gill in 1842.

✪ **Madura foot:** Foot lesion of mycetoma is **called madura foot.**

➢ **Definition:** Chronic granulomatous lesion of subcutaneous & deeper tissues with multiple sinuses, discharging pus or granules.

➢ **Etiological agents:** Two etiological types.

A. **Actinomycetoma:** Mycetoma caused by bacteria.

i. **Aerobic bacteria:**

- *Nocardia asteroids*
- *N. brasiliensis*
- *N. caviae*
- *Streptomyces somaliensis*
- *Actinomadura madurae*

} Yellowish-white colour grains

- *Actinomadura pelletieri:* Red colour grains. It is the most common cause of Mycetoma in India in West coast.
- *Nocardiopsis dassonvillei*: Cream colour grains.

ii. **Anaerobic bacteria:**

- *Actinomyces israelii*
- *Actinomyces bovis*

} Yellowish **called sulfur granules**

B. **Eumycetoma (mycotic mycetoma):** Mycetoma caused by fungus.

i. **Black grains fungi:**

- *Madurella mycetomatis.*
- *Madurella grisea.*
- *Exophiala* (formerly *Phialophora*) *jeanselmei.*
- *Cuvularia geniculata.*

ii. **White grains fungi:**

- *Pseudoallescheria boydii.*
- *Aspergillus nidulus.*
- *Acremonium falciforme.*
- *Fusarium graminiarum.*

➢ **Pathogenicity:**

✪ **Reservoir & source of infection:** Fungus present in soil or wooden sticks.

✪ **Mode of transmission:** By trauma or thorn prick injury which allows the entry of microbes.

✪ **Portal of entry:** Skin

✪ **Sites:** Most commonly on foot **[fig.-1(a)]**, but also present on hands, shoulders, scalp or buttocks.

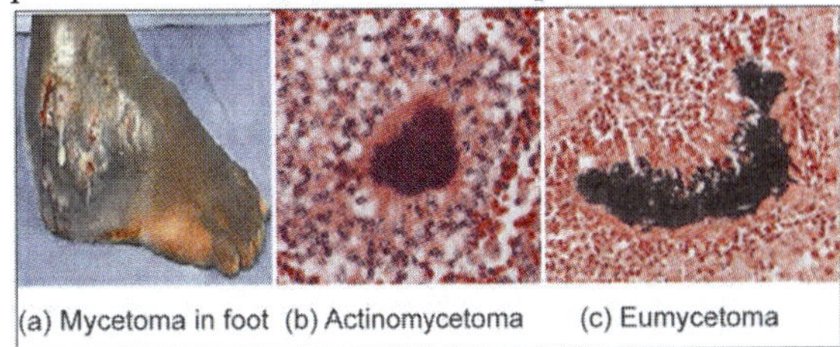

(a) Mycetoma in foot (b) Actinomycetoma (c) Eumycetoma

Figure-1: Mycetoma

✪ **Precipitating factors (epidemiological determinants):**

1. **Occupation:** common in farmers, carpenters & field workers.
2. **Age:** In adults between 20-40 years.
3. **Sex:** More in male.
4. **Areas:** More in rural areas than urban.
5. **Poor hygiene:**

✪ **Pathogenesis:** Mycetoma is present with granulomatous lesions & sinus that discharging the granules. Granules, centrally contains organism (bacteria or fungi) which looks gram positive surrounded by deposition of Ag-Ab complex in periphery which looks gram negative.

✪ **Clinical features:** Lesion is painless. It is a triad of

- Granulomatous swelling (tumefaction).
- Sinus.
- Discharge of grains or granules. Grains are different in colour according to causative agent as mentioned earlier. Pus discharge is present due to secondary bacterial infections.

✪ **Complications:**

- Secondary bacterial infections.
- Local spread occus in surrounging tissues like involvement of underlying fasciae & bones causing osteolytic or osteosclerotic bony lesions. No lymphatic or blood spread in distant sites.
- Recurrence after treatment.

➢ **Differential diagnosis:**

1. Leprosy.
2. Benign tumour.
3. Botryomycosis.
4. Actinomycosis.
5. Dermatophytosis.
6. Granuloma.
7. Tuberculosis.

➢ **Laboratory diagnosis:**

✪ **Specimens:** Grains, discharge or tissue from lesion.

✪ **Testing:**

A. Macroscopic:

- Colour: → **Follow etiological agents**
- Consistency & size: Thin & < 1μm in actinomycetes while thick & larger in mycetoma.

B. Microscopy:

- KOH, gram stain, modifies ZN stain (for *Nocardia* spp.) & histopathological stains are useful.
- Actinomycetoma **[fig.-1(b)]** is identified by filamentous gram positive bacilli. Granule contains, centrally gram positive filaments (due to bacterial colonies) & peripherally gram negative materials (due to Ag-Ab complex by host defence mechanism) giving club shape or sun ray appearance.
- Eumycetoma **[fig.-1(c)]** is identified by hypha & spore formation.

C. Culture: It is done for bacteria & fungus.

- Actinomycetoma: BHIA, LJ medium or blood agar
- Eumycetoma: SDA with antibiotics. Cultivation technique is same as like other fungi.

D. Serological tests: Like ELISA, precipitation, RIA, CFT, agglutination etc.

E. Skin test: Also a useful test.

F. Animal inoculation: Guinea pig & mice are useful.

G. Special tests: Like slide culture, teased mount are useful for identification of fungus.

➢ **Prevention:**

- Improvement of hygiene.
- Avoiding traumatic injury.
- Removal of risk factors.
- Health education.

➢ **Treatment:**

- Surgical removal of lesion.
- Eumycetoma: Poor response to antifungal drugs. Useful drugs are ketoconazole, itraconazole or AMB.
- Actinomycetoma is treated by Welsh regimen (co-trimoxazole & amikacin).
- Recurrence is common after treatment.

II. Sporotrichosis

➢ **Synonym:** Rose Gardner's or rose thorn disease, because it can be spread by rose.

➢ **Definition:** It is a chronic pyogranulomatous lesion of skin & subcutaneous tissues which may be fixed or spread to lymph nodes or other organs.

➢ **Etiological agent:**

- *Sprothrix schenckii.*
- It is a dimorphic fungi which grow as yeast phase at 37^0C in tissue & as mycelial phase at 22^0C in environment.

➢ **Pathogenicity:**

✪ **Reservoir & source of infection:** Fungi found as saprobes in soil, plants, wood, bark, leaves, straw & other dead materials.

✪ **Mode of transmission:**

- It introduced by trauma by wooden stick.
- Inhalation of conidia may elicit the lung's lesion.

✪ **Incubation period:** 8-30 days (average 3 weeks).

✪ **Portal of entry:** Skin.

✪ **Sites:** Skin, subcutaneous tissue & lymphatics of feet & hands are common sites. Rarely in lungs & in other organs.

✪ **Precipitating factors (epidemiological determinants):**

a. Agent factors (virulence factors):

1. **Fungal dimorphism:** As described in *H capsulatum.*
2. **Enzymes:** Fungus releases the proteinase I (serine proteinase) & proteinase II (aspartic proteinase) which helps in fungal invasion.

b. Host factors:

1. **Age:** Common in young adults.
2. **Sex:** Three times more in males than females due to outdoor job.
3. **Occupation:** Common in person exposed to soil or plants like gardeners, farmers, carpenters, field workers, mine workers, florists & forest workers.

c. Environmental factors:

- Fungus is common in tropical & subtropical countries with high humidity (65%) & moderate temperature (25-28^0C).
- It is reported from Central South America & South Africa.
- In India it is endemic in sub Himalayan holly areas of North - East states ranging from Himachal

Pradesh to Assam. Other endemic areas northern Karnataka & southern Maharashtra.

✪ **Pathogenesis:** Formation of granulomatous lesion with yeast cells in center surrounded by eosinophilic material & Ag-Ab complex deposition **called asteroid body [fig.-2(b)]**. Deposition of eosinophilic material around yeast cells is due to immune phenomenon of body **called Splendore-Hoeppli phenomenon**.

✪ **Clinical features:**

a. **Fixed cutaneous sporotrichosis:**
- Granulomatous nodule at inoculation site in skin & subcutaneous tissue.
- Nodules followed by ulcer & necrosis.
- It is the most common form of sporotrichosis.
- It remains fixed & no spread by lymph, hence **called 'fixed cutaneous sporotrichosis'.** It is common in endemic areas like Mexico, where peoples show the strong immunity against it.

b. **Lymphocutaneous sporotrichosis:**
- Cutaneous lesion spread along to course of lymphatic vessels to lymph node **called 'lymphocutaneous sporotrichosis'.**
- Enlarged lymph nodes extending centripetally, like beaded chain **[fig.-2(a)]**.

c. **Pulmonary sporotrichosis:** It may occur as primary infection due to inhalation of conidia.

✪ **Complications:** Very rarely nodules spread by haematogenous route to meninges, brain, bones, joints, kidneys etc. **called 'disseminated sporotrichosis'.**

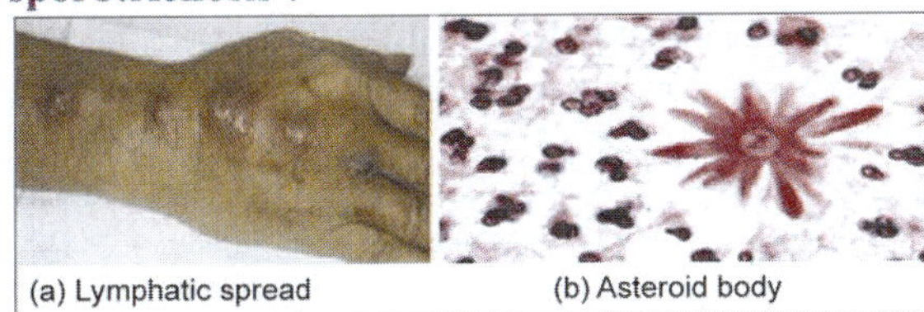

Figure-2: Images of sporotrichosis

➢ **Laboratory diagnosis:**

✪ **Specimens:** Skin scraping, discharge or tissue from granulomatous lesion.

✪ **Testing:**

A. **Microscopy:**

i. **Wet mount preparation:**

a. **Direct 10% KOH :**
- **Yeast phase morphology:**
- It present as round, spherical yeast cells or as cigar shaped body as shown in **fig.-3(a).**

ii. **Differential stains:**

a. **Gram stain:** Gram positive yeast cells.

b. **Histopathological stains:** H &E, PAS & GGMS stain shows asteroid body **[fig.-2(b)].**

B. **Culture:**
- **Routine media:** SDA with antibiotics.
- **Cultivation technique:** Follow chapter → Laboratory diagnosis of fungal infections (section →flow chart-1).
- **C/Cs on SDA:** Creamy-white colony in 2-5 days may turn in to brown-black colour in 10-14 days.
- **Identification of culture growth by LCB/PHOL stain:**

1. **From yeast phase plate:** Round-spherical or cigar shape yeast cell as shown in **fig.-3(a).**
2. **From mycelia phase plate:** Shows hyaline septate hyphae & conidiophores with arrangement of conidia in chain giving **flower like pattern** as shown in **fig.-3(b).**

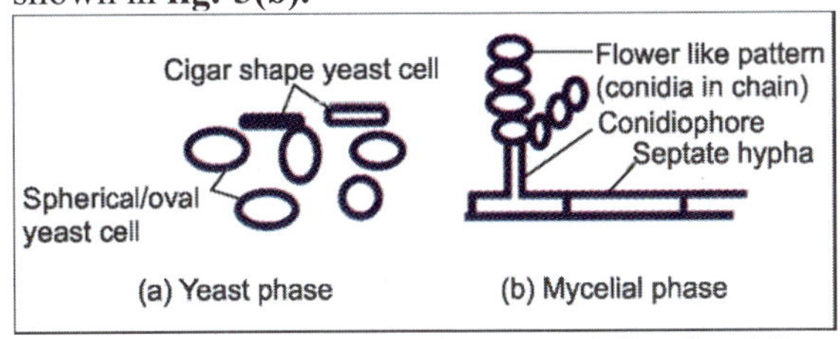

Figure-3: Schematic diagram of *S. schenkii*

C. **Serological tests:** Like agglutination test, CFT, immunodiffusion test etc.

D. **Molecular method:**
- **Advantages:** High sensitivity & specificity.
- **Disadvantages:** High cost & not available in peripheral centre.
- **Methods:** DNA probe, hybridisation & PCR.

E. **Skin test:** By using sporotrichin-Ag of mycelial phase or peptido-rhamno-mannan Ag of yeast phase.

F. **Animal inoculation:** Mice & rats are susceptible.

G. **Special tests:** Teased mount, slide culture cellophane tape mount & exo-antigen tests are useful.

➢ **Prevention:** Preventive measures are same as mycetoma.

➢ **Treatment:**
- Surgical removal of localised lesion.
- Ketoconazole, itraconazole or terbinafine are the drug of choice.
- Fungus is sensitive to temperature above 39^0C, so hyperthermic treatment is successful for disseminated lesions.

III. Chromomycosis

➢ **Meaning:** Chromo = coloured (black) + mycosis = fungal infection (black fungus).

➢ **Definition:** It is a chronic granulomatous infection of skin & subcutaneous tissues caused by black fungi (phaeoid fungi or dematiaceous fungi).

➢ **Etiological agents:** Two variants

A. **Chromoblastomycosis (verrucous dermatitis):**

✪ **Properties:** Caused by yeast phase of fungi & characterised by presence of black yeast cell with dividing septum **called sclerotic bodies** or

muriform cells or **medlar bodies** or **copper pennies bodies** as shown in **fig.-4.** Sclerotic bodies are dark brown, about 5-12μm is size with multiple internal transverse septa, chest nut in appearance, pathognomic features of chromoblastomycosis & not seen in any other phaeoid fugal infection.

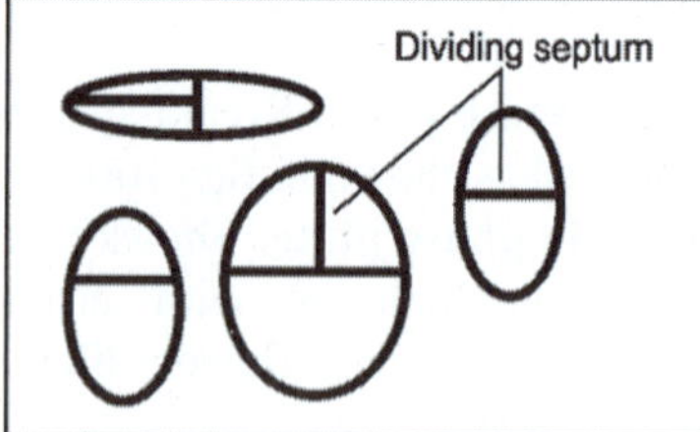

Figure-4: Sclerotic bodies

- **Following fungus are responsible**

1. *Fonsecaea compacta.*
2. *Fonsecaea pedrosoi.*
3. *Phialophora verrucosa.*
4. *Cladophialophora* (formerly *Cladosporium*) *carrionii.*
5. *Rhinocladiella aquaspersa.*

B. Phaeohyphomycosis:

- **Properties:** Caused by mycelial (hyphae) phase of fungi & characterised by presence of black hyphae & no sclerotic bodies.
- **Following fungus are responsible**

1. *Wangiella dermatitidis.*
2. *Exophiala jeanselmei.*
3. *Cladophialophora* (formerly *Cladosporium*) *bantiana.*
4. *Nattrassia magniferae.*

➢ **Pathogenicity:**

- **Reservoir & source of infection:** All fungus found as saprobes in soil, plants, wood, bark, leaves, straw & other dead materials.
- **Mode of transmission:** It introduced by wooden stick injury.
- **Portal of entry:** Skin.
- **Sites:** Skin & subcutaneous tissue of feet & hands are common sites.
- **Precipitating factors (epidemiological determinants):**

1. **Age:** More in young adults.
2. **Sex:** More in males due to outdoor job.
3. **Occupation:** Common in person exposed to soil or plants like gardeners, farmers, carpenters & field workers, mine workers, florists & forest workers.

- **Pathogenesis, clinical features & complication:**

A. Chromoblastomycosis

- Nodular, verrucous, tumoral, plaques & cicatricial skin lesion.
- It raised about 1-3cm above the skin level with irregular surface & gives a cauliflower like appearance **hence called verrucous dermatitis.**
- It shows the presence of sclerotic bodies.
- Not dissemination but local spread may occur.
- Sometimes it produces oral ulcer with local lymphadenopathy.

B. Phaeohyphomycosis:

- Granulomatous lesion with abscess, giant cells & histiocytes.
- Presence of black hyphae.
- Disseminated to other organs (complication).

➢ **Diagnosis:**

- **Specimens:** Skin scraping, discharge or tissue from lesion.
- **Testing:** Microscopy revealed black hyphae & sclerotic bodies, while culture gives black colonies.

➢ **Prevention:** Same as mycetoma.

➢ **Treatment:**

- Surgical removal of localised lesion.
- Flucytosine alone or along with itraconazole or AMB are the drugs of choice.
- Fungus is sensitive to high temperature, so hyperthermic treatment is also an alternate.
- Local application of cryotherapy (liquid nitrogen) or laser therapy is useful.

IV. Rhinosporidiosis & oculosporidiosis

➢ **Meaning:**

- Rhino = nose + sporidiosis = sporozoan infection.
- Oculo = eye + sporidiosis = sporozoan infection.

➢ **Definition:** Chronic pyogranulomatous lesion by *Rhinosporidium* of nose **called rhinosporidiosis** & & of eye **called oculosporidiosis.**

➢ **Etiological agent:** *Rhinosporidium seeberi* → its taxonomical status is uncertain, whether to put in fungus or in parasite.

➢ **Taxonomy:** Taxonomy is unclear & classified as parafungal agent.

➢ **Life cycle:**

- It enters as spore about 6-8μm in size.
- Spores undergoes to form large (200-250μm), thick double wall structure **called sporangium** containing about 12,000-16,000 endospores.
- Sporangium rupture after maturation to release the endospores, produce another infection as shown in **fig.-5**.

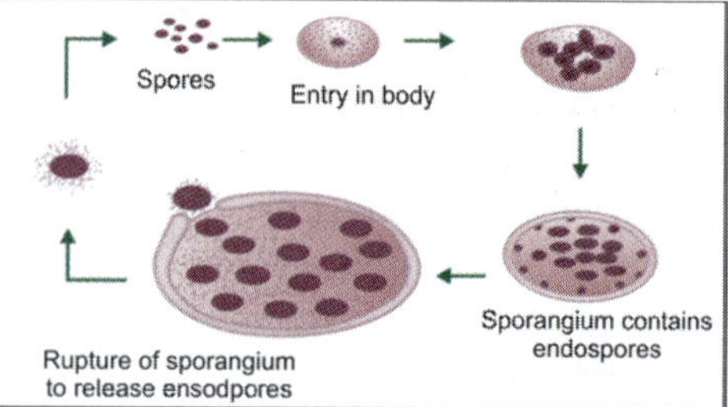

Figure-5: Life cycle of *R. seeberi*

➢ **Pathogenicity:**

- **Reservoir & source of infection:** Water.
- **Mode of transmission:** Hydrophilic fungi habitat in fresh or stagnant water and introduced by direct contact with water.

- **Incubation period:** 1-10 months.
- **Portal of entry:** Nasal or ocular mucosa.
- **Sites:** Nose & eyes.
- **Precipitating factors (epidemiological determinants):**

1. **Age:** No age is exempt but more common between 2nd & 4th decade of life.
2. **Sex:** Male female ratio is 3:1 to 4:1.
3. **IDDs:** It is reported from patient of AIDS.
4. **Distribution:** Endemic areas are South India (coastal areas like Tamil Nadu, Kerala, Andhra Pradesh & Pondicherry) & Sri Lanka. Isolated cases are reported from East Africa, South America, North America & Europe.

- **Pathogenesis & clinical features:**

a. **Rhinosporidiosis:** Chronic granulomatous lesion of nasal cavity characterised by development of polyp. Granuloma contains central sporangium surrounded by inflammatory cell **called spherules**.

b. **Oculosporidiosis:** Chronic granulomatous lesion of eye (more in palpebral conjunctiva & rare in other parts) characterised by development of polyp.

- **Complications:**

- Disseminated lesion in other organs like bone due to blood spread.
- Recurrence after treatment.

➢ **Diagnosis:**

- **Specimens:** Biopsy from lesion.
- **Testing:**

A. **Microscopy:**

- Routine microbiological stains are not useful.
- Histopathological stains like PAS stain, GGMS stain & MGG stain are useful for **spherules**.

B. **Culture & animal inoculation test:** Several attempts has been made for cultivation of *R. seeberi* in cell free media, cell containing media & animal culture, but successful reports are not achieved.

C. **Serological tests & skin test:** Are not useful.

➢ **Prevention:** Same as mycetoma.

➢ **Treatment:**

- Surgical removal of lesion or electro-cauterisation
- Dapsone 100mg orally given for 1 year to prevent the recurrence.
- Antimony compound like neostibasan also given.
- Despite all efforts recurrence is common.

V. Lobomycosis

➢ **Synonym:** Jorge Lobo's disease or Keloidal blastomycosis.

➢ **Definition:** It is chronic granulomatous infection of skin & subcutaneous tissue without involvement of mucosa or deeper tissues.

➢ **Etiological agent:** *Loboa loboi* (*Lacazia loboi*).

➢ **Pathogenicity:**

- **Reservoir & source of infection:** Water.
- **Mode of transmission:** Hydrophilic fungi habitat in water and introduced by direct contact of abraded skin with infected water.
- **Incubation period:** Very long about 2.5 years.
- **Portal of entry:** Skin.
- **Sites:** Skin & subcutaneous tissues of lower limb, ears, upper limb & face.
- **Precipitating factors (epidemiological determinants):**

1. **Age:** More in young adults.
2. **Sex:** More in males due to farm activities. Male to female ratio is 20:1.

- **Pathogenesis:** Formation of granulomatous lesion with yeast cells in center surrounded by eosinophilic material & Ag-Ab complex deposition **called asteroid body**. Deposition of eosinophilic material around yeast cells is due to immune phenomenon of body **called Splendore-Hoeppli phenomenon**.
- **Clinical features:** Chronic granulomatous infection of skin & subcutaneous tissue without involvement of mucosa or deeper tissues which may present as keloid or verrucous type.
- **Complications:**

- Local & lymphatic spread occurs in surrounding tissue while disseminated lesion in other organs likely less.
- Recurrence after treatment.

➢ **Diagnosis:**

- **Specimens:** Biopsy from lesion.
- **Testing:**

A. **Microscopy:**

i. **Wet mount preparation:**

a. **Direct 10% KOH:**

- It present as round, spherical, budding yeast cells.
- Yeast cells are also arranged in chain of 4-7 cells **called blastoconidia** as shown in **fig.-6.**

ii. **Differential stains:**

a. **Gram stain:** Gram positive yeast cells.

b. **Histopathological stains:** Fungi contain melanin & stain by Masson-Fontana stain & show the asteroid body.

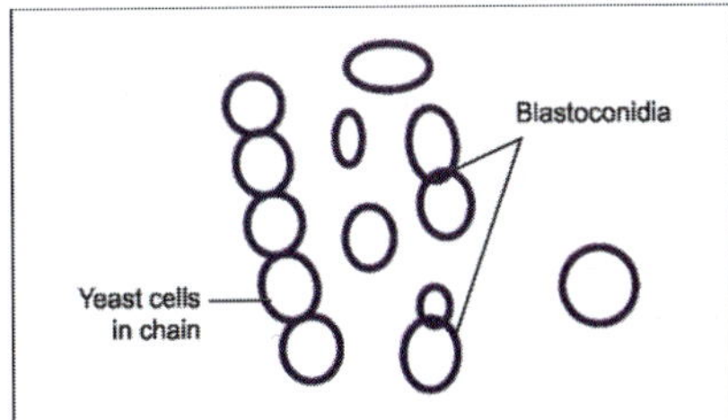

Figure-6: Schematic diagram (yeast cells & blastoconidia) of *L. loboi*

B. **Culture:** It is not cultivated on cell free media.

C. **Serological tests & skin tests:** Are not useful methods.

D. **Animal inoculation:** Mouse is best useful.

➢ **Prevention:** Same as mycetoma.

➢ **Treatment:**
- Surgical removal of localised lesion.
- Clofazimine produced good result in some patient either alone or with itraconazole.

VI. Subcutaneous zygomycosis

➢ **Synonym:** Entomophthoromycosis or Entomophthoramycosis because all the fungi are belong to order *entomopthorales.*

➢ **Meaning: Entomo (Greek) = insect,** because primary pathogens of insect.

Features	*C. coronatus*	*B. ranarum*
Reservoir & source	Both are present on decaying vegetation & in soil & insects	
Mode of transmission	Inhalation of spores	By insect bite
Portal of entry	Mucosa	Skin
Sites	Nose, paranasal sinuses, lips	Trunk & buttocls
Precipitating factors	Both are opportunistic fungi, cause infection only in immunodeficient persons.	
Pathogenesis	Eosinophulic infiltration occurs around centrall located hyphae in both fungus **called Splendore-Hoeppli phenomenon**	
C/Fs	Painless, mucosal nodules, which may enlarge in size	Painless subcutaneous nodules, which may enlarge in size
Complication	Locally spread to involve to entire face with disfigurement of face	Dissemination may occurs in GIT, lungs & retroperitoneal tissues but very rare

Table-1: Differences between *C. coronatus* & *B. ranarum*

➢ **Etiological agents:** Caused by fungus from Zygomycetes group like *Conidiobolus coronatus* & *Basidiobolus ranarum.*

➢ **Pathogenicity:** Written in **table-1** with differences between two species.

➢ **Diagnosis:**

✪ **Specimens:** Biopsy from lesion.

✪ **Testing:** Difficult to isolate in culture. Histo-pathological stain shows non-septate hyphae.

➢ **Prevention:** Same as mycetoma.

➢ **Treatment:**
- Oral potassium iodide alone or with surgical excision of lesion gives better result.
- Hyperbaric oxygen is believed to accelerate the healing process.

Systemic mycoses

❖ **Definition:** These are the fungal infections of different systems.

❖ **Properties:**
- All the systemic fungi are dimorphic.
- All the dimorphic fungi can grow on SDA with antibiotics like gentamicin to prevent the bacterial growth & cycloheximide to prevent the fungal contamination.
- They are endemic in different regions, so **called endemic mycosis** (few authors defined only Coccidioidomycosis as endemic mycosis).

❖ **Examples:**

I. Histoplasmosis
II. Blastomycosis
III. Coccidioidomycosis
IV. Paracoccidioidomycosis

I. Histoplasmosis

➢ **Synonym:** Following are other names.
- Darling's disease, as disease was 1st described by Samuel Darling in 1905.
- Cave disease.
- Spelunker's lung.
- Caver's disease.
- Ohio valley disease.
- Reticuloendotheliosis.

➢ **Definition:** Granulomatous infection of RE system.

➢ **Etiological agent:** Caused by *Histoplasma capsulatum* (species name is misnomer, infact fungus has no capsule). It is a dimorphic fungus with following three variants.

1. *H. capsulatum* var. *capsulatum*: Causing classical histoplasmosis in human.
2. *H. capsulatum* var. *duboisi:* Causing African histoplasmosis in human.
3. *H. capsulatum* var. *farciminosum:* Causing histoplasmosis (epizootic) in animal.

➢ **Pathogenicity:**

✪ **Reservoir & source of infection:** Present in soil with high nitrogen contents especially in birds (chicken coops, pigeon roosts) or bat dropping.

✪ **Mode of transmission:** By inhalation of spores. Person to person spread does not occur.

✪ **Incubation period:** 10-16 days.

✪ **Portal of entry:** Respiratory system.

✪ **Sites:** Pulmonary & extra-pulmonary like skin, subcutaneous tissues, liver, spleen, nodes etc.

✪ **Precipitating factors (epidemiological determinants):** Three types.

a. **Agent factors (virulence factors):** It is dimorphic fungus has two forms like mycelium & yeast phase, possess different antigenic & surface features, and require different host mechanisms to contain it.

b. **Host factors:**

1. **Age:** In young adults.

2. **Sex:** More in males due to outdoor job.
3. **Occupation:** Accidental transmission occurs in laboratory workers while handling the culture.
4. **IDDs:** Like AIDS.

c. **Environmental factors:**

1. **Endemicity:**
- Fungus is distributed word wide.
- It is endemic in USA, particularly in states bordering the Ohio River Velley & the lower Mississippi river.
- In India it is endemic in West Bengal along the Ganga river.

✪ **Pathogenesis:**
- It includes acute as well as chronic inflammation.
- Inhaled spore, engulfed by macrophage but evade the host defence due to dimorphism & change to yeast phase & elicits the immune response resulting formation of granuloma like tuberculosis contains yeast cells, giant cells, epitheloid cells with or without caseation necrosis.
- Granuloma healed with fibrosis and calcification.
- Unlike latent tuberculosis, histoplasmosis once heals rarely reactivates.

✪ **Clinical features:**

A. **Classical histoplasmosis:**
- Acute pulmonary histoplasmosis: Minor respiratory features like cough, fever & flu like illness. Chest X-ray findings are normal in 40–70% of cases.
- Chronic pulmonary histoplasmosis: Granulomatous lesion in lungs **called histoplasmoma** & may simulates the tuberculosis. Chest X-ray suggest pulmonary infiltrate with hilar or mediastinal lymphadenopathy.
- Others: Dissemination of infection occurs in patient with low CMI in organs like skin, subcutaneous tissues, oral cavity (common in India) lymph nodes, liver, spleen etc.

B. **African histoplasmosis**: More in skin, subcutaneous tissue & bones.

✪ **Complications:** In absence of proper treatment and especially in individuals IDDs, complications can arise like
- Recurrent pneumonia.
- Respiratory failure.
- Fibrosis.
- Mediastinitis: Fibrosing mediastinitis is a serious complication and can be fatal.
- Superior vena cava syndrome.
- Pulmonary vessel obstruction.
- Progressive fibrosis of lymph with structural lung disease has higher probability of developing chronic cavitary histoplasmosis.
- After healing of lesions, hard calcified lymph nodes can erode the walls of airway causing haemoptysis.
- Dissemination of infection in organs.
- Anaemia & high fatality.

➢ **Diagnosis:**

✪ **Specimens:** BAL, sputum, biopsy from lesion or other suitable specimens.

✪ **Testing:**

A. **Microscopy:**

i. **Wet mount preparation:**

a. **Direct 10% KOH:**
- **Yeast phase morphology:** It present as round, spherical yeast cells about 2-4μm in classical while in African histoplasmosis they are larger about 7-15 μm inside the mononuclear or polymorphonuclear cells. [**fig.-7(a)**].

ii. **Differential stains:**

a. **Gram stain:** Gram positive yeast cells.

b. **Histopathological stains:** Giemsa & PAS stain shows granulomatous lesion with intracellular fungi.

iii. **Flourescent stains:** It is also useful.

B. **Culture:**

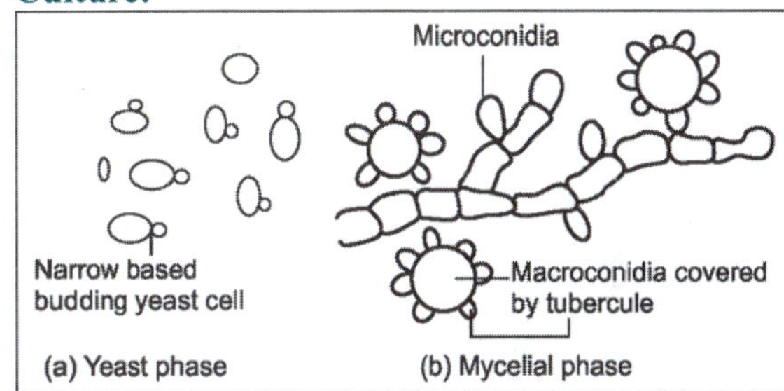

Figure-7: Schematic diagram of *H. capsulatum*

- **Routine media:** SDA with antibiotics.
- **Cultivation technique:** Follow chapter → Laboratory diagnosis of fungal infections (section →flow chart-1)
- **C/Cs on SDA:**

1. **Yeast phase:** Mucoid –cream colour colony may turn in to brown colour in 10-14 days.
2. **Mycelia phase:** Initially white colony later becomes brown.

- **Identification of culture growth by LCB/PHOL stain:**

1. **From yeast phase plate:** Round-spherical, narrow based budding yeast cell as shown in **fig.-7(a).**
2. **From mycelia phase plate:** Shows hyaline septate hyphae side by microconidia & with macroconidia surrounded by a finger like projections or tubercles **called tuberculate spores** as shown in **fig.-7(b).**

C. **Serological tests:** Like agglutination test, CFT immunodiffusion test.

D. **Molecular methods:**
- **Advantages:** High sensitivity & specificity.
- **Disadvantages:** High cost & not available in peripheral centre.
- **Methods:** DNA probe, hybridisation & PCR.

E. **Skin test:** Detection of DTH by using **histoplasmin-Ag** of mycelial phase.

F. **Animal inoculation:** Mouse is an ideal model.

G. **Special tests:** Teased mount, slide culture, cellophane tape mount & exo-antigen tests are also useful.

➢ **Prevention:**
- Avoiding visit of bird reservoirs.
- Use of PPE by laboratory workers.

➢ **Treatment:**
- AMB is given for acute & disseminated lesions.
- Itraconazole is effective in chronic cavitary pulmonary lesions.

II. Blastomycosis

➢ **Synonym:** North American Blastomycosis, as it is endemic in North American continents.

➢ **Definition:** It is a chronic pyogranulomatous infection especially of lungs & skin.

➢ **Etiological agent:** Caused by *Blastomyces dermatitidis* (Teleomorphic / sexual state *Ajellomyces dermatitidis*).

➢ **Pathogenicity:**

✪ **Reservoir & source of infection:** Exactly not known but spores may present in moist soil.

✪ **Mode of transmission:** By inhalation of spores.

✪ **Incubation period:** 45 days.

✪ **Portal of entry:** Respiratory system.

✪ **Sites:** Pulmonary & extra-pulmonary like skin, bone, genitor-urinary system, breast etc.

✪ **Precipitating factors (epidemiological determinants):** Three types.

a. **Agent factors (virulence factors):** Fungal dimorphism as described with *H capsulatum*

b. **Host factors:**

1. **Age:** In young adults.
2. **Sex:** Male to female ratio is 6:1.
3. **IDDs:** Like AIDS, leukemia/lymphoma & steroid therapy may favour the infection.

c. **Environmental factors:**

1. **Endemicity:**
- Fungus is endemic in North American continents.
- In India it is isolated from bronchial aspirates of a patient in Delhi & also from the lungs of insectivorous bats.

✪ **Pathogenesis:** Inhaled spore, change to yeast phase & elicits the immune response resulting formation of pyogranulomatous lesion in lungs. Later it disseminate to other sites by blood.

✪ **Clinical features:** Pyogranulomatous lesion in lungs **called pulmonary Blastomycosis.**

✪ **Complications:**
- Disseminated lesions occur in other organs due to haematogenous spread like skin (cutaneous blastomycosis), bone, genitor-urinary system, breast etc.
- Relapse is common.

➢ **Diagnosis:**

✪ **Specimens:** BAL, sputum, biopsy from lesion or other suitable specimens.

✪ **Testing:**

A. **Microscopy:**

i. **Wet mount preparation:**

a. **Direct 10% KOH :**

- **Yeast phase morphology:** Round, spherical, thick, double wall, broad based budding yeast cells gives figure of 8 appearance & about 7-20µm in size. **[fig.-8(a)].**

ii. **Differential stains:**

a. **Gram stain:** Gram positive yeast cells.

b. **Histopathological stains:** Giemsa & PAS stain shows fungus surrounded by granuloma.

iii. **Flourescent stains:** is also useful.

H. **Culture:**

- **Routine media:** SDA with antibiotics.
- **Cultivation technique:** Follow chapter → Laboratory diagnosis of fungal infections (section →flow chart-1)
- **C/Cs on SDA:**

1. **Yeast phase:** Cream colour colony becomes tan colour in old culture.
2. **Mycelia phase:** Same as like yeast phase.

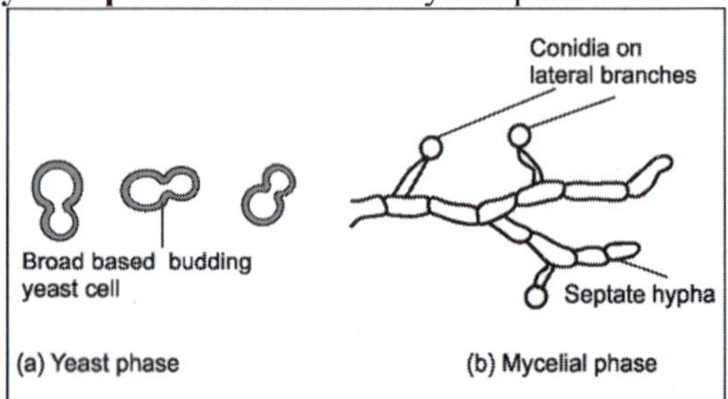

Figure-8: Schematic diagram of *B. dermatitidis*

- **Identification of culture growth by LCB/PHOL stain:**

1. **From yeast phase plate:** Broad based budding yeast cell as shown in **fig.-8(a).**
2. **From mycelia phase plate:** Shows hyaline septate hyphae with microconidia on tip of lateral branches as shown in **fig.-8(b).** Also shows the chlamydospores.

B. **Serological tests:** like agglutination test, CFT, immunodiffusion test etc.

C. **Molecular methods:**

- **Advantages:** High sensitivity & specificity.
- **Disadvantages:** High cost & not available in peripheral centre.
- **Methods:** DNA probe, hybridisation & PCR.

D. **Skin test:** Detection of DTH by using **blastomycin-Ag** of mycelial phase.

E. **Animal inoculation:** Mouse, rat, guinea pig, & hamster are susceptible.

F. **Special tests:** Teased mount, slide culture, cellophane tape mount & exo-antigen tests are also useful.

➢ **Prevention:**
- Avoid visiting the suspected places.

- Live recombinant vaccine is developed by using surface antigen (**called BAD antigen → *B. dermatitidis* adhesin**), which is immunogenic in animals & under trial for human use.

➢ **Treatment:**
- AMB is given in all cases.
- Itraconazole is effective in pulmonary & extra-pulmonay cases.
- Follow up for 1 year is needed after treatment to know about relapse.

III. Coccidioidomycosis

➢ **Synonym:** Following are other names.
- San Joaquin Velley fever.
- Desert rheumatism.
- California fever.
- Also **called Kok-see** in local language.

➢ **Definition:** Primarily granulomatous infection of respiratory system.

➢ **Etiological agent:** Caused by *Coccodioides immitis* (Im+mitis = not + mild, because of serious nature).

➢ **Pathogenicity:**

✪ **Reservoir & source of infection:** Spores are present in alkali soil of desert. Fungus produces the large numbers of arhthroconidia which are dispersed in air by recurring winds.

✪ **Mode of transmission:** By inhalation of spores. Person to spread is not reported.

✪ **Incubation period:** About 2 weeks.

✪ **Portal of entry:** Respiratory system.

✪ **Sites:** Pulmonary & extra-pulmonary, almost all sites except GIT.

✪ **Precipitating factors (epidemiological determinants):** Three types.

a. Agent factors (virulence factors):
1. **Fungal dimorphism:** As described in *H capsulatum.*
2. **Large size spherule:** Difficult to kill by host cells.

b. Host factors:
1. **Age:** In young adults.
2. **Sex:** More in male than female.
3. **IDDs:** Immunodeficient persons are also at risk.

c. Environmental factors:
1. **Season:** Infection is common during dry summer seasons & fall succeeding rainy winter & spring.
2. **Endemicity:** Fungus is endemic in Northern Mexico, Arizona, California, Nevada, Texas & Utah.

✪ **Pathogenesis:**
- Spore change to spherules which elicits the neutrophilic reaction to produces the abscess.
- Spherules also stimulate the granulomatous reaction with infiltration by giant cells, lymphocytes, plasma cells, & epitheloid cells.
- Few persons develop the hypersensitivity reaction.
- Calcification may occur in pulmonary lesion.
- 5% patients move to lung cavities.
- Dissemination occurs by blood in almost all organs except GIT.
- Spherules rupture to release the endospores.

✪ **Clinical features:**
- **Pulmonary coccidioidomycosis:**
- Acute stage: Flu like symptoms like fever, cough, headache, malaise etc.
- Chronic stage: About 90% turns to chronic stage with granulomatous lesion **called coccidioidoma**.

✪ **Complications:**
- Calcification in pulmonary lesion.
- Lung cavities develop in 5 % cases.
- Disseminated coccidioidomycosis: Infection spread from lungs via blood to involve almost all body parts except skin.
- Relapse is common.

➢ **Diagnosis:**

✪ **Specimens:** BAL, sputum, biopsy from lesion or other suitable specimens.

✪ **Testing:**

A. Microscopy:

a. Histopathological stains: Giemsa, GGMS & PAS stain shows spherules [**fig.-9(b)**] with granuloma formation. When spherule becomes mature it ruptures to release endospores. Spherules develop in tissue (lungs) not in culture. Barrel shaped spores **called arthrospores** are also present in tissues.

B. Culture:
- **Routine media:** SDA with antibiotics.
- **Cultivation technique:** Follow chapter → Laboratory diagnosis of fungal infections (section →flow chart-1)
- **C/Cs on SDA:**
- It grows as mold at 25^{0}C & at 37^{0}C.
- Spherules develops in tissue (lungs) not in culture
- It produce white-tan colour colony.
- **Identification of culture growth by LCB/PHOL stain:**

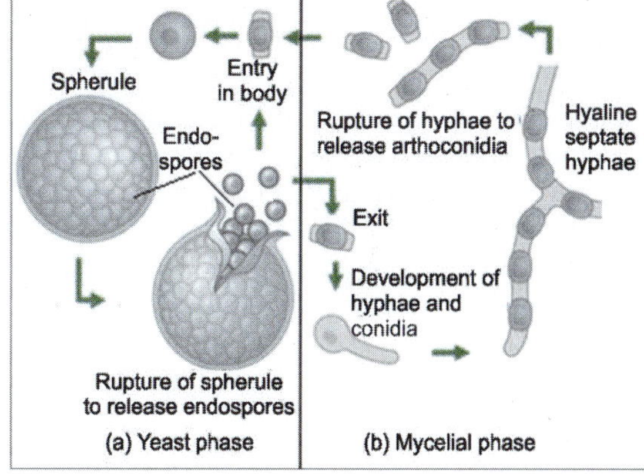

Figure-9: Schematic diagram of *C. immitis*

1. **Yeast phase:** No yeast (spherule) phase develops in culture but it develops in body.

2. **Mycelial phase plate:** Shows hyaline septate hyphae with arthrospores (barrel shaped spores) as shown in **fig.-9(a).** Rupture of hyphae release the arhthroconidia which are infectious.

C. **Serological tests:** Like agglutination test, CFT immunodiffusion test etc.

D. **Molecular methods:**

- **Advantages:** High sensitivity & specificity.
- **Disadvantages:** High cost & not available in peripheral centre.
- **Methods:** DNA probe, hybridisation & PCR.

E. **Skin test:** Detection of DTH by using **coccidiodin-Ag** of mycelial phase & **spherulin**-Ag from spherules.

F. **Animal inoculation:** Mouse, rat, guinea pig, & hamster are susceptible.

G. **Special tests:** Teased mount, slide culture, cellophane tape mount & exo-antigen tests are also useful.

➢ **Prevention:**
- Avoid visiting the suspected places.
- Immunity develop following primary infection provide the lifelong protection.
- Vaccine is developed useful for person living in endemic areas.

➢ **Treatment:**
- It is a self limiting condition.
- Itraconazole is effective in all cases except diffuse pneumonia where AMB is recommended.
- Relapse is major issue following treatment.

IV. Paracoccidioidomycosis

➢ **Synonym:** Following are other names.
- South American Blastomycosis, because common in South American countries.
- Lutz Splendore de Almeida disease.

➢ **Definition:** Acute or chronic granulomatous endemic systemic fungal infection primarily involving lungs & disseminated to other tissues.

➢ **Etiological agent:** Caused by *Paracoccidioides brasiliensis.*

➢ **Pathogenicity:**

✪ **Reservoir & source of infection:** It is a saprophytic fungus & spores are present in soil.

✪ **Mode of transmission:** By inhalation of spores.

✪ **Incubation period:** Clinical illness develops after several years of exposure.

✪ **Portal of entry:** Respiratory system.

✪ **Sites:** Pulmonary & extra-pulmonary.

✪ **Precipitating factors (epidemiological determinants):** Three types.

a. **Agent factors (virulence factors):**

1. **Fungal dimorphism:** As described in *H capsulatum.*

b. **Host factors:**

1. **Age:** About 90% infection occurs in adult between 20-50 years of age.
2. **Sex:** Less in female due to inhibitory effect of oestrogen for conversion of mycelial phase to yeast phase.
3. **IDDs:** Like AIDS may favour the infection.

c. **Environmental factors:**

1. **Humidity & temperature:** High humidity & temperature around 23^{0}C growth of fungus.
2. **Endemicity:** Endemic in Brazil & other South American countries.

✪ **Pathogenesis:** After entry spore changed to yeast cells to establish the infection. Acute stage is present with non-specific inflammatory response while chronic stage present with granulomatous reaction.

✪ **Clinical features:**

- **Pulmonary paracoccidioidomycosis:**
- Acute (juvenile) form: Pneumonia.
- Chronic (adult) form: Granulomatous lesion.

✪ **Complications:**
- Disseminated coccidioidomycosis: Infection spread from lungs via blood to other organs like skin, bone, genitor-urinary system, breast, CNS etc.
- Disseminated coccidioidomycosis is difficult to treat & relapse is common.

➢ **Diagnosis:**

✪ **Specimens:** BAL, sputum, biopsy from lesion or other suitable specimens.

✪ **Testing:**

A. **Microscopy:**

i. **Wet mount preparation:**

a. **Direct 10% KOH :**

- **Yeast phase morphology:** Round, spherical, multiple based budding yeast cells **like Mariner's wheel** or **Pilot's wheel** as shown in **fig.-10(a).**

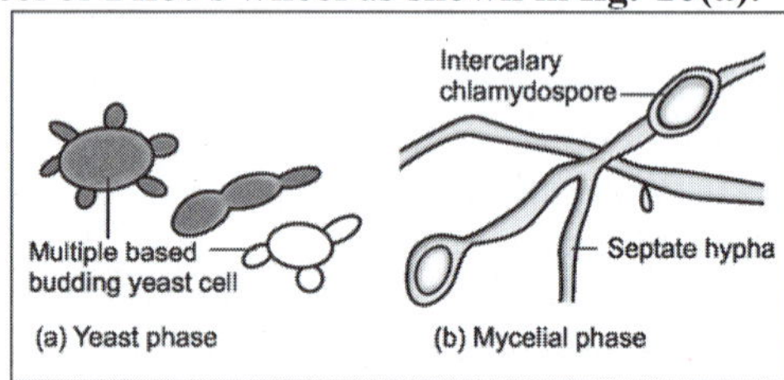

Figure-10: Schematic diagram of *P. brasiliensis*

ii. **Differential stains:**

a. **Gram stain:** Gram positive yeast cell.

b. **Histopathological stains:** H & E stain & GGMS stain shows fungus with granulomatous lesion.

iii. **Flourescent stains:** Also a useful stain for diagnosis.

B. **Culture:**

- **Routine media:** SDA with antibiotics.
- **Cultivation technique:** Follow chapter → Laboratory diagnosis of fungal infections (section →flow chart-1)
- **C/Cs on SDA:**

1. **Yeast phase:** Off-whit to cream, rough to pasty in appearance.
2. **Mycelia phase:** White to tan & yellow-brown on reverse.

- **Identification of culture growth by LCB/PHOL stain:**

1. **From yeast phase plate:** Round, spherical, multiple based budding yeast cells **like Mariner's wheel or Pilot's wheel** are present as shown in **fig.-10(a).**
2. **From mycelia phase plate:** Shows hyaline septate hyphae with intercalary chlamydospores [**fig.-10(b)**].

C. **Serological tests:** Like agglutination test, CFT, immunodiffusion test etc.

D. **Molecular methods:**

- **Advantages:** High sensitivity & specificity.
- **Disadvantages:** High cost & not available in peripheral centre.
- **Methods:** DNA probe, hybridisation & PCR.

E. **Skin test:** Detection of DTH by using **paracoccidioidin-Ag**.

F. **Animal inoculation:**

- Mouse, rat, guinea pig & hamster are susceptible.
- Nine banded armadillo (*Dasypus novemcinctus*) is the naturally infected animal & may provide clue to understand the patho-physiology of fungus.

G. **Special tests:** Teased mount, slide culture, cellophane tape mount & exo-antigen tests are also useful.

➢ **Prevention:**

- Avoid visiting the suspected places.
- DNA based vaccine is developed but not useful for human.

➢ **Treatment:**

- Itraconazole is effective in all cases except seriously ill where AMB is recommended.
- Relapse is major issue following treatment.

Opportunistic mycoses

❖ **Definition:** These are the fungal infections in host with IDDs.

❖ **Properties:** It may be endogenous or exogenous in origin.

❖ **Examples:**

I. Candidiasis
II. Cryptococcosis
III. Pneumocystosis
IV. Penicilliosis
V. Aspergillosis
VI. Zygomycosis
VII. Others

I. Candidiasis

Follow chapter → Superficial mycoses

II. Cryptococcosis

➢ **Synonym:** Previously **called torulosis** or **called European blastomycosis** (originally reported from Europe).

➢ **Definition:** Acute, subacute or chronic form of fungal infection primarily involving lungs, brain & disseminated to other tissues.

➢ **Etiological agents:**

✪ **Most common pathogen:** *Cryptococcus neoformans* with three varieties

- *C. neoformans* var.*neoformans.*
- *C. neoformans* var. *grubii.*
- *C. neoformans* var. *gatii.*

✪ **Others:** Rare human pathogens.

- *Cryptococcus albidus.*
- *Cryptococcus laurentii.*

➢ **Pathogenicity:**

✪ **Reservoir & source of infection:**

- It is a saprophytic fungus found in house dust & soil.
- It is associated with Eucalyptus tree.
- It is present in pigeon's faeces because contain nitrogen which is essential growth factor for fungus.
- Pigeons are not suffered by disease.

✪ **Mode of transmission:** By inhalation of blastospores.

✪ **Incubation period:** 2-4 weeks.

✪ **Portal of entry:** Respiratory system.

✪ **Sites:** Pulmonary & extra-pulmonary sites.

✪ **Precipitating factors (epidemiological determinants):**

a. **Agent factors (virulence factors):**

1. **Capsule:**

- It is polysaccharide in nature & inhibits the phagocytosis.
- Five different serotypes of *C. neoformans* based on polysaccharide capsule like A, B, C, D & AD. However many authors mentioned only four serotype from A-D. For laboratory diagnosis these serotypes are nor important & all isolates are reported simply as *Cryptococcus neoformans.*
- Capsular antigen is poorly antigenic & anti-capsular antibody is neither protective nor prevent recurrence. Protective role offered by CMI.

2. **Ability to produce melanin:** Melanin protects the fungus from

- Intracellular killing by phagocytes.
- High temperature.
- UV light.
- Antibiotics like amphotericin B.
- Reduced state of iron.

3. **Ability to produce mannitol:** Mannitol protect the fungus from intracellular killing by phagocytes.

4. **Ability to survive at high temperature:** About 41-43^{0}C.
5. **Urease production:** Convert urea in to ammonia which acts as nitrogen source.
6. **Phospholipase production:** Help in fungal invasion.

b. Host factors:

1. **Age:** Common between 30-60 years & uncommon in children.
2. **Sex:** More in male.
3. **Immunosuppressive disease or conditions:** Like
   - Long term steroid therapy.
   - Antibiotic therapy.
   - DM.
   - Immunosuppressive therapy.
   - Renal transplantation.
   - Malignancy.
   - AIDS: It is the 4th most common cause of CNS infection in AIDS patient. It may occur at any stage of AIDS but most common when CD4 count fall < 100/cmm.
4. **Fungal predilection of CNS:** Because of following reasons
   - Presence of specific receptors of yeast cells on nerve cells.
   - Presence of nitrogen sources like asparigine & creatinine in CSF.
   - Absence of inhibitory factors like present in serum.

c. Environmental factors:

1. **Temperature:** Higher temperature about 41-43^{0}C favour the growth of fungus.
2. **Distribution:** Var. *neoformans* is common in Europe & var. *gattii* is common in Vancouver.

✪ **Pathogenesis:**

- It is the only fungus having capsule.
- It primarily infect lung-lymph node complex.
- Later yeast cells spread to CNS by crossing the blood brain barrier either via direct migration through endothelium or carried inside the macrophages as **"Trojan horse".**

✪ **Clinical features:** Pulmonary cryptococcosis characterised by pneumonia.

✪ **Complications:**

- **CNS cryptococcosis:**
  - Meningitis or meningo-encephalitis: Features include fever, headache, sensory & memory loss, cranial nerve paresis & loss of vision due to optic nerve involvement. Loss of vision may be rapid (sudden) or slow. Neck rigidity & stiffness are found in one third of patient. Kernig's & Brudzinski's sign are usually negative but may be positive in few patients.
  - Granulomatous lesion or ICSOL (Intra Cranial Space Occupying Lesion) in brain **called cryptococcoma**.
- **Generalised cryptococcosis:** Dissemination via blood to other organs like skin, bone, prostate, eyes etc. Least invasion occurs in GIT, liver & kidneys.
- **Relapse:** It is the common problem.

➢ **Diagnosis:**

✪ **Specimens:** Sputum, CSF or other suitable specimens.

✪ **Testing:**

A. Microscopy:

i. Wet mount preparation:

a. Negative staining:

- Indian ink (60-70% sensitivity) or 10% Nigrosin shows round / oval budding yeast cells with capsule as shown in **fig.-11.**
- Capsule is twice as thick as the diameter of yeast cells.

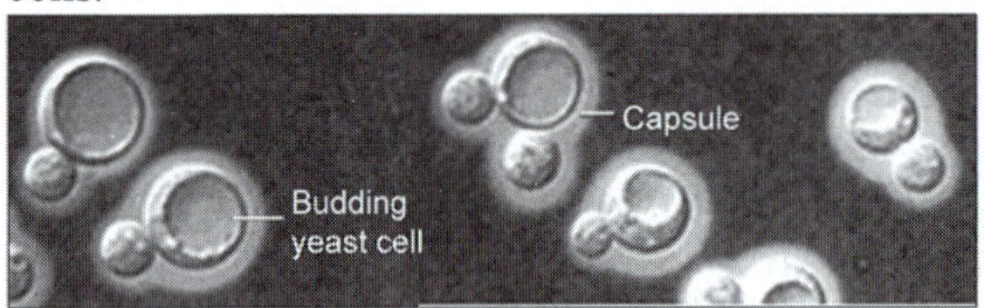

Figure-11: Capsule of *C. neoformans* under Indian ink preparation

ii. Differential stains:

a. Gram stain: Gram positive yeast cells.

b. Histopathological stains:

- HE, PAS & GGMS stains fungus in tissue section
- Mayer's mucicarmine stain: Capsule stains deep rose in colour.
- Masson Fontana Silver (MFS) stain: To demonstrate melanin production by fungus. Fungus stains black & nuclei in red.
- Alcian blue stain: Demonstrate the capsule of fungus.

iii. Flourescent stains: Also a useful stain.

B. Culture:

- **Routine media:** SDA with antibiotics.
- **Selective media:**
  - Bird seed (niger seed) agar: } Brown colour colony
  - Sunflower seed agar: }
- **Cultivation technique:** Follow chapter → Laboratory diagnosis of fungal infections (section →flow chart-1)
- **C/Cs on SDA:**
  - Mucoid, cream-to buff colour colony.
  - Mucoid colony is due to polysaccharide capsule.
- **Identification of culture growth by LCB/PHOL stain:** Round, budding yeast cells with capsule. No hyphae (mycelium) or pseudohyphae.

C. Biochemical test:

- Assimilation of inositol.
- Urease test is positive.
- May be nitrate positive.

D. Serological tests:

- Capsular Ag is detected by latex agglutination test (95% sensitivity) from CSF & serum.
- Other tests are: CFT, immunodiffusion test etc.

E. Molecular methods:

- **Advantages:** High sensitivity & specificity.
- **Disadvantages:** High cost & not available in peripheral centre.
- **Methods:** DNA probe, hybridisation, PCR & RFLP.

F. Animal inoculation: Mouse is susceptible.

G. Antifungal sensitivity testing: Report the result with drug sensitivity pattern.

➤ **Prevention:**

- General measure: Avoid visiting the suspected places like bird reservoirs.
- Chemoprophylaxis: Prophylactic use of fluconazole in AIDS patient to avoid the risk of Cryptococcosis.
- Immunoprophylaxis: Vaccine contains major capsular components like glucuronoxylomannan is developed provide protection in mice & also effective in human.

➤ **Treatment:**

- Induction therapy: Started with AMB & flucytosine
- Maintenance therapy: Fluconazole is given to prevent the relapse.

III. Pneumocystosis

➤ **Meaning:** Pneumo = air (suggest lungs) + cystis = cyst like structure.

➤ **Synonym:** Pnemo Cystis Pneumonia (PCP), *P. jirovecii* pneumonia (PJP).

➤ **Definition:** It is an opportunistic fungal infection characterised by primary atypical (interstitial) pneumonia.

➤ **Etiological agent:** Caused by *Pneumocystis jirovecii* (previously it was labelled as *P. carinii*).

- **Taxonomy:**
  - Initially protozoa: Initially it was classified as protozoa based on morphology, resistant to antifungal drugs (because no ergosterol in cell wall), sensitive to antiprotozoal drugs & no growth on fungal media but in cell culture media.
  - Now fungus: Now it is classified as fungus as *Ascomycetes*, because

- Cell wall contains β-1,3 glucans which is responsible for staining with histopathological stains as described below.
- Contains chitins in cell wall & produces the enzyme chitinase as like other fungi.
- rRNA study, protein synthesis elongation factor (EF3) & thymidylate synthase are homologous to the ascomycetes.
- Sporozoites (intracystic bodies) of cyst structure are simulating the ascospores of ascomycetes.
- Mitochondria are with laminar cristae as in ascospores of ascomycetes while protozoal mitochondria are tubular & vesicuar cristae.
- However, still is controversial to classify it as fungus & better to classify as **atypical fungus** under the new phylum **called *Protomycota.***

- **Nomenclature**

- It was 1st identified from the lungs of guinea pig by Chagas in 1909 & from the lungs of rat by Antonio Carinii in 1910 (*Pneumocystis carinii* is considered as rat species) & after 2nd world war it was identified from the lung of infant in Central & Eastern Europe by Otto Jirovec & Joseph Vanek (*Pneumocystis jirovecii* is considered as human species).
- When the name *P. jirovecii*, replaced the *P. carinii*, at first it was felt that *P. jirovecii* pneumonia (PJP) should replace *P. carinii* pneumonia (PCP). However, the term PCP remain continue with **P**neumo **C**ystis (jirovecii) **P**neumonia, because it was used by many physician.

- **Life cycle:** Three stages as shown in **fig.-12.**

a. Trophozoite: Thin wall, amoeboid shaped & 1-5μm in size. Containing tubular projection **called filopodia** (glycoprotein in nature) for attachment with host cells.

b. Pre-cyst: Intermediate stage with 5-8μm length & oval shape. Few filopodia.

c. Mature cyst: Thick wall, 8μm in size & spherical shaped. It contains 8 nuclei (intra-cystic bodies / sporozoites) & its rupture release the sporozoites which start new cycle.

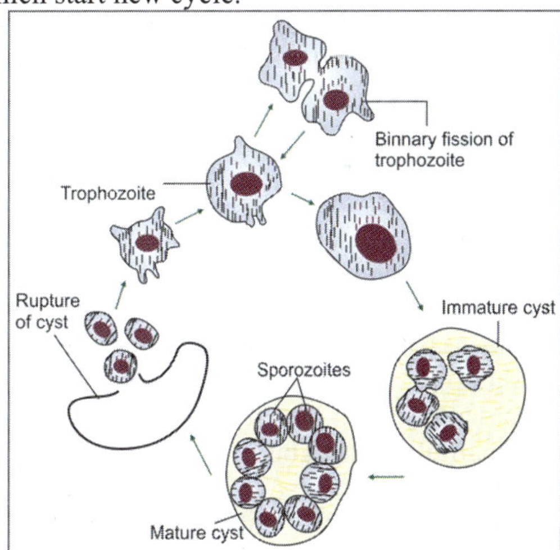

Figure-12: Life cycle stage of *P. jirovecii*

➤ **Pathogenicity:**

✪ **Reservoir & source of infection:** Uncertainty about source & reservoir, but fungi present in animals, in human & free in the environment.

✪ **Mode of transmission:**

- By inhalation of trophozoites.
- Congenital transmission also reported.

✪ **Incubation period:** 4-8 weeks.

✪ **Portal of entry:** Respiratory system.

✪ **Sites:** Pulmonary & extra-pulmonary sites.

- **Precipitating factors (epidemiological determinants):**
1. **Age:** Common in old age
2. **Immunosuppressive disease or conditions:** Like
- Steroid therapy.
- DM.
- Immunosuppressive therapy.
- Organ or bone marrow transplantation.
- Malignancy like leukemia, lymphoma etc.
- Cushing syndrome.
- Congenital disease like hypogammaglobulinemia.
- AIDS: Pneumonia occurs in patient when $CD4^+$ count fall <200/cmm.
- Protein energy malnutrition like marasmus.
- **Pathogenesis:** Inhaled trophozoite attaches with alveolar epithelium & initiate the eosinophilic infiltration in alveoli or in interstitial space, **called primary atypical (interstitial) pneumonia.**
- **Clinical features:** Primary atypical (interstitial) pneumonia characterised by fever, nonproductive cough & shortness of breath.
- **Complications:**
- Secondary bacterial infection in lungs.
- Extra- pulmonary pneumocystosis: Lymph node, spleen, pancreas, eye ("cotton wool" spot in fundus), liver, heart etc.

➢ **Diagnosis:**
- **Key points for diagnosis of PCP:**
- $CD4^+$ count <200/cmm.
- Both trophozoite & cyst are the diagnostic features. Trophozoites are more in numbers than cysts with 10:1 ratio. Trophozoites are 1-5μm in size while cysts are 8μm in size.
- Positivity of PCP in induced sputum is 60%.
- It also based on radiological study, clinical presentation & histopathological examination of BAL or lung biopsy.
- **Specimens:** Sputum, BAL or other suitable specimens.
- **Testing:**

A. **Microscopy:**

a. **Histopathological stains:**

1. **Stains for cyst wall:** Are best useful & stain the wall of cyst but stains neither the trophozoites nor the nuclei (sporozoites) of cyst. Cysts are appearing in cluster of 2-8 bodies.

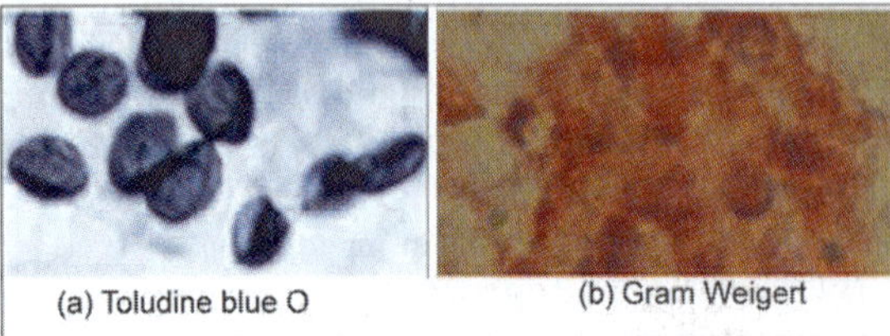

Figure-13: Stains for cyst wall of PCP

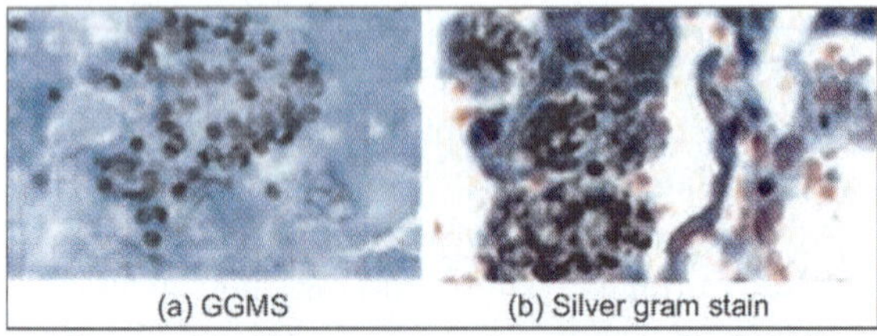

Figure-14: Silver stains for cyst wall of PCP

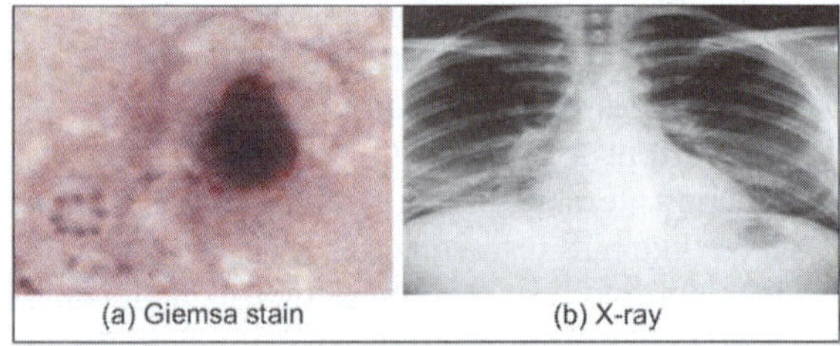

Figure-15: Giemsa stains (a) & X-ray (B) findings for PCP

- Toludine blue O: Blue coloured cyst as shown in **fig.-13(a).**
- Gram-Weigert stain: Appearance of cyst is shown in **fig.-13(b).**
- Silver stains: Like GGMS [**fig.-14(a)**] & silver gram stain [**fig.-14(b)**], which stains the cyst in black coloured.
- Cresyl echt violet stains.

2. **Stains for trophozoites & sporozoites (internal nuclei) of cyst:** They don't stain the cyst wall but stain the sporozoites of cyst appear negatively stained. Also stains the trophozoites (1-5μm).
- Giemsa stain: It stains the nuclei in pink colour & cytoplasm in blue colour as shown in **fig.-15(a)**.
- Trichrome stain.
- Papanicolaou stain.
- MGG stain.

b. **Flourescent stains:** Are also useful.

B. **Culture:** No growth on media but can grow in several cell lines like A549 & WI-38.

C. **Serological tests:** Like agglutination test & CFT.

D. **Molecular method:**
- **Advantages:** High sensitivity & specificity.
- **Disadvantages:** High cost & not available in peripheral centre.
- **Methods:** Nested-PCR.

E. **Animal inoculation:** Mouse is susceptible.

F. **Other tests:**
1. **Pulmonary Function Test (PFT):** It revealed the reduction in the vital capacity & total lung capacity.
2. **Chest X-ray:** Wide spread pulmonary infiltration (Mottling of lung fields) & opacification (whiteness) in lower lungs on both sides as shown in **fig.-15(b)**.

➢ **Prevention:**
- **Types of chemoprophylaxis:** Two types.

1. **Primary prophylaxis:** Patient with $CD4^+$ count <200/cmm or with oral thrush or with unexplained fever >100F for > 2 weeks but never had PCP.
2. **Secondary prophylaxis:** HIV infected patient with history of PCP. (Lifelong prophylaxis is given to the HIV patient).

- **Commonly used drugs:**

- Co-trimoxazole.
- Dapsone.
- Aerosolised pentamidine.

➢ **Treatment:** The most effective treatment for PCP is a combination of two drugs.

1. Co-trimoxazole (trimethoprim &sulfamethoxazole).
2. Pentamidine.
3. Clindamycin-primaquine.
4. Trimethoprim –dapsone.
5. Trimetrexate-leucovorin.
6. Aerosolized pentamidine.
7. Prednisone.

IV. Penicilliosis

◊ **Etiological agent:** Caused by *Penicillium* with more than 250 species.

Penicillium marneffei

- *Penicillium marneffei* is most pathogenic.
- *Penicillium marneffei* is the only dimorphic fungus; other species are not dimorphic & can grow at 25^0C as mold.
- Cells are multiply by binary fission not by budding.
- It produces brick-red pigment.
- It is a common laboratory contaminant.
- Present in environment & grow on various substances like bread, jam, fruit, vegetables etc.

➢ **Pathogenicity:**

✪ **Reservoir & source of infection:** Conidia (spores) are present in soil. Natural infection occurs in human & bamboo rats [*Rhizomys sinensis* (Vietnam), *R.pruiosus* (China) *R. sumatrensis* & *Cannomys badius*].

✪ **Mode of transmission:**

- By inhalation of spores.
- In Southern China it is acquired by man due to ingestion of infected rat/rat's meat.
- Direct inoculation in skin.

✪ **Incubation period:** 4 weeks.

✪ **Portal of entry:** Respiratory system.

✪ **Sites:** Pulmonary & extra-pulmonary sites.

✪ **Precipitating factors (epidemiological determinants):** Three types.

a. **Agent factors (virulence factors):**

1. **Fungal dimorphism:** As described in *H capsulatum.*

b. **Host factors:**

1. **IDDs:** Cases are increased in numbers following discovery of HIV-AIDS. It may causes fulminant disease in person with IDDs.

c. **Environmental factors:**

1. **Environmental season:** Disease is more likely to occur following the rainy season.
2. **Distribution:** It is endemic in South East Asian countries like Thailand, Vietnam & India (Manipur).

✪ **Pathogenesis:** After entry spores target the RE system, with formation of three patterns as follows.

1. **Granulomatous:** Centrally yeast cells with transverse septa but without budding are surrounded by inflammatory cells.
2. **Suppurative:** Abscess formation.
3. **Necrosis:** With little or no granuloma.

✪ **Clinical features:**

- Intracellular in RE system.
- Granulomatous & suppurative lesion in lungs.

✪ **Complications:**

- Extra - pulmonary sites like lymph node, liver, spleen etc.
- Pericarditis or pericardial effusion.
- Peritonitis.
- Osteomyelitis.
- Endophthalmitis.
- Relapse.

➢ **Diagnosis:**

✪ **Specimens:** Sputum, BAL or other suitable specimens.

✪ **Testing:**

A. **Microscopy:**

a. **Histopathological stains:**

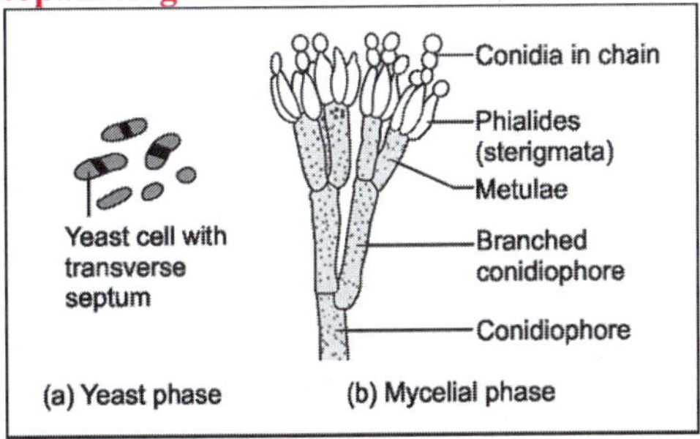

Figure-16: Schematic diagram of *P. marneffei*

- H & E, PAS & GGMS stain shows granulomatous lesion in tissue.
- Yeast cells are present in macrophages.
- Yeast cells are round, spherical, elongated with curved end & transverse septum but without budding **[fig.-16(a)]** giving '**sausage –like appearance**'.

b. **Flourescent stains:** Are also useful.

B. **Culture:**

- **Routine media:** SDA with antibiotics.
- **Cultivation technique:** Follow chapter → Laboratory diagnosis of fungal infections (section →flow chart-1)

- **C/Cs on SDA:**
1. **Yeast phase:** Cerebriform, convoluted colonies becomes pink-white.
2. **Mycelia phase:** Greyish-white colonies & red on reverse due to red pigment production.
- **Identification of culture growth by LCB/PHOL stain:**
1. **From yeast phase plate:** Yeast cells are round, spherical, elongated with curved end & transverse septum **[fig.-16(a)]** giving **'sausage –like appearance'**.
2. **From mycelia phase plate:** Shows hyaline septate hypha with conidiophores, verticilis (branched conidiophores ?) metulae, phialides & conidia which are basipetal in nature & arranged in chain giving **brush like appearance → fig.-16(b).**

C. **Serological tests:** Like agglutination test, CFT immunodiffusion test etc.

D. **Molecular method:**
- **Advantages:** High sensitivity & specificity.
- **Disadvantages:** High cost & not available in peripheral centre.
- **Methods:** PCR.

E. **Animal inoculation:** Bamboo rat is susceptible.

F. **Special tests:** Teased mount, slide culture, cellophane tape mount & exo-antigen tests are also useful.

➢ **Prevention:** Nothing particular. Antibiotics may prescribe to AIDS patient to prevent the infection.

➢ **Treatment:**
- Antifungal sensitivity test indicates that itraconazole & ketoconazole are highly sensitive; AMB is moderate while fluconazole is least sensitive.
- Lifelong maintenance therapy is given with itraconazole to prevent the relapse.

Other species of *Penicillium*

- Other species are occurs as laboratory contaminants.
- Rarely they are causing disease in human like
1. Superficial disease: Otomycosis, keratitis & onychomycosis.
2. Invasive disease: Endophthalmitis & endocarditis.
3. Allergic fungal disease: Follow chapter → Miscellaneous topics in Mycology (section →Allergic fungal disease)
4. Food poisoning: Aflatoxin is produced by *P puberulum.*

V. Aspergillosis

➢ **Meaning:** from **aspergillum** means **perforated globe used to sprinkle the holy water**, as chain like arrangement of conidia, radiating from central structure resemble to aspergillum.

➢ **Definition:** Systemic fungal infection occurs in immunocompetent & immunodeficient individuals.

➢ **Etiological agents:**
- Caused by *Aspergillus* with more than 185 species.
- 23 are pathogenic for human & three are most pathogenic like *A. flavus, A. fumigatus* & *A. niger.*
- It is a common laboratory contaminant & it is difficult to differentiate it from true pathogen.
- Present in environment & grow on various substances like bread, jam, fruit, vegetables etc.

➢ **Pathogenicity:**

✪ **Reservoir & source of infection:** It is a saprophytic fungi & spores are present in soil, environment & on decaying vegetation.

✪ **Mode of transmission:**
- By inhalation of spores (conidia), specially working with decaying vegetation like moldy hay.
- Direct entry by traumatised skin.

✪ **Incubation period:** Allergic illness develops after 6-9 months of exposure. Exact time for invasive aspergillosis is unknown.

✪ **Portal of entry:** Respiratory system or skin.

✪ **Sites:** Pulmonary & extra-pulmonary.

✪ **Precipitating factors (epidemiological determinants):**

a. **Agent (virulence) factors:** Small size of spores (<5μm) evades the host response.

b. **Host factors:**
1. **Occupation:** Common in farmers.
2. **Immunodeficiency status:** Like
- Diabetes mellitus.
- AIDS may favour the infection.
- Prolonged treatment with antibiotics, steroid & cytotoxic drugs may favour the infection.

✪ **Pathogenesis & clinical features:** After entry, spore establish following types of diseases.

A **Pulmonary aspergillosis:** Following three categories.

i. **Allergic: Called allergic broncho pulmonary aspergillosis** with following subtypes.
- Type-I hypersensitivity: Asthma (atopy type).
- Type-III hypersensitivity: Extrinsic alveolitis.
- Combined Type-I & III hypersensitivity.

ii. **Non-invasive:** In the lungs fungal mass is surrounded by dense fibrous wall **called aspergilloma (fungus ball).** It present with haemoptysis. Common in patient with old tuberculosis or bronchiectasis. Surgical removal is necessary.

iii. **Invasive:** At first it cause the pneumonia & later disseminate to other organs like skin, CNS, paranasal sinuses, CVS, kidneys, heart , bones etc.

B **PNS (paranasal sinuses) aspergillosis:** Most common agent is *A flavus*. It includes nasal & paranasal sinuses with following four categories.

i. **Allergic:**
- Present with rhinitis, nasal discharge, nasal blockage etc.
- Mostly combined Type-I & III hypersensitivity.

ii. **Non-invasive:** Characterised by aspergilloma (fungus ball) formation in sinuses. It present as chronic sinusitis. Surgical removal is necessary.

iii. **Invasive:** Present as facial mass (like a neoplastic growth or polypoid growth) & proptosis. It disseminate through bone to orbit & finally to brain (**called rhinocerebral aspergillosis**). Rhinocerebral aspergillosis may present with proptosis or polypoid lesion in nose.

iv. **Fulminant:** It is angio invasive, rapidly destructive & often fatal.

C **Food poisoning:** Pre formed toxin production in food causing food poisoning.

D **Other disease:** In addition to above mentioned lesion *Aspergillus* spp. cause following lesions either primarily or secondary due to distant spread.

- CNS aspergillosis.
- Endocarditis: Common following cardiac surgery.
- Ear: Otomycosis, mastoiditis etc.
- Eye: Oculomycosis like mycotic keratitis.
- Nail: Onychomycosis.
- Cutaneous aspergillosis.
- Osteomyelitis.

✪ **Complications:** Intracranial aneurysm & other invasive disease are the major issues.

➢ **Diagnosis:**

✪ **Specimens:** BAL, sputum, CSF, biopsy from lesion or other suitable specimens.

✪ **Testing:**

A. **Microscopy:** KOH [**fig.-17(a)**] & histopathological stain shows the hyaline septate hyphae. Flourescent stain is also useful.

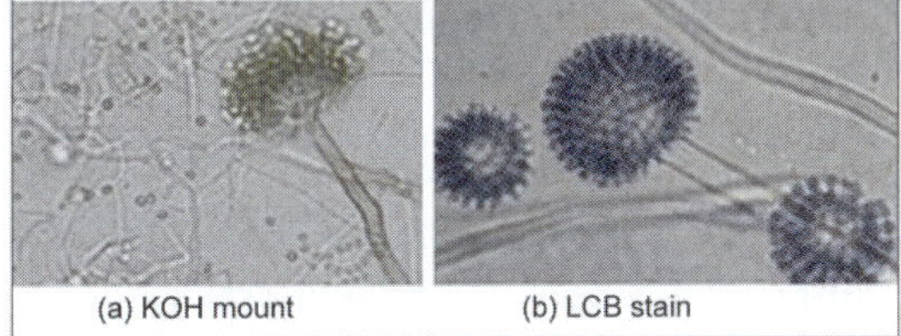

Figure-17: KOH & LCB stains of *Aspergillus*

B. **Culture:**

- **Routine media:** SDA with antibiotics.
- **Cultivation technique:** **Follow chapter → Laboratory diagnosis of fungal infections** (section →flow chart-1)
- **C/Cs on SDA:**

- *A. fumigatus*: Dark green colony [**fig.-18(b)**].
- *A. niger*: Black colony [**fig.-18(c)**].
- *A. flavus*: Yellow-green colony [**fig.-18(a)**].

- **Identification of culture growth by LCB [fig.-17(b)] / PHOL stain:** Shows hyaline septate hyphae with conidiophores, vesicle, phialides & chain like arrangement of conidia. Hyphae showing dichotomous branches, where conidiophores & stem are equal in size (3-6μm) & at acute/narrow angle of 45^0 (V shaped). Follow **fig.-19 & 20** for schematic diagram of *Aspergillus.*
- **Selective medium:** Czapek-Dox agar: To differentiate the *Aspergillus* spp.

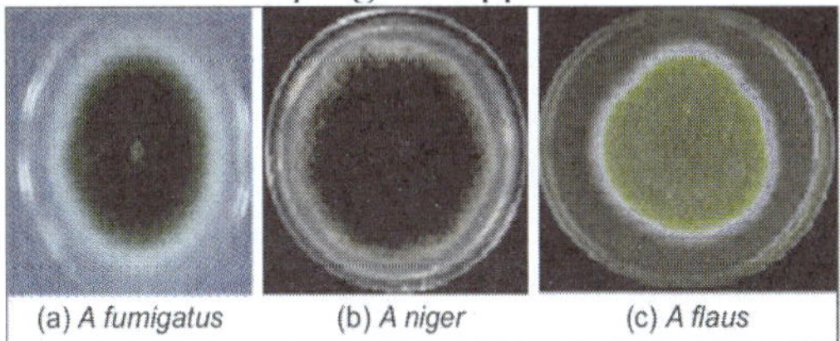

Figure-18: C/Cs of *Aspergillus spp.*

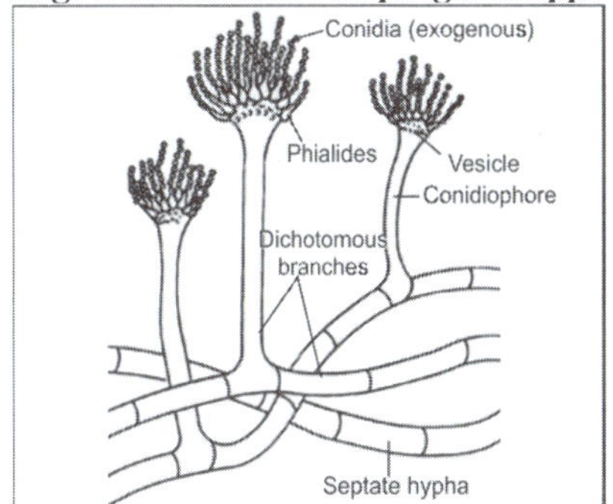

Figure-19: Schematic diagram of *Aspergillus*

C. **Serological tests:** Like Agglutination test, RIA, ELISA & immunodiffusion tests are useful.

D. **Skin test:** To detect the type-I & type-III hypersensitivity.

E. **Molecular method:**

- **Advantages:** High sensitivity & specificity.
- **Disadvantages:** High cost & not available in peripheral centre.
- **Methods:** PCR.

F. **Animal inoculation:** Rabbit & mouse are susceptible.

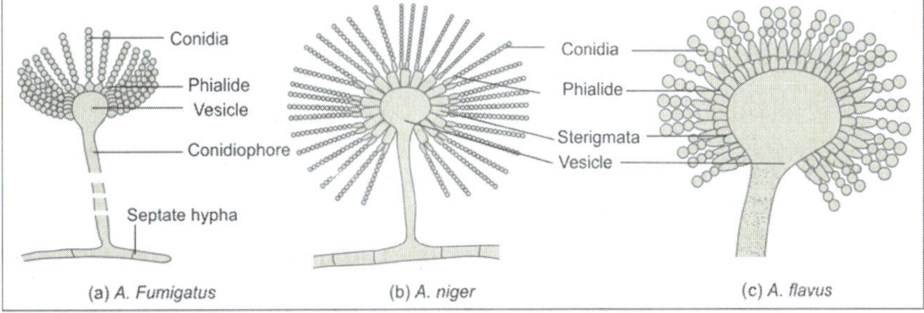

Figure-20: Schematic diagram of different *Aspergillus* spp.

G. Test to detect fungal metabolites:
- **Gag Liquid Chromatography:** To detect the fungal metabolites like D-mannitol.
- **G-test:** To detect β-1, 3-D-glucan.

H. Special tests: Slide culture is useful for better species identification.

I. Antifungal sensitivity test: Report the result with drug sensitivity pattern.

➢ **Prevention:** Reduction of environmental exposure.

➢ **Treatment:** It has high mortality rate. Following are the answers
- Surgery: Surgical removal of fungal ball.
- Chemotherapy: AMB is the drug of choice. Azoles like voriconazole or itraconazole are also useful.
- Immunotherapy: Interferon-α, G-CSF & GM-CSF.

VI. Zygomycosis

◊ **Definition:** It is an acute or chronic infection caused by several fungal agents belongs to phylum Zygomycota.

◊ **Types:** Two main types.

A. Subcutaneous Zygomycosis: → Vide supra

B. Systemic Zygomycosis: → Vide infra

Systemic Zygomycosis

➢ **Synonym:**
- Mucormycosis: Because all the fungi are belong to order Mucorales.
- Phycomycosis: Because all the fungi are belong to class Phacomysetes (Zygomycetes).

➢ **Etiological agents:** These are the common laboratory contaminants & also caused confusion in diagnosis. Caused by fungus from different genus like

1. *Mucor racemosus.*
2. *Rhizomucor pusillus.*
3. *Rhizopus arrhizus.*
4. *Rhizopus microspores.*
5. *Absidia corymbifera.*
6. *Apophysomyces elegans.*
7. *Cunninghamella bertholletiae.*
8. *Saksenaea vasiformis.*
9. *Cokeromyces recurvatus.*
10. *Syncephalastrum recemosum.*

➢ **Pathogenicity:**

✪ **Reservoir & source of infection:** These are saprophytic fungus & spores are present in soil, in environment, on decaying vegetation & on leaf littre.

✪ **Mode of transmission:**
- By inhalation of spores (conidia), specially working with decaying vegetation like moldy hay.
- Direct entry by percutaneous inoculation.
- By ingestion of spores.

✪ **Incubation period:** The incubation period is measured in days. The clinical course can progress from normal to symptomatic in a week and from sinus opacification to uncal herniation and death in just a few days.

✪ **Portal of entry:** Respiratory system, skin or GIT.

✪ **Sites:** Pulmonary & extra-pulmonary.

✪ **Precipitating factors (epidemiological determinants):**

a. Agent (virulence) factors:
1. Angio-invasive nature.
2. Ability to grow at & above the body temperature.
3. Dormant spores evade the body defence.
4. *Rhizopus* have high active ketone reductase enzyme, which help to survive in high acidic condition like diabetic ketoacidosis.

b. Host factors:

1. Immunosuppressive disease or conditions: Like
- Steroid therapy.
- DM: Acidosis favours the growth of *Rhizopus*, while normal serum inhibits the growth.
- Organ transplantation.
- Immunosuppressive therapy.
- Malignancy like leukemia, lymphoma etc
- HIV-AIDS.
- Patient on dialysis & iron overloaded, who are being treated with deferoxamine (iron chelator) are more susceptible to zygomycosis.

✪ **Pathogenesis:** Inhaled spores evade the host defence & change to mycelial form which have more predilection for elastic lamina of small & large arteries (Angio invasion) causing thrombosis, haemorrhage & infarction.

✪ **Clinical features:** Following are the primary lesions of zygomycosis.

i. Rhinocerebral zygomycosis:
- It is the most common & fulminant variety.
- Most common agent is *Rhizopus arrhizus.*
- It spread from nasal mucosa to turbinate bones, paranasal sinuses, orbit & palate with extension in to brain where massive invasion in to blood vessels causes major infarct.
- It present with brownish blood stained nasal discharge, black eschar on palate, fixed & dilated pupil, global proptosis & ptosis due to dysfunction of cranial nerves especially 5th & 7th.
- If left remain untreated, may cause the death within a week.
- It is more common in patient with DM or ketoacidosis, leukemia & lymphoma.

ii. Pulmonary zygomycosis:
- Occurs following inhalation of sporangiospores.
- Present with chest pain, dyspnoea & haemoptysis.

iii. Cutaneous zygomycosis: It is primary due to direct inoculation of fungus in to skin or secondary due to blood spread.

iv. **Gastrointestinal zygomycosis:** It is primary due to direct ingestion of fungal spores via food or secondary due to blood spread.

✪ **Complications:**

i. **Local spread:**

- From nasal mucosa enter in orbit via cribriform plate **called orbital zygomycosis.**
- It present with chemosis, periorbital cellulitis, ophthalmoplegia, proptosis, ptosis, abrupt visual loss, orbital pain & fascial hyposthesia.
- Fungi may invade the blood vessels & causing vasculitis & thrombosis.
- Precipitating factors are same as of rhinocerebral zygomycosis because it spread from nose.

ii. **Haematogenous spread:** Dissemination via blood to other organs like heart, bones, kidneys, eyes etc.

➢ **Diagnosis:**

✪ **Specimens:** BAL, sputum, CSF, biopsy from lesion or other suitable specimens.

✪ **Testing:**

a. **Microscopy:** KOH & histopathological stain shows the hyaline non-septate hyphae (co-enocytic hyphae). Flourescent stain is also useful.

b. **Culture:**

- **Routine media:** SDA with antibiotics.
- **Cultivation technique:** Follow chapter → Laboratory diagnosis of fungal infections (section →flow chart-1)
- **C/Cs on SDA:**
  - Almost same colony by different species.
  - Grey-white, thick-cottony fluffy surface.
- **Identification of culture growth by LCB/PHOL stain:** Shows irregular, broad (10-20μm), hyaline, non-septate (co-enocytic) or sparsely septate hyphae. Hyphae showing obtuse branches, where conidiophores & stem are at wide – angle or right angle of 45-90^0 (L-shaped) & at irregular interval with sporangiophores. Round sporangium contains endospores **called sporangiospores** as shown in **fig.-21.** Rhizoids are present in *Rhizopus.* Due to absence of septa/cross wall, fluid from hyphae free to escape & during handling of tissue hyphae collapse or wrinkle giving ribbon like appearance.

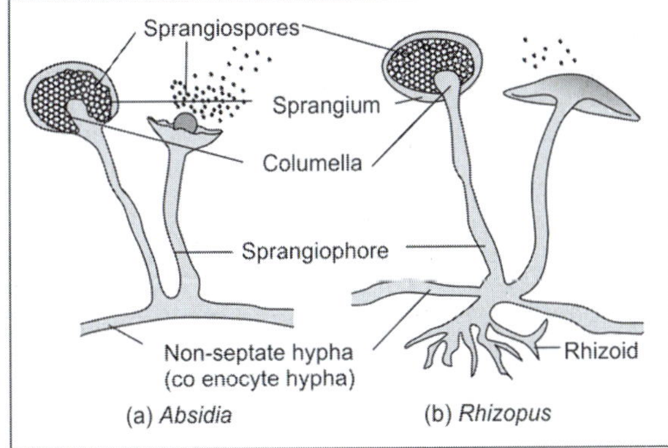

Figure-21: Schematic diagram of Zygomycetes

c. **Serological tests:** Like agglutination test, RIA, ELISA & immunodiffusion tests are useful.

d. **Molecular method:**

- **Disadvantages:** High cost & not available in periphery.
- **Advantages:** High sensitivity & specificity.
- **Methods:** PCR

e. **Animal inoculation:** Rabbit & mouse are susceptible.

➢ **Prevention:** Prevented by avoiding the exposure of spores.

➢ **Treatment:** Surgery & antifungal drugs are useful.

➢ **Morphological differences between *Aspergillus* & Zygomycetes:** → Table-2

Features	*Aspergillus*	Zygomycetes
Hyphae	Septate	Aseptate
Branches	Dichotomous branches, where conidiophores & stem are at acute / narrow angle of 45^0 (V shaped)	Obtuse branches, where conidiophores & stem are at wide – angle or right angle of 45-90^0 (L shaped)
Spores	Exogenous in chain	Endogenous in a sporangium
Rhizoides	Absent	Present in spme species

Table-2: Morphological differences between *Aspergillus* & Zygomycetes

VII. Other Opportunistic mycoses

i. ***Trichosporon beigelii*:** Produce white piedra & other systemic lesion.

ii. ***Fusarinm graminiarum.***

iii. ***Geotrichum candidum.***

iv. ***Blastoschizomyces capitatus.***

v. ***Saccharomyces cerevisiae* (Baker's yeast or Brewer's yeast).**

vi. ***Rhodotorula* spp.**

Question bank

Case study

1) A 30 year old male occupationally farmer present with granulomatous swelling on leg with sinuses discharge granules. Granules are collected for gram stain which revealed centrally gram positive bacterial filaments. Identify the organism & answer the following

a) Name the probable clinical disease in given case.
b) Write the etiological agents of clinical disease in given case.
c) Write the pathogenicity of clinical disease in given case.
d) Write the laboratory diagnosis of clinical disease in given case.

2) A 30 year old female, resident of Himachal Pradesh, prickled her left finger while pruning rose bushes develop a granulomatous nodule at the site of injury. Later she developed series of similar lesions on the left hand. Tissue is collected from granulomatous nodule & cultured on SDA. Microscopy of

culture growth revealed cigar shaped yeast cells. Identify the organism & answer the following

a) Name the clinical disease & causative agent in given case.
b) Write the pathogenicity of causative agent
c) Write the laboratory diagnosis of causative agent

3) A 30 year old male, resident of West Bengal, associated with chicken coops, present with tuberculosis like features like chronic cough, haemoptysis & lymphadenopathy. Chest X ray show the pulmonary infiltrate. Lymph node aspirate cultured on SDA in two plates, one incubated at 25^{0}C & other at 37^{0}C. Microscopy of culture growth at 37^{0}C revealed hyaline septate hyphae with microconidia & tuberculate macroconidia. Identify the organism & answer the following

a) Name the clinical disease & causative agent in given case.
b) Write the pathogenicity of causative agent.
c) Write the laboratory diagnosis of causative agent.

4) A 22 year old male, brought to emergency with headache, neck rigidity & sudden loss of vision. Lumber puncture is performed & CSF is collected. Microscopy performed with indian ink which revealed capsulated budding yeast cells. Identify the organism & answer the following

a) Name the clinical disease & causative agent in given case.
b) Write the pathogenicity of causative agent.
c) Write the laboratory diagnosis of causative agent.

5) A 25 year old female, visited the hospital with complains of rhinitis, nasal discharge & nasal blockage. She has history of asthma & allergy. On examination multiple ethmoidal polyps are noted. Biopsy is taken from the lesion, cultured on two plates of SDA & incubated at room temperature & at 37^0. Septate hyphae with dichotomous branching at 45^0 angle are identified under the microscopy from culture growth. Identify the organism & answer the following

a) Name the clinical disease & causative agent in given case.
b) Write the pathogenicity of causative agent.
c) Write the laboratory diagnosis of causative agent.

6) A 30 year old male, brought to emergency with bloody nasal discharge & obital swelling. Patient given history of diabetes. Discharge is collected & tested by culture on SDA. Aseptate broad hyphae are identified under the microscopy from culture growth. Identify the organism & answer the following

a) Name the disease & most common species in given case.
b) Write the pathogenicity of causative agent.
c) Write the laboratory diagnosis of causative agent.

Essay/Full question

1) Deep mycoses.
2) Opportunistic mycoses.

Short notes

1) Mycetoma.
2) Sporotrichosis.
3) Histoplasmosis.
4) Cryptococcosis.
5) Aspergillosis (Aspergilloma).
6) Zygomycosis.

Short questions for theory/viva questions

1) Name the four fungi/bacteria causing mycetoma.
2) Write four examples of subcutaneous mycoses / systemic mycoses / opportunistic mycoses.
3) Write four examples of dimorphic fungi.
4) What are asteroid bodies & sclerotic bodies?
5) What is Splendore-Hoeppli phenomenon?
6) What are dichotomous branches of hyphae? Name the fungus with such haphae.
7) Comment: Cryptococcus is carminophilic fungus.
8) Comment: *Pneumocystis* is classified as fungus.
9) Write four morphological differences between *Aspergillus* & zygomycetes.

MCQs for chapter review

Subcutaneous mycoses

1) Actinomycotic mycetoma is caused by - (PGI-05, May-13)
(a) *Actinomyces* (b) *Nocardia* (c) *Streptomyces* (d) Madura mycosis (e) *Staphylococcus*

2) Causative organism in Madura mycosis mycetoma is(AI-96)
(a) *Nocardia* (b) Dimorphic fungus (c) *Aspergillus* (d) Dermatophytes

3) Mycetoma foot can be caused by following (PGI, Nov-13, May-10)
(a) *Cladosporium* (b) *Phialophora jeanselmei* (c) *Madura mycetomatis* (d) *Allesheria boydii*

4) Colour of granules in mycetoma caused by *Actinomyces* spp.
(a) Black (b) Yellow (c) Red (d) Brown

5) Colour of granules in mycetoma caused by *A. pelleiterri*
(a) Black (b) Yellow (c) Red (d) Brown

6) The most common cause of Mycetoma in India (PGI -97)
(a) *Nocardia braziliensis* (b) *Actinomedua maduraei* (c) Piedra (d) Tinea cruris

7) Yellow black granules are seen in which fungal infection
(a) Mucormycosis (b) Mycetoma (c) Aspergillosis (d) Rhinosporidiosis

8) Which of the following is the most predominant constituent of sulfur granules of actinomycosis- (AIIMS, May- 04)
(a) Organisms (b) Neutrophils and monocytes (c) Monocytes and lymphocytes (d) Eosinophils

9) The granules discharged in mycetoma contains- (AIIMS, May- 02)
(a) Bone specules (b) fungal colonies (c) Pus cells (d) Inflammatory cells

10) True about mycetoma (PGI, Dec -08, 04)
(a) Commonly occurs on hands (b) Commonly erodes bone (c) Drain through lymphatics (d) Inflammatory cells

11) Which of the following is false about mycetoma (AI - 95)
(a) Can affect lower and upper extremities (b) Caused by actinomycetes and filamentous fungi (c) Diagnosis is by examination of pus (d) Uncommon in India

12) Discharging sinus is seen in
(a) Sprotrichosis (b) Cryptococcosis (c) Histoplasmosis (d) Mycetoma

13) True about madura mycetoma (PGI, June- 05)
(a) Fungal infection (b) Presented as non-painful nodular lesion for many months (c) Discharging sinus (d) Bone involvement seen

14) A plant prick can produce sporotrichosis. All are true statements about sporotrichosis
(a) Is a chronic mycotic disease that typically involves skin, subcutaneous tissue and regional lymphatics (b) Most cases are acquired via cutaneous inoculation (c) Enlarged lymph nodes extending centripetally as a beaded chain are a characteristic finding (d) Is a occupational disease of butchers, doctors

15) A gardner has multiple vesicles on hand and multiple eruption along the lymphatics. Most common fungus responsible is? (AIIMS, Nov- 08)
(a) *Sprothrix schenckii* (b) *Cladosporium* (c) *Histoplasma* (d) *Candida*

16) A farmer from the sub Himalayan region presents with multiple leg ulcers. The most likely causative agent is (AIIMS, Nov- 12, AI-12)

(a) *Trichophyton rubrum* (b) *Cladosporium* species (c) *Sprothrix schenckii* (d) *Aspergillus*

17) Cigar body is seen in
(a) Cryptococcosis (b) Histoplasmosis (c) Sprothrichosis (d) Aspergillosis

18) Asteroid body and cigar shaped globi may be produced by (AIIMS -87)
(a) *Sporothrix* (b) Sporotrichosis (c) *Phialophora* (d) *Aspergillus*

19) A series of ulcer in lower extremities in sub Himalayan area is often caused by (AI -97, 12)
(a) *Trichophyton rubrum* (b) *Pseudoallescheria boydii* (c) *Cladosporium* (d) *Sporothrix schenckii*

20) Causative organism of chromoblastomycosis (AIIMS, May -93)
(a) *Cladosporium* (b) *Blastomyces* (c) *Sporothrix* (d) *Histoplasma capsulatum*

21) Sclerotic bodies 3-15µm in size, multiseptate chest nut brown colour seen in
(a) Rhinosporidiosis (b) Chromoblastomycosis (c) Phacohyphomycosis (d) Histoplasmosis

22) Sclerotic bodies is seen
(a) *Sporothrix* (b) Blastomycosis (c) Chromoblatomycosis (d) *Coccicidioides*

23) Which is not a fungus
(a) Rhinosporidiosis (b) Sporotrichosis (c) Torulosis (d) Candidiasis

24) Rhinosporidiosis is caused by (PGI -06)
(a) Fungus (b) Bacteria (c) virus (d) Protozoan (e) Parasite

25) True about *Rhinosporidium seeberi*
(a) Fungi (b) Bacteria (c) Ketoconazole - treatment (d) Present in coastal India

Systemic mycoses

26) The medium of choice for culturing yeast form of dimorphic fungi is
(a) Brain heart infusion (b) Sabouraud's (c) Sabouraud's plus antibiotics (d) Any medium incubated at 35-37^{0}C

27) Systemic infection is caused by all fungi except-
(a) *Cryptococcus* (b) *Histoplasma* (c) Dermatophytes (d) *Paracoccidioides*

28) Systemic fungal infections can be caused by the following (AIIMS-85)
(a) *Cryptococcus neoformans* (b) *Histoplasma capsulatum* (c) *Paracoccidioides brasiliensis* (d) *Naegleria fowleri* (e) *Isospora belli*

29) Endemic fungal infection is caused by all of the following except (PGI, Dec -05)
(a) *Coccidioides immitis* (b) *Cryptococcus* (c) Histoplasmosis (d) *Aspergillus* (e) *Blastomyces*

30) True about *Histoplasma capsulatum* (PGI -97)
(a) Dimorphic fungus (b) Causative organisms of moniliasis (c) Causative organism of velly fever (d) Capsulated

31) Darling disease is caused by
(a) *Histoplasma* (b) *Candida* (c) *Cryptococcus* (d) *Rhizopus*

32) What is true about histoplasmosis (AIIMS, May -08)
(a) In early stage it is indistinguishable from TB (b) Culture is not diagnostic (c) Hyphal forms are infectious form (d) Person to person spread occurs by droplet infection

33) 'Tuberculate spores' are characteristic features of (PGI, May -10)
(a) *Candida* (b) *Histoplasma* (c) *Coccidioidomyces* (d) *Cryptococcus*

34) Histoplasmosis is spread by
(a) Human (b) Water (c) Soil (d) None

35) *Blastomyces* is characterised by all except
(a) Yeast like fungus (b) Commonly involves lung and skin (c) Dimorphic fungus (d) Common in South America

36) Valley fever or Desert rheumatism is caused by
(a) *Coccidioides immitis* (b) *Cryptococcus* (c) Histoplasmosis (d) *Aspergillus*

37) In tissue *Coccidioides immitis* produces (AIIMS-84)
(a) Spherules and endospores (b) Encapsulated yeast cells (c) Fine, delicate hyphae (d) Coarse, septate hyphae

38) *Coccidioides immitis* is identified in tissue on the basis of the following (AIIMS-97)
(a) Budding yeast cells with pseudohyphae (b) Yeast like forms with very large capsules (c) Arthospores (d) Endosporulating spherules

39) Following is not matched
(a) *H. capsulatum* - Narrow based budding yeast cells
(b) *B. dermatitidis* - Broad based budding yeast cells
(c) *H. capsulatum* - Yeast cells gives figure 8 appearance
(d) *C. immitis*- Arthospores & Endosporulating spherules
(e) *P. braziliensis* - Multiple based budding yeast cells

Opportunistic mycoses

40) *Cryptococcus neoformans* is a (AI-99)
(a) Protozoa (b) Fungus (c) Parasite (d) Mycoplasma

41) *Eucalyptus camaldulensis* is associated with the transmission of (PGI-99)
(a) *Blastomyces dermatitidis* (b) *Histoplasma* (c) *Cryptococcus* (d) *Coccidioides immitis*

42) Primary site of infection of cryptococcosis is?
(a) Adrenal (b) Bone (c) Central nerve system (d) Lung

43) *Cryptococcus* is least likely to cause infection of (AI-95)
(a) Skin (b) Bone (c) Brain (d) Kidney

44) *Cryptococcus* has predilection for (PGI-98)
(a) Lungs (b) Meninges (c) Liver (d) GIT

45) Virulence factor of *C. neoformans* includes all except
(a) Polysaccharide capsule (b) Production of protease (c) Ability to make melanin (d) Urease production

46) Phagocytosis of *C. neoformans* is inhibited by (PGI-83)
(a) Cryptococcal capsular material (b) The size of yeast cell (c) The cell wall (d) Toxins produced by the organism

47) Cryptococcal meningitis is common in (PGI-00)
(a) Renal transplant patient (b) Agammaglobulinemia (c) Neutropenia (d) IgA deficiency

48) The capsule of *Cryptococcus neoformans* in a CSF sample is best seen by
(a) Gram stain (b) Indian ink preparation (c) Giemsa stain (d) Methenamine silver stain

49) *Cryptococcus* can be readily demonstrated by
(a) Albert;s stain (b) Indian ink preparation (c) Giemsa stain (d) Gram's stain (e) ZN stain

50) Latex agglutination study of the antigen in CSF helps in the diagnosis of (AI-00)
(a) *Cryptococcus* (b) Candidiasis (c) Aspergillosis (d) Histoplasmosis

51) All are true regarding cryptococcal infection except (AI-98, AIIMS, Sept-96)
(a) Occurs in immunodeficient states (b) Capsular antigen in CSF is a rapid method of detection (c) Anti-capsular antibody is protective (d) Urease +Ve

52) True about *Cryptococcus neoformans* is all except (AIIMS-96)
(a) Capsular antigen is detected in CSF (b) Common in immunocompromised patient (c) Anti-capsular antibody prevents recurrence (d) Strongly positive mucicarmine stain of the organism in tissue is diagnostic

53) Which is false regarding *Cryptococcus neoformans* (AI-95)
(a) Grows at 5^{0}C and 37^{0}C (b) It has 4 serotypes (c) Urease negative (d) Causes superficial skin infection

54) Which of the following features is used for identification of *Cryptococcus neoformans*? (AI-95)
(a) Oxidase +Ve (b) Dextran fermentation (c) Hydrolyse urea (d) Grows at 42^{0}C

55) **All are true about *Cryptococcus* except**
(a) Polysaccharide capsule (b) Reproduce by budding (c) Pseudohyphae (d) Mycelium has a narrow base

56) **The important organism causing meningitis in immunocompromised patient is** (AI-91)
(a) *Histoplasma* (b) *Cryptococcus* (c) *Coccidioidomycosis* (d) *Candida albicans*

57) ***Pneumocystis carinii* is** (PGI -03)
(a) Bacteria (b) Fungus (c) Virus (d) Parasite

58) ***Pneumocystis carinii* is primarily a pathogen of**
(a) Rabbit (b) Human (c) Rat (d) Dog

59) ***Pneumocystis carinii* infects**
(a) Human (b) Monkeys (c) Rat (d) Cats

60) ***Pneumocystis carinii* is a fungus because** (PGI -00)
(a) rRNA, mitochondrial protein gene sequence and presence of thymidylate synthase (b) Cell wall contains glucans (c) Antifungal are effective against *P. carinii* (d) Commonest infection in AIDS

61) ***Pneumocystis carinii* is diagnosed by**
(a) Sputum examination for trophozoites and cyst under microscope (b) Culture (c) Positive serology (d) Growth on artificial media

62) ***Pneumocystis carinii* is diagnosed by** (AIIMS-92)
(a) Silver nitrate staining (b) Leishmann staining (c) Fontana's staining (d) Acid fast staining

63) **Which is false about *Penicillium marnefei***
(a) Black colonies (b) Dimorphic fungus (c) Amphotericin B used for treatment (d) Causes fulminant infection in immunocompromised patients

64) ***Penicillium marnefei* is seen in**
(a) Tuberculosis (b) AIDS (c) Diabetes (d) Kala azar

65) **Bronchopulmonary aspergillosis is mediated by**
(a) Type I hypersensitivity (b) Type III hypersensitivity (c) Type II hypersensitivity (d) Both a and b

66) **What is the most probable entry of a *Aspergillus*** (AIIMS-80)
(a) Puncture wound (b) Blood (c) Lungs (d) Gastro intestinal tract

67) ***Aspergillus* causes all except**
(a) Bronchopulmonary allergy (b) Otomycosis (c) Dermatophytosis (d) Oculomycosis

68) **A diabetic patient present with blood nasal discharge, orbital swelling and pain. Culture of periorbital swelling showed branching septate hyphae. Which of the following is the most probable organism involved** (AI-12)
(a) *Mucor* (b) *Candida* (c) *Aspergillus* (d) *Rhizopus*

69) **Acute angled septate hyphae are seen in**
(a) *Aspergillus* (b) *Mucor* (c) *Pencillium* (d) *Candida*

70) **Aspergilloma has**
(a) Septate hyphae (b) Pseudohyphae (c) Metachromatic hyphae (d) No hyphae

71) **Aseptate hyphae are not seen in**
(a) *Rhizopus* (b) *Mucor* (c) *Aspergillus* (d) None

72) **Mucormycosis** (PGI, Dec -02)
(a) Angio invasion (b) Lymph invasion (c) Septate hyphae (d) Long term deferoxamine is the precipitating factor (e) It may lead to blindness

73) **Orbital mucormycosis is a complication of**
(a) AIDS (b) Steroid therapy (c) Cushing's disease (e) Diabetic ketoacidosis

74) **Vascular invasion is a characteristic feature of** (AIIMS-80)
(a) Candidiasis (b) Mucormycosis (c) Blastomycosis (e) Sporotrichosis

75) **A diabetic patient present with pus from eye. Colonies of isolated organism are black with microscopic feature of non septate hyphae and obtuse branching. Diagnosis is**
(a) Aspergillosis (b) Candidiasis (c) Mucormycosis (d) Histoplasmosis

76) **Vascular involvement and thrombosis is seen in**
(a) Coccidioidomycosis (b) Aspergillosis (c) Mucormycosis (d) Histoplasmosis

Answers of MCQs & explanation

1) (a), (b) & (c)
2) (a) & (c)
3) (b), (c) & (d)
4) (b)
5) (c)
6) (b)
7) (b)

Follow section (**mycetoma → etiological agents)** for explanation

8) (a)
9) (b)
10) (b)
11) (d)
12) (d)
13) (a), (b) (c) & (d)

Follow section, **subcutaneous mycoses (mycetoma → pathogenicity)** for explanation

14) (d)
15) (a)
16) (c)
17) (c)
18) (a) & (b)
19) (d)

Follow section, **subcutaneous mycoses (sporotrichosis)** for explanation

20) (a)
21) (b)
22) (c)

Follow section, **subcutaneous mycoses, chromomycosis [chromoblastomycosis (verrucous dermatitis)]** for explanation

23) (a)

- Torulosis, is the former name for cryptococcosis
- Sporotrichosis & candidiasis are fungi
- Rhisporidiosis is not fungi but parafungal agent

24) (a)
25) (d)

Follow section, **subcutaneous mycoses (rhinosporidiosis)** for explanation

26) (c)
27) (a) & (c)
28) (b) & (c)
29) (b) (c) & (d)

Follow section, **systemic mycoses (properties & examples)** for explanation

30) (a)

- Moniliasis is caused by *Candida* spp.
- Valley fever is caused by *C immitis* while *Histoplasma* causes valley disease
- For explanation of option (d), follow section, **systemic mycoses (Histoplasmosis → etiological agent)**

31) (a)

- Follow section, **systemic mycoses (histoplasmosis → synonym)** for explanation

32) (a) Partially correct

- Histoplasmosis, not in early (acute) stage, but in late (chronic) stage is indistinguishable from TB
- Culture is the most diagnostic method
- Not the hyphal but spores are infectious
- Person to person spread does not occurs

33) (b)
34) (c)

Follow section, **systemic mycoses (histoplasmosis)** for explanation

35) (d)

- *Blastomyces* is common in North America
- Follow section, **systemic mycoses (blastomycosis)** for explanation of other options

36) (a)
37) (a)
38) (c) & (d)

Follow section, **systemic mycoses (coccidioidomycosis)** for explanation

39) (c)

- *B. dermatitidis* has broad based budding yeast cells which are giving figure 8 appearance
- Follow section, **systemic mycoses** for explanation of other options

40) (b)
41) (c)
42) (d)
43) (d)
44) (a) & (b)
45) (b)
46) (a)
47) (a)
48) (b)
49) (c) & (d)
50) (a)
51) (c)
52) (c)
53) (a) & (c)
54) (c) & (d)
55) (c) & (d)

(40–55) Follow section, **opportunistic mycoses (cryptococosis)** for explanation

56) (b)

- All options are known to produce meningitis, but for immunocompromised patient, agent is *Cryptococcus*

57) (b)
58) (c)
59) (c)
60) (a) & (b)
61) (a)
62) (a)

(57–62) Follow section, **opportunistic mycoses (pneumocystosis)** for explanation

63) (a)
64) (b)

(63–64) Follow section, **opportunistic mycoses (penicilliosis)** for explanation

65) (a) & (b)
66) (c)
67) (c)
68) (c)
69) (a)
70) (a)

(65–70) Follow section, **opportunistic mycoses (aspergillosis)** for explanation

71) (c)

- Aseptate (co-enocytic) hyphae are the features of *Zygomycets* (*Rhizopus* & *Mucor*) while *Aspergillus* has septate hyphae

72) (a)
73) (e)
74) (b)
75) (c)

(72–75) Follow section, **opportunistic mycoses (zygomycosis)** for explanation

76) (b) & (d)

- Fulminant paranasal sinuses aspergillosis is angio invasive, rapidly destructive & often fatal
- For option 'c' Follow section, **opportunistic mycoses (zygomycosis → pathogenesis).**

79 Miscellaneous topics in Mycology

Learning heading & subheadings

- Otomycoses
- Oculomycoses
- Allergic fungal diseases
- Fungal food poisoning

Otomycoses

❖ **Definition:** Subacute or chronic superficial fungal infection of external auditory canal.

❖ **Etiological agents:** Two etiological types,

A. **Molds / filamentous fungi:** *Aspergillus* is the most common cause.
- *Aspergillus flavus.*
- *Aspergillus fumigates.*
- *Aspergillus niger.*
- *Aspergillus terreus.*
- *Penicillium* species.
- *Pseudoallescheria boydii.*
- *Dermatophytes:* Also reported as otomycotic agent.

B. **Yeast like:**
- *Candida albicans.*
- *Candida tropicalis.*
- *Candida krusei.*
- *Malassezia sympodialis* (causes malignant otitis externa).

❖ **Pathogenicity:**

♣ **Reservoir & source of infection:** Water & external objects entering in the ear are the reservoir & source of infection.

♣ **Mode of transmission:** Entry of water, oil or other external objects may carry the microorganisms in ear.

♣ **Precipitating factors (epidemiological determinants):**

a. **Agent factors:** Organisms are penetrating very deep in the layers of skin; hence long term treatment is required.

b. **Host factors:**

1. **Age:** Common between 2nd & 3rd decade of life.
2. **Occupation:** People exposed to external atmosphere are more prone to get the disease.
3. **Entry of water:** During swimming, bathing or wetting rain.
4. **Poor hygiene:** It is common in patient with poor hygiene & who are not cleaning the ear following swimming or bathing.
5. **Disease:** Local in ear or systemic like IDDs.
6. **Local application:** Of oil, ear drops etc.
7. **Hormonal changes:** During pregnancy or menstruation are also responsible for infection.
8. **Malnutrition:** Are also the favouring factors for otomycosis.
9. **Socio-economic status:** Common in people with poor socio-economic status.

c. **Environmental factors:** Common in rainy season

♣ **Pathogenesis:** Organisms are penetrating very deep in the layers of skin; hence long term treatment is required. They also invite the secondary bacterial infections.

♣ **Clinical features:**
- Itching, little pain, irritation & discharge.
- Feeling of blocked ear due to collection of discharge or fungal growth.
- Cotton like growth: Cotton like growth may be identified in ear on examination which may be white (in *C. albicans*), green (in *A. fumigates*) or black (in *A. niger*).
- Hyperemic or oedematous skin or bleeding from ear present sometimes.

♣ **Complications:**
- Secondary bacterial infections.
- Deafness.
- Local penetration in mastoid bone or even in brain.

❖ **Differential diagnosis:** Otomycosis should be differentiated from
- Bacterial otitis externa.
- Furunculosis.
- Other local ear diseases.

❖ **Laboratory diagnosis:**

♣ **Specimens:** Ear discharge.

♣ **Testing:**

A. **Microscopy:**

i. **Direct 10% KOH:** It revealed fungal hyphae or yeast cells.

ii. **Gram stain:** Budding yeast cells & pseudohyphae are present un case of *Candida albicans.*

iii. **Immunofluoresent microscopy:** Also a useful method.

B. **Culture:**

- **Routine media:** SDA with antibiotics.
- **Cultivation technique:** Follow chapter → Laboratory diagnosis of fungal infections (section →flow chart-1).
- **C/Cs:** Creamy white colony by *C. albicans*, green colony by *A. fumigates* & black colony by *A. niger.*
- **LCB/PHOL stain:** Hyaline septate hyphae indicate the *Aspergillus* species.
- **Spores producing media:** Corn meal agar to identify the chlamydospores of *Candida albicans.*

❖ **Prevention:**

- **Improvement in hygiene:** Cleaning the ear following swimming or bathing by using sterile ear buds.
- Avoiding the application of antibacterial drops, oil or unsterile objects in ear.
- Special care during bathing & swimming.

❖ **Treatment:** Two types treatment

A **Local:** Antifungal drops like

- 1% clotrimazole & tolnaftate.
- 1% salicylic acid.
- 2% acetic acid.
- 1% gentian violet.
- Hamycin.
- Nystatin.

B **Systemic:** Antibacterial to control the secondary bacterial infection & analgesic to relieve the pain.

Oculomycoses

❖ **Definition:** It is the fungal infection of eyes.

❖ **Types:** Three types.

I. **Fungal keratitis**

II. **Endophthalmitis**

III. **Infection of ocular adnexa**

I. Fungal keratitis

✪ **Synonym:** Keratomycosis or mycotic keratitis.

✪ **Definition:** It is the invasive fungal infection of corneal stroma.

✪ **Etiological agent:** Majority of cases are caused by *Aspergillus, Fusarium & Candida* species.

A. **Molds or filamentous:** Total ⅓ cases of keratomycosis are caused by filamentous fungi, where *Aspergillus* (order of *Aspergillus* species is as mentioned below) is the most common cause followed by *Fusarium* spp. & phaeoid fungi.

- *Aspergillus fumigates.*
- *Aspergillus flavus.*
- *Aspergillus glucans.*
- *Aspergillus niger.*
- *Fusarium solani.*
- *Fusarium oxysporum.*
- *Penicillium* species.
- *Pae udoallescheria boydii.*
- *Paecilomyces* species.

B. **Phaeoid fungi:** 3rd common cause of keratomycosis after *Aspergillus & Fusarium.*

- *Curvularia* species.
- *Bipolaris* species.
- *Alternaria* species.
- *Exserohilum* species.
- *Aureobasidium pullulans.*
- *Fonseca pedrosoi* var. *cladosporium.*

C. **Yeast like:**

- *Candida albicans.*
- *Candida tropicalis.*
- *Candida krusei.*

✪ **Pathogenicity:**

♣ **Reservoir & source infection:** Fungi are present free in environment or on decaying vegetation.

♣ **Mode of transmission:** Following traumatic injuries in eyes.

♣ **Precipitating factors (epidemiological determinants):**

a. **Agent factors:**

- *Candida* species causes more localised & lesion looks like collar button.
- *Fusarium* is more aggressive & less responsive to treatment than *Aspergillus.*
- Phaeoid fungi are low virulent & produces the protracted infection.

b. **Host factors:**

1. **Age:** Middle age due to maximum activities.
2. **Sex:** More in male due to outdoor work.
3. **Earlier bacterial infection**
4. **Corneal injuries:** Following surgery like keratoplasty, wearing contact lens or vegetative in origin at farm.
5. **Local used of steroids for long term**
6. **Occupation:** Most common in agriculture workers following trauma with vegetative material contaminated by fungi.

c. **Environmental factors:**

1. **Season:** Peak in harvesting season.
2. **Distribution:**

- **USA:** *Fusarium* is most common in South East USA (Florida) & & *Candida* are most common in Northern USA.
- **India:** *Aspergillus* is the most common.

- **Pathogenesis:** Fungi are not able to penetrate the intact cornea, hence trauma inoculate the fungi in corneal. Fungal spores colonise the injured tissues & develop the hypopyon corneal ulcer. Hyphae invade from the ulcer bed to deep in corneal stroma leading to lesion with oedema & coagulative necrosis. Leucocyte infiltration with feathery border to lesion.
- **Clinical features:**
  - Mostly unilateral.
  - Pain, irritation, burning or foreign body sensation.
  - Redness of eye.
  - Blurred vision.
  - Photophobia.
  - May be discharge form eye.
  - Examination: Hypopyon corneal ulcer with oedema in corneal stroma.
- **Complications:** Blindness: 2nd major cause after cataract for blindness.
- **Differential diagnosis:** Fungal keratitis should be differentiated from viral, bacterial, parasitic (*Acanthamoeba*) & caused by *Pthium insidiosum.*
- **Laboratory diagnosis:**
- **Specimens:** Corneal scraping or discharge
- **Testing:** Two plates are inoculated by "C" or "S" shaped streak, to differentiate the growth from the contaminants. Other methods & finding are same as that of otomycosis.

Prevention:

- Avoiding the application of steroid drops in eye.
- Special care in wearing the contact lens & during work with vegetative material.
- Wearing goggles to prevent the injury.

Treatment: Two types treatment.

A. **Local drops:** Antifungal drops like
- 5% Pimaricin (natamycin).
- Nystatin, AMB or flucytosine lavage can be tried.

B. **Systemic drugs:** Oral fluconazole.

C. **Surgery:** Debridement of damaged tissues.

Allergic fungal diseases

Types: Two types.

i. **Id reaction:**

1. Candid: Follow chapter → Superficial mycoses
2. Dermatophytid: Follow chapter → Superficial mycoses

ii. **Systemic disease:**

- **Farmer's lung:** It is caused by fungi (**table-1**) & bacteria like
  - *Micromonospora (Thermocactinomyces / Saccharomonospiria) vulgaris & M candidus*
  - *Micropolyspora faenia (faenia rectivirgula)*
- **Other disease & agents: → Table-1**

Diagnosis: Diagnosis of specific reagin Ab (IgE).

Prevention:

- Avoiding exposure to allergen.
- Removal of mold laden object fungal growth on wall due to humidity or water leakage.
- Reducing humidity <50% may be beneficiary in reducing the fungal allergen.
- Dehumidifier or air conditioner can reduces both bacteria & mold, but care should be taken to avoid the contamination of conditioner or dehumidifier, otherwise they may form the new source of allergen.

Treatment: Anti-allergic drugs are useful. No role of antifungal drugs.

Disease	Source	Fungus
Farmer's lung	Stored hay	*A. flavus, A. niger A. fumigates, Penicillium rubrum, P. simplicissimum*
Maple bark stripper's lung	Maple tree bark	*Cryptostroma corticale*
Cheese washer's disease	Cheese	*Penicillium casei*
Maltster's lung	Barely malt	*Aspergillus clavatus*
Sequoiosis	Redwood sawdust	*Aureobasidium pullulans*
Suberosis	Cork	*Penicillium frequentans*
Wood pulp worker's disease	Wood pulp	*Alternaria* species
Bronchial asthama	-	Species of *Bipolaris, Alternaria , Penicillium & Aspergillus*
Allergic fungal rhinosinisitis	-	
Allergic broncho pulmonary aspergillosis	-	*Aspergillus* species
Scopulariopsis	-	*Scopulariopsis brumpti*
Lycoperdonosis	-	*Lycoperdono* species

Table-1: Allergic fungal disease, source & fungus

Fungal food poisoning

Types: Two types.

i. **Mycotoxicoses:**

➢ **Definitions:**
- **Mycotoxicoses:** Clinical illness due to ingestion of mycotoxin only.
- **Mycotoxin:** It is a toxin produced by fungus.

➢ **Examples:**

1. **Aflatoxins:**

- Acronym has been derived from ***A**spergillus **fla**vus* **toxin.**
- It has four types like B_1, B_2 G_1 & G_2 based on green (G) & blue (B) fluorescence produced under ultraviolet light on thin layer chromatographic plates.
- B_1 & B_2 are produced by *Aspergillus flavus,* G_1 & G_2 are produced by *Aspergillus parasiticus.* It also produced by *Aspergillus nominus* & *Penicillium puberulum.*
- It is ingested along with groundnut, peanut, corn, cotton-seed & tree nut.
- In human it causing Reye's syndrome (characterised by encephalopathy & fatty degeneration of viscera), hepatitis, hepatomegaly, renal disease etc.
- Aflatoxin B_1 is classified as group 1 human carcinogen by IARC & responsible to produce the renal & liver cancer.

2. **Fumonisins:**
- Produced by *Fusarium* species especially by *Fusarium moneliforme*, which is the common contaminant in maize & maize based products.
- It is responsible for major toxicological effects in animals like pigs (porcine oedema), rats (hepatotoxicity) & horses (equine leuco encephalomalacia).
- Fumonisins is classified as class 2B human carcinogen by IARC & responsible to produce the oesophageal cancer, in endemic regions of South Africa particularly in Transkei & also in parts of China. It also causing liver cancer in rat.

3. **Tricothecene:**
- Produced by *Fusarium* species mainly by *Fusarium graminearum* & rarely by *Fusarium sporotrichioides.* It also produced by other genera like *Trichoderma, Trichothecium, Myrothecium* & *Acremonium (Cephalosporium).*
- There are four types of trichothecene but type A is medically significant.
- It is ingested along with maize & soughum.
- Toxin is responsible for cardiomyopathy, alimentary toxic aleukia (necrotic lesion of oral cavity, oesophagus & stomach with marked leucopenia) & immunodepression.
- It is not the carcinogen but synergise the effect of aflatoxin.
- It was used in biological warfare in Laos **called yellow rain.**

4. **Ochratoxin:**
- Produced by *Aspergillus ochraceous, Aspergillus niger* & *Penicillium verrucosum.*
- It **called ochratoxin**, because originally it was identified from *Aspergillus ochraceous.*
- There are different types of ochratoxin but type A is medically significant.
- It is ingested along with cereals (like wheat, oats), peanut, peas, meat, milky powder, hay etc.
- It is identified as nephrotoxic (endemic nephropathy in different areas), carcinogen, immunosuppressant, mutagen & teratogen in all experimental animals.
- Ochratoxin A is identified urinary tract carcinogen by IARC.

5. **Cyclopiazonic acid:**
- It is produced by *Aspergillus flavus, Aspergillus oryzae* & also by *Penicillium cyclopium.*
- It is ingested along with groundnut & corn mostly as a contaminant with aflatoxin, however it does not augment the action of other toxin.
- In human it causing symptoms of "**kodua poisoning**" which actually occurred due to consumption of kodo millet (*Paspulum scrobiculatum*) & characterised by giddiness, sleepiness & tremors recover after 1-3 days.
- It also producing other symptoms like anorexia, weight loss, dehydration, convulsion & death.

6. **Zearalenone:**
- It is an estrogenic toxin produced by *Fusarium graminearum.*
- It is the common contaminant in maize, wheat & sorghum.
- It causing genital disorders in animals & in human it causing precocious pubertal changes.
- It's having carcinogenic property to produce cervical cancer in human.

7. **Other toxins:** Like **patulin, nitropropionic acid** etc. are able to produce the mycotoxicoses in human & animals.

ii. Mycetism (mycetismus, muscarinism or mushroom poisoning):

➢ **Definition:** Clinical illness due to ingestion of mycotoxin along with fungus.

➢ **Examples:**

1. *Claviceps* spp.: Ergot poisoning.
2. *Coprine* spp.: Coprine poisoning.
3. *Inocybe* spp.: Muscarine poisoning.

❖ Diagnosis:

➢ **Specimens:** Toxins are present in urine, bile, stool, milk & food stuff.

➢ **Testing methods:**

i. **Culture:** By using primary foetal bovine kidney cells.

ii. **Serological tests:** ELISA, RIA & precipitation based tests are useful.

iii. **Molecular method:** DNA-DNA homology & RFLP.

iv. **Animal inoculation:** Duckling, rat, rabbit & trout are useful animals.

v. **Chromatography:** GLC & HPLC.

❖ Prevention: Three ways.

1. **Decontamination:** Removal of fungal growth from the stored grains by hand picking.
2. **Detoxification:** Conversion of aflatoxoin B1 to less active metabolites like aflatoxoin M1 by using physical, chemical or microbiological methods.
3. **Legislation:** Strict rule for overuse of mycotoxin in food above permitted level.

❖ **Treatment:** Specific antidote for particular mycotoxin is not available, so symptomatic treatment is given.

Question bank

Case study

1) A 25 year male, who is regular visiting the swimming pool present in ENT OPD with greening discharge from ear. On examination of discharge by microscopy & culture septate hyphae with exospores are identified. Identify the disease & organism & answer the following
   a) Name the clinical condition & the most common causative agent in given case.
   b) Describe the other etiological agents of clinical condition, in given case.
   c) Write treatment of clinical condition, in given case.
2) A 30 year male, who is occupationally farmer visit the eye clinic with complain of discharge, red eye & photophobia. On examination corneal ulcer is identified. Corneal scraping is done & examined by microscopy & culture on SDA which revealed fungus with septate hyphae. Culture produces dark green colonies. Identify the disease & organism & answer the following
   a) Name the clinical condition & the most common causative agent in given case.
   b) Describe the other etiological agents of clinical condition, in given case.
   c) Write treatment of clinical condition, in given case.

Short notes

1) Otomycosis.
2) Oculomycosis.
3) Allergic fungal disease.
4) Fungal food poisoning.

Short questions for theory/viva questions

1) Name the four fungi causing otomycosis.
2) Name the four fungi causing mycotic keratitis.
3) Define: Mycetism & mycotoxicoses.

MCQs for chapter review

Otomycosis

1) **White discharge from ear indicate infection with**
   (a) *C. albicans* (b) *A. fumigate* (c) *A. niger* (d) *M. furfur*
2) **Which of the following is the most common etiological agent in paranasal sinuses** (AIIMS, May-06)
   (a) *Aspergillus* spp. (b) *Histoplasma* (c) *Conidiobolus coronatus* (d) *Candida albicans*

Oculomycosis

3) **Common fungus causing corneal ulcer** (PGI, June-01)
   (a) *Aspergillus* (b) *Mucor* (c) *Fusarium* (d) *Sporothrix*
4) **Branched septate hyphae found on corneal smear in a case of corneal ulcer is** (AIIMS, June-00)
   (a) *Candida* (b) *Mucor* (c) *Aspergillus* (d) *Histoplasma*
5) **In a patient, corneal ulcer scraping reveals narrow angled septate hyphae, which of the following is likely etiological agent** (AI-02)
   (a) *Mucor* (b) *Aspergillus* (c) *Histoplasma* (d) *Candida*

Allergic fungal diseases

6) **Farmer's lung is caused by** (PGI -87)
   (a) Micromonospore faenia (b) Aspergillosis (c) *Histoplasma capsulatum* (d) All of above

Fungal food poisoning

7) **Aflatoxins are produced by** (AI-11)
   (a) *Aspergillus flavus* (b) *Aspergillus niger* (c) *Aspergillus fumigatus* (d) *Candida*

Answers of MCQs & explanation

1) **(a)**
- Follow section **(otomycosis →clinical features)** for explanation
2) **(a)**
- *Aspergillus* is the most common etiological agent of infection in paranasal sinuses.
3) **(a) & (c)**
4) **(c)**
5) **(b)**
- (3–5) *Aspergillus* spp., *Fusarium* spp. & phaeoid fungi are common pathogen of keratitis, but *Aspergillus* is the most common etiological agent of keratitis (corneal ulcer), which shows hyaline septate hypha with conidiophores, vesicle, phialides & chain like arrangement of conidia. Hyphae showing dichotomous branches, where conidiophores & stem are equal in size (3-6μm) & at acute/narrow angle of 45^0 (V-shaped)
6) **(b)**
- Actual name of bacteria causing farmer's lung is *Micropolyspora faenia, Micromonospora candidus & Micromonospora vulgaris*
- Fungi causing farmer's lung are mentioned in **table-1**
7) **(a)**
- Aflatoxin = ***A****spergillus* ***fla****vus* **toxin**
- For other species producing aflatoxin follow section, **fungal food poisoning (mycotoxicoses → aflatoxins)**

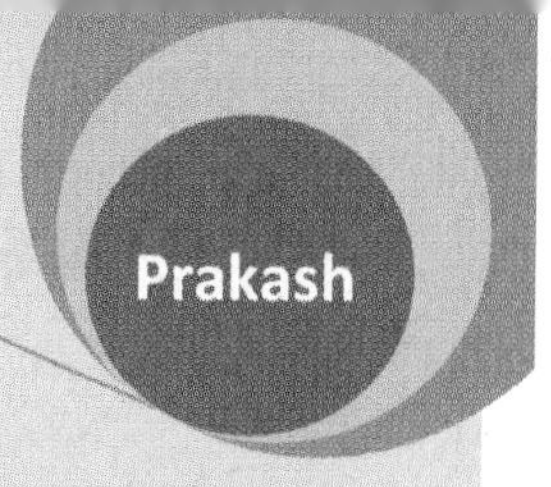

Section VI

Parasitology

Preview of Parasitology

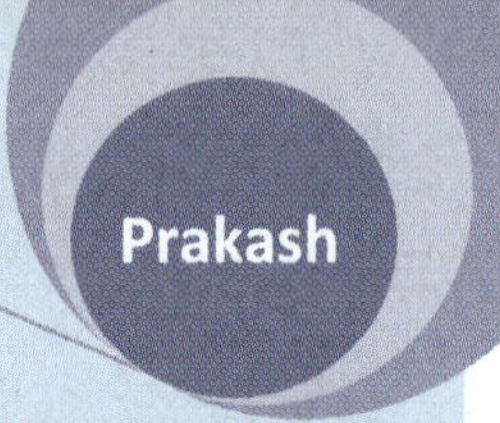

In Parasitology system almost all parasites are written with following headings & subheadings with use of specific bullets & numberings.

- **History:**
- **Geographical distribution:**
- **Habitat:**
- **Morphology:** With appropriate figures.
- **Culture:** Mainly in Protozoa.
- **Resistance:**
- **Immunity:**
- **Life cycle:**
  - **Hosts:**
  - **Methods of reproduction:** Only in Protozoa.
  - **Cycles:** With appropriate figures & flow charts.
- **Pathogenicity:**
  - **Disease name:**
  - **Reservoir of infection:**
  - **Source of infection:**
  - **Mode of transmission:**
  - **Incubation period:**
  - **Portal of entry:**
  - **Site:**
  - **Exit form:**
  - **Infective form:**
  - **Precipitating factors:**
  - **Pathogenesis:**
  - **Clinical features:**
  - **Complications:**
- **Laboratory diagnosis:**
  - **Specimens:**
  - **Testing methods:**

I. Direct methods

A. **Macroscopy:** Mainly in Metazoa.
B. **Microscopy:**
C. **Culture:** Mainly in Protozoa.

II. Indirect methods

A. **Cell count:** Like blood picture, urine picture etc.
B. **Immunological tests:**
C. **Serological tests:**
D. **Molecular methods:**
E. **Other methods:**

- **Prevention:**
- **Treatment:**

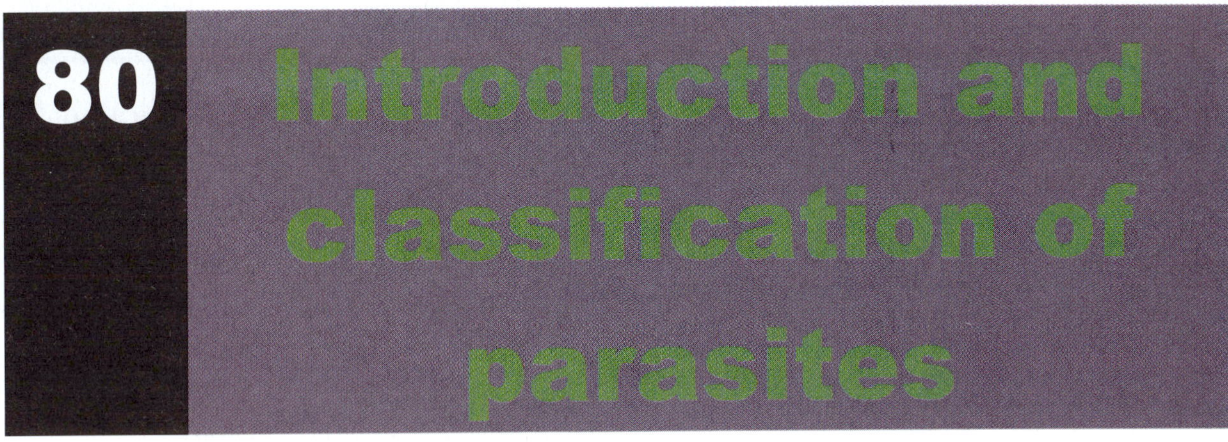

80 Introduction and classification of parasites

Learning heading & subheadings

- Parasite
- Host
- Life cycle

Parasite

❖ **Meaning:** Parasite word derived from **parasitos (Greek) = eater at the court (meat eater).**

❖ **Definitions:** Living organism which receives nourishment & shelter from other organism is **called parasite.**

❖ **Nomenclature:** Parasites have Latinized name, hence written in **Italics** (**Italics**= typed letter that slant to right). It consist two parts. 1st **part** is genus name starts with capital letter & 2nd **part** is species name starts with small letter like *Giardia lamblia.*

❖ **Classification:** Different types are as follows.

A. According to habitat: Two types.

1. **Ecto-parasite:** Parasite living outside on the body surface of the host **called ecto-parasite** like
   - **Itch mite:** *Sarcoptes scabiei* (*Acarus scabiei*).
   - **Louce:** Three types.
     - Head louse: *Pediculus capitis (Pediculus humanus capitis*).
     - Body louse: *Pediculus corporis (Pediculus humanus corporis*).
     - Pubis or crab louse: *Pthirus pubis.*
2. **Endo-parasite:** Parasite living inside the body of the host **called endo-parasite**.

B. According to visit to host: Following are types

1. **Temporary parasite:** Visit the host for short time.
2. **Permanent parasite:** Whole life passes as a parasitic life.
3. **Facultative parasite:** Lives the parasitic life when the opportunity arises.
4. **Obligatory parasite:** Can't exist without parasitic life.
5. **Occasional (accidental) parasite:** Attacks on unusual host.
6. **Wandering (abcrrant) parasite:** Happen to reach a place where it can't live.

C. Morphological classification: Based on their cellular structure, all parasites of medical importance are fall in two broad categories like protozoa & metazoa (helminths or worms) as shown in **flow chart-1, table-1 & table-2.**

D. Systemic classification:

- **Based on:** Conventional scheme of classification
- **General scheme of classification:** Kingdom (sub kingdom) → phylum (subphylum) → class (super class/subclass) → order (suborder) → family (super family/subfamily) → genus →species (sub species).
- **Parasites of medical importance are fall in to two kingdoms:**

1. **Protista:** Eukaryotic, microscopic & unicellular organisms **called protozoa** are fall in to protista as shown in **table-3.**
2. **Animalia:** Eukaryotic, macroscopic & multicellular organisms **called metazoa** are fall in to animalia as shown in **table-4.**

E. Pathogenic classification:

- **Based on:** Ability of species to produce diseases.
- **Types:**

1. **Pathogenic:**
2. **Nonpathogenic:**

} Described in respective chapter

Host

❖ **Definition:** Living organism which harbours the parasite **called host.**

❖ **Classification:** Different types are as follows.

i. Definitive (primary) host:

- Host which harbours the adult or sexual stage of parasite **called definitive host.**
- In major cases man is the definitive host.

ii. Intermediate (secondary) host:

- Host which harbours the larval or asexual stage of parasite **called intermediate host.**
- In major cases man is the definitive host, however in few parasitic infection man acts as an **intermediate host** like
  - *Plamodium* spp. (malaria).
  - *Babesis* spp. (babesiosis).
  - *Echinococcus granulosus* (hydatid disease).
  - *Toxoplasma gondii* (toxoplasmosis).
  - *Sarcocystis lindemanni* (sarcocystosis).
- In some parasitic infections two intermediate hosts are required **called first & second intermediate host** respectively like in *D. latum.*

iii. Paratenic host (carrier / transport host): Host where parasite remains viable without further development **called paratenic host.**

iv. Accidental / incidental host: Host in which parasite is not found usually but enters accidentally & host will be considered as dead end host like

1. Free living amoebae: *N. fowleri, Acanthamoeba* spp. & *B. mandrillaris.*
2. Invasive or muscular *Sarcocystis (S. lindamanni).*
3. *Spirometra* species.
4. *Echinococcus granulosus* in man.
5. *Multiceos multiceps.*
6. *Trichina spiralis.*
7. *Angiostrongylus* species.
8. *Capillaria hepatica.*

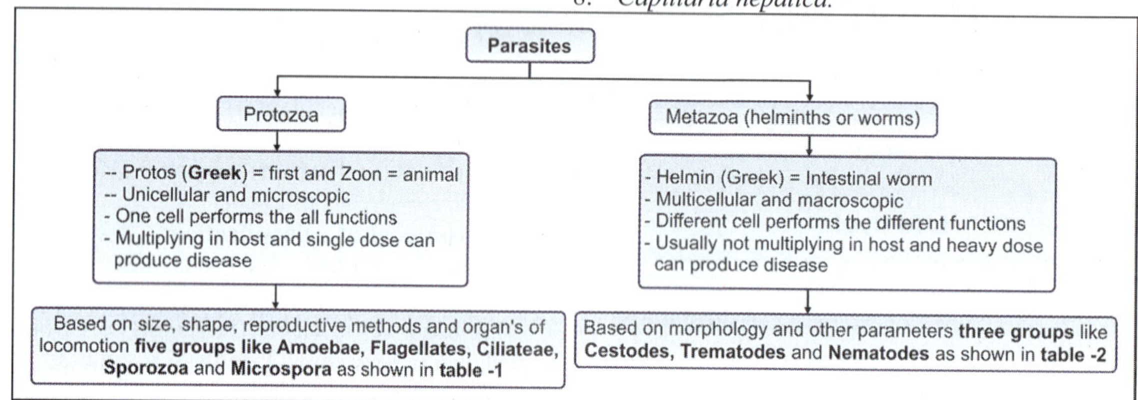

Flow chart-1: Morphological classification of parasites

Features	Amoebae	Flagellates	Ciliateae	Sporozoa	Microspora
Organ of locomotion	Pseuopodium	Flagella	Cilia	Non-motile	Non-motile
Examples	*E. histolytica, E. coli, N. fowleri* etc.	**(1) Oral/genital flagellates:** *Giardia, Trichomonas* **etc.** **(2) Haemo-flagellates:** *Leishmania & Trypanosoma*	*B. coli*	**(1) Blood inhabiting:** *Plasmodium, Babesia* **(2) GIT inhabiting:** *Isospora, Toxoplasma* etc.	*Pleistophora, Nosema, Enterocytozoon, Encephalitozon* etc.

Table-1: Morphological classification of parasites (protozoa)

Features	Cestoda	Trematoda	Nematoda
General features			
Common name	Tape worms or cestodes	Flukes or trematodes	Round worm or nematodes
Adult stage			
Shape	Tape like	Leaf like	Cylindrical
Segments	Segmented	Unsegmented	Unsegmented
Sexes	Not separate, hermaphrodite (monoecious)	Not separate / hermaphrodite (monoecious) except *Schistosoma*	Separate (diecious)
Head	Suckers often with hooks	Suckers, no hooks	No suckers, No hooks well developed buccal capsule for adhesion
GIT	Absent	Present but incomplete (No anus)	Present & complete with anus
Body cavity (Coelom)	Absent	Absent	Present
Female	Oviparous	Oviparous	Oviparous / vivi (larvi) parous / ovivivi parous
Egg stage			
Opeculum	Present in Pseudophylidea & absent in Cyclophylidea	Present in monoecious trematodes & absent in diecious trematodes	Absent
Larval stage			
Larval forms	Cysticercus, Cyticercoid, Hydatid cyst, Coenurus, Coracidium, Procercoid, Plerocercoid	Miracidium, Redia, Cercaria, Metacercaria. Redia, Sporocyst	Rhabditiform larvae, Filariform larvae. Microfilaria
Example	*D. latum* etc.	*S. haematobium* etc.	*A. lumbricoides* etc.

Table-2: Morphological classification of parasites (metazoa)

9. *Gnathostoma* spp.
10. Others: Normally cycle is continuing; but when parasite enters in certain tissues, man will be act as dead end host.
- *Taenia solium:* When larvae enter beyond the intestine.
- *E. histolytica:* When trophozoites enter beyond the intestine (extra-intestinal amoebiasis).

Life cycle

❖ **Definition:** Sequential change in growth, development & multiplication of parasite **called life cycle.**

❖ **Types:** Following are the types.

I. According to reproductive methods & types of host:

A. Sexual cycle / cycle in definitive host: Development & multiplication occurs by sexual methods.

B. Asexual cycle / cycle in intermediate host: Development & multiplication occurs by asexual methods.

II. According to numbers of host:

A. Direct (simple) cycle:

- **Definition:** When parasites require only single host to complete the cycle **called direct cycle.**
- **Examples:** Follow **table-5.**

B. Indirect (complex) cycle:

- **Definition:** When parasites require two or more host to complete the cycle **called indirect cycle.**
- **Subtypes:**

1. Requires two hosts
- In this cycle one host act as definitive while other acts as intermediate host.
- Examples: → **Table-6**

2. Requires three hosts
- Some parasites requires three hosts, of this one act as definitive while other two acts as intermediate hosts **called 1st intermediate host & 2nd intermediate host.**
- Examples: → **Table-7**

Kingdom: → Protista **Subkingdom:** → Protozoa							
Phylum	**Class**	**Sub-class**	**Order**	**Suborder**	**Family**	**Genus**	**Species**
Sarcomastigophora	**Subphylum** (Sarcodina) **Superclass** (Rhizopoda) **Class** (Lobosea /Amoebae)		Amoebida	Tubulina	Entamoebidae	*Entamoeba*	Pathogenic & non-pathogenic species are mentioned in **respective chapters**
						Endolimax	
						Iodamoeba	
				Acanthopodina	Hartmannellidae	*Acanthamoeba*	
	Class (Heterolobosea)		Schizopyrenida		Vahlkampfiidae	*Naegleria*	
	Subphylum (Mastigophora) **Class** (Zoomastigophora)		Trichomonadida		Trichomonadidae	*Trichomonas*	
						Dientamoeba	
						Retortomonas	
			Diplomonadida	Deploomonadida	Hexamitidae	*Giardia*	
				Enteromonadida		*Enteromonas*	
			Retortamonadida			*Chilomastix*	
			Kinetoplastida	Trypanosomatina	Trypanosomatidae	*Trypanosoma*	
						Leishmania	
Ciliophora	Kinetofrgaminophorea	Vestibuliferia	Trichostomatida	Trichostomatina		*Balantidium*	
Apicomplexa	Sporozoa		Haemosporida	Haemosporina	Haemosporidae	*Plasmodium*	
						Laverania	
			Piroplasmida	Piroplasmina	Piroplamidae	*Babesia*	
		Coccidia	Eucoccidia	Eimeriina	Eimeriidae	*Isospora*	
					Sarcocystidae	*Cyclospora*	
						Toxoplasma	
						Sarcocystis	
					Cryptosporidae	*Cryptosporidium*	
Microspora			Microsporida			*Enterocytozoon*	
						Encephalitozoon	
						Microsporidium	
						Nosema	
						Pleistophora	

Table-3: Systemic classification of protozoa

Kingdom → Animalia

Subkingdom: → Metazoa or Helminths

Phylum	Class	Subclass	Order	Suborder	Family	Genus	Species
Platyhelminths	Cestoda		Pseudophylidea		Diphylobothriidae	*Diphylobothrium*	Pathogenic & non-pathogenic species are mentioned in respective chapters
						Spirometra	
			Cyclophylidea		Taeniidae	*Taenia*	
						Echinococcus	
					Hymenolepidae	*Hymenolepis*	
					Dilepididae	*Dypilidium*	
	Trematoda	Digenea (So **called** because di (two) + genetic (generation), means required two hosts for cycle	Prosostomata	Strigeata	Schistosomatidae	*Schistosoma*	
				Amphistomata	Fasciolidae	*Fasciolopsis*	
						Fasciola	
				Distomata	Heterophyidae	*Heterophyes*	
						Metagonimus	
					Echinostomatidae	*Echinostoma*	
						Paryphostomum	
					Paraphistomatidae	*Watsonius*	
						Gastrodiscoides	
					Opisthorchidae	*Clonorchis*	
						Opisthorchis	
					Triglotrematidae	*Paragonimus*	
Nemathelminths	Nematoda	Aphasmidia (No caudal Chemo-receptors)	Enoplida		Trichinellidae	*Trichinella*	
					Trichuridae	*Trichuris*	
						Capillaria	
		Phasmidia (Caudal Chemo-receptors)	Rhabditidia		Ascarididae	*Ascaris*	
					Ancyclostomatidae	*Ancyclostoma*	
						Necator	
					Strogyloididae	*Strongyloides*	
					Oxyuridae	*Enterobius*	
					Angiostrogylidae	*Angiostrongylus*	
			Spirurida		Onchocercidae (Acanthocheilonematidae)	*Wucheria*	
						Brugia	
						Onchocerca	
						Dipetalonema	
						Mansonella	
						Dirofilaria	
						Loa	
					Dracunculidae	*Dracunculus*	
					Gnathostomatidae	*Gnathostoma*	

Table-4: Systemic classification of metazoa

Parasites	Host
Protozoa	
E histolytica	Man
G lamblia	Man
T vaginalis	Man
B coli	Pig & man
I belli	Man
C parvum	Man
C cayetanensis	Man
Microspora	Man
Metazoa	
A lumbricoides	Man
A duodenale	Man
N americanus	Man
S stercoralis	Man
T trichuria	Man

Table-5: Parasites with direct (simple) life cycle

❖ **Clinical significances:** Ideas of life cycle help

- To know the growth & development of parasite.
- To know the clinical disease produced by parasites.
- To diagnose the parasite in laboratory.
- To treat & to prevent the parasitic disease.

❖ Role of man in parasitic life cycle:

- **Normal (natural) life cycle:** Life cycles of many parasites normally continue between man & external environment or other host like animal, vector etc., all such life cycles are described with **green arrows** (↓) in respective chapters.
- **Dead end life cycle:**
  - Many parasites once enter in man, can't continue their life cycle & man act as **dead end,** all such life cycles are described with **red arrows** (↓) in respective chapters.
  - **Red arrows** (↓) also given where parasites, (especially trophozoites) are released in external environment where they get disintegrate.
- **Life cycle with autoinfection in man:** Life cycles of parasites in which autoinfection in man is possible are described with **sky blue arrows** (↓) in respective chapters.

- **Other type of life cycles:** All other type life cycles in man like exoenteric cycle in *T gondii*, retrograde cycle in *E vermicularis* etc. are described with **black arrows** (↓) in respective chapters. These cycles allows the continuation of life cycle but these are not occurs normally or naturally.
- In certain parasitic life cycle, either naturally or accidentally man acts as both definitive host (harbours adult/sexual stage) as well as intermediate host (harbours larval/asexual stage) like in *H nana*, *T solium* & *T. spiralis*.

Parasites	Definitive host	Intermediate host
Protozoa		
Plamodium spp.	Mosquito	Man
Babesia spp.	Hard (*Ixodid*) tick	Man
T gondii	Cat	Man/animals
S. bovihominis	Man	Cattle
S. suihominis	Man	Pig
S. lindamanni	Cat or dog	Man
Metazoa		
T saginata	Man	Cattle (cow)
T solium	Man	Pig
E granulosus	Dog	Man
H nana (direct cycle)	Man/rat	Man/rat
H nana (indirect cycle)	Man	Flea
D caninum	Man	Flea
Schistosoma spp	Man	Snail
F buski	Man	Snail
G hominis	Man	Snail
F hepatica	Man	Snail
A costaricensis	Man	Slug
W bancrofti	Man	Mosquito
B malayi	Man	Mosquito
O volvulus	Man	Black fly
L loa	Man	Deer fly
Mansonella spp.	Man	Mosquito
D medinensis	Man	Cyclops

Table-6: Parasites requires two hosts

Parasites	Definitive host	1st Intermediate host	2nd Intermediate host
Metazoa			
D latum	Man	Cyclops or diaptomus	Fish
H hetrophyes	Man	Snail	Fish
M yokogawai	Man	Snail	Fish
Echinostoma spp.	Man	Snail	Mollusc
C sinensis	Man	Snail	Fish
O felineus	Man	Snail	Fish
P westermanii	Man	Snail	Crab/cray fish
G spinigerum	Animal	Cyclops	Fish

Table-7: Parasites requires three hosts

Question bank

Essay/Full question

1) Types of parasites.

Short notes

1) Differences between cestodes & trematodes.
2) Differences between cestodes & nematodes.
3) Differences between trematodes & nematodes.
4) Systemic classification of protozoa.
5) Systemic classification of metazoan (helminths).

Short questions for theory/viva questions

1) What is ecto-parasite? Write two examples.
2) Write two differences between protozoa & metazoan.
3) Name the 4 parasites in which man act as an intermediate host.
4) Name the four parasites in which man act as dead end host.
5) Define definitive host & intermediate host.
6) Name two parasites in which man act as both definitive host & intermediate host.

MCQs for chapter review

Parasite

1) **Nematodes are differentiated from other worms by** (PGI, May-13, Dec-05)
(a) Segmentation absent (b) Separate coelomic cavity (c) As Sexes are separate (d) They are cylindrical (e) GIT is formed completely
2) **Operculated eggs are seen in**
(a) Nematodes (b) Cestodes (c) Trematodes (d) Protozoa
3) **Alimentary canal is absent in**
(a) Cestodes (b) Trematodes (c) Nematodes (d) None of above
4) **Cylindrical worms are**
(a) Tape worms (b) Flukes (c) Round worms (d) Cestodes
5) **True about trematodes**
(a) Two hosts required (b) Segmented (c) Anus present (d) Body cavity present

Host

6) **Definitive host is one**
(a) In which sexual multiplication takes place (b) In which asexual multiplication takes place (c) Harbours adult form (d) Harbours larval form
7) **Man acts as an intermediate host in**
(a) *L. donovani* (b) *Plamodium* spp. (c) *E. granulosus* (d) b+c
8) **Man is secondary host for**
(a) Malaria (b) Tuberculosis (c) Filariasis (d) relapsing fever

Life cycle

9) **Simple life cycle requires**
(a) One host (b) Two host (c) Three host (d) Four host
10) **Simple life cycle seen in** (PGI, Dec -06)
(a) *Ascaris* (b) *T solium* (c) *Toxoplasma* (d) *Giardia* (e) *Schistosoma*
11) **Two hosts required in** (PGI, Dec -02)
(a) *T solium* (b) *E histolytica* (c) *T saginata* (d) *Giardia* (e) *Toxoplasma*
12) **The intermediate host for *T saginata***
(a) Man (b) Cow (c) Dog (d) Pig
13) **Which of the following parasites passes through three hosts**
(a) *Fasciola hepatica* (b) *Fasciola buski* (c) *Schistosoma haematobium* (d) *Clonerchis sinensis*

14) **Crab is the intermediate host for**
(a) *Clonerchis sinensis* (b) *Paragonumus westermanii* (c) *Fasciola hepatica* (d) *Schistosoma haematobium*

15) **Fish acts as intermediate host in** (PGI-04)
(a) *D latum* (b) *Clonerchis sinensis* (c) *H diminuta* (d) *H nana*

16) **Man is definitive host for**
(a) Echinococcosis (b) Malaria (c) Filariasis (d) Rabies (e) Leishmaniasis

Answers of MCQs & explanation

1) **(a), (b), (c), (d) & (e)**
2) **(b) & (c)**
3) **(a)**
4) **(c)**

(1–4: Follow **table-2** for explanation)

5) **(a)**
- Option a: Follow **table-4** for explanation (trematodes are classified under class ***Digenea***)
- Option b, c & d: Follow **table-2** for explanation

6) **(a) & (c)**
- Follow section, **host (classification → definitive host)** for explanation

7) **(b) & (c)**
8) **(a)**

(7–8: Follow section, **host (classification → intermediate host)** for explanation)

9) **(a)**
10) **(a) & (d)**

(9–10: Follow section, **life cycle (table-5)** for explanation)

11) **(a), (c) & (e)**
12) **(b)**

(11–12: Follow section, **life cycle (table-6)** for explanation)

13) **(d)**
14) **(b)**
15) **(a) & (b)**

(13–15: Follow section, **life cycle (table-7)** for explanation)

16) **(a) & (e)**
- In echinococcosis & malaria man is the intermediate host
- In filariasis & leishmaniasis, man allows the sexual stage of life cycle hence it s definitive host
- Rabies is viral disease, does not required like definitive & intermediate host.

81 Laboratory diagnosis of parasitic infections

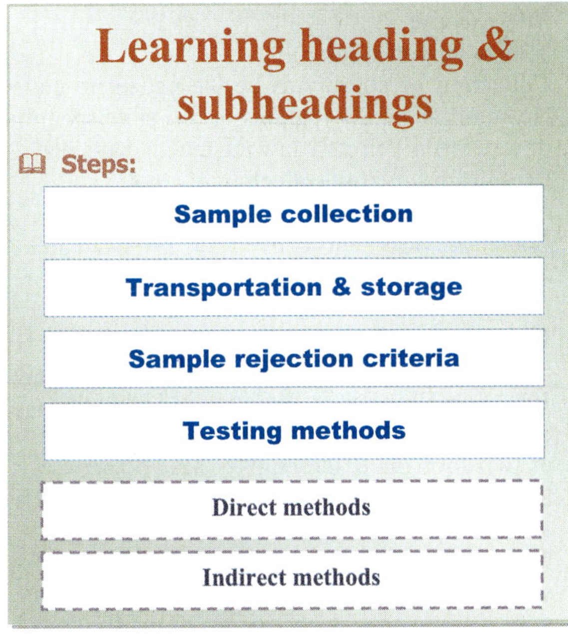

Steps: Following are the different steps employed for diagnosis of parasitic infections

- ◊ **Sample collection:**
- ◊ **Transportation & storage:**
- ◊ **Sample rejection criteria:**
- ◊ **Testing methods:**

Sample collection

❖ **Precautions:** Following are the precautions to be taken before collecting the sample

- Take all the aseptic precautions
- Wearing the PPEs (Personal Protective Equipments) like disposable gloves, eye shields, apron, cap, mask & shoes cover.
- Collect at right time.
- Use disposable needle & syringe.
- Container should be sterile, leak proof & securely fastened.
- Filling the request form with complete data.
- If spillage of sample then wipe it with 10% sodium hypochlorite.
- Proper waste disposal of hazardous material.

❖ **Samples & indications:** Collect the following samples in sterile container.

➢ **Blood:**

- *Typanosoma* spp.
- *Leishmania* spp. in macrophages.
- *Plasmodium* spp. in RBCs.
- *Babesia* spp.
- *Toxoplasma gondii.*
- Microfilariae free in blood.
- Blood → centrifuge → separate serum → for serological testing.

➢ **Stool (GIT parasites):**

✪ **Trophozoites or cyst stage:**

- *E. histolytica.*
- *E. coli.*
- *G. lamblia.*
- *B. coli.*

✪ **Oocyst**

- *Isospora belli.*
- *Cryptopsoridium parvum.*

✪ **Spores like yeast cells:** *Microsporidia.*

✪ **Adult stage:**

- Round worm.
- Hook worm.
- Thread worm.
- Whip worm.

✪ **Larval stage:** *S. stercoralis.*

✪ **Egg stage:**

- Round worm **(bile stained).**
- Hook worm.
- Thread worm.
- Whip worm **(bile stained).**
- *Taenia* spp. **(bile stained).**
- *H. nana.*
- *Fasciolopsis buski.*
- *Fasciola* spp.
- *Schistosoma mansoni & S. japonicam.*
- *Dipylidium* spp.
- *D. latum.*

✪ **Segments of adult stage:**

- *Taenia* spp.
- *D. latum* & other tape worm species.

➢ **Urine:**

- Trophozoite: *T. vaginalis.*
- Eggs: *S. haematobium.*
- Larvae: Microfilariae.

➢ **Sputum (pulmonary parasites / lung parasites):**
- Trophozoites of *E. histolytica.*
- Scolex & hooklets of *E. granulosus* when hydatid cyst ruptures.
- Eggs of *P. westermanii.*
- Larvae of round worm (*Ascaris lumbricoides,* hook worm spp. (*Ancyclostoma duodenale* & *Necator americanus*), *Toxocara canis*, *Toxocara cati* & *S stercoralis.*

➢ **CSF:**
- *E. histolytica.*
- Trophozoites of *N. fowleri.*
- *Acanthamoeba* species.
- *T. brucei.*
- *H. cyst.*
- *A. cantonensis.*

➢ **Perianal swab:** By using **NIH swab** for
- *E. vermicularis.*
- *T. saginatum.*
- *S. mansoni.*

➢ **Aspiration of materials:**
- H. cyst fluid: To examine the scolex & hooklets.
- Amoebic abscess: To examine the trophozoites.
- Hydrocele: To examine the microfilariae.

➢ **Biopsy specimens:**
- Spleen puncture: *L. donovani.*
- Bone marrow: *L. donovani, T.brucei* etc.
- Lymph node: *L. donovani, T. brucei* & microfilariae.
- Muscle: *C. cellulosae, T. spiralis* & *T. cruzi.*
- Skin snip/biopsy: *Leishmania donovani* (dermal leishmanoid), *L. brasiliensis* & *Onchocercus volvulus.*
- Rectal biopsy: *S. haematobium* & *S. mansoni.*
- Liver biopsy: *S. mansoni* & *S. japonica.*

Transportation & storage

❖ **Transportation:**
- Transport the samples with triple layer packing & biohazard symbol.
- More details about triple layer packing & biohazard symbol: **Follow chapter → Laboratory diagnosis of bacterial infections**

❖ **Storage:** For detection of motility of parasite immediate transport is required. If there is delay in transport of sample, then it should be stored in refrigerator.

Sample rejection criteria

- More details: **Follow chapter → Laboratory diagnosis of bacterial infections**

Testing methods

❖ **Testing methods:** Two types like direct & indirect are described below

Direct methods

I. Macroscopic examination: Stool is examined macroscopically for adult stage & segments of adult stage.

II. Microscopy:

A. Microscopy of stool:

➢ **Collection of stool:** Advice the patient to collect the stool (about 20-40grams or 5-6 table spoonfuls of water stool) directly in wide mouth container.

➢ **Precautions during collection of stool:**
- Do not mix with urine.
- Container does not contain or pre-treated with antiseptics.
- Oil or barium should not be given to the patient.

➢ **Preservation of stool:**

i. **5% Fomalin:** For preservation of protozoan cysts.

ii. **10% Fomalin:** For preservation of helminthic eggs & larvae. 1-2g stool can be preserved with 8-10ml of 10% formalin & thoroughly shake before use.

iii. **Sodium acetate Acetic acid Fomalin (SAF):** Less toxic than PVA.

iv. **Merthiolate Iodine Formalin (MIF):** 2.35 ml of stock MF (Merthiolate –Formaldehyde) is mixed with 0.15ml of stock iodine (Lugol's iodine). Faeces with pea size added to this mixture. Acts as both fixative & stain. Permanent slide can't be made.

v. **Schaudin's fixative:** Contains mercuric chloride.

vi. **Poly Vinyl Alcohol (PVA) or modified Schaudin's fixative::** For preservation of protozoan cysts & trophozoites. PVA has long shelf life (6-12 months). Permanent slide can be made. For preservation 3 parts of PVA are added to one part of faeces. Mercuric chloride has been replaced with cupric sulphate.

➢ **Transportation of stool:**
- Transport within 30 minutes, as motile protozoa can die & unidentifiable after that.
- Transport in leak proof container with triple layer packing.

➢ **Examination of stool:**

i. **Wet mount preparation:**

a. **Normal saline (NS) & 1% iodine preparation (routine method):**

✪ **Preparation of iodine solution:** Two main steps.

1. **Preparation of Lugol's iodine (5%):**

- **Reagents:**

Iodine crystal/powder: 5g
Potassium iodide: 10g
Distilled water: 100ml

- **Steps:**
- Dissolve the potassium iodide with distilled water.
- Add the iodine crystal slowly.
- Filtered the solution & stored in amber colour bottle.

2. **Preparation of 1% iodine (weak iodine solution):**

- **Steps:** For parasitic examination 1% iodine is recommended by Dobell & O'Connor, which is prepared by diluting Lugol's iodine about five times with distilled water.
- **Disadvantages:** Deteriorates very quickly, hence it should be prepared every two week.

✪ **Steps of preparation of NS & iodine smear: →Fig.-1**

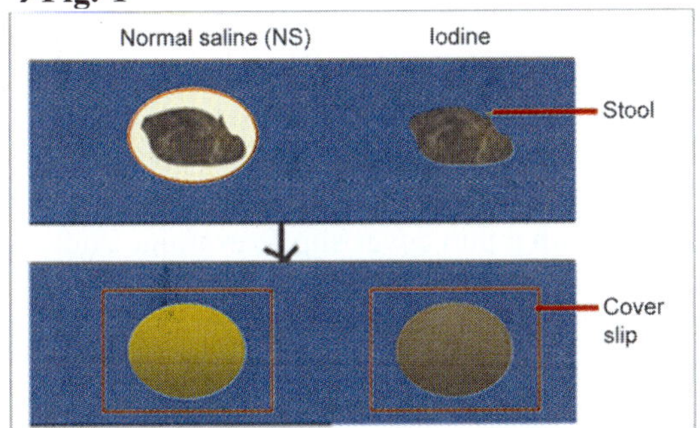

Figure-1: Normal saline & iodine preparation

- Take one clean glass slide.
- Put one drop of NS on one side & iodine on other.
- Add one drop of stool material in NS & iodine.
- Mix with wooden stick & remove large undigested food particles.
- Put cover slip& examined under the microscope.

✪ **Method (direction) of smear examination:**

- Start from low power & when eggs are found move to high power for details microscopic study.
- Start from one side & move to opposite side as shown in **fig.-2.**

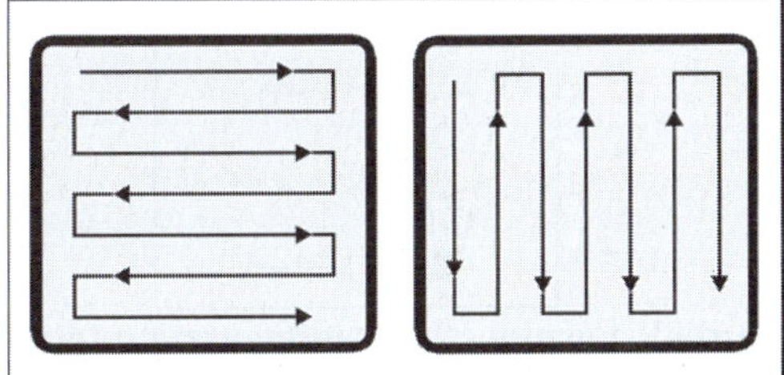

Figure-2: Direction of smear examination

b. **Buffered Methylene Blue (BMB) preparation:**

- Indicated for amoebic trophozoites but not for cyst.
- Used only on fresh samples but not on preserved samples.

c. **Hanging drop preparation:**

- It is useful to detect the motility of bacteria & also of parasites.
- Organs of locomotion & motile parasites: **Follow chapter → General properties of protozoa.**

ii. **Concentration methods:**

✪ **Indication:** Due to less numbers of parasites in stool, routine method like normal saline (NS) & 1% iodine preparation is not useful. This method is then necessary to selectively concentrate the protozoan cysts, heliminthic eggs & larvae, thus it increasing the sensitivity of copro-microscopic techniques.

✪ **Types:** Following different types concentration methods are useful.

a. **Flotation:**

- **Principle:** Faeces is suspended in a solution of high specific gravity than of parasitic eggs, so that parasitic eggs & cysts float up & get concentrated at surface.
- **Common floatation fluids/solutions:**
- Saturated solution of common salt (400 gm NaCl / 1000 ml water) with specific gravity of 1.18-1.20.
- Saturated sugar/sucrose solution (500 gm sugar / 1000 ml water) with specific gravity of 1.25.
- Saturated solution of sodium nitrate (400 gm sodium nitrate / 1000 ml water) with specific gravity of 1.18
- Glycerine.
- Zinc sulphate solution (32.5% solution) with specific gravity of 1.18
- A.E.X. (Acid HCl of with specific gravity of 1.03 + Ether + Xylol equal parts) solution.
- Magnesium sulphate solution.
- **Uses & limitations:** All the eggs are float except unfertilised eggs of *A. lumbricoides*, larvae of *S stercoralis*, eggs of *T. saginata* & *T. solium* & eggs of intestinal flukes.
- **Methods:**

1. **Willi's (Leviation) simple floatation technique by using saturated salt solution:**

- o Steps:
- About 2 ml of saturated salt is taken in flat bottom tube (or penicillin tube).
- Add 1 g of faeces.
- Fill the tube completely with salt solution up to brim. Care should be taken to see that not a drop of the contents overflows.
- Apply a slide over the tube, so that it is in direct contact with the surface of solution without any intervening bubbles.
- Allow it to stand for 10-15 minutes by which time all the eggs would have floated up.
- Remove the slide without jerking & reversed to bring the wet surface on top, put cover slip & then examined under the low power of the microscope for eggs.
- o Advantages:
- Light infections are detected by this technique invariably. Only eggs are clearly visible without the hindrance of faecal and fibres material.

- This method is useful in the examination of few nematodes only like round worm, hook worm & whip worm & thread worm.
- Disadvantages:
  - This method is not useful for protozoan cysts, eggs of cestodes, eggs of trematodes & unfertilised eggs of *A. lumbricoides*.
  - Different solution with different specific gravity is needed to float the eggs of different kinds of parasites.
  - The eggs may distort if kept in a floatation solution for long time.
  - Any delay in examination may cause salt crystal to develop, interfering in examination.

2. **Zinc sulphate Centrifuge Flotation technique**
- History: Discovered by Faust *et at* in 1939.
- Steps:
  - A fine suspension is made by adding 1 g of freshly passed faeces to the 10 ml of luke warm distilled water. Strain through wire gauze (40 meshes to an inch) to remove coarse faecal materials.
  - Filtrate is collected in Wassermann tube & centrifuged at the rate of 2500 rpm for one minute.
  - Poured off the supernatant fluid & add the water to the sediment. It is shaken well, centrifuged & repeat the process for 2-3 times till the supernatant fluid become clear, which is then poured off.
  - Add the 3-4 ml zinc sulphate solution to the sediment, sediment is stirred & further zinc sulphate solution is added to fill the tube up to the top. Again centrifuged the tube at the rate of 2500 rpm/minute for one minute.
  - Remove the surface film by a platinum wire loop of 5mm size, on to a clean glass slide, put cover slip & then examined under the low power of the microscope for eggs.
  - Add the one drop of iodine before putting the cover slip for protozoan cysts.
- Advantages: This method is useful in the examination of protozoan cysts, eggs of nematodes & small tape worms.
- Disadvantages:
  - This method is not useful for large cestodes, eggs of most trematodes & unfertilised eggs of *A. lumbricoides* & larvae of nematodes.

3. **Sheather's sugar floatation method:** This method is useful for oocyst of *Cryptosporidium* spp. & oocyst of *Isospora belli*
4. **Lane's direct centrifugal floatation (DCF) method**

b. Sedimentation:

- **Principle:** Faeces is suspended in a solution of low specific gravity than of parasitic eggs, so that parasitic eggs & cysts sediment & get concentrated at bottom either spontaneously or after centrifugation.
- **Common floatation fluids/solutions:**
  - Simple tap water.
  - Formol ether (Formalin-Ethyl Aceatate).
- **Methods:**

1. **Simple sedimentation technique by using tap water:**
- Steps:
  - Add about 2 g faeces in a suitable container.
  - Add water about 3/4th in to the faecal material.
  - Thoroughly emulsify the faecal material. Strained the emulsion through a sieve (tea strainer) to remove all the coarser particles in a cone shaped tube (urine analysis flask). 0.5% glycerine in water can be used for emulsifying the faeces instead of plain water.
  - Centrifuge at 2,000 rpm for 2 minutes. All the eggs get packed at the bottom of the tube along with the sediment.
  - The supernatant fluid is then poured off.
  - A drop of the sediment is placed on the slide, covered with a thin cover slip & examine under low power microscope.
- Advantages: This method is the most reliable one by which one can recover the eggs of three types of worms like trematodes, cestodes & nematodes.
- Disadvantages: Presence of too many faecal materials and fibres may hinder the visualization of egg.

2. **Formol ether sedimentation technique:**
- Synonym: Formalin-Ethyl Acetate sedimentation technique.
- Steps: → **Fig.-3**

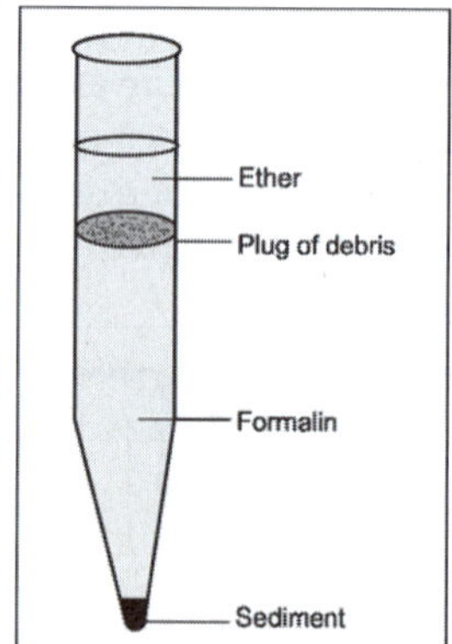

Figure-3: Formol ether sedimentation technique

  - Add about 2 g faeces in a suitable container.
  - Add about 10 ml of water in to the faecal material.
  - Thoroughly emulsify the faecal material. Strained the emulsion through a sieve (tea strainer) to remove all the coarser particles in a cone shaped tube.
  - Centrifuge at 2,000 rpm for not less than 10 minutes. All the eggs get packed at the bottom of the tube along with the sediment.
  - The supernatant fluid is then poured off and washes the sediment with 10 ml of saline solution.

Centrifuge again & repeat washing until supernatant is clear.

- After the last wash, decant the supernatant and add 10 ml of 10% formalin to the sediment. Mix and let stand for 5 minutes to effect fixation.
- Add 1 to 2 ml of ethyl acetate, Stopper the tube and shake vigorously.
- Centrifuge at 1500 rpm for 10 minutes.
- Four layers should result like a top layer of ether (ethyl acetate), plug of debris, layer of formalin (formal water) & sediment.
- Detach the plug of debris from the side of the tube by an applicator stick. Carefully decant the top three layers.
- With a pipette, mix the remaining sediment which contains eggs, with the small amount or remaining fluid and transfer one drop, each to a drop of saline and iodine on a glass slide. Apply the cover slip and examine under low power microscope.

o Advantage:

- Formalin fixes the eggs, larvae, oocysts, and spores, so that they are no longer infectious, as well as preserves their morphology.
- This method is useful for helminthic eggs & protozoan cysts.

o Disadvantage: Ether is explosive & inflammable, which is over come by sing ethyl acetate

c. Other concentration methods:

1. Baermann's method (Baermanization): **Follow chapter → Nematodes: Intestinal nematodes.**
2. Water-emergency semi-concentration technique.
3. Kato-Katz preparation.

➢ **Microscopic appearance of parasites under normal saline & iodine preparation present in stool: →Fig.-4-14, 15(b) & 15(c)**

➢ **Artefacts in stool:** Following material present in stool are looks like parasite **called artefacts.**

- Yeasts.
- Air bubbles.
- Charcot-Layden crystals.
- Plants.
- Cells like leukocytes, RBCs, muscle cells, epithelial cells, pus cells, fat cells etc.
- Undigested food materials.
- Hair or other fibers.

➢ **Eggs counting technique in stool:**

✪ **Indications:**

1. Epidemiological survey.
2. Therapeutic monitoring by estimating numbers of worm infecting patients.

✪ **Techniques:**

a. Stoll's method: Most popular method.

- Transfer 4g faeces to Stoll's flask containing 60ml, 0.1N NaOH.
- Add the several glass of beads to make a uniform suspension.
- Close the flask with rubber stopper & shake vigorously.
- Take exactly 0.15ml suspension by pipette over slide.
- Put cover slip over it & examine under microscope.
- Count the total number of eggs in entire smear.
- Numbers of eggs per gram of faeces is obtained by multiplying the count of two such preparation by 100 (It is roughly estimated that 100eggs can be passed by one female per gram of faeces per day.
- Exact numbers depends on consistency of stool & correction factors (CF) applied as follows.

1. Mushy formed stool: CF is 1.5
2. Mushy stool: CF is 2.
3. Mushy diarrhoeic stool: CF is 3.
4. Franky diarrhoeic stool: CF is 4.
5. Watery stool: CF is 5.

b. Direct smear technique: Rarely useful.

➢ **Permanent stained smear of stool:**

✪ **Indications:** Normal saline is useful to detect the motility; iodine increases the amount of details that can be seen in most cysts, while concentration techniques are useful when cyst & eggs numbers are very less in specimens. Permanent stains are essential for cytological details.

✪ **Fixatives:** Commonly used fixatives are

1. **Schaudin's fixatives:** Best fixative.
2. **PVA (Poly Vinyl Alcohol):**

✪ **Stains:** Commonly used stains are

1. **Gomori's Trichome stain:** Stains nucleus in red & cytoplasm in bluish green.
2. **H & E (Haematoxylin & Eosin) stain:** provides excellent contrast between nucleus & cytoplasm.

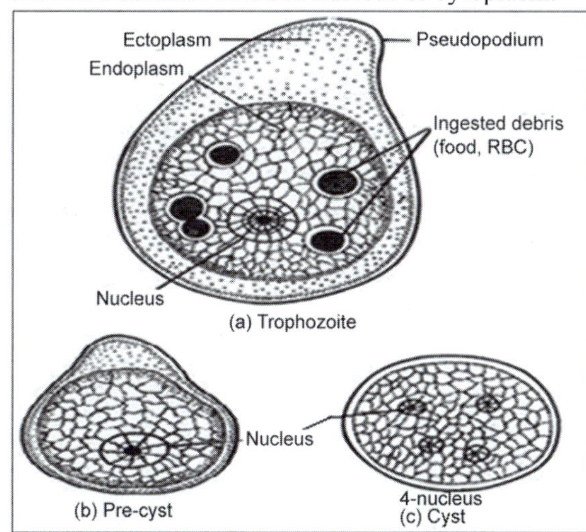

Figure-4: Morphology of *E. histolytica*

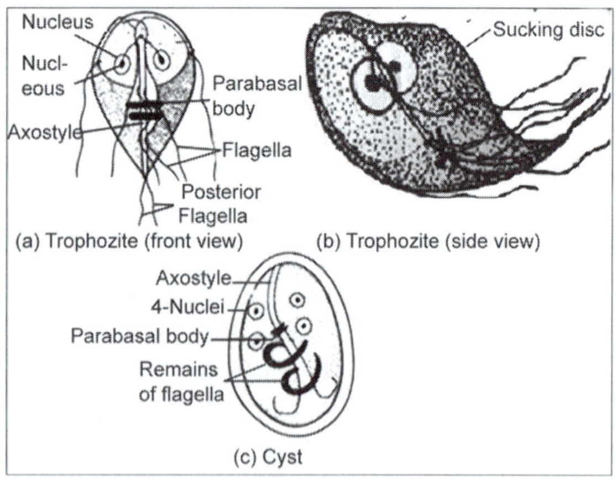

Figure-5: Morphology of *G. lamblia*

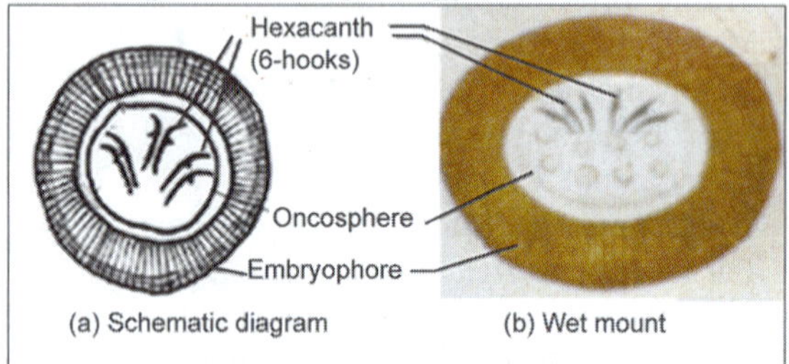

Figure-6: Egg of *Taenia* spp.

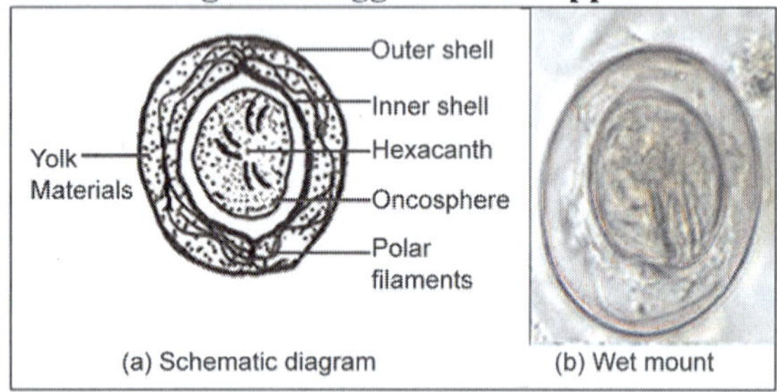

Figure-7: Egg of *H. nana*

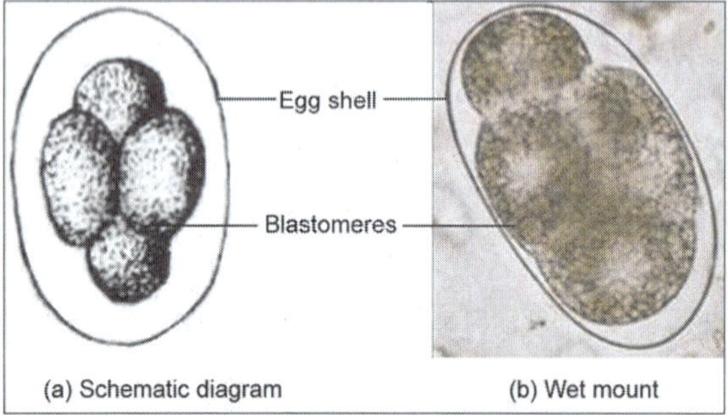

Figure-8: Egg of *A. duodenale*

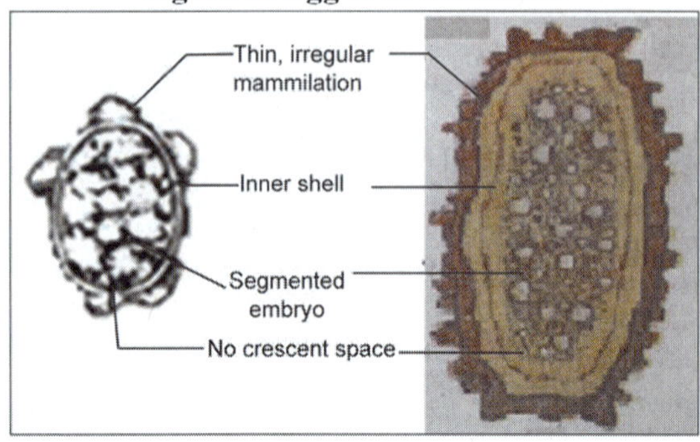

Figure-9: Unfertilised egg of *A. lumbricoides*

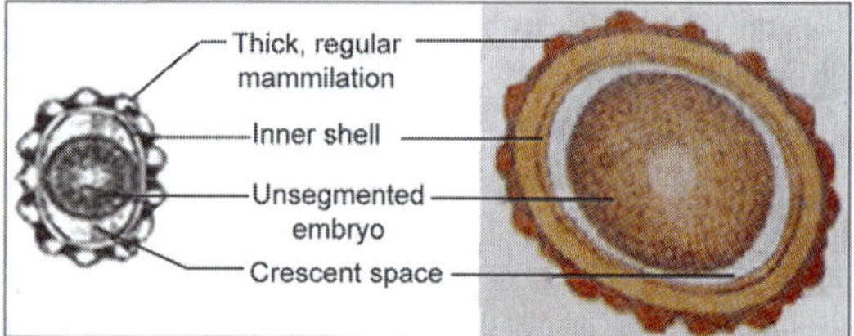

Figure-10: Fertilised egg of *A. lumbricoides*

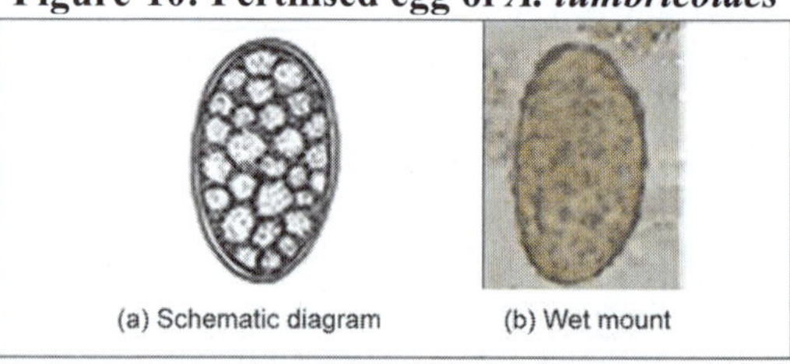

Figure-11: Unfertilised –decorticated egg of *A. lumbricoides*

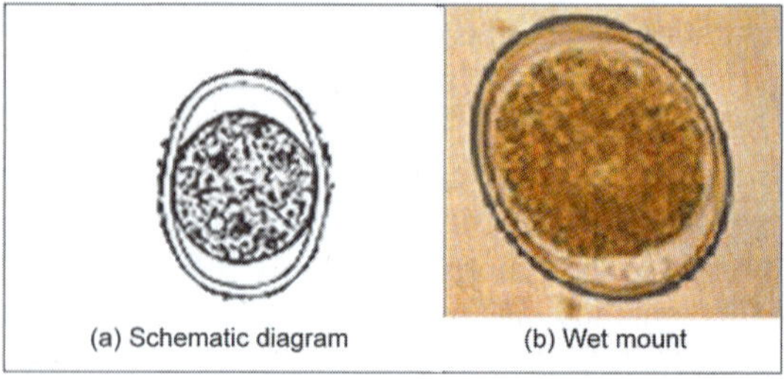

Figure-12: Fertilised –decorticated egg of *A. lumbricoides*

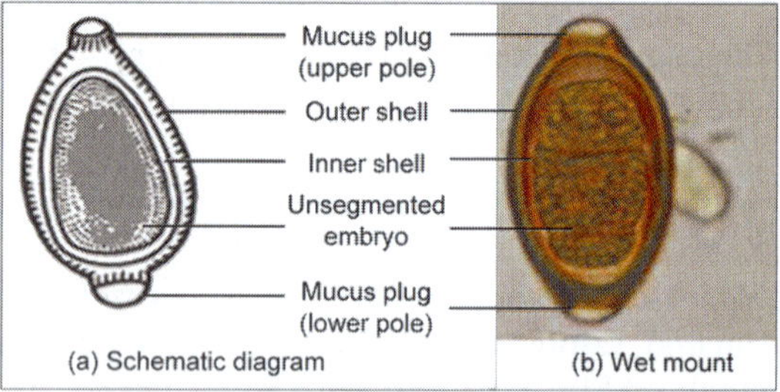

Figure-13: Egg of *T. trichuria*

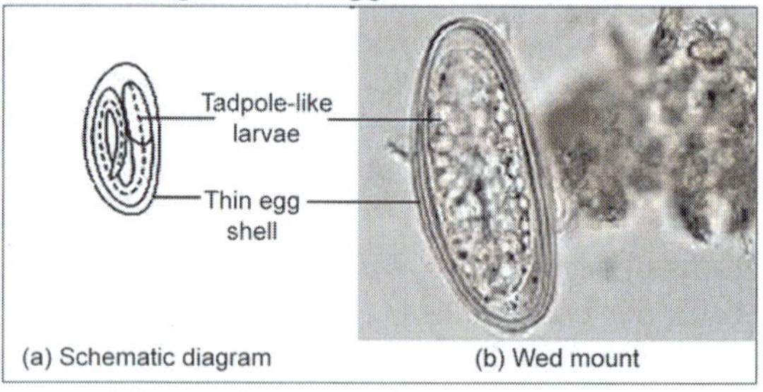

Figure-14: Egg of *E. vermicularis*

B. Microscopy of urogenital specimen: Like urine or urethral discharge.

i. Wet mount direct from sample:

✪ **Steps:**

- Take clean glass slide.
- Put one drop of sample on one side (centrifuge the sample if required).
- Put cover slip& examined under low power.

✪ **Microscopic appearance of parasites present in urogenital specimens: → Fig.-15(a) &16**

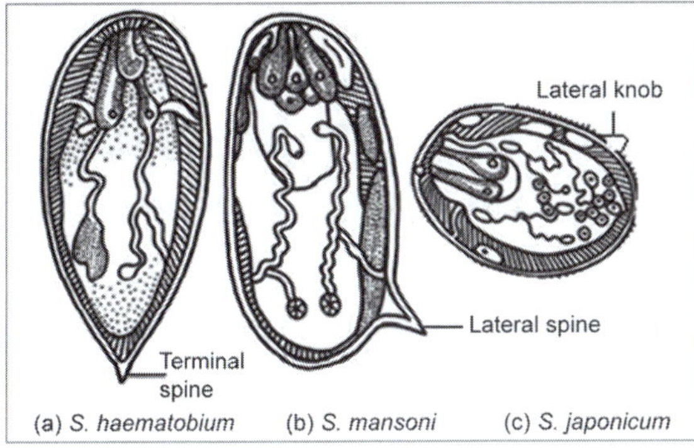

Figure-15: Eggs of *Schistosomes*

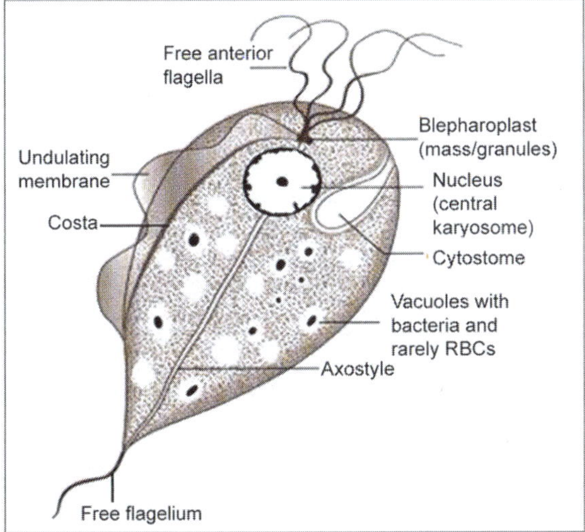

Figure-16: Morphology of *T. vaginalis*

C. Peripheral Blood Smear (PBS) microscopy:

- For *Typanosoma* spp.: **Follow chapter → Blood and tissue flagellates**
- For *Leishmania* spp. in macrophages: **Follow chapter → Blood and tissue flagellates**
- For *Plasmodium* spp. & *Babesia* spp.: **Follow chapter → Blood inhabiting sporozoa**
- For microfilariae: **Follow chapter → Nematodes: Somatic (tissue) nematodes**
- For *Toxoplasma gondii:* **Follow chapter → Gastrointestinal sporozoa**

D. Other microscopical technique:

i. Modified Z.N. satin:

- For acid-fast parasite.
- More details: **Follow chapter → Microscopy and staining.**

ii. Trichrome stain: For *Microsporidia* spp.

iii. Fluorescence microscopy: For *Cyclospora* spp., *Toxoplasma gondii* etc.

III. Culture:

- Some protozoa can grow over artificially prepared media. Culture methods in details for each parasite are described in **respective chapters.**
- Few important media or culture techniques with parasites are listed in **table-1.**

Parasite	Culture medium
E. histolytica	Different polyaxenic & monoaxenic media
G. lamblia	Diamond medium
T. vaginalis	Trypticase serum medium
Leishmania spp. & *T. cruzi*	Novy, mcNeal and Nicolle (NNN) medium
B. coli	Balamuth medium
Plasmodium spp.	RPMI1640 (Rose Park Memorial Institute) medium
T. gondii	Tissue or animal or egg culture
Microspora spp.	Cell culture media
Hook worm spp., Pseudohook worm spp. & *S. stercoralis*	Coproculture

Table-1: Culture media of parasites

IV. Xenodiagnosis: It based on diagnosis of microorganisms from the body of vector by allowing vector to bite the infected person in *T. cruzi* & *W. bancrofti.*

Indirect methods

I. Cytological examination of body fluids: Eosinophilia & cell counting is done from different body fluids like blood, CSF etc. It helps in diagnosis.

II. Serological tests: Based on different principle like ELISA, Precipitation, RIA, CFT, Agglutination, Haemagglutination etc.

III. Skin tests: Two types as follows.

i. Based on immediate type of hypersensitivity: Like

1. Casoni's test in *H. cyst.*
2. Skin test for *T. spiralis.*
3. Skin test for wucheriasis.
4. Mazzotti's test for *O. Volvulus.*

ii. Based on delayed type of hypersensitivity: Like

1. Skin test for trypanosomes.
2. Leishmanin test: Positive in African kala azar.
3. Frenkel's test: For *T. gondii.*
4. Scratch test: For *A. lumbricoides.*

IV. Molecular methods:

- **Advantages:** High sensitivity & specificity.
- **Disadvantages:** High cost & not available in peripheral centre.
- **Methods are**
  - Hybridisation.
  - PCR.
  - Real time PCR.

V. Radiological methods: Like X-ray, USG, CT-scan & MRI are useful.

Question bank

Essay/Full question

1) Laboratory diagnosis of parasitic infections.

Short notes

1) Stool examination in Parasitology.
2) Blood examination in Parasitology.
3) Parasitic culture.

Short questions for theory/viva questions

1) Name the four parasites present in peripheral blood.
2) Name the four parasites present in CSF.
3) Name the four protozoa present in stool.
4) Name the culture media for following parasites: *G. lamblia*, *T. vaginalis*, *Leishmania* spp. & *Plasmodium* spp.

MCQs for chapter review

Sample collection

1) Larval form in stool is found in (PGI, Dec-01, May-10 & 13)
(a) *Strongyloides* (b) *Ancyclostoma duodenale* (c) *Ascaris lumbricoides* (d) *Necator americanus* (e) *Trichuris trichuria*

2) Parasite / parasites present in sputum is/are
(a) *E. granulosus* (b) *E. histolytica* (c) None of above (d) a+b

3) Which of the following is best diagnosed by muscle biopsy
(a) *T. spiralis* (b) *E. granulosus* (c) *L. donovani* (d) All of above

4) In which parasitic infestation sputum examination is not of much value (AIIMS, Dec-94)
(a) *Trichuris trichuria* (b) *Strongyloides* (c) *Ancyclostoma duodenale* (d) *Paragonimus westermanii*

5) Sputum examination is not useful in diagnosis of (AIIMS-96, AI-98)
(a) *Trichuris trichuria* (b) *Ancyclostoma duodenale* (c) *Paragonimus* (d) *Strongyloides*

6) Skin snip is used in the diagnosis of
(a) Trichinosis (b) Strongyloidiasis (c) Schistosomiasis (d) Onchocerciasis

7) Which of the following does not pass through the lungs (AI-96)
(a) Hook worm (b) *Ascaris* (c) *Strongyloides* (d) *Enterobius vermicularis*

8) Parasite causing lung infestation are (PGI, Dec-03)
(a) *H. nana* (b) *Paragonimus westermanii* (c) *Taenia saginata* (d) *E. granulosus* (e) *E. multilocularis*

Testing methods

9) Protozoan cysts are stored in
(a) Saline (b) Phenol (c) Sodium hypochlorite (d) Formalin

10) Hanging drop method/preparation is used for
(a) *T vaginalis* (b) *Plasmodium* (c) *Toxoplasma* (d) *Cryptosporidium*

11) On microscopic examination eggs are seen, but on saturation with salt solution, no eggs are seen. The eggs are likely to be of (AIIMS-98)
(a) *Trichuris trichuria* (b) *Taenia solium* (c) *Ascaris lumbricoides* (d) *Ancyclostoma duodenale*

12) All float in a saturated salt solution except (AIIMS, May-95)
(a) *Chlonerchis sinensis* (b) Fertilise eggs of *Ascaris* (c) Larvae of *Strongyloides* (d) *Trichuris trichuria*

13) The egg of which helminth, can be concentrated in saturated salt solution. (AIIMS, May-93)
(a) *Taenia saginata* (b) *Taenia solium* (c) Unfertilise egg of *Ascaris* (d) *Ancyclostoma duodenale*

14) In formol ether concentration technique, which layer contain parasites
(a) Ether (b) Faecal debris (c) Formal water (d) Sediment

Answers of MCQs & explanation

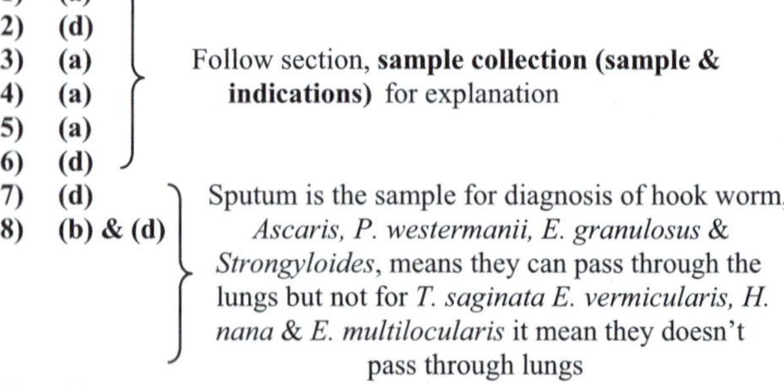

1) (a)
2) (d)
3) (a)
4) (a)
5) (a)
6) (d)

Follow section, **sample collection (sample & indications)** for explanation

7) (d)
8) (b) & (d)

Sputum is the sample for diagnosis of hook worm, *Ascaris, P. westermanii, E. granulosus* & *Strongyloides*, means they can pass through the lungs but not for *T. saginata E. vermicularis, H. nana* & *E. multilocularis* it mean they doesn't pass through lungs

9) (d)

- Follow section, **testing methods (direct methods → microscopy of stool → preservation of stool)** for explanation

10) (a)

- Follow section, **testing methods (direct methods → microscopy of stool → wet mount preparation → hanging drop preparation)** for explanation

11) (b)
12) (a) & (c)
13) (d)

Follow section, **testing methods (concentration methods → Willi's (Leviation) simple floatation technique by using saturated salt solution)** for explanation

14) (d)

- Follow section, **testing methods (concentration methods → formol ether sedimentation technique)** for explanation

82 General properties of protozoa

Learning heading & subheadings

- Meaning:
- Variation in species:
- Morphology:
- Methods of reproduction
- Life cycle:

❖ **Meaning:** Protozoa word derived from **Protos (Greek) = first + Zoon = animal.**

❖ **Variation in species:** There are about 65,000 known species of protozoa. 10, 000 are parasitic & 17 are medically important.

❖ **Morphology:**

➢ **Size:** Microscopic in size & visible under high power microscope. Largest protozoan is *B coli*.

➢ **Structure:** Unicellular & single cell perform the all functions. Structure of protozoa consist cytoplasm, nucleus & other materials.

A. **Cytoplasm:** It is divided in two portions.

i. **Endoplasm:** → **Fig.-1**

✪ **Definition:** Internal, granular portion of cytoplasm **called endoplasm**.

✪ **Functions:**

- Nutrition.
- Excretion.
- Reproduction.

✪ **Contains:**

- Nucleus.
- Contractile vacuoles.
- Food debris.
- Endoplasmic reticulum.
- Golgi bodies.
- RBCs in some parasite.

ii. **Ectoplasm:** → **Fig.-1**

✪ **Definition:** External, clear, hyaline portion of cytoplasm **called ectoplasm**.

✪ **Functions:**

- Protection.
- Locomotion.
- Sensory.

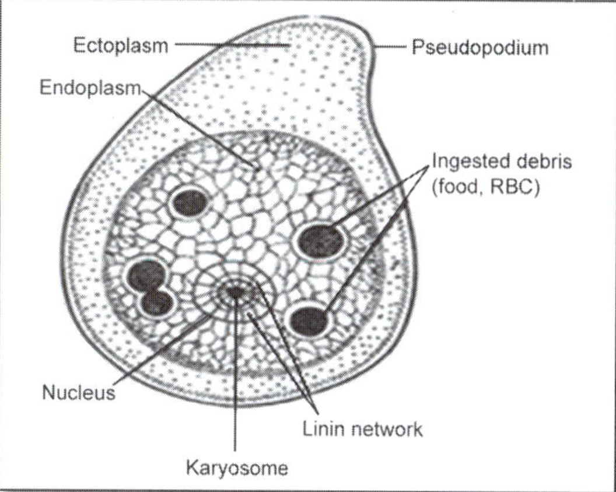

Figure-1: Pseudopodium in *E. histolytica*

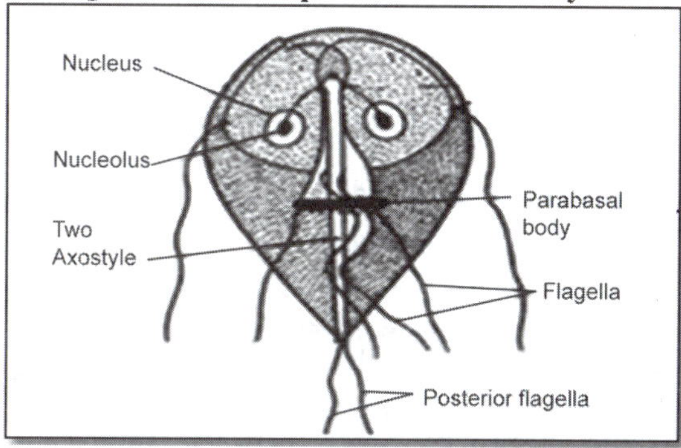

Figure-2: Flagella in *G. lamblia*

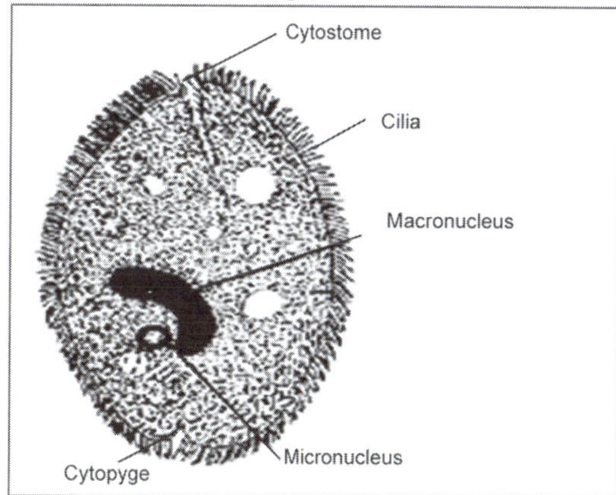

Figure-3: Cilia in *B. coli*

✪ **Structures developed from ectoplasm:**

a. **Organs of locomotion:** Three types as follows.

1. **Pseudopodia:** → **Fig.-1**

- It is a prolongation of ectoplasmic process.
- Helps in ingestion of food.
- Temporary.
- Seen in Rhizopodea (***E. histolytica***).
- Speed of locomotion: 0.2-0.3μm per seconds.

83 Amoebae

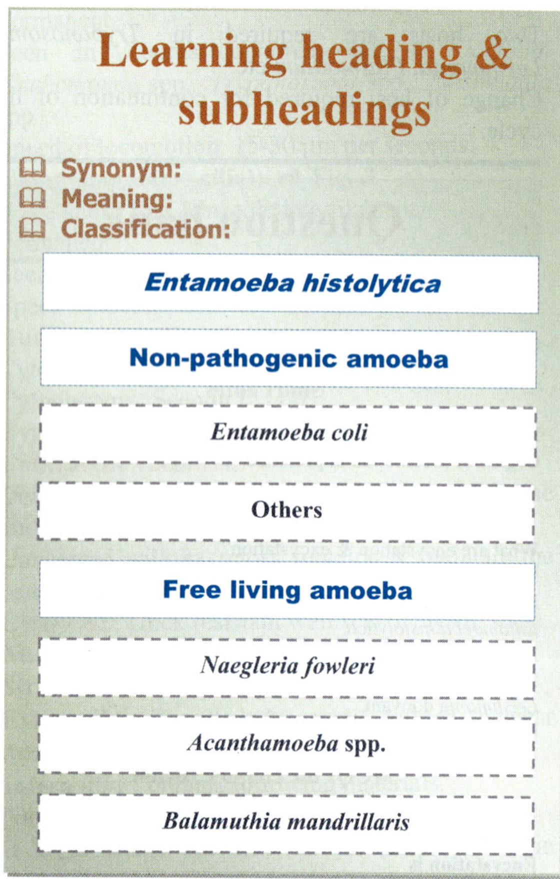

Learning heading & subheadings
Synonym:
Meaning:
Classification:
Entamoeba histolytica
Non-pathogenic amoeba
Entamoeba coli
Others
Free living amoeba
Naegleria fowleri
Acanthamoeba spp.
Balamuthia mandrillaris

Synonym: Ameba/Amoeba are singular & Amebas or Amoebas/Amoebae are plural.

Meaning: From **amoibe (Greek) = change**, as the organism have habit to change the shape constantly.

Classification:

I. **Systemic classification:** Follow chapter → Introduction and classification of parasites. (section →**Table-3)**

II. **Pathogenic classification:** Two groups.

A. **Gastrointestinal amoebae:** Two subgroups according to site of infection.

i. **Pathogenic:** *Entamoeba histolytica* (intestinal in large intestine & extra- intestinal).

ii. **Non- pathogenic:**

a. **Mouth:** *Entamoeba gingvalis.*

b. **Intestinal:**

1. ***Entamoeba:*** *E. coli, E. hartmanni & E. polecki.*
2. ***Endolimax:*** *E. nana.*
3. ***Iodamoeba:*** *I. butchlii.*
4. ***Dientamoeba:*** *D. fragilis.*

B. **Free leaving amoebae:** Following are **pathogenic** species.

1. ***Naegleria:*** 18 species, only *N. fowleri* is pathogenic.
2. ***Acanthamoeba:*** *A. culbertsoni, A. castellanii,A. hatchetti, A. polyphaga, A.rhysodes, A.astronyxis, A.divionensis & A. healyi.*
3. ***Balamuthia:*** *B. mandrillaris.*

Entamoeba histolytica

History:

- *E. histolytica* was 1st described by **Losch** from stool of Russian suffering with dysentery in 1875.
- **Koch** reported the trophozoites in hepatic capillaries of patients of amoebic dysentery with hepatic abscess in 1887.
- **Boek & Drobhlav** described the polyaxenic medium for cultivation in 1925.
- **Diamond** described the axenic medium with successful *in-vitro* cultivation in 1965.

Geographical distribution: World-wide. More in tropics & sub-tropics than temperate zone.

Habitat: Large intestine.

Morphology: Unicellular & single cell performs the all functions. It is studied in stained **[iodine & Iron-Haematoxylin (I &H)]** & unstained **[Normal Saline (NS)]** preparation with three stages like trophozoite, pre-cyst & cyst.

I. Trophozoite stage

➢ **Synonym:**
- Tropic stage.
- Active stage.
- Growing stage.
- Feeding stage.
- Vegetative stage.

➢ **Size:** Average from 18-40μm.

➢ **Shape:** Not fixed, because of constantly changing position of pseudopodium.

➢ **Motility:**

✪ **Type:** Showing crawling or gliding motility due to pseudopodium. Movement is jerky & unidirectional due to formation of new pseudopodium at different site, when whole cytoplasm moves in to the direction of new pseudopodium. In a culture test tube trophozoites are crawl by side of tube. Motility & pseudopodium formation is inhibited at low temperature.

✪ **Speed:** 0.2-3μm per second.

➢ **Structure:** It consist cytoplasm & nucleus.

A. **Cytoplasm:** It is divided in two portions.

i. Endoplasm: → Fig.-1(a)

✪ **Definition:** Internal, granular portion of cytoplasm **called endoplasm**.

✪ **Functions:**
- Nutrition.
- Excretion.
- Reproduction.

✪ **Contains:**
- RBCs **called erythrophagocytosis.** Only intestinal amoebae having RBCs in cytoplasm & it is the diagnostic feature.
- WBCs.
- No bacteria.
- Food debris.
- Nucleus.

ii. Ectoplasm: → Fig.-1(a)

✪ **Definition:** External, clear, hyaline portion of cytoplasm **called ectoplasm.**

✪ **Functions:**
- Protection.
- Locomotion.
- Sensory.

✪ **Structures developed from ectoplasm: → Fig.-1**

a. Organelles of locomotion: Called pseudopodia.
- It is a prolongation of ectoplasmic process.
- Helps in ingestion of food.
- Temporary.
- Speed of locomotion: 0.2-0.3μm per seconds.

b. Cyst-wall: Thick resistant wall seen in cystic stage.

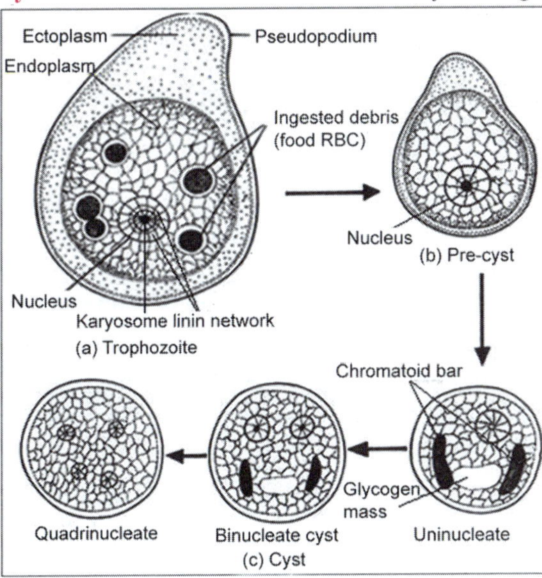

Figure-1: Morphology of *E. histolytica*

B. Nucleus:

✪ **Size:** 4-6μm.

✪ **Shape:** Spherical.

✪ **Numbers:** Single nucleus is present.

✪ **Structure: → Fig.-1 (a)**

i. Unstained preparation: Not visible due to motility, but when motility decrease, it observed with faint outline & eccentric position.

ii. Stained preparation:

1. **Nucleolus (karyosome):**
- It is a small dot like, centrally located, concentrated chromatin material.
- Located either centrally or peripherally.

2. **Linin network:** Space between karyosome & nuclear membrane is filled by radially (spoke like) arranged fine threads **called linin network** which gives cartwheel appearance.
3. **Nuclear membrane:** Nucleus bounded by thin & well defined nuclear membrane which is lines by fine chromatin granules.
4. **Nuclear sap:** Fluid present in nucleus.

✪ **Functions:**
- Control all activities of cell.
- Essential for cell division, growth & replication.
- Takes part in fertilisation & hereditary transmission of genetic information.

II. Pre-cyst stage

➢ **Size:** 10-20μm.

➢ **Shape:** Oval.

➢ **Numbers:** Single nucleus is present.

➢ **Structure: → Fig.-1 (b)**

A. Cytoplasm:

i. Ectoplasm: Blunt pseudopodium.

ii. Endoplasm: Endoplasm is free of RBCs & other ingested food debris.

B. Nucleus:

✪ **Size:** Smaller than trophozoite, but larger than cyst.

✪ **Shape:** Spherical.

✪ **Structure:** Same as nucleus of trophozoites **[fig.-1(b)].**

III. Cyst stage

➢ **Synonym:**
- Inactive stage.
- Resistant stage.
- Resting stage.

➢ **Size:** Variable, from smaller about 6-9μm to larger about 12-15 μm.

➢ **Shape:** Spherical.

➢ **Structure: → Fig.-1 (c)**

✪ **Structure of immature cyst:**

A. Cytoplasm:

- **Nature:** It is clear & hyaline. Free of RBCs & other ingested food debris.
- **Contains:**

1. **Chromatoid bars or chromodial bars:**
   - Numbers: 1-4.
   - Size: Variable from ½ to 2/3 the size of cyst.
   - Life: Disappear in mature cyst.
   - Staining reaction:
     - Iodine: Remains unstained.
     - NS: Seen as rounded ends.
     - I & H stain: Seen in black colour.

2. **Glycogen mass:**
- Number: 1
- Life: Disappear in mature cyst.
- Staining reaction:
- Iodine: Stains in brown colour.
- NS: Not seen.
- I & H stain: Remains unstained.

B. **Nucleus:**
- **Size:** Smaller than trophozoites & pre- cyst.
- **Shape:** Spherical.
- **Numbers:** Immature cyst is uninucleate but nucleus divides by binary fission to develop in to binucleate & quadrinucleate bodies. Mature cyst is quadrinucleate in nature.
- **Structure:** Same as trophozoites.

✪ **Structure of mature cyst:** Immature cyst passed in faeces & becomes mature over the soil.

A. **Cyst wall:**
- Thick & highly resistant.
- Help to cyst to survive in unfavourable condition.

B. **Cytoplasm:**
- **Nature:** It is clear & hyaline. Free of RBCs, ingested food debris, chromatoid bars & glycogen mass.

C. **Nucleus:**
- **Size:** Smaller than trophozoites & pre- cyst.
- **Shape:** Spherical.
- **Numbers:** Quadrinucleate.
- **Structure:** Same as trophozoites.

❖ Culture:

i. **Culture on media:** Three types of media.

a. **Axenic culture:** It is culture in which single species or variant or strain is present and free of other microbes or contaminants.

1. **Boeck & Drbohlav's medium:** Contains solidifies blood agar (or egg slopes) & Locke's solution.
2. **Nelson's medium**
3. **Craig's medium**
4. **Balamuth's medium**
5. **Robinson's medium**
6. **Cleverland & Sander's medium**
7. **St. Jhonson's medium**
8. **Diamond's medium**

b. **Monoaxenic culture:** It is culture in which single species or variant or strain can grow in presence of other microbes.

1. **Philip's medium:** Contains thyoglycollate preparation, horse serum & *T. cruzi.*
2. **Shaffer & Frye's medium:**
- Contains thyoglycollate preparation & penicillin inhibited *Streptobacilli.*
- Bacilli are living but not multiplying.

c. **Polyaxenic culture:**

ii. **Culture in animals:**
- **Uses:** To study the
- Pathogenicity.
- Effect of amoebicidal drugs.
- **Animals:**
- Experimental amoebiasis can be produced in **cats, dogs & monkeys.**
- **Kittens:** Fatal within 2-3 days with production of extensive sloughing & colonic ulcer.
- **Pups (Dogs):** Lesion is similar to human amoebiasis but animal lives longer than kittens.
- **Hamsters:** Production of hepatitis.
- **White rats:** Production of caecal ulcer after intra-caecal injection.
- **Guinea pigs:** Production of colonic ulcer after intra-ileal injection.

❖ Resistance:
- Trophozoites are killed by drying, heating & disinfection.
- Trophozoites survive for 5 hrs at 37^{0}C & even if enter from fresh stool they are killed by stomach acidity; hence infection is not transmitted by trophozoites.

❖ Immunity:
- Specific antibodies are formed in invasive amoebiasis, which are detected by CFT, precipitation test, immobilisation test & immunofluorescent microscopy.
- Antibodies are not protective against re-infection.

❖ Life cycle:
➢ **Host:** Man is the only host.

➢ **Methods of reproduction:**

✪ **Methods of transformation:** Two types as mentioned below **(flow chart-1).**

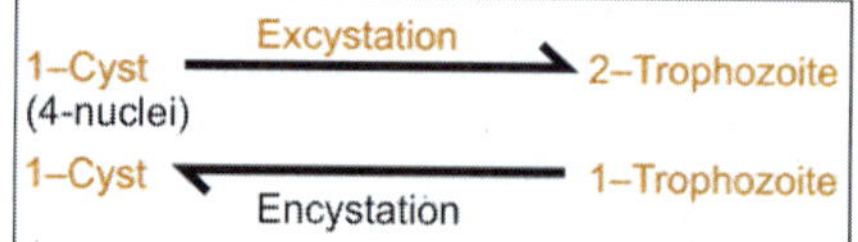

Flow chart-1: Excystation & Encystation

a. **Encystation:**
- **Definition:** Transfer of trophozoite (active) to cyst (inactive) **called encystation.**
- **Properties:**
- Encystation is not a reproductive process, but a process of protection.
- It takes place inside the lumen of intestine.
- It occurs in few hours & mature cyst last for 2 days inside the lumen.
- It not occur intestinal wall, liver, lungs, brain etc.
- One trophozoite gives one cyst.
- Mature cyst is quadrinucleate in nature.

b. **Excystation:**
- **Definition:** Transfer of cyst (inactive) to trophozoite (active) **called excystation.**
- **Properties:**

- It takes place inside the lumen of intestine of infected person.
- Mature cyst is quadrinucleate in nature.
- Each nuclei divides by binary fission, which gives birth to eight amoebulae.
- Each amoebulae is capable to develop in to trophozoites.

✪ **Methods of multiplication:** Occurs only in trophozoite stage. Trophozoite divides by binary fission every 8 hours. 1st nucleus is divides by binary fission (asexual method) & then cytoplasmic body.

➢ **Cycles:** Three stages of life cycle are described in **figure-2 & flow chart -2.**

➢ **Summary: → Flow chart -3.**

❖ Pathogenicity:

➢ **Disease name: Called amoebiasis.**

➢ **Reservoir of infection:**
- Natural infection occurs in men & monkeys.
- Man is the commonest reservoir.
- In China, dog is the possible reservoir.

➢ **Source of infection:**
- Contaminated food & water from faeces.
- Cyst of ***E. histolytica*** also found in dropping of cockroaches, which also serve a source of infection.

➢ **Mode of transmission:**
- Fluid borne (water): Faecal contamination of drinking water.
- Food borne: Eating of uncooked vegetable & fruits, which are fertilised with infected human faeces.
- Fomites borne.
- Fingers borne.
- Flies (vector borne): House flies, cockroaches & rodents are capable to transmit the cyst from faeces to open food stuff.
- Also transmitted by sexual intercourse. In developed countries sexual transmission is reported. It is transmitted by oral-rectal route.

➢ **Incubation period:** Variable, but generally 4-5 days.

➢ **Exit form:** Trophozoites or cyst in faeces.

➢ **Infective form:** Mature quadrinucleate cyst.

➢ **Portal of entry:** GIT.

➢ **Site:**
- Intestinal: Large intestine.
- Extra intestinal: Liver, lungs, spleen, brain, skin etc.

➢ **Precipitating factors (epidemiological determinants):**

i. **Agent factors (virulence factors):**

a. **Lectin mediated adherence protein:** Helps in contact with target cells.

b. **Toxins:** Like enterotoxin or cytotoxin induces tissues damage has been studied in certain studies.

c. **Enzymes:**

1. **Histiolysin:** It brings the destruction & necrosis of tissues & slough formation. Organisms receive the nourishment by absorption of dissolved tissue juice.
2. **Other enzymes:** Like hyaluronidase, trypsin, pepsin, amylase etc. may induce tissues destruction.

d. **Amoebapore:**
- It is a pore (hole) forming protein.
- It polymerise in target cell membrane → producing holes in cell membrane → cell lysis (cytolysis).

e. **Motility:** Helps in deeper penetration.

f. **Infective dose:** Direct relation between the numbers of cyst ingested & disease development.

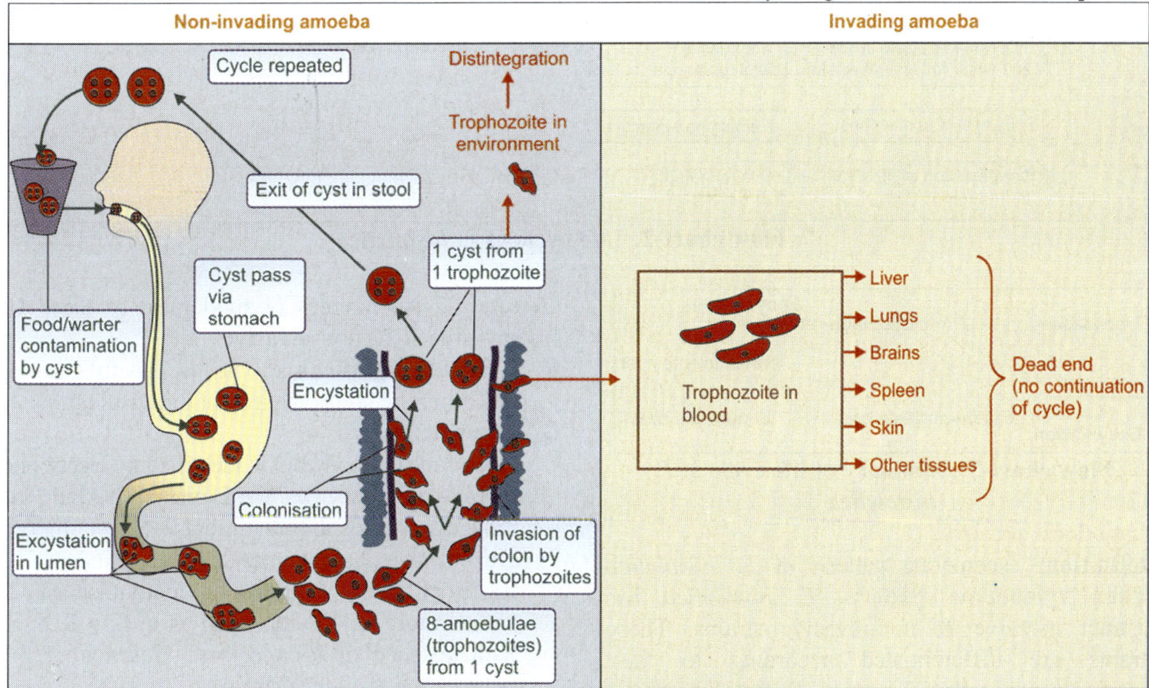

Figure-2: Life cycle of *E. histolytica*

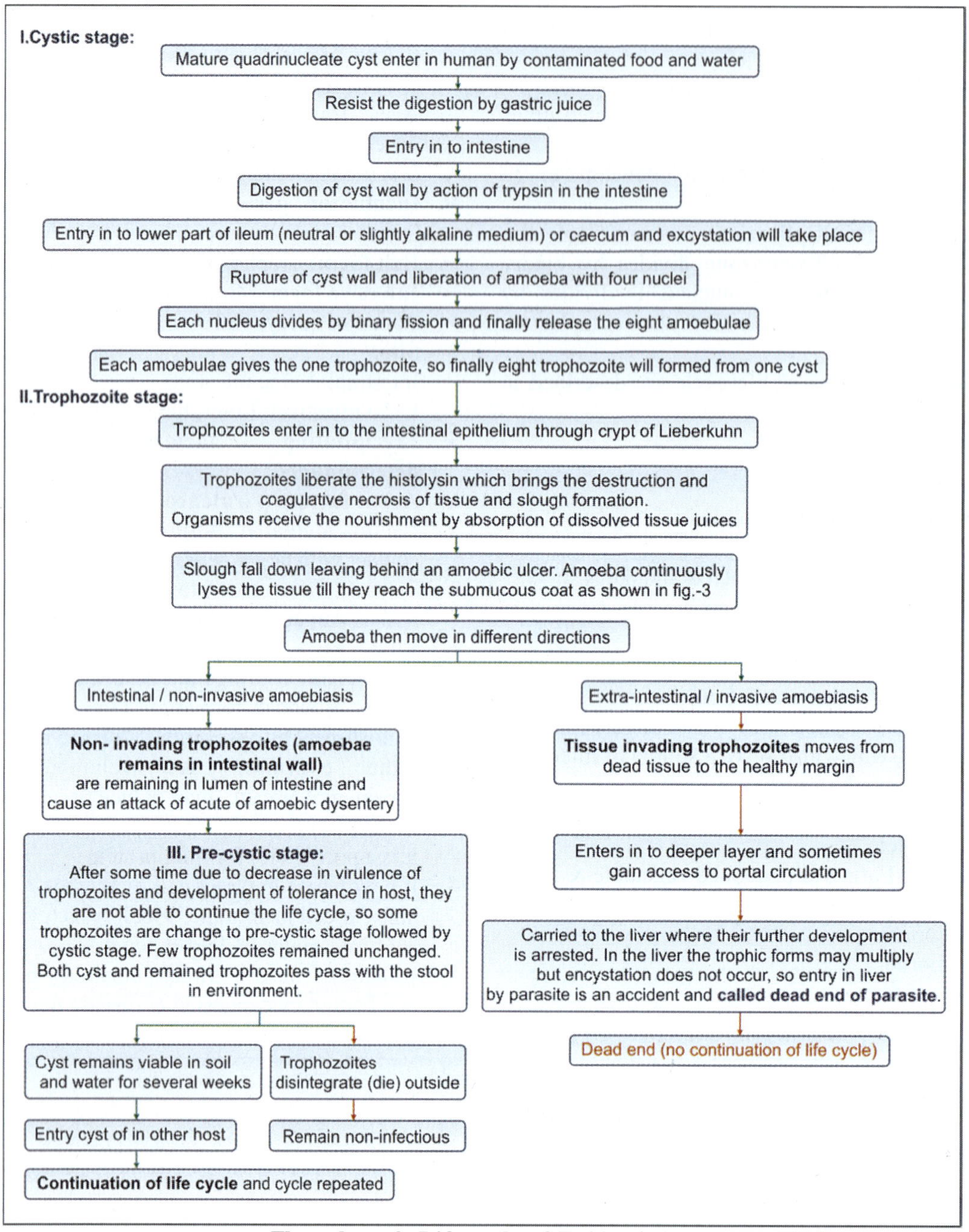

I. Cystic stage:

Mature quadrinucleate cyst enter in human by contaminated food and water

↓

Resist the digestion by gastric juice

↓

Entry in to intestine

↓

Digestion of cyst wall by action of trypsin in the intestine

↓

Entry in to lower part of ileum (neutral or slightly alkaline medium) or caecum and excystation will take place

↓

Rupture of cyst wall and liberation of amoeba with four nuclei

↓

Each nucleus divides by binary fission and finally release the eight amoebulae

↓

Each amoebulae gives the one trophozoite, so finally eight trophozoite will formed from one cyst

II. Trophozoite stage:

Trophozoites enter in to the intestinal epithelium through crypt of Lieberkuhn

↓

Trophozoites liberate the histolysin which brings the destruction and coagulative necrosis of tissue and slough formation. Organisms receive the nourishment by absorption of dissolved tissue juices

↓

Slough fall down leaving behind an amoebic ulcer. Amoeba continuously lyses the tissue till they reach the submucous coat as shown in fig.-3

↓

Amoeba then move in different directions

↓

Intestinal / non-invasive amoebiasis

↓

Non- invading trophozoites (amoebae remains in intestinal wall) are remaining in lumen of intestine and cause an attack of acute of amoebic dysentery

↓

III. Pre-cystic stage: After some time due to decrease in virulence of trophozoites and development of tolerance in host, they are not able to continue the life cycle, so some trophozoites are change to pre-cystic stage followed by cystic stage. Few trophozoites remained unchanged. Both cyst and remained trophozoites pass with the stool in environment.

↓

Cyst remains viable in soil and water for several weeks → Entry cyst of in other host → **Continuation of life cycle** and cycle repeated

Trophozoites disintegrate (die) outside → Remain non-infectious

Extra-intestinal / invasive amoebiasis

↓

Tissue invading trophozoites moves from dead tissue to the healthy margin

↓

Enters in to deeper layer and sometimes gain access to portal circulation

↓

Carried to the liver where their further development is arrested. In the liver the trophic forms may multiply but encystation does not occur, so entry in liver by parasite is an accident and **called dead end of parasite.**

↓

Dead end (no continuation of life cycle)

Flow chart-2: Life cycle of *E. histolytica*

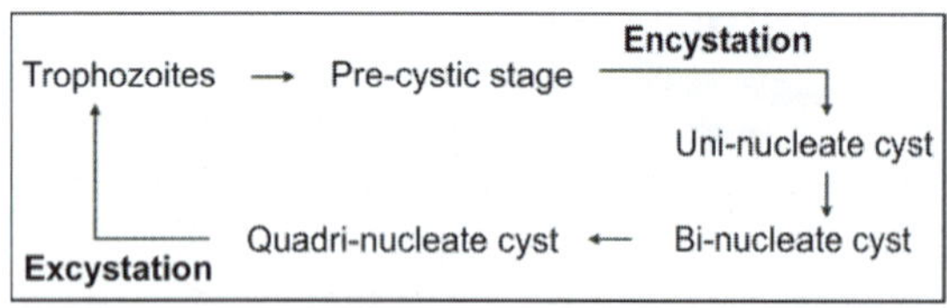

Flow chart-3: Summary of life cycle of *E. histolytica*

g. Zymodeme pattern:

- **Definition:** Isoenzyme pattern of *E. histolytica* **called zymodeme pattern**. *E. histolytica* has distinct invasive & non-invasive strains. These strains are differentiated according to their isoenzyme (zymodeme) pattern. *E. histolytica* have total 22 isoenzymes (zymodemes) of these 10 are invasive & 12 non-invasive.
- **Clinical significance:** It is useful to detect wheather the strain is virulent or avirulent.
- **Identification:**
  - Isoenzyme (zymodeme) is identified by electrophoretic mobility of 4 enzymes like L-malate (NADP + oxido-reductase), phosphoglucomutase (most important), glucose phosphate isomerise & hexokinase.
  - Electrophoresis of phosphoglucomutase can show one or more of 4 bands such as α, β, γ & δ. Strain with absence of α-band with presence of β-band indicate the virulence strain.

ii. Host factors influencing the virulence:

1. **Age:** More in adults than in children.
2. **Sex:** More in male than in female.
3. **Diet:**
   - Low iron → restriction of trophozoite growth → restriction of disease.
   - High protein → restriction of disease.
   - Vitamin C deficiency, high carbohydrate, high lipid → precipitate the infection.
4. **Immunosuppressive status:** Like
   - Late pregnancy.
   - Diabetes.
   - Malignancy.
   - Steroid therapy.
   - Immunosuppressive drugs.
   - Anti-metabolites
5. **Co-infection:** By bacteria enhance the pathogenicity & evidenced by
   - Better growth of amoebae in culture in presence of bacteria like *Streptobacilli* (also in presence of parasite like *T. cruzi*).
   - Reduction of intensity of disease with antibiotics.
   - No growth of amoebae in germ free animals.
6. **Resistant host:** Minimal injuries /superficial ulcers are produced, if parasite enters in to resistant host.
7. **Others are like:** Poverty/poor socio-economic status, poor hygiene etc.

➢ **Pathological types of amoebiasis:** Two types like intestinal / primary / non-invasive amoebiasis **and** extra-intestinal / secondary / invasive amoebiasis (metastatic amoebiasis).

Intestinal / primary / non-invasive

✪ **Definition:** Infection limited to large intestine **called intestinal (primary) amoebiasis.**

✓ **Note: Amoebic dysentery.**

- It is defined as increase the frequency of stool with presence of blood & mucus in stool with tenesmus.
- Term **amoebic dysentery** neither used as synonym as amoebiasis nor it denotes the full picture of intestinal lesion.
- It is a clinical feature of intestinal amoebiasis due to extensive intestinal ulceration and there are large numbers of cases of intestinal amoebiasis without amoebic dysentery symptoms.

✪ **Pathogenesis: →Flow chart-4 & fig.-3**

✪ **Subtypes (pathology):** Two types like acute & chronic.

A. Acute: Macroscopic & microscopic of features acute amoebic ulcers are described below.

i. Macroscopic features:

- **Sites: Fig.-4**

a. Generalised: Ulcer is distributed through the whole length of large gut & up to internal anal sphincter.

b. Localised: Two levels

1. **Ileo-caecal region:** It is the most common site. Ileo-caecal valve, caecum, ascending colon, appendix are involved. It is found twice then sigmoido-rectal region.
2. **Sigmoido-rectal region:** Sigmoido colon & rectum are involved.

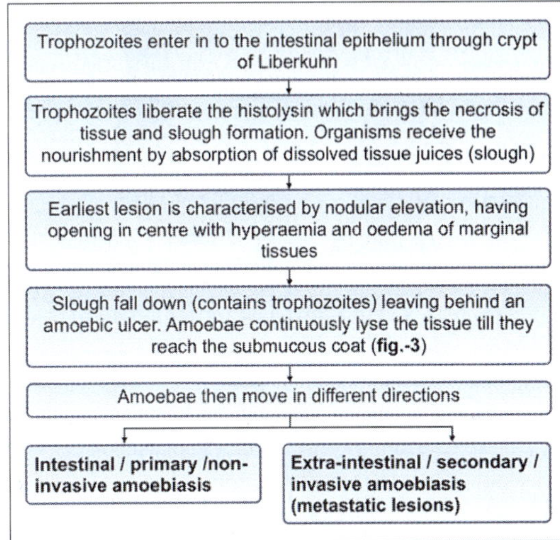

Flow chart-4: Pathogenesis of *E. histolytica*

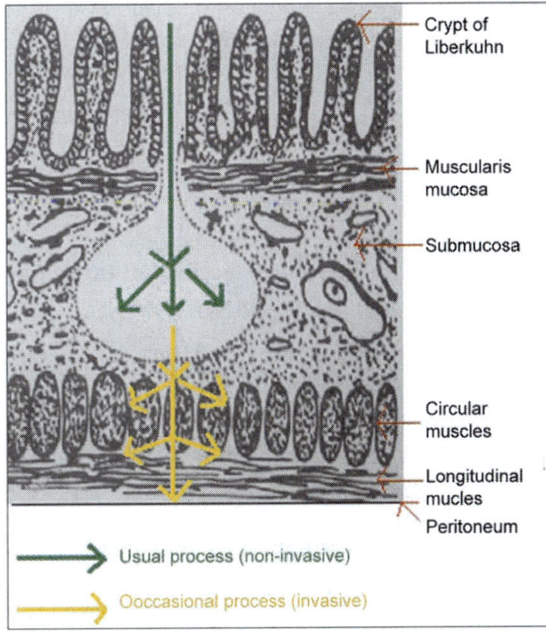

Figure-3: Amoebic ulcer (flask shape)

- **Size:** Varying from pin's head to one inch or greater in diameter.
- **Shape:** Round to oval. **Flask shape ulcer (water bottle or water decanter or undermined ulcer)** indicates the process of tissue necrosis as shown in **fig.-3.**

- **Margin:** Ragged & undermined, being formed by overhanging mucous membrane. On vertical section it appears in flask-shape.
- **Base:** Formed by muscular coat.

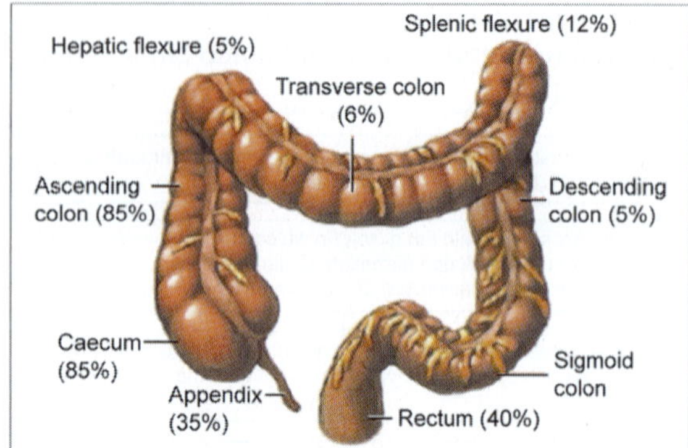

Figure-4: Distribution of amoebic ulcer

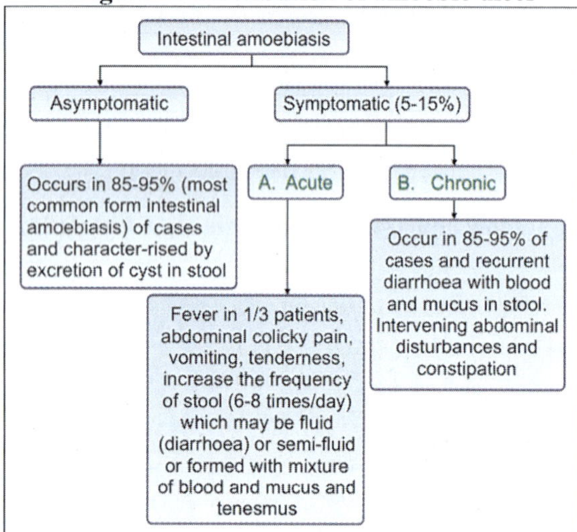

Flow chart-5: Clinical features of intestinal amoebiasis

- **Contains:** Yellowish-black slough (necrosed tissues & trophozoites).
- **Extension of ulcers:**
  - Superficial ulcer: Do not extend beyond the muscularis mucosae.
  - Deep ulcer:
    - Do not extend beyond the submucous coat & extend laterally in surrounding tissues.
    - However, sometimes it extends beyond the submucous coat & even serous layer & produces complications (**complications →Vide infra**).
- **Healing of ulcers:**
  - Superficial ulcer: Heal without scar.
  - Deep ulcer: Heal with scar.

ii. Microscopic features:

- **Early ulcers:** If a section is made through the middle of early ulcer, following features would be present.
  - Centre: Coagulative necrosed tissues.
  - Periphery: Trophozoites, either single or in groups.
- **Advanced ulcers:**
  - Trophozoites migrates away from the site of actual ulcer, invades the intermuscular spaces to reach the peritoneal coat.
  - Parasites also invading the small venules, causing hyperplasia of endothelial cells & thrombosis of blood vessels.

B. Chronic: Chronic stage is different from acute as follows & depends on resisting power of host.

- **Size:** Small size ulcer.
- **Extension:** Superficial ulcer involving the mucosa.
- **Healing of ulcers:** Healed with marked scaring of intestinal wall.

✪ **Clinical features:** Two type cases **(flow chart-5).**

✪ **Complications of intestinal amoebiasis:**

A. Acute:

1. Perforation.
2. Local peritonitis.
3. Generalised peritonitis.
4. Haemorrhage.
5. Pericaecal or pericolic abscess.
6. Gangrene of large gut.
7. Amoebic appendicitis.
8. Excessive scaring of healed ulcers leads to
   - Thickening of intestinal wall.
   - Stricture formation.
   - Partial intestinal obstruction.

B. Chronic:

1. Due to **marked scaring** there is a thinning, dilatation & sacculation of wall.
2. **Localised thickening** of intestinal wall leading to narrowing of the lumen of the gut.
3. **Generalised thickening** rendering the palpable gut
4. Formations of **granulomatous tumour like mass called amoebic granuloma or amoeboma** simulating the carcinoma of bowel, which is differentiated with presence of trophozoites in biopsy specimens.

Extra-intestinal / secondary / invasive amoebiasis (metastatic amoebiasis)

♣ **Intestinal lesions in metastatic amoebiasis**

- Small superficial ulcers with thickening of intestinal wall.
- Latent ulcer in caecum.
- Pigmented / non-pigmented scar, representing the sites of previous ulcer.

♣ **Sites of metastatic amoebiasis**

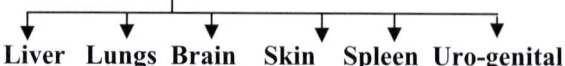

I. Hepatic amoebiasis (Amoebic liver abscess)

✪ **Incidence:** It is the most common form intestinal amoebiasis. Average 5% case in *E. histolytica* infection produces the hepatic amoebiasis.

✪ **Pathogenesis: → Flow chart-6**

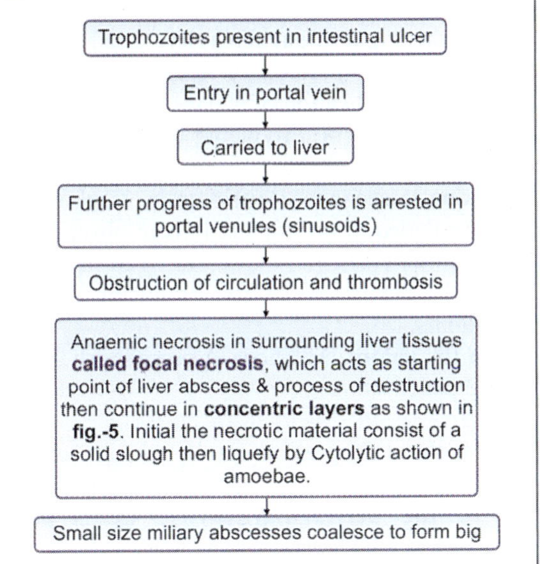

Flow chart-6: Pathogenesis hepatic amoebiasis

✓ **Note: Diffuse Amoebic hepatitis**

- Non-specific hepatomegaly present in patients of amoebic dysentery with enlarged tender liver, right upper quadrant pain, intermittent fever & leucocytosis **called diffuse amoebic hepatitis**.
- Liver biopsy does not reveal the presence of *E. histolytica.*
- Enlargement of liver is due to periportal inflammation & congestion by **bacteria** carried to liver by blood stream from ulcerated gut.

✪ **Subtypes (pathology):** Two subtypes

A. **Amoebic hepatitis:** Only inflammation of liver & no pus detected in liver.

B. **Amoebic liver abscess:** Liver abscess is not the pus formation (no suppuration) but a mixture of sloughed liver tissues & blood **called anchovy sauce pus**. It is bacteriologically sterile.

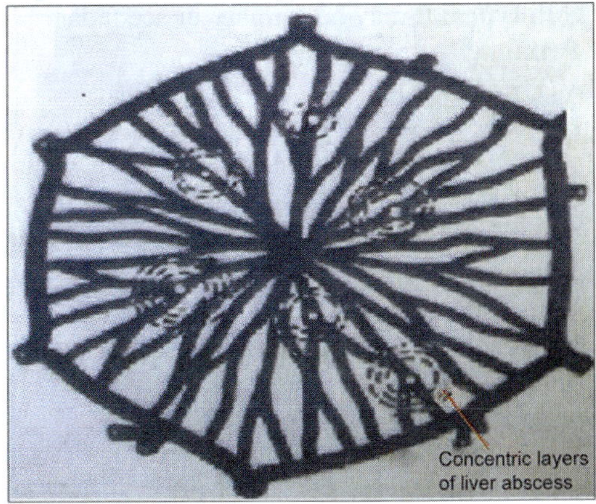

Figure-5: Concentric layers of liver abscess

i. **Macroscopic features of liver abscess:**

- **Sites:**
  - Most common site: Postero-superior surface of **right lobe** liver.
  - Rarely in left lobe but more important because of more chances of rupture due to less liver mass.
- **Size:**
  - Small in size. Average size is 10-15 cm.
  - Sometimes multiple small abscesses (miliary abscess) coalesce to form big sized abscess, which may hold litre of pus.
- **Numbers:** In > 80% cases solitary abscess.
- **Colour:** Chocolate-brown.
- **Consistency:** Semifluid or grumous.
- **Smell:** Offensive smell.
- **Wall of abscess cavity:** It is ragged & shaggy& formed by necrotic liver tissues which gradually merge in to healthy tissues with intervening zone of hyperaemia.

ii. **Microscopic features of liver abscess:** When a cut section made through the margin of liver abscess & examined microscopically shows the following three zones (**fig.-5**).

1. **Central zone:** Cytolysed granular material & no amoeba.
2. **Intermediate zone:** RBCs, WBCs, Degenerated liver cells & few trophozoites of *E. histolytica.*
3. **Peripheral zone:**
   - Congested capillaries necrosed liver cells & amoebae (multiplying).
   - In long standing cases it may consists the lymphocytes, monocytes & connective tissues cell.

✪ **Clinical features:**

a. **Symptoms:**

- **Onset:** Sudden.
- **Pain & tenderness:** In right hypochondrium due to stretching of liver capsule.
- **Referred pain:**
  - In right shoulder due to irritation of phrenic nerve which supply the under surface of diaphragm.
  - Also referred pain in lower abdomen & in right iliac region.
- **Fever:**
  - High, continuous fever with chills, rigor & sweating.
  - It can be remittent or intermittent or absent.
- **Jaundice:** Rarely present & mild if present.
- **GIT:** No diarrhoea/ dysentery.
- **General symptoms:**
  - Emaciation.
  - Shallowness of the skin.

b. **Signs:** Following are findings.

1. **Liver:**

- **Inspection:** Movement on right side of chest during respiration is decrease or absent.
- **Palpation:**
  - Liver is **tender & palpable** below the costal margin.

- **Dullness** of liver which may extend upwards.
- **Rigidity** on upper part of right rectus which may interfere with enlarged liver's palpation.
- **Compensatory hypertrophy** of left lobe of liver in case of large abscess.

2. **GIT:** Tenderness & thickening of bowel may elicited on abdominal palpation.
3. **Lungs:**

- Collapse of base of right lung due to growing liver abscess.
- Occasionally presence of right pleural effusion.

✪ **Complications (course & termination):**

- **Healed with**: Encysted mass/ fibrosis / calcification.
- **Infection:** Secondary bacterial infection occurs
  - Via blood stream.
  - During aspiration.
  - During surgery.
  - Following spontaneous rupture.
- **Haematogenous spread:** In distant organs like brain, kidney etc.
- **Termination:** Continuous growth & termination in neighbouring tissues as described below (**fig.-6**).

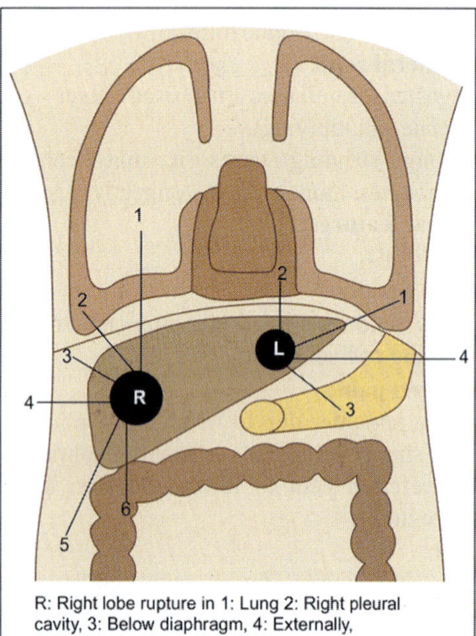

R: Right lobe rupture in 1: Lung 2: Right pleural cavity, 3: Below diaphragm, 4: Externally, 5: Peritonal cavity and 6: Colon
L: Left lobe rupture in 1: Left pleural cavity, 2: Pericardial cavity, 3: Stomach and 4: Externally

Figure-6: Rupture of right (R) & Left (L) side liver abscess

a. Rupture of right side liver abscess:

1. **In to the lungs:**

- Presence of anchovy-sauce pus in sputum with viscid consistency & chocolate brown colour (like haemoptysis).
- Liver cells & trophozoites are revealed microscopically from sputum.

2. **In to the right pleural cavity:** Leads empyema thoracis. Pleuro-pulmonary termination is the most common complication of hepatic amoebiasis.
3. **Below diaphragm:** Producing subphrenic abscess
4. **Externally in to skin:** Granulomatous lesions of skin due to secondary infection by trophozoites of *E. histolytica* from ruptured liver abscess **called granuloma cutis.**
5. **In to the peritoneal cavity:** Producing generalised peritonitis.
6. **In to the colon:** Diarrhoea & presence of anchovy-sauce pus in stool.

b. Rupture of left side liver abscess:

1. **In to the left pleural cavity:** Leads empyema thoracis.
2. **In to the pericardial cavity:** Leads purulent pericarditis which is fatal in nature.
3. **In to the stomach:**

- Presence of anchovy-sauce pus in vomiting with viscid consistency & chocolate brown colour (like haematemesis).
- Liver cells & trophozoites are revealed microscopically from vomitus.

4. **Externally:** Through anterior abdominal wall in epigastric region.

c. Rupture of inferior surface liver abscess:

1. **In to the transverse colon / duodenum:** Diarrhoea & presence of anchovy-sauce pus in stool.
2. **In to the peritoneal cavity:** Causing a fatal peritonitis.

d. Rupture of posterior surface liver abscess: In to inferior vena cava, which is very are but fatal.

e. Other sites of rupture: Are common bile duct, pelvis of kidney & perinephric tissues of lumbar region.

II. Pulmonary amoebiasis

✪ **Sub types:** It may be primary or secondary.

A. Primary:

- Very rare.
- It is due to direct entry of trophozoites from gut wall by portal circulation in to the pulmonary capillaries.
- Numbers: Single or multiple abscesses in lungs.

B. Secondary

- Very common.
- It is due to rupture of liver abscess in to lungs.
- Site: Lower lobe of right lung.
- Numbers: Mostly single abscess.

III. Cerebral amoebiasis

- Very common.
- It is due to complication of hepatic or lung amoebiasis or both.

- Site: one of the cerebral hemisphere.
- Numbers: Mostly single abscess.
- Size: Variable.

IV. Cutaneous amoebiasis

- It is due to rupture of underlying visceral abscess.
- Common sites arc drainage of liver abscess, colostomy wound, peri-anal region etc.
- Characterised by rapidly spreading necrotising granulomatous lesions of skin & subcutaneous tissues **called granuloma cutis.**
- Rapidly improve with anti-amoebic treatment.

V. Splenic amoebiasis

- It is **primary** from splenic flexure of colon or **secondary** from liver abscess.

VI. Uro-genital amoebiasis

- Very common.
- Entry of amoeba by recto-vesical fistula or recto-vaginal fistula.
- Present with amoebic vaginitis or amoebic ulcer on penis.

❖ Differential diagnosis (D/D):

D/D of intestinal amoebiasis

It should be differentiated from following disease.

1. **Bacillary dysentery:**
- Caused by bacteria Entero Invasive E. coli (EIEC), *C. jejuni*, *V. parahaemolyticus* & *Shigella* spp.
- Both types are differentiated by stool examination as shown in **fig.-7 & table -1.**

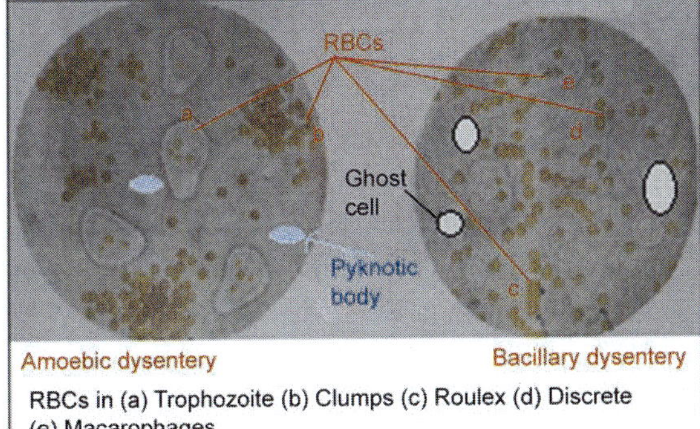

Figure-7: Microscopic appearance of stool in amoebic & bacillary dysentery

2. ***Entamoeba coli*:**
- *E. histolytica* also differentiated from normal commensals like *Entamoeba coli*. (→ **Vide infra**)
- Presence of *Entamoeba coli* in stool creates confusion in diagnosis & starting of unnecessary treatment for non-pathogenic organisms.

3. **Other parasitic dysentery:** *B. coli, S. mansoni, S. japonicum, S. intercalatum , H. heterophyes & Trichuris trichuria, S stercoralis* etc. are also allow the presence of blood & mucus in stool.
4. **Psedomembranous colitis.**
5. **Ulcerative colitis.**
6. **Crohn's disease.**
7. **Haemorrhoids.**
8. **Neoplastic growth.**

Features	Amoebic dysentery	Bacillary dysentery
	Macroscopy of stool	
Numbers	6-8 motions/day	>10 motions/day
Amount	Copious	Small
Odour	Offensive	Odourless
Colour	Dark red	Bright red
Nature	Blood & mucus with faeces	Blood & mucus, no faeces
Reaction	Acid	Alkaline
Consistency	Not adherent to container	Adherent to the bottom of container
	Microscopy of stool by normal saline	
RBCs	In clumps, reddish-yellow in colour	Discrete / in rouleaux, bright red in colour
Pus cells	Scanty	Numerous
Macrophages	Very few	Large & numerous, contain RBC, so mis-taken as *E. histolytica*
Eosinophils	Present	Scarce
Cyst /motile trophozoites	Present	Absent
Ghost cells	Nil	Numerous
Pyknotic bodies	Very common	Nil
C L crystals	Present	Absent

Table -1: Differences between amoebic & bacillary dysentery

✓ **Note: Ghost cells, Pyknotic bodies & CL crystals**

1. **Ghost cells:** It is an enlarged eosinophilic epithelial cells with eosinophilic cytoplasm without nucleus.
2. **Pyknotic bodies:** Condensed nuclear/ chromatin materials of epithelial cells, macrophages or pus cells in amoebic dysentery.
3. **CL crystals:**

- **Full form:** Charcoat-Layden crystals.
- **Definition:** Breakdown products of eosinophils & basophils.
- **Mechanism of production**:
  - Lysophospholipase which is present in eosinophils, convert it in to CL crystals.
  - Their presence indicates that immune response has taken place which may be due to parasitic infection or allergic reactions.
  - Their presence in stool may not correlate with eosinophilia in blood.
- **Morphology:**

- **Shape:** Slender, hexagonal or bipyramidal or diamond or whetstone shaped.
- **Size:** Different in size from 5-50 μm.

▪ **Diagnosis:**

o Specimens:
- Parasitic infection: Stool
- Asthma: Sputum.

o Methods:
- Normal Saline (NS): Diamond or whetstone shaped, clear & refractile as shown in **figure-8.**
- Trichrome stain: Stain in red-purple colour as shown in **figure-9.**

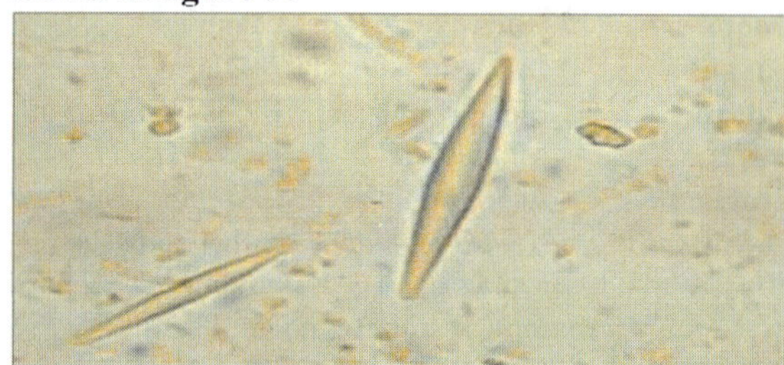

Figure-8: CL crystals under NS preparation

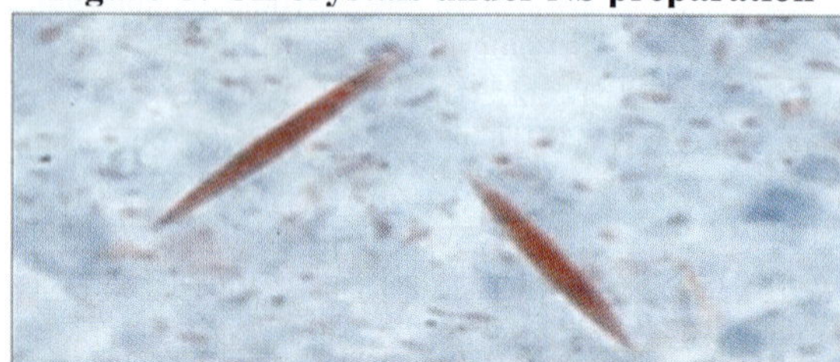

Figure-9: CL crystals under Trichrome stain

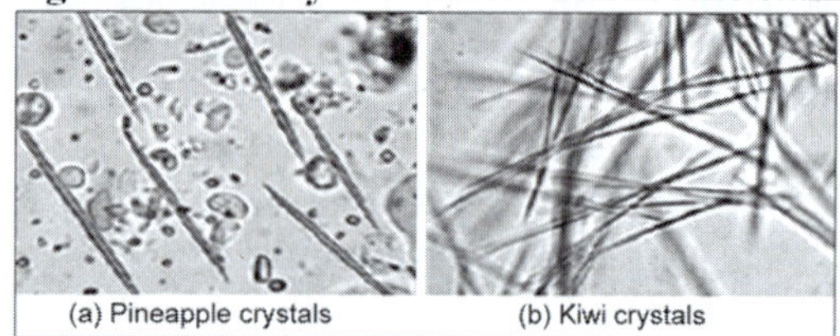

(a) Pineapple crystals (b) Kiwi crystals

Figure-10: CL crystals of fruit juices

▪ **Interpretation:** CL crystals are detected in following conditions.

▫ Frequently present in exudates & granuloma containing eosinophils.

▫ **Parasitic infection** like
- *E. histolytica:* In stool
- *A. duodenale:* In stool.
- *Trichuris trichuria:* In stool.
- *A. lumbricoides:* In sputum.

▫ **Allergic reaction:** Like asthma.

▫ **False positive:** Fruit juices like pineapple [**fig.-10(a)**] & kiwis [**fig.-10(b)**] crystals and vegetables like aspargas sometimes looks like CL crystals & should be differentiated with history of ingestion of juice or vegetables.

D/D of extra-intestinal amoebiasis

I. D/D of hepatic amoebiasis

1. Viral hepatitis.
2. Alcoholic hepatitis.
3. Cirrhosis of liver.
4. H. cyst.
5. Malignancy of liver.
6. Pyogenic liver abscess.
7. Subphrenic abscess.
8. Pleurisy.

II. D/D of pulmonary amoebiasis

1. Bacterial lung abscess.
2. H. cyst of lungs.
3. Malignancy of lungs.
4. Granulomatous lesions of lungs.

❖ **Carrier:**

➢ **Synonym:** Also **called cyst passer.**

➢ **Types:** Following two types.

a. **Healthy (contact) carrier:** Who contains the organisms but never suffered from amoebic dysentery (Health remains intact).

b. **Convalescent carrier:** Who recovered from acute clinical attack of amoebic dysentery.

➢ **Diagnosis:** Diagnosed by microscopy. It is non-invasive, so serological tests are not useful.

❖ **Laboratory diagnosis:** It is described under two broad heading like intestinal & extra-intestinal amoebiasis.

Diagnosis of intestinal amoebiasis

↓

Flow chart-7

Diagnosis of extra-intestinal amoebiasis

I. Diagnosis of hepatic amoebiasis

A. **Direct:**

➢ **Specimens:**

- **Aspiration of pus or liver biopsy material:** For diagnosis of *E. histolytica* material should be taken from the abscess wall by scraping & not from the abscess contents.
- **Stool**

➢ **Testing methods:**

a. **Trophozoites detection:** Motile trophozoites are detected by microscopy from pus (**anchovy sauce pus**) or biopsy material.

b. **Cyst:** From stool by microscopy.

B. **Indirect:**

a. **Blood:** Leucocytosis, (15, 000 – 30, 000 cmm).

b. **Serological tests:**

- **Detection of specific antibody:**

1. **ELISA test:**
- Most sensitive (99%) & most specific (90%)
- It becomes negative within 6 months of successful treatment

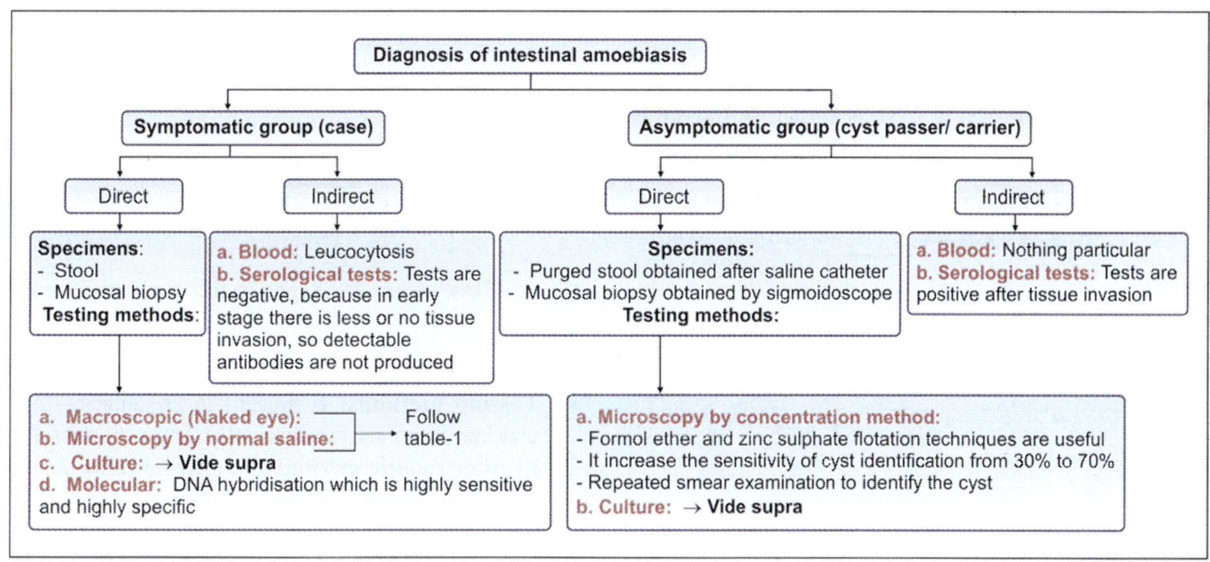

Flow chart-7: Diagnosis of intestinal amoebiasis

2. **Indirect haemagglutination test & latex agglutination test:**
- Highly sensitive but less specific & often give false positive result.
- Both remain positive for 10 years of successful treatment, so differentiate between recent & remote infection.

3. **Gel diffusion precipitation test & counter current immunoelectrophoresis test:** Both become negative within 6 months of successful treatment.
4. **CFT:** Availability of highly specific Ag is the problem with this test.
5. **Cellulose acetate membrane precipitation test.**
6. **Precipitin test.**
7. **Immunofluorescent (Goldman) test.**

- **Inhibition of trophozoite's motility by specific antiserum:** By immobilisation test.

c. **Immunological test:**

1. **Intradermal skin test:**
- Intradermal introduction of 0.1 ml antigen of *E. histolytica.*
- Erythema produced after 3 hrs, reaching maximum in size about 9-10cm in 20-24 hrs & disappear in next 24-48 hrs.
- Antigen is prepared from trophozoites of *E. histolytica* grown on axenic culture & from cyst of *E. invadens* (snake amoeba).

2. **PCA (Passive Cutaneous Anaphylaxis) test:** Positive in guinea pig skin.

II. Diagnosis of pulmonary amoebiasis

- **Specimens:** Sputum or Aspiration of pus from abscess or lung biopsy material.
- **Testing methods:**

a. **Trophozoites detection:** Motile trophozoites are detected by microscopy from pus (**anchovy sauce pus**) or biopsy material.
b. **Cyst:** From stool by microscopy.

❖ Prevention:
- Prevention of contamination of food & water by human excreta.
- Detection & treatment of carrier & their exclusion from food handling occupation. Carriers are treated by luminal amoebicides.
- Health education.

❖ Treatment:
A. **Oral rehydration & electrolyte replacement.**
B. **Amoebicides drugs:** Three types of drugs

i. **Luminal/intestinal amoebicides:** Diloxanide furoate, iodoquinol, paromycin & tetracycline.
ii. **Extra - intestinal (tissue) amoebicides:** Chloroquine (1g/day for 2 days followed by 5g/day for 3 weeks), emetine etc.
iii. **Mixed:** Metronidazole, tinidazole & ornidazole are the drug of choice for intestinal & extra- intestinal (tissue) amoebiasis.

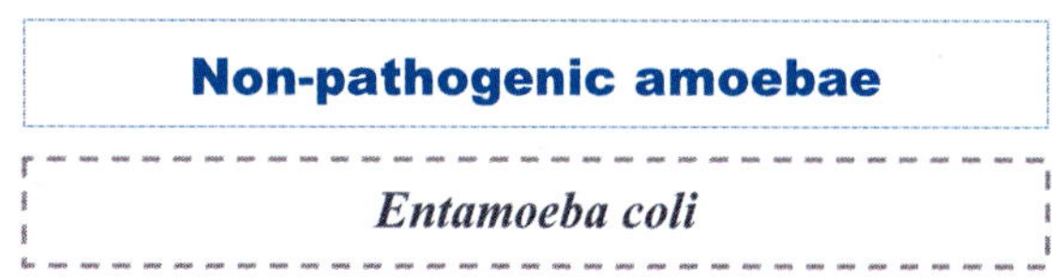

❖ History:
- E. coli was 1st described by **Lewiss** in 1870 & **Cunnigham** in 1871 in Kolkatta.
- **Grassi** reported its presence in intestine of healthy person in 1878.

❖ Geographical distribution: World-wide.

❖ **Habitat:** Large intestine.

❖ **Morphology:** Unicellular & single cell performs the all functions. Three morphological stages like trophozoite, pre-cyst & cyst as shown in **fig.-11 & table-2.**

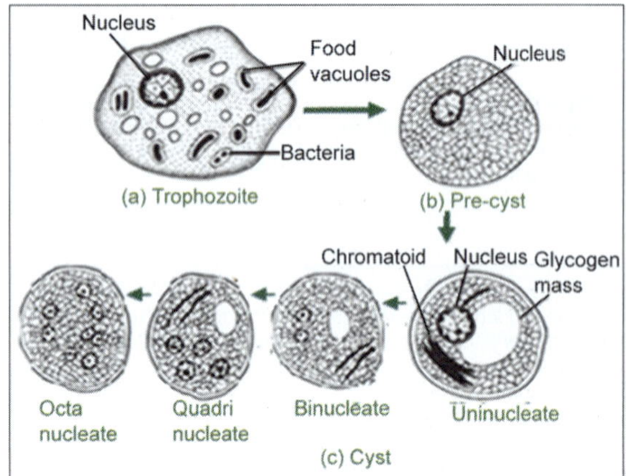

Figure-11: Morphology of *E. coli*

Features	*E. histolytica*	*E. coli*
Trophozoite		
(a) NS preparation from fresh stool		
Size	18-40μm	20-40μm
Motility	Active	Sluggish
Cytoplasm	Clearly defined in to ectoplasm & endoplasm	Ill defined, ectoplasm scarcely seen
Cytoplasmic inclusion	- RBCs, WBCs & tissue debris - No bacteria	- Bacteria & other materials - No RBCs
Nucleus	Not visible in NS preparation	Visible in NS preparation
(b) Iodine preparation (Nuclear character)		
Karyosome	Central	Eccentric
Linin network	Fine	Coarse
Nuclear membrane	Delicate	Thick
Chromatin granules	Fine & lined to nu -clear membrane	Coarse & lined to nuclear membrane
Cyst		
(a) NS preparation from fresh stool		
Size	6-15μm	15-20μm
Chromatoid bars	Rounded	Filamentous, thread like & pointed ends
(b) Iodine preparation		
Nucleus	1-4	1-8
Glycogen mass	Visible in uninucleate stage	Visible in bi or quadric- nucleate stage

Table -2: Differences between *E. histolytica* & *E. coli*

❖ **Pathogenicity:** Transmitted by faeco-oral route & non-pathogenic.

❖ **Life cycle:**

- Octanucleate cyst ingested by food or water.
- Cyst produces eight trophozoites **(flow chart-8).**
- Trophozoites converted in to cyst, which pass through faeces & cycle will repeat.

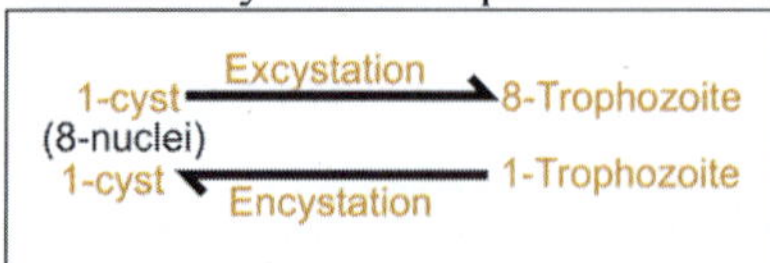

Flow chart-8: Stages in life cycle of *E. coli*

❖ **Diagnosis:**

➢ **Specimens:** Stool.

➢ **Testing methods:** It present in dysenteric stool & differentiated morphologically from *E. histolytica* by **microscopic method** as shown in **table-2.**

Others

❖ **Details of other non-pathogenic amoebae:** → **Table-3**

❖ **Life cycle:** →**Flow chart-9**

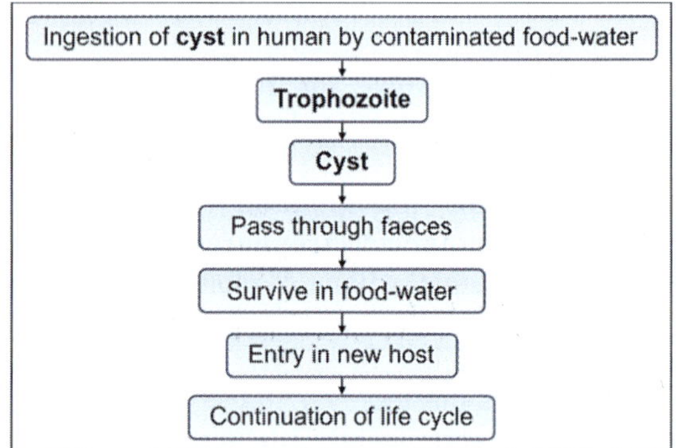

Flow chart-9: Life cycle of non-pathogenic amoeba

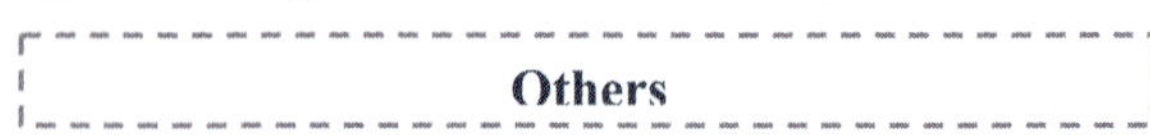

Free living amoebae

❖ **Meaning:** Living free in fresh water, mud & moist soil so **called free living amoebae.**

❖ **Synonym:**

1. **Opportunist amoebae:**
2. **Amphizoic amoebae:** As living free (exozoic) & in the body of host (endozoic).

❖ **History:**

- New concept was reported by Fowler & Carter in 1965.
- Few cases reported from Australia, USA, New Zealand, Britain & Czecholslovakia.
- 2 cases were reported in India from Kolkatta by Ghosh & Pan.

❖ **Classification:** →**Vide supra**

Features	E. gingivalis	E. hartmanni	E. polecki	E. nana	I. butchlii	D. fragilis
Trophozoites						
History	Gross, 1849 Brumpt,1913	von Prowazek, 1912	von Prowazek, 1912	Wenyon & O,Conner, 1917 Brug, 1918	von Prowazek, 1912 Dobell, 1919	Jeps & Dobell, 1918
Figure-12	(a)	(b)	(c)	(d)	(e)	(f)
Size	10-20μm	4-12μm	8-25μm	5-10μm	8-20μm	5-8μm
Motility	Active	Sluggish	Sluggish	Sluggish	Sluggish	
Cytoplasm	Divided in ectoplasm & endoplasm	Divided in ectoplasm & endoplasm	Divided in ectoplasm & endoplasm	Divided in ectoplasm & endoplasm		Fragile cytoplasm
Cytoplasmic inclusion	- Bacteria, food vacuoles - No RBCs	- Bacteria - No RBCs	- Bacteria - No RBCs	- Bacteria - No RBCs	- Bacteria, yeast &food particles - No RBCs	- Bacteria & food particle - No RBCs
Other features	Multiple pseudo-podium	Same as like *E. histolytica*, but smaller in size, so called small race of *E. histolytica*		Trophozoite & cyst are in same size		So called, because it is bi-nucleate & cytoplasm is fragile
Mature cyst						
Figure-13	No cyst stage	(a)	(b)	(c)	(d)	No cyst stage
Size		5-10μm	10-20μm	5-10μm	5-10μm	
Nuclei		1-4	1	4	1	
Chromatoid bars		Rounded ends	Pointed ends	Absent	Absent	
Glycogen mass		Diffuse	Diffuse	Absent	Rarely seen	
Nucleus						
Figure-14	(a)	(b)	(c)	(d)	(e)	(f)
Karyosome	Central	Central	Central	Large, irregular mass is connected with one small mass	- Central in position - Large mass surrounded by refractile globules	Karyosome is divided in 6-chromatin granules
Chromatin granules	Coarse (Ring like deposit)	Fine	Fine, symmetrical	Not clearly visible	Not clearly visible	

Table-3: Details of other non-pathogenic amoebae

Naegleria fowleri

- **Synonym:** Brain eating amoeba.
- **Habitat:** CNS system.
- **Morphology:**

I. Trophozoite stage

- **Types:** Two types of trophic forms **[fig.-15(a)].**

a. **Amoeboid form:**

- **Size:** Average from 10-35μm μm.
- **Shape:** Elongated.
- **Motility:** Actively motile.
- **Cytoplasm:** Having pseudopodia **called lopopodia.**

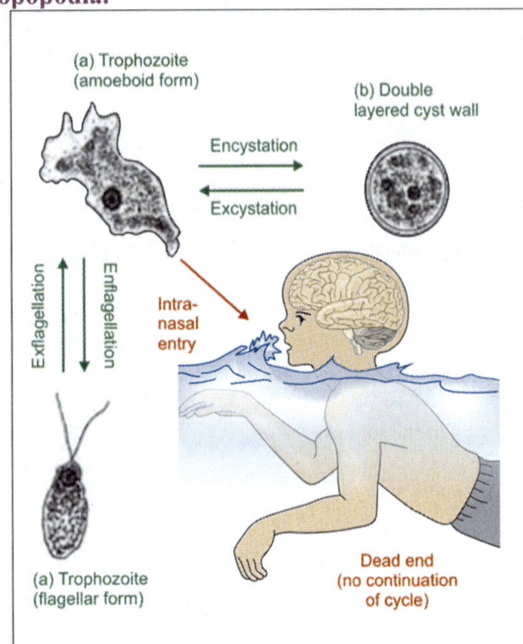

Figure-15: Morphology & life cycle of *N. fowleri*

- **Nucleus:**
  - Spherical with central karyosome (endosomes).
  - Visible in stained preparation.
- **Features:** Can multiply & convert in to cyst form.

b. **Flagellate form:**

- **Shape:** Pear shape.
- **Motility:** With two flagella at anterior end.
- **Nucleus:** Spherical with endosomes.
- **Features:** Not able to multiple & comes back to amoeboid form to produce cyst stage.

II. Cystic stage

- **Size:** -10 μm.
- **Shape:** Spherical or oval shape.
- **Nucleus:** Spherical with central karyosome (endosomes) as shown **fig.-15(b).**
- **Features:**
  - Smooth double layered cyst wall.
  - It is not present in tissues.

- **Life cycle:**
  - Cyst stage never form in human body.
  - Entire life cycle completed in external environment & all life cycle stages are **shown in fig.-15.**
  - Man is infected accidently by amoeboid trophozoite form by contact of nasal mucosa with contaminated swimming pool water, which produces the disease in man with **dead end** of cycle.

- **Pathogenicity:**

- **Disease name:** **Called Primary Amoebic Meningo-encephalitis (PAM).** Also **called terramoebiasis.**
- **Mode of transmission:**

1. **Direct contact** of nasal mucosa with contaminated swimming pool water [Others swimming pool originated microbes are *M. balnei* (*M. marinum*) causing **swimming pool granuloma** on prominence like elbows, nose etc. & *C. trachomatis* causing **swimming pool conjunctivitis.**
2. **Inhalation** of dust particles containing the cyst **or** air of air-cooler.

- **Incubation period:** 1-7 days.
- **Precipitating factors:**

1. **Age:** Mostly in children & young adults.
2. **Humidity:** Amoebas are common in air of air cooler & live symbiotically with *Legionella* & *Listeria.* Also transmitted by inhalation of air of air-cooler.

- **Pathogenesis: →Flow chart-10**

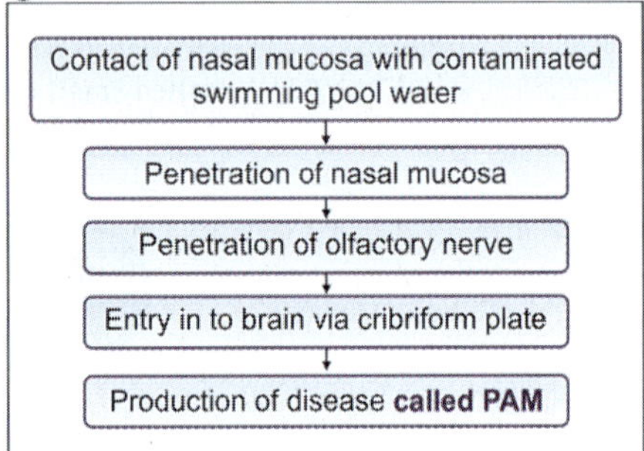

Flow chart-10: Pathogenesis of *N. fowleri*

- **Clinical features:**

1. **Acute purulent PAM:**
   - Acute purulent PAM. Severe headache, fever, vomiting, stiff neck, seizure & coma.
   - Most fatal & patients are die within a week (average in 5 days).
2. **Allergic alveolitis:** Present with humidifier fever due to inhalation of air from air cooler.

- **Complications:** Cranial nerve palsies of 3rd, 4th & 6th nerve. Most patients die within a week.

- **Differential diagnosis:** Disease should be differentiated from each & every case of meningitis.
- **Laboratory diagnosis:**

- **Specimens:** CSF & brain biopsy.
- **Testing methods:**

1. **Microscopy by normal saline:**
   - To identify the motile trophozoites.
   - Sugar & protein level is higher than the bacterial meningitis in CSF. Cyst is not present in tissues.
2. **Culture:** Grow in proteose peptone glucose medium or non nutrient agar seeded with

Escherichia coli as a food source. Both trophozoites & cyst can grow in culture.

- **Prevention:** Avoiding contact with contaminated water.
- **Treatment:**
- High dose of amphotericin B & rifampicin. amphotericin B can be given intravenously or direct instillation in brain.
- Miconazole & sulfadiazine shows the limited success only when administered in early stage.

Acanthamoeba spp.

- **Important species:**
- **Species name→ Vide supra.**
- *A. culbertsoni* is most pathogenic for human.
- **Habitat:** Found freely in soil & lakes. Eye & brain are natural habitat in human.
- **Morphology: → Fig.-16**

I. Trophozoite stage

- **Size:** Average from 15-45µm.
- **Shape:** Oval.
- **Motility:** Sluggishly motile.
- **Cytoplasm:** Showing the multiple pointed pseudopodia **called spiny amoeba** or **acanthopodia** & having no flagellate form.
- **Nucleus:** Same as like *N. fowleri.*
- **Features:**
- Present in tissues.
- It can multiply & convert in to cyst form.

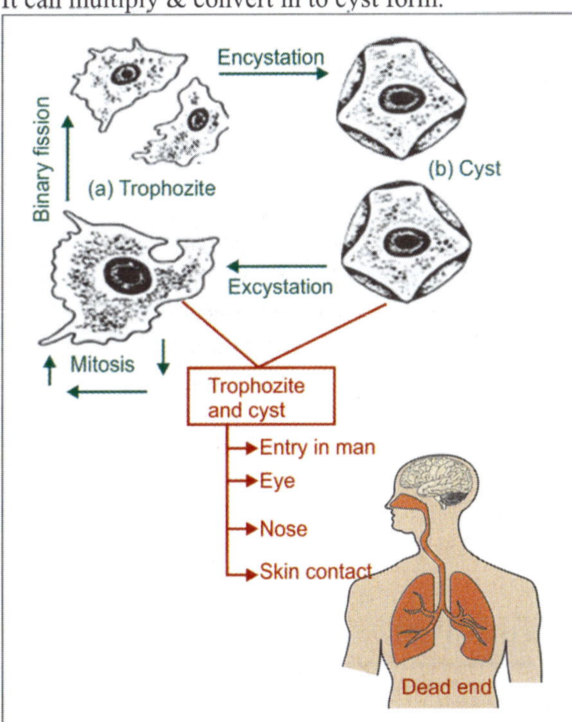

Figure-16: Morphology & life cycle of *Acanthamoeba*

II. Cystic stage

- **Size:** 8-25 µm.
- **Shape:** Spherical.
- **Nucleus:** Same as like *N. fowleri.*
- **Features:**
- Smooth double cyst wall.
- Inner wall is smooth & outer wrinkled.
- Present in tissues.
- **Life cycle:** Stages are shown in **fig.-16.**
- **Pathogenicity:**
- **Mode of transmission:**

1. **Direct contact** with contact lenses or to traumatised skin.
2. **Also by inhalation, ingestion**

- **Incubation period:** Few weeks to several months.
- **Precipitating factors:** Wearing contact lenses (especially soft one) during swimming or cleaning it with home-made saline or poor disinfectant.
- **Clinical features:**

1. **Eye:**
- Ulcerative keratitis **called chronic amoebic keratitis** & corneal ulceration.
- Trophozoites are present in tissues.
2. **Skin:** Ulceration.

Features	*Naegleria*	*Acanthamoeba*
Trophozoite		
- Size **- Psedopodia** **- Flagellate**	- Smaller - Single & **called lopopodia** - Present	- Larger - Multiple & **called spiny amoeba** - Absent
Cyst		
- Size **- Surface**	- Smaller - Smooth	- Larger - Wrinkled
Nucleus		
Mitosis	Nucleolus divides & nuclear membrane persist	Nuclear membrane dissolves
Pathogenicity		
Disease	PAM	GAM
Portal of entry	Nose	Eye/ respiratory tract
Precipitating factor	Swimming in contaminated water	Immunodeficiency disease/AIDS
Clinical course	Acute	Subacute/chronic
Pathology	Acute inflammation	Granulomatous inflammation
Laboratory diagnosis		
Tissues	Only trophozoite	Cyst & trophozoite
CSF	Predominantly PMNs	Predominantly leucocytes
Serological test	Most species die rapidly so rare useful	Immonofluorescence or immuno-peroxidase staining

Table-4: Differences between *Naegleria* & *Acanthamoeba*

3. **GAM (Granulomatous Amoebic Meningo-encephalitis):** Unlike *Naegleria* it is secondary by blood invasion of trophozoite from mucosa/ulcer of skin or from lower respiratory tract infection.
4. **Opportunistic infection:** Occurs in sinuses & lungs in immunocompromised/AIDS patient.

✪ **Differential diagnosis from *Naegleria*:**
- Flood the culture plate containing the distilled water or buffer with *Naegleria* & *Acanthamoeba* & examined for development of flagellate form of *Naegleria*.
- More differences are shown in **table-4**.

➢ **Laboratory diagnosis:**

✪ **Specimens:** CSF, corneal scraping.

✪ **Testing methods:**

a. Microscopy by normal saline:
- To identify the motile trophozoites.
- Protein & PMNs count is higher in CSF.

b. Culture:

1. **Culture in media**

- **Media:** Nutrient agar + *Escherichia coli* + *E. aerogenes / Kleb pneumoniae.*
- **Inoculation:** Culture plate is inoculated with drop of CSF.
- **Incubation:** At 37^0C or 42^0C in an aerobic condition for 24 hrs.
- **Result:** Culture plate can be examined with dissecting microscope under 10 × magnification.

2. **Animal culture:** Intranasal inoculation in mice develops brain infection,

c. Serological test: Follow **table-4.**

➢ **Prevention:** Improvement of hygiene specially of wearing contact lenses.

➢ **Treatment:**
- No specific treatment is available for GAM.
- Multi drugs like fluconazole, sulfadiazine, rifampicin & pentamidine shown the limited success.
- Corneal lesions are treated by biguanide or chlorhexidine with or without diamidine agent. In severe case keratoplasty is also indicated when vision is under threat.

Balamuthia mandrillaris

➢ **Habitat:** Found freely in soil & water. Eye & brain are natural habitat in human.

➢ **Morphology:** → **Fig.17**

I. Trophozoite stage

- **Size:** Average from 12-60µm.
- **Shape:** Irregular.
- **Motility:** Actively motile.
- **Cytoplasm:** Showing the broad pseudopodia.
- **Nucleus:** Same as like *Acanthamoeba.*
- **Features:** Present in tissues, can multiply & convert in to cyst form.

II. Cystic stage

- **Size:** 6-20 µm.
- **Shape:** Spherical.
- **Nucleus:** Same as like *Acanthamoeba.*
- **Features:**
- Smooth double cyst wall.
- Inner wall is smooth & outer irregular.
- Present in tissues.

➢ **Life cycle (fig.-17):** Same as like *Acanthamoeba.*

➢ **Pathogenicity:**

✪ **Mode of transmission: Direct contact** with contact lenses or to traumatised skin.

✪ **Precipitating factors:** Wearing contact lenses.

✪ **Clinical features:**
1. Eyes: Keratitis.
2. CNS: GAM (Granulomatous Amoebic Meningo-encephalitis).

➢ **Laboratory diagnosis:**

✪ **Specimens:** CSF & corneal scraping.

✪ **Testing methods:**

a. Microscopy by normal saline:

b. Culture: Also useful.

c. Serological test: Like ELISA.

d. Molecular: Like PCR.

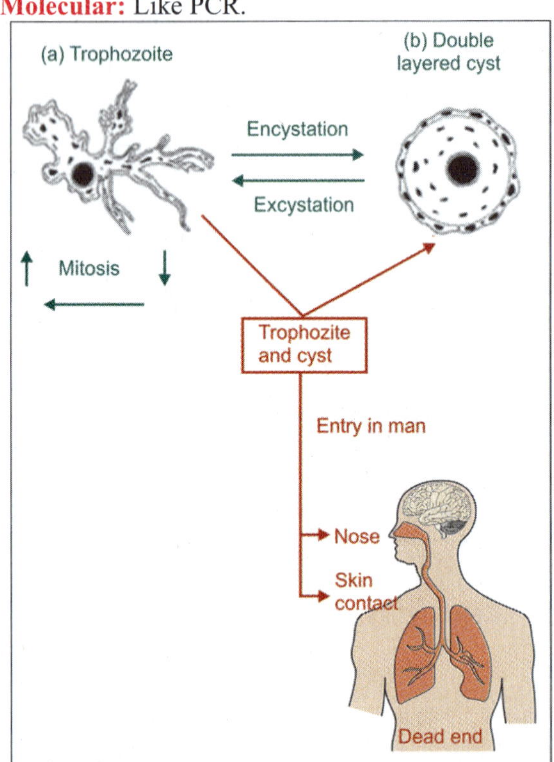

Figure-17: Morphology & life cycle of *B. mandrillaris*

Question bank

Case study

1) A female came with complain of abdominal pain & diarrhoea. Stool examination revealed presence of blood, mucus, motile trophozoites & RBCs in clumps. Identify the case and answer the following.

a) Name & draw the properly labelled diagram of morphological stages of causative agent.
b) Describe the life cycle of causative agent.
c) Describe the Pathogenicity of causative agent.
d) Describe the lab. diagnosis of causative agent.

Essay/Full question

1) *E. histolytica.*
2) Free living amoebae.

Short notes

1) Morphology/life cycle / pathogenicity / laboratory diagnosis of *E. histolytica.*
2) Differences between amoebic & bacillary dysentery.
3) Differences between *E. histolytica* & *E. coli.*
4) Hepatic amoebiasis.
5) Extra-intestinal amoebiasis.
6) CL crystals.

Short questions for theory/viva questions

1) Comment: Motility of *E. histolytica* is unidirectional.
2) Comment: Infection of *E. histolytica* is not transmitted by trophozoites.
3) What is zymodeme pattern in *E. histolytica*?
4) Name the four enzymes useful in zymodeme pattern in *E. histolytica.*
5) What is granuloma cutis?
6) What is diffuse amoebic hepatitis?
7) What is Anchovy sauce pus?
8) What is pyknotic body?
9) Name the four parasites causing dysentery.
10) Name the free living amoebae.
11) Name the two microbes transmitted by contaminated swimming pool water.
12) What is spiny amoeba?

MCQs for chapter review

Classification

1) **All of the following amoebae live in the large intestine except**
(a) *E. coli* (b) *E. nana* (c) *E. gingivalis* (d) *E. butchlii*
2) **Non pathogenic amoebae is/are**
(a) *E. histolytica* (b) *E. coli* (c) *Acanthamoeba* (d) *E. hartmanni* (e) *Balamuthia*

Entamoeba histoytica

3) **Which of the following is true about mature cyst of *E. histolytica*** (AI-96)
(a) Endoplasm and ectoplasm are clearly defined (b) Eight chromatoid bodies (c) Shows chromatoid bodies and glycogen mass (d) Nuclear structure retains characteristics of trophozoite
4) **Which is true of trophozoite of *E. histolytica*** (AI-93)
(a) Has eccentric karyosome (b) Nuclear membrane with chromatin (c) Shows erythro-phagocytosis (d) Presence of bacteria inside cell
5) **All are true about *Entamoeba histolytica* except** (AI-91)
(a) Cysts are 8 nucleated (b) Cysts are 4 nucleated (c) Trophozoites are colonise in the colon (d) Chrmoatoid bars are stained by iodides
6) **All are seen in cyst of *Entamoeba histolytica* except**
(a) Glycogen mass (b) Chromatoid bars (c) Eccentric nucleus (d) Refractile nucleus
7) **Culture medium used for *Entamoeba histolytica* is**
(a) Blood agar (b) Philip's medium (c) CLED medium (d) Trypticase serum
8) **The main reservoir for *Entamoeba histolytica* is** (AI-91)
(a) Man (b) Dirty water (c) Ponds
9) **Amoebiasis is transmitted by all except** (AIIMS, Nov-10)
(a) Cockroaches (b) Faeco-oral (c) Vertical transmission (d) Oro-rectal
10) **Pathogenicity of *E. histolytica* is indicated by**
(a) Zymodeme pattern (b) Size (c) Nuclear pattern (d) ELISA test
11) **True about amoebic colitis is** (PGI, June-02)
(a) Caused by *E. histolytica* (b) Cyst contains 8 nuclei (c) Flask shaped ulcers are present (d) Caecum is most commonly affected (e) Is premalignant
12) **Diffuse amoebic hepatitis is caused by**
(a) *E. histolytica* (b) Bacteria (c) a+b (d) None of above
13) **Most common extra hepatic complication of amoebic hepatitis is**
(a) Meningitis (b) Lung abscess (c) Nephritis (d) Encephalitis
14) **Which of the following statement is false** (AIIMS-02)
(a) The presence of ingested erythrocytes is seen only in *E histolytica* (b) Young adult male of low socio economic status are most commonly affected by invasive amoebiasis (c) A low iron content in the diet predispose to invasive amoebiasis (d) The pathogenic and non pathogenic strains of *E histolytica* can be differentiated by the electrophoretic study of zymodemes
15) **Charcoat-Layden crystals in stool are seen in**
(a) Bacillary dysentery (b) Amoebic dysentery (c) Giardiasis (d) Cholera
16) **Parasite having Charcoat-Layden crystals but no pus cells**
(a) *Giardia* (b) *Taenia* (c) *E. histolytica* (d) *Trichomonas*
17) **Charcoat-Layden crystals are derived from**
(a) Macrophages (b) Eosinophils (c) Basophils (d) Neutrophils
18) **Commonest site of extra intestinal amoebiasis is**
(a) Brain (b) Liver (c) Spleen (d) Lungs
19) **Regarding cutaneous amoebiasis which is not true**
(a) It is a spreading necrotising inflammation of the skin and subcutaneous tissue (b) Rapid improvement with anti-amoebic treatment occur. (c) Can occur in peri-anal region (d) Infection reaches the skin through the blood stream
20) **Investigation of choice for amoebiasis is**
(a) ELISA (b) Colonoscopy (c) Microscopy (d) Microscopy + ELISA
21) **Invasive amoebiasis can be best diagnosed by** (AIIMS, Nov-01)
(a) ELISA (b) Counter current immunoelectrophoresis (c) Indirect haemagglutination test (d) Complement fixation test
22) **Significant titre of IHA is seen in all types of amoebiasis except** (AIIMS-98)
(a) Acute amoebic dysentery (b) Brain abscess (c) Liver abscess (d) Cyst passer
23) **Amoebic liver abscess can be diagnosed by demonstrating** (AI-91)
(a) Cysts in sterile pus (b) Trophozoite in the pus (c) Cysts in the intestine (d) Trophozoite in the faeces
24) **Diagnostic test for amoebic hepatitis is** (AI-90)
(a) Indirect haemagglutination test (b) Isolation from pus (c) Isolation from wall of cavity (d) Cyst in stool
25) **A patient present with lower gastro intestinal bleed. Sigmoidoscopy shows ulcer in the sigmoido colon. Biopsy from area show flask shaped ulcer. Which of the following is the most important treatment.** (AIIMS-05)
(a) Intravenous ceftriaxone (b) Intravenous metronidazole (c) Intravenous steroids and sulphasalazine (d) Hydrocortison enemas

Non pathogenic amoebae

26) **Mature cyst of *Entamoeba histolytica* differs from *Entamoeba coli, in the following except*** (AI-91)
(a) Size is 6-15 microns (b) Nuclei are 1 to 4 in number (c) Karyosome is central in position (d) Chromatoid bars seen

Free living amoebae

27) **A 30 year old patient presented with features of acute meningo-encephalitis in the casualty. His CSF on wet mount microscopy revealed motile unicellular microorganisms. The most likely organism is** (AIIMS, May-05)
(a) *Naegeria fowleri* (b) *Acanthamoeba culbertsoni* (c) *Entamoeba histolytica* (d) *Trypanosoma cruzi*

28) **Acute primary meningo-encephalitis true is** (AIIMS-08 AI-91)
(a) Meningitis caused by *Acanthamoeba* species is acute in nature (b) Diagnosis is by demonstration of trophozoite in CSF (c) Caused by faeco-oral transmission (d) More common in tropical climate

29) **Most fatal (fulminant) amoebic encephalitis is caused by**
(a) *E. histolytica* (b) *Naegleria* (c) *E. dispar* (d) *Acanthamoeba*

30) **Selective medium for *Naegleria fowleri* is**
(a) Nutrient agar rich with *E. coli* (b) NNN medium (c) Non-nutrient agar rich with *E. coli* (d) Diamond media

Answers of MCQs & explanation

1) **(c)**
2) **(b) & (d)**
} Follow section, **classification** for explanation

3) **(d)**
4) **(b) & (c)**
5) **(a) & (d)**
} Follow section, ***Entamoeba histolytica* (morphology)** for explanation

6) **(d)**
- Glycogen mass, chromatoid bars & eccentric nucleus are present in initial cystic stage. Follow section, ***Entamoeba histoytica* (morphology → cyst stage)** for explanation

7) **(b)**
- Follow section, ***Entamoeba histoytica* [culture characteristics (C/Cs)]** for explanation

8) **(a)**
9) **(c)**
10) **(a)**
11) **(a), (c) & (d)**
12) **(b)**
13) **(b)**
} Follow section, ***Entamoeba histoytica* (pathogenicity)** for explanation

14) **(c)**
- Option 'a': Follow section, ***Entamoeba histoytica* (morphology → trophozoite stage)** for explanation
- Option 'b' & 'c': Follow section, ***Entamoeba histoytica* (pathogenicity → host factors)** for explanation
- Option 'd': Follow section, ***Entamoeba histoytica* [pathogenicity → agent factors (virulence factors)]** for explanation

15) **(b)**
16) **(c)**
17) **(c)**
} Follow section, ***Entamoeba histolytica* [differential diagnosis (D/D) → CL crystals]** for explanation

18) **(b)**
- Follow section, ***Entamoeba histoytica* (extra-intestinal amoebiasis → hepatic amoebiasis → incidence)** for explanation

19) **(d)**
- Follow section, ***Entamoeba histoytica* (extra-intestinal amoebiasis → cutaneous amoebiasis)** for explanation

20) **(d)**
21) **(a)**
22) **(d)**
23) **(b)**
24) **(a)**
} Follow section, ***Entamoeba histolytica* (diagnosis)** for explanation

25) **(b)**
- Follow section, ***Entamoeba histoytica* (treatment)** for explanation

26) **(d)**
- Follow section, **non-pathogenic amoebae (*Entamoeba coli*)** for explanation

27) **(a)**
28) **(b)**
29) **(b)**
30) **(c)**
} Follow section, **free living amoebae (*Naegeria fowleri*)** for explanation

84 Intestinal, oral and genital flagellates

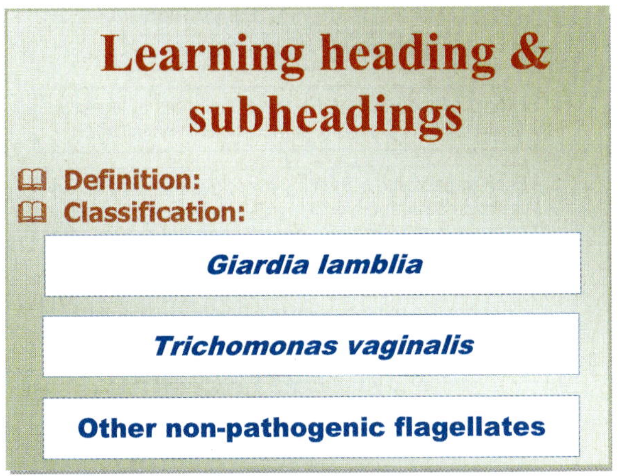

Definition: Parasites possess flagella as organ of locomotion are **called flagellates.**

Classification:

I. **Systemic classification:** **Follow chapter → Introduction and classification of parasites.** **(Table-3)**

II. **Pathogenic classification:** Two groups.

A. **Intestinal:**

i. **Pathogenic:** *Giardia lamblia* (duodenum & upper part of jejunum).

ii. **Non- pathogenic:**

1. ***Trichomonas:*** *T. hominis* (caecum).
2. ***Chilomastix:*** *C. mesnili* (caecum).
3. ***Enteromonas:*** *E. hominis* (colon).
4. ***Retortamonas (Embadomonas):*** *R. intestinalis* (colon).

B. **Oral:**

i. **Non- pathogenic:** *Trichomonas tenax* (mouth).

C. **Genital:**

i. **Pathogenic:** *Trichomonas vaginalis* (vagina & urethra).

Giardia lamblia

❖ **Synonym:**

- *Giardia intestinalis.*
- *Giardia duodenalis.*
- *Lamblia intestinalis.*

❖ **History:**

- It was discovered by Leeuwenhoeck in 1681 in his own stool.
- Lamb (1859) & Alexeieff (1914) also contributed in discovery of this parasite.

❖ **Geographical distribution:** Worldwide.

❖ **Habitat:** Duodenum & upper part of jejunum.

❖ **Morphology:** It exist in two morphological phase like trophozoite & cyst **(fig.-1).**

I. Trophozoite stage

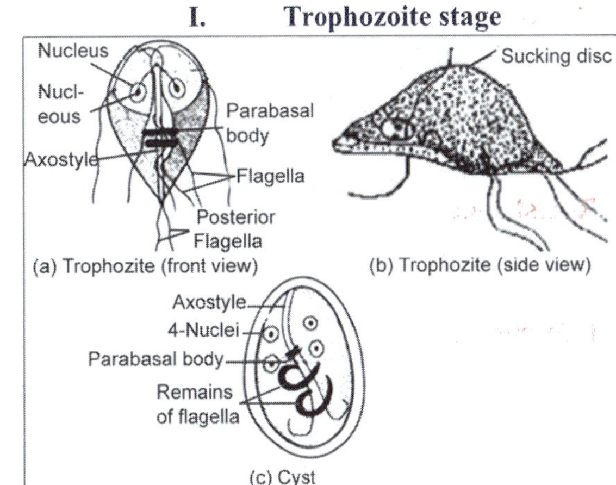

Figure-1: Morphology of *G. lamblia*

➢ **Size:** 14μm ×7μm.

➢ **Shape:**

- **Front view [fig.-1(a)]:** Tennis/badminton racket or tear shape with broad anterior end & pointed posterior end.
- **Side view [fig.-1(b)]:** Longitudinally split pear.

➢ **Motility:** Resembles a falling leaf.

➢ **Structure:**

- **Ends:** Anterior end is broad & posterior end is pointed.
- **Surfaces:** Dorsal surface is convex & ventral surface is concave with disc like structure **called sucking disc or ventral disc**, provides the organ of adhesion.
- **Organs:** Bilaterally symmetrical & all the organs are paired.
- **Contains:**
  - **Axostyles:** Centrally two **axostyles** which divide the trophozoite in two equal half.
  - **Parabasal body or median body:** Two sausage shaped parabasal bodies.
  - **Flagella:** Four pairs of flagella.

- **Nuclei:** Two nuclei with central karyosome (Nucleolus) which give **monkey face appearance** of parasite under microscope.

II. Cyst stage

- **Size:** 12µm in length& 7µm in breadth.
- **Shape:** Oval.
- **Structure: → Fig.-1 (c)**
- **Axostyles:** Lies more diagonally & forms the dividing line.
- **Parabasal body or median body:** Two sausage shaped parabasal bodies.
- **Axoneme:** Remains of flagella **called axoneme** & sucking disc seen inside the cytoplasm.
- **Nuclei:** Four nuclei with central karyosome.
- **Properties:** Acid environment & wet condition favours the encystation.

❖ **Culture:** Karapetyan has discovered the cultivation method of *Giardia* with yeast & *C. guilliermondi*. It grows well on a medium contains chick embryo extract, human serum, Hottinger's digest (tryptic meat digest) & Hank's solution.

❖ **Resistance:** Chlorination of water is ineffective to remove the cyst from water. Cyst is removed from water by boiling & filtration by membrane filter.

❖ **Life cycle:**

- **Host:** Man is the only host.
- **Methods of reproduction:** Two types (methods of transformation) as shown in **flow chart-1.**

a. **Excystation:** One cyst gives two trophozoites.
b. **Encystation:** One trophozoite gives one cyst.

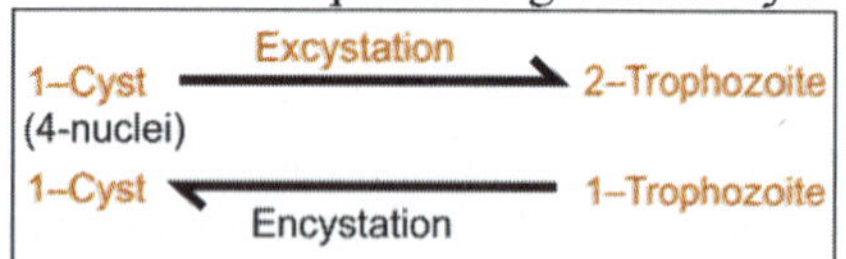

Flow chart-1: Excystation & encystation

- **Cycles:** Two stages of life cycle are described in **flow chart -2 & fig.-2.**

❖ **Pathogenicity:**

- **Disease name: Called giardiasis.**
- **Nature of disease:** It is endemic & one of the agents responsible for traveller's diarrhoea.
- **Reservoir of infection:** Mainly human & other wild & domestic animals.
- **Source of infection:** Food & water.
- **Mode of transmission:**
  - **Ingestion:** By ingestion of contaminated food & water. It is transmitted from man to man & also from animal to man.
  - Also transmitted by **sexual intercourse** like male homosexual.
- **Incubation period:** Average 10 days.
- **Exit form:** Trophozoite & cyst.
- **Infective form:** Cyst.
- **Infective dose:** Ingestion of up to 10 (range 10-100) cysts is enough to cause infection.
- **Portal of entry:** GIT.
- **Sites:** Duodenum & upper part of jejunum.

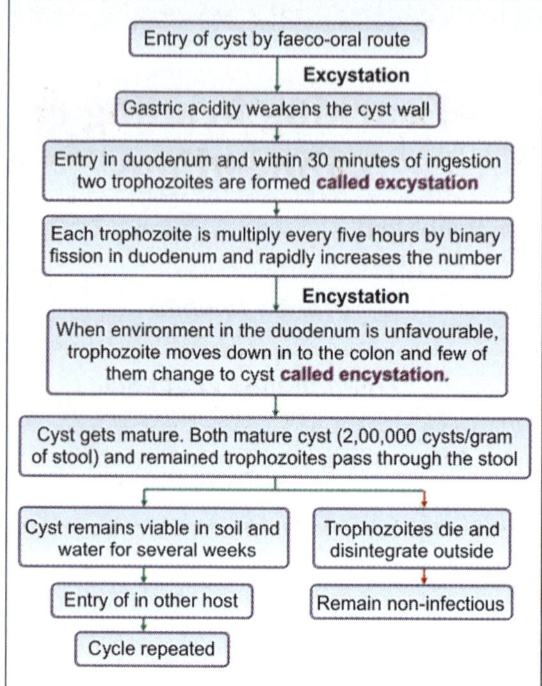

Flow chart-2: Life cycle of *G. lamblia*

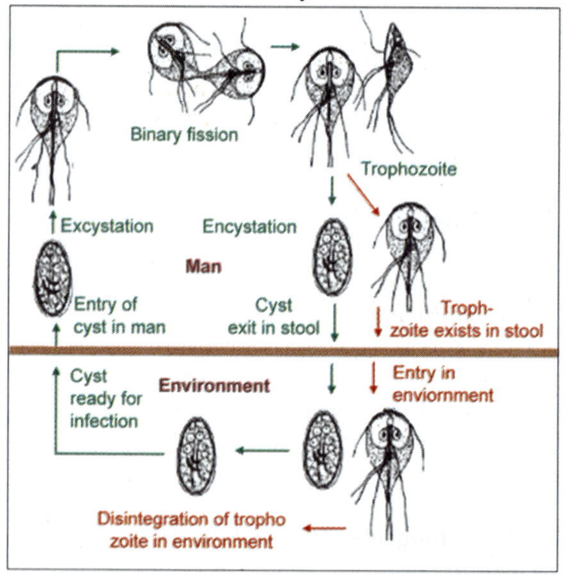

Figure-2: Life cycle of *G. lamblia*

- **Precipitating factors (epidemiological determinants):**

a. **Agent factors (virulence factors):**

1. **Sucking disc:**

- It is the organ of adhesion. It does not invade the tissue but remains tightly adhere to the intestinal epithelium.
- Parasite attaches to the convex surface of epithelium & cause the intestinal disturbances

leading to malabsorption of fat (**called steatorrhoea**) in children & in adults.

2. **Toxin:** Causing allergic manifestations.

b. **Host factors:**

1. **Age:** Common in paediatric age.
2. **Blood group:** Group A is more prone to disease.
3. **Habit:** Common in cannabis users.
4. **Diseases:**

- Achlorhydria or hypochlorhydria, chronic pancreatitis (leads to deficiency of pancreatic enzymes) & malnutrition.
- IDDs: Recurrent giardiasis is associated with selective IgA deficiency, X-linked & autosomal recessive agammaglobulinemia, hypogammaglobulinemia, Combined (Common) Variable Immuno Deficiency Disease (CVIDD), AIDS etc.

➢ **Pathogenesis:**

- In majority of cases morphology of bowel remains unaltered, but in chronic cases flattened villi present with clinical picture resemble to tropical sprue & gluten sensitive enteropathy.
- Villous architecture may damage by cell apoptosis & increased lymphatic infiltration in lamina propria.

➢ **Clinical features: → Flow chart-3**

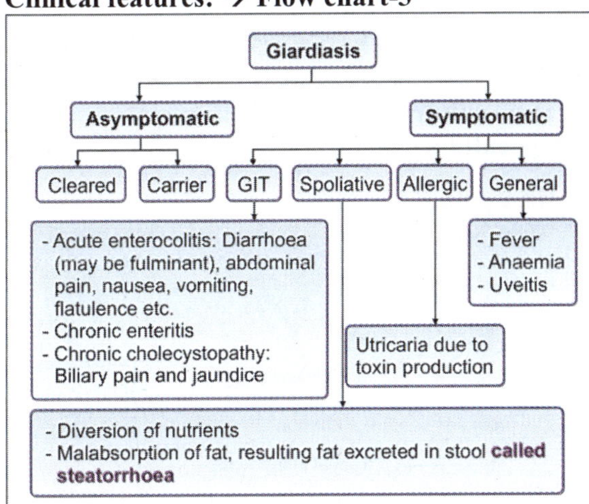

Flow chart-3: Clinical features of giardiasis

❖ **Laboratory diagnosis:**

➢ **Specimens:**

- **Stool:**
  - Collected after defecation or by purgation.
  - Contains both cyst & trophozoite.
- **Bile A:** Collected from duodenum by aspiration method or by using gelatin capsule **called entero test** (also **called string test**).
- **Bile B:** Collected from biliary tract, because to avoid the acidity of duodenum, trophozoite often enters in to the biliary tract (gall bladder).
- **Mucosal biopsy:** From duodenum & proximal jejunum. Jejunal wash is not useful.

✓ **Note: Entero test**

- **Synonym:** String test or E-test in short.
- **Apparatus: → Fig.-3**
- **Steps: Flow chart-4**

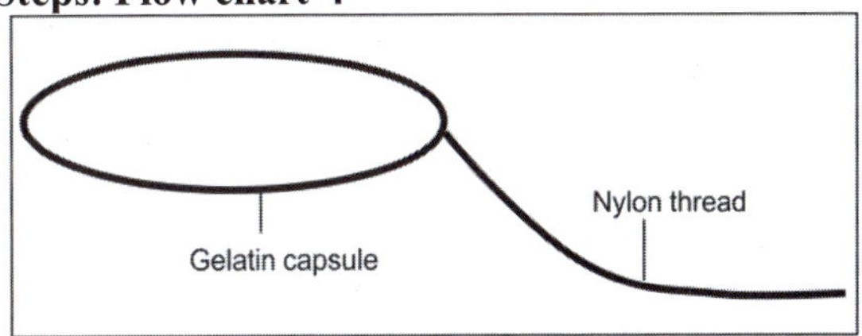

Figure-3: Device of entero test

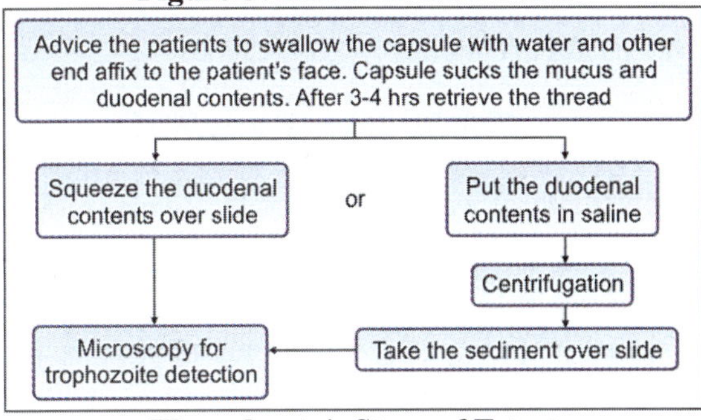

Flow chart-4: Steps of E-test

- **Uses:** For detection of

1. Trophozoite of *G. lamblia.*
2. Larvae of *S. stercoralis.*
3. Eggs of liver flukes like *C. sinensis*, *O. felineus*, *F. hepatica.*
4. Oocyst of *C. parvum.*

➢ **Testing methods:**

I. Direct tests

A. **Macroscopy of stool:** Pale or yellow colour stool due to presence of fat.

B. **Microscopy by normal saline preparation:** It is considered as gold standard for detection of trophozoite or cyst or both.

1. **For Trophozoite:** Motile trophozoite will be detected under normal saline preparation with leaf like motility in fresh stool.
2. **For Cyst:** Cysts are sheds intermittently in stool, so 2-3 specimens are collected at 4-5 hours interval & examined for cyst under normal saline preparation.
3. **No RBCs & pus cells:** *Giardia* is not causing dysentery, so RBCs & pus cells are absent.

C. **Culture: →Vide supra**

II. Indirect tests

A. **Serological tests:** ELISA & Counter Immuno Electrophoresis (CIE) are useful test but lack of sensitivity & specificity.

B. **Molecular test:** DNA probe & PCR are useful.

❖ **Prevention:**

- Prevention of contamination of food & water by human faeces.

- Hand washing before eating & proper disposal of diaper.
- Boiling & filtration of water to remove the cyst.
- Health education.

❖ **Treatment:** Only symptomatic cases need treatment.

i. **Oral amoebicides:** Paromycin for pregnant woman
ii. Tinidazole (2g single dose) & metronidazole (250mg TDS for 5-7 days) are the drugs of choice. Tinidazole is more effective than metronidazole. Cure rate with metronidazole is > 90%.
iii. Furazolidone & nitazoxamine: Fewer side effects, so useful in children.

Trichomonas vaginalis

❖ **History:** It was 1st observed by Donne in 1836 in vaginal secretion.

❖ **Geographical distribution:** Prevalent in the sexually active age groups in all climates & racial groups.

❖ **Habitat:** Humans is the only known host.

- **Female:** Present in vagina, cervix, Bartholin's gland, urethra & in urinary bladder.
- **Male:** Mostly in the anterior urethra & rarely in prostate & preputial sac.

❖ **Morphology:** **No cystic stage,** only trophozoite stage which has following properties **(fig.-4)**.

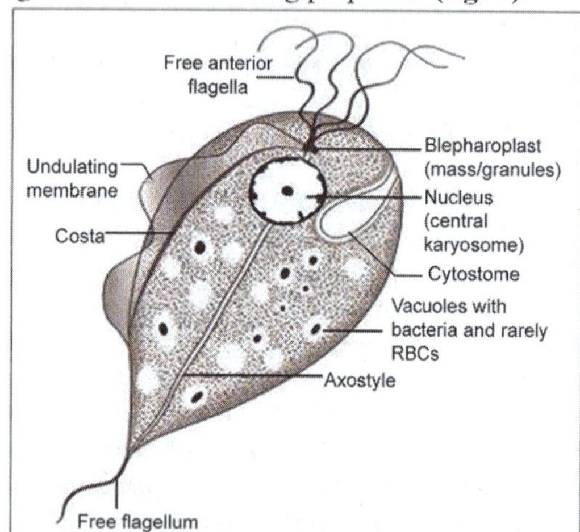

Figure-4: Trophozoite of *T. vaginalis*

➢ **Size:** 10-12μm in length & 5-10μm in breadth.
➢ **Shape:** Oval or pear shape.
➢ **Motility:** Wobbling (side to side) / rotator or jerky movement.
➢ **Structure:**

✪ **Ends:** Anterior end is broad & posterior end is pointed.
✪ **Contains:**

- **Axostyles:** It runs the middle of the body & ends in posterior pointed end.
- **Flagella:**
  - 3 to 5 free anterior flagella.
  - One thicker flagellum passes backwards along the body of parasite with formation of membrane like structure **called undulating membrane.** It covers the ½ -$^{1}/_{3}$ of the body & becomes free at posterior end.
- **Costa:** Undulating membrane is supported at the base by thick rod like structure **called costa.**
- **Nuclei:** Single nucleus situated at the anterior end.
- **Cytostome (mouth):** It is a cleft like depression lies near by nucleus.

❖ **Methods of reproduction:** **No cystic stage,** only trophozoite, which divide by binary fission.

❖ **Culture:** It is the gold standard if microscopy is negative.

A. **Cell free media:** Most sensitive (>95%) if performed properly by using following media.
- Bushly's medium.
- Feinberg-Whittington medium.
- Roiron's medium.
- Johnson-Trussel's medium.
- CPLM (Cysteine Peptone Liver Maltose) medium.
- Plastic envelope medium.

B. **Tissue culture media:** } Also useful
C. **Egg culture:**

❖ **Life cycle:**

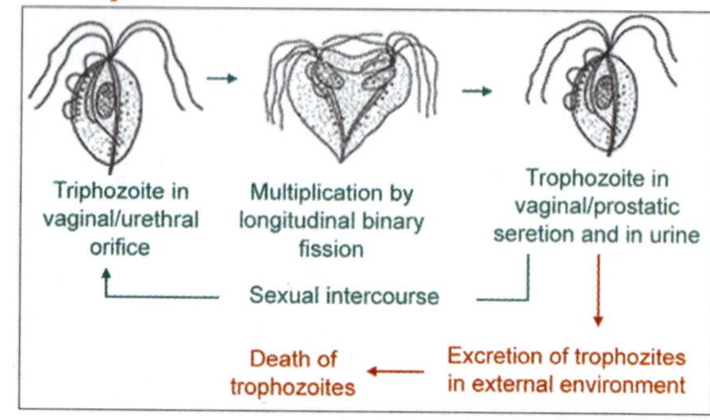

Figure-5: Life cycle of *T. vaginalis*

➢ **Host:** Man is the optimum host.
➢ **Methods of reproduction:** Parasite does not have a cyst form. It multiplies by binary fission.
➢ **Cycle:** Trophozoites live in urogenital tract and multiply by binary fission as shown in **fig.-5.** Cycle is maintained by sexual transmission from person to person. Few trophozoites are excreted with urine in external environment, but they do not survive.

❖ **Pathogenicity:**

➢ **Disease name: Called trichomoniasis.**
➢ **Reservoir of infection:** Asymptomatic male will be act as reservoir of infection.

- **Source of infection:** Genital materials will be act as source of infection.
- **Mode of transmission:**
  - By sexual intercourse (other parasite transmitted by sexual intercourse are *G. lamblia, E. histolytica, C. parvum*).
  - Fomites borne like toilet articles or cloths.
  - Vertical: From infected birth canal to infant.
- **Incubation period:** 4-28 days.
- **Infective & exit form:** Trophozoites.
- **Portal of entry:** Genital organs.
- **Sites:** Follow habitat.
- **Precipitating factors (epidemiological determinants)**

a. **Agent factors (virulence factors):**

1. **Obligate parasite:** Can't live without close association with vaginal, urethral or prostatic tissues.
2. **Liberation of enzymes & other metabolites:** Like cysteine protease, lactic acid & acetic acid.

b. **Host factors:**

1. **Age:** Common in adult.

- **Pathology:** It causes petechial haemorrhage (**strawberry mucosa**), metaplastic changes & desquamation of vaginal epithelium.
- **Clinical features: → Flow chart-5**

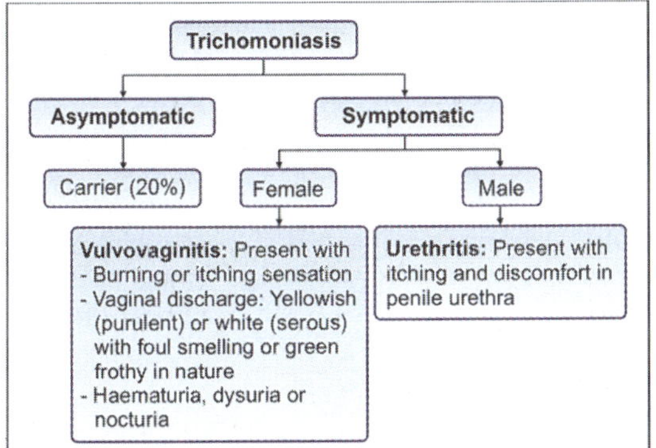

Flow chart-5: Clinical features of trichomoniasis

- **Complications: →Flow chart-6**

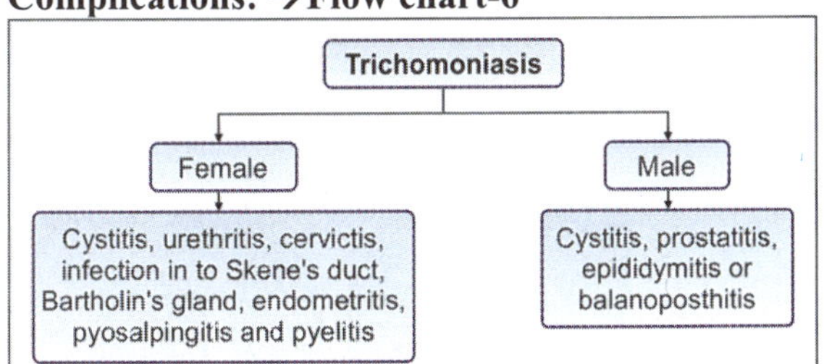

Flow chart-6: Complications of trichomoniasis

Features	*T. vaginalis*	*C. albicans*	*G. vaginalis*
Discharge	Yellowish-white	White	Grey & offensive
pH	>4.5	<4.5	>4.5

Table-1: D/D of *T. vaginalis*

❖ Differential diagnosis (D/D): → Table-1

✓ **Note: Normal vaginal pH** → From puberty to menopause is 3.0-3.5

❖ Laboratory diagnosis:

- **Specimens:**
  - **Vaginal discharge:** Collected from the posterior fornix.
  - **Urethral secretion:** In male, massage the prostate & collect the specimen from urethral orifice.
  - **Urine:** Collect in sterile test tube → centrifugation → Use the sediment for testing.
- **Testing methods:**

I. Direct tests

A. **Microscopy:**

i. **Wet mount by normal saline:** Prepare the smear from specimens & examine under the low power for motile trophozoite.

ii. **Staining:** By using Papanicolaou stain, Giemsa stain, Gram stain, Periodic Acid Schiff stain, Leishman stain, Diff-quick method or by Acridine-Orange stain.

B. **Culture: →Vide supra**

II. Indirect tests

A **Serological tests:** ELISA is useful to detect the 65-kda surface polypeptide Ag of *T. vaginalis*.

B **Molecular test:** DNA probe & PCR are useful.

❖ Prevention:

- Similar measures as required to prevent the venereal diseases like wearing condom etc.
- Sex education.
- Testing of partner for *T. vaginalis*.

❖ Treatment: Only symptomatic cases need treatment.

- Metronidazole: 2g single dose or 500mg BD for 5-7 days is the drug of choice. Increase the dose or administered by IV route in unresponsive cases. It is safe 2nd % 3rd trimester.

Other non-pathogenic flagellates

↓

Table-2 & fig.-6-9

Figure-6: Trophozoite of *T. hominis* & *T. tenax*

Features	*T. hominis* (*T intestinalis*)	*T. tenax* (*T. buccalis*)	*C. mesnili*	*E. hominis*	*R. intestinalis* (*E. intestinalis*)
History	Davine, 1854		Wenyon, 1910 Alexeieff, 1912	Da Fonseca, 1915	Wenyon & O'Conor, 1917
Habitat	Ileo-caecal region & feeds the bacteria	Mouth	Caecum	Colon	Colon
			Trophozoites		
Figure	Fig.-6 (a)	Fig.-6(b)	Fig.-7(a)	Fig.-8(a)	Fig.-9(a)
Size	5-15μm × 7-10μm	5-10μm in length	10-15μm × 5-6μm	8μm × 4μm	5μm × 3μm
Shape	Pyriform	Pyriform	Pear	Pear	Oval
Flagella	3-5 anterior flagella	4-anterior flagella	3-anterior flagella & 4th lies within cytostome	3-anterior flagella & 4th posterior adherent with body & becomes free in the end	1-anterior flagella & 2nd pass through cytostome, before becomes free
Nucleus	Single situated near anterior end	Single situated near anterior end	Single situated near anterior end	Single situated near anterior end	Single situated near anterior end
Cytostome	Present	Present	Present	Absent	Present
Axostyle	Present	Present	Absent	Absent	Absent
Undulating membrane	Along the entire length of parasite	Along the entire length of parasite	Absent	Absent	Absent
Motility	Jerky	Jerky	Rotatory	Jerky	Jerky
			Cyst		
Figure	No cyst stage	No cyst stage	Fig.-7(b)	Fig.-8(b)	Fig.-9(b)
Size			7-10μm × 4-6μm	8μm × 4μm	4-5μm × 4-6μm
Shape			Lemon	Oval	pear
Nucleus			One with central karyosome	1-4 nuclei situated at opposite pole	1 nuclei situated in the centre
Other features			- Projection at anterior end **called nipple** - Remnant of cytostome present	It mimics a *E. nana*	Nucleus is surrounded by fibril **called bird's beak appearance**
			Mode of transmission		
Route	Faeco-oral route	Kissing, salivary droplet or by fomites	Faeco-oral route	Faeco-oral route	Faeco-oral route

Table-2: Non pathogenic flagellates

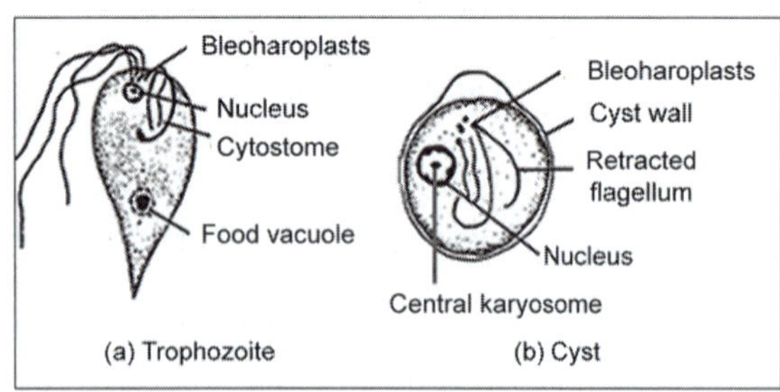

Figure-7: Morphology of *C. mesnili*

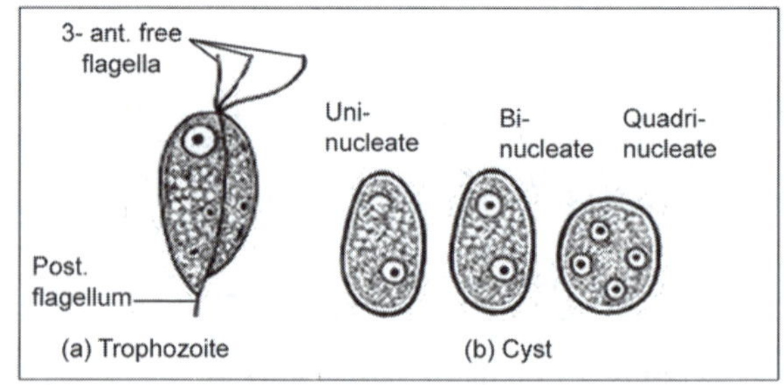

Figure-8: Morphology of *E. hominis*

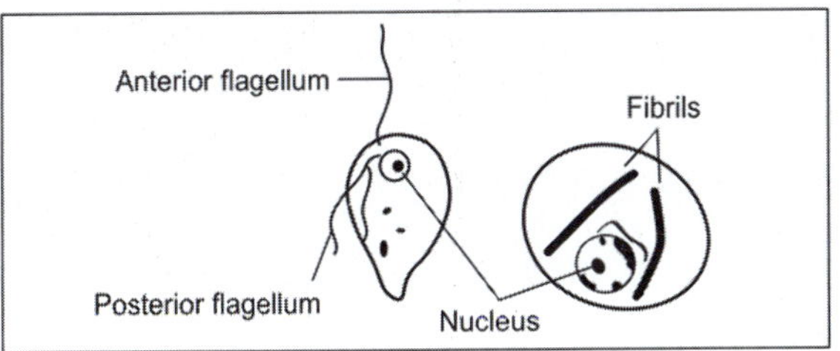

Figure-9: Morphology of *E. intestinalis*

Question bank

Case study

1) A 10 years girl presents with abdominal pain, nausea, vomiting with fever. Microscopical examination of stool revealed pear shaped organisms about 14μm ×7μm in size & falling leaf like motility without pus cells & RBCs. Identify the organism & answer the following

a) Name the causative agent & draw the diagram of morphology of causative agent.
b) Describe the life cycle of causative agent.
c) Write the pathogenicity & laboratory diagnosis of causative agent.

Short notes

1) *Giardia lamblia.*
2) *T. vaginalis.*
3) E-test.

Short questions for theory/viva questions

1) Name the type of motility for *Giardia lamblia* & *Trichomonas vaginalis.*
2) Name the four parasites in transmitted by sexual intercourse.

MCQs for chapter review

Giardia lamblia

1) **Normal habitat of *Giardia* is** (AIIMS-90)
(a) Duodenum and jejunum (b) Stomach (c) Caecum (d) Ileum
2) **How many pairs of flagella does *Giardia lamblia* possess**
(a) 1 (b) 2 (c) 3 (d) 4
3) **Recurrent giardiasis is associated with** (AIIMS-00,97)
(a) Severe combined immuno deficiency (b) Common variable immuno deficiency (c) Di George syndrome (e) C8 deficiency
4) **A case of giardiasis present with**
(a) Nausea and vomiting (b) Abdominal pain (c) Steatorrhoea and flatulence (d) All of the above
5) **True about giardiasis**
(a) Only cyst is infective (b) Reside in caecum (c) Only man to man transmission (d) Exist in one phases
6) **True about *Giardia* is** (AIIMS, May-94)
(a) May causes traveller's diarrhoea (b) *Giardia* inhabits ileum (c) Trophozoites are infective form (d) None of the above
7) **The following is true of giardiasis except** (AI-92)
(a) Complement fixation test is diagnostic (b) Stool contain only cysts (c) Habitat is colon (d) Trophozoites and cysts are found in duodenum
8) **Which of the following is true about *Giardia*** (PGI -95)
(a) CFT is diagnostic (b) Trophozoites and cysts are seen in man (c) Live in lower intestine (d) Invades normal mucosa
9) **Which of the following is true with *Giardia lamblia*** (PGI, Nov-13, Dec-05)
(a) Malabsorption commonly seen (b) Trophozoite form is binucleate (c) Diarrhoea is seen (d) Jejunal wash fluid is diagnostic (e) Is a free living nematode

Trichomonas vaginalis

10) **Following is the feature of *Trichomonas vaginalis***
(a) Trophozoite is the largest among all protozoa (b) Cyst is absent (c) Habitat in genital organs (d) Transmitted sexually

Answers of MCQs & explanation

1) **(a)**
- Follow section, ***Giardia lamblia* (habitat)** for explanation
2) **(d)**
- Follow section, ***Giardia lamblia* (morphology → trophozoite stage)** for explanation
3) **(b)**
- Follow section, ***Giardia lamblia* (pathogenicity → host factors)** for explanation
4) **(d)**
- Follow section, ***Giardia lamblia* (pathogenicity → clinical features & flow chart-3)** for explanation
5) **(a)**
6) **(a)**
7) **(a), (b) & (c)**
8) **(b)**

(5–8: All options are explained in respective section of ***Giardia lamblia***)

9) **(b) & (c)**
- Most cases are asymptomatic & malabsorption seen rarely
- Jejunal wash fluid is not diagnostic, biopsy is useful.
- It is a protozoan.
10) **(b), (c) & (d)**
- Largest protozoan is *Balantidium coli*
- Follow section, ***Trichomonas vaginalis*** for explanation

85 Blood and tissue flagellates

Learning heading & subheadings

- Synonym:
- Classification:
- Morphological parts:
- Reproduction:
- Staining reaction:

Trypanosoma spp.

- *Trypanosoma brucei gambiense*
- *Trypanosoma brucei rhodesiense*
- *Trypanosoma brucei zambiense*
- *Trypanosoma cruzi*

Leishmania spp.

- *Leishmania donovani*
- *Leishmania tropica*
- *Leishmania braziliensis*

Synonym: Also called **haemoflagellates.**

Classification:

I. Systemic classification: Follow chapter → Introduction and classification of parasites **(section →Table-3)**

II. Pathogenic classification: Two pathogenic groups like *Trypanosoma* & *Leishmania* mentioned below.

A ***Trypanosoma:*** **→ Flow chart-1.**

B ***Leishmania:*** Three pathogenic species.

i. ***Leishmania donovani:*** Causing kala azar or dum dum fever (visceral leishmaniasis.

✓ **Notes:**

- **Other species of *Leishmania* causing kala azar:** *L. infantum. L. chagasi, L. canis* were identified earlier, but later it was found that all were identical to *L. donovani.*
- **Ecological types of kala azar: → Vide infra**

a. Old World kala azar: It includes Indian, Mediterranean & African kala azar.

b. New World kala azar: Includes American kala azar.

- **Above species & types are not widely in use**

ii. ***Leishmania tropica:*** Causing oriental sore (cutaneous leishmaniasis).

iii. ***Leishmania brasiliensis:*** Causing espundia (muco-cutaneous leishmaniasis).

> **Mnemonic:**
> - **dv** → **d**ono**v**ani = **dv** → **d**um dum / **v**isceral
> - **oc** → tr**o**pi**c**a = **oc** → oriental sore/**c**utaneous
> - **en** → brasili**en**sis = **en** →**e**spundia **n**asopharyngeal / mucocutaneous

Morphological parts: →Fig.-1

- **Body:** Two types.
  - **Flagellar:** Elongated, narrow & curved with free flagellum.
  - **Aflagellar:** Round or oval without free flagellum.
- **Nucleus:** Single & centrally located.
- **Kinetoplast:** Extra-nuclear DNA containing body having mitochondrial structure.
- **Basal body:** Starting point of flagellum.
- **Axoneme or axial filament:** Part of flagella lying inside the body.
- **Undulating membrane:**
  - Folding of flagella around the body before becomes free from body.
  - Numbers of folds depend on the length of parasite.

Reproduction:

- **Methods of reproduction:** Multiply by longitudinal binary fission. **No sexual cycle** is known. It begins with division of kinetoplast, basal body & nucleus. Flagellum with undulating membrane remains with one half of basal body while new one develops from other. Cytoplasmic body then splits longitudinally from anterior end.
- **Reproductive stage:** Nomenclature of stage is based on flagellar characteristic like starting point, its course & point of becoming free from body.

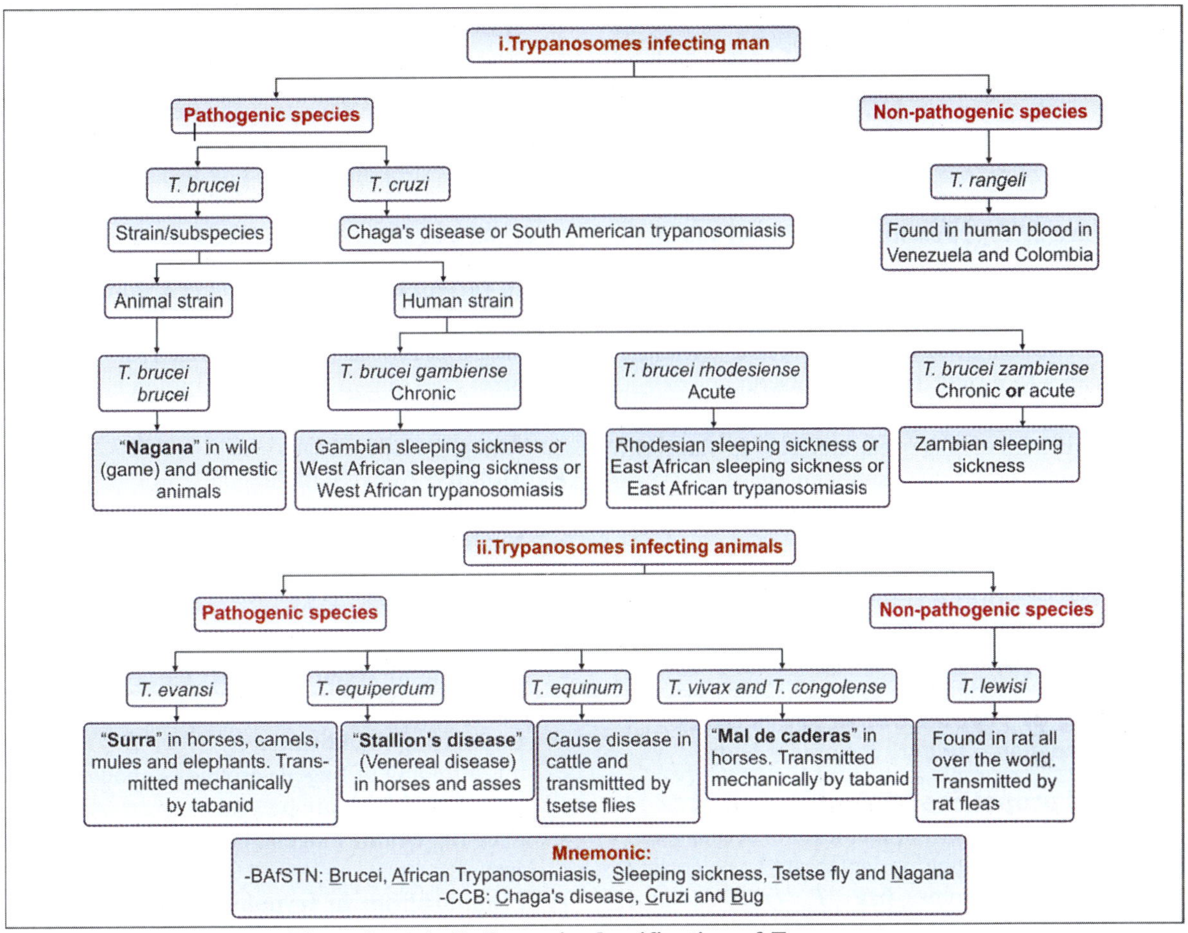

i. Trypanosomes infecting man

- **Pathogenic species**
  - *T. brucei* → Strain/subspecies
    - Animal strain → *T. brucei brucei* → "**Nagana**" in wild (game) and domestic animals
    - Human strain
      - *T. brucei gambiense* Chronic → Gambian sleeping sickness or West African sleeping sickness or West African trypanosomiasis
      - *T. brucei rhodesiense* Acute → Rhodesian sleeping sickness or East African sleeping sickness or East African trypanosomiasis
      - *T. brucei zambiense* Chronic **or** acute → Zambian sleeping sickness
  - *T. cruzi* → Chaga's disease or South American trypanosomiasis
- **Non-pathogenic species**
  - *T. rangeli* → Found in human blood in Venezuela and Colombia

ii. Trypanosomes infecting animals

- **Pathogenic species**
  - *T. evansi* → "**Surra**" in horses, camels, mules and elephants. Transmitted mechanically by tabanid
  - *T. equiperdum* → "**Stallion's disease**" (Venereal disease) in horses and asses
  - *T. equinum* → Cause disease in cattle and transmittted by tsetse flies
  - *T. vivax and T. congolense* → "**Mal de caderas**" in horses. Transmitted mechanically by tabanid
- **Non-pathogenic species**
  - *T. lewisi* → Found in rat all over the world. Transmitted by rat fleas

Mnemonic:
-BAfSTN: Brucei, African Trypanosomiasis, Sleeping sickness, Tsetse fly and Nagana
-CCB: Chaga's disease, Cruzi and Bug

Flow chart-1: Pathogenic classification of *Trypanosma*

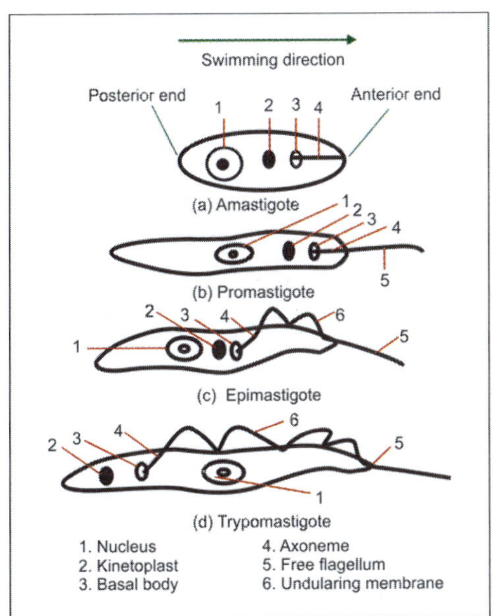

Figure-1: Morphological parts & developmental stages of haemoflagellates

i. Amastigote stage: → Fig.-1 (a)

- **Meaning:** A= without + Mastigote [from mastix (Greek)] = whip.
- Also **called aflagellar stage.**
- Oval or spherical in shape & contains nucleus, kinetoplast (**antenuclear**), basal body & axoneme but no free flagellum.
- Occurs in *Leishmania* in human.

ii. Promastigote stage: → Fig.-1 (b)

- Elongated in shape & contains nucleus, kinetoplast (**antenuclear**), basal body, axoneme & free flagellum but no undulating membrane.
- Occurs in *Leishmania* in culture & vector.

iii. Epimastigote stage: → Fig.-1 (c)

- Elongated in shape & contains nucleus, kinetoplast (near to the nucleus, so **called juxtranuclear kinetoplast**), basal body, axoneme, undulating membrane & free flagellum.
- Occurs in *Trypanosoma.*

iv. Trypomastigote stage: → Fig.-1 (d)

- Elongated in shape with blunt posterior end & pointed anterior end.
- Contains nucleus, kinetoplast (**post-nuclear**), basal body, axoneme, undulating membrane & free flagellum.
- Occurs in *Trypanosoma.*

🕮 Staining reaction:

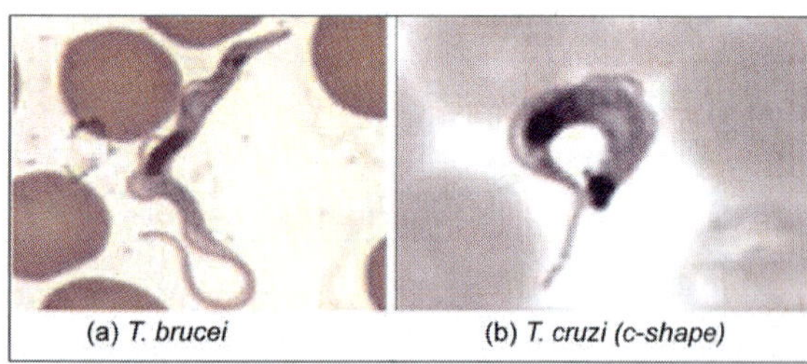

Figure-2: Trypomastigotes in blood smear

a. **For body fluid:**
- **Smear preparation:** By thin & thick films.
- **Stains:** Romanowsky's stain like Giemsa, Leishman's & Wright's stains are useful.
- **Examination:** Cytoplasm & undulating membrane stains blue, kinetoplast red, nucleus & flagellum appears pink (dark red) as shown in **fig.-2.**

b. **For tissues:** Haematoxylin & Eosin (H & E) stain.

Trypanosoma spp.

Trypanosoma brucei gambiense

❖ **Meaning of *Trypanosoma* :** From **Greek** word **Trypanon = to bore & Soma = body.**

❖ **General properties of *Trypanosoma*:**

➢ **Reproductive stage:** All members of trypanosome exist as trypomastigote in vertebrate hosts (man & animal), while some like *T. cruzi* assumes amastigote forms in vertebrate hosts.

➢ **Pleomorphism:** Trypomastigote stage of *T. brucei* exhibits variation in size & shape at different stage of its life cycle with short stumpy, intermediate, long slender & metacyclic forms.

➢ **Hosts:** Life cycle passes in two types of hosts.

1. **Vertebrate host:** Man & animal.
2. **Insect host:** Like tsetse fly & ruduvid bug.

➢ **Modes of reproduction**

1. **Anterior station (called salivaria):** Trypomastigotes are carried to midgut of tsetse fly & proceed forward to salivary glands (foregut). Transmission occurs by bite of tsetse fly. E.g. *T. brucei* subgroup.
2. **Posterior station (called stercoraria):** Trypomastigotes are carried to midgut of bug & proceed backward to hind gut. Transmission occurs by ingestion of faeces of the vector as in *T. lewisi* or by rubbing the faecal material against the wound caused by bite of vector as in *T. cruzi.*

❖ **History:**

- *T. brucei* was discovered by David Bruce in 1890 from cattle suffered with "**nagana**" in Zululand.
- Human strain was discovered in Gambia by Forde & Dutton in 1902.

❖ **Geographical distribution:** West & Central Africa.

❖ **Habitat:**

- It is a connective tissues parasite.
- Invades more in lymph node & less in the brain.
- African sleeping sickness is a disease of CNS. It consumes plenty of glucose from tissues.

❖ **Morphology:**

A. **In vertebrate host:** Man, game & domestic animal.

i. **Trypomastigote stage:** Normal form in vertebrate host with following features **[fig.-1(d) / fig.-3(a)].**

➢ **Size:** 16-42μm in length & 1-3μm in breadth.

➢ **Shape:** Elongated in shape with blunt posterior end & pointed anterior end.

➢ **Motility:** Actively motile.

➢ **Structure:**

- **Nucleus:** Large oval & central in position.
- **Kinetoplast:** Situated near posterior end **called postnuclear kinetoplast.**
- **Basal body:** Starting point of flagellum.
- **Axoneme or Axial filament:** Part of flagella lying inside the body.
- **Undulating membrane:**
  - It is a folding of flagella around the body of parasite
  - Usually 3-4 folds are present.
- **Free flagellum:** Flagella become free from anterior end.

➢ **Pleomorphism in trypomastigote stage:** It exist variation in size & shape with following different forms.

1. **Intermediate form:** Stage occurs between short stumpy & trypomastigote forms **called intermediate form [fig.-3(b)].**
2. **Short stumpy form:** It is short, stumpy form about 10μm in length & 5μm in breadth with small or no free flagellum **[fig.-3(c)].**

B. **In insect host:** Tsetse fly.

i. **Epimastigote form:**

➢ **Structure:** It develops from long slender form in salivary gland **[fig.-1(c) or fig.-3(e)].**

➢ **Pleomorphism:**

1. **Long slender form:** It is long, slender form about 20μm in length & 3μm in breadth with long free flagellum **[fig.-3(d)].**
2. **Metacyclic form:** Form similar to short stumpy form developed in vector from epimastigote stage & responsible for human infection, so **called infective form** also **[fig.-3(f)].**

✓ **Notes: Latent forms or occult visceral form of trypomastigote.**

- **Sites:** Choroid plexus & lungs
- **History:**

- Non-flagellate latent form of trypomastigote was 1st observed in capillaries of internal organs in vertebrate host by Fantham in 1911.
- Non-flagellate latent form (**called amastigote** →Vide supra) & flagellate latent form (**called spheromastigote** → small, spherical form with undulating membrane & short free flagellum): Were found in choroid plexus of rat inoculated with trypomastigote of Botswana strain of *T. brucei* by Ormerod & Venkatesan in 1971.

▪ **Clinical significance:** Responsible for recurrence.

❖ Culture:

i. Culture on media: Long slender form (mid-gut form of fly) grows over medium contains Ringer's solution, with sodium chloride, Tyrode's solution & citrated human blood.

ii. Culture in animals:

✪ **Uses:**
- In diagnosis when trypomastigote are scanty or difficult to find in blood smear.
- To maintain the strain.

✪ **Animals:**
- It causes the overwhelming parasitaemia in **rats, mice & Guinea pigs** & kills the animal in few days.
- **Rabbit:** Produce chronic infection & animal die in 4-5 weeks.

❖ Antigenic variant:

- Infection lasting for long time in spite of strong antibodies response, due to antigenic variation in parasite occurs every 3-4 days by selection of mutation.
- It depends on host defence, when fails it multiply unchecked.
- It is possible by change in outer protein coat **called Variant Surface Glycoprotein (VSG).**
- Each VSG is immunogenic but antigenically different from previous VSG.
- Antibodies are formed against each type but when titre rise homologous variant will disappear with emergence of new variant.
- Each variant is followed by fever & leucocytosis (Monocytosis, no neutrophilia).

❖ Immunity:

- Produce strong antibodies (Abs) response like IgG & IgM against antigens (Ags) of trypomastigote, but these are not specific & non-protective.
- Serum antibody **called ablastin** prevents the multiplication of trypomastigote.
- It suppresses the immune response which allows the bacterial infection.

❖ Life cycle:

➢ **Hosts:**

A. Vertebrate host: Man, game & domestic animals.

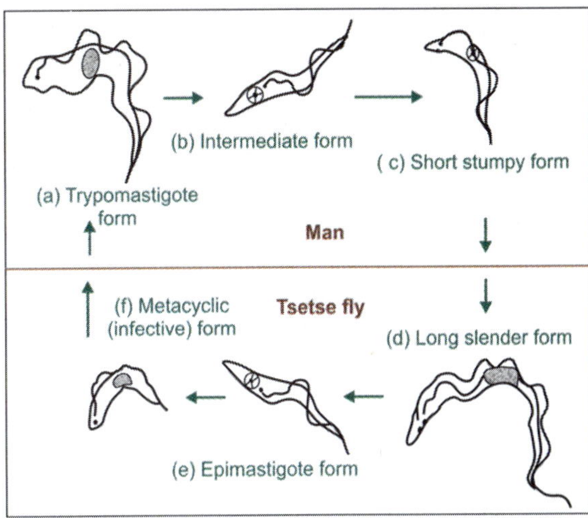

Figure-3: Life cycle of *T. brucei*

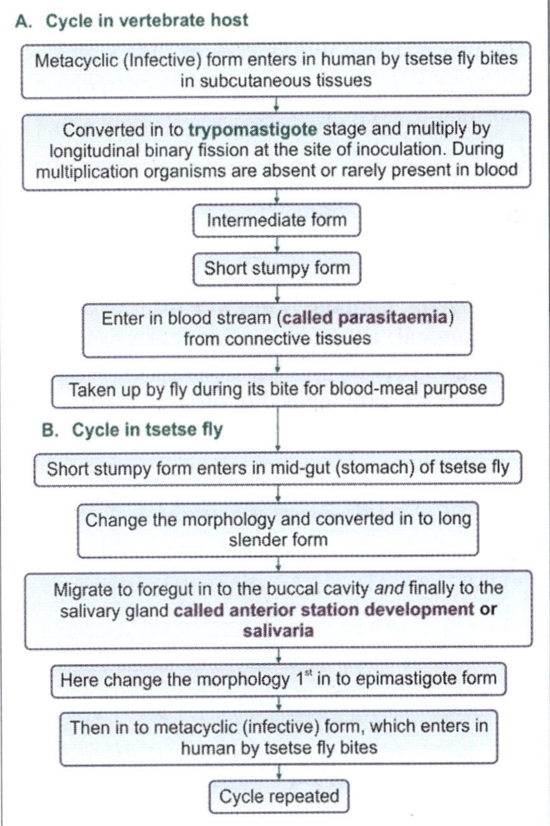

Flow chart-2: Life cycle of *T. brucei*

B. Insect host: Tsetse fly.

✪ **Species:**

1. **Animal strain:** Transmitted by *Glossina morsitans*
2. **Gambiense strain:** Transmitted by *G. palpalis, G. pallidipes & G. tachinoides.*
3. **Rhodesiense strain:** Transmitted by *G. morsitans, G. swynertoni & G. pallidipes.*

✪ **Features:**
- Both male & female fly can transmit the infection.

- It takes 20 days to produce infective stage & once infected remains infective for rest of life (extending up to 185 days).
- No evidence of hereditary transmission in fly.
- Fly produce single larva & about 6-12 larvae in whole life, so reproduction in limited.
- **Method of reproduction:** Longitudinal binary fission.
- **Cycles: → Fig.-3 & flow chart-2**

❖ Pathogenicity:

- **Type of disease:** It is a chronic disease.
- **Disease name: Called Gambian sleeping sickness or West African sleeping sickness or West African trypanosomiasis.**
- **Reservoir / source of infection:** Animal reservoir is still not known in gambiense strain, man himself is the reservoir of infection for gambiense strain.
- **Mode of transmission:**
  - By bites of tsetse fly: **Species → vide supra.**
  - By both male & female in daylight usually in early morning & evening.
- **Exit form:** Short stumpy form.
- **Infective form:** Metacyclic form.
- **Portal of entry:** Skin.
- **Sites: →Follow habitat**
- **Pathogenesis:**

i. **Pathogenic damage is not due to:**

a. **Mechanical:** By motility of organisms.

b. **Allergic reaction:** As organism is non-toxic.

ii. **Pathogenic damage is due to:**

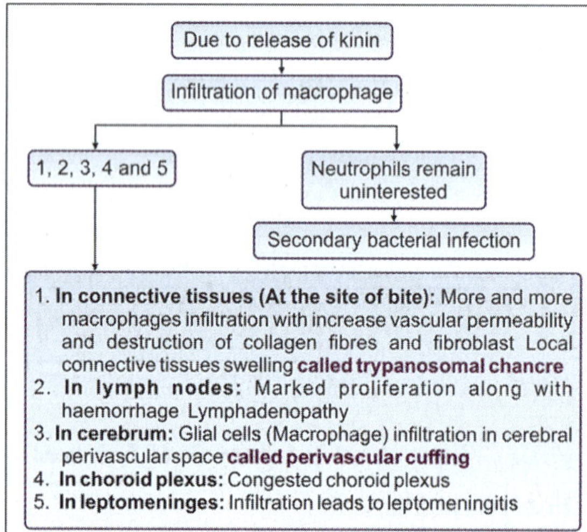

Flow chart-3: Inflammatory reaction

a. **Mutant of VSG:** Abs are formed which destroy most of the trypomastigote, but mutant of VSG escape this destruction & produce new wave of parasitaemia characterised by fever.

b. **Auto-immune reaction:** Large numbers of non specific Abs like IgM & IgG are formed which are not able to sensitise the Ags of trypomastigote, but instead damage the normal tissues.

c. **Inflammatory reaction: → Flow chart-3**

- **Clinical features:** In gambiense strain symptoms develops after 2 years of bite.
- ✪ **History:** History of tsetse bite is often available.
- ✪ **Trypanosomal chancre:**
  - Local, painful, connective tissue induration at the site of bite.
  - Contains trypomastigote.
  - 25-100mm in size & heals in 1-2 weeks without suppuration.
- ✪ **Fever:** Intermittent fever with severe headache, loss of nocturnal sleep, feeling of oppression.
- ✪ **Skin:** A fleeting, circinate erythematous rashes appear on chest & shoulders, which observe easily in person with fair skin & difficult in coloured skin.

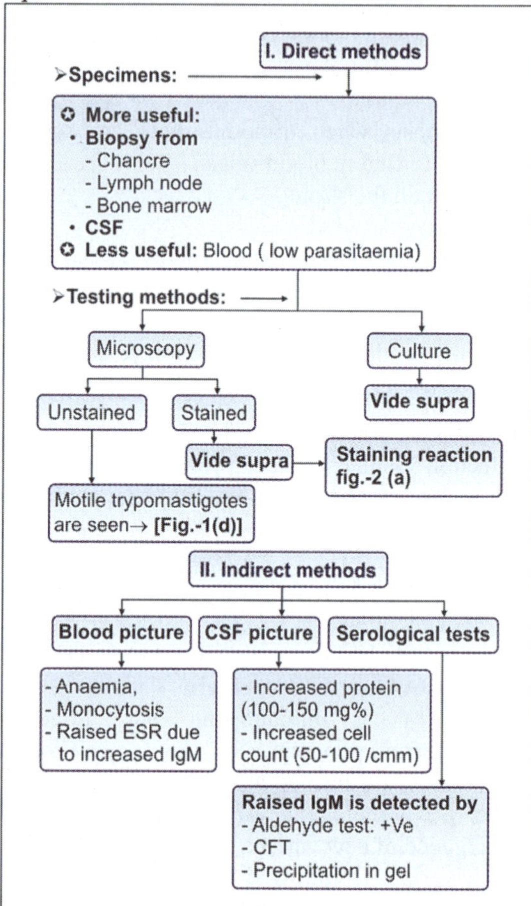

Flow chart-4: Lab. diagnosis of *gambiense*

- ✪ **Lymphadenopathy:** More in gambiense strain than other. At 1st enlargement of local lymph node & later generalised, especially posterior triangle **called Winterbottom's sign.**
- ✪ **CNS features**
  - Pressure on the palm or over the ulnar nerve may be followed by severe pain within short time after the pressure is released **called Keranadel's sign.**
  - Meningoencephalitis with classical sleeping sickness.
  - Less in gambiense strain & more in rhodesiense.

✪ **Final stage**

- Patient becomes thin & wasted accompany by various sign of malnutrition.
- Patient survive longer naturally unlike rhodesiense strain.
- Patient die sooner or later if remains untreated.

❖ **Laboratory diagnosis:** → **Flow chart-4**

❖ **Prevention:** Control of fly by using insecticides, traps etc.

❖ **Treatment:**

- Before CNS involvement: Pentamidine is the drug of choice & given in the dose of 3-4 mg/kg of body weight by IM route for 7-10 days.
- After CNS involvement: Eflornithine is the drug of choice.

Trypanosoma brucei rhodesiense

❖ **History:** Was discovered in Rhodesia by Stephens & Fanthom in 1909.

❖ **Geographical distribution:** East & Central Africa.

❖ **Habitat:**

- It is a connective tissues parasite.
- Invades less in lymph node & more in the brain.
- African sleeping sickness is a disease of CNS. It consumes plenty of glucose from tissues.

❖ **Morphology & culture:** Same as gambiense strain.

❖ **Immunity:** Similar to gambiense strain, but produce **heterophile antibody** which agglutinates the sheep RBCs & useful to screen this type.

❖ **Life cycle:**

➢ **Hosts:**

A. Vertebrate host: Man, game & domestic animal.

B. Insect host: Tsetse fly by *G. morsitans, G. swynertoni* & *G. pallidipes.*

➢ **Cycles:** Same as gambiense strain.

❖ **Pathogenicity:**

➢ **Type of disease:** It is an acute disease.

➢ **Disease name:** **Called Rhodesian sleeping sickness or East African sleeping sickness or East African trypanosomiasis.**

➢ **Reservoir/ source of infection:** Wild animal like antelope & domestic like cattle acts as reservoir of infection for rhosiense strain.

➢ **Mode of transmission:** By bites of tsetse fly (**Species: → Vide supra**).

➢ **Sites: →Follow habitat**

➢ **Clinical features:** In rhodesiense strain symptoms develops after 2 weeks of bite. Similar to gambiense strain but

✪ **Lymphadenopathy:** Less.

✪ **CNS features:** More.

✪ **Final stage:** Patient dies earlier if remains untreated.

❖ **Laboratory diagnosis:** → **Flow chart-5**

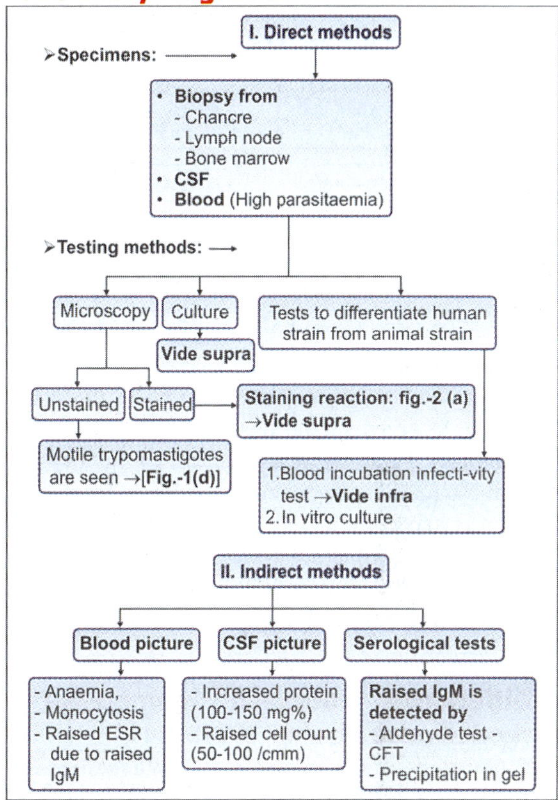

Flow chart-5: Lab. diagnosis of *rhodesiense*

✓ **Notes: Blood incubation infectivity test**

- **History:** Test was developed by Rickma & Robson in 1970.
- **Principle:** Human blood rendered the animal strain non-infective.
- **Steps: → Flow chart-6**
- **Result & interpretation:**
  - Positive: Development of parasitaemia in **both** the rats indicates human strain, because infectivity remains unimpaired by human blood.
  - Negative:
    - **Test strain:** No parasitaemia in rat, because animal strain become non-infective by human blood.
    - **Control strain:** Parasitaemia in rat.
- **Uses:** Used to differentiate between animal stain (*brucie*) & human stain (*rhodesiense*).

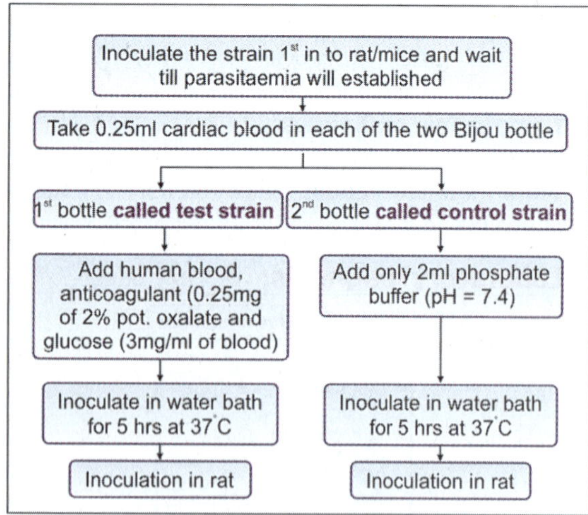

Flow chart-6: Blood incubation infectivity test

❖ **Prevention:** Control of fly by using insecticides, traps etc.

❖ **Treatment:**

- Before CNS involvement: Suramin is the drug of choice & given in the dose of 20 mg/kg of body weight by IV route at an interval of 5-7 days with total 5 injections. It not cross the blood brain barrier but it is nephrotoxic.
- After CNS involvement: Melarsoprol (mel-B) is the drug of choice, as it cross the blood brain barrier. It given in the dose 2-3 mg/kg/day (maximum 40 mg) for 3-4 days.

❖ **Differences between gambiense & rhodesiense strain:** → Table -1

Features	Gambiense	Rhodesiense
History	Vide supra	Vide supra
Geographical distribution	West & Central Africa	East & Central Africa
More habitat	In lymph nodes	In CNS
Disease name	Called Gambian sleeping sickness	Called Rhodesian sleeping sickness
Type of disease	Chronic & features occur 2 years after bite	Acute & symptoms develop 2 weeks after bite
Reservoir	Man	Animal
Mode of transmission	By tsetse fly like *G. Palpalis, G. Pallidipes & G. Tachinoides*	By tsetse fly like *G. morsitans, G. swynertoni & G. Pallidipes*
Lymph features	More	Less
CNS features	Less	More
Death	Late	Early

Table -1: Differences between gambiense & rhodesiense strain

Trypanosoma brucei zambiense

- **Chronic form:** It is like gembiense strain & found in East Africa.
- **Acute form:** It is like rhodesiense & found in Tanzania, Uganada & Kenya.
- **Clinical features:** In zambiense strain symptoms develops after 2 weeks of bite. Patient overcomes the infection naturally & acts as health carrier.

Trypanosoma cruzi

❖ **Synonym:** *Schizotrypanum cruzi.*

❖ **History:**

- *T. cruzi* was discovered by Carlos Chaga in 1909, while he was medical students.
- He named the organism as *T. cruzi* from the name of his mentor & disease **called Chaga's disease**.

❖ **Geographical distribution:** South & Central America.

❖ **Habitat:** Two forms present in human.

i. **Trypomastigote stage:** Present in peripheral blood
ii. **Amastigote stage:** Intra cellular form present in muscles (striated → heart & skeletal), nervous system & RE system.

❖ **Morphology:**

A. **In human:** Two forms present in human.

i. **Trypomastigote stage:** Present in blood with following features **[fig.-1 (d)]**.

➢ **Size:** 20μm in length & 1-3μm in breadth.
➢ **Shape:** Elongated but unusual forms like **C-shape [fig.-2 (c)]**, **U-shape or S-shape** appears in stained film.
➢ **Motility:** Actively motile.
➢ **Structure:**

- **Nucleus:** Large oval & central in position.
- **Kinetoplast:** Situated near posterior end **called postnuclear kinetoplast.**
- **Basal body:** Starting point of flagellum.
- **Axoneme or axial filament:** Part of flagella lying inside the body.
- **Undulating membrane:**
  - It is a folding of flagella around the body of parasite
  - Usually 3-4 folds are present.
- **Free flagellum:** Flagella become free from anterior end.

➢ **Pleomorphism in trypomastigote:** two forms appear in peripheral blood.

1. **Long slender form:**
2. **Short stumpy form:**

➢ **Multiplication:** Not take place in this stage.
➢ **Progress:** It is taken up by vector or enters in cell where it continuously lives as an amastigote forms.

ii. **Amastigote stage:** Present in cells (intracellular) with following features **[fig.-1 (a)]**.

- **Size:** 2-4μm diameter.
- **Shape:** Oval.
- **Motility:** Non- motile as it is without flagella.
- **Structure:**
- **Nucleus:** Large oval & central in position.
- **Kinetoplast:** Situated near anterior end **called antetnuclear kinetoplast.**
- **Basal body:** Starting point of flagellum.
- **Axoneme or axial filament:** Part of flagella lying inside the body.
- **Undulating membrane & free flagellum:** Not present.
- **Multiplication:** Take place in this stage only by binary fission.

B. In vector: Two forms present in vector.

i. Amastigote stage:

ii. Epimastigote stage:

❖ Culture:

i. Culture on media: Grow in NNN (Novy, McNeal & Nicolle) medium or in other modified media.

ii. Culture in animals:

- **Uses:** In diagnosis when trypomastigote are not found in patient's blood.
- **Animals: Guinea pig** is inoculated with patient's blood.

❖ Immunity:

Produce serum antibodies (Abs), but ineffective as the organisms are intracellular.

❖ Life cycle:

- **Hosts:**

A. Vertebrate host: Man.

B. Insect host: Reduviid bug like *Panstrongylus megistus, Triatoma infestans & Rhodnius prolixus.*

- **Method of reproduction:** Longitudinal binary fission.
- **Cycles: → Fig.-4 & Flow chart-7.**

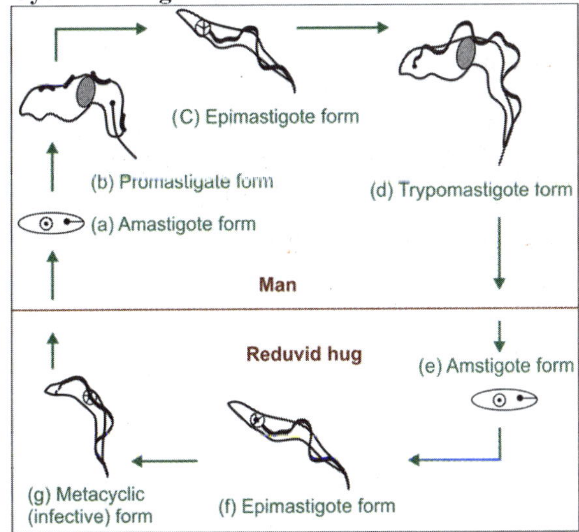

Figure-4: Life cycle of *T. cruzi*

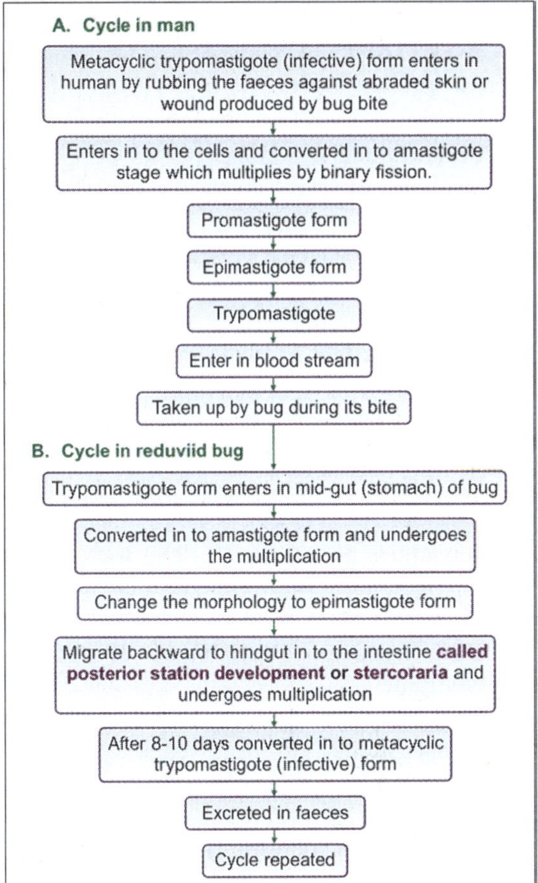

Flow chart-7: Life cycle of *T. cruzi*

❖ Pathogenicity:

- **Disease name: Called Chaga's disease or South American trypanosomiasis.**
- **Reservoir/ source of infection:**
  - Animal reservoir: Like armadillo, opossum, cat, dog, bat & wood rat.
  - Man is the secondary host.
- **Mode of transmission:**

a. Direct:

1. **Direct contact:** Direct contact of infected body fluid with abraded skin/mucosa (in hospital worker).
2. **Vertical or mother to baby:** By placenta.

b. Indirect (vehicle borne):

1. **Fluid borne:** Transfusion of blood or blood products.
2. **Vector borne:** Metacyclic (infective) form enters in human by rubbing the bug's faeces against abraded skin or wound produced by bite of reduviid bug (**species: → Vide supra**).
3. **Unclean hands & fingers:** Rubbing the exposed mucosa or conjunctive with contaminated fingers.

- **Incubation period:** 7-14 days.
- **Exit form:** Trypomastigote form.
- **Infective form:** Metacyclic trypomastigote form.
- **Portal of entry:** Skin or conjunctiva.
- **Sites: → Follow habitat**

➢ **Clinical features:** Two clinical types.

a. **Acute:** Occurs in infants & children.

✪ **At the site of entry:**

- **In skin:**
  - Unilateral facial swelling.
  - Swelling of skin at the site of entry **called chagoma.**
  - Sometimes chagoma present on facial skin because of feeding preference of reduvid bug **called kissing bug.**
- **In conjunctiva:** Swelling of conjunctiva at the site of entry **called Roman's sign.**

✪ **General features:** Fever, enlargement of spleen & lymph node, anaemia & lymphocytosis.

✪ **Final stage**

- It last for 20-30 days.
- Sometimes patient die (5-10%) with symptoms of meningo-encephalitis or myocardial failure.

b. **Chronic:** Occurs in adults & adolescent.

✪ **CVS features:** Heart block & Adams-Stokes syndrome.

✪ **CNS features:** Spastic paralysis & psychological changes. It may last for 12 years.

➢ **Complications:** Dilatation of organs due to damage to muscle & nerve that controls the tone, particularly in hollow organ like

- **GIT:**
  - Oesophagus: Megaoesophagus.
  - Colon: Megacolon.
- **Heart:**
  - Cardic myopathy
  - Herniation of endocardium at apex of left ventricle
- **Lungs:** Dilatation of pulmonary conus.

❖ Laboratory diagnosis: → Flow chart-8

❖ Prevention:

- Control of bug by using insecticides.
- Elimination of bug's breeding places by improvement in housing quality & environment.
- Bug bite is avoided by using mosquito net or repellents.

❖ Treatment:

- No specific & effective treatment is available.
- Nifutrimox & benzinidazole have been used for acute & chronic stages with some success. They kill extracellular parasites but not intracellular.
- Nifutrimox is given orally in the dose of 8-10 mg/kg of body weight in 4 divided doses for 90-120 days.
- Benzinidazole is given orally in the dose of 5-10 mg/kg of body weight in for 60 days.

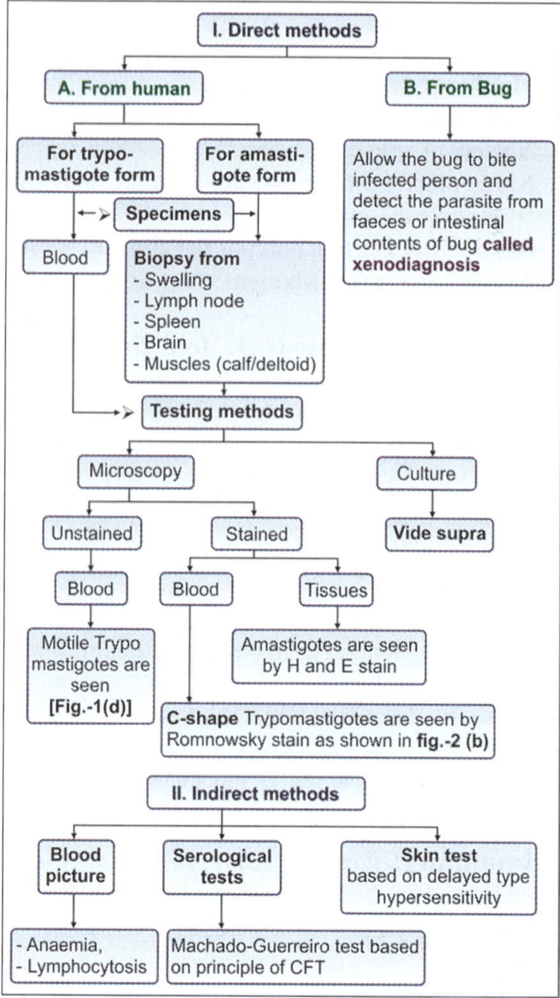

Flow chart-8: Lab. diagnosis of *T. cruzi*

Leishmania spp.

Leishmania donovani

❖ History:

It was discovered simultaneously by two persons. Sir William Leishman in May-1903 in London, from his name genus **called *Leishmania*** & Donovan in Madras (Chennai) in July 1903, from his name species **called *donovani.***

❖ Geographical distribution:

➢ **In World:** South America, Russia, South Europe (Mediterranean countries), Africa & China.

➢ **In India:** It is endemic along the coastal area of Ganges & Brahmaputra & in Bihar, Orissa, Madras & Eastern part of Uttar Pradesh.

❖ Habitat:

A. **In vertebrate host:** Amastigote (aflagellar) stage is present (in RE system).

B. **In vector (sand fly) & in culture:** Promastigote (flagellar) stage is present.

❖ Morphology:

A. In vertebrate host: Man, dog & hamster.

i. Amastigote (aflagellar) stage: Present inside the cells of RE system with following features [**fig.-1 (a)**]. Its intracellular form **called LD (*Leishmania donovani*) body** as shown in **fig.-7.**

- **Size:** 2-4µm diameter at long axis.
- **Shape:** Oval.
- **Motility:** Non- motile as it is without flagella.
- **Structure:**
  - **Nucleus:** Large oval & central in position.
  - **Kinetoplast:** Situated near anterior end **called antetnuclear kinetoplast.**
  - **Basal body:** Starting point of flagellum.
  - **Axoneme or axial filament:** Inner part of flagellum.
  - **Undulating membrane & free flagellum:** Absent
  - **Vacuole:** Clear unstained space lying alongside the axoneme.
- **Multiplication:** Take place by binary fission.

B. In vector (sand fly) & in culture:

i. Promastigote (flagellar) form: →**Fig.-1 (b)**

- **Size:** 5-10µm in length & 2-3µm in breadth.
- **Shape:** Elongated pear shaped body.
- **Motility:** Actively motile.
- **Structure:**
  - **Nucleus:** Large oval & central in position.
  - **Kinetoplast:** Situated near anterior end **called antetnuclear kinetoplast.**
  - **Basal body:** Starting point of flagellum.
  - **Axoneme or axial filament:** Part of flagella lying inside the body.
  - **Vacuole:** Light stained space lying alongside the axoneme.
  - **Free flagellum:** Present, but sometimes it is absent.
  - **Undulating membrane:** Absent.
- **Multiplication:** Take place by binary fission.

❖ Culture:

i. Culture on media: Promastigote stage is developed on culture media.

a. Monophasic media:

1. **Schneider's insect tissue culture medium:**
2. **Grace's insect medium:**
3. **Solid medium:**
   - Prepared by J C Ray in 1932.
   - Contains agar, glucose, beef heart infusion, peptone, amino acid, glycerine & rabbit's blood.
4. **Liquid medium: →HO-MEM (Eagle's minimal essential medium):**
   - It is a semi-defined liquid medium contains Spinner's salt & 10% foetal calf serum.
   - It transforms amastigote form of *Leishmania* to promastigote form in 48 hrs in 60-80% cases.

b. Biphasic media:

1. **Brain heart infusion agar:**
2. **Tobies medium:**
3. **NNN [Novy, McNeal (1904) & Nicole (1908)] medium:**

- **Medium:**
  - ✪ **Ingredients:**
    - **Solid part:**
      - **Two parts of salt agar** (prepared by adding 14 g agar & 6 g NaCl in 900ml distilled water).
      - **One part of defibrinated rabbit's blood.**
    - **Liquid part:** Water of condensation.
  - ✪ **Preparation:**
    - Add the rabbit's blood with liquid agar during cooling & mix by rotating the tube between the palms.
    - Allow to settle in sloping position, so medium can solidify in slant as shown in **fig.-5.**
- **Specimens to be cultivated:**
  - ✪ **Blood:**
    - Collect 1-2 ml of blood & dilute with 10ml citrated solution (0.85% saline with 2% sodium citrate).
    - Either centrifuge or allow to settle 22^{0}C overnight
    - Cellular deposit is inoculated in water of condensation of NNN medium.
  - ✪ **Biopsy from spleen, bone marrow& lymph nodes** (In case of African & Chinese form).
- **Cultivation technique & result: → Flow chart-9**

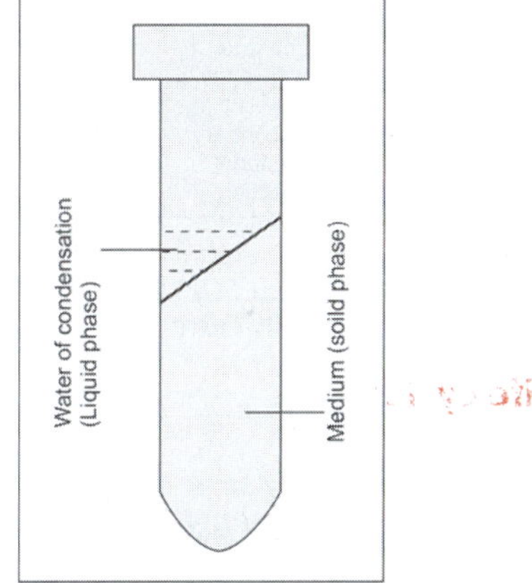

Figure-5: NNN medium

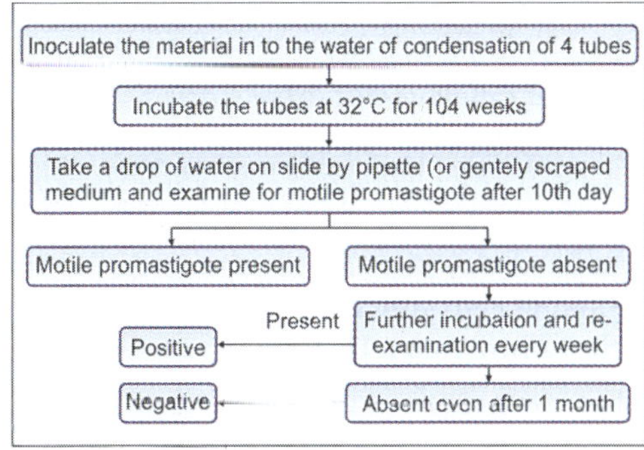

Flow chart-9: Cultivation technique & result

- **Disadvantages:**
  - Chances of contamination during examination.
  - Slow & taking long time about 1 month.

- **Advantages of using 4 tubes:** One tube remains un opened up to 1month, which avoids the chances of contamination.

ii. Culture in animals:

- **Uses:**
- For diagnosis & research purpose.
- To test the efficacy of leishmanicidal drugs.

Animals:

- **Rats, mice & guinea pigs** are not useful.
- **Hamster (small rodents):** Intraperitoneal inoculation kills the hamster (*Cricetulus griseus*) in 2-3 months & parasite can be seen in organs like liver & spleen.

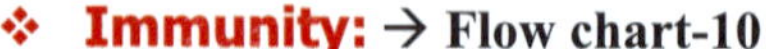

Immunity: → Flow chart-10

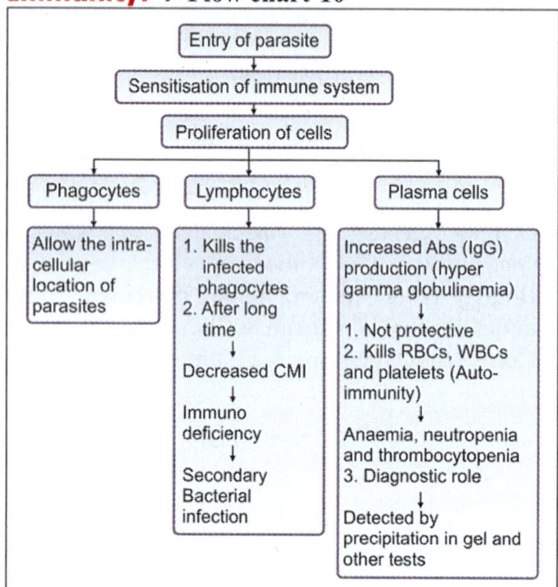

Flow chart-10: Immunity in *L. donovani*

Life cycle:

- **Hosts:**

A. Vertebrate host: Man & dog.

B. Insect host: Sand fly like

In World:

- In South America: *Lutzomyia longipalpis.*
- In South Europe (Mediterranean countries): *Phlebotomus pernicious* in Italy & Silicy.
- In Russia: *Phlebotomus arpaklensis.*
- In Africa (Sudan & East Africa): *Ph. martini.*
- In China: *Ph. chinensis & Ph. sergenti* var. *mongolensis.*

In India: *Phlebotomus argentipus.*

- **Method of reproduction:** Binary fission.
- **Cycles: Flow chart-11 & fig.-6.**

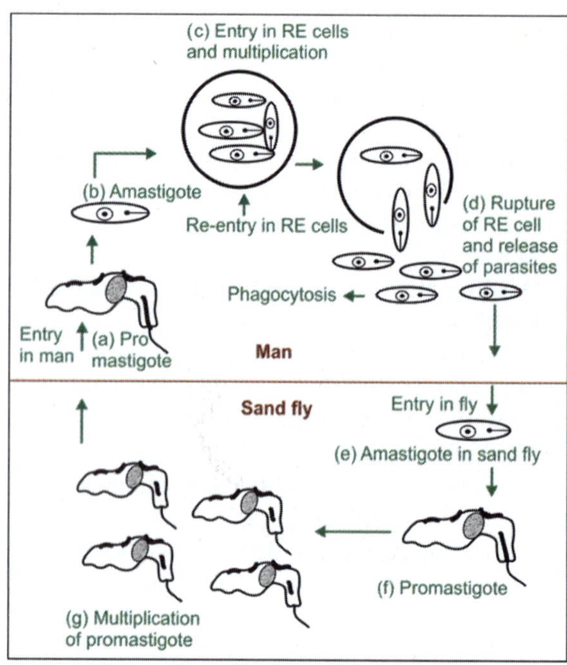

Figure-6: Life cycle of *L. donovani*

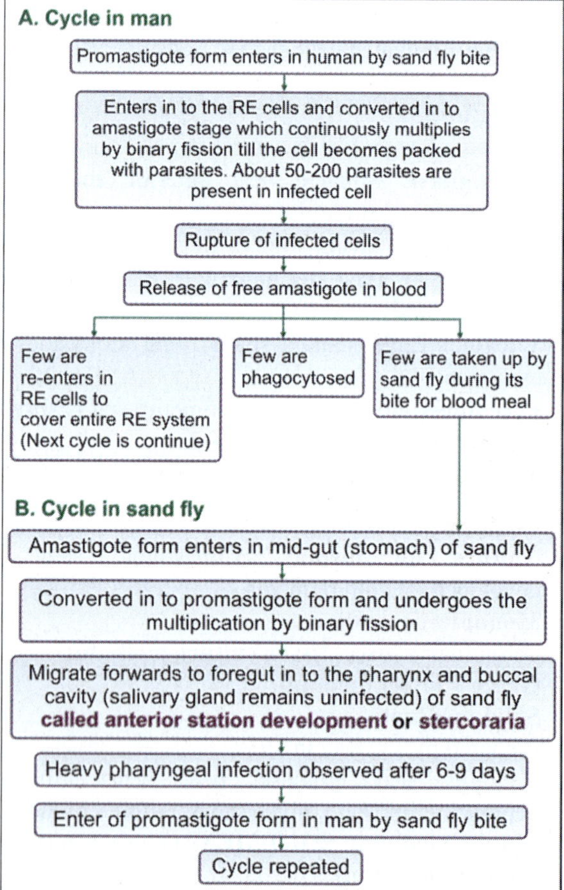

Flow chart-11: Life cycle of *L. donovani*

Pathogenicity:

- **Disease name: Called visceral leishmaniasis.**
- **Synonym:** Also **called kala azar or dum dum fever.**

- **Meaning:** Kala azar is an Indian terminology. Here **Kala =Black** and also **deadly** while **Azar = Illness** which indicates blackening of skin and fatal nature of illness.
- **Reservoir of infection with ecological types of kala azar:**
- Rodent reservoir: African kala azar.
- Canine reservoir: Mediterranean or Infantile or Chinese or South American kala azar.
- Jackls reservoir: Russian kala azar.
- Human reservoir: Indian kala azar (case of acute visceral leishmaniasis).
- **Source of infection:** Sand fly.
- **Mode of transmission:**

a. **Direct:**

1. **Sexual transmission:**
2. **Vertical or mother to baby (congenital):** By placenta.
3. **Inoculation under skin / mucosa:** By accidental inoculation of culture in laboratory.

b. **Indirect (vehicle borne):**

1. **Fluid borne:** Transfusion of blood or blood products.
2. **Vector borne:**

- By bite of sand fly: **Species → vide supra.**
- Pharynx & buccal cavity of sand fly are completely blocked by presence of promastigote **called blocked sand fly**. They are not present in salivary gland.
- Bites of such blocked sand fly transmit the infection in wound produced by proboscis.
- To take the blood meal fly has to empty the pharynx & buccal cavity.
- **Incubation period:** Generally 3-6 months, but sometimes exceed up to 1-2 years.
- **Exit form:** Amastigote form.
- **Infective form:** Promastigote form.
- **Portal of entry:** Skin.
- **Sites: → Follow habitat**
- **Clinical types:** Two clinical types.

a. **Acute:** Early case of kala azar of 2-6 weeks duration **called acute kala azar.**

b. **Chronic:** Case of kala azar after 2-6 weeks duration **called chronic kala azar.**

- **Pathological changes in different systems:**

a. **Spleen:**

✪ **Macroscopic:**

- Spleen is the most commonly affected organ.
- Enlarged spleen & thickened capsule.
- Soft consistency & easily friable by pressure with thumb.
- Cut surface shows congestion with dull red or chocolate colour.

✪ **Microscopic:**

- Vascular space are widely dilated & filled with blood.
- RE cells are increased in number (hyperplasia) & size & filled with amastigote form of parasite.
- Sinus lining cells (**Called littoral cells**) do not contain any parasite.
- No evidence of fibrosis, but increase the reticulin fibrils to support the proliferating cells.
- Increase plasma cells.
- Malpighian corpuscles are disappearing, due to hyperplasia.

b. **Liver:**

✪ **Macroscopic:**

- Enlarged liver.
- Cut surface shows congestion & nutmeg appearance.

✪ **Microscopic:**

- Sinusoids are dilated & filled with blood.
- Kupfer's cells are increased in number (hyperplasia) & size & filled with amastigote form of parasite.
- Liver cells do not contain any parasite.
- No evidence of fibrosis, but increase the reticulin fibrils to support the proliferating cells.

c. **Lymph node:**

- Enlarged nodes are observed in African & Chinese form.
- Only two cases with lymphadenopathy are observed in Indian kala azar (Sen Gupta-1961, Sne Gupta & Mukherjee-1968).
- Cells are increased in number (hyperplasia) & size & filled with amastigote form of parasite.

d. **GIT:** Intestinal ulcer due to secondary infection but not due to *L. donovani.*

e. **Bone marrow:**

- RE cells are increased in number (hyperplasia) & size & filled with amastigote form of parasite.
- Increase plasma cells.
- Leucoblastic elements are increased, resulting leucopenia (neutropenia).

f. **Blood picture:** Pancytopenia is the feature.

✪ **Haemoglobin (Hb) concentration:** 5-10g/100ml.

✪ **RBCs count:**

- **Anaemia**: Decrease RBCs count, but less compared to neutrophils. It is due to
- Autoimmunisation: Destruction of RBCs by anti – RBCs antibodies.
- Reduction of survival time of RBCs up to 50%.
- Sequestration & destruction of RBC in spleen.

✪ **WBCs count:**

- **Total count:** Is 3000/cmm & sometimes reduce up to 1000/cmm.
- **Neutropenia:** Due to
- Destruction of WBCs by anti –WBCs antibodies.
- Increased leucoblastic elements in bone marrow.
- **Agranulocytosis:** It is an extreme reduction of granulocytes, although not common but reported in some cases.

- **Lymphocytosis & monocytosis:** Due to proliferation.
- **Platelets count:** Thrombocytopenia is due to destruction of platelets by anti – platelets antibodies.
- **WBC to RBC ratio:**
- **Normal:** 1:750.
- **In kala azar:** Altered to 1:1000 to 1:2000.
- **Clinical features:**
- **Skin:**
- **At the site of entry:**
- Nodular swelling developed in skin at the site of sand fly bite **called leishmanioma.**
- 1-1½ inch in diameter.
- Last for 1-3 weeks.
- It observed in Sudan, Middle Asia & Kenya.
- It also observed after artificial inoculation of culture from human, gerbil or ground squirrel strain of *L. donovani.*
- It is not observed in India & South America.
- **Other part of skin:**
- It becomes dry, rough, harsh & pigmented (black colour).
- In African kala azar warty eruption of skin & mucocutaneous lesion may appear.
- **Skin appendages:** Hair becomes brittle& falls out.
- **Fever:**
- It may be continuous or remittent type, becoming remittent in later stage.
- 20% of cases show the double rise in 24 hrs.
- Waves of pyrexia may be followed by apyrexia.
- **Splenomegaly:** It reaches below the coastal margin & often fills the entire abdomen.
- **Lymphadenopathy:** Observed in African & Chinese form.
- **Hepatomegaly:**
- Enlarged but not as much as spleen.
- No jaundice, unless liver is enlarged greatly.
- **General features:**
- There is no malaise or apathy.
- Emaciation & patient remains unaware about fever
- Epistaxis may present.
- **Final stage:** 75-95% chances of death if remains untreated due to following complications.

✓ **Note: Visceral leishmaniasis triad:** Few authors described fever, splenomegaly & hepatomegaly as visceral leishmaniasis triad.

- **Complications:** Immunosuppressive effect leads the following complications which may produce death.
- Amoebic dysentery.
- Bacillary dysentery.
- Pneumonia.
- Pulmonary tuberculosis.
- Cancrum oris in case of sever neutropenia.
- Other septic infections.

Differential diagnosis:

- **Fungal:** Chromoblastomycosis, lobomycosis, deep fungal infection.
- **Bacterial:** Rhinoscleroma, tropical pyoderma, cutaneous diphtheria and other mycobacterioses (e.g. *Mycobacterium marinum* infection of the skin &*Mycobacterium avium intracellulare*)
- **Viral:** Orf.
- **Inflammatory diseases:** Pyogenic granuloma, nummular dermatitis & plaque psoriasis.
- **Malignancy:** Metastases, psoriasis & keloids.
- **Ulcers:** Traumatic ulcers & stasis ulcers.
- **Cutaneous and Muco-cutaneous leishmaniasis:**
- Based on clinical picture.
- Also differentiated by laboratory test **called Adler's test → Vide infra**

Laboratory diagnosis:

Diagnosis chronic kala azar

I. Direct methods

- **Specimens:**
- **Blood:**
- **Biopsies:** From following organs.

1. **Biopsy from spleen:**
   - **Advantage:** Most useful specimen.
   - **Disadvantage:** Chances of bleeding which may continue from soft & enlarged spleen leading to death.
   - **Positivity:** 98%.
2. **Biopsy from bone marrow:** Collected from sternum or iliac crest.
   - **Advantage:** Most useful when spleen is not enlarged.
   - **Disadvantage:** Gives negative result when parasites are scanty.
   - **Positivity:** 50-85%.
3. **Biopsy from lymph nodes:**
   - **Advantage:** In case of African & Chinese form
   - **Positivity:** 98%.

- **Testing methods:**

A. **Microscopy:**

- **Preparation of smear:**

i. **From Blood:**

a. **Thin film:** Less useful because of scanty parasites & chances of false negative result.
b. **Thick film:** As recommended for *Plasmodium* spp.
c. **Centrifugation of blood:** Use the sediment to prepare the smear.
d. **Straight leucocytic edge:**

- When thin film is being drawn & before the blood is almost exhausted, the spreading slide is abruptly lifted off.
- This will not produce a film with tail but a straight edge, which will contains large numbers of WBCs.

- This area is necessary to examine the amastigotes.

ii. **From biopsies:** Rub the tissues over the slide & then fix with methanol.

✪ **Staining of smear:**

- Stain by Giemsa or Leishman stain and examine under oil immersion lenses.
- Intracellular amastigote is examined **called LD body** as shown in **fig.-7.**
- Cytoplasm appears blue, kinetoplast red & nucleus appears pink (violet) as shown in **fig.-7(b)** in inset.

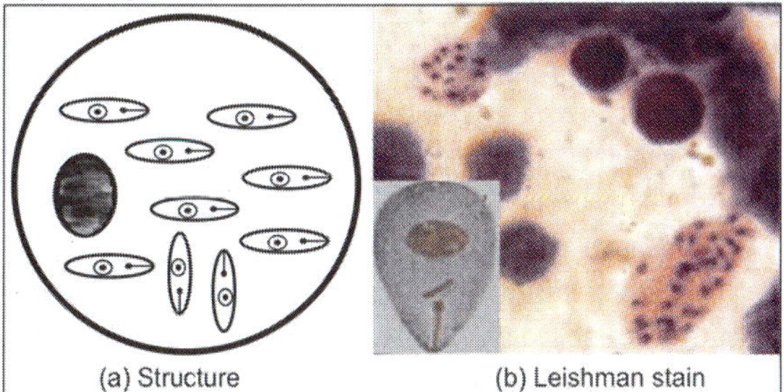

Figure.-7: LD body

✪ **Grading of smear:** Grading of smear is done on the basis of numbers of amastigotes in smear as mentioned in **table-2.**

Grade	No. of amastigotes	No. of fields
0	0	1000
1	1-10	1000
2	1-10	100
3	1-10	10
4	1-10	1
5	>10-100	1
6	>100	1

Table-2: Grading of smear

B. **Culture: → Vide supra**

C. **Test to differentiate cutaneous and muco-cutaneous leishmaniasis from kala azar:**

i. **Adler's test:**

✪ **Principle:** It based on inhibition of development of promastigote form in Locke's serum agar by using specific antiserum.

✪ **Use:** To differentiate *L. donovani, L. tropica* & *L. brasiliensis* by using sera.

✪ **Disadvantage:** It also possible by heterologous serum.

II. Indirect methods

➢ **Specimens:**

✪ **Blood/serum:**

✪ **Solution contains antigen for skin test:**

➢ **Testing methods:**

A. **Blood picture: → Vide supra**

B. **Serological tests:**

i. **Non- specific tests:**

a. **Aldehyde test (Napier):**

✪ **Principle:** Based on precipitation reaction, to detect the increase the gamma globulin in serum.

✪ **Testing methods:**

- Mix 1-2 ml serum with 40% formalin in a test tube
- Allow to stand for 20 minutes.

✪ **Result:**

- **Positive:** Jellification of milk-white opacity like a white of hard-boiled egg within 2-20 minutes **called strong positive.**
- **Negative:** No jellification.

✪ **Interpretation:**

- **Positive:**
  - Visceral leishmaniasis: Becomes positive after 3 months (12 weeks).
  - Other conditions giving positive results are: African trypanosomiasis (*T. brucei*), *S. japonicum*, *S. haematobium* & multiple myeloma & cirrhosis.
- **Negative:** Cutaneous leishmaniasis.

b. **Antimony test (Chopra et al):**

✪ **Principle:** Based on precipitation reaction, to detect the increase the gamma globulin in serum.

✪ **Testing methods:**

- Mix 1-2 ml serum (whole serum or 1:10 diluted) with 4% urea stibamine solution in a test tube.
- Allow to stand for few minutes.

✪ **Result:**

- **Positive:** Formation of precipitate (flocculant).
- **Negative:** No precipitation.

✪ **Interpretation:**

- **Positive:** Visceral leishmaniasis.
- **Negative:** No visceral leishmaniasis.

✪ **Disadvantage:** Less reliable than aldehydes test.

c. **Non- specific CFT with WKK antigen:**

✪ **Principle:**

- Sharing the common antigens by *Leishmania* & *M. tuberculosis* is the basis of this test.
- **Called non- specific**, as the antigen used in the test is not prepared from the *Leishmania* itself, but from human tubercle bacilli (*M. tuberculosis*) **called Kedrowsky's strain.**
- Antigen is prepared by **W**itebusky, **K**ligenstein & **K**uhn, hence **called WKK antigen.**
- WKK antigen detect the certain antibodies present in serum of kala azar patient by using principle of CFT.

✪ **Interpretation:**

- **Positive:**
  - Visceral leishmaniasis: Becomes positive in initial 3 weeks of the infection & useful in acute infection.
  - Other conditions giving positive results are: Lepromatous leprosy, pulmonary tuberculosis & tropical pulmonary eosinophilia.

ii. **Specific tests:**

a. **Specific CFT:** Two ways to prepare the antigen.

1. Prepared from promastigote form of *L. donovani* by Ghosh & Ray in1951.
2. Prepared from infected hamster's spleen or liver by Chung & Chang in 1951.

b. Indirect haemagglutination test:

c. Immunochromatographic test:

d. ELISA:

e. Immunofluorescent test:

C. Skin (allergic) test:

i. Leishmanin test:

- **Synonym:** Montenegro reaction.
- **Principle:** Based on delayed type hypersensitivity.
- **Steps:** 0.1-0.2ml killed culture contains 6-10million promastigote/ml is injected intradermally & examine for result.
- **Result:**
- **Positive:**
- Development of induration after 72 hrs.
- Test becomes positive after 6-8 weeks of recovery of kala azar.
- **Negative:** No induration.
- **Interpretation:**
- **Positive:** Positive in African kala azar but not in Mediterranean & Indian kala azar.
- **Negative:** Untreated case of kala azar & Post Kala azar Dermal Leishmaniasis (PKDL).

Diagnosis of acute azar → Flow chart-12

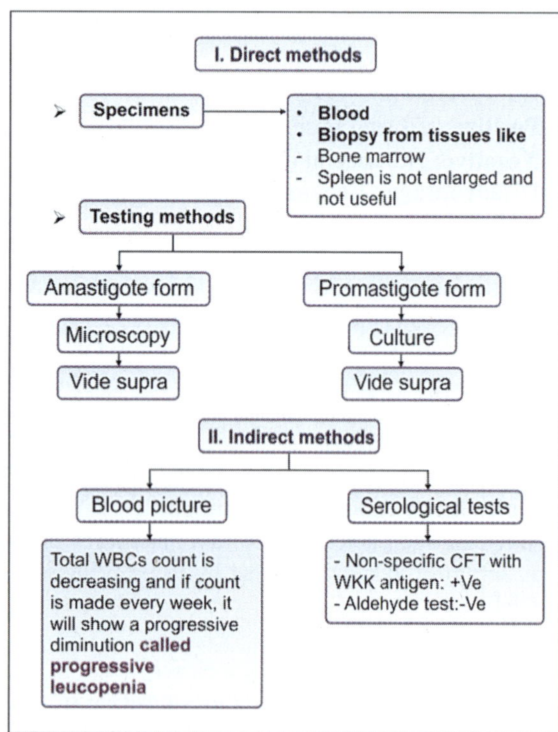

Flow chart-12: Lab. diagnosis of acute kala azar

Post Kala azar Dermal Leishmaniasis (PKDL):

- **Synonym:** Dermal leishmanoid.
- **Definition:** Non-ulcerative cutaneous lesion occurs in kala azar patients, 1-2 years after completion of treatment for original disease, where visceral infection disappears & skin infection persists.
- **Incidence:** It's not occurs commonly, but seen in 2-10% cases.
- 10% in Indian kala azar, mostly in Bengal, less in Chennai (Madras) & Assam.
- 2% in African kala azar.
- Rare in Chinese kala azar.
- Not in Mediterranean kala azar.
- **Clinical features:** Three types of lesions.

a. Depigmented patches:

- Early lesion.
- Sites: trunk, limbs & rare on face.
- Properties: No complete loss of pigment.

b. Erythematous patches:

- Early lesion.
- Sites: Butterfly distribution on nose, cheeks & chin **called butter fly erythema.**
- Properties: Photosensitive & becomes prominent in middle of the day.

c. Yellowish pink nodules:

- Replace the early lesion & occasionally appear from beginning.
- Sites: Mostly on face & mucosa of tongue & eye, however, it can appear anywhere.
- Properties: Soft & painless granulomatous ulcer, which differentiate it from espundia & oriental sore.
- **Complications:**
- Recurrence of kala azar occurs in case associated with PKDL.
- These cases are resistant to antimony treatment.
- Incidence is 1 in 700 cases.
- It was reported by Sen Gupta & Mukherjee in 1968.
- **Differential diagnosis:**
- Leprosy.
- Espundia.
- Oriental sore.
- **Diagnosis:**
- **Specimens:** Biopsies from nodular lesion, but not from depigmented lesion as it does not contain parasites.
- **Testing methods:** Microscopy to detect the amastigote form.
- **Treatment:**
- Pentavalent antimonial compound used in double dose, cures the condition.
- If second dose is required, then should not be repeated within 2 months of 1st course.

Prevention:

- Control of sand fly by using insecticides.
- Elimination of animal reservoir.
- Sand fly bite is avoided by using thick full sleeve clothes, mosquito net or repellents.

Treatment:

a. Antiparasitic pentavalent antimonial agents:

- **Preparation:** Two types like sodium stibogluconate & meglumine antimonite.

- **Dose:** 20mg/kg/day by IV/IM route for 20-30 days
- **Effectiveness:** It is the drug of choice in most part of the world with > 90% cure rate except in Bihar, India.

b. **Liposomal amphotericin B:**
- **Dose:** 3mg/kg/day.
- **Effectiveness:** Higher dose can improve the cure without toxicity. It is the only drug approved by US FDA & used extensively to treat visceral leishmaniasis in all part of the world.

c. **Amphotericin B:**
- **Dose:** 0.75 – 1.0mg/kg on alternate day for 15 infusion.
- **Effectiveness:** It is the 1st line drug in Bihar, India especially when antimonial compound are fail.

d. **Oral miltefosine:**
- **Dose:** 50mg/day for patient having weight < 25 kg & 50mg two times in a day for patient having weight >25 kg for 25 days.
- **Effectiveness:** It is the 1st oral drug approved for treatment leishmaniasis.

e. **Paromomycin:** 11.0mg/kg/day for 21 days.

f. **Pentamidine:** Intramuscular pentamidine is effective against visceral leishmaniasis, but this drug is associated with persistent diabetes mellitus and disease recurrence.

g. **Sitamoquine:** It is the 8 aminoquinolone analogue, which is active orally for visceral leishmaniasis, but causes nephotoxicity.

Leishmania tropica

History:
- 1st it was observed in 1885 by Cunningham in the tissue of Delhi boil in Calcutta, but misinterpreted.
- Its morphology was accurately defined by Russian surgeon Borovsky (1898) & Wright (1903).
- It was Luhe, who gave the name *L. tropica.*

Geographical distribution:
- **In World:** Along the coast of Mediterranean sea.
- **In India:**
  - It never coexists with kala azar.
  - In India kala azar present in western part, while infection of *L. tropica* occurs in Central & Western part.

Habitat:
A. **In vertebrate host:** Amastigote (aflagellar) stage is present in cells of RE system of skin **called clasmatocytes.**

B. **In vector (sand fly) & in culture:** Contains the promastigote (flagellar) stage.

Morphology: Same as *L. donovani.*

Culture:
i. **Culture on media:** Promastigote stage can be developed in NNN medium & can be maintain indefinitely by subculture.

ii. **Culture in animals:**
- **Animals used to produce local lesion (oriental sore):** Spermophile (*Citillus citillus*).
- **Animals used to produce visceral lesion:** Syrian hamster & mice can produces visceral lesion by intraperitoneal inoculation.

Immunity:
- Some degree of natural immunity present in people of endemic area and single attack can gives life-long acquired immunity.
- Infection can bc cleared by Cell Mediated Immunity (CMI), but also developed delayed type of hypersensitivity.
- Humoral immunity is not significant here.

✓ **Notes: Two conditions in which CMI failed to clear the local lesions**

1. **Leishmaniasis tegumenteria diffusa**
- **Synonym**: Also **called leishmaniasis diffusa** or **diffuse cutaneous leishmaniasis.**
- **Causes & distribution:**
  - *L. tropica*: In Ethiopia.
  - *L. pifanoi*: In South America with malignant form of lesion → **Vide infra.**
- **Pathogenesis:** It is due to deficiency of CMI to leishmanin antigen and characterised by nodular lesion which looks like lepromatous leprosy.
- **Clinical features:**
  - Nodular lesion which is neither destructive nor erosive and present as single lesion on skin which spread to covers the face, ears, extremities, buttock & entire body.
- **Diagnosis:**
  - Leishmanin reaction: Negative.
  - Histology:
    - Lesion contains Histiocytes but no lymphocytes and plasma cells.
    - Parasites are numerous (amastigote) inside the macrophages & also extracellular.
  - Blood & bone marrow examination: Also contains amastigote form.
- **Treatment:** Poor response to antimonial compound, but pentamidine & amphotericin B are effective but with serious side effect.

2. **Leishmaniasis recideva**
- **Causes & distribution:** *L. tropica minor* in Asia.
- **Pathogenesis:** It is a delayed type hypersensitivity reaction (Infective type) occurs after healing of Oriental sore and characterised by granulomatous swelling which looks like lupus vulgaris (cutaneous tuberculosis).
- **Clinical features:** Nodular or popular lesion present on skin.

- **Diagnosis:**
  - Leishmanin reaction: Positive.
  - Histology:
    - Granulomatous swelling contains lymphocytes & epitheloid cells.
    - Numerous parasites but not seen in the epitheloid cells.

❖ Life cycle:

➢ **Similar to *L. donovani*:**

- Similar to *L. donovani* except that amastigote form develops in skin (**cells called clasmatocytes**) and do not in viscera.
- Amastigote form in man & promastigote form in sand flies divide by binary fission.

➢ **Hosts:**

A. **Vertebrate host:** Man & dog.

B. **Insect host:** Sand flies like.

✪ **In World:**

- In North Africa & Mediterranean area: *Phlebotomus papatesii.*
- In Persia: *Ph. sergenti.*
- In Central Asia: *Ph. caucasicus & Ph. papatesii.*

✪ **In India:** *Phlebotomus sergenti.*

❖ Pathogenicity:

➢ **Disease name:** Produces local lesion in skin **called oriental sore or cutaneous leishmaniasis or Old World Cutaneous Leishmaniasis (OWCL) or tropical sore or Chiclero's disease or Delhi boil or Baghdad boil or Aleppo button or Aleppo evil.**

➢ **Mode of transmission:**

a. **Direct:** Transmission by direct contact is possible.

b. **Indirect (Vehicle borne):**

- By bite of sand fly: **Species → vide supra**
- Also by crushing the infected sand fly against wounded skin.

➢ **Reservoir of infection**: Dog of endemic area.

➢ **Source of infection**: Rodents (*Rhombomys opimus*)

➢ **Incubation period:** Generally few days – 6 months & in some cases it may extend up to 1or 2 years.

➢ **Exit form:** Amastigote form.

➢ **Infective form:** Promastigote form.

➢ **Portal of entry:** Skin.

➢ **Sites: → Follow habitat**

➢ **Pathology & clinical features:** Nodular granulomatous swelling developed at the site of skin bite with following features.

✪ **Macroscopic:**

- **Size:** One inch.
- **Site:** Exposed part of body like face or extremities.
- **Numbers:** Single or 2-3.
- **Ulceration:** In majority of cases it ulcerates with clear cut margin & raised indurated edge surrounded by red areola.
- **Healing:** Spontaneous or slowly in 6 months with production of white scar.

✪ **Microscopic (histology):** Granulomatous lesion contains monocytes / macrophages with parasites inside, lymphocytes, plasma cells & fibroblast.

➢ **Clinical types:** Two clinical types of cutaneous lesion as mentioned in **table-3.**

Features	*Leishmania tropica minor*	*Leishmania tropica major*
Distribution	Urban Middle East & Mediterranean area: N. Africa, North - West India, Pakistan	Rural Central Asia & Iran
Incubation period	2 months to >year	2-6 weeks
Type	Dry (Non-ulcerating)	Moist (ulcerating)
Site	Facial	Extremities
Protection	Can't protect against major	Can protect against minor

Table-3: Clinical types of leishmania tropica

❖ Laboratory diagnosis:

I. Direct methods

➢ **Specimens:** Biopsies or tissues from the edge of indurated swelling.

➢ **Testing methods:**

A. **Microscopy:**

✪ **Preparation of smear from specimens**

✪ **Staining of smear:**

- Stain by Leishman stain and examine under oil immersion lenses.
- Intracellular amastigote is examined in macrophage of skin (**cells called clasmatocytes**).

B. **Culture: → Vide supra**

II. Indirect methods

➢ **Testing methods:**

A. **Blood picture:** Normal cell count.

B. **Serological tests:** Are not useful (Normal Ig & aldehydes test is negative).

C. **Skin (allergic) test:**

i. **Leishmanin test/reaction:** Positive skin test after intra-cutaneous injection of suspension of promastigote of *Leishmania tropica.*

❖ **Prevention:** Same as kala azar.

❖ **Treatment:** Same as kala azar.

a. **Pentavalent antimonial resistant:** Treated by pentamidine.

b. **Local:** Application of paste consists 10% charcoal in sulphuric acid or liquid nitrogen.

Leishmania brasiliensis

❖ History:

- It was 1st observed in 1911 by Carini.
- It was defined as a new species by Vianna in 1911.

❖ **Geographical distribution:** Central & South America.

❖ **Habitat:**

A. **In vertebrate host:** Amastigote (aflagellar) stage is present in cells of RE system of skin, nasal mucosa & buccal mucosa.

B. **In vector (sand fly) & in culture:** Contains the promastigote (flagellar) stage.

❖ **Morphology:** Morphologically similar to *L. donovani* and *L. tropica.*

❖ **Culture:**

i. **Culture on media:** Promastigote stage can be developed in NNN medium.

ii. **Culture in animals:** Syrian hamster produce only local lesion & even intraperitoneal inoculation can't produces visceral lesion.

iii. **Culture in chick embryo:** Also grow in chorio-allentoic membrane (CAM)

❖ **Immunity:** Cell Mediated Immunity (CMI) develops after metastasis in skin (**cells called clasmatocytes**) & mucosa (**monocytes**).

❖ **Life cycle:**

➢ **Similar to *L. donovani*:**

- Similar to *L. donovani* except that amastigote form develops in skin and mucosa.
- Amastigote form in man & promastigote form in sand flies divide by binary fission.

➢ **Hosts:**

A. **Vertebrate host:** Man.

B. **Insect host:** Sand fly like *Lutzomyia.*

❖ **Pathogenicity:**

➢ **Disease name:** Produces local lesion in skin & mucosa **called espundia or muco-cutaneous leishmaniasis.**

➢ **Mode of transmission:**

a. **Direct:** Transmission by direct contact is possible.

b. **Indirect (vehicle borne):** By bite of sand fly (**Species: → Vide supra**).

➢ **Incubation period:** Few days – few weeks.

➢ **Reservoir of infection:** Small forest rodents.

➢ **Portal of entry:** Skin.

➢ **Clinical features:** Granulomatous swelling with following features.

✪ **Macroscopic:**

- **Site:** Granulomatous swelling developed at the site of skin bite.
- **Ulceration:** Lesion is enlarging radially forming an ulcer with clear cut margin & weeping surface.
- **Spread:** In 5% of cases it extends to nasal or buccal mucosa either by direct spread or by blood.

✪ **Microscopic (histology):** Granulomatous lesion contains monocytes / macrophages with parasites inside, lymphocytes, plasma cells & necrosis of tissues.

➢ **Clinical types:** In 1961, Pessoa subdivided the disease in to following clinical types based on biological strains of *L. brasiliensis.*

a. ***L. brasiliensis brasiliensis*:**

➢ **Severity:** Malignant form.

➢ **Distribution:** Most prevalent in South & Central America.

➢ **Features:**

- It is a papulo-pustular swelling, affecting skin of face, ears, elbows & knees.
- It also affects the eyes.
- It spread to oro-nasal mucosa causing destructive & mutilating erosion & sometimes with destruction of nasal septum.
- It healed with scarring producing typical tapir nose. **called camel nose**

b. ***L. brasiliensis guyanensis*:**

➢ **Severity:** Benign form.

➢ **Features:** It's affecting oro-nasal mucosa.

c. ***L. brasiliensis peruwiana*:**

➢ **Severity:** Benign form almost disappeared.

➢ **Features:**

- It is dry papular lesion present singly **called single sore** or **uta** in peru (local name).
- It's not affecting oro-nasal mucosa.

➢ **Reservoir:** Domestic dog.

➢ **Transmission:** By bite of sand fly like *Lutzomyia noguchi.*

d. ***L. brasiliensis pifanoi*:**

➢ **Severity:** Malignant form.

➢ **Features:**

- It produces the lesion similar to lepromatous leprosy **called leishmaniasis diffusa** or **diffuse cutaneous leishmaniasis** (**vide supra**).
- By many scientists it is not accepted s valid subspecies.

e. ***L. brasiliensis mexicana*:**

➢ **Severity:** Benign form.

➢ **Features:**

- It is single papular lesion present on skin at the site of bite like face, ear & hand **called bay sore.**
- It's not affecting oro-nasal mucosa.
- It healed with production of scar.
- Person recovered from *L. tropica* is immune to *L.maxicana.*

❖ **Laboratory diagnosis:**

I. Direct methods

➢ **Specimens:** Biopsies or tissues from the edge of lesion of skin or mucosa.

➢ **Testing methods:**

A. **Microscopy:**

✪ **Preparation of smear from specimens**

✪ **Staining of smear:**

- Stain by Leishman stain and examine under oil immersion lenses.
- Intracellular amastigote is examined in macrophage of skin & mucosa.
- Amastigote are very few in bay sore & uta.

B. Culture: → Vide supra

II. Indirect methods

➢ **Testing methods:**

A. Blood picture: Normal cell count.

B. Serological tests: Are useful like ELISA.

C. Skin (Allergic) test:

i. Leishmanin test/reaction: Positive skin test after intradermal injection of suspension of promastigote of *Leishmania brasiliensis*.

❖ **Prevention:**

- General measures are same as kala azar.
- Polyvalent vaccine: It is prepared by using 5 *Leishmania* strain & successful reports are achieved of removal of cutaneous leishmaniasis from Bihar, India.

❖ **Treatment:** Same as kala azar.

a. Pentavalent antimonial resistant: Moderately effective.

b. Amphotericin B: Bets alternative drug.

c. Glucocorticoid: In case of respiratory complication.

Question bank

Case study

1) A 55 years old male presents with nodular swelling over feet. Examination revealed pallorness, splenomegaly, oedema feet. Haemogram revealed anaemia, 5% Hb, neutropenia & agrnulocytosis. Blood microscopy shows the LD body. Identify the organism & answer the following

a) Name the causative agent.
b) Describe the life cycle of causative agent.
c) Write the pathogenicity causative agent.
d) Describe the lab. diagnosis of causative agent.

Essay/Full question

1) Blood and tissue flagellates.
2) *Trypanosoma.*
3) *Leishmania.*

Short notes

1) Classification of haemoflagellates.
2) Morphology / life cycle / pathogenicity/Lab. diagnosis of *T. brucei* or *T.cruzi.*
3) Morphology / life cycle / pathogenicity/Lab. diagnosis of *L. donovani.*
4) Post kala azar dermal leishmanoid.
5) Oriental sore.
6) Espundia.

Short questions for theory/viva questions

1) Name two haemoflagellates & two intestinal flagellates.
2) Write the vector of *T. brucei* & *T. cruzi.*
3) What are Winterbottom's sign & Keranadel's sign?
4) What is Roman's sign?
5) Write the difference between gambiense & rhodesiense strain.
6) What is blood incubation infectivity test?

MCQs for chapter review

Classification

1) Animal disease produced by *T. brucei* is known as
(a) Chaga's disease (b) Nagana (c) Sleeping sickness (d) None of above

2) Mucocutaneous leishmanisasis is caused by (PGI-97)
(a) *L. braziliensis* (b) *L. tropica* (c) *L. donovani* (d) *L. orientalis*

3) Oriental sore is caused by
(a) *L. donovani* (b) *L. tropica* (c) *L. brasiliensis* (d) *L. infantum*

4) Nasopharyngeal leishmanisasis is due to
(a) *Leishmania braziliensis* (b) *Leishmania tropica* (c) *Leishmania chagasis* (d) *Leishmania donovani*

Trypanosoma

5) Tse tse fly transmit
(a) *Trypanosoma brucei* (b) *T cruzi* (c) Kala azar (d) Oriental sore

6) Sleeping sickness is transmitted by (PGI-86)
(a) Tse tse fly (b) House fly (c) Sand fly (d) Simulium fly

7) Winter bottom's sign in sleeping sickness refers to
(a) Unilateral conjunctivitis (b) Posterior cervical lymphadenopathy (c) Narcolepsy (d) Transient erythema

8) Vector of *T cruzi*
(a) Reduvid bug (b) Tse tse fly (c) Sand fly (d) Hard tick

9) Reduvid bug is a vector for the transmission of (AIIMS-05)
(a) Relapsing fever (b) Lyme's disease (c) Scrub typhus (d) Chaga's disease

10) Roman's sign present in
(a) *L. donovani* (b) *T. brucei* (c) *L. infantum* (d) *T. cruzi*

Leishmania

11) Aflagellar stage of *L. donovani* is known as
(a) Amastigote stage (b) Promastigote stage (c) a+b (d) None

12) Amastigote forms are seen in (PGI, June-01)
(a) *Leishmania donovani* (b) *Toxoplasma gondii* (c) *Leishmania major* (d) *Entamoeba*

13) Amastigote form is seen in
(a) RE system (b) WBC (c) RBC (d) Macrophage

14) The most important reservoir of leishmaniasis in India is
(a) Dogs (b) Rodents (c) Acute visceral leishmaniasis (d) Case of post kala azar dermal leishmaniasis

15) Double rise of temperature in 24 hours is seen in case of
(a) Kala azar (b) Malaria (c) TB (d) Hodgkin's lymphoma (e) Brucellosis

16) Which of the following is most severely affected in kala azar
(a) Spleen (b) Liver (c) Adrenal gland (d) Bone marrow

17) The followings tests help in laboratory diagnosis of kala azar except (AI-02)
(a) Bone marrow examination (b) Immobilisation test (c) Blood smear examination (d) Aldehyde test

18) In case of kala azar aldehydes test becomes positive after
(a) 2 weeks (b) 4 weeks (c) 8 weeks (d) 12 weeks

19) Drug not used in visceral leishmaniasis (AIIMS, Nov-09)
(a) Sitamoquine (b) Paromycin (c) Miltefosine (d) Hydroxy chlorquine

20) **Visceral leishmaniasis** (PGI, May-13, Dec-02)
(a) Caused by *L. tropica* (b) Post leishmaniasis dermatitis is common (c) Antimonial are useful drugs (d) Diagnosed by blood smear (e) Vector is *Phlebotomus sergenti*

21) **The followings are true of kala azar except**
(a) Persistent hyper gamma globulinemia (b) Pancytopenia (c) Cancrum oris can occur (d) Full treatment prevents post kala azar dermal leishmaniasis

22) **True about visceral leishmaniasis** (PGI, Dec-02)
(a) Neutropenia (b) Eosinophilia (c) Hyper gamma globulinemia (d) Skin hyperpigmentation (e) Lymphadenopathy

Answers of MCQs & explanation

1) **(b)**
2) **(a)**
3) **(b)**
4) **(a)**
} Follow section, **classification** for explanation

5) **(a)**
6) **(a)**
} All the strains of *T cruzi* are transmitted by tse tse fly but species are different

7) **(b)**

- Follow section, ***Trypanosoma brucei gambiense* (pathogenicity →clinical features)** for explanation

8) **(a)**
9) **(d)**
} Follow section, ***Trypanosoma cruzi* (pathogenicity →mode of transmission & life cycle)** for explanation

10) **(d)**

- Follow section, ***Trypanosoma cruzi* (pathogenicity →clinical features)** for explanation

11) **(a)**
12) **(a) & (c)**
13) **(a) & (d)**
} Follow section, ***Leishmania donovani* & *Leishmania tropica* (morphology & table-3)** for explanation

14) **(c)**

- Follow section, ***Leishmania donovani* (pathogenicity → Reservoir of infection with ecological types of kala azar)** for explanation

15) **(a)**
16) **(a)**
} Follow section, ***Leishmania donovani* (pathogenicity →clinical features)** for explanation

17) **(b)**
18) **(d)**
} Follow section, ***Leishmania donovani* (diagnosis)** for explanation

19) **(d)**

- Follow section, ***Leishmania donovani* (treatment)** for explanation

20) **(c), (d) & (e)**
21) **(d)**
22) **(a), (c), (d) & (e)**
} Follow section, ***Leishmania donovani*** for explanation

86 Ciliatea

Learning heading & subheadings

- Definition:
- Classification:

Balantidium coli

Definition: Thin, delicate & hair like process covers the body of parasites **called cilia** & such parasites **called ciliatea.**

Classification:

I. **Systemic classification:** **Follow chapter → Introduction and classification of parasites** **(Section →Table-3)**

II. **Pathogenic classification:** *Balantidium coli.*

Balantidium coli

❖ **History:**

- It was 1st described by Malmsten in 1857 from the stool of two dysenteric patients.
- It was also discovered by Leuckart in 1861 & by Stein 1862, who classified the species in to the genus *Balantidium*.

❖ **Geographical distribution:** Worldwide.

❖ **Habitat:** Large intestine (caecum & colon).

❖ **Morphology:** It exist in two forms **(fig.-1).**

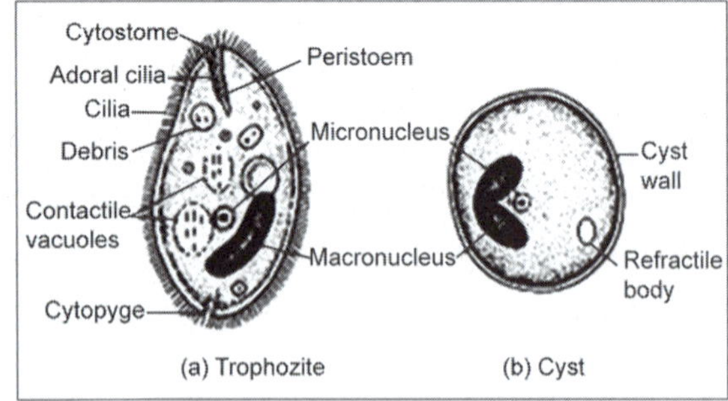

Figure-1: Morphology *B. coli*

I. Trophozoite stage

➢ **Found in:** In dysenteric stool.
➢ **Size:** 60-70µm in length & 40-50µm in breadth. It is the largest protozoan.
➢ **Shape:** Oval.
➢ **Motility:** Resembles a 'thrown football'.
➢ **Structure:** → **Fig.-1 (b)**

✪ **Ends:** Narrow anterior end & broad posterior end.

✪ **Surfaces:**

- Surface is covered with thin, delicate & hair like process **called cilia.**
- Cilia are shorter over entire body but longer at mouth part.
- Cilia are acts as organ of locomotion.

✪ **Contains:** Body organs, cytoplasm & nucleus.

A. **Organs:** Following are the features of alimentary system.

- **Peristome:**
  - Anterior end present with a groove like structure **called peristome.**
  - Cilia present at the peristome **called adoral cilia.**
  - It represents the mouth **called cytostome** & terminating in to a short funnel shaped gullet **called cytopharynx.**
  - It extends up to one third of body.
- **Cytopyge:** At the posterior end there is a anus (but no intestine) **called cytopyge.**
- **Nutrition:** It eats the intestinal bacteria, RBCs & epithelial cells,

B. **Cytoplasm:** Divided in two portions **[fig.-1 (a)].**

i. **Endoplasm:** → **Fig.-1(a)**

- **Definition:** Internal, granular portion of cytoplasm **called endoplasm**.
- **Functions:**
  - Nutrition.
  - Excretion.
  - Reproduction.
- **Contains:**
  - RBCs.
  - WBCs.
  - Food debris from host's gut & tissue debris.
  - Two nucleuses.
  - Two contractile vacuoles: one near the posterior end & 2nd in middle of the body.

ii. **Ectoplasm:** It presents as external thin layer.

C. **Nucleus:**

- **Numbers:** Two nuclei.
- **Location & shape:** Lager one is kidney- shape & situated in the middle of the body **called macronucleus** & smaller is spherical & situated in the concavity of macronucleus **called micronucleus.**

II. Cyst stage

➢ **Found in:** In chronic cases & carrier.
➢ **Size:** 50-60µm.
➢ **Shape:** Spherical or oval.
➢ **Structure:** → **Fig.-1 (b)**

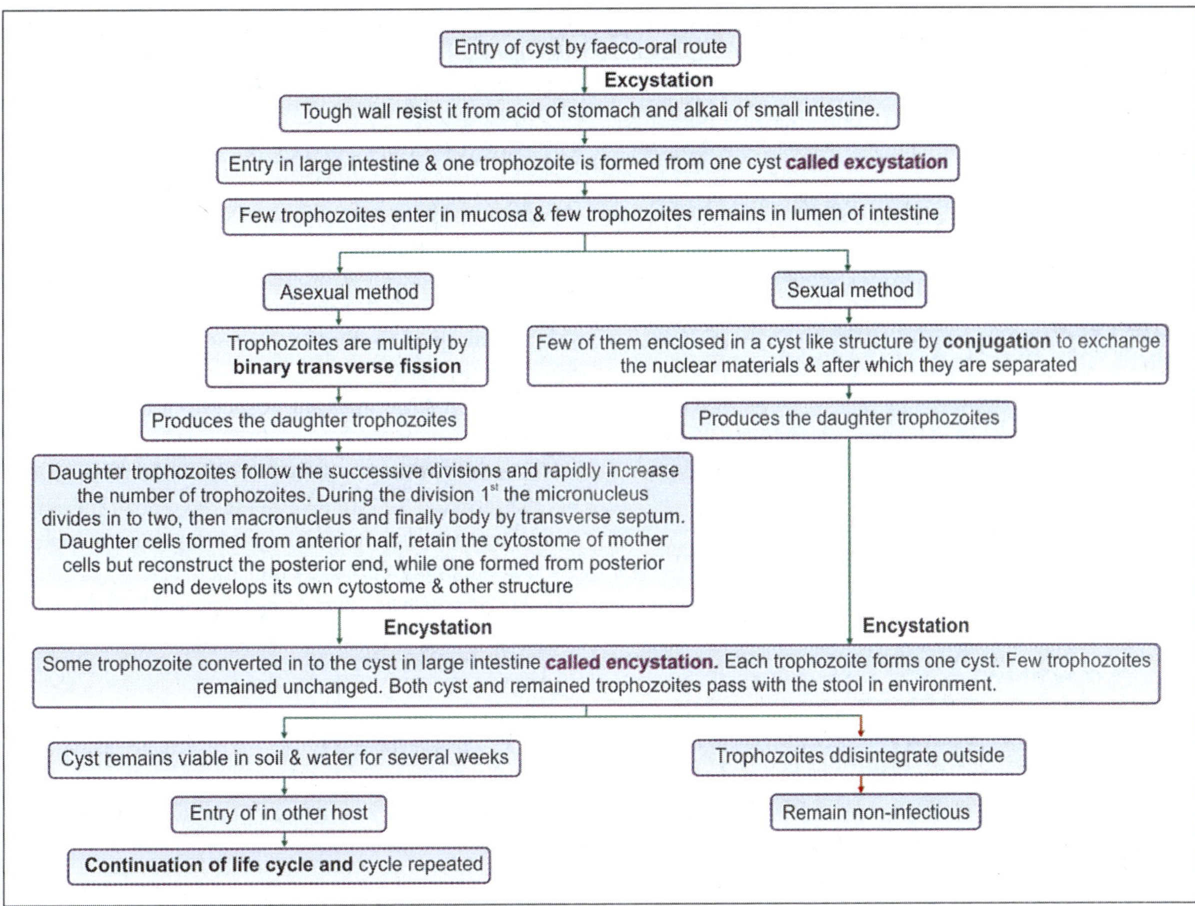

Flow chart-1: Life cycle of *B. coli*

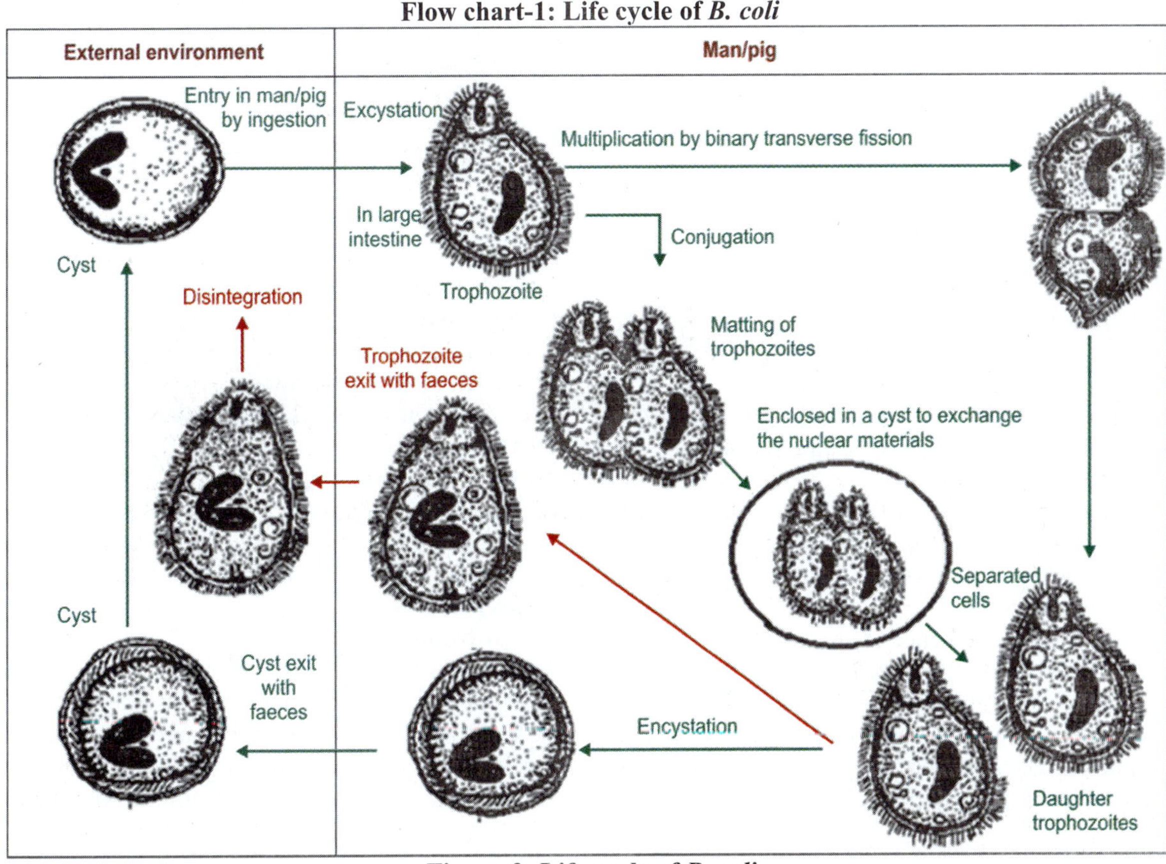

Figure-2: Life cycle of *B. coli*

- **Cyst wall:** Cyst surrounded by thick transparent double layered wall.
- **Contains:**
- Cytoplasm is granular & contains the two nuclei & refractile body.
- Contractile vacuoles remain active for some time during encystment.

❖ **Culture:** *B. coli* can be grows in media of *E. coli.*

❖ **Life cycle:**

➤ **Host:** Only one host is pig, while man is the incidental host; however it having two stage of life cycle of which trophozoites exist in host (in pig or in man) & cystic stage in environment.

➤ **Method of reproduction:** Two types.

a. **Asexual method:** Binary transverse fission.

b. **Sexual method:** By conjugation.

➤ **Cycles: → Flow chart-1, 2 & fig.-2**

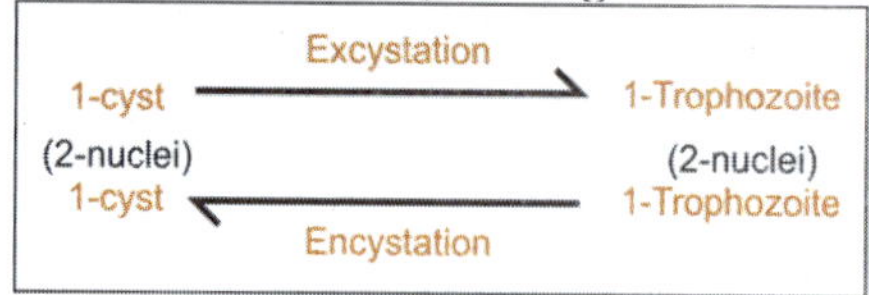

Flow chart-2: Excystation & encystation

❖ **Pathogenicity:**

➤ **Disease name:** **Called balatidiasis or ciliate dysentery.**

➤ **Reservoir of infection:**
- Mainly pig, however parasite is non-pathogenic to pig.
- Rarely monkey & chimpanzee are also the reservoirs.

➤ **Source of infection:** Food & water.

➤ **Mode of transmission:**
- **Ingestion:** By ingestion of contaminated food & water contains cyst from pig/man.
- **Contact:** By occupation contact with pig.
- It transferred from pig to pig, pig to man, man to man or man to pig.
- Cyst is the infective (transmitting) stage.

➤ **Incubation period:** Few days to week.

➤ **Exit form:** Trophozoites & cyst in faeces.

➤ **Infective form:** Cyst.

➤ **Portal of entry:** GIT.

➤ **Sites: → Follow habitat**

➤ **Precipitating factors (epidemiological determinants):**

i. **Agent factors (virulence factors):**

1. **Tough cyst wall:** Protects it from gastric acid of stomach & high alkalinity of small intestine.
2. **Enzymes:** Parasite secretes an enzyme **called hyaluronidase**, which degrades the intestinal mucosa and facilitates penetration.

ii. **Host factors:**

1. **Concurrent infection:** Presence of *T. trichuria* in intestine, encourage the tissue invasion by *B. coli.*
2. **Nutritional:** Like absence of starchy food in intestine.

- Parasite thrives mainly on starchy food found in plenty in pig's intestine.
- **Hoare** stated that presence of abundant fat in pig's intestine renders it harmless, while scarcity in human makes it pathogenic for man.

➤ **Pathology:** *Balantidium* ulcer has following pathological findings.

✪ **Macroscopic:**
- **Sites:** In large intestine (caecum or colon).
- **Size:** Varying from small to large.
- **Shape:** Similar to amoebic ulcer like **flask shape**
- **Extension of ulcers:** May extend mucosa, sub mucosa & sometimes up to muscularis mucosae. Parasite is not able to enter the liver.

✪ **Microscopic:** Presence of necrosed tissues in ulcer.

➤ **Clinical features: → Flow chart-3**

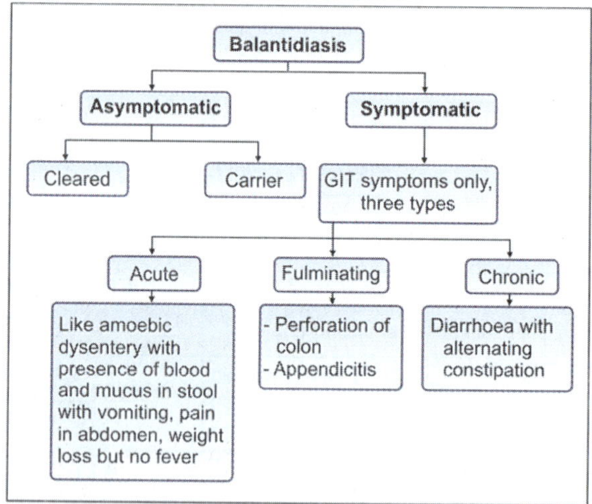

Flow chart-3: Clinical features of balantidiasis

❖ **Laboratory diagnosis:**

➤ **Specimens:**
- **Stool:**
- Collected after defecation.
- Contains both cysts & trophozoites.
- **Mucosal biopsy:** Collected by sigmoidoscope.

➤ **Testing methods:**

A. **Macroscopy of stool:** Presence of blood & mucus in stool.

B. **Microscopy of stool by normal saline preparation:**

1. **For trophozoites:**

- Motile trophozoites will be detected under normal saline preparation in fresh stool.
- **Disadvantage:** Major drawback of stool examination is that parasites shed intermittently & undergoes the rapid degeneration. Trophozoites are not found in stool after 6 hours of its passage.

- **Rate of detection:** Rate of detection of trophozoites to cysts in stool is 9:1.

2. **For cysts:** Cysts are also present in stool.

C. **Culture: →Vide supra**

D. **Serological tests:** Are not useful tests.

Question bank

Case study

1) A female patient with abdominal pain, diarrhoea, vomiting without fever. Stool examination revealed presence of blood, mucus & trophozoites with thrown football like motility. Identify the organism & answer the following.

a) Name the causative agent & describe the morphology of causative agent.
b) Describe the life cycle of causative agent.
c) Write the pathogenicity causative agent.

Essay/Full question

1) *B. coli.*

Short notes

1) Life cycle / pathogenicity / laboratory diagnosis of *B. coli.*

Short questions for theory/viva questions

1) Name the method of reproduction for *B. coli.*
2) Name the organ of locomotion for following parasites.
   - *B. coli* - *E. histolytica*
   - *T. cruzi* - *G. lamblia*
3) Name the type of motility for following parasites.
   - *B. coli* - *T. vaginalis*
   - *E. histolytica* - *G. lamblia*

MCQs for chapter review

Morphology

1) **Numbers of nuclei in the cyst of *B coli***
   (a) 2 (b) 4 (c) 6 (d) 8

Answers of MCQs & explanation

1) **(a)**
- Follow section, ***Balantidium coli* (morphology → cyst stage)** for explanation

87 Blood inhabiting sporozoa

Learning heading & subheadings

- Introduction:
- Classification of sporozoa:

Plasmodium spp.

Babesia spp.

Introduction:

- Reproduction in this group of parasites take place by asexual method (**called schizogony**) & sexual method (**called sporogony**) **called alteration of generation.**
- Products of schizogony **called merozoites** & productss of sporogony **called sporozoite.**
- Bothe these methods are take place in different host **called alteration of host.**

Classification of sporozoa:

I. Systemic classification: **Follow chapter → Introduction and classification of parasites** **(Section → Table-3).**

II. Pathogenic classification: Two groups.

A. Blood inhabiting sporozoa: Following are **pathogenic** species.

i. *Plasmodium:* Around 172 species under the genus *Plasmodium,* few of them are listed below.

a. Common species infecting man:

✪ **Benign tertian malaria:** Less dangerous & recur after 48 hrs or 3rd day.

1. *P. vivax:*
- Described by Grassi & Feletti in 1890.
- Causing vivax malaria.
- **Meaning:** From **vivere = to live**, indicates the activity of movement (especially amoeboid form).

2. *P. ovale:*
- Described by Stephens in 1922.
- Causing ovale tertian type /ovale malaria.
- **Meaning:** Because it is oval in shape & also makes the infected RBCs in oval shape.

✪ **Malignant tertian malaria:** More dangerous (most virulent) & recur after 48 hrs or 3rd day.

1. *P. falciparum*:
- Described by Welch in 1897.
- **Meaning:** From **falx = sickle,** because having sickle shaped gametocytes.

✪ **Benign quartan malaria:** Less dangerous & recur after 72 hrs or 4th day.

1. *P. malariae*:
- Described by Laveran in 1880 (Noble Prize in 1907) & Grassi & Feletti in 1890.
- Causing malariae malaria.

b. Rare species infecting man:

✪ **Benign tertian type:**
- *P. cynomolgi:* Mayer (1907).
- *P. cynomolgi bostianellii:* Garnham (1959).

✪ **Ovale tertian type:**
- *P. simium:* Fonseca (1951).

✪ **Quartan type:**
- *P. inui:* Halberstadter & Von Prowazek (1907).
- *P. brasilianum:* Gonder & von Berenberg - Gossler (1908).
- *P. shortii:* Bray (1963).

✪ **Quotidian type:**
- *P. knowlesi:* Sinton & Mulligan (1932).

ii. *Babesia:* *B. bovis, B. divergens, B. microti, B. canis, B. equi.*

✓ **Note:** Few persons divided the genus ***Plasmodium*** in to two sub genus as follows

1. ***Plasmodium:*** *P. vivax, P. malariae & P. ovale.*
2. ***Laverania:*** *P. falciparum.*

B. Gastrointestinal sporozoa:
- Following are **pathogenic** species.
- More details: **Follow chapter → Gastrointestinal sporozoa.**

i. *Isospora:* *I. belli, I. hominis & I. natalensis.*
ii. *Cyclospora:* *C. cayetanensis.*
iii. *Toxoplasma:* *T. gondii.*
iv. *Cryptosporidium:* *C. parvum.*
v. *Sarcocystis:* *S. suihominis, S. bovihominis & S. lindermanii.*
vi. Unclassified: *Pneumocystis carinii.*

Plasmodium spp.

❖ History:

- In 1880, In Algeria Alpnonse Laveran, a French army surgeon, discovered the malarial parasite in RBC of patient. Name of discoverers & year of discovery of important species of *Plasmodium* were described earlier with the pathogenic classification.

- In 1886 Golgi in Italy described the asexual development of the parasites in RBCs (erythrocytic schizogony), hence it also **called Golgi cycle.**
- In Russia, in 1891, Romanowsky developed the staining method of malarial parasite.
- In Secundarabad, India, in 1897, Ronald Ross identified the developing stage of malarial parasite in mosquito & he described the mode of transmission. This led to discovery of mosquito control measures to eradicate the malaria. Ronald Ross got Noble prize in 1902.

I. Human cycle or schizogony cycle or asexual cycle or golgi cycle

Entry of sporozoites in man by the bite of mosquitoes (female anopheles) and later they pass by following four stages

A.Pre-erythrocytic schizogony:

- Sporozoites before entering in to the RBCs, they enter in to liver cells **called pre-erythrocytic schizogony**.
- During this stage parasites are not found in blood, patients is asymptomatic without any clinical findings or pathological changes and transfusion of blood during this stage does not allows the transmission of malaria, hence **called sterile blood**. Sporozoites are multiply by asexual method (**called schizogony**) and converted in to pre-erythrocytic schizont (mature liver schizont) and merozoites.
- **Duration of stage:** 8 days in *P. vivax*, 9 days *P. ovale*, 6 days *P. falciparum* and 14-16 days *P. malariae.*
- Liberated parasites **called merozoites** (also **called cryptozoites**) which are two types.

Larger one **called macromerozoites** re-enters in liver to start exo-erythrocytic schizogony.

Smaller one **called micromerozoites** enters in to RBCs by a process of invagination to start erythrocytic schizogony

Parasites reside in RBCs and pass through the following stages

B. Erythrocytic schizogony:

- Few micromerozoites are converted in to trophozoite (Also **called ring forms**) schizont merozoites.
- During this stage patient feels the clinical attack of malaria **called overt malaria** & can transmit the infection.
- **Duration of stage**: In *P. vivax*, *P. oval* and *P. falciparum* last for 48 hrs and in *P. malariae* for 72 hrs.
- **Duration of presence of asexual forms in thick blood smear after completion of pre-erythrocytic stage**: After 12 days in *P. vivax* and After 9 days in *P. falciparum.*
- Cycle is continue for considerable time by re-entry of merozoites in RBCs or may end due to exhaustion of asexual reproductive capacity of parasites or spontaneous destruction.

C. Gametogony:

- Few micromerozoites are converted in to male and female gametocytes. (These are immature and still in the RBCs of capillaries of internal organs like spleen & bone marrow).
- Gametocytes become mature in 4 days and available free in peripheral blood and can transmit the infection to others, so **called carrier stage of malaria.**
- Gametocytes do not cause any febrile illness and this stage is for continuation of life cycle (mosquito cycle) after taking entry in mosquito. They are most numerous about 1000/cmm, in early stage of infection (not increased with time).

D. Exo-erythrocytic schizogony:

- After the establishment of erythrocytic schizogony, this stage disappear in *P. falciparum* so no relapse while in *P. vivax*, *P. oval* & probably in *P. malariae* it persist in liver and responsible for relapse.
- This stage never arises from erythrocytic schizogony but it provides the asexual parasites in absence of fresh infection to start the erythrocytic schizogony. Liberated (micromerozoites) parasites **called merozoites** (also **called phanerozoites**) which are again of two types like micro and macro.
- Many micromerozoites remain dormant in liver for very long time **called hypozoites** are responsible for latent infection / recrudescence. (**Note:** Latent infection in *P. falciparum* is due to dormant form of parasite remain in RBCs)

II. Mosquito cycle or sporogony cycle or sexual cycle

- Ingestion of mature microgametocytes (**called male gametocytes**) and macrogametocytes (**called female gametocytes**) along with blood in midgut (stomach) of mosquito by bite. One microgametocytes produces 4-8 microgametes by a process **called ex-flagellation** & one macrogametocytes produces only one macrogametes.

Microgamates attract towards the macrogamates by a process of chemotaxis and resulting fusion cells **called zygot**

After 24 hrs, zygot lengthens and converted in to a form **called ookinete** (Still outside the stomach's mucosal cells)

Release the proteolytic substances, enters in to the mucosal cells and becomes intra-cellular **called oocyst**

Oocyst undergoes the meiotic and mitotic divisions (sexual methods) to increase the number of intra-cellular oocyst

Mucosal cells are ruptures and release free oocyst (extra-cellular) in body cavity of mosquito **called sporozoite**

Sporozoites enter in to circulation and distributed in all organs of mosquito (except ovary) with maximum concentration in salivary duct which enters in man by bite to repeat the cycle

Flow chart-1: Life cycle of *Plasmodium* species

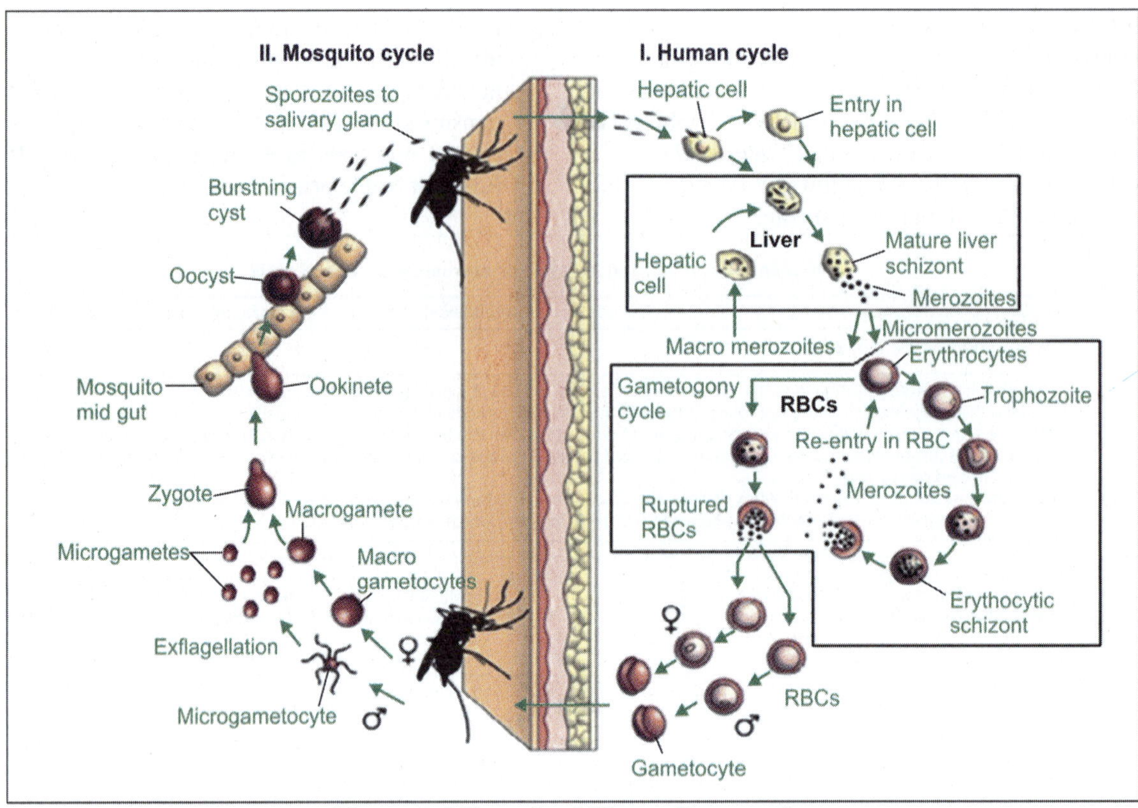

Figure-1: Life cycle of *Plasmodium* species

❖ **Geographical distribution:** Worldwide, mostly in tropical zone extending from 40^0S to 60^0N.

- *P. vivax:* Most prevalent in tropical & subtropical zone like Asia, North America, & Central & South America.
- *P. falciparum:* Up to 80% cases of malaria are due to this species. It is most prevalent in tropical & subtropical zone of Africa, Asia and Central & South America. In India about 50% cases by *P. falciparum*, 4-8% are mixed & rest by *P. vivax.*
- *P. malariae:* It responsible for around 25% of malaria cases and most prevalent in tropical Africa.
- *P. ovale:* It responsible for around 10% of malaria cases and not reported in India.

❖ **Habitat:** Liver, RBCs & later carried to all the organs by blood.

❖ **Life cycle:**

➢ **Hosts:**

✪ **Definitions:**

- *Plasmodium* parasites reproduce by asexual method (**called schizogony**) in intermediate host & by sexual method (**called sporogony**) in definitive host **called alteration of generation.**
- Products of schizogony **called merozoites** & products of sporogony **called sporozoites.**
- Bothe these methods are take place in different host **called alteration of host.**

✪ **Types of host & types of cycle:** Both are two types

I. **Intermediate host:** It is man and cycle **called human cycle** or **schizogony cycle** or **asexual cycle.**

II. **Definitive host:** It is mosquito (female anopheles) and cycle **called mosquito cycle** or **sporogony cycle** or **asexual cycle.**

➢ **Methods of reproduction:** Two types.

a. **Asexual method:** Occurs in human cycle **called schizogony.**

b. **Sexual method:** Occurs in mosquitoe cycle (female anopheles) **called sporogony.**

➢ **Cycle:** Two types as mentioned in **flow chart-1 & fig.-1.**

➢ **Salient features of life cycle:**

I. **Human cycle:**

✪ **Infective form for human:** Sporozoite.

✪ **Phases of human cycle:** Mainly two phases.

A. **Inside the liver:**

1. **Pre-erythrocytic schizogony:** Sterile blood & no clinical attack of malaria.
2. **Exo-erythrocytic schizogony:** Sterile blood & no clinical attack of malaria but cause relapse.

B. **Inside the RBCs:**

1. **Erythrocytic schizogony:**

- Inoculation is positive (case) & clinical attack of malaria (overt malaria).
- Method of entry of merozoites in to RBCs is not clear, because the envelopes remain intact after the merozoites have entered.

2. **Gametogony:** Inoculation is positive (carrier) & it can infect the mosquito.

✪ **Summary of human cycle:**

A. **For:** *P. vivax, P. malariae & P. ovale* **(flow chart-2).**

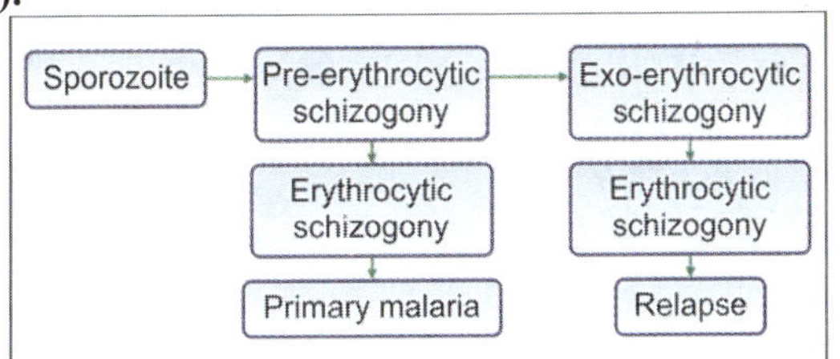

Flow chart-2

B. **For:** *P. falciparum* **(flow chart-3).**

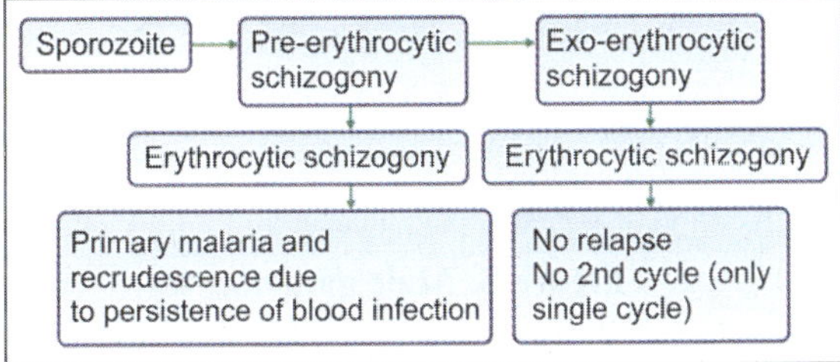

Flow chart-3

II. **Mosquito cycle:**

✪ **Infective form for mosquito:** Male & female gametocyte.

✪ **Other features:**

- It starts in human with formation of gametocytes & enters in mosquito for further maturation.
- Female *anopheles* mosquito ingested by sexual asexual forms, but only sexual forms follows the further development while rest will die immediately.
- To infect the mosquito, human blood should contain at least 12 gametocytes per mm^3 of blood & female gametocytes must be in excess of the male gametocytes.
- Presence of sporozoites in the salivary gland of mosquito is to be taken as a positive proof for epidemiological survey of malaria.
- **Mix infection:** Different malarial species can develop in same mosquito at a time & such mosquito can give rise mixed infection & it is common in *P. falciparum & P. vivax.*

❖ **Culture:**

i. **Culture on media:**

➢ **Aim:** Culture technique is to identify the erythrocytic stage of parasites, so in fact it's not a culture method but concentration method.

➢ **Types:**

a. **Brass & Jone's technique:**

- Invented in 1912.
- Cultivation done in artificial medium.
- **Drawback:** It could not maintain the parasite for more than one cycle.
- Later it was improved by Black in 1945.

b. **Trager &Jensen's technique:**

➢ **Indication:**

1. To differentiate the trophozoite of *P. falciparum & P. vivax.*
2. To obtain the erythrocytic stage for the study of antigenic structure.
3. To prepare the antigen for sero-epidemiological purposes.
4. To anti-malarial drug sensitivity testing.
5. To prepare the vaccine

➢ **History:** In 1976, Trager & Jensen's successfully cultivated the malarial parasite (*P. falciparum*) by continuous culture technique to obtain the erythrocytic stage.

➢ **Medium:** RPMI 1640 (Rose Park Memorial Institute) medium.

➢ **Advantage:**

1. It is a continuous culture & maintains the parasite for more than one cycle.
2. It also useful for other plasmodium species.

➢ **Technique (steps):**

- RBCs infected with malarial parasites are cultivated in petri dish supplemented with human or rabbit or calf serum.
- Plate is incubated in candle jar to provide the 3% CO_2 & 10% O_2.
- Fresh RBCs will be added periodically to maintain the continuous culture & further multiplication of parasites. These parasites retain their infectivity.

ii. **Culture in animals:** Human malarial species can infect the animal & several animal species can be transferred to man (*P. cynomolgi bostianellii* of monkey).

❖ **Morphology:** It exists in two hosts.

➢ **Morphological stages:**

I. **Morphological stages in human:**

A. **Inside the liver:**

i. **Sporozoites:** Entry in human by mosquito bites & multiplies by schizogony.

ii. **Pre-erythrocytic schizonts:** Variable in size.

iii. **Merozoites:**

- End products of schizogony.
- They come out from liver cells.

B. **Inside the RBCs:**

i. **Trophozoites (ring forms):**

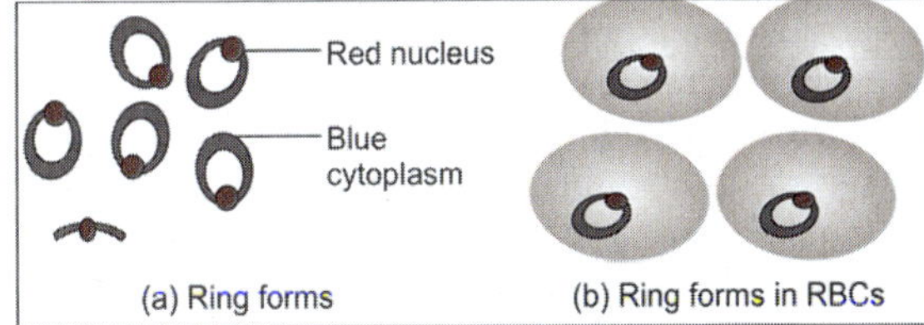

Figure-2: Ring forms of trophozoites

- **Types:** Two forms.

1. **Early (young) forms:**

- It contains blue cytoplasmic ring, red nuclear mass (**fig.-2**) & unstained area **called nutrient vacuole.**
- Portion of the cytoplasm of RBCs, unoccupied by the parasites undergoes degenerative changes & gives dotted or stippled appearance (**called Schuffner's dots** in *P. vivax,* **called Maurer's dots** in *P. falciparum,* **called Ziemann's dots** in *P. malariae* & **called James's dots** in *P. ovale*).

2. **Late (growing/mature) forms:** In a later stage they are active & produces different forms in different species as follows.

- With amoeboid movement inside the RBCs by pseudopodium like process in *P. vivax* **called amoeboid forms.**
- In *P. falciparum,* it remains like ring forms but with enlarge size. Late trophozoite stage & schizonts are present in the capillaries of internal organs hence not identified in peripheral blood smear.
- In *P. malariae,* it stretches within the RBCs & gives the band like appearance **called band forms.**
- In *P. ovale,* it gives ribbon like appearance **called ribbon forms.**

ii. Schizonts:

- **Meaning:** From Greek word schizein = dividing.
- **Definition:** Initial stage of malarial parasites in RBCs **called schizonts.**
- **Types:** Two types.

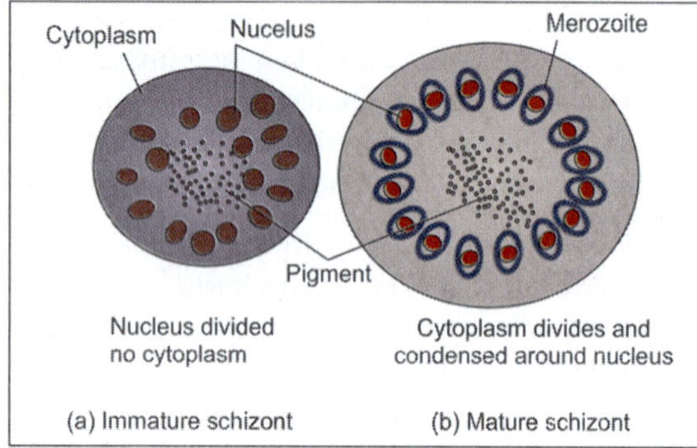

Figure-3: Schizonts

1. **Immature schizonts [fig.-3(a)]:** Initial stage, when only nucleus divides not the cytoplasm.
2. **Mature schizonts [fig.-3(b)]:**

- Later stage, when cytoplasm divides & condenses around the nucleus.
- Ultimately newly formed nucleus along with surrounding cytoplasm covered by cell membrane.
- Pigments are present in cytoplasm.

iii. Merozoites: →**Fig.-4**

- **Definition:** Newly formed parasites containing nucleus along with surrounding cytoplasm released after rupture of host cell **called merozoites.**
- **Shape:** Oval shape.
- **Size & numbers per cells:** Varies depending on the species of malarial parasites.

iv. Gametocytes:

- **Definition:** When malarial parasites enter in RBCs, instead of merozoites few are converted in to sexual forms **called gametocytes.**
- **Types:** Two types as shown in **table -3.**

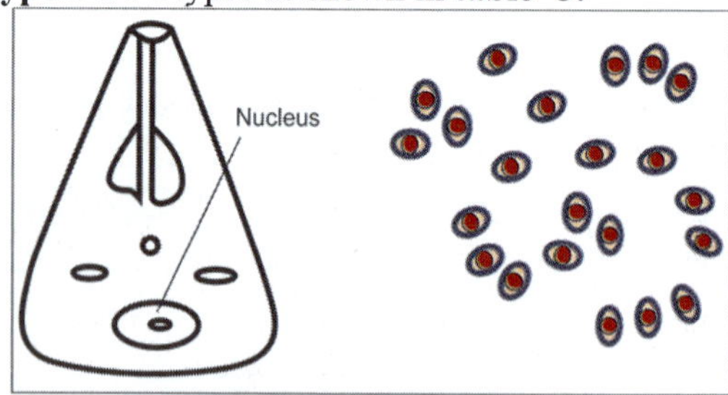

Figure-4: Merozoites

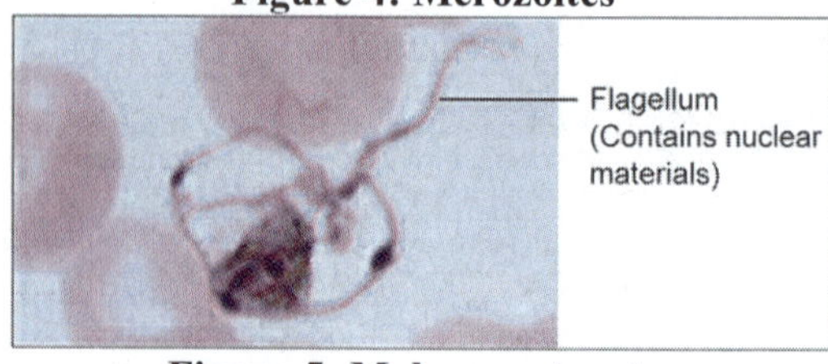

Figure-5: Male gametocytes

II. Morphological stages in mosquito:

i. Male gametes:

- **Synonym:** Microgametes.
- **Definition:** After removal of flagella, (**called exflagellation**) male gametocytes **(fig.-5)** are converted in to a form, **called male gametes.**
- **Method of development:** By exflagellation.
  - **Meaning:** Casting of cilia or flagella.
  - **Definition:** Formation of microgametes by extrusion of nuclear material present in peripheral process resembling flagella **called exflagellation.**
  - One male gametocytes will produces 6-8 male gametes.

ii. Female gametes:

- **Synonym:** Macrogametes, because comparatively larger in size.
- One female gametocyte will produces one female gamete.

iii. Zygote:

- Microgametes are attracting toward the macrogametes by a process of chemotaxis.
- Fusion take place between microgametes & macrogametes and resulting body **called zygote.**
- It developed in 20 minutes -2 hrs after mosquito's blood meal in mid gut (extracellular).

iv. Ookinete:

- **Synonym:** Formerly **called vermicule.**
- **Definition:** Zygote lengthens & matures to form structure **called ookinete.**
- **Mechanisms of entry in to mucosal cells:**
  - Howard (1906) suggested that mucosal cells engulf the ookinete.
  - Garnham *et al* (1962) suggested that it enters in to the mucosal cells by secretion of proteolytic substances from anterior end.

- **Shape:** Elongated.
- **Size:** 10-12μm in length.
- **Structure:** → Fig.- 6

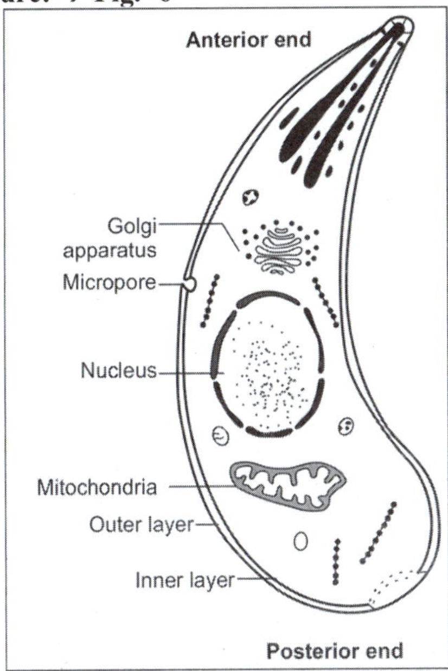

Figure-6: Ookinete

- **History:** It was defined by Garnham *et al* (1962) under electron microscope.
- **Layers:** Two layers with outer corrugated & inner smooth layer.
- **Anterior end:** Inner layer appears more dense & to split **called mouth.**
- **Peripheral fibrils:** Hollow structure with 55-65 in numbers.
- **Nucleus:** Granular with nucleolus.
- **Cytoplasm:** Crystalloid in nature & contains mitochondria, lysosomes & black pigments.

v. Oocyst:

- **Definition:** Ookinete enters inside the mucosal cells of mid gut of mosquito, which **called oocyst.**
- **Shape:** Spherical mass.
- **Size:** 6-12μm in length.
- **Structure:** It contains single vesicular nucleus & pigment granules.

vi. Sporozoite:

- **Shape:** Slender banana shaped.
- **Size:** 10-12μm in length.
- **Structure:** → Fig.- 7

- **History:** It was defined by Garnham *et al* (1960) under electron microscope.
- **Layers:** Two layers with outer corrugated & inner strong layer.
- **Anterior end:** Cup like depression **called apical cup.**
- **Peripheral fibrils:**
  - Hollow structure.
  - Contractile or tensile in nature.
  - Function: Locomotion.
  - Numbers:

1. *P. vivax:* 11 (10+1).
2. *P. ovale:* 13 (12+1).
3. *P. falciparum:* 15 (14+1).
4. *P. cynomolgi bastianellii:* 11 (10+1).

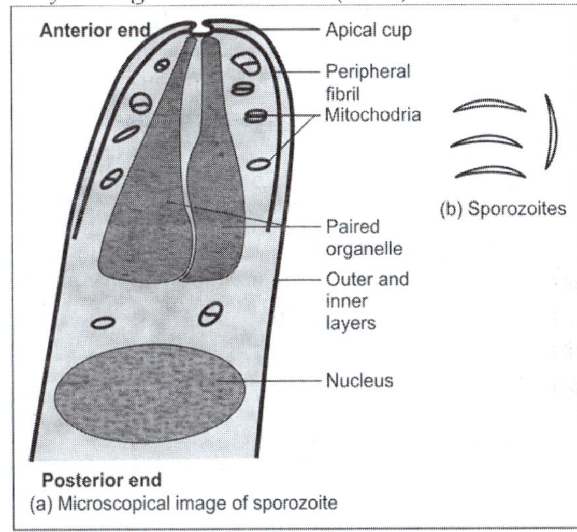

Figure-7: Sporozoite

- **Paired organelles:** Contains the proteolytic enzymes for penetration in to host cells.
- **Nucleus:** Present in well marked pit.
- **Cytoplasm:** Contains mitochondria (Source of energy), lysosomes & black pigments.

➢ **Comparison of morphological stages in each species:**

A. **Pre-erythrocytic schizogony: Table-1**
B. **Erythrocytic schizogony: Table-2 & fig.-8**
C. **Gametogony: Table-3 & & fig.-9**
D. **Exo-erythrocytic schizogony: Table-4**

Features	*P. vivax*	*P. falciparum*	*P. malariae*	*P. ovale*
Duration	Single cycle last for 8 days	Single cycle last for 6 days	15 days	9 days
Pre-erythrocytic schizonts	42μm in diameter	60μm in length & 30μm in breadth	- 22μm in diameter (This stage was not observed in man, but observed by Garnham in 1951 in chimpanzee after intravenous inoculation of sporozoites)	70-80μm in length & 40-50μm in breadth
Merozoites	12,000 (numbers)	40,000	2,000	15,000

Table-1: Pre-erythrocytic schizogony

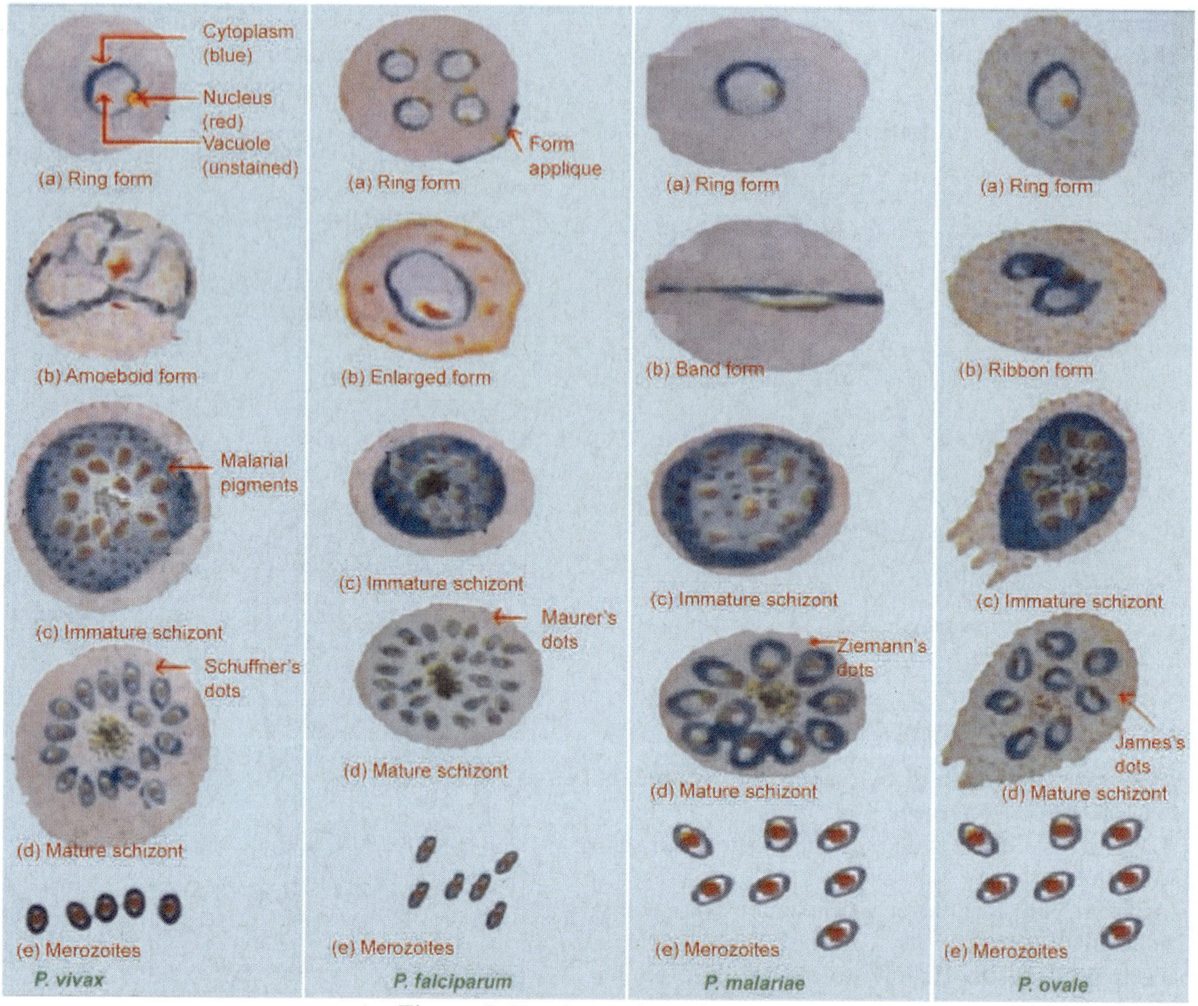

Figure-8: Erythrocytic schizogony

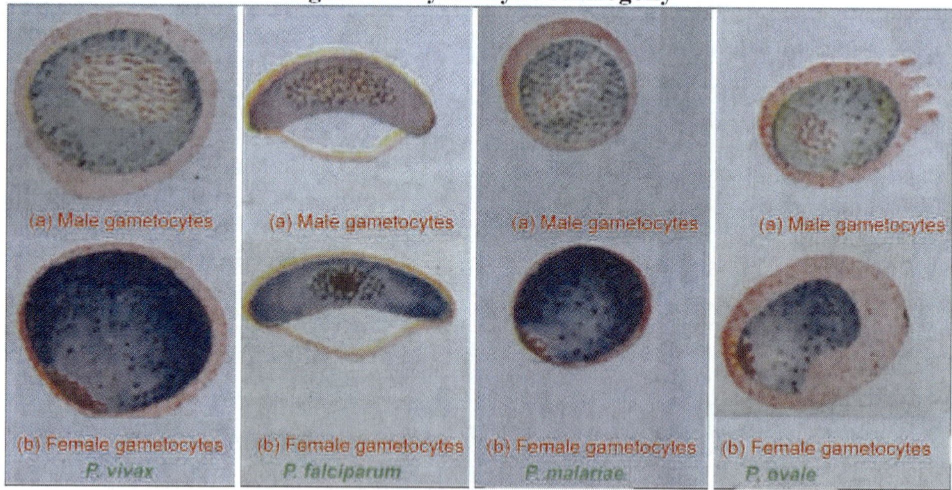

Figure-9: Gametogony

✓ **Note:** In *P. falciparum* late trophozoite stage & schizonts are present in the capillaries of internal organs, hence not identified in peripheral blood smear & also it's difficult to estimate the parasitic burden by peripheral blood smear examination. All infected RBCs adhere to venous wall & to other RBCs causing rosette formation.

Features	*P. vivax*	*P. falciparum*	*P. malariae*	*P. ovale*
Type of RBCs infected	Young RBCs & reticulocyte. 1-2% of total RBCs are infected. One parasite will infect one RBC	Young & old RBCs & reticulocytes. Multiple (2-6) parasites infect one RBC	Mature & older RBCs. 1% of total RBCs are infected	Young RBCs
Changes in infected RBCs	- **Size:** Double than normal - **Shape:** Irregular /Rhomboidal - **Colour:** Pale / Colourless - **Unoccupied cytoplasm:** It becomes stippled / dotted **called Schuffner's dots,** which stains pink by Leishman's stain	- **Size:** Unaltered - **Shape:** Crenated appearance at periphery in a cells containing large size ring - **Colour:** Reddish violet - **Unoccupied cytoplasm** Becomes stippled / dotted **called Maurer's dots** & stains brick red by Leishman's stain	- **Size, shape & colour:** Unaltered - **Unoccupied cytoplasm:** It becomes stippled /dotted **called Ziemann's dots,** which stains brick red by Leishman's stain	- **Size:** 24% enlargement than normal - **Shape:** Oval with fimbriated edge - **Colour:** Eosinophilic - **Unoccupied cytoplasm:** Becomes stippled / dotted **called James's dots** which stains in violet colour
Duration	2 days (48 hrs)	36-48hrs	3 days (72 hrs)	2 days (48 hrs)
Development	Parasite pass through trophozoite → schizont → merozoite	Parasite pass through trophozoite → schizont → merozoite	Pass via trophozoite → schizont → merozoite	Parasite pass through trophozoite → schizont → merozoite
Trophozoites	• **Types:** Two types **1. Early / young form: Called ring form** - **Shape:** Ring shape - **Size:** 2.5-3μm - **Leishman's stain:** Blue cytoplasmic ring & red nucleus, situated at thinner part of the ring & central unstained area of parasite **called vacuole** **2. Late (growing / mature) form: called amoeboid forms** - Active amoeboid movement inside the RBCs by pseudopodium like process hence the name - Yellowish brown pigment production	• **Types:** Two types **1. Early / young form: Called ring form** - **Shape:** Ring shape - **Size:** 1.25-1.5μm - **Leishman's stain:** Blue cytoplasmic ring & red nucleus, situated beyond the ring or outside the ring & central unstained area of parasite **called vacuole.** Parasite often attach to the margin/edge of host cell with nucleus & few part of cytoplasm remain outside **called form appliqué or accole** **2. Late (growing / mature) form:** No active amoeboid form but enlarged ring (4μm) with dark brown/black pigment	• **Types:** Two types **1. Early / young form: Called ring form** Same as like P. vivax **2. Late (growing / mature) form: called band forms** - Parasite often stretch within the RBCs & assuming the band like appearance - Dark brown or black colour pigment production	• **Types:** Two types **1. Early / young form: Called ring form** Same as like P. vivax **2. Late (growing / mature) form: called ribbon forms** - Parasite gives ribbon like appearance - Coarse & dark brown colour pigment production
Schizont	• Parasites lose all vacuoles, amoeboid activities & becomes round in shape • Pigments are scattered throughout the cytoplasm • **Types & other details:** **1. Immature:** } Vide **2. Mature:** } supra - Size: 9-10μm - RBCs burst to release the daughter cell **called merozoites**	• Parasites lose all vacuoles. • Pigments are arranged in the central part of cytoplasm • **Types & other details:** - Like *P. vivax* but smaller size (4.5-5μm) - RBCs burst to release the daughter cell **called merozoites**	• **Types & other details:** - Like *P. vivax* but smaller size (6.5-7μm) - When maturation is completed, RBCs unable to hold the weight & burst to release the daughter cell **called merozoites**	• **Types & other details:** - Like *P. vivax* but smaller size (6.2μm) - When maturation is completed, RBCs unable to hold the weight & burst to release the daughter cell **called merozoites**
Merozoite	- Oval mass of cytoplasm with central nucleus - **Size:** 1.5-1.75μm length & 0.5μm breath - **Numbers:** 12-24	- Oval mass of cytoplasm with central nucleus - **Size:** 0.5-0.7μm in diameter - **Numbers:** 18-24	- Oval mass of cytoplasm with central nucleus - **Size:** 2-2.5μm - **Numbers:** 6-12	- Oval mass of cytoplasm with central nucleus - **Size:** 2-2.5μm - **Numbers:** 8

Table-2: Erythrocytic schizogony

Features	*P. vivax*		*P. falciparum*		*P. malariae*		*P. ovale*	
Pre - patent period	- Gametocytes appear in peripheral blood after 16 days of inoculation of sporozoites or 4-5 days after the initial appearance of the asexual parasites in thick smear or from the 1st day of fever.		Gametocytes appear in peripheral blood after 21 days of inoculation of sporozoites or 10 days after the initial appearance of the asexual parasites in thick smear.		Gametocytes appear in peripheral blood few days after the 1st attack of fever			
Survival of game-tocytes in human blood	If not taken up by mosquito, it will not survive longer than a week in human blood.		If not taken up by mosquito, it will survive up to 30-60 days or longer in human blood.					
Features			- Gametocytes are sickle shape **called crescent** - They are larger than the size of RBCs & can stretch from one side & their remain can present as arched rim on concave side		-Female is comparatively large - No enlargement of host cell			
Types of gameto-cytes	Male (Gives 1 gametes)	Female (Gives 6-8 gametes)	Male	Female	Male	Female	Male	Female
Also called	**Micro-gameto cyte**	**Macro-gameto cyte**	**Micro-gametocyte**	**Macro-gametocyte**	**Microgame tocyte:** Male is comparative ly smaller & other features are same as like *P. vivax*	**Macrogam etocyte:** Female is comparative ly large & other features are same as like *P. vivax*	**Microgame tocyte:** Same as like *P. vivax* & *P. malariae* but small size of infected cell with irregular outlines& gametocytes	**Macroga metocyte:** Same as like *P. vivax* & *P. malariae* but small size of infected cell (oval shaped) & gametocyt es
Shape	Oval	Oval	Sickle shape & blunt ends	Sickle shape, pointed ends				
Size	Smaller, 9-10μm	Larger, 9-12μm	Smaller, 8-10μm by 2-3μm	Larger, 10-12μm by 2-3μm				
Cytoplasm	Stain light blue	Stain deep blue	Stain light blue	Stain deep blue				
Nucleus	Compact & small	Diffuse & large	Spread as fine granules over wide area	Condensed in small compact mass in centre				

Table-3: Gametogony

Features	*P. vivax*	*P. falciparum*	*P. malariae*	*P. ovale*
	- Morphology is similar to erythrocytic schizogony. - This stage is not observed in human liver, it was observed by Rodhain (1956) in the liver of chimpanzee, 9 months after intravenous inoculation of sporozoites of *P. vivax,* - It is responsible for relapse	Not occurs in this species & no chances of relapse	Nothing is known about this phase, but relapse can occur & parasite can persist for 32 years or 55 years or even for life (Garnham, 1966)	This stage is discovered in liver but relapse do not occur (?)

Table-4: Exo-erythrocytic schizogony

❖ Immunology:

➢ **Immunity:** Two main types of immunity

I. **Innate / native immunity (biological resistance against malaria):**

✪ **Definition:** Resistance to malarial infection in a species/race/individual due to genetic or constitutional make-up.

- **Examples:** Some individual living in the endemic (Like Africa) areas producing innate resistance against malaria, by following mechanisms. Increase in the incidence of below mentioned conditions in the population, spared the death due to malaria

1. **Haemoglobin S (Hb S) gene:** Genetical abnormalities in RBCs (sickle cell anaemia) provide protection against *P. falciparum*.
2. **Thalassaemia gene:** Interference with synthesis of normal Hb & persistence of foetal haemoglobin (Hb F) provide protection against *P. falciparum*.

3. **Glucose -6-Phosphate Dehydrogenase (G6PD) enzyme's deficiency:** Enzyme required for parasites to utilise glucose (glycolysis).
4. **Duffy blood group antigen (alleles Fy^a & Fy^b):** It provides receptors for attachment of *P. vivax*. Its absence resist merozoite invasion.
5. **Ovalocytosis gene:** Where RBCs are rigid & resist merozoite invasion.
6. **HLA:** Possession of class-I HLA-BW53 & class-II HLA-DRBI 1302, are believed to be protects against malaria.
7. **Deficiency of Para Amino Benzoic Acid (PABA):**
- PABA is required for metabolism of parasite during erythrocytic phase.
- It's absence in mother's milk, provide protection to child against malaria.

II. Acquired immunity:

✪ **Definition:** Resistance to malarial infection that an individual acquired during life.

✪ **Types:**

A. Active immunity: Resistance developed due to antigenic stimulation.

i. Natural:

- **Definition:** Resistance developed due to malarial infection.
- **Examples:**

a. Humoral immunity: It is specific against particular species of parasites.

♣ **Antigens:**

- Properties of antigens:
  - Soluble in nature.
  - Present in sera of patients & detected by Ouchterlony double diffusion precipitation method.
  - Also can be extracted from infected RBCs.
- Types: In 1969, Wilson et al classified following three types of antigens of *P. falciparum* according to heat susceptibility.

1. **Labile (L) antigen:** Destroyed by heating at 56^0C for 30 minutes. It is further divided in to two sub classes like La (4 antigens) & Lb (3 antigens).
2. **Resistant (R) antigen:** Tolerate 56^0C for 30 minutes.
3. **Stable (S) antigen:** Not destroyed by heating at 100^0C for 5 minutes.

♣ **Antibodies:** Antibodies are following two types, reported by Mc Gregor & Wilson in 1971.

1. **Protective antibodies:**

- Properties of antibodies:
  - Antibody to La Antigen is protective type.
  - IgG in nature, it can cross the placenta & provides the congenital immunity (→**Vide infra**).
- Actions of antibodies: Following are the antibodies produced in response to *Plamsmodium* infection.
  - Antibodies against merozoites: Preventing reinvasion of RBCs.
  - Antibodies against erythocytic schizonts: Promoting the phagocytosis of parasites cells or intracellular death of parasites.
  - Antibodies against sporozoites are also believed to be produced.
  - Children in malarial endemic area, who suffer repeatedly by malarial parasites from the age of few months, will develop the immunity by 6 years of age due to presence of toxic product. However this immunity is not long lasting because the toxic product can neutralised. It doesn't provide the protection against the reinfection but minimise the severity of symptoms.

2. **Diagnostic antibodies:**
- IgM & IgG in nature.
- Diagnosed by precipitation test.

b. Cell mediated immunity: T cells play an important role in CMI.

ii. Artificial: Development of artificial active immunity against malarial parasites by using vaccine is still under trial.

B. Passive immunity: Resistance transmitted in readymade form.

i. Natural:
- New born infant below 6 months is protected by transfer of readymade IgG antibodies of La antigen (**called congenital immunity**) from immune mother via milk or placenta.
- Almost all new born infant in Gambia, Hyperendemic *P. falciparum* area showed specific IgG antibodies in their sera.

ii. Artificial: Development of artificial passive immunity against malarial parasites by using immunoglobulin is still under trial.

➢ **Phagocytosis:** Macrophages of liver & spleen phagocytose the infected cells, parasites & malarial pigments.

➢ **Premunition:**

- Synonym: Infection immunity or concomitant immunity.
- Definition: "Relative resistance offered by host to re-infection already harbouring the microbes."
- Properties:
  - Immunity to re-infection lasts as long as active infection is present, once active infection cured patients become susceptible to subsequent infection by same organisms.
  - However, Shortt & Garnham reported that immunity in malaria may be complete or last for some time even after disappearance of parasites.

➢ **Hypersensitivity:**
- Type –III hypersensitivity reaction **called malarial nephrosis** occurs in *P. falciparum* infection.
- It is due to deposition of antigen - antibody complex in glomerular capillary basement membrane.

- Glomerular injury caused by complement activation (β_1, C globulin) & release of enzymes from granules of leucocytes (Reported by Giglioli 1962 & Cameron 1972).

➢ **Autoimmunity:** Development of auto-antibody to RBCs in pregnant women in *P. falciparum* infection **called autoimmune haemolytic anaemia**

➢ **Immunodeficiency:**

1. **No development of antitoxin to TT:**
   - Immunosuppressive effect of malarial parasites has been reported by McGregor I.A. & Burr M. in 1962, in their following experiments.
   - Tetanus Toxoid (TT) failed to produce antitoxin in Gambian (type of *T. brucei*) children with malaria.
2. **Burkit's lymphoma:**
   - Hyperendemic malaria prevalent in **Africa** is impairing the immune system of children & co-infection with Epstein –Barr Virus (EBV) produces the Burkit's lymphoma.
   - Immunosuppressive effect of malarial parasite allows the virus proliferation & interference with immune mechanisms to neoplastic cells.
3. **Antagonism between malaria & visceral Leishmaniasis:** Such antagonism increases the immunologically competent cells.
4. **Secondary bacterial infection:** Due to immunodeficiency status.

➢ **Tolerance:** Cessation of clinical phenomenon despite parasitaemia due to active immunity by cellular & humoral mechanisms & also due to concomitant presence of parasites.

❖ Pathogenicity:

➢ **Disease name:** Disease **called malaria** & according to nature of fever produced by each species the disease is further designated as follows.

✪ **Benign tertian malaria:** Less dangerous & fever recur after 48 hrs or 3rd day.

- **Vivax malaria:** Produced by *P. vivax.*
- **Ovale malaria:** Produced by *P. ovale.*

✪ **Malignant tertian malaria:** More dangerous & fever recur after 48 hrs or 3rd day.

- **Falciparum malaria:** Produced by *P. falciparum.*

✪ **Benign quartan malaria:** Less dangerous & fever recur after 72 hrs or 4th day.

- **Malariae malaria:** Produced by *P. malariae.*

➢ **Meaning:** Malaria derived from italic word **mal = bad & aria = air,** far back in 1753, as it was believed to be caused by foul emanations from marshy soil.

➢ **Nature & history of disease:**

- It occurs in endemic & epidemic (periodic cases with sharp rise) forms.
- WHO classified the following types of endemicity based on spleen rate or parasite rate in children (2-9 years) & adults.

a. **Hypoendemic:** Transmission is low. Spleen or parasite rate is < 10%.
b. **Mesoendemic:** Transmission is moderate. Spleen or parasite rate is 11-50%.
c. **Hyperendemic:** Transmission is intense but seasonal. Spleen or parasite rate is 51-75%.
d. **Holoendemic:** Transmission is of high intensity. Spleen or parasite rate is >75%.

- In India, malaria is continues to be major public health problem. In India, about 27% people lives in high transmission (>1 case / 1000 population) & 58% people lives in low transmission (0-1 case / 1000 population) area.

➢ **Reservoir of infection:**

- Human species of malaria are not harboured by any lower animals; hence man particularly children acts as a reservoir for human infection.
- In some part of Africa, chimpanzees may act as reservoirs for *P. malariae.*

➢ **Source of infection:** Mosquitoes.

➢ **Mode of transmission:** It is discussed with natural & therapeutic type of malaria.

A. **Natural malaria:** Two ways of classification.

i. **According to mode/route of entry of parasites:** Following two categories.

a. **Direct:**

1. **Injection:**
   - By contaminated (through blood) needles or syringes in intravenous (IV) drug users.
   - Injection of secretion of salivary glands containing sporozoites will also induce the infection.
2. **Vertical or transplacental:** Placental defect allow the transmission of malarial parasites from mother to baby **called congenital malaria.** Healthy placenta acts as a barrier for malarial parasites.

b. **Indirect:**

1. **Vector borne:**

✪ **History: Vide supra (history)**

✪ **Vector's name:** Female *Anopheles* mosquito.

✪ **Vector's species:** More than 10 species of *Anopheles* mosquito are responsible for the transmission in India by bite.

- *A. cu<u>l</u>cifacies* (In rura<u>l</u> area, **Mnemonic: ll**).
- *A. stephe<u>n</u>si* (In urba<u>n</u> area, **Mnemonic: nn**).
- *A. philipinensis.*
- *A. fluviatilis.*
- *A. varuna.*
- *A. minimus.*
- *A. annularis.*
- *A. leucosphyrus (A. balabacensis).*
- *A. sundaicus.*
- *A. jeyporiensis candidiensis.*

✪ **Method of introduction:**

- Female *Anopheles* mosquito act as a definitive host for malarial parasites.
- It sucks the parasites from human blood during its bite for blood meal purpose.

- Parasite takes 8-10 days for development in mosquito, its presence in salivary gland & to be infective for man. This period **called extrinsic incubation period** (**definition:** →Time taken by vector to become infective after receiving the microorganisms **called extrinsic incubation period**). It depends on environmental conditions.
- During the act of bite mosquito's proboscis pierce the skin & salivary secretion containing the sporozoites is introduced directly in to blood through the puncture wound. However parasites cannot be found in blood after about half an hour.

2. **Vehicle borne:**
- Transfusion of blood containing asexual forms of erythrocytic schizogony **called trophozoite induced malaia** or **merozoite induced malaia.**
- Storage of blood may reduce the infectivity of malarial parasites.
- Infectivity is highest with *P. falciparum* & *P. malariae*, while not more than 2% in *P. vivax*.

ii. **According to entry of morphological stages of parasites:**

✪ **Types:** Following two categories.

a. **Sporozoite induced malaria:**
1. **Injection:** Injection of secretion of salivary glands containing sporozoites will also induce the infection
2. **Vector borne:** Transmission by mosquito bite.

b. **Trophozoite induced malaria:**
1. **Injection:** By contaminated (through blood) needles or syringe in intravenous (IV) drug users.
2. **Vertical or transplacental:** Placental defect allow the transmission of malarial parasites from mother to baby **called congenital malaria.**
3. **Vehicle borne:** Transfusion of blood or blood products.

✪ **Differences between sporozoite & trophozoite induced malaria:** Follow **table- 5.**

Features	Sporozoite induced malaria	Trophozoite induced malaria
Pre - erythrocytic (PE) stage	Present	Absent
Incubation period	Long	Short
Exo - erythrocytic (EE) stage	May be present	Absent
Relapse	May occur	No relapse
Schizonticidal drugs	No radical cure, because of presence of EE stage	Radical cure, because no EE stage

Table- 5: Induction of malaria

B. **Therapeutic malaria:**

✪ **Definition:** Introduction of artificial malarial infection to the man **called therapeutic malaria.**

✪ **Indication:** Mostly in case of neurosyphilis (generalised paralysis of insane) caused by *T. pallidum*.

✪ **Plasmodium species:** *P. vivax* is used for introduction of therapeutic malaria.

✪ **Method of introduction:** Two types of methods.

a. **Sporozoite induced therapeutic malaria:**
1. **Injection:** Injection of secretion of salivary glands containing sporozoites will also induce the infection
2. **Vector borne:** By allowing the laboratory-bred infected mosquito bite to the recipient.

b. **Trophozoite induced therapeutic malaria:**
1. **Vehicle borne:** Transfusion of blood or blood products of infected donor.

➢ **Pre-patent period:**

✪ **Definition:** Time taken by microbes to appear first in blood after infection **called pre-patent period**.

✪ **Pre-patent period in different species: →Table-3**

✪ **Clinical significance:**
- After entry in body parasites are enter in liver & not detected in blood. Patient remains **asymptomatic** during this time. Parasites appear in blood after few days of infection.
- It is a part of intrinsic incubation period.

➢ **Intrinsic incubation period (incubation period):**

✪ **Definition:** Interval between entry of microorganisms & appearance of 1st clinical features **called incubation period**.

✪ **Incubation period in different species:**
- In *P. vivax*: 8-17 (average 14) days.
- In *P. falciparum* (shortest): 9-14 (average 12) days.
- In *P. malariae* (longest): 18-40 (average 28) days to 6 weeks.
- In *P. ovale*: 16-18 (average 17) days.

✪ **Effective factors:** It depends on many factors like
- **Numbers of parasites injected:** Long incubation period about 38 weeks has been noticed in European stain of *P. vivax* & *P. falciparum* which indicates that numbers of sporozoites injected may have relation with incubation period.
- **Use of antimalarial drugs:** Long incubation period also noticed in person who used antimalarial drugs.

➢ **Exit form:** Gametocytes.

➢ **Infective form:** Sporozoites.

➢ **Portal of entry:** Skin.

➢ **Site:** First in liver cells then in RBCs.

➢ **Precipitating factors (epidemiological determinants):** Occurrence of malaria depends on chain of following factors. Breaking of this chain at any point can prevent the spread of malaria.

a. **Agent (virulence) factors:** Parasite factors include numbers of sporozoites injected & other virulence factors are described with pathogenesis (**flow chart-4**).

- **Features:** It present with high fever, convulsion, dehydration due to vomiting & excessive sweating.

➢ **Relapses in malaria:** Two types.

a. **Recrudescence (latent infection):**

✪ **Definition:** It is a latent (dormant) form of malarial parasites, which activate after 1 year or longer due to impairment of immunity or by any other stimuli.

✪ **Types & reasons:**

1. **Erythrocytic form in *P. falciparum*:** Latent form present in RBCs & activates after 1 year.
2. **Liver form in *P. vivax, P. ovale & P. malariae*:**

- Latent form present in liver **called hypnozoites,** which activate later to produce recrudescence.
- Meaning: Term **"hypnozoite"** is derived from the **Greek** words **hypnos = sleep** & **zoon = animal.**

a. **Recurrence (true relapse):**

✪ **Definition:** It is a repeated attack of malaria.

✪ **Reasons:** It occurs in *P. vivax, P. ovale* & *P. malariae* (?) due to presence of exoerythocytic stage but not in *P. falciparum* due to absence of exoerythocytic stage.

✓ **Note:** As like **relapsing fever** by *Borrelia* species.

➢ **Complications of malaria:**

In general complications by *Plamodium* spp.

↓

Flow chart-4

Complications by *P. falciparum*

Two major complications by *P. falciparum* like pernicious malaria & black water fever.

A. **Pernicious malaria:**

✪ **Definition:** Series of phenomenon occurs during the course of *P. falciparum* infection & if not effectively treated, threatens the life of patient within 1-3 days.

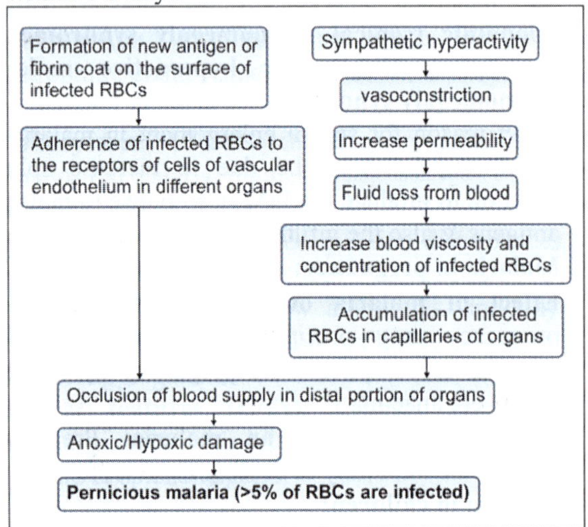

Flow chart-5: Pathogenesis of pernicious malaria

✪ **Pathogenesis:** It is an anoxic damage in internal organs due to capillary blockage & due to decreased effective circulating blood volume by different mechanisms as shown in **flow chart-5.**

✪ **Clinical types & pathological changes in different system:** Following are three different types.

i. **Cerebral type:**

a. **Brain in cerebral malaria:**

✪ **Macroscopic:** Cut section shows the following features.

- **Colour:** Slate-grey or black due to deposition of pigments.
- **Haemorrhage:** Multiple small haemorrhages in white matter.
- **Infarct:** Small infarct in brain substances.

✪ **Microscopic:**

1. **Initial stage: →Fig.- 15**

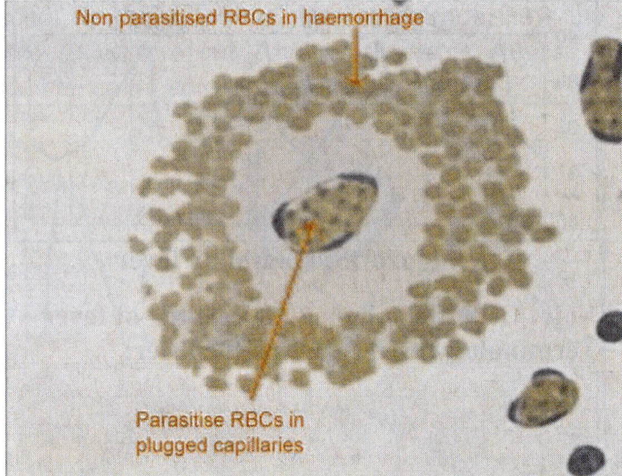

Figure-15: Initial stage in cerebral malaria

- **Dilatation & congestion:**
  - Dilatation & congestion of cerebral capillaries & plugged with parasitized RBCs.
  - It is more in grey matter than white matter.
  - Capillary blood contains parasites with erythrocytic (like trophozoites & schizonts) & gametogony stages.
- **Haemorrhage:** Present around the plugged capillaries **called ring haemorrhage,** which contains non parasitised RBCs.
- **Nerve tissue:** There are scattered areas showing degeneration of nerve tissue, **called soft areas.**

2. **Later stage (reparative stage): →Fig.- 16**

- **Macrophages (glial cells):**
  - Reparative work start in soft areas with infiltration by glial cells **[fig.-16(a)]** & produce the granulomatous structure **called malarial granuloma of Durck [fig.- 16(b)].**
  - All the glial cells are arranged radially around the occluded blood vessels.
  - In advanced cases granuloma terminated in to multiple sclerosis & remains as sequel. Patients may present with psychotic syndrome after recovery from such illness.

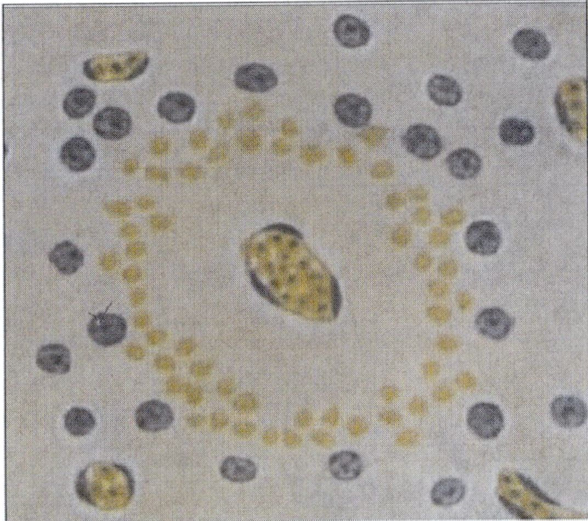

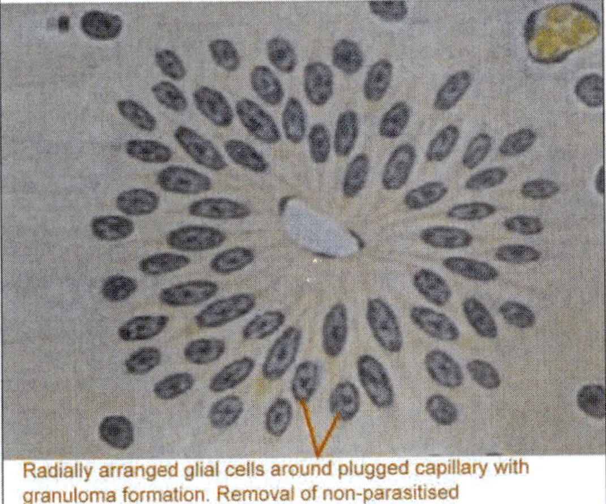

Radially arranged glial cells around plugged capillary with granuloma formation. Removal of non-parasitised
(b) Granuloma formation

Figure-16: later stage in cerebral malaria

ii. Algid type (Algid = Frozen / Cold):

a. Gastro intestinal:

- Slate grey colour mucosa with haemorrhage but no ulceration.
- Capillaries of mucosa & submucosa are packed with parasitized RBCs but capillaries of muscular & serous layer contains very few parasitized RBCs.

b. Adrenal:

- Necrosis of zona fasciculata & haemorrhage with congestion in zona reticulate.
- Capillaries are packed with parasitized RBCs & pigmented phagocytes.

iii. Septicaemic type:

a. Blood: Heavy parasitaemia leading to presence of erythrocytic schizogony & gametogony in blood & anaemia.

b. Heart:

- Macroscopic examination does not show any abnormalities.
- Coronary blood vessels are packed with parasitized RBCs.
- Cardiac muscles show the fatty degeneration & necrosis.

c. Lungs:

- Cut section shows the evidence of haemorrhage & oedema.
- Alveolar capillaries are congested & packed with parasitized RBCs.
- Alveoli contain extra-vasated RBCs & pigmented phagocytes.

✪ **Clinical features:** Following three types according to involvement of organs.

i. Cerebral type: Present with hyperpyrexia, coma & paralysis.

ii. Algid type: Present with cold clammy skin with vascular collapse leading to peripheral circulatory failure with following intestinal varieties.

a. Gastro intestinal:

1. **Gastric/vomitus type:** Present with vomiting.
2. **Choleric type:** Present with watery diarrhoea.
3. **Dysenteric type:** Present with blood & mucus in stool.

b. Adrenal: Peripheral circulatory failure resulting death. It is due to adrenal damage or independent.

iii. Septicaemic type: Present in following forms.

1. **Fever form:** High continuous typhoid like fever.
2. **Haemorrhagic form:** Leading to anaemia.
3. **Cardiac form:** Cardiac syncope.
4. **Pulmonary form:** Pneumonia or pulmonary oedema.
5. **Renal form:** Nephritis or renal failure.

✪ **Laboratory diagnosis:**

- **Specimens & diagnostic features:**

1. **Blood:**
   - Heavy parasitaemia with presence of erythrocytic schizogony & gametogony in blood.
   - Anaemia.
   - Mild leucopenia: total count is 5200/cmm.
2. **Biopsy of internal organs:** It shows the capillary blockage by parasitized RBCs & other changes as described earlier.

✪ **Treatment:**

- Start an intravenous therapy with quinine & antibiotics without delay.
- Blood transfusion including a erythrapheresis and plasmapheresis.

B. Black water fever:

✪ **Definition:** It is a manifestation of *P. falciparum* infection occurs in previously infected patients & characterised by sudden intravascular haemolysis (haemolytic crisis) followed by fever & haemoglobinuria.

✪ **Etiology:** Following are the precipitating factors.

1. **Inadequate quinine therapy:** Occurs in *P. falciparum* infection in non-immune (non-indegenous) individual who resided in malarious countries for 6 months to 1 year & have inadequate prophylactic plus therapeutic dose of quinine for repeated clinical attack.

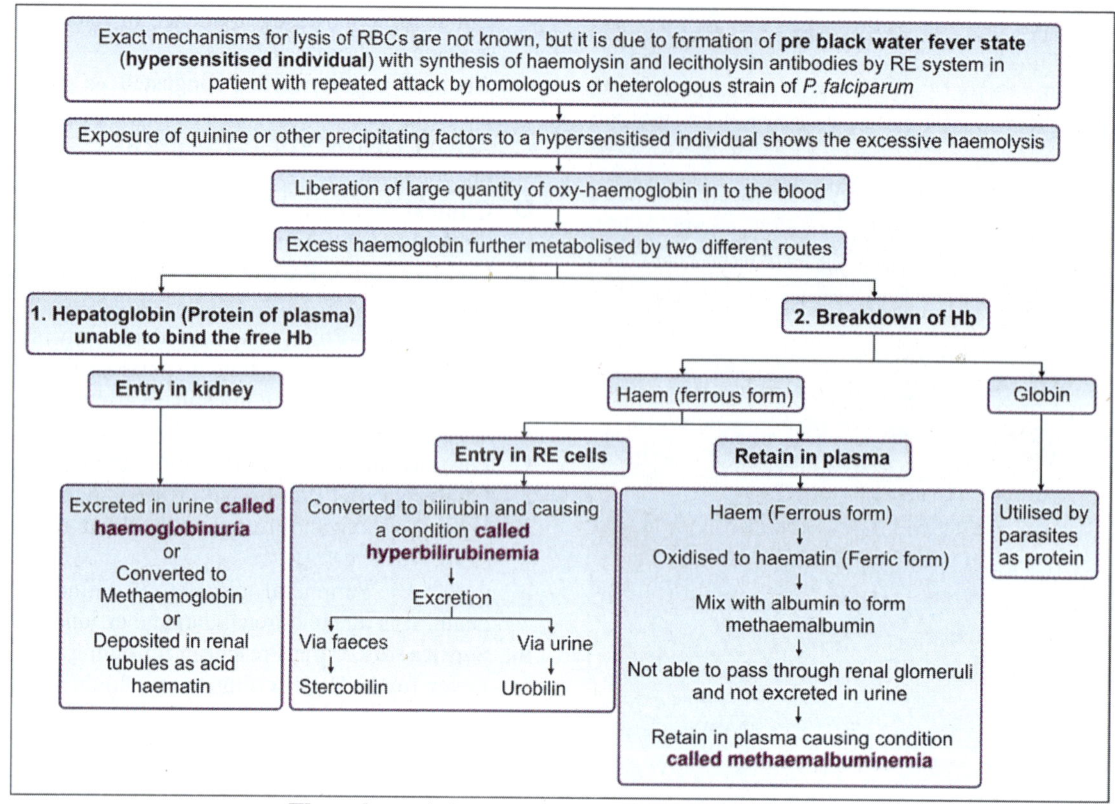

Flow chart-6: Pathogenesis of black water fever

2. **Other contributory factors are**
- Cold.
- Sun exposure.
- Trauma.
- Pregnancy.
- Fatigue.
- Parturition.
- X-ray treatment of spleen.
- Person with G6PD deficiency are also susceptible to this infection.

✪ **Pathogenesis: → Flow chart-6**

✪ **Pathological changes in different system:**

a. Kidneys:
- **Macroscopic:**
  - **Size:** Large.
  - **Colour:** Dark in colour due to congestion & pigmentation.
- **Microscopic:**
  - Degenerative changes in distal convoluted tubules which are blocked with eosinophilic granules (Haemoglobin cast).
  - Parasitised RBCs may or may not be detected in renal capillaries.

b. Liver:
- **Macroscopic:**
  - **Size:** Large.
  - **Colour:** Yellow in colour due to haemosiderin.
  - **Consistency:** Soft.
- **Microscopic:** Necrotic changes in central zone.

c. Gall bladder: Filled with dark green viscid bile.

d. Spleen: Larger in size & dark in colour due to pigmentation.

e. Blood picture:
- **Parasites:** Parasites are not present in blood during haemolytic crisis, but re-appear within a week.
- **Haematology (cytology):**
  - Hb concentration: <10 gm/dl.
  - RBCs counts: 1-2million per cmm. Normocytic anaemia. Polychromasia & basophilic stippling of RBCs.
  - WBCs counts: Moderate degree of neutrophilic leucocytosis.
- **Pigments:** It includes
  - Haemoglobin.
  - Methaemalbumin.
  - Bilirubin (indirect Van den Bergh positive).
  - Absence of methamoglobin.
- **Biochemical reaction:**
  - Increased blood urea.
  - Decreased blood cholesterol.
  - Plasma hepatoglobin is reduced.

f. Urine picture:
- **Parasites:** Not present.
- **Cytology:** No RBCs in urine.
- **Pigments:** It includes.
  - Haemoglobin (red colour of urine).
  - Methaemoglobin: Dark brown / black colour of urine.

- Urobilin with positive testing.
- Absence of methaemalbumin.
- **Biochemical reaction:**
- Colour: Red to brown.
- pH: Acidic pH.
- Amorphous deposit at bottom, when allow to settle.
- Haemoglobin cast: Present.
- Haemetin crystals: Present.

✪ **Clinical features:**
- Fever with rigor.
- Aching pain in the loin region.
- Bilious vomiting (green colour).
- Black urine.
- Icterus.
- Circulatory collapse.
- Acute renal failure (uraemia).
- Acute liver failure.

✪ **Sequelae:**
- Anaemia.
- Pigment calculi.

✪ **Laboratory diagnosis:**
- **Blood picture:** } →**Vide supra**
- **Urine picture:** }

✪ **Prevention:**
- Avoid quinine & use other antimalarial drugs.
- Leave the endemic area & never return back.

✪ **Treatment:**
- Start the chloroquine & in resistant area like South East Asia other drug is advisable.
- Renal failure is the cause of death in black water. Fever; hence patients are treated with artificial kidney or peritoneal dialysis.
- Blood transfusion.
- Intravenous glucose drip is given, but risky in patient with oliguria or anuria.
- Alkalies are also advisable, but toxic to kidney's functions.

❖ Laboratory diagnosis of malaria:

➢ **Specimen & time of collection:**
- Blood is an ideal sample.
- In *P. falciparum,* parasites are present in blood (highest parasite density about 250000 – 300000 per ml than other species) during pyrexial period, so it is good to collect the blood at the height of fever in case of *P. falciparum,* while in case of *P. ovale, P. vivax* & *P. malariae* parasites can be demonstrated during febrile & afebrile period.

➢ **Testing methods:** Two types methods, like direct & indirect.

I. Direct methods

A. Microscopy:

✪ **Types, preparation & staining of smears:** Three types of smears as described below.

i. Thin smear:

- **Indication:** For identification & differentiation of species of parasite.
- **Steps of smear preparation: → Fig.-17**
- Wipe the pulp of finger or ear lobe with alcohol & allowed to dry.
- Prick the pulp of finger or ear lobe with sterile needle or lancet.
- Take a drop of blood on slide at a distance about half an inch from the right side.
- Hold the spreader (slide or cover slip) at 45^0 angle in contact with drop of blood & lower it to 30^0 angle.
- Push the spreader to the left till the blood is exhausted, which makes the tail of tongue shaped smear in centre of slide.
- Allow drying & labelled with pencil.

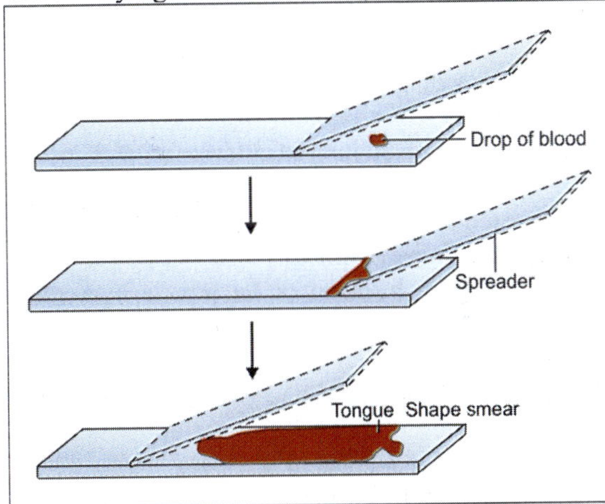

Figure-17: Thin smear

- **Faulty technique:** Do not follow the following steps.
- To large drop of blood.
- Holding the spreader at greater than 45^0 angle.
- Spreading the smear to fast.
- **Properties of ideal smear:**

1. Even & uniform surface.
2. Tail end near about centre of the slide.
3. Consists single layer of RBCs.
4. Margin of the smear do not extend to the sides of the slides.

- **Fixation of smear:**
  - Not required: For Leishman's stain & Field's stain (because already alcohol present in stain, which acts as fixative also).
  - Required: For Giemsa's & JSB stain by following methods.
- For Giemsa stain: Fix with methyl alcohol or ethyl alcohol for 2-3 minutes & dry it.
- For JSB stain: Fix with methyl alcohol for 1-2seconds & dry it.
- **Staining methods:**

a. Leishman's stain:

- History: Named after its discoverer, the Scottish pathologist William Boog Leishman.
- Preparation of stain:
  - Clean all the required container with methyl alcohol
  - Add 100ml methyl alcohol in graduated glass cylinder.
  - Add the 0.15gm powder or 0.15gm tablets of Leishman stain (contains methylene blue & eosin).
  - Mix well till the powder/tablets is dissolved.
  - Incubate at 37^{0}C to dissolve the powder/tablets very rapidly.
  - Store at room temperature in dark.
  - Label it as toxic & flammable.
- Principle of stain: The stain contains chemical like methylene blue & eosin. With ageing or exposure to acids, alkalis or ultraviolet light, a number of oxidation products are formed from methylene blue like methylene blue eosinate, methylene azure eosinate, which gives following colour contrast.
  - Eosin stains RBCs pink.
  - Methylene blue stains the cytoplasm of parasites in blue.
  - Eosin stains nucleus (chromatin material) in red.
- Steps of staining of smear:
  - Pour the stain by drop or by pipette over the dry film & keep for 30 seconds.
  - Dilute the stain with twice its volume of distilled water with neutral/alkaline pH (7-7.2) & keep for 10-15 minutes.
  - Cover it to prevent drying.
  - Wash the slide with tap water & clean the reverse side with sterile cotton wool.
  - Keep the slide in upright position to drain & dry.
  - Examine under oil immersion lens.
- Criteria for ideal staining of smear: Stained slide has bluish violet tinge.
- Uses: To differentiate & to identify
  - *Plasmodium* spp.
  - *Trypanosoma* spp.
  - *Leishmania* spp.
  - Microfilariae.
  - Body cells.

b. Giemsa's stain:

- Steps of staining of smear:
  - Fix the smear with methyl or ethyl alcohol for 3-5 minutes & allowed to dry.
  - Dilute the stain by adding one drop to 1ml of distilled water with neutral/alkaline pH (7-7.2).
  - Pour the diluted stain by drop or by pipette over the dry film & keep for 30-45 minutes.
  - Wash the slide with tap water & clean the reverse side with sterile cotton wool.
  - Keep the slide in upright position to drain & dry.
  - Examine under oil immersion lens.
- **Advantages of thin smear:** Better identification of species, because of clear morphology.
- **Disadvantages of thin smear:** Less sensitive compare to thick smear, because of less numbers of parasites.

ii. Thick smear:

- **Indication:** For rapid detection of parasite.
- **Techniques of smear preparation:** Two ways.

a. By using four drops of blood: →Fig.-18.

- History: This technique was invented by James in 1920.
- Steps:

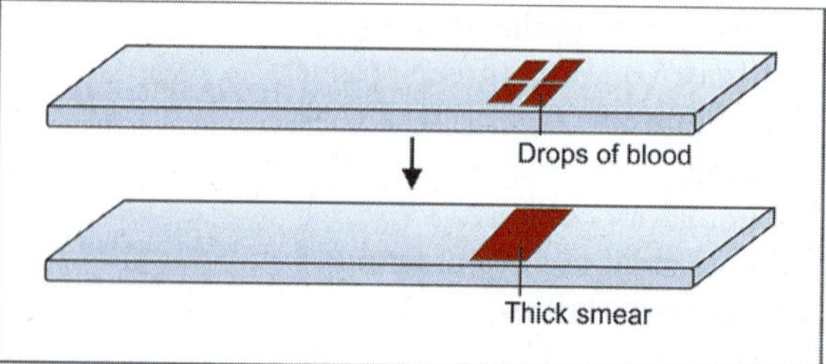

Figure-18: Thick smear with four drops of blood

  - Take four drops of blood on slide.
  - Joining the corners of the drops by using needle or corner of other slide to make an area of a half-inch as shown in **fig.-18.**
  - Labelled with pencil.
  - Allow the smear to dry in horizontal position (at room temperature it takes 30 minutes for drying, which is accelerated by putting the slide in the incubator).

b. By using single large drop of blood: →Fig.-20(b).

- Steps:
  - Take a one large drop of blood on slide.
  - Spread it by using needle or corner of other slide to make an area of a half-inch.
  - Labelled with pencil.
  - Allow the smear to dry in horizontal position (at room temperature it takes 30 minutes for drying, which is accelerated by putting the slide in the incubator).
- **Properties of ideal smear:**
  - It allows the newsprint to be read or wrist watch to be seen through the dry smear.
  - Contains 15-40 WBCs per oil immersion field.
- **Dehaemoglobinisation of smear:**
- Not required: For Field's stain.
- Required: For Leishman's stain & Giemsa's stain by following methods.
  - Flood the smear with the mixture of glacial acetic acid & tartaric acid.
  - Drain off the fluid, as soon as the dehaemoglobinisation is over, which is indicated by the greyish white colour of the film.
  - It is then fixed with methyl alcohol for 3-5minutes.
  - Finally wash the slide by putting it in the vertical position in neutral or slightly alkaline distilled water for 5-10 minutes to remove the minor element of acid.

- Take out the slide when it becomes the white, allow drying followed staining.
- o Preparation of mixture of glacial acetic acid & tartaric acid: Mixture contains 4 parts of 2% glacial acetic acid & 1 part of 2% tartaric acid.

- **Staining methods:**

a. Leishman's stain: } **Vide supra**
b. Giemsa's stain:

c. Field's stain:

- o History: Invented by Field in 1941.
- o Advantages:

1. It is a quick stain.
2. Not required fixation.

- o Reagents: It consist two solutions.

1. Solution A

- Distilled water	500ml
- Methylene blue	0.8g
- Azure I (Azure B)	0.5g
- Disodium hydrogen phosphate (anhydrous)	5g
- Potassium dihydrogen phosphate (anhydrous)	6.25g

2. Solution B

- Distilled water	500ml
- Yellow eosin (water soluble)	1g
- Disodium hydrogen phosphate (anhydrous)	5g
- Potassium dihydrogen phosphate (anhydrous)	6.25g

- o Preparation of stain:
- Dissolve the phosphate salts then add the stain.
- Solution of Azure I may be facilitated by grinding in a mortar with the phosphate solvent.
- Each of prepared solution is filtered & ready for use after 24 hours.
- o Maintenance of stain:
- Repeat the filtration if there is a precipitate.
- Eosin solution should be renewed after development of greenish colour.
- Keep the stain in a jar with wide neck enough to allow the insertion of glass slide.
- Depth of solution is about 3 inches, which is maintained by adding the new stain at time to time.
- o Steps of staining of smear:
- Place the thick smear in solution A for 1-2 seconds (or till the haemoglobin is removed or no any evidence of green colour left).
- Removed the slide & wash with clean water until the stain stop to flow from the film & glass slide is free from stain.
- Place the smear in solution B for 1second.
- Removed the slide & wash with clean water.
- Allow to dry in vertical position.

d. JSB (Jaswant Singh & Bhattcharji) stain:

- o History: Invented by Jaswant Singh & Bhattcharji in 1944.
- o Advantages: Useful for thick & also for combined smear.
- o Reagents: It consist two solutions.

1. Solution I

- Water	500ml
- Methylene blue	0.5g
- Potassium dichromate	0.5g
- 1% Sulphuric acid	3ml
- 1% Potassium hydroxide	10ml

2. Solution II

- Water	500ml
- Eosin (water soluble)	1g

- o Steps of staining of thick smear:
- Place the thick smear in solution I for 10 seconds.
- Removed the slide & wash for 2 seconds with acidulated water with pH 6.2-6.6 adjusted by adding 5% citric or acetic acid.
- Stain the smear with solution II for 1 second,
- Wash with acidulated water in same jar for 5 seconds.
- Place smear again in solution I for 10 seconds.
- Wash the smear as above for 10 seconds or till the smear gives pink background.
- Allow to dry in vertical position & examine.

- **Advantages of thick smear:**

1. More sensitive compare to thin smear, because of more numbers of parasites.
2. One field is equal to 50 fields of thin film, hence it is a quick diagnostic method & useful for mass survey.
3. It also guide for treatment, to know the efficacy of antimalarial drugs.

- **Disadvantages of thick smear:**

1. Species identification can be difficult due to
   - Unclear morphology or unfamiliar setting of parasites.
   - Absence/destruction of RBCs or absence of the outlines of host-RBCs.
2. RBCs are destroyed (or remain unstained) & only elements seen in the smear are stained parasites & WBCs. So relationship of RBCs with parasites or any morphological changes in RBCs are not observed.

iii. Combined smear:

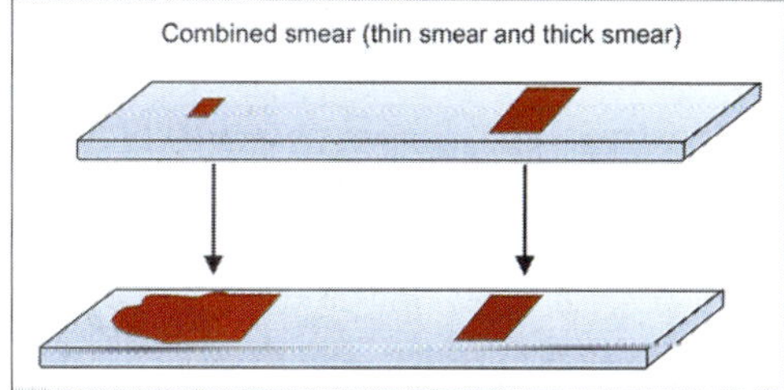

Figure-19: Combined smear

- **History:** Recommended by Sinton in 1925.
- **Indication:** For surveillance work.
- **Techniques of smear preparation:**

- Two drops of blood are taken on slide, one half an inch & second inch from the right end of slide.
- Draw the line with pencil inbetween.
- Make a thick smear from former & thin from later as shown in **fig.19.**

- **Staining:** By using any one of following methods.

a. **Leishman's stain:** First dehaemoglobinise the thick film then poured the undiluted Leishman stain over thin film & after dilution stain is flood over thick film.

b. **Giemsa's stain:** First fix the thin part with methyl alcohol & after drying the whole slide is flooded with diluted Giemsa stain & allow to remains for half to two hours.

c. **JSB (Jaswant Singh & Bhattcharji) stain:**

- Fix the thin smear in a methyl alcohol for 1-2 seconds & dry.
- Place the whole slide in solution I for 30 seconds.
- Removed the slide & wash for 2 seconds with acidulated water (pH 6.2-6.6).
- Stain with solution II for 1 second.
- Wash with acidulated water in same jar for 4 seconds.
- Place smear again in solution I for 30 seconds.
- Wash the smear as above for 10 seconds or till the smear gives pink background.
- Allow to dry in vertical position & examine.

✪ **Comparison of smears: →Fig.-20.**

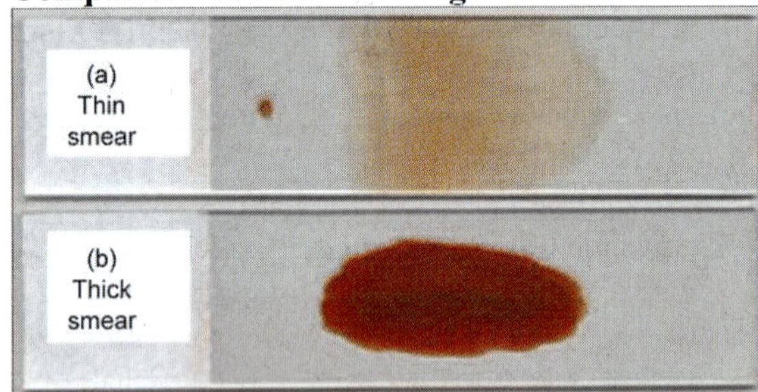

Figure-20: Comparison of thin & thick smear (thick smear → From single large drop of blood)

✪ **Examination of smears:**

✪ **Rules to be adopted: →Flow chart-7**

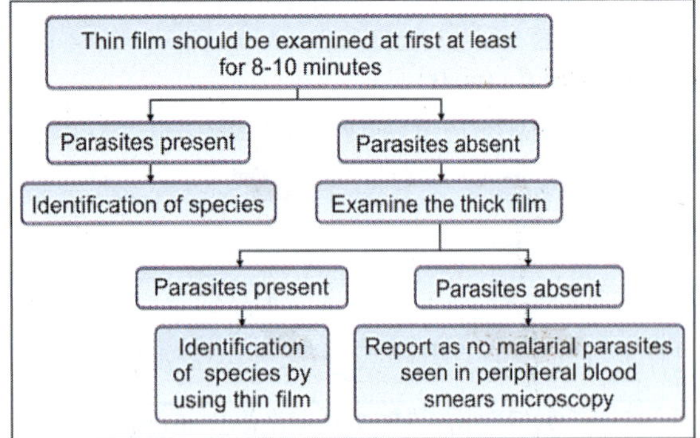

Flow chart-7: Rules for smear examination

✪ **Remarks on the smear examination:**

i. **Thin smear:** Before any slide declared as negative for malarial parasites by thin film, it is desirable to keep following things in mind.

- Area to be examined is upper & lower margins of "tail end", because parasites are maximum in numbers at there.
- Minimum 100 fields should be examined at least for 8-10minutes. It is accepted that in non immune person, at least one parasite is present in 100 fields.

i. **Thick smear:** Thick film is neither a method of choice nor a substitute of thin film. It is a supplementary or actually a concentration method for detection of parasites, as it contains the large numbers of parasites in given field than thin film.

✪ **Examination of smears & appearance of parasites:**

i. **Thin smear: → Fig.-7 & 8**

- **Common features:**
  - Cytoplasm: Blue in colour.
  - Nucleus: Red in colour.
  - Central unstained portion **called vacuole.**
  - Pigment granules: Different in colour.
  - Portion of the cytoplasm of RBCs, unoccupied by the parasites gives dotted or stippled appearance as pink dots (**called Schuffner's dots** in *P. vivax,* **called Maurer's dots** in *P. falciparum,* **called Ziemann's dots** in *P. malariae* & **called James's dots** in *P. ovale*).
  - Round gametocytes in all species, except crescent/sickle shape in *P. falciparum.*
- **Other notable features:**
  - RBCs are almost double in size in *P. vivax.*
  - Multiple invasions of RBCs by ring forms or presence of ring form on surface of RBCs (**called appliqué from or accole form**) in *P. falciparum.*

ii. **Thick smear:** Because of dehaemoglobinisation & lack of fixation, the morphology of the parasite is altered.

- **Trophozoites (early ring form):** Rings are broken & detached nucleus. Variable morphological pattern & certain terms are employed by Field & Fleming in 1938.
  - Comma shape: Curved cytoplasm with red nucleus.
  - Swallow or Gull's wing: Blue cytoplasm on either side of red nucleus like two wings.
  - Exclamatory mark (!): Blue cytoplasmic line with red nucleus at below.
- **Schizonts & gametocytes:** Retain the normal appearance; however appear smaller with irregular outlines.
- **Pigments:** Seen more clearly.
- **RBCs:**
  - Absence of stippling appearance or all dots like Maurer's dots etc.
  - Occasionally in *P. vivax,* outlines of enlarged RBCs (Ghost's cells) with Schuffner's dots are observed.

- **WBCs:** Tattered cytoplasm with deep purple nuclei.
- **Platelets:** Stain purple having woolly texture & outline.

✪ **Grading of smear:** Grade the smear by counting the average numbers of parasites observed per thick film field (100X) as shown in **table-6.**

Grade	Numbers of parasites	Numbers of fields
+	1-10	100
++	11-100	100
+++	1-10	1
++++	> 10	1

Table-6: Grading of malarial smear

✪ **Concentration technique:**
- **Aim:** To increase the chance of parasitic detection
- **Method:**
  - Blood is centrifuged at high speed after collection.
  - Separate the sediment & mix with normal serum.
  - Prepare the smear & examine for parasites.
- **Advantage:** It increases the positivity rate.
- **Disadvantage:** It changes the morphology of parasites.

✪ **Counting of parasites:**
- **Methods:**

a. **By using the WBCs numbers:**
- Count the numbers of parasites against the pre-determined numbers of WBCs in thick film. By this way parasites per µl of blood can be calculated.
- Usually WBCs count are 200, but it can be more in case of low parasitaemia
- Taking WBCs count at 8000/cmm (normal value), the parasite count would be done with following formula.

$$\frac{\text{Number of parasites counted}}{\text{Numbers of WBCs counted}} \times 8000$$

b. **By using the RBCs numbers:** Count the numbers of parasites against the pre-determined numbers of RBCs in thin film. By this way parasites per µl of blood can be calculated by using the same formula.

- **Numbers of parasites in blood:**
  - After pre-patent period: 10 parasites per mm^3 of blood.
  - After intrinsic incubation period: 50 parasites per mm^3 of blood.

✪ **Difficulties in detecting the parasites:** False negative microscopy may be possible in conditions like
- Blood films taken after antimalarial drugs.
- Blood films taken during apyrexial period.
- Blood films taken in initial stage in 2-3 days.

✪ **Difficulties in identifying the species:** It is possible when only few ring forms are available in smear.

B. **Culture: →Vide supra**

II. Indirect methods

A. **Blood picture: →Vide supra** (follow pathological changes in different system).

B. **Serological tests:**

✪ **Indications:** Not useful in diagnosis of acute case, but useful to
- Study the immunological aspects of population living in highly endemic areas.
- To screen blood donor.
- To detect the latent (recrudescence) infection.

✪ **Tests:**

i. **Non- specific tests:**

a. **Melanin flocculation test (Henry's):**

✪ **Principle:** Based on flocculation reaction, to detect the increase the globulin in serum.

✪ **Disadvantages:** Less useful, because false positive result may occurs in
- African Trypanosomiasis.
- Visceral leishmaniasis.
- Hepatitis.

ii. **Specific tests:**

a. **Complement Fixation Test (CFT):** In hyper-endemic area, positive result found in children in whom parasites may or may not be present & also in adult in whom parasites are present.

b. **Passive haemagglutination test:**
- Applicable in *P. falciparum.*
- Positive result indicates recent infection.
- Infected RBCs are agglutinated with homologous antiserum.

c. **Immunofluorescence test:** Both direct & indirect tests are useful.

d. **Gel precipitation test:**
- Applicable by using antigen of *P. falciparum.*
- Highly positive in hyperendemic areas.

e. **Immuno Chromatographic Test (ICT):** Applicable in case of *P. falciparum* by using following antigens.

1. **HRP-2 (Histidine Rich Protein -2) antigen:** Like ParaSight F test & ICT Malaria Pf test,
2. **pLDH (parasite Lactate De-Hydrogenase) antigen:** OptiMAL test.

C. **Molecular tests:** DNA probe & PCR for malaria are also useful.

❖ Prevention:

➢ **General measures (mosquito control measures):**
- More details: Follow chapter → Medical Entomology

➢ **Chemoprophylaxis:**

✪ **Indications:**
- Non immune travellers.
- Non immune persons living in endemic areas for temporary periods like army persons, labour forces etc.
- Pregnant women: *P. falciparum* has serious risk in pregnancy. Start the prophylaxis in 1st trimester & continue till 1 month after delivery.

- **Drugs:** Drugs are used before development of erythrocytic stage.

A. **Causal prophylaxis:** It targets the pre erythrocytic stage in liver. Following drugs are useful as causal prophylaxis.
- Proguanil: For *P. falciparum.*
- Primaquine: For all species.

A. **Suppressive prophylaxis:** These drugs are schizonticides, which suppress the erythrocytic phase & thus prevent the clinical attack of malaria. Following drugs are useful as suppressive prophylaxis.
- Chloroquine.
- Proguanil.
- Primaquine.
- Mefloquine.
- Doxycycline.

➢ **Immunoprophylaxis:** By using malaria vaccine.

- **Introduction:** Most of the vaccine are directed to the *P. falciparum* as it is the most pathogenic species, however vaccine are also developed against *P. vivax, P. ovale* & *P. malariae.*
- **Types:** Following two main types.

A. **Under trial vaccines:** Following four types.

i. **Anti-sporozoite vaccine:**
- **Aim:** Prepared to prevent the human infection at first step by blocking the liver invasion by parasites.
- **Contains:** Vaccine is still under trial & it is prepared by using the following antigens.
  - CS (Circum Sporozoite) protein.
  - TRAP (Thromboplastin Related Anonymous Protein).
  - LSA-1 (Liver Stage Antigen-1).
  - LSA-2 (Liver Stage Antigen-2).
  - SALSA (Sporozoite And Liver Stage Antigen).

ii. **Anti-asexual blood stage vaccine:**
- **Aim:**
  - Prepared to reduce the morbidity & mortality with reduction in severity & complication of disease in children below 5 years of age in endemic country like Africa.
  - Priority is given by WHO to develop such vaccine.
- **Contains:** Vaccine is still under trial & it is prepared by using the following surface antigens of erythrocytic stage (trophozoites, schizonts & merozoites)
  - MSP-1 (Merozoite Surface Protein-1).
  - MSP-3.
  - GLURP (Glutamate Rich Protein)
  - RAP 1/2 (Rhoptry antigen).
  - AMA-1 (Apical Membrane Antigen-1).
  - EBA-175 (Erythrocyte Binding Antigen-175).
  - PfHRA-2 (*P. falciparum* Histidine Rich Protein -2).
  - SERA (Serine Rich Antigen).
  - pf 126.
  - pf 140 (Ag2).
  - pf 332.
  - pf EMP (*P. falciparum* Erythrocyte Membrane Protein).

iii. **Antigametocytes vaccine:**
- **Aim:** Prepared to block the transmission by arresting the development of parasites in mosquito.
- **Principle:** Human blood contains the anti-gametocytes antibody which ingested by mosquito & prevents the fertilisation.
- **Contains:** Vaccine is still under trial & it is prepared by using the pfs25 antigens.

iv. **Multi stage targeting vaccine:**
- **Aim:** Prepared to target the parasite at multiple stages. Vaccine is differs from previous vaccine.
- **History:** It was prepared by CDC (Centre for Disease Control & prevention) in Atlanta, Georgia.
- **Contains:** It is recombinant, multivalent vaccine & prepared by combining the 25 different antigens from *P. falciparum* in to a single recombinant protein. All the antigens are identified as immunogenic in previous vaccine trial & able to activate the B cells, T cells & other cells.

B. **In use vaccines:** Following two categories.

i. **Spf 66 vaccine:**
- Synthetic polypeptide vaccine developed by Patarroyo et al from sporozoite antigens.
- Moderate success achieved in Colombia, Tanzania & Gambia.

ii. **Candidate molecules vaccine:** Antigametocyte vaccine prepared to block the transmission.

❖ **Treatment:** Drugs are divided in following three categories.

A. **Clinical cure:** It targets the erythrocytic stage (schizonticidal) to terminate the clinical attack of malaria. Following two types of drugs are useful.

i. **Fast acting drugs:** Chloroquine, amodiaquine, quinine, mefloquine, halofantrine, lumefantrine, atovaquone & artemisin are used single to treat the malaria.

ii. **Slow acting drugs:** Proguanil, pyrimethamine, sulphonamides & tetracycline are used in combination to treat the malaria.

B. **Radical cure:** It targets the exo erythrocytic stage in liver, so it totally removes the parasite from the body & no chances of relapse or recrudescence. Drug of choice for radical cure is primaquine.

C. **Gametocidal:** It removes the male & female gametocytes from the blood & interrupts the transmission in mosquito. Following are gametocidal drugs.
- Quinine & chloroquine: For *P. vivax* but not for *P. falciparum.*
- Primaquine & artemisin: For all species.
- Proguanil & pyrimethamine: Gametes exposed to these drugs are failing to the life cycle in mosquito.

❖ **World malaria day:** 25th April of every year is celebrated as world malaria day with an aim to control it.

Babesia spp.

❖ **Synonym:** Formerly it called *Piroplasma*

❖ **Introduction:**
- It is an intracellular parasite, morphologically resembles to ring form of *Plasmodium* & creates confusion in diagnosis.
- Babesiosis is the zoonosis & human is the accidental host.

❖ **Species:**

✪ **Common species:** More than 100 species are known in this category like
- *B. bovis:* Cattle species of Europe.
- *B. divergens:* Unguate species of Europe.
- *B. microti:* Rodent species of rural Mexico.
- *B. canis:* Dog species.
- *B. equi:* Horse species of Europe.

✪ **Human species:** *B. divergens* & *B. microti* are human pathogens in North America & Europe.

❖ **History:**
- It was 1st discovered by the Romanian bacteriologist Victor Babe□ in 1888 from sheep & cattles, but he misinterpreted it as bacteria called *Haematococcus bovis*.
- In 1893, Theobald Smith and Fred Kilborne identified it as parasite & labelled as Babesia.
- Later, Victor Babe□, Smith & Fred Kilborne identify the tick as a vector for transmission.
- First human case was identified in 1957.

❖ **Geographical distribution:** Human cases have been reported from USA, Africa & Europe.

❖ **Habitat:** RBCs.

❖ **Morphology:** It exists in three forms **(figure-1).**

I. Sporozoite stage

➢ It is an infective forms & present in saliva of infected ticks, transmitted to human/animal during bite by ticks.

➢ It enters in RBCs & change to trophozoite form.

II. Trophozoite stage

➢ **Found in:** RBCs.

➢ **Size:** 2-4μm in diameter.

➢ **Shape:** Ring form.

➢ **Structure:**
- It contains small chromatin dot & scanty cytoplasm
- It feeds on haemoglobin, but do not produce any pigments & also no schizonts stage.
- Multiply by budding to form merozoites.

III. Merozoite stage

➢ Present in RBCs in group of four (tetrad structure) & giving an appearance called maltese cross form. Tetrad morphology, which can be seen under Giemsa's stain of a thin blood smear, is unique to *Babesia*, & serves as a distinguishing feature from *P. falciparum*.

➢ During the growth, few of merozoites are converted in to gametocytes.

➢ When RBCs packed with parasites, it burst to release the merozoites & gametocytes in to blood.

❖ **Culture:** Intraperitoneal inoculation of blood in hamsters or gerbils followed by preparation of thin film after a month to identify the *Babesia* in RBCs.

❖ **Life cycle:**

➢ **Host:** Two types.

I. **Intermediate host:** Vertebrate animals like mice, cattle, ungulate etc. are the natural host. Man is the accidental host.

II. **Definitive host:** Hard ticks like *Ixodid dammini* & *I. ricinus*.

➢ **Cycles:** Two types as shown in **flow chart-8 & fig.-21.**

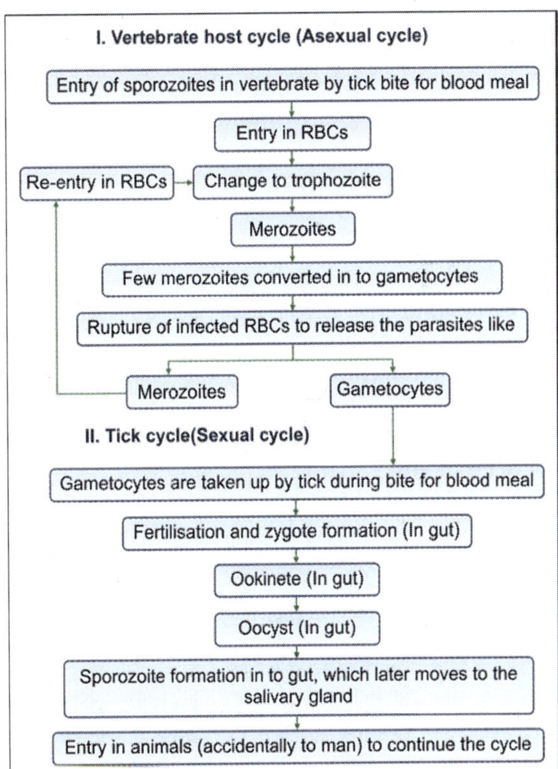

Flow chart-8: Life cycle of *Babesia*

❖ **Pathogenicity:**

➢ **Disease name:** It is a zoonosis called babesiosis.

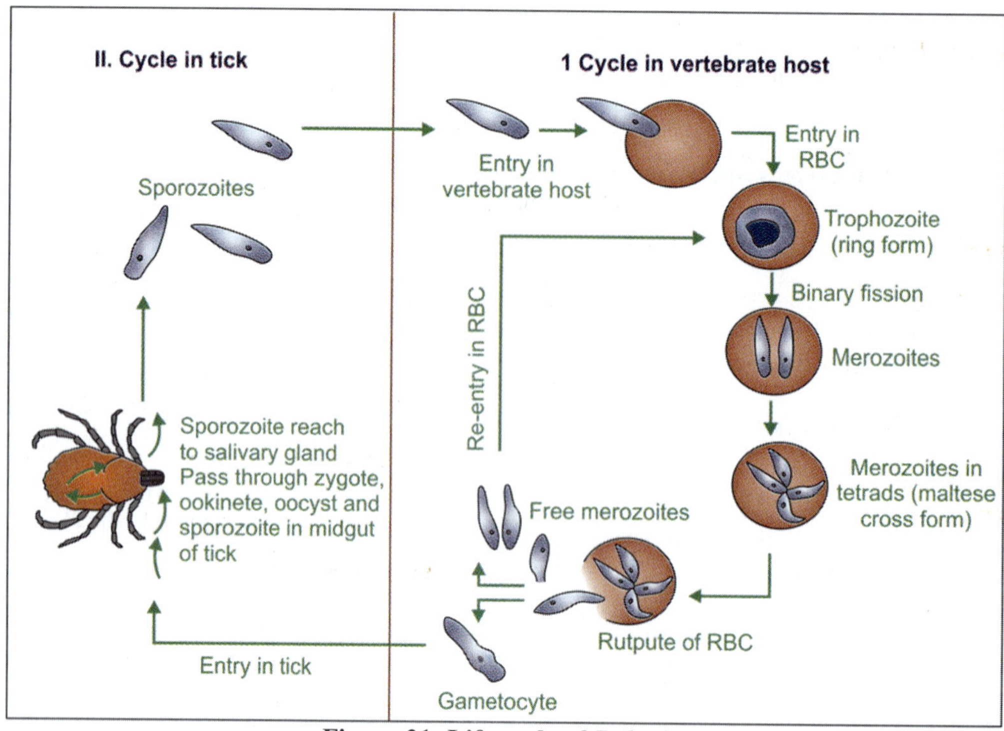

Figure-21: Life cycle of *Babesia*

- **Synonym:** Also **called piroplasmosis, Texas cattle fever, red water fever, tick fever** or **Nantucket fever.**
- **Reservoir / source of infection:**
- Natural reservoirs are mainly animals like rodents.
- Transovarian transmission of parasites occurs from mother Tick to the offspring, so Tick can act as source & also reservoir of infection.
- **Mode of transmission:**
- **Vector borne:**
- **Vector's name:** By bite of hard ticks of genera *Ixodid* & *Dermacentor*.
- **Vector's species:** Like *I. dammini* & *I. ricinus.*
- **Fluid borne:** By blood transfusion.
- **Incubation period:** 1-4 weeks.
- **Exit form:** Gametocytes.
- **Infective form:** Sporozoites.
- **Portal of entry:** Skin.
- **Site:** RBCs.

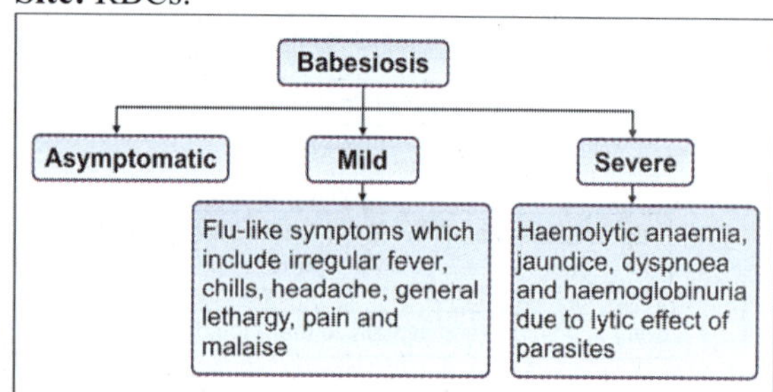

Flow chart-9: Clinical features of babesiosis

- **Precipitating factors:** Like splenectomy.
- Immunocompetent with healthy spleens often recover without treatment.
- Splenectomised patients are more susceptible to the disease & the course of infection often ends fatally within 5-8 days of symptom onset.
- Parasitemia levels can reach up to 85% in patients without spleens compared to 1-10% in individuals with spleens and effective immune systems.
- **Clinical features: →Flow chart-9.**

Differential diagnosis:

1. **Malaria: Vide infra** (follow staining methods)
2. **Lyme disease:** As two infections are co-exist & transmitted by same vector.

Laboratory diagnosis:

- **Specimens:** Blood.
- **Testing methods:**

A. Microscopy:

- **Smears:** By using thin & thick smears as described in ***Plasmodium.***
- **Staining methods & examination:**
- Cytoplasm of trophozoite (ring form) stain blue while chromatin (nucleus) dot in red by Giemsa's or Leishman's stain as shown in **fig.-22.**
- It creates confusion with ring form of *P. falciparum* which is separated by absence of pigments & no schizonts, tetrads morphology (**called maltese cross form**) & tick borne transmission.
- Under polarising microscope maltese cross form is seen in *Cryptococcus neoformans, Aspergillus nidulus,* starch granules & lipid (cholesterol) droplets.

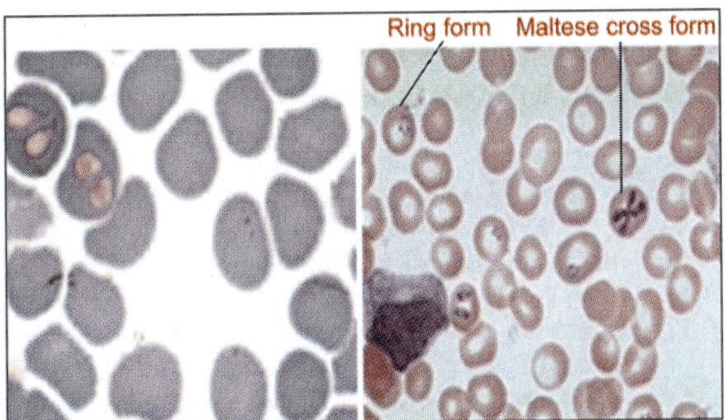

Figure-22: Staining reaction of *Babesia*

B. Culture: Vide supra

C. Serological tests: ELISA & rapid agglutination test are most useful. Cross reactivity may occur with *P. falciparum*.

❖ Prevention:

- Control of tick by using insecticides.
- Tick bite is avoided by using repellents or wearing clothes with full sleeves.
- Avoid the blood transfusion from the person with high Ab titre or with history of symptomatic babesiosis.

❖ Treatment:

- Babesiosis by *B microti* is the self limiting condition & most of the patients are recovering without any specific treatment.
- In acute case, atovaquine 750 mg twice daily with azithromycin 500 g/day for 7-10 days or alternatively clindamycin 300-600 mg, 4 times in a day with quinine 650 mg 3-4 time in a day is effective.
- In fulminant case exchange transfusion is advised.

Question bank

Case study

1) A 24 years male presents with high grade fever with chills & rigor which subside with profuse sweating. Blood examination revealed anaemic picture with amoeboid form of parasites in RBCs. Identify the organism & answer the following.

a) Name the causative agent & name the vector responsible for its transmission.
b) Describe the life cycle of causative agent.
c) Write the pathogenicity causative agent.
d) Describe the lab. diagnosis of causative agent.

2) A female patient admitted with malignant tertian type of fever history. Blood examination revealed anaemic picture with sickle shaped gametocytes in RBCs. Identify the organism & answer the following.

a) Name the causative agent & name the vector responsible for its transmission.
b) Describe the life cycle of causative agent.
c) Write the pathogenicity causative agent.
d) Describe the lab. diagnosis of causative agent.

Essay/Full question

1) Blood inhabiting sporozoa.
2) *P. vivax*.
3) *P. falciparum*.

Short notes

1) Classification of sporozoa.
2) Morphology / life cycle / pathogenicity / laboratory diagnosis of *P. vivax* or *P. falciparum*.
3) Different modes of transmission of *Plasmodium* spp.
4) Black water fever.
5) Pernicious malaria.
6) Differences between *P. vivax* & *P. falciparum*.
7) Malaria vaccine.
8) Babesiosis.

Short questions for theory/viva questions

1) What is alteration of generation & alteration of host in sporozoa?
2) Name the end products of sporogony & schizogony in malarial parasites.
3) Comment: *P. falciparum* not showing relapse.
4) Comment: In *P. falciparum* infection peripheral blood smear showing only gametocytes & ring forms **or** In *P. falciparum* late trophozoite stage & schizonts not identified in peripheral blood smear.
5) Comment: Anaemia & splenomegaly are common in patient of malaria.
6) What is hypnozoite? Write its clinical significance.
7) Mention the sites (organs/cells) in which malarial parasite remain in dormant form to produces the latent infection.
8) What is "therapeutic malaria"?
9) Name the fever for following parasites.
P. vivax, *P. falciparum P. malariae* & *P. ovale*.
10) Write four differences between trophozoite & sporozoite induced malaria.
11) What is "maltese cross form"?
12) Name two blood inhabiting sporozoa.
13) Name the plasmodium species causing following type fever.
- Benign tertian fever - Ovale tertian fever
- Malignant tertian fever - Benign quartan fever

MCQs for chapter review

Classification of sporozoa

1) **Most virulent *Plasmodium* species causing malaria is**
(a) *P. ovale* (b) *P. vivax* (c) *P. falciparum* (d) *P. malariae*

Plasmodium spp.

2) **Causative agent of malaria**
(a) Protozoa (b) Mosquito (c) Bacteria (d) Virus
3) **Malarial parasite was discovered by**
(a) Ronal Ross (b) Paul Muller (c) Laveran (d) Pampana
4) **The scientists who discovered the transmission of malaria by *Anopheles* mosquito**
(a) Laveran (b) Paul Muller (c) Ronal Ross (d) Pampana
5) **The mostcommon cause of malaria in India**
(a) *P. ovale* (b) *P. vivax* (c) *P. falciparum* (d) *P. malariae*
6) **In malaria sexual cycle is**
(a) Sprozoites to gametocytes (b) Gametocytes to sporozoites (c) Occurs in human (d) Responsible for relapse
7) **In malaria, pre-erythrocytic schizogony occurs in**
(a) Lungs (b) Liver (c) Spleen (d) Kidney
8) **In transmission of malaria mosquito bite transfers** (PGI-79)
(a) Sprozoite (b) Merozoites (c) Hypnozoite (d) Gametocyte
9) **The infective stage form of malarial parasite for vertebrate host is**
(a) Gametocyte (b) Sprozoites (c) Zygote (d) Merozoite

10) **Which is the infective stage for mosquito in case of *Plasmodium vivax*** (AIIMS, Nov-09)
(a) Gametocyte (b) Sprozoites (c) Zygote (d) Merozoite

11) **Which form of malarial parasite is present in saliva of infective mosquito**
(a) Ring form (b) Schizont (c) Gametocyte (d) Sprozoite

12) **In which type of malarial parasite is the exo-erythrocytic stage is absent** (PGI-96)
(a) *P. ovale* (b) *P. vivax* (c) *P. falciparum* (d) *P. malariae*

13) **Malaria carrier contain**
(a) Sprozoites (b) Gametocytes (c) Merozoites (d) Trophozoites

14) **In *Plasmodium falciparum* the number of cycle the parasite undergoes in the liver is**
(a) O (b) 1 (c) 2 (d) 3 (e) 5

15) ***Plasmodium vivax* attacks**
(a) Reticulocytes (b) Young RBCs (c) Old RBCs (d) Dead RBCs

16) **True about *P falciparum* includes all except**
(a) Duration of erythrocytic cycle is 48 hours (b) Exo-erythrocytic phase is absent (c) Parasitic burden can be estimated by peripheral parasitaemia (d) Causes rosette formation

17) ***Plasmodium falciparum* infection of man is characterised by** (AI -97)
(a) The erythrocytes are increased in size (b) All stages of erythrocytic schizogony are seen in peripheral blood (c) Multiple infection of erythrocytes are seen (d) Each erythrocytes cycles last 72 hours

18) **Stages seen in peripheral smear of *falciparum* malaria** (PGI, Nov-13, Dec -05)
(a) Schizonts (b) Gametocytes (c) Accole (d) Ring form (e) Trophozoite

19) **In *Plasmodium falciparum* following are seen in blood except** (PGI -97)
(a) Schizonts (b) Mature trophozoites (c) Mature Gametocytes (d) None

20) **Stages of *falciparum* not seen in PBS is** (PGI -99)
(a) Schizonts (b) Gametocytes (c) Ring form (d) Double ring

21) **Not seen in the peripheral smear in *Plasmodium falciparum* infection** (PGI -97)
(a) Accole (b) Maurer's dots (c) Schuffner's dots (d) Schizonts

22) **Schizonts of *P. falciparum* are not seen in peripheral blood smear because**
(a) Killed by antibodies (b) Absent in life cycle (c) Present in capillaries of internal organs (d) None of above

23) **A patient diagnose to have malaria, smear shows all stages of schizonts, 14-20 merozoites, yellowish-brown pigment. The type of malaria is** (AIIMS -01)
(a) *P. falciparum* (b) *P. malariae* (c) *P. vivax* (d) *P. ovale*

24) **RBCs are enlarged in infection with** (AIIMS -02)
(a) *P. vivax* (b) *P. malariae* (c) *P. ovale* (d) *P. falciparum*

25) **Band shaped trophozoites are seen in**
(a) *P. vivax* (b) *P. malariae* (c) *P. ovale* (d) *P. falciparum*

26) **Multiple infection of RBCs us seen in**
(a) *P. vivax* (b) *P. malariae* (c) *P. ovale* (d) *P. falciparum*

27) **Which of the following is true about malaria** (AI -96)
(a) Size of RBC is enlarged in *vivax* infection (b) Size of RBC is enlarged in *flaciparum* infection (c) Schuffner's dots are seen in *malariae* (d) Relapse is seen in *flaciparum* infection

28) **Which of the following is true about *P. falciparum* malaria**
(a) James dots are seen (b) Accole forms are seen (c) Relapses are frequent (d) Longest incubation period

29) **In malaria reservoir, parasite remains as**
(a) Merozoite (b) Sporozoite (c) Trophozoite (d) None

30) **Shortest incubation period in malaria**
(a) *P. vivax* (b) *P. falciparum* (c) *P. malariae* (d) *P. ovale*

31) **Most common *Anopheles* vector for transmission of malaria in urban area is**
(a) *A. stephensi* (b) *A. gambiae* (c) Both (d) None

32) **Malarial pigment is formed by** (AIIMS, May -94)
(a) Parasite (b) Bilirubin (c) Haemoglobin (d) Any of the above

33) **Chronic complication of malaria** (PGI, Dec -02)
(a) Splenomegaly (b) Nephrotic syndrome (c) Pneumonia (d) Hodgkin's disease

34) **Splenic rupture is most common in infection with**
(a) *P. vivax* (b) *P. malariae* (c) *P. ovale* (d) *P. falciparum*

35) **Complication in malaria are commonly with**
(a) *P. vivax* (b) *P. malariae* (c) *P. ovale* (d) *P. falciparum*

36) **Pernicious malaria is a complication seen in infection with**
(a) *P. vivax* (b) *P. malariae* (c) *P. ovale* (d) *P. falciparum*

37) **Cerebral malaria is caused by *Plasmodium***
(a) *falciparum* (b) *ovale* (c) *malariae* (d) *vivax*

38) **Parasitaemia is highest in**
(a) *P. vivax* (b) *P. falciparum* (c) *P. malariae* (d) *P. ovale*

39) **Which of the following is detected by the antigen detection test used for the diagnosis of *P. falciparum* malaria** (AIIMS-04)
(a) Circum sporozoite protein (b) Merozoite surface antigen (c) Histidine Rich Protein-I (HRP-I) (d) Histidine Rich Protein-II (HRP-II)

40) **Thin blood smear of malaria is used to identify** (AIIMS, May -93)
(a) Schizont (b) Gametocyte (c) *Plasmodium* parasite (d) Type of parasite

41) **JSB stain is used for which parasite**
(a) Malaria (b) Filaria (c) Kala azar (d) Sleeping sickness

42) **What is the treatment of choice for benign tertian malaria?**
(a) Sulphamethaxozole - pyrimethamine (b) Quinine (c) Mefloquine (d) Choroquine

43) **Malarial parasite – which statement is false regarding communicability** (AIIMS, Nov -06)
(a) Gametocytes appear in blood 4-6 days after asexual phase in *P vivax* (b) Gametocytes appear in blood 10-12 days after asexual phase in *P flaciparum* (c) The number of gametocytes increase in blood with time (d) The number of gametocytes increase by 1000 times

44) **Malarial parasites** (AIIMS -84)
(a) Has man as its intermediate host (b) Has life cycle that alternate between man and tse tse fly (c) Has 4 important species in man (d) Can be easily culture in the laboratory

45) **Which is true of malaria** (AI-93)
(a) Rods forms are seen in *P. malariae* (b) RBC size is more in *P. vivax* (c) Relapse seen in *P. falciparum* (d) Male and female mosquito transmit the disease

Babesia spp.

46) **True about babesiosis** (PGI, June-03)
(a) Caused by *Babesia microti* (b) Reside in RBC (c) Reside in WBC (d) Chloroquine is the treatment of choice (e) It is filarial parasite

47) **Babesiosis is transmitted by**
(a) Tick (b) Mites (c) Flea (d) Mosquito

48) **Maltese cross is characteristic of** (AI -09)
(a) *Cryptococcus neoformans* (b) *Babesia microti* (c) Blastomycosis (d) *Penicillium marnefeii*

49) **Maltese cross seen on polarising microscope in** (AIIMS, May -10)
(a) *Cryptococcus neoformans* (b) *Penicillium marnefeii* (c) *Blastomyces* (d) *Candida albicans*

Answers of MCQs & explanation

1) **(c)**
- Follow section, **classification of sporozoa (malignant tertian malaria)** for explanation

2) **(a)**
- Malaria is caused by *Plasmodium* which is a protozoa

3) (c)
4) (c)
Follow section, ***Plasmodium* spp. (history)** for explanation
5) (c)
- Follow section, ***Plasmodium* spp. (geographical distribution)** for explanation

6) (b)
7) (b)
8) (a)
9) (b)
10) (a)
11) (d)
12) (c)
Follow section, ***Plasmodium* spp. (life cycle & flow chart-1)** for explanation
13) (b)
14) (b)
- Follow section, ***Plasmodium* spp. (life cycle → Summary of human cycle → flow chart-3)** for explanation

15) (a) & (b)
16) (c)
17) (c)
18) (b), (c) & (d)
19) (a) & (b)
20) (a)
21) (c) & (d)
22) (c)
23) (c)
24) (a) & (c)
25) (b)
26) (d)
Follow section, ***Plasmodium* spp. (morphology & table-2) & note** for explanation

27) (a)
- Option a, b & c: Follow section, ***Plasmodium* spp. (morphology & table-2)** for explanation
- Option d: Follow section, ***Plasmodium* spp. (life cycle)** for explanation

28) (b)
- ***P. falciparum***
  - Contains Maurer's dots
  - Has no exo-erythrocytic phase, hence no relapse
  - Has shortest incubation period

29) (d)
- Follow section, ***Plasmodium* spp. (pathogenicity → reservoir & source of infection)** for explanation

30) (b)
- Follow section, ***Plasmodium* spp. (pathogenicity → incubation period)** for explanation

31) (a)
- Follow section, ***Plasmodium* spp. (pathogenicity → mode of transmission → indirect → vector borne)** for explanation

32) (c)
33) (a) & (b)
34) (d)
Follow section, ***Plasmodium* spp. (pathogenicity → pathogenesis & virulence factors & flow chart-4)** for explanation

35) (d)
36) (d)
37) (a)
Follow section, ***Plasmodium* spp. (pathogenicity → complications)** for explanation
38) (b)
- Follow section, ***Plasmodium* spp. (laboratory diagnosis → Specimen & time of collection)** for explanation

39) (d)
40) (d)
41) (a)
Follow section, ***Plasmodium* spp. (laboratory diagnosis)** for explanation
42) (d)
- Follow section, ***Plasmodium* spp. (treatment)** for explanation

43) (c)
- Option a & b: Follow **table-3**
- Option c & d: Follow life cycle (**flow chart-1**)

44) (a) & (c)
- Malarial parasite
  - Has life cycle that alternate between man and mosquito
  - Can't be easily culture in the laboratory

45) (b)
- Band (not rod) forms are seen in *P. malariae*
- RBC size is more in *P. vivax* & *P. ovale*
- Relapse not seen in *P. falciparum*
- Only female mosquito transmit the disease

46) (a) & (b)
47) (a)
48) (a) & (b)
49) (a)
Follow section, ***Babesia* spp.** for explanation

88 Gastrointestinal sporozoa

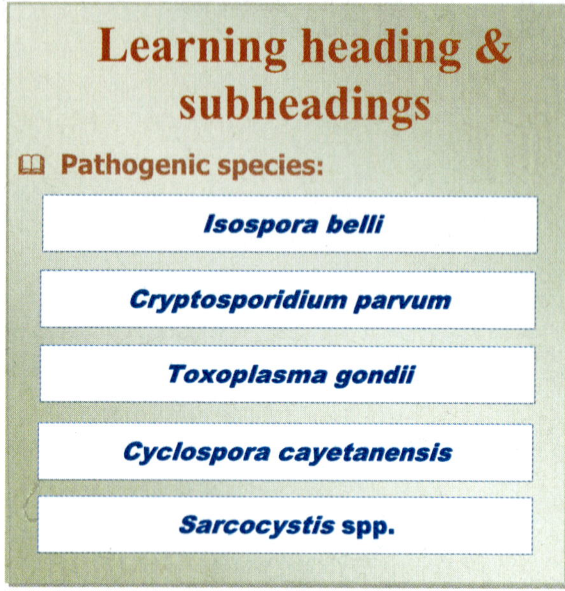

Pathogenic species: Following are **pathogenic** species of gastrointestinal sporozoa.

i. ***Isospora:***
- *I. belli:* Wenyon-1923, most important pathogen.
- *I. natalensis:* Rarely isolated.
- *I. hominis*: Rivolta- 1878 & Dobell- 1919, now classified under *Sarcocystis.*

ii. ***Cryptosporidium:*** So, far 8 species are identified as shown in **table-1** & human pathogen is *C. parvum.*

Species	Host
C. parvum	Domestic mouse
C. baileyi	Chicken
C. felis	Cat
C. meleagridis	Turkey
C. muris	Domestic mouse
C. nasorum	Fish
C. serpentis	Corn snake, rat snake
C. wrairi	Guinea pig

Table-1: Species of *Cryptosporidium*

iii. ***Toxoplasma:*** *T. gondii.*

iv. ***Cyclospora:*** *C. cayetanensis.*

v. ***Sarcocystis:*** Two broad groups of species according to habitat.

a. Intestinal:
- *S. bovihominis* (in cattle also **called *S. hominis***).
- *S. suihominis* (in pig).

b. Invasive or muscular: *S. lindemanni* in skeletal & cardiac muscles (in lymph nodes & vessels also).

Isospora belli

❖ **Meaning:** Word **belli** came from **bellum means war,** as it caused infection among troops in Middle East during First World War.

❖ **Geographical distribution:** Central & South America, Africa & South-East Asia.

❖ **Habitat:** Small intestine (lower part of ileum).

❖ **Morphology:** Morphological stage **called oocyst,** which pass through the followings stages.

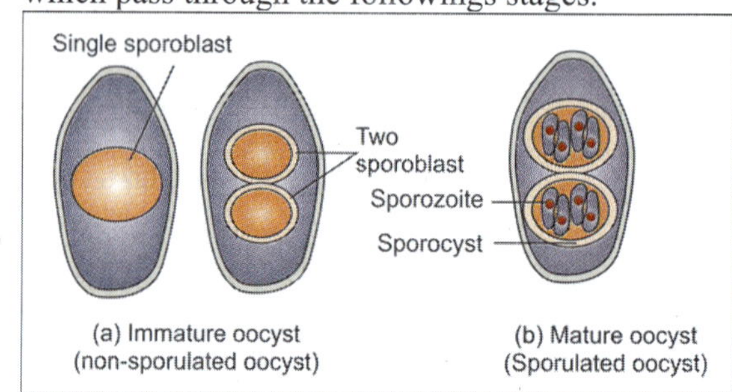

Figure-1: Morphology of *I. Belli*

A. Immature (non-sporulated) oocyst: →Fig.-1 (a)

➢ **Development & structure:**
- Zygote change to oocyst, which contains single sporoblast **called immature oocyst** & passes through faeces over soil.
- Sporoblast undergoes division in external environment to produce the two sporoblasts.

B. Mature (sporulated) oocyst: →Fig.-1 (b)

➢ **Development & structure:**
- Immature oocyst undergoes to further development in external environment.
- Each sporoblast undergoes division to produce four sporozoites, so finally 8-sporozoites are produced.
- Sporozoites are arranged in two groups, each contains four sporozoites in a specialised structure **called sporocyst** (**Greek → Sporos = seed**) within oocyst & such oocyst **called mature oocyst.**
- Mature oocyst is an infective form & digested by digestive juices to release the eight sporozoites.

➢ **Time required for maturation:** 1-5 days.

➢ **Size:** Mature oocyst is 20-30μm in length & 10-20μm in breadth.

➢ **Shape:** Elongated.

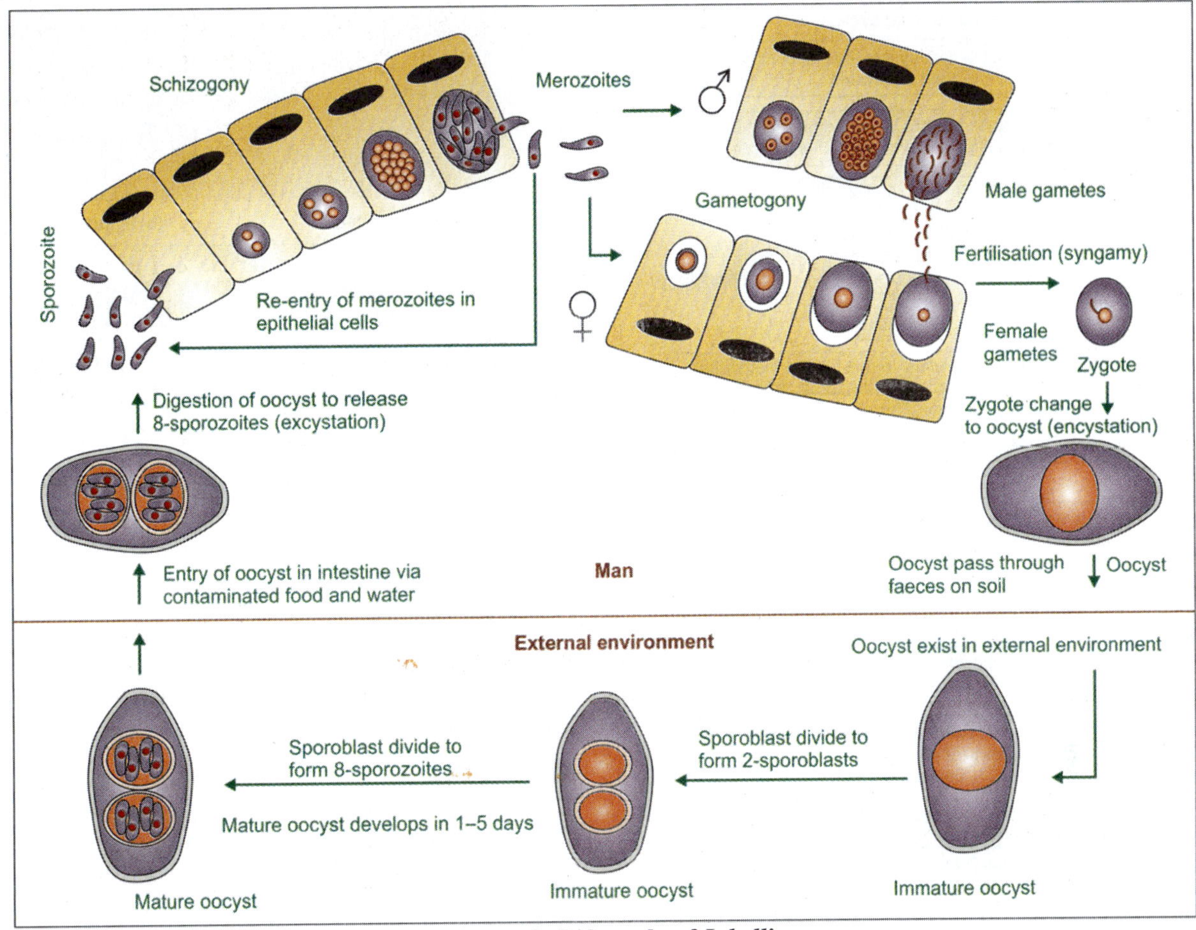

Figure-2: Life cycle of *I. belli*

❖ Life cycle:

- **Hosts & methods of reproduction:** Both asexual (schizogony) & sexual (gametogony followed by syngamy) stages are occurs in man.
- **Cycles:** Two types **(flow chart-1 & fig.-2).**

❖ Pathogenicity:

- **Disease name: Called isosporiasis.**
- **Reservoir of infection:** Man is the only reservoir & no any animal reservoir is known.
- **Source of infection:** Food & water.
- **Mode of transmission:**
  - **Ingestion:** By ingestion of contaminated food & water contains oocyst.
  - **Sexual transmission:** By oral-anal sex.
- **Incubation period:** 1-4 days.
- **Exit form:** Oocyst with single sporoblast.
- **Infective form:** Oocyst with 2 sporocysts (eight sporozoites).
- **Portal of entry:** GIT.
- **Site:** Small intestine (lower part of ileum).
- **Precipitating factor:**
  - Most common in AIDS patient.
  - Existence of *Isospora* infection in patients for more than 1 month indicates AIDS.
- **Clinical features: → Flow chart-2.**

❖ Laboratory diagnosis:

I. Direct methods

- **Specimens:**
  - **Stool:**
    - Preserve the stool in 2.5% potassium dichromate solution.
    - It kills the bacteria & helps in clear identification of *Isospora* after 24-48 hours.
  - **Duodenal aspirate:**
  - **Mucosal biopsy:**
  - **Muscle biopsy:** In case of extra-intestinal infection.
- **Testing methods:**

A. **Microscopy:** To examine the oocyst.

i. **Normal saline (NS) & iodine (I) preparation: →Fig.-3**
  - In fresh stool oocyst with nucleus can be identified.
  - In old stool unsporulated (immature) or sporulated (mature) oocyst can be identified.

ii. **Modified ZN stain: →Fig. -4**

iii. **Flourescent microscopy:** By using auramine dye.

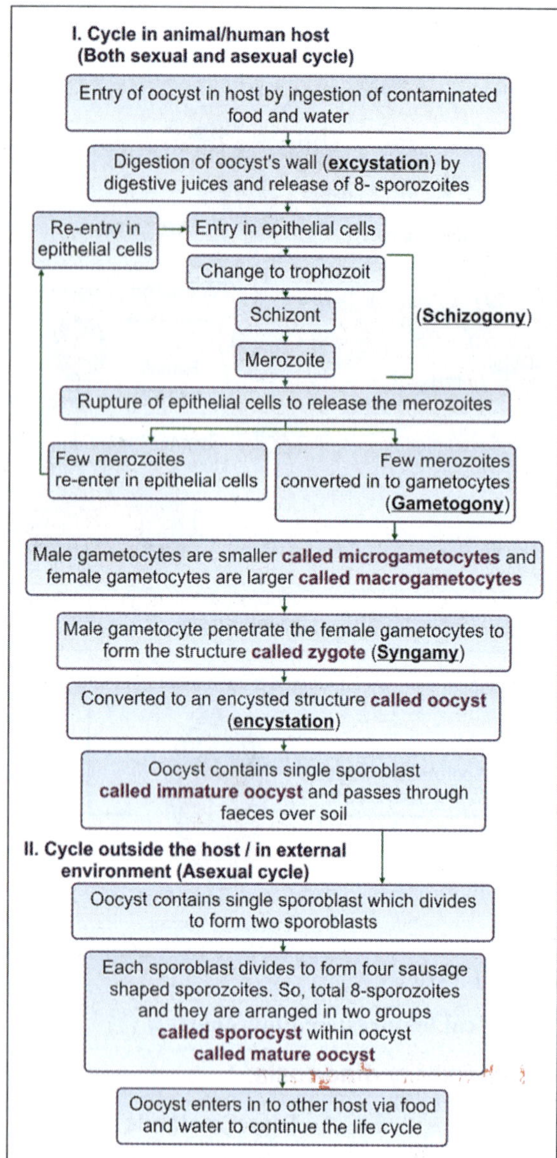
I. Cycle in animal/human host
(Both sexual and asexual cycle)
Entry of oocyst in host by ingestion of contaminated food and water
Digestion of oocyst's wall (excystation) by digestive juices and release of 8- sporozoites
Re-entry in epithelial cells
Entry in epithelial cells
Change to trophozoit
Schizont
Merozoite
(Schizogony)
Rupture of epithelial cells to release the merozoites
Few merozoites re-enter in epithelial cells
Few merozoites converted in to gametocytes (Gametogony)
Male gametocytes are smaller called microgametocytes and female gametocytes are larger called macrogametocytes
Male gametocyte penetrate the female gametocytes to form the structure called zygote (Syngamy)
Converted to an encysted structure called oocyst (encystation)
Oocyst contains single sporoblast called immature oocyst and passes through faeces over soil
II. Cycle outside the host / in external environment (Asexual cycle)
Oocyst contains single sporoblast which divides to form two sporoblasts
Each sporoblast divides to form four sausage shaped sporozoites. So, total 8-sporozoites and they are arranged in two groups called sporocyst within oocyst called mature oocyst
Oocyst enters in to other host via food and water to continue the life cycle

Flow chart-1: Life cycle of *I. belli*

✓ **Note: Two modes of epithelial cells infection**

1. Fresh sporozoites from ruptured oocyst.
2. Infection by merozoites.

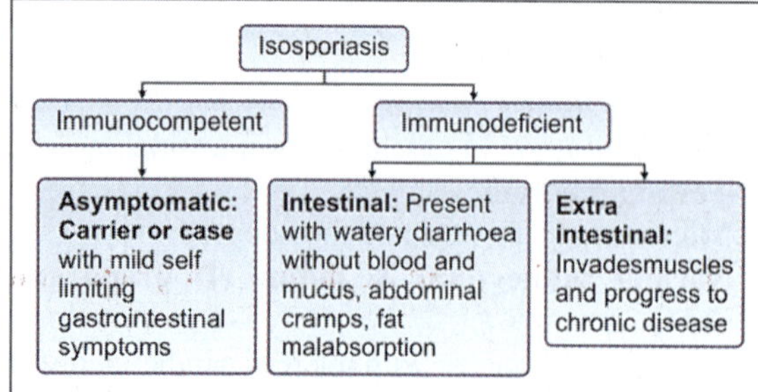
Isosporiasis
Immunocompetent
Immunodeficient
Asymptomatic: Carrier or case with mild self limiting gastrointestinal symptoms
Intestinal: Present with watery diarrhoea without blood and mucus, abdominal cramps, fat malabsorption
Extra intestinal: Invadesmuscles and progress to chronic disease

Flow chart-2: Clinical features of isosporiasis

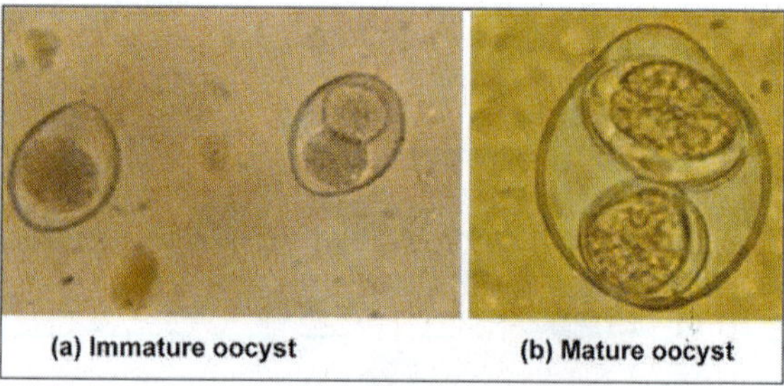
(a) Immature oocyst
(b) Mature oocyst

Figure-3: Oocyst under NS & I preparation

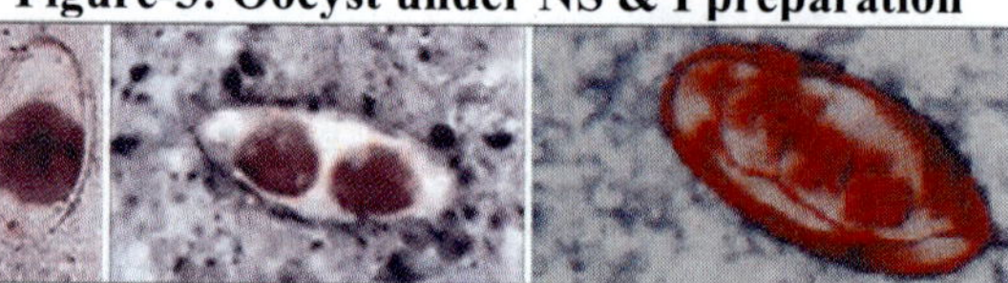

Figure-4: Different oocyst under ZN preparation

II. Indirect methods

- **Specimens:**
- **Stool:** Presence of high fat, fatty acid crystals & Charcot-Leyden (CL) crystals.
- **Blood:** Eosinophilia.

❖ **Prevention:** Measures are directly toward the stopping the transmission. Proper washing of hands, fruits, vegetables etc. before eating.

❖ **Treatment:** Self limiting diarrhoea. Treatment is required in AIDS patient with cotrimoxazole (trimithoprim-sulfamethoxazole). Alternative drug is pytimethamine.

Cryptosporidium parvum

❖ **History:**

- It was first reported by Tyzzer in 1907 in the gastric crypt of laboratory mouse.
- It was first reported in 1971 as an animal pathogen causing diarrhoea.
- First human case was identified in children in 1976 causing self limited diarrhoea.
- Incidences are increase with increasing immunosuppressive diseases like AIDS.
- Massive water borne outbreak of was reported in Milwaukee, USA in 1993, affected around 4,00,000 people.

❖ **Geographical distribution:** It is an animal pathogen, distributed worldwide.

❖ **Habitat:** Small intestine (Distal part of jejunum, ileum & colon).

❖ **Morphology:** Morphological stage **called oocyst,** which having following two types.

A. Thin walled oocyst: →Fig.-5(a)

- It develop from zygote,
- It is not excreted in to external environment & penetrate the epithelial cells to produce autoinfection (internal reinfection).

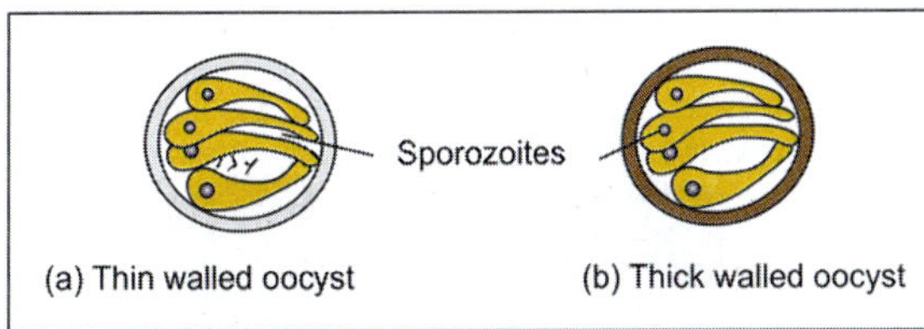

Figure-5: Morphology of C. *parvum*

B. Thick walled oocyst: →Fig.-5(b)

➢ **Types, development & structure:**

1. **Immature (unsporulated) oocyst:** Initial it is immature & excreted in to external environment for further maturation.
2. **Mature (sporulated) oocyst:**
   - Oocyst undergoes further development in external environment and produces four sporozoites.
   - **Size:** 4-5µm in diameter.

❖ Life cycle:

➢ **Hosts & methods of reproduction:** Both asexual (schizogony) & sexual (gametogony followed by syngamy) stages are occurs in man.

➢ **Cycles:** Two types **(flow chart-3 & fig.-6)**

✓ **Note: Three modes of epithelial cells infection**

1. Fresh sporozoites from ruptured oocyst.
2. First generation merozoites.
3. Second generation merozoites.

❖ Pathogenicity:

➢ **Disease name: Called cryptosporidiosis.**

➢ **Reservoir of infection:** Man & animal are the known reservoirs.

➢ **Source of infection:** Food & water.

➢ **Mode of transmission:**

- **Ingestion:** By ingestion of contaminated food & water contains oocyst.
- **Sexual transmission:** By oral-anal sex.
- **Autoinfection: → Flow chart-3**

➢ **Incubation period:** 1-12 days.

➢ **Exit form:** Thick walled oocyst.

➢ **Infective form:** Thin & thick walled oocyst.

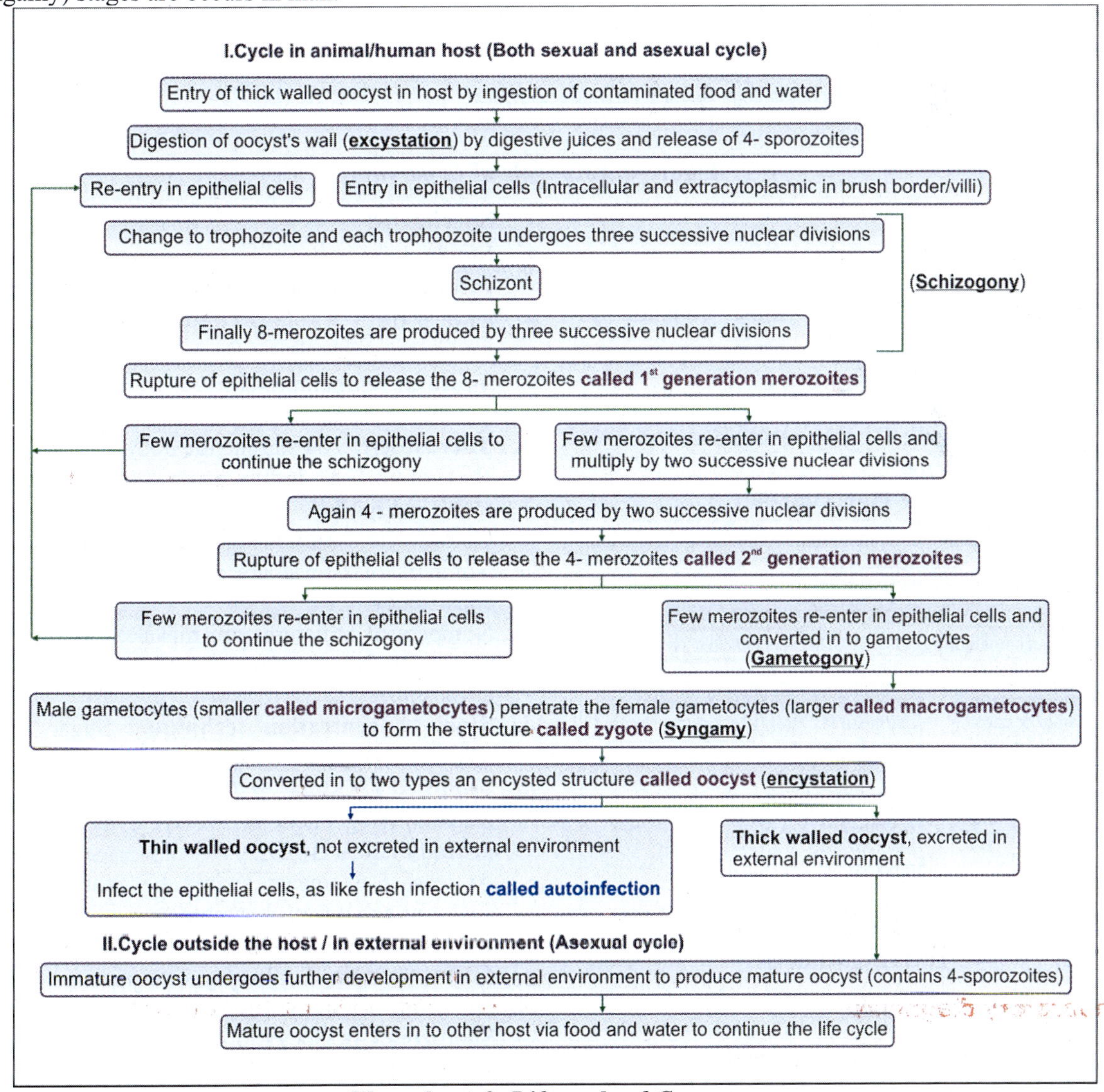

I.Cycle in animal/human host (Both sexual and asexual cycle)

Entry of thick walled oocyst in host by ingestion of contaminated food and water
↓
Digestion of oocyst's wall (**excystation**) by digestive juices and release of 4- sporozoites
↓
Entry in epithelial cells (Intracellular and extracytoplasmic in brush border/villi) | Re-entry in epithelial cells
↓
Change to trophozoite and each trophoozoite undergoes three successive nuclear divisions
↓
Schizont
↓
Finally 8-merozoites are produced by three successive nuclear divisions
(**Schizogony**)
↓
Rupture of epithelial cells to release the 8- merozoites **called 1st generation merozoites**
↓
- Few merozoites re-enter in epithelial cells to continue the schizogony (→ Re-entry in epithelial cells)
- Few merozoites re-enter in epithelial cells and multiply by two successive nuclear divisions
↓
Again 4 - merozoites are produced by two successive nuclear divisions
↓
Rupture of epithelial cells to release the 4- merozoites **called 2nd generation merozoites**
↓
- Few merozoites re-enter in epithelial cells to continue the schizogony (→ Re-entry in epithelial cells)
- Few merozoites re-enter in epithelial cells and converted in to gametocytes (**Gametogony**)
↓
Male gametocytes (smaller **called microgametocytes**) penetrate the female gametocytes (larger **called macrogametocytes**) to form the structure **called zygote** (**Syngamy**)
↓
Converted in to two types an encysted structure **called oocyst** (**encystation**)
↓
- **Thin walled oocyst**, not excreted in external environment → Infect the epithelial cells, as like fresh infection **called autoinfection**
- **Thick walled oocyst**, excreted in external environment

II.Cycle outside the host / In external environment (Asexual cycle)

Immature oocyst undergoes further development in external environment to produce mature oocyst (contains 4-sporozoites)
↓
Mature oocyst enters in to other host via food and water to continue the life cycle

Flow chart-3: Life cycle of C. *parvum*

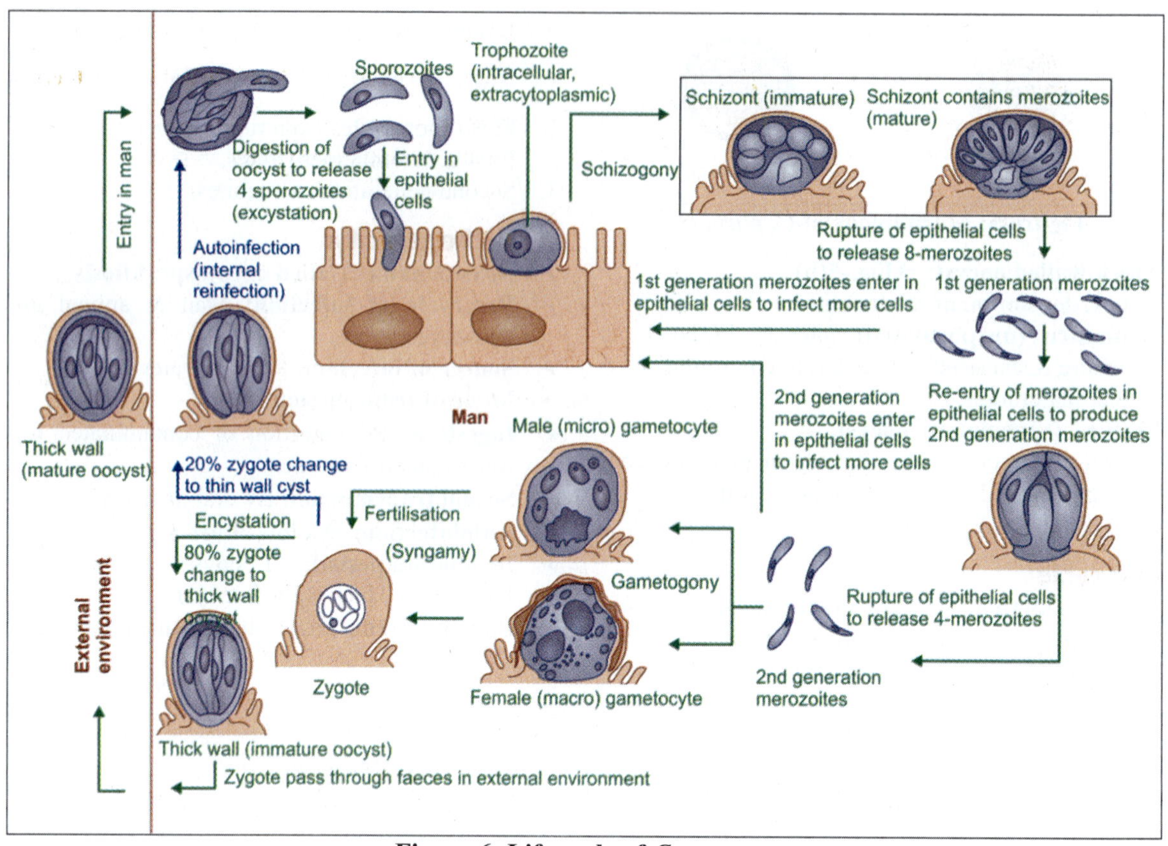

Figure-6: Life cycle of *C. parvum*

- **Portal of entry:** GIT.
- **Site:** Small intestine.
- **Precipitating factor:**

1. **Immunodeficiency disease:** Most common in AIDS patient.
2. **Animal handlers:** At risk.
3. **Homosexual person:** At risk.
4. **Resistant cyst wall:** Highly resistant cyst wall to chlorination & ozone.

- **Clinical features:** → **Flow chart-4**

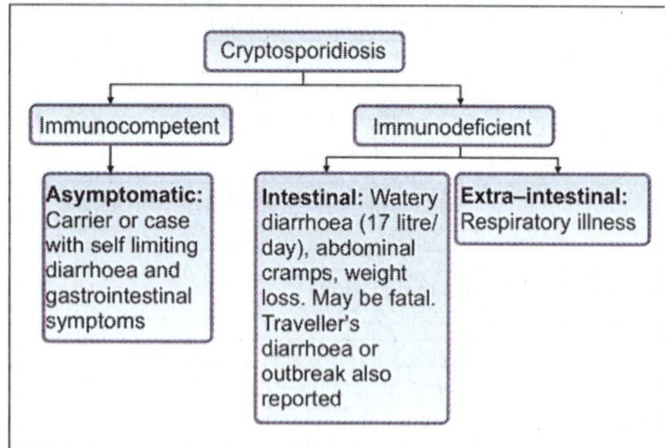

Flow chart-4: Clinical features of cryptosporidiosis

❖ Laboratory diagnosis:

I. Direct methods

- **Specimens:**
  - **Stool.**
  - **Intestinal, gall bladder or biliary tract biopsies.**
  - **Entero test:** →Follow chapter → Intestinal, oral and genital flagellates for more details.
  - **Sputum:** Formalin fixed.
- **Testing methods:**

A. Microscopy: To examine the oocyst.

i. Wet mount & iodine preparation from fresh stool: →**Fig.-7**

- Oocyst with 4-5µm in size can be identified.
- Numbers of oocyst are more in stool with water consistency.
- Numbers of structures are mistaken as oocyst like yeast cell, fungal spore, cyst of *B. coli* & oocyst of *Cyclospora.*

ii. Stool concentration technique: Sugar flotation (Sheather's) technique is useful.

iii. Modified ZN stain: →**Fig.-8**

- Decolourising agent is 3% HCL in 95% ethanol instead of 20% H_2SO_4.
- At least 5-6 smears should be examined before declaring the negative sample.

iv. Flourescent microscopy: Is also useful.

v. Giemsa's stain: For biopsy specimens.

vi. Di Amidino Phenyl Indole (DAPI) stain:

- Sporozoites of oocyst are not visualised by above methods.
- It stain the nuclei of sporozoites in oocyst.

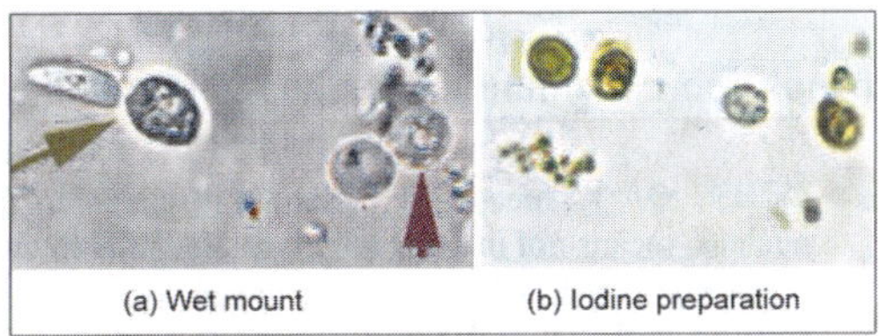

Figure-7: Oocyst under wet mount & iodine preparation

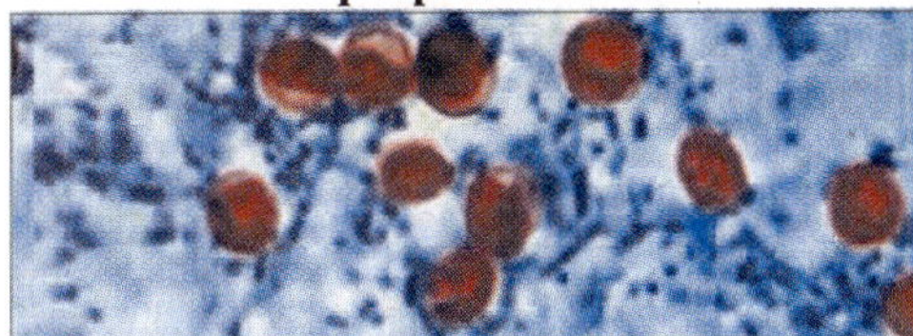

Figure-8: Oocyst under ZN preparation

II. Indirect methods

A. Serological test:
- Antibodies are detected from serum by ELISA.
- It attain the significant titre in 8-10 weeks & persist for about one year.

B. Molecular test: Like PCR.

❖ **Prevention:** Proper washing of hands, fruits, vegetables etc. before eating.

❖ **Treatment:**
- No any drug is effective.
- Treatment with nitazoxanide or parmomycin may be partially effective in AIDS patient.

Toxoplasma gondii

❖ **History & Meaning:**
- Genus name came from two words: **Tox (Greek) = Arc/Bow & Plasma = form**, because of arc shape.
- It was first identified in 1908 by Nicolle & Manceaux from the small rodent **called gundi** (scientific name: → *Ctenodactylus gundi*) of Africa, hence the species name is ***gondii.***
- Only one species is known, but strain to strain variation may appear.

❖ **Geographical distribution:**
- Distributed worldwide.
- About 30-40% population of different countries are sero-positive, but incidence is higher, about 75-80% in France & Scandinavia.

❖ **Habitat:** Small intestine & many organs.

❖ **Morphology:** Three morphological stages.

A. Oocyst:

➢ **Development, structure & subtypes:**

1. Immature (non sporulated) oocyst: →Fig.-9 (a)
- Develops only in the definitive host of family ***Felidae*** (domestic or wild cats) but not in intermediate hosts (like man or other animals/birds).
- Zygote change to oocyst, which contains single sporoblast & passes through faeces over soil.
- Freshly passed oocyst is not infective.
- Sporoblast undergoes division in external environment to produce the two sporoblasts, such structure **called immature oocyst.**

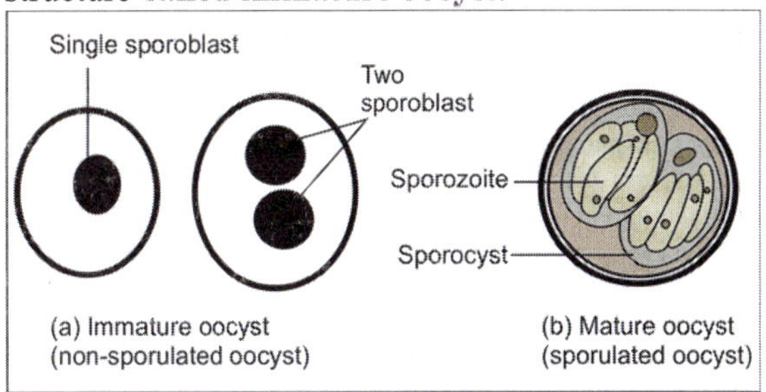

Figure-9: Oocyst of *T. gondii*

2. Mature (sporulated) oocyst: →Fig.-9(b)
- Each sporoblast follows the successive divisions to form four sausage shaped sporozoites. So, total 8-sporozoites & they are arranged in two groups in a specialised structure **called sporocyst** within oocyst. Such oocyst **called mature oocyst.**
- Mature oocyst enters in to other host like cat, man & other animals to produce infection.
- Mature oocyst is an infective form & digested by digestive juices in human intestine to release the eight sporozoites.
- Oocyst do not sporulate below 4^0C or above 37^0C
- Dry heat (>66^0C) or boiling renders the oocyst non-infectious.

➢ **Time required for maturation:** 1-5 days.

➢ **Size:** Mature oocyst is 10-12μm in size.

➢ **Shape:** Spherical or oval.

B. Pseudocyst: →Table-2 & fig.-10 (a).

C. Tissue cyst: → Table-2 & fig.-10 (b).

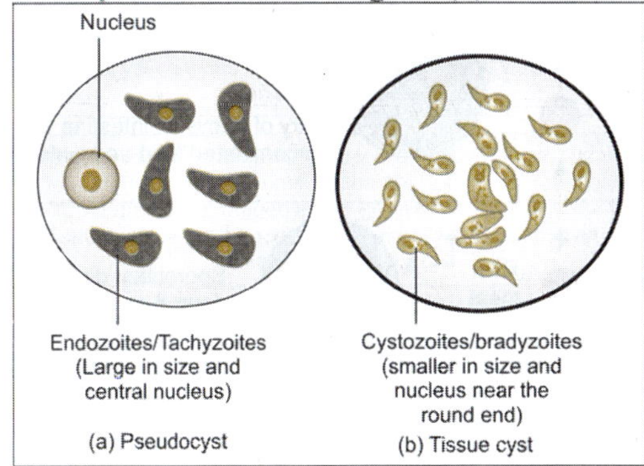

Figure:10 (a) Pseodocyst & (b)Tissue cyst of *T. gondii*

❖ **Culture:**

i. Tissue culture: It can grow in presence of living cells.

ii. Animal culture: Animal culture can be done in mice, guinea pigs & hamsters.

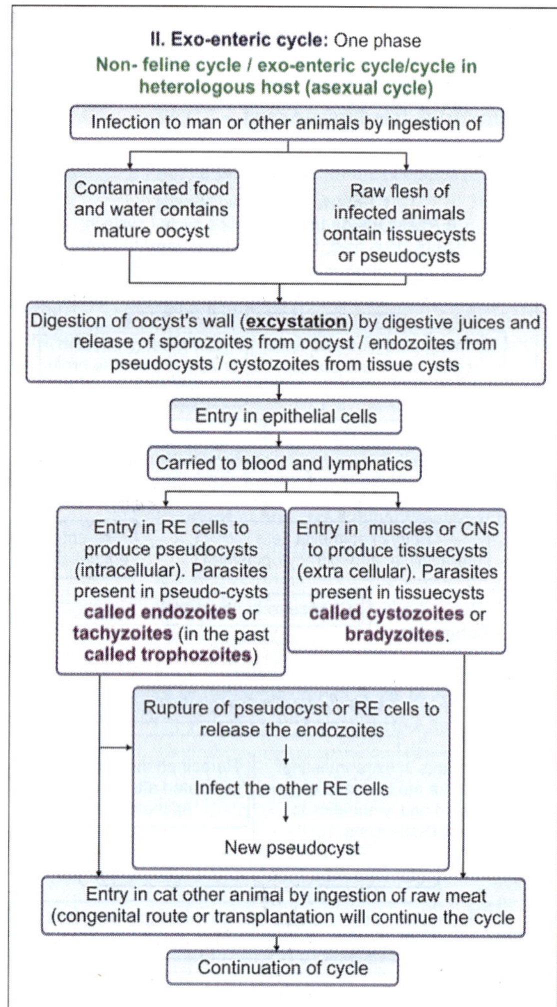

Flow chart-6: Exo-enteric cycle of *T. gondii*

❖ Pathogenicity:

➢ **Disease name:** It is a zoonosis (zoonotic disease) & transmitted from animals to humans. It is also a reverse zoonosis (anthroponosis or anthroponotic disease) & transmitted from humans to animals. Disease **called toxoplasmosis.**

➢ **Reservoir of infection:**
- Both definitive host (domestic or wild cats) & intermediate host are the reservoirs.
- Sheep & swine are the source of human infection
- Dog does not play any role in human infection.

➢ **Source of infection:** Infected tissues or food-water.

➢ **Mode of transmission:** Following are two modes.

a. Direct:

1. **Direct contact:** Contact with infected tissues. *Toxoplasma* can enter through abraded skin.
2. **Inoculation under skin:** By infected needle or syringe.
3. **Transplacental (vertical or congenital):**

- One of the agent among ToRCH list → **Follow chapter → Infection and infectious diseases** for more details.
- Incidence of foetal transmission is less in 1st trimester, but one happened infection is more sever. Incidence is highest in 3rd trimester but foetal risk is not severe.
- Transmitted by placenta & also by mother's milk.

b. Indirect:

1. **Food & water borne (ingestion):**

- By ingestion of contaminated food & water contains oocyst from cat's faeces. Freshly passed oocyst (contains sporoblast & **called immature oocyst**) is not infective, if becomes infective only after getting maturation (contains 8 sporozoites & **called mature oocyst**) in external environment either in water or soil.
- Ingestion of raw meat or eggs (pseudocyst also found in ovary of hen) of infected animal contains pseudocyst or tissue cyst.
- Ingestion of milk from infected mother to children

2. **Inhalation:** Bronchial secretions also contains parasites & responsible for respiratory illness.
3. **Blood or organ transplantation:**
4. **Vector borne:** Flies, cockroaches & earth worms can act as non infected transporter.

➢ **Incubation period:** In adults, it is from 10 -23 days after the ingestion of undercooked meat & from 5-20 days after the ingestion of oocysts.

➢ **Exit form:** Oocyst from cat only.

➢ **Infective form:** Three infective forms.

1. **Mature oocyst:** Not freshly passed but mature oocyst, which contains 8-sporozoites (arrange in two groups within a specialised structure **called sporocyst**).
2. **Pseudocyst:** Contains endozoites or tachyzoites (in the past **called trophozoites**).
3. **Tissue cyst:** Contains cystozoites or bradyzoites.

➢ **Portal of entry:** GIT.

➢ **Sites:** It starts infection from small intestine (common in ileum) & later disseminated in many organs like liver, spleen, lymph nodes, brain, spinal cord, bone marrow, eyes, lungs, heart muscles, skeletal muscles & placenta.

➢ **Precipitating factor:**

1. **Immunodeficiency disease:** Especially AIDS, aggravate the symptoms.
2. **Animal or meat handlers:** At risk.
3. **Pregnancy:** Mother is mostly asymptomatic & chances of foetal infection are

- **First trimester:** 10%.
- **Second trimester:** 30%.
- **Third trimester:** 60%.

4. **Age:** Especially children & adults.

➢ **Pathogenesis:**
- Parasites settle in vacuole in RE cells. Here it may die or survive by preventing the fusion of lysosomes with vacuole to form phagolysosome with help of parasitic factors **called membrane active substances.**

- RE cell enlarge with plenty of parasites in side & make a structure **called pseudocyst,** which is surrounded by area of necrosis & inflammatory cells like monocytes, plasma cells & lymphocytes.

➢ **Clinical features:**

A. Toxoplasmosis in immunocompetent: Flow chart-7.

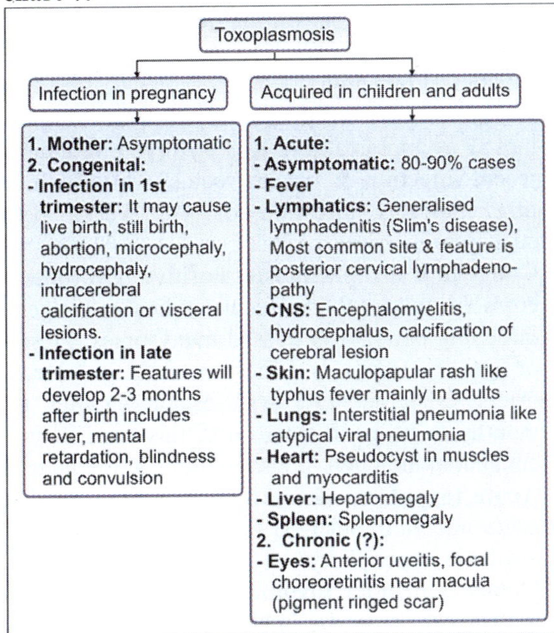

Flow chart-7: Clinical features of toxoplasmosis

B. Toxoplasmosis in immunodeficient:

✪ **Features:**
- High & prolonged fever.
- No response to antibiotics.
- Diffuse encephalitis.
- Others symptoms includes paralysis, blindness, myocarditis or death.

✪ **Pathogenesis:** It occurs in AIDS or patients with immuno-suppressive therapy when CD4 count fall below 100/cmm, by following two ways.
- Endogenous: Due to activation of previous infection **called recrudescent** (**table-2**).
- Endogenous: Due to entry of new parasites **called opportunistic infection.**

✪ **Diagnosis:**
1. **CSF testing:** Contains neutrophils, mononuclear cell & tachyzoites stained by Giemsa stain.
2. **Serological tests:** Positive IgG & radiological findings indicates *Toxoplasma* infection.

✪ **Treatment:** Symptoms subside with antitoxoplasmic treatment.

➢ **Recrudescence (latent infection) in toxoplasmosis:** Tissue cyst remains latent for long time & reactivated in immunodeficiency time.

❖ Laboratory diagnosis:

I. Direct methods

➢ **Specimens:**
- **CSF:**
- **Muscle biopsies:** Skeletal or cardiac muscles.
- **Tissue biopsies:** From liver, spleen, lymph node, bone marrow etc.
- **Cat's faeces:**

➢ **Testing methods:**

A. Microscopy:

i. Histopathological stains: Like
1. **Alkaline methylene blue dye test: →Vide infra**
2. **Giemsa's [fig.12 (a)] or Wright's stain:** It stain cytoplasm blue, nucleus reddish purple & para-nuclear body in red colour.
3. **Periodic Acid Schiff (PAS) stain:** Bradyzoites contain large amount polysaccharide & strongly react with PAS stain.
4. **Wet mount from cat's faeces: → Fig.12(b)**

ii. Flourescent microscopy (Goldman's test):
- It detect the parasites from tissue.
- Parasites appears brightly fluorescent **(fig.-13)** when treated with fluorescin tagged globulin fraction of homologous antiserum.

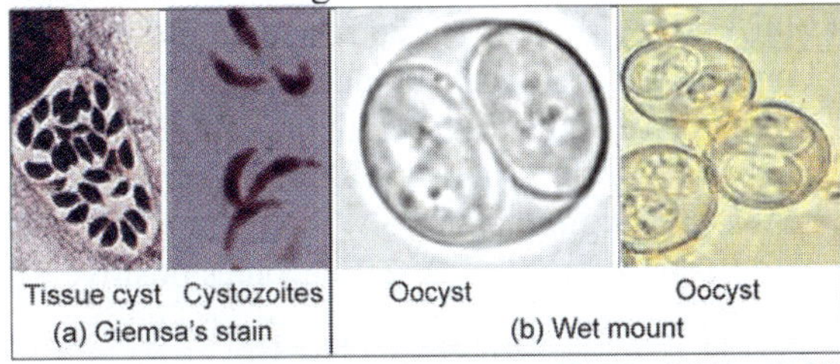

Figure-12: Microscopic appearance of *T. gondii*

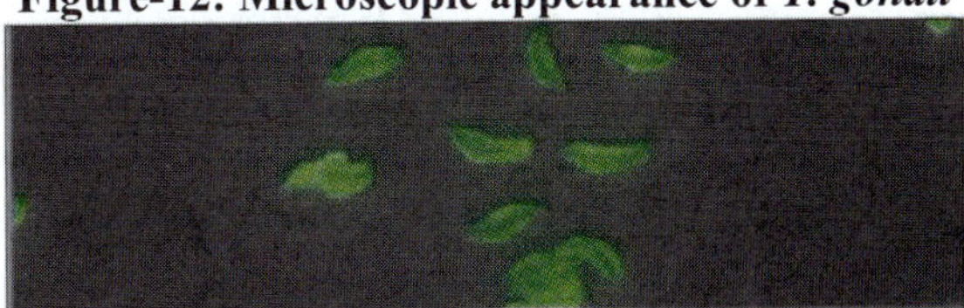

Figure-13: Fluorescent microscopy of *T. gondii*

B. Culture: → Vide supra

II. Indirect methods

A. Blood picture: It resemble to infectious mononucleosis (glandular fever).
- Leucocytosis (12,000/cmm of blood) with increase lymphocytes & monocytes.
- Atypical lymphocytes as like glandular fever.
- In many cases 20% rise in eosinophils count has been noticed.
- Low platelets count.

B. CSF picture: In case of meningo-encephalitis
- Colour: Yellow.
- Protein: Increased.
- Leucocytes: Increase in large numbers.

C. Serological test:

✪ **Types:**

i. Alkaline methylene blue dye (Sabin & Feldman's) test:

- **History:** Described by Sabin & Feldman in 1948.
- **Principle:** It based on inhibition of alkaline methylene blue dye's staining of tachyzoites by specific antiserum finally examined under microscope.
- **Reagents:**

1. **Antigen (suspension of tachyzoites):** *T.gondii* is cultivated in mice peritoneal cavity.
2. **Antibody:** Patient's serum.
3. **Alkaline methylene blue dye: pH = 11.0**
4. **Accessory (complement) factor:** Human serum.

- **Steps:**
  - Equal volume contains suspension of tachyzoites, accessory factor & patient's serum is mixed in a tube with serial dilution & incubated at 37^0C in a water bath for one hour.
  - Add one drop of alkaline methylene blue to each tube & re-incubated.
  - One drop of suspension from each tube is examined under microscope.
- **Examination & results:**
  - Tachyzoites are killed if patient's serum contains anti toxoplasma antibody in presence of complement (complement mediated lysis)
  - Dilution of the test serum at which 50% of tachyzoites are stained (hence not killed), is reported as significant titre
  - Significant titre is 1:4 & test becomes positive after 1-2 weeks
- **Disadvantages:**
  - It was 1st serological test described for *Toxoplasma* but having historical value only.
  - False positive test is reported in *T. vaginalis, Trypanosoma lewisii* & *Sarcocystis.*

ii. Indirect Haem Agglutination (IHA) test:

- **Advantages:** Most sensitive test & useful to detect the prevalence.
- **Disadvantages:** It becomes positive after long time & remains positive for long time.

iii. Latex agglutination (Fulton's) test: Significant titre is 1:16.

iv. ELISA: Widely used test currently for IgM & IgG.

v. Neutralisation (Sabin & Ruchman's) test:

- It based on neutralisation reaction.
- Intracutaneous injection of patient's serum with living *Toxoplasma* in to rabbit.
- Positive result: No reaction like erythema with oedema at the injection site after 3-5 days.

vi. CFT (Sabin & Warren's test):

- Complement antibody develops after 3-4 weeks & sooner gets negative.
- Antigen prepared from chick embryo culture
- Significant titre: 1:8.

D. Immunological (skin) test:

i. Frenkel's test:

- It based on delayed type of hypersensitivity (DTH).
- Toxoplasmin antigen is injected intradermally.
- Erythema & induration about 10 mm in size after 48 hrs indicates positive reaction.

E. Molecular test: Detection of parasite DNA from patient's serum.

✪ **Interpretation of results of serological test:** It is very difficult to interpret the serological result of *Toxoplasma,* because of high prevalence of *Toxoplasma* antibodies in population due to past & subclinical infection.

1. **Toxoplasmosis in pregnant women:** Mother is mostly asymptomatic & IgM positive titre indicates recent infection & risk to foetus, while high IgG titre indicates infection of 4-8 weeks before conception.
2. **Congenital toxoplasmosis:** Positive IgM (does not cross the placenta) in foetus indicates congenital infection, but IgM is missed many times. Presence of IgG in foetus is either maternal or infection origin. Maternal IgG will disappear after 6-10 months & its persistence after this time indicates congenital infection. It also requires X-ray help.
3. **Acute toxoplasmosis:** Positive IgM titre indicates acute infection, but IgM tests are expensive & not available in periphery.
4. **Ocular (chronic) toxoplasmosis:** IgG is required to diagnose the ocular infection.
5. **Toxoplasmosis in immunodeficient patient:** Positive IgG & radiological findings indicates *Toxoplasma* infection.
6. **CSF antibodies titre:** It is not helpful in diagnosis.

❖ Prevention:

➢ **General measures:**

- Measures are directly toward the stopping the transmission.
- Risk group should avoid contact with cat or cat's faeces.
- No female workers of child bearing age with negative Dabin-Feldman dye test are allowed to work in *Toxoplasma* laboratory especially with culture test.
- Proper washing of hands, fruits, vegetables etc. before eating.
- Screening of blood & blood products before transfusion.

➢ **Chemoprophylaxis:**

- It required especially in AIDS patient with CD4 count < 100/cmm.
- Trimithoprim-sulfamethoxazole is the drug of choice, if not tolerates then shift to dapsone-pyrimethamine.
- Discontinue the prophylaxis if CD4 count is > 200/cmm & ART is effective.

➢ **Immunoprophylaxis:** A genetically engineered vaccine is under trial.

❖ Treatment:

- **Treatment to pregnant woman:** Spiramycin is the drug of choice.
- **Treatment in neonate:** Oral pyrimethamine (1mg/kg/day) plus sulfadiazine (100mg/kg/day) with folic acid for 1 year. Steroid also given to reduce the risk of chorioretinitis.
- **Treatment in adults & young children:**

- Oral pyrimethamine 50 mg 3-4 times in 1st day followed by 25 mg/day for 2-4 weeks.
- Oral sulfadiazine 2 g stat followed by 1 g 6 hourly for 2-4 weeks.
- Steroid (prednisolone) also given to reduce the risk of ocular features.
- Folic acid & vitamin B complex should be given along with.

Cyclospora cayetanensis

❖ History & meaning:

- First human case was reported in 1985 in Peru.
- The species name refers to the **Cayetano Heredia University** in Lima, Peru, where early epidemiological and taxonomic work was done.

❖ Geographical distribution:

- Distributed worldwide in many animals like reptiles, birds & animals.
- In human it is a cause of traveller's diarrhoea.
- It is reported from Nepal, India & South America.

❖ Habitat: Small intestine (duodenum & jejunum).

❖ Morphology: Morphological stage **called oocyst**, which pass through the followings stages.

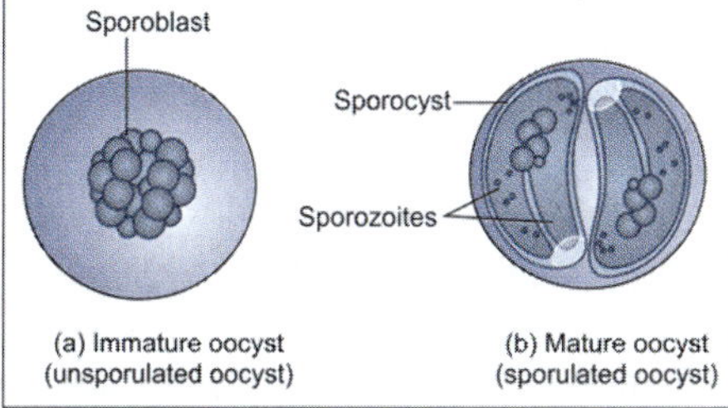
Sporoblast
Sporocyst
Sporozoites
(a) Immature oocyst
(unsporulated oocyst)
(b) Mature oocyst
(sporulated oocyst)

Figure-14: Oocyst of *C. cayetanensis*

A. Immature (non-sporulated) oocyst: →Figure 14 (a)

➤ **Development & structure:**

- Zygote change to oocyst, which contains single sporoblast **called immature oocyst** & passes through faeces over soil.

B. Mature (sporulated)oocyst: →Fig.-14 (b)

➤ **Development & structure:**

- Immature oocyst undergoes to further development in external environment.
- Sporoblast undergoes successive division to produce four sporozoites which are arranged in two groups, in a specialised structure **called sporocyst** within oocyst & such oocyst **called mature oocyst**
- Mature oocyst is an infective form & digested by digestive juices in human intestine to release the four sporozoites.

➤ **Time required for maturation:** 7-15 days.

➤ **Size:** Mature oocyst is 8-10μm in diameter.

➤ **Shape:** Spherical.

❖ Life cycle: Similar to *I. belli.*

➤ **Hosts & methods of reproduction:** Both asexual (schizogony) & sexual (gametogony followed by syngamy) stages are occurs in man.

➤ **Cycles:** Two types **(flow chart-8 & fig.-15).**

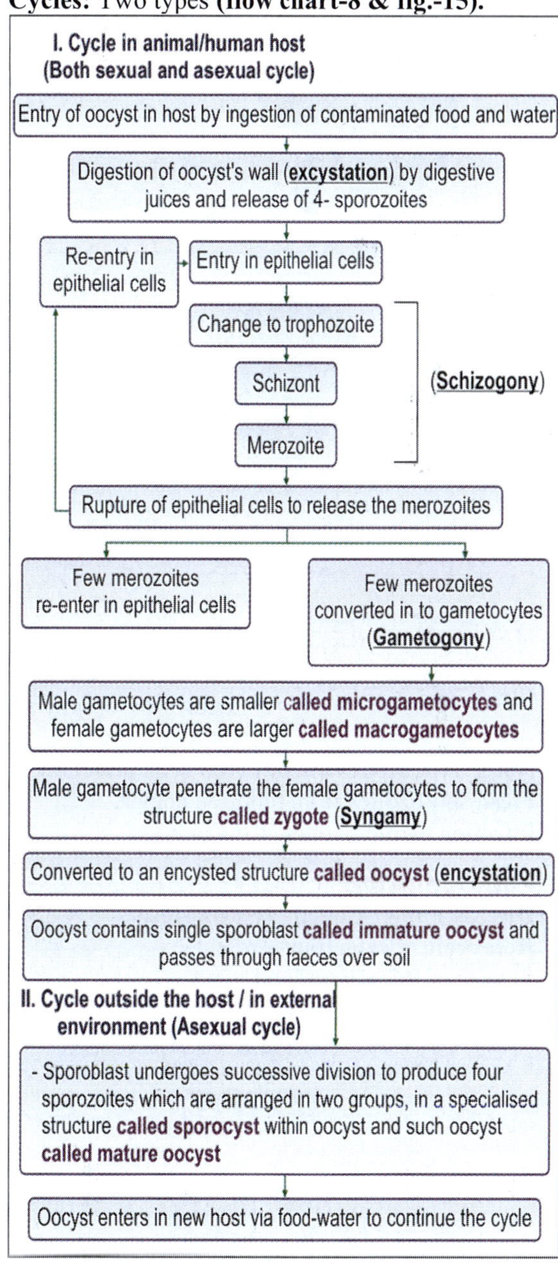
I. Cycle in animal/human host
(Both sexual and asexual cycle)
Entry of oocyst in host by ingestion of contaminated food and water
Digestion of oocyst's wall (excystation) by digestive juices and release of 4- sporozoites
Re-entry in epithelial cells
Entry in epithelial cells
Change to trophozoite
Schizont
Merozoite
(Schizogony)
Rupture of epithelial cells to release the merozoites
Few merozoites re-enter in epithelial cells
Few merozoites converted in to gametocytes (Gametogony)
Male gametocytes are smaller called microgametocytes and female gametocytes are larger called macrogametocytes
Male gametocyte penetrate the female gametocytes to form the structure called zygote (Syngamy)
Converted to an encysted structure called oocyst (encystation)
Oocyst contains single sporoblast called immature oocyst and passes through faeces over soil
II. Cycle outside the host / in external environment (Asexual cycle)
- Sporoblast undergoes successive division to produce four sporozoites which are arranged in two groups, in a specialised structure called sporocyst within oocyst and such oocyst called mature oocyst
Oocyst enters in new host via food-water to continue the cycle

Flow chart-8: Life cycle of *C. cayetanensis*

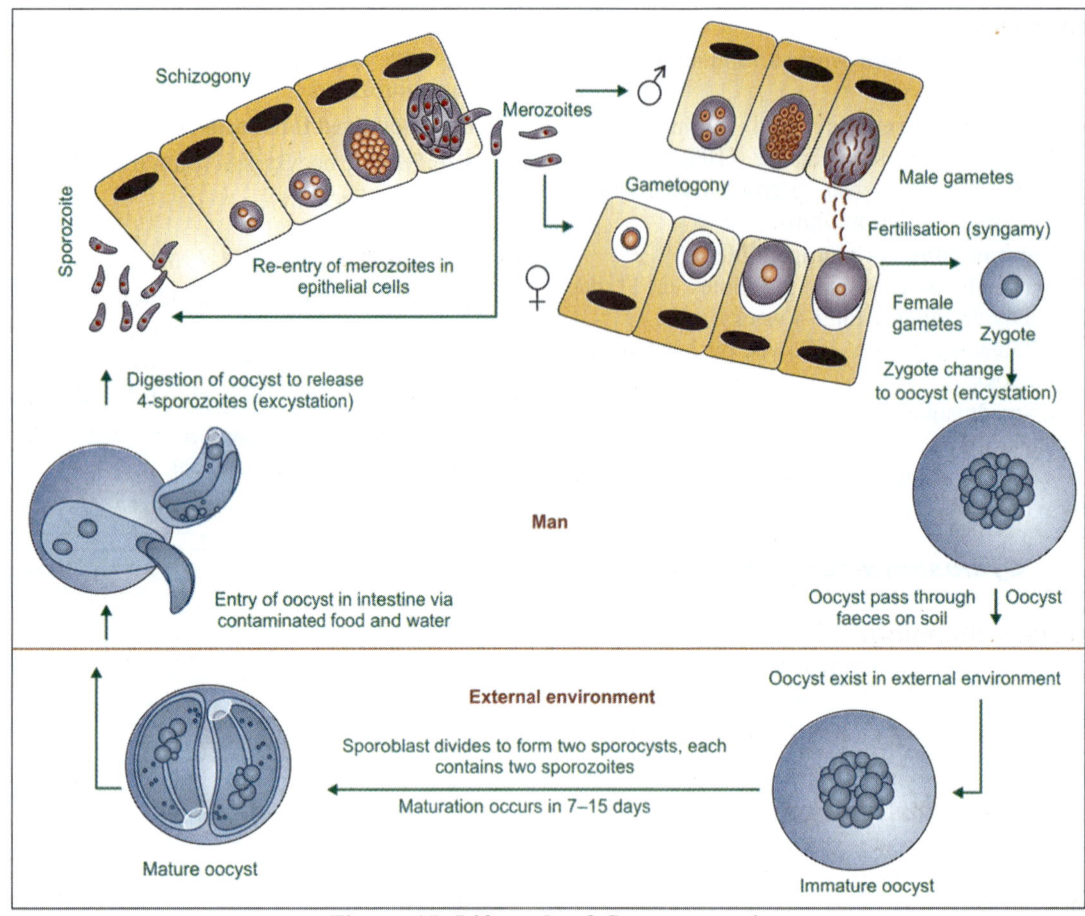

Figure-15: Life cycle of *C. cayetanensis*

Parasites	Size	No. of sporocysts	Sporozoites		Acid fast	Maturation time
			Per sporocyst	Total		
I. belli	20-30 µm × 10-20 µm	2	4	8	Yes	1-5 days
C. parvum	4-5 µm	-	-	4	Yes	-
C. cayetanensis	8-10 µm	2	2	4	Variable	7-15days

Table-3: Comparison of oocysts of different parasites

✓ **Note: Two modes of epithelial cells infection**

1. Fresh sporozoites from ruptured oocyst.
2. Infection by merozoites.

❖ Pathogenicity:

- **Disease name:** **Called cyclosporiosis.**
- **Reservoir of infection:** Animal.
- **Source of infection:** Food-water.
- **Mode of transmission:** By ingestion of contaminated food-water contains sporulated oocyst.

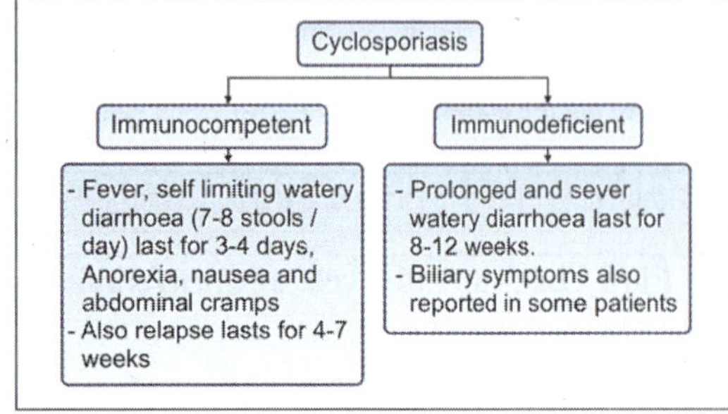

Flow chart-9: Clinical features of cyclosporiosis

- **Incubation period:** 2-11 days.
- **Portal of entry:** GIT.
- **Site:** Small intestine (duodenum & jejunum).
- **Infective form:** Oocyst with 2 sporocysts (total four sporozoites).
- **Exit form:** Oocyst with single sporoblast.
- **Precipitating factor:** Common in immunodeficient / AIDS patient.
- **Clinical features: → Flow chart-9.**

❖ Laboratory diagnosis: By using direct methods.

- **Specimens:** Stool.
- **Testing methods:**

A. Microscopy: To examine the oocyst.

i. Wet mount preparation:

- Spherical oocyst 8-10µm in diameter is present as shown in **fig.-16**.
- Oocyst is differentiated from *I. belli* & *C. parvum* as shown in **table-3.**

ii. Modified ZN stain:

- It is variable in acid fast properties as shown in **fig.-17.**
- It used to differentiate from other related oocyst as shown in **fig.-18.**

iii. Auto-flourescence:

- Cyclospora are fluorescent in nature under UV microscope **called auto-flourescence** as shown in **fig.-19**.
- This nature could be taken in to consideration while performing immunofluorescent microscopy for *C. parvum* & *Giardia.*

iv. Stool concentration method: Oocyst can be concentrated by modified zinc sulphate flotation technique.

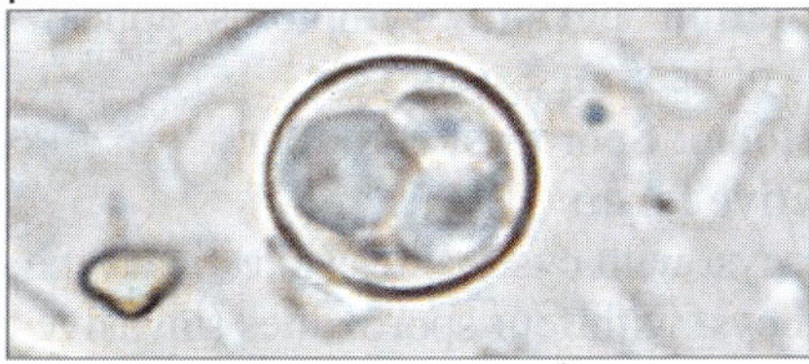

Figure-16: Oocyst under wet mount preparation

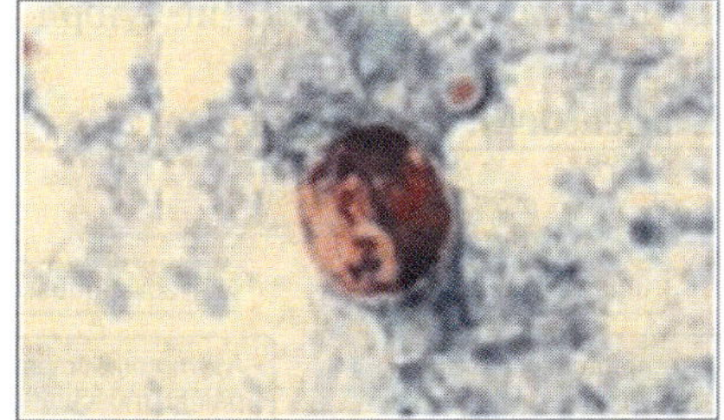

Figure-17: Oocyst under ZN preparation

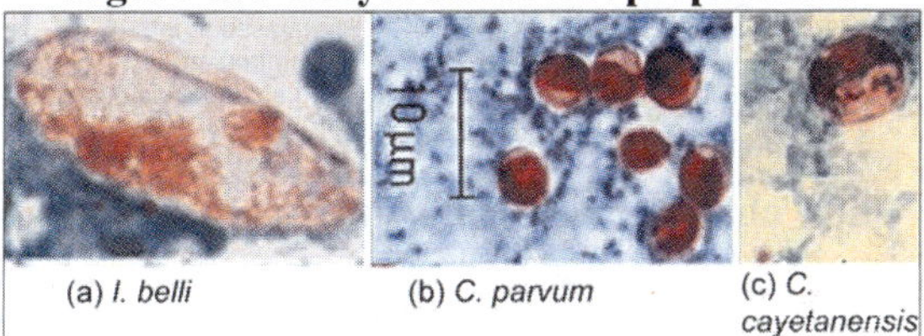

Figure-18: Different oocyst under ZN preparation

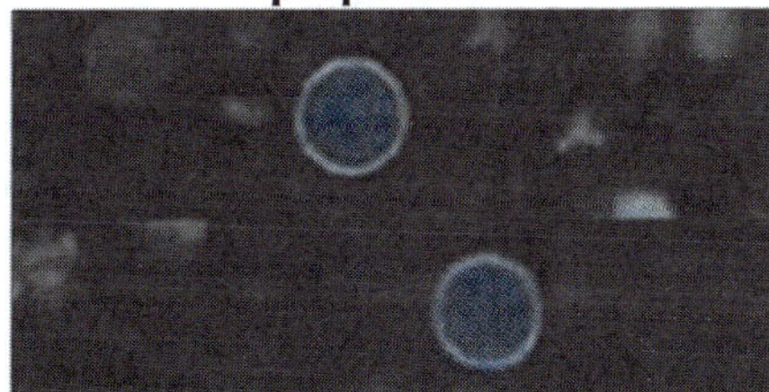

Figure-19: Auto-fluorescence in oocyst

❖ **Prevention:** Proper washing of hands, fruits, vegetables etc. before eating.

❖ **Treatment:** Cotrimoxazole is the effective drug. Long term suppressive therapy is required in AIDS patient.

Sarcocystis spp.

❖ **Meaning:** Genus name came from the **sarx (Greek) = meat + kystis (Greek) = cyst/bladder**

❖ **History:**

- It was observed first time by Miescher 1843 & initially **called miescher tube.**
- The first human infection was reported by Lindemann in 1868. Although several additional reports were subsequently published. Later the species was named as *S. lindemanni* by Rivolta.
- *I. bovihominis* (Rivolta- 1878 & Dobell- 1919): Initially it was classified as *Isospora hominis*, now classified under *Sarcocystis hominis (S. bivihiminis*).

❖ **Geographical distribution:** Distributed worldwide in human & animals like reptiles, birds, animals etc.

❖ **Morphology:** Three morphological stages.

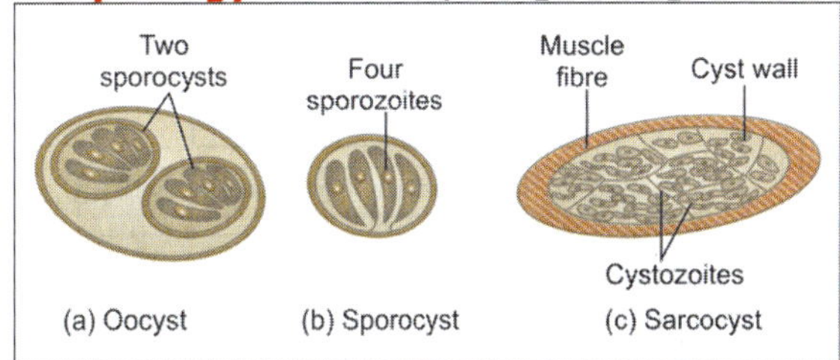

Figure-20: Morphology of *Sarcocystis*

A. Oocyst: →Fig.-20 (a)

➢ **Development & structure:**

- Zygote differentiated to oocyst, which contains two sporocysts & four sporozoites in each sporocyst (total eight sporozoites).
- Oocyst excysted to release the sporocyst, which passes through faeces over soil.

➢ **Size:** 19 µm × 13µm in diameter.

➢ **Shape:** Oval.

B. Sporocyst: →Fig.-20 (b)

➢ **Structure:** Contains 4 banana shaped sporozoites.

➢ **Size:** 13-16 µm × 8-10µm in diameter.

➢ **Shape:** Oval or spherical.

C. Sarcocyst or muscular cyst: →Fig.-20 (c)

➢ **Structure:** It is a tissue cyst with thick wall present in muscles & contains parasites **called cystozoites or bradyzoites** which are 7-16µm long.

➢ **Size:** 300 µm × 100µm in diameter. It present parallel to the long axis of muscle fibres.

➢ **Shape:** Tongue or spindle shape.

❖ **Life cycle:** Different in different species.

Intestinal *(S. bovihominis & S. suihominis)*

➢ **Hosts & methods of reproduction**

I. Definitive host: Man is the definitive host, which harbours the sexual (gametogony followed by syngamy) stage.

II. Intermediate host: Cattle in case of *S. bovihominis* & pig in case of *S. suihominis* are the intermediate hosts, which harbours the asexual stage.

size is 12-15 nm (d) AFB +ve cyst (e) Treatment is metronidazole

4) ***Cryptosporidium* cyst identified by which stain in stool sample**
(a) PAS (b) H and E (c) Giemsa (d) Acid fast stain

5) **In human cryptosporidiosis is present as** (PGI-03)
(a) Meningitis (b) Diarrhoea (c) Pneumonia (d) Hepatitis

Toxoplasma gondii

6) **Tachyzoites are seen in** (PGI-97)
(a) *Toxoplasma* (b) *Toxocara* (c) Pulmonary eosinnophilia (d) *Ascaris*

7) **Definitive host for *Toxoplasma***
(a) Man (b) Dog (c) Cat (d) Rat

8) **Intermediate host for *Toxoplasma* are all except**
(a) Human (b) Sheep (c) Cat (d) Pig

9) **Oocyst of *Toxoplasma* is found in** (AIIMS, Dec-97)
(a) Cat (b) Dog (c) Mosquito (d) Cow

10) **True about *Toxoplasma gondii* is, it is carried by** (AIIMS-97)
(a) Cats (b) Dogs (c) Rats (d) Cows

11) **Route of transmission of *Toxoplasma***
(a) Blood (b) Faeces (c) Urine (d) None

12) **Cat is an agent for transmission of following disease in**
(a) *Isospora hominis* (b) *Fasciola hepatica* (c) *Toxoplasma gondii* (d) *Chilomestix mesnili*

13) **Infective form of *Toxoplasma gondii* is**
(a) Oocyst (b) Bradyzoite (c) Tachyzoite (d) All of the above

14) **Sabin Feldman dye test is used to demonstrate infection with**
(a) Filaria (b) *Toxoplasma* (c) *Histoplasma* (d) *Ascaris*

15) **Toxoplasmosis in the foetus can be best be best confirmed by** (AIIMS, May-09)
(a) IgM antibodies against *Toxoplasma* in the mother (b) IgM antibodies against *Toxoplasma* in the foetus (c) IgG antibodies against *Toxoplasma* in the mother (d) IgG antibodies against *Toxoplasma* in the foetus

16) **All of the following statements about toxoplasmosis are true except** (AI-97, 01)
(a) Oocyst in freshly passed cat's faeces is infective (b) May spread by organ transplantation (c) Maternal infection acquired after 6 months has high risk of transmission (d) Arthralgia, sore throat and abdominal pain are the most common manifestations

17) **All true regarding toxoplasmosis except** (AIIMS, Nov-93)
(a) Subclinical in most cases among adults (b) Intracerebral calcification in children (c) IgM antibody in new born suggest congenital infection (d) Not effective in 3rd trimester in pregnancy

18) **True about toxoplasmosis is all except** (AIIMS, Nov-01)
(a) In adult toxoplasmosis is usually asymptomatic (b) IgG antibodies are diagnostic in congenital toxoplasmosis (c) Is a anthroponotic disease (d) Encephalitis is uncommon (rare) in immunocompetent individuals

19) **True about toxoplasmosis** (PGI, May-13, Dec-03)
(a) Due to ingestion of sporocyst with meat (b) Due to ingestion of oocyst from cat's faeces (c) Spiramycin given pregnancy (d) Due to bite of *Anopheles* mosquito (e) Mostly symptomatic

Cyclospora cayetanensis

20) **Following is not the property of *Cyclospora cayetanensis***
(a) Autofluorescence (b) Acid fastness (c) Transmitted by faeco oral route (d) Oocyst contains 4 sporocysts

21) **25 year old male presented with diarrhoea for 6 months. On examination the causative agent was found to be acid fast with 12 micro meter diameter. The most likely agent is** (AIIMS, May-09)
(a) *Cryptosporidium* (b) *Isospora* (c) *Cyclospora* (d) *Giardia*

22) **Acid fast organism with oocyst of size 5 µm on stool examination, causing diarrhoea in HIV positive patient**
(a) *Cryptosporidium* (b) *Isospora belli* (c) *Microsporidia* (d) *Blastocystis hominis*

Answers of MCQs & explanation

1) **(a), (b) & (c)**
- Oocyst of ***Isospora belii*** contains 2 sporocyst & each sporocyat contains 4 sporozoites (total 8 sporozoites in oocyst)

2) **(c)**
3) **(b) & (d)**
4) **(b)**
5) **(d)**
} Follow section, ***Cryptosporidium parvum*** for explanation

6) **(a)**
- Follow section, ***Toxoplasma gondii* (morphology & table-2)** for explanation

7) **(c)**
8) **(c)**
9) **(a)**
10) **(a)**
} Follow section, ***Toxoplasma gondii* (life cycle)** for explanation

11) **(a) & (b)**
12) **(c)**
} Follow section, ***Toxoplasma gondii* (pathogenicity → mode of transmission)** for explanation

13) **(d)**
- Follow section, ***Toxoplasma gondii* (pathogenicity → infective form)** for explanation

14) **(b)**
15) **(b)**
} Follow section, ***Toxoplasma gondii* (laboratory diagnosis)** for explanation

16) **(a) & (d)**
- Option a, b & c: Follow section, ***Toxoplasma gondii* (pathogenicity → mode of transmission & infective form)** for explanation
- Most common manifestations of toxoplasmosis is cervical lymphadenopathy.

17) **(d)**
- Option a & b: Follow section, ***Toxoplasma gondii* (pathogenicity → clinical feature & flow chart-7)**
- Option c: Follow section, ***Toxoplasma gondii* (life cycle)** for explanation
- Option d: Follow section, ***Toxoplasma gondii* (pathogenicity → mode of transmission)** for explanation

18) **(b)**
- Option a & d: Follow section, ***Toxoplasma gondii* (pathogenicity → clinical feature & flow chart-7)**
- IgM antibodies are diagnostic in congenital toxoplasmosis
- Option c: Follow section, ***Toxoplasma gondii* (pathogenicity → disease name)** for explanation

19) **(b) & (d)**
- Option a, b & d: Follow section, ***Toxoplasma gondii* (pathogenicity → mode of transmission)** for explanation
- Option c: Follow section, ***Toxoplasma gondii* (treatment)** for explanation

20) **(d)**
- Oocyst of *Cyclospora cayetanensis* contains 2 sporocyst & each sporocyst have two sporozoites (total 4 sporozoites in mature oocyst)

21) **(c)**
- All options except *Giardia* are acid fast
- Oocyst is the diagnostic form present in stool. Its size help to differentiate the option a, b & c as per **table-3**.

22) **(a)**
- Oocyst is the diagnostic form present in stool. Its size help to differentiate the option a & b as per **table-3**.
- *Microsporidia* & *Blastocystis hominis* are not containing oocyst.

89 Microspora and unclassified protozoa

Learning heading & subheadings

- **Microspora**
- **Unclassified protozoa**
  - *Blastocystis homonis*

Microspora

❖ **Taxonomy:**

- Taxonomic status is still unclear, few workers classified it as fungus, while protozoa by few.
- They are true eukaryotes, as they possess membrane bound nucleus & other cellular features, but they are unusual eukaryotes in that they contains 70S ribosome, no mitochondria & golgi membrane.

❖ **History:**

- It was Pastuer who identify the Microspora (*Nosema bombycis*) as a causative agent of **pebrine (Silkworm disease)** in 1863 in France.
- Microspora had been known as an animal pathogen for a very long time, it's role as human pathogen was identified in 1980 & advancing with AIDS.

❖ **Classification:**

I. **Systemic classification:** Follow chapter → Introduction and classification of parasites. **(Section →Table-3)**

II. **Pathogenic classification:**

- Million of species are known under the title of Microspora, almost all are animal pathogen.
- Only 9 genera & 13 species are known as human pathogen especially in immunodeficient persons **called opportunistic pathogens.**
- Few genera & species as human pathogens are mentioned in **table-1.**

❖ **Geographical distribution:** Worldwide.

❖ **Habitat:** Intestine & dissemination in other tissues as shown in **table-1**. Obligate intracellular parasite present free in cytoplasm or extracytoplasmic within the parasitophorous vacuole. It survive outside the host in free environment.

❖ **Morphology:** Morphological stage **called spore,** as shown in **fig.-1** with following features.

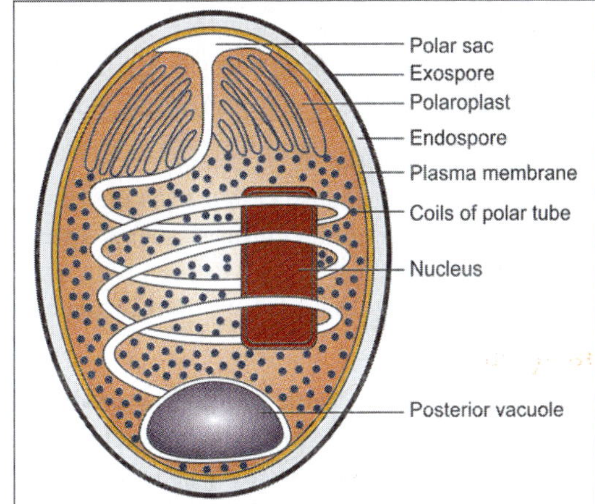

Figure-1: Spore of Microspora

➢ **Staining reaction:** Gram positive & acid fast in nature.

➢ **Size:** Up to 6μm in diameter.

➢ **Shape:** Variable like spherical, oval or rod shaped.

➢ **Structure:**

✪ **Nucleus:** Uninucleate or binucleate (diplokaryon).

✪ **Spiroplasm:**

- Contains tubular structure **called polar tube** or **polar filament** or **spiroplasm** which is 1.1 – 1.6μm in length & 0.7 – 1.0μm in breath.
- During infection sporoplasm is injected in to the host cells by extrusion mechanism.
- It is coiled up in the posterior half of the spore.

✪ **Polaroplast:** The anterior part of the polar filament is surrounded by a structure **called polaroplast.**

✪ **Vacuole:** Behind the polar filament, there is a posterior vacuole.

Genus	Species	Non human host	Clinical features in immunodeficient patients	Clinical features in immunocompetent patients
			Common	
Enterocytozoon	*E. bieneusi*	Pigs, non human primates	Chronic diarrhoea, wasting syndrome Cholangitis, AIDS cholengiopathy, cholecystitis, pneumonia, chronic sinusitis	Traveller's diarrhoea
Encephalitozon	*E. cuniculi* (three strain I, II & III)	Mammals, rabbits, mice, blue foxes, dogs	Sinusitis, keratoconjunctivitis, bronchitis, pneumonia, hepatitis, encephalitis	Not described
	E. hllem	Parrots	Sinusitis, keratoconjunctivitis, cystitis, bronchitis, pneumonia, urethritis	Not described
	E. intestinalis	Goats, donkeys, pigs, cows, dogs	Sinusitis, bronchitis, pneumonia, nephritis, chronic diarrhoea, cholangiopathy	Self limiting diarrhoea Asymptomatic carrier
			Uncommon	
Microsporidium	*M. africanum*	Not identified	Not described	Corneal ulcer, keratitis
	M. ceylonensis	,,	Not described	Corneal ulcer, keratitis
Nosema	*N. connori*	,,	Disseminated infection	Not described
	N. ocularum	,,	Not described	Keratitis
Pleistophora	*P.ronneafier*	,,	Myositis (Skeletal)	Not described
Brachiola	*B. vesicularum*		Myositis (Skeletal)	Not described
	B. conori		Myositis (Smooth & cardiac)	Not described
Trachi-pleistophora	*T. anthropo-phthera*	,,	Disseminated infection (Brain)	Not described
	T. hominis	,,	Sinusitis, keratoconjuctivitis, myositis	Not described
Vittaforma	*V. corneae*	,,	Keratitis	Not described

Table-1: Classification, non human host & clinical features of Microspora

✪ **Cell wall:** Consisting of three layers like
1. **Outer:** It is electron-dense **called exospores.**
2. **Middle:** Wide, containing chitin & seems structure less **called endospores.**
3. **Internal:** It is thin **called plasma membrane.**

❖ Life cycle:

➢ **Methods of reproduction:** Spores are produce by asexual method **called sporogony** which may be either binary fission **called merogony** or multiple fissions **called schizogony.**

➢ **Cycles:** →**Flow chart-1 & fig.-2.**

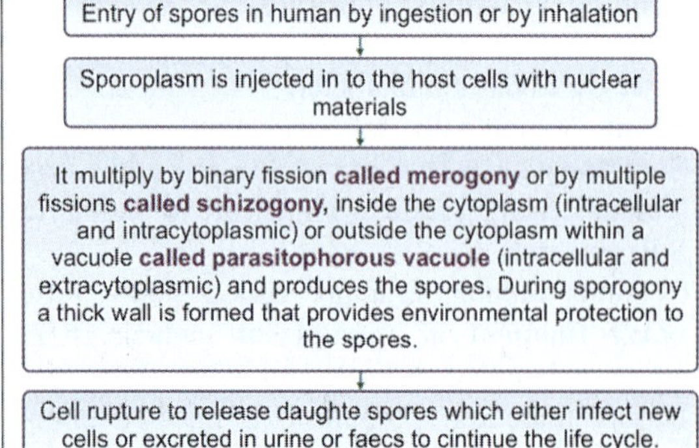

Entry of spores in human by ingestion or by inhalation
Sporoplasm is injected in to the host cells with nuclear materials
It multiply by binary fission called merogony or by multiple fissions called schizogony, inside the cytoplasm (intracellular and intracytoplasmic) or outside the cytoplasm within a vacuole called parasitophorous vacuole (intracellular and extracytoplasmic) and produces the spores. During sporogony a thick wall is formed that provides environmental protection to the spores.
Cell rupture to release daughte spores which either infect new cells or excreted in urine or faecs to cintinue the life cycle.

Flow chart-1: Life cycle of Microspora

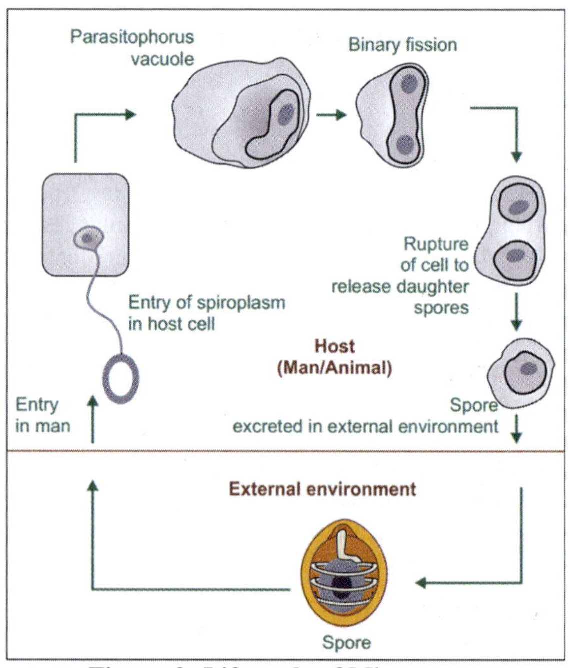

Figure-2: Life cycle of Microspora

❖ Pathogenicity:

➢ **Disease name: Called microsporidiosis.**

➢ **Reservoir of infection:** Exactly unknown but many vertebrate & invertebrate animals are reservoirs.

➢ **Source of infection:** Food & water contaminated by excreta of vertebrate & invertebrate animals.

➤ **Mode of transmission:**

- **Ingestion:** By ingestion of contaminated food & water contains spores that have been shed in the urine & faeces of infected man & animals.
- **Inhalation:** Is also possible route.

➤ **Infective & exit form:** Spore.

➤ **Portal of entry:** GIT or respiratory tract.

➤ **Sites:** Intestine & dissemination in other tissues.

➤ **Precipitating factor:** Most common in patient with AIDS & CMI defect.

➤ **Clinical features: → Table-1**

❖ Laboratory diagnosis:

I. Direct methods

➤ **Specimens:** Stool, urine, CSF, biopsy from infected tissues.

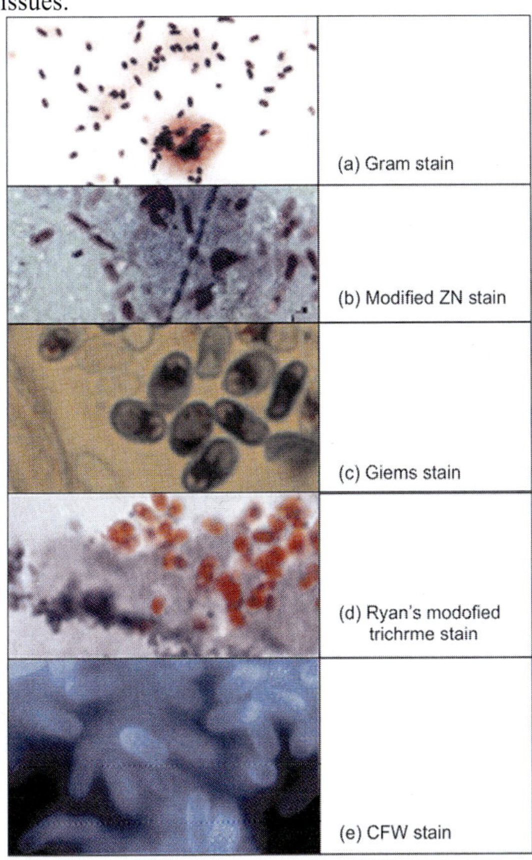

Figure-3: Microspora under different stains

➤ **Testing methods:**

A. Microscopy: To examine the spores.

i. Gram stain: Gram positive spores are appear as shown in **fig.-3 (a).**

ii. Modified ZN stain: Spores are acid fast (1% H_2SO_4) as shown in **fig.-3 (b)**.

- The acid-fast spores appeared bright red on a blue background, and a posterior vacuole and central diagonal strip within the spores were often visible.
- Bacteria and other cell debris appeared blue, owing to methylene blue counter stain.

iii. Giemsa stain: The darkly stained spores could be identified as shown in **fig. -3(c).**

iv. Ryan's modified trichrome stain: Appear red in colour as shown in **fig. -3(d).**

v. Calco Fluor White (CFW) stain: Spores are seen as white oval bodies, often clustered in groups, against a relatively dark background as shown in **fig.-3(e).** Spores displayed variable fluorescence intensities.

B. Culture: Microspora can be cultured in following cells.

- Monkey kidney cells.
- Rabbit kidney cells.
- Human foetal lung fibroblast.

II. Indirect methods

A. Serological tests: Under trial.

B. Molecular tests: Under trial.

❖ Prevention: Avoid the use of contaminated food & water.

❖ Treatment:

- No any specific & effective drug.
- Intestinal microsporidiasis is treated with Metronidazole or albendazole.
- For superficial keratoconjunctivitis, topical therapy with fumagilin suspension can be used.

Unclassified protozoa

Blastocystis homonis

❖ Taxonomy: Initially it was considered as an alga, then yeast & since 1982 a protozoan.

❖ Habitat: Human intestine.

❖ Morphology: Four morphological forms.

1. Vacuolated form:

- Most common form.
- About 8 µm (range 5-32 µm).
- It has large central vacuole & thin rim of cytoplasm contains 2-4 nuclei.
- It multiplies by binary fission.

2. Granular form:

- Second most common form.
- Multiply by endodyogeny & endosporulation.

3. Amoeboid form:

- It is non motile.
- A research study has reported that amoeboid forms are produced only in cultures taken from symptomatic individuals, with asymptomatic individuals producing exclusively vacuolar forms.

4. Cyst form:

- It is the infective form.

- Immature cyst released from host which gets mature in external environment & infects the other host.

❖ **Life cycle:** → **Fig.-4**

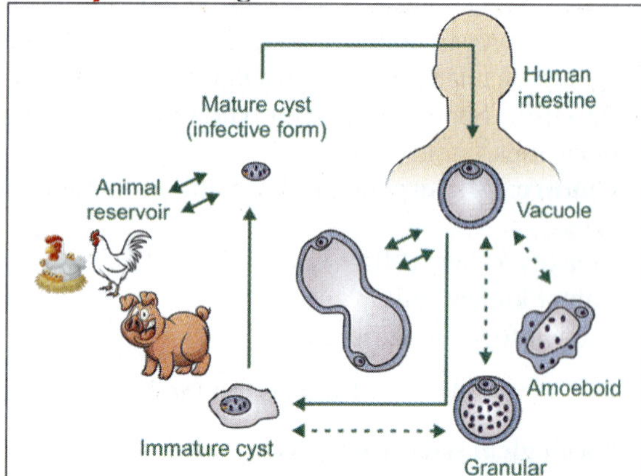

Figure-4: Life cycle of *Blastocystis homonis*

❖ **Pathogenicity:**

➢ **Disease name: Called blastocytosis.**

➢ **Reservoir of infection:** Like hens & other as shown in **fig.-4.**

➢ **Source of infection:** Food & water contaminated by excreta of hens & others.

➢ **Mode of transmission:**

- **Ingestion:** By ingestion of contaminated food & water contains mature cyst.

➢ **Infective:** Mature cyst.

➢ **Exit form:** Immature cyst.

➢ **Portal of entry:** GIT.

➢ **Sites:** Intestine.

➢ **Clinical features:** Causes diarrhoea.

❖ **Treatment:** Iodoquinol & Metronidazole are effective drugs.

Question bank

Short notes

1) Microspora.

Short questions for theory/viva questions

1) Name the methods of reproduction for *Microspora.*
2) Draw the morphological diagram of *Microspora.*

MCQs for chapter review

Microspora

1) **Causative agent of Silk worm disease was identified by**
(a) Pasteur (b) Jener (c) Koch (d) Philpis
2) **Which of the following is true with Microsporidia** (PGI, Dec-05)
(a) It is fungus (b) It is protozoan (c) It is bacteria (d) It is associated with diarrhoea in HIV

Answers of MCQs & explanation

1) **(a)**
- Follow section, ***Microspora*** (**history**) for explanation

2) **(b) & (d)**
- Follow section, ***Microspora*** (**taxonomy & pathogenicity**) for explanation

90 General properties of metazoa

Learning heading & subheadings

- ❖ Synonym:
- ❖ Meaning:
- ❖ Classification:
- ❖ General morphological features:
- ❖ Methods of reproduction:

❖ **Synonym:** Term metazoan also **called helminths** or **worms.**

❖ **Meaning:** Helminths is a **Greek** word derived from **helmin = worm**, originally referred to intestinal worms.

❖ **Classification:** →**Flow chart-1**

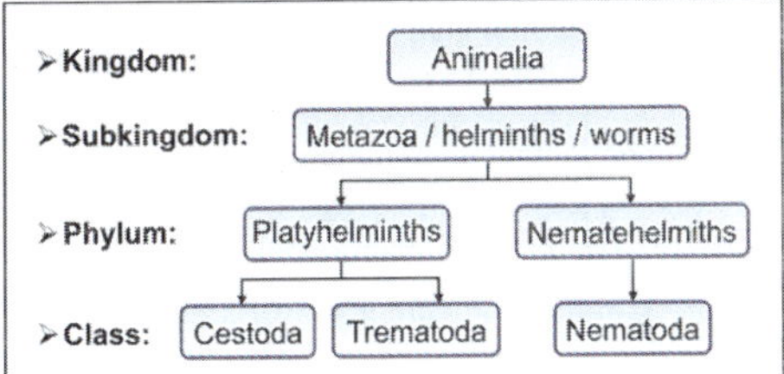

Flow chart-1: Classification of metazoa

❖ **General morphological features:**

I. Adult stage

➢ **Numbers of cell:** Multicellular & bilaterally symmetrical.

➢ **Size:** Male is usually smaller than female.

➢ **Germ layers:** They have three germ layers **called treploblastic genera**.

➢ **Covering:** Helminths have tough outer protective covering **called cuticle** or **tegument** which may be armed with spines or hooks & resistant to intestinal digestion.

➢ **Organs of adhesion:** Many helminths have suckers &/or hooks on head for attachment to host cells.

➢ **Organs for locomotion:**

- They do not have organs of locomotion, but have suckers, assist in movement.
- Locomotion is mainly due to muscular contraction & relaxation.

➢ **Mouth:** It contains teeth or cutting plates.

➢ **Nervous system:** It is primitive in many worms.

➢ **Excretory system:** Better developed.

➢ **Reproductive system:**

- In many worms both male & female reproductive organs are present in single individual **called monoecious** or **hermaphrodite** while in some both male & female species are separate **called diecious.**
- In monoecious worms self or cross fertilisation take place.
- Male die after fertilising the female in diecious worms.
- **Parthenogenic helminth:** Female laying eggs or larvae without mating to male **called parthenogenic helminth** like in *S. stercoralis*.

II. Egg (ovum) stage

➢ **Numbers:** About 2, 00, 000 eggs are produced per female per day.

➢ **More details:** Discussed in respective chapters.

III. Larval (embryonic or maggot) stage

➢ **More details:** Discussed in respective chapters.

❖ **Methods of reproduction:** Reproductive organs & methods are described in respective chapters.

➢ **Cestodes:** **Follow chapter → Cestodes: General features and classification.**

➢ **Trematodes:** **Follow chapter → Trematodes: General features and classification.**

➢ **Nematodes:** **Follow chapter → Nematodes: General features and classification.**

Question bank

Short questions for theory/viva questions

1) What is tegument in helminths?
2) What are monoecious & diecious parasites?

MCQs for chapter review

General morphological features

1) **Maggots word to which stage of parasite**
(a) Adult (b) Egg (c) Larval (d) None

Answers of MCQs & explanation

1) **(c)**
- Follow section, **general morphological features (larval stage)** for explanation

91 Cestodes: General features and classification

Learning heading & subheadings

- Synonym:
- Meaning:
- Habitat:
- Morphology:
- Differences between Pseudophyll idea & Cyclophyllidea:
- Classification:

❖ **Synonym:** **Tape worm** because dorso-ventrally flat & broad as like a measure tape.

❖ **Meaning:** Cestodes originated from **Kestos (Greek) = ribbon** or **girdle + edios = appearance,** as the parasites are ribbon or measure tape in shape.

❖ **Habitat:** Small intestine & also in tissues.

❖ **Morphology:**

I. Adult stage

➢ **Shape:** They are dorso-ventrally flat & broad as like a measure tape hence **called tape worm[fig.-1(a)].**

➢ **Size:** Segmented & few millimetre to several metres in length**[fig.-1(a)].**

➢ **Morphological parts:** Three parts.

A. **Scolex (head):**Contains following organs.

✪ **Suckers:→ Fig.-1(b) & (c).**

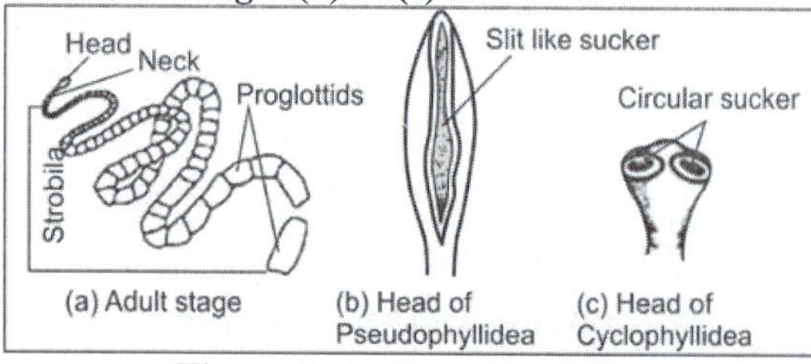

Figure-1: Sucker of cestodes

- It is an organ for adhesion with host cells.
- It may be slit like as in Pseudophyllidea**called bothria**or cup (circular) like as in Cyclophyll idea **called acetabula.**

✪ **Hooks:**

- It is also an organ for adhesion with host cells.
- Parasite with hooks **called armed tape worm**& which lacks**called unarmed tape worm.**

✪ **Rostellum:**

- Beak like projection on the head **calledrostellum.**
- It present in some tape worm like *Taeniasolium.*
- It is surrounded by hooks
- Its having characteristic shape in each family.

B. **Neck:**It is the part behind head from which segments (proglottids) of the body are generated continuously.

C. **Strobila (body or trunk):**Some authors used it for entire worm - head, neck & trunk.It is composed of chain of segments **called proglottids.**

✪ **Proglottids (segments):**

- **Types:** Three types according to maturity with following order from front to backwards.

1. **Immature:** Male & female organs are not differentiated.
2. **Mature:**Male & female organs are differentiated & male organs are appear first.
3. **Gravid:** Uterus is filled with eggs with disappearance or atrophy of other organs.

- **Nervous system &excretory system:** Are present.
- **Alimentary canal:** Absent.
- **Body cavity:** Absent.
- **Reproductive system:→Fig.-2& fig.-3.**

○ Definition:In cestodes both male & female reproductive organs are present in single individual **called monoecious** or **hermaphrodite.**

○ Reproductive organs:

A. **Female reproductive organs:**Present on ventral surface with following organs.

1. **Ovary:**

- Numbers: Single or paired.
- Lobes: Bilobed.
- Site: Lying behind equatorial plane of each segments.
- Function: It discharge the ova in the oviduct which connect the spermatic duct with the ootype.

2. **Vagina:**
- Course: Extend from genital pore to the ootype& inner end contains the receptacle for storage of sperms **called seminal receptacle** followed by constricted tubule **called spermatice duct.**
- Function: It provide route for entrance of sperm.

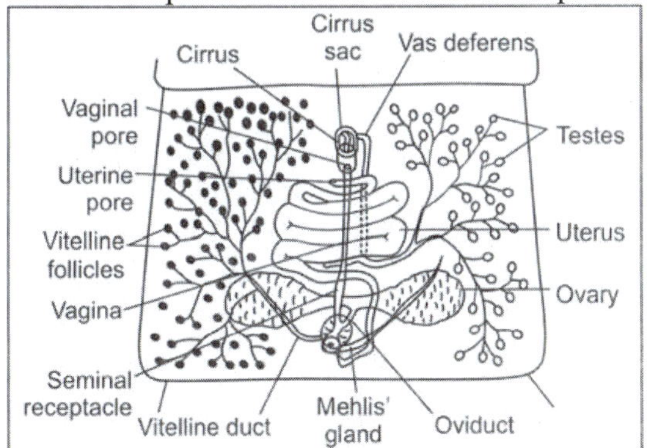

Figure-2: Reproductive system of Pseudophyllidea

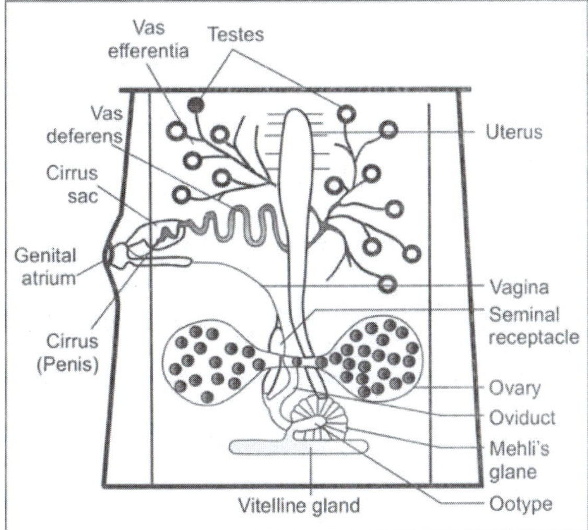

Figure-3: Reproductive system of Cyclophyllidea

3. **Uterus:**
- Course: Straight tube arises from ootype.
- In Pseudophyllidea uterus is non-branching & in Cyclophyllidea it may sometime contains branches.
- It may be open in Pseudophyllidea (uterine pore present) or like blind sac as in Cyclophyllidea (uterine pore absent).
- Function: Contains eggs when gravid.

4. **Ootype:**
- Site: Situated posteriorly in the middle of each segments.
- Function: It provides platform for fertilisation of eggs.

5. **Vitelline/yolk glands (vitellaria):** It scattered throughout the segment in Pseudophyllidea or remains as a single mass in Cyclophyllidea.

6. **Mehli's gland:**
- Synonym: Also **called shell gland.**
- Site: Very small organ surrounding the ootype& contains unicellular glands which open separately in to the ootype.

B. Male reproductive organs: Present on dorsal surface & mature prior to female system with following organs.

1. **Testes:**
- Numbers& lobes: Remains as multiple follicle.
- Site: It scattered throughout the segment.
- Function: It produces the sperms && each testes connected to vas deferens via small tubules **called vas efferentia.**

2. **Vas deferens:**
- Course: It is a convoluted tubule that begins from the centre of each segment & ascends upward to open in to the common genital pore in Pseudophyllidea or passes laterally to open in to the genital atrium (common genital pore) in Cyclophyllidea.
- Function: It enlarge for storage of sperms **called seminal vesicle.**

3. **Cirrus sac & cirrus (penis):**
- A sac like structure at the end of vas deferens **called cirrus.**
- It contains a muscular organ **called cirrus**or **penis.**

- Genital atrium:
- Synonym: Common genital pore.
- Site: It present on the mid-ventral surface in Pseudophyllidea& laterally in Cyclophyllidea.
- Function: It provides place for common opening of penis & vagina.

- Fertilisation:
- Definition: Mating of sperm with ovum.
- Types: Two types.

1. **Self fertilisation:**When take place in a same segment.
2. **Cross fertilisation:** When take place between the segments of same or other worm.

II. Eggstage

- **Development:** Formed in ootype& surrounded by protective covering.
- **Morphological features:**

A. Eggs of Pseudophyllidea:→ Fig.-4

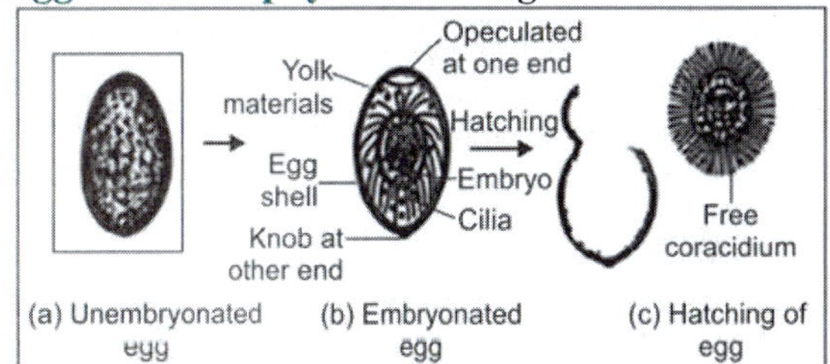

Figure-4: Egg stage ofPseudophyllidea

i. **Unembryonated eggs:** Initial not containing the embryo & passed with faeces in water for further maturation.

ii. Embryonated eggs:

- **Size:** 70µm × 45µm.
- **Shape:** Oval &operculated at one end & small knob at other end.
- **Colour:** Brown colour (bile stained).
- **Covering:** Single covering **called egg shell.**
- **Yolk material:** Present in abundant amount.
- **Embryo:**
  - Initial not present but formed later within 1-2 weeks of egg's escape from host.
  - Single egg gives the single embryo.
  - Embryo is unsegmented**called coracidium.**
  - Coracidium released free in water on hatching of egg & taken up by cyclops.
- **Cilia around embryo:** Present.

B. Eggs of Cyclophyllidea:→ Fig.-5

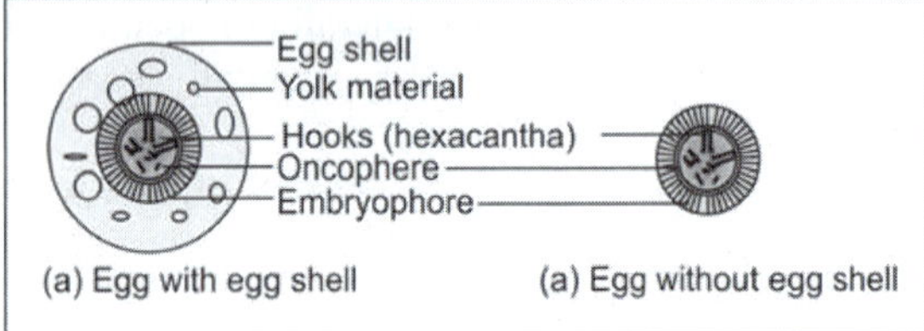

Figure-5: Egg stage ofCyclophyllidea

- **Size:** 31- 43µm in diameter.
- **Shape:**Spherical &non-operculated.
- **Covering:** Two covering as follows.

1. Outer:

- It is thin **called egg shell.**
- Sometime it ruptures before the eggs are excreted with faeces.

2. Inner:

- It is thick **called embryophore.**
- It becomes very thick after rupture of egg shell & radially striated to protect the inner oncosphere.

- **Space between two coverings:** Taken up by yolk material.
- **Embryo:**
  - Initially contains embryo **called oncopshere** when laid down.
  - Contains 6- hooklets (3- pairs) **called hexacanth.**
- **Cilia around embryo:** Absent.

III. Larval stage

A. Larvae of Pseudophyllidea:→ Fig.-6

Figure-6: Larval stage of Pseudophyllidea

- **Form:**Solid forms of larva are present.
- **Stages, name& hosts:** 1st stage develops free in water **called coracidium**while 2nd stage in cyclops(1^{s} intermediate host) **called procercoid**& 3rd stage in fish/frog/snake (2nd intermediate host) **called plerocercoid**or **sparganum.**

B. Larvae of Cyclophyllidea:→ Fig.-7

- **Form:**Vesicular /bladder forms of larva are present.
- **Name:Called cysticercus**(in *T. solium*&*T. saginata*) or**hydatid cyst** (in *E. granulosus*)or**cysticercoid**(in *H. nana*) or **coenurus**(in *M.multiceps*)discussed in respective chapters.

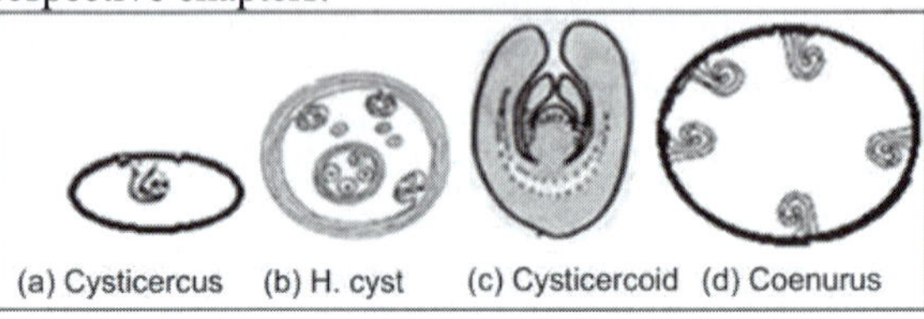

Figure-7: Larval stage of Cyclophyllidea

❖ Differences between Pseudophyllidea & Cyclophyllidea: →Table-1

Features	Pseudophyllidea	Cyclophyllidea
Suckers	Slit like **called bothria**	Circular shape **called acetabula**
Uterus	No branching	May or may not be branching
Uterine pore (opening)	Present	Absent
Vitelline glands	Scattered	Single mass
Vas deferens	Ascend upward	Pass laterally
Genital atrium	Present on mid ventral surface. Allows the three opening of vas deferens, vagina & uterus	Present laterally. Allows the two opening of vas deferens & vagina
Egg's shape	Oval &operculated	Spherical &Nonoperculated
Covers of egg	Single	Two
Embryo formation	Not present initially in eggs & formed later	Present since beginning
Cilia around embryo	Present	Absent
Larva	Solid form **called coracidium, procercoid&plerocercoid**	Vesicular/bladder form **called CysticercusorHydatid cyst** or **Cysticercoid** or **Coenurus**

Table-1: Differences between Pseudophyllidea&Cyclophyllidea

❖ Classification:

I. Systemic classification: Follow chapter → Introduction and classification of parasitesfor more details.

II. Pathological classification: Following are the pathogenic species & further classified on the basis of morphological stage infecting man.

A. Pseudophyllidea:→ Table-2

B. Cyclophyllidea:→ Table-3

Genus	Species	Definitive host	Intermediate host
	Adult stage		
Diphyllobothrium	*D. latum*	Man, dog, cat	Cyclops & fish
	Larval stage		
Spirometra	*S. mansoni*	Cat & dog	Cyclops, Frog, fish, snake
	S. proliferum	Cat & dog	Cyclops, Frog, fish, Snake

Table-2: Pseudophyllideancestodes

Genus	Species	Definitive host	Intermediate host
	Adult stage		
Taenia	*T. saginata*	Man	Cow
	T.solium	Man	Pig, Man
Hymenolepis	*H. nana*	Man, Rat	Rat flea, human flea (?)
	H. diminuta	Rat, Man	Rat flea, Beetle
Dypylidium	*D.caninum*	Dog, Cat, Man	Dog flea, Cat flea, Human flea
	Larval stage		
Echinicoccus	*E. granulosus*	Dog, Wolf, Jackal	Sheep, Cattle, Goat, Man
	E. multilocularis	Fox, Dog, Dingo, Wolf	Man, Field mouse, Tundra vole
Taenia	*Cysticercuscellulosae* of *T. solium*	Man	Pig, Man
Multiceps	*Coenurus*of *M. multiceps*	Fox, Dog, Wolf	Sheep, Cattle, Goat, Man

Table-3: Cyclophyllideancestodes

Question bank

Short notes

1) Difference between Pseudophyllidea&Cyclophyllidea.
2) Pathological classification of cestodes.
3) Systemic classification of cestodes.

Short questions for theory/viva questions

1) What is armed tape worm?
2) What is unarmed tape worm?
3) Name the larval stages of Pseudophyllidea.
4) Name the larval stage for following parasites.
   - *T. solium* - *T. saginata*
   - *E. granulosus*- *H. nana* - *M .multiceps*

MCQs for chapter review

Morphology

1) **Acetabulum of cestodesrefers to**
   (a) Hook (b) Sucker(c) Rostellum (d) Proglotid
2) **The following eggs have hexacanth embryo except**
   (a) *T solium*(b) *T saginata* (c) *Chlonorchis nana* (d) *Hnana*
3) **Larval form of *Taenia* is referred to as**
   (a) Cysticerus (b) Cysticercoid (c) *Echinococcosis* (d) Coenurus
4) ***Cysticeruscellulosae* seen in**
   (a) *T saginata* (b) *T solium*(c) *D latum* (d) *S haematobium*

Classification

5) **Which of the following is not a cestodes**
   (a) Diphyllobo-thrium*latum* (b) Taenia*saginata*(c)*Schistosomamansoni* (d) *Echinicoccusgranulosus*

Answers of MCQs & explanation

1) **(b)**
- Follow section **morphology (adult stage) & table-1** for explanation
2) **(c)**
- Follow section **morphology (egg stage → eggs of Cyclophyllidea)** for explanation
3) **(a), (b) & (d)**
- Echinococcosis is the disease name caused by *E granulosus.*
- Cysticercusis the larval stage in *T. solium*&*T. saginata*, cysticercoid is the larval stage in *H. nana (Taenia nana)* &coenurusis the larval stage in *M. multiceps (Taeniamulticeps*).
4) **(b)**
- *Schistosomahaematobium* is trematode. Follow section **morphology (larval stage → larvae of Cyclophyllidea→name)** for explanation.
5) **(c)**
- *Schistosomamansoni* is trematode while all others are cestodes. Follow section **classification (table-2 & table-3)** for explanation.

92 Cestodes: Pseudophyllidea

Learning heading & subheadings

- General features:
- Classification:

Diphyllobothrium latum

Spirometra spp.

General features:

➢ **Adult stage:**

- **Suckers:** Two slit like suckers or groove **called bothria.**
- **Uterus:** No branching.
- **Uterine pore:** Uterine opening or pore is present through which eggs are come out.
- **Vitelline glands:** Scattered through the segment & consist many acini.
- **Vas deferens:** Ascend upward.
- **Genital atrium:**
  - Present on mid ventral surface.
  - There are three genital opening in each segment.
  1. Male orifice of vas deferens.
  2. Female orifice of vagina.
  3. Female orifice of uterus.

➢ **Egg stage:**

- **Shape:** Oval & operculated. Eggs are developing only in water. They are immature when oviposited.
- **Cover:** Single.
- **Embryo formation:** Not present initially in eggs & formed later.
- **Cilia around embryo:** Present.

➢ **Larval stage:**

- **Form:** Solid form of larva is present.
- **Stages, name & hosts:** 1st stage develops free in water **called coracidium** while 2nd stage in cyclops (1^{s} intermediate host) **called procercoid** & 3rd stage in fish/frog/snake (2nd intermediate host) **called plerocercoid** or **sparganum.**

Classification:

I. **Systemic classification:** Follow chapter → Introduction and classification of parasites **(Section → table-4).**

II. **Pathological classification:** Following are the pathogenic species.

i. ***Diphylobothrium latum***

ii. ***Spirometra* species:** Following are different species.

- *S. mansoni* (Cobbold, 1882).
- *S. ranarum.*
- *S. mansonoides.*
- *S. erinacei.*
- *S. proliferum* (Ijima, 1905).
- *S. erinacei.*

Diphyllobothrium latum

❖ **Common name:**

1. **Fish tape worm:** As it transmitted by eating the raw fish. It is not occurs in India, as Indian does not have habit to eat raw fish.
2. **Broad tape worm:** Related to morphology.

❖ **Meaning:** **Di = Two + Bothria = Slit like suckers (Sucking organs).**

❖ **Synonym:** *Taenia lata, Bothriocephalus latus* & *Dibothriocephalus latus.*

❖ **History:**

- It was 1st identified by Dunus in 1592.
- Life cycle was 1st worked out by Janicki & Rosen in 1917.

❖ **Geographical distribution:**

- Central Europe, America, Japan, & Central Africa.
- Not reported from India.

❖ **Habitat:** Adult worm lives in small intestine (ileum) of man & in dog, cat, fox or other fish eating mammals.

❖ **Morphology:** Three morphological stages like adult, egg & larval are described below.

I. Adult stage

➢ **Time of maturation:** Plerocercoid larva transformed to sexually mature adult stage in 5-6 weeks in definitive host.

➢ **Colour:** Yellowish grey/ Ivory in colour with dark central marking caused by egg filled uterus.

- **Shape:** They are dorso-ventrally flat & broad as like a measure tape hence **called tape worm.**
- **Size:** 3 to 10 metres in length.
- **Life span:** 5-13 years.
- **Parts:** Three parts as shown in **(fig.-1).**

A. Scolex (head): → Fig.-1(b).

- **Shape:** Elongated & spoon (almond / lancet) shape.
- **Size:** 2-3mm × 1mm.
- **Suckers**: Two slit like suckers **called bothria** one is on the dorsal & other is on the ventral surface.
- **Rostellum:** Absent.
- **Hooklets:** Absent.

B. Neck:

- It is a thin part behind head from which segments (proglottids) of the body are generated continuously.
- It is much longer than the head.

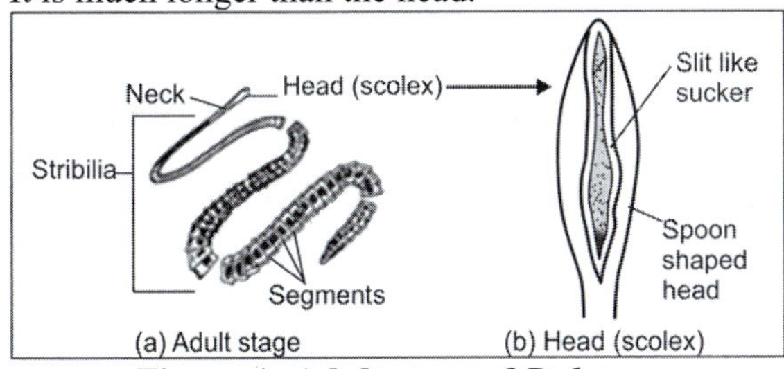

Figure-1: Adult stage of *D. latum*

C. Strobila (body or trunk): It is composed of chain of segments **called proglottids** having following features.

- **Proglottids (segments):**
- **Numbers:** 3,000 - 4,000.
- **Size (mature segment):** 2-3mm × 10-20mm. Greater in breadth than length.
- **Types:** Three types according to maturity with following order from front to backwards.

1. **Immature:** Male & female organs are not differentiated.
2. **Mature:** Male & female organs are differentiated & male organs are appear first.
3. **Gravid:** Uterus is filled with eggs with disappearance or atrophy of other organs.

- **Terminal segments:** Shrunken & empty due to constant discharging of eggs through uterine pore. Later dried segment break up from strobila in chain & passed in faeces.
- **Reproductive system: → Fig.-2**
  - Definition: In cestodes both male & female reproductive organs are present in single individual **called monoecious** or **hermaphrodite.**
  - Reproductive organs:

A. Female reproductive organs:

1. **Uterus:** Large & remains coiled in the centre of each segment in the form of each rosette.
2. **Ovary, Ootype, Mehli's gland & other organs:** As shown in **fig.-2.**

B. Male reproductive organs: As shown in **fig.-2.**

- Genital atrium: It comprises the opening of vas deferens, vagina & uterus.

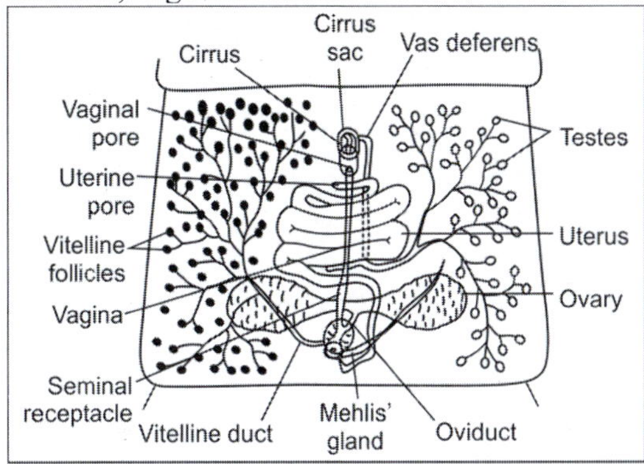

Figure-2: Reproductive system of *D. latum*

II. Egg stage

- **Development:** Formed in ootype & surrounded by protective covering.
- **Morphological features: → Fig.-3**

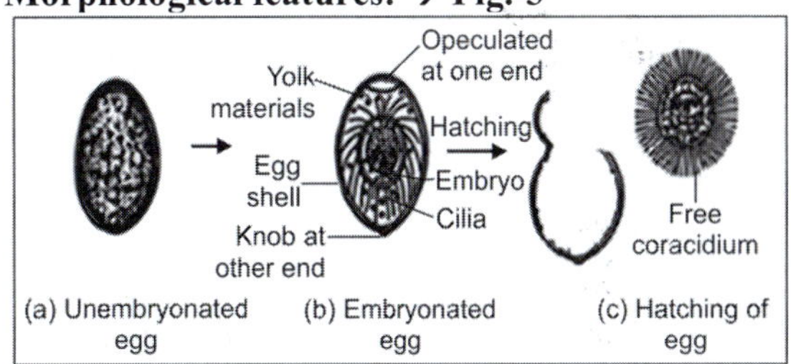

Figure-3: Egg stage of *D. latum*

i. **Unembryonated eggs:** Initial not containing the embryo & passed with faeces in water for further maturation.

ii. **Embryonated eggs:**

- **Size:** 70µm × 45 µm.
- **Shape:** Oval & operculated at one end & small knob at other end.
- **Colour:** Brown colour (bile stained).
- **Covering:** Single covering **called egg shell.**
- **Yolk material:** Present in abundant amount.
- **Embryo:**
  - Initial not present but formed later within 1-2 weeks of egg's escape from host.
  - Single egg gives the single embryo.
  - Embryo is unsegmented **called coracidium.**
  - Coracidium released free in water on hatching of egg & taken up by cyclops.

III. Larval stage

Single egg gives the single embryo. It passed by following three stages.

A. First stage: →Fig.-4 (a)

- Name: **Called coracidium.**
- Host: Present free in water.
- Hooklets: Contains 3 pairs of hooklets (hexacanth).
- Size: 40-55 µm in diameter.
- Shape: Spherical.

- Cilia: Surrounded by ciliated epithelium.
- Time of development: Eggs release the coracidium within 2-4 weeks.

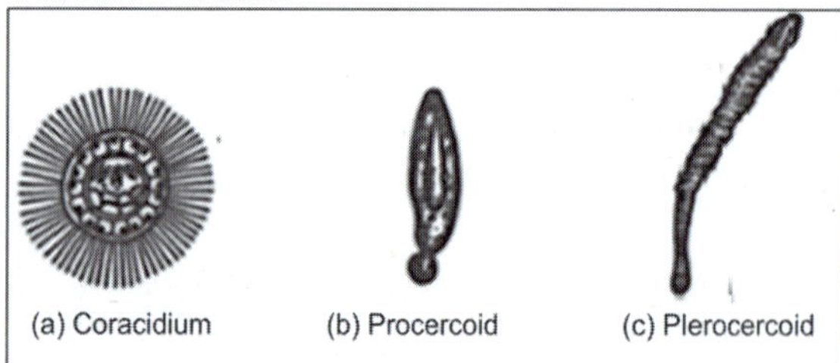
(a) Coracidium
(b) Procercoid
(c) Plerocercoid

Figure-4: Larval stage of *D. latum*

B. Second stage: →Fig.-4 (b)
- Name: **Called procercoid.**
- Host: Present in cyclops. Cyclops does not contain more than two larvae at a time.
- Hooklets: Spherical caudal appendages contain 3 pairs of useless hooklets.
- Size: About 500 -550μm in length.
- Shape: Elongated.
- Time of development: Coracidium transformed to procercoid form within 3 weeks in cyclops.

C. Third stage: →Fig.-4 (c)
- Name: **Called plerocercoid** or **sparganum.**
- Host: Present in fish.
- Colour: White.
- Size: About 6mm (small body) or 1-2cm in length (large body).
- Shape: Elongated & flattened. It's having wrinkled surface & rudimentary scolex.
- Time of development: Procercoid transformed to plerocercoid form within 1-3 weeks in fish.
- Clinical significance: It is the infective form.

❖ Life cycle:

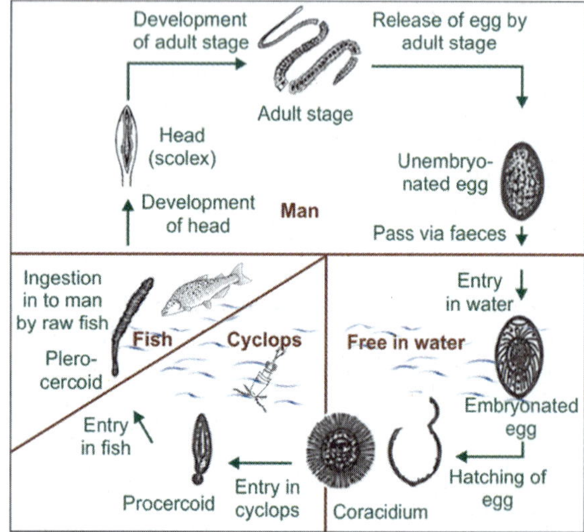
Development of adult stage
Release of egg by adult stage
Adult stage
Head (scolex)
Unembryo-nated egg
Development of head
Man
Pass via faeces
Ingestion in to man by raw fish
Fish
Cyclops
Entry in water
Free in water
Plero-cercoid
Embryonated egg
Entry in fish
Hatching of egg
Procercoid
Entry in cyclops
Coracidium

Figure-5: Life cycle of *D. latum*

➢ **Types of host:** Two types.

I. Definitive host: Man, dog & cat.

II. Intermediate hosts: Larval stage developed in two different aquatic animals.

1. **First intermediate host:** Cyclops or diaptomus.
2. **Second intermediate host:** Fresh water fish, pike, trout, salmon, perch & other fish.

➢ **Cycles:** As shown in **flow chart-1 & fig.-5.**

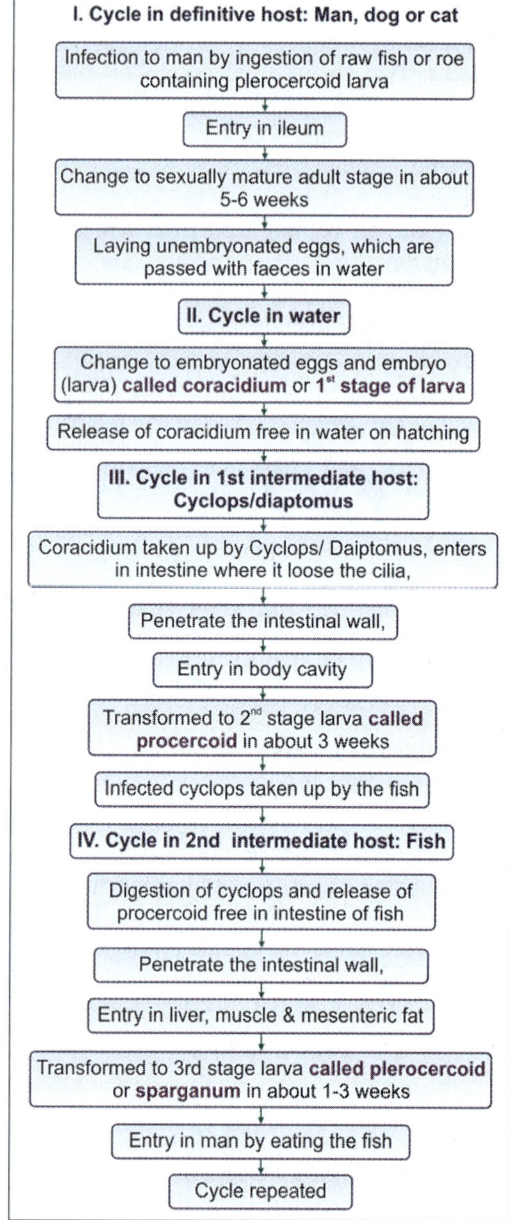
I. Cycle in definitive host: Man, dog or cat
Infection to man by ingestion of raw fish or roe containing plerocercoid larva
Entry in ileum
Change to sexually mature adult stage in about 5-6 weeks
Laying unembryonated eggs, which are passed with faeces in water
II. Cycle in water
Change to embryonated eggs and embryo (larva) called coracidium or 1st stage of larva
Release of coracidium free in water on hatching
III. Cycle in 1st intermediate host: Cyclops/diaptomus
Coracidium taken up by Cyclops/ Daiptomus, enters in intestine where it loose the cilia,
Penetrate the intestinal wall,
Entry in body cavity
Transformed to 2nd stage larva called procercoid in about 3 weeks
Infected cyclops taken up by the fish
IV. Cycle in 2nd intermediate host: Fish
Digestion of cyclops and release of procercoid free in intestine of fish
Penetrate the intestinal wall,
Entry in liver, muscle & mesenteric fat
Transformed to 3rd stage larva called plerocercoid or sparganum in about 1-3 weeks
Entry in man by eating the fish
Cycle repeated

Flow chart-1: Life cycle of *D. latum*

❖ Pathogenicity:

➢ **Disease name: Called diphyllobothriasis.**

➢ **Reservoir of infection:** Animal like bears, minks, canine family (dog, fox) & feline (cat).

➢ **Source of infection:** Fish.

➢ **Mode of transmission:** By ingestion of raw fish contains third stage of larva **called plerocercoid** or **sparganum**. It is not destroyed by ordinary salting, pickling or smoking.

➢ **Exit form:** Unembryonated egg.

- **Infective form:** Third stage of larva **called plerocercoid** or **sparganum.**
- **Portal of entry:** GIT.
- **Site:** Small intestine (ileum).
- **Precipitating factor:** Infection is precipitated in patients having hereditary or racial tendency.
- **Clinical features:**
- **Asymptomatic:**
- **GIT:**
  - Abdominal pain.
  - Diarrhoea.
  - Intestinal obstruction by adult worm.
  - Cholangitis due to migrating proglottids.
- **Anaemia: Called bothriocephalus anaemia** with following two types.

1. **Pernicious anaemia:**
   - Hypothesis given by Wardle & Green in 1941.
   - Unsaturated fatty acids liberated by *D. latum* interfere with intrinsic factors (of castle) which lead to pernicious anaemia.
2. **Megaloblastic anaemia:**
   - Hypothesis given by Von Bonsdorff in 1956.
   - When *D. latum* present in proximal part of jejunum, it utilises the vitamin B_{12} as nutritional material & causing the vitamin B_{12} deficiency.
   - About 40% of patients have low serum vitamin B_{12} & about 2% progress to megaloblastic anaemia.

- **CNS:** Numbness, paresthesia & loss of vibration sense due to vitamin B_{12} deficiency.
- **Blood:** Early eosinophilia.

❖ Laboratory diagnosis:

I. Direct methods

- **Specimens:** Stool.
  - *D. latum* is viable in refrigerated stool for one year.
  - Stool can be preserved by using 10% formalin.
- **Testing methods:**

A. **History:** Of raw fish eating is present.

B. **Macroscopic (naked eye) examination:** To rule out the presence of adult stage or segments.

C. **Microscopy:**

i. **For eggs:**

a. **Wet mount by using normal saline & iodine:** **→Fig.-6**
   - It shows the bile stained (brown colour) operculated egg with knob at the bottom.
   - Careful examination is needed to reveal the operculum.
   - When operculum is not examined easily, tapped the cover slip of wet mount & pressure may open the operculum.

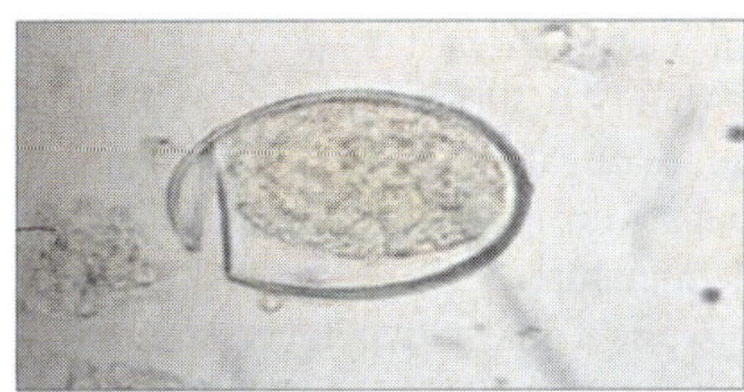

Figure-6: Egg of *D. latum* under wet mount

b. **Concentration technique:** In case of negative result by wet mount method.

ii. **For segments:** A segment has been identified under the microscope by knowing the characters of uterus & position of uterine pore.

D. **Isozyme technique:**
   - Useful to identify the segment.
   - Disadvantage: Available at reference centre.

II. Indirect methods

A. **Blood picture:** Eosinophilia.

B. **Serological tests:** ELISA & latex agglutination are positive in late cases.

❖ Prevention:

- Proper cooking of fish.
- Deep freezing (-10°C for 24-48 hours) of fish, if it is consumed to be raw.
- Periodical deworming of cats & dogs.
- Avoiding the faecal contamination of water.

❖ Treatment:

- Praziquantel: Single dose 10mg/kg is effective.
- Parenteral B12 is given of deficiency is present.

Spirometra spp.

❖ History:
History of discovery of different species is described with classification **(vide supra).**

❖ Geographical distribution:

- *S. mansoni* found in many parts of Asia like Japan, China, Vietnam, Taiwan, Korea & Thailand.
- *S. mansonoides* from America.
- Few cases reported from India also.

❖ Habitat:

- Naturally (adult worm) habitat in intestine of dog & cat. Dog & cat are infected by third stage of larva.
- Man is the accidental host & harbours the larval stage in peritoneum, subcutaneous tissue, eyes, muscles, brain & abdominal viscera.

❖ Morphology:
Similar to *D. latum* with following important features.

- Adult stage not occurs in man, but in dog or cat.
- Man is the accidental host & infected by 2nd or 3rd stage of larva.
- **Sparganum (3rd stage of larva):** Have following important features to keep in mind for diagnosis.

- Colour: Creamy –white.
- Size: About 10-30mm × 2-7mm.
- Shape: Elongated & flattened. Anterior end is without scolex (head) & marked by vertical groove.
- Motile in nature.
- Body wall: Consist two layers of muscles & one layer of tegument.
- Life span: Can live for more than 9 years in human
- Clinical significance: Infective form for man.

✓ **Note: Developmental variation in *S. proliferum***

- Sparganum found in granulomatous nodule/cyst often proliferate to give **supernumary buds** which eventually detach themselves & develop in to larva.

❖ Life cycle:

➢ **Types of host:** Three types.

I. **Definitive host:** Dog / cat.

II. **Intermediate hosts:** Larval stage develops in two different aquatic animals.

1. **First intermediate host:** Cyclops.
2. **Second intermediate host:** Frog / snakes / fish.

III. **Accidental host:** Man.

➢ **Cycles:** Two main types of cycle as shown in **flow chart-2 & fig.-7.**

I. **Cycle between definitive & intermediate hosts:** Cycle is continuing between dog/cat, cyclops & frog / snake / fish.

II. **Cycle in accidental host (cycle in man):**

- Man is the accidental host & act as dead end host & does not allow the continuation of cycle.
- It start from definitive host (dog/cat), pass through intermediate hosts (cyclops & frog/snakes/fish) & end in accidental host (man).

❖ Pathogenicity:

➢ **Disease name:** Man is infected by second & third stage of larva, but disease is produced by 3rd stage of larva **called sparganosis.**

➢ **Reservoir of infection:** Dog /cat.

➢ **Source of infection:** Cyclops / fish / frog.

➢ **Mode of transmission:** By following routes.

a. **Direct contact:** By applying the raw flesh to skin sore or eye sore or vagina as poultices (in China as custom). Wounded skin allows the entry of parasites.

b. **Indirect:** By ingestion mode as follows.

- **Water borne:** By drinking the water contains infected cyclops with 2nd stage of larva **called procercoid.**
- **Food borne:**
  - By eating the raw fish / frog contains 3rd stage of larva **called plerocercoid** or **sparganum.**
  - Human infection also occurs by ingestion of pork (Pig's meat) containing plerocercoid larvae (in case of *S. mansoni*).

➢ **Exit form:** Unembryonated egg is exit from dog/cat. Man is the dead end host for parasites.

➢ **Infective form:** Second & third stage of larva.

➢ **Portal of entry:** GIT & skin.

➢ **Sites:** Peritoneum, subcutaneous tissue, muscles, eyes, brain & abdominal viscera.

➢ **Precipitating factor:** Common in Chinese people due to customs of applying frog's flesh as poultices to skin sore or eye sore or vagina.

➢ **Pathogenesis:** It is characterised by granulomatous nodule with infiltration of lymphocytes, macrophages, eosinophils, neutrophils, plasma cells, giant cells. Charcoat – Layden crystals & multinucleated giant cells may be seen.

➢ **Clinical features:**

- **Granulomatous nodule / cyst:** In peritoneum, subcutaneous tissue, muscles, eyes, brain & abdominal viscera.
- **Eye swelling:** It should be differentiated from Chaga's disease (Romana's sign).

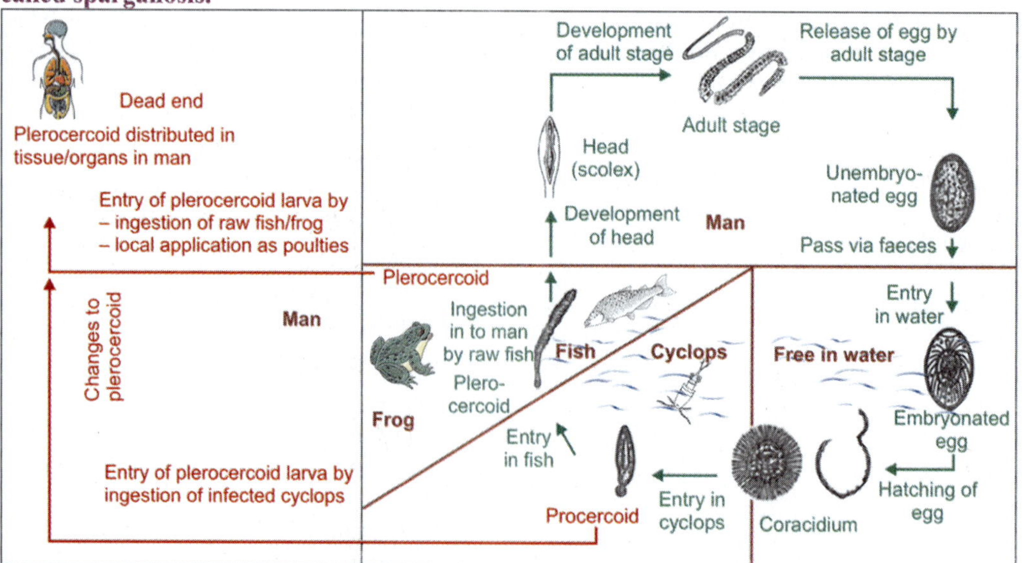

Figure-7: Life cycle of *Spirometra*

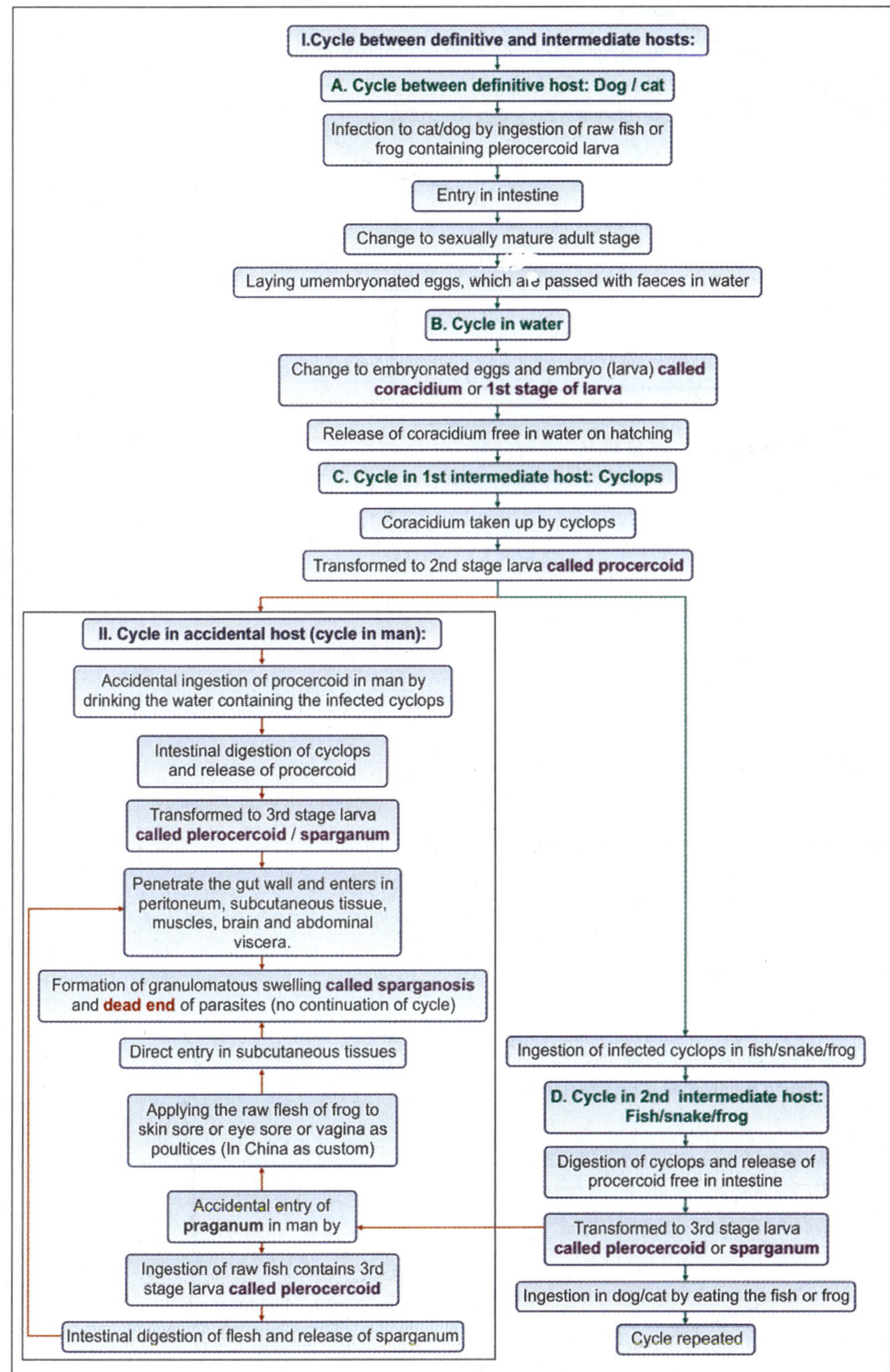
I.Cycle between definitive and intermediate hosts:
A. Cycle between definitive host: Dog / cat
Infection to cat/dog by ingestion of raw fish or frog containing plerocercoid larva
Entry in intestine
Change to sexually mature adult stage
Laying umembryonated eggs, which are passed with faeces in water
B. Cycle in water
Change to embryonated eggs and embryo (larva) called coracidium or 1st stage of larva
Release of coracidium free in water on hatching
C. Cycle in 1st intermediate host: Cyclops
Coracidium taken up by cyclops
Transformed to 2nd stage larva called procercoid
II. Cycle in accidental host (cycle in man):
Accidental ingestion of procercoid in man by drinking the water containing the infected cyclops
Intestinal digestion of cyclops and release of procercoid
Transformed to 3rd stage larva called plerocercoid / sparganum
Penetrate the gut wall and enters in peritoneum, subcutaneous tissue, muscles, brain and abdominal viscera.
Formation of granulomatous swelling called sparganosis and dead end of parasites (no continuation of cycle)
Direct entry in subcutaneous tissues
Applying the raw flesh of frog to skin sore or eye sore or vagina as poultices (In China as custom)
Accidental entry of praganum in man by
Ingestion of raw fish contains 3rd stage larva called plerocercoid
Intestinal digestion of flesh and release of sparganum
Ingestion of infected cyclops in fish/snake/frog
D. Cycle in 2nd intermediate host: Fish/snake/frog
Digestion of cyclops and release of procercoid free in intestine
Transformed to 3rd stage larva called plerocercoid or sparganum
Ingestion in dog/cat by eating the fish or frog
Cycle repeated

Flow chart-2: Life cycle of *Spirometra*

Laboratory diagnosis:

I. Direct methods

- **Specimens:** Tissue removal or biopsy from nodule.
- **Testing methods:**

A. **Macroscopic (naked eye) examination:** To rule out the presence of sparganum. It is looks like narrow tape worm & differentiated from adult stage of other tape worms by absence of suckers & hooklets.

B. **Species identification:** It can be done by allowing the cat or dog to eat live sparganum & subsequently identification of adult worm.

E. **Microscopy:** Histological examination is useful.

II. Indirect methods

A. **Blood picture:** Eosinophilia in 30-40% cases.
B. **Serological tests:** Agar gel diffusion & Indirect Haem Agglutination (IHA) tests are positive.

❖ **Prevention:**
- Proper cooking of fish.
- Proper boiling & filtering the drinking water.
- Periodical deworming of cats & dogs.
- Avoiding the faecal contamination of water from infected animals.

❖ **Treatment:** Surgical removal of nodule.

Question bank

Essay/Full question

1) Pseudophyllidea.
2) *D. latum.*

Short notes

1) Life cycle / pathogenicity / laboratory diagnosis of *D. latum.*
2) *Spirometra.*
3) Sparganosis.

Short questions for theory/viva questions

1) Write the two mechanisms for development of anaemia in *D. latum* infection.
2) Name the four parasites in which cyclops act as intermediate host or cyclops required to complete the life cycle.
3) Write the name of 1st, 2nd & 3rd stages of larva of *D. latum.*

MCQs for chapter review

Diphylobothrium latum

1) **Second intermediate host of *Diphylobothrium latum* is** (PGI-86)
(a) Cyclops (b) Man (c) Snail (d) Fresh water fish
2) **Vitamin deficiency due to *Diphylobothrium latum* infection**
(a) B1 (b) B2 (c) B4 (d) B12
3) ***Diphylobothrium latum* is causative organism of**
(a) Megaloblastic anaemia (b) Iron deficiency anaemia (c) Peptic ulcer (d) None

Answers of MCQs & explanation

1) **(d)**
- Follow section, ***Diphylobothrium latum*** **(life cycle → types of host)** for explanation

2) **(d)**
3) **(a)**
} Follow section, ***Diphylobothrium latum*** **(pathogenicity → clinical features)** for explanation

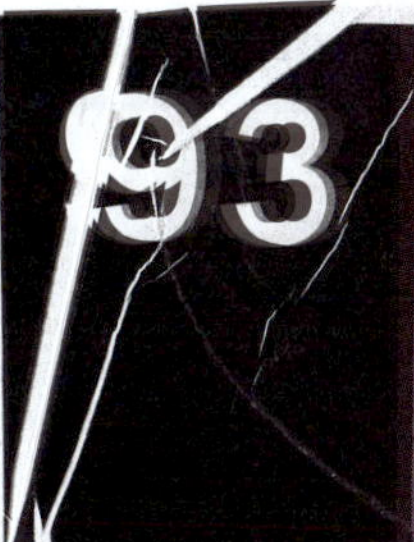

Cestodes: Cyclophyllidea

Learning heading & subheadings

- General features:
- Classification:

Taenia spp.
- *Taenia saginata saginata*
- *Taenia saginata asiatica*
- *Taenia solium*

Echincoccus spp.
- *Echinococcus granulosus*
- *Echinococcus multilocularis*
- *Echinococcus vogeli*
- *Echinococcus oligarthus*

Hymenolepis spp.
- *Hymenolepis nana*
- *Hymenolepis diminuta*

Dypylidium caninum

Multiceps spp.
- *Multiceps multiceps*

General features:

➤ **Adult stage:**
- **Suckers:** Four cup like suckers called acetabula.
- **Uterus:** Branching uterus is present.
- **Uterine pore:** Uterine opening or pore is absent & eggs are released by rupture of ripe segments. I Taenidae, Dilepidide ripe segments are detach from the main body & passed in the faeces.
- **Vitelline glands:** Present as single mass.
- **Vas deferens:** Passes laterally to open in to genit atrium.
- **Genital atrium:**
  - Present on lateral side.
  - There are two genital opening in each segment.
  1. Male orifice of vas deferens.
  2. Female orifice of vagina.

➤ **Egg stage:**
- **Shape:** Spherical, non-operculated. Eggs a mature when oviposited. They are expelled rupture of ripe segments.
- **Covering:** Two covering as follows.
  1. **Outer:**
     - It is thin called egg shell.
     - Sometime it ruptures before the eggs are excreted.
  2. **Inner:**
     - It is thick called embryophore.
     - It becomes very thick after rupture of egg shel radially striated to protect the inner oncosphere.
- **Space between two coverings:** Taken up by y material.
- **Embryo formation:**
  - Initial (when laid down) embryo calle oncosphere.
  - Contains 6 hooklets (3 pairs) called hexacanth.
- **Cilia around embryo:** Absent

➤ **Larval stage:**
- **Form:** Vesicular / bladder form of larva are present
- **Name:** Called cysticercoid (in *H. nana*) or cysticercus (in *T. solium* & *T. saginata*) or coenurus (in *M. multiceps*) or hydatid cyst (in *E. granulosus*) discussed in respective chapters.

Classification:

I. **Systemic classification:** F[illegible] → Introduction and classif[illegible] (Section → Table 4) for mo

II. **Pathological classificat[illegible]** pathogenic species.

i. ***Taenia* species:** Followi
- *Taenia saginata:* Two s

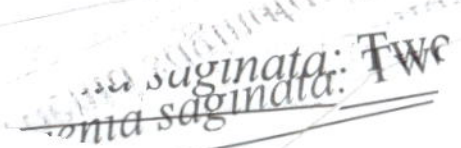

- *T. saginata saginata* & *T. saginata asiatica.*
- *Taenia solium.*
- **Echinococcus species:** Two species like
  - *Echinicoccus granulosus.*
  - *Echinicoccus multilocularis.*
- **Hymenolepis species:** Two species like
  - *Hymenolepis nana.*
  - *Hymenolepis diminuta.*
- ***Dypylidium caninum***
- **Multiceps species:** Three species like
  - *M. multiceps.*
  - *M. serialis (Taenia serialis)*: Definitive hosts are same as *M. multiceps* but intermediate host includes rabbits or rodents.
  - *M. glomeratus (Taenia glomeratus)*: Definitive host is unknown & intermediate host is gerbil.

Taenia spp.

Taenia saginata saginata

Meaning: From Taenia (Greek) ≡ tape or band, as it is dorso-ventrally flat like measure tape.

Common name:

- **Beef tape worm:** As it is transmitted by eating the raw beef (beef ≡ cow's meat) contains *Cysticercus bovis* (larval stage). Such infected beef looks like human measles so **called measly beef or beef measles** (beef + larva ≡ measly beef).
- **Unarmed tape worm:** Word is related to morphology like unarmed means without hooklets while tape worm means dorso-ventrally flat & broad adult stage as like a measure tape.

Synonym: *Taeniarhynchus saginata.*

History:

- Tapeworm infections have been recorded in history from 1500 B.C. and have been recognized as one of the earliest human parasites.
- *T. saginata* was differentiated from *T. solium* infection by the late 1700s by Goeze.
- Exact life cycle of *T. saginata* was discovered around 1863 when the cattle were identified as the immediate host by Leuckart.

Geographical distribution:

- World wide.
- In India it is common in Mohammedans (Non-vegetarian), due to custom of eating beef, but not in Hindu (vegetarian), as no rule of eating beef.

Habitat: Adult worm lives in small intestine (upper jejunum) of man & moves against peristaltic movements.

Morphology: Three morphological stages like adult, egg & larval are described below.

I. Adult stage

- **Time of maturation:** Larva transformed to sexually mature adult stage in 2-3 months in definitive host.
- **Colour:** White & semitransparent.
- **Size:** 5 to 10 metres in length (may be up to 24m).
- **Shape:** Like a measure tape.
- **Life span:** 10 years.
- **Morphological parts:** Three parts like head, neck & strobila (body/trunk) as shown in fig.-1(a).

A. Scolex (head): ⇒ Fig.-1(b)

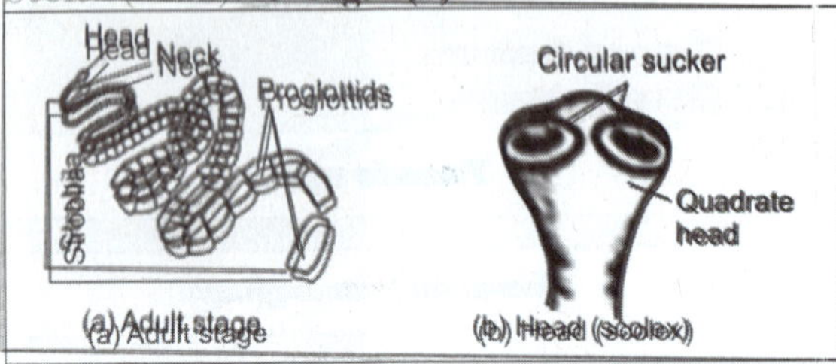

Figure-1: Adult stage of *T. saginata*

- **Shape:** Quadrate in shape.
- **Size:** Larger & about 1-2mm in diameter.
- **Suckers:** Four circular suckers **called acetabula** which may be pigmented.
- **Rostellum:** Absent.
- **Hooklets:** Absent.

B. Neck: It is long, narrow about 0.5mm wide & fragile.

C. Strobila (body or trunk): It is composed of chain of segments **called proglottids** having following features.

- **Proglottids (segments):** ⇒ Fig.-2

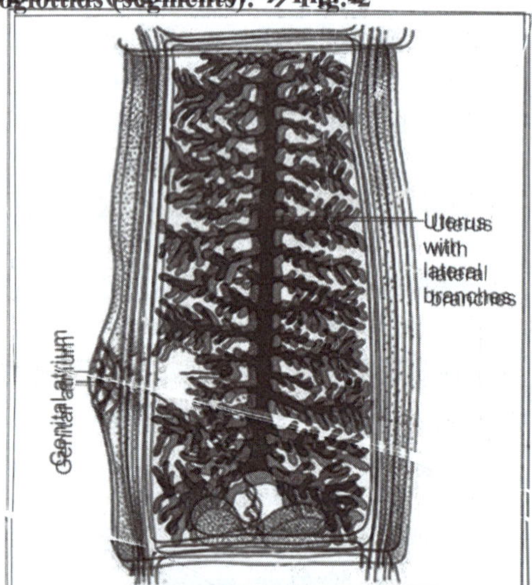

Figure-2: Segment of *T. saginata*

- **Numbers:** 1,000 - 2,000.
- **Size (gravid segment):** 22mm × 5mm. Length is 3-4 times greater than breadth.
- **Types:** Three types according to maturity with following order from front to backwards.

1. **Immature:** Male & female organs are not differentiated.
2. **Mature:** Male & female organs are differentiated & male organs are appear first.
3. **Gravid:** Uterus is filled with eggs.

- **Expulsion of eggs:** Expelled singly & may force anal sphincter. Free gravid segment while crawling out of anal orifice oviposits in the peri-anal skin, which are collected by NIH swab.
- **Reproductive system:**
  - Definition: In cestodes both male & female reproductive organs are present in single individual **called monoecious** or **hermaphrodite.**
  - Reproductive organs:

A. Female reproductive organs:

1. **Uterus:** 15-30 lateral branches on each side, thin & dichotomous (sub-branches).
2. **Ovary:** Two ovaries without any accessory lobe.
3. **Vagina:** Vaginal sphincter present.
4. **Ootype, Mehli's gland & other organs:** Present.

B. Male reproductive organs:

1. **Testes:** 300-400 follicles.
2. **Vas efferentia, vas deferens & cirrus (penis):** Are also present.

- Genital atrium: Present near the posterior end of lateral margin of each segment & alternates irregularly between right & left margins.

II. Egg stage

- **Development:** Formed in ootype & surrounded by protective covering.
- **Colour:** Brown colour (Bile stained).
- **Size:** 31- 43 μm in diameter.
- **Shape:** Spherical & non-operculated.
- **Life span:** Live about 8 weeks on field.
- **Morphological features:** → **Fig.-3**

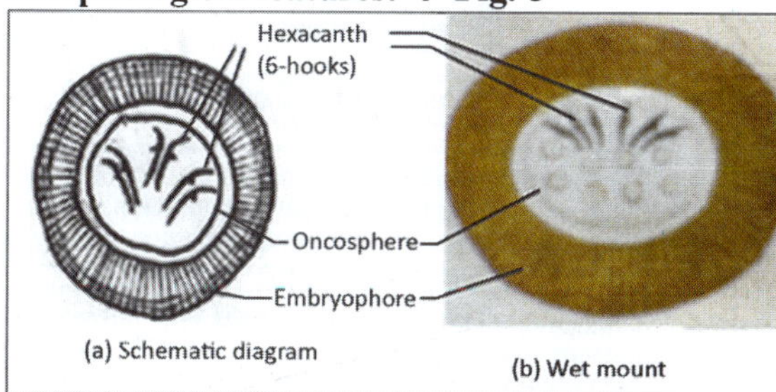

Figure-3: Egg of *T. saginata*

- **Covering:** Two covering as follows.

1. **Outer:**
   - It is thin **called egg shell.**
   - Sometime it ruptures before the eggs are excreted, but when present it represents the remnant of yolk mass.
   - It causes the eggs to clump together.
2. **Inner:**
   - It is thick **called embryophore.**
   - It becomes very thick after rupture of egg shell & radially striated to protect the inner oncosphere.

- **Embryo:**
  - Initially contains embryo when laid down.
  - Embryo **called oncopshere** with 14- 20 μm in size
  - Contains 6 hooklets (3 pairs) **called hexacanth,** which helps to penetrate the gut wall in intermediate host.
- **Cilia around embryo:** Absent.
- **Other features:**
  - Does not float in saturated common salt solution.
  - Infective only to cattle.
  - Acid fast under modified ZN stain. Only way to differentiate it from the egg of *T. solium.*

III. Larval stage

- **Development:** It develops in muscles of intermediate host (cow / buffalo) & matures further when ingested by man. It does not occur in man.
- **Size:** 3-4 mm in length × 5-10 mm in breadth.
- **Shape:** Oval.
- **Life span:** Live for 8 months in muscles of cattle.
- **Morphological features:** → **Fig.-4**

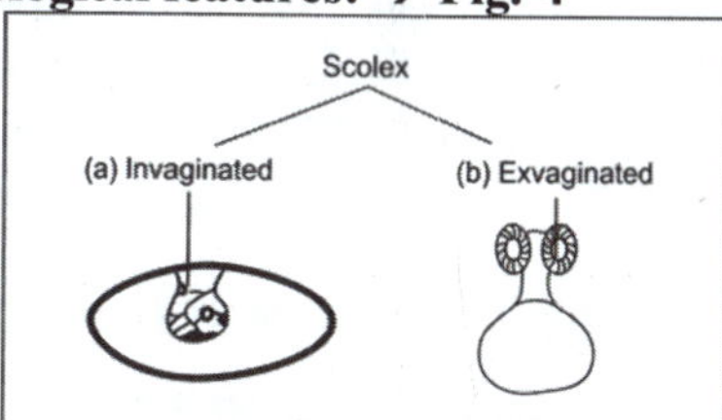

Figure-4: Larva of *T. saginata*

- Name: **Called *Cysticercus bovis*** (taxonomically not correct).
- Hooklets: Absent.
- Scolex (Future head of adult worm): It is invaginated from one side **[fig.-4(a)]**, later exvaginated **[fig.-4(b)]** in definitive host.
- Time of development: Eggs develop the *Cysticercus* within 60-70 days.

❖ Life cycle:

- **Types of host:** Two types.

I. Definitive host: Man (adult stage).

II. Intermediate host: Cow / buffalo (larval stage).

- **Cycles:** Two types as shown in **flow chart-1 & fig.-5.**

❖ Pathogenicity:

- **Disease name: Called intestinal taeniasis.**
- **Reservoir of infection:** Man.
- **Source of infection:** Cattle (beef).
- **Mode of transmission:** By ingestion of raw beef contains *C. bovis* (measly beef or beef measles).
- **Exit form:** Embryonated eggs / segments.
- **Infective form:** Larvae **called *Cysticercus bovis.***
- **Portal of entry:** GIT.

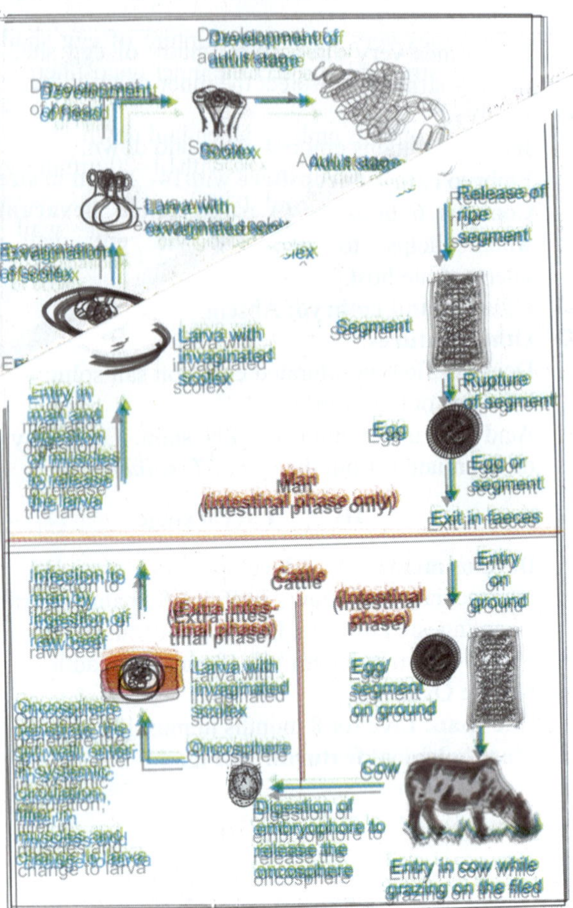

Figure-5: Life cycle of *T. saginata*

I. Cycle in definitive host: Man (intestinal phase only)

- Infection to man by ingestion of raw beef containing *Cysticercus bovis* (called measly beef or beef measles)
- Entry in intestine
- Digestion of muscle mass and larva becomes free in intestine
- Exagination of scolex on contact with bile
- Anchors to the gut wall by its scolex and change to sexually mature adult stage in about 2-3 months
- Release of ripe (gravid) segments from adult stage
- Rupture of segment to lay the eggs
- Segments (sometimes) and eggs are passed with the faeces on the ground

II. Cycle in intermediate host: Cattle

A. Intestinal phase

- *Entry of eggs in cattle (cow/buffalo) while grazing in the field*
- *Digestion of embryophore and release of oncospheres free in intestine*

B. Extra intestinal phase

- *Oncospheres penetrate the gut wall with the help of hooks*
- *Entry in portal circulation*
- Liver
- Right side of heart
- Lungs
- Left side of heart
- Systemic circulation
- The naked oncospheres are filtered out from the blood in to the muscles like tougue, neck, shoulder, hamstring and cardiac
- Oncospheres are losing their hooks and further develops to form *Cysticercus bovis* in 60-70 days, which enter in man by ingestion of raw beef. Each oncosphere give rise to single *Cysticercus*.
- Cycle repeated

Flow chart-1: Life cycle of *T. saginata*

- **Site:** Small intestine (upper jejunum).
- **Clinical features:** Only by adult stage as below.
- **Asymptomatic:**
- **GIT:** Abdominal discomfort like indigestion, diarrhoea with alternating constipation, intestinal obstruction & appendicitis has been observed.
- **Anaemia:**

Laboratory diagnosis:

I. Direct methods

- **Specimens:**
  - Stool: Segments of adult worm present in stool.
  - Eggs collection from perianal region by using.
    1. NIH (cellophane) swab method.
    2. Cellulose (Scotch) tape method.
  - Muscle biopsy from slaughtered animal.
- **Testing methods:**

A. History: Of beef eating is present.

B. Macroscopic (naked eye) examination:

i. For segments:

- White segments are present against yellowish stool
- Sometimes segments are also present in clothes of patient.

ii. For scolex: Species differention can be made by macroscopic examination of scolex (If adult stage is available) after antihelmintic treatment.

C. Microscopy:

i. For eggs:

a. Wet mount by using normal saline & iodine:

- It shows the bile stained (brown colour) eggs as shown in fig.-3(b).

b. Concentration technique: In case of negative result by wet mount method.

1. **Immature:** Male & female organs are not differentiated.
2. **Mature:** Male & female organs are differentiated & male organs are appear first.
3. **Gravid:** Uterus is filled with eggs.

- **Expulsion of eggs:** Expelled singly & may force anal sphincter. Free gravid segment while crawling out of anal orifice oviposits in the peri-anal skin, which are collected by NIH swab.
- **Reproductive system:**
  - Definition: In cestodes both male & female reproductive organs are present in single individual **called monoecious** or **hermaphrodite.**
  - Reproductive organs:

A. Female reproductive organs:

1. **Uterus:** 15-30 lateral branches on each side, thin & dichotomous (sub-branches).
2. **Ovary:** Two ovaries without any accessory lobe.
3. **Vagina:** Vaginal sphincter present.
4. **Ootype, Mehli's gland & other organs:** Present.

B. Male reproductive organs:

1. **Testes:** 300-400 follicles.
2. **Vas efferentia, vas deferens & cirrus (penis):** Are also present.

- Genital atrium: Present near the posterior end of lateral margin of each segment & alternates irregularly between right & left margins.

II. Egg stage

- **Development:** Formed in ootype & surrounded by protective covering.
- **Colour:** Brown colour (Bile stained).
- **Size:** 31- 43 µm in diameter.
- **Shape:** Spherical & non-operculated.
- **Life span:** Live about 8 weeks on field.
- **Morphological features:** → **Fig.-3**

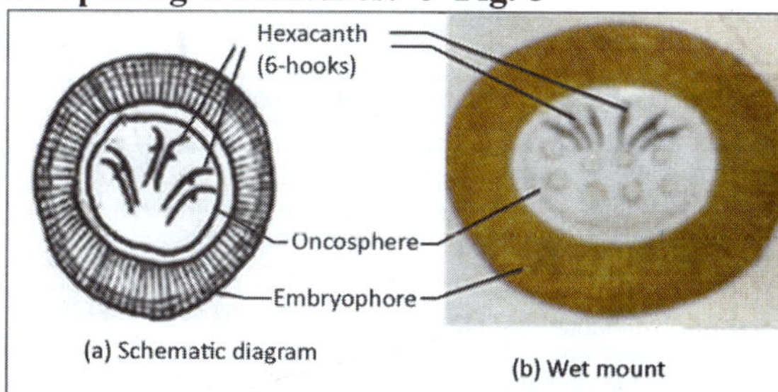

Figure-3: Egg of *T. saginata*

- **Covering:** Two covering as follows.

1. **Outer:**
   - It is thin **called egg shell.**
   - Sometime it ruptures before the eggs are excreted, but when present it represents the remnant of yolk mass.
   - It causes the eggs to clump together.
2. **Inner:**
   - It is thick **called embryophore.**
   - It becomes very thick after rupture of egg shell & radially striated to protect the inner oncosphere.

- **Embryo:**
  - Initially contains embryo when laid down.
  - Embryo **called oncopshere** with 14- 20 µm in size
  - Contains 6 hooklets (3 pairs) **called hexacanth,** which helps to penetrate the gut wall in intermediate host.
- **Cilia around embryo:** Absent.
- **Other features:**
  - Does not float in saturated common salt solution.
  - Infective only to cattle.
  - Acid fast under modified ZN stain. Only way to differentiate it from the egg of *T. solium.*

III. Larval stage

- **Development:** It develops in muscles of intermediate host (cow / buffalo) & matures further when ingested by man. It does not occur in man.
- **Size:** 3-4 mm in length × 5-10 mm in breadth.
- **Shape:** Oval.
- **Life span:** Live for 8 months in muscles of cattle.
- **Morphological features:** → **Fig.-4**

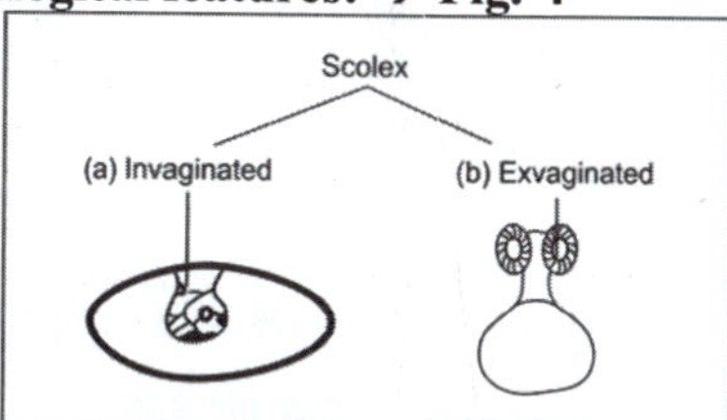

Figure-4: Larva of *T. saginata*

- Name: **Called *Cysticercus bovis*** (taxonomically not correct).
- Hooklets: Absent.
- Scolex (Future head of adult worm): It is invaginated from one side **[fig.-4(a)]**, later exvaginated **[fig.-4(b)]** in definitive host.
- Time of development: Eggs develop the *Cysticercus* within 60-70 days.

❖ Life cycle:

- **Types of host:** Two types.

I. **Definitive host:** Man (adult stage).
II. **Intermediate host:** Cow / buffalo (larval stage).

- **Cycles:** Two types as shown in **flow chart-1 & fig.-5.**

❖ Pathogenicity:

- **Disease name: Called intestinal taeniasis.**
- **Reservoir of infection:** Man.
- **Source of infection:** Cattle (beef).
- **Mode of transmission:** By ingestion of raw beef contains *C. bovis* (measly beef or beef measles).
- **Exit form:** Embryonated eggs / segments.
- **Infective form:** Larvae **called *Cysticercus bovis.***
- **Portal of entry:** GIT.

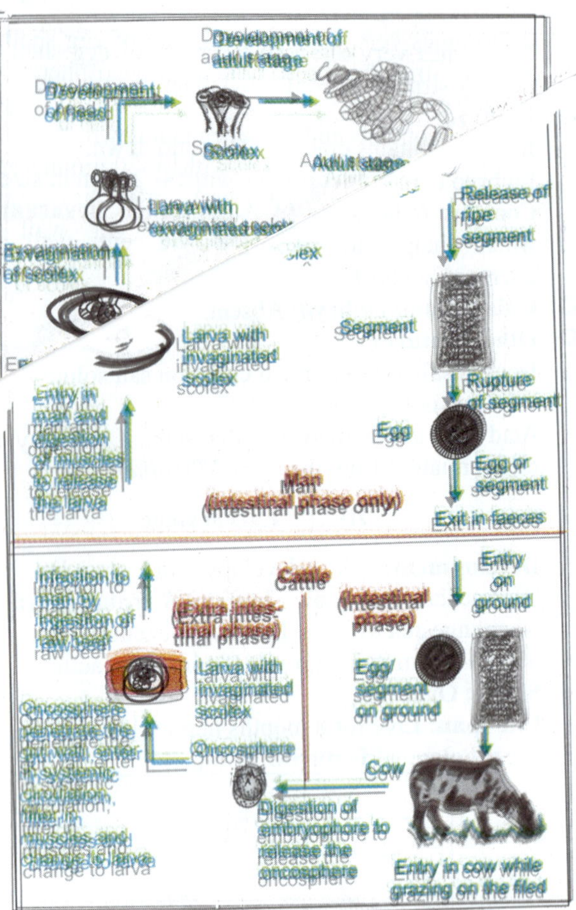
Development of adult stage
Development of head
Scolex
Adult stage
Larva with evaginated scolex
Release of ripe segment
Evagination of scolex
Larva with invaginated scolex
Segment
Rupture of segment
Entry in man and digestion of muscles to release the larva
Egg
Egg or segment
Man (intestinal phase only)
Exit in faeces
Infection to man by ingestion of raw beef
Cattle
(Extra intestinal phase)
(Intestinal phase)
Entry on ground
Larva with invaginated scolex
Egg/ segment on ground
Oncosphere penetrate the gut wall enter in systemic circulation, filter in muscles and change to larva
Oncosphere
Cow
Digestion of embryophore to release the oncosphere
Entry in cow while grazing on the filed

Figure-5: Life cycle of *T. saginata*

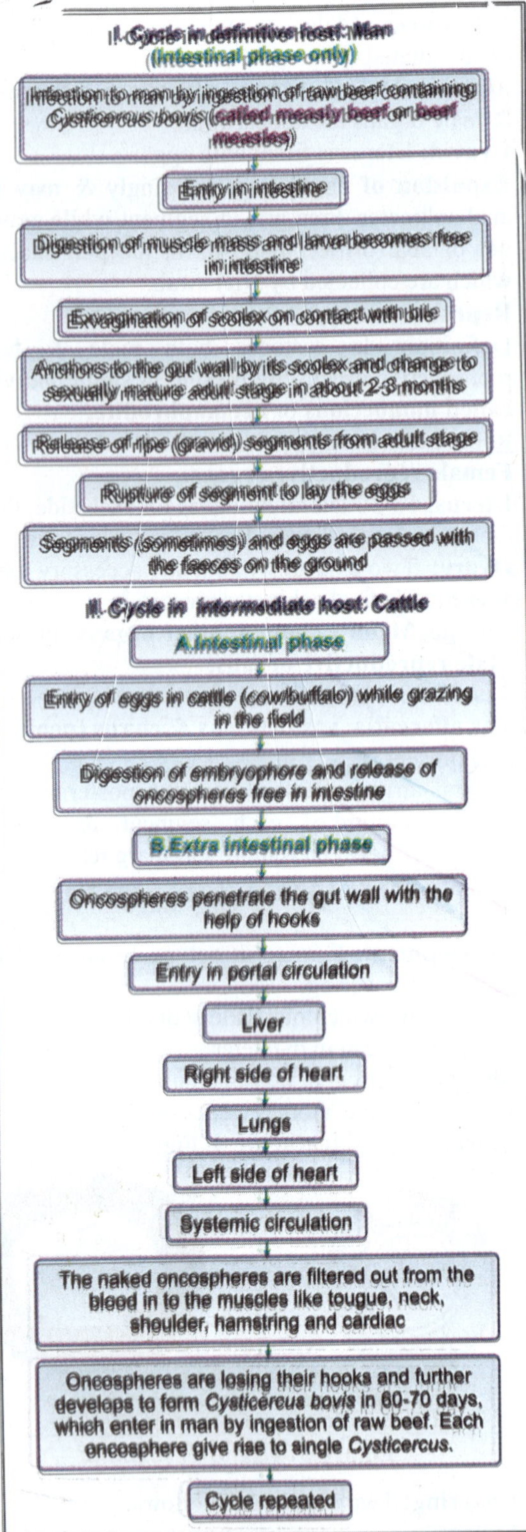
I. Cycle in definitive host: Man
(Intestinal phase only)
Infection to man by ingestion of raw beef containing Cysticercus bovis (called measly beef or beef measles)
Entry in intestine
Digestion of muscle mass and larva becomes free in intestine
Exvagination of scolex on contact with bile
Anchors to the gut wall by its scolex and change to sexually mature adult stage in about 2-3 months
Release of ripe (gravid) segments from adult stage
Rupture of segment to lay the eggs
Segments (sometimes) and eggs are passed with the faeces on the ground
II. Cycle in intermediate host: Cattle
A. Intestinal phase
Entry of eggs in cattle (cow/buffalo) while grazing in the field
Digestion of embryophore and release of oncospheres free in intestine
B. Extra intestinal phase
Oncospheres penetrate the gut wall with the help of hooks
Entry in portal circulation
Liver
Right side of heart
Lungs
Left side of heart
Systemic circulation
The naked oncospheres are filtered out from the blood in to the muscles like tougue, neck, shoulder, hamstring and cardiac
Oncospheres are losing their hooks and further develops to form Cysticercus bovis in 60-70 days, which enter in man by ingestion of raw beef. Each oncosphere give rise to single Cysticercus.
Cycle repeated

Flow chart-1: Life cycle of *T. saginata*

- **Site:** Small intestine (upper jejunum).
- **Clinical features:** Only by adult stage as below.
  - **Asymptomatic:**
  - **GIT:** Abdominal discomfort like indigestion, diarrhoea with alternating constipation, intestinal obstruction & appendicitis has been observed.
  - **Anaemia:**

Laboratory diagnosis:

I. Direct methods

- **Specimens:**
  - Stool: Segments of adult worm present in stool.
  - Eggs collection from perianal region by using.
    1. NIH (cellophane) swab method.
    2. Cellulose (Scotch) tape method.
  - Muscle biopsy from slaughtered animal.
- **Testing methods:**

A. History: Of beef eating is present.

B. Macroscopic (naked eye) examination:

i. For segments:

- White segments are present against yellowish stool
- Sometimes segments are also present in clothes of patient.

ii. For scolex: Species differention can be made by macroscopic examination of scolex (If adult stage is available) after anthelmintic treatment.

C. Microscopy:

i. For eggs:

a. Wet mount by using normal saline & iodine:

- It shows the bile stained (brown colour) eggs as shown in fig.-3(b).

b. Concentration technique: In case of negative result by wet mount method.

ZN stain: Egg of *T. saginata* is acid fast, while of *T. solium* is non acid fast.

For segments:

Species differention [as shown in **table-1]** can be made by microscopic examination of segments.

It can be pressed between two slides & examined by hand lens.

Isozyme technique:

Useful to identify the segment.

Disadvantage: Available at reference centre.

II. Indirect methods

Serological tests: ELISA & IHA are useful test, but only disadvantage is that they are not able to differentiate *T. saginata* from *T. solium* & subspecies *T. saginata saginata* from *T. saginata asiatica.*

Molecular tests: Both DNA probe & PCR are useful methods to diagnose & to make a difference between species & subspecies.

Prevention:

Periodical checking of beef for presence of larvae.

Proper cooking of beef.

Critical thermal point for larvae is 56^0C for 5 min.

Avoiding the faecal contamination of soil, water & food.

Treatment:

Praziquantel: Single dose 10mg/kg is the drug of choice.

Niclosamide 2g single dose is another effective drug.

Taenia saginata asiatica

It is similar to *T. saginata saginata* on the basis of morphology, molecular studies & pathology, however differentiated as follows.

Identified from Asian countries like Taiwan, Korea, Phillipines & few other parts.

Adult stage has two rows of rudimentary hooks.

Smaller than *T. saginata saginata.*

Intermediate host is pig (not cattle).

Larval (*Cysticercus bovis*) stage is located in pig's liver (not in muscle).

Taenia solium

Common name:

Pork tape worm: As it is transmitted by eating the raw pork (pork = pig's meat) contains *Cysticercus cellulosae* (larval stage). Such infected pork looks like human measles so **called measly pork** or **pork measles** (pork + larva = measly pork).

Armed tape worm: Word is related to morphology like armed means with hooklets on head while tape worm means dorso-ventrally flat & broad adult stage as like a measure tape.

❖ **Meaning:** Originated from **Sol (Latin) = sun,** as the hooks around rostellum gives **sun (sun rays)** like appearance.

❖ **Synonym:** *Taenia cucurbitiana.*

❖ **History:** It was discovered by Linnaeus in 1758.

❖ **Geographical distribution:** World - wide distributed & common in pork eater, however it may occurs in vegetarian due to consumption of contaminated food & water contains eggs.

❖ **Habitat:**

- Adult worm lives in small intestine (upper jejunum) of man.
- Larval stage lives in brain, eye, subcutaneous tissues & muscles.

❖ **Morphology:** Three morphological stages like adult, egg & larval are described below.

I. Adult stage

➢ **Time of maturation:** Larva transformed to sexually mature adult stage in 2-3 months in definitive host.

➢ **Colour:** White & semitransparent.

➢ **Size:** 2 to 3 metres in length.

➢ **Shape:** Like a measure tape.

➢ **Life span:** 25 years.

➢ **Morphological parts:** Three parts like head, neck & strobila (body/trunk) as shown in **fig.-6.**

A. Scolex (head): → **Fig.-6(b)**

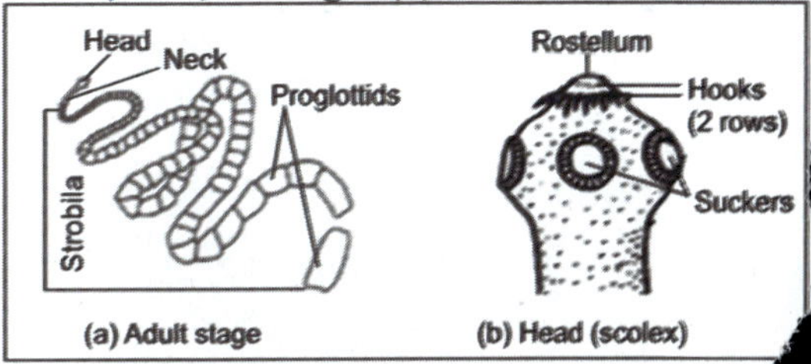

Figure-6: Adult stage of *T. solium*

✪ **Shape:** Globular in shape.

✪ **Size:** Smaller & 1mm in diameter (pin head si

✪ **Suckers:** Four circular suckers **called ace** which are not pigmented.

✪ **Rostellum (beak like projection from** Present.

✪ **Hooklets:** Present around rostellum in with alternating large & small hooks. with surrounding hooks are shaped like Arabian poniards.

B. Neck: Short & 0.5mm wide.

C. Strobila (body or trunk): It is compos of segments **called proglottids** having features.

✪ **Proglottids (segments): → Fig.-7**

- **Numbers:** <1,000 (800-900).
- **Size (gravid segment):** 12mm × 6mm. Length is twice than breadth.
- **Types:** Three types according to maturity with following order from front to backwards.

1. **Immature:** Male & female organs are not differentiated.
2. **Mature:** Male & female organs are differentiated & male organs are appear first.
3. **Gravid:** Uterus is filled with eggs.

- **Expulsion of eggs:** Expelled in chain of 5-6 & passively.
- **Reproductive system:**

o Definition: In cestodes both male & female reproductive organs are present in single individual **called monoecious** or **hermaphrodite.**

o Reproductive organs:

A. **Female reproductive organs:**

1. **Uterus:** 5-10 lateral branches on each side, thick & dendritic (no sub-branches).
2. **Ovary:** Two in numbers with an accessory lobe.
3. **Vagina:** Vaginal sphincter absent.
4. **Ootype, Mehli's gland & other organs:** Are also present.

C. **Male reproductive organs:**

1. **Testes:** 150-200 follicles.
2. **Vas efferentia, vas deferens & cirrus (penis):** Are also present.

o Genital atrium: Present near the middle of lateral margin of each segment & alternates irregularly between right & left margins.

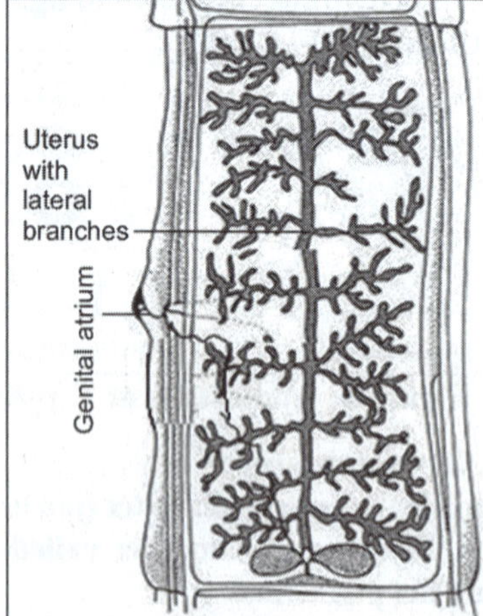

Figure-7: Segment of *T. solium*

II. Egg stage

to *T. saginata* (**fig.-3**) but non-acid fast.

III. Larval stage

ment: It develops in muscles of iate host like pig & matures further when ingested by man. It also occurs in brain, eye, subcutaneous tissues & muscles of man.

➢ **Size:** 5 mm in length × 10 mm in breadth.

➢ **Shape:** Oval.

➢ **Life span:** Live for 8 months in muscles of pig.

➢ **Morphological features: → Fig.-4**

- Name: **Called *Cysticercus cellulosae*** (taxonomically not correct).
- Hooklets: Present.
- Scolex (future head of adult worm): It is invaginated from one side **[fig.-4(a)]**, later exvaginated **[fig.-4(b)]** in definitive host.
- Time of development: Eggs develop the *Cysticercus* within 60-70 days.
- Contains: It contains fluid rich in salt & albuminous materials.

❖ Life cycle:

➢ **Types of host:** Two types.

I. **Definitive host:** Man. Harbours the adult stage.

II. **Intermediate hosts:**

A. **Pig:** Harbours the larval stage.

B. **Man:** Sometimes man also act as an intermediate host & harbours the larval stage.

➢ **Cycles:** Two types as shown in **flow chart-2 & fig.-8.**

❖ Pathogenicity:

➢ **Disease name:** Disease produced by adult **called intestinal taeniasis** & by larvae **called cysticercosis.**

➢ **Reservoir of infection:** Man.

➢ **Source of infection:** Pig (pork).

➢ **Mode of transmission:**

1. **Larva stage:** By **ingestion** of raw pork contains *C. cellulosae* (measly pork or pork measles).
2. **Egg stage:**

- **Autoinfection:** Entry of gravid segments in stomach from intestine by
  - Reversal of peristalsis (regurgitation).
  - Poor personal hygiene (may be by finger contamination/oral faecal route).
- **Ingestion:** Ingestion of contaminated food & water contains eggs.

➢ **Exit form:** Embryonated eggs / segments.

➢ **Infective form:** In *T. solium* man is infected by both, larvae & eggs, & pathological lesions are due to adult plus larval stage while *T. saginata* only egg stage is infective & pathological lesions are due to only adult stage, hence *T. solium* is more dangerous than *T. saginata.*

➢ **Portal of entry:** GIT.

➢ **Site:** Small intestine (upper jejunum) for adult stage infection & brain, eye, subcutaneous tissues, muscles for larval stage infection.

➢ **Clinical types & features:** Two types.

A. **Adult stage disease:** Same as *T. saginata.*

B. Larval stage disease: As below.

- **Disease caused by larva: Called cysticercosis.**
- **Clinical subtypes & features:** Most common sites are subcutaneous tissues & muscles. Following are the clinical subtypes according to involvement of different organs.

i. **Subcutaneous cysticercosis:** Present as palpatory nodule or inspector swelling. Mostly asymptomatic.

ii. **Muscular cysticercosis:** May be present as acute myositis.

iii. **Ocular cysticercosis:**

- Located in vitreous humour, subretinal space & conjunctiva.
- It produce blurred or loss of vision, iritis, uveitis & palpebral conjunctivitis.

iv. **Cysticercosis of brain:**

- It also **called neurocysticercosis.**
- It is the most common parasitic CNS lesion worldwide. It is the 2nd most common cause of Intra Cranial Space Occupying Lesion (ICSOL) after tuberculosis in India.
- It is the most serious form. Brain parenchyma is most common sites of neurocysticercosis.

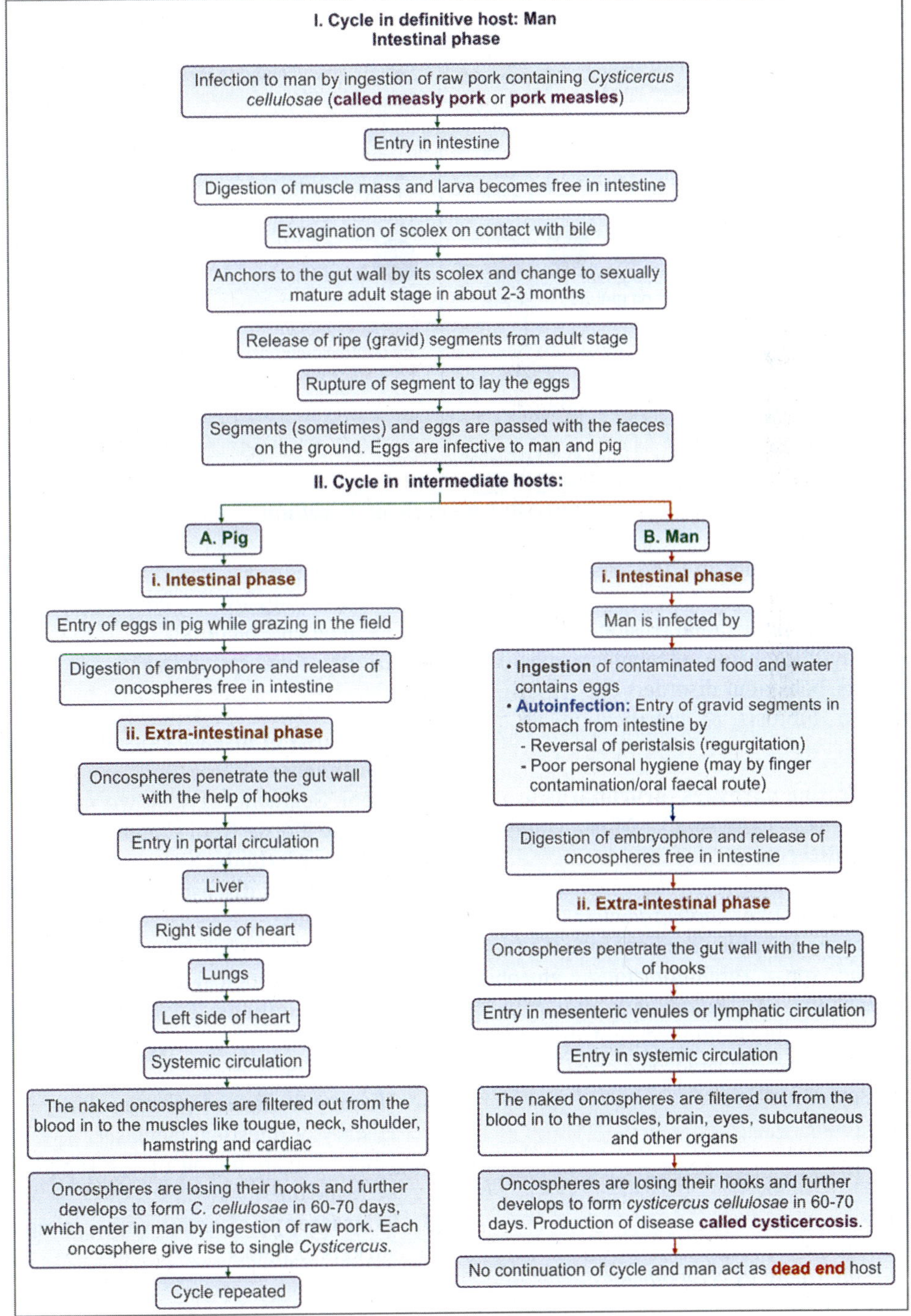

I. Cycle in definitive host: Man
Intestinal phase
Infection to man by ingestion of raw pork containing Cysticercus cellulosae (called measly pork or pork measles)
Entry in intestine
Digestion of muscle mass and larva becomes free in intestine
Exvagination of scolex on contact with bile
Anchors to the gut wall by its scolex and change to sexually mature adult stage in about 2-3 months
Release of ripe (gravid) segments from adult stage
Rupture of segment to lay the eggs
Segments (sometimes) and eggs are passed with the faeces on the ground. Eggs are infective to man and pig
II. Cycle in intermediate hosts:
A. Pig
i. Intestinal phase
Entry of eggs in pig while grazing in the field
Digestion of embryophore and release of oncospheres free in intestine
ii. Extra-intestinal phase
Oncospheres penetrate the gut wall with the help of hooks
Entry in portal circulation
Liver
Right side of heart
Lungs
Left side of heart
Systemic circulation
The naked oncospheres are filtered out from the blood in to the muscles like tougue, neck, shoulder, hamstring and cardiac
Oncospheres are losing their hooks and further develops to form C. cellulosae in 60-70 days, which enter in man by ingestion of raw pork. Each oncosphere give rise to single Cysticercus.
Cycle repeated
B. Man
i. Intestinal phase
Man is infected by
• Ingestion of contaminated food and water contains eggs
• Autoinfection: Entry of gravid segments in stomach from intestine by
- Reversal of peristalsis (regurgitation)
- Poor personal hygiene (may by finger contamination/oral faecal route)
Digestion of embryophore and release of oncospheres free in intestine
ii. Extra-intestinal phase
Oncospheres penetrate the gut wall with the help of hooks
Entry in mesenteric venules or lymphatic circulation
Entry in systemic circulation
The naked oncospheres are filtered out from the blood in to the muscles, brain, eyes, subcutaneous and other organs
Oncospheres are losing their hooks and further develops to form cysticercus cellulosae in 60-70 days. Production of disease called cysticercosis.
No continuation of cycle and man act as dead end host

Flow chart-2: Life cycle of *T. solium*

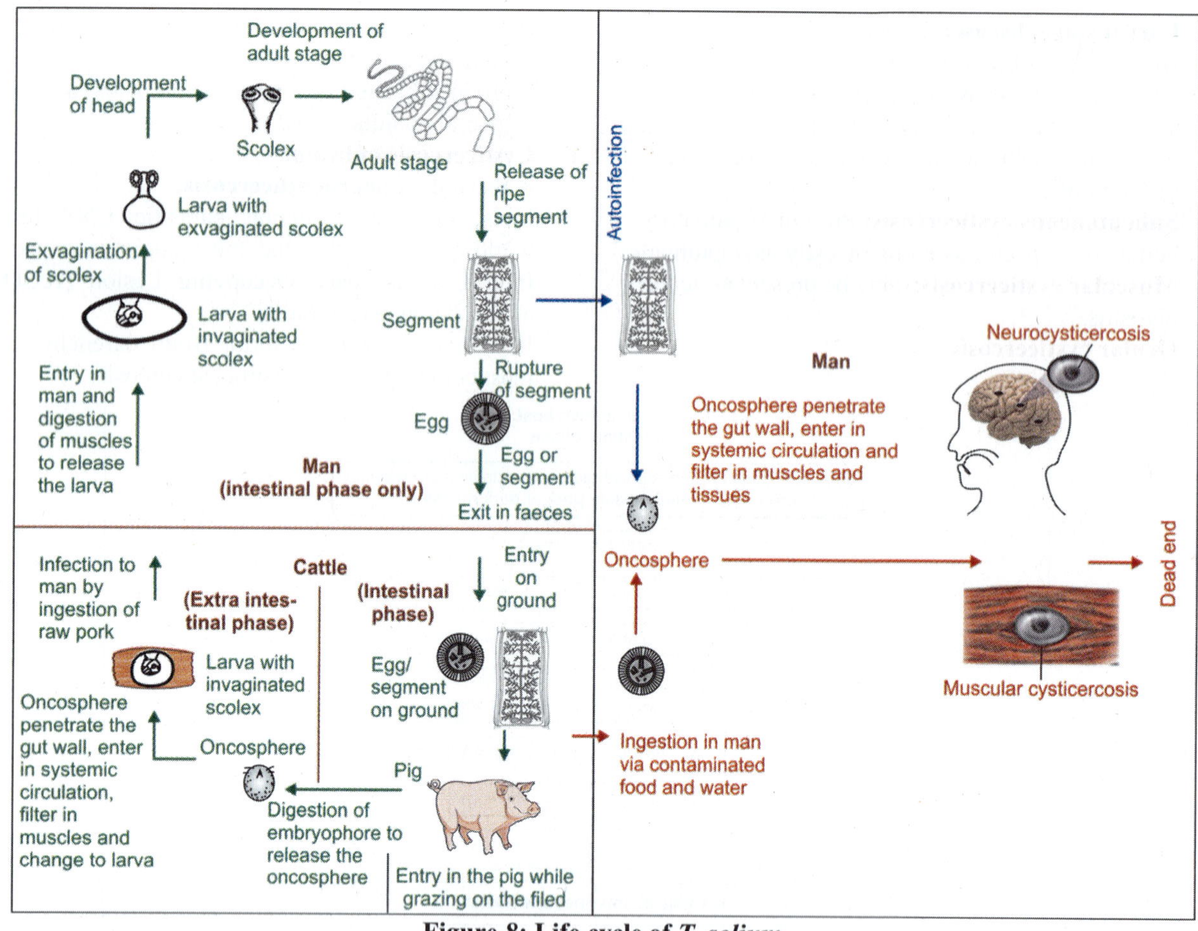

Figure-8: Life cycle of *T. solium*

- It is the causative agents in 70% cases of adult epilepsy.
- It also causes rise in intracranial tension, psychiatric disturbances, hydrocephalus, meningoencephalitis, transient paresis, behaviour disorders etc.

✪ **Complications:** Fibrosis & calcification in 5-6 years.

✓ **Note: CNS infecting parasites (neuroparasites)**

- *Taenia solium* (*C. cellulosae*): Most common **called neurocysticercosis.**
- *Entamoeba histolytica.*
- Free living amoebae like *Naglria fowleri* (acute & purulent primary ameobic meningoencephalitis), *Acanthamoeba* spp. (granulomatous ameobic meningoencephalitis) & *Balamuthia mandrilaris* (granulomatous ameobic meningoencephalitis).
- *Trypanosoma brucei* & *Trypanosoma cruzi.*
- *Plasmodium* spp.
- *Toxoplasma gondii.*
- *Spirometra* spp.
- *Echinococcus granulosus* (hydatid cyst), *E multilocularis.*
- *Multiceps multiceps.*
- *Schistosoma* spp. (more by *S japonicum*).
- *Paragonimus westermanii.*
- *Loa loa.*
- *Angiostrongylus cantonensis* (eosinophilic meningoencephalitis).
- *Gnathostoma spinigerum.*

❖ Laboratory diagnosis:

➢ **Diagnosis of disease caused by adult stage:**

✪ **Specimens:**

- Stool: Segments of adult worm present in stool.
- Muscle biopsy from slaughtered animal.

✪ **Testing methods:** Same as *T. saginata.*

➢ **Diagnosis of disease caused by larval stage:**

✪ **Specimens:**

- Biopsy from infected organs.
- CSF for serological tests.

✪ **Testing methods:** Two types as below.

I. Direct method

A. History & clinical examination:

- History of intestinal taeniasis.
- Clinical examination of eye (ophthalmoscopy) can be made out.

B. Microscopy: Larva with invaginated scolex, suckers & hooks.

Features	*T. saginata*	*T. solium*
Common name	- Beef tape worm -Unarmed tape worm	- Pork tape worm - Armed tape worm
Subspecies	Two like saginata & asiatica	No subspecies
Synonym	*Taeniarhynchus saginata*	*Taenia cucurbitiana*
Geographical Distribution	In beef eater (Non –vegetarian) & not in vegetarian	In pork eater (Non –vegetarian) & in vegetarian
Habitat	Only intestine	Intestine & tissues
Size	5 to 10 metres	2 to 3 metres
Life span	10 years	25 years
Scolex (Head)		
Figure	**Figure-1(b)**	**Figure-6(b)**
Shape	Quadrate	Globular
Size	Larger, 1-2mm in diameter	Smaller, 1mm in diameter
Suckers	Four circular suckers which may be pigmented	Four circular suckers which are not pigmented
Rostellum	Absent	Present
Hooklets	Absent	Present
Neck	Long, narrow	Short
Proglottids (Gravid segments)		
Figure	Figure-2	Figure-7
Numbers	1,000 – 2,000	<1,000 (800-900)
Size	22mm × 5mm, length is 3-4 times more than breadth	12mm × 6mm Length is twice than breadth.
Expulsion of eggs	Singly & force to anal sphincter.	Expelled in chain of 5-6 & passively
Uterus	15-30 lateral branches on each side, thin & dichotomous	5-10 lateral branches on each side, thick & dendritic
Ovary	Two without any accessory lobe	Two with an accessory lobe
Vagina	Sphincter present	Sphincter absent
Testes	300-400 follicles.	150-200 follicles.
Genital atrium	Present near the posterior end of lateral margin	Present near the middle of lateral margin
Eggs (Figure-3)		
Stain	Acid fast	Non acid fast
Infective to man	No	Yes
Larva (Figure-4)		
Name	*C. bovis*	*C. cellulosae*
Size	3-4mm × 5-10mm	5 mm × 10 mm
Host	Cattle only	Pig & man
Hooklets	Absent	Present
Hosts & other differences		
Definitive	Man	Man
Intermediate	Cattle only	Pig & man
Infection	Only by larva	By larva & eggs
Disease	Intestinal taeniasis	Intestinal taeniasis & cysticercosis

Table-1: Differences between *Taenia* spp.

II. Indirect methods

A. **Blood picture:** Eosinophilia.
B. **Serological tests:** Antigen or Antibody can be detected by ELISA from serum or CSF.
C. **Molecular tests:** Are useful methods.
D. **Radiological:**

1. **X-ray:** Soft tissue X-ray demonstrates the calcified cyst in thigh, subcutaneous tissues or brain.
2. **CT scan:** It revealed disc or ring like calcified cyst in brain.
3. **MRI:** More useful to detect the non-calcified cyst in brain, ventricle or in spine.

❖ Prevention:

- Periodical checking of pork for presence of larvae.
- Other measures are same as *T saginata.*

❖ Treatment:

➢ **Intestinal lesions:** Same as *T saginata.*

➢ **Treatment of cysticercosis:**

✪ **Lesion in subcutaneous tissues or muscles:** It should be excised.

✪ **Neurocysticercosis:**

- **Asymptomatic:** No treatment required.
- **Symptomatic:**
  - Praziquantel 50mg/kg in 3 divided doses for 20-30 days & albendazole, 400 mg BD for 30 days.
  - Steroid to avoid the inflammatory reaction caused by dead larvae.
  - Antileprotic is advised until the brain reaction is subsided.
  - Surgery is indicated in case of hydrocephalus.

❖ Differences between *T. saginata* & *T. solium*: → Follow table-1

Echinococcus spp.

Echinococcus granulosus

❖ Common name:

1. **Dog tape worm:** As dog is the definitive (optimum) host.
2. **Hydatid worm:** Name given from the larval stage name called **hydatid cyst** which cause the human disease.
3. **Hyper tape worm:**

❖ Synonym: *Taenia echinicoccus.*

❖ History:

- Ancient disease, known since the time of Hippocrates & other physician.
- Adult stage was described by Hartmann in 1695 from dog's intestine & larval stage was described by Goeze in 1782.

❖ Geographical distribution:

- World wide.
- It is common in sheep & cattle raising countries like Africa, Australia, South America, Europe, China, Middle East & India.
- It is common in temperate than tropical countries.

❖ **Habitat:**

- Adult stage: Found in small intestine (duodenum & jejunum) of carnivorous animals like dog, fox, jackal & wolf.
- Larval stage: Found in tissues of man & herbivorous animals like sheep, goat, cattle, pig & horse.

❖ **Morphology:** Three morphological stages like adult, egg & larval are described below.

I. Adult stage

➢ **Time of maturation:** Larva transformed to sexually mature adult stage in 6-7 weeks in definitive (canine) host.
➢ **Colour:** White & semitransparent.
➢ **Size:** 3 to 6 mm in length.
➢ **Shape:** Like a measure tape.
➢ **Life span:** 6-30 months in canine host.
➢ **Morphological parts:** Three parts like head, neck & strobila (body/trunk) as shown in **fig.-9.**

A. Scolex (head): → Fig.-9

✪ **Shape:** Pyriform in shape.
✪ **Suckers:** Four circular suckers.
✪ **Rostellum:** Present & prominent.
✪ **Hooklets:** Present around rostellum in two circular rows.

B. Neck: It is shorter than rest of worms (3mm×6mm).

C. Strobila (body/trunk): It is composed of 3-4 segments **called proglottids** with following features.

✪ **Proglottids (segments): → Fig.-9**

- **Numbers:** 3-4
- **Size (gravid segment):** 2-3mm × 0.6mm. Length is 3-4 times greater than breadth.
- **Types:** Three types according to maturity with following order from front to backwards.

1. **1st segment:** It is immature & contains male & female organs, which are not differentiated.
2. **2nd segment:** It is mature. Male & female organs are differentiated. Male organs are appearing first.
3. **3rd segment:** It is gravid & uterus is filled with eggs.
4. **4th segment:** Rarely seen & gravid when present.

- **Reproductive system:**
  - Definition: In cestodes both male & female reproductive organs are present in single individual **called monoecious** or **hermaphrodite.**
  - Reproductive organs: All the female & male reproductive organs are shown in **fig.-9.**
  - Genital atrium: Present on the lateral margin of each segment.

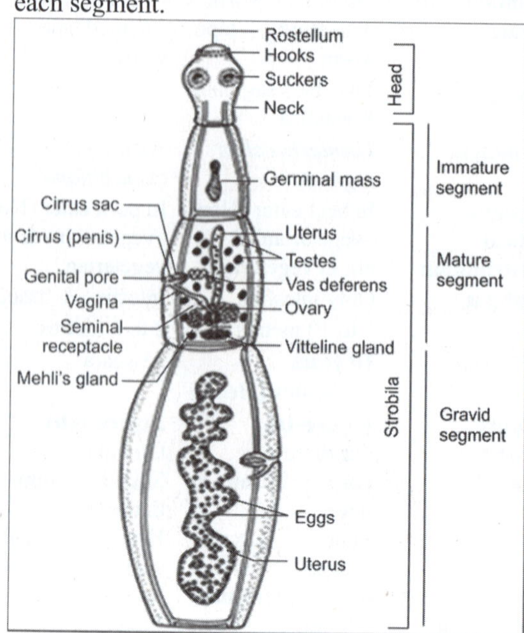

Figure-9: Adult stage of *E. granulosus*

II. Egg stage

➢ **Colour:** Brown colour (bile stained).
➢ **Size:** 32-36μm × 25-32 μm.
➢ **Shape:** Oval.
➢ **Morphological features:** Same as *T. saginata* **(fig.-3).**

III. Larval stage

➢ **Development:** It is a vesicular body with invaginated scolex develops in intermediate host like man & herbivorous animals like sheep, goat, cattle, pig & horse.
➢ **Size:** Variable with 0.5-1 cm in diameter.
➢ **Shape:** Oval or spherical.
➢ **Life span:** It may continue to develop for many years.
➢ **Morphological features: → Fig.-10**

- **Name:** Larva is a vesicular body with invaginated scolex present in a cystic structure **called hydatid** or **hydatid cyst.**
- **Meaning:** From **hydatis (Greek) = drop of water,** because containing fluid.
- **Time of development:** Eggs develop the hydatid in about 6 months.
- **Layers:** Oncosphere secrets following two layer from inner to outer.

a. Endocyst:

- Synonym: Also **called inner layer** or **germinal layer.**
- Size: Very thin 22-25 μm in thickness.
- Contains: It is cellular & consists of a number of nuclei embedded in protoplasmic mass.
- Functions:

Gives brood capsules with scolices. Scolices are present with hooks & invaginated, which later exvaginated in definitive host to form adult stage.
Forms the ectocyst.
Secretes the hydatid fluid.

Ectocyst:

Synonym: Also **called outer layer** or **cuticular layer** or **laminated layer** or **hyaline layer.**
Size: 1mm in thickness.
Appearance: It is elastic & appears like hard-boiled egg.
Function: Protective role & exposing the inner layer on incision or rupture.

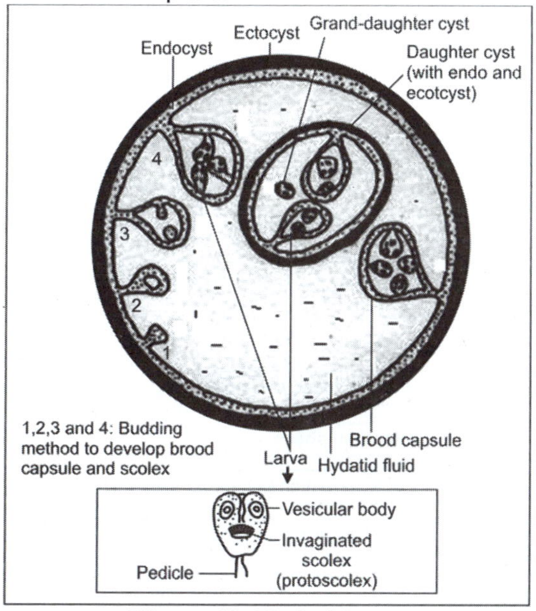

Figure-10: Hydatid cyst

Hydatid fluid: Have following composition & features.
Colour: May be clear & colourless or sometimes pale yellow.
pH: 6.7 & slightly acidic.
Specific gravity: Low, 1.005-1.010
Contains:
Biochemical substances: Sodium chloride, sodium sulphate, sodium phosphate and sodium & calcium salts of succinic acid (**called Fehling reducing substances**).
Hydatid sand: These are granular material in form of liberated brood capsules, free scolices & loose hooks, present at the bottom of larva.
Clinical significances:
Toxigenic: Highly toxic & when absorbed in systemic circulation it gives allergic or anaphylaxis reactions.
Antigenic: Antigenic in nature & used for Casoni's test.
Development of brood capsules:
Brood capsules sprout from endocyst by budding method.

- It starts with small spherical bud which becomes vacuolated & transformed in to vesicle.

- **Development of scolices:**

- Scolex also developed by budding method from brood capsule.
- They are 5-20 in numbers.
- Also **called protoscolices.**
- It represents the development of future head of adult worm.
- It remains invaginated & present with suckers & hooks.
- In growing hydatid cyst all stages of scolex are present from small bud to fully developed scolex with suckers & hooks.
- It is attached to the brood capsule by pedicle or remains free as grains of hydatid sand.

❖ Life cycle:

➢ **Types of host:** Two types.

I. **Definitive host:** Carnivorous animals like dog (optimal/ideal host), fox, jackal & wolf.

II. **Intermediate host:**

- Herbivorous animals like sheep (optimal/ideal host), goat, cattle, pig & horse.
- Man (children) is the accidental or dead end host.

➢ **Cycles:** Two types as shown in **flow chart-3 & fig.-11.** Natural cycle continue between carnivorous animal & herbivorous animal.

❖ Pathogenicity:

A. **Adult stage disease:**

- Adult stage present in dog & does not cause any illness.
- 100-1000 parasites are present in dog that can be examined at post-mortem examination.
- Eggs are passed in faeces.

B. **Larval stage disease:** As below

➢ **Disease name:** It is a zoonosis & human disease is present with unilocular cyst **called hydatid disease,** or **hydatidosis** or **echinococcal disease** or **echinococcosis.**

➢ **Reservoir of infection:** Dog.

➢ **Source of infection:** Food is the source for human infection.

➢ **Mode of transmission:** Eggs enter in man by

- Ingestion of food contaminated with faeces of infected canine. It not enters by water, as the heavy eggs sink at the bottom.
- Eating in a same dish with dog.
- Direct contact (may by finger contamination during handling or fondling of dog by children).

➢ **Exit form:** Man act as dead end host & eggs are exit from definitive host (dog).

➢ **Infective form:** Eggs.

➢ **Portal of entry:** GIT.

➢ **Sites:**

- Liver (most common site & mostly in right lobe): 65-70%.
- Lungs (2nd most common site after liver & mostly lower lobe of right lung): 20%.
- Brain: 5%.
- Kidneys: 2%.
- Spleen: 2%.
- Bones: 1%.
- Pelvic organs, muscles & other tissues: 1-3%.

➢ **Precipitating factors:** Common in childre farmers, shepherds & shoe maker.

➢ **Pathology & pathogenesis:**

✪ **Numbers of cyst:** It mostly cause uni-locular cyst

✪ **Rate of growth:** In man it is very slow & at the er of a year it is approximately 4 cm in diameter brood capsules & scolices begin to appear.

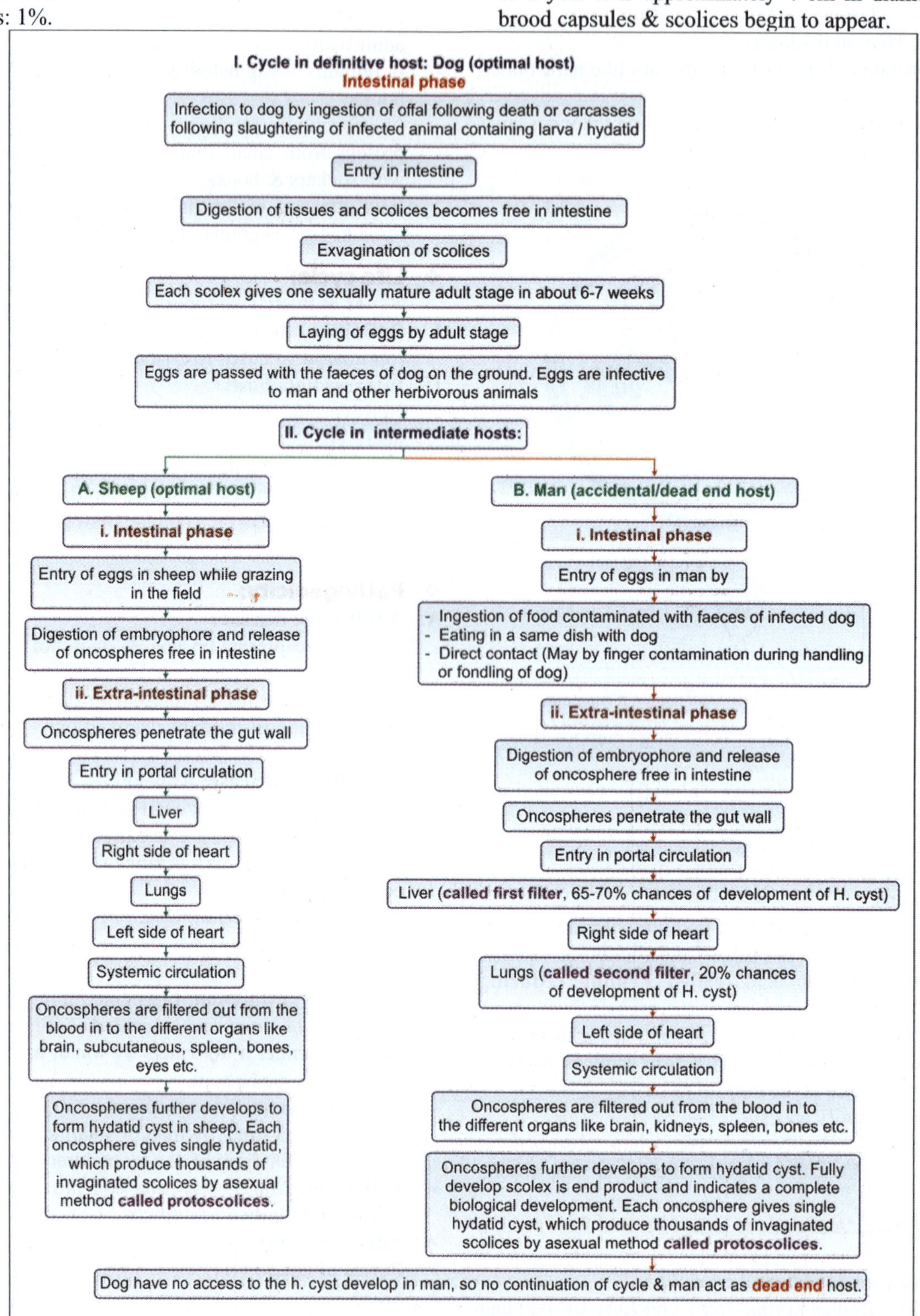

Flow chart-3: Life cycle of *E. granulosus*

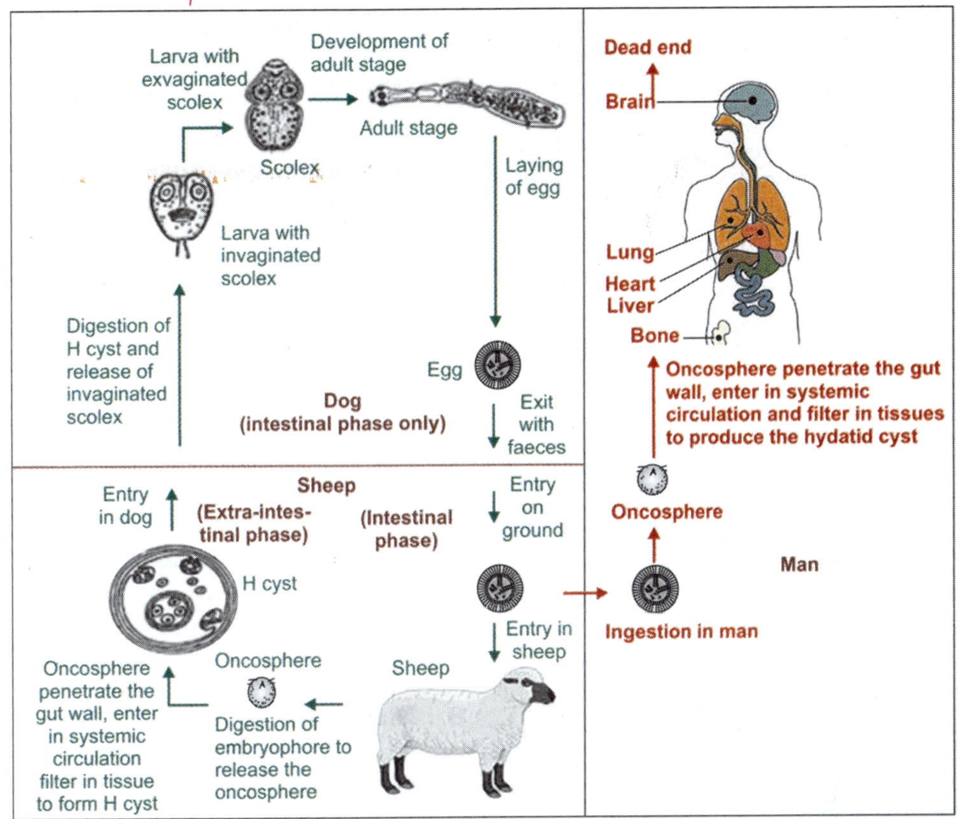

Figure-11: Life cycle of *E. granulosus*

✪ **Variation of hydatid cyst:** During its growth it shows following variations.

i. **Acephalocyst:**

- **Synonym:** Sterile cyst.
- **Host:** It found in large numbers in cattle.
- **Structure & development:** Sometimes brood capsule is not developed & if developed, it is without scolices **called acephalocyst.**

ii. **Endogenous daughter cyst:**

- **Host:** It develop after many years & particularly in man.
- **Structure:** It also present with endocyst & ectocyst.
- **Mechanisms of development:** It develops in mother cyst probably.

1. By detachment of fragment of germinal layer or
2. By regressive changes or regressive metamorphosis of the young brood capsule & scolex.

- It is the characteristic of cestodes "to migrate against the law" with transformation of scolex in daughter cyst in a same host without passing to the adult stage.
- This phenomenon was observed very early by Naunyn in 1862 & enunciated by Van Beneden.
- Normally, fully developed scolex is the end product which changes to adult stage when entered in definitive host. It is not able to go regressive changes to produce daughter cyst.
- Experimental work had been confirmed by Deve in 1925, shows that *E. granulosus* does not follow the general biological rule of development & shows the regressive changes to produces the daughter cyst.

iii. **Grand-daughter cyst:** It develops in daughter cyst.

iv. **Exogenous cyst:**

- **Site:** Mostly found in bony hydatid.
- **Mechanisms:** →**Flow chart-4.**

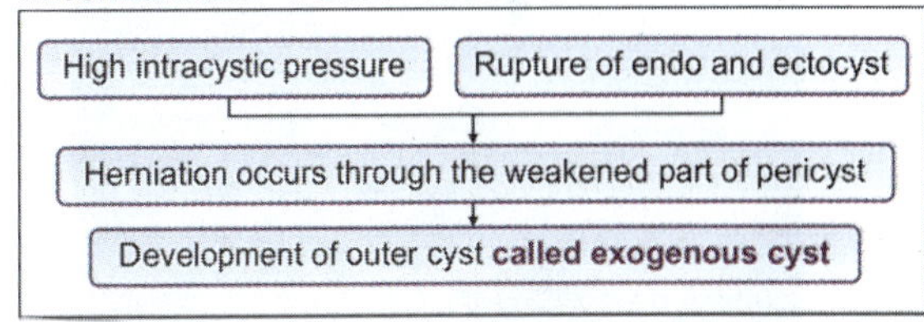

Flow chart-4: mechanism of exogenous cyst

v. **Pericyst:**

- **Synonym:** Also **called adventitial layer.**
- **Development of pericyst**
  - Development of hydatid cyst from oncosphere is prevented by body defence mechanism with cellular infiltration of monocytes, lymphocytes & giant cells around it.
  - Many of embryos have been destroyed, while those escapes will develop in to the hydatid cyst.
  - Cellular infiltration is replaced by fibroblast & new blood vessels, which ultimately transferred in to new fibrous layer around cyst **called pericyst.**
- **Clinical significances:**

- Pericyst is not the morphological part of hydatid cyst. It gradually merged in to surrounding healthy tissues & provides channel for nutrition of parasites
- In older cyst, pericyst may be calcified or sclerosed & parasites within it may die or degenerate owing to lack of nutrition.

➢ **Clinical features:** Depends on its size, location & integrity.

- **Size:**
  - Smaller size is asymptomatic.
  - Larger size produces pressure symptoms on surrounding organs.
- **Location:**
  - Superficial: Asymptomatic & inspectory swelling
  - Deep: Palpatory nodule in organs like liver **(cut section in fig.-12)**, lungs, spleen kidneys etc. & detected at the time of autopsy **(fig.-13)**. **Liver cyst** produces the hepatomegaly, pain in right hypochondrium & obstructive jaundices. **Lung cyst** produces the cough, chest pain, haemoptysis, dyspnoea & pneumothorax.

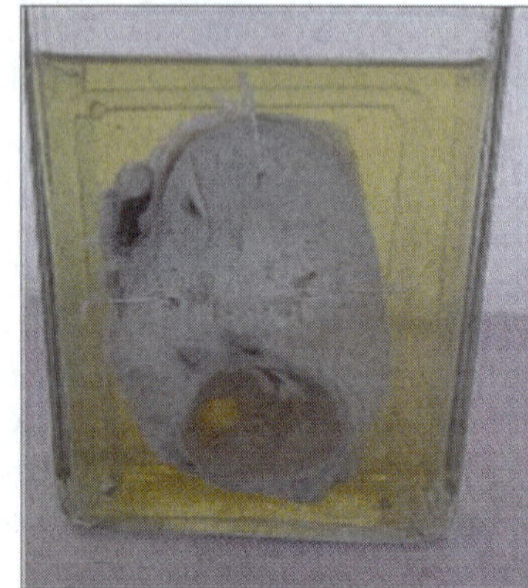

Figure-12: Cut section of hydatid cyst in liver

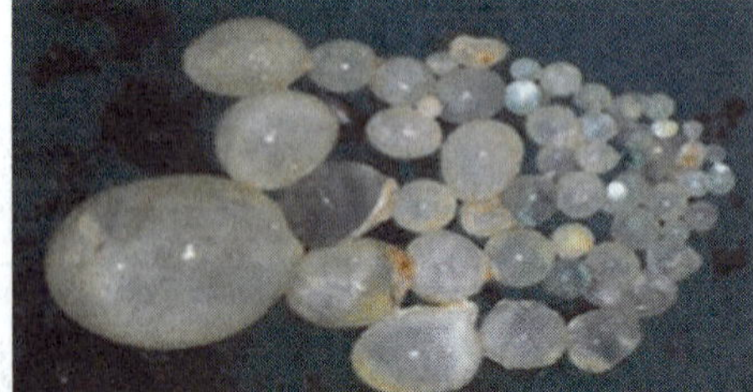

Figure-13: H. cyst in liver after surgery

- **Integrity:**
  - Intact cyst: Asymptomatic or pressure symptoms.
  - Ruptured cyst: Allergic like utricaria or anaphylaxis.

➢ **Complications:**

1. **Cure or evacuation of cyst**: It is due to inflammatory reaction.
2. **Rupture of cyst:**
   - Spontaneous rupture of cyst in surrounding organs & producing disseminated lesions.
   - Like liver cyst rupture in lungs or body cavity.
3. **Suppuration:** Pus formation by secondary bacterial infection.
4. **Calcification:** Pulmonary hydatid cyst almost never calcified unlike mediastinal cyst.
5. **Sclerosis:**
6. **Death:** 10% of all diagnosed cases are fatal.

❖ Laboratory diagnosis:

➢ **Specimens:**

- **Hydatid fluid:**
  - Fluid aspiration is not advised generally, because spillage of fluid during aspiration may cause allergic reaction.
  - Fluid is collected from surgically removed cyst.
- **Urine:** } Scolices & hooks are present
- **Sputum:** } when cysts are rupture

➢ **Testing methods:** Two types as below.

I. Direct methods

A. History & clinical examination:

- It is very difficult to diagnose the hydatid cyst by direct methods.
- History taking & clinical examination are the supportive methods:

B. Microscopy: Scolices & hooks are identified under the microscope [by ZN, trichrome or Lacto Phenol Blue (LCB) stain→?] in case of ruptured cyst.

II. Indirect methods

A. Blood picture: Eosinophilia (20-25%).

B. Immunological test: → Casoni's test

✪ **History:** Introduced by Casoni in 1911.

✪ **Principle:** It based on immediate type of hypersensitivity reaction.

✪ **Antigen:**

- Fresh hydatid fluid obtained by operation from human case.
- It also obtained from after slaughtering.
- It is sterilised by Seitz filter or membrane filtration.

✪ **Other reagents:** Normal saline for control.

✪ **Steps:**

a. **Test arm:** Intradermal injection of 0.5ml hydatid fluid in one arm.

b. **Control arm:** Intradermal injection of 0.2ml normal saline in other arm.

✪ **Result:**

i. **Positive:**

a. **Test arm:**

- Primary reaction: A large wheal about 5 cm in diameter with multiple fingers like projection **called pseudopodia** is present within half an hour & it fades in hour.
- Secondary reaction: Sometimes secondary reaction with oedema & induration appears after 8 hours.

b. **Control arm:** No reaction.

ii. **Negative:** No reaction in any arm.

✪ **Interpretation:**

i. **Positive test:** It indicates the hydatid cyst in patient.

ii. **Negative test:** No hydatid cyst in patient.

✪ **Disadvantage:**
- Non specific test & not used now a days.
- It is replaced by serological tests.

C. **Serological tests:** Antigen or antibody can be detected by
- ELISA.
- CFT.
- IHA.
- Immuno electrophoresis.
- Flocculation based test like bantonite or latex particle coated with hydatid fluid antigen.

D. **Molecular tests:** Are useful methods.

E. **Radiological:**

1. **X-ray:** Liver & lung cyst are characterised by sharp outline & bone cyst gives mottled appearance. Calcified cyst is diagnosed easily.
2. **USG:**
3. **CT scan:**
4. **MRI:**
5. **Intra Venous Pyelogram (IVP):**

} are most useful methods

❖ Prevention:
- Periodical deworming of pet dog.
- Avoid contact or kissing to infected dog & hand washing after touching the dog.
- Ensure that pet dog can't eat the animal offal.

❖ Treatment:

➢ **Chemotherapy:**
- Benzimidazole is restricted to residual, post surgical & inoperable cyst.
- Albendazole & praziquantel have proved with good results.

➢ **PAIR:**

✪ **Full form:** Puncture, Aspiration, Injection & Re aspiration.

✪ **Indications:**
- Cysts with internal echoes on ultrasound (snow flake sign).
- Multiple cysts.
- Cyst with detached laminar membrane.

✪ **Contraindications:**
- Superficial cysts.
- Cysts with multiple thick internal septal divisions (honey combing pattern).
- Cyst communicating with biliary tree.

✪ **Basic steps:**
- Puncture of cyst guided by ultrasound or CT.
- Aspiration of cyst fluid.
- Injection of scolicidal (agent which kills the scolex/head of larvae) solution like 95% ethanol alternatively hypertonic saline.
- Re-aspiration of fluid after 5 minutes.

✪ **Precautions:**
- Great care to avoid the spillage of hydatid fluid.
- Sterilise the cavity with 0.5% silver nitrate or 2.7% NaCl for prophylaxis of secondary peritoneal echinococcosis develop after spillage of fluid.
- Albendazole, 2 mg/kg BD start 4 days before & continue for 4 weeks.

✪ **Other scolicidal agents & side effects:**
- Cetrimide: Acidosis.
- 95%Alcohol: Cholangitis.
- Hypertonic saline: Hypernatraemia.
- Sodium hypochlorite: Hypernatraemia.
- H_2O_2.

➢ **Surgery:**

✪ **Indications:**
- Cyst communicating with biliary tree.
- When PAIR is not possible.

✪ **Types of surgery:**
- Laparoscopic surgery: For hydatid cyst in liver.
- Percutaneous thermal ablation of the germinal layer of cyst using radiofrequency ablation device.
- Pericystectomy.
- Lobectomy or wedge resection: For pulmonary cyst.

✪ **Follow up treatment:** Pre & post operative albendazole for 2 years after surgery is recommended.

✪ **Disadvantages:** Recurrence.

Echinococcus multilocularis

❖ Synonym: *E. alveolaris.*

❖ History:
- Multilocular disease was first recognised & differentiated from unilocular hydatid cyst by Virchow in 1855.
- Leuckart discovered the causative agent in 1863.
- Life cycle was discovered by Thomas in 1954

❖ Geographical distribution: Disease is prevalent in certain part of Europe.

❖ Habitat: Most commonly involved organ is liver.

❖ Morphology: Three morphological stages like adult, egg & larval are described below.

➢ **Adult stage:** Same as *E. granulosus*, but smaller in size about 1.2-3.7mm in length.

➢ **Egg stage:** Same as other *Taenia* species, but more resistant to cold & other environmental conditions.

➢ **Larval stage: → Fig.14**
- Multilocular larval stage.
- Cyst is sterile without scolices (protoscolices).
- No capsule unlike hydatid cyst.
- Germinal layer is hyperplastic & folded or budded.
- Hyaline layer very thin is less conspicuous.
- Persistent reaction by eosinophil & endothelial cells around the cyst.
- Contains less or no fluid.

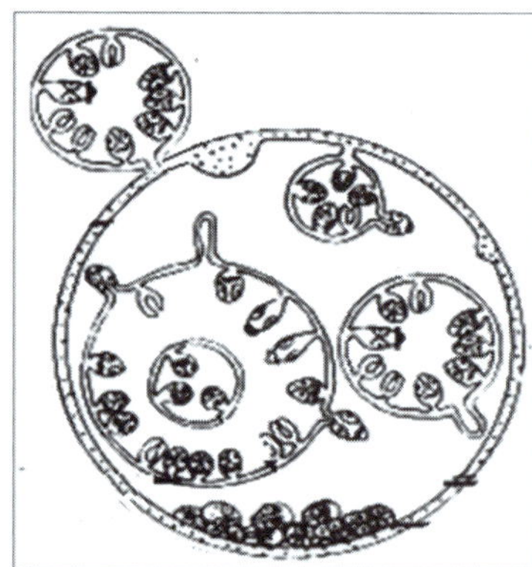

Figure-14: Multi-locular hydatid cyst

❖ Life cycle:

➢ **Types of host:** Two types.

I. **Definitive host:** Carnivorous animals like fox (optimal) , dog & wolf.

II. **Intermediate hosts:**

- Mouse (optimal) & tundra vole.
- Man is the accidental or dead end host.

➢ **Cycles:**

- It is similar to *E. granulosus* & cyst developed in mouse ingested in to fox, which develop the adult stage. Adult stage laying eggs, pass through faeces over soil & taken up by mouse to repeat the cycle.
- Man is dead end host & infected by eating fruits & vegetable contaminated by faeces of fox.

❖ Pathogenicity:

➢ **Disease name:** It is a zoonosis & human disease is present with multi-locular cyst **called multilocular hydatid cyst** or **alveolar hydatid cyst.**

➢ **Mode of transmission:** Eggs enter in man by

- Ingestion of fruits & vegetables contaminated with faeces of infected canine.
- Inhalation of faecal dust carrying eggs, especially in trappers who handle pelts.

➢ **Portal of entry:** GIT.

➢ **Site:** Mostly in liver, lungs & rarely in brain.

➢ **Infective form:** Eggs.

➢ **Exit form:** Embryonated eggs.

➢ **Pathology & pathogenesis:**

- Hyaline layer of cyst is very thin & cyst is not limited by hyaline membrane.
- Germinal layer is budded (folded) & form many daughter cyst internally as well as externally, hence **called multilocular cyst.**

➢ **Clinical features:**

- Cyst is very slow growing & it takes around 30 years to produce the symptoms.
- Due to exogenous cyst formation, it mimics a carcinoma.
- Liver cyst may produce the symptoms like pain in right upper quadrant & hepatomegaly.
- Malignant hydatid disease: Multilocular cyst mimics clinically & prognosis wise to malignancy, hence the name.

➢ **Complications:**

1. Calcification.
2. Portal hypertension.
3. Cirrhosis.
4. It is a lethal disease.

❖ Laboratory diagnosis:

It is a sterile cyst & laboratory methods are not useful. Better diagnosed by **serological** & **radiological** methods.

❖ Prevention:

Proper washing vegetable before eating.

❖ Treatment:

➢ **Chemotherapy:** Albendazole for indefinite time where surgery is not possible.

➢ **Surgery:** Surgical removal of cyst with post operative albendazole for 2 years is recommended.

Echinococcus vogeli

❖ History & geographical distribution:

15 cases have been reported from Costa Rica, Panama, Columbia, Equador & Venezuela.

❖ Habitat:

Most commonly involved organ is liver.

❖ Morphology:

All the stages are same as E. granulosus with following differences.

- Size of adult stage: 4-11mm in length.
- Larval stage is intermediate between hydatid cyst & multilocular hydatid cyst & present with brood capsules & protoscolices.

❖ Life cycle:

➢ **Types of host:** Two types.

I. **Definitive host:** Carnivorous animals like bush dog (*Speothos venaticus*).

II. **Intermediate hosts:** Rodent like paca (*Cuniculus paca*). Man is the accidental host.

❖ Pathogenicity:

➢ **Disease name:** It is a zoonosis & human disease **called polycystic hydatid cyst.**

➢ **Clinical features:** Liver cyst present with pain in right upper quadrant, hepatomegaly & jaundice.

❖ Laboratory diagnosis:

1. **Microscopical methods:** Aspiration of fluid from cyst & examination under microscope for brood capsules & protoscolices.
2. **Serological tests:** Are more useful.
3. **Radiological methods:** Are more useful.

Echinococcus oligarthus

❖ **History & geographical distribution:** 55 cases have been reported from Central & South America.

❖ **Habitat:** Most commonly involved organ is liver.

❖ **Morphology:** Adult stage: 1.9-2.9mm in length.

❖ **Life cycle:**
➢ **Types of host:** Two types.
I. **Definitive host:** Wild cats like jaguar & puma.
II. **Intermediate hosts:** Rodent like paca or spiny rats or opossum. Man is the accidental host.

❖ **Pathogenicity:**
➢ **Disease name:** It is a zoonosis & human disease **called multivesicular (polycystic) hydatid cyst.**
➢ **Clinical features:** Liver cyst present pain in right upper quadrant, hepatomegaly & jaundice.

❖ **Laboratory diagnosis:**
1. **Microscopical methods:** Aspiration of fluid from cyst & examination under microscope for brood capsules & protoscolices.
2. **Serological tests:** Are more useful.
3. **Radiological methods:** Are more useful.

Hymenolepis spp.

Hymenolepis nana

❖ **Meaning:**
- Originated from **hymen (Greek) = membrane & lepis = shell** or **shell** or **outer covering,** as outer egg shell looks like membrane.
- *H. nana* from **nanus = dwarf or short.**

❖ **Common name: Dwarf tape worm** because of short size.

❖ **Synonym:** *Taenia nana, Vampirolepis nana.*

❖ **History:** It was first discovered by Bilharz in 1857.

❖ **Geographical distribution:**
- World – wide.
- Most common in warm than cold climates, in school children & in institutional population.

❖ **Habitat:** Adult worm lives in small intestine (proximal ileum) of man/rat. Larva in fleas.

❖ **Morphology:** Three morphological stages like adult, egg & larval are described below.

I. Adult stage

➢ **Time of maturation:** Larva transformed to sexually mature adult stage in 1-2 weeks.
➢ **Colour:** White & semitransparent.
➢ **Size:** 1 to 4 cm in length × 1mm in diameter.
➢ **Shape:** Like a measure tape.
➢ **Life span:** Very short about 2 weeks.
➢ **Numbers:** 1,000 & maximum up to 8,000.
➢ **Morphological parts:** Three parts like head, neck & strobila (body/trunk) as shown in **fig.-15 (a).**

A. **Scolex (head):** → **Fig.-15(b).**
✪ **Shape:** Globular in shape.
✪ **Size:** 0.3mm in diameter (1/3rd of *T. solium*).
✪ **Suckers:** Four circular suckers.
✪ **Rostellum:** Present.
✪ **Hooklets:** Present in single row & around 20-30 in numbers. Rostellum with hooks gives tuning fork like appearance.

B. **Neck:** It is long & slender.

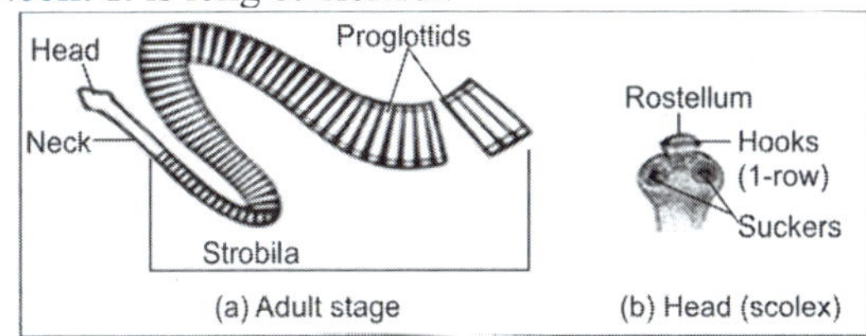

Figure-15: Adult stage of *H. nana*

C. **Strobila (body or trunk):** Contains chain of segments **called proglottids** having following features.
✪ **Proglottids (Segments):** → **Fig.-16.**

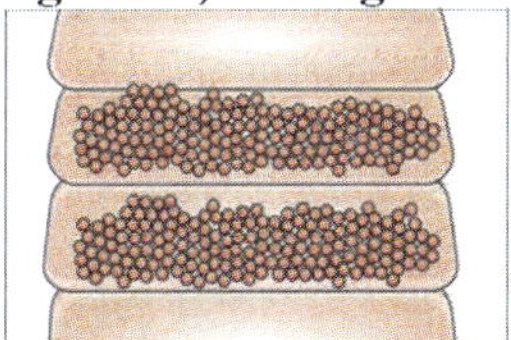

Figure-16: Segment of *H. nana*

- **Numbers:** Around 200.
- **Size (gravid segment):** 0.3mm × 0.9mm. Breadth is 3-4 times greater than length.
- **Types:** Three types according to maturity with following order from front to backwards.

1. **Immature:** Male & female organs are not differentiated.
2. **Mature:** Male & female organs are differentiated & male organs are appear first.
3. **Gravid:** Uterus is filled with eggs.

- **Expulsion of eggs:** Released by disintegration of gravid segment.
- **Reproductive system:**

o Definition: In cestodes both male & female reproductive organs are present in single individual **called monoecious** or **hermaphrodite.**
o Reproductive organs:

A. **Female reproductive organs:**
1. **Uterus:** Transverse sac with lobulated wall. Gravid uterus filled with 80-100 eggs.
2. **Ovary:** Bilobed coarsely granular ovary lies posteriorly between the testes.
3. **Ootype, Mehli's gland & other organs:** Are also present.

B. Male reproductive organs:

1. **Testes:** 3 in numbers.
2. **Vas efferentia, vas deferens & cirrus (penis):** Are also present.

- Genital atrium: Marginal & Present on same side.

II. Egg stage

- **Colour:** Colourless (non bile stained).
- **Size:** 30- 40 µm in diameter.
- **Shape:** Spherical or oval.
- **Life span:** Survive about 10 days in external environment.
- **Morphological features:** → **Fig.-17**

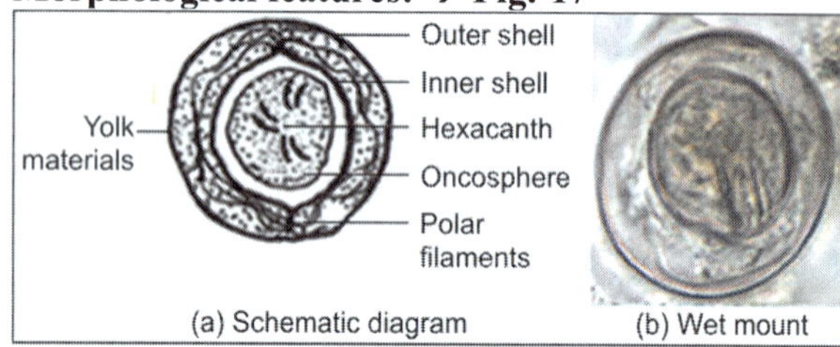

Figure-17: Egg of *H. nana*

- **Covering:** Two covering as follows.

1. **Outer:** It is thin **called egg shell.**
2. **Inner:** It is thick **called embryophore.**

- **Space between two covers:** Filled by yolk materials & polar filaments.
- **Embryo:** Eggs contain embryo **called oncopshere** with 6 hooklets (3 pairs) **called hexacanth.**
- **Other features:** Float in saturated common salt solution.

III. Larval stage

- **Development:** It develops in small intestine of host in 4 days.
- **Shape:** Pyriform.
- **Morphological features:** → **Fig.-18**
  - Name: **Called cysticercoids.**
  - Hooklets: Present.
  - Scolex: It is invaginated from one side.
  - Time of development: Eggs develop the *Cysticercercoid* in 4 days.

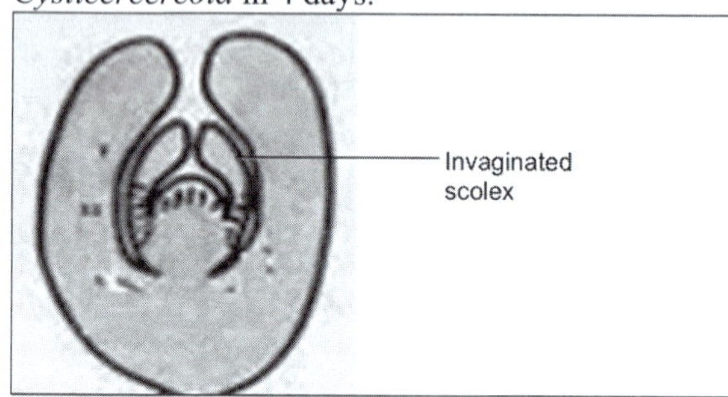

Figure-18: Larva of *H. nana*

❖ Life cycle:

- **Cycles & hosts:** As mentioned below **(fig.-19).**

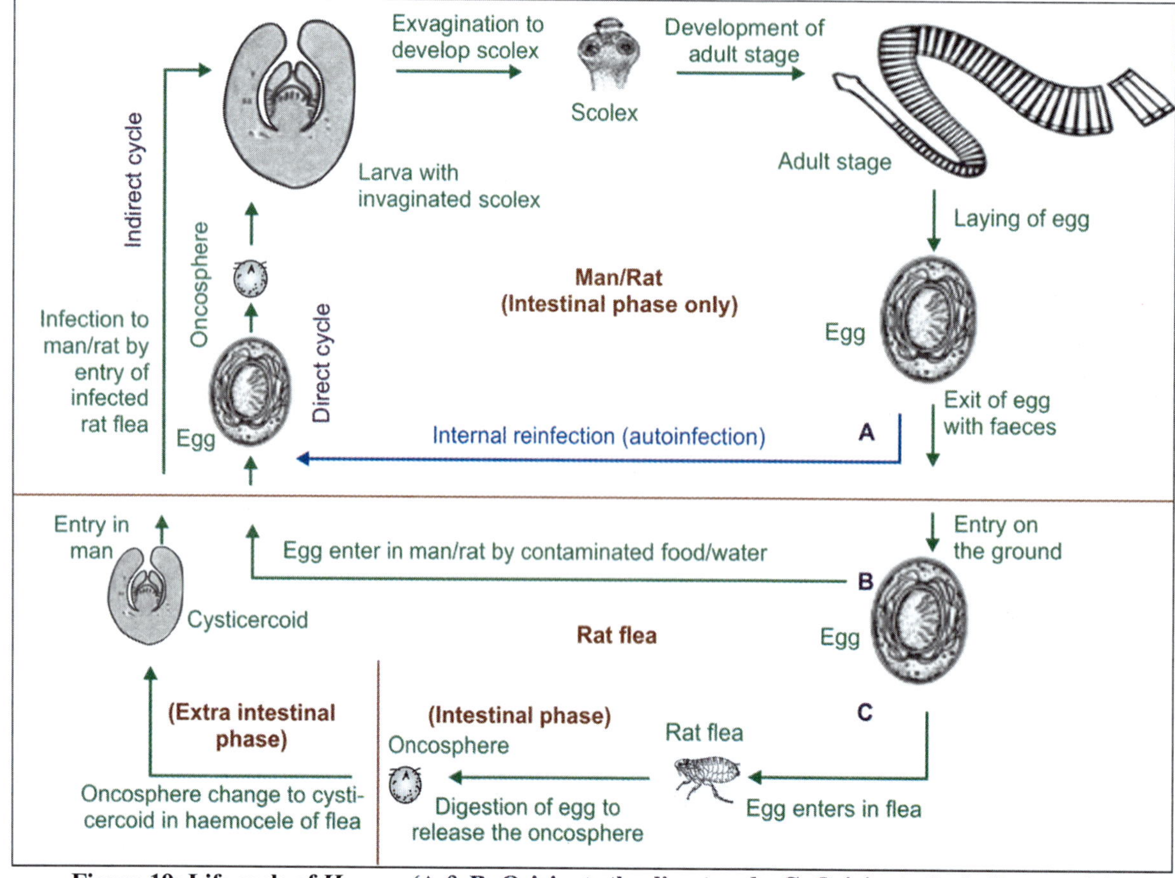

Figure-19: Life cycle of *H. nana* (A & B: Originate the direct cycle, C: Originate the indirect cycle)

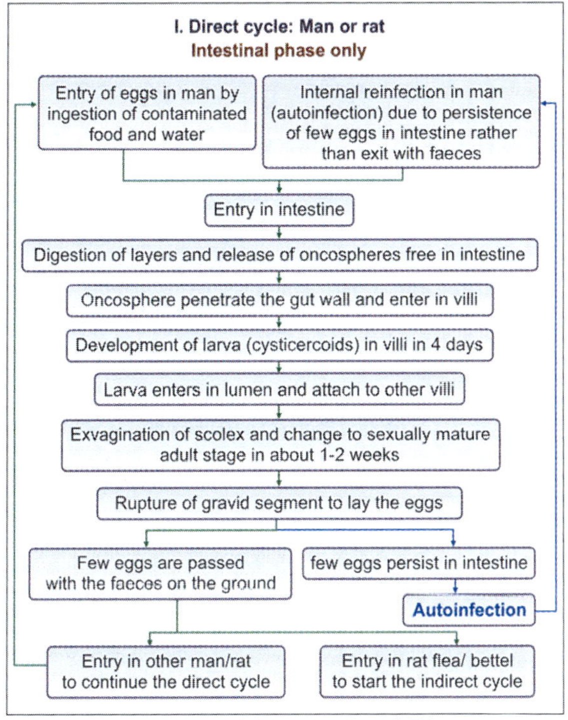

Flow chart-5: Direct cycle of *H. nana*

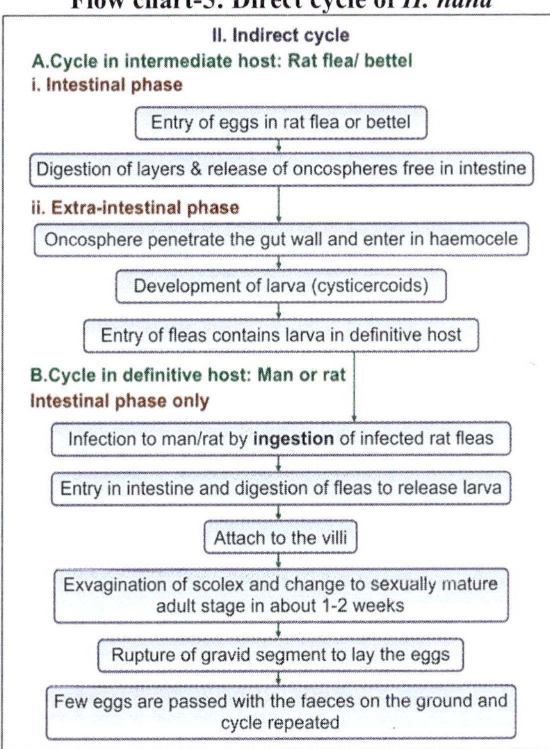

Flow chart-6: Indirect cycle of *H. nana*

I. **Direct cycle:** Man or rat act as definitive host (adult stage) & intermediate host (larval stage) as shown in **flow chart -5.**

II. **Indirect cycle:** As shown in **flow chart -6.** This cycle is true in Argentina.

✓ **Note: Strain of *H. nana*:** In above cycle strain mentioned is able to infect human to rat & vice versa also, however few authors says that human strain can infect rat but not vice versa.

A. **Definitive host:** Man or rat (adult stage).

B. **Intermediate host:** Rat flea (*Xenopsylla cheopis*) or beetle (larval stage).

❖ Pathogenicity:

- **Disease name: Called hymenolepiasis** or **hymenolepidosis** or **dwarf tape worm disease.**
- **Reservoir & source of infection:** Man.
- **Mode of transmission:**
  - Entry of eggs in man by **ingestion** of contaminated food & water.
  - Internal reinfection in man **(autoinfection)** due to persistence of few eggs in intestine rather exits.
  - Infection to man / rat by **ingestion** of infected rat fleas/bettles contains cysticercoids (larva) in haemocele.
- **Exit form:** Embryonated eggs.
- **Infective form:**
  - Embryonated eggs.
  - Larva **called cysticercoids.**
- **Portal of entry:** GIT.
- **Site:** Small intestine (proximal ileum).
- **Precipitating factors:**
  - Age: Most common in children.
  - Climate: Common in warm than cold climates.
  - Locality: Common in institutional population.
  - Immunity: Immunosuppression can cause dissemination of infection.
- **Clinical features:** Only by adult stage as below.
- **Asymptomatic:**
- **GIT:** Minor symptoms like abdominal pain or diarrhoea.

❖ Laboratory diagnosis:

I. Direct methods

- **Specimen:** Stool (eggs are infectious & unpreserved stool can be handled with care).
- **Testing methods:**

A. **Macroscopic (naked eye) examination:** For segments which are rarely or not available.

B. **Microscopy:**

a. **Wet mount by using normal saline & iodine:** It shows the non bile stained (colourless) egg as shown in **fig.-17(b).**

b. **Concentration technique:** In case of negative result by wet mount method.

II. Indirect methods

A. **Serological test:** ELISA test has been developed with 80% sensitivity.

❖ Prevention:

- Avoid the use of contaminated food & water.
- Rodent & flea control.

❖ **Treatment:**
- Praziquantel: Single dose 25mg/kg is the drug of choice for adult & larval stage.
- Nitazoxanide 500mg BD is another effective drug.

Hymenolepis diminuta

❖ **Meaning:** Word diminuta is misnomer (inappropriate) as it is larger than *H. nana*.

❖ **Common name:** Rat tape worm.

❖ **History:** It was first discovered by Rudolph in 1819 & later by Blanchard in 1891.

❖ **Geographical distribution:** Worldwide.

❖ **Habitat:**
- Adult worm lives in small intestine (upper three quarters of ileum) of rat, mice or man.
- Larva in fleas.

❖ **Morphology:** Three morphological stages like adult, egg & larval are described below.

I. Adult stage

➢ **Colour:** White & semitransparent.
➢ **Size:** 20 to 60 cm in length × 4mm in diameter.
➢ **Shape:** They are dorso-ventrally flat & broad as like a measure tape hence **called tape worm.**
➢ **Morphological parts:** Three parts like head, neck & strobila (body/trunk).

A. **Scolex (head):**
✪ **Size:** 0.2-0.4mm.
✪ **Suckers:** Four suckers.
✪ **Rostellum:** Present.
✪ **Hooklets:** Absent.

B. **Neck:** It is long & slender.

C. **Strobila (body or trunk):** Contains chain of segments **called proglottids** having following features.

✪ **Proglottids (segments):**
- **Numbers:** Around 800-1000.
- **Size (gravid segment):** 0.75mm × 2.5mm. Breadth is greater than length.
- **Other features:** Are same as *H. nana*.

II. Egg stage

➢ **Colour:** Bile stained.
➢ **Size:** Larger than *H. nana* about 60- 80 µm in diameter.
➢ **Morphological features:**
✪ **Covering:** Two covering as follows.
1. **Outer:** It is thin & yellow colour.
2. **Inner:** It is thick & with two knob like structure **called embryophore.**

✪ **Space between two covers:** Does not contain polar filaments.
✪ **Embryo:** Eggs contain embryo **called oncopshere** with 6 hooklets (3 pairs) **called hexacanth.**

III. Larval stage

➢ **Development:** Cysticercoid develops in rat flea.

❖ **Life cycle:**
➢ **Hosts:**
A. **Definitive host:** Man or rat (adult stage).
B. **Intermediate host:** Rat flea (*Xenopsylla cheopis*) or flour beetle or ear wigs (larval stage).

➢ **Cycles:** Following two types of cycle as shown in **flow chart-7.**

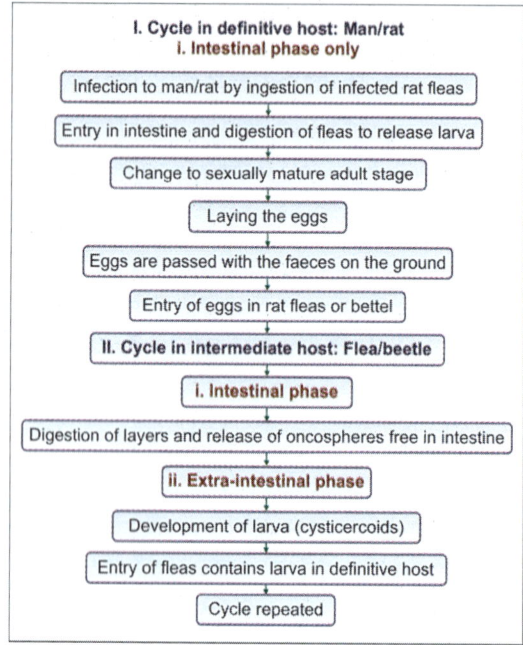

Flow chart-7: Life cycle of *H. diminuta*

❖ **Pathogenicity:**
➢ **Disease name: Called hymenolepiasis diminuta.**
➢ **Reservoir of infection:** Rat.
➢ **Source of infection:** Rat fleas / bettles contain cysticercoids (larva).
➢ **Mode of transmission:** Accidental infection to man by **ingestion** of infected rat fleas / bettles.
➢ **Exit form:** Embryonated eggs.
➢ **Infective form:** Larva **called cysticercoids.**
➢ **Portal of entry:** GIT.
➢ **Site:** Small intestine (upper three quarters of ileum).
➢ **Precipitating factors:** Most common in children.
➢ **Clinical features:** Only by adult stage as below.
- **Asymptomatic:**
- **GIT:** Minor symptoms like abdominal pain or diarrhoea.

❖ **Laboratory diagnosis:**

I. Direct methods

➢ **Specimen:** Stool
➢ **Testing methods:**

A. **Macroscopic (naked eye) examination:** Not useful because segments are not break away from strobila & absent in stool.

B. **Microscopy:**

a. **Wet mount by using normal saline & iodine:** It shows the bile stained eggs without polar filaments.

b. **Concentration technique:** In case of negative result by wet mount method.

II. Indirect methods

A. **Serological test:** Not useful.

Dipylidium caninum

❖ **Meaning:**

- Originated from **dis (Greek) = two + pylis = gate** or **entrance,** as parasite have bilateral genital pores in each segment (Two entrance).
- Caninum from **canine = dog**, indicates dog species.

❖ **Common name:** Double pored dog tape worm.

❖ **History:**

- Linnaeus (1758) & Ralliet (1892) contributed in discovery of parasite.
- Most of the cases occurred in European countries.
- Chowdhary & Bandyopadhyay from Kolkatta, India reported the cases with adult 2 adult parasites in children in 1862.

❖ **Geographical distribution:** Worldwide.

❖ **Habitat:** Adult worm lives in small intestine of man/dog/cat. Larva in dog fleas / cat fleas.

❖ **Morphology:** Three morphological stages like adult, egg & larval are described below.

I. Adult stage

➢ **Time of maturation:** Larva change to sexually mature adult stage in 20 days in definitive host.

➢ **Colour:** White & semitransparent.

➢ **Size:** 10 to 17 cm in length.

➢ **Shape:** Like a measure tape.

➢ **Morphological parts:** Three parts like head, neck & strobila (body/trunk) as shown in **fig.-20 (a).**

A. **Scolex (head): → Fig.-20(b)**

✪ **Suckers:** Four elliptical suckers.

✪ **Rostellum:** Refractile rostellum is present.

✪ **Hooklets:** Present in 3-4 rows giving rose thorns like appearance.

B. **Neck:** It is short & thin.

C. **Strobila (body or trunk):** Contains chain of segments **called proglottids** having following features.

✪ **Proglottids (segments): → Fig.-21**

- **Shape:** Melon seeds in shape.
- **Numbers:** Around 200.
- **Size (gravid segment):** Elongated 23mm × 8mm.
- **Reproductive system:**

○ Reproductive organs:

- **Numbers:** Each segment present with two set of reproductive organs.
- **Uterus:** Sac like & when gravid, break up in numbers of egg capsules containing 8-20 eggs in each **called egg pocket.**
- **Expulsion of eggs:** Eggs are passed in faeces with segments which may disintegrate either in bowel or later after evacuation.

○ Genital atrium: Two pores situated on lateral side.

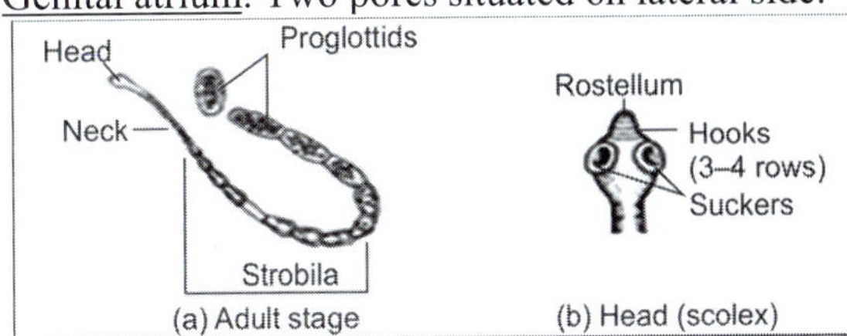

Figure-20: Adult stage of *D. caninum*

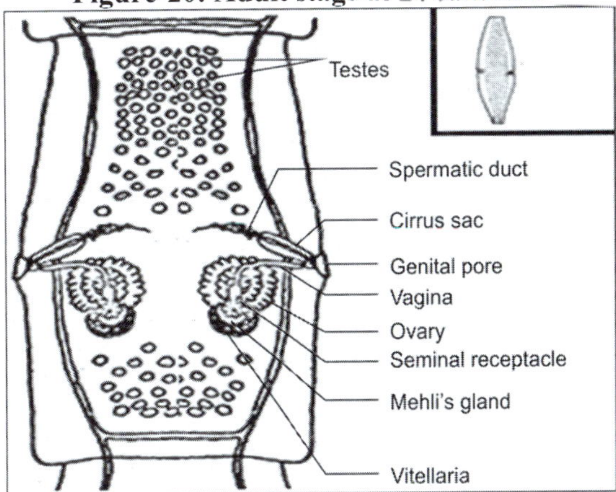

Figure-21: Segment of *D. caninum*

II. Egg stage

➢ **Egg capsule:** Gravid uterus break up in numbers of egg capsules containing 8-20 eggs.

➢ **Size:** 20-35μm in diameter.

➢ **Morphological features:** All the eggs are covered by capsule **called egg pocket** as shown in **fig.-22.**

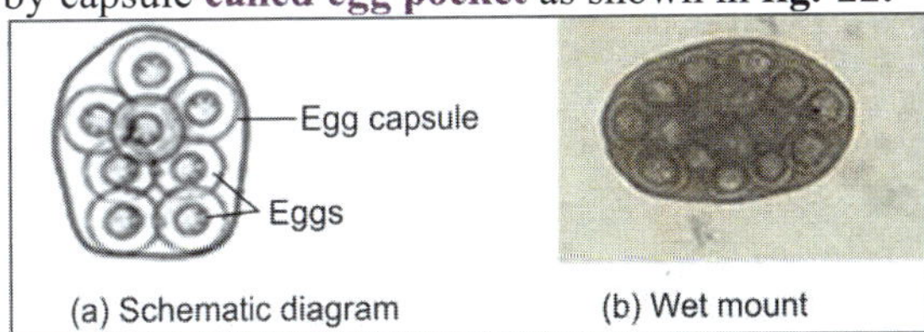

Figure-22: Egg of *D. caninum*

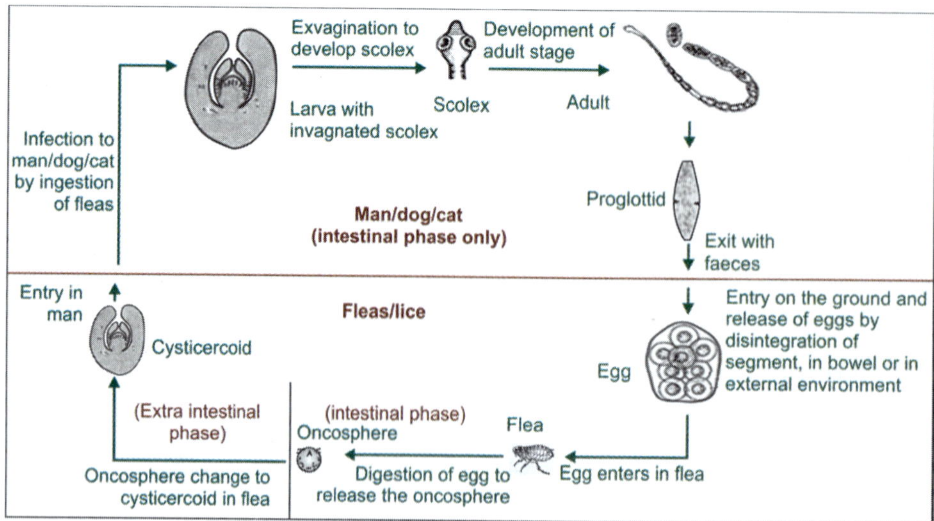

Figure-23: Life cycle of *D. caninum*

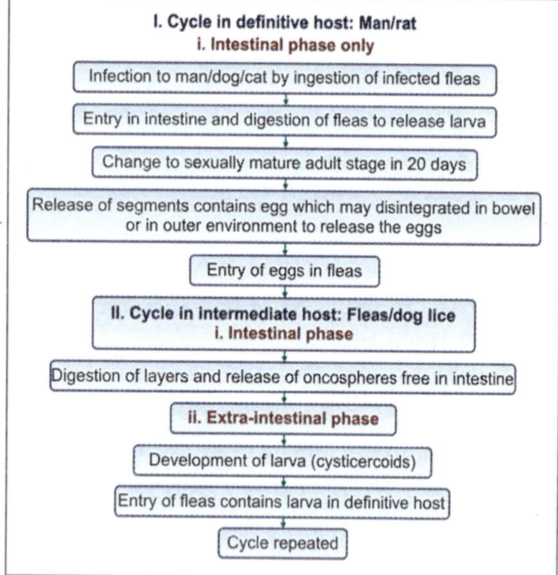

Flow chart-8: Life cycle of *D. caninum*

III. Larval stage

- **Development:** Cysticercoid develops in dog/cat flea.

❖ Life cycle:

- **Hosts:**

A. Definitive host: Man or dog or cat (adult stage).

B. Intermediate host: Dog flea (*Ctenocephalus canis*) or cat flea (*C. felis*) or human flea or dog lice (larval stage).

- **Cycles:** Following two types of cycle as shown in **figure-23** & **flow chart-8.**

❖ Pathogenicity:

- **Disease name: Called dipylidiasis.**
- **Reservoir of infection:** Animals like dog or cat.
- **Source of infection:** Fleas or lice.
- **Mode of transmission:** Accidental infection to man by **ingestion** of infected fleas especially in children during fondling cats or dogs.
- **Infective form:** Larva **called cysticercoids.**
- **Exit form:** Proglottids or eggs.
- **Portal of entry:** GIT.
- **Site:** Small intestine.
- **Precipitating factors:** Most common in children.
- **Clinical features:** Only by adult stage as below.

- **Asymptomatic:**
- **GIT:** Minor symptoms like abdominal pain or diarrhoea or pruritus ani (due to motile proglottids).

❖ Laboratory diagnosis:

I. Direct methods

- **Specimen:** Stool.
- **Testing methods:**

A. Macroscopic examination: For segments.

B. Microscopy:

a. Wet mount by using normal saline & iodine: It shows the characteristic egg pocket as shown in **Fig.-22**

b. Concentration technique: It is useful in case of negative result by wet mount method.

II. Indirect methods

A. Serological test: Rarely useful.

❖ Prevention: Flea control.

❖ Treatment: Praziquantel is the drug of choice.

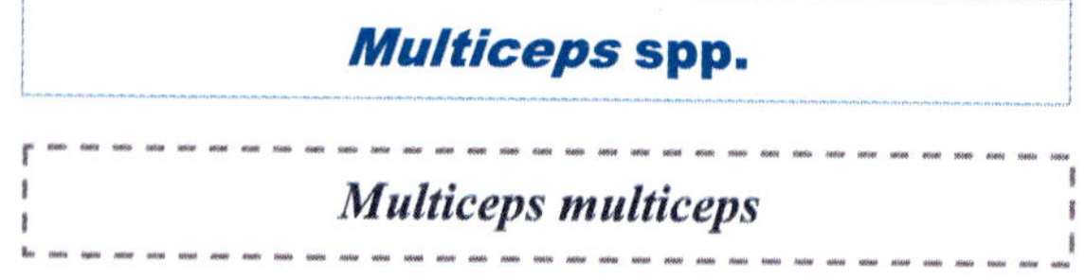

❖ **Meaning:** Contains multiple protoscolices hence the name Multiceps.

❖ **Synonym:** *Taenia multiceps.*

❖ **History:** Luke contributed in discovery of parasites.

❖ **Geographical distribution:** Human coenurosis is most common in Africa, Europe & USA.

❖ **Habitat:**

- Adult worm lives in small intestine (proximal ileum) of definitive hosts.
- Larva present in brain, spinal cord & subcutaneous tissues in man & in other intermediate hosts.

❖ **Morphology:** Three morphological stages like adult, egg & larval are described below.

I. Adult stage

- **Size:** 40 to 60 cm in length.
- **Morphological parts:** Three parts like head, neck & strobila (body/trunk).

A. Scolex (head):

- **Shape:** Pyriform in shape.
- **Suckers:** Four suckers.
- **Rostellum:** Present.
- **Hooklets:** Present in two rows (22-32 large & small hooks. Large 150-170 µm long & small 90-130 µm long.

B. Neck:

C. Strobila (body or trunk): Contains chain of segments called proglottids & uterus in gravid segment has 18-26 branches.

II. Egg stage

- **Size:** 30- 40 µm in diameter & other features are same as *Taenia* species.
- **Shape:** Spherical or oval.

III. Larval stage

- **Development:** It develops in small intestine of intermediate host & penetrates the tissues.

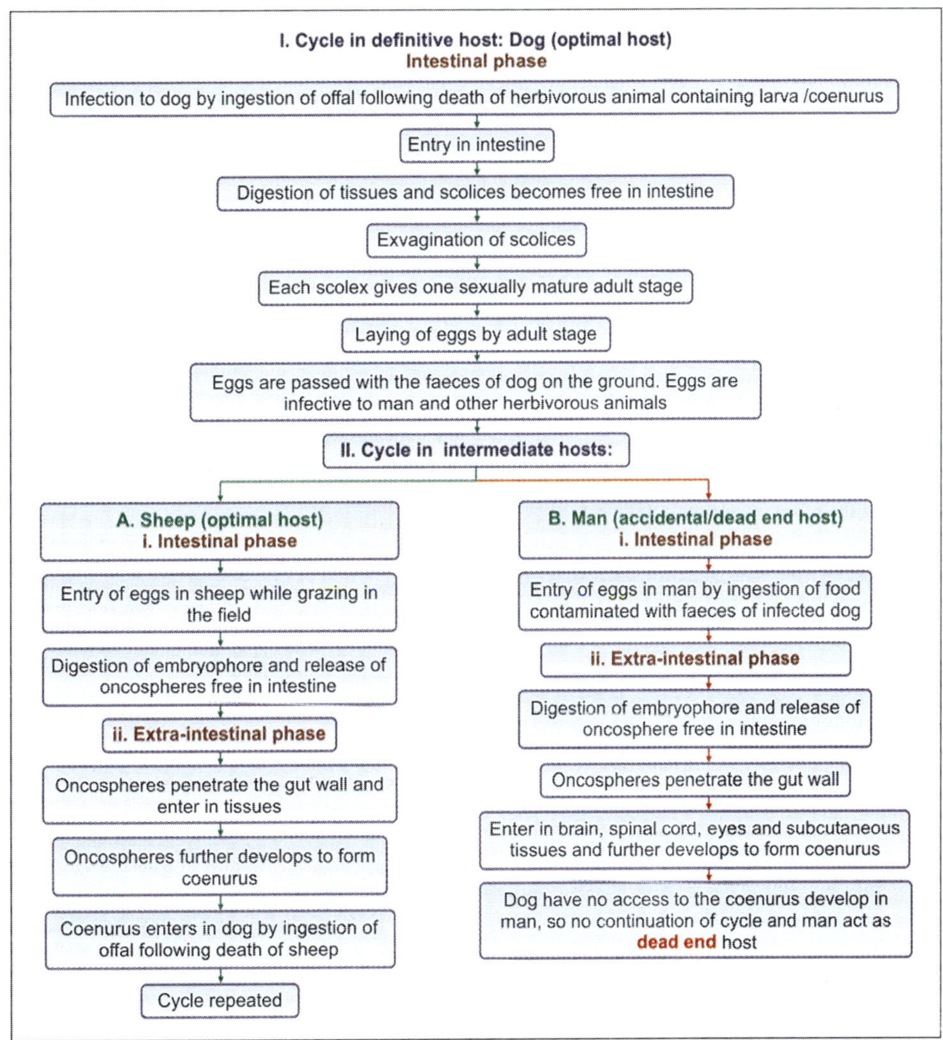
I. Cycle in definitive host: Dog (optimal host)
Intestinal phase
Infection to dog by ingestion of offal following death of herbivorous animal containing larva /coenurus
Entry in intestine
Digestion of tissues and scolices becomes free in intestine
Exvagination of scolices
Each scolex gives one sexually mature adult stage
Laying of eggs by adult stage
Eggs are passed with the faeces of dog on the ground. Eggs are infective to man and other herbivorous animals
II. Cycle in intermediate hosts:
A. Sheep (optimal host)
i. Intestinal phase
Entry of eggs in sheep while grazing in the field
Digestion of embryophore and release of oncospheres free in intestine
ii. Extra-intestinal phase
Oncospheres penetrate the gut wall and enter in tissues
Oncospheres further develops to form coenurus
Coenurus enters in dog by ingestion of offal following death of sheep
Cycle repeated
B. Man (accidental/dead end host)
i. Intestinal phase
Entry of eggs in man by ingestion of food contaminated with faeces of infected dog
ii. Extra-intestinal phase
Digestion of embryophore and release of oncosphere free in intestine
Oncospheres penetrate the gut wall
Enter in brain, spinal cord, eyes and subcutaneous tissues and further develops to form coenurus
Dog have no access to the coenurus develop in man, so no continuation of cycle and man act as dead end host

Flow chart-9: Life cycle of *M. multiceps*

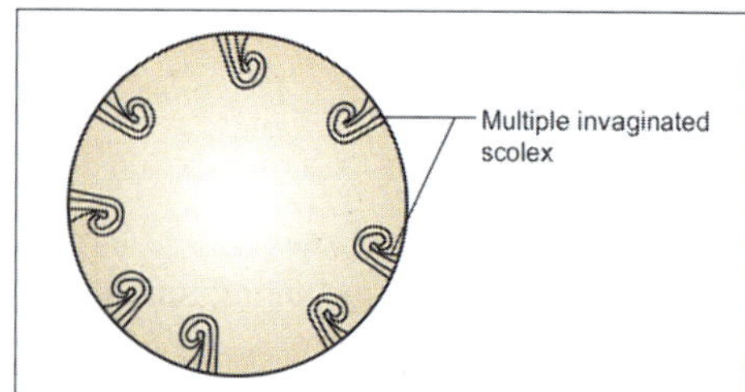

Figure-24: Larva of *M. multiceps*

- **Shape:** Spherical or oval.
- **Size:** 3cmm in diameter.
- **Morphological features:** → **Fig.-24**
- Name: **Called coenurus.**
- Scolex: Multiple in numbers & invaginated from one side.

❖ Life cycle:

- **Hosts:**

A. Definitive host: Carnivorous animals like dog or wolf or fox (adult stage).

B. Intermediate host:

- Herbivorous animals like sheep, cattle, horse or other ruminant.
- Man is the accidental intermediate host.
- **Cycles:** Natural cycle continues between carnivorous animal & herbivorous animal, while man act as dead end host as shown in **flow chart-9.**

❖ Pathogenicity:

- **Disease name: Called coenurosis.**
- **Reservoir of infection:** Dog.
- **Source of infection:** Food & water contaminated with faces of dogs.
- **Mode of transmission:** Accidental infection to man by **ingestion** of food & water contaminated with faces of dogs contains eggs.
- **Exit form:** Man act as dead end host & eggs are exit from definitive host (dog).
- **Infective form:** Larva **called coenurus.**
- **Portal of entry:** GIT.
- **Sites:** Brain, spinal cord, eyes & subcutaneous tissues.
- **Clinical features:** Only by larval stage, which produce the space occupying lesions.
- **Asymptomatic:**
- **Pressure symptoms:** Headache, vomiting, paresis, seizures etc.

❖ Laboratory diagnosis:

I. Direct methods

- **Specimen:** Biopsies from infected tissues.
- **Testing methods:**

A. History & clinical examination: Supportive method.

B. Microscopy: Histological examination of biopsy material to identify the coenurus.

II. Indirect methods

A Serological test: Very useful methods.

B Radiological methods: X-ray, CT-scan, MRI & USG are useful methods.

❖ **Prevention:** Avoid the faecal contamination of food.

❖ **Treatment:** Surgical removal of space occupying lesion.

Question bank

Case study

1) A 24 years male presents with abdominal discomfort since 10 days. He is giving history of beef ingestion. Stool examination revealed bile stained, spherical & hexacanth containing egg. Identify the organism & answer the following
a) Name the causative agent.
b) Describe the life cycle of causative agent.
c) Write the pathogenicity causative agent.
d) Describe the lab. diagnosis of causative agent.

2) A 40 year old patient admitted with complains of pain in right hypochondrium. Occupationally patient is farmer. Ultrasonography reported the cyst in right lobe of liver. Identify the organism & answer the following.
a) Name the causative agent & draw the diagram of larval stage of causative agent.
b) Describe the life cycle of causative agent.
c) Write the pathogenicity of causative agent.
d) Describe the lab. diagnosis of causative agent.

Essay/Full question

1) *T. saginata.*
2) *T. solium.*
3) *E. granulosus.*

Short notes

1) Morphology / life cycle / pathogenicity / laboratory diagnosis of *T. saginata* or *T. solium* or *E. granulosus.*
2) Differences between *T. saginata* & *T. solium.*
3) Cysticercosis.
4) Hydatid cyst.
5) Casoni's test or Casoni's reaction.
6) *H. nana.*
7) *D. caninum.*
8) *M. multiceps.*
9) Multilocular hydatid cyst.

Short questions for theory/viva questions

1) Comment: *T. solium is more* dangerous than *T. saginata.*
2) Comment: Diagnostic aspiration of hydatid fluid from hydatid cyst is generally not advised.
3) What is measly beef (beef measles) & measly pork (pork measles)?
4) What is acephalocyst & pericyst in H. cyst?
5) Write two mechanisms of development of daughter cyst in H. cyst.
6) Name two parasites causing unilocular & multilocular hydatid cyst.
7) What is egg pocket & egg capsule?
8) What is malignant hydatid disease?

MCQs for chapter review

Taenia solium

1) **Man is both definitive and intermediate host for**
(a) *T solium* (b) *T saginata* (c) *E granulosus* (d) *Dicroftis hominis*
2) **Consumption of uncooked pork is likely to cause which of the following helminthic disease**
(a) *T solium* (b) *T saginata* (c) *H nana* (d) *H cyst*
3) **Neurocysticercosis following are true except** (PGI -98)
(a) Not acquired by eating contaminated vegetables (b) Caused by regurgitation of larvae (c) Acquired by orofaecal route (d) Acquired by eating pork
4) **The most commonly affected tissue in cysticercosis is** (PGI -79, AIIMS-81)
(a) Brain (b) Eye (c) Muscles (d) Liver
5) **The following regarding cysticercosis are true except** (PGI -95)
(a) Commonest sites are meninges and cerebral ventricle (b) Calcification is common (c) Causes focal neurological complication (d) Found in subcutaneous tissues
6) **Which of the following is the most common location of intracranial neurocysticercosis** (AIIMS -03)
(a) Brain parenchyma (b) Subarachnoid space (c) Spinal cord (d) Orbit
7) **Commonest parasite of CNS in India is** (AI -99)
(a) Schisosomiasis (b) Cysticercosis (c) *Trichinella spiralis* (d) Hydatid cyst
8) **Which of the following is the most common central nervous system parasitic infection** (AIIMS -03)
(a) Echinococcosis (b) Spaganosis (c) Paragonimiasis (d) Neurocysticercosis
9) **Neurocysticercosis is caused by**
((a) *T solium* (b) *T saginata* (c) *D latum* (d) *Ascaria lumbricides*
10) **Which of the following is not a neuroparasite** (AI -05)
(a) *Taenia solium* (b) *Acanthamoeba* (c) *Naegleria* (d) *Trichinella spiralis*
11) **Parasitic encephalitis is caused by** (PGI, Dec -05)
(a) *Naegleria* (b) *Acanthamoeba* (c) *Balamuthia* (d) *Gnathostoma*
12) **Primary amoebic meningo encephalitis is caused by**
(a) *Naegleria fowleri* (b) *Entamoeba histolytica* (c) *Endolimax nana* (d) *Dientamoeba fragilis*
13) **Eosinophilic meningo encephalitis is caused by** (PGI-00)
(a) *Gnathostoma* (b) *Naegleria* (c) *Toxocara canis* (d) *Angiostrongylus cantonensis*
14) **Drug of choice in cerebral cysticercosis is** (PGI-00)
(a) Piperizine (b) Pyevinium (c) Thiabendazole (d) Mebendazole (e) None

Echinococcus granulosus

15) **Hydatid disease of liver is caused by** (AIIMS -03)
(a) *Strongyloides* (b) *Echinococcus granulosus* (c) *Taenia solium* (d) *Trichinella spiralis* (e) *Echinococcus multilocularis*
16) **Definitive host of hydatid disease (*Echinococcus granulosus*) is**
(a) Man (b) Dog (c) Horse (d) sheep
17) **Intermediate host of hydatid disease** (AIIMS, May-03)
(a) Man (b) Dog (c) Cat (d) Foxes
18) **Most common site for hydatid cyst**
(a) Lung (b) Liver (c) Brain (d) Kidney
19) **Least common site for calcified hydatid cyst** is
(a) Lung (b) Mediastinum (c) Extraperitoneal site (d) Liver
20) **Which of the following show regressive metamorphosis**
(a) Hydatid cyst (b) Cysticercoid (c) *Cysticercus bovis* (d) *Cysticercus cellulosae*
21) **A company executive, who travel worldwide present with upper abdominal mass and +ve Casoni's test/ The organism is** (AI-00)
(a) *Echinococcus* (b) *Entamoeba histolytica* (c) Hepatitis (d) Ascariasis

Echinococcus multilocularis

22) **The following infection resemble malignancy** (JIPMER -02)
(a) *Echinococcus granulosus* (b) *E. multilocularis* (c) *E vogeli* (d) *E oligarthus*
23) **What is malignant hydatid disease** (JIPMER -02)
(a) Malignant change in to hydatid cyst (b) Infection with *E. multilocularis* (c) Hydatid disease in immunocompromised host (d) None of the above

Hymenolepsi nana

24) **Dwarf tape worm refer to** (AIIMS -84)
(a) *Echinococcus* (b) *Loa loa* (c) *Hymenolepis nana* (d) *Schistosoma haematobium*
25) **The egg which of the following parasites consist of polar filaments arising from either end of the embryophore**
(a) *Taenia saginata* (b) *Taenia solium* (c) *Echinococcus granulosus* (d) *Hymenolepis nana* (e) *Diphylobothrium latum*

Answers of MCQs & explanation

1) **(a)**
- Follow section, ***Taenia solium*** **(life cycle)** for explanation
2) **(a)**
- Follow section, ***Taenia solium*** **(pathogenicity → mode of transmission)** for explanation
3) **(a) & (d)**
- Follow section, ***Taenia solium*** **(life cycle → flow chart-2 & pathogenicity → mode of transmission)** for explanation

4) **(c)**
5) **(a)**
6) **(a)**
7) **(b)**
8) **(d)**

} Follow section, ***Taenia solium*** **(pathogenicity → clinical types & features → larval stage disease)** for explanation

9) **(a)**
10) **(a)**
11) **(a), (b), (c) & (d)**
12) **(a)**
13) **(d)**

} Follow section, ***Taenia solium*** **(pathogenicity →notes)** for explanation

14) **(e)**
- Follow section, ***Taenia solium*** **(treatment)** for explanation.

15) **(b) & (e)**
16) **(b)**
17) **(a)**
18) **(a)**
19) **(a)**
20) **(a)**
21) **(a)**

} Follow section, ***Echinococcus granulosus*** for explanation

22) **(b)**
23) **(b)**

} Follow section, ***Echinococcus multilocularis*** **(pathogenicity → clinical features)** for explanation

24) **(c)**
25) **(d)**

} Follow section, ***Hymenolepis nana*** for explanation

94 Trematodes: General features and classification

Learning heading & subheadings

- ❖ Synonym:
- ❖ Meaning:
- ❖ Habitat:
- ❖ Morphology:
- ❖ Mode of transmission of trematodes:
- ❖ Life cycle:
- ❖ Classification:
- ❖ Differences between diecious & monoecious trematodes:

❖ **Synonym:** **Fluke** from **Floc (Anglo-saxon) = flat fish,** because it is dorso-ventrally flat & unsegmented like flat fish or leaf of tree.

❖ **Meaning:** Trematodes originated from **trema (Greek) = hole + edios = appearance,** as the parasite have large conspicuous suckers with hole in middle.

❖ **Habitat:** Intestine, blood, liver & lungs.

❖ **Morphology:**

I. Adult stage

➢ **Shape:**

A. Diecious (non-hermaphrodite) trematodes: It includes *Schistosomes* which are not flattened & leaf like, but cylindrical as like round worm as shown in **fig.-1.**

B. Monoecious (hermaphrodite) trematodes: They are dorso-ventrally flat, like a leaf of tree or flatfish hence **called flukes** as shown in **fig.-2.**

➢ **Size:** Unsegmented & 1 millimetre to several centimetres in length.

➢ **Organs: → Fig.-1 & 2**

✪ **Tegument:**

- **Definition:** Body of parasite is covered with noncellular layer **called tegument** or **called cuticle**.
- **Structure:**

a. Under light microscope:

- It looks as homogenous layer about 7-16 μm in thickness.
- It showing affinity for basic stains.
- It may partially or completely cover with spines or tubercles or ridges.

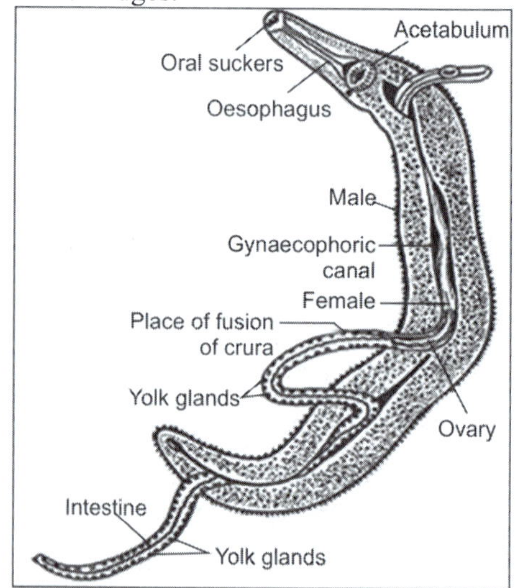

Figure-1: Adult stage of diecious trematodes

b. Under electron microscope: Two zones can be seen.

1. **Outer zone:** Thrown in folds to form microvilli.
2. **Inner zone:** It contains mitochondria, endoplasmic reticulum & glycogen granules.

- **Functions:**

1. **Absorption:** It plays a role in absorption of carbohydrate.
2. **Excretion:** It also plays a role in excretion of excessive mucus & other metabolites.

✪ **Suckers:**

- **Definition:** It is a strong muscular cup shaped depression.
- **Function:** Act as an organ for adhesion with host cells.
- **Numbers:** Two in number, so species **called distomata** (**Greek** word from **di = two + stomata = mouth).**

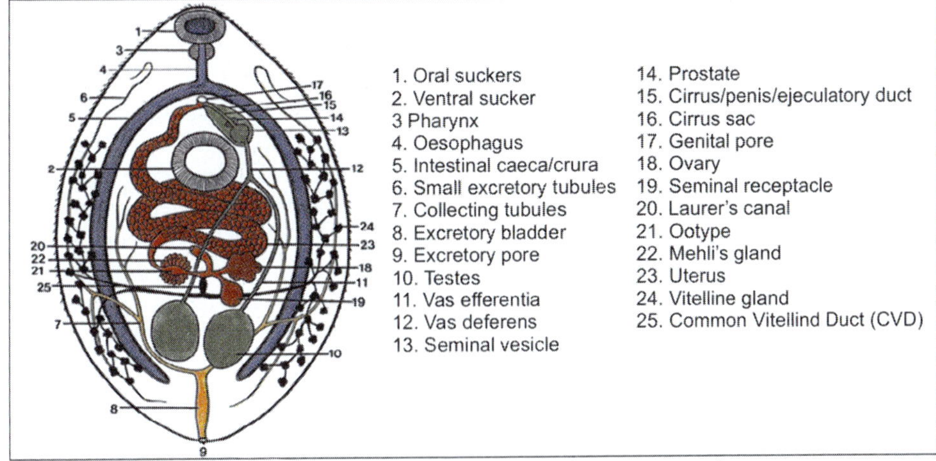

Figure-2: Adult stage of monoecious trematodes

- **Types:** Two types.

1. **Oral sucker:** One is surrounding the oral cavity **called oral sucker.**
2. **Ventral sucker or acetabula:** Another one is present on ventral surface **called acetabula** (Latin word meaning a shallow vinegar vessel or cup) or **called ventral sucker.**

✪ **Body cavity:** Absent.

✪ **Gastrointestinal system:**

- It is present but without anus so **called incomplete**
- Mouth: Situated anteriorely in the centre of oral sucker.
- Prepharynx: Present.
- Pharynx: Bulbous & muscular.
- Oesophagus is bifurcated in front of ventral sucker in to two tube like structure **called intestinal caeca** or **called crura** which may be simple (*C. sinensis*) or branched (*F. hepatica*) or curved in middle without branches (*F. buski*) or reunite to form the single caecum (*Schistosomes species*). Crura are lined by epithelial cells.

✪ **Excretory system:** Present with following contains

- **Collecting tubules:** Excretory system contains small tubules which are united to form the collecting tubules.
- **Flame cells:** Tubules are present with ciliated cells **called flame cells** & they provide the basis for species identification.
- Tubules open posteriorly in excretory pore via excretory bladder.

✪ **Nervous system:** Present with following features.

- Primitive in nature & of low grade.
- It includes lateral ganglia connected by dorsal commisure.
- Sense organs are almost lacking.

✪ **Gynaecophoric canal:** Present only in diecious flukes.

✪ **Reproductive system:**

- **Definition:** In trematodes both male & female reproductive organs are present in single individual **called monoecious** or **hermaphrodite** except *Schistosomes* in which separate male & female species are available **called diecious.**
- **Features:**
  - Highly developed & complete in each individual.
  - Reproductive organs lie between the two branches of the intestine.
- **Reproductive organs:**

A. Female reproductive organs: Consists following organs.

1. **Ovary:**
   - Numbers: Single.
   - Site: Lying in front of testes.
   - Function: It discharge the ova in the oviduct.
2. **Laurer's canal (rudimentary vagina):**
   - It represents the rudimentary vagina & inner end contains the receptacle for storage of sperms **called seminal receptacle.**
   - Function: It may not open or if opened then opening present on dorsal surface & act as vagina for entrance of sperm & cross fertilisation.
3. **Uterus:**
   - Course: Tortuous tube emanate from the ootype & ends in genital atrium.
   - Terminal part **called metaterm**, which in absence of Laurer's canal act as vagina.
   - Function: Contains eggs when gravid.
4. **Ootype:**
   - Function: It provides platform for fertilisation of eggs.
5. **Vitelline / yolk glands (vitellaria):**
   - Site: It scattered lateral to intestinal crura & connected to vitelline ducts which are join to form common vitelline duct (common yolk channel) which open in the ootype.
   - Function: It produces the shell material.
6. **Mehli's gland:**
   - Synonym & function: Also **called shell gland** because material from the ovi duct, seminal receptacle & common vitelline duct comes in Mehli's gland where egg shell has been formed.

- Site: Very small organ surrounding the ootype & contains unicellular glands which open in to the ootype.

B. Male reproductive organs: Consists following organs.

1. **Testes:**
- Numbers: Two (except in schistosomes).
- Site: Present in the posterior region of the body.
- Function: It produces the sperms & each testis connected to vas deferens via small tubule **called vas efferentia.**
2. **Vas deferens:**
- Number: Single.
- Function: It enlarge later for storage of sperms **called seminal vesicle** & followed by a constriction **called ejaculatory duct** (cirrus / penis).
3. **Prostate:** Constricted part of vas deferens surrounded by prostate.
4. **Cirrus (penis):** Terminal part of vas deferens modified in a muscular organ **called cirrus** or **penis.**
5. **Cirrus sac:**
- A sac like structure at the end of vas deferens **called cirrus.**
- It contains a seminal vesicle, prostate & cirrus.

- **Genital atrium:**
- Function: It provides place for common opening of ejaculatory duct & uterus.
- Opening: Opening **called genital pore** which present on ventral surface near acetabulum.

- **Fertilisation:**
- Definition: Mating of sperm with ovum.
- Types: Two types.
1. **Self fertilisation:**
2. **Cross fertilisation:**

II. Egg stage

- **Development:** Formed in ootype & surrounded by protective covering.
- **Morphological features:**

A. Eggs of diecious trematodes: → Fig,-3

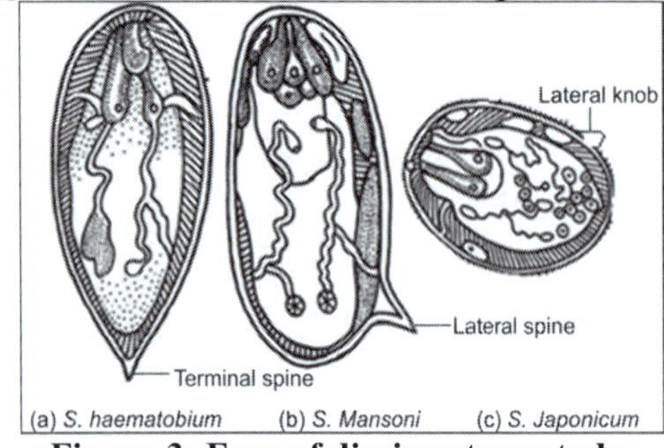

Figure-3: Eggs of diecious trematodes

- **Size:** 70-140μm × 50-90 μm.
- **Shape:** Oval & non-operculated.
- **Colour**: Yellowish - brown colour.
- **Covering:** Surrounded by transparent & brownish yellow protective covering.
- **Embryo:**
- Initially contains ciliated embryo when laid **called miracidium.**
- Miracidium released free in water on hatching of egg & taken up by intermediate host (snail).
- **Spine:** Spine or lateral knob is characteristic of the species & useful for identification.
- **Yolk material:** Present in abundant amount.

B. Eggs of monoecious trematodes: → Fig.-4

- **Shape:** Oval or spherical & operculated at one end.
- **Covering:** Surrounded by transparent & brownish yellow protective covering.
- **Embryo:** In some egg miracidium present at the time of laying while in some it develop after laying.
- **Spine:** Not contains spine or knob except terminal hook in *C. sinensis.*

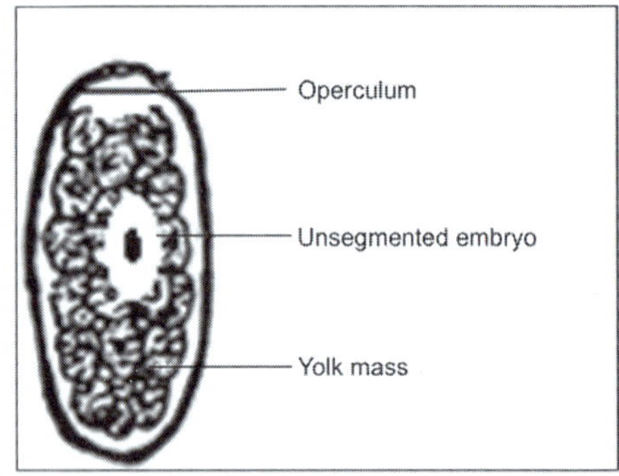

Figure-4: Egg of monoecious trematodes (*F. buski*)

III. Larval stage

A. Larva of diecious trematodes:

- **Form:** Solid forms of larva are present.
- **Stages, names & hosts:**

i. Miracidium: →Fig.-5(a)

- **Definition:** It is the 1st larval stage of trematodes
- **Meaning:** Greek word meaning little boy.
- **Host:** Eggs contains ciliated embryo **called miracidium** which released free in water on hatching of egg & taken up by intermediate host (snail).

ii. Sporocyst:

- **Definition:** It is the 2nd larval stage of trematodes
- **Meaning: Sporos (Greek) = seed & kystis (Greek) = cyst or bladder.**
- **Hosts:** It occurs in molluscs or snail.
- **Multiplication:** Asexual multiplication take place in this stage & it pass through 1st **[fig.-5(b)]** & 2nd generation sporocyst **[fig.-5(c)].**

iii. Cercaria: →Fig.-5(d)

- **Definition:** It is the 3rd larval stage of trematodes
- **Meaning: Kerkos (Greek) = tail.**
- **Host:** It occurs in molluscs/snail & later release free in water.

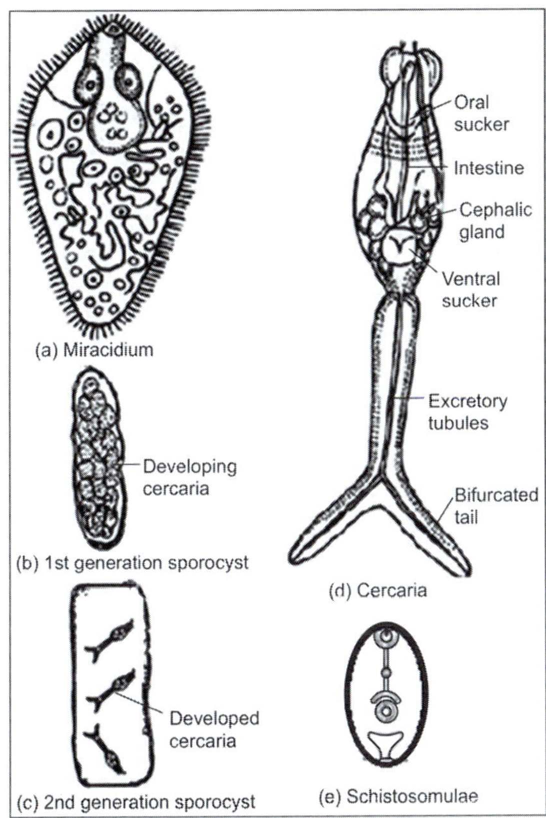

Figure-5: Larva of diecious trematodes

- **Structure:** It possesses suckers, intestine like that of adult worm, body & tail.
- **Development:** From single miracidium multiple cercaria can develop.
- **Types:** According to nature of tail it's having following types as shown in **fig.-6.**

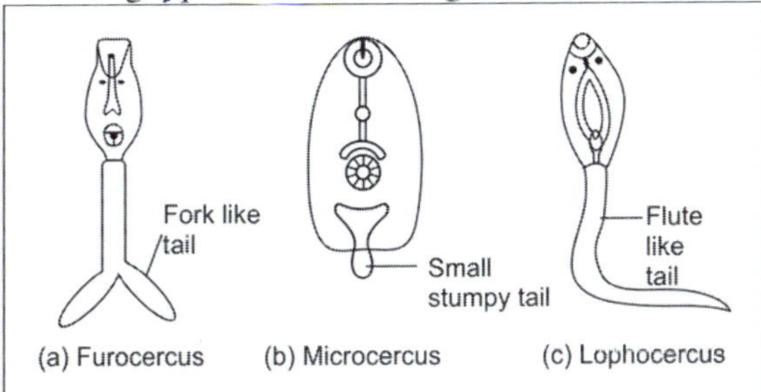

Figure-6: Types of cercaria

a. **Furocercus cercaria:** Fork like / bifurcated tail (as in schistosomes).

✓ **Note:** Types b-c (**vide infra**) are belong to monoecious trematodes.

b. **Microcercus cercaria:** Small stumpy tail (as in *Paragonimus*).
c. **Lophocercus cercaria:** Flute like tail (as in *Metagonimus, Clonorchis, Fasciolopsis, Fasciola & Heterophyes*).
d. **Pleurolophocercus cercaria:** Long powerful tail with a pair of fin fold (as in *Opisthorchis*).

iv. **Schistosomulae:** →**Fig.-5(e)**

- **Definition:** Cercaria penetrates the skin of definitive host & loses the tail **called schistosomulae.** It is the final larval stage.
- **Host:** It develops in definitive host.
- **Structure:** Same as cercaria but without tail & infective to definitive hosts.

B. Larva of monoecious trematodes:

i. **Miracidium:** →**Fig.-7(a)**

- **Definition:** It is the 1st larval stage of trematodes.
- **Meaning:** Greek word meaning little boy.
- **Host:** Eggs contains ciliated embryo **called miracidium** which released free in water on hatching of egg & taken up by 1st intermediate host (snail).

ii. **Sporocyst:** →**Fig.-7(b)**

- **Definition:** It is the 2nd larval stage of trematodes.
- **Meaning: Sporos (Greek) = seed & kystis (Greek) =□cyst or bladder.**
- **Hosts:** It occurs in snail.
- **Multiplication:** Asexual multiplication does not take place in this stage, so no formation of 1st & 2nd generation sporocyst.

iii. **Redia:**

- **Definition:** It is the 3rd larval stage of trematodes.
- **Meaning:** Named after Italian naturalist **Fransesco Redi.**
- **Host:** It occurs in snail.
- **Multiplication:** Asexual multiplication take place in all trematodes & pass through 1st **[fig.-7(c)]** & 2nd generation of redia **[fig.-7(d)].**
- **Structure:** It contains oral sucker, pharynx, a sac like intestine & birth pore through which next generation escape.
- **Future development:** It contains germ cells which develop in to 2nd generation of redia (**also called daughter redia**) or in to final larval stage **called cercaria.**

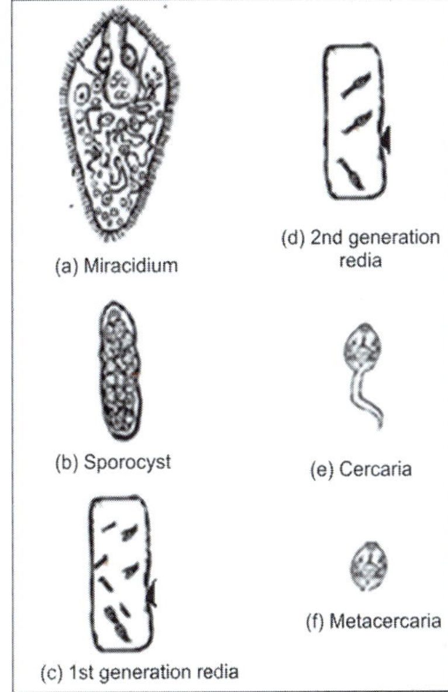

Figure-7: Larva of monoecious trematodes

iv. **Cercaria:** →**Fig.-7(e)**
- **Definition:** It is the 4th larval stage of trematodes
- **Meaning: Kerkos (Greek) = tail.**
- **Host:** It occurs in snail & later release free in water.
- **Structure:** It possesses suckers, intestine like that of adult worm, body & tail.
- **Development:** From single miracidium multiple cercaria can develop.
- **Types:** → Vide supra

v. **Metacercaria** or **adolescearia:** →**Fig.-7(f)**
- **Definition:** It is the final larval stage of trematodes without tail & encysted in animals like molluscs, fish, crab, ants or on water plants **called metacercaria** or **called adolescaria.**
- **Host:** It encysted in 2nd intermediate host like molluscs, fish, crab, ants or free on vegetables.
- **Structure:** Same as cercaria but without tail & infective to definitive hosts.

❖ Mode of transmission of trematodes:

a. **Direct:**
- **Infective stage:** Cercaria enters directly via skin & loses the tail after entering in body **called schistosomulae.**
- **Examples:** *S. haematobium*, *S. mansoni* & *S. japonicum.*

b. **Indirect:**
- **Infective stage:** Metacercaria via food.
- **Examples:**

1. **By eating the vegetable (water plant):** *F. buski, W. watsoni, G. hominis, F. hepatica* & *F. gigantica.*
2. **By eating the fish:** *H. heterophyes, M. yokogawai* & *C. sinensi.*
3. **By eating the molluscs:** *Echinostoma* species.
4. **By eating the ants:** *D. dendriticum.*
5. **By eating the crab or crayfish:** *P. westermani.*

❖ Life cycle: Worm passes its life cycle in two different hosts.

I. **Definitive host:** Man who harbours the adult stage.
II. **Intermediate hosts:** Larval stage developed in two different aquatic animals.

1. **First intermediate host:** Snail or molluscs required for development.
2. **Second intermediate host:** Water fish or crab or crayfish or ant required for encystment.

➢ **Cycles:** Summarise in **flow chart-1.**

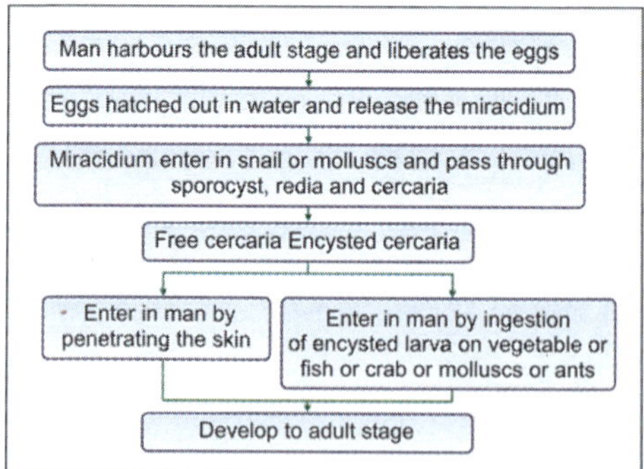

Flow chart-1: Summary of life cycle of flukes

❖ Classification:

I. **Systemic classification:** Follow chapter → Introduction and classification of parasites **(section →table-4)** for more details.
II. **Pathological classification:** Pathogenic species are further classified on the basis of reproductive organs & habitat as below.

A. **Diecious (non-hermaphrodite) trematodes:** Male & female species are separate & habitat in blood.

i. **Vesical venous plexus:** *S. haematobium.*
ii. **Rectal & portal venous plexus:** *S. mansoni*, *S. japonicum.*

B. **Monoecious (hermaphrodite) trematodes:** Male & female species are not separate & single species can harbours both male & female reproductive organs with following habitat.

i. **Intestinal trematodes (intestinal flukes):**
a. **Small intestine:** *F. buski*, *H. heterophyes*, *M. yokogawai*, *E. ilocanum*, *E. malayanum*, *E. revolutum*, *P. supraryfex* & *W. watsoni.*
b. **Large intestine:** *G. hominis.*

ii. **Hepatic trematodes (liver flukes):** *C. sinensis*, *O. felineus*, *F. hepatica*, *F. gigantica*, *D. dendriticum* & *E. pancreaticum.*
iii. **Pulmonary trematodes (lung flukes):** *P. westermani.*

❖ Differences between diecious & monoecious trematodes: → Table-1

Features	Diecious	Monoecious
Adult stage		
Sex	Separate	Nor separate
Shape	Cylindrical like round worm (**fig.-1**)	Leaf like (**fig.-2**)
Gynaeco-phoric canal	Present	Absent
Egg stage		
Figure	**Fig.-2**	**Fig.-4**
Egg's shape	Non-peorculated	Operculated
Spine	Present	Absent
Embryo formation	Miracidium present at the time of laying	In some eggs miracidium present at the time of laying while in some at develop later
Larval stage		
Figure	**Fig.-5**	**Fig.-7**
Larva	No redia	Redia present
Infective stage	Cercaria which lose the tail **called schistosomulae** (tail less after infection)	Metacercaria (Tail less before infection)

Table-1: Differences between diecious & monoecious trematodes

Question bank

Short notes

1) General features of trematodes.
2) Cercaria.
3) Classification of trematodes.

Short questions for theory/viva questions

1) Write the different modes of transmission of trematodes.
2) What are metacercaria & schistosomulae?
3) Write the difference between diecious & monoecious trematodes.

MCQs for chapter review

Morphology

1) **Schistosomulae of trematodes refers to**
(a) Cercaria without tail (b) Cercaria with tail (c) Cercaria with bifurcated tail (d) Cercaria with short stumpy tail

Classification

2) **Diecious trematode is**
(a) *S. haematobium* (b) *C. sinensis* (c) *F. hepatica* (d) None of above

Answers of MCQs & explanation

1) **(a)**
- Follow section, **morphology (larval stage → cercaria & schistosomulae)** for explanation

2) **(a)**
- Follow section, **classification** for explanation

95 Trematodes: Diecious trematodes

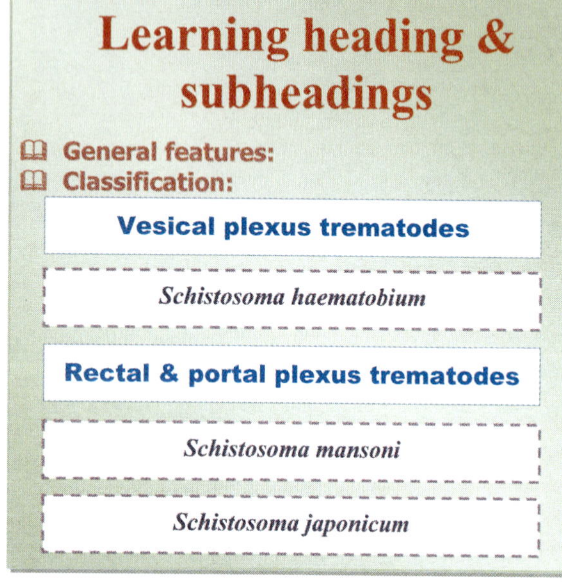

General features: → Table-1

Classification:

I. **Systemic classification:** Follow chapter → Introduction and classification of parasites **(Section → table-4)** for more details.

II. **Pathological classification:** Male & female species are separate hence **called diecious** or **called non hermaphrodite trematodes**. Following are the important pathogenic spp. as per their habitat.

i. **Vesical plexus trematodes:** *Schistosoma haematobium.*

ii. **Rectal & portal plexus trematodes:** *Schistosoma mansoni* & *Schistosoma japonicum.*

Vesical plexus trematodes

Schistosoma haematobium

❖ **Common name:** → **Table-1**

❖ **Meaning:** **Schisto (Greek) = split + soma (Greek) = body,** it looks vertically split because of presence of gynaecophoric canal in male.

❖ **Synonym:** Initially genus was known as *Bilharzia,* from the name of Theodor Bilharz, who 1st discovered the parasite in the mesenteric vein of Egyptian in 1851 from Cairo. Later name changes to *Schistosoma* with above mentioned meaning.

❖ **History:**

- Theodor Bilharz, who 1st discovered the parasite in the mesenteric vein of Egyptian in 1851 from Cairo
- Life cycle was 1st worked out by Leiper in Bulinus in Egypt in 1915.

❖ **Geographical distribution:** → **Table-1**

❖ **Habitat:** → **Table-1**

❖ **Morphology:** Three morphological stages like adult, egg & larval stages. Few important features of diecious trematodes are given below. For more details, **follow chapter → Trematodes: General features and classification.**

I. Adult stage

➢ **Time of maturation:** Schistosomulae transformed to sexually mature adult stage in 3 weeks in definitive host.

➢ **Size:** Female is larger & stout than male.

➢ **Shape:** Unlike other tramatodes, *Schistosomes* are not flattened & leaf like, but cylindrical as like round worm as shown in **fig.-1.**

➢ **Life span:** 20-30 years.

✪ **Organs:** Following are the important organs as shown in **fig.-1.**

✪ **Tegument:** Body of parasite is covered with acellular layer **called tegument** or **called cuticle.**

✪ **Suckers:**

- **Definition:** It is a strong muscular cup shaped depression & armed with delicate spines.
- **Function:** Act as an organ for adhesion with host cells.
- **Numbers:** Two in number, so species **called distomata** (**Greek** word from **di = two** & **stomata = mouth).**

Features	*S. haematobium*	*S. mansoni*	*S. japonicum*
Common name	Vesical blood fluke	Manson's blood fluke	Oriental blood fluke
Geographical distribution	- Parts of Africa & middle east - India: Few cases reported from Ratnagiri district of Maharashtra by Gadgil & Shah in 1951.	- Various part of Africa & America	- Parasite of far East - Found in China, Japan, Philippines & Shah state of Burma
Habitat (Fig.-8)	- **Common site:** Adult worm lives in **vesical plexus (pelvic plexus)** supplying urinary bladder (inferior mesenteric vein) - **Ectopic sites:** Lungs, brain, spinal cord (due to outflow phenomenon in case of heavy infection)	- **Common site:** Adult worm lives in **rectal plexus** supplying sigmoido-rectal area (inferior mesenteric vein) - **Ectopic sites:** Liver (portal vein), lungs & spinal cord	- **Common sites: (1)** Superior mesenteric vein supplying ileo-caecal area (superior mesenteric vein) **(2) Rectal plexus** (haemorrh-oides) **(3)** Liver (**portal vein / plexus)** - **Ectopic sites:** Lungs & brain
	Adult stage (Fig. - 1)		
	Male		
Size	Size	Size	Size
Cuticula	Cuticula	Cuticula	Cuticula
Testes	Testes	Testes	Testes
	Female		
Size	Size	Size	Size
Ovary	Ovary	Ovary	Ovary
Uterus	Contains 20-30 eggs	Contains 1- 3 eggs	Contains ≥ 50 eggs
	Egg stage (Fig. - 2)		
Size	$150\mu m \times 50\mu m$	$150\mu m \times 60\mu m$	$100\mu m \times 65\mu m$
Spine	Terminal	Lateral	Lateral knob
ZN staining	Non acid fast	Acid fast	Acid fast
	Larval stage (Fig. - 3)		
Cephalic gland	2 pairs oxyphilic & 3 pairs basophilic	2 pairs oxyphilic & 4 pairs basophilic	5 pairs oxyphilic & no basophilic
	Hosts		
Intermediate	Snail (*Ferrissia* etc.)	Snail (*Biomphalaria* etc.)	Snail (*Oncomelania*)
Definitive	Man	Man	Man & domestic animals

Table-1: General features & differences between major *Schostosomes*

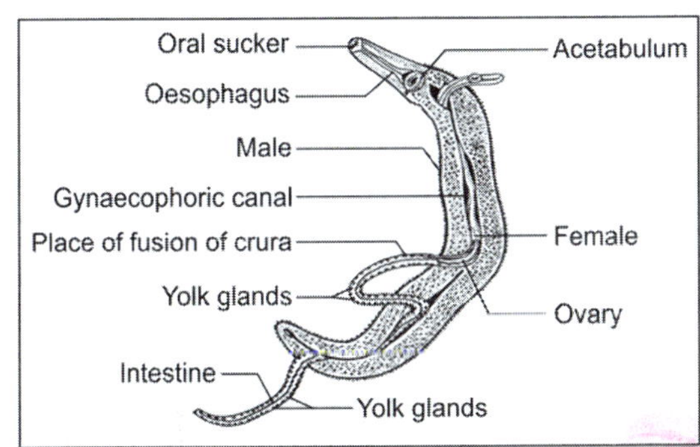

Figure-1: Adult stage of *Schistosomes*

- **Types:** Two types.

1. **Oral sucker:** It is small & surrounding the oral cavity **called oral sucker.**
2. **Ventral sucker or acetabula:** Another one is larger & present on ventral surface **called acetabula (Latin word meaning a shallow vinegar vessel or cup)** or **called ventral sucker.**

✪ **Body cavity:** Absent.

✪ **Gastrointestinal system:**

- It is present but without anus so **called incomplete.**
- Mouth: Situated anteriorely in the centre of oral sucker.
- Pharynx: Muscular pharynx is lacking.
- Oesophagus is bifurcated in front of ventral sucker in to two tube like structure **called intestinal caeca** or **called crura** which reunite to form the single caecum.
- Length of reunited intestine is variable with different species.

✪ **Excretory system:** Present.

✪ **Nervous system:** Present.

✪ **Reproductive system:**

- Both male & female species are separate.
- Testes are 3-4 in numbers.
- Laurer's canal (rudimentary vagina): Absent.

✪ **Gynaecophoric canal:**

- Lateral margin of males are folded ventrally with a canal like structure **called gynaecophoric canal.**
- Function: Helps to hold the female during copulation.
- Both male & female are live together in gynaecophoric canal **called coupled worm.**

II. Egg stage

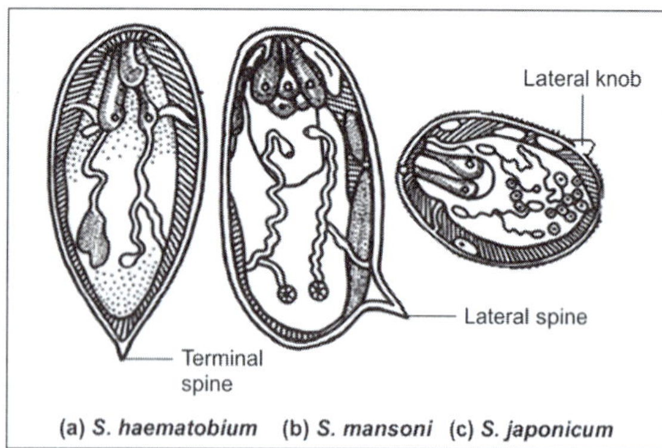

Figure-2: Egg stage of *Schistosomes*

- **Development:** Formed in ootype.
- **Morphological features: → Fig.-2(a).**
- **Shape:** Oval & non-operculated.
- **Size:** 150μm ×50μm.
- **Covering:** Surrounded by transparent & brownish yellow protective covering.
- **Embryo:** Initially contains ciliated embryo when laid **called miracidium.**
- **Spine:** Terminal spine is characteristic of the species & for useful foe identification.
- **Egg laying:**
- **Sites:**
  - Common site: In small venules of vesical plexus & pelvic plexus.
  - Ectopic site: Very rare & in mesenteric portal system, pulmonary arterioles & ectopic sites.
- **Mechanism: →Flow chart-1**

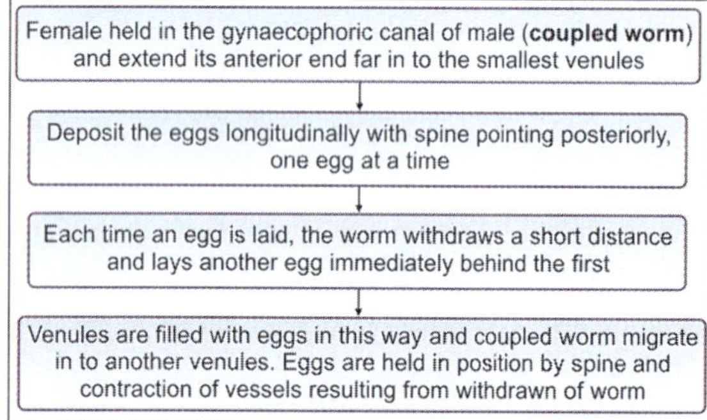

Flow chart-1: Mechanism of eggs laying

- **Mechanism of eggs expulsion:**
- **From vesical plexus:**
  - Eggs laid in the vesical plexus are makes their way through the vessels & mucosa of bladder. Entre in to the cavity & escape with urine, usually at the end of micturition.
  - It mostly expelled in mid day than other time with unknown reasons.
- **From ectopic site:**
  - Eggs laid in the ectopic sites are generally died & evoke local tissue reactions.
  - They are found in biopsy of local tissues & rarely expelled in local material like faeces or sputum.

III. Larval stage

Single egg gives the single miracidium, which produces multiple cercariae. It passes by following three stages.

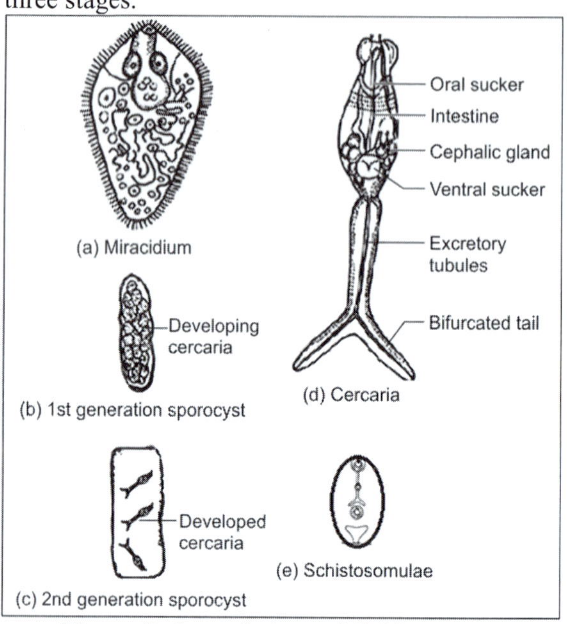

Figure-3: Larval stage of *Schistosomes*

- **Form:** Solid forms of larva are present **(fig.-3).**
- **Stages, names & hosts:**

A. Miracidium: → Fig.-3(a)

- **Definition:** It is the 1st larval stage of trematodes
- **Meaning:** Greek word meaning little boy.
- **Host:** Eggs contains ciliated embryo **called miracidium** which released free in water on hatching of egg & taken up by snail.

B. Sporocyst:

- **Definition:** It is the 2nd larval stage of trematodes.
- **Meaning: Sporos (Greek) = seed & kystis (Greek) =cyst or bladder.**
- **Hosts:** It occurs in snail.
- **Multiplication:** Asexual multiplication take place in this stage, it passes through 1st **[fig.-3(b)]** & 2nd **[fig.-3(c)]** generation sporocyst.

C. Cercaria: → Fig.-3(d)

- **Definition:** It is the 3rd (final) larval stage of trematodes.
- **Meaning: Kerkos (Greek) = tail.**
- **Host:**
  - It occurs in snail & later release in water.
  - It remains free in water & never encysted.
- **Structure:** It possesses suckers, intestine like that of adult worm, body & fork like tail, **so called furocercus cercaria**.
- **Development:** From single miracidium multiple cercariae can develop.
- **Mode of entry of cercaria in man:** By penetrating the skin.

D. Schistosomulae: → Fig.-3(e)

- **Definition:** Cercaria penetrates the skin of definitive host & loses the tail **called schistosomulae.** It is the final larval stage.
- **Host:** It develops in definitive host.
- **Structure:** Same as cercaria but without tail & infective to definitive hosts.

✓ **Note:** There is no redia stage in *Schistosomes.*

❖ Immunity:

- **Acquired immunity:**
  - Developing schistosomula are more susceptible to the immune response & death occurs due to destruction of tegument.
  - Adult worms are the long lasting worms & immunity develops in endemic areas after long time.
- **Premunition (concomitant/ infection immunity):**
  - Definition: Development of immunity to reinfection in presence of active adult infection.
  - History: Determined by Smithers & Terry in 1969.
- **Hypersensitivity:**
  - Toxic metabolites by schistosomulae: Produces anaphylaxis (immediate type hypersensitivity).
  - Toxic metabolites by eggs: Come out through the pores & elicits the cellular infiltration & granuloma formation (delayed type hypersensitivity).

❖ Life cycle:

➢ **Types of host:** Two types.

I. **Definitive host:** Man.

II. **Intermediate hosts:** Fresh water snail with following species.

1) **In Africa:** *Bulinus (Physopsis) truncates.*
2) **In Morocco & Portugal:** *Planorvarius metidjensis.*
3) **In India:** *Ferrissia tenuis.*

➢ **Cycles:** As shown in **flow chart-2 & fig.-4.**

❖ Pathogenicity:

➢ **Disease name: Called schistosomiasis.**

➢ **Synonym:** Also **called bilharziasis** or **urinary schistosomiasis** or **schistosomiasis haematobia** or **endemic haematuria.**

➢ **Virulence factors:**

1. **Cytolytic secretion by cercaria from cephalic gland:** Causing local lesion **called swimmer's itch.**
2. **Toxic metabolites by schistosomulae:** Produces anaphylaxis (immediate type hypersensitivity).
3. **Toxic metabolites by eggs:** Come out through the pores & elicits the cellular infiltration & granuloma formation (delayed type hypersensitivity).
4. **Mechanical by spine of egg:** It erodes the blood vessels & cause haemorrhages.

➢ **Reservoir of infection:** Man.

➢ **Source of infection:** Water.

➢ **Mode of transmission:** Cercaria enters by penetrating the skin.

➢ **Exit form:** Embryonated eggs.

➢ **Infective form:** Cercaria.

➢ **Portal of entry:** Skin.

➢ **Sites:** Follow habitat in **table-1.**

I. Cycle in definitive host: Man
Infection to man by direct penetration of intact skin by cercaria

↓

After entry in man, cercaria cast off their tail **called schistosomulae** and gain access to peripheral circulation→ Right side of heart→lungs and pass few days in capillary bed of lungs→left side of heart→systemic circulation→abdominal aorta→mesenteric artery→pass through the capillary bed of intestine and finally enter in portal circulation

↓

Reach in liver in 5 days

↓

Change to sexually differentiated male and female adult stages in intrahepatic portion of portal blood stream within 5 days

↓

Parasites are move against the blood flow and migrating in to the inferior mesenteric vein→rectal venous plexus→pelvic vein and→finally enter in the vesical plexus of veins. After initial exposure through skin parasite takes 1-3 months to take entry in vesical plexus

↓

Sexually mature worms are copulate and fertilised female lay the embryonated eggs in vesical plexus

↓

Eggs laid in the vesical plexus are makes their way through the vessels and mucosa of bladder. Entre in to the cavity and voided with the urine in water

↓

II. Cycle in intermediate host: Snail

↓

Hatching of eggs to release the ciliated larva **called miracidium**

↓

Miracidium move freely in water in search of snail

↓

Miracidium enter in to the snail, penetrate in to the soft tissues and make its way to the liver

↓

In the liver, miracidium loose the cilia and other organs and in the course of 4-8 weeks undergoes the development

↓

Transformed to 1st generation sporocyst and 2nd generation sporocyst

↓

Finally converted in to the fork tailed larvae **called cercariae** (final stage of larva and infective form)

↓

Rupture of sporocyst

↓

Cercariae leave the snail and release free in water (live for 3 days in free form)

↓

Entry in man by penetrating the skin

↓

Cycle repeated

Flow chart-2: Life cycle of *S. haematobium*

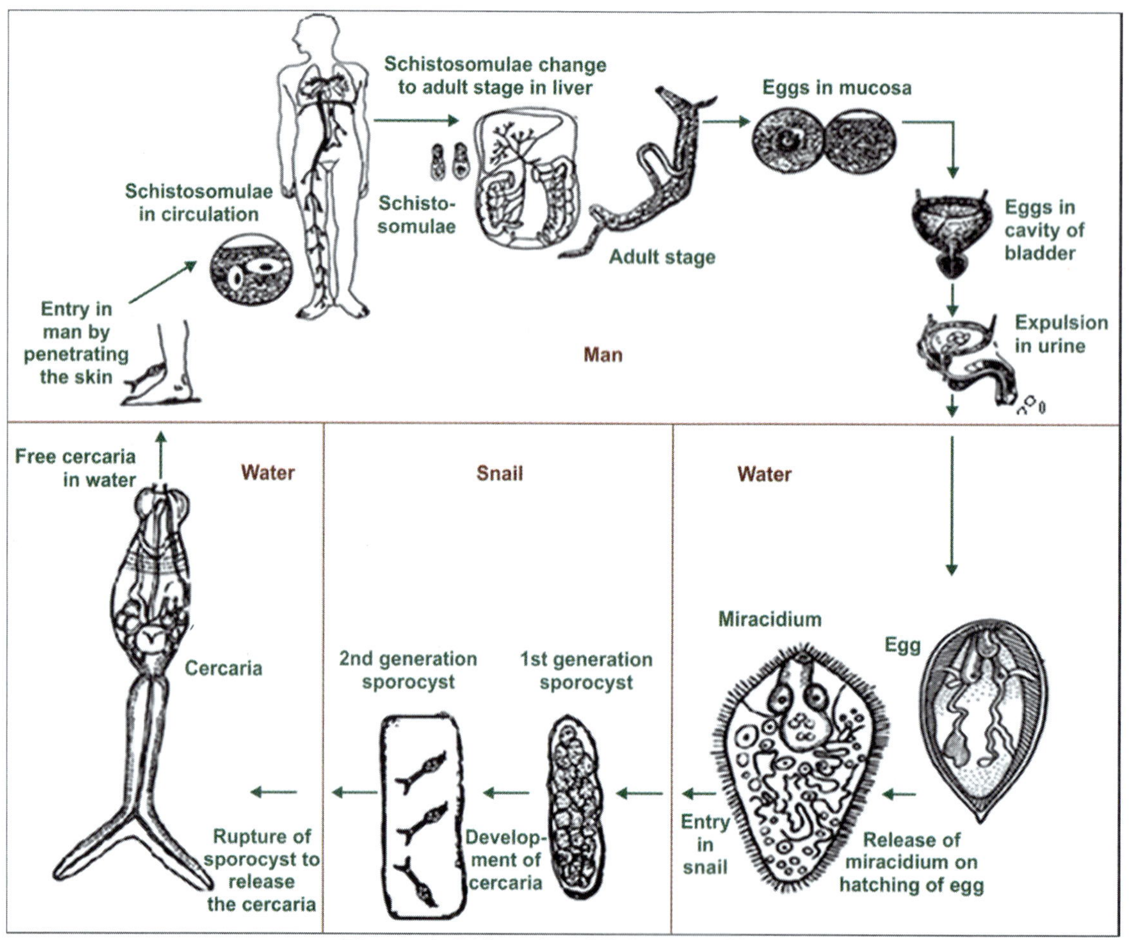

Figure-4: Life cycle of *S. haematobium*

- **Pathogenesis: →Flow chart-3.**

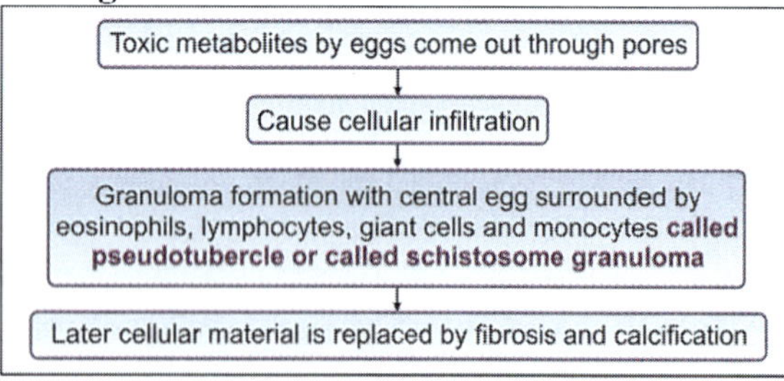

Flow chart-3: Pathogenesis of *S. haematobium*

- **Clinical features:** Three types (**flow chart-4).**
- **Complications:** Occurs after very long time.

a. **Squamous cell carcinoma of bladder:** Close association between vesical schistosomiasis & cancer of urinary baldder has been observed in endemic areas.

b. **Ectopic lesions:** Due to out flow phenomenon in heavy infection. Eggs & worms are escape in to pelvis vein & carried to lungs & sometimes from portal circulation to brain & spinal cord.

1. **Lungs:**

- Granulomatous lesion with fibrosis.
- Pulmonary endarteritis.
- Obstruction of pulmonary blood flow.

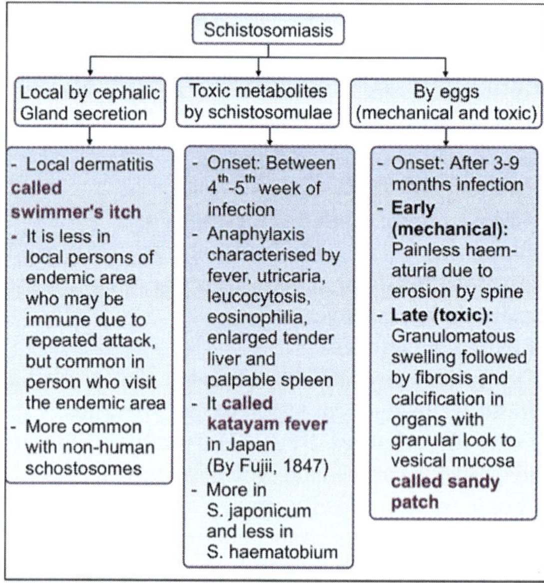

Flow chart-4: Clinical features of *S. haematobium*

- Pulmonary hypertension.
- Chronic cor pulmonale.

2. **Brain:** Space occupying lesion (more in *S. japonicum*).

3. **Spinal cord:** Transverse myelitis like syndrome (more in *S. haematobium* & in *S. mansoni*).

c. **Fibrosis/calcification:** Occurs in egg granuloma.

❖ Laboratory diagnosis:

➢ **Specimens:**

✪ **Urine:**

- Eggs are present in end part of micturition, so not the mid stream but last few drops of urine should be collected.
- Miracidium can be found if urine is left to stand for few hours without preservatives.
- Urine can be preserved by using 10% formalin.
- For egg counting 24 hours urine is collected to which add 10% of formalin (0.5ml per 100ml urine).

✪ **Mucosal biopsy:**

- Piece of vesical mucosa is removed by cystoscope.
- Excised tissue is divided in two pieces.
- One piece is compressed between two slides & examined for eggs under low power.
- Put other piece in fixative for histological study.

➢ **Testing methods:**

I. Direct methods

A. **Macroscopic (naked eye) examination:** Reddish or cloudy urine due to presence of blood.

B. **Microscopy:**

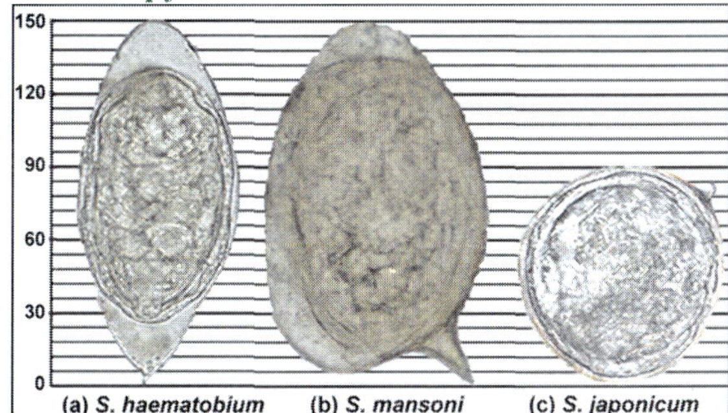

Figure-5: Eggs of *Schistosomes* under wet mount

a. **Wet mount direct from centrifuged urine:** Egg is identified by terminal spine as shown in **fig.-5.**

b. **Immunofluorescent microscopy:** By using antigen from cercaria & miracidium.

II. Indirect methods

A. **Blood picture:** Eosinophilia.

B. **Allergic / skin test:** Fairley's intradermal skin test is positive in all forms of schistosomiasis.

C. **Serological tests:**

i. **Non specific tests:** Aldehyde test: It is positive due to high globulin value.

ii. **Specific test:**

a. **Slide precipitation test:** Plasma card test, which is positive after mixing one drop of blood from finger prick with a drop of antigen on slide.

b. **CFT:** Positive with cercarial antigens prepared from infected snail's liver.

c. **Tests performed from patient's serum:**

1. **Circum Oval Precipitin test (COP) of Oliver & Gonzalez (1954):** Precipitin formation around egg of schistosomes.
2. **Miracidium immobilisation test of Senterfit (1953):**
3. **Cercarein Hullen Reaction (CHR) of Vogel & Mining:** Development of membrane around cercaria.

D. **Radiological:** For calcified egg granuloma.

❖ Prevention:

- Eradication of intermediate host (snail).
- Prevention of water contamination by the urine of case.
- Avoiding swimming, bathing & washing in contaminated water.

❖ Treatment: Praziquantel (40mg/kg/day, single dose) is the drug of choice. Metriphonate is the other alternative drug of choice (7.5mg/kg/week for 3 weeks).

Schistosoma intercalatum

Same as *S. haematobium* with following difference

- **History & distribution:** It was recognised in 1934 by Fisher & occurs in human in Western & Central Africa. Eggs were recovered from the faeces of man in the Congo basin.
- **Habitat:** Adult worm habitat the intestinal venous plexus (mesenteric & portal vein) than vesical plexus. Lay the egg which penetrate the intestinal wall, enter in lumen & cause dysentery.
- **Eggs:** 175μm × 60μm & egg shell is acid fast in nature. About 20μm long terminal spine.
- **Snail hosts:** *Bulinus africanus* & *B. globosus.*

Rectal & portal plexus trematodes

Schistosoma mansoni

❖ Common name: → **Table-1**

❖ Meaning: Species name given by Sambon from the name of Manson, who identifies the parasite, 1st in America.

❖ History:

- Theodor Bilharz reported that *S. haematobium* produces eggs with terminal & lateral spine in 1851.
- Manson 1st identified this parasite in Amercia.
- It identified as separate species by Sambon in 1901 with only lateral spine egg & species name given from the name of initial worker Manson.

- Further confirmed by Leiper in Bulinus in Egypt in 1915 by his experimental work.

❖ **Geographical distribution:** →**Table -1**

❖ **Habitat:** →**Table -1**

❖ **Morphology:** Morphologically it is similar to *S. haematobium* with difference as shown in **table -1.**

❖ **Life cycle:**

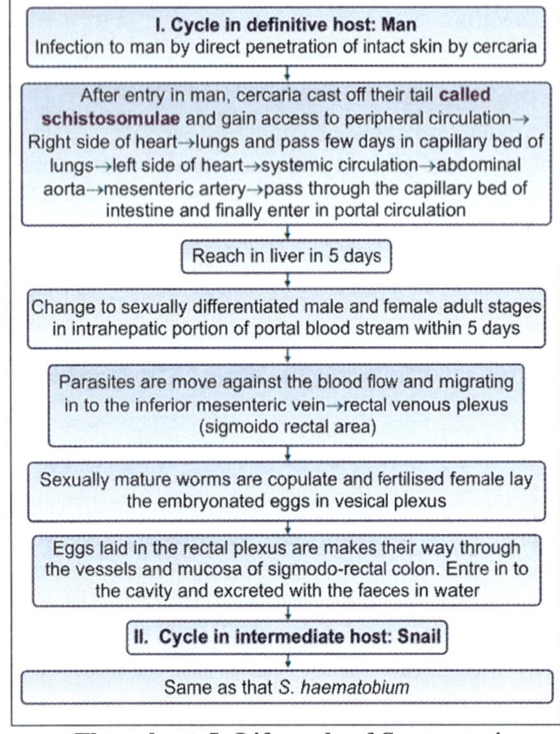

Flow chart-5: Life cycle of *S. mansoni*

➢ **Types of host:** Two types.

I. Definitive host: Man.

II. Intermediate hosts: Fresh water snail with following species.

1. **In Africa:** *Biomphalaria alexendrina.*
2. **In America:** *Australorbis glabratus.*

➢ **Cycles:** Cycle in intermediate host is same as that of *S. haematobium* while cycle in definitive host is little different as shown in **flow chart-5 & fig.-6.**

❖ **Pathogenicity:**

➢ **Disease name: Called schistosomiasis mansoni.**

➢ **Synonym:** Also **called intestinal bilharziasis** or **schistosoma dysentery.** Visceral form also **called visceral schistosomiasis** or **Egyptian plenomegaly.**

➢ **Virulence factors:** Same as *S. haematobium.*

➢ **Reservoir of infection:** Man.

➢ **Source of infection:** Water.

➢ **Mode of transmission:** Cercaria enters by penetrating the skin.

➢ **Exit form:** Embryonated egg.

➢ **Infective form:** Cercaria.

➢ **Portal of entry:** Skin.

➢ **Sites:** Follow habitat in **table-1.**

➢ **Clinical features:** Three types as shown in **flow chart-6.**

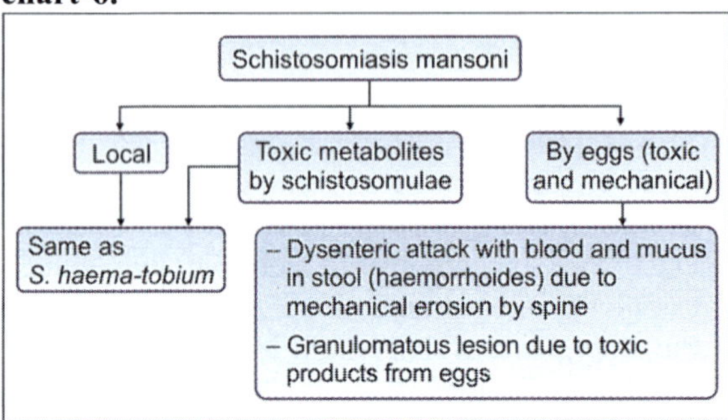

Flow chart-6: Clinical features of *S. mansoni*

➢ **Complications:** Occurs after very long time.

a. Ectopic lesions:

1. Liver:

- Hepatomegaly.
- Periportal cirrhosis.
- Portal hypertension which leads splenomegaly & haematemesis.

2. Lungs: Cor pulmonale.

3. Spinal cord: Transverse myelitis like syndrome (more in *S. haematobium* & in *S. mansoni*).

❖ **Laboratory diagnosis:**

➢ **Specimens:**

✪ **Stool:**

✪ **Mucosal biopsy:**

- Piece of rectal mucosa is removed by simoidoscope.
- Excised tissue is divided in two pieces.
- One piece is compressed between two slides & examined for eggs under low power.
- Other piece: Put in fixative for histological study.

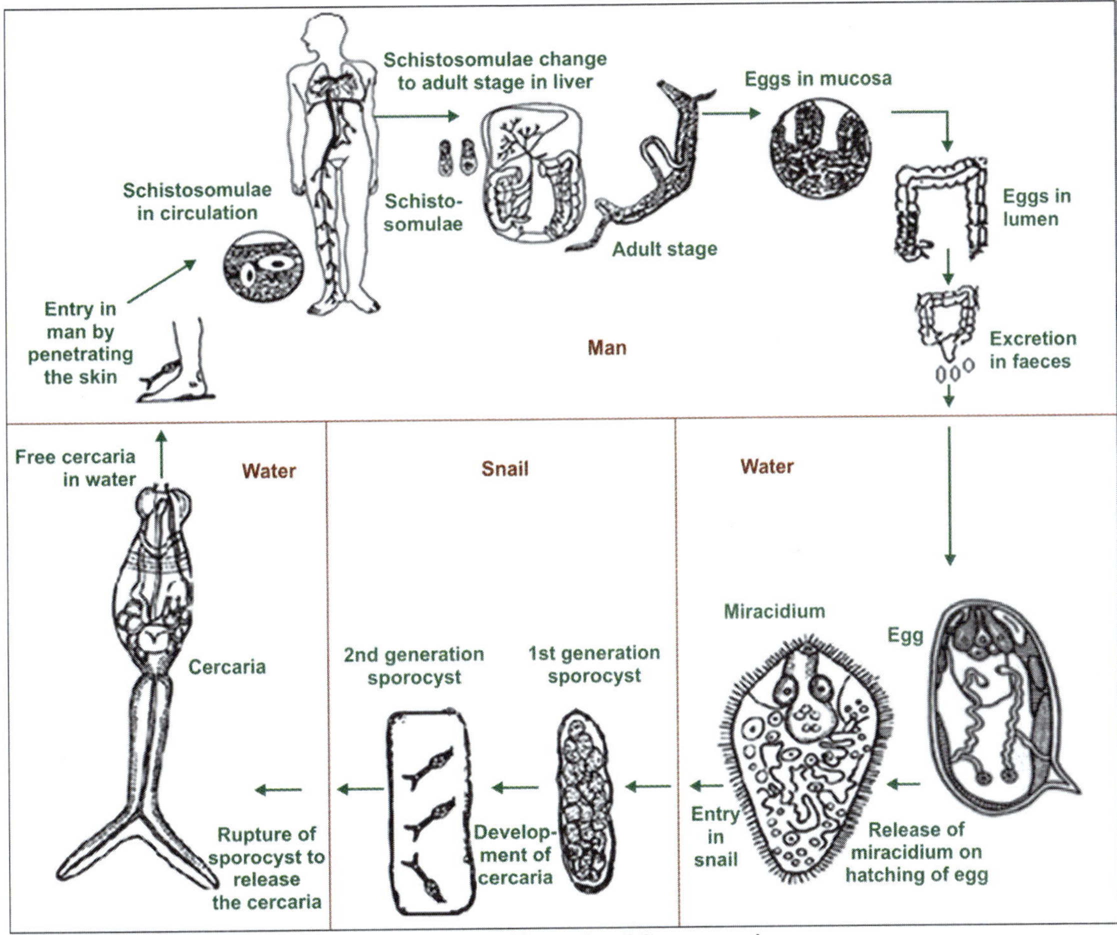

Figure-6: Life cycle of *S. mansoni*

✪ **Liver & lung biopsy:** Tissues are digested with potash solution & examine for presence of eggs.

➢ **Testing methods:**

I. Direct methods

A. Macroscopic (naked eye) examination: For presence of blood & mucus in stool.

B. Microscopy:

a. Wet mount from stool by using normal saline & iodine: Egg is identified by lateral spine as shown in **Fig.-5.**

b. Immunofluorescent microscopy: By using antigen specific antigens.

II. Indirect methods

Indirect tests are same as *S. haematobium.*

❖ **Prevention:**

- Prevention of water contamination by the faeces of case.
- Other measures are same as *S. haematobium.*

❖ **Treatment:**

- Praziquantel (40mg/kg/day, single dose) is the drug of choice.
- Oxamniquine is also effective. It damages the tegument of male worm & there by, makes the worm more susceptible to immune system of host.

Schistosoma japonicum

❖ **Common name:** → **Table-1**

❖ **History:**

- Fujii mentioned the Katayam disease (schistosomiasis japonica) occurring in man in 1847
- Adult stage (female) was recovered by Fujinami in the portal vein of a man at autopsy in 1904.
- Egg stage was identified by Katsurada in the human faeces in 1904.
- Life cycle was worked out by Miyairi & Suzuki in 1913-14.

❖ **Geographical distribution:** →**Table -1**

❖ **Habitat:** →**Table -1**

❖ **Morphology:** Morphologically it is similar to *S. haematobium* with difference as shown in **table -1.**

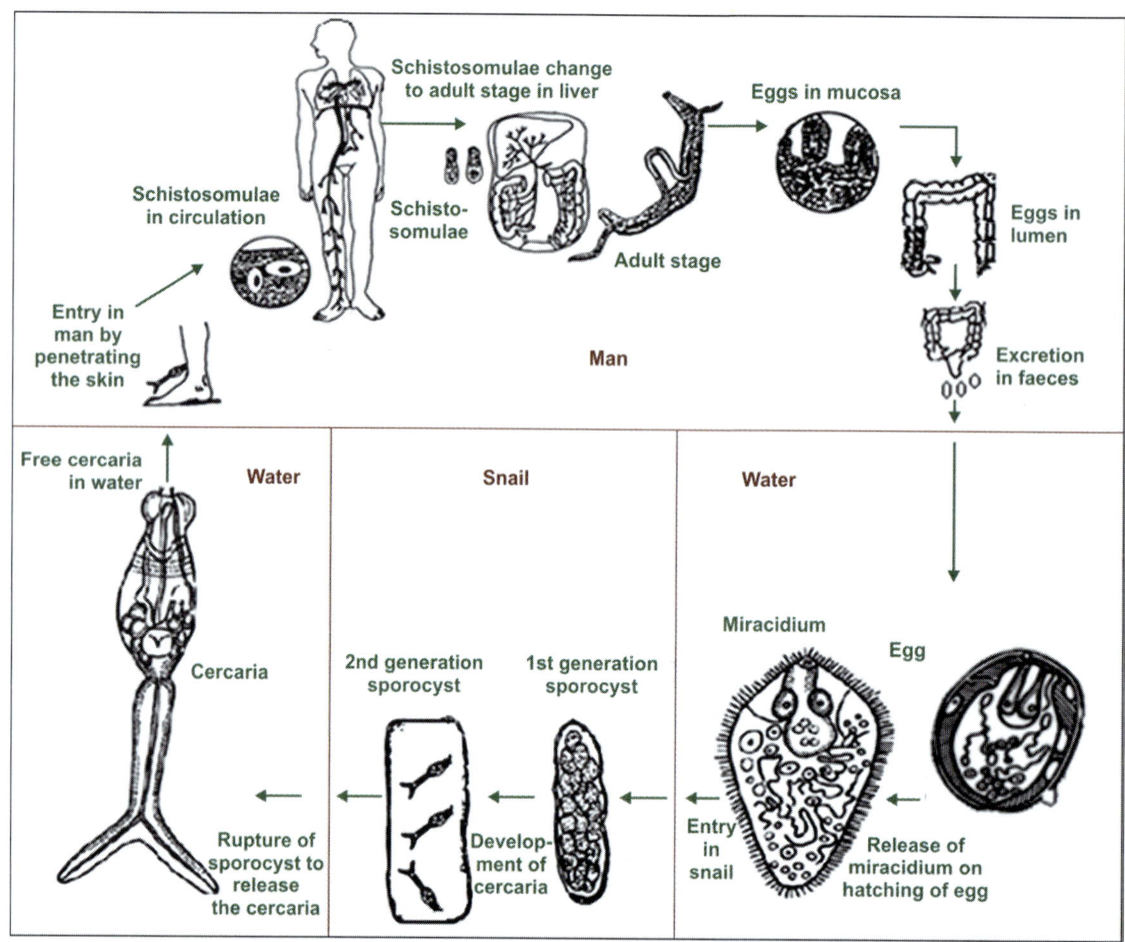

Figure-7: Life cycle of *S. japonicum*

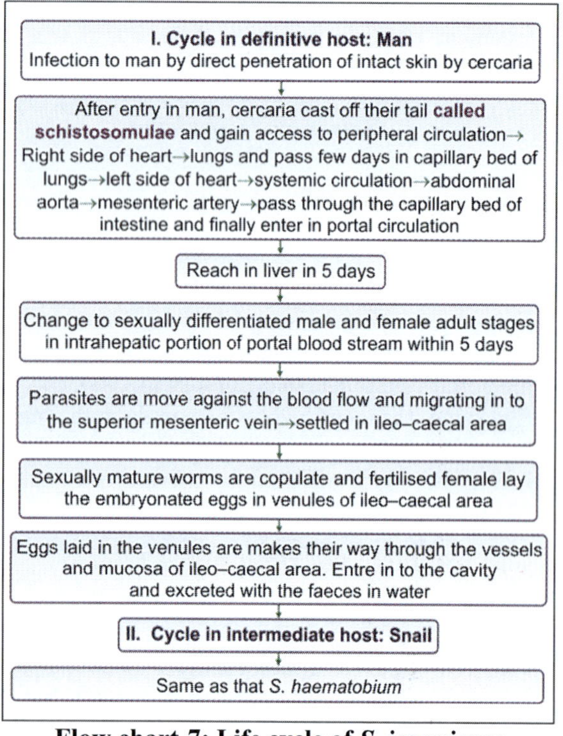

Flow chart-7: Life cycle of *S. japonicum*

❖ Life cycle:

- **Types of host:** Two types.

I. Definitive host: Man. Domestic animal like cat, dog, pig, cattle & field mice serve as reservoir of infection.

II. Intermediate hosts: Fresh water amphibian snail of genus *Oncomelania* (*Katayama* or *Blanfordia*).

- **Cycles:** Cycle in intermediate host is same as that of *S. haematobium* while cycle in definitive host is little different as shown in **flow chart-7 & fig.-7.**

❖ Pathogenicity:

- **Disease name:** **Called schistosomiasis japonica.**
- **Synonym:** Also **called intestinal & hepatic schistosomiasis of the orient** or **katayama disease.**
- **Virulence factors:** Same as *S. haematobium.*

1. **Toxic metabolites by schistosomulae:** Produces anaphylaxis (immediate type hypersensitivity).
2. **Toxic metabolites by eggs:** Come out through the pores & elicits the cellular infiltration & granuloma formation (delayed type hypersensitivity).
3. **Mechanical by lateral knob of egg:** It erodes the blood vessels & cause haemorrhages.
4. **Numbers of eggs:** Lesions are more conspicuous because of heavy load of eggs.

- **Reservoir of infection:** Domestic animals as mentioned above.

- **Source of infection:** Water
- **Mode of transmission:** Cercaria enters by penetrating the skin.
- **Portal of entry:** Skin.
- **Site:** Follow habitat in **table-1.**
- **Infective form:** Cercaria.
- **Exit form:** Embryonated eggs.
- **Clinical features:** Lesions produced in *japonicum* are more pronounced than *mansoni*, because of larger output of eggs. Common symptoms are involving the ileo-caecal region, but due to close proximity to liver chances of liver involvement are greater. Features are shown in **flow chart-8.**

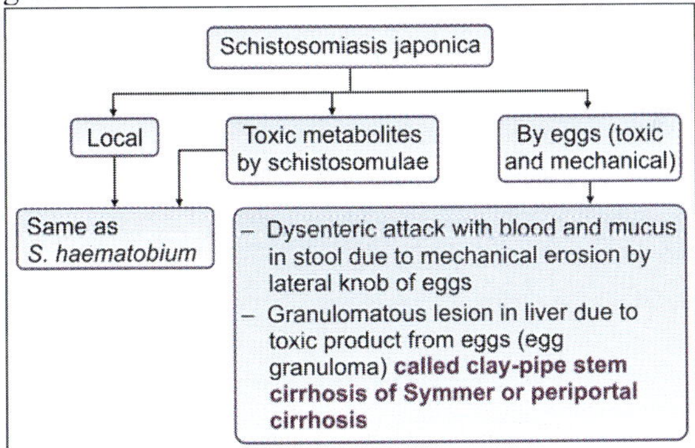

Flow chart-8: Clinical features of *S. japonicum*

- **Complications:** Occurs after very long time.

a. **Due to egg granuloma of liver:** Portal hypertension which leads to oesophageal varices, splenomegaly etc.

b. **Ectopic lesions:**

1. **Lungs:** Cor pulmonale.
2. **Brain:** Space occupying lesion.

❖ Laboratory diagnosis: Same as *S. haematobium.*

❖ Prevention: Same as *S. mansoni.*

❖ Treatment:

- More resistant to treatment.
- Praziquantel is the drug of choice.
- A prolonged course of intravenous tartar emetic gives good result.

Schistosoma mekongi

Same as *S. japoncium* with following difference

- **History & distribution:** It was recognised in 1978 in the Mekong river basin in Laos & Cambodia. It is endemic in Khong Island & people living the raft houses in the Mekong river in Southern Laos & Northern Cambodia.
- **Habitat:** Adult worm habitat the intestinal venous plexus (mesenteric vein).
- **Eggs:** Smaller in size about 30-35μm × 55-65μm & egg shell is acid fast in nature. Lateral knob also present.
- **Hosts:**
- Definitive: Man & dog.
- Intermediate: Aquatic snail of genus *Trienla aperta*
- **Pathogenicity:** Dysentery, hepatomegaly, splenomegaly, dilated superficial abdominal veins are common findings.

❖ Anatomical aspect & portal system: →Fig. - 8

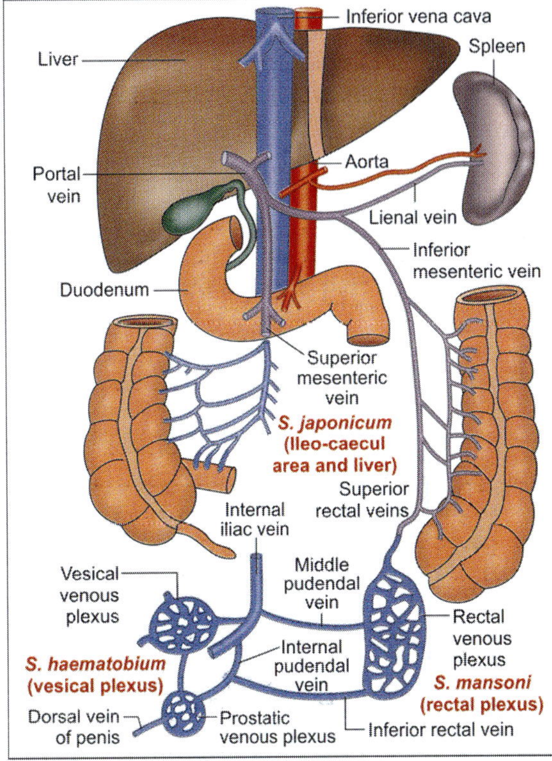

Figure-8: Anatomical aspect & portal system

Question bank

Case study

1) A 35 year man came with complain of local skin lesion & painless haematuria. He is giving history of swimming in water. Urine examination revealed non acid fast egg with terminal spine. Identify the case and answer the following.

a) Name & draw the properly labelled diagram of egg of causative agent.
b) Describe the life cycle of causative agent.
c) Describe the pathogenicity of causative agent.
d) Describe the lab. diagnosis of causative agent.

Essay/Full question

1) *Schistosoma haematobium.*
2) *Schistosoma mansoni.*

Short notes

1) Write difference between *Schistosoma haematobium* and *Schistosoma mansoni.*
2) Life cycle / pathogenicity/ laboratory diagnosis of *Schistosoma haematobium.*

Short questions for theory/viva questions

1) What is gynaecophoric canal? Write its function.
2) Write the mechanisms of eggs laying & eggs expulsion in *Schistosomes.*
3) Name the four parasites causing dysentery.
4) Name the larval stage of *Schistosomes.*

MCQs for chapter review

General feature

1) Natural habitat of *Schistosoma* (blood flukes) (PGI-80)
(a) Veins of the urinary bladder (b) Portal & pelvic veins (c) Vesical plexus (d) All of the above

2) Terminal spine eggs are seen in (PGI-95)
(a) *Schistosoma haematobium* (b) *Schistosoma mansoni* (c) *Schistosoma japonicum* (d) *Chlonorchis sinensis*

3) Water host required for schistosomiasis
(a) Fish (b) Cyclops (c) Snails (d) Crabs

Schistosoma haematobium

4) Painless haematuria is seen as one of the manifestation in the infection caused by
(a) *Schistosoma japonicum* (b) *Schistosoma mansoni* (c) *Schistosoma haematobium* (d) *Plasmodium falciparum*

5) Katayam fever is caused by
(a) *F hepatica* (b) *C sinensis* (c) *S. haematobium* (d) *A lumbricoides*

6) Fairley's test is done
(a) Cysticercosis (b) LGV (c) Schistosomiasis (d) Filariasis

Answers of MCQs & explanation

1) (d)
2) (a)
3) (c)
} Follow section, **general features (table-1)** for explanation

4) (c)
5) (c)
} Follow section, ***Schistosoma haematobium* (pathogenicity → clinical features → flow chart-4)** for explanation

6) (c)
- Follow section, ***Schistosoma haematobium* (laboratory diagnosis → indirect methods → allergic / skin test)** for explanation

96 Trematodes: Monoecious trematodes

Learning heading & subheadings

Classification:

Small intestinal trematodes

Fasciolopsis buski

Heterophyes heterophyes

Metagonimus yokogawai

Echinostoma spp.

Paryphostomum supraryfex

Watsonius watsoni

Large intestinal trematodes

Gastrodiscoides hominis

Hepatic trematodes

Clonorchis sinensis

Opisthorchis spp.

Fasciola spp.

Dicrocoelium dendriticum

Eurytrema pancreaticum

Pulmonary trematodes

Paragonimus spp.

Classification:

I. **Systemic classification:** Follow chapter → Introduction and classification of parasites **(section→ table-4)** for more details.

II. **Pathological classification:**

A. **Monoecious (hermaphrodite):** Male & female species are not separate (hence **called monoecious**) & single species can harbours both male & female reproductive organs. Following are the pathogenic species according to their habitat.

i. **Intestinal trematodes (intestinal flukes):**

a. **Small intestine:** *Fasciolopsis buski*, *Hetrophyes heterophyes*, *Matagonimus yokogawai*, *Echinostoma ilocanum, Echinostoma malayanum, Echinostoma revolutum, Paryphostomum supraryfex* & *Watsonius watsonis.*

b. **Large intestine:** *Gastrodiscoides hominis.*

ii. **Hepatic trematodes (liver flukes):** *Clonorchis sinensis*, *Opsthorchis felineus*, *Fasciola hepatica, Fasciola gigantica, Dicrocoelium dendriticum* & *Erytrema pancreaticum.*

iii. **Pulmonary trematodes (lung flukes):** *Paragonimus westermani* & other species.

Small intestinal trematodes

Fasciolopsis buski

❖ **Common name:**

1. **Giant or large intestinal fluke:** Because it is the largest intestinal fluke infecting man.
2. **Ginger worm:** This name is common in because it appear like slice of ginger.

❖ **Synonym:** Initially it was known as *Distoma buski.*

❖ **History:** It was 1st discovered in the duodenum of East Indian sailor in 1843 by Busk.

❖ **Geographical distribution:** This Asiatic trematode distributed in China, Thailand, Malaysia, Bengal, Assam & other oriental region.

❖ **Habitat:** Adult stage lives in small intestine of man & pig.

❖ **Morphology:**

I. Adult stage

- **Development:** Metacercaria change to adult worm in 3 months time.
- **Shape:** Elongated, flat & oval in shape. Anterior end is narrower than posterior **[fig.-1].**
- **Size:** Largest trematodes with 2-7.5cm in length & 8-20mm in breadth with 0.5-3mm in thickness.
- **Life span:** Not more than 6 months.
- **Organs (fig.-1):** Few important points are discussed below. For more details, **follow chapter → Trematodes: General features and classification.**

✪ **Tegument:** Body of parasite is covered with noncellular layer **called tegument** or **called cuticle.**

✪ **Suckers:**

- **Definition:** It is a strong muscular cup shaped depression.
- **Function:** It is an organ for adhesion to host cells.
- **Numbers:** Two in number, so species **called distomata** [**di = two (Greek) + stomata = mouth].**
- **Types:** Two types.

1. **Oral sucker:** One is surrounding the oral cavity **called oral sucker**.
2. **Ventral sucker or acetabula:** Another one is present on ventral surface **called acetabula** or **called ventral sucker.** It is larger than oral sucker & lies close to the oral sucker.

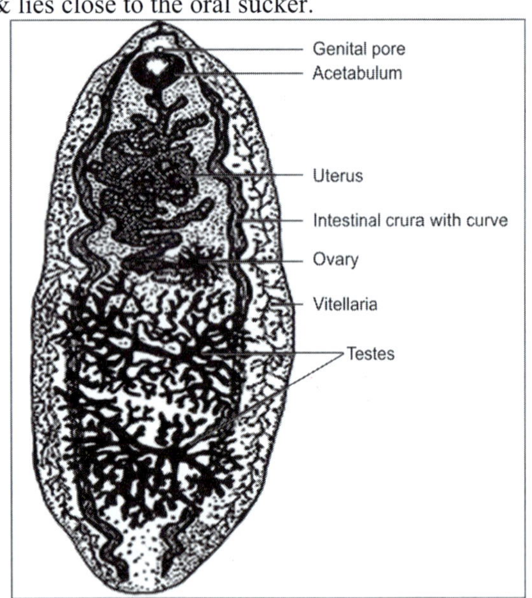

Figure-1: Adult stage of *F. buski*

✪ **Body cavity:** Absent.

✪ **Gastrointestinal system:**

- It is present but without anus so **called incomplete**
- Oesophagus is bifurcated in to two tube like structure **called intestinal caeca** or **called crura.**
- Crura are present with two characteristic curves in middle.
- Crura do not bears any branches.

✪ **Excretory system:** Present.

✪ **Nervous system:** It has no cephalic cone as in *F. hepatica.*

II. Egg stage

- **Numbers of eggs laid by adult worm:** 25, 000 egg per worm per day.

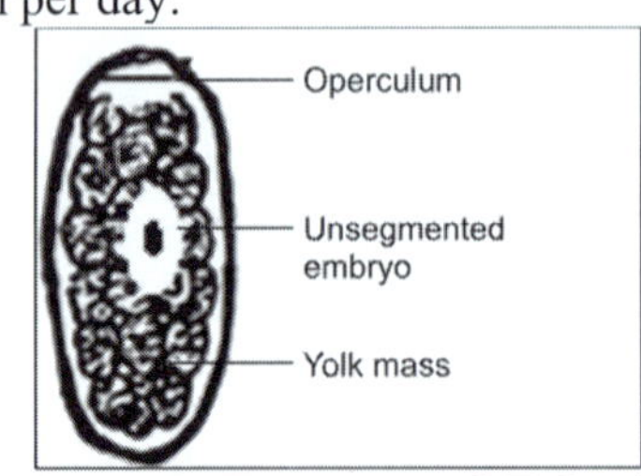

Figure-2: Egg stage of *F. buski*

- **Morphological features: → Fig.-2**

✪ **Size:** 130-140μm × 80-85 μm.

✪ **Shape:** Oval or spherical & with small operculum.

✪ **Colour**: Yellowish - brown colour (bile stained).

✪ **Covering:** Single covering **called egg shell.**

✪ **Yolk material:** Present in abundant amount.

✪ **Embryo:**

- Initially it is unsegmented, nonciliated & surrounded by yolk mass.
- Eggs mature freely in water to develop the ciliated embryo **called miracidium.**

III. Larval stage

✪ **Form:** Solid forms of larva are present.

✪ **Stages, names & hosts:**

- On hatching egg release the ciliated embryo free in water, **called miracidium.**
- Miracidium enters in snail of genus *Segmentina* (intermediate host) & pass through the stages of sporocyst → 1st & 2nd generation of redia →cercaria (lophocercus type) as shown in **fig.-3.**
- Single egg gives the single miracidium, which produces multiple cercariae.
- It encysts on water plants **called metacercaria** or **adolescaria** & ingested by definitive host.

❖ Life cycle:

- **Hosts:** Worm passes its life cycle in two different hosts.

I. **Definitive host:** Man & pig, (adult stage).
II. **Intermediate hosts:** Small flatty coiled aquatic snail of genus *Segmentina* (larval stage).

- **Cycles:** As shown in **flow chart-1 & fig.-3.**

❖ Pathogenicity:

- **Disease name: Called fasciolopsiasis.**
- **Virulence factors:**

1. **Toxic metabolites by adult worms:** Produces allergic reaction with oedema & eosinophilia.
2. **Mechanical injury:**

- **Reservoir of infection:** Pig.
- **Source of infection:** Water.
- **Mode of transmission:**

1. **Ingestion:** Ingestion of aquatic plant as raw food stuff like water chestnut or water caltrop.
2. **Peeling** of water chestnut /water caltrop with teeth.

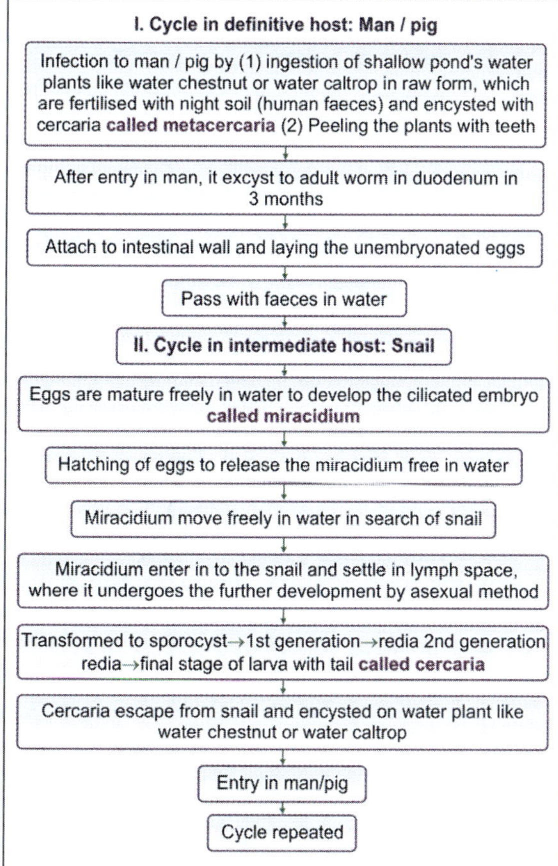

Flow chart-1: Life cycle of *F. buski*

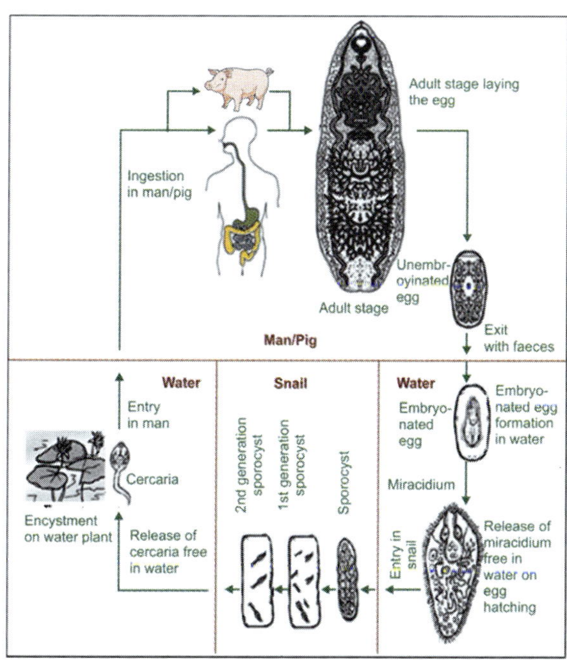

Figure-3: Life cycle of *F. buski*

- **Exit form:** Unembryonated eggs.
- **Infective form:** Encysted cercaria **called metacercaria** or **adolesceria.**
- **Portal of entry:** GIT.
- **Site:** Small intestine.
- **Clinical features:** As shown in **flow chart-2.**

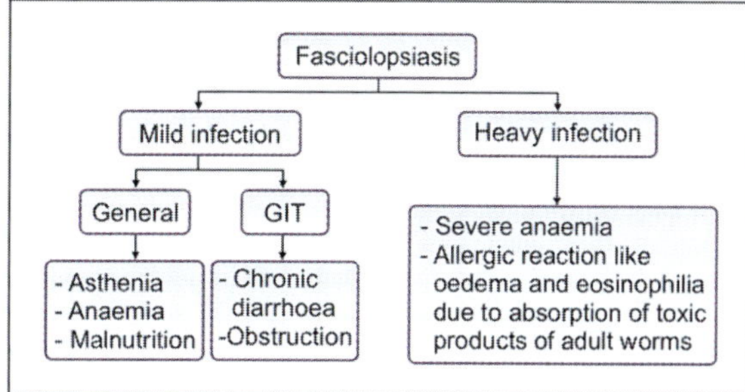

Flow chart-2: Clinical features of *F. buski*

❖ Laboratory diagnosis:

- **Specimen:** Stool.
- **Testing methods:**

I. Direct methods

A. **History taking:** History of residence in endemic area is useful in diagnosis.

B. **Macroscopic:** Adult worms can be demonstrated after purgatives.

C. **Microscopy:**

a. **Wet mount:**

- To examine the egg.
- Eggs of *F. buski, Echinostoma* species, *G. hominis* & *F. hepatica* are indistinguishable.

II. Indirect methods

A. **Blood picture:** Eosinophilia in heavy infection.

❖ Prevention:

- Eradication of intermediate host (snail).
- Prevention of water contamination by the faeces of case.
- Washing of food & vegetables before eating.

❖ Treatment:

- Praziquantel is the drug of choice.
- Hexylresorcinol & tetrachlorethylene are also useful drugs.

Heterophyes heterophyes

❖ **Common name:** Von Siebold's fluke, Dwarf fluke.

❖ **Meaning:** It is the smallest fluke hence **called dwarf fluke.**

❖ **History:** Infection was 1st reported by Bilharz in 1851.

❖ **Geographical distribution:** Prevalent in Egypt, Iran, Israel, Sudan, Turkey & Far East like China, Korea, Japan, Taiwan, Philippines & India.

❖ **Habitat:** Adult stage lives in small intestine of fish eating mammals like man, cat, dog, wolf, bird & fox.

❖ **Morphology:** Three morphological stages like adult, egg & larval stages.

I. Adult stage

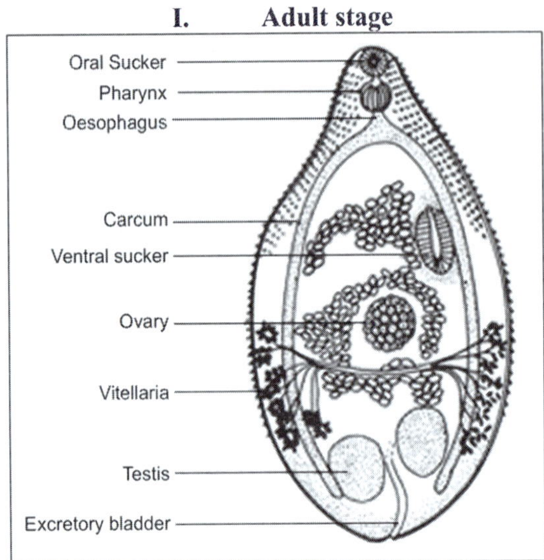
Oral Sucker
Pharynx
Oesophagus
Carcum
Ventral sucker
Ovary
Vitellaria
Testis
Excretory bladder

Figure-4: Adult stage of *H. heterophyes*

- **Development:** Metacercaria change to adult worm in 15-20 days.
- **Size:** 1.5mm×0.3mm.
- **Shape:** Flattened dorso-ventrally with narrow anterior end & rounded posterior end.
- **Life span:** 2 months.
- **Organs (fig.-4):** For more details, **follow chapter → Trematodes: General features and classification.**

II. Egg stage

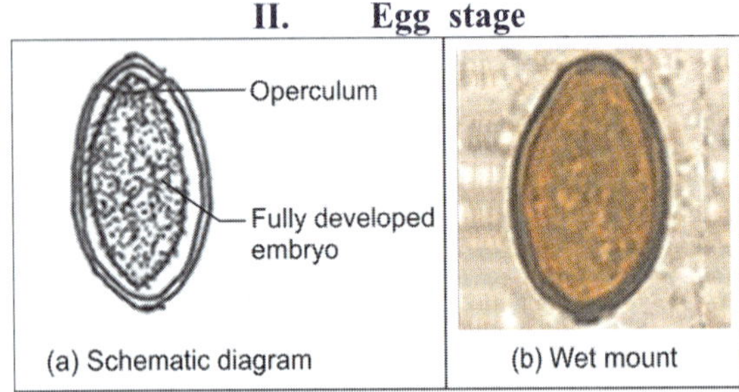
Operculum
Fully developed embryo
(a) Schematic diagram
(b) Wet mount

Figure-5: Egg stage of *H. heterophyes*

- **Morphological features:** → **Fig.-5 (a).**
- **Shape:** Oval & operculated.
- **Size:** 28-30µm ×16-18µm.
- **Colour**: Yellowish - brown colour (bile stained).
- **Covering:** Surrounded by transparent & brownish yellow protective covering.
- **Embryo:** Ciliated embryo present initially when laid **called miracidium.**

III. Larval stage

- **Form:** Solid forms of larva are present.
- **Stages, names & hosts:**
  - On hatching egg release the ciliated embryo free in water, **called miracidium.**
  - Single egg gives the single miracidium, which produces multiple cercariae.
  - Miracidium enters in snail of genus *Pirenella conica* or *Ceithidea* (1st intermediate host) & pass through the stages of sporocyst → 1st & 2nd generation of redia → cercaria (lophocercus type) as shown in **fig.-6.**
  - Cercaria release free in water & encyst in fish like mullet & tilapia (2nd intermediate host) **called metacercaria** or **adolescaria** & ingested by definitive host.

❖ **Life cycle:**

- **Types of host:** Two types.

I. Definitive host: Man, cat, dog, wolf, bird & fox.

II. Intermediate hosts:

A. 1st intermediate host: Marine & brackish water snail like *Pirenella conica* or *Ceithidea.*

B. 2nd intermediate host: Fish like mullet (*Mugil cephalus*) & tilapia.

- **Cycles:** As shown in **flow chart-3 & fig.-6.**

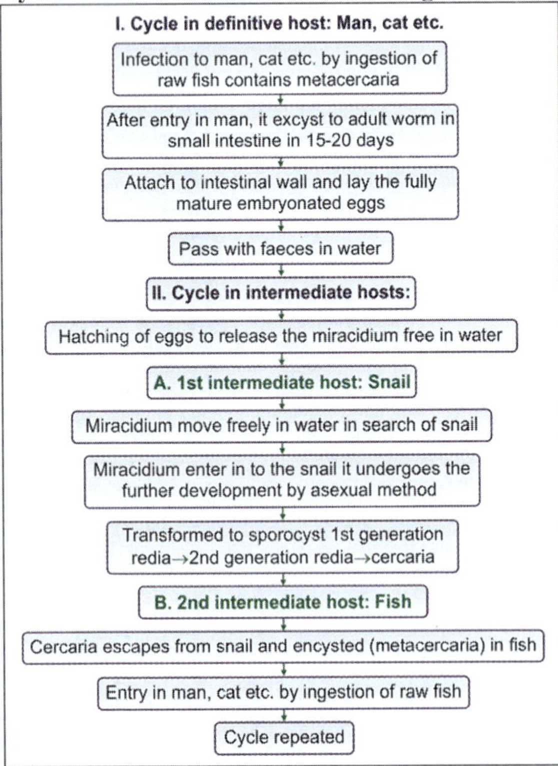
I. Cycle in definitive host: Man, cat etc.
Infection to man, cat etc. by ingestion of raw fish contains metacercaria
After entry in man, it excyst to adult worm in small intestine in 15-20 days
Attach to intestinal wall and lay the fully mature embryonated eggs
Pass with faeces in water
II. Cycle in intermediate hosts:
Hatching of eggs to release the miracidium free in water
A. 1st intermediate host: Snail
Miracidium move freely in water in search of snail
Miracidium enter in to the snail it undergoes the further development by asexual method
Transformed to sporocyst 1st generation redia→2nd generation redia→cercaria
B. 2nd intermediate host: Fish
Cercaria escapes from snail and encysted (metacercaria) in fish
Entry in man, cat etc. by ingestion of raw fish
Cycle repeated

Flow chart-3: Life cycle of *H. heterophyes*

❖ **Pathogenicity:**

- **Disease name: Called heterophyiasis.**

- **Reservoir of infection:** Cat, dog, wolf, bird & fox.
- **Source of infection:** Fish.

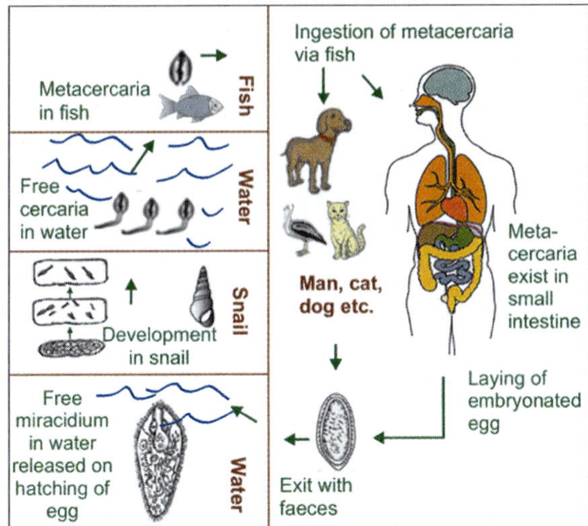

Figure-6: Life cycle of *H. heterophyes*

- **Mode of transmission:** Ingestion of raw fish like mullet & tilapia contains metacercaria.
- **Exit form:** Embryonated eggs.
- **Infective form:** Metarcaria.
- **Portal of entry:** GIT.
- **Sites:**

1. **Common site:** Small intestine & extra-intestinal like heart, brain & spinal cord.
2. **Ectopic sites:** Brain, spinal cord & heart.

- **Clinical features: → Flow chart-4.**

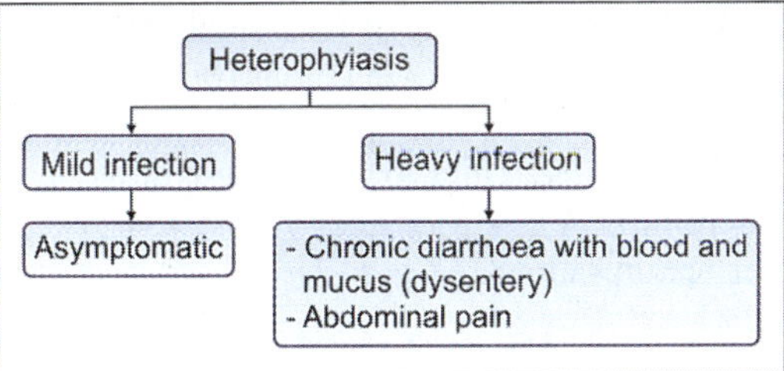

Flow chart-4: Clinical features of *H. heterophyes*

- **Complications:** Adult worms penetrate the gut & laying the eggs, which are carried to brain, spinal cord & heart via blood & lymphatics as like emboli with following manifestation.

1. Granuloma formation.
2. Death: 15% of fatal heart diseases in Philippines are due to heterophyiasis.

❖ **Laboratory diagnosis:**

- **Specimen:** Stool.
- **Testing methods:** Only direct methods are useful.

A. **History taking:** Food history is useful in diagnosis

B. **Macroscopic:** Adult worms absent or can be demonstrated in heavy infection.

C. **Microscopy:**

a. **Wet mount:**

- Bile stained eggs are present as shown in **fig.-5(b)**.
- Eggs of *H. heterophyes, M. yokogawai* & *C. sinensis* (terminal hook) are indistinguishable.

b. **Concentration method:** Formol ethyl acetate sedimentation method is useful.

Metagonimus yokogawai

❖ **Common name:** Yokogawa's fluke.

❖ **History:** Parasite was 1st reported by Katsurada in 1911.

❖ **Geographical distribution:** Prevalent in Far East (like Korea, Japan, China, & Fomosa) & in Egypt, Siberia & Balkan states.

❖ **Habitat:** Adult stage lives in small intestine (particularly in upper & middle part of jejunum & rarely in duodenum, ileum & caecum) of fish eating mammals like man, cat, dog, bird (pelican) & pig.

❖ **Morphology:** Three morphological stages like adult, egg & larval stages.

I. Adult stage

- **Size:** 2mm×0.5mm.
- **Organs & other features:** Same as *H. heterophyes* but little larger & ventral sucker located laterally on right side of mid line as shown **in fig.-7.**

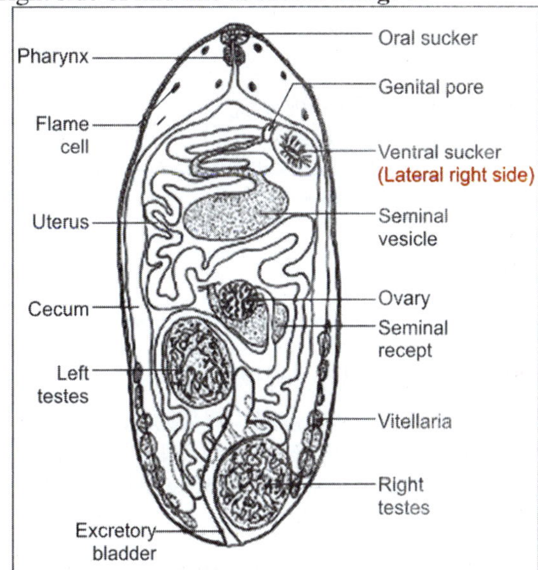

Figure-7: Adult stage of *M. yokogawai*

II. Egg stage

III. Larval stage

Both egg stage & larval stage are indistinguishable from *H. heterophyes.*

❖ **Life cycle:**

- **Types of host:** Two types.

I. **Definitive host:** Man, cat, dog, bird (pelican) & pig.

II. **Intermediate hosts:**

A. **1st intermediate host:** Fresh water snail like *Melania* species.

B. **2nd intermediate host:** Fresh water (sweet) Fish like *Plectoglossus altivelis.*

➢ **Cycles:** Same as *H. heterophyes.*

❖ **Pathogenicity:**

➢ **Disease name:** **Called metagonimiasis.**

➢ **Reservoir of infection:** Cat, dog, bird (pelican) & pig.

➢ **Source of infection:** Fish.

➢ **Mode of transmission:** Ingestion of raw fish like *Plectoglossus altvalis* contains metacercaria.

➢ **Exit form:** Embryonated eggs.

➢ **Infective form:** Metacercaria.

➢ **Portal of entry:** GIT.

➢ **Sites:**

1. **Common site:** Small intestine (particularly in upper & middle part of jejunum & rarely in duodenum, ileum & caecum) & extra-intestinal like heart, brain, spinal cord.
2. **Ectopic sites:** CNS.

➢ **Clinical features:** Mild diarrhoea.

➢ **Complications:** Sometime eggs are carried to brain, spinal cord & heart via blood & lymphatics as like emboli which later cause granuloma formation.

❖ **Laboratory diagnosis:**

- Same as *H. heterophyes.*
- Species identification can be made on the basis of adult worm examination.

Echinostoma spp.

Echinostoma ilocanum

❖ **Common name:** Garrison's fluke.

❖ **Meaning:** Genus name ***Echinostoma*** = **Spiny mouth,** as having spine surrounding to oral sucker & Species ***ilocanum*** **from ilocanan population** in which it is common.

❖ **History:** Eggs of parasite was 1st discovered by Garrison in 1907 in a native prisoner in Manila (Philippines) & obtained the adult worms after the administration of drug filix mas.

❖ **Geographical distribution:** Prevalent in **ilocanan population** of Luzon province, the Manila-Philippines, Japan, China, Indonesia, Taiwan & India (Assam).

❖ **Habitat:** Adult stage lives in small intestine of man, dog & rat.

❖ **Morphology:** Three morphological stages like adult, egg & larval stages.

I. Adult stage

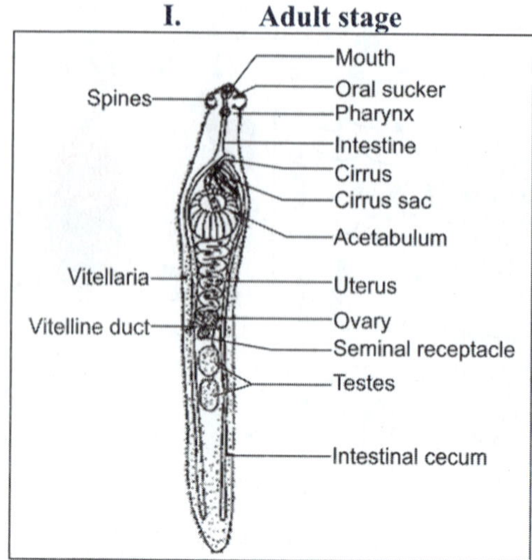

Figure-8: Adult stage of *E. ilocanum*

➢ **Size:** 20mm×2mm.

➢ **Colour:** Reddish gray in appearance.

➢ **Organs (fig.-8):** Oral sucker is surrounded by spine; hence the genus name is *Echinostoma.* For more details, **follow chapter → Trematodes: General features and classification.**

II. Egg stage

- **Size:** 90-125μm × 55-75 μm.
- **Shape:** Oval or spherical & with small operculum.
- **Colour**: Yellowish - brown colour (bile stained).
- **Other features:**

- Contains ciliated embryo when laid down **called miracidim.**
- Other features are same as *F. buski.*

III. Larval stage

- **Form:** Solid forms of larva are present.
- **Stages, names & hosts:**

- On hatching egg release the ciliated embryo free in water, **called miracidium.**
- Miracidium enters in snail (1st intermediate host) & pass through the stages 1st & 2nd generation of redia →cercaria (no sporocyst).
- Single egg gives the single miracidium, which produces multiple cercariae.
- It encyst in molluscs (2nd intermediate host) **called metacercaria** or **adolescaria** & ingested by definitive host.

❖ **Life cycle:**

➢ **Types of host:** Two types.

I. **Definitive host:** Man, dog & rat.

II. **Intermediate hosts:**

A. **1st intermediate host:** Snail.

B. 2nd intermediate host: Molluscs.

- **Cycles:** Same as *H. heterophyes* except that 2nd intermediate host is molluscs & no stage of sporocyst formation.

❖ **Pathogenicity:**

- **Disease name:** **Called echinostomiasis.**
- **Reservoir of infection:** Man, dog, & rat.
- **Source of infection:** Molluscs.
- **Mode of transmission:** Ingestion of molluscs contains metacercaria.
- **Exit form:** Embryonated eggs.
- **Infective form:** Metacercaria.
- **Portal of entry:** GIT.
- **Site:** Small intestine.
- **Clinical features:**
  - Mild infection: Asymptomatic.
  - Heavy infection: Produce nausea, severe diarrhoea, abdominal pain, distension etc.

❖ **Laboratory diagnosis:**

- Same as *H. heterophyes.*
- Species identification can be made on the basis of adult worm examination.

Echinostoma malayanum

- History: Discovered by Leiper in 1911.
- Common name: It was 1st reported from Singapore & Kuala Lumpur, hence **called Malayan fluke.**
- Habitat & distribution: Common intestinal parasite of tribes living in the Sino-Tibetian frontier (Bare, 1930).

Echinostoma revolutum

- History: Discovered by Forhlichr in 1802.
- Host: Parasite of duck, geese & fowl. Human infection is accidental.

Paryphostomum supraryfex

- Distribution: It is reported from India.
- Host: Parasite of pig & clinically similar to *F. buski.*

Watsonius watsoni

❖ **History:** Only one case was found in Africa.

❖ **Geographical distribution:** Prevalent in Africa Japan & Malaysia.

❖ **Habitat:** Adult stage lives in small intestine in man & monkey.

❖ **Morphology:** Three morphological stages like adult, egg & larval stages.

I. Adult stage

- **Size:** 8-10mm× 4-5mm.
- **Shape:** Pear shaped & flat dorso-ventrally.
- **Organs:** Body is ventrally concave near the posterior sucker.

II. Egg stage
III. Larval stage

Egg & larval stages are same as *F. buski.*

❖ **Life cycle:** It has not been worked out yet.

❖ **Pathogenicity:** One case with severe diarrhoea resulting death was found in Africa.

❖ **Laboratory diagnosis:** Based on identification of eggs in stool.

Large intestinal trematodes

Gastrodiscoides hominis

❖ **Synonym:** *Amphostomum hominis.*

❖ **History:** It was discovered in 1876, by Lewis & Mc Connell in the caecum of Indian patient.

❖ **Geographical distribution:** Prevalent in India (Bengal, Assam, Bihar, Orissa), Cochin-China Malaya & Indian immigrants to British Guiana.

❖ **Habitat:** Adult stage lives in large intestine in man, monkey, pig, deer & mouse.

❖ **Morphology:** Three morphological stages like adult, egg & larval stages.

I. Adult stage

- **Size:** 5-10mm× 4-6mm (broad at the widest part)
- **Shape:** Pyriform shaped & flat dorso-ventrally.
- **Organs (fig.-9):** Body is divided in two portions.

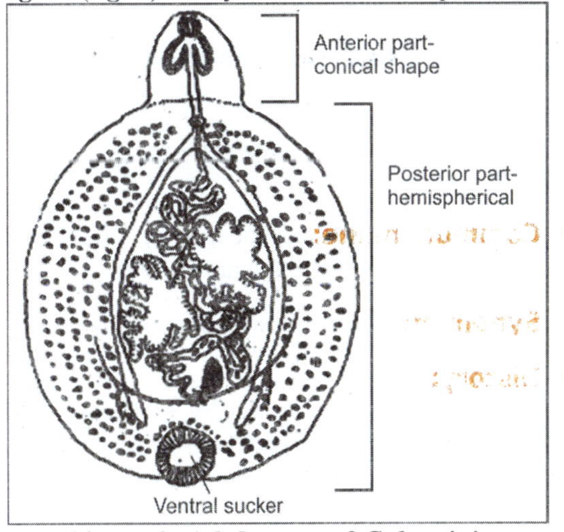

Figure-9: Adult stage of *G. hominis*

A. Anterior part: Conical.

B. Posterior part:

- Hemispherical.
- Hollowed out ventrally to form a concave disc.
- Acetabulum (ventral sucker) is postero-terminal & situated ventrally.
- Notch at the posterior end.
- Other organs are same as other monoecious trematodes.

II. Egg stage

- 130 µm × 60 µm & greenish grey.
- Other details are same as *F. buski*.

III. Larval stage

Same as *F. buski*.

❖ **Life cycle:**

➢ **Types of host:** Two types.

I. **Definitive host:** Man, pig, monkey, deer & mouse

II. **Intermediate hosts:** Planorbid snail like *Helicorbis coenosus* (larval stage).

➢ **Cycles:** Same as *F. buski*.

❖ **Pathogenicity:**

➢ **Disease name: Called gastrodiscoidiosis.**

➢ **Reservoir of infection:** Man, monkey, pig, deer & mouse,

➢ **Source of infection:** Water vegetables.

➢ **Mode of transmission:** Ingestion of raw vegetable like water chest-nut contains metacercaria.

➢ **Exit form:** Unembryonated egg.

➢ **Infective form:** Metacercaria.

➢ **Portal of entry:** GIT.

➢ **Site:** Large intestine.

➢ **Clinical features:** Mucoid diarrhoea.

❖ **Laboratory diagnosis:**

- It is made by identifying the eggs in stool.
- Eggs are same as *F. buski* but narrower & greenish gray instead of yellowish brown.

Hepatic trematodes

Clonorchis sinensis

❖ **Common name:** Chinese liver fluke, Oriental liver fluke, Distoma of China.

❖ **Synonym:** *Opisthorchis sinensis.*

❖ **History:**

- Parasite was 1st discovered by McConnel in 1857 from the autopsy of a Chinese carpenter in the Calcutta Medical College Hospital.
- Life cycle was worked out by Faust & Khaw in 1927.

❖ **Geographical distribution:**

- Prevalent in Far East like China, Korea, Japan, South & North Vietnam & Formosa.
- It also prevalent in USA, France, Canada & Australia among Asian refugee from endemic area.

❖ **Habitat:** Adult stage lives in biliary tract & sometimes in pancreatic duct.

❖ **Morphology:** Three morphological stages like adult, egg & larval stages.

I. Adult stage

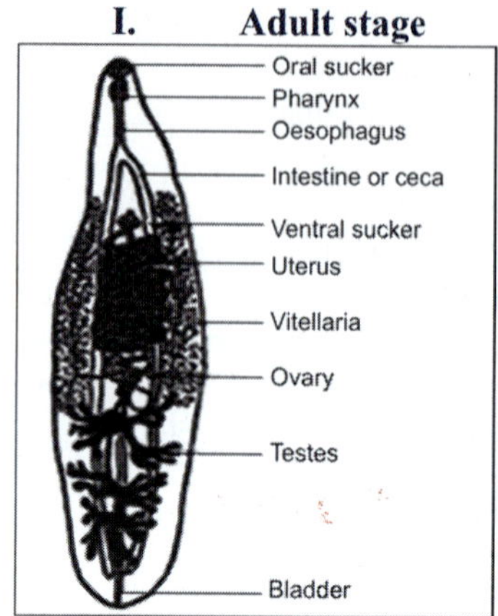

Figure-10: Adult stage of *C. sinensis*

➢ **Development:** Metacercaria change to adult worm in 1 month.

➢ **Size:** Variable, 10-25mm×2-3mm.

➢ **Shape:** Flattened dorso-ventrally with narrow anterior end & rounded posterior end.

➢ **Life span:** 20-30 years.

➢ **Organs (fig.-10):** Few important points are discussed below. For more details, follow chapter → Trematodes: General features and classification.

✪ **Suckers:** Oral sucker is larger & ventral sucker is located at the junction of the anterior & middle third of the body.

✪ **GIT:** Blind intestinal caeca are simple & extend to the caudal region.

✪ **Reproductive system:**

- Two in numbers & in large size.
- Deeply branches & located in the posterior third of the body, one behind the other.

II. Egg stage

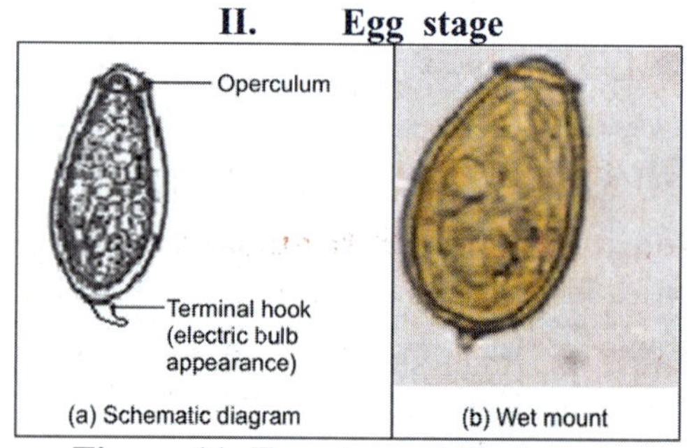

Figure-11: Egg stage of *C. sinensis*

➢ **Morphological features: → Fig.-11(a)**

✪ **Shape:** Flask shaped & operculated.

✪ **Size:** 35µm ×20µm.

- **Colour**: Yellowish - brown colour (bile stained).
- **Covering:** Surrounded by protective covering.
- **Embryo:** Contains ciliated embryo when laid **called miracidium.**
- **Other features:**
  - It contains hook like spine at the end give electric bulb like appearance.
  - Does not hatch in water but in snail.
  - Does not float in saturated common salt solution
  - Infective to snail only.

III. Larval stage

- **Form:** Solid forms of larva are present.
- **Stages, names & hosts:**

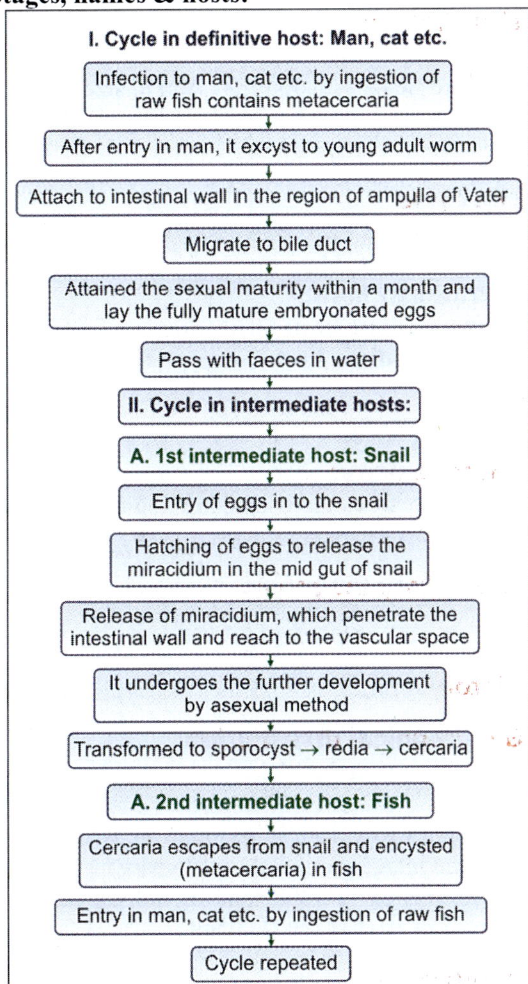

I. Cycle in definitive host: Man, cat etc.
Infection to man, cat etc. by ingestion of raw fish contains metacercaria
After entry in man, it excyst to young adult worm
Attach to intestinal wall in the region of ampulla of Vater
Migrate to bile duct
Attained the sexual maturity within a month and lay the fully mature embryonated eggs
Pass with faeces in water
II. Cycle in intermediate hosts:
A. 1st intermediate host: Snail
Entry of eggs in to the snail
Hatching of eggs to release the miracidium in the mid gut of snail
Release of miracidium, which penetrate the intestinal wall and reach to the vascular space
It undergoes the further development by asexual method
Transformed to sporocyst → redia → cercaria
A. 2nd intermediate host: Fish
Cercaria escapes from snail and encysted (metacercaria) in fish
Entry in man, cat etc. by ingestion of raw fish
Cycle repeated

Flow chart-5: Life cycle of *C. sinensis*

- Egg are hatched in snail of genus *Bulimius, Parafossarulus* & *Alocina* (1st intermediate host) & release the ciliated embryo **called miracidium.**
- Miracidium pass through the stages of sporocyst → redia → cercaria (lophocercus type) as shown in **fig.-12.**
- Single egg gives the single miracidium, which produces multiple cercarias.
- Cercaria release free in water & encyst in fresh water fish of genus *Cyprinoid* (2nd intermediate host) **called metacercaria** or **adolescaria** & ingested by definitive host.

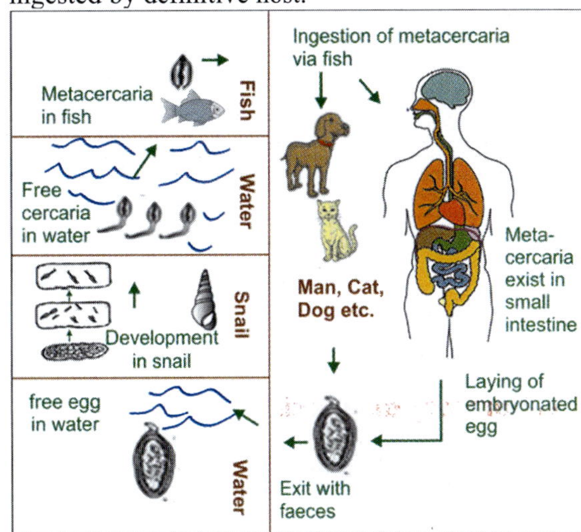

Figure-12: Life cycle of *C. sinensis*

❖ Life cycle:

- **Types of host:** Two types.

I. Definitive host: Man, cat, dog, pig & rat.

II. Intermediate hosts:

A. 1st intermediate host: Snail (*Bulimius suchsianus, Parafossarulus manchouricus* & *Alocina longicornis*).

B. 2nd intermediate host: Fresh water fish of genus *Cyprinoid.*

- **Cycles:** As shown in **flow chart-5 & fig.-12.**

❖ Pathogenicity:

- **Disease name:** **Called clonorchiasis.**
- **Virulence factors:**

1. **Mechanical:**
   - Irritation of mucosa of biliary tract → hyperplasia.
   - Obstruction of bile flow → jaundice & secondary infection.
2. **Toxic metabolites:** Responsible for hyperplasia of mucosa.

- **Reservoir of infection:** Cat, dog, pig & rat.
- **Source of infection:** Fish.
- **Mode of transmission:** Ingestion of raw fish like cyprinoid contains metacercaria.
- **Exit form:** Embryonated eggs.
- **Infective form:** Metacercaria.
- **Portal of entry:** GIT.
- **Sites:**

1. **Common site:** Biliary tract.
2. **Rare site:** Pancreatic duct.

- **Clinical features:** → **Flow chart-6**
- **Complications:** It occurs after long term (chronic) infection like

1. **Secondary infection:** Hyperplasia of duct → narrowing of lumen → blockage of biliary tree → obstruction of bile flow → secondary bacterial infection (also by heavy infection).

2. **Stone:** Intrahepatic calculi formation.
3. **Cancer of bile duct: Called cholangiocarcinoma** which epidemiologically related to China.

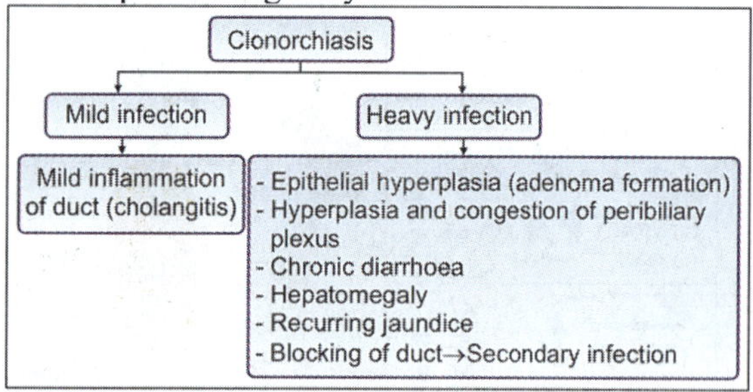

Flow chart-6: Clinical features of *C. sinensis*

❖ **Laboratory diagnosis:**

➢ **Specimens:**

1. **Stool:** Eggs are not present in case of biliary obstruction.
2. **Aspirated bile:** Collected by entero (string) test. **Follow chapter → Intestinal, oral and genital flagellates** for more details.

➢ **Testing methods:**

I. Direct methods

A. Microscopy:

a. Wet mount:

- Bile stained eggs are present as shown in **fig.-11(b)**
- Eggs of *H. heterophyes, M. yokogawai* & *C. sinensis* (terminal spine) are indistinguishable.

b. Concentration method:

- Does not float in saturated common salt solution due to operculum.
- It sediment with normal tap water concentration method.

II. Indirect methods

A. Blood picture: Leucocytosis with eosinophilia.

B. Allergic /skin test: Intradermal test gives immediate type of hypersensitivity.

C. Serological tests: Antigen is prepared from *C. sinensis*.

1. Precipitation test.
2. CFT.
3. Indirect Haem Agglutination (IHA) test.

❖ **Prevention:**

- Eradication of intermediate host (snail & fish).
- Prevention of water contamination by the faeces of case.
- Avoid the use of raw fish.

❖ **Treatment:**

- Praziquantel (25mg/kg, 3 doses in 1 day) is the drug of choice.
- Surgical intervention is necessary in case of obstructive jaundice.

Opisthorchis spp.

Opisthorchis felineus

❖ **Common name:** Cat liver fluke.

❖ **History:** Rivolta 1884 & Blanchard 1895.

❖ **Geographical distribution:**

- It has been reported from Prussia, Poland, Siberia & Japan.
- Chandler found that 60% of cat in Kolkata (India) were infected with the parasites & human cases were reported from India.

❖ **Habitat:** Adult stage lives in biliary & pancreatic duct.

❖ **Morphology:** Same as *C. sinensis* but

- Testes are not branched.
- Eggs are small with 30μm ×11μm in size.
- Cercarias are with long tail with pair of fin fold (pleurolophocercus type).

❖ **Life cycle:**

➢ **Types of host:** Two types

I. Definitive host: Man, cat, dog, pig & fox.

II. Intermediate hosts:

A. 1st intermediate host: Snail (*Bithynia leachi*)

B. 2nd intermediate host: Fresh water fish of genus *Cyprinoid*

➢ **Cycles:** Same as *C. sinensis*.

❖ **Pathogenicity:** Same as *C. sinensis* but cholangio carcinoma is epidemiologically related to North –East Thailand.

❖ **Laboratory diagnosis:** Same as *C. sinensis*.

Opisthorchis viverini

❖ **History:** Poirier, 1886; Stiles & Hasall, 1896.

❖ **Geographical distribution:**

- It is prevalent in the Mekong river valley in Laos & Thailand.
- Prevalence was 100% in some areas of Laos & Thailand in age group below 10 years.
- It is estimated in 1992 that 10 million people are infected in North East Thailand.

❖ **Habitat:** Adult stage lives in distal bile duct.

❖ **Morphology:**

➢ Same as *C. sinensis* but

- Adult worm is smaller in size about 8-12mm in length.
- Eggs are small with 25μm ×15μm in size.
- Cercarias are with long tail with pair of fin fold (pleurolophocercus type).

➢ Differentiation from *O. felineus*

- Greater proximity of ovary & testis.
- Few cluster of Vitellaria.

❖ **Life cycle:**

- **Types of host:** Two types.

I. **Definitive host:** Man & cat.

II. **Intermediate hosts:** Same as *C. sinensis*.

- **Cycles:** Same as *C. sinensis*.

Pathogenicity:

- **Clinical features:** It produces diarrhoea, pain the right hypochondrium & mild jaundice.
- **Complication:**
- Periportal fibrosis of liver.
- Inflammation of biliary canaliculi.
- Epithelial hyperplasia.

Laboratory diagnosis: Same as *C. sinensis*.

Opisthorchis noverca

- History: Braun, 1902.
- Common name: It was 1st reported from Pariah dog, pig & man in India.

Fasciola spp.

Fasciola hepatica

Common name: Sheep liver fluke & Common liver fluke.

History:

- It was 1st discovered by Jehan De Brie in 1379.
- Life cycle was worked out by Leuckart & Thomas in 1883, independently to one another.

Geographical distribution: Cosmopolitan.

Habitat: Adult stage lives in biliary tract of man & herbivorous animals like sheep, goat & cattle.

Morphology: Three morphological stages like adult, egg & larval stages.

I. Adult stage

- **Development:** Metacercaria change to adult worm in 3-4 months.
- **Size:** 3 cm×1.5cm.
- **Shape:** Leaf like.
- **Colour:** Brown to pale grey in colour.
- **Life span:** In sheep 5 years & in man 9-13 years.
- **Organs (fig.-13):** Few important points are discussed below. For more details, follow chapter → Trematodes: General features and classification.
- **Suckers:** Two suckers as follows.

1. **Oral sucker:** It is smaller & anterior end bearing the oral sucker form a conical projection (cephalic cone).
2. **Ventral sucker:** It is located in line with the two shoulders formed by the broadening of the conical projection posteriorly.

- **GIT:** Both the intestinal caeca bears the numbers of lateral branches.

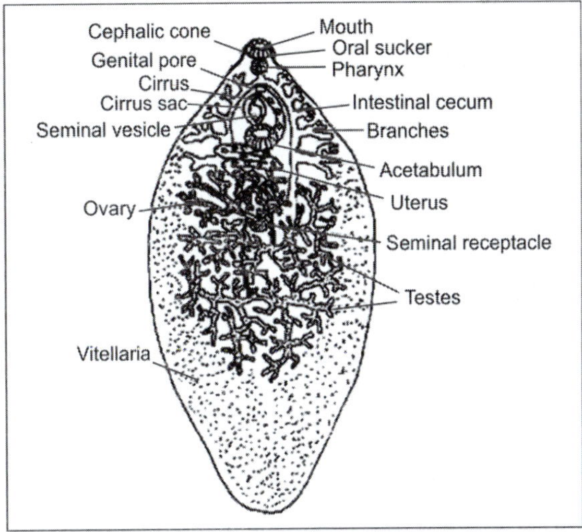

Figure-13: Adult stage of *F. hepatica*

II. Egg stage

- **Morphological features: → Fig.-14(a)**
- **Shape:** Ovoid & operculated.
- **Size:** 140µm ×80µm.
- **Colour**: Yellowish - brown colour (bile stained).
- **Covering:** Surrounded by protective covering.
- **Embryo:** It contains unsegmented ovum surrounded by yolk mass initially & miracidium formed later in water.
- **Other features:**
- Hatch in water to release the miracidium.
- Does not float in saturated common salt solution.
- Excreted with bile duodenum & then passed out along with faeces.

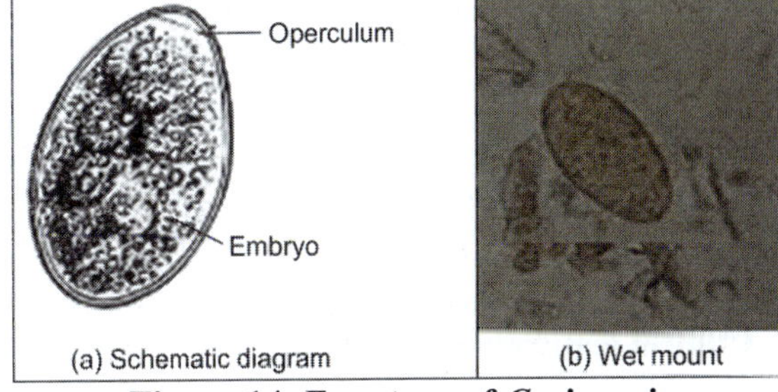

Figure-14: Egg stage of *C. sinensis*

III. Larval stage

- **Form:** Solid forms of larva are present.
- **Stages, names & hosts:**
- On hatching egg release the ciliated embryo free in water, **called miracidium.**
- Miracidium enters in snail of genus *Lymnaea truncatula* (intermediate host) & pass through the stages of sporocyst → 1st & 2nd generation of redia → cercaria (lophocercus type) as shown in **fig.-15.**
- Single egg gives the single miracidium, which produces multiple cercariae.

- It encyst in blades of grass or water-cress **called metacercaria** or **adolescaria** & ingested by definitive host.

❖ Life cycle:

➢ **Types of host:** Two types.

I. **Definitive host:** Man, sheep, goat & cattle.

II. **Intermediate hosts:** Amphibian snail (*Lymnaea truncatula*).

➢ **Cycles:** As shown in **flow chart-7 & fig.-15.**

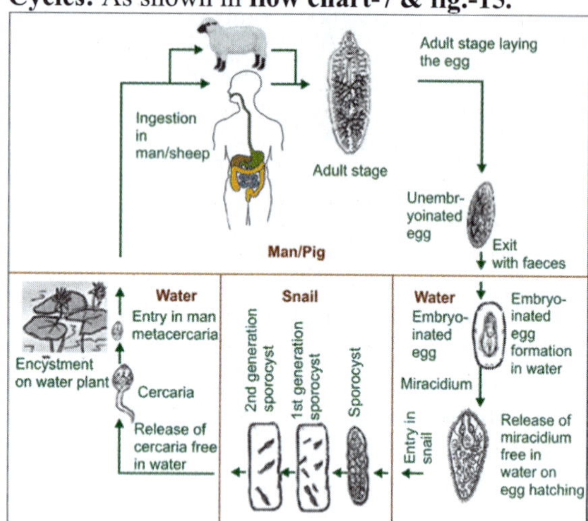

Figure-15: Life cycle of *F. hepatica*

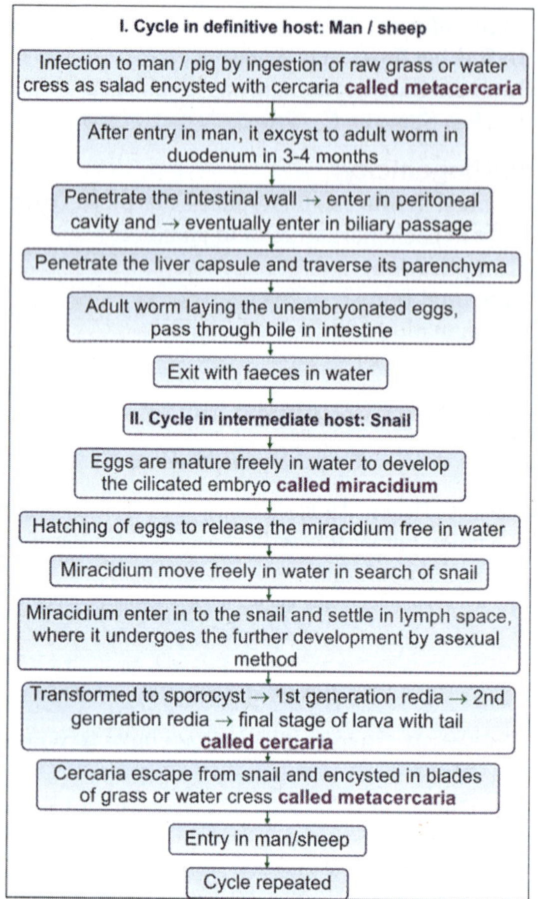

Flow chart-7: Life cycle of *F. hepatica*

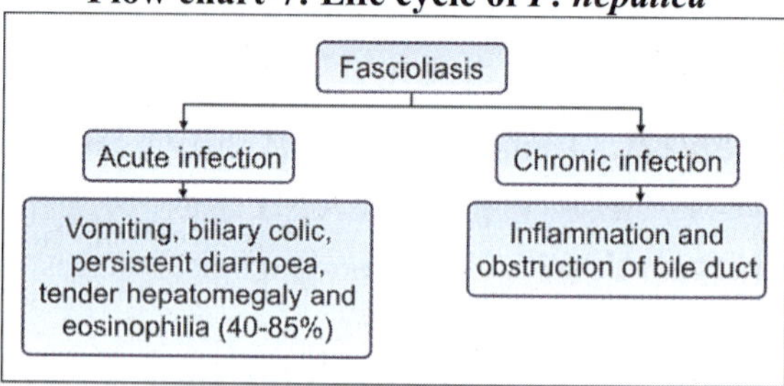

Flow chart-8: Clinical features of *F. hepatica*

❖ Pathogenicity:

➢ **Disease name: Called fascioliasis (liver rot in animal → Vide infra).**

➢ **Reservoir of infection:** Sheep, goat & cattle.

➢ **Source of infection:** Raw grass or water cress as salad encysted with cercaria **called metacercaria.**

➢ **Mode of transmission:** Ingestion of raw grass or water cress as salad contains metacercaria.

➢ **Exit form:** Embryonated eggs.

➢ **Infective form:** Metacercaria.

➢ **Portal of entry:** GIT.

➢ **Sites:**

1. **Common site:** Biliary tract.
2. **Ectopic sites:** During migration larva may enter in lungs, cutaneous tissues etc.

➢ **Clinical features: → Flow chart-8**

➢ **Complications:** During migration larva may enter in lungs & cutaneous tissues with production of abscess or fibrotic lesion.

❖ Laboratory diagnosis:

➢ **Specimens:**

1. **Stool:** Eggs are present. It also contains *Fasciola* copra antigen.
2. **Aspirated bile:** Collected by entero (string) test **Follow chapter → Intestinal, oral and genital flagellates** for more details.
3. **Pus in case of ectopic lesion:** It may contain the worms.

➢ **Testing methods:**

I. Direct methods

A. Microscopy:

a. Wet mount:

- Bile stained eggs are present as shown in **fig.-14(b).**
- Eggs of *F. buski* are indistinguishable.

b. Concentration method:

- Does not float in saturated common salt solution due to operculum.
- It sediment with normal tap water concentration method.

II. Indirect methods

A. Blood picture: Eosinophilia (40-85%).

B. Allergic /skin test: Intradermal test gives immediate type of hypersensitivity.

C. Serological tests: Antigen is prepared from *F. hepatica*.

1. **ELISA:** Positive after 2 weeks of infection & negative after treatment.
2. **Immuno Electrophoresis test:**
3. **CFT:**
4. **Indirect Haem Agglutination (IHA) test:**
5. **Latex agglutination test:**

❖ **Prevention:**
- Eradication of intermediate host (snail).
- Prevention of water contamination by the faeces of case.
- Washing of vegetables before eating.

❖ **Treatment:**
- Oral triclabendazole (10mg/kg, single dose) is the drug of choice.
- Bithionol (30-50 mg for 10-15days) is the other option.

✓ **Note: Halzoun & Liver rot**

Halzoun

- **Meaning:** Actual meaning is suffocation.
- **History & cause:** Common in Syria (Lebanon) due to ingestion of raw liver of sacrificial goat. Initially it was believed that it was due to invasion of immature *F. hepatica* & commonly **called pharyngeal fascioliasis**, but now it is considered due to nymph of *Linguatula serrata* (Tongue shaped animal parasite belong to **pentastome** subclass).
- **Features:** Present with acute dysphagia & laryngeal obstruction.

Liver rot

- **Definition:** Animal infection *F. hepatica* **called liver root.**
- **Causes:** It is due to migration of metacercaria & their localisation in biliary passages.
- **Features:**
- Liver: Extensive damage to liver & portal cirrhosis.
- Biliary tract: Due to mechanical irritation & production of toxic metabolites it causes obstruction of bile flow (obstructive jaundice), dilatation & thickening of bile duct, fibrosis & adenoma due to epithelial hyperplasia.

Fasciola gigantica

❖ **Meaning:** Size of egg is larger than *F. hepatica* hence species **called gigantic.**

❖ **Geographical distribution:**
- Infection rate is high China, Iraq & Northe East Thailand (50% cattle, 45% goats & 33% water buffalo).
- Sporadic cases have been reported from Zimbabwe, Uganda, Tashkent, Iraq, Vietnam & Hawai.

❖ **Habitat:** Common in herbivorous animals like cattle, goats, camels, water buffalo etc.

❖ **Morphology:** Same as *F. hepatica,* with following differences.
- Lanceolate shape.
- Less distinct cephalic cone.
- Large size egg about 160-190μm ×70-90μm.

❖ **Life cycle:** Same as *F. hepatica* but intermediate host is fully aquatic snail instead of amphibian snail.

❖ **Pathogenicity:** Same as *F. hepatica.*

❖ **Laboratory diagnosis:** Same as *F. hepatica.*

Dicrocoelium dendriticum

❖ **Common name:** Lancet fluke, because of its shape.

❖ **Geographical distribution:**
- Prevalent in Europe, North Africa, Northern Asia & Far east in sheep.
- Human infections were reported from Europe, Middle East & China.

❖ **Habitat:** Common in biliary tract of man & herbivorous animals like sheep, deer etc.

❖ **Morphology:**
- Adult is lancet shape, flat, transparent & 5-15mm ×1.5-2.5mm in size.
- Eggs are thick shelled, operculated, about 38-45μm × 22-30μm in size & golden brown in colour.

❖ **Life cycle:**
➢ **Types of host:** Two types.

I. **Definitive host:** Man & herbivorous animals like sheep, deer etc.

II. **Intermediate hosts:**

A. **1st intermediate host:** Land snail.

B. **2nd intermediate host:** Ants of genus *Formica.*

➢ **Cycles:** As shown in **flow chart-9.**

❖ **Pathogenicity:** Human infection is spurious.

Eurytrema pancreaticum

❖ **Common name:** Pancreatic fluke.

❖ **Geographical distribution:** Human infection is noticed in China & Japan.

❖ **Habitat:** Common in pancreatic duct of cattle, sheep, camel & monkeys.

❖ **Morphology:**
- Adult is 8-16mm ×5-9mm in size.
- Egg are same as *D. dendriticum.*

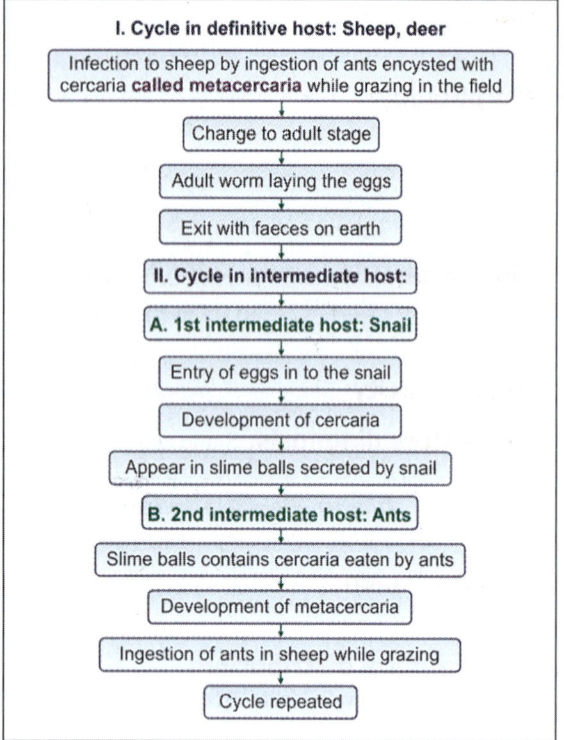

I. Cycle in definitive host: Sheep, deer
Infection to sheep by ingestion of ants encysted with cercaria called metacercaria while grazing in the field
Change to adult stage
Adult worm laying the eggs
Exit with faeces on earth
II. Cycle in intermediate host:
A. 1st intermediate host: Snail
Entry of eggs in to the snail
Development of cercaria
Appear in slime balls secreted by snail
B. 2nd intermediate host: Ants
Slime balls contains cercaria eaten by ants
Development of metacercaria
Ingestion of ants in sheep while grazing
Cycle repeated

Flow chart-9: Life cycle of *D. dendriticum*

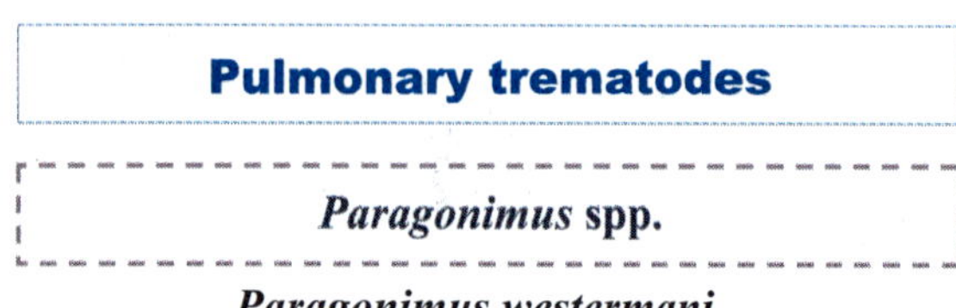

Pulmonary trematodes

Paragonimus spp.

Paragonimus westermani

- **Common name:** Oriental lung fluke or lung distome.
- **Synonym:** *Distoma westermani.*
- **Meaning:** Species name given from the name **Westerman**, director of Amsterdam zoo by Kerbert in 1878.
- **History:** Infection was 1st reported by Naterer in 1828 & later by Kerbert in 1878 from Bengal tiger that died in zoo of Amsterdam. Species name given from Amsterdam.
- **Geographical distribution:** Prevalent in Far East in China, Korea, Japan, Formosa & India (Bengal. Assam & South India). It also reported from Nepal, parts of Africa & South America.
- **Habitat:** Adult stage lives in lungs of man, cat, tiger & leopard.
- **Morphology:** Three stages like adult, egg & larval stages.

I. Adult stage

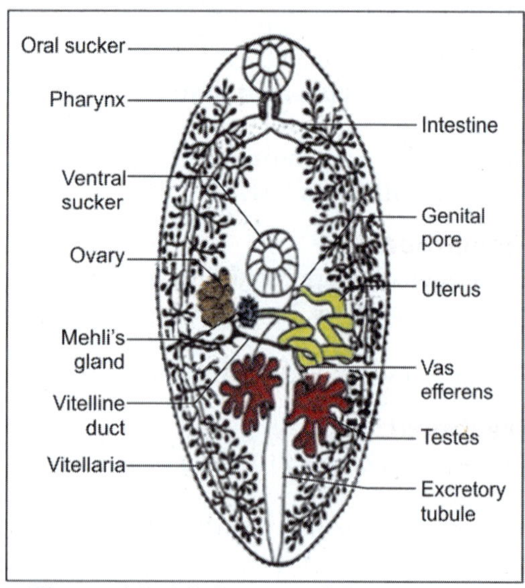

Oral sucker
Pharynx
Ventral sucker
Ovary
Mehli's gland
Vitelline duct
Vitellaria
Intestine
Genital pore
Uterus
Vas efferens
Testes
Excretory tubule

Figure-16: Adult stage of *P. westermani*

- **Development:** Metacercaria change to adult worm in 2 -3 months.
- **Size:** 8-12mm in length, 4-6mm in breadth & 3-5mm in thickness.
- **Shape:** Egg shaped with anterior end is broader than posterior end.
- **Life span:** 6-7 years.
- **Organs (fig.-16):** Few important points are discussed below. For more details, follow chapter → Trematodes: General features and classification.
  - **Tegument:** Covered with spines.
  - **Suckers:** Oral sucker is situated anteriorly & ventral sucker is located in the middle of the body.
  - **Gastrointestinal system:** Crura do not bears any branches & ends blindly in caudal (posterior) area.
  - **Excretory system:** Excretory vesicle is large & extends from posterior to anterior region & divide the body in to two equal half.

II. Egg stage

- **Morphological features: → Fig.-17 (a)**
  - **Shape:** Oval & flat operculated.
  - **Size:** 80µm ×55µm.
  - **Colour**: Golden - brown colour (bile stained).
  - **Covering:** Surrounded by transparent & brownish yellow protective covering.
  - **Embryo:**
    - Initially (when laid) it contains unsegmented embryo surrounded by yolk mass.
    - Miracidium develop later after releasing in water.

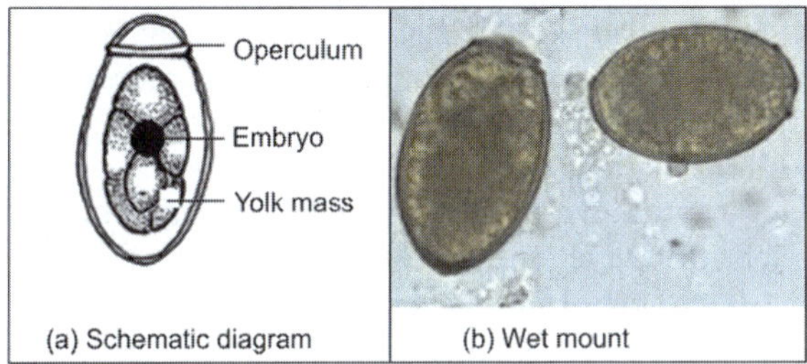

Figure-17: Egg stage of *P. westermani*

III. Larval stage

- **Form:** Solid forms of larva are present.
- **Stages, names & hosts:**
  - On hatching egg release the ciliated embryo free in water, **called miracidium.**
  - Miracidium enters in fresh water snail of genus *Melania liberta* (*Semisulcospira liberta*) or *Brotia* (1st intermediate host) & pass through the stages of sporocyst → 1st & 2nd generation of redia →cercaria (microcercus type) as shown in **fig.-18.**
  - Cercaria release free in water & encyst in crab or crayfish (2nd intermediate host) **called metacercaria** or **adolescaria** & ingested by definitive host.
  - Single egg gives the single miracidium, which produces multiple cercariae.

❖ Life cycle:

- **Types of host:** Two types.

I. Definitive host: Man, cat, tiger & leopard.

II. Intermediate hosts:

A. 1st intermediate host: Fresh water snail of genus *Melania liberta* (*Semisulcospira liberta*) or *Brotia.*

B. 2nd intermediate host: Crab or crayfish.

- **Cycles:** As shown in **fig.-18 & flow chart-10.**

❖ Pathogenicity:

- **Disease name: Called paragonimiasis.**
- **Reservoir of infection:** Cat.
- **Source of infection:** Crab or crayfish.
- **Mode of transmission:**
  - Ingestion of raw crab or crayfish contains metacercaria.
  - Strips of raw crab meat soaked in alcohol **called drunken crab** a popular delicacy in China.
- **Incubation period:** Highly variable from 2-20 days too few months.
- **Infective form:** Metacercaria.
- **Exit form:** Unembryonated eggs.
- **Portal of entry:** GIT.

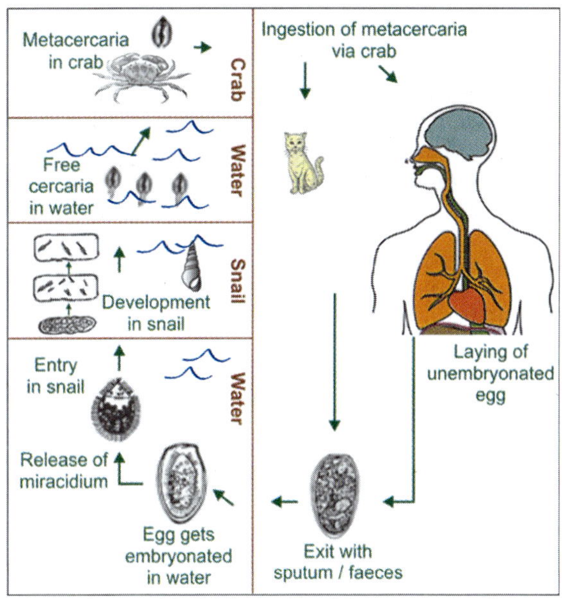

Figure-18: Life cycle of *P. westermani*

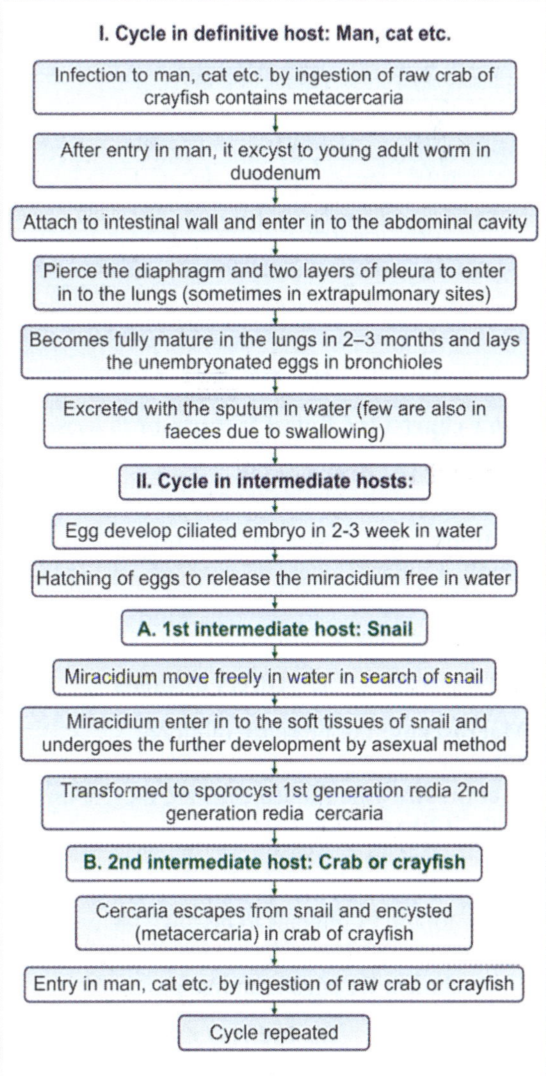

Flow chart-10: Life cycle of *P. westermani*

➢ **Sites:**
1. **Common site:** Lungs.
2. **Ectopic sites:** Extra-pulmonary may be generalised (skin, lymph nodes etc.) or localised in abdomen (liver, intestine, peritoneum) & brain.

➢ **Pathogenesis & virulence factors: → Flow chart-11**

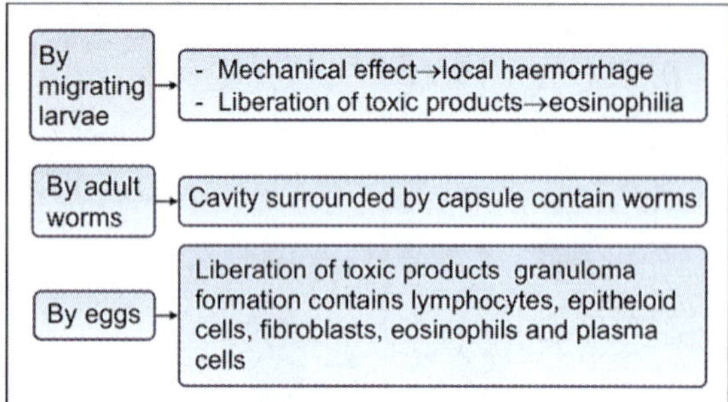

Flow chart-11: Pathogenesis of *P. westermani*

➢ **Clinical features: → Flow chart-12**

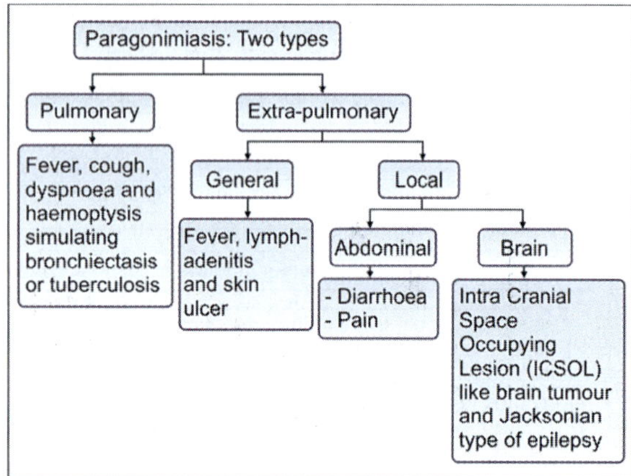

Flow chart-12: Clinical features of *P. westermani*

❖ Laboratory diagnosis:

➢ **Specimens:**
1. **Sputum:**
2. **Stool:** Contains eggs in case of swallowing of sputum.

➢ **Testing methods:**

I. Direct methods

A. **Macroscopy:** For presence of blood.
B. **Microscopy:**
a. **Wet mount:** Bile stained eggs are present as shown in **fig.-17(b).**
b. **Concentration method:**
- Mix the equal volume of sputum with 3-4% NaOH.
- Leave for 10-15 minutes to dissolve the mucus.
- Centrifuge at 2000rpm for 5 minutes.
- Use sediment for eggs examination.

II. Indirect methods

A. **Blood picture:** Eosinophilia present constantly.
B. **Allergic / skin test**: Intradermal test gives immediate type of hypersensitivity.
C. **Serological tests:** IgG & IgM antibodies are present against the antigen of *P. westermani* are detected by ELISA & CFT.
D. **Radiological methods:**
i. **X-ray:** Reveals the abnormal nodular, cystic, ring or infiltrative type shadow.
ii. **CT- scan:** Help to diagnose the pulmonary of cerebral cyst. "Soap bubble" like appearance present in cerebral cyst.

❖ Prevention:

- Eradication of intermediate host (snail & crab / crayfish).
- Prevention of water contamination by the sputum or faeces of case.
- Proper cooking of crab or crayfish & washing of hands after handling such foods.

❖ Treatment:

- Praziquantal (25mg/kg, TDS for 1-2 days) is the drug of choice.
- Bithinol & niclofolan are the other options.

Other pathogenic species of *Paragonimus*

P. mexicanus, P. africanus, P. uterobilateralis, P. heterotremus, P. kellicotti, P. miyazakii, P. philipinensis, P. skrjabini, P. hueitengenesis etc.

Question bank

Case study

1) A young male present with history of cough, haemoptysis, fever & dyspnoea. He took anti-tuberculous treatment for 6 months without sign of improvement. Sputum microscopy revealed the bile stained eggs. Identify the case and answer the following.

a) Name & draw the properly labelled diagram of egg of causative agent.
b) Describe the life cycle of causative agent.
c) Describe the Pathogenicity of causative agent.
d) Describe the lab. diagnosis of causative agent.

Essay/Full question

1) Small intestinal trematodes.
2) Hepatic trematodes.

Short notes

1) Morphology / life cycle / pathogenicity / laboratory diagnosis of *F. buski* or *H. hetrophyes* o *C. sinensis* or *F. hepatica* or *P. westermani.*

Short questions for theory/viva questions

1) Write the scientific name of following parasites.
(a) Ginger worm (b) Dwarf fluke (c) Chinese liver fluke (d) Cat liver fluke (e) Sheep liver fluke (f) Oriental lung fluke
2) What is halzoun?
3) What is liver rot?
4) What is drunken crab? Write its clinical significance.

5) Name the parasites transmitted by ingestion of following foods.
(a) Water chest nut (b) Molluscs (c) Ants (d) Crab

MCQs for chapter review

Classification

1) **Which is not a liver flukes** (PGI, Nov-10)
(a) *Paragonimus* (b) Whip worm (c) *Chlonorchis sinensis* (d) *Gnathestoma spinigerum* (e) *Opisthorchis*

2) **All are inhabitants of liver except** (AI-94)
(a) *F. hepatica* (b) *F. buski* (c) *Chlonorchis sinensis* (d) *Opsthorchis felineus*

3) **Liver is a target organ for** (AIIMS, June-97)
(a) *Fasciola buski* (b) *Paragonimus westermanii* (c) *Chlonorchis sinensis* (d) *Schistosoma haematobium*

Hepatic trematodes

4) **A man on return a country complains of pain in abdomen, jaundice, with increased alkaline phosphatase and conjugated hyperbilirubinemia. USG shows blockage in biliary tree. What could be the cause** (AIIMS, May-09)
(a) *Fasciola buski* (b) *Chlonorchis sinensis* (c) *Strongyloides* (d) *Ancyclostoma*

Pulmonary trematodes

5) **Which organism can be isolated from stool & sputum**
(a) *Paragonimus* (b) *Fasciola* (c) *Chlonorchis* (d) *P carinii*

Answers of MCQs & explanation

1) **(a), (b) & (d)**
- Follow section, **classification (hepatic flukes**) for explanation

2) **(b)**
- Follow section, **classification (intestinal flukes & hepatic flukes**) for explanation

3) **(c)**
- Ooption a, b & c: Follow section, **classification** for explanation
- Option d: *Schistosoma haematobium* is targeting the vesical plexus

4) **(b)**
- Follow section, ***Chlonorchis sinensis* (pathogenicity →complications)** for explanation

5) **(a)**
- Follow **respective section** for explanation
- *P carinii* (now *P jiroveci*) fungus is identified from sputum but not from stool

97 Nematodes: General features and classification

Learning heading & subheadings

- ❖ Synonym:
- ❖ Meaning:
- ❖ Habitat:
- ❖ Morphology:
- ❖ Mode of transmission of nematodes:
- ❖ Life cycle:
- ❖ Classification:

❖ **Synonym:** **Round worm** as they are cylindrical like a tube.

❖ **Meaning:** Nematodes originated from **Nema (Greek) = Thread + edios = appearance,** as they are elongated, unsegmented, cylindrical & tapered at both the ends.

❖ **Habitat:** Intestine & tissues.

❖ **Morphology:**

I. Adult stage

➢ **Shape:** They are elongated, unsegmented, cylindrical & tapered at both the ends. Posterior end of male species is curved or coiled ventrally.

➢ **Size:**
- Great variation in size from smallest (*T. spiralis* & *S. stercoralis*) less than 5mm & longest (*D. medinensis*) about 1 metre in length.
- Male is smaller than female.

➢ **Organs:**

✪ **Cuticle:**
- **Definition:** Body of parasite is covered with acellular layer **called cuticle.**
- **Nature:** It may be smooth, bossed (rough), spiny, or striated.
- **Structure:** From outer to inner it's have following four layers as shown in **fig.-1.**

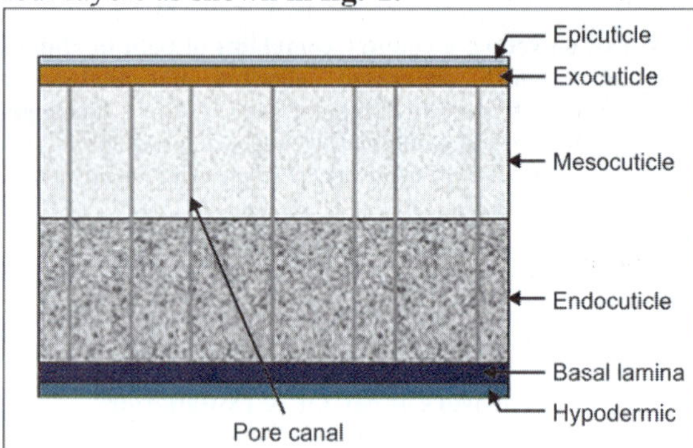

Figure-1: Structure of cuticle

1. Epicuticle.
2. Exocuticle.
3. Mesocuticle.
4. Endocuticle.

- **Functions:** Protection & other metabolic role.
- **Variation:**

1. **Cervical alae:** Wing like expansion of the cuticula near the mouth.
2. **Cervical papillae:** Protuberance of the cuticula near oesophagus.

✪ **Basal lamina (fig.-1):** It separates the cuticle from underlying tissues.

✪ **Body wall musculature:**
- All the muscles are spindle shaped & longitudinally oriented.
- Each cell is divided in to contractile & non-contractile portion.
- Myofibrils are located in the contractile potion, while mitochondria with glycogen granules, nucleus & lipids are located in the non-contractile potion.

✪ **Body cavity:** Present & contains all viscera.

✪ **Gastro Intestinal Tract (GIT): → Fig.-2.**
- It is present with anus so **called complete.**
- It present with oral aperature, mouth cavity, oesophagus, intestine & subterminal anus.
- Mouth cavity contains teeth or cutting plates.
- In case where mouth cavity is absent, the oral aperture is directly continuous with the oesophagus.

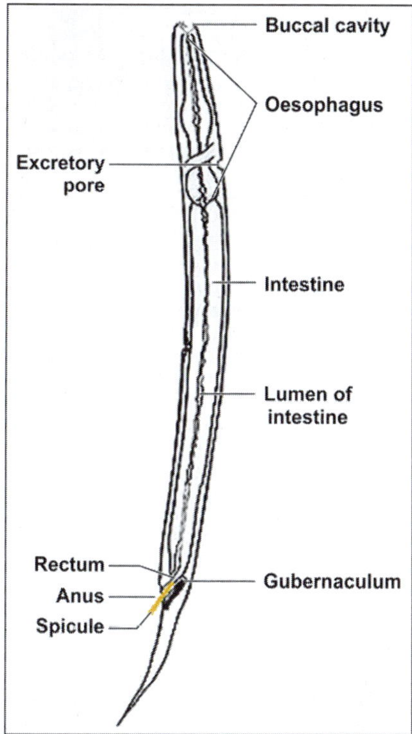

Figure-2: GIT of nematodes

✪ **Excretory system:** Present but rudimentary.

✪ **Nervous system:**

- Present but rudimentary.
- It consists two following parts.

o <u>Commissure</u>: Two major nerve commissure like

1. Circumoesophageal commissure (**fig.-3**): Around oesophagus.
2. Rectal commissure (**fig.-4**): Around rectum.

o <u>Sensory papillae</u>: Following two types & present on the cuticle.

1. Amphids: As shown in **fig.-3.**
2. Phasmids: As shown in **fig.-4.**

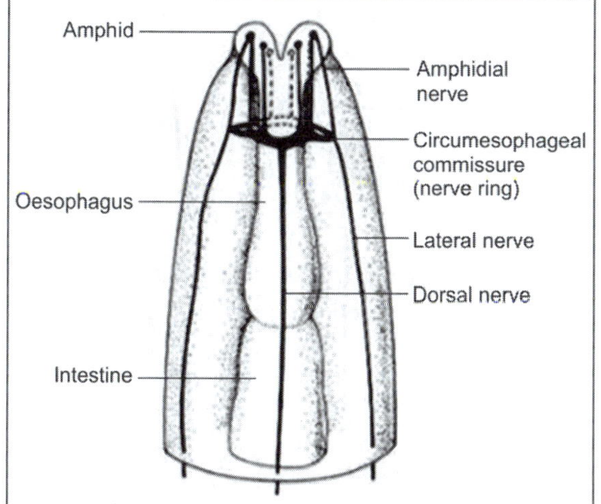

Figure-3: Circumoesophageal commissure & Amphid

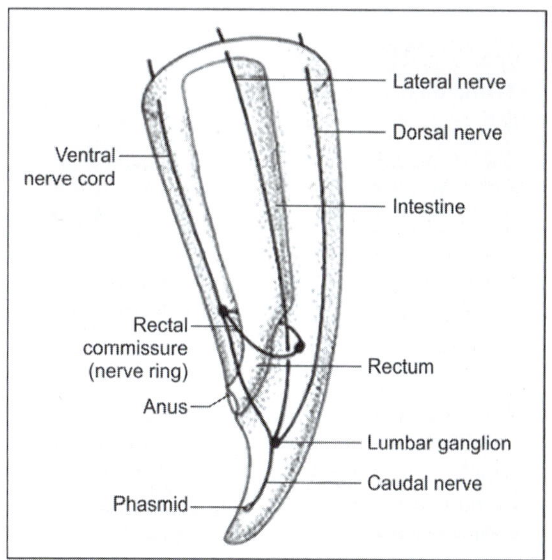

Figure-4: Rectal commissure & phasmid

✪ **Reproductive system:**

- **Definition:** In all nematodes both male & female species are separate so **called diecious.**
- **Features:**

- Highly developed & complete in each individual.
- Reproductive organs lie in body cavity.

- **Reproductive organs:**

A. **Female reproductive organs: → Fig.-5 (a).**

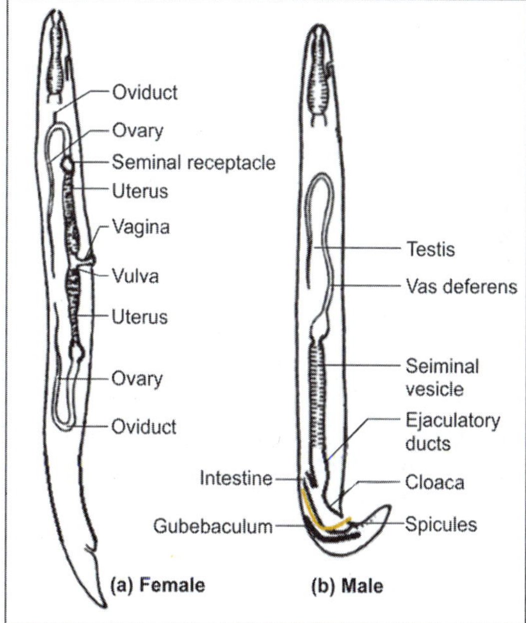

Figure-5: Reproductive system of nematodes

- It is a single or double or multiple convoluted tubes which consists organs like ovary, oviduct, seminal receptacle, uterus, vagina & vulva.
- Genital pore open in the middle of the body or near the mouth.
- When species have two or more tube they unite in a common duct before terminating in to genital pore.

- Female nematodes are divided in following three types based on production of progeny.
1. **Oviparous:** Female laying eggs **called oviparous** like
   - Eggs contains unsegmented embryo: *A. lumbricoides* & *T. trichuria*
   - Eggs contains segmented embryo: *A. duodenale* & *N. americanus.*
   - Eggs contains larva: *E. vermicularis.*
2. **Viviparous:** Female giving birth to larva **called viviparous** like *D. medinensis, W. bancrofti, B. malayi* & *T. spiralis.*
3. **Ovi-viviparous:** Female laying eggs contains rhabditiform larva which immediately hatch out **called ovi-viviparous** like *S. stercoralis.* Rhabditiform larva present in freshly passed stool.

B. Male reproductive organs: → Fig.-5 (b).

- It is a single convoluted tube which differentiated in to testes, vas deferens, seminal vesicle & ejaculatory duct.
- Genital duct forms a common passage with intestine **called cloaca.**
- Accessory copulatory organs: Like
1. **Spicule:** It is rod like & protrucible.
2. **Gubernaculum:** An elevation on the dorsal wall of cloaca which guide the spicule during copulation.
3. **Copulatory bursa (Bursa copulatrix):** Umbrella like expansion of the cuticula surrounding the cloaca of the male nematode of certain species. It is supported by fleshy rays comparable with the ribs of umbrella.

II. Egg stage

➢ **Types of eggs:** Two types as follows.

A. Bile stained eggs: It includes *A. lumbricoides* & *T. trichuria.*

B. Non-bile stained eggs: It includes *A. duodenale, N. americanus* & *E. vermicularis.*

✓ **Note: Other bile stained eggs**

- **Cestodes:**
1. **Pseodophullodean cestodes:** *D. latum.*
2. **Psyclophullodean cestodes:** *T. saginatum, T. solium, E. granulosus* & *D.caninum.*
- **Trematodes:**
1. **Only monoecious trematodes:** *F. buski, H. heterophyes, M. yokogawai, E. ilocanum, E. malayanum, E. revolutum, P. supraryfex, W. watsonis, G. hominis, C. sinensis, O. felineus, F. hepatica, F. gigantica, D. dendriticum* & *P. westermani* (other species also).

III. Larval stage

➢ **Types of larva:** Two types as follows.

A. Rhabditiform larva: Oesophagus is short compared to the length of larva & posterior end is dilated like a bulb as shown in **fig.-6(a).**

B. Filariform larva: Oesophagus is long compared to the length of larva & posterior end is not dilated (no bulb) as shown in **fig.-6(b).**

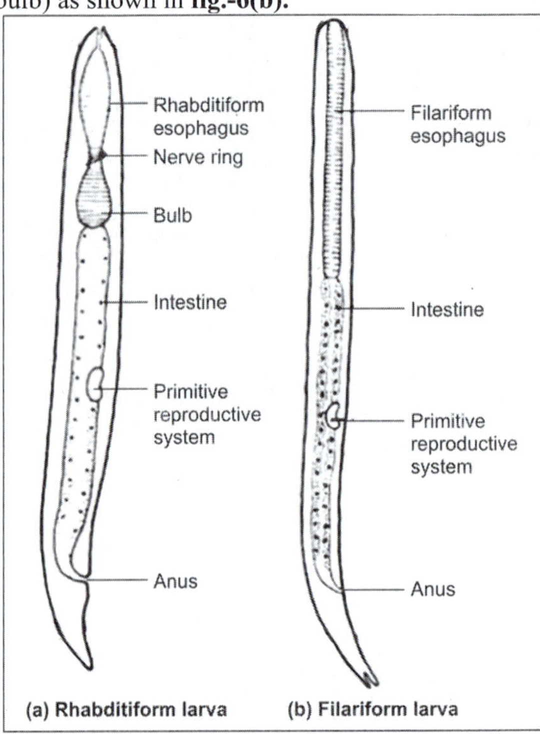

Figure-6: Larvae of nematodes

❖ Mode of transmission of nematodes:

a. Direct transmission:

- **Infective stage:** Filariform larva enters directly via penetrating the skin.
- **Examples:** *A. duodenale, N. americanus* & *S. stercoralis.*

b. Indirect transmission:

1. **By ingestion**
- **Water / food:**
  - **Infective stage:** Embryonated eggs contaminating the food & water.
  - **Examples:** *A. lumbricoides, T. trichuria* & *E. vermicularis.*
- **Pig's flesh:**
  - **Infective stage:** Encysted embryos present in flesh.
  - **Examples:** *T. spiralis.*
2. **By inhalation (air borne):**
   - **Infective stage:** Embryonated eggs present in dust.
   - **Examples:** *A. lumbricoides* & *E. vermicularis*
3. **By vector (vector borne):**
- **Mosquito bite:**
  - **Infective stage:** Microfilariae are present in mosquito.
  - **Examples:** *W. Bancrofti* & *B .malayi* (superfamily Filarioidea).
- **Cyclops ingestion via water:**

- **Infective stage:** Larvae present in cyclops.
- **Examples:** *D. medinensis* (superfamily Dracunculoidea).

❖ Life cycle:

➢ **Superfamily Filarioidea & Dracunculoidea:** Worm pass its life cycle in two different hosts.

I. **Definitive host:** Man who harbours the adult stage

II. **Intermediate hosts:** Arthropod like mosquito for Filarioidea & cyclops for Dracunculoidea who harbours the larval stage.

➢ **Other superfamily of nematodes:**

- Worm passes its life cycle in one host with development in external environment.
- Man is the optimum host in all nematodes except *T. spiralis* where pig is the optimum host & man is the alternative.

❖ Classification:

I. **Systemic classification:** **Follow chapter → Introduction and classification of parasites (section → table-4)** for more details.

II. **Pathological classification:** Following are the pathogenic species & further classified on the basis of habitat.

A. **Intestinal nematodes:**

i. **Small intestinal nematodes:** *T. spiralis, A. lumbricoides, A. duodenale, N. americanus, Trichostrogylus* species, *S. stercoralis* & *C. philippinensis.*

ii. **Large intestinal nematodes:** *T. trichuria* & *E. vermicularis.*

iii. **Arteries & arterioles of ileo- caecal part:** *Angiostrongylus costaricensis.*

B. **Somatic (tissues) nematodes:** Following are the two main types of disease produced by tissue nematodes.

i. **Filariasis:** Filariasis is a broad terminology further classified on the basis of habitat by different species.

a. **Lymphatic filariasis:** *W. bancrofti, B. malayi* & *B. timori.*

b. **Subcutaeous filariasis:** *O. volvulus, L. loa,* & *M. strptocerca.*

c. **Serous cavity filariasis:** *M. perstans* & *M. ozzardi.*

d. **Zoonotic filariasis:** *B. pahangi, D. immitis, D. tenuis* & *D. repens.*

ii. **Other diseases:** Further classified on the basis of habitat by different species.

a. **Diseases in lungs:** Larva of
- *S. stercoralis.*
- *A. lumbricoides.*
- *A. duodenale.*

b. **Diseases in liver:** *C. hepatica.*

c. **Diseases in brain:** *A. cantonensis.*

d. **Diseases in brain & other tissues:** *Gnathostoma* spp.

e. **Diseases in subcutaeous tissues:** *D. medinensis.*

Question bank

Short notes

1) General propertied of nematodes.
2) Bile stained eggs & their morphology.

Short questions for theory/viva questions

1) Nam e accessory copulatory organs in nematodes.
2) Write four name of bile stained eggs.
3) Write the two differences between filariform larvae & rhabditiform larvae.
4) Name the parasite transmitted by arthropod.

MCQs for chapter review

Morphology

1) **Which of the following is viviparous**
(a) *Strongyloides stercoralis* (b) *Trichinella spiralis* (c) *Enterobius* (d) *Ascaris*
2) **Ovi viviparous nematode is**
(a) *Ascaris lumbricoides* (b) *Dracunculus medinensis* (c) *Strongyloides stercoralis* (d) *Enterobius vermicularis*
3) **Rhabditiform larvas in freshly passed stool are seen in**
(a) *Ascaris lumbricoides* (b) *Toxoplasma* (c) *Strongyloides stercoralis* (d) *Enterobius vermicularis*
4) **Which of the following produces bile stained eggs?**
(a) *Ancyclostoma duodenale* (b) *Taenia solium* (c) *Enterobius vermicularis* (d) *Necator americnus*

Mode of transmission of nematodes

5) **Filariform larvae is infective in**
(a) *Enterobius vermicularis* (b) *Ascaris lumbricoides* (c) *Necator americnus* (d) *Trichuris trichuria*

Answers of MCQs & explanation

1) **(b)**
2) **(c)**
3) **(c)**

} Follow section, **morphology (adult stage → female reproductive organs)** for explanation

4) **(b)**

- Follow section, **morphology (egg stage) & note** for explanation

5) **(c)**

- Follow section, **mode of transmission of nematodes (direct transmission)** for explanation

98 Nematodes: Intestinal nematodes

Learning heading & subheadings

Classification:

Small intestinal nematodes

- *Trichenella spiralis*
- *Ascaris lumbricoides*
- Hook worm spp.
- *Trichostrogylus* spp.
- *Strongyloides* spp.
- *Capillaria* spp.

Large intestinal nematodes

- *Trichuris trichuria*
- *Enterobius vermicularis*

Nematodes in arteries & arterioles of ileo- caecal region

- *Angiostrongylus* spp.

Classification:

I. **Systemic classification:** Follow chapter → Introduction and classification of parasites **(section →table-4)** for more details.

II. **Pathological classification:** Following are the pathogenic species & further classified on the basis of habitat in different part of intestine.

i. **Small intestinal nematodes:** *T. spiralis, A. lumbricoides, A. duodenale, N. americanus, Trichostrongylus* species, *S. stercoralis, S. fuelleborni* & *C. philippinensis.*

ii. **Large intestinal nematodes:** *T. trichuria* & *E. vermicularis.*

iii. **Nematodes in arteries & arterioles of ileo- caecal region:** *Angiostrongylus costaricensis*

Small intestinal nematodes

Trichinella spiralis

❖ **Common name:** Trichina worm.

❖ **Meaning:** **Trichos (Greek) = hair + ella (suffix) = spiral**, indicates very thin parasite with spirally coiled larvae.

❖ **History:**

- Tidemann, who 1st discovered the disease in Germany in 1821.
- Later disease has been also defined by Peacock & Own in 1825.
- Larval stage was 1st worked out by Herrick & Janewil in human blood in 1909.

❖ **Geographical distribution:** Common in Europe & USA. Also reported from some parts of Africa, China & Syria but not from India.

❖ **Habitat:** Adult parasite habitat the small intestine & stay for short period, later fertilised female buried in the duodenal or jejuna mucosa & laying the embryo in circulating blood, which ultimately encyst in striated muscles (not smooth or cardiac muscles) of animal (pig or rat) & man.

❖ **Morphology:** Two morphological stages like adult & larval stages. Few important features of parasite are given below. For more details, follow chapter → Nematodes: General features and classification.

I. Adult stage

- **Time of maturation:** Larva transformed to sexually mature adult stage in 2 days in definitive host after ingestion.
- **Size:** Female is larger than male as shown in **fig.-1.**
  - Female: 3-6mm ×0.06mm.
  - Male: 1.4-1.6mm ×0.04mm.
- **Shape:** They are elongated, unsegmented, & cylindrical as shown in **fig.-1.**
- **Life span:**
  - Male die after fertilising the female about one week after infection.
  - Female may live for 4 months.
- **Organs:**
- **Spicule & copulatory bursa:** Absent.
- **Papillae:** Two conspicuous papillae present on either side near the tail end.
- **Type of female:** It is viviparous & laying the embryo.

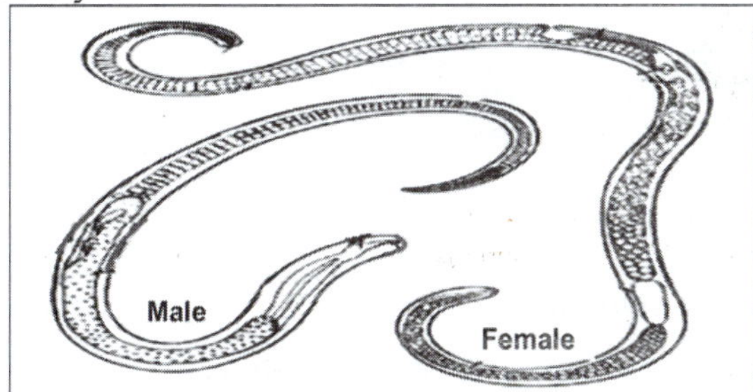

Figure-1: Adult stage of *T. spiralis*

II. Larval stage

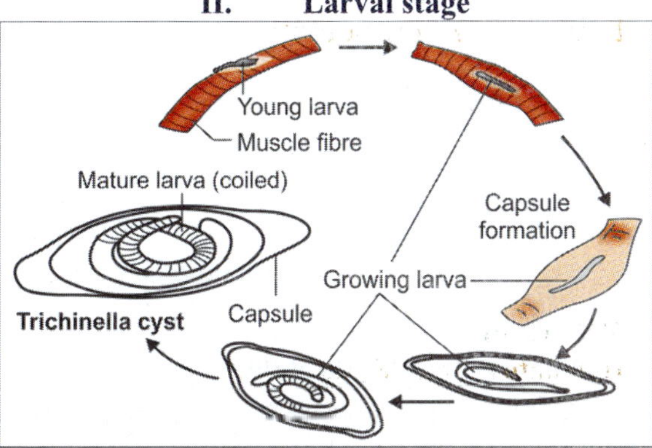

Figure-2: Larval stage of *T. spiralis*

- **Form:** Solid forms of larva are present within a capsule in muscles **called tichinella cyst** as shown in **fig.-2.**
- **Host:**
  - Larvae are present in striated muscles (not smooth or cardiac muscles) like deltoid, biceps, gastrocenemius, diaphragm, intercostals & pectoralis major.
  - Usually one larva is present per cyst, but thousands of larvae are present per gram of muscles.
- **Development of trichinella cyst:** → **Fig.-2**
- **Development of capsule around larva:**
  - Encapsulation of larva begins on 21st day & completed in 3 months.
  - A blunt ellipsoid lemon shaped sheath (0.4-0.25mm) develops around tightly coiled larva.
  - It is due to host reaction.
  - Long axis of capsule is parallel to long axis of muscle fibre.
  - Calcification starts after 6-18 months.
- **Development of larva within capsule:**
  - Initially very small about 100μm×6μm in size & continuously develop in host & achieve the maximum size about 1000μm in 35 day.
  - It is present in coiled form.

❖ Immunity:

- **Acquired immunity:**
  - Experimental removal of adult worms in mice is possible by CMI.
  - Antibodies (IgE) are increased but not protective & useful for serological testing.
- **Hypersensitivity:** Immediate type hypersensitivity developed by antigen from larvae.

❖ Life cycle:

- **Types of host:**
  - Whole cycle is possible in one host only like pig, rat or man (both **definitive** & **intermediate host).**
  - Pig is the optimum host.
  - Change of host is required to continue the cycle.
  - Cycle is continuing between pig to pig or pig to rat or rat to rat.
  - Man is the alternative host & acts as **dead end** host
- **Cycles:** As shown in **flow chart-1 & fig.-3.**

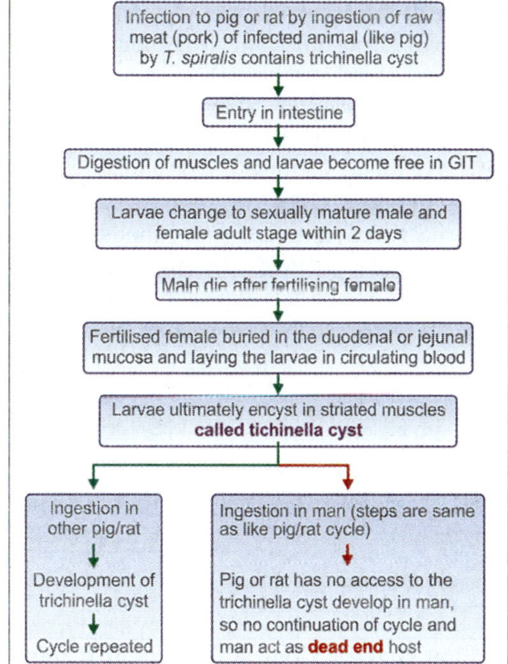

Flow chart-1: Life cycle of *T. spiralis*

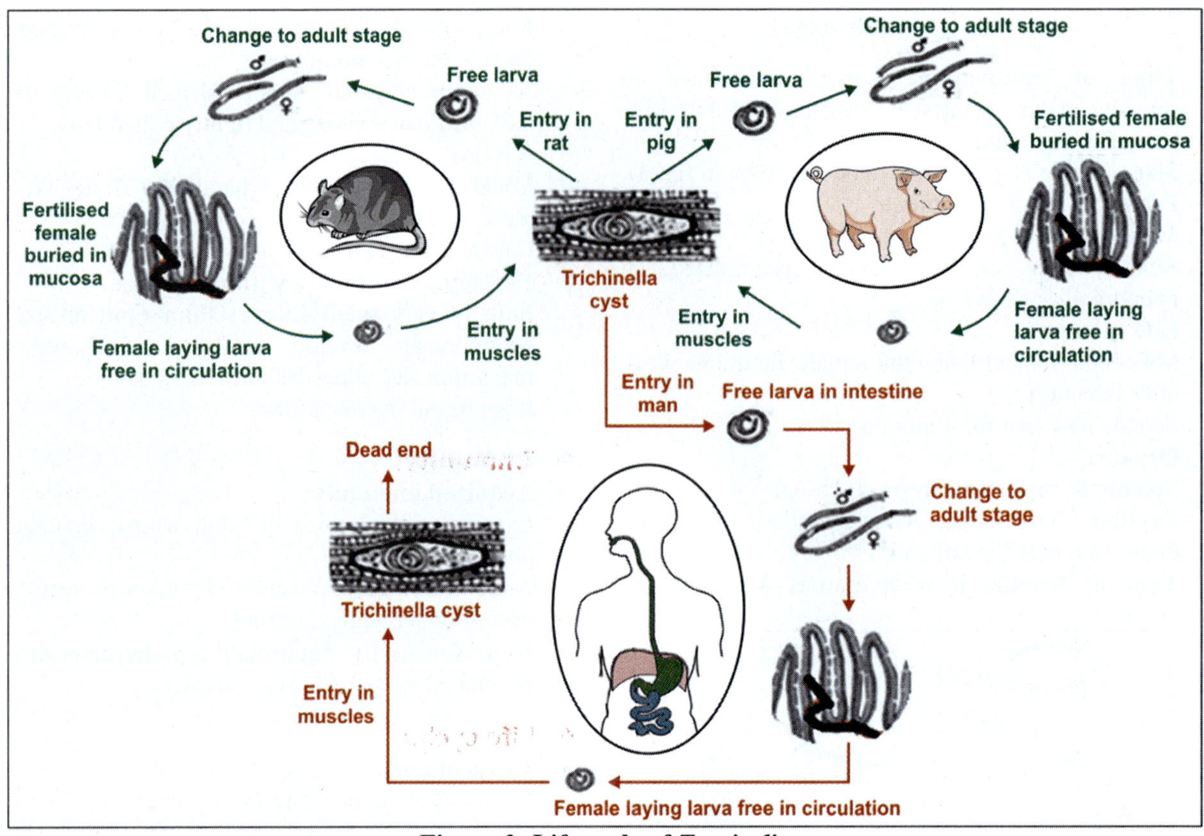

Figure-3: Life cycle of *T. spiralis*

❖ Pathogenicity:

- **Disease name: Called trichinosis.**
- **Synonym:** Also **called trichinelliasis** or **trichiniasis.**
- **Reservoir of infection:** Pig.
- **Source of infection:** Meat of pig contains cyst.
- **Mode of Transmission:** Ingestion of raw meat (muscles) of infected animals.
- **Incubation period:** 5-7 days.
- **Exit form:** Trichinella cyst contains larvae.
- **Infective form:** Trichinella cyst contains larvae.
- **Portal of entry:** GIT.
- **Sites:** Striated muscles (not smooth or cardiac muscles) like deltoid, biceps, gastrocenemius, diaphragm, intercostals & pectoralis major.
- **Clinical features:** Two types (**flow chart-2).**

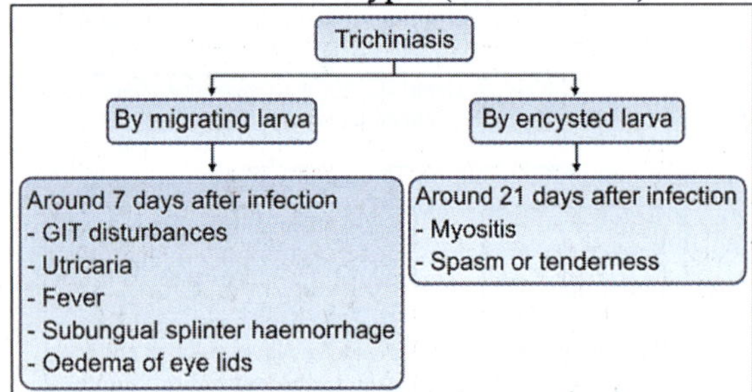

Flow chart-2: Clinical features of *T. spiralis*

- **Complications:**

1. Fatal toxaemia leads to respiratory or cardiac failure.
2. Calcification of cyst.

❖ Laboratory diagnosis:

- **Specimens:**
  - **Muscle biopsy:**
  - **Stool:** For presence of adult stage or for larvae, but rarely recovered.
- **Testing methods:**

I. Direct methods

A. Microscopy:

i. Haematoxylin & Eosin stain:

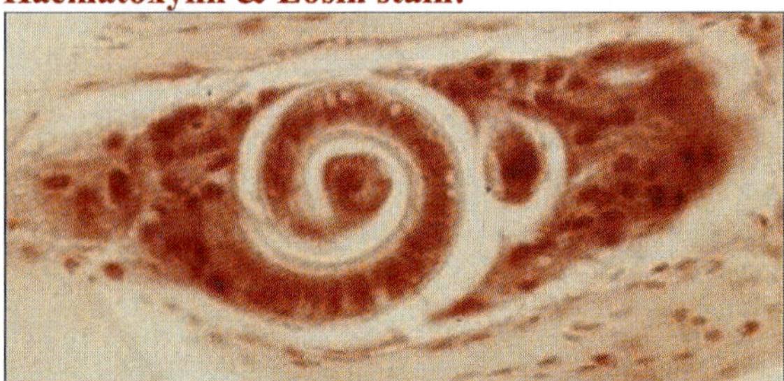

Figure-4: Larva of *T. spiralis* under H & E stain

- Part of muscle tissue is digested in gastric juice.
- Remaining portion is stained by H & E stain to rule out the presence of larvae as shown in **fig.-4.**

ii. Immunofluorescent microscopy:

- By using antigen which is prepared from rat larvae.
- Test is developed by Sadum *et al* in 1962.
- It is positive after 48 days of infection.

II. Indirect methods

A. Blood picture: Eosinophilia (15-50%).

B. Allergic /skin test:

- It based on immediate type of hypersensitivity.
- It is done with Bachman's antigen, prepared from larvae of rabbit's muscles.
- 0.1 ml of 1in 10,000 dilution of antigen is injected intradermally & checks the results.
- Result: Test is positive within 15-20 minutes with development of erythematous patches & persists for 10-20 years.

C. Serological tests: Significant titre developed after 3rd week of infection & persists for 3 years.

i. CFT:

ii. Precipitation test:

iii. Bentonite flocculation test

iv. Latex particle agglutination test: Developed by Innella & Render in 1959.

D. Radiological tests: X-ray shows the calcified cyst.

❖ **Prevention:**

- Proper cooking of pork.
- Best ways is stopping the feeding of pork.

❖ **Treatment:**

- Mild case: Supportive treatment like bed rest, antipyretic & analgesics.
- Moderate case: Albendazole (400mg, BID for 8 days) or mebendazole (200-400mg, TDS) is the drug of choice.
- Severe case: Prednisolone is added to albendazole or mebendazole.

Ascaris lumbricoides

❖ **Common name:** Common round worm.

❖ **Meaning:** Ascaris derived from **Askaris (Greek) = Intestinal worm**.

❖ **History:** Linnaeus, 1758.

❖ **Geographical distribution:** Cosmopolitan.

❖ **Habitat:** Adult parasite habitat in jejunum (85%) & ileum (15%) of man.

❖ **Morphology:** Three morphological stages like adult, egg & larval stages. Few important features of parasite are given below. For more details, follow chapter → Nematodes: General features and classification.

I. Adult stage

➢ **Time of maturation:** Larva (present within ingested egg) transformed to sexually mature adult stage in 6-10 weeks in definitive host after ingestion.

➢ **Colour:** Fresh worms are light brown to pink in colour which gradually changes to white.

➢ **Size:** It is the largest intestinal nematode. Female is larger & stouter than male as shown in **fig.-5.**

- Female: 20-40cm ×3-6mm.
- Male: 15-30cm ×2-4mm.

➢ **Shape:** It is rounded, elongated, unsegmented, & cylindrical as shown in **fig.-5.** Tapers at both the ends and anterior end being thinner than posterior end.

➢ **Life span:**

- Male die after fertilising the female.
- Female may live for less than a year in human.

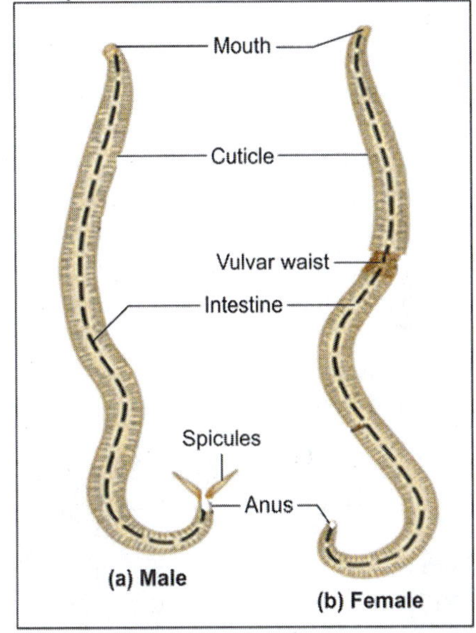

Figure-5: Adult stage of *A. lumbricoides*

➢ **Organs:**

✪ **Mouth:** Opens at the anterior end & possesses three finely toothed lips, one dorsal & two ventral.

✪ **Anterior end:** Same in male & female as shown in **fig.-6.**

✪ **Posterior (tail) end: → Fig.-7**

- **In male:** Curved ventrally in the form of a hook having conical tip.
- **In female:** Neither curved nor pointed but conical & straight.

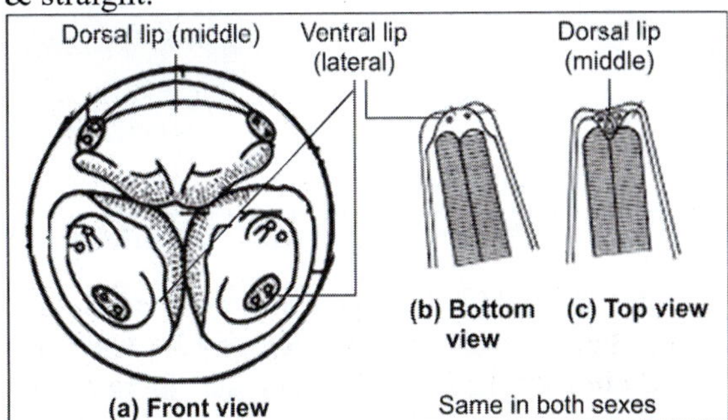

Figure-6: Anterior end of *A. lumbricoides*

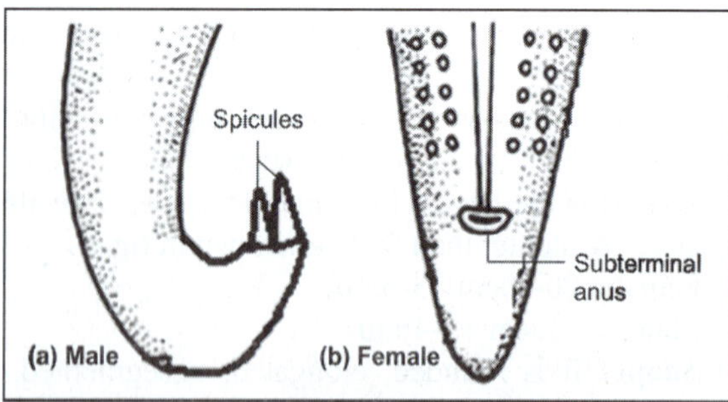

Figure-7: Posterior end of *A. lumbricoides*

- **GIT:**
  - **In male:** Anus with ejaculatory duct opens in cloaca.
  - **In female:** Anus is subterminal & opens directly on the ventral aspect in the form of transverse slit.
- **Reproductive organs:**
  - **In male:** Genital pore opens in to the cloaca.
  - **In female:** Vulva opens at the junction of anterior & middle third of the body on the midventral aspect. This section of the worm is narrower **called vulvar waist.**
- **Spicules:** In male genital pore opens in to the cloaca from which two curved copulatory spicules protrude.

➢ **Type of female:** It is an oviparous & laying the 200,000 eggs /day contains unsegmented embryo.

II. Egg stage

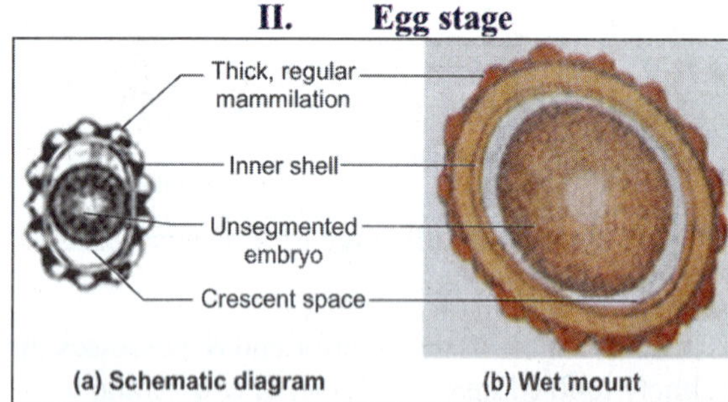

Figure-8: Fertilised eggs of *A. lumbricoides*

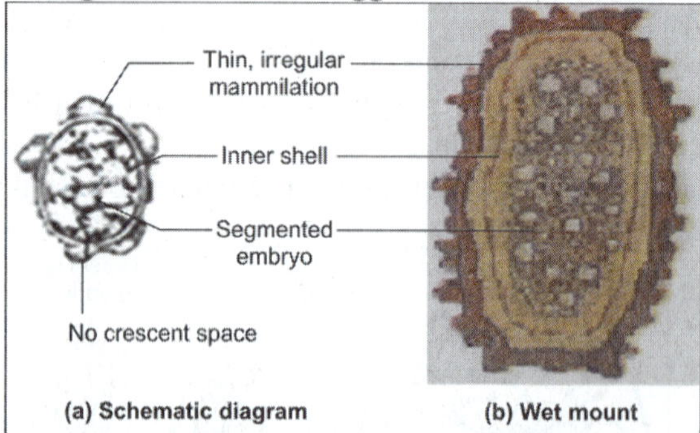

Figure-9: Unfertilised eggs of *A. lumbricoides*

➢ **Types & morphological features:** Female laying two types of eggs, but sometimes 3rd type **called decorticated egg** also present due to removal of albuminous coat.

A. **Fertilised egg:** Laid by fertilise female **(fig.-8).**

- **Shape:** Spherical or oval.
- **Size:** 60-75μm ×40-50μm.
- **Colour**: Golden - brown colour (bile stained).
- **Covering:** Two coverings.
  - i. **Outer:** It is thick protective covering with outer albuminous coat which is thick & thrown in to uniform or regular rugosities or mammillations.
  - ii. **Inner:** It is thin.
- **Embryo:** Unsegmented embryo (nucleus is concealed by large amount of yolk granules) present inside the inner shell & it leaves clear space at both poles of egg **called crescent space** or **called crescent area.**
- **Other features:** Floats in saturated common salt solution.

B. **Unfertilised egg:** Laid by unfertilised female **(fig.-9).**

- **Shape:** Elliptical (elongated).
- **Size:** 80μm ×55μm.
- **Colour**: Yellowish - brown colour (bile stained).
- **Covering:** Two coverings.
  - i. **Outer layer:** It is thick protective covering with outer albuminous coat which is thin & thrown in to irregular rugosities or mammillations.
  - ii. **Inner layer:** It is thin.
- **Embryo:** Segmented embryo present inside the inner shell without leaving clear space at any poles.
- **Other features:** Does not float in saturated common salt solution (heaviest among all helminthic eggs).
- **Clinical significance:** Its presence indicates that host is harbouring only female or mating between male & female has not been occurred.

C. **Decorticated egg:** Sometimes both fertilise **(fig.-10)** & unfertilise **(fig.-11)** eggs can lose albumin coat **called decorticated egg.**

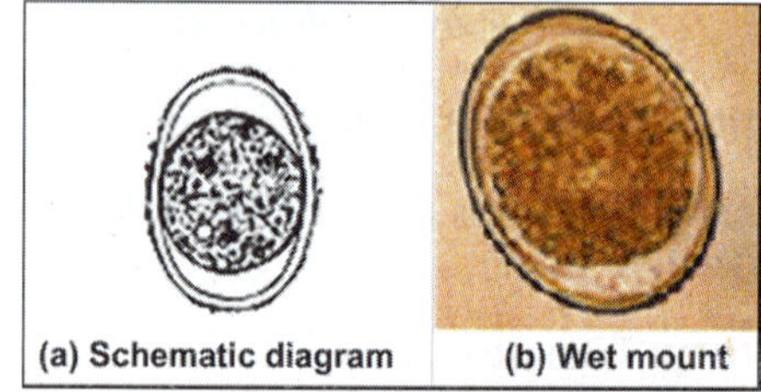

Figure-10: Fertilised –decorticated eggs of *A. lumbricoides*

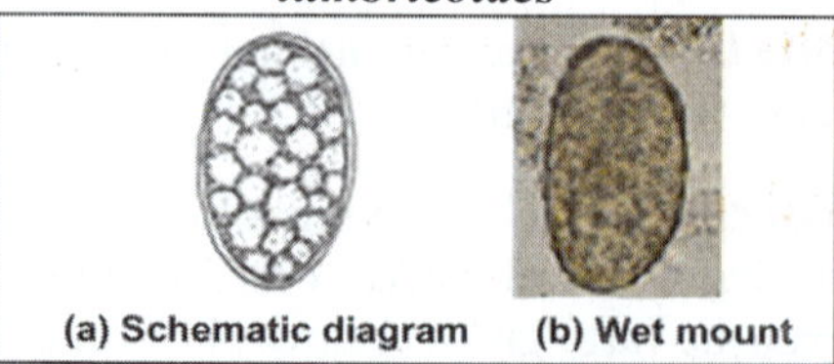

Figure-11: Unfertilised –decorticated eggs of *A. lumbricoides*

➢ **Differences between fertilised & unfertilised eggs of *A. lumbricoides*: →Table-1**

Features	Fertilise egg	Unfertilise egg
Figure	Fig.-8	Fig.-9
Size	60-75μm ×40-50μm	80μm ×55μm
Shape	Oval/spherical	Elliptical/elongated
Albuminous coat	Thick & regular rugosities	Thin & irregular rugosities
Embryo	Unsegmented	Segmented
Crescent space	Present	Absent
Common salt solution	Float	Does not float

Table-1: Differences between fertilised & unfertilised eggs of *A. lumbricoides*

III. Larval stage

➢ **Form:**

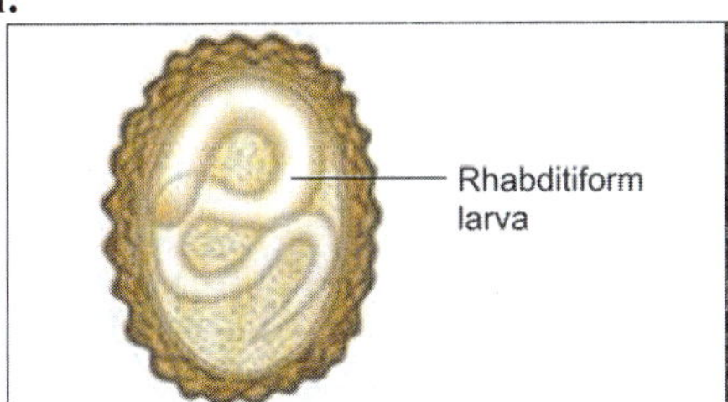

Figure-12: Larva of *A. lumbricoides*

- Rhabditiform larva developed from the unsegmented embryo within the egg shell (**fig.-12**) in 10-14 days depending on the humidity & atmospheric conditions.
- Egg containing larva is infective to man.
- On ingestion egg shell rupture to release the rhabditiform larva in jejunum.

➢ **Host:** It develops over the soil (outside the human).

➢ **Size**: 0.25mm ×14μm.

❖ Immunity:

- **Acquired immunity:**
  - Protective antibodies are developed against antigens of migrating larva which are released during moulting stage.
  - Antibodies lower the worm burden.
  - Antibodies are diagnosed by CFT or precipitation based tests.
- **Hypersensitivity:** It develops hypersensitivity reaction detected by increase in eosinophilic count & skin (**scratch**) test.

❖ Life cycle:

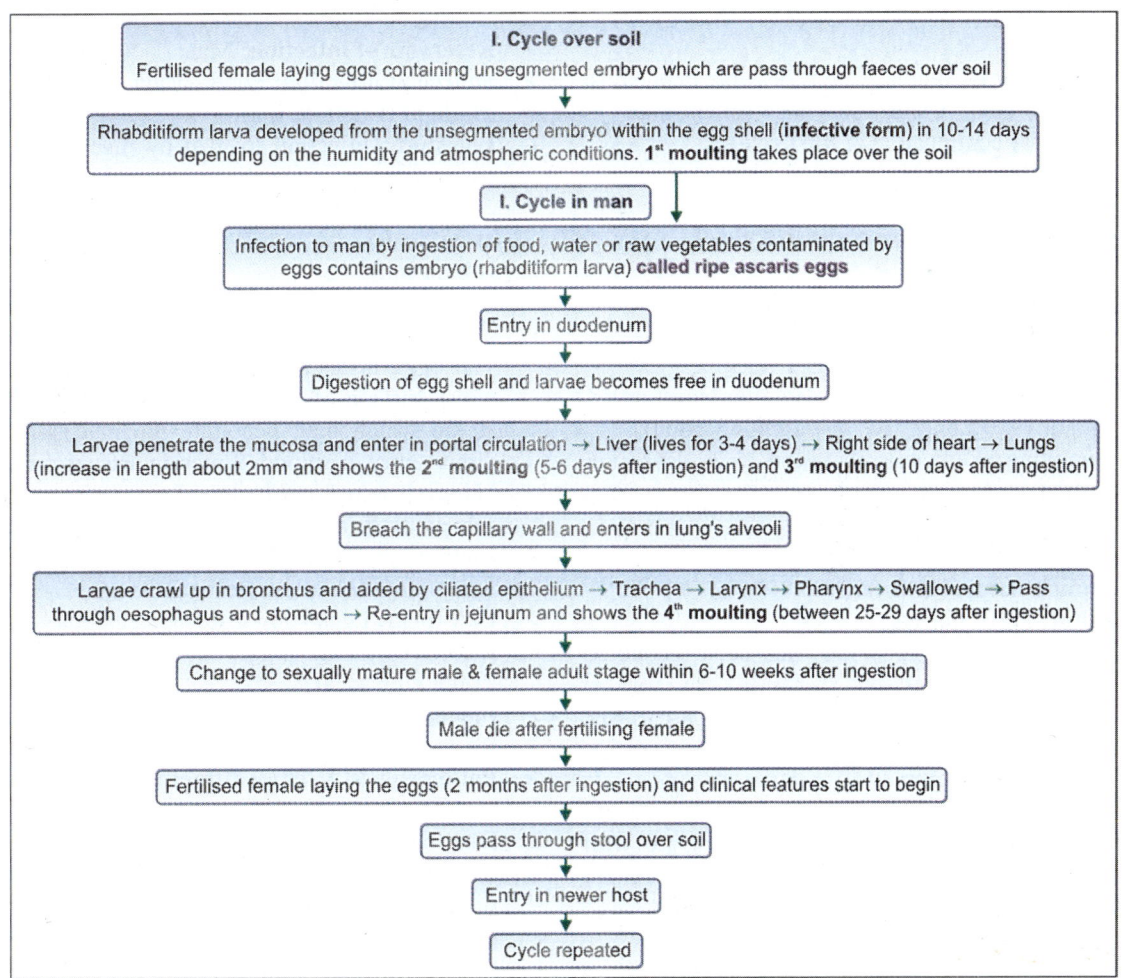

I. Cycle over soil
Fertilised female laying eggs containing unsegmented embryo which are pass through faeces over soil

↓

Rhabditiform larva developed from the unsegmented embryo within the egg shell (**infective form**) in 10-14 days depending on the humidity and atmospheric conditions. 1st **moulting** takes place over the soil

↓

I. Cycle in man

Infection to man by ingestion of food, water or raw vegetables contaminated by eggs contains embryo (rhabditiform larva) **called ripe ascaris eggs**

↓

Entry in duodenum

↓

Digestion of egg shell and larvae becomes free in duodenum

↓

Larvae penetrate the mucosa and enter in portal circulation → Liver (lives for 3-4 days) → Right side of heart → Lungs (increase in length about 2mm and shows the 2nd **moulting** (5-6 days after ingestion) and 3rd **moulting** (10 days after ingestion)

↓

Breach the capillary wall and enters in lung's alveoli

↓

Larvae crawl up in bronchus and aided by ciliated epithelium → Trachea → Larynx → Pharynx → Swallowed → Pass through oesophagus and stomach → Re-entry in jejunum and shows the 4th **moulting** (between 25-29 days after ingestion)

↓

Change to sexually mature male & female adult stage within 6-10 weeks after ingestion

↓

Male die after fertilising female

↓

Fertilised female laying the eggs (2 months after ingestion) and clinical features start to begin

↓

Eggs pass through stool over soil

↓

Entry in newer host

↓

Cycle repeated

Flow chart-3: Life cycle of *A. lumbricoides*

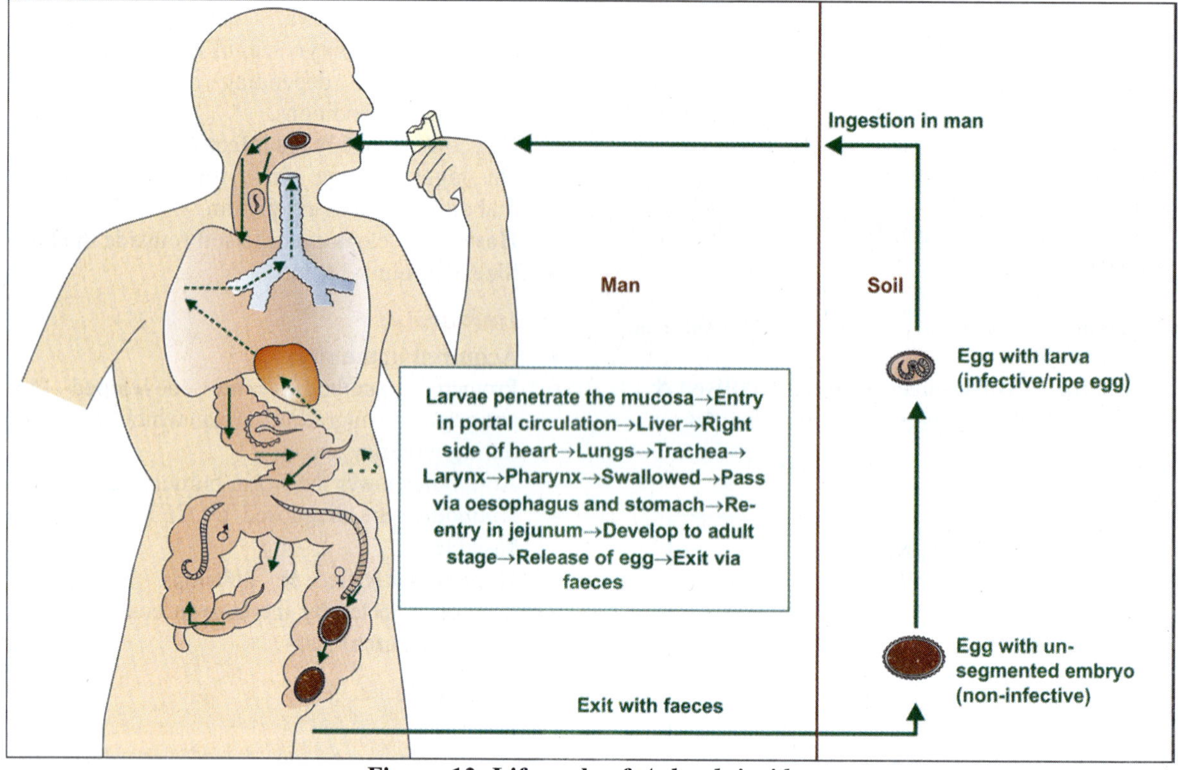

Figure-13: Life cycle of *A. lumbricoides*

➢ **Hosts:**

I. **Definitive host:** Whole cycle is possible in one host only like man. Change of host (other man) is required for continuation of life cycle.

II. **Intermediate host:** Not required.

➢ **Cycles:** Following two types of cycle.

I. **Cycle over soil:** } **Flow chart-3 & fig.-13.**

II. **Cycle in man:**

➢ **Moulting:** Larvae produce the total four moulting at following places.

- 1st moulting → Outside the host over soil.
- 2nd moulting →Lungs (5th -6th day after ingestion).
- 3rd moulting →Lungs (10th day after ingestion).
- 4th moulting → Intestine (between 25-29 days after ingestion).

✓ **Notes: *Ascaris suum***

- **Common name:** Pig ascaris.
- **Habitat:** Pig & gorilla.
- **History:** Eggs of pig ascaris has been recovered from human sources, but it has no any role in pathology & epidemiology of human ascariasis. Crew & Smith (1971) reported a child case that passed the adult worm.
- **Morphology:** Triangular teeth (described by Sprent in 1972) while in *A. lumbricoides* they are with concave sides. It is the only way to differentiate human & pig ascaris.

❖ Pathogenicity:

➢ **Disease name: Called ascariasis.**

➢ **Reservoir of infection:** Man.

➢ **Source of infection:** Food –water.

➢ **Mode of transmission:**

1. **Ingestion:** Infection to man by ingestion of food, water or raw vegetables contaminated by eggs contains embryo (rhabditiform larva) **called ripe ascaris eggs.**
2. **Inhalation:**

- Desiccated eggs in the dust are inhaled & reach to pharynx.
- The eggs instead of swallowed, it may hatch on moist surface of upper air passage & release the larvae which may penetrate the mucosa & takes direct entry in blood. Enter in tissues like brain, kidneys, spinal cord etc. where they are unable achieve the maturity & most of them are destroyed.

➢ **Incubation period:** 60-75 days (by adult stage). Symptoms start after releasing the eggs.

➢ **Exit form:** Eggs with unsegmented embryo.

➢ **Infective form:** Eggs with rhabditiform larva **called ripe ascaris eggs.**

➢ **Portal of entry:** GIT

➢ **Sites:** Jejunum (85%) & ileum (15%).

➢ **Pathogenesis & clinical features:** Divided in two categories.

I. **Due to migrating larvae:**

A. **Lungs:**

- It produces the fever, cough & dyspnoea **called Loeffler's syndrome** or **eosinophilic pneumonia.**
- Sputum is blood tinged may contain larvae & CL crystals.

- Symptoms cleared within 1-2 weeks, however sometimes it may be fatal.

B. General:
- Utricarial rash.
- Eosinophilia (20%).
- In heavy infection larvae enter in blood then to organs where they are destroyed or produce the local symptoms **called visceral larvae migrans.**
- They are also excreted in urine in heavy infection.

II. Due to adult stage: As worm habitat the jejunum, the symptoms are mostly related to GIT.

A. Spoliative actions:

i. Protein Energy Malnutrition (PEM): Parasite required high protein & vitamin rich diet; this effect may contribute to develop Protein Energy Malnutrition (PEM) in host.

ii. Vitamin A deficiency: Causing night blindness.

iii. Anti-enzymatic actions:
- **Types:** Following two types.

a. Anti peptic:

b. Anti tryptic:
- **Effects:** Following two types.
- It protects the worm from digestion by enzymes.
- Reduces the absorption of nutritional materials (malabsorption) & develop the malnutrition.

B. Toxic actions: It is due liberation of toxic fluid **called ascaron** or **ascarase**. It is albumoses (proteose) in nature & produces the following features.
- Typhoid like fever.
- Utricaria.
- Oedema of face.
- Conjunctivitis.
- Irritation of upper air passage.

C. Mechanical actions: Following two types.

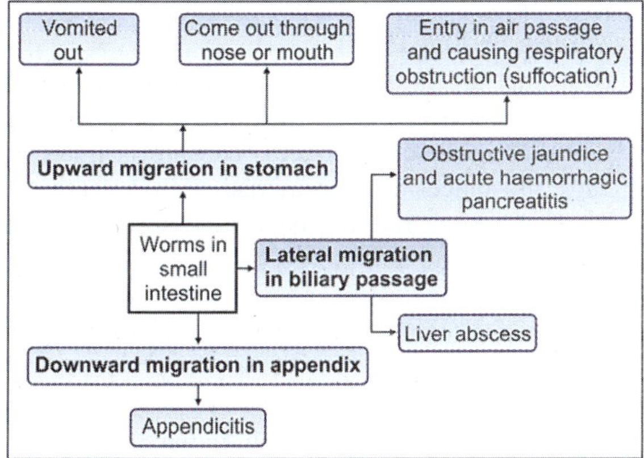

Flow chart-4: Features of ectopic ascariasis

i. Local:
- Intussusception.
- Ulcer in intestinal mucosa.
- Multiple adult parasites can produce the intestinal obstruction mostly in young children because of small size of intestinal lumen.

ii. Ectopic ascariasis (wanderlust): From small intestine it migrates to distant sites **called ectopic ascariasis** as shown in **flow chart-4.**

❖ Laboratory diagnosis:

➤ **Specimens:**
- **Stool:** For presence of adult stage or eggs. Administration of anthelmintic treatment may expuled the worms on stool.
- **Vomitus:** For presence of adult stage.
- **Bile:** Obtained by duodenal intubation for egg stage.
- **Sputum or gastric washing:** For larval stage.

➤ **Testing methods:**

I. Direct methods

A. Macroscopic examination: Of stool & vomitus for presence of adult stage.

B. Microscopy: For presence of eggs & larvae.

i. Wet mount by using normal saline & iodine: It shows the bile stained (brown colour) fertilised/unfertilised/decorticated eggs as shown in **fig.-8(b), 9(b), 10(b) &11(b).**

ii. Concentration technique:
- Useful in case of negative result by wet mount method.
- Unfertilised eggs do not float in common salt solution while fertilise can.

II. Indirect methods

A. Blood picture: Eosinophilia (20%).

B. CL crystals: Present in sputum.

C. Allergic / skin test: Called scratch test.
- Positive with variable results.
- It is done with *Ascaris* antigen.

D. Serological tests: Helpful in extra intestinal ascariasis like Loeffler's syndrome. *Ascaris* antibodies can be detected by

i. CFT.

ii. Precipitation test.

iii. IHA test.

iv. ELISA.

E. Radiological tests: Presence of *Ascaris* has been detected by barium emulsion, which being ingested by the worm within 4-6 hours & produce string like shadow or gut in gut appearance.

❖ Prevention:
- Prevention of faecal contamination of soil, water & food.
- Washing of vegetable before eating.
- *Ascaris* eggs are highly resistant to & can be killed by treating the vegetable with 200ppm of iodine for 15 min. It also kills the larvae.

❖ Treatment:
- Pyrental pamoate: 11mg/kg OD maximum 1 g. Safe in pregnancy.

- Albendazole: 400mg with single dose.
- Mebendazole: 200 mg for 3days or 500 mg single dose.
- Ivermectin: 150-200mg/kg single dose.
- Latter 3 are not safe in pregnancy.
- Partial obstruction are treated with IV fluid, nasogastric suction & piperizine.
- Complete obstruction required surgery.

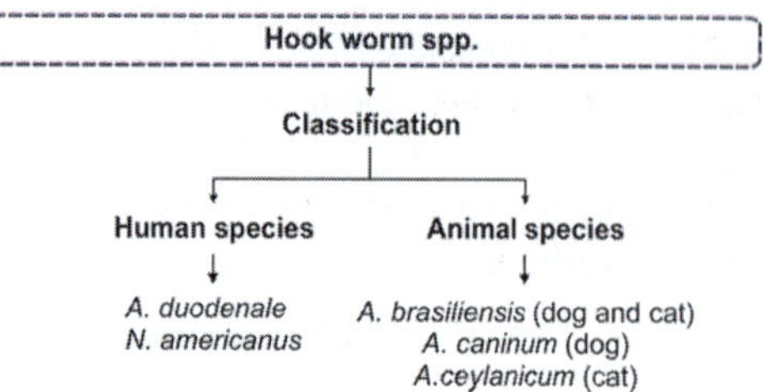

Ancyclostoma duodenale

❖ **Common name:** Old world hook worm.

❖ **Meaning:** **Ankylos (Greek) = hooked + stoma (Greek) = mouth** as anterior end of worm is bent slightly dorsally like hook hence **called hook worm.**

❖ **History:**
- Parasite was first discovered by Italian physician Angelo Dubini in 1838.
- Mode of transmission, life cycle & pathogenesis was worked out by looss in 1898.

❖ **Geographical distribution:** It is widely distributed in all tropical & subtropical countries.

❖ **Habitat:** Adult parasite habitat in jejunum, rare in duodenum & rarely in ileum (jejunum > duodenum > ileum) of man.

❖ **Morphology:** Three morphological stages like adult, egg & larval stages. Few important features of parasite are given below. For more details **follow chapter → Nematodes: General features and classification.**

I. Adult stage

➢ **Time of maturation:** Larva transformed to sexually mature adult stage in 3-4 weeks in definitive host after injection.
➢ **Colour:** It is greyish white in colour.
➢ **Size:** Female is larger than male (**fig.-14).**
- Female: 12.5mm ×0.6mm.
- Male: 8mm ×0.45mm.

➢ **Shape:** It is rounded, elongated, unsegmented, & cylindrical as shown in **fig.-14.**
➢ **Life span:** Adult worm lives about 3-4 years in human.

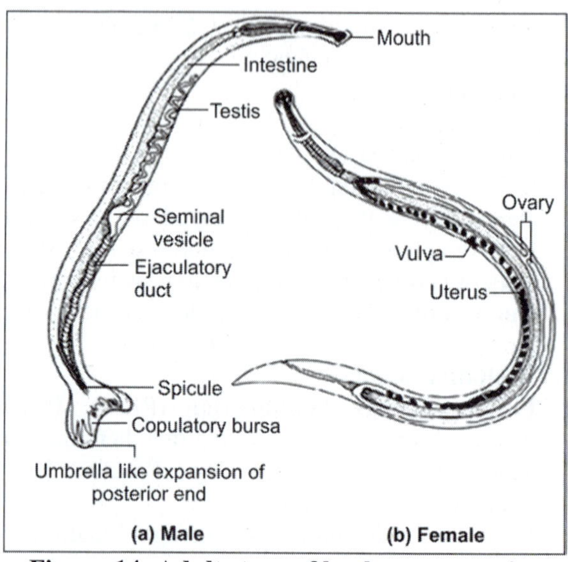

Figure-14: Adult stage of hook worm species

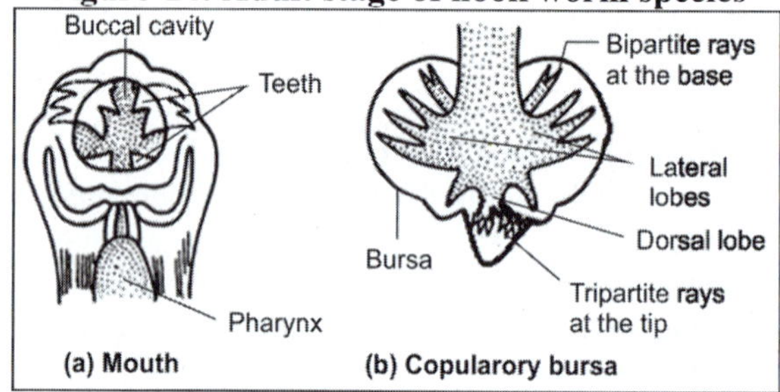

Figure-15: Mouth & bursa of *A. duodenale*

➢ **Organs:**

✪ **Anterior end (fig.-14):** It bent slightly dorsally like hook in the direction of general body curvature.

✪ **Posterior (tail) end: → Fig.-14**
- **In male:** Expanded in umbrella like fashion (copulatory bursa).
- **In female:** Tapering & not expanded.

✪ **Mouth: → Fig.-15 (a)**
- Oral aperture is not terminal but directed towards the dorsal surface.
- Large & conspicuous buccal capsule is lined with hard substances & is provided with 6 teeth from that 4 are hook like on the ventral surface & 2 are knob like (triangular plates) on the dorsal surface.

✪ **GIT:** Contains five glands, one of them is oesophageal gland which secretes the anticoagulant substances.

✪ **Reproductive organs:**
- **In male:** Genital pore opens in to the cloaca.
- **In female:** Genital pore opens at the junction of posterior & middle third of the body, owing to the position of genital pore worms assume the Y-shape appearance during copulation as shown in **fig.-16**.

✪ **Copulatory bursa [fig.-15 (b)]:** Consists of three lobes & each lobe contains chitinous rays (total 13 rays).
- **One dorsal lobe:**

- Contains 3-rays like 1 dorsal & 2 externodorsal.
- Rays are present at tip & **called tripartite.**

• **Two lateral lobes:**

- Contains 10-rays like 3 lateral pairs & 2 ventral pairs.
- Rays are present at base & **called bipartite.**

➢ **Type of female:** It is an oviparous & laying the 25,000-30,000 eggs /day & 15-18 million eggs in whole life. Eggs contains segmented embryo.

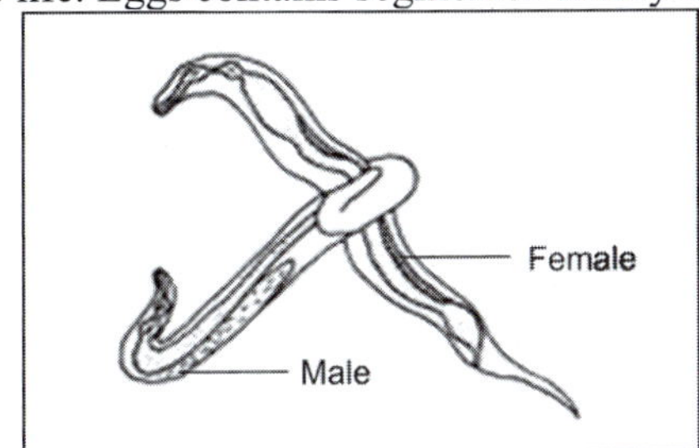

Figure-16: Y-shape appearance during copulation

II. Egg stage

➢ **Morphological features:** Laid by fertilise female **(fig.-17).**

✪ **Shape:** Elliptical or oval.

✪ **Size:** 65µm ×40µm.

✪ **Colour**: Colourless (non-bile stained).

✪ **Covering:** Covered by thin hyaline membrane **called egg shell.**

✪ **Embryo:**

- Contains embryo with four segments **called blastomeres.**
- Clear space present between shell & blastomeres.

✪ **Other features:** Floats in saturated common salt solution.

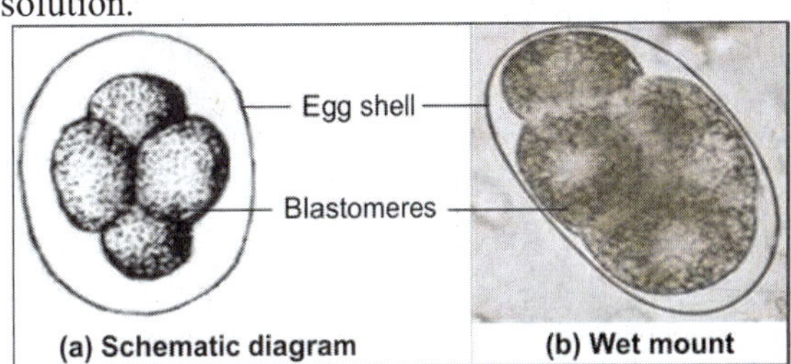

Figure-17: Eggs of *A. duodenale*

III. Larval stages

➢ **Form:** Two forms. **Follow chapter → Nematodes: General features and classification** for more details.

A. Rhabditiform larva:

- Rhabditiform larva developed from the segmented embryo within the egg shell in 2 days.
- It is 250 µm in length & releases over soil on hatching of egg.
- Moults twice on 3rd & 5th day & changes to filariform larva.
- Oesophagus: Bulbous.

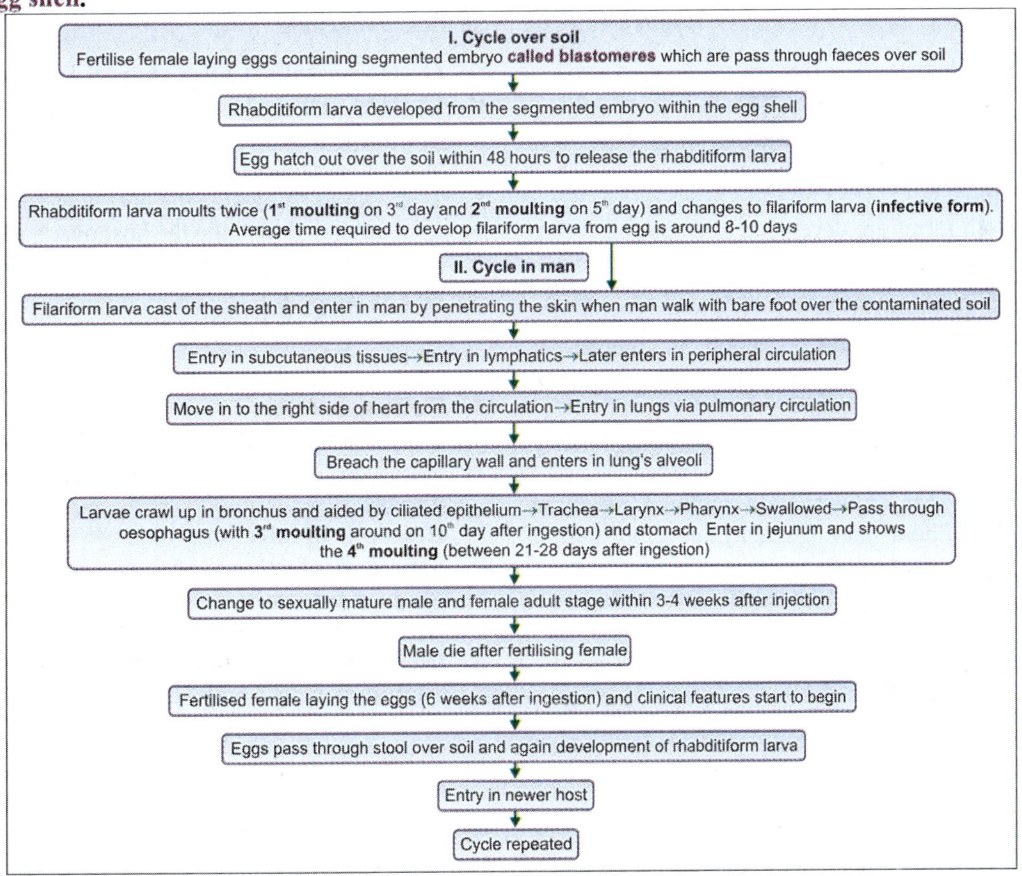

I. Cycle over soil
Fertilise female laying eggs containing segmented embryo called blastomeres which are pass through faeces over soil
Rhabditiform larva developed from the segmented embryo within the egg shell
Egg hatch out over the soil within 48 hours to release the rhabditiform larva
Rhabditiform larva moults twice (1st moulting on 3rd day and 2nd moulting on 5th day) and changes to filariform larva (infective form). Average time required to develop filariform larva from egg is around 8-10 days
II. Cycle in man
Filariform larva cast of the sheath and enter in man by penetrating the skin when man walk with bare foot over the contaminated soil
Entry in subcutaneous tissues→Entry in lymphatics→Later enters in peripheral circulation
Move in to the right side of heart from the circulation→Entry in lungs via pulmonary circulation
Breach the capillary wall and enters in lung's alveoli
Larvae crawl up in bronchus and aided by ciliated epithelium→Trachea→Larynx→Pharynx→Swallowed→Pass through oesophagus (with 3rd moulting around on 10th day after ingestion) and stomach Enter in jejunum and shows the 4th moulting (between 21-28 days after ingestion)
Change to sexually mature male and female adult stage within 3-4 weeks after injection
Male die after fertilising female
Fertilised female laying the eggs (6 weeks after ingestion) and clinical features start to begin
Eggs pass through stool over soil and again development of rhabditiform larva
Entry in newer host
Cycle repeated

Flow chart-5: Life cycle of *A. duodenale*

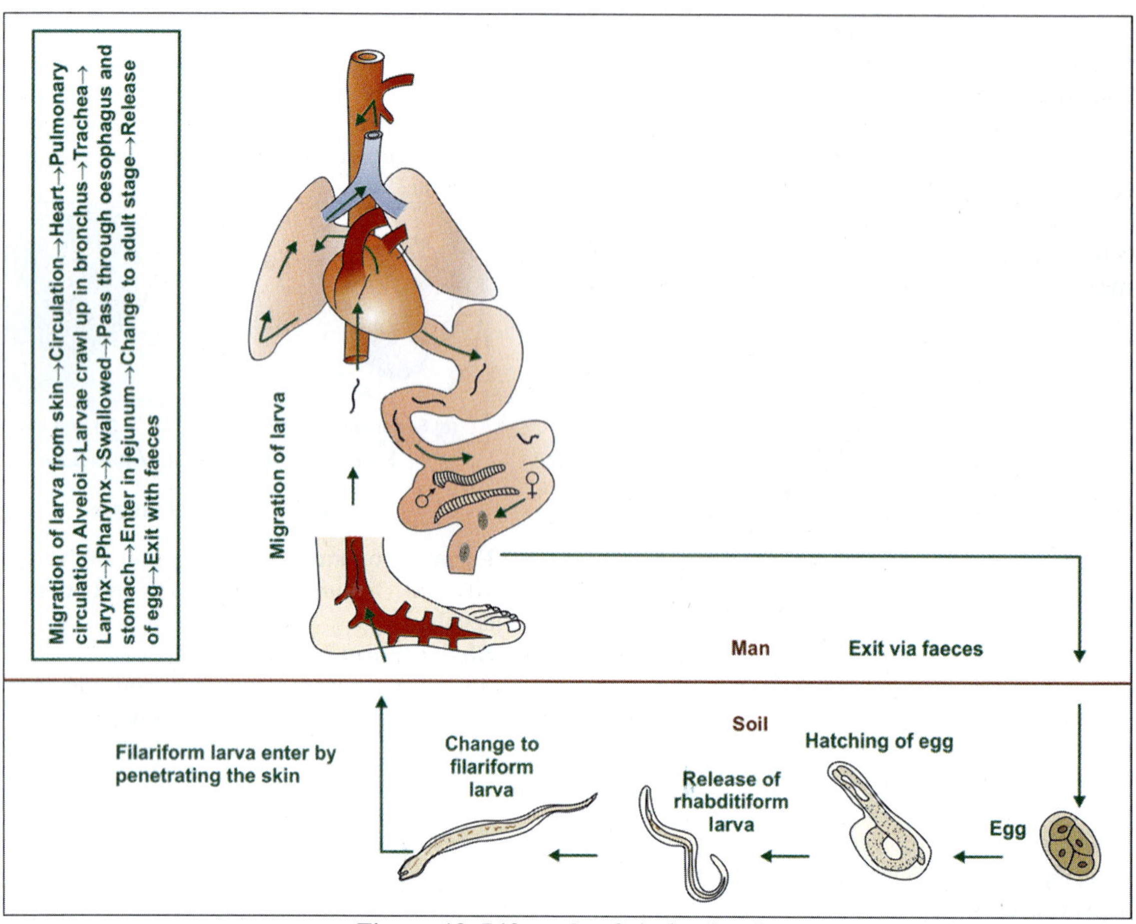

Figure-18: Life cycle of *A. duodenale*

B. Filariform larva:
- It is 500-600 μm in length.
- It is an infective stage & develops within 8-10 days.
- Oesophagus: Not bulbous.
- Tail: Pointed tail.

➤ **Host:** Both forms are developed over the soil.

❖ Immunity:

- **Acquired immunity:**
- Small repeated natural infection in human & experimental infection in dog by *A. caninum* may develop complete immunity.
- Asymptomatic patients may acts as carrier & may develop partial immunity.
- In endemic area patients with minimal intestinal infection without anaemia may develop partial immunity.
- Patients with heavy intestinal infection with anaemia may fail to develop resistance.

❖ Life cycle:

➤ **Hosts:**

I. **Definitive host:** Whole cycle is possible in one host only like man. Change of host (other man) is required for continuation of life cycle.

II. **Intermediate host:** Not required.

➤ **Cycles:** Following two types of cycle.

I. **Cycle over soil:** } **Flow chart-5 & fig.-18.**
II. **Cycle in man:** }

➤ **Moulting:** Larvae produce the total four moulting at following places.
- 1st moulting → outside the host over soil (3rd day).
- 2nd moulting → outside the host over soil (5th day).
- 3rd moulting → oesophagus (around on 10th day after ingestion).
- 4th moulting → Intestine (between 21-28 days after ingestion).

❖ Pathogenicity:

➤ **Disease name:** **Called ancyclostomiasis.**

➤ **Synonym:** Also **called uncinariasis** or **hook worm disease.**

➤ **Reservoir of infection:** Man.

➤ **Source of infection:** Soil.

➤ **Mode of transmission:**

I. **Direct:**

A. **Direct contact of sole with contaminated soil:**
- Filariform larvae enter in man by penetrating the skin when man walk with bare foot over the contaminated soil.
- Common entry points are:

1. Thin skin between toes.
2. Dorsum of feet.

3. Inner side of soles.

B. Direct contact of hands with contaminated soil: It is possible in gardeners & miners.

C. Direct contact of any part of skin with contaminated soil: Filariform larvae can penetrate the any part of skin which is thin.

II. Indirect:

A. Ingestion: →Water borne

- Ingestion of water contaminated by filariform larvae can allow the infection.
- Infection by this route is very rare.
- Okamoto (1961) & Higo (1962) have demonstrated that filariform larvae can develop in to adult stage without lung passage when swallowed.

➤ **Exit form:** Egg contains blastomeres.

➤ **Infective form:** Filariform larvae.

➤ **Portal of entry:** Skin.

➤ **Sites:** Adult parasite habitat in jejunum, rare in duodenum & rarely in ileum.

➤ **Pathogenesis & clinical features:** Divided in two categories.

I. Due to migrating larva:

A. Skin:

i. At the site of entry:

- Lesion **called ground itch** or **ancyclostome dermatitis** or **itchy dermatitis.**
- It is characterised by severe itching with development of erythematous popular rash.
- Self limiting lesion lasting for 2-4 weeks.
- More common with *N. americanus* than *A. duodenale*.

ii. In between the layers of skin:

- Condition **called cutaneous larva migrans** or **creeping eruption.**
- It is characterised by reddish itchy papule along the path traversed by them.
- Larvae of animal species can't penetrate below the level of stratum germinatum of skin & they can migrate in between the layers of skin in aimless manner for several weeks or months or years (up to 2 years). They form the tunnel like structure where roof has been formed by stratum germinatum & floor by stratum cornium.
- Larvae migrate very slowly at speed of 1-2 cm/day.
- Human species can enter in to the circulation, while animal species can die.
- Path left by larvae becomes dry & crusty.
- More common with animal hook worm species than human hook species.
- Maplestone had observed such lesion in Indian tea-garden coolies due to larvae of *N. americanus* in 1933.

B. Lungs: Bronchitis & bronchopneumonia may occur when larvae enter in alveolar space after breaking the pulmonary capillaries.

C. General: Marked eosinophilia.

II. Due to adult stage: Worm attaches to the intestinal mucosa by powerful buccal capsule & produces the following effects.

A. Acute infection: Produce intestinal symptoms.

- Dyspepsia.
- Epigastric tenderness simulating duodenal ulcer
- Perverted taste for earth, mud of lime **called geophagy** or **pica.**
- Constipation or fatty diarrhoea (steatorrhoea) with unknown pathogenicity.
- Pigmentation of mucosa at the bleeding points after long time.
- Achlorhydria or hypoacidity.
- Worms found to be attached to the mucosa, if intestinal examination done within 3 hours of death of patients & free in lumen, when examination delayed.

B. Chronic infection: Produce anaemia with following features.

✪ **Types & mechanisms of anaemia:**

i. Iron deficiency (hypochromic microcytic) anaemia: It is due to following actions of parasites.

- **Spoliative:** Withdrawal of blood by worms as a diet. Worm thrives on plasma (main source of nutrition) & RBCs passes out from the worm practically unchanged in to the lumen of host's intestine.
- **Mechanical:**

- Chronic blood loss from punctured sites. Blood loss is continuing due to secretion of anticoagulant substance by worms.
- Roche *et al* estimated 0.2 ml blood loss per parasite per day by *A. duodenale* & 0.03 ml blood loss per parasite per day by *N. americanus*.
- It is estimated that 0.76 mg iron loss per day by *A. duodenale* & 0.45 mg iron loss per day by *N. americanus*.
- Darling estimated about 1% of haemoglobin loss by 12 worms.

ii. Megaloblastic (macrocytic) anaemia: Due to deficiency of B_{12} or folic acid.

iii. Dimorphic anaemia: Due to deficiency of iron & B_{12} or folic acid.

✪ **Effects of anaemia:**

- Low iron leads to achlorhydria or hypoacidity.
- Shallow appearance of skin (light yellow).
- Pale mucosa of tongue, lips & eye lids.
- Oedema of face (puffy face), lower eye lids, feet & ankle.
- Spoon shaped nail **called koilonychias.**
- Dry lustrelcss hair.
- Protuberant abdomen.
- Hyperkinetic circulation may lead circulatory failure.
- Retardation of growth & development in children.
- Fatty changes in liver.

- Erythroblastic reaction in marrow & the yellow marrow transformed in to a red formative marrow.

❖ Laboratory diagnosis:

➤ **Specimens:**

✪ **Stool:** For presence of adult stage or eggs.

✪ **Bile:** Obtained by duodenal intubation & useful for adult stage or egg stage.

✪ **Blood & bone marrow biopsy:** To detect the effects of anaemia.

➤ **Testing methods:**

I. Direct methods

A. Macroscopic examination: For presence of adult stages.

B. Microscopy: For presence of eggs.

i. Wet mount by using normal saline & iodine: It shows the colourless (non-bile stained) eggs as shown in **figures-17(b).**

ii. Concentration technique:

- Useful in case of negative result by wet mount method.
- Eggs do not float in common salt solution.

C. Culture / coproculture:

✪ **Definition:** Culture technique from stool to obtain the larvae of nematodes by hatching the eggs **called coproculture.**

✪ **Aims:**

- To diagnose the larvae.
- To differentiate the larvae of different nematodes.
- To acquire the large numbers of larvae for research purpose.

✪ **Indications:** Useful to diagnose the larvae of

- Hook worm species like *A. duodenale* & *N. americanus.*
- Pseudohook worm species like *Trichostrogylus colubriformis* &*Trichostrogylus orientalis.*
- Strogyloides stercoralis.

✪ **Precautions:** Faecal specimens to be culture should not be refrigerated.

✪ **Types of methods:** Following are types.

i. Harada -Mori technique:

✪ **Principles:** Based on tendency of larvae to move from dry atmosphere to moisture area.

✪ **Steps: → Fig.-19(a):**

- About 500mg of faeces is smeared in middle or upper two third of thick filter paper by using the spatula.
- It is done evenly & as thin as possible.
- Lower one third of the paper is clean completely & dips in the water for absorbing the moisture.
- With a pipette add 3-4 ml of sterile water to the tube.
- Place filter paper in to the tube.
- Incubate at room temperature (25-28^{0}C) for 4-7 days, during which larvae develop on the filter paper & swim down in to the water.

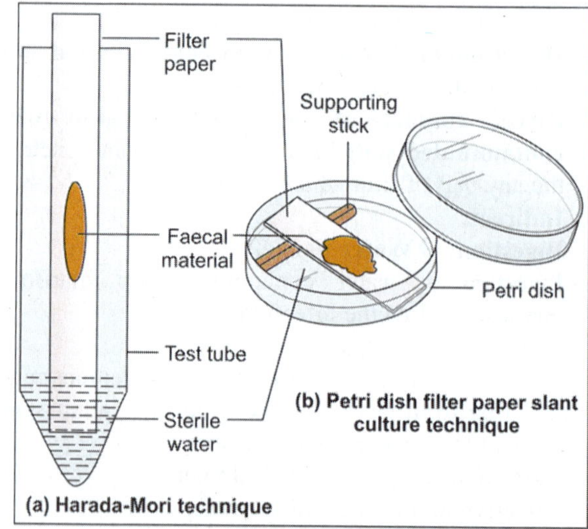

Figure-19: Culture technique

✪ **Examination:** Larvae can be examined by following two techniques.

1. **Magnifying lens:** Larvae can be examined outside at the bottom of tube by magnifying lens.
2. **Microscope:** Take one drop with pipette over slide & examined under microscope for presence of larvae.

ii. Petri dish filter paper slant culture technique:

✪ **Principles:** Same as Harada-Mori technique.

✪ **Steps:** Same as Harada-Mori technique, but petri dish is used instead of tube & filter paper is placed in slanting position with supporting stick instead of vertical position as shown in **fig.-19(b).**

✪ **Examination:** Larvae can be examined under microscope by following two techniques.

1. **By direct way:** Put whole petri dish under microscope & examine for the presence of larvae.
2. **By preparing the slide:** Take one drop with pipette over slide & examined under microscope for presence of larvae.

iii. Charcoal culture technique: It is also a useful method to collect the larvae.

II. Indirect methods

A. Blood picture:

Features	Micro-cytic anaemia	Macro-cytic anaemia	Di-morphic anaemia
RBC(million/mm^3)	2.9	0.73	1.3
Hb (%)	4.64	3.48	3.77
PCV (%)	21	10	16
MCV in femtolitre	72	137	123
MCH in picogram	16	47	24
MCHC (%)	22	34	23

Table-2: Anaemic picture in hook worm disease

- Eosinophilia.
- Anaemic picture: → **Table -2.**

B. Occult blood: Present in stool.

C. C.L. crystals: Present in stool.

D. Bone marrow biopsy: Erythroblastic reaction in marrow & the yellow marrow transformed in to a red formative marrow.

E. Radiological tests: Chest X-ray shows the pulmonary infiltration during migration of larvae.

III. Specific diagnosis

A. Species differentiation:

i. Differentiation between *A. duodenale* & *N. americanus*: →Table-3

ii. Differentiation between larvae of hook worm species & *Strogyloides*:

- If stool examination done after 24 hours & larva develop within eggs it indicates hook worm species, not the *Strogyloides.*
- Further differentiation can be done as per **table-4 & fig.-21** after obtaining larvae by coproculture.

iii. Difference between hook worm species & other species that can be mistaken as hook worm:

a. Adult stage differentiation: →**Flow chart-6**

Features	*A. duodenale*	*N. americanus*
Meaning	**Ankylos (Greek) = hooked + stoma (Greek) = mouth** as anterior end of worm is bent slightly dorsally like hook hence the name hook worm.	**Necator (Latin) = murderer + americanus = America**
Common name	Old world hook worm	- New world hook worm - American hook worm
Geo-graphical distribution	Tropical & subtropical countries	It diagnosed from Texas in 1902 by Stiles, but origin was Africa & later spread to India, Sri Lanka, Far East, Australia & Africa
	Adult stage	
Size	Large & thick	Small & thin
Life span	2-7 years	4-20 years
Anterior end	Bends in the same direction as the body curvature	Bends in the opposite direction as the body curvature
Buccal capsule	6 teeth, 4 hook like on ventral surface & 2 knob like on dorsal surface	4 chitinous plates, 2 on ventral surface & 2 on dorsal surface
Copulatory bursa	Total 13 rays & single dorsal ray which divided at the tip	Total 14 rays & single dorsal ray which divided at the base
Posterior end of female	Spine present	No spine
Vulval opening	Behind the middle of the body	In front of the middle of the body
	Larval stage →Fig.-20 & 21(a) & 21(b)	
Head	Conical	Round
Buccal cavity **- Length** **- Lumen** **-Chitinous wall** **-Oral depression**	- Short, 10-10.5μ - Larger - Thinner & bounded by one line dorsally & two less prominent lines ventrally converge anteriorly - Fine lines joins the oral depression & the anterior end of the buccal structure	- Long, 15-16μ - Shorter - Thicker & dorsal & ventral walls are of equal thickness; diverge anteriorly - No visible lines between the oral depression & the anterior end of the buccal structure
GIT **- O-I junction** **-Lumen** **- Posterior end of intestine**	- No gap at Oesophago-Intestinal (O-I) junction - Anterior dilatation of intestinal lumen less prominent - Small refractive body (ampuliform dilatation) present	- An apparent gap at Oesophago-Intestinal (O-I) junction - Anterior dilatation of intestinal lumen more prominent - Refractive body (ampuliform dilatation) Absent
Genital pore	Behind the mid-point of end of oesophagus & anus	In front of the mid-point of end of oesophagus & anus
Cuticular striae	Less prominent	More prominent
	Pathogenicity	
Risk	More dangerous (Reasons →**Vide infra**)	More dangerous
Blood loss	0.2 ml per parasite per day	0.03ml per parasite per day
Iron loss	0.76mg per parasite per day	0.45mg per parasite per day

Table-3: Differences between *A. duodenale* & *N. americanus*

Features	Hook worm	Strogyloides
Oesophagus	Extended up to 25% of total body length	Extended up to 40% of total body length
Sheath	Present	Absent
Tail	Pointed	Forked

Table-4: Differences between larvae of hook worm species & *Strogyloides*

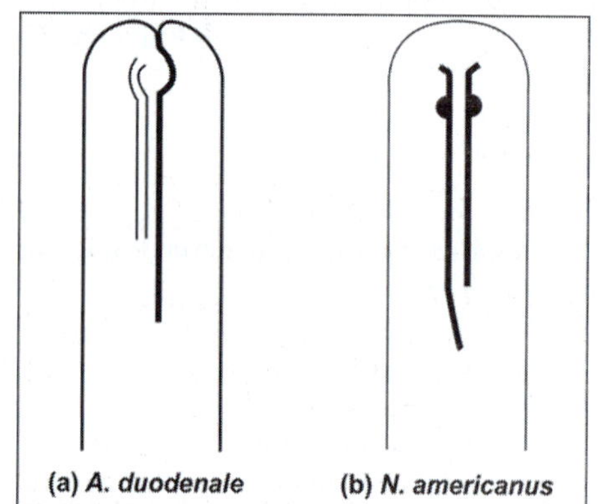

Figure-20: Buccal cavity of larvae of hook worm species

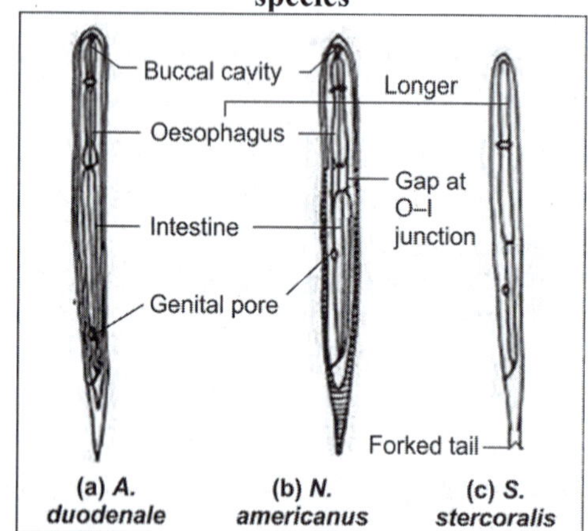

Figure-21: Filariform larvae of hook worm species & *Strongyloides*

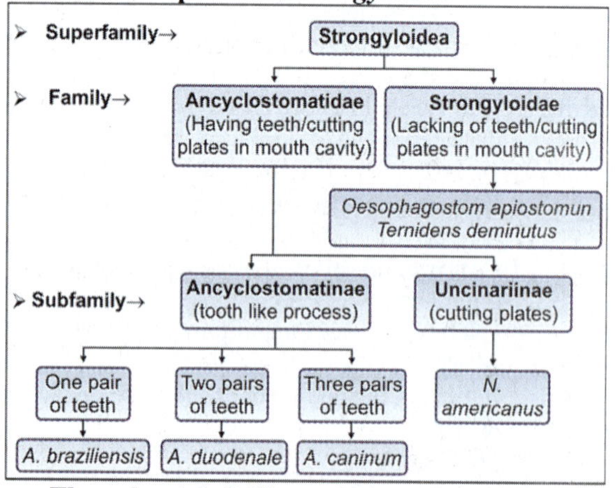

Flow chart-6: Differentiation of species of superfamily Strongyloidea

b. Egg stage differentiation: Following species can be differentiated.

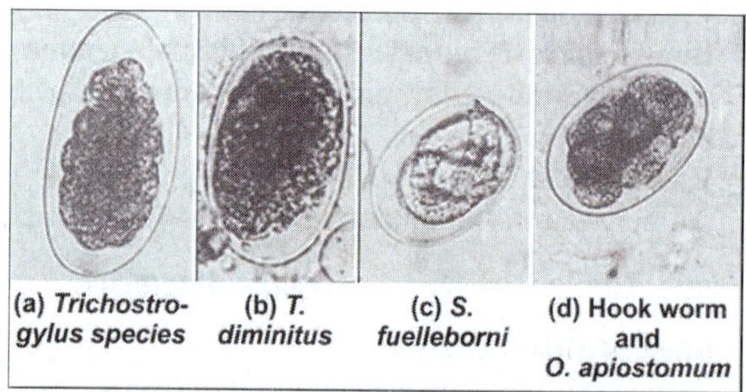

Figure-22: Eggs can be mistaken as hook worm

1. ***Trichostrongylus species:* → Fig.-22(a)**
- Size: Longer & thinner than hook worm egg about 85-115μm in length.
- Shape: Elongated & pointed at one or both ends.
- Embryo: Segmented about 16-32 blastomeres.

2. ***Ternidens deminutus:* → Fig.-22(b)**
- Size: Larger about 85 μm in length.
- Embryo: Segmented but numbers are more.

3. ***Strongyloides fuelleborni:* → Fig.-22(c)**
- Size: Smaller than hook about 35-50μm in length.
- Shape: Oval.
- Colour: Colourless.
- Embryo: May contains partially developed larva.
- Eggs pass in faeces rather than larvae.

4. ***Oesophagostom apiostomum:* → Fig.-22(d)**
- Same as hook worm but pass in faeces in advance stage of development.

❖ Prevention:

- Prevention of faecal contamination of soil.
- Wearing shoes at the time of walking & gloves while working in garden.

❖ Treatment:

➢ **Specific treatment of worm:**
- Albendazole: 400mg, single dose.
- Mebendazole: 500 mg single dose.
- Pyrental pamoate: 11mg/kg OD for 3 days. Safe in pregnancy.
- Thiabendazole is less effective.
- Tetrachlorethylene is effective but toxic.
- Bephenium hydroxynaphthoate is active against *Ancycloctoma* but not against *Necator.*

➢ **Treatment of anaemia:** Oral administration of iron in mild anaemia but in severs case required packed cell transfusion. When haemoglobin is very low 1st clear the anaemia then give the anthelmintics.

Necator americanus

- General morphology, life cycle, pathogenicity & laboratory diagnosis are same as *A. duodenale.*
- *A. duodenale* is more dangerous than *N. americanus* because it cause more blood loss in intestinal infection due to

1. Larger size.
2. Armed with teeth.
3. More migratory so leaving more bleeding points.

- Differences between *A. duodenale* & *N. americanus* are shown in **table-3.**

A. brasiliensis

- **History:** Gomes De Faria, 1910.
- **Geographical distribution:** In Malaysia, Brazil & India.
- **Habitat:** Parasite of dog & cat. In man it habitat only skin & no intestinal lesion.
- **Morphology:**
  - Small adult worm.
  - Buccal capsule have small orifice & ventral dental plate contains one pair of large teeth.
- **Life cycle:** Same as *A. duodenale.*
- **Pathogenicity:** No intestinal lesion, but wanders in between the layers of skin causing lesion **called creeping eruption** or **cutaneous larva migrans.**

A. ceylanicum

- **Geographical distribution:** In Sri Lanka.
- **Habitat:** Parasite of civet cat. In man it habitat intestine & no skin lesion.
- **Morphology:** Same as *A. brasiliensis* & sometimes considered as biological variant of *A. brasiliensis* var *ceylanicum.*
- **Pathogenicity:** In man it habitat intestine & no skin lesion.

A. caninum

- **History:** Ercolani, 1859 & Hall, 1913.
- **Geographical distribution:** Cosmopolitan.
- **Habitat:** Parasite of dog. In man it habitat only skin & no intestinal lesion.
- **Morphology:** Buccal capsule have largest orifice & ventral plates contains 3 teeth, innermost being the smallest & outermost being the largest.
- **Life cycle & Pathogenicity:** Same as *A. braziliensis.*

Trichostrongylus species

- **Common name:** Pseudohook worm.
- **Species:** Total 12 species, but species infecting man are *Trichostrongylus colubriformis* & *Trichostrongylus orientalis.*
- **Geographical distribution:**
  - Present in Australia, Indonesia, Iran, Iraq, Japan & USSR.
  - About 15% population of sheep & goat in Kashmir, India is infected by *Trichostrogylus* species.
- **Habitat:** Adult parasite habitat in small intestine in man. Normally it is a parasite of herbivorous animals like sheep, goat, cow etc.
- **Morphology:** Three morphological stages like adult, egg & larval stages.

I. Adult stage

- Reddish colours.
- Lacking buccal capsule.
- Remain buried in mucosa & never found in stool.
- Male is 4-5 mm long while female is 4-6 mm long.

II. Egg stage

- **Vide supra** →For more details **follow section → laboratory diagnosis of *A. duodenale.***

III. Larval stage

- Eggs released through faeces over soil & moults twice to form larvae (3rd stage).
- Larval stage is the infective stage & enters in human via contaminated vegetables or plants.

- **Life cycle:**
  - It completes its life cycle in single host.
  - Larvae enter in human via contaminated vegetables or plants.
  - On reaching the intestine it transformed to male & female adult stage after two more moultings.
  - Female laying eggs which pass through faeces over soil & cycle gets repeated.
- **Pathogenicity:**
  - **Disease name: Called pseudo hook worm disease**
  - **Reservoir of infection:** Herbivorous animals like sheep, goat, cow etc.
  - **Source of infection:** Contaminated vegetables or plants.
  - **Mode of transmission:** Larvae enter in human via contaminated vegetables or plants.
  - **Exit form:** Eggs.
  - **Infective form:** Larvae (3rd stage).
  - **Portal of entry:** GIT.
  - **Sites:** Small intestine.
  - **Pathogenesis:** Mechanical damage via penetration of anterior part (head) of adult stage in to the mucosa causing traumatic damage & intestinal bleeding.
  - **Clinical features:**

a. **Mild infection:**
- Mostly asymptomatic.
- Rarely features of epigastric discomfort.

b. **Heavy infection:**
- Anaemia.
- Eosinophilia.

- Prolonged diarrhoea.
- Emaciation & oedema.

❖ **Laboratory diagnosis:**

➢ **Specimens:**

✪ **Stool:** It contains eggs but not adult stage because it is embedded in mucosa & not excreted in stool.

➢ **Testing methods:**

A. **Microscopy:** For presence of eggs & it should be differentiated from hook worm eggs as described earlier.

B. **Culture / coproculture:** Harda-Mori technique is useful to obtain the larvae & to differentiated from related genera.

Strongyloides spp.

Strongyloides stercoralis

❖ **Synonym:** *Anguillula stercoralis* or *Anguillula intestinalis.*

❖ **Meaning:** **Strongylus (Greek) = round + edios = appearance (resembling) + stercoralis = faeces,** as this minute cylindrical (round) worm was first identified in diarrheic stool of French soldier in Cochin, China by Normand in 1876.

❖ **History:**

- Parasite was first discovered in diarrheic stool of French soldier in Cochin, China by Normand in 1876.
- Life cycle & pathogenesis was worked out by Stiles & Hassal in 1902.

❖ **Geographical distribution:** It is distributed world-wide but common in Brazil, Far East (China Philippines) & Africa (tropical & temperate countries).

❖ **Habitat:**

- Female parasite habitat in mucosa of duodenum & jejunum. It can be demonstrated post-mortem by mucosal biopsy under low power microscopy.
- Male have no penetrating power & habitat in lumen only.

❖ **Morphology:** Three morphological stages like adult, egg & larval stages. Few important features of parasite are given below. For more details, **follow chapter → Nematodes: General features and classification.**

I. Adult stage

➢ **Time of maturation:** Larva transformed to sexually mature adult stage in 15-20 days in definitive host after injection.

➢ **Size:** In parasitic cycle females are readily identified but not the males.

- Male: 0.6mm ×40-50μm.
- Female: It is larger & narrower than male with 2.5mm ×0.05mm in size.

➢ **Shape:** They are rounded, elongated, unsegmented, & cylindrical as shown in **fig.-23.**

➢ **Life span:** Adult worm lives about 3-4 months in human, but because it can cause autoinfection may survive longer up to 20-30 years.

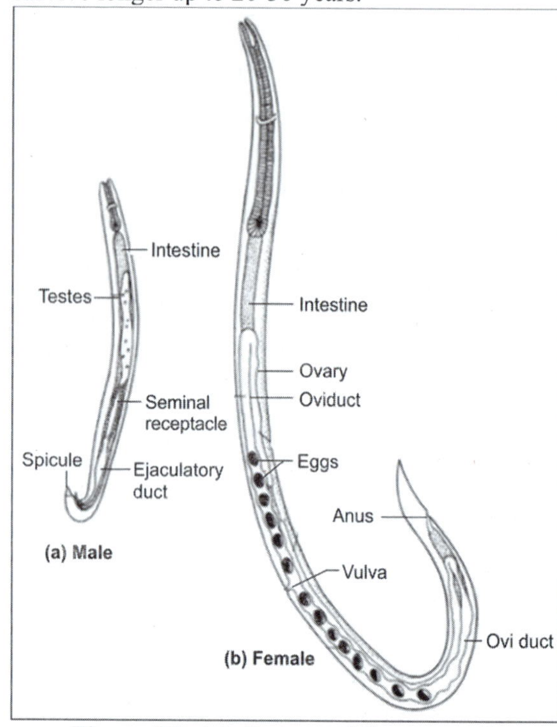

Figure-23: Adult stage of *S. stercoralis*

➢ **Organs:**

✪ **Mouth:**

- Male have conspicuous buccal cavity.
- Till date male was discovered by Kreis only in 1932 but other has failed.

✪ **Anterior end:** Rounded.

✪ **Posterior (tail) end:** Pointed.

✪ **GIT:**

- Muscular oesophagus extends through the anterior third of body.
- Intestine extends through the posterior two thirds.
- Anus open mid-ventrally, a short distance in front of the caudal tip.

✪ **Reproductive organs:**

- **In male:**
  - Genital pore opens in to the cloaca.
  - Copulatory spicules which penetrate the female during copulation are located on each side of the gubernaculum.
- **In female:**
  - Female contains paired uteri, vagina & vulva.
  - Genital pore opens at the junction of posterior & middle third of the body.

- Gravid uterus contains 8-10 eggs arranged antero-posteriorly.

➢ **Type of female:**

- It is an ovi-viviparous & laying eggs contains larva which immediately hatch out.
- It also **called parthenogenetic female** as it laying eggs without fertilisation by male.

II. Egg stage

➢ **Morphological features:** Laid by fertilise female **(fig.-24).**

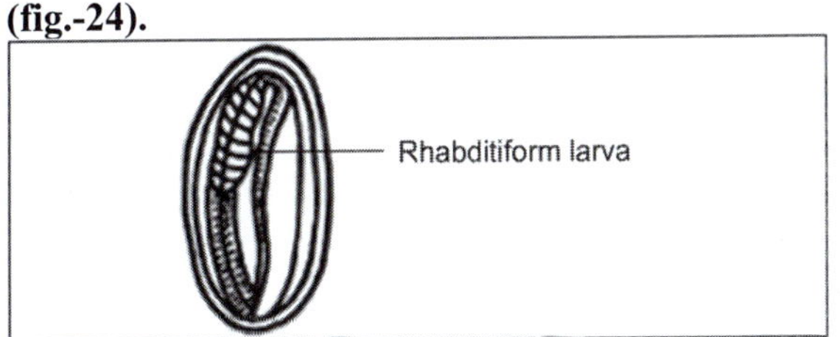

Figure-24: Egg of *S. stercoralis*

✪ **Shape:** Elliptical or oval.

✪ **Size:** 55µm ×30µm.

✪ **Covering:** Covered by thin hyaline membrane.

✪ **Embryo:**

- Eggs contains rhabditiform larva.
- Eggs are immediately hatched out to release it in the intestine; hence it is the larvae not the eggs are present in stool.

III. Larval stage

➢ **Form:** Two forms. Follow chapter → Nematodes: General features and classification for more details.

A. Rhabditiform larva:

- Size: 200-250 µm × 16µm.
- Oesophagus: Bulbous.
- Moult twice on soil to change to filariform larva.
- It is the exit form & present in stool.
- Host: It develops in human intestine & also over soil from hatching of eggs.

B. Filariform larva:

- Size: 500-600 µm × 20µm.
- Oesophagus: Not bulbous.
- Tail: Forked (notched) as shown in **fig.-21(c).**
- It is an infective stage & develop within 3-4 days.

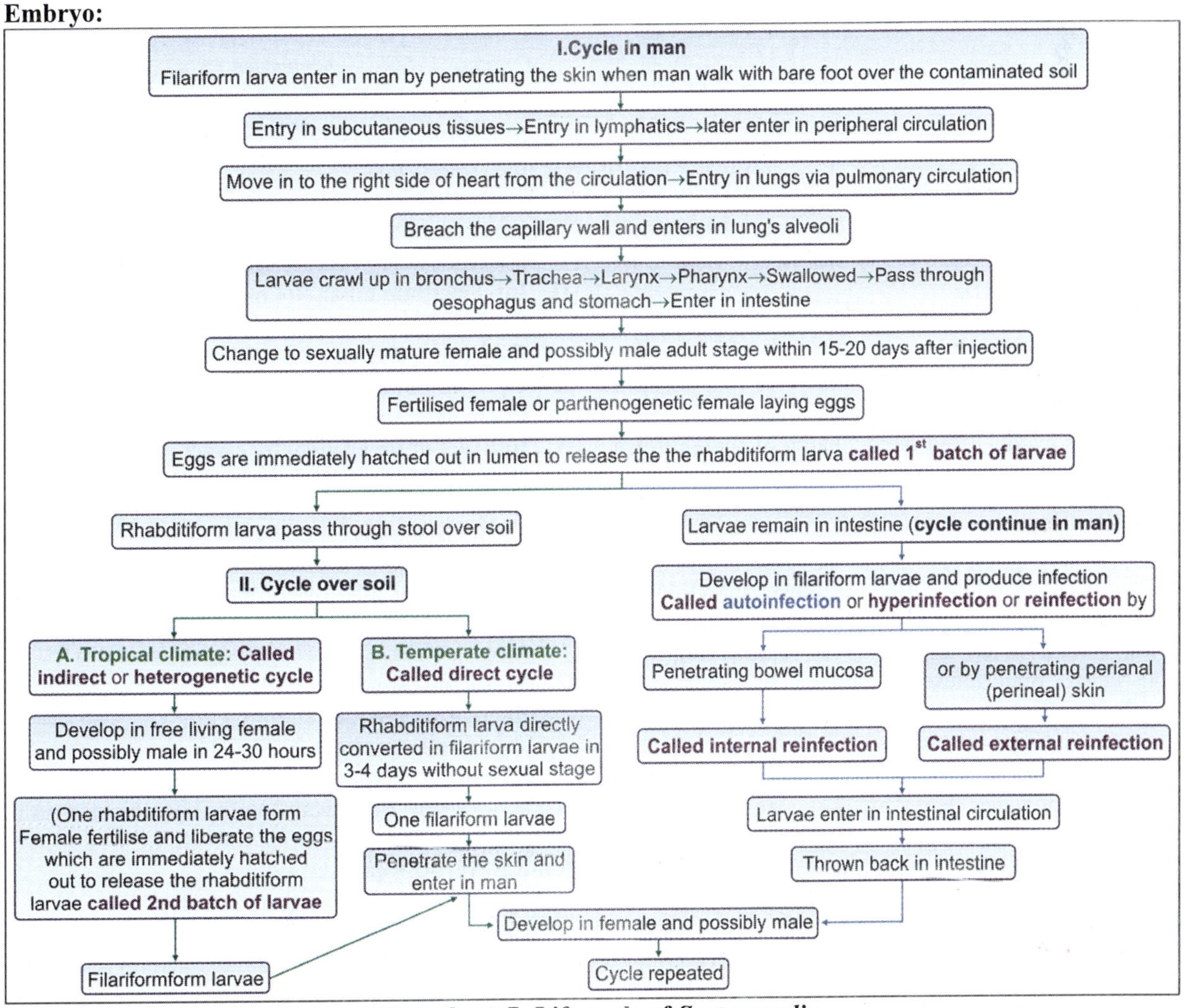

I.Cycle in man
Filariform larva enter in man by penetrating the skin when man walk with bare foot over the contaminated soil

↓ Entry in subcutaneous tissues→Entry in lymphatics→later enter in peripheral circulation

↓ Move in to the right side of heart from the circulation→Entry in lungs via pulmonary circulation

↓ Breach the capillary wall and enters in lung's alveoli

↓ Larvae crawl up in bronchus→Trachea→Larynx→Pharynx→Swallowed→Pass through oesophagus and stomach→Enter in intestine

↓ Change to sexually mature female and possibly male adult stage within 15-20 days after injection

↓ Fertilised female or parthenogenetic female laying eggs

↓ Eggs are immediately hatched out in lumen to release the the rhabditiform larva **called 1st batch of larvae**

Branch 1: Rhabditiform larva pass through stool over soil

↓ **II. Cycle over soil**

- **A. Tropical climate: Called indirect** or **heterogenetic cycle**
  ↓ Develop in free living female and possibly male in 24-30 hours
  ↓ (One rhabditiform larvae form Female fertilise and liberate the eggs which are immediately hatched out to release the rhabditiform larvae **called 2nd batch of larvae**
  ↓ Filariformform larvae → Penetrate the skin and enter in man
- **B. Temperate climate: Called direct cycle**
  ↓ Rhabditiform larva directly converted in filariform larvae in 3-4 days without sexual stage
  ↓ One filariform larvae
  ↓ Penetrate the skin and enter in man
  ↓ Develop in female and possibly male

Branch 2: Larvae remain in intestine (**cycle continue in man)**

↓ Develop in filariform larvae and produce infection **Called** autoinfection or **hyperinfection** or **reinfection** by

- Penetrating bowel mucosa ↓ **Called internal reinfection**
- or by penetrating perianal (perineal) skin ↓ **Called external reinfection**

↓ Larvae enter in intestinal circulation

↓ Thrown back in intestine

↓ Develop in female and possibly male

↓ Cycle repeated

Flow chart-7: Life cycle of *S. stercoralis*

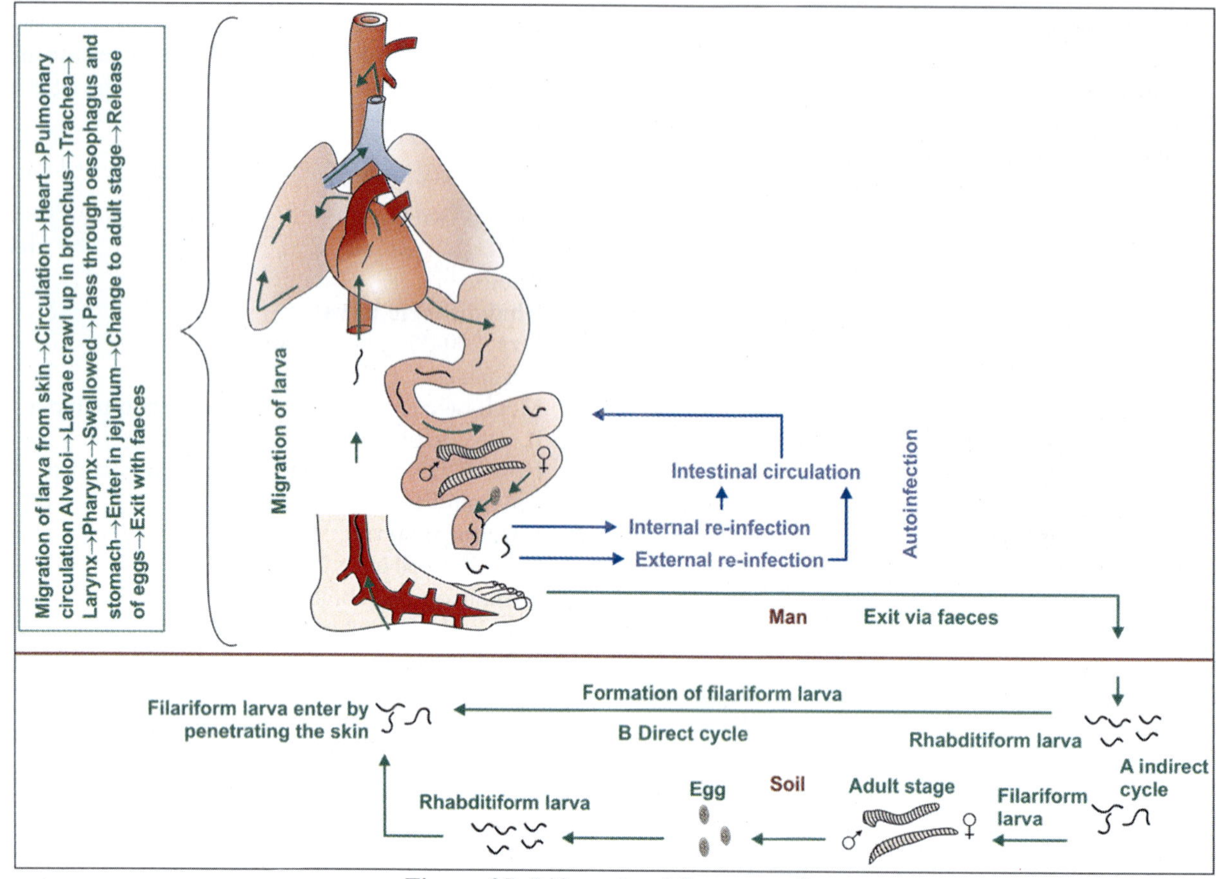

Figure-25: Life cycle of *S. stercoralis*

- Host & development: It develops from rhabditiform larvae by following three modes as shown in **flow chart-7.**

1. **Hyperinfection:** From the 1st batch of rhabditiform larvae in human.
2. **Direct cycle:** From the 1st batch of rhabditiform larvae over the soil in temperate climate.
3. **Indirect cycle:** From the 2nd batch of rhabditiform larvae over the soil in tropical climate.

❖ Immunity:

- **Acquired immunity:**
  - Immunity develops after primary infection in human which prevents the reinfection & also prevents tissue invasion by larvae & adult stage.
  - It is an opportunistic pathogen & adult stage causing infection in immunocompromised host with extensive tissue damage.
  - Serum antibodies are developed which are detected by CFT; however they may cross react with filarial antigens.
- **Hypersensitivity:** It develops after reinfection & characterised by eosinophilia with utricaria.

❖ Life cycle:

➢ **Hosts:**

I. **Definitive host:** Whole cycle is possible in one host only like man. Change of host (other man) is not required for continuation of life cycle, as it undergoes the hyperinfective form (autoinfection).

II. **Intermediate host:** Not required

➢ **Cycles:** Following two types of cycle as shown in **flow chart-7 & fig.-25.**

I. **Cycle in man:**

II. **Cycle over soil:** Two subtypes.

A. **Indirect** or **heterogenetic cycle:**

B. **Direct cycle:**

❖ Pathogenicity:

➢ **Disease name: Called strongyloidiasis.**

➢ **Reservoir of infection:** Man.

➢ **Source of infection:** Soil & human itself in case of autoinfection.

➢ **Mode of transmission:**
- Internal & external autoinfection can also occur as shown in **flow chart-7.**
- Filariform larvae enter in man by penetrating the skin when man walk with bare foot over the contaminated soil.

➢ **Exit form:** Rhabditiform larvae.

➢ **Infective form:** Filariform larvae.

➢ **Portal of entry:** Skin.

➢ **Sites:** Adult stage habitat in duodenum & jejunum.

➢ **Precipitating factors:** Autoinfection is precipitated by

- Steroid therapy.
- AIDS.
- Malignancy.

➢ **Pathogenesis & clinical features:** Divided in two categories as shown in **flow chart-8.**

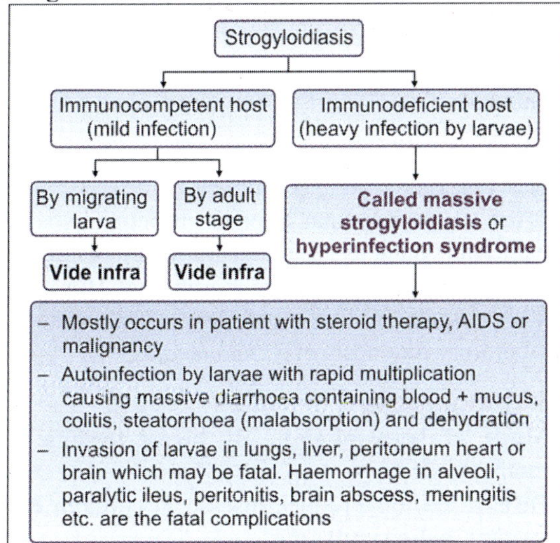

Flow chart-8: Pathogenesis & clinical features of *S. stercoralis*

I. By migrating larvae:

A. Skin:

i. At the site of entry:

- Lesion **called ground itch** or **itchy dermatitis.**
- It present with severe itching than *A. duodenale.*

ii. In between the layers of skin:

- Normally it complete the life cycle in human but due to repeated attack host mount an immune response which prevents larvae to complete the life cycle & larvae limited only to skin. They traverse in between the layers of skin in serpigenous or linear fashion & produce lesion **called cutaneous larva migrans** or **creeping eruption** or **larva currens.**
- Currens (Latin) meaning running/race, as larvae are moves rapidly at speed of 3-4 cm/hour hence **called larva currens (racing larva)**. This term given in 1958.
- The track is start from anus & extend up to buttock, thigh or groin
- It is characterised by reddish itchy papule along the path traversed by larvae.
- Lesion last for few weeks.
- It also produced by other species of *Strogyloides.*

iii. Lungs: Migrating larvae produce alveolar haemorrhage, bronchopneumonia & eosinophilic infiltration in lungs.

iv. General: Moderate eosinophilia (10-25%) in 60-80% of patients.

II. By adult stage: Minimal invasion by adult stage which may be asymptomatic or present with mild diarrhoea, abdominal pain (simulating peptic ulcer), gastro intestinal bleeding & mild chronic colitis.

➢ **Complication:** Migrating larvae carrying bacteria along with, causing gram negative bacteremia (Woodruff, 1968).

❖ Laboratory diagnosis:

➢ **Specimens:** Following specimens can be examined to detect the rhabditiform larvae.

- ✪ **Stool:**
- ✪ **Bile or duodenal washing:** Collected by E- test.
- ✪ **Sputum:**
- ✪ **Mucosal biopsy:**
- ✪ **CSF, ascetic fluid & urine:** In immunodeficient patients with dissemination of larvae.

➢ **Testing methods:**

I. Direct methods

A. Microscopy: For presence of rhabditiform larvae.

i. Wet mount by using normal saline & iodine:

ii. Concentration technique:

a. Formol-ether concentration technique:

- More sensitive than wet mount method.
- Larvae sediment at bottom of fluid.

b. Baermann's method:

- ✪ **Synonym:** Baermannization.
- ✪ **Principle:** Based on tendency of larvae to move from colder to warmer area.
- ✪ **Baermann's apparatus →Figure-26**
- ✪ **Steps:**

- Take one funnel & fix on a stand.
- Funnel is about 10 cm in diameter with a short rubber tube which is screw clamped.
- Insert one round metal sieve in the funnel.
- Funnel is filled with warm water (42^0C) up to sieve level.
- Appropriate amount of fresh faeces is placed in cheese cloth, which is placed on the sieve.
- Incubate the whole preparation at warm temperature for 30 minutes & examine for larvae.

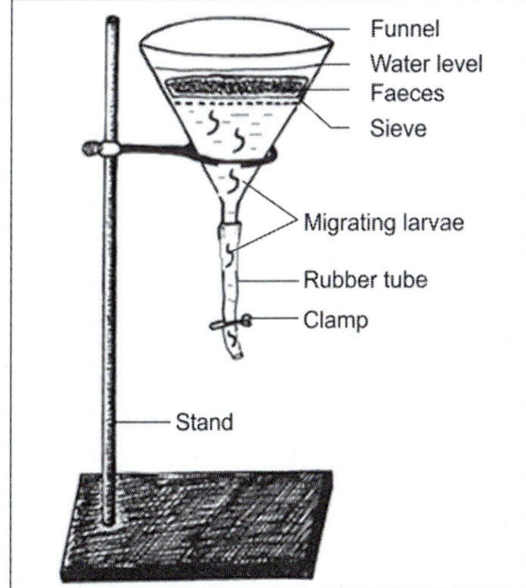

Figure-26: Baermann's apparatus

✪ **Result & examination:**
- During incubation larvae migrate to the bottom of fluid.
- Loose the clamp, take a drop of fluid on slide, put the cover slip & examine under the low power microscope for presence of motile larvae.

✪ **Advantage:** Most sensitive method.

c. **Water emergency semi-concentration technique:**

✪ **Principle:** Same as baermannization.

✪ **Steps:**
- Transfer fresh faeces (not more than 2 hours old) in a petridish.
- Make a central depression in faecal material by using a stick.
- Filled the depression with warm water (not more than 37^{0}C).
- Incubate the whole preparation in incubator at 35-37^{0}C for 1½- 3 hours & examine for larvae.

✪ **Result & examination:** During incubation larvae migrate from faecal area to fluid area & examine the larvae by following two ways of slide preparation.

1. **Direct method:**
- Take a drop of fluid on slide by Pasteur pipette or by plastic bulb pipette.
- Put the cover slip & examine under the low power microscope for presence of motile larvae.

2. **Centrifugation method:**
- Transfer all fluid in conical tube.
- Centrifuge the fluid.
- Take a drop of fluid on slide by Pasteur pipette or by plastic bulb pipette.
- Put the cover slip & examine under the low power microscope for presence of motile larvae.

B. **Culture / coproculture:** Same as *A. duodenale*.

II. Indirect methods

B. **Blood picture:** Moderate eosinophilia (10-25%) in 60-80% of patients.

C. **Serological tests:**
- Serum antibodies are developed which are detected by CFT; however they may cross react with filarial antigens.
- ELISA & immonoblot test are other useful tests.
- Antigen is prepared from immunosuppressed rats, monkeys or dogs, infected with *Strogyloides ratti.*

❖ **Prevention:**
- Prevention of faecal contamination of soil.
- Wearing shoes at the time of walking & gloves while working in garden.

❖ **Treatment:**
- All cases whether symptomatic or not are treated by ivermectin 200 mg/kg daily for 2 days is more effective than albendazole 400mg daily for 3 days.
- For disseminated disease ivermectin should be continue for 5-7 days.

Strongyloides fuelleborni

Same as *S. stercoralis* with following differences.

❖ **Geographical distribution:** Two subspecies.
- ***S. fuelleborni fuelleborni*** is reported from Africa.
- ***S. fuelleborni kellyi*** is reported from Papua New Guinea.

❖ **Habitat:**
- It is a parasite of dog & monkey.
- It can cause intestinal infection in human specially babies as young as 2 months old & young children.

❖ **Morphology:** Egg stage morphology **[fig.-22(c)]. Vide supra** → For more details follow section, laboratory diagnosis of *A. duodenale.*

❖ **Pathogenicity:**
- **Mode of transmission:** By breast feeding from mother to child.
- **Disease name:** Produce disease in children **called swollen belly syndrome.**
- **Clinical features:**
  - It is acute & fatal in nature.
  - Present with protein losing enteropathy, abdominal pain & diarrhoea.
- **Co-infection:** Some time it present with *S. stercoralis* in same person.

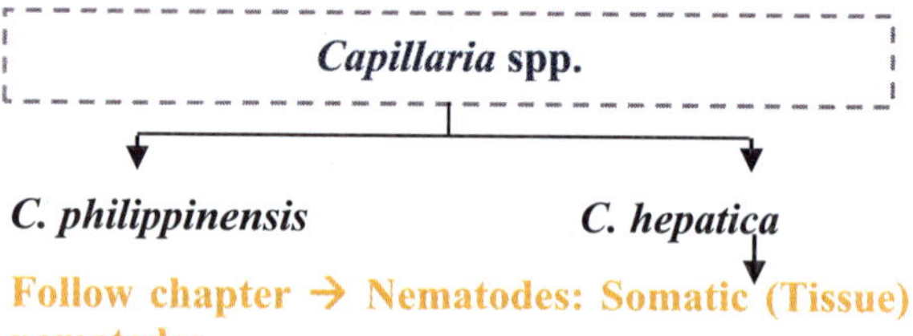

Follow chapter → Nematodes: Somatic (Tissue) nematodes

Capillaria philippinensis

❖ **Meaning:** Species so called because first discovered from a fatal case in Philippines in 1963.

❖ **History:** Chitwood et al, 1968 contributed in discovery of parasite.

❖ **Geographical distribution:** Initially restricted to the Philippines & Thailand, later spread to Japan, Iran, Egypt, Taiwan, Indonesia & Columbia.

❖ **Habitat:** Adult parasite habitat the small intestine particularly jejunum.

❖ **Morphology:** Three morphological stages like adult, egg & larval stages. Few important features of parasite are given below.

I. Adult stage

Same like *T. trichuria* but in smaller size.
- Female: 2.5-3.5mm in length.
- Male: 2.3-3.17 mm in length.

II. Egg stage

Eggs are same in appearance to *T. trichuria* & could be differentiated as per **table-5 & fig.-27.**

Features	*C. philippinensis*	*T. trichuria*
Size	45μm × 21μm	50μm × 25μm
Shape	Barrel shaped but less elliptical	Barrel shaped but more elliptical
Covering	Striated	Smooth
Mucus plug	Bipolar & flattened	Bipolar & protuberant
Embryo	May or may not be embryonated & if present may be Unsegmentd or with 2 segments	Contains unsegmented embryo

Table-5: Egg of *C. philippinensis* & *T. trichuria*

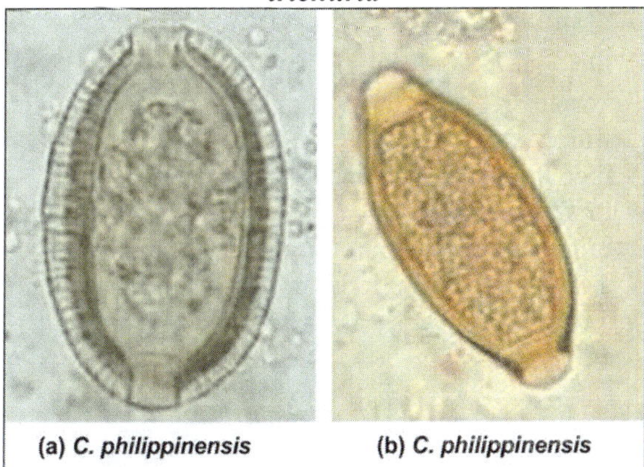
(a) *C. philippinensis* (b) *C. philippinensis*

Figure-27: Egg of *C. philippinensis* & *T. trichuria*

III. Larval stage

Larval stage present in fresh or salt water fish.

❖ Life cycle:

- **Hosts:** Cycle continue between fish-bird-fish. Man is the accidental host & develops all stages in intestine.

I. **Definitive host:** Fish eating birds.

II. **Intermediate host:** Fresh or salt water fish.

- **Cycles:**
- Cycle is not fully worked out.
- Man is infected by ingestion of partially cooked or pickled fish contains larvae. Larvae change to adult stage, which burrowed the jejunal mucosa. Female laying eggs which pass through stool over soil. All the stages develop in human host.
- **Internal autoinfection:** Due to penetration of bowel mucosa by liberated larvae.
- Larvae develop from the eggs which is infective form & taken up by fish.
- Such fish taken up by bird (accidentally by man), where larvae change to sexually mature male & female adult stage. Female laying eggs which pass through stool over soil to continue the cycle

❖ Pathogenicity:

- **Disease name: Called intestinal capillariasis.**
- **Mode of transmission:**
- Man is infected by ingestion of partially cooked or pickled fish contains larvae.
- Internal autoinfection can also occur.
- **Reservoir of infection:** Fish eating birds.
- **Portal of entry:** GIT.
- **Sites:** Adult parasite habitat in jejunum.
- **Infective form:** Larval stage.
- **Pathogenesis & clinical features:**

a. **Mild infection:** Colicky abdominal pain, intestinal gurgling (borborygmi), Chronic watery diarrhoea with frequency of 8-10 stools per day, muscle wasting & oedema.

b. **Heavy infection:**

- **Spoliative action:** Heavy worm burden covers the intestinal mucosa, receive nutrition from intestinal contents, and derange intestinal function & produces following effects.
- Protein loosing enteropathy.
- Malabsorption of fat & sugar.
- Reduction of plasma level of potassium, sodium & calcium.
- **Mechanical action:** Heavy worms causing lymphatic obstruction of intestinal wall & produces oedema & even death also.

❖ Laboratory diagnosis:

- **Specimens:** Adult, larval & egg stage can be diagnosed from following specimens.
- **Stool:**
- **Bile or duodenal aspirates:**
- **Mucosal (jejunal) biopsy:**
- **Testing methods:**

I. Direct methods

A. **Macroscopy:** For presence of adult stage.

B. **Microscopy:**

iii. **Wet mount by using normal saline & iodine:** Eggs are same in appearance to *T. trichuria* & should be differentiated as per **table-5 & fig.-27.**

iv. **Concentration technique:**

a. **Formol-ether concentration technique:**

- More sensitive than wet mount method.
- Larvae sediment at bottom of fluid.

II. Indirect methods

A. **Blood picture:**

- Eosinophilia.
- Reduction of plasma level of potassium, sodium & calcium.

B. **Stool picture:** Presence of fat (fatty acid) & protein in stool.

C. **Serological tests:**

- Serum antibodies are developed which are detected by ELISA, IHA & gel diffusion technique.

- Cross reaction with other parasite may occur.

❖ **Prevention:** Avoid the use of raw fish meat.

❖ **Treatment:** Mebendazole is effective drug.

Large intestinal nematodes

Trichuris trichuria

❖ **Synonym:** *Trichuris intestinalis, Trichuris hominis, Trichocephalus dispar & Ascaris tricuhria.*

❖ **Common name:** Whip worm.

❖ **Meaning:**

- **Scientific name:**
  - ***Trichuris trichuria:*** **Trichuris** from **trichos (Greek) = hair + oura = tail,** means tail of hair.
  - ***Trichocephalus dispar:*** **Trichocephalus** from **Trichos (Greek) = hair + cephalus = head,** means head of hair.
- **Common name:** Whip worm, because its anterior three fifth is very thin & hair like while posterior two fifth is thick & stout like handle of whip.

❖ **History:** It was first discovered by Linnaeus in 1771.

❖ **Geographical distribution:**

- Distributed world-wide.
- Common in warm moist region & areas with poor sanitation.
- Because of common environmental requirement it may co-exist with *Ascaris lumbricoides.*

❖ **Habitat:** Adult parasite habitat the large intestine particularly in caecum & also in appendix.

❖ **Morphology:** Three morphological stages like adult, egg & larval stages. Few important features of parasite are given below. For more details **follow chapter → Nematodes: General features and classification.**

I. Adult stage

➢ **Time of maturation:** Eggs transformed to sexually mature adult stage within 4 weeks in definitive host after ingestion.

➢ **Colour:** It is flesh in colour.

➢ **Size:** Female is larger than male as shown in **fig.-28**

- Female: 4-5cm in length.
- Male: 3-4cm in length.

➢ **Shape:** Rounded, elongated, unsegmented, & cylindrical as shown in **fig.-28.**

➢ **Life span:** Adult worm lives for 10 years or longer in human bowel.

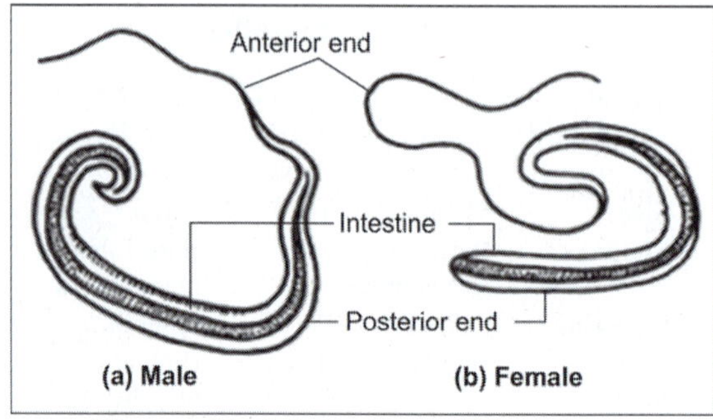

Figure-28: Adult stage of *T. trichuria*

➢ **Organs:**

✪ **Anterior end: → fig.-28**

- Anterior three fifth is very thin & hair like.
- It is embedded in mucous membrane.
- It contains oesophagus which is a minute channel contains secretory cells in single column.

✪ **Posterior (tail) end: → Fig.-28**

- Posterior two fifth is thick & stout like handle of whip.
- It contains the intestine & sex organs.
- In male caudal extremity is coiled ventrally.
- In female caudal extremity is in comma / arc shape.

➢ **Type of female:** It is an oviparous & laying the 5,000-7000 eggs / day contains unsegmented embryo.

II. Egg stage

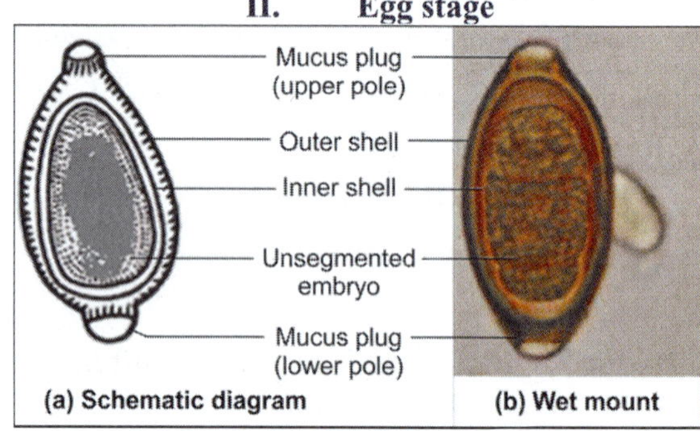

Figure-29: Egg of *T. trichuria*

➢ **Morphological features:** Laid by fertilise female **(fig.-29).**

✪ **Shape:** Barrel.

✪ **Size:** 50μm ×25μm.

✪ **Colour**: Brown colour (bile stained).

✪ **Covering:** Two layers.

- Outer shell: Thick & bile stained, but absent at both poles which is taken by a mucous **called mucus plug.**
- Inner shell: Thin.

✪ **Embryo:** Contains unsegmented embryo present inner to inner shell.

✪ **Other features:** Floats in saturated common salt solution.

III. Larval stage

➢ **Form:**

- Rhabditiform larva developed from the unsegmented embryo within the egg shell **(fig.-30)** depending on the humidity & atmospheric conditions.
- In tropical climates it develop in 3-4 weeks while in temperate climates it develop in 6-12 months
- Freshly passed eggs are not infective but eggs containing rhabditiform larva are infective to man
- On ingestion egg shell rupture to release the rhabditiform larva

➢ **Host:** It develop over the soil (outside the human)

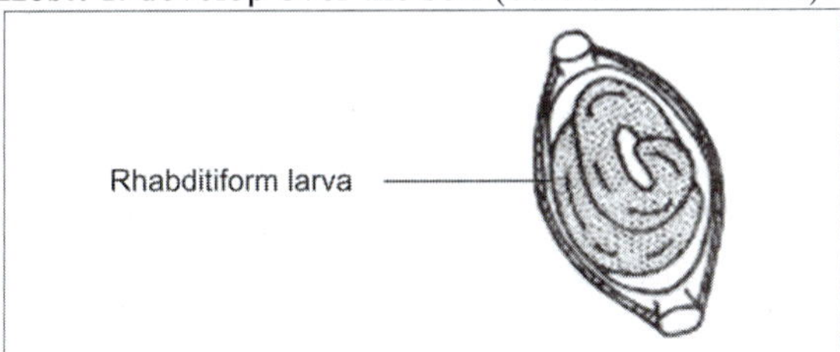

Figure-30: Larva of *T. trichuria*

❖ Life cycle:

➢ **Hosts:**

I. **Definitive host:** Whole cycle is possible in one host only like man. Change of host (other man) is required for continuation of life cycle.

II. **Intermediate host:** Not required.

➢ **Cycles:** Following two types of cycle

I. **Cycle in man:** } **Flow chart-9 & fig.-31**
II. **Cycle over soil:** }

❖ Pathogenicity:

➢ **Disease name:** **Called trichuriasis.**

➢ **Synonym:** Also **called trichocephaliasis** or **whip worm infection.**

➢ **Reservoir of infection:** Man.

➢ **Source of infection:** Contaminated food & water.

➢ **Mode of transmission:** Infection to man by ingestion of food or water contaminated by eggs contains rhabditiform larva.

➢ **Exit form:** Eggs containing unsegmented embryo.

➢ **Infective form:** Freshly passed eggs are not infective but eggs containing rhabditiform larva are infective to man.

➢ **Portal of entry:** GIT.

➢ **Sites:** Adult parasite habitat in caecum & also in appendix.

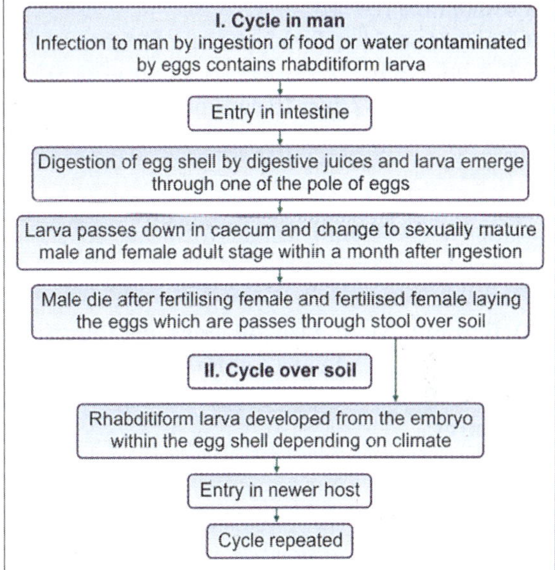

I. Cycle in man
Infection to man by ingestion of food or water contaminated by eggs contains rhabditiform larva
Entry in intestine
Digestion of egg shell by digestive juices and larva emerge through one of the pole of eggs
Larva passes down in caecum and change to sexually mature male and female adult stage within a month after ingestion
Male die after fertilising female and fertilised female laying the eggs which are passes through stool over soil
II. Cycle over soil
Rhabditiform larva developed from the embryo within the egg shell depending on climate
Entry in newer host
Cycle repeated

Flow chart-9: Life cycle of *T. trichuria*

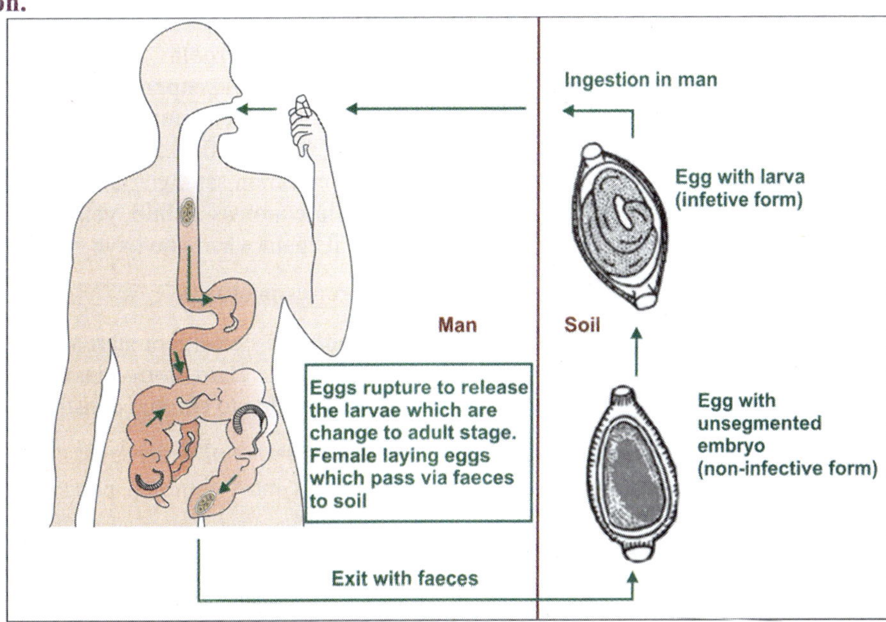

Figure-31: Life cycle of *T. trichuria*

➤ **Pathogenesis:**

1. **Mechanical:**
- Anterior part of adult stage penetrates in to the mucosa causing intestinal bleeding.
- Mechanical obstruction of appendix by heavy worm burden responsible for mucosal irritation & appendicitis.
- Heavy blood loss (0.005ml/day/worm) may cause anaemia.

1. **Liberation of toxic products:** Causing
- Toxic irritation of nerve ending of rectum & responsible for rectal prolapsed.
- Eosinophilia (25%).

➤ **Clinical features:** Two types of infections.

a. **Mild infection:**
- **Definition:** Less than 10 eggs per direct stool smear **called mild infection.**
- **Features:**
- Mostly asymptomatic.
- Rarely present with features of acute appendicitis like abdominal pain etc.

b. **Heavy infection:**
- **Definition:** More than 50 eggs per direct stool smear **called heavy infection** or **massive trichuriasis.**
- **Features:**
- Anaemia.
- Malnutrition.
- Rectal prolapse.
- Bloody diarrhoea (blood & mucus in stool **called whip worm dysentery**).

❖ **Laboratory diagnosis:**

➤ **Specimens:** Adult & egg stage can be diagnosed from following specimens.

✪ **Stool:**

✪ **Mucosal (rectal) biopsy:**
- Collected by sigmoidoscope.
- Sigmoidoscopy may show white bodies of worm hanging from the inflamed mucosa **called coconut cake rectum.**

➤ **Testing methods:**

I. Direct methods

A. **Macroscopy:**
- For presence of adult stage in stool.
- In heavy infection stool also contains blood & mucus.

B. **Microscopy:**

i. **Wet mount from stool by using normal saline & iodine:** It revealed bile stained eggs as shown in **fig.-29(b).**

ii. **Concentration technique:** Floats in saturated common salt solution.

II. Indirect methods

A. **Blood picture:**
- Eosinophilia (25%).
- Features of anaemia in heavy infection.

B. **Stool picture:** Presence of CL crystals in stool.

C. **Serological tests:** Not useful.

❖ **Prevention:**
- Washing of vegetable before eating.
- Avoiding the faecal contamination of soil.

❖ **Treatment:** Mebendazole (100 mg 12 hourly for 3-5 days) or albendazole (400 mg single dose) are effective with 70-90& cure rats.

Enterobius vermicularis

❖ **Synonym:** Formerly called *Oxyuris vermicularis.*

❖ **Common name:** Thread worm, seat worm & pin worm.

❖ **Meaning:**
- **Scientific name:**
- ***Oxyuris vermicularis:*** From **Oxyuris = sharp tail,** Feature of female worm.
- ***Enterobius vermicularis:*** From **Enteron (Greek) = intestine + bios = life + vermiculus = small worm,** means tail of hair.
- **Common name:**
- **Thread worm:** Because resemble to short piece of white thread.
- **Pin worm:** Because sharp tail like feature of female worm.

❖ **History:**
- Eggs of *Enterobius vermicularis* are detected in 10,000 year old **coprolith (vide infra)** making it an oldest identified human parasite.
- Life cycle was first described by Leuckart in 1865
- One common saying about this disease is "You had this infection as a child, you have it now or you will get it again when you have children".

✓ **Note: Coprolith**
- **Synonym:** Fecalith or stercolith.
- **Definition:** Hard stony mass of dried faeces in the intestine due to chronic constipation.

❖ **Geographical distribution:**
- World's most common parasite specially infecting children.
- Distributed world-wide.
- Common in developed countries & in temperate climate than tropical countries.

❖ **Habitat:** Adult parasite habitat the large intestine particularly in caecum & also in appendix. It remains on the surface of mucosa & occasionally enters in submucosa.

❖ **Morphology:** Three morphological stages like adult, egg & larval stages. Few important features of parasite are given below. For more details follow chapter → Nematodes: General features and classification.

I. Adult stage

- **Time of maturation:** Eggs transformed to sexually mature adult stage within 2 weeks to 2 months in definitive host after ingestion.

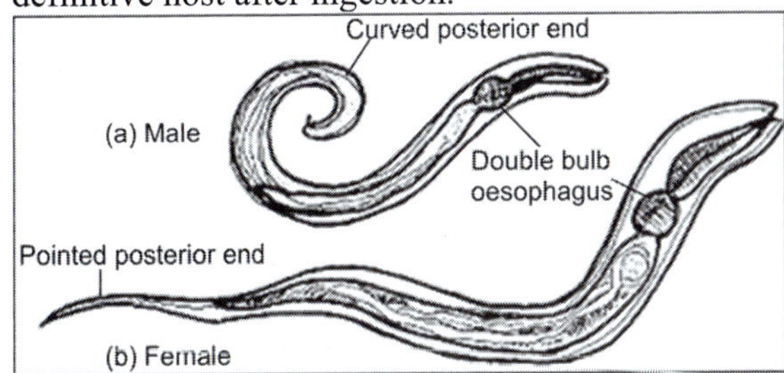

Figure-32: Adult stage of *E. vermicularis*

- **Colour:** It is white in colour.
- **Size:** Female is larger than male as shown in **fig.-32.**
  - Female: 2-4mm × 0.1-0.2mm.
  - Male: 8-12mm × 0.3-0.5mm.
- **Shape:** It is spindle in shape as shown in **fig.-32.** It looks like short white thread.
- **Life span:** Male dies after fertilising female, while female adult worm lives for 37-100 days.
- **Organs:**
- ✪ **Anterior end:** Both, in male & female anterior end is expanded like wings **called cervical alae.**
- ✪ **Posterior (tail) end:**
  - Male: Posterior third of body is curved **(fig.-32)** & sharply truncated.
  - Female: Posterior end is straight & drawn out in to a long, tapering & finely pointed end **(fig.-32)** which is nearly one third of the length of the worm.
- **GIT:**
  - No buccal cavity.
  - Posterior end of oesophagus is dilated like a bulb **called double bulb oesophagus (fig.-32).**
- **Type of female:** It is an oviparous & laying thousand of eggs /day contains tadpole-like larvae.

II. Egg stage

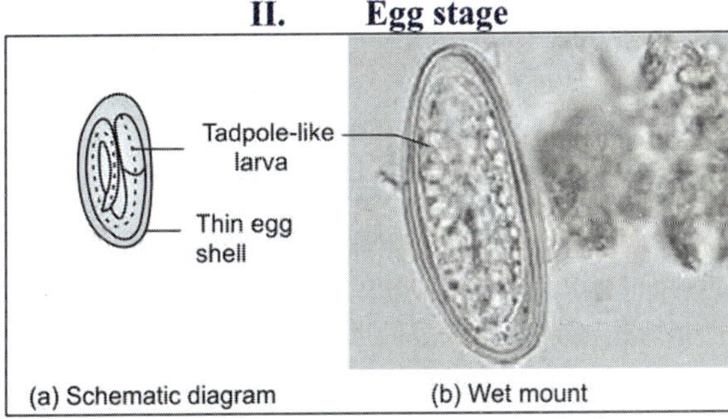

Figure-33: Egg of *E. vermicularis*

- **Morphological features:** Laid by fertilise female **(fig.-33).**
- ✪ **Shape:** Plano-convex (flat on ventral side & convex on dorsal side).
- ✪ **Size:** 50-60μm ×30μm.
- ✪ **Colour**: Colourless (non bile stained).
- ✪ **Covering:** Surrounded by transparent shell.
- ✪ **Embryo:** Contains coiled tadpole-like larva.
- ✪ **Other features:** Floats in saturated common salt solution.

III. Larval stage

- **Form:**
  - Eggs contains tadpole-like larvae are ingested by human host & larvae becomes free on digestion of egg shell.
- **Hosts:** It develop in human intestine.

❖ **Life cycle:**

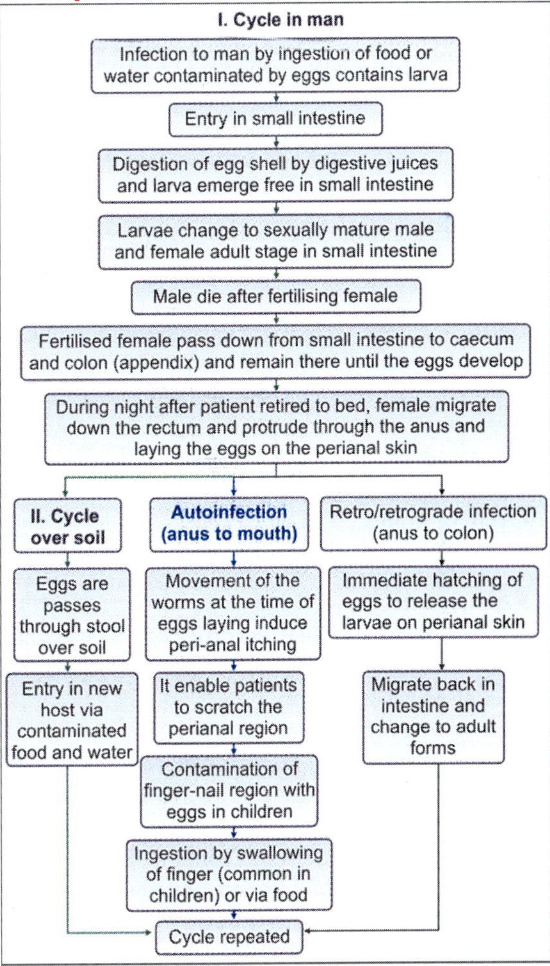

Flow chart-10: Life cycle of *E. vermicularis*

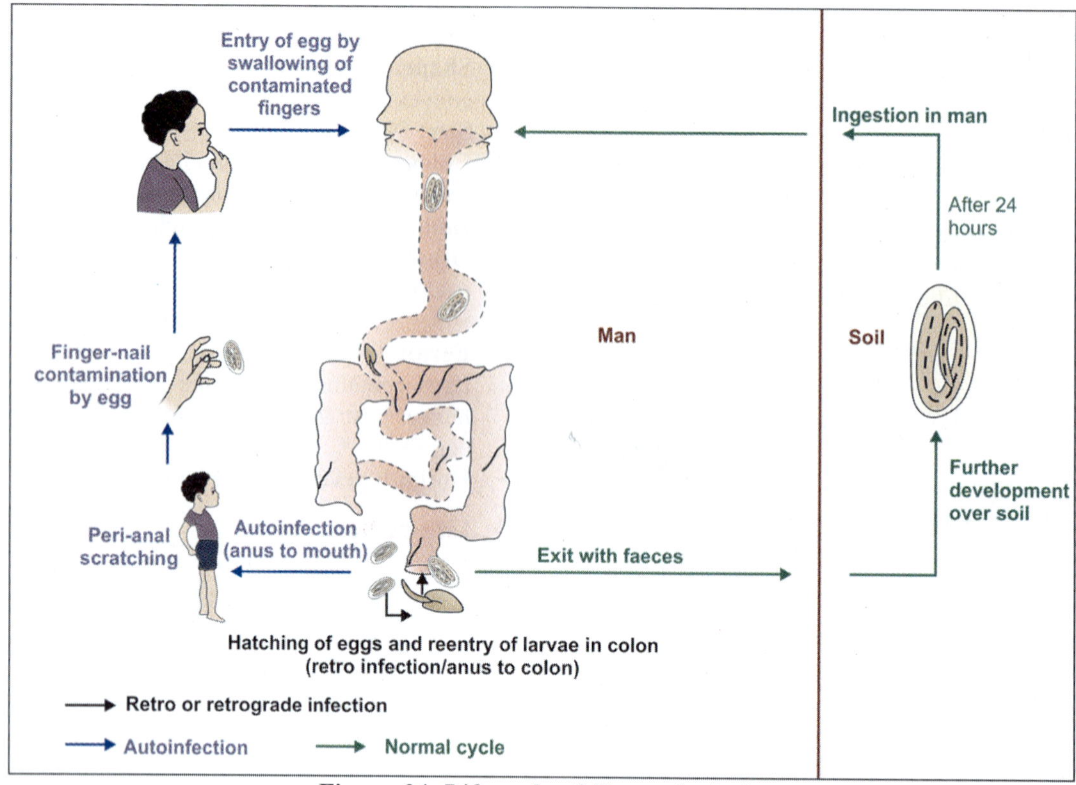

Figure-34: Life cycle of *E. vermicularis*

- **Hosts:**

I. **Definitive host:** Whole cycle is possible in one host only like man. Change of host (other man) is not required for continuation of life cycle, due to autoinfection or retrograde infection.

II. **Intermediate host:** Not required.

- **Cycles:** Following two types of cycle.

I. **Cycle in man:**
II. **Cycle over soil:** } **Flow chart-10 & fig.-34**

❖ Pathogenicity:

- **Disease name: Called enterobiasis** or **oxyuriasis** or **thread worm infection** or **pin worm infection** or **seat worm infection.**
- **Reservoir of infection:** Man.
- **Source of infection:** Food & water.
- **Mode of transmission:** Following four routes.

1. **Ingestion:** Man is infected by ingestion of contaminated food & water contains eggs.
2. **Inhalation:** Especially in infected places.
3. **Auto-infection (anus to mouth):→ Flow chart-9**
4. **Retro/retrograde infection (anus to colon): → Flow chart-9**

- **Exit form:** Eggs.
- **Infective form:** Eggs.
- **Portal of entry:** GIT.
- **Sites:** Adult parasite habitat in caecum & also in appendix.
- **Precipitating factors:**

1. **Age:** Children are the common victims.
2. **Hygiene:** Common in person with poor hygiene.
3. **Climate:** Common in developed countries & in temperate climate than tropical countries.

- **Pathogenesis:** Causes mechanical damage as below
  - It remains on the surface of mucosa & occasionally enters in submucosa.
  - Mechanical irritation of anal mucosa by female worm at the time of eggs laying is responsible for itching **called pruritus ani.**
- **Clinical features:**
  - Mostly asymptomatic.
  - Itching & eczema around the skin of anus & perineum.
  - In 2% it produces the acute appendicitis.
  - Nocturnal enuresis.
  - Abdominal pain & weight loss may occur following heavy infection.
- **Complications:** Migrating female sometimes enters in female genital tract & causing.
  - Urethritis.
  - Salpingitis.
  - Peritonitis after taking entry in peritoneal cavity by fallopian tube.

❖ Laboratory diagnosis:

Indirect methods are not useful. Adult & egg stags can be diagnosed by following direct methods.

I. Adult stage diagnosis:

- **Testing methods:**

A. Macroscopic examination of stool:

- **Collection method & time:**
  - It is collected during normal defecation or by purgation with enema.
  - Early morning time is preferable.
- **Preservation:** Preserve the specimens in alcohol or in 10% formaldehyde, for examination.
- **Macroscopic findings:** Presence of white colour adult worm in stool is examined by adult patients himself or by parents in case of paediatric patients.

B. Direct examination of peri-anal region: Migrating female can be noticed in peri-anal region at the time of eggs laying.

II. Egg stage diagnosis:

➢ **Specimens & testing methods:**

A. Stool specimen:

- **Collection & time:** } Same as like adult stage diagnosis
- **Preservation:** }
- **Microscopic examination:**

i. **Wet mount from stool by using normal saline & iodine:** It revealed non-bile stained eggs as shown in **fig.-33(b).**

ii. **Concentration technique:** Floats in saturated common salt solution.

B. Peri-anal swab: It is collected by following two methods.

i. **NIH swab:**

- **Full form:** National Institute of Health swab.
- **History:**
  - In 1876 Heller recommended the perianl swabbing to collect the materials around perianal region for the enterobiasis diagnosis by using spatulas, curettes, glass slides & rods or by other convenient methods. However, all these measures were not satisfactory.
  - In 1937 Hall invented the cellophane anal swab, commonly **called NIH swab.**
- **NIH swab's apparatus: → Fig.-35**

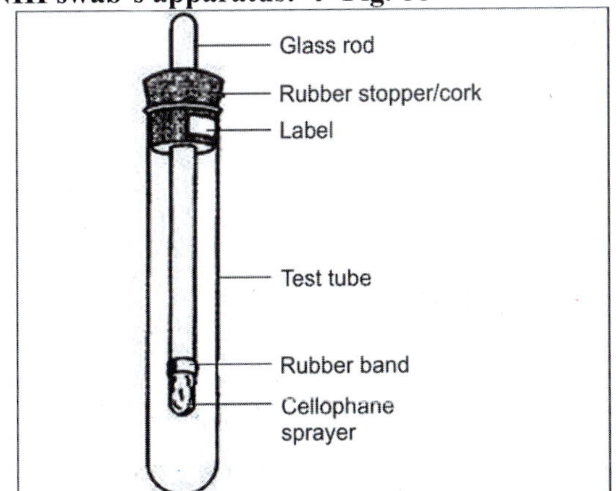

Figure-35: NIH swab's apparatus

- It constitutes a glass rod about 8-10cm× 4mm in size.
- One end of rod is covered with cellophane sprayer (so, **called cellophane sprayer end**) about 1 inch square & held in place by rubber band. This end is inner end & used for swabbing.
- Outer end is passes through rubber cork (stopper) & with which test tube is closed.

- **Time of specimen collection:**
  - An early-morning sample, before the patient has bathed, or used the toilet, is optimal.
  - Up to six successive day morning samples should be collected before a negative result is issued.
- **Swabbing technique:**
  - 1st label the specimen.
  - Remove the glass rod & rub the perianal region with cellophane sprayer end.
  - After swabbing, rod with cellophane sprayer put inside the test tube & sent to the laboratory for smear preparation & testing.
- **Smear preparation technique:**
  - Put a drop of saline over glass slide & hold the cellophane end of rod over it.
  - Push the rubber end up by using forceps until the cellophane is released.
  - With the rod still held in position, the cellophane is spread out & smoothened in such a way that the material adhering to the cellophane comes to lis in direct contact with glass slide.
  - Put a drop of saline over it & placed a cover slip.
  - The eggs thus lie between the glass slide and cellophane.
- **Method of smear examination:** Follow chapter → Laboratory diagnosis of parasitic infections
- **Uses & appearances of eggs:** It is used to collect the peri-anal swab for following parasitic infections.
  - *E. vermicularis:* → **Fig.-33(b).**
  - *T. saginatum:* } →Follow respective chapter.
  - *S. mansoni:* }

✓ **Note: NIH**

- **Full form:** National Institute of Health.
- **Locations:** It is an agency of the Department of Health and Human Services & located in Bethesda, Maryland, USA.
- **Work areas:**
  - It is the primary concerned with biomedical and health-related research.
  - It conducts its own scientific research through its Intramural Research Program (IRP) and provides major research funding to non-NIH research facilities through its Extramural Research Program (ERP).
- **Centres:** It comprises 27 separate institutes & centres for research.

ii. **Scotch cellulose tape method:**

- **Synonym:** Cellophane tape method.

- **Time of specimen collection:** Same as NIH swab.
- **Swabbing technique: → Fig.36 (a-c)**
- Take a cellulose tape about 3-4 inches × ¾ inches in size **[fig.36 (a)].**
- Held it with thumb & index finger on one end of wooden tongue depressor with outer sticky side **[fig.36 (b)].**
- Swabbing is done by placing it on one side & then on other side of anal orifice. **[fig.36 (c)].**

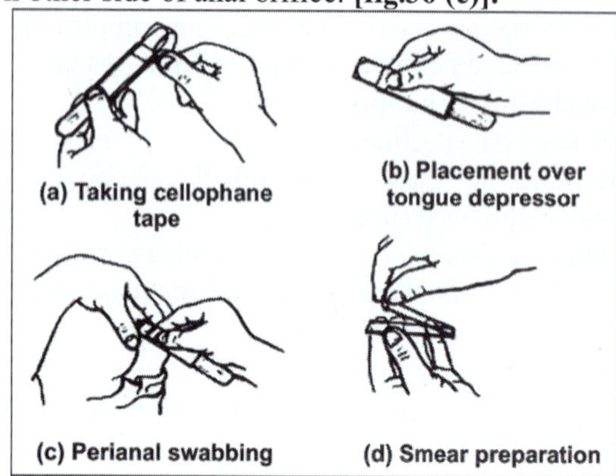

Figure-36: Scotch cellulose tape method

- **Smear preparation technique: → Fig.36 (d)**
- Put a drop of toluene over glass slide for clearing
- Remove the cellulose tape & put on a glass slide with adhesive side down.
- **Method of smear examination:** **Follow chapter → Laboratory diagnosis of parasitic infection.**
- **Uses & appearances of eggs:** Same as NIH swab.

❖ Prevention:

- Frequent washing of hands, cleaning of finger nail region, regular bathing, washing of clothes & bed linen.
- Avoiding the faecal contamination of soil.

❖ Treatment:

- Pyrental pamoate: 11mg/kg OD maximum 1 g. Safe in pregnancy.
- Albendazole: 400mg, single dose.
- Mebendazole: 100 mg single dose.
- Piperizine once daily for 1 week.
- Repeat the treatment to prevent the autoinfection
- Usually pin worm affect the many members of family, so treatment should be given to all members.

Nematodes in arteries & arterioles of ileo- caecal region

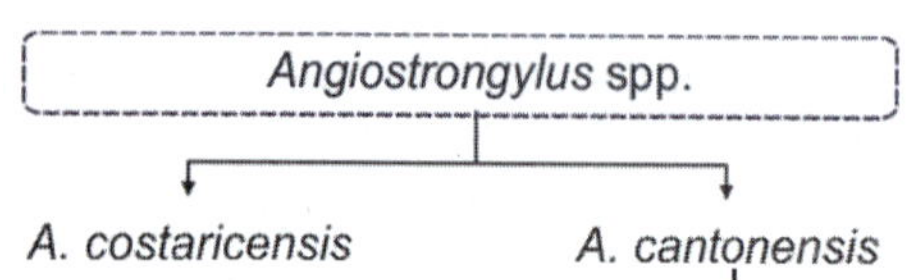

Follow chapter → Nematodes: Somatic (tissue) nematodes

Angiostrongylus costaricensis

❖ Geographical distribution:
Human cases were reported from Costa Rica, Mexico & Central & South America.

❖ Habitat:
Adult parasite habitat in the mesenteric arteries of cotton rats, black rats, number of other rodents & man. Pathology in man is due to both the adults and the eggs.

❖ Morphology:
Three morphological stages like adult, egg & larval stages. Few important features of parasite are given below.

I. Adult stage

- **Size:** Female is larger than male.
- Male: 16-19mm ×0.26mm.
- Female: 21-25 mm × 0.32mm.
- **Shape:** It is transparent filariform body with both ends tapering.

II. Egg stage

- **Morphological features:** Laid by fertilise female.
- **Shape:** Oval.
- **Size:** 72µm ×46µm.
- **Colour**: Colourless (non bile stained).
- **Covering:** Surrounded by delicate hyaline shell.
- **Embryo:** Initially eggs are not embryonated when laid, but embryonated after 6 days.

III. Larval stage

- **Forms & hosts:** Three forms of larvae.

1. **1st stage larva:** It released on hatching of eggs in ileum of rat & excreted with faeces over soil.
2. **2nd stage larva:** 1st stages taken up by slug & moults twice to develop 2nd & 3rd stage of larva.
3. **3rd stage larva:** Develops in slug & infective form for man.

❖ Life cycle:

- **Types of host:**

I. **Definitive host:** Rat.
II. **Intermediate host:** Slug (*Limax maximus*).

- Rat is the optimum host.
- Man is the alternative host & acts as dead end host.
- **Cycles:** As shown in **flow chart-11 & fig.-37.**

❖ Pathogenicity:

- **Disease name:** It is a rat pathogen & human disease **called abdominal angiostrogyliasis** or **eosinophilic gastroenteritis.**
- **Reservoir of infection:** Rat.
- **Source of infection:** Raw slug or food.
- **Mode of transmission:** Man is infected by ingestion of raw slug or food contaminated with slug (3rd stage of larvae).
- **Exit form:** 1st stage of larvae.

- **Infective form:** 3rd stage of larvae.
- **Portal of entry:** GIT.
- **Sites:** Adult parasite habitat in mesenteric arteries of man.

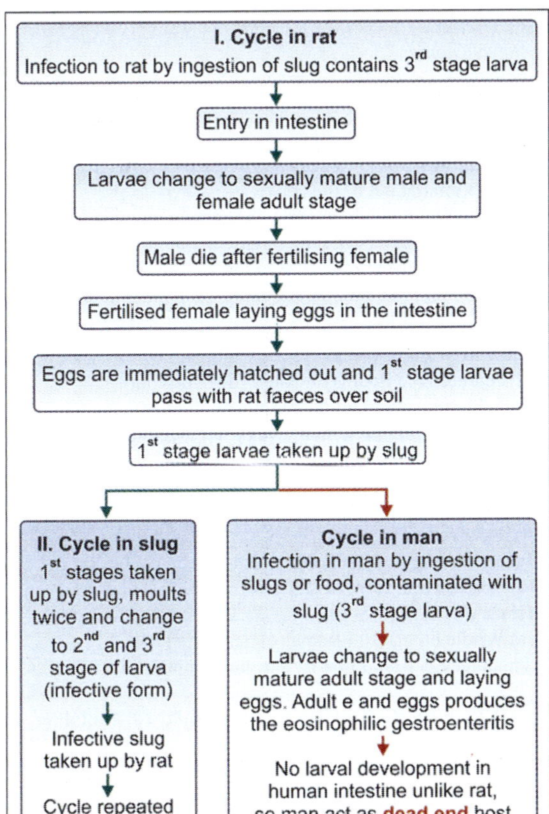

Flow chart-11: Life cycle of *A. costaricensis*

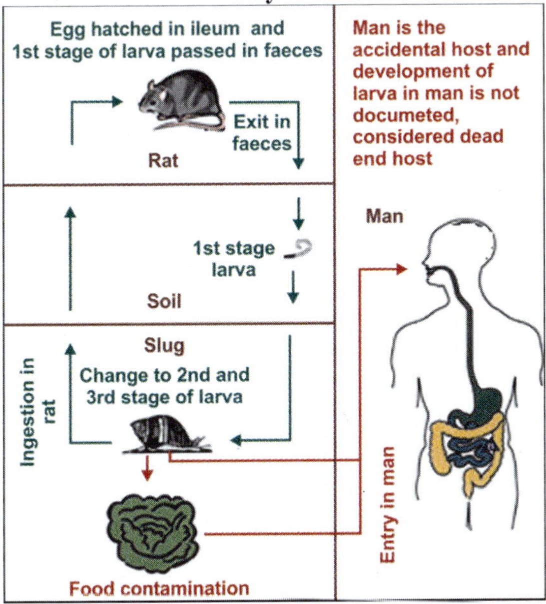

Figure-37: Life cycle of *A. costaricensis*

- **Pathogenesis:**
- Pathology in man is due to both the adults and the eggs.
- Adults in the ileo-caecal arterioles cause an inflammatory (eosinophilic) response in humans. –
- The intestinal wall is also affected. In humans there is a thickening of the intestinal wall (ileum, appendix and caecum).
- In cotton rats with heavy infestations there is a yellow discolouring of the serial surface of the intestinal walls.
- **Clinical features:**

a. **Human infection:**
- Abdominal pain which presents as a palpable mass on clinical examination or simulating appendicitis.
- Anorexia, diarrhoea & vomiting.

b. **Cotton rat infection:**
- In the Cotton rat the adult worms causes local haemorrhages.

❖ Laboratory diagnosis:

- **Specimens:**
- **Stool:** For presence of egg stage or for larvae.
- **Mucosal biopsy or local tissues:**
- **Testing methods:**

I. Direct methods

A **Microscopy:**

i. **Normal saline & iodine preparation from stool:** For eggs or larvae

ii. **Microscopical examination of tissues:** Also shows the presence of eggs or larvae.

II. Indirect methods

A **Blood picture:** Eosinophilia.

B **Biopsy material or Tissue:** Eosinophilia.

C **Serological tests:** ELISA is positive sometimes.

❖ Differences between *A. costaricensis* & *A. cantonensis*: → Table-6

Features	*A. costaricensis*	*A. cantonensis*
Habitat	Mesenteric artery	Pulmonary artery
Intermediate host	Slug	Snail
Pathogenic lesion	By adult & egg stage	By larval stage

Table-6: Differences between *A. costaricensis* & *A. cantonensis*

Question bank

Case study

1) A 40 year female came with complain of fever, cough & dyspnoea. Macroscopic stool examination shows the presence of adult worm with posterior end curved ventrally in the form of a hook having conical tip. Microscopic stool examination revealed bile stained egg with unsegmented embryo. Identify the case and answer the following.

a) Name & draw the properly labelled diagram of egg of causative agent.
b) Describe the life cycle of causative agent.
c) Describe the Pathogenicity of causative agent.
d) Describe the lab. diagnosis of causative agent.

2) A 40 year man came with complain of local skin lesion & pain in abdomen. Stool examination revealed non-bile stained egg with embryo with segments. Blood examination shows the anaemic picture. Identify the case and answer the following.

a) Name & draw the properly labelled diagram of egg of causative agent.
b) Describe the life cycle of causative agent.
c) Describe the Pathogenicity of causative agent.
d) Describe the lab. diagnosis of causative agent.

Essay/Full question

1) Small intestinal nematodes.

Short notes

1) Eggs of *Ascaris lumbricoides* (morphology & types).
2) Life cycle / pathogenicity / laboratory diagnosis of *Ascaris lumbricoides.*
3) Ectopic ascariasis.
4) Life cycle / pathogenicity / laboratory diagnosis of *Ancyclostoma duodenale.*
5) Coproculture.
6) Difference between *A. duodenale* & *N. americanus.*
7) Life cycle / pathogenicity / laboratory diagnosis of *Strogyloides stercoralis.*
8) Life cycle / pathogenicity / laboratory diagnosis of *Trichuris trichuria.*
9) Life cycle / pathogenicity / laboratory diagnosis of *E. vermicularis.*
10) NIH swab.

Short questions for theory/viva questions

1) What is trichinella cyst?
2) What vulvar waist in *Ascaris lumbricoides*?
3) Write the four differences between fertilise & unfetilise eggs of *Ascaris lumbricoides.*
4) What is decorticated egg of *Ascaris lumbricoides*?
5) What is ripe egg of *Ascaris lumbricoides*?
6) What is Loeffler's syndrome?
7) What is Y-shape appearance of hook worm?
8) What is blastomere?
9) What is coproculture & coprolith?
10) Comment: Blood loss by *A. duodenale* is more than *N. americanus* in intestinal infection or *A. duodenale* is more dangerous than *N. americanus.*
11) Define: Blastomere & blastospore.
12) Difference between larvae of hook worm & *strogyloides.*
13) Write 4 names of parasites which eggs can be mistaken as hook worm's eggs.
14) What is parthenogenetic parasite? Write one example.
15) Write different modes of formation of filariform larvae in *strogyloides stercoralis.*
16) Name the two nematodes transmitted by penetrating the skin.
17) What is larva currens?
18) What is swollen belly syndrome?
19) Write the four differences between eggs of *Capillaria philippinensis* & *Trichuris trichuria.*
20) Draw the morphological labelled disgram of eggs of *A. lumbricoides, A. duodenale, T. trichuria* & *E. vermicularis.*
21) Write different modes of transmission of *E. vermicularis.*
22) Name the two nematodes transmitted by inhalation route.

MCQs for chapter review

Classification

1) **Small intestinal helminths are** (PGI-11)
(a) *Ascaris* (b) *Necator* (c) *Trichuris* (d) *Enterobius* (e) *Ancyclostoma*
2) **Which of the following resides in caecum?**
(a) *Trichuris trichuria* (b) *A lumbricoides* (c) *Strongyloides* (d) *Ancyclostoma*

Ascaris lumbricoides

3) **Ascariasis causes**
(a) Appendicitis (b) Intestinal obstruction (c) Bile duct obstruction (d) All of the above
4) **Specific diagnosis of ascariasis is made by** (PGI, Dec-04)
(a) Adult worm in stool (b) Egg detection (c) Antigen detection (d) Antibody detection (e) Skin test

Hook worm spp.

5) **Habitat of hook worm**
(a) Jejunum (b) Ileum (c) Colon (d) Duodenum
6) ***Ankylostoma duodenale* commonly lives in**
(a) Upper $\frac{1}{3}$rd of duodenum (b) Lower $\frac{1}{3}$rd of duodenum (c) Jejunum (d) Ileum
7) ***Ankylostoma* enters the human body by**
(a) Ingestion (b) Inhalation (c) Penetration of skin (d) Inoculation
8) **Infective stage of hook worm is**
(a) Trophozoite form (b) Filariform larva (c) Cyst (d) None
9) **Hook worm thrives on**
(a) Whole blood (b) Plasma (c) Serum (d) RBC
10) **The average blood loss in ankylostomiasis per worm is** (PGI-79)
(a) 0.2 ml/day (b) 2 ml/day (c) 0.33 ml/day (d) 1 ml/day

Strogyloides spp.

11) **Parasitic intestinal infestation seen in immunosuppressed patient is**
(a) Giardisis (b) Ascariasis (c) Liver fluke (d) Schistosomiasis (e) *Strongyloides*
12) **The cause of larva currens**
(a) *Strongyloides stercoralis* (b) *Necator americanus* (c) *Ancyclostoma duodenale* (d) *H nana*
13) **Infection with colitis is caused by** (PGI-00)
(a) *Enterobius vermicularis* (b) *Trichuris trichuria* (c) *Strongyloides* (d) *Clonorchis*

Trichuris trichuria

14) **Mucus plug at each pole of eggs is present in**
(a) *T. spiralis* (b) *A. lumbricoides* (c) *T. trichuria* (d) *E. vermicularis*
15) **Chronic dysentery, abdominal pain and rectal proplapse in children is caused by**
(a) *Enterobius vermicularis* (b) Ascariasis (c) *Trichuris trichuria* (d) *Trichinella spiralis*

Enterobius vermicularis

16) **Seat worm is** (AIIMS, 80,84)
(a) *Enterobius* (b) *Dracunculus* (c) *Ancyclostoma* (d) *Necator*
17) **Child having perianal pruritus is due to eggs of following**
(a) *Enterobius vermicularis* (b) *Ascaris* (c) *Ancyclostoma duodenale* (d) *Strongyloides stercoralis*
18) **Most common presenting symptoms of thread worm infection amongst the following is** (AI-97)
(a) Abdominal pain (b) Rectal prolapse (c) Utricaria (d) Vaginitis

Answers of MCQs & explanation

1) **(a), (b) & (e)**

- Follow section, **classification** for explanation

2) **(a)**
- Follow section, **classification** for explanation
- Also follow section, ***Trichuris trichuria*** **(habitat)** for more explanation

3) **(d)**
- Follow section, ***Ascaris lumbricoides*** **(pathogenicity → clinical features & flow chart-4)** for explanation

4) **(a) & (b)**
- Follow section, ***Ascaris lumbricoides*** **(laboratory diagnosis)** for explanation

5) **(a), (b) & (d)**
6) **(a), (b), (c) & (d)**

} Follow section, ***Ancyclostoma duodenale*** **(habitat)** for explanation

7) **(c)**
- Follow section, ***Ancyclostoma duodenale*** **(pathogenicity → mode of transmission)** for explanation

8) **(b)**
- Follow section, ***Ancyclostoma duodenale*** **(pathogenicity → infective form)** for explanation

9) **(b)**
10) **(a)**

} Follow section, ***Ancyclostoma duodenale*** **(pathogenicity → pathogenesis & clinical features → due to adult stage)** for explanation

11) **(e)**
12) **(a)**
13) **(c)**

} Follow section, ***Strongyloides stercoralis*** **(pathogenicity → pathogenesis & clinical features & flow chart-8)** for explanation

14) **(c)**
- Follow section, ***Trichuris trichuria*** **(morphology → egg stage)** for explanation

15) **(c)**
- From the given options only option 'a' is right. Follow section, ***Trichuris trichuria*** **(pathogenicity → clinical features)** for explanation

16) **(a)**
- Follow section, ***Enterobius vermicularis*** **(common name)** for explanation

17) **(c)**
- Follow section, ***Enterobius vermicularis*** **(pathogenicity → pathogenesis)** for explanation

18) **(a)**
- From the given options only option 'a' is right. Follow section, ***Enterobius vermicularis*** **(pathogenicity → clinical features)** for explanation

99 Nematodes: Somatic (tissue) nematodes

Learning heading & subheadings

Classification:

- **Filariasis**
  - Lymphatic filariasis
  - Subcutaneous filariasis
  - Serous cavity filariasis
  - Zoonotic filariasis
- **Other diseases**
  - Disease in liver
  - Disease in brain
  - Disease in brain & other tissues
  - Disease in subcutaneous tissues

Classification:

I. Systemic classification: Follow chapter → Introduction and classification of parasites (section →table-4) for more details

II. Pathological classification: Following are the two main types of disease produced by tissue nematodes.

i. Filariasis: Filariasis is a broad terminology further classified on the basis of habitat by different species.

a. Lymphatic filariasis: *W. bancrofti, B. malayi* & *B. timori.*

b. Subcutaeous filariasis: *O. volvulus, L. loa,* & *M. strptocerca.*

c. Serous cavity filariasis: *M. perstans* & *M. ozzardi*

d. Zoonotic filariasis: *B. pahangi, D. immitis, D. tenuis* & *D. repens.*

✓ **Note: Non-lymphatic filariasis**

- From the above list subcutaneous, serous & zoonotic are considered as non lymphatic filariasis.

ii. Other diseases: Further classified on the basis of habitat by different species.

a. Diseases in lungs: Larva of

- *S. stercoralis:*
- *A. lumbricoides:*
- *A. duodenale :*

} Follow chapter → Nematodes: Intestinal nematodes

b. Diseases in liver: *C. hepatica.*

c. Diseases in brain: *A. cantonensis.*

d. Diseases in brain & other tissues: *Gnathostoma* spp.

e. Diseases in subcutaeous tissues: *D. medinensis.*

Filariasis

General aspects of filariasis

◊ **Definition:** Infection by any worms from the Superfamily Filarioidea **called filariasis** but it is limited to *W. bancrofti* & *B .malayi* (also newer species like *B. timori*).

◊ **Meaning:** From **filum (Latin) = thread** caused by slender thread like worms.

◊ **Taxonomy:** Filarial parasites are belongs to the **Super family filarioidea**, which has four families, but pathogenic spp. are belongs to **Achantho-cheilonematidae family.**

◊ **Morphology:**

I. Adult stage

➢ **Size:**

- Adult worms are 80-100 mm×0.25-0.30 mm in size, except female of *onchocercus.*
- Female is larger than the male.

➢ **Shape:** Slender thread **(filum)** like worms.

- **Organs:**
- **GIT:** Worms possess simple lipless mouth, cylindrical oesophagus without bulb & simple intestine that may be atrophied at posteriorly.
- **Tail end:** Tail of male worm has perianal papillae & unequal spicules but no caudal bursa.
- **Life span:** Many years.
- **Differential character of adult stages:** → Flow chart-1

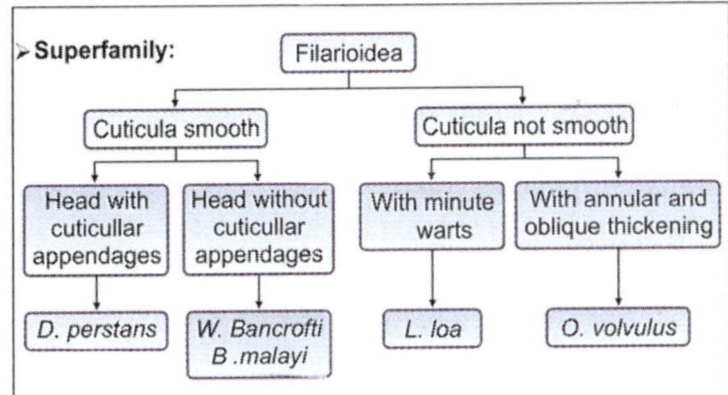

Flow chart-1: Differential characters of adult worms

II. Larval stage

- **Name:** Female is viviparous giving birth to the larvae **called microfilariae.**
- **Size:** About 290 µm× 6-7 µm.
- **Shape:** Vermiform in appearance.
- **Organs:**
- **Sheath:**
  - In some species microfilariae retain their egg membrane which develops in to sheath **called sheathed microfilariae** & which are lacking **called unsheathed microfilariae.**
  - It is longer than the length of larvae so microfilariae can move to & fro within the sheath.
- **Special cells:** These are the precursor of body organs or organelles.
- **Nuclei:** Present along the length of microfilariae & interrupted by spaces or by special cells.
- **Periodicity:**
- **Types, definitions & examples:** Depending on presence of microfilariae in blood, filarial worms can exhibit following type periodicity.

1. **Nocturnal periodicity:**
   - Microfilariae present in blood during night between 10pm-4am.
   - Example: *W. bancrofti.*
2. **Diurnal periodicity:**
   - Microfilariae present in blood during day.
   - Example: *B .malayi.*
3. **Nonperiodic:**
   - Microfilariae constantly present in blood during night & day.
   - Example: *O. volvulus.*
4. **Subperiodic or nocturnal subperiodic:**
   - Microfilariae constantly present in blood during day but detected in late afternoon or during the night.
   - Example: *B .malayi.*

- **Mechanisms:** Exactly not known but may be due to night feeding habit of intermediate host.
- **Hosts:** Microfilariae complete its development in arthropod to achieve infective form for human.
- **Life span:** 3-36 months.
- **Staining properties:** → **Vide infra**
- **Distribution:** While examining blood films following thing should keep in mind.
  - Africa: *Mf. Bancrofti, Mf. perstans* & *Mf. loa.*
  - South America: *Mf. Bancrofti, Mf. perstans* & *Mf. ozzardi.*
  - India: *Mf. Bancrofti* & *Mf. malayi.*
  - Brazil: *Mf. lewisi.*
- **Differential types:** Microfilariae are differentiated on the basis of presence or absence of sheath, periodicity, numbers of nuclei at tail end & habitat as shown in **fig.-1.**

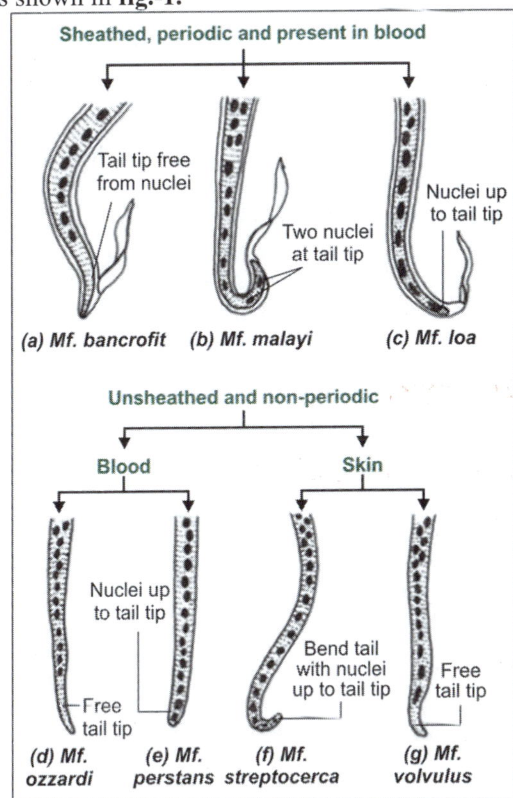

Figure-1: Differential types of microfilariae

- **Immunology:** Following types of immune reaction occurs in man.
- **Acquired immunity:**
  - Acquired immunity develops only against dead parasites but not against live & able to remove microfilaria from body not the adult stage. CMI plays dominant role than AMI.
  - Both cellular & humoral response can develop.

- It lowers the microfilariae density in man in the age group of 15-20 years. In onchocerciasis microfilariae density does not decrease with age.
- High level of antibodies in occult filariasis prevents the entry of microfilariae (*W. Bancrofti, B .malayi* & other animal parasites) in peripheral blood.
- A significant rise of serum IgM observed in wucheriasis & IgE in onchocerciasis.
- Antibodies are diagnosed by CFT, haemagglutination test etc. by using antigen prepared from *D. immitis.*
- Usually positive in occult filariasis & may cross react with *A. lumbricoides, S. stercoralis* & *Schistosoma species*.

➢ **Hypersensitivity:** Immediate type hypersensitivity develops & detected by intradermal test in onchocerciasis (**called Mazzotti's test**) & wucheriasis.

◊ **Life cycle:**

I. **Definitive host:** Man.

II. **Intermediate host:** Vectors (insects).

◊ **Mode of transmission:** Transmitted by blood sucking insects.

◊ **Clinical types:** Different types of filariasis like lymphatic, subcutaneous, serous cavity & zoonotic described in details as follows.

Lymphatic filariasis

Wucheria bancrofti

❖ **Synonym:** *Filaria bancrofti, Wucheria pacifica, Filaria sanguinis hominis.*

❖ **Common name:** Bancroft's filaria.

❖ **Meaning:** **Genus name** given from the **Wucherer** who found the parasite in chylous urine & **species name** came from the **Bancroft** who found the adult female.

❖ **History:**

- **Filariasis** has been known since antiquity.
- **Elephantiasis** has been defined in India by Sushratha & in Persia by Rhazes & Avicenna.
- **"Malabar leg"** was applied to the condition by Clarke in Cochin in 1709.
- Larval stage **called microfilariae** was 1st identified by Demarquay in 1863 in the hydrocele fluid from Havana, Cuba. Wucher identified it in chylous urine in 1866 & Lewis identified it in blood in 1872 in Kolkata.
- Adult female was described by Bancroft in 1876 & the adult male was described by Bourne in 1888.
- Manson identified the Culex mosquito as vector in China in 1878. (1st human disease identified as vector borne). Manson also noticed the nocturnal periodicity of microfilariae in peripheral blood in 1879.

❖ **Geographical distribution:** Parasites are confirmed to tropical & subtropical areas.

- **In world:** Common in West Indies, Puerto Rico, Africa, Southern China, Japan, Pacific Islands & South America.
- **In India:** It is prevalent along the coast of big rivers & also in Rajasthan, Bihar, Uttar Pradesh, Punjab & Delhi.

❖ **Habitat:** Adult parasite habitat the lymphatic vessels & lymph nodes in man. It's not a zoonotic disease, so not habitat in the animals.

❖ **Morphology:** Two morphological stages like adult & larval stages. Few important features of parasite are given below.

I. Adult stage

➢ **Time of maturation:** Larva transformed to sexually mature adult stage in 5-18 months in definitive host after injection.

➢ **Size:** Female is larger than male as shown in **fig.-2.**

- Female: 8-10cm ×0.2-0.3mm.
- Male: 2.5-4cm ×0.1mm.

➢ **Shape:** Long thread or hair like body with both the ends are tapering as shown in **fig.-2.**

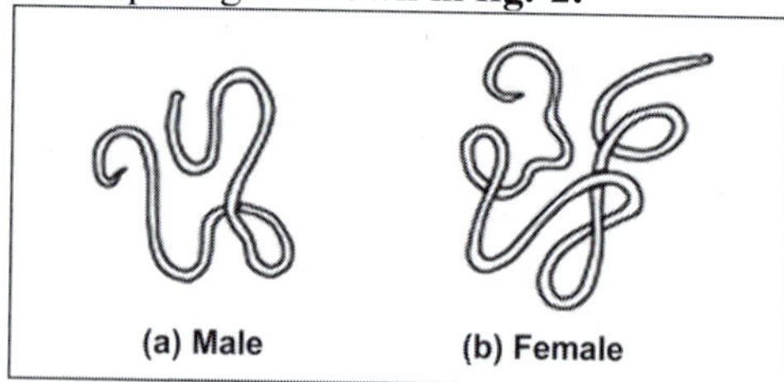

Figure-2: Adult stage of *W. bancrofti*

➢ **Colour:** Transparent & creamy-white in colour.

➢ **Life span:**

- Male die after fertilising the female about one week after infection.
- Female may live for 5-10 years.

➢ **Ends:**

✪ **Head end:** The head end terminating in a slightly rounded swelling.

✪ **Tail end:**

- Female: Narrow & abruptly pointed.
- Male: Curved ventrally & contains two spicules of unequal length.

➢ **Numbers:** Male & female remains coiled together & separated with difficulties. Female's numbers are more than males.

➢ **Type of female:** It is viviparous & laying the embryo.

II. Larval stage (microfilaria)

➢ **Form:** Solid forms of larvae are present **called microfilariae** as shown in **fig.-3.**

➢ **Size:** 290μm×6-7 μm.

- **Shape:** Long body with blunt head & pointed tail end.
- **Colour:** Transparent & colourless.
- **Life span:** In human body it can live for 70 days.
- **Host:** It develops in human & later enters in mosquito.
- **Motility:** It is very active & move through & against the blood flow.
- **Morphology & staining properties:**

a. **Wet mount from samples (unstained preparation):** Actively motile microfilariae are seen under low or high power microscopy.

b. **Stained preparation:** Following morphological features are examined by Romanowsky's stain under oil immersion lens.

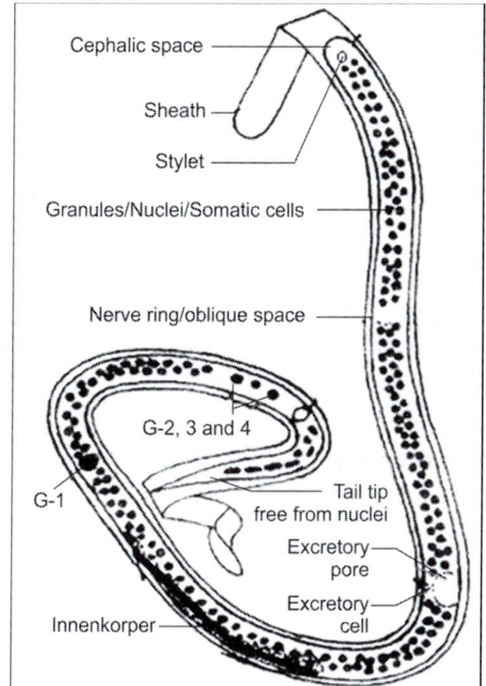

Figure-3: Schematic diagram of microfilaria of *W. bancrofti*

- **Sheath:**
  - It is a structureless sac, seen best when projecting beyond the extremities of embryo.
  - It represents the egg shell.
  - It is longer (359µm) than the length of larva, so larva can move to & fro within the body.
- **Cuticulla:** It is lined by subcuticullar cells.
- **Ends:**
  - Head end: Blunt.
  - Tail end: Pointed.
- **Stylet:** It seen with vital stain.
- **Nuclei or granules or somatic cells:**
  - Appear as granules in central axis of body & extend from the head to tail end except the terminal tip (terminal 5%).
  - They are broken at certain places & making the landmark for identification of species. It includes

1. **Cephalic space:** They are absent at head end **called cephalic space.**
2. **Nerve ring:** It is an oblique space.
3. **Anterior V-spot:** Represent the rudimentary excretory system.
4. **Posterior V-spot or tail-spot:** Represent the terminal part of GIT (anus/cloaca).

- **G-cells or genital cells:** G-2, 3 & 4 are situated just in front of anal pore while G-1 further front.
- **Innenkorper of fulleborn or Central body of Manson or internal body of Manson:**
  - It extends from anterior V-spot to G-cells.
  - It represents the rudimentary alimentary canal.

- **Periodicity:**
- **In India & China:**
  - Microfilariae showing **nocturnal periodicity** & present in blood during night between 10pm-4am.
  - During day time they are residing in capillaries of lungs, kidneys, heart & artery such as carotid.
  - Exactly mechanisms for such are not known but may be due to night feeding habit of its intermediate host (*Culex fatigans*).
- **In Pacific Island:**
  - Microfilariae are **nonperiodic or subperiodic** & present in blood during day plus night.
  - In Polynesian island *Aedes polynesiensis* act as intermediate host, which can bite at any time.
  - In Melanesian island *Anopheles punctulatus* act as intermediate host, which can bite at any time.
- **Density required to infect the mosquito:** At least 15 microfilariae per drop of blood are required to infect the mosquito.

✓ **Note: Nonperiodic or subperiodic microfilariae**

- ***W. pacifica***: Some authors mentioned the distinct species ***W. pacifica*** for nonperiodic or subperiodic microfilariae, which is prevalent in Pacific Island, but this name is not widely accepted.

Immunity:

- **Humoral immunity:** No role.
- **Cell mediated immunity:** Play the dominant role.

Life cycle:

- **Types of host:**

I. **Definitive host:** Man. No animal host or reservoir is known.

II. **Intermediate host:** Female mosquito (mosquito also act as an intermediate host in *Brugia* spp., *Mansonella* spp. & *Dirofilaria* spp.)

- **In India:** *Culex fatigans* (*Culex quinquefasciatus*).
- **In Pacific Island:**
  - **In Polynesian Island:** *Aedes polynesiensis.*
  - **In Melanesian island**: *Anopheles punctulatus.*
- **Cycles:** Whole cycle is possible between man & mosquito as shown in **flow chart-2 & fig.-4.**

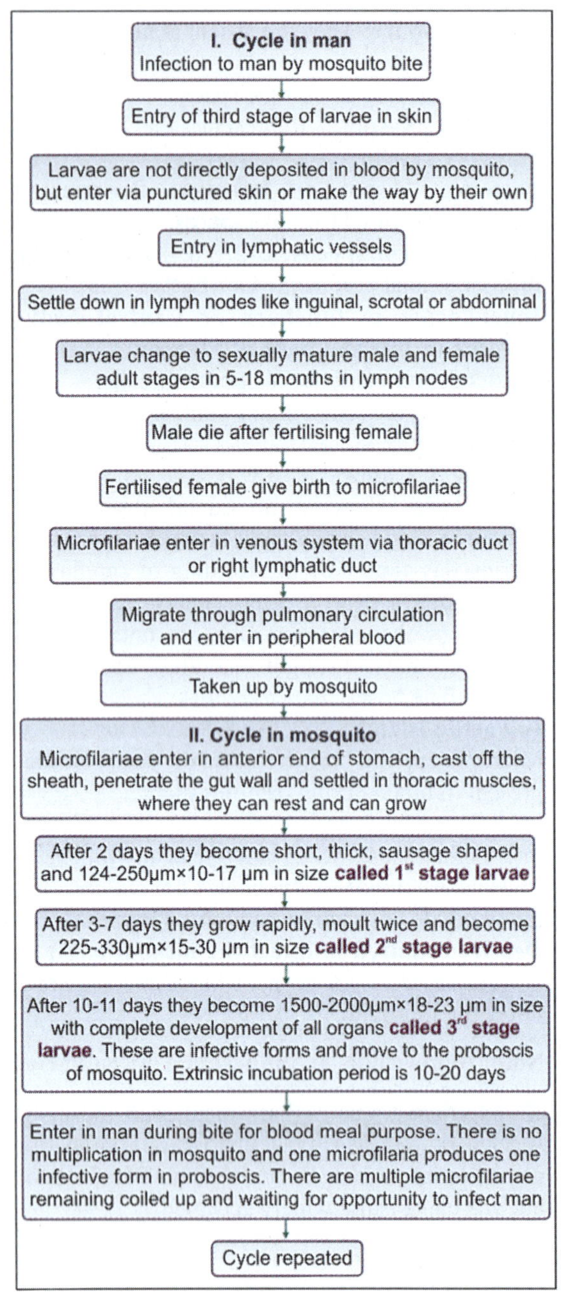

I. Cycle in man
Infection to man by mosquito bite
Entry of third stage of larvae in skin
Larvae are not directly deposited in blood by mosquito, but enter via punctured skin or make the way by their own
Entry in lymphatic vessels
Settle down in lymph nodes like inguinal, scrotal or abdominal
Larvae change to sexually mature male and female adult stages in 5-18 months in lymph nodes
Male die after fertilising female
Fertilised female give birth to microfilariae
Microfilariae enter in venous system via thoracic duct or right lymphatic duct
Migrate through pulmonary circulation and enter in peripheral blood
Taken up by mosquito
II. Cycle in mosquito
Microfilariae enter in anterior end of stomach, cast off the sheath, penetrate the gut wall and settled in thoracic muscles, where they can rest and can grow
After 2 days they become short, thick, sausage shaped and 124-250μm×10-17 μm in size called 1st stage larvae
After 3-7 days they grow rapidly, moult twice and become 225-330μm×15-30 μm in size called 2nd stage larvae
After 10-11 days they become 1500-2000μm×18-23 μm in size with complete development of all organs called 3rd stage larvae. These are infective forms and move to the proboscis of mosquito. Extrinsic incubation period is 10-20 days
Enter in man during bite for blood meal purpose. There is no multiplication in mosquito and one microfilaria produces one infective form in proboscis. There are multiple microfilariae remaining coiled up and waiting for opportunity to infect man
Cycle repeated

Flow chart-2: Life cycle of *W. bancrofti*

✓ **Note: Incubation periods**

- **Extrinsic incubation period:**
- Time taken by vector to become infective after receiving the microorganisms **called extrinsic incubation period.**
- It totally depends on atmospheric temperature, humidity & to certain extent on type of mosquito.
- It is about 10-20 days in *W. bancrofti.*
- **Biological incubation period or pre-patent period:**

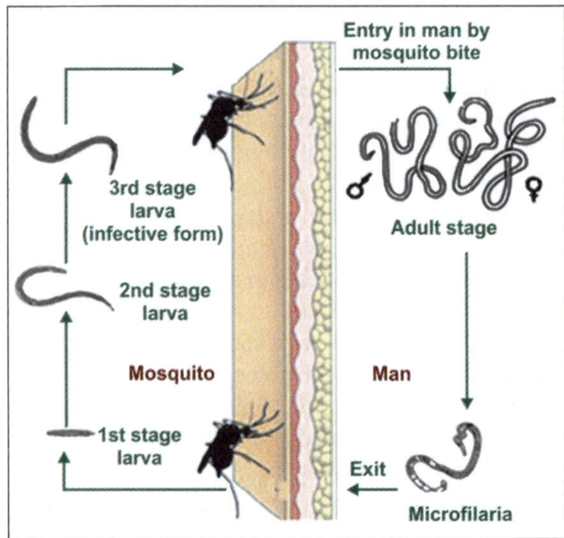

Figure-4: Life cycle of *W. bancrofti*

- Time taken by microbes to appear first in blood after infection **called pre-patent period**.
- It is about 1-1½ years in *W. bancrofti.*
- **Intrinsic Incubation period or Clinical incubation period or Incubation period:**
- Interval between entry of microorganisms & appearance of 1st clinical features **called incubation period**.
- Commonly it is referred as **incubation period.**
- It is about 8-16 months in *W. bancrofti.*

❖ Pathogenicity:

- **Disease name: Called wucheriasis.**
- **Synonym:** Also **called Bancroft's filariasis** or **called lymphatic filariasis** or commonly **called filariasis.**
- **Reservoir of infection:** Man.
- **Source of infection:** Mosquito.
- **Mode of transmission:**
- **Route:** By female mosquito bite.
- **Species:** → Vide supra.
- **Infective dose:**
- It is not know, but many larvae fail to penetrate the skin by themselves & many are destroyed by immunological mechanisms.
- A very large number of infected mosquito bites are required to transmit the infection, perhaps about 15,000 infective bites per person.
- **Incubation period:** 8-16 months.
- **Exit form:** Microfilariae.
- **Infective form:** Third stage of larvae.
- **Portal of entry:** Skin.
- **Sites:** Lymphatic system, mostly inguino-scrotal region & mostly unilateral.
- **Precipitating factors (epidemiological determinants):**

1. **Agent (virulence) factors:** Like liberation of toxic products by live/dead adult stage & microfilariae.

2. **Vector factors:** Like density, life span, choice of host, resting habit, breeding habit, time of biting & resistance to insecticides.
3. **Host factors:**
- **Age:** Morbidity increase with increasing age. More common in older age.
- **Sex:** More in male than female because of outdoor visit & better covering of clothes in female.
- **Human habit:** Sleeping outside & not using mosquito repellents like net, cream etc.
- **Migration:** Migration to endemic areas increases the spread.
4. **Environmental factors:**
- **Climate:** Temperature between 22-38^{0}C & humidity >70% increase the risk.
- **Drainage:** It is associated with bad drainage.
- **Town planning:** Lack of town planning may aggravate the breeding of mosquitoes.

➢ **Clinical types:** Clinical outcome of filariasis is varies in different person as follows.

I. Person from endemic areas:
- It is mostly asymptomatic, even with high microfilarial density in peripheral blood (20,000/ml).
- Such person can tolerate the microfilaria & does not mount any immune response.

II. Person from non-endemic areas: It progress to disease with classical & occult filariasis as below.

A. Classical filariasis:
- **Definition:** It is an acute inflammation of lymphatic vessels.
- **Pathogenesis:**, **Stage of disease**, **Clinical features:** → **Flow chart-3**
- **Pathology:** Below changes seen in lymphatic system.
- Adult worms which are present in lymph nodes are aggravating the eosinophilic infiltration by releasing toxic metabolites which reduce nutrition supply to the worm causing death.
- The tissue surrounding the dead worms undergoes necrosis & worms are undergoes to degeneration or calcification.
- Dead worms (not the live worms) allow the response from RE system indicated by degeneration of dead worms by macrophages & giant cells.
- Eosinophilic infiltration which was appeared earlier start to disappear & replaced by macrophages & giant cells.

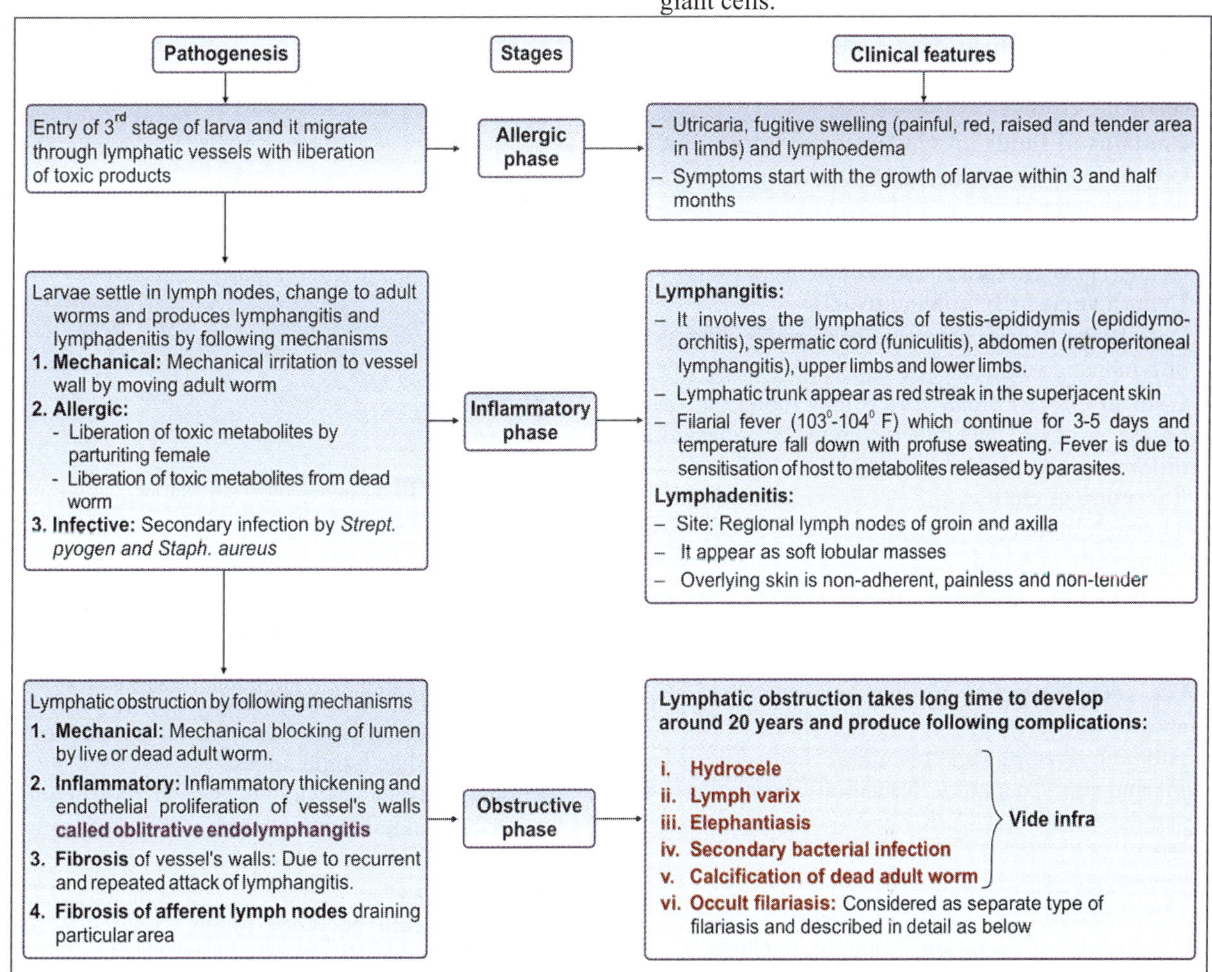

Flow chart-3: Pathogenesis, stage of disease, & clinical features of classical filariasis

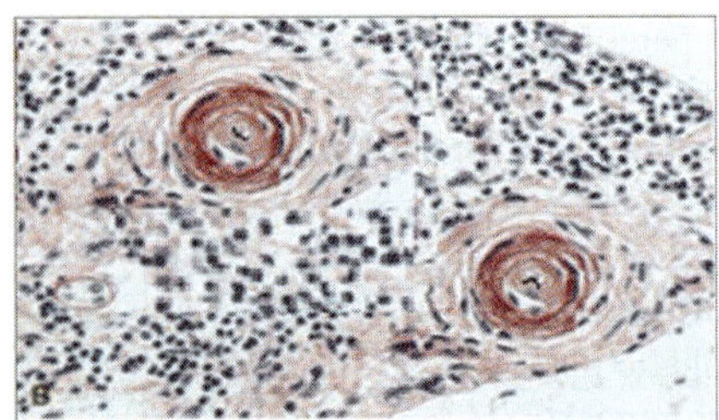

Figure-5: "Parasitic onion" around dead worms

- Fibroblasts begin to appear & form the concentric layers around the nucleus of dead worm, whose presence may not be determined later due to formation of scar tissue.
- New capillaries start to develop in fibrous layer.
- Such pathological layers formation around dead worms **called "parasitic onion"** as shown in **fig.-5.**
- Besides the lymph nodes other organs of RE system like liver & spleen do not take any active part in wucherial infection & they are spared to deal with disposal of microfilariae circulating in blood.

✪ **Complications:**

i. **Hydrocele:**

- **Definition:** It is defined as collection of fluid in scrotum.
- **Mechanisms:** It is due to obstruction of paraaortic lymph nodes which cause interference of fluid drainage from tunica vaginalis, epididymis & spermatic cord.
- **Contains of fluid:** Live microfilariae are present in hydrocele fluid but not able to survive longer & they die in the fluid.
- **Geographical variation:** Common in East Africa, China, Japan but rare in Pacific Islands & India.

ii. **Lymph varix or lymphangiovarix:**

- **Definition:** It is an abnormal irreversible dilatation of lymphatic vessels.
- **Clinical effects:** Small vessels may rupture in large vessels & chyle may either excreted or collected in different body cavities as follows.

a. **Excretion of chyle:**

1. **Through urine:**

o <u>Urine without blood</u>:

♣ **Name: Called chyluria.**

♣ **Appearance:** Milky white (**fig.6**).

♣ **Contains:** Chylous urine contains

- Fat cells: Detected by fat solvents like ether, chloroform or xylol.
- Albumin: Precipitated on boiling.
- Fibrinogen: Coagulum formation when allow to stands.
- RBCs.
- Lymphocytes.
- Microfilariae.

♣ **Geographical variation:** Common in China, Japan & South India but rare in Africa & Pacific Islands.

o <u>Urine mixed with blood</u>: **Called haematochyluria.**

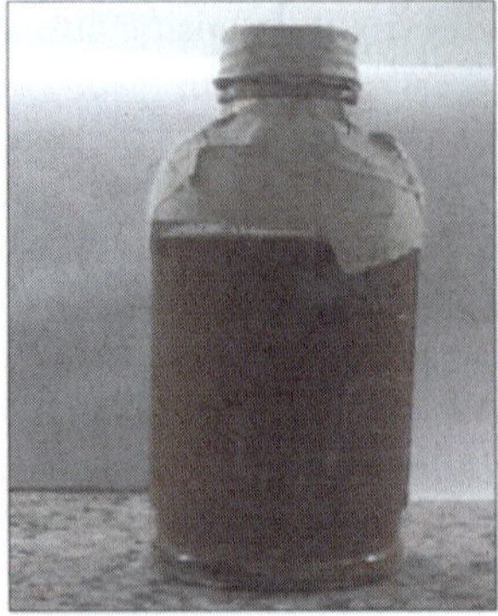

Figure-6: Chylous urine

2. **Through faeces: Called chylous diarrhoea.**

b. **Collection of chyle:** In different body cavities as follows.

1. **In peritoneal cavity: Called chylous ascites.**
2. **In pleural cavity: Called chylothorax.**
3. **In any body cavity: Called chylocele.**

✓ **Note: Chyle**

▪ **Meaning:** From **chylous (Greek) = Juice.**

▪ **Definition:** It is a milky body fluid consisting lymph & lipid digested in intestine.

iii. **Elephantiasis:**

- **Definition:** It is defined as hyperplasia (solid oedema) & hypertrophy of skin & subcutaneous tissues.
- **Sites:**
- It includes legs **[fig.-7(a)]**, scrotum **[fig.-7(b)]**, penis, labia, clitoris, vulva, breast **[fig.-7(c)]** & forearms.
- It not includes the liver, lungs & spleen.

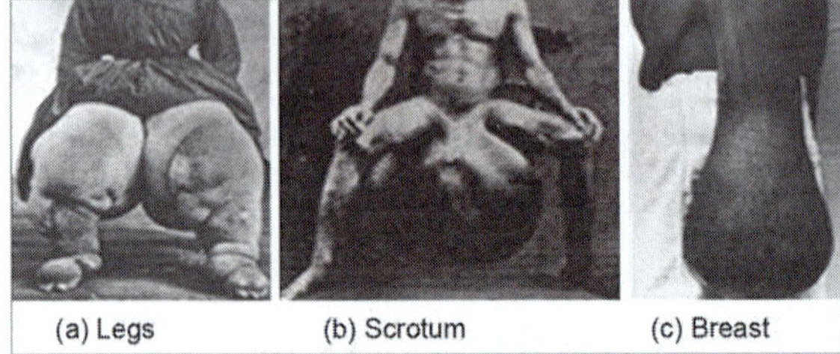

(a) Legs (b) Scrotum (c) Breast

Figure-7: Elephantiasis

- **Pathogenesis:**
- It is due to presence of protein in the exudates which stimulate the connective tissues for excessive growth.
- Eliphantiasis of legs is due to obstruction of inguinal or iliac lymph nodes.
- Eliphantiasis of scrotum is due to obstruction of superficial inguinal lymph nodes.
- **Pathology:**

o <u>Macroscopy:</u>

- Overlying skin becomes rough, fissured & even papillomatous.

- Cut section of skin appears thickened, dense & fibrous. Subcutaneous tissues show a blubbery (oedematous) appearance with presence of dilated & thickened lymphatics & veins. Underlying muscles & bone does not reveal any changes.
- Hair becomes rough & sparse.

o Microscopy:

- Hyperplasia & hypertrophy of skin & subcutaneous tissues with granuloma formation (parasitic onion) including eosinophils, plasma cells, monocytes, giant cells & fibroblast around dead or clacified worms.
- Lymphatics vessel's walls show the inflammatory thickening & endothelial proliferation called **oblitrative endolymphangitis.**
- Also thrombus formation in lymphatics.
- Blood microscopy: Microfilariae are absent in peripheral blood due to death of adult worms or failure of entry in blood due to lymphatic obstruction.

- **Geographical variation:** Elephantiasis of leg & scrotum is common in China, India & Pacific but rare in West Africa.

iv. **Secondary bacterial infection:** By *Strept. pyogen & Staph. aureus.*
- Septic Lymphangitis.
- Abscess.
- Septicaemia.

v. **Calcification of dead adult worn**

B. Occult filariasis:

✪ **Synonym:** Also called **Meyers - Kowenaar syndrome.**

✪ **Definition:** It is hypersensitive reaction characterised by massive eosinophilia (30-80%) around dead microfilariae or their products.

✪ **Pathogenesis:** →Flow chart-4

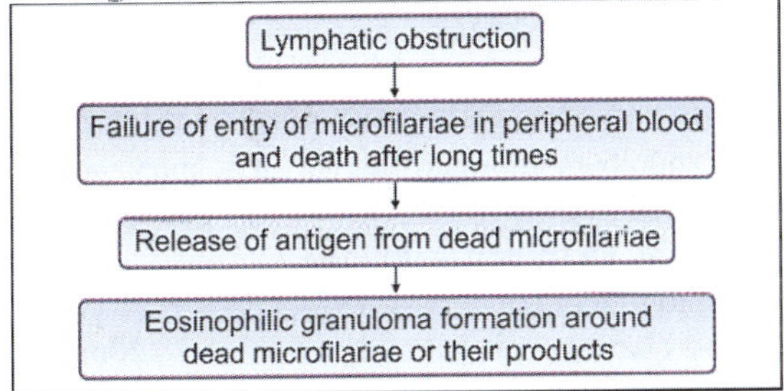

Flow chart-4: Pathogenesis of occult filariasis

✪ **Clinical features:**

- **Lymph nodes:** Generalised enlargement of lymph nodes.
- **Liver & spleen:** Hepato-spleenomegaly.
- **Lungs:** Condition in lungs called **topical pulmonary eosinophilia** or called **eosinophilic lung** or called **Weingarten's syndrome** which have following peculiarities.
  - Low grade fever.
  - Loss of weight.
  - Paroxysmal (sudden & recurrent) cough with scanty sputum with or without blood.
  - Dyspnoea (not expiratory).
  - Also with splenomegaly.
  - Chest X-ray: Increased broncho-vascular marking or diffuse miliary mottling in the lungs.
  - Lung biopsy: Eosinophilic infiltration with microfilariae. Difficult to identify the species.

✪ **Pathological changes in tissues:** It shows the eosinophilic granuloma around dead microfilaria or their products.

✪ **Geographical variation:** Common in India, Sri Lanka. South East Asia, China, Philippines, Brazil & Africa.

✪ **Laboratory diagnosis of occult filariasis:**

- **Blood picture:**
  - Eosinophilia: 30-80%.
  - Absolute count: 3000-5000per cmm.
  - No microfilariae are in peripheral blood.
- **Specific diagnosis of lung features:** Vide supra.
- **Serology:**
  - Increased IgE.
  - Increased IgM detected by CFT.

➢ **Differences between classical filariasis & occult filariasis:** →Table-1

Features	Classical filariasis	Occult filariasis
Cause	Adult worm	Microfilariae
Mecha-nisms	Allergic, inflammatory & obstructive	Allergic
Organs involved	Lymphatic system (lymphatic vessels & lymph nodes)	Lymphatic system, liver, lungs, spleen
Micro-filariae	In blood	In tissues not in blood
Treat-ment	No response to any drugs	DEC is effective
Serology	CFT negative	CFT positive

Table-1: Differences between classical filariasis & occult filariasis

❖ Laboratory diagnosis of classical filariasis: Two type methods.

I. Direct methods

A. Adult stage diagnosis:

i. **Lymph node biopsy:** Adult stage is present but chances of lymphatic obstruction, so not recommended.

B. Larval stage (microfilariae) diagnosis:

i. **From mosquito:** Method called **xenodiagnosis.**

- **Steps:**
  - Allow the mosquito to bite the infected person.
  - Examine the microfilariae in the stomach blood of mosquito.
- **Disadvantage:** Rarely useful method.

ii. **From human:**

➢ **Most commonly used specimens:** Peripheral blood.

✪ **Advantages of blood examination:** It is useful for
- Survey work.
- Differentiation of species.
- Next day examination because microfilariae remain viable for 1-2 days in blood.

✪ **Collection:** It depends on periodicity & stage of disease as shown in **flow chart-5.**

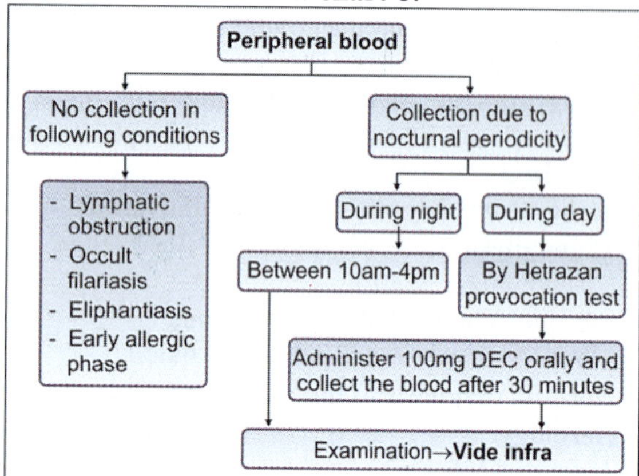

Flow chart-5: Collection of peripheral blood

✪ **Types, preparation & staining of smears:** Two types of smears as described below.

a. Wet mount from samples (unstained smear):
- **Steps:**
  - Take 2-3 drops of blood on clean glass slide.
  - Add equal volume of water to lyse the RBCs.
  - Put the cover slip & examined under the low power
  - Apply the vaseline to the rim of cover slip & put the preparation at room temperature for next day examination.
- **Examination:** Actively motile microfilariae are seen under low or high power microscopy.

b. Stained smears:

1. Thin smear:
- **Steps of smear preparation:**
- **Faulty technique:**
- **Properties of ideal smear:**

} Follow chapter → **Blood inhabiting sporozoa** (Section →*Plasmodium* spp.)

- **Fixation of smear:**
  - **Not required:** For Leishman's stain.
  - **Required:** For Giemsa.
- **Staining methods:** By Leishman's stain & Giemsa's stain.
- **Advantages of thin smear:** Better identification of species, because of clear morphology.
- **Disadvantages of thin smear:** Less sensitive compare to thick smear, because of less numbers of parasites.

2. Thick smear:
- **Techniques of smear preparation:** Follow chapter → **Blood inhabiting sporozoa (Section →*Plasmodium* spp.)**
- **Dehaemoglobinisation of smear:** After preparing the thick smear, kept covered & dehaemoglobinised next morning by putting in distilled water.
- **Fixation of smear:** By methyl alcohol.
- **Staining methods:** Romanowsky's stain like Leishman's stain, Giemsa's stain, haematoxylin & eosin stain or by polychrome methylene blue.
- **Advantage of thick smear:** More sensitive compare to thin smear, because of more numbers of parasites.
- **Disadvantage of thick smear:** Species identification can be difficult.

✪ **Examination of smears:**

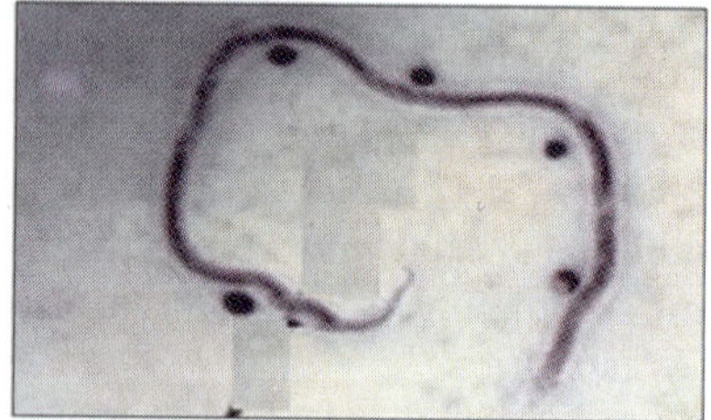

Figure-8: Microfilaria under Romanowsky's stain

- Thin & thick smears are examined under oil immersion lens.
- Appearance of microfilariae under Romanowsky's stain is shown in **fig.-8.**

➢ **Other useful specimens are:**

✪ **Chylous urine:** 10-20ml of the first early morning urine is collected.

✪ **Exudate from lymph varix:**

✪ **Hydrocele fluid:**

➢ **Counting of microfilariae:**

1. By using thick smear
- Take about 20μl blood by haemoglobinometer pipette on a glass slide & proceed like thick smear.
- Total numbers of microfilariae in a thick smear is multiplied by 50 will give the number per ml of blood.

2. Counting chamber technique
- Given by Denham *et al* in 1971.
- Exact quantity of haemolysed blood ($20mm^3$) is examined.

3. Millipore membrane or nucleopore filtration concentration technique:
- Given by Bell, 1967, Desowitz & Southgate, 1973
- It is performed by using millipore membrane or nucleopore filter.
- Exact quantity of heparinised blood (10ml) is passed through filter.
- Microfilariae released from heparinised blood are examined fresh or after staining.
- Advantage: More sensitive so blood can be collected during day time for screening.

- Disadvantages: Cost & required large quantity of blood.

➢ **Concentration technique:**

- **Methods:** Following are different types methods according to agent used for dehaemoglobinisation like distilled water, formalin, saponin, citrated saline or acetic acid.

1. **Centrifugation technique:**
   - Take a large quantity of blood (5-10 ml) in test tube.
   - Blood is centrifuged at a speed of 2,000 rpm for 2-5 minutes.
   - Discard the supernatant & sediment is examined for microfilariae by thick smear preparation.
   - Dehaemoglobinise the smear with **distilled water.**
2. **Knott's concentration technique:** Knott, 1939.
   - One ml of blood is mixed with 9 ml of 2-5% **formalin.**
   - Mixture is centrifuged at a speed of 2,000 rpm for 5 minutes.
   - Discard the supernatant & sediment is examined for microfilariae.
3. **Schuffner & snilder's concentration technique:**
   - 20 drops of blood are placed in 10 ml saline.
   - Add few drops of 10% **saponin** to haemolyse the RBCs.
   - Mixture is centrifuged, discard the supernatant & sediment is examined for microfilariae.
4. **Bhaduri's concentration technique:**
   - 5 ml of blood is placed in 10 ml of a 2.5% **citrated saline.**
   - Next morning blood is dehaemoglobinised by adding 1% saponin drop by drop in mixture till the haemolysis is complete.
   - Add a drop of heparin.
   - Mixture is centrifuged, discard the supernatant & sediment is examined for microfilariae.
5. **By using acetic acid:**
   - Take a 1-2ml of blood in test tube containing 5-10ml of a 2% **acetic acid.**
   - Blood is centrifuged in next morning.
   - Discard the supernatant & sediment is examined for microfilariae by thick smear preparation.
6. **Millipore membrane or nucleopore filtration concentration technique:** → **Vide supra**

- **Advantage:** It increases the positivity rate.
- **Disadvantages:**
  - It changes the morphology of parasites.
  - Cumbersome technique not useful in field.
  - Large quantity of blood (5-10 ml) is required

➢ **Microfilariae survey work:** It is done by

1. Counting chamber technique.
2. Millipore membrane or nucleopore filtration concentration technique.

II. Indirect methods

A. **Blood picture:** Eosinophilia (5-51%).

B. **Allergic /skin test:**
- It based on immediate type of hypersensitivity.
- Antigen is prepared from extract of microfilariae, adult worm& 3rd stage of larvae of *B. malayi* or *D. immitis.*
- Less useful, because of low sensitivity.

C. **Serological tests:** Following two types of tests.

i. **Antibody detection tests:**

➢ **Disadvantages:** Less sensitivity & less specificity.

➢ **Tests:**

a. **CFT:** CFT is negative in classical filariais, but positive in occult filariasis.

b. **ELISA:**
- It detects the IgG4 antibody against WbSXP-1 antigen of *W. bancrofti.*
- Test developed by Bhunia *et al* 2003.

c. **Immunodiffusion test**

d. **IHA**

ii. **Antigen detection tests:**

➢ **Advantages:** High sensitivity & less specificity.

➢ **Disadvantages:** Cross reactivity with intestinal nematodes.

➢ **Tests:**

a. **ELISA:**

b. **Immuno Chromatographic Test (ICT):**
- It detects the filarial antigen from blood, serum or plasma.
- Sample is collected at any time when microfilariae are not in blood.
- Test is positive up to 18 months or more following treatment.

D. **Molecular tests:** PCR which provides sensitivity 10 folds greater than direct methods & 100% specific.

E. **Radiological tests:** More useful for adult stage.

i. **X-ray:** It shows the calcified worms.

ii. **High frequency ultrasound & doppler within the scrotum, breast & spermatic cord:**
- Motile adult parasites are seen **called filaria dance sign.**
- Adult worms are examined in 80% cases in spermatic cord.

❖ Laboratory diagnosis of occult filariasis:

→ **Vide supra**

❖ Prevention:

➢ **General measures (mosquito control measures):** Follow chapter → Medical Entomology

➢ **Chemoprophylaxis:**

✪ **Indications:** For carrier.

✪ **Drugs:** Di Ethyle Carbamazine (DEC, hetrazan), 6 mg/kg/day of body weight is given orally to the carrier for 12 days (6 days in a week for 2 weeks).

➢ **Immunoprophylaxis:** No specific vaccine is available.

❖ Treatment:

➢ **Di Ethyle Carbamazine (DEC, hetrazan):**

- **Indication:** DEC is the drug of choice for occult filariasis (larval stage not for adult stage).
- **Dose:** With above mentioned dose.
- **Administration:** 3 ways.

1. **Mass therapy:**
   - Used in endemic areas to all people with or without microfilariae disease.
   - Treatment must be repeated every 2 years.
   - DEC is given alone or in combination with ivermectin or albendazole.
2. **Selective therapy:** Used in all microfilariae positive people.
3. **DEC medicated salt:** 1 g common salt is medicated with 1-4 g of DEC for filaria control programme in Lakshadweep Island.

- **Side effects:** Mazzotti reaction.
- **Contraindication:** Pregnancy, children < 2 years & seriously ill patients.

Features	*W. bancrofti*	*B. malayi*
Adult worm		
Size	Larger	Smaller
Microfilaria		
Size	290µm×6-7 µm	230µm×6 µm
Shape	Long body with blunt head & pointed tail end	Long body with secondary curve & blunt head & bulb like tail end
Stylet	Single at anterior end	Double stylets at anterior end
Nuclei	Appear clean	blurred hence counting is difficult
Cephalic space	Length & breadth are equal	Twice as long as broad
Tail tip	Free from nuclei	Two nuclei at tail tip with one at the end & second at midway between the tip & posterior column of nuclei
Periodicity	Nocturnal periodicity	- Nocturnal - Diurnal - Subperiodic
Development	Completed in 10-20 days	Completed in 6-8 days
Hosts		
Definitive	Only man	Man & Animal
Intermediate	*Culex*	*Mansonian*
Pathogenicity		
Eliphantiasis	More	Less
Chyluria	More	Absent
Scrotal swelling (hydrocele)	More	Less/absent

Table-2: Differences between *W. bancrofti* & *B. malayi*

➢ **Other drugs:**

- **Ivermectin:**
  - It kills the microfilariae not adults.
  - It is used in Africa not in India.
  - Dose: 12µg/kg.
- **Tetracycline:** It inhibits the endosymbiotic bacteria (*Wohlbachia* species) that are essential for the fertility of the worms.

➢ **Surgery:** Required for elephantiasis & hydrocele.

❖ Differences between *W. bancrofti* & *B. malayi*: → Table-2

Brugia species **→ Flow chart-6.**

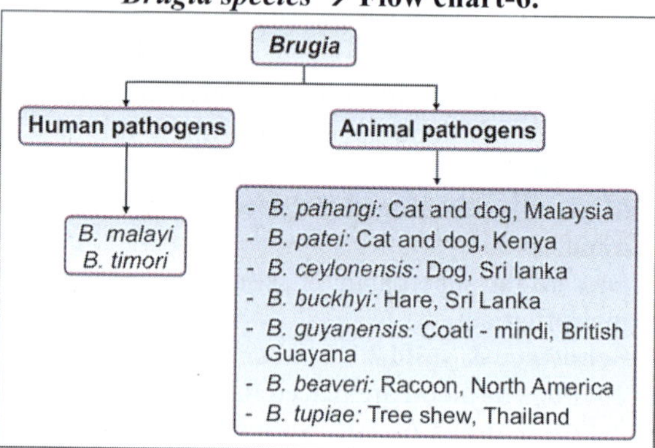

Flow chart-6: *Brugia species*

Brugia malayi

❖ Synonym: *Wucheria malayi.*

❖ Common name: Malayan filaria.

❖ Meaning: **Genus name** given from the **Brug** who found the new type of microfilariae in the blood of natives Sumatra in 1927.

❖ History:

- Microfilaria was 1st identified by Brug in 1927.
- Adult worm was described by Rao & Maplestone in India in 1940.

❖ Geographical distribution:

- **In world:** Common in South Korea, China, Malaysia, Thailand, Vietnam, Indonesia, Borneo, Burma & Koshima Island (Japan).
- **In India:** It is prevalent in Kerala (In Quilon, Allepy, Kottayam, Ernakulam & Trichur districts) Orissa, Madhya Pradesh, West Bengal & Assam.

❖ Habitat: Adult parasite habitat the lymphatic vessels & lymph nodes in man. Its zoonotic disease & animal reservoir are present like dogs, cats & monkeys.

❖ Morphology: Same as *W. bancrofti* with following differences.

I. Adult stage

- Adult female is indistinguishable from *W. bancrofti*.
- Adult male is differs in minor details.

II. Larval stage (microfilaria)

↓

Table-2

❖ **Life cycle:** Same as *W. bancrofti* with following differences.

➤ **Types of host:**

I. Definitive host: Man. Animal reservoirs are present like dogs, cats. & monkeys.

II. Intermediate host: Female Mosquito.

✪ **Extrinsic incubation period:** Larval development completed in mosquito in 6-8 days **called extrinsic incubation period.**

✪ **Species in India:** *Mansonia annulifera, M. indiana, M. uniformis* & also *Anopheles barbirostris*.

❖ **Pathogenicity:** It occurs alone or with *W. bancrofti*. Pathogenicity is same as *W. bancrofti* with following differences.

➤ **Disease name: Called malayan filariasis** or **called brugian eliphantiasis.**

➤ **Reservoir of infection:** Man & animals.

➤ **Mode of transmission:**

- **Route:** By female mosquito bite.
- **Species:** → Vide supra.

➤ **Exit & infective forms:** Same as *W. bancrofti*.

➤ **Portal of entry:** Skin.

➤ **Site:** Lymphatic system.

➤ **Clinical features:**

- Lymphangitis & elephantiasis are more in lower limbs.
- Elephantiasis of genitalia is very rare.
- Absence of chyluria.
- Scrotal swelling is very rare.

❖ **Laboratory diagnosis:** Same as *W. bancrofti* with characteristic identification of microfilariae.

❖ **Prevention:**

➤ **General measures (mosquito control measures):**

- Certain plants like *Pistia*, in Sri Lanka & India are associated with breeding of Mosquitoes. Removal of such plants can be effectively reduced the transmission.
- Follow chapter → Medical Entomology

➤ **Chemoprophylaxis:** Same as *W. bancrofti*.

➤ **Immunoprophylaxis:** No specific vaccine is available.

❖ **Treatment:** Same as *W. bancrofti*

Brugia timori

❖ **Meaning: Genus name** given from the **Brug,** 1927 & species name came from the Timor, Island.

❖ **History:** It was 1st identified in Timor, Island in 1964.

❖ **Geographical distribution:** It is prevalent in Timor & Flores, Island of Eastern Indonesia.

❖ **Other details:** Same as *B. malayi* with following differences.

➤ **Microfilariae:**

- Larger about 230μm in length.
- 5-8 nuclei in tail tip.
- Sheath fails to take Giemsa stain.
- Mostly nocturnal periodicity.

➤ **Life cycle:**

✪ **Types of host:**

I. Definitive host: Man. No Animal reservoirs.

II. Intermediate host: Female Mosquito like *Anopheles barbirostris* which is breeds in rice fields & is a night feeder.

➤ **Pathogenicity:** Lesions are milder than other with following features.

- Lymphangitis & abscess formation in lymph nodes & lymphatic vessels along the saphenous vein leading to scar & lymphatic trunk becomes thickened like scar.
- Minimal elephantiasis.

Subcutaneous filariasis

Onchocercus volvulus

❖ **Synonym:** *O. caecutiens* or *Filarial volvulus*.

❖ **Common name:** Convoluted filaria.

❖ **Meaning: Genus name** given from the **Onkos (Greek) = Hook + Kerkos (Greek) = tail** because parasite have hooked tail.

❖ **History:**

- Microfilaria was 1st identified by O'Neil in 1875.
- Adult worm was 1st identified by Leuckart in 1893. in nodules removed from the chest & scalp of West African native.

❖ **Geographical distribution:** It is reported from Africa (Congo basin & Volta river basin), Central America (Guatemala, Venezuela & Mexico) & South Arabia.

❖ **Habitat:** Adult parasite habitat in subcutaneous connective tissues of man.

❖ **Morphology:** Two morphological stages like adult & larval stages. Few important features of parasite are given below.

I. Adult stage

➤ **Time of maturation:** Larva transformed to sexually mature adult stage in 12-15 months in definitive host after injection.

- **Size:** Female is larger than male as shown in **fig.-9.**
- Female: 50cm × 0.4mm in its greatest diameter.
- Male: 3cm ×0.13mm.
- **Shape:** Elongated & posterior end turn like hook as shown in **fig.-9.**

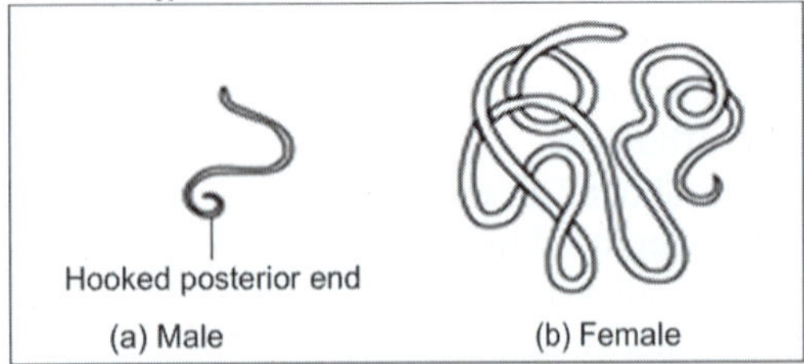

Figure-9: Adult stage of *O. volvulus*

- **Colour:** Whitish, opalescent & transverse stria on the cuticula.
- **Life span:**
- Male die after fertilising the female.
- Gravid female may live long for 15 years.
- **Cuticula:** It is thick & raised in well marked annular & oblique thickenings.
- **End:** Posterior end is like hook hence the name *Onchocerca.*
- **Type of female:** It is viviparous & laying the embryo.

II. Larval stage (microfilaria)

- **Size:** 300μm × 6-8μm.
- **Sheath:** Unsheathed.
- **Nuclei:** Tail tip is free from nuclei **[fig.-1(g)].**
- **Periodicity:** Non-periodic.
- **Host:** It present in skin, subcutaneous lymphatics, conjunctiva & rarely in blood of man.
- **Life span:** It lives for about 1 year.

❖ Life cycle:

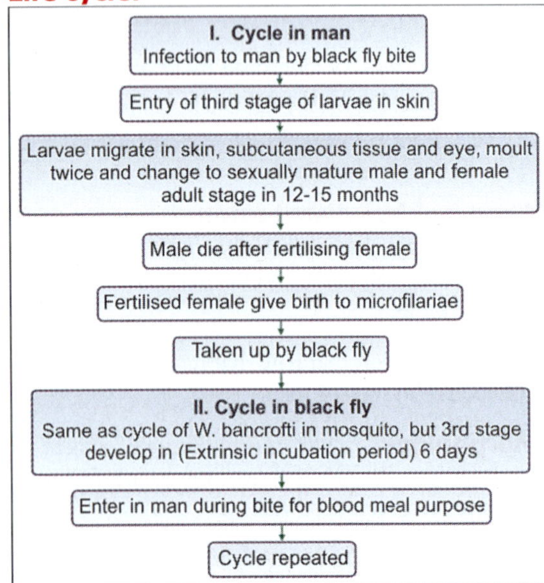

I. Cycle in man
Infection to man by black fly bite
Entry of third stage of larvae in skin
Larvae migrate in skin, subcutaneous tissue and eye, moult twice and change to sexually mature male and female adult stage in 12-15 months
Male die after fertilising female
Fertilised female give birth to microfilariae
Taken up by black fly
II. Cycle in black fly
Same as cycle of W. bancrofti in mosquito, but 3rd stage develop in (Extrinsic incubation period) 6 days
Enter in man during bite for blood meal purpose
Cycle repeated

Flow chart-7: Life cycle of *O. volvulus*

- **Types of host:**

I. **Definitive host:** Man. Animal reservoirs are not present.
II. **Intermediate host:** Day biting female black fly.

- **Extrinsic incubation period:** Larval development completed in black flies in 6 days **called extrinsic incubation period.**
- **Species:**
- **In Africa:** *Simulium damnosum* (commonly **called buffalo gnat**) & *S. naevei.*
- **In Central & South America:** *S. ochraceum* (In Mexico & Guatemala) & *S. metallicum* (in Venezuela).
- **Cycles:** Whole cycle is possible between man & female black flies as shown in **flow chart-7.**

❖ Pathogenicity:

- **Disease name: Called onchocerciasis.**
- **Synonym:**
- Also **called river blindness** as the vector is breed in fast flowing river & disease is common along the course of river.
- Also **called blinding filaria** as it is the 2nd major cause of blindness in the world.
- **Reservoir of infection:** Man only.
- **Mode of transmission:**
- **Route:** By female black fly bite.
- **Species:** → Vide supra.
- **Incubation period:** One year.
- **Exit form:** Microfilariae.
- **Infective form:** Third stage of larvae.
- **Portal of entry:** Skin.
- **Site:** Subcutaneous tissues.
- **Pathogenesis:** Lesions are due to hypersensitivity reactions to the dead adult worm or microfilariae.
- **Clinical features & pathology:** Two types.

I. **Lesions due to adult worms:** Mostly affect skin or subcutaneous tissues.

A **Subcutaneous nodules:**

- **Name: Called onchocercoma.**
- **Size:** Few millimeter to centimetre (up to 6 cm).
- **Numbers:** Single to multiple. Average 3-6 but may be up to 15 in numbers.
- **Sites:** It may depend on habit of fly bite.
- **In Africa:** More on trunk & limbs than on the head as the fly bite commonly on trunk & limbs.
- **In Central & South America:** Particularly over the scalp as the fly bite commonly on head & neck.
- **Associated symptoms:** It raised above the skin surface, painless & non-suppurative.
- **Pathology:** Nodule have two parts.
- **Central:** Honeycombed central area contains adult worms of both sexes. If worms are dead may initiate clacification & foreign body giant cell reaction.
- **Peripheral:** Surrounded by concentric mass of fibrous tissues.

B **Skin lesions:** It includes

- Severe dermatitis **called Sowdah** or **onchodermatitis.**
- Pruritus.
- Depigmentation & hyperpigmentation **called leopard skin.**
- Atrophy.
- Fibrosis.

II. Lesions due to microfilariae:

- Mostly affect the eyes from surrounding lesion by wandering microfilariae.
- It present with simple conjunctivitis, small round opacities & pannus in the anterior quadrant of the cornea, keratitis, retinitis, iridocyclitis, secondary granuloma, optic atrophy & eventually blindness.

➢ **Complications:**

- **Hydrocele or lymph scrotum:**
- **Elephantiasis:** Common in scrotum or legs.
- **Hanging groin:**
  - Seen in Africa.
  - Atrophied & inelastic skin of groin hangs sown in a fold containing enlarged & sclerosed femoral or inguinal lymph nodes.
  - Skin looks like leopard skin.
- **Calcification:** Of dead worms.
- **Abscess:** Due secondary bacterial infection.
- **Dwarfism:** Due to invasion of pituitary by microfilariae.

❖ **Laboratory diagnosis:** Two type of methods.

I. Direct methods

➢ **Specimens & testing methods:**

A Adult stage diagnosis:

i. By biopsy from subcutaneous nodules: Adult stage can be detected from subcutaneous lesion.

B Larval stage (microfilariae) diagnosis:

i. Skin snip preparation:

- **Sample collection:**
  - Maximum microfilariae density is present in iliac crest or trapezius (infrascapular) region. Sample is collected during day time.
  - It is collected by raising the skin with a needle & shaving the epidermal layer with razor.
  - Skin snip is teased in water or saline & incubated for several hours.
- **Examination:** After sufficient incubation sample is examined by dissecting microscope for unsheathed microfilariae.

ii. Eye examination & conjunctival biopsy:

1. **Slip lamp examination of eye:** It revealed the microfilariae in anterior chamber of eye.
2. **Conjunctival biopsy:** Unsheathed microfilariae are examined under microscope.

iii. Other specimens: Unsheathed microfilariae are also present in urine, CSF, blood, sputum or lymph collected specially after DEC treatment.

III. Indirect methods

A. Blood picture: High eosinophilia.

B. Allergic /skin test: Called Mazzotti's test.

- It based on immediate type of hypersensitivity.
- Appearance of pruritic papular rash within 24 hours of oral administration of 100 mg DEC.
- Reaction is due to killing of microfilariae by drug.

C. Serological tests: Following are antibody detecting tests.

i. ELISA: It is more sensitive & detects the antibody against specific onchocercal antigen.

ii. Immuno Chromatographic Test (ICT): It detect the IgG4 antibody against OV16 antigen of *O. Volvulus.*

D. Molecular tests: PCR from skin snip is highly sensitive & specific.

E. Radiological tests: X-ray shows the calcified worms.

❖ **Prevention:**

➢ **General measures:** Control of vector.

➢ **Chemoprophylaxis:** In 1974, WHO launched the control programme in West Africa using aerial larvicides & ivermectin to the patients. This is believed to have prevented the blindness in millions of children.

➢ **Immunoprophylaxis:** No specific vaccine is available.

❖ **Treatment:**

➢ **Ivermectin:**

- Drug of choice in areas coendemic with *L loa.*
- It kills the microfilariae not adults.
- Dose: 150μg/kg, yearly or semiannually.

➢ **Other drugs:**

- **DEC:**
- **Suramin:**
- **Tetracycline:** It inhibits the endosymbiotic bacteria (*Wohlbachia* species) that are essential for the fertility of the worms.

➢ **Surgery:** Required for removal of nodules.

L. loa

❖ **Synonym:** *Microfilaria diurnal* or *Filaria oculi humani.*

❖ **Common name:** African eye worm.

❖ **Meaning:**

- **Genus name** given from the local West African name for worm.
- **Common name** given because of habit of adult worm to live sub-conjunctival tissues of man.

❖ **History:** It was 1st identified in eye of Negro girl in West Indies in 1770.

- **Nuclei:** Nuclei are present up to tail tip **[fig.-1(e)].**
- **Periodicity:** Non periodic.
- **Host:** It present in the blood in man.

❖ **Life cycle:**

- **Types of host:**

I. **Definitive host:** Chimpanzee, Gorilla & Man.
II. **Intermediate host:** Midges specially *Culicoides* spp.

✪ **Species:** *C. grahami* & *C. austeni.*

- **Cycles:** Mosquito steps are same as other filaria.

❖ **Pathogenicity:**

- **Mode of transmission:** By bite of midges of *Culicoides* spp.
- **Reservoir of infection:** Chimpanzee & gorilla.
- **Clinical features:**
  - Mostly asymptomatic but may cause oedema or allergic reaction in the skin.
  - May cause calabar swelling like *Loa loa.*

❖ **Laboratory diagnosis:** Identification of microfilariae in the peripheral blood.

❖ **Prevention:**

- **General measures (midges control measures):** Follow chapter → Medical Entomology
- **Immunoprophylaxis:** No specific vaccine is available.

❖ **Treatment:** Doxycycline (200 mg BID for 6 weeks) is the effective drug. It inhibits the endo-symbiotic bacteria (*Wohlbachia* species) that are essential for the fertility of the worms.

Mansonella ozzardi

❖ **Common name:** Ozzard's filaria.

❖ **History:** Following scientists contributed in discovery of parasite.

- Manson, 1897.
- Faust, 1929.

❖ **Geographical distribution:** West Indies & parts of Central & South America.

❖ **Habitat:** Adult parasite habitat in the mesenteric tissues in man.

❖ **Morphology:**

I. Adult stage

- **Size:**
  - Male is inadequately known & a single incomplete male worm has been found.
  - Female is 7cm × 0.25mm in size.
- **Cuticula:**
  - Appears smooth.
  - Posterior end is pointed & possesses a pair of flap like papillae.
- **Type of female:** Viviparous & laying the embryo.

II. Larval stage (microfilariae)

- **Size:** 224µm × 4-5µm.
- **Sheath:** Unsheathed.
- **Nuclei:** Tail tip is devoid of nuclei **[fig.-1(d)].**
- **Periodicity:** Non periodic.
- **Host:** They are present in the blood in man.

❖ **Life cycle:**

- **Types of host:**

I. **Definitive host:** Man.
II. **Intermediate host:** Midges specially *Culicoides furens.*

- **Cycles:** Mosquito steps are same as other filaria.

❖ **Pathogenicity:**

- **Mode of transmission:** By bite of midges like *Culicoides furens.*
- **Clinical features:**
  - Asymptomatic.
  - Lymph node swelling.
  - Occasionally hydrocele.

❖ **Laboratory diagnosis:** Identification of microfilariae in the peripheral blood.

❖ **Prevention:**

- **General measures (midges control measures):** Follow chapter → Medical Entomology
- **Immunoprophylaxis:** No specific vaccine is available.

❖ **Treatment:**

- **Ivermectin:** Single dose 6 mg is effective.

Zoonotic filariasis

These are natural parasites of animals, but accidentally larvae are enter in man by arthropod bite, which are change to adult worm but not able to release the microfilariae. Later, adult worm die & inflammatory reaction around the adult worm give all clinical manifestations.

Brugia pahangi

- It is a dog & cat parasite in Malaysia.
- In human causing lymphangitis & lymphadenitis.

Brugia beaveri

- It is a parasite of racoon in North America.
- In human causing tender mass in cervical, axillary or inguinal region.

Dirofilariae immitis

- Commonly **called dog heart worm.**
- It located in the right heart or branches of pulmonary artery in man.

- Dead parasite becomes embolus & blocks the small branches of pulmonary artery to produce infarct.
- Healed infarct appears as "coin lesion" under X-ray which can be mistaken as malignancy.
- There are no direct laboratory methods to diagnose the parasite.
- Indirectly diagnosed by serological tests & eosinophilia, a supportive role.
- X- ray method is insufficient.

Dirofilaria repens

- It is a parasite of dog.
- In human causing subcutaneous or subconjunctival nodules, so called *dirofilariae conjunctivae.*

Other *Dirofilaria* spp. as human pathogen

D. tenuis, D. uris, D. striata & D. subdermata.

Other diseases

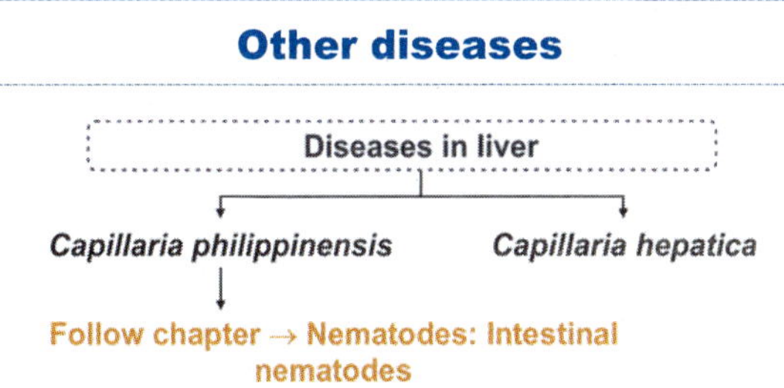
Diseases in liver
Capillaria philippinensis
Capillaria hepatica
Follow chapter → Nematodes: Intestinal nematodes

Capillaria hepatica

❖ **Meaning:** Species so called because infect the liver capillaries.

❖ **History:** 1st case was reported 1923 in a 20 years old British soldier in India at autopsy.

❖ **Geographical distribution:** Cases have been reported from USA, England, Nigeria & South America.

❖ **Habitat:** Adult parasite habitat the liver parenchyma in human. Naturally it habitat in rat, squirrel, pig, chimpanzee, dog & monkey.

❖ **Morphology:** Morphologically indistinguishable from *C. philippinensis*

❖ **Life cycle:**

➢ **Hosts:** Cycle continue between rat & other predators. Man is the accidental host & act as dead end host, as no access of human tissue to animals.

I. Definitive host: Rat, squirrel, pig, chimpanzee, dog & monkey

II. Intermediate host: Not required

➢ **Cycle: → Flow chart-9**

❖ **Laboratory diagnosis:**

➢ **Specimens:**

✪ **Liver biopsy:** For eggs

➢ **Testing methods:**

I. Direct methods

A. Microscopy of liver tissue: Revealed eggs in liver parenchyma & Morphologically indistinguishable from *C. philippinensis*

II. Indirect methods

A. Blood picture: Eosinophilia.

B. Serological tests: Not useful.

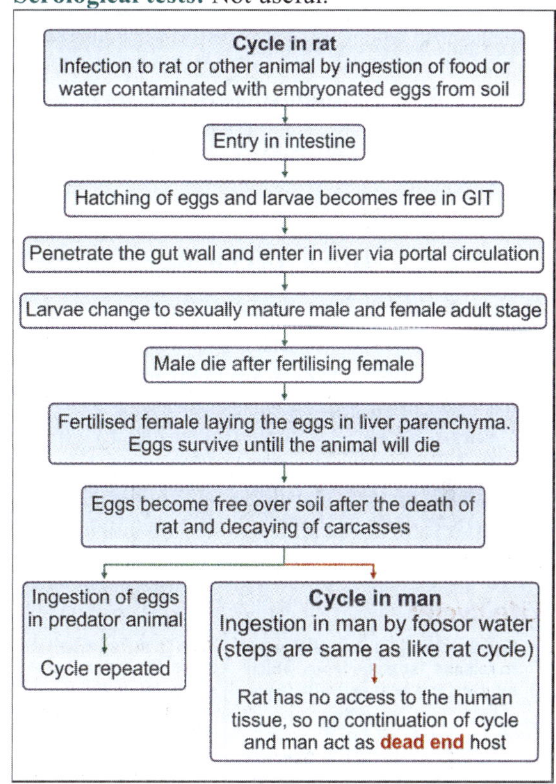
Cycle in rat
Infection to rat or other animal by ingestion of food or water contaminated with embryonated eggs from soil
Entry in intestine
Hatching of eggs and larvae becomes free in GIT
Penetrate the gut wall and enter in liver via portal circulation
Larvae change to sexually mature male and female adult stage
Male die after fertilising female
Fertilised female laying the eggs in liver parenchyma. Eggs survive untill the animal will die
Eggs become free over soil after the death of rat and decaying of carcasses
Ingestion of eggs in predator animal
Cycle repeated
Cycle in man
Ingestion in man by foosor water (steps are same as like rat cycle)
Rat has no access to the human tissue, so no continuation of cycle and man act as dead end host

Flow chart-9: Life cycle of *C. hepatica*

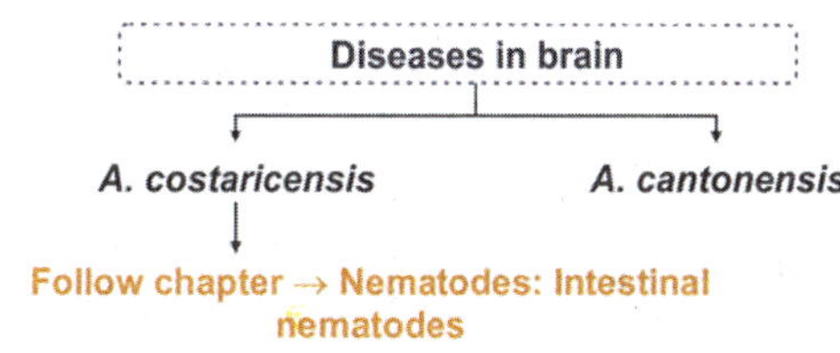
Diseases in brain
A. costaricensis
A. cantonensis
Follow chapter → Nematodes: Intestinal nematodes

Angiostrongylus cantonensis

❖ **Synonym:** *Pulmonema cantonensis.*

❖ **Common name:** Rat lung worm.

❖ **History:**

- Disease was 1st discovered from the CSF of a patient with eosinophilic meningitis by Nomura and Lim in Taiwan in 1944-45.
- Life cycle was worked out by Mackerass & Sanders in 1955.

❖ **Geographical distribution:**

- Hundreds of cases were reported from Taiwan, Thailand, Indonesia & Pacific islands.

- Human infection has also been recovered from India, Egypt, Cuba & USA.

❖ **Habitat:** Adult parasite habitat in branches of pulmonary artery in rat. Pathology in man is due to larval stage which habitat brain.

❖ **Morphology:** Three morphological stages like adult, egg & larval stages. Few important features of parasite are given below.

I. Adult stage & Egg stage

- Adult & egg stage are same as *A. costaricensis*.
- More details: **Follow chapter → Nematodes: Intestinal nematodes.**

II. Larval stage

➢ **Forms & hosts:** Three forms of larvae.

1. **1st stage larva:** It released on hatching of eggs in pulmonary artery of rat & excreted with faeces over soil.
2. **2nd stage larva:** 1st stage taken up by snail & moults twice to develop 2nd & 3rd stage of larva.
3. **3rd stage larva:** Develops in snail/molluscs & infective form for man. It also infects prawns, crabs & frogs.

❖ **Life cycle:**

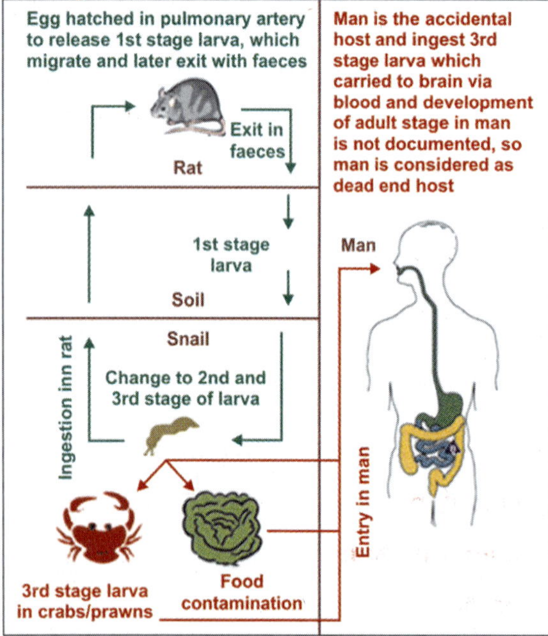

Figure-10: Life cycle of *A. cantonensis*

➢ **Types of host:**

I. **Definitive host:** Brown rat (*Rattus norvegicus*) & the black rat (*Rattus rattus*).

II. **Intermediate host:** Snail or molluscs (*Thelidomus aspera*).

➢ **Cycles:** As shown in **flow chart-10 & fig.-10.**

- Rat is the optimum host.
- Man is the alternative host & acts as dead end host.

❖ **Pathogenicity:**

➢ **Disease name:** It is a rat pathogen & human disease **called cerebral angiostrogyliasis** or **eosinophilic meningoencephalitis.**

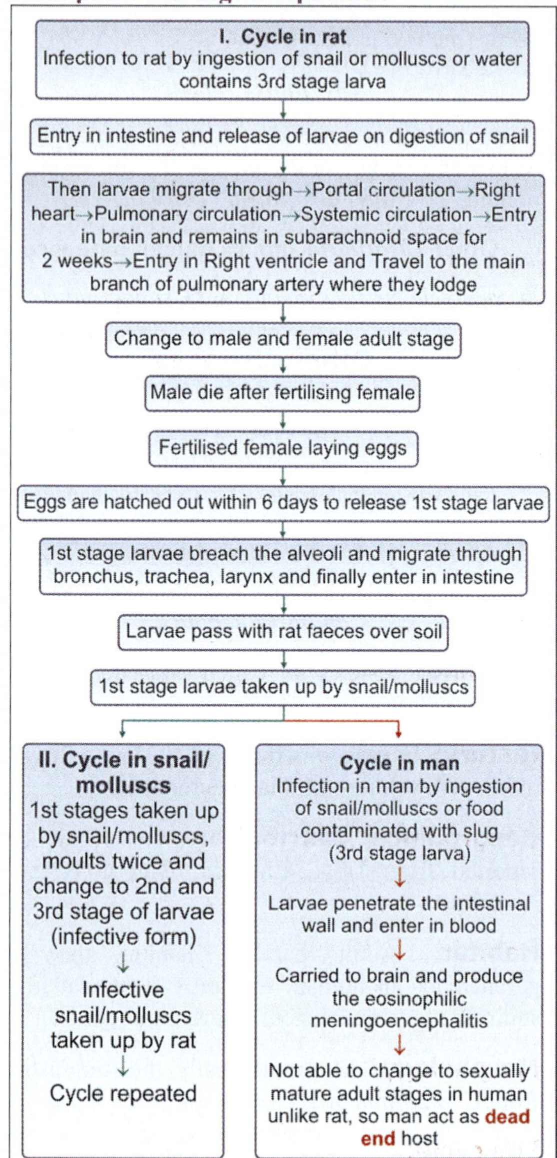

Flow chart-10: Life cycle of *A. cantonensis*

➢ **Reservoir of infection:** Rat.

➢ **Source of infection:** Raw slug or food.

➢ **Mode of transmission:** Man is infected by ingestion of raw snail or food contaminated with slug (3rd stage of larvae) or crab/prawn.

➢ **Incubation period:** 2-3 weeks.

➢ **Exit form:** 1st stage of larvae.

➢ **Infective form:** 3rd stage of larvae.

➢ **Portal of entry:** GIT.

➢ **Sites:** Adult parasite habitat in branches of pulmonary artery in rat. In man larvae habitat the brain.

➢ **Pathogenesis:**

- Pathology in man is due to the larval stage.
- Larvae affect the meninges & superficial plus deeper tissue of brain.
- It cause damages by following ways.

1. Direct mechanical damage to neural tissue migratory larvae.
2. Toxic by-products such as nitrogenous waste.
3. Antigens released by dead and living parasites.
4. Inflammatory (eosinophilic) response in humans.

➢ **Clinical features:**

- Fever is often minor or absent but the presence of high fever suggests severe disease.
- Headaches: A bitemporal character in the frontal or occipital lobe.
- Meningismus: Neck stiffness.
- Photophobia: Sensitivity to light.
- Nausea with or without vomiting.
- Paresthesias: Tingling, prickling or numbing of skin
- Hyperesthesia: Severe sensitivity to touch.
- Bladder dysfunction with urinary retention.
- Vertigo.
- Blindness.
- Paralysis localized to one area.
- General paralysis often ascending in nature starting with the feet and progressing upwards to involve the entire body.
- Convulsion.
- Coma.
- Death (rare).

➢ **Complication:** Ocular damage is the possibility.

❖ Laboratory diagnosis:

➢ **Specimens:**

✪ **CSF:** For presence of larvae.

✪ **Brain biopsy:**

➢ **Testing methods:**

I. Direct methods

A Microscopy:

i. Wet mount from CSF: Shows the presence of larvae.

ii. Microscopical examination of brain tissues: Also shows the presence of larvae.

II. Indirect methods

A CSF picture: Chemical analysis of the CSF typically resembles the findings in "aseptic meningitis" with

- Slightly elevated protein levels.
- Normal glucose levels.
- Significantly decreased glucose is an indicator of severe meningoencephalitis and may indicate a poor prognosis.

B Blood picture: Eosinophilia (90%).

C Brain biopsy: Eosinophilia.

D Serological tests:

- ELISA, IHA are useful tests.
- Antigen is prepared from larvae of *A. cantonensis* present in the brain of case.

❖ Prevention:

➢ **General measures:** Removal of intermediate host (snail or molluscs).

➢ **Immunoprophylaxis:** No specific vaccine is available.

❖ Treatment:

Anthelmintics are not useful as the disease is caused by dead larvae. Drug even may enhance the disease due to destruction of more larvae.

Diseases in brain & other tissues

Gnathostoma spinigerum

❖ **History:** Owen, in1836.

❖ **Geographical distribution:** Central East Asia, Japan, China, New Guinea & India.

❖ Habitat:

- It is zoonotic parasite which habitat in domestic animals (dogs, cats & swine) & wild animals (tigers, dog, raccoons, otters & opossums).
- In human cause accidental infection by larval stage **called visceral larvae migrans,** which migrate in different tissues like brain, spinal cord, mouth, pharynx, intestine, eyes, cervix & subcutaneous tissues.

❖ **Morphology:** Three morphological stages like adult, egg & larval are described below.

I. Adult stage

➢ **Time of maturation:** Larva transformed to sexually mature adult stage in 18 months in animals

➢ **Size:** Female is larger than male.

- Female: 25-54m × 3mm.
- Male: 21-25mm ×2mm.

➢ **Shape:** It curved ventrally at both the ends **[fig.11 (a)]**.

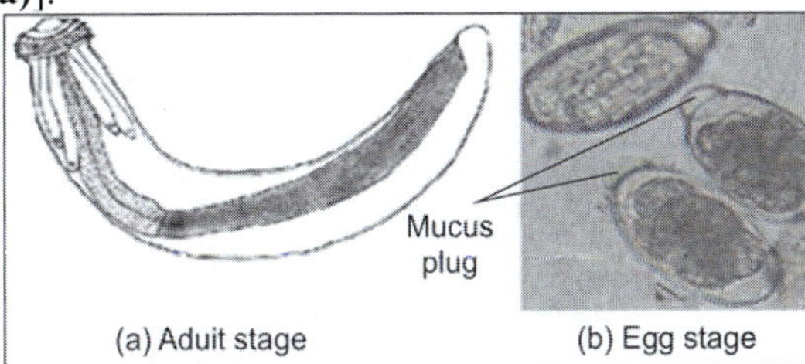

Figure-11: Adult stage of *G. spinigerum*

➢ **Head end:** It possesses 4-8 transverse rows of sharp hooklets on a distinct head bulb.

- **Organs:** Female contains single vulva situated in the middle of the body.
- **Type of female:** Oviparous laying eggs.

II. Egg stage

- **Morphological features:** → **Fig.11 (b)**
- **Size:** 70μm × 40 μm.
- **Shape:** Oval & transparent.
- **Colour:** Brown colour (bile stained).
- **Mucus plug:** Present at one pole.
- **Embryo:**
  - Freshly passed eggs are not embryonated.
  - Eggs are present in granulomatous lesion in animal & passed through faeces in water.

III. Larval stage

- **Forms & hosts:** Three forms of larvae.

1. **1st stage larva:** It released on hatching of eggs in water.
2. **2nd stage larva:** 1st stage taken up by cyclops (1st intermediate host) & develop to 2nd stage of larva in 15 days.
3. **3rd stage larva:** 2nd stage taken up by fish/frog (2nd intermediate host) & develop to 3rd stage of larva which is the infective form.

Life cycle:

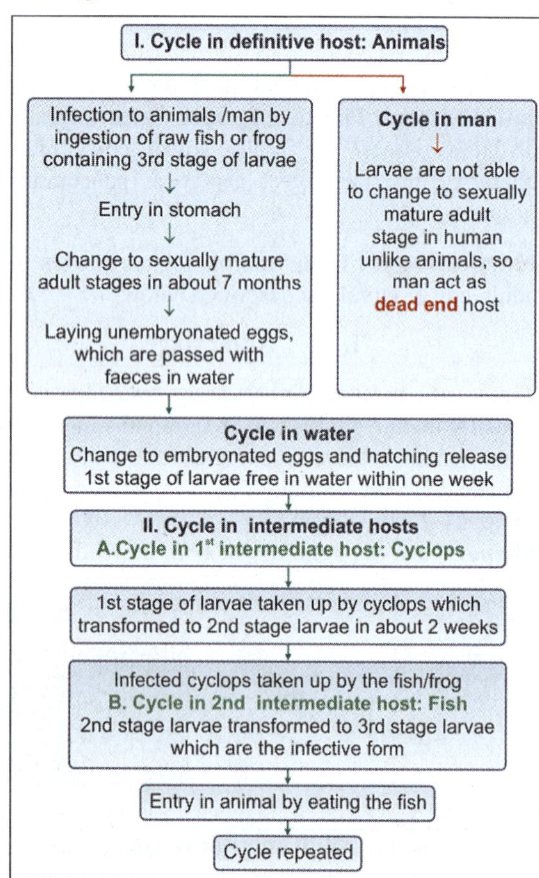

Flow chart-11: Life cycle of *G. spinigerum*

- **Types of host:** Two types.

I. **Definitive host:** Domestic & wild animals.
II. **Intermediate hosts:** Larval stage developed in two different aquatic animals.
A **First intermediate host:** Cyclops.
B **Second intermediate host:** Fresh water fish or frog.

- **Cycles:**
  - Whole cycle is possible between animals & intermediate host as shown in **flow chart-11.**
  - Man is accidental host & acts as dead end host.

Pathogenicity:

- **Disease name:** **Called gnathostomiasis.**
- **Mode of transmission:** By ingestion of raw fish / frog contains third stage of larva.
- **Reservoir of infection:** Animal.
- **Source of infection:** Fish/frog.
- **Exit form:** Unembryonated eggs.
- **Infective form:** Third stage of larvae.
- **Portal of entry:** GIT.
- **Site:** Brain & other tissues.
- **Clinical features:**
  - **Cutaneous larva migrans:** Larva migrate through skin & subcutaneous tissues & producing the fugitive swelling & a condition **called cutaneous larva migrans.**
  - **Visceral larva migrans:** Larva migrate in brain, eyes & other tissue & producing the granulomatous lesions **called visceral larva migrans.**

Laboratory diagnosis:

I. Direct methods

- **Specimens:** Biopsy from tissues.
- **Testing methods:** Microscopical examination shows the presence of larvae.

IV. Indirect methods

A. **Blood picture:** Eosinophilia.
B. **Skin tests:** Intradermal skin test by using the antigen from larvae or adult stage is useful.
C. **Serological tests:** ELISA & precipitation tests are useful measures.

Prevention:

- **General measures:** Removal of intermediate hosts like cyclops & fish/frogs.
- **Immunoprophylaxis:** No specific vaccine is available.

Treatment:

- **Albendazole / mebendazole:** Effective drugs.
- **Surgery:** Incision of lesion & removal of larva.

Gnathostoma hispidum

- Fedtscenka, in 1873.
- It is a pig parasite.

- Adult worms are larger & have 12 hooks on the cephalic bulb.
- Human cases are reported from India, Canton & Japan.

Diseases in subcutaeous tissue

Dracunculus medinensis

❖ **Synonym:** *Fulleborne medinensis, Gordius medinensis, Filaria medinensis, Vena Medina.*

❖ **Common name:** Guinea worm, serpent worm, medina worm, dragon worm & fiery serpent.

❖ **Meaning:**

- **Common name** is given from the name of African country, **Guinea Bisau** from where it was detected in 16th century.
- **Scientific name: Genus name** from the **Dragon/Dracon (Greek) = Serpent & species name** came from the **Makka Medina** where it was common.

❖ **History:**

- Worm is known from the ancient times.
- Galen had given the disease name as **dracontiasis** in 130-200 AD.
- Avicena, Arabian physician had given the parasite name as ***Vena Medina*** in 980-1037 AD as it was common in Medina.
- In the Bible the worm is referred with common name as **"fiery serpent".**

❖ **Geographical distribution:**

- It is prevalent in 13 countries of Africa including Sudan with highest incidences, Niger etc.
- It was eradicated from India & South East Asia region by 2000 & these countries are certified as Guinea worm free by WHO.

❖ **Habitat:** Adult female habitat in the subcutaneous tissues of legs, arms & back in man.

❖ **Morphology:** Two morphological stages like adult & larval stages. Few important features are given below.

I. Adult stage

➢ **Time of maturation:** Larva transformed to sexually mature adult stage in 3-4 months in definitive host after ingestion.

➢ **Size:** Female is larger than male as shown in **fig.-12.**

- Female: 0.6-1metre×1.5-1.7mm (longest nematode).
- Male: 12-30mm ×0.4mm.

➢ **Shape:** Cylindrical like a thread as shown in **fig.-12.**

➢ **Colour:** Milky-white in colour.

➢ **Life span:**

- Male live for not more than 6 months & die after fertilising the female. Male has been discovered from experimental animals but not from man except one case in India.
- Female may live for 1 year.

➢ **Ends:**

✪ **Head end:** The head end rounded.

✪ **Tail end:** In female it is tapered & forms a hook.

➢ **Type of female:** It is viviparous & laying the embryo for a period of 3 weeks until the uterus of gravid female becomes empty.

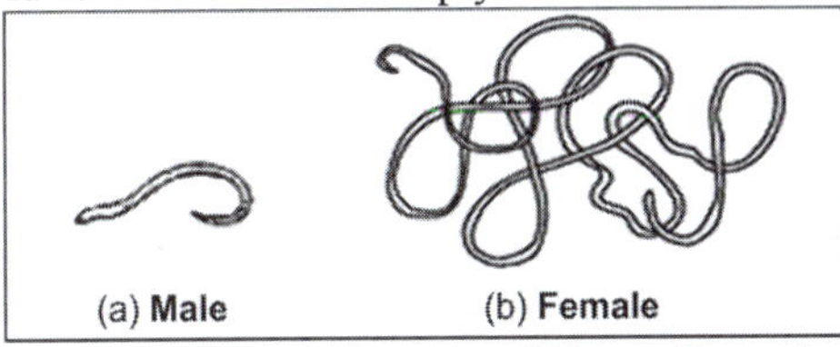

Figure-12: Adult stage of *D. medinensis*

II. Larval stage

➢ **Form:** Solid forms of larvae are present.

➢ **Size:** 650-750μm×17-20 μm at the widest part.

➢ **Shape:** Long body with blunt head & pointed tail.

➢ **Colour:** Transparent & colourless.

➢ **Life span:** In released free in water by gravid female & live for 4-5 days unless taken up by cyclops.

➢ **Host:** It develops in human, released free in water by gravid female & later enters in cyclops.

❖ **Life cycle:**

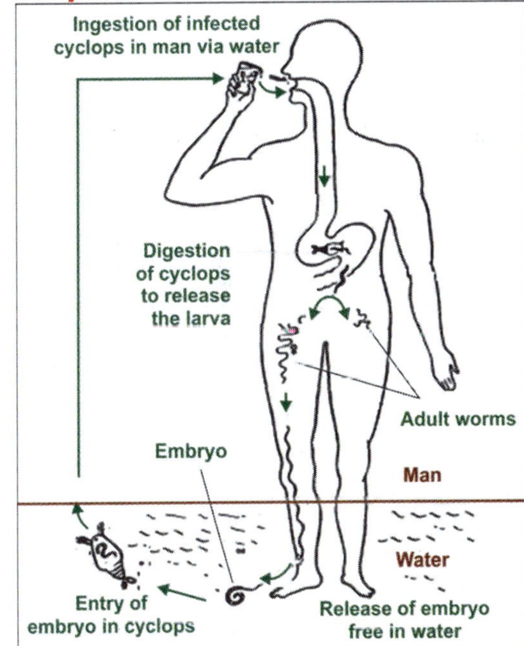

Figure-13: Life cycle of *D. medinensis*

➢ **Types of host:**

I. Definitive host: Man.

II. Intermediate host: Cyclops.

- **Extrinsic incubation period:** Larval development completed in cyclops in 7 days **called extrinsic incubation period.**
- **Species:**
- **In India:** *Mesocyclops leuekarti.*
- **Other species:** *Mesocyclops hyalinus, Thermocyclops vermifer, Encyclops serrulatus, Tropocyclops multivolor* etc.
- **Cycles:** As shown in **flow chart-12 & fig.-13.**

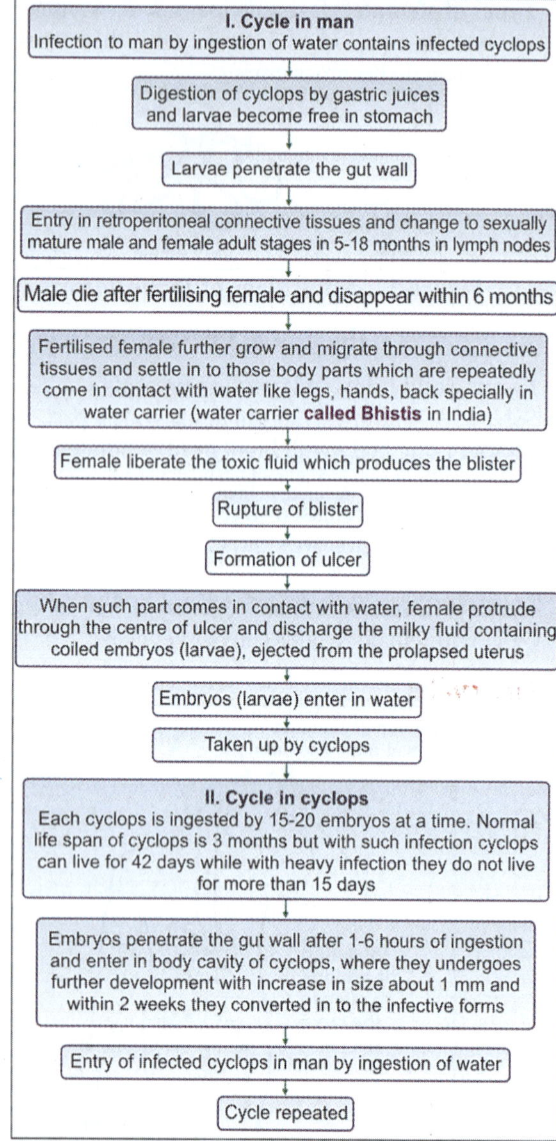

I. Cycle in man
Infection to man by ingestion of water contains infected cyclops
Digestion of cyclops by gastric juices and larvae become free in stomach
Larvae penetrate the gut wall
Entry in retroperitoneal connective tissues and change to sexually mature male and female adult stages in 5-18 months in lymph nodes
Male die after fertilising female and disappear within 6 months
Fertilised female further grow and migrate through connective tissues and settle in to those body parts which are repeatedly come in contact with water like legs, hands, back specially in water carrier (water carrier called Bhistis in India)
Female liberate the toxic fluid which produces the blister
Rupture of blister
Formation of ulcer
When such part comes in contact with water, female protrude through the centre of ulcer and discharge the milky fluid containing coiled embryos (larvae), ejected from the prolapsed uterus
Embryos (larvae) enter in water
Taken up by cyclops
II. Cycle in cyclops
Each cyclops is ingested by 15-20 embryos at a time. Normal life span of cyclops is 3 months but with such infection cyclops can live for 42 days while with heavy infection they do not live for more than 15 days
Embryos penetrate the gut wall after 1-6 hours of ingestion and enter in body cavity of cyclops, where they undergoes further development with increase in size about 1 mm and within 2 weeks they converted in to the infective forms
Entry of infected cyclops in man by ingestion of water
Cycle repeated

Flow chart-12: Life cycle of *D. medinensis*

❖ Pathogenicity:

- **Disease name:** **Called dracunculiasis** or **dracunculosis** or **draconcutiasis** or **guinea worm disease.**
- **Reservoir of infection:** Man.
- **Source of infection:** Water contains infected cyclops.
- **Mode of transmission:** By ingestion of contaminated water contains infected cyclops which is neither boiled nor filtered.
- **Exit form:** Coiled embryos.
- **Infective form:** Larvae.
- **Portal of entry:** GIT.
- **Sites:** Subcutaneous tissues of legs, arms & back.
- **Precipitating factors:** Common in Bhistis.
- **Pathogenesis:** Symptoms are due to release of toxic fluid by female during parturition responsible for allergic manifestation &blister formation.
- **Clinical features:**

1. **Allergic reactions:** Burning or itching sensation at affected areas.
2. **Blister formation:**
   - Initially present as red spot & later change to bleb or blister.
   - Body parts which are repeatedly come in contact with water like legs (in between the metatarsal bones or on the ankles), hands & back especially in water carrier (Bhistis).
3. **Ulcer:**
   - Rupture of blister producing the ulcer.
   - Size: 0.5-0.25 inches in diameter.
   - Centre: In centre hole is present through which head of the worm will protrude, when parts come in contact with water.
   - Toxic fluid present in ulcer is sterile, yellow in colour & contains embryo, monocytes, eosinophils & neutrophils.

- **Complications:**

1. **Secondary bacterial infection in ulcer:** Sometimes it may lead to tetanus.
2. **Worms travel to unusual sites:** Like in spinal canal, pericardium or in the eyes with serious effects.
3. **Calcification:** Present in dead worm which may cause arthritis, fibrosed joints or compression of spinal cord.

❖ Laboratory diagnosis: Two type of methods.

I. Direct methods

- **Specimens & testing methods:**

A **Adult stage diagnosis:** It examined direct over ulcer site & removed by following methods.

- **Removal of worms:**
- **Indications:** For.
  - Diagnosis of disease.
  - Prevention of disease.
  - Treatment of disease.
- **Methods:**

1. **By rolling over wooden stick: →Fig.-14**
   - Worm is removed by rolling over match stick or similar object.
   - Chances of breaking of worm; so remove it very slowly & roll it inch by inch daily.
   - It takes about 15-20 days.
   - Method is safe & effective.

2. **Surgical removal under anaesthesia:** It is also an useful method.

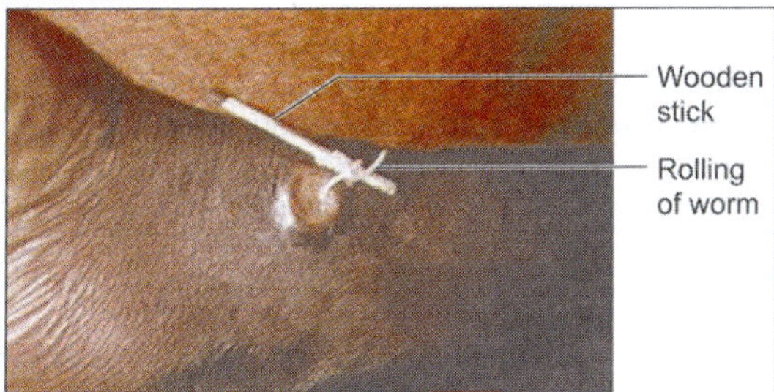

Figure-14: Removal of adult worm by rolling over wooden stick

- **Examination:** By naked eye.

B Larval stage diagnosis:

- From milky fluid collected from ulcer.
- If fluid is not present than bath the ulcer with sterile water which later collected as specimen.
- Larvae can be examined under microscope.

II. Indirect methods

A Blood picture: Eosinophilia.

B Intradermal skin test: Positive with guinea worm antigen.

C Serological tests: ELISA, CFT & other methods are developed to diagnose the antibodies.

D X-ray examination: It may reveal calcified worm.

❖ Prevention:

➢ **General measures:**

- Destruction of cyclops by using abate (temephos).
- Boiling or filtering the water by clothes is the best way to prevent the disease.
- Not allowing the infected person to bath in water.
- Because of simple life cycle, localised distribution & absence of animal reservoir, guinea worm disease is easy to eradicate. Global eradication of disease is imminent.

➢ **Immunoprophylaxis:** No specific vaccine is available.

❖ Treatment:

➢ **Drugs:**

- Antihistaminic & steroids are useful to prevent the allergic reaction.
- Albendazole, niridazole & thiabendazole are effective in treatment.

➢ **Removal of adult worm: → Vide supra**

Question bank

Case study

1) A 55 years male presents with pain & swelling on left arm with fever. Examination revealed lymphangitis & enlargement of axillary lymph nodes. Blood picture shows the microfilariae with tail tip free from nuclei. Identify the organism & answer the following.

a) Name the causative agent & draw the diagram of microfilaria of causative agent.
b) Describe the life cycle of causative agent.
c) Write the pathogenicity causative agent.

Essay/Full question

1) Lymphatic filariasis.
2) Subcutaneous filariasis.

Short notes

1) Microfilariae.
2) Microfilariae of *W. bancrofti.*
3) Life cycle / pathogenicity / lab. diagnosis of *W. bancrofti* or *D. medinensis.*
4) Classical filariasis.
5) Occult filariasis.
6) Complications of wucheriasis.
7) Differences between *W. bancrofti* & *B. malayi.*
8) Darcunculiasis.

Short questions for theory/viva questions

1) Name the four parasites in which microfilariae are present in peripheral blood.
2) Name the four parasites present in CSF.
3) Name the four parasites in which mosquito act as intermediate host.
4) What is "parasitic onion" in wucheriais?
5) Difference between classical filariasis & occult filariasis.
6) What is hetrazan provocation test?
7) Name the four parasites in which fish act as a source of infection.

MCQs for chapter review

Classification

1) **Lymphatic filariasis is caused** (PGI, Nov-10)
(a) *W bancrofti* (b) *Brugia malayi* (c) *Schistosoma* (d) *B timori* (d) *Onchocercus voluvulus*

2) **Which is non lymphatic filariasis**
(a) *Loa loa* (b) *Wucheria bancrofti* (c) *Brugia malayi* (d) *Brugia timori*

General aspect of filariasis

3) **Nocturnal periodicity of microfilaria is in relation with their occurrence in**
(a) Peripheral blood (b) Urine (c) Lymph (d) Internal organs

4) **Sheathed microfilariae is/are** (PGI, Dec-04)
(a) *W bancrofti* (b) *Loa loa* (c) *M perstans* (d) *B malayi*

5) ***Wucheria bancrofti* true is**
(a) Unsheathed (b) Tail tip free from nuclei (c) Non periodic (d) All

6) **One of the following microfilariae does not posses nuclei up to tail tip**
(a) *W bancrofti* (b) *Loa loa* (c) *M perstans* (d) *B malayi*

Lymphatic filariasis

7) **The organism most commonly causing genital filariasis in most part of Bihar and eastern UP is** (AI-03)
(a) *Wucheria bancrofti* (b) *Brugia malayi* (c) *Onchocerca vouvulus* (d) *Dirofilaria*

8) **Which is false about *Wucheria bancrofti*** (AI-90)
(a) Causes filariasis (b) Body is long and slender (c) Terminal nuclei absent (d) Man and *Anopheles* are hosts

9) **False regarding filariasis is** (AIIMS, Nov-03)
(a) Morbidity increase with age in endemic areas (b) Humoral immunity plays dominant role (c) Usually unilateral (d) Man is the only host for filariasis

10) **All are true regarding filariasis except** (AIIMS, feb-03)
(a) Man is intermediate host (b) Caused by *Wucheria bancrofti* (c) Involves lymphatic system (d) DEC is used in treatment

11) **In which stage of filariasis are microfilariae seen in peripheral blood** (AI-01)
(a) Tropical eosinophilia (b) Early adenolymphatic stage (c) Late adenolymphatic stage (d) Elephantiasis

12) **Meyers Kowenaar syndrome is s synonym for** (PGI-88)
(a) Tropical pulmonary eosinophilia (b) Larva migrans (c) Occult filariasis (d) Cutaneous allergic reaction to ascariasis

13) **Which is not a feature of tropical eosinophilia**
(a) Eosinophilia more than 3000/mm^3 (b) Microfilariae in tissues (c) Microfilariae in blood (d) Lymphadenopathy

14) **Hydrocele and oedema in foot occur in** (PGI, Nov-11)
(a) *W bancrofti* (b) *B malayi* (c) *B timori* (d) *Onchocerca vouvulus* (d) Guinea worm

15) **All of the following are true about *Brugia malayi* except** (AI-95)
(a) The intermediate hosts in India are *Mansoni* (b) The tail is free from nuclei (c) Nuclei are blurred, so counting is difficult (d) Adult worm is found in lymphatic system

Subcutaneous filariasis

16) **River blindness is caused by**
(a) *Onchocerca* (b) *Loa loa* (c) *Ascaris* (d) *B. malayi*

17) **Kallu a 30 year old man, presented with subcutaneous itchy nodules over the left iliac crest. On examination they are firm, non tender and mobile. Skin scraping contains microfilariae and adults worms of** (AIIMS, May-01)
(a) *Loa loa* (b) *Onchocerca vouvulus* (c) *Brugia malayi* (d) *Mansonella perstants*

18) **Calabar swelling is produced by**
(a) *Onchocerca vouvulus* (b) *Loa loa* (c) *Brugia malayi* (d) *Wucheria bancrofti*

Dracunculus medinensis

19) **Dragon or serpent worm is** (AIIMS-01)
(a) *Enterobius* (b) *Trichuris* (c) *Dracunculus* (d) *T.solium*

20) **Dracunculosis infection occurs through**
(a) Ingestion of water containing cyclops (b) Ingestion of water containing parasite (c) Ingestion of fish (d) Penetration of skin

21) **Definitive host for guinea worm is** (AIIMS-93)
(a) Man (b) Cyclops (c) Snail (d) Cyclops & man

22) **Cyclops are intermediate host for**
(a) Kala azar (b) Schistosomiasis (c) *Dracunculus medinensis* (d) Taeniasis

23) **The slender rhabditiform larvae of which of the following helminths move about in water and are ingested by species of cyclops**
(a) *D latum* (b) *D medinensis* (c) *W bancrofti* (d) *S. mansoni*

Answers of MCQs & explanation

1) **(a), (b) & (d)**
2) **(a)**
} Follow section, **classification** for explanation

3) **(a)**
4) **(a), (b) & (d)**
5) **(b)**
6) **(a)**
} Follow section, **general aspect of filariasis (morphology → larval stage → periodicity different types, & fig.-1)** for explanation

7) **(a)**
- Follow section, **lymphatic filariasis (*Wucheria bancrofti* → geographical distribution)** for explanation

8) **(d)**
- Follow section, **lymphatic filariasis (*Wucheria bancrofti* → life cycle → types of host)** for explanation

9) **(d)**
- Follow section, **lymphatic filariasis [*Wucheria bancrofti* → option 'a' → host factors (age), option 'b' immunity, option 'c' → sites & option 'd' → life cycle]** for explanation.

10) **(e)**
- Follow section, **lymphatic filariasis [*Wucheria bancrofti* → option 'a' → life cycle, option 'b' already explained, option 'c' → sites & option 'd' → treatment]** for explanation

11) **(a)**
- Tropical eosinophilia (feature of occult filariasis), late adenolymphatic stage & elephantiasis are features of obstructive phase (**flow chart-3**), where microfilariae are not able to come out from tissue in to the blood due to obstruction of lymphatic vessels & remain in tissues only.

12) **(a)**
13) **(c)**
} Follow section, **lymphatic filariasis (*Wucheria bancrofti* → pathogenicity → occult filariasis)** for explanation

14) **(a)**
- Hydrocele and oedema in foot are the feature of *W bancrofti* from the given options. Follow section, **lymphatic filariasis (table-2)** for explanation

15) **(b)**
- Follow section, **lymphatic filariasis (*Brugia malayi* → habitat & table-2)** for explanation

16) **(a)**
- Follow section, **subcutaneous filariasis (*Onchocerca vouvulus* → pathogenicity → synonym)** for explanation

17) **(b)**
- Follow section, **subcutaneous filariasis (*Onchocerca vouvulus* → laboratory diagnosis)** for explanation

18) **(b)**
- Follow section, **subcutaneous filariasis (*Loa loa* → pathogenicity → synonym)** for explanation

19) **(b)**
- Follow section, ***Dracunculus medinensis* (common name)** for explanation

20) **(a)**
- Follow section, ***Dracunculus medinensis* (pathogenicity → mode of transmission)** for explanation

21) **(a)**
22) **(c)**
23) **(b)**
} Follow section, ***Dracunculus medinensis* (life cycle & flow chart-12)** for explanation. Cyclops is also an intermediate host in D latum but it carry the procercoid larvae not the rhabditiform larvae

100 Miscellaneous topics in Parasitology

Learning heading & subheadings

Larva migrans

❖ **Definition:** When certain helminths (Mainly non human like zoophilic helminths) enters in human, their further progress is arrested at certain stage & they migrate in aimless manner in human body with production of clinical lesions **called larva migrans.**

❖ **Types:** Two types according to mode of entrance.

I. **Cutaneous larva migrans:** Migration takes place in the skin.

II. **Visceral larva migrans:** Migration take place in the deeper tissues or organs.

Cutaneous larva migrans

➢ **Synonym:** Also **called creeping eruption** or **ground itch.**

➢ **Etiological agents:**

A **Rapidly moving larvae:**

i. ***Strongyloides stercoralis:*** Follow chapter → Nematodes: Intestinal nematodes

B **Slowly moving larvae:**

i. ***Ancyclostoma braziliensis:***

ii. ***Ancyclostoma caninum:***

iii. ***Gnathostoma spinigerum:***

(i–iii) For more details follow chapter → Nematodes: Somatic (tissue) nematodes

iv. **Maggots (blow fly larvae):**

✪ **Definition:** Human disease caused by migrating fly maggots **called myiasis.**

✪ **Agents:**

- Female fly of genus *Hypoderma bovis* (cattle botfly), *Gastrophilus intestinalis* (horse botfly) & *Dermatobia hominis* (human botfly), *Chrysomyia* (Old World blow fly), *Chochiliomyia* (New World screw-worm fly), *Cordylobia* (mango fly), *Wohlfarhtia* etc. deposit either eggs or larvae (maggots) directly in different body parts like nose, eye, ear, intestine etc.
- Larvae scttle on surface for easy oxygen exchange.
- Larvae produce the pathological changes.
- It may cause the secondary bacterial infection also.

➢ **Common sites:** Feet, legs, thighs, buttocks & back.

➢ **Clinical features:**

- Serpigenous tunnel formation at the path traversed by larvae.
- Intense irritation & inflamed larval track with cellular reaction, especially of eosinophils.
- Mostly all larvae will die.

➢ **Diagnosis:**
- Based on clinical ground.
- Rarely larvae found in local biopsy & also rarity of eosinophilia.
- Serological tests are not useful.

➢ **Prevention:** Body is protected from larvae by using protective clothes & repellents, screening, sanitary improvement etc.

➢ **Treatment:**
- **Local:**
  - 15% Thiabendazole cream in a hydro soluble base is effective.
  - Freezing of advancing part of the eruption with ethyle chloride is effective.
  - Surgical removal of lesions.
- **Oral:** Thiabendazole (25 mg/body weight) twice daily for 2 days.

Visceral larva migrans

➢ **Etiological agents:**

A ***Angiostrongylus costaricesis:*** For more details **follow chapter → Nematodes: Intestinal nematodes**

B ***A. cantonensis:***
C ***Gnathostoma spinigerum:***
D ***Brugia patei:***
E ***Brugia pahangi:***
F ***Dirofilaria immitis:***

For more details **follow chapter → Nematodes: Somatic (tissue) nematodes**

E. ***Anisakis* spp.:**

✪ **Definition:** Human disease caused by *Anisakis species* **called anisakiasis** or **herring worm.**

✪ **Agents:**
- These are parasites of family *Anisakidae* like *Ascaris.*
- Human infection is from four genus *Anisakis, Pseudoterranova, Contracaecum* & *Phocanema.*

✪ **Distribution:** It is prevalent in Japan, Netherland & USA.

✪ **Hosts:**
- Definitive host (Adult stage) for these parasites are sea mammals like dolphins, whales etc.
- Shrimps is the 1st intermediate (2nd larval stage) host & fish is the 2nd intermediate (3rd larval stage) host.

✪ **Pathogenicity:**
- **Mode of transmission:** Human infection is due to ingestion of raw fish.
- **Pathogenesis:** On entering the human GIT, larvae penetrate the stomach wall & produce the eosinophilic granuloma.
- **Clinical features:** Epigastric pain nausea & vomiting.

✪ **Diagnosis:**
- Endoscopic biopsy for presence of larvae.
- ELISA is also useful.

✪ **Treatment:**
- Surgical removal of granuloma.
- Thiabendazole is effective.

F. ***Toxocara canis & Toxocara cati:***

✪ **Definition:** Human disease caused by *Toxocara species* **called toxocariasis.**

✪ **Agents:** These are parasites of dog (*Toxocara canis*) & cat (*Toxocara cati*).

- **Mode of transmission:** Human infection is from ingestion of eggs, contains 2nd stage larvae.
- **Pathogenesis:**
  - In intestine eggs are hatched to release the larvae which invade the intestinal wall & enter in liver, spleen, lungs, eyes, brain & in other organs.
  - Further progress of larvae is arrested by formation of granuloma.
  - Granuloma contains eosinophils, neutrophils, giant cell & macrophages.
- **Clinical features:** Fever, enlargement of liver, & spleen, pneumonitis, endophthamitis, space occupying lesion in brain, convulsion etc.

✪ **Diagnosis:**
- Biopsy for presence of larvae.
- Clinical examination eye.
- Serological tests are positive.

✪ **Treatment**: DEC & thiabendazole are effective.

❖ Common topics between CLM & VLM:
- Man always acquires the infection as an accidental host & parasites are not able to complete their life cycle in man so man act as dead end host.
- Infection may be asymptomatic or present with overt disease like inflammation or granuloma formation.
- Both are widespread in tropical & subtropical countries especially in children.

❖ Differences between CLM & VLM: →Table-1

Features	CLM	VLM
Organs involved	Skin	Organs like liver, lungs, spleen
Portal of entry	Skin	Ingestion
Eosinophilia	Mild	High
Serology	Negative	Positive
Treatment	Thiabendazole	DEC& prednisolone

Table-1: Differences between CLM & VLM

Sexually transmitted parasites

- *Entamoeba histolytica.*
- *Giardia lamblia.*

- *Trichomonal vaginalis.*
- *Isospora belli.*
- *Cryptosporidium parvum:* By oral-anal sex.

Parasites with congenital transmission

- *Toxoplasma gondii.*
- *Tryapamosoma cruzi.*
- *Plasmodium* spp.

Parasites present in blood film

➢ **Protozoa:**
- *Leishmania* spp.
- *Tryapamosoma* spp.
- *Plasmodium* spp.
- *Babesia* spp.

➢ **Metazoa/helminths:** Microfilariae of following helminths are present in blood.
- *Wucheria bancrofti.*
- *Brugia* spp.
- *Loa loa.*
- *Mansonella ozzardi.*
- *Mansonella perstans.*

Parasites enter through skin

➢ **From soil:**
- Hook worm spp.: *Ancyclostoma duodenale, Ancyclostoma braziliensis, Ancyclostoma caninum & Necator americanus.*
- *Strongyloides* spp.: *S. stercoralis & S. fulleborne*

➢ **From water:**
- *Acanthamoeba* spp.: *A. culbertsoni, A. castellanii,A. hatchetti, A. polyphaga, A.rhysodes, A.astronyxis, A.divionensis & A. healyi.*
- *Schistosoma* spp.: *S. haematobium, S. mansoni & S. japonicum.*

Parasites causing anaemia

➢ **Parasites & types of anaemia:**

✪ **Protozoa:**
- *Leishmania donovani*: Autoimmune haemolytic anaemia.
- *Plasmodium* spp.: Autoimmune haemolytic anaemia.
- *Babesia* spp.: Haemolytic anaemia.

✪ **Metazoa:**
- **Cestodes:**
  - *Diphylobothrium latum*: Megaloblastic anaemia
  - *Taenia saginata & Taenia solium*
- **Trematodes:** *Fasciolopsis buski*
- **Nematodes:**
  - *Trichuris trichuria* : Iron deficiency anaemia.

- Hook worm spp.: Follow chapter → Nematodes: Intestinal nematodes

Parasites causing auto-infection

❖ **Synonym:** Reinfection.

❖ **Definition:** Reinfection by pathogen that is already present in body or infection caused by transfer of pathogen from one part of body to another.

❖ **Types:** Two types.

A. **Internal reinfection:** Reinfection by parasites from inner side of body.
B. **External reinfection:** Reinfection by parasites from surface of body.

❖ **Examples:** Parasites with mode of auto-infection are described below.

1. ***Cryptosporidium parvum:*** Thin walled oocyst, not excreted in external environment but infect the epithelial cells, as like fresh infection.
2. ***Taenia solium:*** Entry of gravid segments in stomach from intestine by
   - Reversal of peristalsis.
   - Poor personal hygiene (May by finger contamination).
3. ***Hymenolepis nana*:** It is due to persistence of few eggs in intestine rather than exit in faeces.
4. ***Strongyloides stercoralis*:** Occurs by two ways.
   - **Internal reinfection:** By Penetration of bowel mucosa by filariform larvae.
   - **External reinfection:** By Penetration of perianal (perineal) skin by filariform larvae.
5. ***Enterobius vermicularis*:**
   - Common in children by anus to mouth route.
   - Scratching the peri-anal region may contaminate the finger with eggs & swallowing of such finger especially in children cause the auto-infection.
6. ***Capillaria philippinensis:*** **Internal reinfection** due to penetration of bowel mucosa by liberated larvae.

❖ **Diagnosis:** Follow respective chapters.

✓ **Note: Life cycle with autoinfection in man**
- Life cycles of parasites in which autoinfection in man is possible are described with **sky blue arrow** arrows (↓) in respective chapters.

Eosinophilia in parasitic infections

❖ **Background:**
- **Normal range of eosinophils:**
  - It is 0-6% (0-4%) of total leucocyte count.
  - Normal count: It is 125∓100 per cubic millimetre.
- **Distribution:**
  - They are produced in bone marrow distributed in blood & tissues.
  - Skin, lungs & gastrointestinal tract are the major sites for eosinophils location.

- It is estimated that 100 eosinophils in tissue for everyone eosinophil in blood.
- **Function:** Eosinophils are one kind of leucocytes that are fighting with parasites & other blood invaders. They are binds with parasites with the help of complement, IgE & IgG. It can protect against the parasitic infection & same time causing allergic disorders.
- **Break down products of eosinophils: Called Charcot-Layden crystals** (for more details, follow chapter →Amoebae).

❖ **Definition:** Increase in eosinophils count of more than 5% of total leucocytes count **called eosinophilia.**

❖ **Causes of eosinophila:**

A. **Allergic disease:** Like asthma.

B. **Parasitic infections:**

Eosinophilia	Parasitic infections
High	Trichinosis, early stage of schistosomiasis, early stage of liver & lung fluke infection & tropical pulmonary eosinophilia
Moderate	Ascariasis, hook worm disease, onchocerciasis, lymphatic filariasis, schistosomiasis & late stage of liver & lung fluke infection
Low	Cysticercosis & hydatidosis

Table-2: Parasites causing eosinophilia

i. **Prozoan infection:** Like *I. belli*

ii. **Helminthic infections:** Almost all parasites are causing eosinophilia. Lumen dwelling parasites like *E. vermicularis*, *T. solium* & *T. saginata* are not causing eosinophilia. Important parasites causing eosinophilia are given in **table-2.**

❖ **Causes of pulmonary eosinophila:**

- Larvae of round worm (*Ascaris lumbricoides*, condition **called Loeffler's syndrome** or **eosinophilic pneumonia**), hook worm spp. (*Ancyclostoma duodenale* & *Necator americanus*) & *Strongyloides stercoralis.*
- Parasites causing visceral larva migrans like *Toxocara canis* & *Toxocara cati.*
- *Paragonimus westermanii.*
- *Wucheria bancrofti* & *Brugia malayi* (condition in lungs **called topical pulmonary eosinophilia** or **called eosinophilic lung** or **called Weingarten's syndrome**).

Role of vector in parasitic infections

❖ **Mode of transmission:** By two ways.

A. **Mechanical:** Parasite not enter in the body of vector but transmitted through contamination of body parts like legs, wings etc.

B. **Biological:** Parasite enters in the body of vector & undergoes metamorphosis to achieve the infective stage & transmitted by vector bite, deposition of excreta on human body or by other routes.

❖ **Examples:** →**Table-3**

Parasites	Common name of vector	Species of vector
Protozoa		
E. histolytica	House fly	Musca spp.
T. brucei	Tsetse fly	*Glossina* spp.
T. cruzi	Reduvid bug	*Panstrongylus megistus, Triatoma infestans & Rhodnius prolixus*
L. donovani	Sand fly	- *Lutzomyia* spp. - *Phlebotomus* spp.
L. tropica	Sand fly	*Phlebotomus* spp.
L. braziliensis	Sand fly	- *Lutzomyia* spp.
Plasmodium spp.	Mosquito	*Female anopheles*
Babesia spp.	Tick	- *Ixodid* spp. & - *Dermacentor* spp.
Helminths		
Cestodes		
*D. latum**	Cyclops	-
H. nana	Rat fles	*Xenopsylla cheopis*
H. diminuta	Rat fles	*Xenopsylla cheopis*
D. caninum	Dog flea or cat flea	*Ctenocephalus canis* or *C. felis*
Trematodes		
*S. haematobium**	Fresh water snail	- *Bulinus truncates,* - *Planorvarius metidjensis,* - *Ferrissia tenuis*
*S. mansoni**	Fresh water snail	*Biomphalaria alexendrina, Australorbis glabratus*
*S. japonicum**	Fresh water amphibian snail	*Oncomelania* (*Katayama* or *Blanfordia*)
*S. mekongi**	Aquatic snail	*Trienla aperta*
*Fasciolopsis buski**	aquatic snail	*Segmentina*
*H. heterophyes**	Marine & brackish water snail like	*Pirenella conica* or *Ceithidea*
*M. yokogawai**	Fresh water snail	*Melania* spp.
C. sinensis*	Planorbid snail	*Helicorbis coenosus*
*O. felineus**	Snail	*Bithynia leachi*
*F.hepatica**	Amphibian snail	*Lymnaea truncatula*
*D. dendriticum**	Land snail	-
*P. westermani**	Fresh water snail	*Melania liberta* (*Semisulcospira liberta*) or *Brotia*
Nematodes		

A. costaricensis	Slug	*Limax maximus*
W. bancrofti	Female mosquito	*Culex spp.* Also by *Aedes & Anophelesnspp*
B. malayi	Female mosquito	*Mansonia* spp. & *Anopheles* spp.
B. timori	Female Mosquito	*Anopheles barbirostris*
O. volvulus	Female black fly	*Simulium* spp.
L. loa	Female mango or deer fly.	*Chrysops* spp.
M. streptocerca	Female Mosquito	*Culicoides* spp.
M. perstans	Female Mosquito	*Culicoides* spp.
M. ozzardi	Female Mosquito	*Culicoides* spp.
A. cantonensis	Snail or molluscs	*Thelidomus aspera*
*G. spinigerum**	Cyclops	-
D. medinensis	Cyclops	*Mesocyclops* spp.

Table-3: Vector borne parasites

* Vector is not responsible for transmission of parasite but required to complete the life cycle.

Neuroparasites

Follow chapter → Cestodes: Cyclophyllidea

Biliary tract parasites

- **Parasites:** Following are the different mechanisms & concerned parasites causing biliary tract infection or obstruction.
- Mechanical obstruction: By adult parasite during ectopic ascariasis by *Ascaris lumbricoides*.
- Intra biliary rupture or pressure: In case of hydatid cyst (*Echinococcus granulosus*).
- Mechanical obstruction, liberation of toxins, secondary bacterial infections, stone formation or cancer production: *Clonorchis sinensis* & *Opisthorchis* spp.
- Mechanical obstruction & inflammation: *Fasciola hepatica*.
- **More details:** Follow **respective chapter** for more explanation & disease produced by all above mentioned parasites.

Parasites causing malabsorption

- **Protozoa:**
- *G lamblia.*
- *C cayetanensis.*
- *I belli.*
- *C parvum.*
- **Metazoa:**
- *Strongyloides.*
- *Capillaria phillipinensis.*

Parasites infecting eyes

- **Protozoa:**
- *Aanthamoeba culbertsoni:* Causing ulcerative keratitis **called chronic amoebic keratitis** & corneal ulceration.
- *Balamuthia mandrillaris:* Causing keratitis.
- *Trypanosoma cruzi:* Swelling of conjunctiva at the site of entry **called Roman's sign.**
- *Toxoplasma gondii:* Anterior uveitis, focal choreoretinitis near macula (pigment ringed scar).
- *Microspora: Like Microsporidium* (Corneal ulcer, keratitis) & *Nosema* (keratitis).
- **Metazoa or helminths or worms:**
- *Spirometra* spp.: Granulomatous nodule/cyst in eye
- Larval stage *Taenia solium* (*Cysticercus cellulosae*): Ocular cysticercosis.
- Larva of *Multiceps multiceps:* Space occupying lesions.
- *Onchocercus volvulus:* It present with simple conjunctivitis, small round opacities & pannus in the anterior quadrant of the cornea, keratitis, retinitis, iridocyclitis, secondary granuloma, optic atrophy & eventually blindness.
- *Loa loa:* Eye lesions includes granuloma in bulbar conjunctiva, painless oedema of the eye lids, proptosis, retionpathy etc.
- *Dirofilariae conjunctivae:* It is a parasite of dog. (*Dirofilaria repens*). In human causing subcuta.

Parasites to be remember

- **Protozoa:**
- Largest protozoa: *Balantidium coli.*
- **Metazoa or helminths or worms:**
- Largest or longest helminth: *Taenia saginata.*
- Largest or longest nematode: *D medinensis.*
- Largest trematode: *F buski.*
- Largest liver fluke: *F hepatica.*
- Smallest or shortest nematodes: *S stercoralis* & *T spiralis.*
- Smallest or shortest cestodes: *H nana.*

Question bank

Short notes

1) Larvae migrans.
2) Autoinfection by parasites.
3) Role of vector in parasitic infections.
4) Eosinophilia in parasitic infections.
5) CL crystals.
6) Neuroparasites.

Short questions for theory/viva questions

1) Name the four parasites causing cutaneous larva migrans.
2) Name the four parasites causing visceral larva migrans.
3) Difference between cutaneous & visceral larva migrans.
4) Name four sexually transmitted parasites.
5) Name four parasites present in peripheral blood.
6) Name the four parasites causing auto-infections.

MCQs for chapter review

Larva migrans

1) Eosinophilic meningo-encephalitis is caused by (PGI-01)
(a) *Gnasthestoma spinigerum* (b) *Naegleria* (c) *Toxocara canis* (d) *Angiostrogylous cantonensis*

2) Cutaneous larva migrans is due to
(a) *Ancyclostoma braziliensis* (b) *W bancrofti* (c) *B malayi* (d) *D medinensis*

3) Visceral larva migrans is associated with (AI-11)
(a) *Strongyloides stercoralis* (b) *Ancyclostoma braziliensis* (c) *Toxocara canis* (d) *Visceral leishmaniasis*

Parasites enters through skin

4) Parasites penetrating through skin for entry in to the body are (PGI, June-01)
(a) *Ancyclostoma duodenale* (b) *Strongyloides* (c) Round worm (d) *Trichuris trichuria*

5) Which of the following parasites does not enter in to the body by skin penetration (AIIMS, Dec-97)
(a) *Dracunculus* (b) *Necator americanus* (c) *Ancyclostoma duodenale* (d) *Strongyloides*

Parasites causing anaemia

6) Parasite causing anaemia
(a) Hook worm (b) Thread worm (c) *Ascaris* (d) Guinea worm

7) Microcytic hypochromic anaemia found in infestation of (PGI, June-06)
(a) *Ancyclostoma* (b) *Ascaris* (c) *Necator* (d) *Diphylobothrium*

8) Megaloblastic anaemia is caused by (AIIMS, Dec-95)
(a) *Diphylobothrium latum* (b) *Schistosoma haematobium* (c) *Echinococcus granulosus* (d) *Taenia solium*

Parasites causing autoinfections

9) Autoinfection is seen with (AIIMS, Nov-01)
(a) *Ancyclostoma* (b) *Enterobius* (c) *Echinicoccus* (d) Ascariasis

10) Autoinfection is seen with (AIIMS, May-09)
(a) *Cryptosporidium* (b) *Strongyloides* (c) *Giardia* (d) *Ascaris*

11) Autoinfection is a mode of transmission in (AI-00)
(a) *Trichinella* (b) Cysticercosis (c) *Ancyclostoma* (d) *Ascaris*

Eosinophilia in parasitic infections

12) Which of the following is not responsible for pulmonary eosinophilia (AIIMS, Dec-94)
(a) *Ascaris lumbricoides* (b) *Paragonimus westermanii* (c) *Wucheria bancrofti* (d) *Babesia microti*

13) Pulmonary eosinophilia is seen in the following parasitic infections except (AI -00)
(a) Babesiosis (b) Hook worm infection (c) Strongyloidiasis (d) Visceral larvae migrans

14) Parasite causing pulmonary eosinophilia syndrome (PGI-98)
(a) *Strongyloides* (b) Enterobiasis (c) Hook worm (d) *Trichinella*

15) Eosinophilic pneumonia caused by *Ascaris lumbricoides* is known as?
(a) Mafucci syndrome (b) Loeffler's syndrome (c) Primary pulmonary eosinophilia (d) Sweet syndrome

Biliary tract parasites

16) Which of the following does not cause biliary tract obstruction? (AI-94)
(a) *Ascaris lumbricoides* (b) *Ancyclostoma duodenale* (c) *Clonorchis sinensis* (d) *Fasciola hepatica*

17) Which of the following may cause biliary obstruction?
(a) *Ancyclostoma* (b) *Enterobius* (c) *Strongyloides* (d) *Clonorchis*

18) A traveller present with conjugated hyperbilirubinemia and on investigation eggs were found in his biliary tract. Likely organism (AIIMS, May-09)
(a) *Clonorchis sinensis* (b) *Fasciola buski* (c) *Gnathostoma* (d) *Ascaris*

Parasites causing malabsorption

19) All cause malabsorption except (AIIMS, May-09, 10)
(a) Giardiasis (b) *Ascaris lumbricoides* (c) *Strongyloides* (d) *Capillaria phillipinensis*

20) Which of the following infestation leads to malabsorption (AIIMS-04, AI-06)
(a) *Giardia lamblia* (b) *Ascaris lumbricoides* (c) *Necator americanus* (d) *Ancyclostoma duodenale*

Parasites to be remember

21) Which of the following organism is biggest (JIPMER-93)
(a) *Balantidium coli* (b) *Entamoeba coli* (c) *Escherichia coli* (d) *Entamoeba histolytica*

22) Largest intestinal protozoan is (AI-96)
(a) *E coli* (b) *Balantidium coli* (c) *Giardia* (d) *T gondii*

23) The largest trematodes infecting man is (AI-96)
(a) *F hepatica* (b) *F buski* (c) *E granulosus* (d) *Clonorchis sinensis*

24) Which worm is longest (PGI-09)
(a) *T solium* (b) *T saginata* (c) Hook worm (d) *A lumbricoides*

Answers of MCQs & explanation

1) (a) & (d)
2) (a)
3) (c)
} Follow section, **larva migrans & respective chapters** for explanation

4) (a) & (b)
- Follow section, **parasites enters through skin** for explanation

5) (a)
- *Dracunculus* enter by by ingestion of raw fish contains third stage of larva. Follow section, **parasites enters through skin** for more explanation

6) (a)
7) (a) & (c)
8) (a)
} Follow section, **parasite causing anaemia** for explanation

9) (b)
10) (a) & (b)
11) (b)
} Follow section, **autoinfection & respective chapters** for explanation

12) (d)
13) (a)
14) (a) & (c)
15) (b)
} Follow section, **Eosinophilia in parasitic infections (pulmonary eosinophilia)** for explanation

16) (b)
17) (d)
18) (a) & (d)
} Follow section, **biliary tract parasites** for explanation

19) (b)
20) (a)
} Follow section, **Parasites causing malabsorption** for explanation

21) (a)
22) (b)
23) (b)
24) (b)
} Follow section, **parasites to be remember** for explanation

Section VII

Medical Entomology

Preview of Medical Entomology

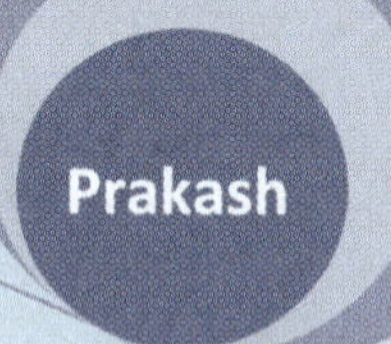

In Medical entomology almost all arthropod are written with following headings & subheadings with use of specific bullets & numberings.

- **Geographical distribution:**

- **Morphology:**
  - **Size:**
  - **Shape:**
  - **Colour:**
  - **Body parts: (in few arthropod only two parts like cephalothorax & abdomen)**
  - **Head:**
  - **Thorax:**
  - **Abdomen:**

- **Life cycle:**
  - **Stages: With appropriate figure**
  - **Life span:**

- **Life styles (habits):**
  - **Breeding sites (habitats):**
  - **Feeding & biting habits:**
  - **Others:**

- **Species & disease transmitted by insect:**

- **Control measures:**

101 Medical Entomology

Learning heading & subheadings

Definition:
Study of the arthropods of medical importance is **called medical entomology.**

Clinical significances:
- Help to fertilise the agricultural products.
- They may damage the agricultural products.
- They are human enemies & carry many microbes. They act as carrier or reservoir or source or vector of microorganism & transmit to human.
- They also cause allergic reaction following bites & induce phobias.

Classification of arthropods:
A. **Morphological classification:** There are 3 classes of arthropods of like **Insecta, Arachnida** & **Maxilopoda** as mentioned in **table-1.**

B. **Systemic classification:** → **Table-2**

Features	Insecta	Arachnida	Maxilopoda
Body parts	3 parts like - Head - Thorax - Abdomen	2 parts like - Cephalo-thorax - Abdomen	2 parts like - Cephalo-thorax - Abdomen
Antennae	1 pair	Absent	2 pairs
Legs	3 pairs	4 pairs	5 pairs
Wings & examples	**- 1 pair:** Mosquitoes, flies & midges **- 2 pairs:** Cockroach & reduviid bug **- Wingless:** Bed bug, louse & flea	Wingless like ticks & mites	Wingless like cyclops
Habitat	Soil	Soil	Water

Table-1: Morphological classification of arthropods

Modes of transmission of arthropod (vector) borne diseases:
Follow chapter → Infection and infectious diseases

Mosquito

❖ **Classification:** →**Flow chart-1**

✓ **Note: Genera in tribe Culicini**
- It includes > 15 genera but medically important are only three like *Culex, Aedes* & *Mansonia.*

❖ **Geographical distribution:** Worldwide.

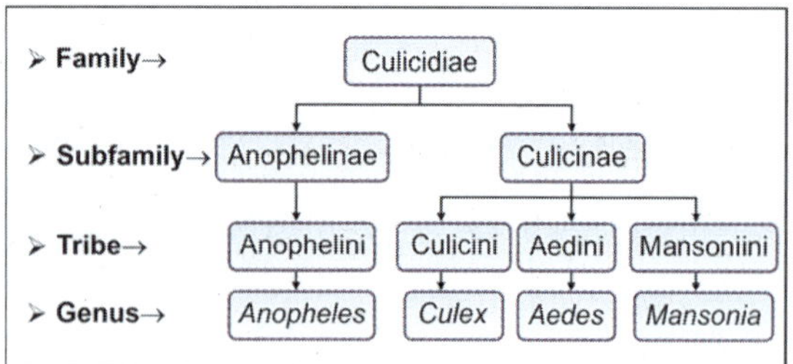

Flow chart-1: Classification of mosquito

❖ **Morphology:** Three main parts of mosquito's body like head, thorax & abdomen.

➢ **Size:** The length of the adult is typically between 3mm and 6mm. The smallest mosquitoes are around 2 mm (0.1 in), and the largest around 19 mm (0.7 in). Mosquitoes typically weigh around 5 mg.

➢ **Shape:** Oval shape.

➢ **Colour:** Mosquitoes are attracted to **dark** colours, so keeping outdoor clothing light will help to avoid bites.

➢ **Body parts**

✪ **Head:**

- **Shape:** Semi-globular.
- **Organs:** 1 pair of eyes, long proboscis (used for biting), 1 pair of palpi & 1 pair of antennae.

✪ **Thorax:**

- **Shape:** Large & rounded.
- **Organs:** 1 pair of wing presents dorsally & 3 pairs of legs present ventrally.

Kingdom → Animalia					
Phylum	**Class**	**Order**	**Family (common name)**	**Genus**	**Species**
Arthopoda	**Insecta**	Diptera	Culicidiae (mosquito)	*Anopheles*	All the species of arthropods, transmitting different microorganisms are mentioned with respective sections
				Culex	
				Aedes	
				Mansonia	
			Muscidae (house fly)	*Musca*	
			Glossinidae (tse tse fly)	*Glossina*	
			Psychodidae (sand fly)	*Phlebotomus*	
				Sergentomyia	
				Lutzomyia	
			Simuliidae (black fly)	*Simulium*	
			Tabanidae (deer fly, horse fly & yellow fly)	*Chrysops* (deer fly)	
				Tabanus (horse fly)	
				Diachlorus (yellow fly)	
			Calliphoridae (blow fly)	*Chrysomya*	
			Ceratopogonidae (midges)	*Culicoides*	
				Forcipomyia	
				Austroconops	
				Leptoconops	
		Blattaria	Blattidiae (cockroach)	*Blatta*	
		Hemiptera	Reduviidae (reduviid bug)	*Triatoma*	
			Cimicidae (bed bug)	*Cimex*	
		Phthiraptera	Pediculidae (head louse & body louse)	*Pediculushumanus capitis* (head)	
				Pediculushumanus corporis (head louse)	
			Phthiridae (pubic louse)	*Phthirus*	
		Siphona-ptera	Pulicidae (flea)	*Xenopsylla*	
				Nosopsylla	
				Ctenocephalus	
				Pulex	
				Tunga	
	Arachnida	Ixodida	Ixodidae (hard tick)	*Dermacentor*	
				Haemaphysalis	
				Amblyoma	
				Ixodes	
				Rhipicephalus	
				Hyaloma	
			Argasidae (soft tick)	*Ornithodorus*	
		Actinedida	Trombiculidae (trombiculid mite)	*Trobicula*	
		Astigmata	Sarcoptidae (itch mite)	*Sarcoptes* (*Acarus*)	
	Maxilopoda (Subphylum → Crustacea)	Cyclopoida	Cyclopidae (cyclops)	*Cyclops*	
				Mesocyclops	
				Thermocyclops	
				Tropocyclops	
				Encyclops	

Table-2: Systemic classification of arthropods

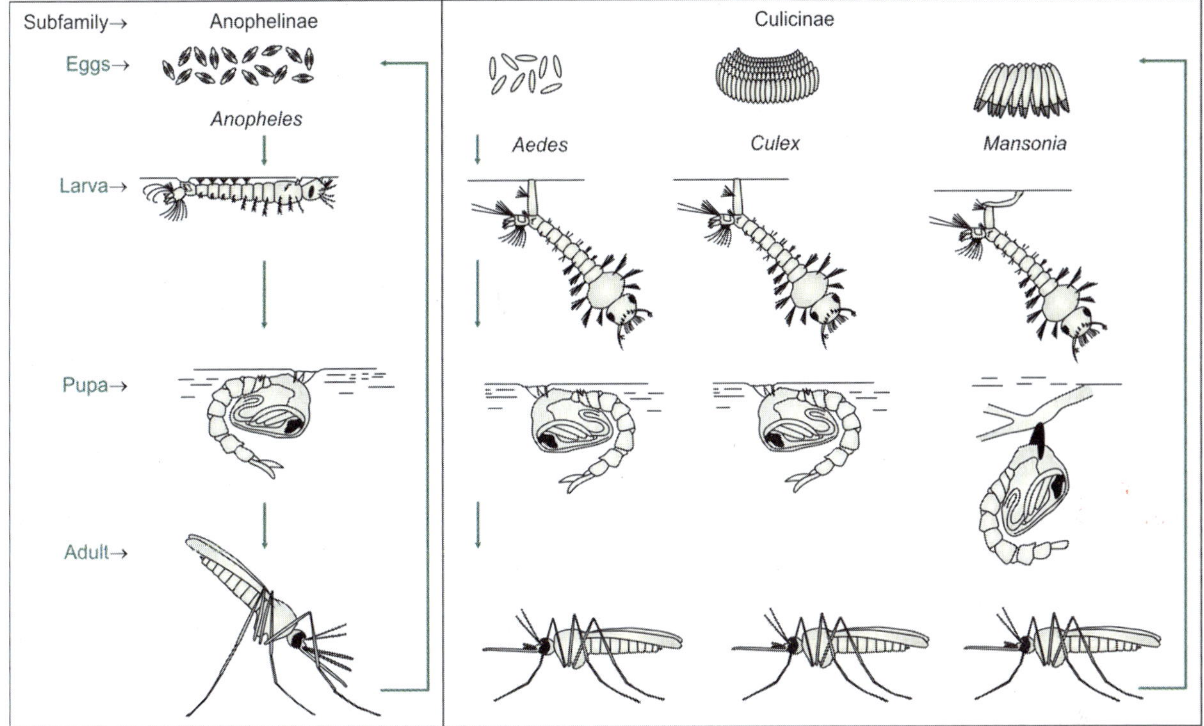

Figure-1: Life cycle of mosquitoes

✪ **Abdomen:**

- **Shape:** Long, narrow & with 10 segments.
- **Organs:** Last 2 segments are modified to form external genitalia.

❖ **Life cycle:** → **Figure-1**

➢ **Stages:** Following four stages of life cycle are occurs in mosquito.

i. Egg (plural → eggs):

- In most species, adult females lay their eggs in stagnant water; some lay eggs near the water's edges. *Culex* & *Anopheles* lay their eggs on the water surface while many *Aedes* lay their eggs on damp soil that will be flooded by water.
- Eggs are laid one at a time or attached together to form "rafts." They float on the surface of the water. In the case of *Culex* species, the eggs are stuck together in rafts of up to 200.
- *Anopheles* & *Aedes*, as well as many other genera, do not make egg rafts, but lay their eggs singly.
- Most eggs hatch into larvae within 48 hours in favourable conditions; others might withstand subzero winters before hatching.
- Water is a necessary part of their habitat.

ii. Larva (plural → Larvae):

- Also **called wiggler.**
- Larval body have three parts like head, thorax & abdomen.
- Larvae feed on algae, bacteria & vegetable matter.
- Larvae shed (moult) their skins four times, growing larger after each moult. The developmental stages **called "instars".**
- Larvae live in the water & come to the surface to breathe. They breaths through siphon tube (air tube) or by breathing opening.
- *Anopheles* larvae do not have a siphon and lie parallel to the water surface to get a supply of oxygen through a breathing opening.
- *Culex, Mansonia* and *Aedes* have siphon tube (situated in 8th segments of abdomen) for breathing.
- *Mansonia* larvae are attached to rootlets of plants through siphon tube to obtain air.
- They suspended in water with head downside.
- During the fourth moult the larvae change into pupae.

iii. Pupa (plural → Pupae):

- Also **called tumbler.**
- The pupal stage is a resting, non-feeding stage of development.
- Pupae are mobile, responding to light changes & after disturbances they move (tumble) with a flip of their tails towards the bottom or protective areas.
- They are in comma shape.
- They have cephalothorax & abdomen.
- They breathe through trumpet shaped breathing tubes on the thorax.
- Pupal stage last for 1-2 days & when development is complete, the pupal skin splits and the adult mosquito (imago) emerges.

iv. Adult (plural → Adults):

- Also called imago.
- The newly emerged adult rests on the surface of the water for a short time to allow itself to dry and all its body parts to harden.
- The wings have to spread out and dry properly before it can fly.
- Blood feeding and mating does not occur for a couple of days after the adults emerge.

➢ **Life span:**
- How long each stage last is depends on temperature & species characteristics.
- Total period from egg to adult stage development is 7-10 days in favourable conditions.
- Life span of adult stage is 2 weeks.

❖ Differences between Anophelinae & Culicinae : → Table-3

Features	Anophelinae	Culicinae
Eggs **- Laid** **- Shape**	- Singly - Boat shape with lateral shaft	- Cluster or in raft - Oval without lateral shaft - Except in *Aedes* laid eggs singly & in cigar shaped
Larvae - Resting habit - Air tube - Plamate hairs	- Parallel to surface - Absent - Present on abdomen	- Hanged at an angle with downside head - Present - ABsent
Pupae	Broad & short air tube	Long & narrow air tube
Adult - Resting habit - Wings - Palpi	- An an angle to surface with downside head - Spotted - Long in both sexes	- Parallel to surface - Not spotted - Short in female

Table-3: Differences between Anophelinae & Culicinae

❖ Life styles (habits):

i. ***Anopheles:*** → **Figure-2**

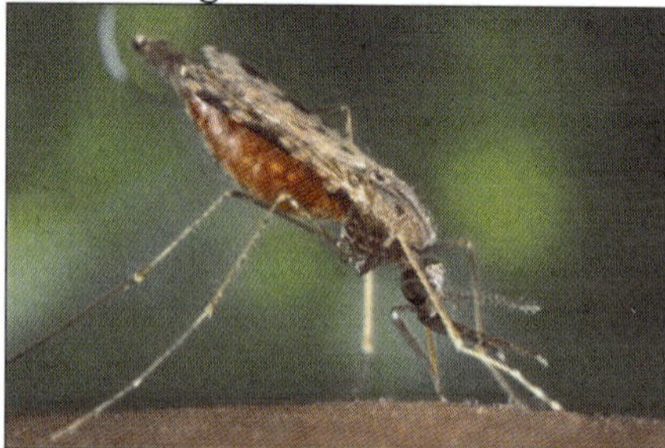

Figure-2: *Anopheles* mosquito

- **Breeding sites (habitats):** *Anopheles* prefers the clean water for breeding.
- **Feeding & biting habits:** *Anopheles* feed in evening or night & indoors or outdoors.
- **Resting habit & identification point:** They rest at right angle to surface with head down.

ii. ***Culex* (nuisance mosquito):** → **Figure-3**

- **Breeding sites (habitats):** *Culex* prefers the dirty water for breeding like stagnant drains, cesspools, septic tank, burrow pits & in fact all types of water collection. Rapid urbanisation without proper drainage facilities increased the spread of *Culex*. Strong winged mosquito can dispersed up to 11 km in urban areas.

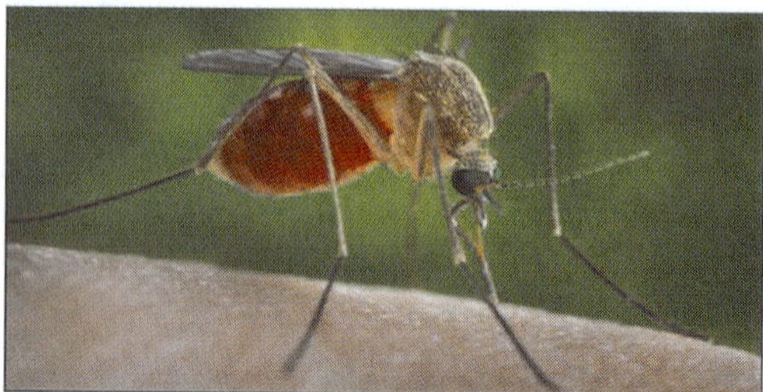

Figure-3: *Culex* mosquito

- **Feeding & biting habits:**
  - They feed in night & doing rest in day times in dark cool place, indoors on walls, under furniture, inside empty pots & in dark corners. Best biting time is midnight, particularly below knee.
  - Males are short lived & they never bite for blood meal & feed on plant juices.
  - Female bite for blood meal every 2-3 days as they required blood for development of eggs.
- **Others:**
  - **Resting habit:** They rest parallel to surface.
  - **Identification point:** *Culex* is identified by the round tips of abdomen.

iii. ***Aedes (Stegomyia):*** → **Figure-4**

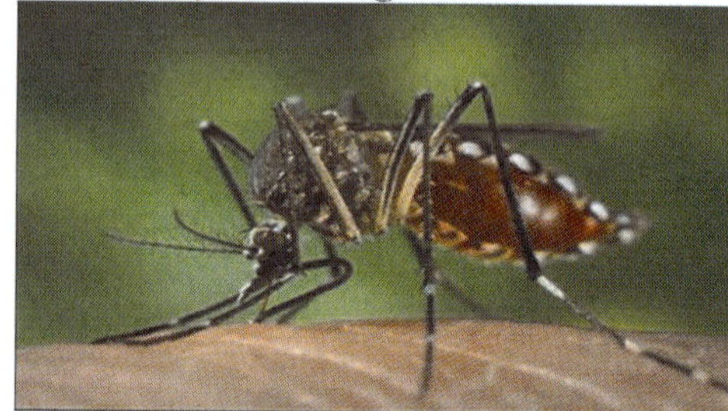

Figure-4: *Aedes* mosquito

- **Breeding sites (habitats):** *Aedes* prefers the artificially collected water sites for breeding like water present in coconut shell, discarded tube/bottles/tins, flower pots, tree holes, tyres etc. *Aedes* mosquitoes are most abundant in rainy seasons & can dispersed up to <100 meters, which helps in the eradication.
- **Feeding & biting habits:** Females bite (ferocious or fearless biters) in day or night & indoors or outdoors.
- **Others:**
  - **Resting habit:** They rest parallel to surface.

- **Identification point:** *Aedes* is identified by the white stripes on black body & legs, (so **called tiger mosquito**).

iv. ***Mansonia:*** → **Figure-5**

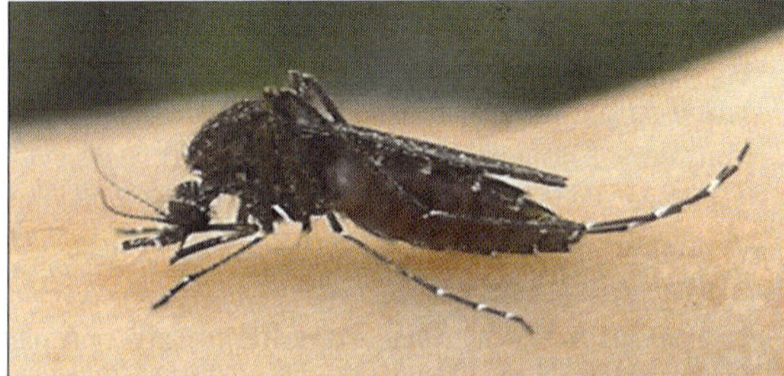

Figure-5: *Mansonia* mosquito

- **Breeding sites (habitats):** *Mansonia* breeds in ponds & lakes containing floating type aquatic plants like *Pistia stratiotes* & water hyacinth. Eggs are laid in star shaped clusters under surface of leaves of these plants. *Mansonian* larvae & pupae are attached to rootlets of these plants through siphon tube to obtain air, which is supplied to rootlets. Pupae comes to surface, becomes adults & escaper. It is very easy to control the *Mansonia* by removing the aquatic plants.
- **Feeding & biting habits:** They feed in night either indoors or outdoors & during day in swamp forests.
- **Others:**
  - **Resting habit:** They rest parallel to surface.
  - **Identification point:** *Mansonia* is very big, black or brown with speckling on the wings or legs.

❖ Species & disease transmitted by mosquitoes:

i. ***Anopheles:*** Total 45 species, of which only few are known to transmit the *Plasmodium* spp. (causing malaria) like

- *A. culcifacies* (In rural area, **Mnemonic: ll**).
- *A. stephensi* (In urban area, **Mnemonic: nn**).
- *A. philipinensis.*
- *A. fluviatilis.*
- *A. varuna.*
- *A. minimus.*
- *A. annularis.*
- *A. leucosphyrus* (*A. balabacensis*).
- *A. sundaicus.*
- *A. jeyporiensis candidiensis.*

ii. ***Culex* (nuisance mosquito):**

- *Culex fatigans* (*Culex quinquefasciatus*): *Wucheria bancrofti* (Bancroft's filariasis) in India.
- Arboviruses: **Follow chapter → Arboviruses and Roboviruses.**

iii. ***Aedes:***

- Arboviruses: **Follow chapter → Arboviruses and Roboviruses.**

iv. ***Mansonia:***

- *Mansonia annulifera, M. indiana, M. uniformis*: *Burgia malayi* (malayan filariasis) in India.

❖ Mosquito control measures:

A. Anti larval measures:

i. Physical or environmental control:

- Elimination or reduction of the number, size & frequency of mosquito breeding sites like filling, levelling & drainage of breeding places.
- Removal of aquatic plants to control the *Mansonia.*

ii. Biological control:

- **Larvicidal fish or mosquito fish:**
  - Uses of fish which eats the larvae like *Gambusia affinis, Lebister reticulates* etc.
  - It can be used in burrow pits, sewage, oxidation ponds, ornamental ponds, cisterns & farm ponds.
- **Larvicidal bacteria:**
  - *Bacillus thuringiensis* subsp. *israelensis* (*Bti*) or S-methoprene under certain circumstances.
  - Commercial products "Mosquito Dunks" and "Mosquito bits" containing *Bti* can be purchased at many hardware/garden stores for homeowner use.

iii. Chemical control:

a. Mineral oils:

- **Examples:** Diesel, kerosene, crude oil etc.
- **Mechanisms of action:**
  - All these oils can spread in water & make a thin film which cut the air supply to the larvae & pupae.
  - Oil has direct toxic effect on larvae.
- **Application:** Life cycle of mosquitoes is 8 days, so it must to apply every week in all breeding places.
- **Disadvantages:** It kills fish & also makes water unfit for drink.

b. Paris green or copper acetoarsenite:

- **Mechanisms of action:** Paris green is stomach poison, so it should be ingested by larvae for desire effect.
- **Application:**
  - Good sample of paris green contains 50% of arsenious oxide
  - It is applied as 2% dust (20-25 microns particles) by using hand blower or rotary blower
  - 2% dust contains 2kg paris green plus 98kg diluents such as soapstone powder or slaked lime in a rotary mixture.
  - Advised dose is 1kg of actual aris green per hectare of water surface.
- **Disadvantages:** It is a crystalline water insoluble powder & it kills the surface larvae like *Anopheles*, for bottom feeding larvae it should be applied in granular form.
- **Advantages** It does not ham fish, man & water quality.

c. Organo phosphorous (OP) compound:

- **Examples & dose:**
  - Abate: 56-112g/hectare.

- Malathion: 224-672 g/hectare.
- Fenthion: 22-112 g/hectare.
- Chlorpyrifors: 11-16g/hectare.
- **Advantages:** They hydrolyse quickly in water.

✓ **Note: Organochlorine compound**
- Like DDT, HCH are not used as larvicides because of long residual effect, water contamination & chances of resistance in the vector mosquitoes.

B. Anti adult measures:

i. Residual spray:

- **DDT**
- Most effective.
- Dose: 1-2g pure DDT / square meter. Effect last for 6-12 months, so it is applied 1-3 times in a year to walls & other surfaces where mosquitoes are rest.
- **DDT resistant areas:** Resistance to insecticides is common, so periodic testing is essential. Following insecticides are useful in DDT resistant areas.
- Malthion: 2g/square meter & effect last for 3 months.
- Gamma-HCH/lindane: 0.5g/square meter & effect last for 3 months.
- Propoxure/OMS33: 2g/square meter & effect last for 3 months.

ii. Space spray: It includes spraying of mist or fog to kill the insects.

- **Pyrethrum extract (pyrethrin)**
- It is extracted from pyrethrum flowers.
- The active ingredient is pyrethrin.
- Dose & application: 1 oz (contains 1% pyrethrin) of the spray solution/ 1000^3 feet area. Close door & windows for half an hour. For small scale it is applied by hand gun with fine nozzle but for large scale aerosol dispenser or power sprayer is required.
- Action: It is the nerve poison & kills insect on mere contact.
- Disadvantage: It has no residual effect, so reinfestation from outside source is occur in short time.
- **Residual insecticides**
- Malathion & fenthion are useful.
- They are spray by ultra low volume (ULV) sprayer.

iii. Genetic control: It include genetic methods (under trial) of mosquito control like
- Sterile male technique.
- Cytoplasmic incompatibility.
- Chromosomal translocations.
- Sex distortion.
- Gene replacement.

C. Protection against mosquito bite:

i. Mosquito net:

- **Types:** Screening windows by using following types wire net can prevent against mosquito bite
- Ordinary net: Less effective.
- Chemically impregnated net: Net impregnated with gamma-cyhalothrin is more effective.
- **Selection of nets:**
- Material should be in white colour for easy detection of mosquito.
- Best pattern is rectangular net.
- Not a single hole or rent in net.
- Number of holes per square inch is 150.
- The size of hole should not be > 0.0475 inch in any diameter.

ii. Mosquito repellents:

- **Preparation:** Mosquito repellents are prepared from different chemicals like diethyltoluamide/deet (outstanding in all purpose & effective for18-20 hours against *Culex fatigans*), indalone, dimethyl phthalate, dimethyl carbate, ethyl hexanediol etc.
- **Application:** Applied on a skin for short term protection.

iii. Screening:
- Screening of building with copper or bronze gauze having 16 meshes to the inch is recommended.
- The size of aperture should not be > 0.0475 inch in any diameter.
- It is costly but gives excellent result.

House fly

❖ **Geographical distribution:** Worldwide.

❖ **Morphology:** Three main parts of body of house fly like head, thorax & abdomen. Following are the main features of *Musca domestica.*

➢ **Size:** Fly is about 8 mm long.

➢ **Shape:** Wings form V shape when they are folded.

➢ **Colour:** Mouse grey in colour.

➢ **Body parts:**

✪ **Head:**
- **Organs:** 1 pair of eyes (close in male while set apart in female), single refractile proboscis (used for sucking foods) & 1 pair of antennae.

✪ **Thorax:**
- **Stripes:** 3-4 longitudinal stripes present in *Musca domestica.*
- **Organs:** 1 pair of wings & 3 pairs of legs. Legs & body are covered with numerous short & stiff hairs, **called tenant hairs** which secrete sticky substances.

✪ **Abdomen:** It is segmented & shows the light & dark marking. The underside of the male is yellowish.

❖ **Life cycle:** → **Figure-6**

➢ **Stages:** Following four stages of life cycle are occurs in house fly.

i. Egg:

- Eggs are white, about 1.2 mm in length, are laid singly but eggs are piled in small groups. Eggs can be seen naked eye.
- Each female fly can lay up to 500 eggs in several batches of 75 to 150 eggs/batch over a three to four day period in moist decaying organic matters **(breeding sites)** like human excreta; animal excreta, manure heaps, garbage & vegetable refuse. *Musca domestica* & *Musca vicinia* breeds on human excreta.
- The number of eggs produced is a function of female size which, itself, is principally a result of larval nutrition.
- Maximum eggs production occur at intermediate temperatures, 25 to 30°C. Often, several flies will deposit their eggs in close proximity, leading to large masses of larvae and pupae.
- Eggs are hatch in 8-24 hours. In India they hatch in 3 hours.
- It has been estimated that mated pair of flies can produce in a single summer not < 325, 923, 200, 000 eggs.

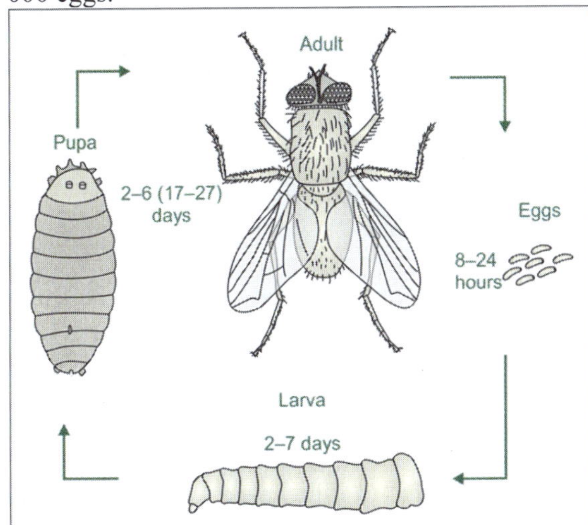

Figure-6: Life cycle of house fly

ii. Larva:

- Also **called maggots.**
- Early instar larvae are 1-2 mm long, typical creamy whitish in colour, cylindrical but tapering toward the head.
- The head contains one pair of dark hooks. The posterior spiracles are slightly raised and the spiracular openings are sinuous slits which are completely surrounded by an oval black border.
- The legless maggots emerge from the eggs in warm weather within eight to 20 hours. Maggots immediately begin feeding on and developing in the material in which the eggs were laid.
- The larvae go through three instars, eats voraciously; moult twice to be mature larvae with 7-12 mm length & greasy, cream-colored appearance.
- High-moisture manure favours the survival of the house fly larva. The optimal temperature for larval development is 35 to 38°C, though larval survival is greatest at 17 to 32°C.
- Larvae complete their development in 2 - 7 days at optimal temperatures, but require 14 - 30 days at temperatures of 12 to 17°C.
- Nutrient-rich substrates such as animal manure provide an excellent developmental substrate.
- When the maggot is full-grown, it can crawl up to 50 feet to a dry, cool place near breeding material and transform to the pupal stage.

iii. Pupa:

- The pupae are about 8 mm long & vary in colour from yellow, red, brown to black. The shape of the pupa is quite different from the larva, being bluntly rounded at both ends.
- Pupae complete their development in 2-6 days at 32 to 37°C, but require 17 -27 days at about 14°C.
- The emerging flies escape from the pupae through the use of an alternately swelling and shrinking sac, **called the ptilinum.**

iv. Adult:

- Pupa changes to adult stage.
- The house fly female usually larger than the male.

➤ **Life span:**

- Complete life cycle from egg to adult takes 5-6 days in summer in India but at other times it may take 8-20 days.
- Fly lives for 15 days in summer & 25 days in winter.

❖ Life styles (habits):

- **Breeding sites (habitats):**
- Breeding sites are mentioned earlier in life cycle under the egg section.
- Normally remain close to breeding sites but adult fly can move up to 4 miles & sometimes even more.
- **Feeding & biting habits:**
- Fly never bites.
- It is attracted toward the food by its sense of smell
- It can't eat solid food. It vomit over solid food, make it liquid followed by sucking.
- Adult fly can delight from sputum, wound discharge & faeces.
- **Others:**
- **Resting habit:** Fly has a tendency to rest on vertical surface / hanging object & can move towards light source.
- **Identification point:** Easy to identify from all morphological points mentioned earlier.

❖ Species & disease transmitted by house fly:

- Major species of flies available in India are *Musca domestica, M vicinia, M nebulo & M sorben.*

- **Mechanical transmission:** Adult fly is restless insect & move to & forth between foods; which allow the **mechanical transmission** of disease like cholera, enteric fever (typhoid & paratyphoid), amoebic dysentery, shigellosis, *E coli* diarrhoea, intestinal helminth diseases, conjunctivitis, trachoma, anthrax, yaws, hepatitis etc.
- **Defecation:** Fly is defecating frequently whole day, so depositing bacteria over food.
- **Vomiting:** Fly vomit frequently, the vomit drop is culture of disease agents.

❖ House fly control measures:

A. Anti larval measures:

i. Physical or environmental control:

- Elimination or reduction of breeding sites.
- Proper collection (in bin with tight lid), transport (without spillage) & disposal (in a sanitary landfill by incineration or deep burial) of house hold wastes.
- No open defecation.
- Use of sanitary latrines.
- Sanitary disposal of animal excreta.
- Keep the poultry house clean, especially from excreta. Keep fan on in poultry house which dry the bird dropping.
- Dung heaps should be covered plastic or other fly proof material. It prevents the egg laying & heat generated from dung is not escape which kills larvae & pupae.

ii. Chemical control: Larvicides like diazinon (0.5%), dichlorovos (2%), dimethoate (2%) or runnel (1%) are applied at breeding sites in the dose of 28-56 litres/ meters^2.

A. Anti adult measures:

i. Physical methods:

a. Protection by screening:

- Screening of house, markets, hospitals etc. with 14 meshes to the inch will keep out houseflies but finer screening will keep away other insects also.
- It is expensive.

b. Fly consciousness programme:

- It improves the health education about flies.
- It required willing co-operation from people & health authorities.

c. Fly net:

- Don't keep food open & cover it with fly net. It reduces the attraction of fly.
- Covers the children sleeping area with fly net.

d. Fly traps:

- Large numbers of flies can be caught with fly traps.
- An attractive breeding & feeding place is provided in a darkened container. When they try to leave, the flies are caught in a sunlit gauze trap covering the opening of the container. This method is suitable for outdoors.

e. Light trap with electrocutor:

- Flies attracted to the light are killed on contact with an electrocuting grid that covers it.
- Blue and ultraviolet light attracts blowflies but is not very effective against houseflies. The method should be tested under local conditions before an investment is made. It is sometimes used in hospital kitchens and restaurants.

f. General measures:

- Prevention of fly contact with slaughter house & dead animals.

ii. Chemical methods:

a. Residual spray: It includes spraying at fly resting sites. It has immediate & long term effect from days to weeks. It is important to know where the flies spend most of their time at night. Only surfaces that have been observed to be used as resting sites should be sprayed.

- **DDT (5%), methoxychlor (5%), lindane (0.5%) & chlordane (2.5%):**
  - Most effective.
  - Dose: Sprayed by 5 lit / 100 square meters.
- **Resistant to above chemicals:**
  - Resistance to insecticides is common, so periodic testing is essential. Insecticides useful in resistant areas are diazinon (2%), dimethiote (2.5%), fenthion (2.5%), malthion (5%) or runnel (5%).
  - The addition of sugar enhances the effectiveness.
  - Care should be taken to avoid the contamination with food & water.

b. Space spray:

- It includes spraying in air. Flies can be quickly killed by mists or aerosols of insecticide solutions or emulsions. The treatment is carried out by spraying with pressurized aerosol spray cans, hand-operated sprayers or small portable power-operated sprayers.
- The principle is to fill a space with a mist of small droplets that are picked up by the insects when they fly.
- Compared with residual spraying of resting surfaces, space-spraying has an immediate effect but it is short-lasting. The risk of the development of insecticide resistance is less. The method can be used indoors, outdoors and for direct spraying of aggregations of flies.
- It is done by using pyrethrin, DDT or HCH.
- Disadvantage: It has no residual effect (short lasting), so reinfestation from outside source is occurs in short time, which is overcome by repeating of spraying.

c. Baits:

- **Preparation:** Toxic baits made use of sugar, water & other fly-attracting liquids like strong poison.
- **Chemical used are:**
  - Sodium arsenite.

- Milk or sweet liquids with 1-2% formaldehyde can still be recommended for killing flies.
- Improvements became possible with the use of OP compound (Dichlorvosa, dimethoatea, trichlorfona, azamethiphos, diazinon, fenchlorvos, malathion & propetamphos) & carbamate compounds (bendiocarb, dimetilana, methomylc & propoxur) that are highly toxic to flies but relatively safe to humans & other mammals.

- **Types of bait**

- Dry scatter baits.
- Liquid sprinkle baits.
- Liquid bait dispensers.
- Viscous paint-on baits.

d. Cords & ribbons:

- Cords or ribbon impregnated with diazinon, dimethiote or fenthion are tried with success.
- These are hung like festoons from ceiling.
- Period of effectiveness is 1-6 months.

e. Fly papers:

- They are made by mixing 2 lbs of resins & one pint of castor oil which should be heated together until the mixture resembles molasses. It should be paint, while hot on paper with ordinary paint brush.
- Mixture can also be applied on wire or other place where the fly can rest.

f. Sticky tapes:

- Commercially available sticky tapes, suspended from ceilings, attract flies because of their sugar content.
- Flies landing on the tapes are trapped in glue. The tapes last for several weeks if not fully covered by dust or trapped flies.

Tse tse fly

❖ **Geographical distribution:** Tse tse flies are found in African continents. Regions infested with flies **called "fly belt".**

❖ **Morphology:** Three main parts of body of tse tse fly like head, thorax & abdomen. Following are the main features.

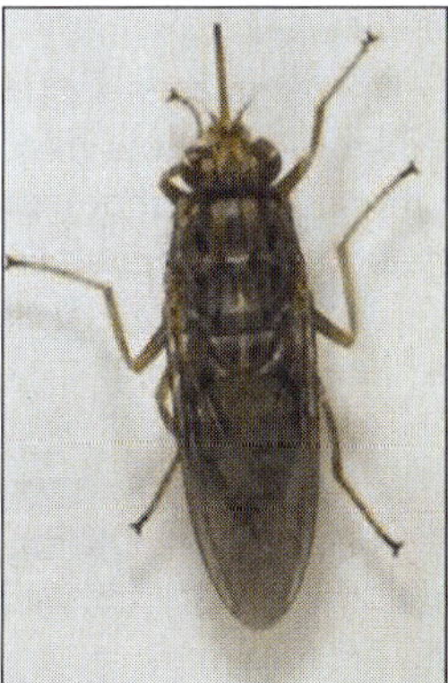

Figure-7: Tse tse fly

➢ **Size:** Fly is about half an inch long.
➢ **Colour:** Yellow or dark brown in colour (**fig.-7**).
➢ **Head:** Single, rigid & non-refractile proboscis used for piercing the skin & sucking the blood
➢ **Body parts:**
✪ **Head:** 1 pair of antennae.
✪ **Thorax:** 1 pair of wings that are folded on the back (overlap each other like blade of scissors) while resting.
✪ **Abdomen:** Also present.

❖ **Life cycle:**

➢ **Stages:** Following four stages of life cycle are occurs in tse tse fly.

i. Egg:

- Egg is produce but not coming out.
- Female tsetse mate just once. After 7 - 9 days it produces a single egg which develops into a larva within her uterus.

ii. Larva:

- About nine days later, the mother produces a larva which burrows (about one inch below the surface) into the ground where it pupates.
- The mother continues to produce a single larva at roughly nine day intervals for her entire life.

iii. Pupa:

- Larva emerges to pupa in few hours.
- Pupal stage last for 20-30 days.

iv. Adult:

- The adult fly emerges from the pupa in the ground after about 30 days. Over a period of 12-14 days it matures, mates and, if it is a female, deposits its first larva.
- Thus, 50 days elapse between the emergence of one female fly and the subsequent emergence of the first of its progeny.
- This life cycle, with a slow reproductive rate and substantial parental investment in the care of young, is a relatively unusual example of an insect with a so-**called 'K-type' life history**.
- This slow rate of reproduction means that tsetse populations can be eradicated by killing just 2-3% of the female population per day.

➢ **Life span:** Fly lives <100 days.

❖ **Life styles (habits):**

- **Breeding sites (habitats):**

- Mother produces a larva which burrows about one inch below the surface into the ground.
- It rarely enters in house, but can travel by road or rail for a long distance to get the blood meal.
- *G. palpalis* & *G. tachinoides:* These species **called "riverine species**', because they inhabit the woodland vegetation near water source.
- *G. morsitans* & *G. pallidipes* : These species **called "savannah species**', because they inhabit the woodland vegetation in savannah country.

- **Feeding & biting habits:**
- Both the sexes can bite, mainly during days for blood meal.
- Fly can bite to man, animals, all type wild games, birds, lizards & snakes.
- **Others:**
- **Resting habit:** When it rest both wings are folded.
- **Identification point:** From colour & folded wings.

❖ **Species & disease transmitted by tse tse fly:** It is a vector of *Trypanosoma brucei* which cause sleeping sickness (African trypanosomiasis) with following types & respective species.

1. **Gambiense & Zambian strain:** Transmitted by *G. palpalis, G. pallidipes & G. tachinoides.*
2. **Rhodesiense strain:** Transmitted by *G. morsitans, G. swynertoni & G. pallidipes.*
3. **Animal strain:** Transmitted by *Glossina morsitans.*

❖ **Tse tse fly control measures:**

i. **Physical or environmental control:**
- Destruction of wild game.
- This method has been given up.
- Removing vegetation where tst tse fly can breed is effective measure. Using alone can give slow result & with insecticides it gives speedy result.

ii. **Chemical control:**
- Insecticides like DDT (25%) & dieldrin (18-20%) are most commonly used chemicals.
- Resistance also reported to these chemicals.
- They can be applied from air craft if large areas to cover.

iii. **Genetic control:** Sterile male release technique is under control.

Sand fly

❖ **Geographical distribution:** Found in the warm countries.

❖ **Morphology:** Three main parts of body of sand fly like head, thorax & abdomen. Following are the main features.

➢ **Size:** Sand fly is about 3-5 long & smaller than mosquito.
➢ **Colour:** Light or dark brown in colour.
➢ **Body parts:**

✪ **Head:**
- 1 pair of hairy antennae & a pair of palpi.
- Single rigid, non-refractile proboscis, used for piercing the skin & sucking the blood.

✪ **Thorax:**
- 1 pair of upright hairy wings. Wings are in lanceolate shape. Winged sand fly, hop about but don't fly. In *Phlebotomus* spp. 2nd longitudinal vein of the wing branched twice, the1st branching take place in the middle.
- 3 pairs of long & slender legs. Legs are out of proportion of body size.

✪ **Abdomen:**
- Contains 10 segments, which are covered by hairs.
- In female the tip of abdomen is rounded & in male it contains claspers, which are conspicuous & attached to the last segment.

❖ **Life cycle:** → **Figure-8**

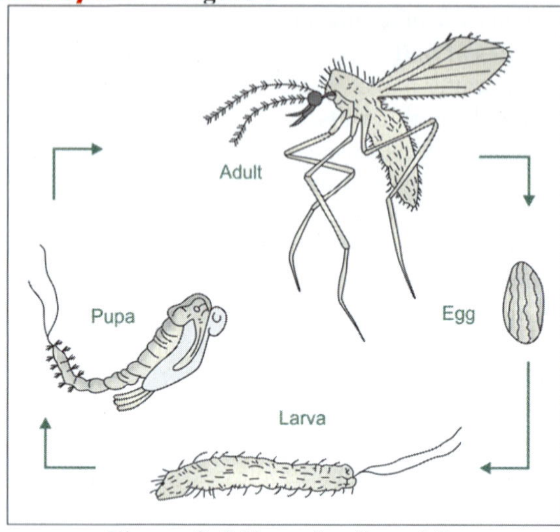

Figure-8: Life cycle of sand fly

➢ **Stages:** Following four stages of life cycle are occurs in sand fly.

i. **Egg:**
- A blood meal is typically required for females to develop eggs.
- Female lay between 30-70 eggs on a moist soil & damp dark places in the cattle sheds & poultry, which hatch within 1-2 weeks.
- At first sand fly eggs are oval-shaped & pale. Once exposed to air, the eggs turn brown.
- The eggs measure 0.31mm long and 0.10mm wide.

ii. **Larva:**
- Caterpillar-like larvae hatch from eggs through a J-shaped crack. Four different stages or instars, of larval development occur over a period of around two weeks, each one larger than the one before. The newly hatched first instar larvae have two rear bristles, or whiskers, while all later larval developments have four rear bristles.
- The larvae are hairy maggots like structure, having large head, thorax and abdomen and two long bristle on last abdominal segment.
- Larvae feed on decaying organic matter and become pupae in about 2 weeks.

iii. **Pupa:**
- To prepare for the pupal stage, larvae attach themselves to a substrate. During this stage, each larva resembles a butterfly chrysalis as it develops into adults and grows wings.
- Sand flies are immobile during this life cycle stage and do not eat.

- Pupae are found in cracks and crevices in the wall.
- The pupal stage develops in 5-10 days & last for 1week.

iv. **Adult:**
- Sand flies emerge from their pupal stage as adults at night, shortly after they develop their wings, which are a characteristic V shaped when erected.
- Sand flies are active during the early morning & evening hours when temperatures are cooler & humidity is lower.

➢ **Life span:**
- The total time from egg to adult takes five weeks.
- The average life of a sand fly is about 2 weeks.

❖ Life styles (habits):

- **Breeding sites (habitats):**
- Moist soil & damp dark places in the cattle sheds & poultry.
- The range of flight is 50 yard from their breeding places, by hoping not by flying.
- **Feeding & biting habits:**
- Only female can bite in the dwelling at night (nocturnal pests), male rely on vegetable juices.
- It takes shelter during day in holes (in trees, dark rooms, store room & stables) and crevices in wall, in dark room and store room etc.
- **Others:**
- **Resting habit:** It can rest with upright wings.
- **Identification point:** Upright hairy wings.

❖ Species & disease transmitted by sand fly:
Sand fly bite is very irritating & painful. It transmits following diseases.

- *Leishmania* spp.: **Follow chapter → Blood and tissue flagellates.**
- Arboviruses (sand fly fever): **Follow chapter → Arboviruses and Roboviruses.**

❖ Sand fly control measures:

i. **Physical or environmental control:**
- Removal of shrubs and vegetation.
- Filling of cracks and crevices in the wall & floor.
- Minimum 50 yards distance of cattle sheds and poultry from human habitations.
- Sandfly are easily controlled because they do not move long distance from their breeding places.

ii. **Chemical control:**
- Single application of DDT (1-2g/m^2) is effective. Its residue may remain effective for a period of 1-2 years.
- Lindane (0.25g/m^2) has been proved effective. Its residue may remain effective for a period of 3 months.
- Spraying should be done in the human dwellings, cattle sheds and poultry.

Black fly

❖ Synonym:
- Because of the hump visible behind their head when viewed in profile, black flies are also **called buffalo gnats** (**fig.-9**).
- Also **called turkey gnats.**

❖ Geographical distribution:
Distributed Worldwide. *Simulium slossonae* is found in Florida. *Simulium indicum* is found in India.

❖ Morphology:
Three main parts of body of black fly like head, thorax & abdomen. Following are the main features.

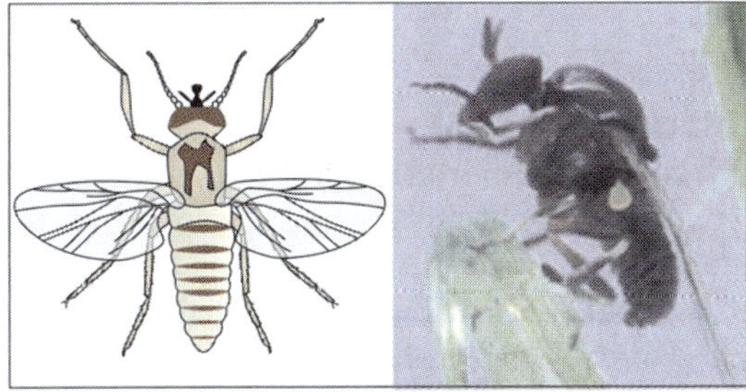

Figure-9: Black flies

➢ **Size:** Black fly is about 1.5-4mm long.

➢ **Colour:** Black in colour with grey to yellow shade (**fig.-9**).

➢ **Body parts:**

✪ **Head:** Short proboscis, used for piercing the skin & sucking the blood.

✪ **Thorax:** 1 pair of large, broad wings & have short stout legs. Thorax is shiny (middle of the fly).

✪ **Abdomen:** Also present.

❖ Life cycle:

➢ **Stages:** Following four stages of life cycle are occurs in black fly.

i. **Egg:** Females lay 200- 800 eggs on vegetation beneath the surface of oxygenated water.

ii. **Larva:**
- Once hatched the larvae have unique hooks that allow them to stay on submerged rocks (stones) or vegetation.
- The larvae feed on passing bacteria, algae and other small organic matter.
- Larvae pass through six stages before reaching the pupal stage.
- Pupal stage last for 3-4week.

iii. **Pupa:**
- As the larvae advance to the pupae stage, they become inactive so it is not necessary for them to feed.
- Pupal stage last for 1-3 week.

iv. **Adult:**
- The pupa becomes an adult and floats to the surface of the water protected in an air bubble.
- Soon after leaving the water, the females will seek blood so they can begin the life cycle again.

➢ **Life span:** The average life cycle is about 3 weeks.

❖ Life styles (habits):

- **Breeding sites (habitats):**
- It breeds below the oxygenated water surface.
- *Simulium indicum* is breed in hill stream.
- It can fly up to 100 miles.
- **Feeding & biting habits:** Female can bite to man, animals for blood.
- **Identification point:** Black colour & shiny thorax.

❖ Species & disease transmitted by black fly:

- *Simulium slossonae* (Florida) & *S. indicum* (India) are vector of *Onchocercus volvulus* (onchocerciasis).

❖ Black fly control measures:

i. **Physical or environmental control:** Difficult to control the adult fly because it can fly up to 100 miles.

ii. **Chemical control:** Larvae are killed by abate in the dose of 0.05-0.1 mg /litre for 10 minutes.

Deer fly

❖ Geographical distribution:

Worldwide. *Chrysops* spp. "**called hydrobionts**" and are found in areas with high water content.

❖ Morphology:

Three main parts of body of deer fly like head, thorax & abdomen. Following are the main features.

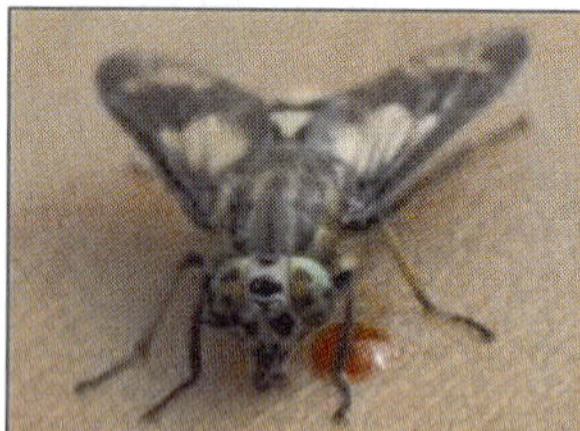
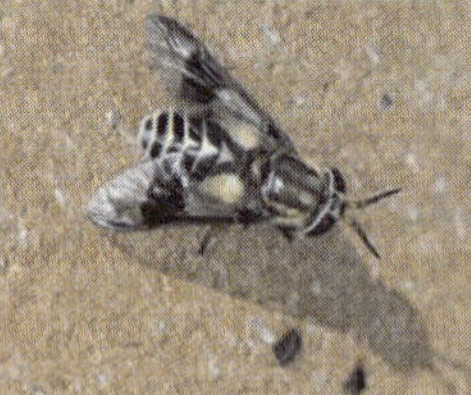

Figure-10: Deer flies

- **Size:** Deer fly is about 9-10 mm long.
- **Colour:** Yellow to black, have stripes on the abdomen, and possess mottled wings with dark patches (**fig.-10**).
- **Body parts:**

✪ **Head:**

- **Shape:** Wide triangular head.
- **Organs:**
- Long & three segmented antennae.
- Bulging eyes. The males are easily differentiated from female flies because eyes are contiguous in the males and widely separated in the females.

✪ **Thorax:**

- Covered with fine hairs.
- 1 pair of broad banded wings.

✪ **Abdomen:**

- Also covered with fine hairs.
- It is yellow or orange with black stripes (**fig.-10**).

❖ Life cycle:

- **Stages:** Following four stages of life cycle are occurs in deer fly.

i. **Egg:**

- Eggs are laid in masses ranging from 100-1000 in layers on a vertical surface such as overhanging foliage, projecting rocks, sticks & aquatic. The vertical surfaces are always directly over water & wet ground favours the development of larvae vegetation. Aquatic vegetation is preferred. The female will not deposit egg masses on vegetation that is too dense.
- A shiny or chalky secretion, which aids in water protection, often covers eggs.
- Eggs are initially a creamy white colour but soon darken to gray and black.
- Eggs are cylindrical in shape & about 1-2.5 mm in length.
- Eggs hatch in 5-7 days, depending upon ambient weather conditions, & the larvae fall to the moist soil & water below.

ii. **Larva:**

- Larvae use a hatching spine to break out of the egg cases. The larvae are aquatic, semi-aquatic or terrestrial.
- The larvae taper at each end and are usually whitish in colour, but also can be brownish or green depending on the species.
- Black bands are found around each segment of the body in many species.
- The larvae breathe through a tracheal siphon located at their posterior end.
- The larvae have a small head & 11-12 additional segments.
- Larvae pass through six to nine stadia.
- Larval stage can last from a few months to year.
- The larvae of *Chrysops* feed upon organic matter in the soil.
- Larvae moves into the upper 2.5 to 5.0 cm of the soil, where it is drier, when it is ready to pupate.
- Within two days after moving to the surface the pupal stage is reached.

iii. **Pupa:**

- The pupae are brown coloured, rounded anteriorly, tapered posteriorly, and have leg & wing cases attached to the body. There is a row of spines encircling each abdominal segment. A pupal "aster" consisting of six pointed projections is located at the apex of the abdomen.
- Pupal stage last for 2-3 week.

iv. **Adult:**

- The adult flies emerge from the pupae via a slit located along the thorax of the case.
- In most species the males emerge before the females. After emergence of both sexes, the flies mate. Mating starts with the male pursuing the

female. Mating is initiated in the air & completed on the ground. The female then deposit egg mass & is ready to seek a host.
- Adult life span is 30 to 60 days.

➢ **Life span:** Most have a year-long life cycle but some larger species may take two or three years.

❖ Life styles (habits):

- **Breeding sites (habitats):**
- Vertical surface like overhanging foliage, projecting rocks, sticks & aquatic which are always directly over water.
- Flies disperse in different areas in minutes.
- **Feeding & biting habits:**
- Female can bite to man, animals for blood. Males do not consume blood. The males are mainly pollen and nectar (juice secreted from flower use prepare the honey by bee) feeders.
- Deer flies will feed on a variety of mammals that include humans, pets, livestock and deer.
- **Others:**
- **Identification point:** Black colour & shiny thorax.

❖ Species & disease transmitted by deer fly:

➢ **Species:** *Chrysops silacea* & *C. dimidiate.*

➢ **Diseases:**

- **Bite wound:**
- Swelling, pain & an itchy red area around the bite.
- Persistent itching and scratching of bite wounds leading to secondary bacterial infections if the bite is not kept clean and disinfected.
- Since deer flies inject anticoagulant-containing saliva during blood feeding, some life threatening serious reactions may occur in people that are highly allergic to the anticoagulant compounds.
- General symptoms may include a rash on the body, wheezing, swelling around the eyes, swelling of the lips and dizziness or weakness.
- **Tularemia:** There is evidence that deer flies in the western U.S. are involved in the transmission of tularaemia (caused by *Francisella tularensis*), also **called deer fly fever** or **rabbit fever**. Compared to ticks, deer flies are minor vectors of tularemia.
- **Loiasis:** Caused by *Loa loa.*

❖ Deer fly control measures:

i. Physical or environmental control:

- For personal protection to prevent bites by wearing long sleeve shirts, pants, and a hat.
- Standard insect repellents are only marginally effective.
- Products that contain high levels of the repellent DEET do provide some protection, but these products can melt plastic materials and are often unpleasant to work with. When flies are swarming, swatting them or running is counterproductive, as these will only serve to attract more flies.
- The use of sticky cloth tape that is placed on the back of caps has been shown to be effective in capturing flies that hover around the head. Use of these products will reduce the numbers of flies, and the bother of flies hovering around the head.
- For pets or livestock, providing a shaded, sheltered area such as a barn, shed or doghouse will give animals a place to escape flies.
- Deer fly traps have been developed to take advantage of the attraction of deer flies to large dark moving objects.

ii. Chemical control:

- No satisfactory chemical control has been developed for deer and horse flies. The wetland habitat that supports the larvae of these insects makes it impractical and environmentally unacccptable to treat breeding sites.
- Adults do not rest on any surface for extended periods, so residual insecticide treatments are not effective.
- Fogging, or the use of aerosol insecticides, will only kill flies that are present at the time of treatment, but more flies can migrate into an area in a matter of minutes.

Horse fly & yellow fly

❖ Species & disease transmitted by flies:

➢ **Species:**
- Horse fly: *Tabanus atratus, T punctifer* & *T nigrovittatus.*
- Yellow fly: *Diachlorus ferrugatus.*

➢ **Diseases:** No any particular disease transmitted to human by these flies.

Midges

❖ Morphology:

Three main parts of body of midges like head, thorax & abdomen. Following are the main features.

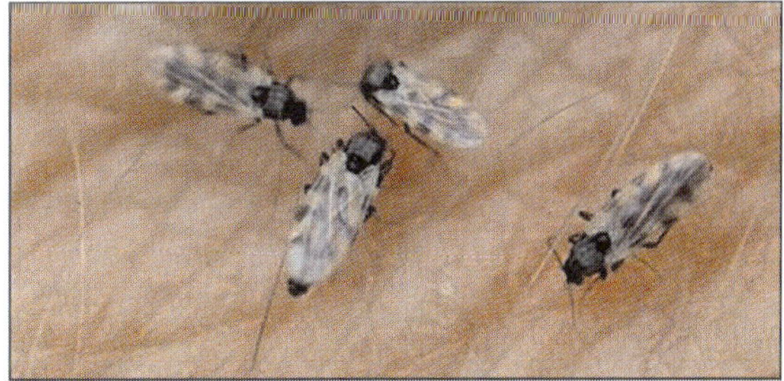

Figure-11: Midges

➢ **Size:** < 2 mm long.

➢ **Colour:** Dark coloured (**fig.-11**).

➢ **Body parts:**

✪ **Head:** Have 1 pair of antennae.

- **Thorax:** Humped thorax with spotted wings which are folded flat, one over the other, on their backs when they are at rest.
- **Abdomen:** It is segmented (**fig.-11**).

❖ Life cycle:

➢ **Stages:** Following four stages of life cycle are occurs in midges.

i. Egg:

- The eggs are laid in wet soil in boggy flushes, mires and in the transition zone at the edge of bogs.

ii. Larva:

- The larvae are narrow and worm-like with a distinct head, and they live in the soil.
- They are omnivorous and their diet includes small animals such as nematodes, other insect larvae, fungi and parts of plants.
- The larvae are semi-aquatic; they drown in open water and desiccate in dry soil. In suitable habitat the larvae can be found in densities of up to about 700 per square metre. The density of larvae can vary markedly over short distances depending upon the water content of the soil.
- The larvae develop slowly to pupae.

iii. Pupa: Pupae change to adult stages. The larvae go through several moults before they pupate.

iv. Adult: The adult emerges and sits on its empty case for a moment to open its wings before buzzing off.

➢ **Stages:**

- Time required from egg to adult stage development is 2-6 weeks, but depend on environmental conditions.
- Adults live for only 3 -12 days.

❖ Life styles (habits):

- **Breeding sites (habitats):** Wet surface especially at tourist places like beaches, mountain & resorts.
- **Feeding & biting habits:** Female can bite to man, animals for blood. Males consume flowers.

❖ Species & disease transmitted by midges:

➢ **Species & diseases:** The species which bite man all belong to the genus *Culicoides.* Following are species & micrororganims transmitted by midges.

- *C. grahami* & *C. austeni: Mansonella strptocerca* (streptocerciasis).
- *C. grahami* & *C. austeni: M. perstans* (non specific manifestation like allergic reaction & swelling).
- *Culicoides furens: M. ozzardi* (non specific manifestation like hydrocele & swelling).

❖ Midges control measures:

Midges can impact the economy of areas especially by tourism disturbances.

i. Physical control:

- Repellents are effective but not perfect.
- Avoiding being bitten.

ii. Chemical control: No satisfactory chemical control has been developed.

Cockroach

❖ Geographical distribution:

Worldwide.

❖ Morphology:

Three main parts of body of cockroach like head, thorax & abdomen. Following are the main features.

➢ **Size:** 5mm -9cm long.

➢ **Shape:** Oval shape.

➢ **Colour:** Reddish brown.

➢ **Body parts:**

- **Head:** 1 pair of antenna.
- **Thorax:** Have 3 pairs of legs & 2 pairs of wings.
- **Abdomen:** Hind gut is loaded with microbes.

❖ Life cycle: →Figure-12

➢ **Stages:** Following three stages of life cycle are occurs in cockroach.

i. Egg case or ootheca (plural → othecae):

- Within three to seven days after mating, American cockroach females produce egg cases **called oothecae**. Each ootheca contains approximately 15 embryos. Adult females produce 6- 14 oothecae in one lifetime.
- After carrying the egg cases on the tip of her abdomen for hours to a couple of days, the female deposits egg cases in a hidden location.
- They are adheres to the surface of its new location through the female's saliva.

ii. Nymph:

- Under optimum conditions & temperatures, nymphs, will emerge within 28-38 days.
- Nymphs undergo metamorphosis & in 10-13 moultings, they changes to adults.

iii. Adult:

- After undergoing their final moult, nymphs are equipped with wings & reproductive capabilities to achieve adult stage.
- Nymphs reach to adults in 9-13 months.

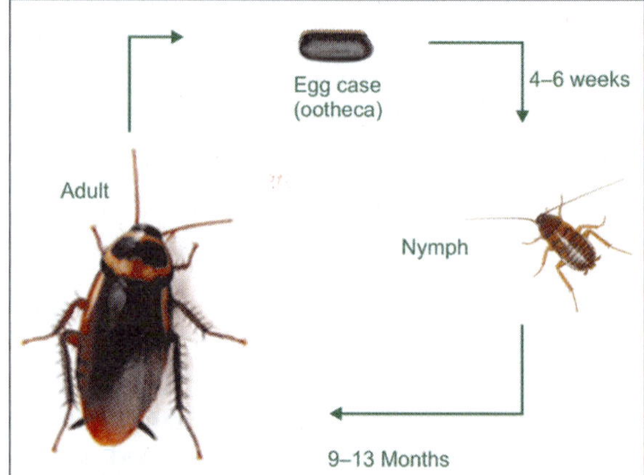

Figure-12: Life cycle of cockroach

➢ **Life span:** American cockroaches live for approximately one year.

❖ **Life styles (habits):**

- **Breeding sites (habitats):**
- American cockroaches normally live outdoors. They prefer warm, damp areas like flowerbeds, and under mulch. In many parts of the USA people **call them "palmetto bugs"** because they live on trees. Indoor cockroaches present in bathrooms, kitchens, laundry rooms and basements.
- Cockroaches are nocturnal insects and are rarely seen during the day.
- **Feeding & biting habits:**
- Cockroaches enter homes to find water or food. They can easily pass under doors & through basement windows.
- Outdoor eats tiny wood particles, fungi and algae.
- Normally non-biters.

❖ **Species & disease transmitted by cockroach:**

➢ **Species & diseases:** *Periplaneta americana* (American cockroach) & *Blatta orientalis* are distributed worldwide & they carry following organism in their hind gut or on the body which are transmitted mechanically by defecating or walking over food.

- *E. histolytica* (cyst).
- Enterobacteria.
- Hepatitis viruses.
- Eggs of nematodes.
- Polio virus.

❖ **Cockroach control measures:**

i. **Physical control:** Covering of food.
ii. **Chemical control:** Following are satisfactory methods.
a. **Cockroach foggers:** Foggers releases a mist of pesticide into the air which kill cockroaches.
b. **Residual spray:** Boric acid is useful.
c. **Cockroach bait:** Prepared from boric acid is useful.
d. **Cockroach gel:** Prepared from different insectisides is useful.
e. **Cockroach trap:** Cockroaches are nocturnal insects and are rarely seen during the day. As such, an infestation can be difficult to identify. One way of confirming the presence of cockroaches is through the use of cockroach traps. Cockroaches can be trapped indoors or outdoors.

Reduviid bug

❖ **Synonym:** Following are the different other name of reduviid bug.

- Kissing bug: Because it bits mainly around eyes & lips.
- Assassin bug: Because it is predator on insects.
- Cone nose bug.
- Triatomine bug.
- Local names in different places are like barbeiros, vinchucas, pitos and chinches.

❖ **Geographical distribution:** Distributed mainly in Latin America & the southern USA. It also available in India but concerned with transmission of any disease.

❖

❖ **Morphology:** Three main parts of body of reduviid bug like head, thorax & abdomen (**fig.-13**). Following are the main features.

➢ **Size:** It is about 25-35mm long.

➢ **Body parts:**

✪ **Head:** 1 pair of antennae.

✪ **Thorax:** 2 pair of wings & 3 pairs of legs.

✪ **Abdomen:** Also present.

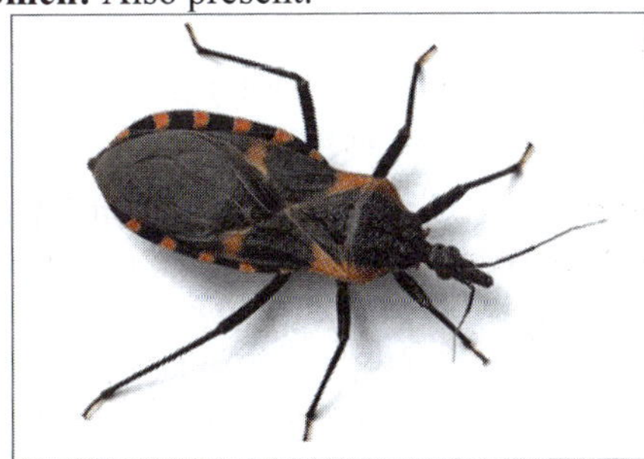

Figure-13: Reduviid bug

❖ **Life cycle:**

➢ **Stages:** Three stages of life cycle like egg, nymph & adult of reduviid bug as mentioned in **fig.-14**.

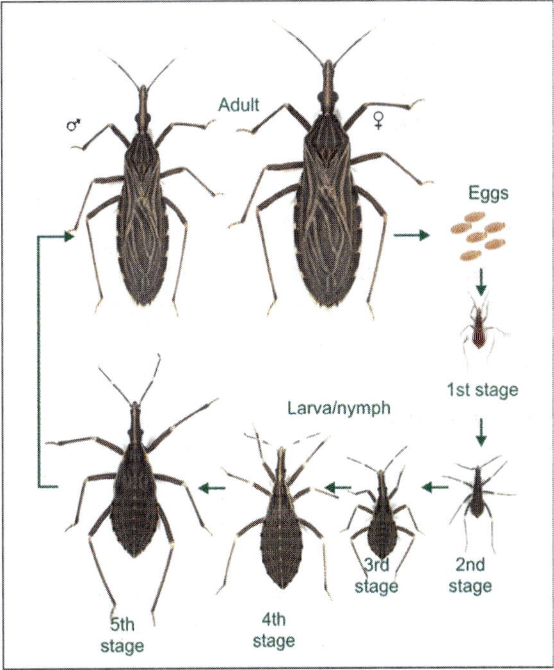

Figure-14: Life cycle of reduviid bug (*Rhodnius prolixus*)

➢ **Life span:**

- The total duration of the life cycle of the triatomine bug, from egg to adult, varies from 4 to 24 months, depending on the species & environmental conditions.
- Life span of adult bug is not clear.

❖ **Life styles (habits):**

- **Breeding sites (habitats):**
  - The adult & immature stages live in the burrows and nests of wild animals, including birds, bats, squirrels, opossums & armadillos, on which they feed during the night by sucking blood when the animals are asleep.
  - A number of species have adapted to living in & near houses, where they feed on humans & domestic animals, including chickens, cattle, goats, cats and dogs.
  - Feeding may take 10–25 minutes.
- **Feeding & biting habits:** Bug bite to man, animals etc. for blood. It rest during the day in dark devices close to their source of blood.

❖ **Species & disease transmitted by reduviid bug:** Reduviid bug like *Panstrongylus megistus, Triatoma infestans, Triatoma dimidiata* & *Rhodnius prolix* are a vector for *Trypanosoma cruzi*, causes Chagas disease (South American trypanosomiasis).

❖ **Reduviid bug control measures:**

i. **Physical or environmental control:**
- Elimination of bug's breeding places by improvement in housing quality & environment.
- Bug bite is avoided by using mosquito net or repellents.

ii. **Chemical control:** Residual spray by using HCH (0.5g/m^2) or dieldrin (1g/m^2) is commonly used to control the bug.

Bed bug

❖ **Geographical distribution:** Bed bugs occur around the world. *Cimex lactularius* occurs in temperate zone & *Cimex hemipterus* occurs in tropical zone.

❖ **Morphology:** Three main parts of body of bed bug like head, thorax & abdomen. Following are the main features.

➢ **Size:** Bed bug is about 8mm long & dorsoventrally flat.

➢ **Colour:** Reddish brown in colour.

➢ **Body parts:**

✪ **Head:** With one pair of antennae.

✪ **Thorax:** Non wings but 3 pair of legs.

✪ **Abdomen:** Also present.

❖ **Life cycle:** →**Figure-15**

➢ **Stages:** Following 3 stages of life cycle are occurs in bed bug.

i. **Egg:**
- A bed bug's life begins with eggs which are grain like and milky white in colour.
- Female bed bugs lay between 1-5 eggs each day & may lay up to 500 eggs within one lifetime.
- Eggs are laid singly or in clusters and are placed within tight cracks or crevices.
- The eggs are approximately 1 mm in length & are comparable in size to two grains of salt. Within two weeks, eggs hatch to produce nymphs.

ii. **Larva / nymph:**
- After hatching of eggs, nymphs begin immediately to feed.
- Nymphs, pass through 5 moults before reaching maturity. Although nymphs appear similar to adults, they are smaller in size.
- Young nymphs are yellow-white in colour, while older nymphs and adults are reddish-brown.
- In order to complete a moulting stage, each nymphs requires a blood meal. At room temperature, nymphs moult and become adults within five weeks.

iii. **Adult:** Upon reaching maturity, bed bug adults often make weekly feedings.

➢ **Life span:** The average life of bed bug is 4-6 months. However, some bed bugs may live up to a year under cool conditions and with no food.

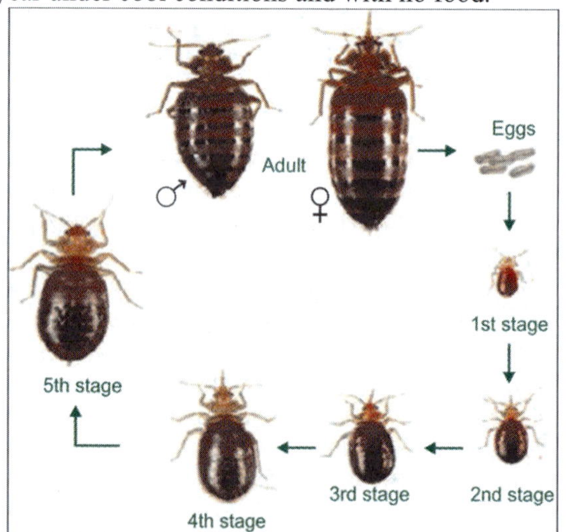

Figure-15: Life cycle of bed bug

❖ **Life styles (habits):**

- **Breeding sites (habitats):** Dorsoventrally flattened bodies that allow them to hide in areas such as floor cracks, carpets, beds and upholstered furniture.
- **Feeding & biting habits:** Bed bugs are nocturnal, that feed on the blood of humans and other warm-blooded animals.

❖ **Species & disease transmitted by black fly:**

- *Cimex lactularius* & *Cimex hemipterus*: Are infected with bacteria & viruses. Hepatitis virus has been reported from West Africa, South America & Ethiopia with evidences.
- Bed bug bite produces inflammation & allergic reaction in host who are sensitive to bed bug saliva.

❖ **Bed bug control measures:**

i. Physical or environmental control:

- Bed bug gives characteristics smell from scent glands, located in its thorax, which helps to access the breeding sites.
- Domestic cleaning is advised.
- Treating of mattresses an hour at a temperature of 45 °C (113 °F) or over, or two hours at less than −17 °C (1 °F) kills them.

ii. Chemical control:

- Insecticides like pyrethroids, dichlovoros & malathion has historically value.
- Resistance or theirs harm full effects does not allow their use.

iii. Biological control: The fungus *Beauveria bassiana* is being researched as of 2012 for its ability to control bed bugs.

Louse

❖ **Types:** Louse (plural → lice) is the permanent ectoparasite. Three main types of louse are (**fig.-16**).

A. **Head louse:** *Pediculus humanus capitis.*
B. **Body louse:** *Pediculus humanus corporis.*
C. **Pubic louse or crab louse:** *Phthirus pubis.*

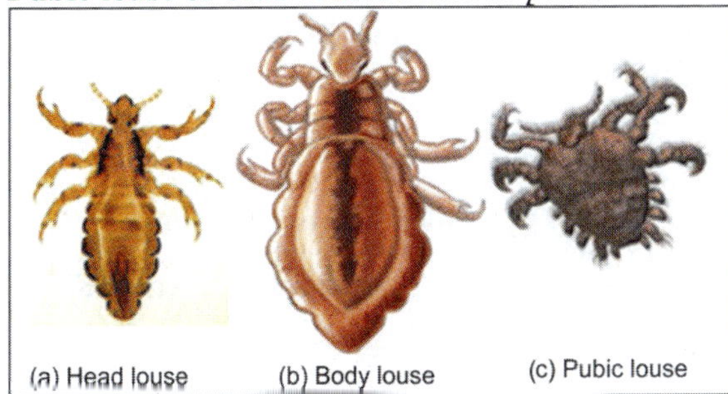

Figure-16: Types of louse

A. Head louse

➢ **Geographical distribution:** Worldwide.

➢ **Morphology:** Head louse (plural → lice) is permanent ectoparasite, whose only known host is human. Three main parts of body of head louse like head, thorax & abdomen. Following are the main features.

✪ **Size & shape:** 1-2mm long. Size & shape is like sesame seed. Females are usually larger than males. Louse looks flat dorso ventrally.

✪ **Colour:** Greyish white. In persons with dark hair, the adult louse will appear darker.

✪ **Body parts:**

- **Head:** 5 pair of joint antennae. Mouth part is doing blood sucking.
- **Thorax:** It is shape almost like a square. Have 3 pairs of legs, which are with claws & help the louse to cling to the hairs & clothes. Wings are absent.
- **Abdomen:** It is elongated with 9 segments. It is pointed in male & bilobed in females.

➢ **Life cycle:** →**Figure-17**

✪ **Stages:** Following three stages of life cycle are occurs in head louse.

i. Egg or nit (plural → nits):

- Nits (head lice eggs) are hard to see & are often confused for dandruff or hair spray droplets.
- Nits are laid ether singly or in groups by the adult female & are cemented at the base of the hair shaft nearest the scalp.
- Female can lay up to 300 eggs at the rate of 4-9 / day.
- They are 0.8 mm by 0.3 mm, oval & usually yellow to white. They are pointed at the end & truncated & pitted at other end.
- Nits take about 1 week to hatch (range 6 to 9 days) in favourable conditions. They will not hatch if temperature is below 22°C.
- Viable eggs are usually located within 6 mm of the scalp.

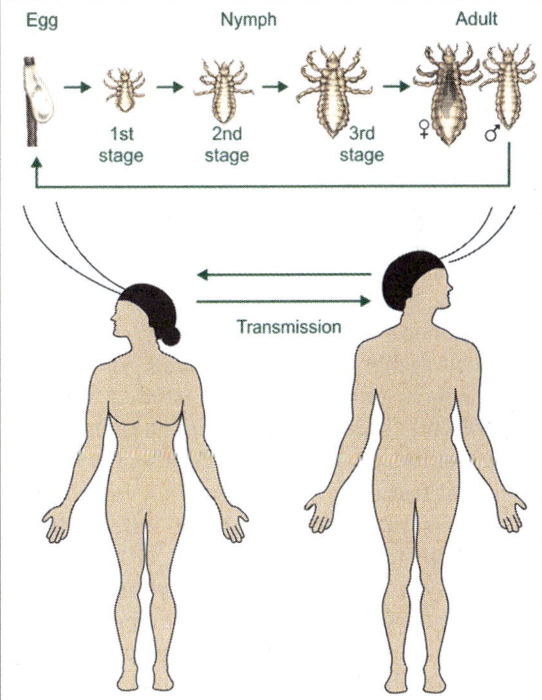

Figure-17: Life cycle of head louse

ii. Nymph or larva:

- The eggs hatch to release nymphs.
- The nymphs look like an adult head lice, but smaller size of a pinhead.

- Nymphs feed on human host, mature after 3 moults & become adults about 7 days after hatching.

iii. **Adult:** Adults develops from the nymphs.

✪ **Life span:** Louse can live up to 30-50 days on a person's head. To live, adult louse needs to feed on blood several times in a day. Without blood meals, the louse will die within 1 to 2 days off the host.

➢ **Life styles (habits):**

- **Breeding sites (habitats):** Human head.
- **Feeding & biting habits:** Adult louse feeds on human blood several times in a day.

➢ **Species & disease transmitted by head louse:** *Pediculus humanus capitis* produce harmful effect by direct infestation & by transmitting different microbes as mentioned below.

✪ **Infestation:**

- **Disease name: Called pediculosis.**
- **Source & reservoir of infestation:** Only human host.
- **Precipitating factors:**
  - Age: Preschool and elementary-age children, 3 to 11 years of age are infested most often.
  - Sex: Females are infested more often than males, probably due to more frequent head to head contact.
  - Socio-economic status: Body lice are also cosmopolitan but are less common and usually seen in settings of poverty, war, overcrowding and homelessness.
- **Modes of transmission:**
  - Direct (by contact): Louse is transmitted by direct head-to-head contact. Contact is common during play (sports activities, playgrounds, at camp, and slumber parties) at school and at home.
  - Indirect (by fomites): Less commonly to head lousee & more common with body louse. Wearing clothing, hats, scarves, coats, sports uniforms, or hair ribbons worn by an infested person; using infested combs, brushes or towels; or lying on a bed, couch, pillow, carpet, or stuffed animal that has recently been in contact with an infested person may result in transmission.
- **Clinical features:**
  - The majority of head louse infestations are asymptomatic.
  - When symptoms are noted they may include a tickling feeling of something moving in the hair, itching, caused by an allergic reaction to louse saliva, irritability & dermatitis.
  - People with long lasting disease have darkened & thickened skin **called Vagabond's disease.**
- **Complication:** Secondary bacterial infection.

✪ **Diseases transmitted by louse:** Head louse can serve as vectors for

- *Rickettsia prowazekii* (epidemic typhus).
- *Bartonella quintana* (trench fever).
- *Borrelia recurrentis* (louse-borne relapsing fever).

➢ **Head louse control measures:**

i. **Physical control:**

- Avoiding contact with infested person.
- Avoid use of items used by infested person.
- Regular checking of child's hair.
- Improvement in hygiene: Regular bath with soap & water, washing all items in hot water & pressed with hot iron.
- Improvement in health education.

ii. **Chemical control:** Lice are resistant to DDT & HCH in many places. Following are satisfactory methods.

a. **Lotion:** Prepared from malthion (0.5%) & keeping for 12-24 hours on hair followed by washing is effective.

b. **Louse dust:** Prepared from carbaryl is effective.

B. Body louse

Body louse is similar to head louse with following differences.

- Size: 2-4 mm long.
- It habitats on body & on clothes.
- It is not known as vector for any organisms.
- It causes pediculosis on body parts with above mentioned features.
- Powder containing 1% malthion is the treatment of choice. It is applied to on inner surface of clothes, socks & on body. About 50 g powder required for one person. After this treatment clothes are not removed. Single application eradicates the all lice, but sometimes 2nd application require after 7 days.
- Dust prepared from carbaryl is also effective.
- "Mass delousing" is carried out for large numbers of people with hand dusters.

C. Pubic louse or crab louse

Crab louse [fig.-12(c)] is similar to head louse with following differences.

- Size: 2 mm long.
- Square body.
- Head impacted on thorax.
- Relatively enormous & powerful legs & claws. The 1st pair of leg is slender than others.
- Very inert & does not move to much away from site of birth.
- It is not known as vector for any organisms.
- Autoclaving of clothes required to control body louse.

Fleas

❖ **Types:** Following are the different types of fleas.

A. **Oriental (tropical) rat flea:** *Xenopsylla cheopis, X astia & X braziliensis.*

B. Northern (temperate) rat flea: *Nosopsylla fasciatus.*
C. Cat flea: *Ctenocephalides / Ctenocephalus felis.*
D. Dog flea: *Ctenocephalides / Ctenocephalus canis.*
E. Human (house) flea: *Pulex irritans.*
F. Sand flea (chigoe flea or jiggers): *Tunga penetrans.*

A. Oriental (tropical) rat flea

➢ **Geographical distribution:** Worldwide.

➢ **Morphology:** Three main parts of body of Oriental rat flea like head, thorax & abdomen. The head & the thorax have rows of bristles (**called combs**). The Oriental rat flea has no genal or pronotal combs, which can be used to differentiate the oriental rat flea from the cat flea, dog and other fleas. Following are the main features.

✪ **Size & shape:** About 2.5 mm long.

✪ **Colour:** Adults vary from light brown to dark brown.

✪ **Body parts:**

- **Head:**
  - 1 pair of antennae.
  - Mouth has two functions: One for squirting saliva or partly digested blood into the bite, and other for sucking up blood from the host. This process mechanically transmits the pathogens.
- **Thorax:**
  - Wings are absent, so it cannot fly.
  - Flea has 3 pairs of small, powerful legs, which help to jump long distances. Flea smell exhaled carbon dioxide from humans & animals & jump rapidly to the source to feed on the newly found host. A flea's leg consists of four parts, the part that is closest to the body is the coxa; next are the femur, tibia, and tarsus. A flea can use its legs to jump up to 200 times its own body length (about 20 inches or 50 cm).
  - Flea can move passively through their host movement, transport vehicles, luggage & movement of goods like hide, grains etc.
- **Abdomen:** Abdomen consists of eight visible segments.

➢ **Life cycle:** →**Figure-18**

✪ **Stages:** Following four stages of life cycle are occurs in fleas.

i. Egg:
- About 15 to 20 eggs per day up to 600 in a lifetime are shed by the female on the ground, on the animals bedding area, on the host (like rat, cat, dog etc.), on the animal hair or anywhere especially where the host rests, sleeps or nests (rugs, carpets, upholstered furniture, cat or dog boxes, kennels, sand boxes etc.) or in the cracks, crevices etc.
- Eggs are small about 0.5mm, ovoid & white in colour.

ii. Larva:
- Eggs hatch into larvae in about 3-4 days.
- Larvae feed on organic debris in the environment or blood in the faeces of adult fleas.
- Larvae pass through 3 moults, which usually last about 9-15 days, but can last up to 200 days in unfavourable conditions. The number of larval instars (moults) varies among the species.
- Larvae are 4.5 mm long and resemble worms; they are slender, white, eyeless, leg less & bear sparse long hairs on their body.
- The larval stages last for 1-2 weeks.

iii. Pupa:
- Larvae eventually form pupae, which are in cocoons that are often covered with debris from the environment (sand, pebbles etc.).
- The pupal stages last for 1-2 weeks.

iv. Adult: Adults hatch from pupae & seek out a warm-blooded host for blood meals. It passes 3-4 weeks from egg to adult stage under favourable conditions.

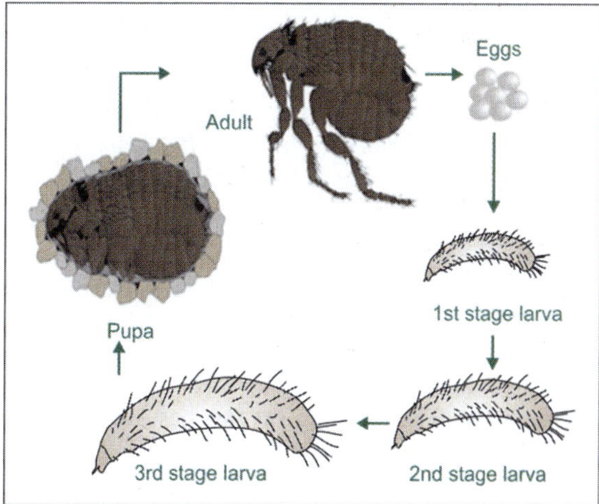

Figure-18: Life cycle of Oriental (tropical) rat flea

✪ **Life span:** An adult can survive for 1 year. It can survive for 4 years in the burrow microclimate.

➢ **Life styles (habits):**

- **Breeding sites (habitats):** Eggs laying sites are the breeding sites of rat flea as mentioned earlier.
- **Feeding & biting habits:** Adults of both sexes feed on blood. They bite *Rattus rattus* (black rat) & other mammals, including humans. They feed once in a day or sometimes oftener. They can live without food for several day/months, but female required blood for eggs production.

➢ **Species & disease transmitted by Oriental (tropical) rat flea:** *Xenopsylla cheopis* is a vector for pathogens like

- **Bacteria:** *Yersina pestis* (plague) & *Rickettsia typhi* / *Rickettsia mooseri* (endemic typhus / murine typhus / flea borne typhus).
- **Parasites:** *Hymenolepis nana* (hymenolepiasis) & *Hymenolepis diminuta* (hymenolepiasis diminuta).

➢ **Rat flea & rodent control measures:**

i. **Flea control :**

a. **Insecticidal spray or dust or powder:**

- Dusting by 10% DDT or HCH or dieldrin is most widely used & cheapest ways to control fleas. When rodents pass over the dust, they pick it up on the fur which kills fleas.
- Flea resistant to DDT or HCH or dieldrin, has been developed which is over come by using carbaryl, diazion (2%) & malthion (5%).
- It is applied to walls & floors up to a height of about 1 foot, over rat runs, rat burrows by using dust blower at about 30 g per burrow & cat plus dog resting places.

b. **Repellents:** Diethyltoluamide & benzyle benzoate are effective. Clothes impregnated with these repel fleas for > 1 week.

iii. **Rodent control:** It is equally important.

B. Northern (temperate) rat flea

➢ **Species & habitat:** *Nosopsylla fasciatus*, found on domestic rats (Norway rat →*Rattus norvegicus*) & house mice. It has occasionally been observed feeding on humans and wild rodents.

➢ **Distribution:** Originated in Europe, but has been transported to temperate regions all over the world

➢ **Morphology:** Elongated body, 3 to 4 mm in length. It has a pronotal ctenidium with 18 to 20 spines (on the first thoracic tergitr), but lacks a genal ctenidium. The northern rat flea has eyes and a row of three setae below it on the heads. Both sexes have a prominent tubercle on the front of the head. The hind femur has 3-4 bristles on the inner surface.

➢ **Life cycle:** Almost same as Oriental (tropical) rat flea with 3 moulting of larval stage.

➢ **Disease transmitted:** It is a minor vector for plague & intermediate host of *Hymenolepis diminuta* (hymenolepiasis diminuta) in South America, Europe & Australia.

C. Cat flea

➢ **Species:** *Ctenocephalides / Ctenocephalus felis*, found on domestic cats. Also found on dogs & humans.

➢ **Distribution:** Worldwide.

➢ **Morphology:** Adults of both sexes range from 1–2 mm long & are usually a reddish-brown colour, although the abdomens of gravid females often swell with eggs causing them to appear banded in cream and dark brown. Like all fleas, the cat flea is compressed laterally allowing it to slip between the sometimes dense hairs of its host just above the top layer of the skin, resulting in an extremely thin insect that may be difficult to observe even if the host's coat is pure white.

➢ **Life cycle:** Almost same as Oriental (tropical) rat flea but larvae pass through four stages of moulting.

➢ **Disease transmitted:**

- Cat fleas can transmit parasites & bacteria to dogs, cats & humans. The most prominent of these are *Rickettsia felis* / feline rickettsiae (endemic typhus / murine typhus / flea borne typhus) & *Dipylidium caninum* (dipylidiasis → intermediate host).
- Very rare pathogens encountered by this flea are *Bartonella henselae* (cat-scratch disease) & *Borrelia burgdorferi* (agent of Lyme disease, but their ability to transmit the disease is unclear).

D. Dog flea

➢ **Species:** *Ctenocephalides / Ctenocephalus canis*, found on dogs. Also found on cats & humans.

➢ **Distribution:** Worldwide.

➢ **Morphology:** The dog flea can be distinguished from the very similar cat flea by its head, which is anteriorly rounded rather than elongate, & the tibiae of its hind legs, which exhibit eight setae-bearing notches rather than six.

➢ **Life cycle:** Almost same as Oriental (tropical) rat flea but larvae pass through three stages of moulting.

➢ **Disease transmitted:** Dog fleas can transmit *Dipylidium caninum* (dipylidiasis → intermediate host).

E. Human (house) flea

➢ **Species:** *Pulex irritans*, found on humans, pig, goat, sheep, cats, babbons, dogs etc.

➢ **Distribution:** Worldwide.

➢ **Morphology:** Both genal and pronotal combs are absent and the adult flea has a rounded head.

➢ **Life cycle:** Almost same as Oriental (tropical) rat flea but larvae pass through three stages of moulting.

➢ **Disease transmitted:**

- Bite of flea cause local itching & swelling.
- Human flea transmits *Hymenolepis nana* (hymenolepiasis) & *Dipylidium caninum* (dipylidiasis → intermediate host).

F. Sand flea (chigoe flea or jiggers)

➢ **Synonym:** Nigua, chica, pico, pique or suthi.

➢ **Species:** *Tunga penetrans* (*Sarcopsylla penetrans* or *Pulex penetrates*) found on humans, cats, birds, monkeys, dogs etc.

- **Distribution:** Tropical and subtropical climates. It is native to Mexico, Central America, South America, West Indies & has been inadvertently introduced by humans to sun Saharan Africa. It has been reported from Western part of India. The fleas normally occur in sandy climates, including beaches, stables and farms. It flourishes in sandy soil.
- **Morphology:** Smallest flea about 1 mm.
- **Life cycle:** Larvae have two stages of moulting. Both males & females feed intermittently on their host, but only mated females burrow into the skin (epidermis) of the host, where they cause a nodular swelling as shown in **fig.-19.**

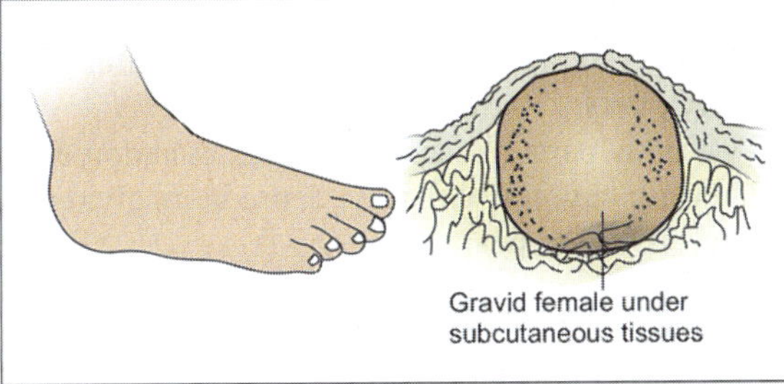

Figure-19: Gravid female of sand flea under subcutaneous tissue.

- **Disease transmitted:**
- **Disease name: Called tungiasis.**
- **Modes of transmission:** It penetrates the skin of its host by legs & proboscis.
- **Clinical features:**
  - Initial 1-2 days: Host may feel an itching or irritation but no pain.
  - Later stage: Inflammation and ulceration may become severe, and multiple lesions in the feet can lead to difficulty in walking. As the flea's abdomen swells with eggs later in the cycle, the pressure from the swelling may press neighbouring nerves or blood vessels. Depending on the exact site, this can cause sensations ranging from mild irritation to serious discomfort.
- **Complication:** Secondary bacterial infections, including tetanus and gangrene.

Ticks

- **Types:** Following are the different types of ticks.

A. **Ixodid tick or hard tick:**
B. **Argasid tick or soft tick:**

A. Ixodid tick or hard tick:

- **Geographical distribution:** Worldwide.
- **Morphology:** Two main parts of body of hard tick flea like cephalothorax & abdomen.
- **Size:** Variable length for different species like *Ixodes* 3.12 mm long & *Amblyoma* 6.35 mm long. Female is larger than male.
- **Shape:** They are ovoid in shape.
- **Colour:** Dark brown.
- **Body parts:**
- **Cephalothorax:**
  - No antennae.
  - Four pairs of legs.
  - Head or capitulum is at anterior side.
- **Abdomen:** Hard tick is covered by chitinous shield **called scutum** on dorsal surface. In male it covers entire back & in female only small part in front.

- **Life cycle:** →**Figure-20**
- **Stages:** Following four stages of life cycle are occurs in hard tick.

i. **Egg:**
- Female lay about 100-1000 eggs at a time & after that it dies.
- Eggs are deposited on the ground & hatched in 1-3 weeks.

ii. **Larva:**
- Larvae posses 3 pairs of legs.
- Larvae are lies in grass & herbiage till it attach to a suitable host.
- After a blood meal they drop off (moult) & change to nymphs after some time.
- The larval stage last for 3-13 day.

iii. **Nymph:**
- Nymphs are resemble to adult & having 4 pairs of legs but have no genital pore.
- Nymphs are attaching to a suitable host. For blood meal.

iv. **Adult:**
- Adult stages have 4 pairs of legs.
- Duration from egg to adult stag is 2 months.

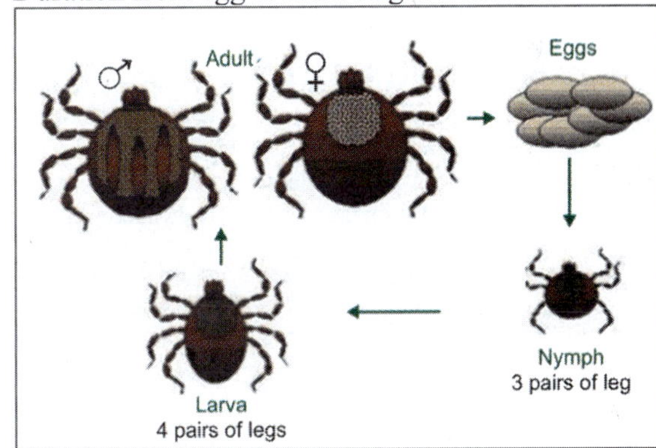

Figure-20: Life cycle of hard tick

- **Life span:** An adult can survive for 1 year or more.

- **Life styles (habits):**
- **Breeding sites (habitats):** Hard ticks are always found on their host like dogs, cattle, deers etc.
- **Feeding & biting habits:** Hard tick feed both during day & night & cant withstand starvation. Larvae, nymphs & adult stages required blood.

➢ **Species & disease transmitted by hard tick louse (for species of hard tick follow respective chapters):**

- *Dermacentor:* Rocky Mountain spotted fever, Colorado tick fever, tularemia, Siberian tick typhus, Omsk haemorrhagic fever and Central European tick-borne encephalitis.
- *Haemaphysalis:* Kyasanur forest disease.
- *Amblyomma:* Tularemia, ehrlichiosis, Rocky Mountain spotted fever & boutonneuse fever.
- *Ixodes:* Lyme disease, babesiosis, human granulocytic ehrlichiosis, and Russian spring-summer encephalitis.
- *Rhipicephalu:* Rocky Mountain spotted fever & boutonneuse fever.
- *Hyalomma:* Siberian tick typhus & Crimean-Congo hemorrhagic fever.

➢ **Tick control measures:**

a. **Insecticidal spray or dust:** Dusting or spraying by DDT or dieldrin or lindane or malthion in animal places gives good result.

b. **Repellents:** Diethyltoluamide & benzyle benzoate or permethrin are effective. Clothes impregnated with these agents should be worn while working in tick infested areas.

B. Argasid tick or soft tick

It is similar to hard tick with few differences as mentioned in **table-4.**

Features	Hard tick	Soft tick
	Morphology	
Scutum	Present	Absent
Head	Situated at anterior end	Lies ventrally, not seen from above
	Life cycle	
Egg	100-1000 laid down at a time	20-100 over long time in different batches
Nymph	One stage	Five stage
	Habits	
Breeding	Always on their host	Hide in crevices & cracks in day
Feeding	Feed in day & night. Cant withstand starvation	Feed in night. Can withstand starvation for year or more
	Others	
Genera & diseases	*Dermacentor* *Haemaphysalis* *Amblyoma* *Ixodes* *Rhipicephalus* *Hyaloma* Diseases: Mentioned in text	*Ornithodorus*: Tick borne relapsing fever
Control	Insecticides	Insecticides plus filling of cracks & crevices

Table-4: Differences between hard tick & soft tick

Mites

❖ **Types:** Following are the different types of mites.

A. **Trombiculid mite:**

B. **Itch mite:**

A. Trombiculid mite

➢ **Geographical distribution:** Over 10,000 species of trombiculid mites have been recorded from throughout the world.

➢ **Morphology:** Two main parts of body of trombiculid mite like caphalothorax & abdomen.

✪ **Size:** Very small about 0.55 -1 mm long.

✪ **Shape:** Spider in shape or figure-eight-shaped.

✪ **Colour:** Adult is usually bright red in colour.

✪ **Body parts:**

- Two body parts like cephalothorax & abdomen.
- They are covered with tiny, dense hairs giving them a velvet-like appearance.

➢ **Life cycle:** →Figure-21

✪ **Stages:** Following four stages of life cycle are occurs in trombiculid mite.

i. **Egg:** Female lays the eggs singly & hatches in about a week.

ii. **Larva:**

- Larvae are **called chiggers.**
- They posses 3 pairs of legs.
- They are very small, pale orange in colour.
- When gorged with blood, they drop down on the ground for moulting to produce the nymph.
- The larval stages last for 1-2 weeks.
- Larvae are infective for human & rodents.
- Larvae feed on serum of warm blooded animals.

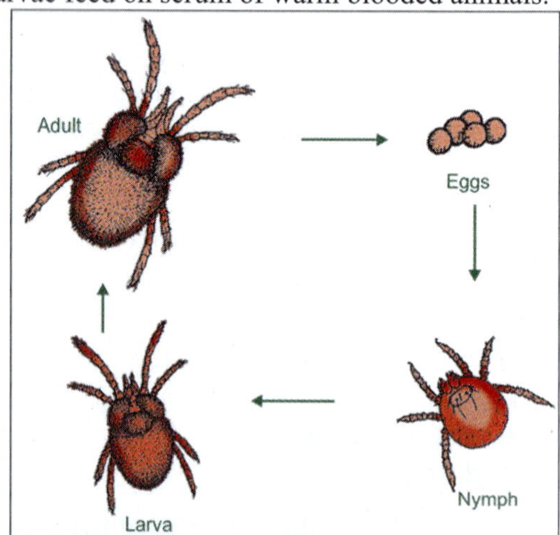

Figure-21: Life cycle of trombiculid mite

iii. **Nymph:**

- Nymphs are brick red in colour & have 4 pairs of legs.
- They live on vegetables juices.
- The nymphal stages last for 1-3 weeks.

iv. Adult:

- Adult stages have 4 pairs of legs with largest 1st pair.
- Duration from egg to adult stag is about 1 month.

✪ **Life span:** An adult can survive for 6 months.

➢ **Life styles (habits):**

- **Breeding sites (habitats):** They live in soil, & are often found when digging in yards, gardens or in compost bins.
- **Feeding & biting habits:**
- Chiggers feed on serum of warm blooded animals.
- Nymphs are feed on vegetable juices.
- Adult mites are independent predators that feed on small insects and their eggs, and are also found to eat plant material.

➢ **Species & disease transmitted by trombiculid mite:** Larvae (**called chiggers**) of trombiculid mite are the vector of *Orientia tsutsugamushi* (scrub typhus or chigger borne typhus). Following are the species of trombiculid mite.

- In India: *Leptotrombidium deliensis.*
- In Japan: *Leptotrombidium akamushi.*

➢ **Trombiculid mite control measures:** Same as hard tick.

B. Itch mite

➢ **History:** In 1867, the Italian biologists Cosimo Bonomo & Diacinto Cestoni showed that scabies is caused by *Sarcoptes scabiei.*

➢ **Geographical distribution:** Worldwide.

➢ **Morphology:**

✪ **Size:** It is very small naked eye visible, ecto-parasite. Female is 0.3–0.45 mm long & 0.25–0.35 mm wide, and male is just over half that size.

✪ **Shape:** Tortoise shaped, ventrally (below) flattened and dorsally (above) convex.

✪ **Colour:** Adult is straw coloured.

✪ **Body parts:**

- No demarcation into cephalothorax or abdomen but body is thrown in folds covered with short bristles.
- Adult scabies mite is eyeless with four pairs of legs (two pairs in front and two pairs behind), & multiple cuticular spines. The front legs end in long, tubular processes **called suckers**, and the hind legs end in long bristles. The male has suckers on all legs except the third pair, which distinguishes it from the female.

➢ **Life cycle: →Figure-22**

✪ **Stages:** Following four stages of life cycle are occurs in trombiculid mite.

i. Egg:

- Upon infesting a human host, the adult female burrows into the stratum corneum (outermost layer of skin), where it deposits 2-4 eggs per day. A female can lay up to 30 eggs, then dies at end of a burrow.
- Eggs are oval & 0.1–0.15 mm long.
- Eggs are hatched in 3-4 days to produce six-legged larvae.

ii. Larva:

- Larvae migrate to the skin surface & then burrow into moulting pouches, usually into hair follicles, where vesicles form (these are shorter and smaller than the adult burrows).
- After 3-4 days, the larvae moult, turning into eight-legged nymphs.

iii. Nymph:

- Nymph moults twice to change into adult mites.
- The nymphal stages last for 6-8 days.

iv. Adult:

- Adult mites then mate when the male penetrates the moulting pouch of the female. Mating occurs only once, as that one event leaves the female fertile for the rest of her life (one to two months).
- The impregnated female then leaves the moulting pouch in search of a suitable location for a permanent burrow. Once a site is found, the female creates her characteristic S-shaped burrow, laying eggs in the process.
- The female will continue lengthening her burrow and laying eggs for the duration of her life.
- Duration from egg to adult stag is about 10-17 days.

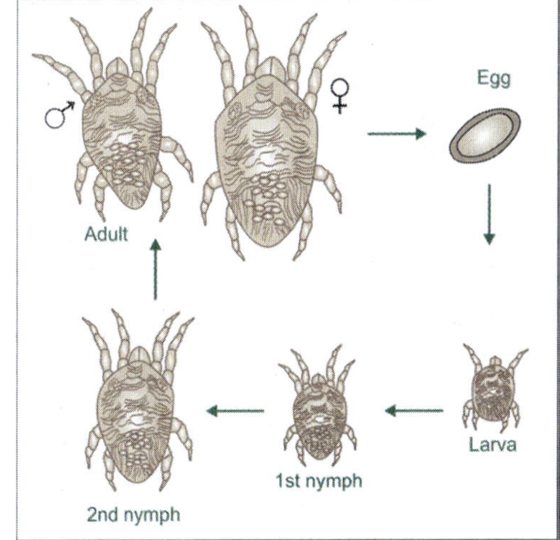

Figure-22: Life cycle of scabies

✪ **Life span:** An adult can survive for 1-2 months.

➢ **Life styles (habits):**

- **Breeding sites (habitats):** Mites are surviving on human fingernails, clothes, towels, bed linens and other household objects. Female parasites burrow in to epidermis where they can breed & cause scabies. They also present on animals like dog, cattle, horse etc. The animal species are different phylogenitically from human species & they can't cause human scabies.

- **Feeding habit:** Males only create burrows to find a mate, and are generally found wandering and feeding on the host's skin. Scabies mites ingest cell liquids and skin cells from their hosts.

➢ **Species & disease by itch mite:** *Satcoptes scabies or Acarus scabies* produce harmful effect by direct infestation as mentioned below. It is not reported as vector for microbes.

- **Disease name: Called scabies.**
- **Synonym:** Mange, crusted scabies, Norwegian scabies, seven-year itch.
- **Source & reservoir of infestation:** Only human host.
- **Precipitating factors:** Common with overcrowding and poor hygiene.
- **Modes of transmission:**
- Direct (by contact): Skin-to-skin contact with infested persons. Theoretically, touching an object that a mite is on is also a mode of transmission; however, this is not at all common.
- Indirect (by fomites): Rarely, it can be transmitted by sharing of clothes and bedding.
- **Incubation period:** Usually 2-6 weeks. However, in individuals with prior exposure to scabies, it is much shorter up to 1-4 days (Markell & Voge).
- **Sites:** Scabies mites are human skin parasites, burrowing into the upper skin layer, never below the stratum corneum (the outermost layer of skin, consisting of only dead cells). Scabies mites penetrate and burrow into the skin more easily where the skin is thin and are found in highest concentrations there, with 63% of mites found on the hands and wrists, 11% on elbows, 9% on feet and ankles, 12% in genital areas, and 2% in armpits. In women mites also affects the breast.
- **Pathogenesis:** The action of the mites moving within the skin and on the skin itself produce an intense itch that may resemble an allergic reaction in appearance. A delayed type IV hypersensitivity reaction to the mites, their eggs, or scybala (packets of faeces) occurs approximately 30 days after infestation. The presence of the eggs produces a massive allergic response that, in turn, produces more itching. Individuals who already are sensitized from a prior infestation can develop symptoms within hours.
- **Clinical features:**
- Superficial burrows [**fig.-23 (a)**], intense pruritus (itching) & a generalized rash.
- Acropustulosis, or blisters and pustules [**fig.-23 (b)**] on the palms and soles of the feet, are characteristic symptoms of scabies in infants.
- In immunocompromised, malnourished, elderly or institutionalized individuals, infestation can cause a more severe form of scabies **called crusted scabies or Norwegian scabies (fig.-24)**. This syndrome is characterized by a scaly rash, slight itching and thickened crusts of skin containing thousands of mites. Norwegian scabies is the form of scabies that is hardest to treat.

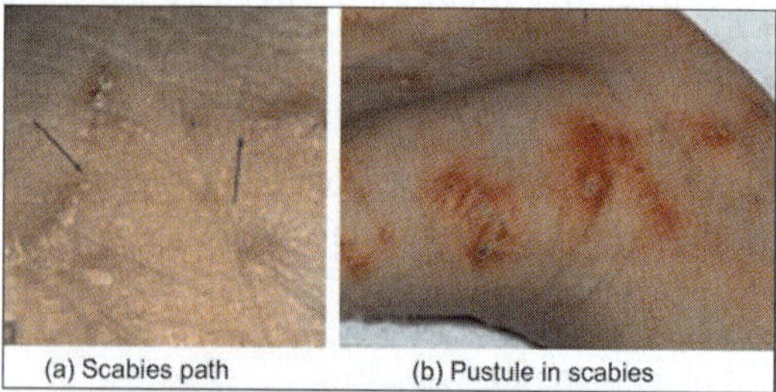

(a) Scabies path (b) Pustule in scabies

Figure-23: Clinical features of scabies

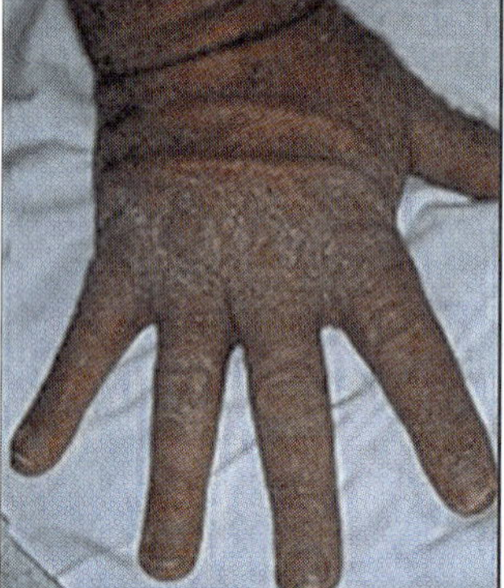

Figure-24: Crusted scabies

- **Complication:** Secondary bacterial infection.
- **Differential diagnosis:** Dermatitis, syphilis, allergic reactions, and other ecto-parasites such as lice and fleas are resembles to scabies.
- **Diagnosis:**

a. **Clinical presentation:** Bets way.

b. **Laboratory tests:**

○ <u>Tests:</u>

1. **Skin scraping & microscopy:** A drop of oil or saline is placed on top of the affected skin area. A scalpel is then used to scrape the area of tissue samples, and the material is examined until the microscope to check for mites or eggs.
2. **Felt-tip marker test:** A washable felt-tip marker is drawn across the rash, followed by an alcohol wipe. This procedure helps identify burrows because the ink penetrates deeply into the skin.

○ <u>Disadvantages</u>: Both tests have rather low sensitivity, as mites are often hard to find. So even if a test is negative, the medical provider may still recommend treatment.

➢ **Treatment:**

1. **The topical medication:**

- 5% Permethrin cream (Elimite) or 10% Crotamiton (Eurax) cream is suggested for infants less than 2 months of age. Bath is given with soap & water before cream application. Creams should be applied to clean, dry skin from the top of the head to the bottom of the feet, with special attention paid to skin folds and the webs of the digits (between the fingers and toes). The topical cream is left on the skin for 10-14 hours, and then washed off in the shower. It is best to apply the cream at bedtime, and then wash it off in the morning.

- 1% Gamma Benzene Hexachloride (Lindane): It is older, less safe than other options & cause neurotoxicity, especially in kids, so not recommended.
- 6% Sulfur: Sulfur ointment is effective, but may require extra applications, is messy, smells bad, and stains clothing.
- 5% Tetmosol: Applied 3 times in a day.

2. **Systemic:**

- Ivermectin, single oral dose of 150-200 micrograms of Ivermectin per kilogram of body weight is effective. This option should not be used by small children or women who are pregnant or breast feeding.
- The intense pruritus (itching): Treated with antihistamines such as Diphenhydramine (Benadryl), Hydroxyzine (Atarax), Cetirizine (Zyrtec) and Promethazine (Phenergan).
- Secondary infection by scratching of the skin: Treated with oral antibiotics or antibiotic ointment.
- For patients with crusted scabies, several applications of lotions, use of Ivermectin pills, and extensive skin care are required for management.
- If scabies symptoms persist two weeks after initial treatment, treatment may be repeated.

✓ **Note: Ectopasites**

- **Itch mite:** *Sarcoptes scabiei* (*Acarus scabiei*).
- **Louce:** Three types
  - Head louse: *Pediculus capitis (Pediculus humanus capitis).*
  - Body louse: *Pediculus corporis (Pediculus humanus corporis).*
  - Pubis or crab louse: *Pthirus pubis.*

Cyclops

❖ **Synonym:** Water fleas.

❖ **Geographical distribution:** Worldwide.

❖ **Morphology:** Three main parts of body of bed bug like head, thorax & abdomen. Following are the main features.

➢ **Size:** Cyclops is about 1mm long.

➢ **Shape:** Pear shaped body with forked tail.

➢ **Colour:** Light green or colourless (?).

➢ **Body parts: → Figure-25**

- **Cephalothorax:** Oval front section which comprise first five thoracic segments. Have 2 pairs of antennae, are used by the males for gripping the females during mating.
- **Abdomen:**
  - The hind part is considerably slimmer and is made up of the sixth thoracic segment and the four legless pleonic segments.
  - Cyclops has 5 pairs of legs.

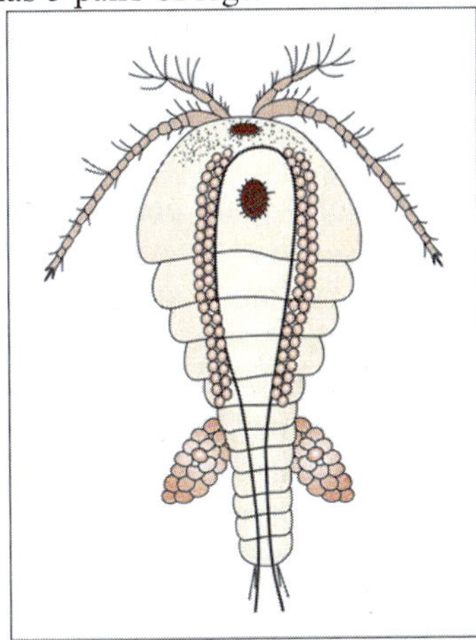

Figure-25: Cyclops

❖ **Life cycle:**

➢ **Stages:** Cyclops has 4 stages of life cycle like egg, larva or nauplii, copepodite & adult.

➢ **Life span:** Cyclops has the capacity to survive unsuitable conditions by forming a cloak of slime. Average lifespan is about 3 months.

❖ **Life styles (habits):**

- **Breeding sites (habitats):** Cyclops has a cosmopolitan distribution in fresh water, but is less frequent in brackish water. It lives along the plant-covered banks of stagnant and slow-flowing bodies of water.
- **Feeding habits:** Cyclops feeds on small fragments of plant material, animals or carrion. It swims with characteristic jerky movements.

❖ **Species & disease transmitted by cyclops:**

- **Species:** *Mesocyclops leukarti* (In India for *Dracunculus medinensis*), *Mesocyclops hyalinus, Thermocyclops vermifer, Encyclops serrulatus* & *Tropocyclops multivolor.*
- **Disease transmitted:** Cyclops act as intermediate host for following parasites.
  - *Dyphylobothrium latum.*
  - *Spirometra* spp.
  - *Dracunculus medinensis.*
  - *Gnathostoma spinigerum.*

❖ **Cyclops control measures:**

i. **Physical or environmental control:**

- Straining of water through piece of fine cloth is sufficient to remove cyclops.

- It can also be killed by boiling water, as it is easily killed by heat at 60 °C.
- Provision of drinking water through piping water supply, use of tube wells & abolition of step wells are effective measures on community level.

ii. Chemical control:

- Chlorine destroys guineaworm larvae and Cyclops in strength of 5 ppm; although this concentration of chlorine gives bad odour and taste to water. Excess chlorine can be removed by dechlorination.
- Lime at dosage of 4 gram per gallon of water can be used.
- Temefos kills cyclops at concentration of 1 mg/litre.

iii. Biological control: Small fish like *Barbel* and *Gambusia* feed on Cyclops. This method was used in Indian state of Karnataka to eradicate dracunculiasis.

Question bank

Essay/full question

1) Vectors & vector borne diseases.

Short notes

1) Ecto-parasites.

Short questions for theory/viva questions

1) What are ecto-parasites? Write two examples.
2) Write scientific name for jiggers & chiggers.
3) Name the four parasites in which cyclops act as intermediate host.

MCQs for chapter review

Mosquito

1) *Anopheles* is a vector of
(a) Relapsing fever (b) Malaria (c) Babesiosis (d) Typhus fever

Sand fly

2) Vector of kala azar is (AIIMS-07)
(a) Flea (b) Tse tse fly (c) Sand fly (d) Mite

Reduviid bug

3) Reduviid bug is vector for the transmission of (AIIMS-05)
(a) Relapsing fever (b) Lyme disease (c) Scrub typhus (d) Chaga's disease

Louse

4) Lice are not vector for - (AIIMS-06, AI-07)
(a) Relapsing fever (b) Q fever (c) Trench fever (d) Epidemic typhus

Ticks

5) Soft tick transmits (AI -08)
(a) Relapsing fever (b) KFD (c) Tick typhus (d) Tularemia

6) Tick is a vector for - (PGI-12)
(a) Crimean congo haemorrhagic fever (b) Rocky mounted spotted fever (c) Endemic typhus (d) Scrub typhus

Mites

7) Mite transmits: - (AI -91)
(a) Scrub typhus (b) Trench fever (c) Endemic typhus (d) Epidemic typhus

8) Scrub typhus is transmitted by (AIIMS, Nov -07)
(a) Reduviid bug (b) Tromiculid mite (c) Enteric pathogen (d) Cyclops

Cyclops

9) *Dracunculus medinensis* is transmitted by
(a) Cyclops (b) House fly (c) Tick (d) Flea

Answers of MCQs & explanation

1) (b)
- Relapsing fever: Either tick borne or louse borne
- Babesiosis: Tick borne
- Typhus fever: Different type of typhus are caused by different species of *Rickettsia* which are transmitted by louse, flea, tick, or by mite

2) (c)
- Follow section, **sand fly** for explanation

3) (d)
- Relapsing fever: Either tick borne or louse borne
- Lyme disease: Transmitted by *Ixodid tick*
- Scrub typhus: It is transmitted by bite of trombiculoid mite's larvae **called chigger** (hence disease **called chigger borne typhus**)

4) (b)
- Lice is the vector for relapsing fever, caused by *B recurrnetis* (also can be tick borne)
- Q fever: caused by *Coxiella burnetii* & transmitted by *Ixodid tick*
- Trench fever caused by *B. quintana* & transmitted by head louse
- Epidemic typhus caused by *R. prowazekii* & transmitted by head louse

5) (a)
6) (a) & (b) } Follow section, **ticks** for explanation

7) (a)
8) (b) } Follow section, **mites** for explanation

9) (a)
- Follow section, **cyclops** for explanation

Prakash

Section VIII
Clinical Microbiology

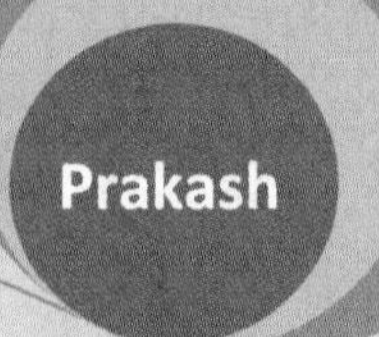

It includes the health care associated (hospital acquired) infection & all systemic infections like

- **Blood stream infections**
- **Respiratory tract infections**
- **Meningitis**
- **Urinary tract infections (UTIs)**
- **Infective endocarditis**
- **Gastroenteritis & food poisoning**
- **Skin & soft tissue infections**
- **Eye infections**
- **Ear infections**
- **Sexually transmitted infections (STIs)**
- **Pyrexia of Unknown Origin (PUO)**
- **Zoonotic infections**
- **Opportunistic infections**

102 Health care associated infections (HCAIs)

Learning heading & subheadings

- ❖ **Synonym:**
- ❖ **Definition:**
- ❖ **Important features:**
- ❖ **Precipitating factors (epidemiological determinants)**
- ❖ **Sources of infection:**
- ❖ **Modes of transmission:**
- ❖ **Classification:**
- ❖ **Nosocomial infection prevention & control programme:**

❖ Synonym:

➢ **Nosocomial infection:** From **nosocomion (Greek) = hospital.**

➢ **Hospital Acquired Infection.**

❖ Definition:

An infection acquired by a hospitalized patient, which was neither present nor in incubation at the time of admission.

❖ Important features:

- This includes infections acquired in the hospital but clinically evident after (48 hrs) discharge.
- It is due to endemic nature of organisms in institute
- It increases morbidity, mortality & actual cost in addition to actual illness.
- It occurs in 5-10% in developed & 25% in developing countries.
- It also includes infection to hospital staff.
- **Iatrogenic infection (physician induced infection):** Infection acquired by patients from physician during diagnosis, treatment & prevention of disease.

❖ Precipitating factors (epidemiological determinants):

Three types.

A. Microbial agent factors: Like

➢ **Bacterial resistance:**

- Emergence of new resistant strains.
- Increased prevalence of multidrug resistant organisms like *Klebsiella, P. aeruginosa* & *Acinetobacter*.

➢ **Antibiotic therapy:** Widespread use of antimicrobials for therapy or prophylaxis.

➢ **Common microbes available in hospital environment:**

i. **Bacteria:** CONS (coagulase negative *Staphylococci*), *E. coli, S. aureus*, β-Hemolytic *Streptococci*, *Klebsiella*, *Proteus* spp., *Pseudomonas* etc.

ii. **Viruses:** HBV, HCB, HIV, RSV, *Rotavirus* spp. & *Enterovirus* spp.

iii. **Fungi:** *C. albicans, Aspergillus* spp. & *C. neoformans.*

iv. **Parasites:**

a. **Protozoa:**

- *Toxoplasma gondii.*
- *Cryptosporidium parvum.*
- *Plasmodium* spp.
- *Babesia* spp.
- *Leishmania donovani.*
- *Trypanosoma* spp.

b. **Helminths:**

- *Taenia solium.*
- *Enterobius vermicularis.*

c. **Ectoparasites:** *Sarcoptes scabiei.*

B. Host factors:

➢ **Age:** Infancy & old age.

➢ **Immune status:** Poor immunity by AIDS, malignancies, leukemia, diabetes mellitus, renal failure, immunosuppressive therapy or radio therapy may activate the normal flora & cause the endogenous infection.

➢ **Malnutrition:**

➢ **Diagnostic and therapeutic interventions:** biopsies, endoscopic examinations, catheterization, intubation/ventilation, suction & surgical procedures, transfusions, dialysis etc.

➢ **Transfer:** Frequent transfers of patients from one unit to another.

C. Environmental factors:

- Crowded conditions within the hospital.

- Poor sterilisation& disinfection practices in hospital.
- Poor hospital administration.

❖ Sources of infection:

A **Endogenous:** Mostly pathogens are the normal flora of body which may activate to produce the infection.

B **Exogenous:** Any part of hospital ecosystem like

- People.
- Food.
- Water.
- Hospital devices: Needle, catheter, suture materials, surgical instruments, hospital bed, bed sheet etc.
- Bio-medical waste sites.

❖ Modes of transmission:

a. Direct:

1. Contact:

- Contact of hand or body surface with other body surface.
- Contact of hand or body surface with inanimate objects.
- Hand contact is the most common mode of transmission of nosocomial infection.
- Diseases which are transmitted by this route include colonization or infection with multi drug resistant organisms (like MRSA), enteric infections and skin infections.

2. Droplet infection:

- Droplet nuclei/particles of saliva or nasopharyngeal secretion arise during coughing, sneezing, speaking or talking enter in to other host directly who is in close contact.
- Such particles are $\geq$ 5 μm in diameter & spread to short distance (< 3 feet) & directly enter in other host. However such larger particle can be filtered by nose.
- Particles $\leq$ 5 μm in diameter are traverse to long distance & produces the air borne (indirect) infection.
- Infection by droplet nuclei is increased in close contact, overcrowding & lack of ventilation.
- Infections transmitted by droplet nuclei are pneumonia, pertusis, diphtheria, influenza type B, mumps, meningitis etc.

3. Inoculation: By IV line.

b. Indirect: Required mediator/vehicle.

1. Inhalation (air borne):

- Some droplet nuclei settle over different object & become part of dust & cause respiratory infection like open /active pulmonary tuberculosis, measles, chicken pox, pulmonary plague and haemorrhagic fever with pneumonia.
- Particles arise during coughing or sneezing from patient & $\leq$ 5 μm in diameter are traverse to long distance & produces the air borne infection.

2. Ingestion (food & water borne): Water / food borne → food poisoning.

❖ Classification:

Overall leading agent of nosocomial infection is *Staph aureus.* Following are the other agents.

A. Urinary Tract Infections (UTIs):

- UTI is the most common type (33%) of nosocomial infection.
- Occurs due to indwelling catheter.
- Common pathogens are: *E. coli, Klebsiella, Proteus, Pseudomonas, Serratia marcescens, E. faecalis, Candida* spp. etc.
- *E. coli* is most common agent of nosocomial UTI.
- *Candida* is most common agent of UTI in ICU.

B. Respiratory Tract Infections (RTIs):

- Pneumonia is the second most common type (15%) of nosocomial infection.
- Occurs due to ventilation, instumentation, aspiration in unconscious patients.
- Common pathogens are: *E. coli, Pseudomonas, Staph aureus, Klebsiella, Proteus* etc.
- GNB like *Pseudomonas* & *E. coli* are most common agent of nosocomial pneumonia.
- *Pseudomonas* (21%), *Staph aureus* (20%), *Enterobacter* spp. (9%), *Klebsiella* spp. (8%), & *Acinatobacter* are most common agent of ventilator associated pneumonia.

C. Soft tissue infection:

- Wound infections (15%) & bed sores.
- Due to surgery, poor aseptic precaution, prolonged hospitalization, prolonged immobilisation etc. are the precipitating factors.
- Pathogens: *Staph aureus, Staph epidermidis, E. coli, C albicans, Enterococcus* etc.
- *Staph aureus* is most common agent of surgical wound infections & surgical wound is the most common reason for establishment of nosocomial infection.
- Common agent causing infection when bowel mucosa is breached (surgically most important): *E coli, Bacteroides* & *Prevotella.*

D. Bacteremia & septicemia:

- It covers 13% of total nosocomial infection.
- Occur due to IV line (IV catheter).
- Common pathogens are: *S. epidermidis* (CONS), *Staph aureus, E. faecalis, Pseudomonas* spp. (most common is *Pseudomonas aeruginosa*), *Candida* spp. etc.
- CONS (30-40%) are the most common agents of bacteremia followed by *Staph aureus* (5-10%), *Pseudomonas aeruginosa* (2-5%).

E. Gastroenteritis:

- Due to contamination of hospital food & water.
- Common pathogens are: *Staph aureus* (enterotoxin). & *Salmonella* food poisoning

diarrhoea due to *E. coli, Cl. difficile* & some *Enterovirus* species.

F. **Others:**

- HBV, HCV, HIV: Due to blood transfusion, haemodialysis or by contaminated needle.
- Tetanus: It is common with poor antiseptic practice during surgery, cutting umbilical cord, injection administration, wound dressing or using materials contaminated by bacterial spores.

❖ Nosocomial infection prevention & control programme:

➢ **Purpose:** To manage the risk associated with the transmission of microorganisms from staff to staff, staff to patient and or visitors, patient and or visitors to staff, equipment and environment.

➢ **Aims & objectives:**

- To interpret, uphold & implement the infection prevention & control policies & procedures in the health care facilities (HCFs).
- To develop written policies & procedures for standards of infection prevention & control practices, cleanliness, sanitation & asepsis in the HCFs.
- To review & analyse data on HCAI in order to take corrective and preventive actions.
- To review & provide input for investigations of HCF related outbreaks.
- To develop a mechanism to supervise infection. control measures in all phases of hospital activities and to promote infection control practices at all levels of the facility.
- To ensure continuing education of employees on infection prevention and control practices.

➢ **Hospital infection control committee & functions:**

✪ **Committee:** Hospital infection control programmes is organised by medical superintendent, for which he/she constitutes hospital infection control committee. It includes following members

- Chairman (medical superintendent).
- Head (officer) of all clinical departments.
- Microbiologists.
- Epidemiologist.
- Hospital administrators.
- Nursing staff.
- Pharmacist.
- CSSD (central sterile supplies department).
- Mortuary.
- Housekeeping.
- Biomedical engineer if available.
- Maintenance in charge of linen, laundry & kitchen.

✪ **Functions of committee:** It acts as advisory committee for superintendent to take all measures for infection control & prevention.

- **Infection surveillance:** 4 key parameters used are
  - Catheter associated UTIs.
  - IV line associated blood stream infections.
  - Ventilator associated pneumonia.
  - Surgical wound infections.
- **System development:** To identify, report, analyse, investigate & control the HCAIs.
- **Antibiogram:** Development of guidelines on antibiotics usage, maintenance of data for sensitive & resistant drugs & follow on actions after detection of drug resistant strain.
- **Training:** Training of different categories of staff on infection prevention & control guideline.
- **Post exposure prophylaxis:** Especially after needle prick injury like HBV vaccination, post exposure prophylaxis of HIV to health care workers.
- **Outbreak management:** Identification of source & corrective measures.
- **Meeting:** All members of committee should meet regularly not less than a month & as often as required. However in emergency (like outbreak) committee should meet promptly.

➢ **Standard precautions:** It includes following

A **Hand hygiene:** Hands of all health care workers can carry microorganisms (bacteria, viruses and fungi) that are potentially infectious to them and others, hence hand washing before & after contact with patient is the best & inexpensive way to prevent the HCAIs. Hand hygiene includes following.

✪ **Nail care:**

- Nails are the area of greatest contamination. Short nails are easier to clean and are less likely to tear gloves.
- Nail varnish/ polish/ extensions/ art and acrylic nails are prohibited, regardless of colour, for staff with direct patient contact or who work in direct patient care area.

✪ **Skin care:**

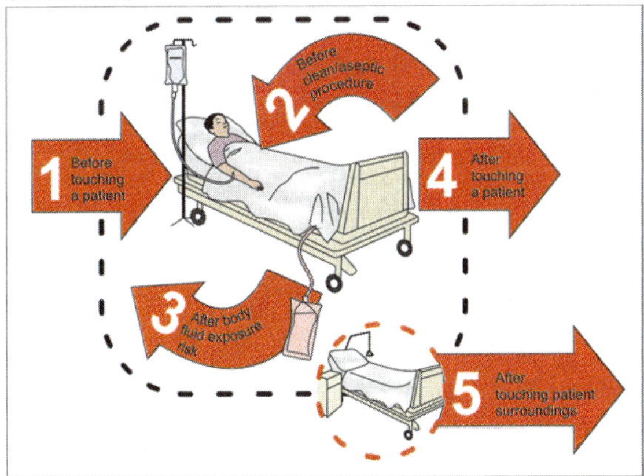

Figure-1: Five moments for hand hygiene

- Ensure the skin on your hands does not become dry or damaged. In these conditions the hands show a

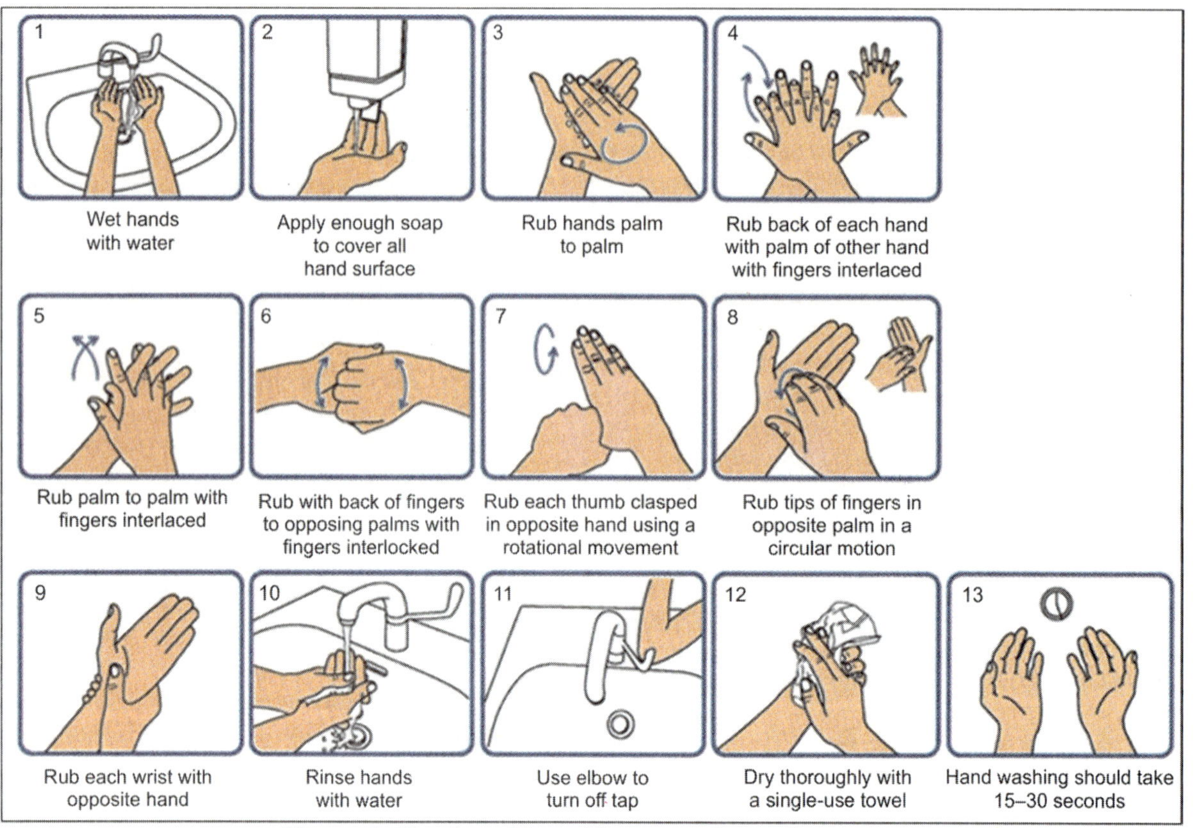

1
Wet hands with water
2
Apply enough soap to cover all hand surface
3
Rub hands palm to palm
4
Rub back of each hand with palm of other hand with fingers interlaced
5
Rub palm to palm with fingers interlaced
6
Rub with back of fingers to opposing palms with fingers interlocked
7
Rub each thumb clasped in opposite hand using a rotational movement
8
Rub tips of fingers in opposite palm in a circular motion
9
Rub each wrist with opposite hand
10
Rinse hands with water
11
Use elbow to turn off tap
12
Dry thoroughly with a single-use towel
13
Hand washing should take 15–30 seconds

Figure-2: Hand washing with soap and running water

1a

1b

Apply a palmful of the product in cupped hand, covering all surfaces.

2

Rub hands palm to palm.

3

Right palm over left dorsum with interlaced fingers and vice versa.

4

Palm to palm with fingers interlaced.

5

Back of fingers to opposing palm with fingers interlocked.

6

Rotational rubbing of left thumb clasped in right palm and vice versa.

7

Rotational rubbing, backwards and forwards with clasped fingers or right hand in left palm and vice versa.

8

Once dry, your hands are safe.

Figure-3: Alcohol based hand rub

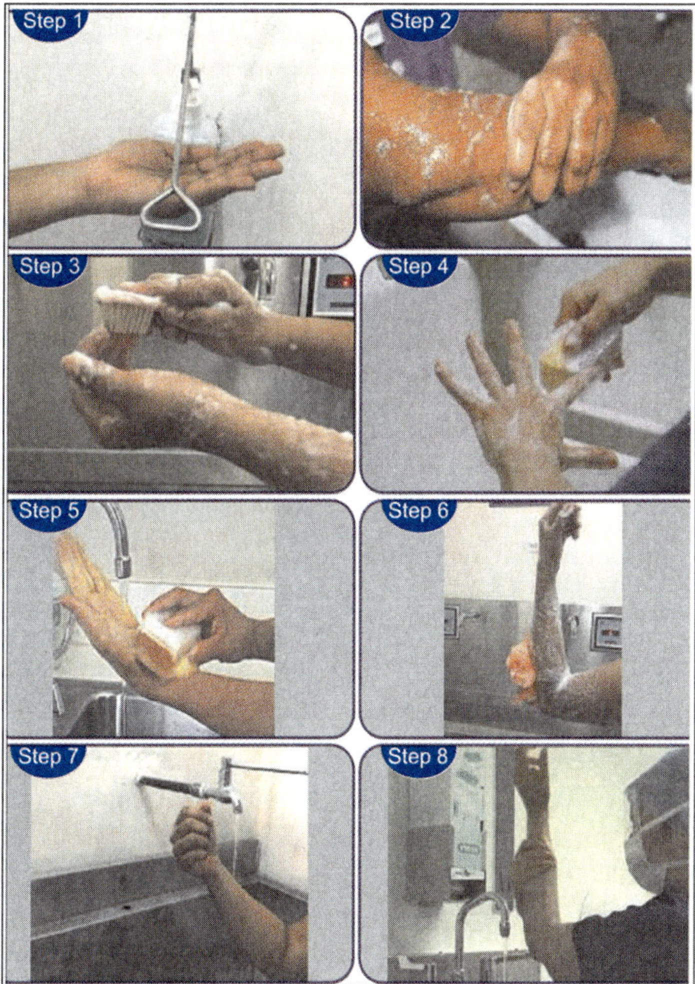

Figure-4: Surgical hand scrub

higher bacterial load and are difficult to remove than with intact skin.

- Hand lotion may be used to prevent skin damage from frequent hand washing.

✪ **"Five moments for hand hygiene" approach (fig.-1):** It came from WHO hand hygiene guide lines.

1. Before touching a patient.
2. Before clean or aseptic procedure.
3. After body fluid exposure risk.
4. After touching a patient.
5. After touching patient's surroundings.

✪ **Types of hand hygiene (hand cleaning):** Three types as follows.

i. Hand washing with soap and running water:

- **Indications:** Wash hands with soap & water when
  - Visibly dirty/contaminated with blood, body fluids etc.
  - After using a rest room.
  - Before and after having food.
  - After arriving and before leaving work place.
- **Effects:** Removes transient microorganisms, soil, blood & other organic material from hands.
- **Steps: → Figure-2**

ii. Alcohol based hand rub:

- **Indications:**
  - Hands are not visibly soiled.
  - Before having direct contact with patients.
  - Before putting on gloves.
  - After contact with patient's intact skin (e.g. after taking pulse, BP, lifting a patient etc.).
  - After contact with inanimate objects (e.g. medical equipment) in the immediate vicinity of the patient.
  - After removing gloves.
  - Hand washing with soap and water is not possible, as long as hands are not visibly soiled.
- **Effects:** It is an antiseptic hand rub. It kills most transient & resident microorganisms, but ineffective if hands are visibly soiled.
- **Steps: → Figure-3**

iii. Surgical hand scrub with antiseptic:

- **Indications:** Before surgical or invasive procedure to reduce the risk of infection to patient if gloves develop tears or holes during procedure.
- **Effects:** It minimise the microorganisms on hands under the gloves.

- **Steps: → Figure-4**
- Remove all jewelleries like rings, watches, bracelets.
- Wash hands & arms with hand wash gel.
- Take 5-10 ml of gel.
- Scrub each side of each finger , between the fingers and the back and front of the hand.
- Proceed to scrub the arms, keeping the hand higher than the arm at all times. This prevents bacteria-laden soap & water from contaminating the hand.
- Wash each side of the arm little above the elbow.
- Repeat the process on the other hand and arm, keeping hands above elbows at all times.
- Rinse hands and arms by passing them through the running water in one direction only, from fingertips to elbow. Do not move the arm back & forth through the water.
- Hands shall be thoroughly dried with single use towel/ tissue paper.
- Proceed to the operating room suite holding hands above elbows.
- **Points to note:**
- Do not dip hands into basins containing standing water even if antiseptic agents have been added.
- Microorganisms can survive & multiply in the solutions.
- Liquid soap shall be used.

B Respiratory hygiene (cough etiquette):

- Cover the nose and or mouth & use handkerchief/ tissue paper while coughing or sneezing.
- Perform hand hygiene when having contact with respiratory secretions & contaminated objects/ materials.

C Wearing personal protective equipments:

- Like apron, gloves, mask, gown, face shield, shocks, boots/shoe cover, goggles, cap etc.
- Steps of wearing & removing gloves are shown in **fig. 5 & fig. 6** respectively.

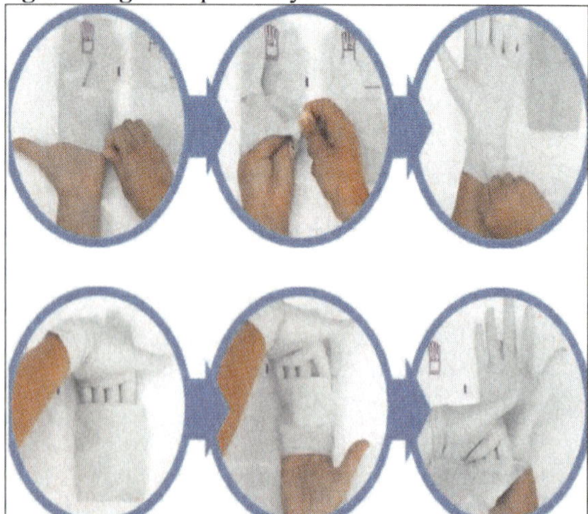

Figure-5: Steps of wearing gloves

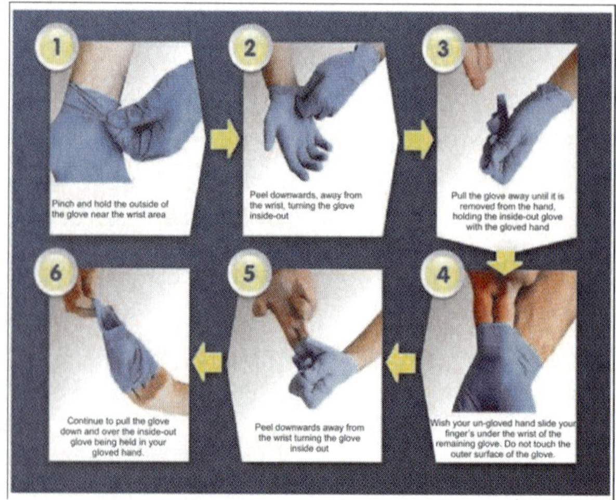

Figure-6: Steps of removing gloves

D Safe injection practise: Use the disposable needle & syringes.

E Post exposure management: Especially for HBV, HCV & HIV.

F Safety of health care workers: It required to prevent the transmission of HBV, HCV & HIV via blood spillage in mucosa or abraded skin or by needle prick injury.

G Environmental control: Measure for preventing infection associated with air, water & other elements.

H Isolation of patients & assessment of infection risk: Diseases requiring isolation

- Severe influenza cases.
- SARS.
- Open case of tuberculosis.
- Anthrax.
- Diphtheria.
- Pertussis.
- Chicken pox.
- Pneumonic plague.
- Patients suffering from multidrug resistant pathogen.
- Patients with low immunity.

I Patient resuscitation: All staff who participate in resuscitation shall adhere to standard precautions throughout the resuscitation.

J Linen: Soiled linens are the source of infection, so required careful handling.

K Sterilisation & disinfection practise: It includes the autoclaving of instrumentation, disinfection of spillage, fumigation of ward, laboratory, operation theatres & other rooms etc.

L Proper collection, handling & disposal of waste: **Follow chapter → Bio Medical Waste (BMW) management**

➢ **Additional precautions:** These precautions are based on mode of transmission of pathogens with following types.

A Transmission based precautions :

i. Contact precautions:

- Implement standard precautions.
- Place patient in a single room / in a room with another similarly infected patients. Consider the epidemiology of the disease and the patient population when determining patient placement.
- Wear clean, non-sterile gloves and gown when entering the room if substantial contacts with the patient, environmental surfaces or items in the patient's room are anticipated.
- Limit the movement and transport of the patient from the room for essential purposes only.
- If transportation is required, use precautions to minimize the risk of transmission.

ii. Droplet precautions:

- Implement standard precautions.
- Place patient in a single room / in a room with a similarly infected patients.
- Wear a mask when working within 1-2 meters of the patient.
- Place a mask on the patient if transport is necessary.
- Special air handling & ventilation are not required to prevent droplet transmission of infection.

iii. Airborne precautions:

- Airborne precautions are used in addition to routine practices for clients/patients/residents known or suspected of having an illness transmitted by the airborne route.
- Implement standard precautions.
- Anyone who enters the room must wear appropriate PPE.
- Airborne infection isolation.
- Requires particulate respirator e.g. N95 shall be worn & use of a negative pressure isolation room.
- Place patient in a single room that has a monitored negative airflow pressure and is often referred to as a "negative pressure room".

B Management of an outbreak:

✪ **Definition:** An outbreak is defined as an unusual or unexpected increase of cases of a known HCAI of the emergence of cases of a new infection.

✪ **Outbreak investigation:**

1. **Step 1:** Constitution outbreak investigation team with various specialities.
2. **Step 2:** Verify the diagnosis, developing a case definition, define the outbreak in terms of time, person and place.
3. **Step 3:** Determine the magnitude of the problem & if immediate control measures are required, such as isolation or cohorting of infected cases, strict hand washing & asepsis shall be applied.
4. **Step 4:** Notification to concerned departments.
5. **Step 5:** Line listing, collection of microbiological records & patient details, epidemic curve preparation, risk factors identification, & reporting to hospital infection control committee.
6. **Step 6:** Identification of cause, mode of transmission etc. by microbiological & epidemiological study.
7. **Step 7:** Implementation of control measures.
8. **Step 8:** Rule out the efficacy of control measures.

C Requirements of isolation: Accommodation for the suspected or confirmed patient, in a room or area designated for infectious diseases.

D Notifiable disease:

✪ **Definition:** Disease where steps are needed to be taken to prevent them from taking the form of epidemic or spreading from one person to another are **called notifiable disease.**

✪ **List of notifiable disease:**

- Dengue.
- Chikungunya.
- Japanese encephalitis (JE).
- Meningococcal meningitis.
- Typhoid fever.
- Diphtheria.
- Cholera.
- Shigellosis.
- Viral hepatitis.
- Leptospirosis.
- Malaria.
- TB.
- H1N1 Flu.
- HIV.
- Syphilis.
- Others.

✪ **Notification:** Health care authority shall notify about the disease noticed in health care facility to concerned departments.

Question bank

Essay/Full question

1) Nosocomial infections (health care associated infections).

Short notes

1) Nosocomial infections prevention & control (programme).

Short questions for theory/viva questions

1) Define hospital acquired infection. Write its sources.
2) Write five moments for hand hygiene.

MCQs for chapter review

1) **A person get infected in a hospital & clinical manifestation appear after he is discharged this is called**
(a) Nosocomial infection (b) Opportunistic infection (c) Epizootic infection (d) Physician induced infection
2) **All the following are true about nosocomial infection except**
(AI-04)

(a) May manifest within 48 hours of admission (b) May develop after discharge of patient from hospital (c) Denote new condition which is unrelated to the patients primary conditions (d) May already present at the time of admission

3) **All the following are true common nosocomial infection except** (AIIMS-03)
(a) *Staph aureus* (b) *P aeruginosa* (c) Enterobactericeae (d) *Mycobacterium*

4) **Most common mode of transmission of nosocomial infection**
(a) Hand contact (b) Droplet infection (c) Blood and blood products (d) Contaminated water

5) **Most common organism involved in nosocomial infection**
(a) *Staph aureus* (b) *E coli* (c) *Legionella* (d) *Strept pneumoniae*

6) **Most common pathogens responsible for nosocomial pneumonia in ICU are** (AI-05)
(a) Gram positive organisms (b) Gram negative organisms (c) *Mycoplasma* (d) Virus infections

7) **Most common organism causing ventilator associated pneumonia**
(a) *Legionella* (b) *Pneumococcus* (c) *Pseudomonas* (d) Coagulase negative *Staphylococcus*

8) **Anaerobic bacteria surgically most important**
(a) *Bacteroides* (b) *Staph aureus* (c) *Pseudomonas* (d) *Pneumococcus*

9) **Most common species of *Pseudomona* causing intravascular catheter related infections is** (AIIMS, Nov-08)
(a) *P cepacia* (b) *P aeruginosa* (c) *P maltophila* (d) *P mallei*

10) **Most common catheter related blood stream infections is** (AIIMS, May-07)
(a) *Candida* (b) Gram negative organisms (c) Coagulase positive *Staphylococcus* (d) Coagulase negative *Staphylococcus*

11) **Which of the following causes highest risk of nosocomial infection to a patient** (AIIMS, May-09)
(a) Patient admitted for elective surgery (b) HIV patient coming in follow up OPD (c) Patient undergoing endoscopy (d) Patient admitted for normal delivery

Answers of MCQs & explanation

1) **(a)**
2) **(d)**
} Follow section, **definition** for explanation

3) **(d)**
- Follow section, **precipitating factors (epidemiological determinants → microbial agent factor)** for explanation

4) **(a)**
- Follow section, **mode of transmission** for explanation

5) **(a)**
6) **(b)**
7) **(c)**
8) **(a)**
9) **(b)**
10) **(d)**
11) **(a)**
} Follow section, **classification** for explanation

103 Systemic infections

Learning heading & subheadings

Blood stream infections

❖ Definition:

- **Bacteremia:** Means entry of bacteria in blood (transient presence) & no multiplication.
- **Septicemia:** Means entry of bacteria in blood, multiplication & clinical sign-symptoms.
- **Pyemia:** Septicemia & abscess in organs like liver, spleen & other tissues.
- **Toxemia:** Clinical sign-symptoms are due to toxin production.

❖ Types of bacteremia: Bacteremia may be

a. **Transient:** It occurs when organisms, often members of the normal flora, are introduced into the blood by –
- Minimal trauma to membranes such as brushing teeth or chewing food.
- Minor events like manipulation of infected tissues, instrumentation of contaminated mucosal surface, and surgery involving non sterile sites (e.g. during dental procedures, after gastrointestinal biopsy etc.)

b. **Continuous:** Bacteria are released in to blood at constant rate from bacterial endocarditis or septic shock.

c. **Intermittent:**
- Bacteria are intermittently found in blood from undrained abscess, meningitis, pneumonia or pyogenic arthritis.
- Bacteria are found in blood about 45 minutes before pyrexia.

❖ Etiological agents:

i. **Bacteria:** *Staph. aureus,* Coagulase negative *Staphylococcus* (CONS), β-hemolytic *Streptococcus, Enterococcus, Pneumococci, E. coli, Klebsiella, Proteus, Salmonella, Pseudomonas, Brucella* etc.

ii. **Viruses:** EBV, CMV, HBV, HCV, HIV etc.

iii. **Fungi:** *C. albicans, Aspergillus* spp., *C. neoformans* & other systemic or opportunistic fungi

iv. **Parasites:** *Plasmodium* spp., microfilariae, *Babesia, Leishmania* spp., *Typanosoma* spp. & *Toxoplasma.*

❖ Mode of transmission & classification:

Two types as per mode of transmission.

A. **Intra vascular infections:** Organisms are enter in blood with CVS from endocarditis, aneurysm, thrombophlebitis & by IV line.

B. **Extra vascular infections:** Organisms are enter in blood by lymphatic system from GIT (25%), respiratory system (20%), abscess (10%), biliary tract (5%), wound site (5%) other or uncertain sites (35%).

❖ **Clinical features:**

- Septicemia.
- Septic shock.
- DIC (Disseminated Intravascular Coagulation).
- Other systemic features.

❖ **Diagnosis:**

➢ **Specimens:** Blood.

➢ **Testing:**

i. **Diagnosis of bacteria:** Follow chapter → Laboratory diagnosis of bacterial infections

ii. **Diagnosis of viruses:** Follow chapter → Laboratory diagnosis of viral infections

iii. **Diagnosis of fungi:** Follow chapter → Laboratory diagnosis of fungal infections

iv. **Diagnosis of parasites:** Follow chapter → Laboratory diagnosis of parasitic infections

Respiratory tract infections

❖ **Anatomy:** Two parts →**Fig.-1**

A. **Upper respiratory tract:** Mouth, nose, nasal cavity, sinuses, pharynx, epiglottis & larynx.

B. **Lower respiratory tract:** Trachea, bronchi, bronchioles, lungs & alveoli.

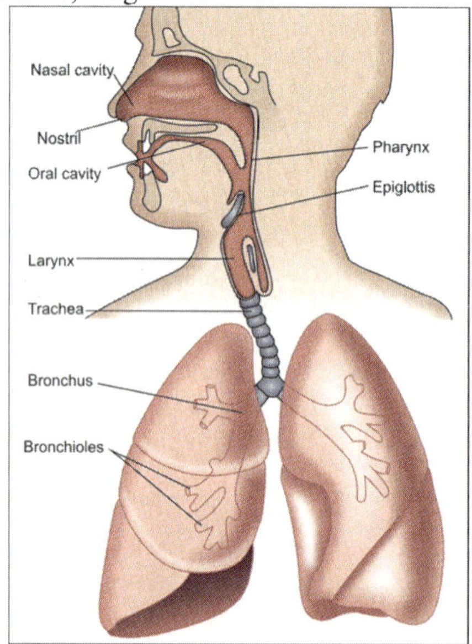

Figure-1: Anatomy of respiratory tract

❖ **Normal defence of respiratory tract:**

- Nasal hair.
- Cilia.
- Mucus.
- Reflex like coughing, sneezing, swallowing.
- Pulmonary Alveolar Macrophages (PAM).
- Secretory IgA against specific pathogens.
- Norma flora

❖ **Etiological agents:**

i. **Bacteria:** *Staph. aureus, Strept. pyogenes,* Group B *β*-haemolytic *Streptococci, Strept. pneumoniae, C. diphtheria, M. tuberculosis, Atypical mycobacteria, N. meningitidis, E. coli, Klebsiella, Proteus, Pseudomonas, H. influenzae, Bordetella, Mycoplasma pneumoniae* etc.

ii. **Viruses:** Adeno virus, *Rhinovirus*, influenza virus (swine flu, bird flu), RSV, parainfluenza virus, EBV, ECHO virus, measles virus, VZV etc.

iii. **Fungi:** *C. albicans, Aspergillus* spp., *C. neoformans* & other systemic or opportunistic fungi.

iv. **Parasites:** *P. westermanii, A. lumbricoides, A. duodenale* & *C. sinensis.*

❖ **Classification:**

A. **Upper respiratory tract:**

- Rhinitis or common cold.
- Sinusitis.
- Acute otitis media (ear infection).
- Streptococcal pharyngitis.
- Diphtheria.

B. **Lower respiratory tract:**

➢ **Bronchitis**

➢ **Pneumonia:** Most common causes for pneumonia.

- Bronchopneumonia: *Staphylococcus aureus.*
- Lobar pneumonia: *Strept. pneumoniae.*
- Primary atypical pneumonia: *Mycoplasma pneumoniae.*
- GNB like *Pseudomonas* & *E. coli* are most common agent of nosocomial pneumonia.
- *Pseudomonas* (21%), *Staph aureus* (20%), *Enterobacter* spp. (9%), *Klebsiella* spp. (8%) & *Acinatobacter* are most common agent of ventilator associated pneumonia.

➢ **Pneumatocele:**

- **Definition:** Thin walled, air-filled cysts that develop within the lung parenchyma result from pulmonary trauma during mechanical ventilation.
- **Features**: It can be single emphysematous lesions but are more often multiple, thin-walled, air-filled, cyst like cavities.
- **Causes:**

- Infectious: Most often, they occur as sequelae to acute pneumonia, commonly caused by *Staph aureus*. However, pneumatocele formation also occurs with other agents, like *Strept pneumoniae, Haemophilus influenzae, Escherichia coli, Strept pyogenes, Serratia marcescens, Klebsiella pneumoniae, Mycobacterium tuberculosis* & adenovirus. Pneumatoceles are generally observed soon after the development of pneumonia but can be observed on the initial chest radiograph.
- Non-infectious: It includes hydrocarbon ingestion, trauma & positive pressure ventilation.

➢ **Lung abscess.**

➢ **Granulomatous lesion:** Like tuberculosis.

➢ **Pleural effusion.**

❖ **Mode of transmission:** Mostly by inhalation.

❖ **Clinical features:** Fever, coughing with or without blood, headache, malaise, anorexia etc.

❖ **Diagnosis:**

➢ **Specimens:** Sputum, BAL & lung biopsy.

➢ **Testing:**

i. **Diagnosis of bacteria:** Follow chapter → Laboratory diagnosis of bacterial infections

ii. **Diagnosis of viruses:** Follow chapter → Laboratory diagnosis of viral infections

iii. **Diagnosis of fungi:** Follow chapter → Laboratory diagnosis of fungal infections

iv. **Diagnosis of parasites:** Follow chapter → Laboratory diagnosis of parasitic infections

Meningitis

❖ **Anatomy of meninges:** Brain has two protective covering like outer bone & inner meninges. Meninges has three layers. From outer to inner are

✪ **Dura mater:**

✪ **Arachnoid mater:** } Collectively called leptomeninges

✪ **Pia mater:**

❖ **Definition:** Meningitis is an inflammation of leptomeninges (inner two layers of meninges).

❖ **Types & etiological agents:** Two types of meningitis.

A. **Septic (purulent or pyogenic) meningitis:**

➢ **Definition:** Characterised by presence of multinucleated cells (PMNs) in CSF.

➢ **Subtypes:**

i. **Acute:** Mostly by bacteria.

✪ **< 1 months (neonates):**

- **Most common:** *E. coli* (34%) > Group B β-Haemolytic *Streptococci* (*Strept. agalactiae,* 30%) > GNB (8%) > *Listeria monocytogenes* (6%).
- **Others:** *Staph. aureus, Strept. Pneumoniae, N. meningitidis, Flavobacter meningosepticum, Pseudomonas* & *H. influenzae.*

✪ **1-11 months (infants):** *N. meningitidis > Strept. pneumoniae > Haemophilus influenzae.*

✪ **1-6 (children) or 1-20 years:** *N. meningitidis > Strept. pneumoniae > H. influenzae.*

✪ **> 20 years (adults):**

- **Most common:** *Strept. pneumoniae*
- **Others:** *N. meningitidis, Staph. aureus, Strept. pneumoniae, Listeria* & GNB.

ii. **Chronic:**

a. **Bacteria:** *Nocardia, Actinomyces, M. tuberculosis, B. abortus, Salmonella* etc.

b. **Fungi:** *C. albicans, Aspergillus* spp., *C. neoformans* & other systemic or opportunistic fungi.

c. **Parasites:** *E. histolytica, T. gondii, C. cellulosae, P. westermanii* & *T. spiralis.*

B. **Aseptic meningitis:** Characterised by presence of mononuclear cells (lymphocytes) in CSF & caused by virus with exception of few bacteria.

a. **Viruses:** HSV-1 & 2, VZV, EBV, CMV, adeno virus, influenza virus, RSV, measles virus, mumps virus, polio virus, *Flavivirus*, *Bunyavirus*, rhabo virus etc.

b. **Bacteria:** *T. pallidum* & *Leptospira.*

❖ **Mode of transmission:**

- Direct spread from surrounding organs.
- Exogenous by trauma to skull/bone.
- Haematogenous route from distant organs.
- Nerve route: Intraneural transmission in case of rabies virus.

❖ **Clinical features:** Severe headache, fever, altered sensorium, neck rigidity & stiffness, positive Kerning's & Brudzinski's sign.

❖ **Diagnosis:**

➢ **Specimens:** CSF & brain biopsy.

➢ **Testing:**

i. **Diagnosis of bacteria:** Follow chapter → Laboratory diagnosis of bacterial infections

ii. **Diagnosis of viruses:** Follow chapter → Laboratory diagnosis of viral infections

iii. **Diagnosis of fungi:** Follow chapter → Laboratory diagnosis of fungal infections

iv. **Diagnosis of parasites:** Follow chapter → Laboratory diagnosis of parasitic infections

Infective endocarditis

❖ **Synonym:** Bacterial endocarditis.

❖ **Definition:** It is an infection of the inner surface of the heart, usually the valves.

❖ **Etiological agents:** There is also a non-infective endocarditis. Following are the infective causes of endocarditis.

A **Bacteria:**

1. ***Streptococci*:**

- Viridans group (30-40%): Most common organism of endocarditis. Species are *Strept sanguis, Strept parasanguis, Strept oralis, Strept mitis, Strept mutans, Strept gordonii* & *Strept mitior* etc.
- *Enterococci*: *E. faecalis, Strept. bovis* etc.

2. ***Staphylococcus* spp.:**

- COPS (10-27%): *Staph. aureus.*
- CONS (1-3%): *Staph. albus* (*Staph epidermidis*).

3. **GNB:**

- 1.5-13% case are from GNB origin.
- *Pseudomonas aeruginosa* is the most common GNB for endocarditis.
- HACEK group of microorganisms.

- Enterobactericeae: Very rare like *S typhi* & others.
- Less commonly reported bacteria responsible for so **called "culture negative endocarditis"** like *Bartonella*, *Chlamydia psittaci* & *Coxiella*. Such bacteria can be identified by serology, culture of the excised valve tissue, sputum, pleural fluid, and emboli, and by PCR or sequencing of bacterial 16S ribosomal RNA.

4. **Others:**

- *Tropheryma whipplei*.
- *Propionibacterium* sp.
- *Citrobacter koseri*.
- *Neisseria bacilliformis* was found in a patient with a bicuspid aortic valve.

B **Fungi:** Fungal endocarditis is a fatal and one of the most serious forms of infective endocarditis.

- *Candida albicans*: It forms biofilms around thick-walled resting structures like prosthetic heart valves & additionally colonizes & penetrates endothelial walls. *C. albicans* is responsible for 24-46% of all the cases of fungal endocarditis, & its mortality rate is 46.6-50%.
- Other fungi demonstrated to cause endocarditis are *Histoplasma capsulatum* & *Aspergillus*. *Aspergillus* contributes to roughly 25% of fungal endocarditis cases.
- Endocarditis with *Tricosporon asahii* has also been reported in a case report.

❖ Predisposing factors:

1. **Age:** Increased incidence of infective endocarditis in persons 65 years of age & older, probably due to increase risk factors.
2. **Sex:** The male to female case ratio is over 2:1.
3. **Heart diseases:** Valvular heart disease including rheumatic disease, congenital heart disease & artificial valves are the risk factors. However, 50% of all cases develop in people with no known history of valvular disease.
4. **Medical & surgical procedures:**

- Viridans *Streptococci* are the primary habitats oral cavity & upper respiratory tract. They enter the bloodstream usually by dental procedures (like tooth extractions) or by genitourinary manipulation
- *Staphylococcus* can enter the blood stream through procedures that cause break in the integrity of skin, like surgery, haemodialysis, during access of long term indwelling catheters or secondary to IV injection of recreational drugs. It infecting normal heart valve & having prosthetic valve.
- *Enterococcus* can enter the bloodstream due to defect in the gastrointestinal or genitourinary tracts.
- *Strept bovis* and *Clostridium septicum*, are part of the natural flora of the bowel, are associated with colorectal cancer. They cause the endocarditis due to breaking down the barrier between the gut & the blood vessels which drain the bowel bacteria.
- HACEK organisms are a group of bacteria that live on the dental gums, and can cause endocarditis due to poor dental hygiene or pre-existing valve disease.
- Electronic pacemakers.
- *Candida albicans* present in IV drug users (IV drug users tend to get their right-sided heart valves infected because the veins that are injected drain in to the right side of the heart), patients with prosthetic valves, and in person with IDDs.

5. **Others:**

- History of infective endocarditis.
- Age-related degenerative valvular lesions.
- Low levels of white blood cells.
- Diabetes mellitus, alcohol abuse, HIV/AIDS etc.

❖ **Pathogenesis:** Damaged part of a heart valve allows the platelet and fibrin deposition which later allow bacteria to take hold and form vegetations.

❖ **Clinical features:** Symptoms may include fever (97%), small areas of bleeding into the skin, heart murmur, feeling tired, and low red blood cell count, night sweats, rigors, spleen enlargement etc.

❖ **Complications:** Valvular insufficiency, heart failure, stroke, glomerulonephritis, which allows for blood and albumin to enter the urine, kidney failure, Osler's nodes (painful subcutaneous lesions in the distal fingers), Roth's spots on the retina, positive serum rheumatoid factor etc.

❖ Classification:

A. **According to duration & clinical presentayion:**

i. **Subacute bacterial endocarditis (SABE):** It is often due to *Streptococci* of low virulence (mainly viridans group) & mild to moderate illness which progresses slowly over weeks and months (>2 weeks) and has low propensity to haematogenously seed extra-cardiac sites.

ii. **Acute bacterial endocarditis (ABE):**

- It is a fulminant illness over days to weeks (<2 weeks), & is more likely due to *Staphylococcus aureus* which has much greater virulence, or disease-producing capacity and frequently causes metastatic infection.
- This classification is now discouraged, because the ascribed associations (in terms of organism and prognosis) were not strong enough to be relied upon clinically. The terms **short incubation** (meaning < about six weeks), and **long incubation** (> about six weeks) are preferred.

B. **According to culture results:** Infective endocarditis may also be classified as **culture-positive** or **culture-negative.**

- The most common cause of a "culture-negative" endocarditis is prior administration of antibiotics.
- Sometimes microorganisms can take a longer period of time to grow in the culture media, such

organisms are said to be *fastidious* because they have demanding growth requirements. Some examples include pathogens like *Aspergillus* species, *Brucella* species, *Coxiella burnetii*, *Chlamydia* species, and HACEK bacteria. Due to delay in growth and identification in these cases, patients may be erroneously classified as "culture-negative" endocarditis.

C. According to heart side:

i. Right side: Patients who intravenously inject opioids such as heroin or methamphetamine may introduce infection which can travel to the right side of the heart, classically affecting the tricuspid valve, and most often caused by *S. aureus*.

ii. Left side: Regardless of cause, left-sided endocarditis is more common in both IV drug users and non-drug users than right-sided endocarditis.

D. According to source:

i. Nosocomial endocarditis: It is a form of healthcare associated endocarditis in which the infective organism is acquired during a stay in a hospital and it is usually secondary to presence of intravenous catheters, total parenteral nutrition lines, pacemakers etc.

ii. Community acquired: From community & outside the hospital.

E. According to valve type:

i. Native-valve endocarditis: It is caused by *Staph aureus*. It is common in IV drug abusers & specially involves the tricuspid valve (right side valve). Few authors suggested that right side valves are commonly infected by *Staph aureus* while left side valves are infected by *Staph aureus, enterococcus & other bacteria.*

ii. Prosthetic-valve endocarditis: It can be

- Early (<1 year of valvular surgery): Nosocomial type due to intraoperative or a postoperative bacterial contamination. Mainly by *Staph epidermidis* as it is capable of growing as a biofilm on plastic surfaces.
- Late (> 1 year following valvular surgery). Late prosthetic valve endocarditis is usually due to community acquired microorganisms. Mainly by viridans group of bacteria.

❖ Diagnosis:

➢ **Specimens:** Three blood samples every 1 hour interval.

➢ **Testing methods:**

A. Blood culture:

B. Echocardiography: Vegetation on the tricuspid valve is present. The transthoracic echocradiogram has a sensitivity is 65% and specificity is 95%.

C. Antibiogram: Drug sensitivity to different organisms.

➢ **Modified Duke criteria for diagnosis of infective endocarditis:** Established in 1994 by the Duke Endocarditis Service and revised in 2000. It includes major & minor criteria.

✪ **Criteria:**

- **Major criteria:**

1. Positive blood culture with typical microorganism, defined as one of the following.

- o <u>Typical microorganism consistent with 2 separate blood cultures:</u>
  - Viridans-group streptococci or
  - *Strept bovis* including nutritional variant strains, or
  - HACEK group, or
  - *Staphylococcus aureus*, or
  - Community-acquired *Enterococci*, in the absence of a primary focus
- o <u>Microorganisms consistent with persistently positive blood cultures:</u>
  - 2 positive blood cultures drawn >12 hours apart, or
  - All of 3 or a majority of 4 separate cultures of blood (with 1st and last sample drawn 1 hour apart)
  - *Coxiella burnetii* detected by at least 1 positive blood culture or IgG antibody titer for Q fever phase 1 antigen >1:800. This was previously a minor criterion.

2. Evidence of endocarditis with positive echocardiogram: Defined as

- Oscillating intra-cardiac mass on valve or supporting structures, in the path of regurgitant jets, or on implanted material in the absence of an alternative anatomic explanation, or
- Abscess, or
- New partial dehiscence of prosthetic valve or new valvular regurgitation (worsening or changing of pre-existing murmur not sufficient).

- **Minor criteria**
  - Predisposing factor: Known cardiac lesion, recreational drug injection.
  - Fever >38 °C.
  - Embolism evidence: Arterial emboli, pulmonary infarcts, Janeway lesions & conjunctival haemorrhage.
  - Immunological problems: Glomerulonephritis, Osler's nodes, Roth's spots, rheumatoid factor.
  - Microbiologic evidence: Positive blood culture (that doesn't meet a major criterion) or serologic evidence of infection with organism consistent with IE but not satisfying major criterion.
  - ~~Positive echocardiogram (that doesn't meet a major criterion)~~ (this criterion has been removed from the modified Duke criteria).

✪ **Diagnosis:** As per Duke criteria diagnosis of infective endocarditis can be **definite, possible, or rejected.**

- **Definite diagnosis:** Following pathological or clinical criteria are met.
  - o <u>One of these pathological criteria:</u>

- Histology or culture of a cardiac vegetation, an embolized vegetation, or intracardiac abscess from the heart finds microorganisms.
- Active endocarditis.

o One of these combinations of clinical criteria:
- 2 major clinical criteria.
- 1 major and 3 minor criteria.
- 5 minor criteria.

- **Possible diagnosis:** Following clinical criteria are met.
  - 1 major and 1 minor criteria.
  - 3 minor criteria are fulfilled.

❖ Prevention:

- Prophylactics should be bactericidal rather than bacteriostatic.
- In some countries like the USA, high risk patients may be given prophylactic antibiotics such as penicillin, amoxycillin (for beta lactamase bacteria) or clindamycin for penicillin allergic patients prior to dental procedures. Such measures are not taken in certain countries like Scotland due to the fear of antibiotic resistance.
- Not all people with heart disease require antibiotics to prevent infective endocarditis. Heart diseases have been classified into high, medium and low risk of developing. Those falling into high risk category require prophylaxis before endoscopies and urinary tract procedures. Diseases listed under high risk include:

1. Prior endocarditis.
2. Unrepaired cyanotic congenital heart diseases.
3. Completely repaired congenital heart disease in their first 6 months.
4. Prosthetic heart valves.
5. Incompletely repaired congenital heart diseases.
6. Cardiac transplant valvulopathy.

- Following are the antibiotic regimens recommended by the American Heart Association.

a. Not allergic to penicillins

1. Oral amoxicillin 1 hour before the procedure.
2. Intravenous or intramuscular ampicillin 1 hour before the procedure.

b. Allergic to penicillins

1. Azithromycin or clarithromycin orally 1 hour before the procedure.
2. Cephalexin orally 1 hour before the procedure.
3. Clindamycin orally 1 hour before the procedure.

- Antibiotics were historically commonly recommended to prevent infective endocarditis in those with heart problems undergoing dental procedures.

❖ Treatment:

- Treatment is generally with intravenous antibiotics.
- The choice of antibiotics is based on results of blood cultures.
- Occasionally heart surgery is required.

Urinary tract infections (UTIs)

❖ Anatomy: Two parts.

A. **Upper urinary tract:** Kidneys & ureters.
B. **Lower urinary tract:** Bladder & urethra.

❖ Normal defence of urinary tract:

- Low urine pH & high urea concentration are inhibitory for microbes.
- If bacteria gain access to the bladder the constant flushing of urine eliminates bacteria.
- Valve like mechanisms at the junction of ureter and bladder prevents the reflux of urine from bladder to upper urinary tract.
- The bladder mucosal surface has anti bacterial properties.

❖ Predisposing factors:

- **Age:** More in paediatric due to faecal contamination. More in female during sexually active stage.
- **Sex:** More in female due to short urethra & proximity to anus.
- **Pregnancy:** Dilatation of ureter, renal pelvis, stasis, hormonal changes, incompetence of vesico-urethral valve.
- **Diseases:** Like stone, urethral stricture, prostate hypertrophy, tumour, vesico-urethral reflux, genital prolapsed, neurogenic bladder, diabetes mellitus, local trauma.
- **Instrumentation:** Like catheterisation.
- **Bacterial:** Pili help in adhesion.

❖ Etiological agents:

i. **Bacteria:** *Staph aureus, Staph epidermidis, Staph. saprophyticus, Enterococci* spp., *M. tuberculosis, N. gonorrhoea, E. coli, Klebsiella, Proteus* spp., *Pseudomonas, Enterobacter, Salmonella, G. vaginalis, Acinetobacter, M. hominis, U. urealyticum, C. trachomatis* etc.
ii. **Viruses:** Adeno virus, herpes simplex virus etc.
iii. **Fungi:** *C. albicans* is most common.
iv. **Parasites:** *T. vaginalis, S. haematobium & E. vermicularis.*

❖ Mode of transmission:

a. Ascending route:

- It is most common route of infection in females.
- From faecal contamination of perineum to urethra & kidneys.
- Common causes are: *E. coli, Klebsiella, Proteus, Serratia, Pseudomonas, C. trachomatis, Staph saprophyticus, N. gonorrhea* & herpes simplex virus.

b. Descending (haematogenous) route:

- Spread from distant site to the kidneys via blood.
- This route accounts for < 5% of UTIs.

- Common causes are: *S. aureus* & *C albicans*.

❖ **Clinical types:**
1. Urethritis.
2. Asymptomatic bacteriuria.
3. Acute urethral syndromes.
4. Cystitis.
5. Pyelonephritis.

❖ **Clinical features:**
- Increase frequency with the feeling of having to urinate even though there may be very little urine to pass.
- Nocturia: Need to urinate during the night.
- Urethritis: Discomfort or pain at the urethral meatus or a burning sensation throughout the urethra with urination (dysuria).
- Pain in the midline suprapubic region.
- Pyuria: Pus in the urine or discharge from the urethra.
- Haematuria: Blood in urine.
- Pyrexia: Mild fever.
- Cloudy and foul-smelling urine.
- Emesis: Vomiting is common.
- Pain: Back, side (flank) or groin pain, abdominal pain or pressure.
- Shaking chills and high spiking fever.
- Night sweats.
- Extreme fatigue.

❖ **Diagnosis:**
➢ **Specimens:** Urine & urethral discharge.
➢ **Testing:**
i. **Diagnosis of bacteria:** Follow chapter → Laboratory diagnosis of bacterial infections
ii. **Diagnosis of viruses:** Follow chapter → Laboratory diagnosis of viral infections
iii. **Diagnosis of fungi:** Follow chapter → Laboratory diagnosis of fungal infections
iv. **Diagnosis of parasites:** Follow chapter → Laboratory diagnosis of parasitic infections

Gastroenteritis & food poisoning

Gastroenteritis

❖ **Definitions:**
➢ **Gastroenteritis:** Inflammation of mucosa of stomach & intestine resulting vomiting, diarrhoea, abdominal pain with or without mucus & blood in stool (dysentery) or fever or dehydration. It is better to describe the gastroenteritis with diarrhoea & dysentery for easy understanding.
➢ **Diarrhoea:** Passage of three or more liquid/semi-solid stools per day, in excess than usual habit for that person (WHO).
➢ **Dysentery:** Presence of blood & mucus in stool often with fever, abdominal pain & tenesmus. Tenesmus means desire of defecation without resulting evacuation.

❖ **Synonym:** Few authors referred gastroenteritis as **infectious diarrhoea.**

❖ **Etio-pathogenetic classification:** Clinical presentation of gastroenteritis is based on mechanism of actions of bacterial toxin as described below. (It also covers the microbes other than bacteria having tendency to causes watery diarrhoea & dysentery but may be by different mechanisms).

a. **Enterotoxicity:**
- Outpouring of electrolytes & fluid in to intestinal lumen responsible for diarrhoea **called watery diarrhoea** or **secretory diarrhoea** or **non-invasive diarrhoea**.
- It is non inflammatory (no RBCs/pus cells in stool)
- It is non invasive to epithelial cells (no systemic features like fever).
- Common agents for **watery diarrhoea** are
1. **Bacteria:** *Vibrio cholerae,* ETEC, EPEC, EAEC, *Staph aureus Clostridium welchii* & *Bacillus cereus.*
2. **Virus:** *Rotavirus*, nor walk virus, adenoviruses, corona virus, *Calcivirus*, *Astrovirus*, *Enterovirus* etc.
3. **Fungus:** *C. albicans* etc.
4. **Parasite:** *Giardia lamblia, I. belli, Cryptosporidium* spp., *Microsporidia* & *Cyclospora* spp.

b. **Cytotoxicity:**
- Disruption of intestinal mucosa leaving raw unprotected mucosa resulting passage of blood & mucus in stool **called bloody diarrhoea** or **dysentery** or **invasive diarrhoea**.
- It is inflammatory (WBCs/pus cells in stool).
- It is invasive to epithelial cells (cell death → bleeding → RBCs & ruptured mucosa in stool) & also extraintestinal in blood & lymph nodes (systemic features like fever).
- Common agents for **dysentery** are
1. **Bacteria: Called bacillary dysentery**
- *Cl. difficile.*
- *Shigella* spp.
- EIEC (Entero Invasive *Escherichia Coli*).
- EHEC (Entero Haemorrhagic *Escherichia Coli*).
- *C. jejuni.*
- *V. parahaemolyticus* (causing dysentery but non toxigenic).
- May be few non typhoidal *Salmonella* spp.
2. **Parasite: Called parasitic dysentery**
- *E. histolytica:* **Called amoebic dysentery.**
- *B. coli.*
- *I. belli.*

- *Schistosoma* spp.: *S. mansoni, S. japonicum, S. intercalatum.*
- *H. heterophyes.*
- *Trichuris trichuria.*
- *Strogyloides stercoralisl.*

c. **Neurotoxicity:**

- Enterotoxin of *S. aureus* acts on autonomic nervous system rather than on Gastro Intestinal (GI) mucosa. It stimulates the vagus nerve & vomiting center. It also knows to stimulate the peristaltic activity.
- Botulinum toxin acts on peripheral nerve system & produces the flaccid paralysis.
- Shiga toxin/shiga like toxin causing paralysis & death on injection in mice/rabbit. Not act directly on CNS but acting on the blood vessels supplying nerves & neurotoxic effect is secondary.

❖ **Mode of transmission:** Mostly by ingestion.

❖ **Diagnosis of gastroenteritis:**

➢ **Specimens:** Stool, vomitus, rectal swab, water-food sample.

➢ **Testing:**

i. **Diagnosis of bacteria:** Follow chapter → Laboratory diagnosis of bacterial infections

ii. **Diagnosis of viruses:** Follow chapter → Laboratory diagnosis of viral infections

iii. **Diagnosis of fungi:** Follow chapter → Laboratory diagnosis of fungal infections

iv. **Diagnosis of parasites:** Follow chapter → Laboratory diagnosis of parasitic infections

✓ **Note: Traveller's diarrhoea**

- **Definition:** Diarrhoea that develop during or shortly after, visiting the endemic areas.
- **Organisms:**

5. **Bacteria:**

- Entero Toxigenic *E coli* (ETEC): Few authors defined ETEC is the most common agent for traveller's diarrhoea.
- Entero Aggregative *E coli* (EAEC): Few authors defined ETEC & EAEC are the most common agents for traveller's diarrhoea.
- *Salmonella.*
- *Shigella.*
- *Vibrio cholerae.*
- *Vibro parahaemolyticus.*
- *Campylobacter jejuni.*
- *Aaeromonas hydrophila.*
- *Plesiomonas shigelloides.*

6. **Viruses:**

- *Rotavirus.*
- Nor walk virus.

7. **Parasites:**

- *Entamoeba histolytica.*
- *Giardia lamblia.*
- *Cryptosporidium* spp.
- *Cyclospora cayetanensis.*

✓ **Note: In addition to above mentioned agents following agents are known to cause diarrhoea**

- *T. solium.*
- *T. saginata.*
- *H. nana.*
- *F. hepatica* (persistent diarrhoea).

Food poisoning

❖ **Synonym:** Food borne illness or food borne disease.

❖ **Definitions:**

➢ **General definition:** Acute gastro-enteritis caused by the ingestion of the food or drink contaminated with either

- Living bacteria and/or bacterial toxins.
- Fungi and/or their toxins.
- Viruses or parasites.
- Inorganic chemical substances.
- Poison delivered from plants or
- Poison delivered from animals.

➢ **WHO definition:** Disease either infectious or toxic in nature, caused by agents that enter the body through the ingestion of food.

➢ **Intra-dietic toxin** or **preformed toxin:** Toxin is already present in food before ingestion **called intra-dietic toxin** or **preformed toxin.** Incubation period is short if toxin is preformed. It is present in *Staph. aureus, B. cereus* (emetic illness) & *Cl. botulinum* (food borne botulism).

❖ **Predisposing factors:**

- Preparing food too far in advance.
- Storing raw food at incorrect temperatures.

Intoxications	Infectious
Food contains preformed toxins	Food contains microbes which infect the body after consumption
Toxins (natural / preformed)	Bacterial / viral / parasitic
No invasion or multiplication	Invade and/or multiply in lining of intestine
IP: Minutes - hours	IP: Hours - days
C/Fs: Intestinal & extra-intestinal	C/Fs: Intestinal
Not communicable	Communicable – spreads from person to person
Factors: Inadequate cooking, improper handling temperatures	Factors: Inadequate cooking, poor personal hygiene, bare hand contact, cross contamination,
Examples: **Table-2**	Examples: **Table-2**

Table-1: Differences between intoxication & infections

- Incorrect cooling of food.
- Incorrect heating of food.
- Inadequate cooking of meats / poultry / fish.
- Frozen food not fully thawed.
- Cross contamination of cooked food by raw food.
- Holding hot and chilled food at incorrect temperatures.
- Contamination of food by food handlers.

❖ General features:

- There is history of the ingestion of a common food.
- Attack of the many persons at the same time.
- Similar C/Fs in majority of the cases, therefore, food poisoning must be suspected when an acute illness with gastrointestinal or neurological manifestation affect two or more persons, who have shared a meal during the previous 72 hours.

❖ Classifications:

I. **According to contains of food:** It may be of two types like infections or intoxication as shown in **table-1 & 2.**

II. **According to etiological agents:**

A. **Bacterial food poisoning:** Bacteria are classified as per incubation period as shown in **table-2.**

B. **Fungal food poisoning:** Follow chapter → Miscellaneous topics in Mycology

C. **Chemical food poisoning:**
- Accidental: By insecticides spray over food in farm.
- Intentional: Flavouring agents or preservatives.
- Products of food processing: Smoking of fleshy food.
- Radionucleotides.

D. **Animal food poisoning:** Fish & marine animal.

Microbes	Symptoms	Source of food
Intoxications (Preformed / intra-dietic toxin, so incubation period is very short)		
IP = 1-6 hours		
Staph. aureus	Nausea, vomiting & diarrhoea. No fever	Meat, fish, milk & milk products
B. cereus (Emetic illness)	Nausea & vomiting. Rarely diarrhoea. No fever	Rice (Chinese restaurant)
IP = 12-36 hours		
Cl. botulinum (food borne botulism)	Vomiting, thirst, constipation, ocular paresis, difficulty in swallowing-in speaking & in breathing	Preserved food- meat or meat product, fish, sea foods, canned vegetables.
Infectious (Toxin formed inside the intestine after ingestion of organisms)		
IP = 8-16 hours		
B. cereus (Diarrheal illness)	Diarrhoea, abdominal pain & fever	Vegetable & cooked meat
Cl. welchii (*Cl perfrigens*)	Abdominal pain/cramps, vomiting & diarrhoea	Meat (like beef & poultry meat) & legumes
IP = More than 16 hours		
Cl. botulinum (infant borne botulism)	Constipation, poor feeding, lethargy, weakness, pooled oral secretion, altered cry, floppiness and loss of head control	It occurs due to ingestion of food like honey contaminated by spore
Entero Haemorrhagic Escherichia coli (EHEC)	Causing mild diarrhea to haemorrhagic colitis, HUS (Haemorrhagic Uremic Syndrome) & food poisoning in children & in elder group in developed countries.	Vegetables (radish/alfalfa) or salad
Salmonella spp. (like *S. typhimurium, S. anatum* etc.)	Cholerae type diarrhoea (passage of ≥1 loose stool) or dysentery type diarrhoea (Blood + mucus in stool) with abdominal pain, vomiting & fever	- Animal product like egg, meat, milk or milk-derivatives. - Also by ingestion of salad/vegetables which are contaminated by manure or poor handling. - Food contamination by dropping of rat, lizard and other small animal.
Infectious but non toxigenic (No toxin formed before or after the ingestion of organisms)		
IP = More than 16 hours		
V. parahaemolyticus	Abdominal pain, nausea, vomiting, diarrhoea & low grade fever.	Ingestion of sea (marine) food like sea-fish, shrimps, crabs or mollusks (Oyster). In Calcutta found in small pond fish

Table-2: Bacterial food poisoning

✓ **Notes:**
- Remember food poisoning by heart because, almost in every year exam there is a MCQ of food poisoning.
- Incubation period help to solve the MCQs based on food poisoning.
- Diarrhoea is present in all except *Cl. botulinum.*

E. **Vegetable food poisoning:**
- *Lathyrus sativus* / Kesari dhal (Lathyrism).
- *Argemone maxicana* / Ujarkanta / Sialkanta / Kutila (Epidemic dropsy).
- *Atropa beladona* / poisonous berries.
- *Lolium temulentum* / Darnel.
- *Paspalam scrobiculatum* / Kodra.
- Cabbage: Specially of *Brassia* family has sulphar containing compound, which inhibit the thyroxine secretion.
- Soya bean: It has trypsin inhibitors, which makes protein unavailable for body.

❖ **Mode of transmission:** Mostly by ingestion.

❖ **Diagnosis:**
➢ **Specimens & testing methods:**
- **Human samples:** Stool, vomitus or rectal swab: Tested by gram staining & culture methods.
- **Water, food & dairy products sample:** Are tested by special methods.

Skin & soft tissues infections

❖ **Mode of transmission:**
1. **Primary skin lesion:** Direct entry of organism due to trauma or by else.
2. **Secondary skin lesion:** Involvement of skin due to underlying systemic disease.

❖ **Types of skin lesion:**
1. **Skin lesion:** Common skin lesions are like macule, papule, pustule, abscess, ulcer, erysipelas, impetigo, cellulitis, nodule, bulla, malignant pustule, pyoderma, ecthyma, wound infections (surgical, burns & accidental) etc.
2. **Nail lesions:** Like paronychia (bacterial nail infection), onychomycoses (fungal nail infection).
3. **Hair follicle:** Folliculitis, furuncle & carbuncle.
4. **Fascia & muscles:** Necrotising fasciitis, fournier gangrene, pyomyositis, myonecrosis, mycetoma etc.

❖ **Laboratory diagnosis:**
➢ **Samples:** Discharge from lesion, pus, skin biopsy, muscles fragments etc.
➢ **Testing methods:** It includes microscopy, culture, biochemical reactions, antibiogram etc.

Fournier gangrene

➢ **Synonym:** Polymicrobial necrotizing fasciitis.

➢ **Definition:** It is a type of necrotizing fasciitis or gangrene affecting the external genitalia (scrotum, penis & vulva). perianal and/or perineum (area between anus & scrotum/vulva) areas.

➢ **History:** It was first described by Baurienne in 1764 & is named after a French venereologist, Jean Alfred Fournier, following five cases he presented in clinical lectures in 1883.

➢ **Precipitating factors:**
1. **Sex:**
- About 1 per 62,500 males are affected a year.
- Males are affected about 40 times more often than females.
- In women: Septic abortions, vulvar or Bartholin gland abscesses, hysterectomy & episiotomy.
- In men: Anal intercourse may increase risk of perineal infection, either from blunt trauma to the area or by spread of rectally carried microbes.
2. **Age:**
- Common in extreme age.
- In children: Circumcision, omphalitis, insect bites, trauma, urethral instrumentation, perirectal abscesses, systemic infections.
3. **IDDs:** HIV, long-term corticosteroid therapy etc.
4. **Diabetes mellitus:** Present in as many as 60% of cases.
5. **Others:** Obesity, alcoholism, vascular disease of the pelvis, malignancy, systemic lupus erythematosus, Crohn's disease & malnutrition.
6. **No temperature effect:** Gangrene is affected by low temperature (hypothermia), but in Fournier gangrene hypothermia doesn't occur.

➢ **Etiological agents:** It is a polymicrobial infection with an average of 4 isolates per case. *Escherichia coli* is the predominant aerobe & *Bacteroides* is the predominant anaerobe. Other agents are, *Staphylococcus*, *Streptococcus* (aerobic & anaerobi), *Enterococcus*, *Pseudomonas*, *Klebsiella, Proteus* & *Candida albicans.*

➢ **Clinical features:**
- Fever, pallor, dehydration & generalized weakness.
- Pain and swelling in the genitals or anal area.
- Foul odour & purulent discharge from the infected tissues.
- Crackling sound (crepitus) when touching the affected area.
- Anaemia.
- It begins as a subcutaneous infection. However, soon necrotic patches appear in the overlying skin which later develops into gangrene.

➢ **Diagnosis:** Three types.

I. **Clinical diagnosis:** Fournier gangrene is usually diagnosed clinically.

II. **Radiological diagnosis:**
- X-rays and ultrasounds may show the presence of gas below the surface of the skin.

- CT scan can be useful in determining the site of origin and extent of spread.

III. Laboratory diagnosis:

➢ **Specimens:** Different body fluid, discharge or biopsy materials, blood etc.

➢ **Testing:**

A. **Bio-chemical diagnosis:** Includes liver function test, Renal function test & other biochemical analysis.

B. **Pathological diagnosis:** Includes haematological & histological diagnosis.

C. **Microbiological diagnosis:** Includes culture, microscopy & other tests.

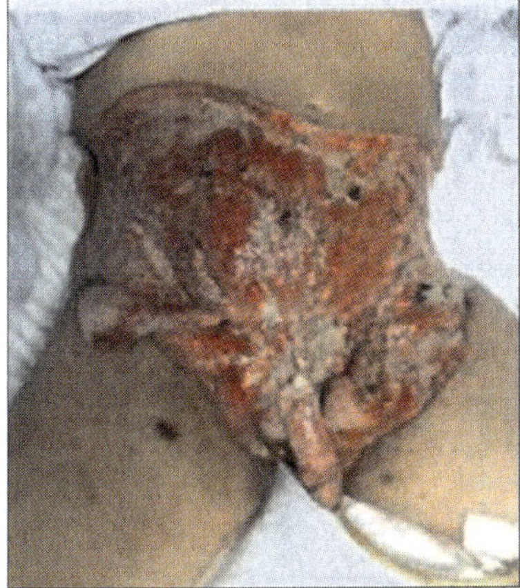

Figure-2: Fournier gangrene after debridment

➢ **Treatment:** Fournier gangrene is a urological emergency requiring IV antibiotics & debridement of necrotic (dead) tissue (**fig.-2**). In addition to surgery & antibiotics, hyperbaric oxygen therapy (HBOT) may be useful and acts to inhibit the growth of and kill the anaerobic bacteria.

Eye infections

❖ **Etiological agents:**

i. **Bacteria infecting eyes:** Follow chapter → Neisseriae, Moraxellaceae and Mimeae

ii. **Viruses infecting eyes (conjunctivitis):** Follow chapter → Picornaviridae

iii. **Fungi infecting eyes (oculomycoses):** Follow chapter → Miscellaneous topics in Mycology

iv. **Parasites infecting eyes:** Follow chapter → Miscellaneous topics in Parasitology

Ear infections

❖ **Types:** Two types of ear infections.

i. **Otitis externa:** Infection/inflammation of external ear by following microbes.

a. **Acute**

1. **Bacteria:**

- *Staph. aureus.*
- *Strept. pyogenes.*
- *Pseudomonas aeruginosa:* Malignant otitis externa.
- Other GNB.

2. **Fungi:**

- *C. albicans:* White discharge.
- *Aspergillus fumigates:* Greenish discharge.
- *Aspergillus niger:* Black discharge.

b. **Chronic:**

- Anaerobes: Most common.
- Aerobes: *Pseudomonas aeruginosa.*

ii. **Otitis media:** Infection/inflammation of middle ear by following microbes.

a. **Acute**

1. **Bacteria:** *Strept. pneumoniae (*Most common in children in 33% cases) > *Haemophilus influenzae* type b *(*2nd most common) > *Moraxella catarrhalis* > *Strept. pyogenes.*

2. **Viruses:**

- Respiratory syncitial virus.
- Influenza virus.

b. **Chronic:**

- Anaerobes: Most common.

Sexually transmitted infections (STIs)

❖ **Synonym:** Venereal diseases or Sexually transmitted diseases (STDs).

❖ **Etiological agents:**

i. **Bacteria:**

1. *Neisseria gonococci:* Disease **called gonorrhoea.**
2. *Shigella* species*:* In male homosexual **called Gey bowel syndrome.**
3. *Klebsiella granulomatis:* Disease **called granuloma inguinale** or **called donovanosis** or **called granuloma venereum.**
4. *Campylobacter jejuni:* By oral-anal sex.
5. *Haemophilus ducreyi:* Disease **called chancroid** or **called soft sore.**
6. *Brucella abortus* & other species.
7. *Gardnerella vaginalis* Disease **called bacterial vaginosis.**
8. *Treponema pallidum:* Disease **called syphilis.**
9. *Mycoplasma hominis.*
10. *Ureaplasma Urealyticum.*
11. *Chlamydia trachomatis:* Two types disease **called genital chlamydiasis** & **called LGV.**

ii. **Viruses:** Like MCV, herpes viruses (like HSV-1, HSV- 2, CMV, KSHV, HPV (most common among the viral etiology), zika virus, HBV, HCV, HTLV-I, HTLV-II, HTLV-III (HIV) etc.

iii. **Fungi:** *C. albicans.*

iv. **Parasites:** *Entamoeba histolytica, Giardia lamblia, Trichomonas vaginalis, Isospora belli* & *Cryptosporidium parvum* (by oral-anal sex).

v. **Ecto- Parasites:** *Sarcoptes scabiei* & *Pthirus pubis.*

❖ **Clinical features:**

i. **Urethral/cervical/vaginal discharge:**

✪ **Purulent watery discharge:** Bacterial.

✪ **Thick white discharge:** Candidiasis.

✪ **Frothy discharge:** Trichomoniasis.

ii. **Ulcer:**

✪ **Chancroid or soft sore:** Non-indurated, tender, irregular swelling on external genitalia which gets ulcerated. Infection is localized spreading to only to regional lymph nodes. Lymph nodes enlarged and painful.

✪ **Chancre / hard chancre:** Painless, ulcerated, indurated swelling with exudative discharges.

✪ **Genital herpes:** Multiple, non-indurated, painful, markedly tender ulcer with moderate to no lymph node swelling.

iii. **Pain:** Lower abdominal pain & fever also.

❖ **Complications:**

- Infertility.
- Ectopic pregnancy.
- Premature labour or abortion.
- PID (Pelvic Inflammatory Disease).
- Cervical carcinoma.

❖ **Diagnosis:**

➢ **Specimens:** Urine, fluid/discharge, swab & blood.

➢ **Testing:**

i. **Diagnosis of bacteria:** Follow chapter → Laboratory diagnosis of bacterial infections

ii. **Diagnosis of viruses:** Follow chapter → Laboratory diagnosis of viral infections

iii. **Diagnosis of fungi:** Follow chapter → Laboratory diagnosis of fungal infections

iv. **Diagnosis of parasites:** Follow chapter → Laboratory diagnosis of parasitic infections

Pyrexia of unknown origin (PUO)

❖ **Synonym:** Fever of Unknown Origin (FUO).

❖ **Definition:** Temperature above 38^0C for more than three weeks & without diagnosis even after one week of investigation.

❖ **Etiological agents:**

A. **Infectious disease:**

i. **Bacteria:** *M. tuberculosis* (most common cause but remain undetected), *Atypical mycobacteria, Salmonella, Brucella, Chlamydiae, Leptospira, Rickettsia, Coxiella, Mycoplasma* etc.

ii. **Viruses:** CMV, Arboviruses, HIV, Enteroviruses etc.

iii. **Fungi:** *C. albicans*, different systemic or opportunistic fungi.

iv. **Parasites:** *Plasmodium* spp., Microfilariae, *Babesia, Leishmania* spp., *Typanosoma* spp. & *Toxoplasma.*

B. **Non- Infectious disease:**

i. **Granulomatous disease**

ii. **Autoimmune disease**

iii. **Hypersensitivity reaction**

iv. **Malignancy**

v. **Trauma**

❖ **Diagnosis:** Three types.

I. **Clinical diagnosis:** Based on pattern of fever, history & clinical examination.

II. **Radiological diagnosis:** X-ray, USG, CT-scan, MRI etc.

III. **Laboratory diagnosis:**

➢ **Specimens:** Different body fluid, discharge or biopsy materials.

➢ **Testing:**

A **Bio-chemical diagnosis:** Includes liver function test, renal function test & other biochemical analysis.

B **Pathological diagnosis:** Includes haematological & histological diagnosis.

C **Microbiological diagnosis:**

i. **Diagnosis of bacteria:** Follow chapter → Laboratory diagnosis of bacterial infections

ii. **Diagnosis of viruses:** Follow chapter → Laboratory diagnosis of viral infections

iii. **Diagnosis of fungi:** Follow chapter → Laboratory diagnosis of fungal infections

iv. **Diagnosis of parasites:** Follow chapter → Laboratory diagnosis of parasitic infections

Zoonotic infections

❖ **Synonym:** Zoonosis or zoonotic disease or anthropozoonoses or anthroponotic diseases (infections).

❖ **Definition:** Infection transmitted from animal to human **called zoonotic infections.**

❖ **Meaning:** Anthro (Greek) = human + zoon (Greek) = animal + nosos (Greek) = disease.

❖ **Predisposing factors:**

✪ **Occupation:** Common in veterinary doctors, animal handlers, agricultural workers, butchers, hunters, non-vegetarian merchants etc.

✪ **Consumer:** All those who are consuming contaminated animal product like milk, meat, eggs etc.

❖ **Etiological agents:**

i. **Bacteria:** *M. bovis, Salmonella* spp., *Brucella* spp., *Francisella tularensis, Leptospira, Rickettsia, Coxiella burnetii, Pseudomonas mallei, Borrelia burgdorferi, Bacillus anthracis* etc.

ii. **Viruses:** Rabies virus, Yellow fever virus, Japanese encephalitis virus, CCHF, Swine flu virus etc.

iii. **Fungi:** *Trichophyton* spp., *Microsporum* spp. & *Histoplasma capsulatum.*

iv. **Parasites:** *Taenia* spp., *Leishmania* spp., *Typanosoma* spp., *Toxoplasma gondii, Plasmodium* spp., *E. granulosus* etc.

❖ Mode of transmission:

a. **Direct:**

- Contact of abraded skin with water infected by animals excreta and contains bacteria like *Leptospira.*
- Direct animal bite: Rabies.

b. **Indirect:**

1. **Inhalation (Air borne):** Inhalation of aerosols from infected wool.
2. **Ingestion (Food & water borne):**
   - Eggs ingestion contains *Salmonella.*
   - Partially cooked beef & pork in *Taenia* spp.
   - Milk of infected animal like *M. bovis.*
3. **Vector borne:** Blood sucking insect can transmit pathogens from animals to humans like CCHF.

❖ Diagnosis:

➢ **Specimens:**

- **Human samples:** According to system infected.
- **Animal samples:**
  - Ear sample, swab soaked in blood: Anthrax.
  - Severed head: Rabies.
  - Pieces of kidney: Leptospirosis.
  - Pooled milk sample: Brucellosis.

➢ **Testing:**

i. **Diagnosis of bacteria:** Follow chapter → Laboratory diagnosis of bacterial infections

ii. **Diagnosis of viruses:** Follow chapter → Laboratory diagnosis of viral infections

iii. **Diagnosis of fungi:** Follow chapter → Laboratory diagnosis of fungal infections

iv. **Diagnosis of parasites:** Follow chapter → Laboratory diagnosis of parasitic infections

Opportunistic infections

❖ Definition:

Infection in immunocompromised (IDDs) host is **called opportunistic infection.**

❖ Etiological agents:

Following are the opportunistic pathogens.

i. **Bacterial:**

- *M. tuberculosis.*
- Non- Tuberculous Mycobacteria (NTM).
- *Salmonella* spp.
- *Campylobacter* spp.
- *Nocardia* spp.
- *Actinomycetes* spp.
- *Legionella* spp.

ii. **Viral:**

- VZV.
- HSV.
- CMV.

iii. **Fungal:**

- *Candida* spp.
- *Cryptococcus neoformans.*
- *Aspergillus* spp.
- *Zygomycetes* spp.
- *Histoplasma capsulatum.*
- *Penicillium marneffei.*
- *Pneumocystis jirovecii/ Pneumocystis carinii* (also classified as parasite by some workers).
- *Trichosporon beigelii.*
- *Geotrichum candidum.*
- *Blastoschizomyces capitatus.*
- *Saccharomyces cerevisiae* (Baker's yeast or Brewer's yeast).

iv. **Parasitic:**

a. **Protozoa:**

1. *Toxoplasma gondii.*
2. *Isospora* (> 1 month duration).
3. *Cryptosporidium parvum* (> 1 month duration).
4. *Cyclospora.*
5. *Microsporidia.*
6. *Entamoeba histolytica.*
7. *Giardia lamblia.*

b. **Metazoa/Helminths:**

1. *Strongyloides stercoralis.*

❖ Diagnosis:

➢ **Specimens:** According to system infected.

➢ **Testing:**

i. **Diagnosis of bacteria:** Follow chapter → Laboratory diagnosis of bacterial infections

ii. **Diagnosis of viruses:** Follow chapter → Laboratory diagnosis of viral infections

iii. **Diagnosis of fungi:** Follow chapter → Laboratory diagnosis of fungal infections

iv. **Diagnosis of parasites:** Follow chapter → Laboratory diagnosis of parasitic infections

Question bank

Short notes

1) Blood stream infections.
2) Respiratory tract infection.
3) Bacterial meningitis.
4) Infective endocarditis.
5) Dysentery.
6) Food poisoning.
7) STDs (STIs).
8) PUO.
9) Zoonosis.
10) Opportunistic infections.

Short questions for theory/Viva questions

1) What is aseptic meningitis? Write two examples of bacteria causing aseptic meningitis.
2) Name four bacteria causing dysentery.

3) What is preformed toxin? Name two bacteria producing preformed toxin.
4) Name four sexually transmitted parasites/bacteria/viruses.
5) Name four parasites / fungi / bacteria causing opportunistic infections.

MCQs for chapter review

Respiratory tract infections

1) **Pneumatoceles are seen in-**
(a) *Klebsiella pneuminiae* (b) *Streptococcus pneumoniae* (c) *Mycoplasma pneumoniae* (d) *Listeria monocytogenes*

Meningitis

2) **Following bacteria are most often associated with acute neonatal meningitis except-** (AI-05)
(a) *E. coli* (b) *Streptococcus agalactiae* (c) *Neisseria meningitidis* (d) *Listeria monocytogenes*

Infective endocarditis

3) **Which of the following is least likely to cause infective endocarditis** (AI-06)
(a) *Staphylococcus albus* (b) *Streptococcus faecalis* (c) *Salmonella typhi* (d) *Pseudomonas aeruginosa*

UTI

4) **Most common organism implicated in the aetiology of urinary tract infection in the community is?**
(a) *E. coli* (b) *Proteus* (c) Pseudomonas (d) *Streptococci*
5) **Most common cause of UTI in young female is?**
(a) *Staph saprophyticus* (b) *E. coli* (c) *Klebsiella* (d) *Proteus*
6) **A 30 year old male present with urethritis. All the following can be the causative agent except** (AIIMS, Nov-04)
(a) *Neisseriae gonorrhoea* (b) *Chlamydia trachomatis* (c) *Trichomonas vaginalis* (d) *Haemophilus ducreyi*
7) **All are common organisms causing UTI except** (AIIMS-92)
(a) *Streptococcus faecalis* (b) *Escherichia coli* (c) *Proteus mirabilis*(d) *Haemophilus influenzae*
8) **Ascending UTI is caused by** (PGI, June-05)
(a) *Salmonella* (b) TB (c) *E. coli* (d) *Chlamydia* (e) *Klebsiella*

Gastroenteritis

9) **Noninvasive diarrhoea can be caused by one of following-** (AI-09)
(a) *Shigella* (b) *B. cereus* (c) *Salmonella* (d) *Y. enterocolitica*
10) **18 year old girl present with watery diarrhoea. Most likely causative agent**
(a) *Rotavirus* (b) *V. cholerae* (c) *Salmonella* (d) *Shigella*
11) **In a patient presenting with diarrhoea and pus cells in stool, the causative organisms can be all except-** (PGI, Dec-01)
(a) *Non cholera vibrio* 01 (b) Enterotoxigenic *E. coli* (c) Enteroinvasive *E. coli* (d) *Shigella dysentery* 1 (e) *Vibrio cholerae*
12) **Micro-organisms invading the GIT causing gastroenteritis** (PGI, Dec-07)
(a) EHEC (b) *Shigella* (c) *Vibrio parahaemolyticus* (d) *Campylobacter* (e) *Salmonella*
13) **A child with fever with RBCs & pus in stool, causative organism is**
(a) ETEC (b) EHEC (c) EPEC (d) EAEC
14) **Pus cells in diarrhoea seen in** (PGI-05)
(a) *Vibrio cholerae* (b) EPEC (c) *Rotavirus* (d) *Shigella* (e) *Campylobacter*
15) **Faecal leucocytes are absent in all the following except**
(a) Giardiasis (b) Cryptosporidiasis (c) *Campylobacter* infection (d) *Clostridium perfrigens* infection

Traveller's diarrhoea

16) **Traveller's diarrhoea is caused by** (AIIMS, Dec-97)
(a) *Shigella* (b) *E. coli* (c) *E.histolytica* (d) Giardiasis
17) **The most common causative organism for traveller's diarrhoea is** (AIIMS, Dec-94)
(a) *E. coli* (b) *Shigella* (c) Norwalk virus (d) *Rotavirus*
18) **In which of the following is true regarding the cause of traveller's diarrhoea**
(a) Giardiasis (b) *E. coli* (c) Amoebiasis (d) Idiopathic without any causative organisms

Food poisoning

19) **A cook prepares sandwitches for 10 people going for picnic. Eight out of them develop severe gastroenteritis within 4-6 hours of consumption of the sandwitches. It is likely that on investigations the cook is found to be the carrier of** (AIIMS, Nov-02)
(a) *Salmonella typhi* (b) *Vibrio cholerae* (c) *Entamoeba histolytica* (d) *Staphylococcus aureus*
20) **A patient present with vomiting. He had eaten rice 6 hours before. The most probable cause is-**
(a) *Bacillus cereus* (b) *Staph. aureus* (c) *Cl. difficile* (d) All of above
21) **Kallu, a 22 year old male had an outing with his friends and developed fever of 38.5^{0}C, diarrhoea and vomiting following eating chicken salad, 24 hours back. Two of his friends developed the same symptoms. The diagnosis is-** (AIIMS-01)
(a) *Salmonella enteritidis* (b) *Bacillus cereus* (c) *Staph. aureus* (d) *Vibrio cholerae*
22) **Most probable cause of food poisoning in a child who has eaten ice cream 16-18 hrs earlier.** (AIIMS-92)
(a) *Staph. aureus* (b) *Clostridium perfrigens* (c) *Clostridium botulinum* (d) *Salmonella typhimurium*
23) **Thirty eight children consumed eatables, procured from a single source at a picnic party. Twenty children developed abdominal cramps followed by vomiting and watery diarrhoea 6-10 hours after the party. The most likely etiology for the outbreak is** (AI-03)
(a) *Rotavirus* infection (b) *Enterotoxigenic E coli* infection (c) Staphylococcal toxin (d) *Clostridium perfrigens* infection
24) **An adolescent male developed vomiting and diarrhoea 1 hour after having food from a restaurant. The most likely pathogen is** (AI-03)
(a) *Clostridium perfrigens* (b) *Vibrio parahaemolyticus* (c) *Staphylococcus aureus* (d) *Salmonella typhimurium*
25) **Food poisoning with diarrhoea within 6 hours.**
(a) *Staph. aureus* (b) *Clostridium perfrigens* (c) *Clostridium botulinum* (d) *V cholerae*
26) **Preformed toxin is important in food poisoning due to all except.** (AIIMS, Nov-01)
(a) *Staph. aureus* (b) *Clostridium botulinum* (c) ETEC (d) *B cereus*
27) **Toxin is implicated as the major pathogenic mechanism in all of the following bacterial diarrhoea except** (AI-04)
(a) *Vibrio cholerae* (b) *Shigella* sp. (c) *Vibrio parahaemolyticus* (d) *Staphylococcus aureus*
28) **Most common organism causing food poisoning in canned food.**
(a) *Staph. aureus* (b) *Clostridium perfrigens* (c) *Clostridium botulinum* (d) *V cholerae*

Fournier gangrene

29) **All causes Fournier gangrene except**
(a) *Staphylococcus* (b) *Streptococcus* (c) *Clostridium* (d) *Bacteroides*

Ear infections

30) A patient with history of discharge from right ear presented with severe earache. This discharge was culture and organism was found to be gram negative cocci. The least like cause.
(a) *Pseudomonas* (b) *Streptococcus pneumoniae* (c) *Staphylococcus* (d) *Haemophilus influenzae*

Sexually transmitted infections (STIs)

31) Which of the following is/are not STD (PGI, May-13, Nov-10)
(a) HAV (b) HPV (c) HIV (d) Varicella zoster virus (e) HTLV-I

32) Genital ulcer is seen in all except (PGI, May-10, Nov-13)
(a) *H aegypticus* (b) *H ducreyi* (c) HSV (d) *Chlamydia* (e) *T pallidum*

33) Which of the following is not a sexually transmitted disease
(a) Hepatitis B (b) Amoebiasis (c) Bacterial vaginosis (d) Yaws

34) A man presents to a STD clinic with urethritis and urethral discharge. Gram stain shows numerous pus cells but no microorganisms. The culture is negative on the laboratory media. The most likely agent is (AIIMS, Nov-02, 07)
(a) *Chlamydia trachomatis* (b) *Haemophilus ducreyi* (c) *Treponema pallidum* (d) *Neisseriae gonorrhoea*

35) A young male presents with UTI, on urine examination pus cells were found but no organisms. Which method would be best used for culture. (AIIMS, Nov-06, 11, May-12, AI-07)
(a) Mac coy cell line (b) Thayer Martine medium (c) LJ medium (d) Levinthal medium

36) Green frothy vaginal discharge is produced by (AIIMS, May-94)
(a) Herpes simplex (b) *Candida albicans* (c) *Trichomonas vaginalis* (d) Normal vaginal flora

37) Treatment of partner is required in all infections except (PGI-00)
(a) *Candida* (b) Herpes (c) *Trichomonas* (d) *Gardnerella*

Pyrexia of unknown origin (PUO)

38) The single most common cause of pyrexia of unknown origin (AIIMS, May-06)
(a) *Mycobacterium tuberculosis* (b) *Salmonella typhi* (c) *Brucella* spp. (d) *Salmonella paratyphi* A

39) A veterinary doctor had pyrexia of unknown origin. His blood culture in special laboratory media was positive for gram negative short bacilli which was oxidase positive. Which one of the following is the likely organism grown in culture. (AI-06)
(a) *Pasteurella* spp. (b) *Francisella* spp. (c) *Batonella* spp. (d) *Brucella* spp.

40) The organism most likely to cause fever of unknown origin in a farmer who raises goats
(a) *Brucella melitensis* (b) *Clostridium novyi* (c) *Histoplasma capsulatum* (d) *Mycobacterium tuberculosis*

Zoonotic infections

41) Anthropozoonosis are all except- (AI-09)
(a) Guinea worm infection (b) Rabies (c) Plague (d) Hydatid cyst

42) Zoonotic disease are all except- (AI-09)
(a) Typhoid (b) Anthrax (c) Rabies (d) Q fever

43) Zoonotic bacterial infection is/are
(a) Bovine tuberculosis (b) Brucellosis (c) a+b (d) None of above

Opportunistic infections

44) Humoral immunodeficiency is suspected in patient and he is under investigation. Which of the following infections would be consistent with the diagnosis (AIIMS-04)
(a) Giardiasis (b) *Pneumocystis carinii* pneumonia (c) Recurrent sinusitis (d) Recurrent subcutaneous abscess

Answers of MCQs & explanation

1) (a) & (b)
- Pneumatocele is commonly caused by *Staph aureus*, which is not given in options. From the given options right answers are *Strept pneumoniae* & *Klebsiella pneumoniae*
- Follow section **respiratory tract infections (pneumatocele)** for more explanation

2) (c)
- Follow section **meningitis (types & etiological agents)** for explanation

3) (c)
- Follow section **infective endocarditis (etiological agents)** for explanation

4) (a)
- *E. coli* is the most common cause of acute UTI (in 80% cases without catheter), neonatal meningitis, intra-abdominal abscess & nosocomial infection
- *E. coli* cause 80-90% of lower UTI (cystitis) in young women

5) (b)
- *E. coli* cause 80-90% of lower UTI (cystitis) in young women

6) (d)
- Follow section, **urinary tract infections (etiological agents)** for explanation

7) (d)
- Follow section **urinary tract infections (etiological agents)** for explanation

8) (c) & (d)
- Follow section **urinary tract infections (mode of transmission → ascending route)** for explanation

9) (b)
- Few authors referred dysentery as invasive diarrhoea, which is caused by *Shigella spp.*, *Cl difficile*, EIEC, ETEC, *C. jejuni*, *V. parahaemolyticus, Y. enterocolitica* & *Salmonella* spp.,

10) (b)
- *Rotavirus* & *V. cholerae* are the agents of watery diarrhoea from the given option, but *Rotavirus* causes watery diarrhoea in children, so *V. cholerae* is the right answer.

11) (a), (b) & (e)
- Given case is of dysentery (pus cells/RBCs in stool) which is caused by many bacteria & parasites, but in given question only bacteria are given as option.
- Follow section **gastroenteritis (etio-pathogenetic classification → cytotoxicity)** for explanation.

12) (a), (b), (c), (d) & (e)
13) (b)
14) (d) & (e)
} Follow section **gastroenteritis (etio-pathogenetic classification → cytotoxicity)** for explanation.

15) (c)
16) (a), (b), (c) & (d)
17) (a)
18) (b)
} Follow section **gastroenteritis (traveller's diarrhoea)** for explanation

19) (d)
- Given case is food poisoning within 6 hours of consumption of sandwitches mostly caused by *B. cereus* or *Staph. aureus*. *B. cereus* is not given in option, so right answer is *Staph. aureus.*
- Follow **table-1 & 2** for more explanation

20) (a)
- Given case is of food poisoning with emetic illness of *B. cereus* which is transmitted by rice from chinese restaurant
- Follow **table-1 & 2** for more explanation

21) (a)
- Given case is of food poisoning with 24 hours incubation period due to consumption of chicken & salad.

Salmonella enteritidis is the right answer from the given options.

- Follow **table-1 & 2** for more explanation

22) (d)

- Given case is of food poisoning with 24 hours incubation period due to consumption of milk products (ice cream) *Salmonella typhimurium* is the right answer from the given options.
- Follow **table-1 & 2** for more explanation

23) (d)

- Given case is of food poisoning with 8-16 hours incubation period. Children are present with abdominal pain/cramps, vomiting & diarrhoea, so agent is *Cl perfrigens*
- Follow **table-1 & 2** for more explanation

24) (c)
25) (a)
26) (c)
27) (c)
28) (d)
} Follow section **gastroenteritis (food poisoning & table-2** for explanation

29) (c)

- Follow section, **skin & soft tissues infections (Fournier gangrene)** for more explanation

30) (d)

- Gram negative cocci or coccobacilliis *H influenzae* which is the 2nd most common bacteria for acute otitis media after *Streptococcus pneumoniae.*
- Follow section, **ear infections** for more explanation

31) (a) & (d)
32) (a)
33) (d)
} Follow section, **sexually transmitted infections (STIs)** & respective chapters for more explanation

34) (a)

- *Haemophilus ducreyi* & *Treponema pallidum* are causing lesion in external genitals
- *Neisseriae gonorrhoea* & *Chlamydia trachomatis* are causing urethritis with pus cells under gram stain. *Chlamydia trachomatis* is gram negative but not identified under gram stain & also not growing on routine laboratory media while *Neisseriae gonorrhoea* can.
- *H ducreyi* can grow on routine laboratory media.
- In *T pallidum* non pathogenic strain can grow over media.
- Follow respective chapters for more details.

35) (a)

- In given UTI case organisms are not identified under microscopical examination but pus cells are noticed, so most probable organism is *Chlamydia trachomatis* which also not growing on routine laboratory media but grow on cell culture media like Mac coy cell line.
- Follow respective chapters for more details.

36) (c)

- Vaginal discharge is a feature of *Candida albicans* & *Trichomonas vaginalis* where it is whitish in initial one while yellowish (purulent) or white (serous) with foul smelling or green frothy in later.

37) (a) & (d)

- Exact reason is not known but may of endogenous infection by these two microbes.

38) (a)
39) (d)
40) (a)
} Follow section, **pyrexia of unknown origin (PUO) → etiological agents** & respective chapters for more explanation

41) (a)
42) (a)
43) (c)
} Follow section, **zoonotic infections** for explanation

44) (a) & (b)

- Follow section, **opportunistic infections (etiological agents)** for more explanation.

104 Oncogenic microbes

Learning heading & subheadings

- Definition:
- Classification:

Oncogenic bacteria

Oncogenic viruses

Oncogenic fungi

Oncogenic parasites

❖ **Definition:** Microorganisms causing cancer are **called oncogenic microbes.**

❖ **Classification:** Microbes causing cancer are

I. **Bacteria: Called oncogenic bacteria.**
II. **Viruses: Called oncogenic viruses.**
III. **Fungi: Called oncogenic fungi.**
IV. **Parasites: Called oncogenic parasites.**

Oncogenic bacteria

1. ***Helicobacter pylori***

- It produces gastric carcinoma & Mucosa Associated Lymphoid Tissue (MALT) lymphoma.
- More details: Follow chapter → Campylobacterales **(section → *Helicobacter*)**.

Oncogenic viruses

➢ **Definition:** Viruses which produces tumour in their natural host or in experimental animals or which induce malignant transformation of cells on culture are **called oncogenic viruses**.

➢ **History:** Viral association with malignancy was 1st described by Rous in 1911, when he identified the fowl sarcoma caused by virus. Later Nobel Prize was given to him in 1966.

➢ **Classification**: Viruses causing cancer are listed in **table-1** (human cancer) **& table-2** (animal cancer).

Family	Species	Cancer (s)
DNA viruses		
Papova-viridae	HPV	- Oropharyngeal cancer (Typ1 16) - Laryngeal or oesophageal carcinoma (Typ1 16 & 18) - Genital cancers: Seen in vulva, vagina, cervix, penis, & anus [Highest risk (16, 18, 31, 45), Other high-risk (33, 35, 39, 51, 52, 56, 58, 59) Probably high-risk (26, 53, 66, 68, 73, 82)]
Herpes-viridae	HHV-1 (HSV-1)	Lip cancer
	HHV-1 (HSV-2)	Cervical cancer
	HHV-4 (EBV)	- Nasopharyngeal carcinoma - Burkit's lymphoma - Lymphoma (Hodgkin's & Non-Hodgkin's lymphoma)
	HHV-5 (CMV)	- Carcinoma of prostate - Kaposi's sarcoma
	HHV-8 (KSHV)	Kaposi's Sarcoma
Hepadn-viridae	HBV	HCC
RNA viruses		
Flavi-viridae	HCV	Hepatocellular carcinoma (HCC)
Retro-viridae	HTLV-I	- Human T cell leukemia / lymphoma - Cutaneous T cell lymphoma
	HTLV-II	T cell malignancy
	HTLV-III (HIV 1 & HIV 2)	AIDS related malignancies like - Kaposi's Sarcoma (KS) - Lymphoma: Hodgkins & non-Hodgkin's type. - Cervical cancer

Table-1: Human oncogenic viruses

➢ **Transformation:**

✪ **Definition:** Conversion of normal cells in to malignant cells **called transformation**.

✪ **Properties of transformed cells:**

a. **Alteration of morphology:**

- Change in shape.
- In fibroblast they becomes shorten, loss of parallel orientation & chromosomal aberration.

b. **Alteration of metabolism:**

- Increased production of organic acids & acid mucopolysaccharide.

c. **Alteration of growth properties:**
- Change in growth rate.
- Indefinites division.
- Loss of contact inhibition, so instead of monolayer formation there is piled up growth & **microtumour formation**.
- Can grow in semi-solid agar or in suspension.

d. **Formation of new Ag (tumour Ags):** **Follow chapter → Immunology of transplantation & malignancy.**

e. **Capacity to induce tumour:** In animals.

Family	Species	Cancer
DNA viruses		
Adeno-viridae	Type 12, 19 & 21	Sarcoma in new borne rodents
Pox-viridae	Rabbit fibroma virus	Rabbit fibroma
	Yaba virus	Benign tumour
Herpes-viridae	Marek's disease virus	Marek's disease
	Lucke's frog tuour virus	Renal adenocarcinoma in frog
	Herpes virus saimiri	Lymphoma or reticular cell carcinoma in owls, monkeys or rabbits
RNA viruses		
Retro-viridae	Rous sarcoma virus	- Avian leukosis complex (Lymphomatosis, myeloblastosis & erythroblastosis) - Sarcoma in fowls
	Murine leukosis virus	Murine leukemia & sarcoma
	Mice mammary tumour virus (Bittner's milk factor or Bittner's virus)	Breast cancer in mice
	Leukosis sarcoma virus	Leukosis & sarcoma in different animals

Table-2: Animal oncogenic viruses

✪ **Types of viruses according to transformation:**

a. **Slow transforming viruses:**
- Low oncogenic potential.
- Transformation occurs after a long latent period.
- Do not transform the culture cells.
- They cause malignancy of blood cells. E.g. leukemia.
- Example of virus: HTLV.
- Replication: Normal.

b. **Acute transforming viruses:**
- Low oncogenic potential.
- Transformation occurs after a short latent period of weeks or months.
- Can transform the culture cells.
- They cause different types of malignancy. E.g leukemia, carcinoma, sarcoma etc.
- Example of virus: Rouse sarcoma Virus, HBV etc.
- Replication: Not normal & may be following types.

1. **Replication defective:** Viruses are not replicate normally because contain additional gene like **viral oncogene (V-onc gene)**, which replace the normal gene of virus & viruses depend on co-infection by helper virus for replication.
2. **Replication competent:** viruses are replicate normally because contain **viral oncogene** {**src** (Pronounced as 'sark') **for Rous rarcoma virus**} and full complement of normal genes like **gag, pol & env genes.**

➢ **Viral oncogenes (V-onc / viral cancer genes):**

✪ **Definition:** Viral genes which are encode for conversion of normal cells in to malignant cells **called oncogenes (V-onc)**.

✪ **Properties:**
- They are not responsible for viral replication.
- Formed by recombination between viral & cell genes.
- Certain genes resembling V-onc are present in cancer cells **called cellular oncogenes (C-onc)** and in normal host cells **called cellular proto-oncogenes.**
- **C-onc** is having all characteristics of prokaryotic cells while V-onc does not have.
- **Proto-oncogenes** are present in normal cells with certain functions like (1) Oncogene-src → tyrosine specific protein kinase (2) Oncogene-sis → platelet derived growth factor (3) Oncogene-myc → DNA binding protein.

➢ **Anti-oncogenes:**

✪ **Definition:** Certain genes suppress the development of tumour **called anti-oncogenes**. Their absence produce tumour.

✪ **Examples:**
1. Rb gene: Its absence produces Retinoblastoma (Rb).
2. P53: Tumour suppressor gene.

✪ **Mechanisms of absence of anti-oncogenes:** It may be due to absence of chromosomes.

➢ **Mechanism of viral oncogenesis:**

a. **DNA viruses:** Integration of viral DNA in to host cell genome, which bring the transformation in host cells. It is like lysogenic conversion in bacterium.

b. **RNA viruses:**
- Introduction of oncogene in to host cells.
- Pre-existing cellular gene alteration.

Oncogenic fungi

➢ **Introduction:** Few fungal toxins which are known to produce the fungal food poisoning are also having oncogenic properties concluded by IARC (International Agency for Research on Cancer).

Fungal food poisoning are classified as **mycotoxicoses** (clinical entity due ingestion of fungal toxin only) & **mycetism / mycetismus / muscarinism or mushroom poisoning** (clinical entity due ingestion of fungal toxin along with fungus).

- **Types:** Following are the fungal toxins causing mycotoxicoses, are known as carcinogens.
- **More details:** Follow chapter → Miscellaneous topics in Mycology.

1. **Aflatoxin:** Aflatoxin B_1 is classified as group 1 human carcinogen by IARC & responsible to produce the renal & liver cancer.
3. **Fumonisins:**
- Fumonisins is classified as class 2B human carcinogen by IARC & responsible to produce the oesophageal cancer, in endemic regions of South Africa particularly in Transkei & also in parts of China.
- It also causing liver cancer in rat.
4. **Ochratoxin:**
- There are different types of ochratoxin but type A is medically significant.
- Ochratoxin A is identified urinary tract carcinogen by IARC.
5. **Zearalenone:** In human it causes cervical cancer.

Oncogenic parasites

- **Types:** Following are the parasites causing cancers.

1. ***Schistosoma haematobium:*** It causing the squamous cell carcinoma of urinary bladder.
2. ***Clonorchis sinensis:*** Causing liver, bile duct (cholangio-carcinoma), gall bladder (?) & pancreas (adenocarcinoma).
3. ***Opisthorchis viverrini:*** Causing bile duct cancer **called cholangio carcinoma.**

- **More details:** Follow → Respective chapters

Question bank

Essay/Full question

1) Oncogenic microbes.

Short notes

1) Oncogenic viruses.

Short questions for theory/viva questions

1) Write two examples of each, DNA & RNA oncogenic viruses with cancer produced by them.
2) Name four fungal toxins causing cancer along with cancer's produced by them.

MCQs for chapter review

Oncogenic viruses

1) **Which is not oncogenic virus** (AIIMS, June-97)
(a) HTLV-1 (b) Herpes simplex (c) Papilloma virus (d) HBV
2) **Oncogenic RNA virus is**
(a) Avian leukosis virus (b) Herpes virus (c) Adeno virus (d) Toga virus
3) **Most common oncogenic RNA virus**
(a) Retrovirus (b) Picornavirus (c) Orthomyxo virus (d) Paramyxo virus
4) **RNA oncogenic virus amongst the following is?**
(a) HIV (b) HTLV (c) HBV (d) Cytomegalo virus
5) **Oncogenic virus** (AIIMS, June-97)
(a) CMV (b) VZV (c) Polio virus (d) EBV
6) **Which of the following has malignant potential** (PGI -05)
(a) HSV-1 (b) EBV (c) CMV (d) Varicella
7) **Which of the following "Oncogenic viruses" is so far not shown to be oncogenic in man**
(a) Hepatitis B virus (b) Epstein Barr virus (c) Herpes simplex virus type 2 (d) Adenovirus (e) Human T cell lymphotropic virus 1

Oncogenic parasites

8) **Pancreatic Ca is caused by** (AI-01)
(a) *Fasciola* (b) *Clonorchis* (c) *Paragonimus* (d) None
9) **Cholangiocarcinoma is caused by** (PGI, June-02)
(a) *Fasciola* infestation (b) *Clonorchis* infestation (c) *Paragonimus* infestation (d) *Ascaris* infestation (e) None of above
10) **Causes of biliary tract carcinoma after ingesting infected fish** (AIIMS, Nov-10)
(a) *Gnathostoma* (b) *Angiostrongylus cantonensis* (c) *Clonorchis sinensis* (d) *H diminuta*

Answers of MCQs & explanation

1) **All options are wrong**
2) **(a)**
3) **(a)**
4) **(a) & (b)**
5) **(a) & (d)**
6) **(a), (b) & (c)**

} Follow section, **oncogenic viruses (table-1)** for explanation

7) **(d)**

- Follow section, **oncogenic viruses (table-2)** for explanation

8) **(b)**
9) **(b)**
10) **(c)**

} Follow section, **oncogenic parasites** for explanation

105 Bioterrorism

Learning heading & subheadings

- Synonym::
- Definitions:
- Classification:
- Properties of bio-weapons:
- Advantages of using bio-weapons for terrorism:
- Disadvantages of using bio-weapons for terrorism:
- Mode of transmission:
- Preparedness before the bioterrorism:
- Warning sign of bioterrorism:
- Steps after attack:

❖ Synonym:
Biological warfare or germ warfare.

❖ Definitions:

- **Bioterrorism:** According to the U.S. Centres for Disease Control and Prevention bioterrorism is defined as "the deliberate release of viruses, bacteria, fungi, toxins or other harmful agents to cause illness or death in people, animals or plants".
- **Bio-weapons or biological agents:** Agents useful for bioterrorism like viruses, bacteria, fungi or toxins are **called bio-weapons** or **biological agents.**

❖ Classification:
CDC, classified the bio-weapons in 3 categories like A, B & C as shown in **table-1.**

- **Category A:** These high-priority agents pose a risk to national security, can be easily transmitted and disseminated from person to person, result in high mortality, have potential major public health impact or require special action for public health preparedness.
- **Category B:** These are moderately easy to disseminate, result in moderate morbidity rates and low mortality rates; and require specific enhancements of CDC's diagnostic capacity and enhanced disease surveillance.
- **Category C:** These are emerging pathogens that could be engineered for mass dissemination in the future because of availability, ease of production and dissemination, and potential for high morbidity and mortality rates and major health impact.

Bioweapon	Disease
Category A	
Bacillus anthracis	Anthrax
Clostridium botulinum toxin	Botulism
Yersinia pestis	Plague
Variola major	Smallpox
Francisella tularensis	Tularemia
- **Flaviviruses:** Like Yellow fever virus. KFD virus, Omsk haemorrhagic fever virus - **Bunyaviruses:** Like CCHF virus, Rift valley fever virus - **Filoviruses:** Like *Ebolavirus*, *Marburgvirus* - **Arenaviruses:** Like lassa virus, machupo virus, junin virus, guanarito virus & Sabia virus	Viral hemorrhagic fevers
Category B	
Brucella species	Brucellosis
Epsilon toxin of *Clostridium perfringens*	Food poisoning
Salmonella species, *E. coli* O157:H7, *Shigella*.	Food poisoning
Burkholderia mallei	Glanders
Burkholderia pseudomallei	Melioidosis
Chlamydia psittaci	Psittacosis
Coxiella burnetii	Q fever
Ricinus communis (castor beans)	Ricin toxin poisoning
Abrin toxin from *Abrus precatorius* (Rosary peas, Gunja, Rati etc.)	Abrin toxin poisoning
Staphylococcal enterotoxin B	Food poisoning
Rickettsia prowazekii	Epidemic typhus
Water safety threat - *Vibrio cholerae* - *Cryptosporidium parvum*	- Cholera - Cryptosporidiosis
- **Alphaviruses:** Like Eastern equine encephalitis virus, Western equine encephalitis virus, Venezuelan equine encephalitis virus - **Flaviviruses:** Like West Nile virus, Saint Louis virus, dengue fever virus	Viral encephalitis
Category C (Emerging agents)	
Nipah virus	Encephalitis
Hantavirus	Haemorrhagic fever renal syndrome
SARS –coronavirus	SARS
H1N1 (a strain of influenza)	Swine flu

Table-1: Bio-weapons & disease

✓ Notes:

- ***Clostridium botulinum* toxin:** Most dangerous & most likely to be used in bioterrorism is toxin of *Clostridium botulinum*, which causes botulism.
- **Yellow rain:**
- ***C. immitis*:**

} Follow chapter → General Properties of fungus

❖ **Properties of bio-weapons:** These are either natural agents or mutated or altered agent with increase virulence, increase drug resistance or with increase communicability to make them more dangerous.

❖ **Advantages of using bio-weapons for terrorism:** Bioterrorism is an attractive weapon because biological agents are

- Relatively easy to obtain.
- Inexpensive.
- Can be easily disseminated.
- Can cause widespread fear and panic beyond the actual physical damage.
- Disrupt the economy.

❖ **Disadvantages of using bio-weapons for terrorism:** Bio-weapons are like two edge sword, as it damage not only to enemies but also to friendly forces.

❖ **Mode of transmission:** Spread via air, water, food or from person to person.

❖ **Preparedness before the bioterrorism:** The American Red Cross, in cooperation with the CDC, has developed a detailed plan that gives people the proper steps to take to prepare in the event there is a bioterrorism attack.

➢ **Storage of all needful items:** The first step starts long before there is an attack. People must have appropriate supplies stored in a safe place in their house, where they work, and even in their cars. List includes following items.

- Water.
- Food.
- Items for infants: Diapers, bottles, pacifiers, powdered milk & medications not requiring refrigeration.
- Items for seniors, disabled people or anyone with serious allergies.
- Kitchen accessories.
- Power supply: A portable battery, powered radio or television and extra fresh batteries.
- A first aid kit.
- Sanitation and hygiene items: Shampoo, deodorant, toothpaste, toothbrushes, comb and brush, lip balm, sunscreen, contact lenses, any medications regularly used, toilet paper, soap, hand sanitizer, liquid detergent, feminine supplies, plastic garbage bags (heavy-duty) and ties (for personal sanitation uses), medium-sized plastic bucket with tight lid, disinfectant and household chlorine bleach.
- Other essential items: paper, pencil, needles, thread, small A-B-C-type fire extinguisher, medicine dropper, whistle, and emergency-preparedness manual.
- Entertainment: including games, books, favourite dolls and stuffed animals for small children.
- A map of the area marked with places you could go and their telephone numbers.
- An extra set of keys and IDs: Including keys for cars and any properties owned and copies of driver's licenses, passports, and work-identification badges.
- Cash, coins, and copies of credit cards.
- Copies of medical prescriptions.
- Matches in a waterproof container.
- A small tent, compass, and shovel.

❖ **Warning sign of bioterrorism:**

➢ **Drug resistance:** Potential clues that raise suspicion for a bioterrorism attack include new types of antibiotic resistance in bacteria, because some biologic agents are modified (weaponised) to make them more lethal.

➢ **Multiples cases:** Unusual numbers of cases of a disease with atypical presentation. Large number of ill or dead people in a small geographic area, multiple dead animals of different species and patients with multiple different diseases, indicating a mixed attack.

➢ **Clinical features:** The symptoms of illness caused by the different bioterrorism agents are frequently very nonspecific. Many of the agents cause a "flu-like" illness. These symptoms would include fever, cough, nausea, vomiting & headache.

❖ **Steps after attack:**

➢ **Right information:** If there has been a bioterrorism attack, the first important step is to get information immediately from the news media as to the right course of action.

➢ **Skin cleaning:** If you think that you have been exposed to a biological agent, the most important thing to do is to quickly remove your clothing and wash off your skin. Most biological agents cannot penetrate intact skin. Showering with soap and water will remove most agents from the skin. If you have already inhaled or ingested the agent, decontamination using soap and water may not help you but might help prevent exposing other family members or co-workers.

➢ **Mask:** If the biological agent has been released into the air but you do not believe (or do not know) you have been exposed, you can utilize masks (HEPA) to help prevent inhalation of the agent.

- **Isolation and quarantine:**
  - Isolation is keeping people known to be ill away from other people. Quarantine is keeping people who may have been exposed away from other people.
- **No outdoor visit:** The problem is that many times we may not know who has been exposed. In these cases, the public health officials will likely recommend that everyone stay in their homes and avoid all public gatherings.
- **Shifting:** For some terrorist attacks, it may be correct to try and leave the area.
- **Communication break:** With bioterrorism, there may be the possibility of person to person transmission of disease (for example, measles, influenza, avian flu, smallpox, plague & viral hemorrhagic fevers). In the case it may be necessary to avoid contact with infected people or just remain inside for a period of time until the infected people are no longer contagious.
- **Follow messages:** The key action is to understand the recommendations from public health officials as delivered through the news media.
- **Testing:** It is very hard to differentiate many of the different diseases initially, and tests to confirm the diagnosis often must be done at specialized state laboratories and may require weeks until the results are received.
- **Supportive treatment:** Many diseases do not even have a treatment other than supportive care which can often be done at home.
- **Drug distribution:** Among the community by government.

Question bank

Short notes

1) Bioterrorism.

Short questions for theory/viva questions

1) Name the four bio-weapons from category A.

MCQs

1) **Most potent and potential agent that can be used for bioterrorism,-** (AI-11)
(a) Plague (b) Smallpox (c) TB (d) *Clostridium botulinum*
2) **Which of the following is not group A bioterrorism**
(a) Small pox (b) Haemorrhagic fever (c) *Salmonella* (d) Botulism
3) **Category A bioterrorism agents are** (AIIMS, Nov-06)
(a) Ebola (b) *Yersinia* (c) *Clostridium botulinum* (d) *Rickettsia* (e) Cholera
4) **Bioterrorism group A agent**
(a) Q fever (b) Typhus fever (c) *Brucella* (d) Anthrax
5) **Micro-organism used as weapon in biological terrorism** (PGI-02)
(a) Small pox virus (b) Rabies virus (c) Ebola virus (d) Influenza C virus (e) Human parvo virus
6) **Which of the following is belongs to category B of bioterrorism**
(a) Cholera (b) Anthrax (c) Plague (d) Botulism

Answers of MCQs & explanation

1) **(d)**
- *Clostridium botulinum* toxin is the most dangerous & most commonly used agent

2) **(c)**
3) **(a), (b) & (c)**
4) **(d)**
5) **(a) & (c)**
6) **(a)**

(2–6) Follow section, **classification (table-1)** for explanation

106 Microbiology of water, milk and air

Learning heading & subheadings

- Microbiology of water
- Microbiology of milk
- Microbiology of air

Microbiology of water

❖ **Drinking water or whole some water:** Water that is fit to use for drinking, cooking, food preparation or washing without any potential to human health & with following properties **called drinking water or whole some water.**

- Biological properties: Free from all pathogenic microorganisms.
- Chemical properties: Free from all chemicals like gases, metals, solvents, pesticides & hydrocarbons
- Physical properties: Should be pleasant for taste, odour & colour.

❖ **Microbiology of water:**

➢ **Water flora (saprobes):** These are the organisms which are normally present in water & non pathogenic to humans. Their presence in water does not warrant threat. They are arising from decomposing organic matter. List of water flora is available in **table-1**.

➢ **Water borne pathogens:**

✪ **Pathogens:** These are the organisms which are concerned with life threatening disease & their presence in water cause major threat for its use.

✪ **Sources:**

- These organisms are arising either due to sewage (faeces, urine etc.) contamination of water from animals or humans source or by soil wash due to rainy water.
- These are either community acquired or hospital acquired.
- List of water pathogens with their source is available in **table-2**.

Micrococcus	*Flavobacter*
Pseudomonas	*Alkaligenes*
Serratia	*Acintobacter*
Bacteriophage	

Table-1: Water flora

Organism	Disease
Sewage source	
Escherichia coli	Diarrhoea
Vibrio cholerae	Cholera
Clostridium perfrigens	Food poisoning & others
Salmonella spp.	Enteric fever & food poisoning
Enterococcus faecalis	Diarrhoea
Proteus spp.	Diarrhoea
Shigella spp.	Dysentery
Pseudomonas	Septicemia
Leptospira spp.	Leptospirosis
Entero viruses	Enteritis
E histolytica	Amoebiasis
G lamblia	Giardiasis
Cestodes like *T saginata, T solium* etc.	Intestinal diseases
S haematobium	Intestinal & urinary illness
Intestinal nematodes like *A lumbricoides, S stercoralis, A duodenale, E vermicularis* etc.	Intestinal diseases
D medinensis	Dracunculiasis
Soil source	
Bacillus spp.	Minor illness
Enterobacter spp.	Septicemia

Table-2: Water borne pathogens

❖ **Indicator organisms:**

➢ **Definitions:** These are the intestinal organisms which contaminate the water.

➢ **Clinical significances:**

- These are present in excess numbers so can be detected easily.

- They are more resistant than other organisms to disinfectants.
- Their presence in water indicate that sewage contamination of water & water supplies need chlorination, however mere presence of these indicator organism does not means the sewage contamination.
- Detection of indicator organism gives ideas about faecal contamination of water (**called faecal pollution**).

❖ Bacteriological examinations of water:

➢ **Aims:** To detect the indicator organism to rule out the faecal contamination.

➢ **Frequency of testing:** From daily to monthly depends on the size of population served.

➢ **Sample collections:**

- Heat sterilised screw capped bottle about 200 ml capacity should be used as container. Collect about 150 ml of water.
- Care should be taken to avoid the environmental or hand contamination of collecting person.
- Add sodium thiosulphate to neutralise the bactericidal effects of residual chlorine.
- Tap water: Water is collected only after running it from tap for 2-3 minutes.
- Water from stream or lake: Open the bottle after immersing it at the depth of 30 cm with mouth facing the current.
- Water from well: It is collected by bottle tide with heavy weight like stone.

➢ **Transport:** Bottle should be properly labelled & sent to the laboratory as soon as at least within 6 hours. If delay is anticipated, the bottle should be kept in ice box & protect from light.

➢ **Indicator organism & testing methods:** Following are the different tests & different microbes.

I. Bacteria

A. Plate count:→ Flow chart-1

B. Detection of coliform bacteria like *E coli*:

✪ **Definition:** Coliform means bacteria which ferment the lactose like *E coli, Klebsiella* etc.

✪ **Tests:**

i. Presumptive coliform count test: → Fig.-1

- **Synonyms:**
  - Most probable number (MPN) test.
  - Multiple tube method.
- **Meaning:**
  - Test is **called presumptive**, because the final result may be due to organism other than coliform category which further required confirmation.
  - Most probable number (MPN) means coliform count per 100 ml of water.
- **Principle:** Water to be tested is diluted serially & inoculated in lactose broth, coliforms if present in water ferment the lactose of medium to produce acid and gas. Acid is indicated by colour change of the medium & gas is indicated by bubbles collection in the inverted Durham tube. The numbers of total coliforms are determined by counting the number of tubes giving positive reaction (i.e both colour change and gas production) and comparing the pattern of positive results (the number of tubes showing growth at each dilution) with standard statistical tables. If the **presumptive test** is negative, no further testing is required, & the water source is considered microbiologically safe. If, however, any tube in the series shows acid & gas, the water is considered unsafe & the **confirmatory test** is performed on the tube displaying a positive reaction.
- **Steps of test:** Done in two steps like screening & confirmatory test as follows.

a. Screening (presumptive) test for coliform

○ Aims:

- To check whether the coliform are present or not in water.
- To check the numbers of coliform per 100 ml of water.
- To check the quality of water.

○ Requirements:

- Medium: Lactose broth or Mac Conkey broth (with pH indicator like bromocresol purple or neutral red or others) or Lauryl tryptose (lactose) broth in single and double strength concentration.

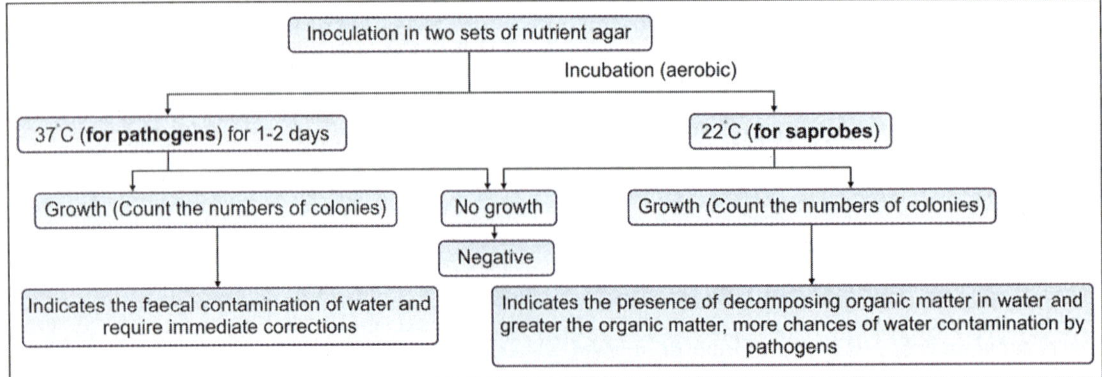

Flow chart-1: Plate count

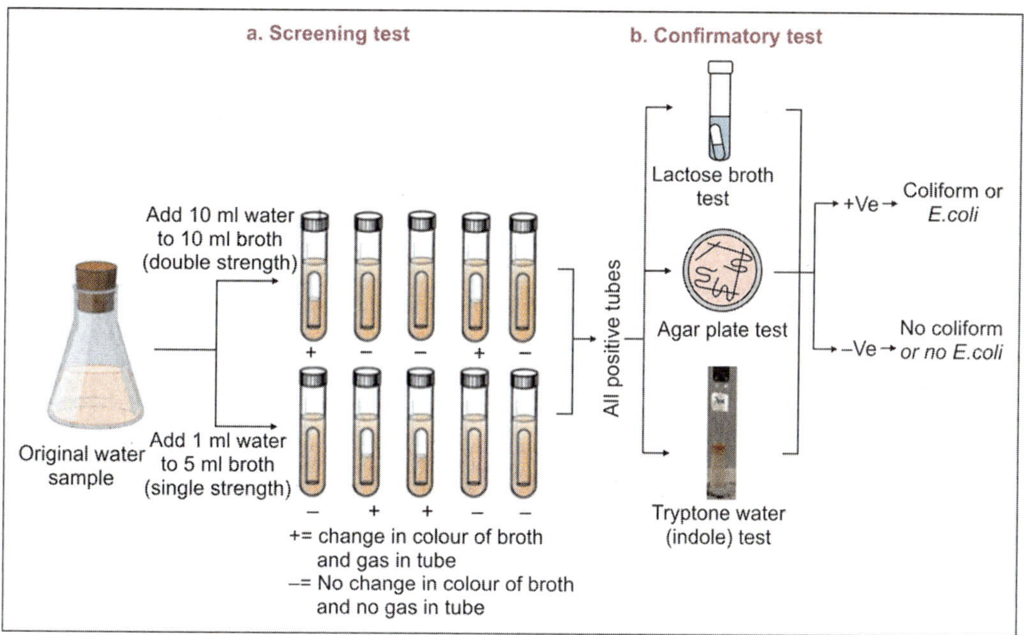

Figure-1: Presumptive coliform count test

- Glass wares: Bottle (50ml), test tubes of various capacities (10ml, 5ml etc.) & Durham tube.
- Others: Sterile pipettes.

o Steps:

- Examine the Durham tubes to make sure that they are full of liquid with no air bubbles.
- Take 1 bottle of double strength (50ml), 5 tubes of double strength (10ml) & 5 tubes of single strength (5ml) for water sample to be tested.
- Using a sterile pipette add 50 ml of water to the bottle containing 50 ml double strength medium. Similarly add 10 ml of water to 5 tubes containing 10 ml double strength medium & add 1 ml of water to 5 tubes containing 5 ml single strength medium.
- Incubate the bottle & tubes at 37°C for 24 hrs.
- If no tubes appear positive re-incubate up to 48 hrs.

o Results:

1. **Presumptive count:**

- Compare the number of tube giving positive reaction (both colour change and gas production in Durham tube) to a standard **McCrady's probability table** (**table-3**) and record the number of bacteria present in it. This is **called presumptive coliform count** or **most probable number (MPN) of coliform** present in tested water.
- Any further positive (positive after re-incubation) is added to the previous figures.
- For example: A water sample tested shows a result of 1-4 (2 × 10 ml positive, 2 × 5 ml positive) gives an MPN value of 4, i.e. the water sample contains an estimated 4 coliforms per 100 ml.

2. **Quality of water:** The MPN is categorises as excellent, satisfactory, intermediate & unsatisfactory as mentioned in **table-4.**

- **Interpretation:**

o -Ve result: If the presumptive test is negative, no further testing is performed, and the water source is considered microbiologically safe.

o +Ve result:

- If any tube in the series shows acid & gas, the test is +Ve & water is considered unsafe and the confirmed test is performed on the tube showing a positive reaction.
- MPN positive always does not indicate the faecal contamination, as some of them may be by environmental contamination, hence it is further tested by confirmatory test.

b. Confirmatory test or Eijkman test or differential coliform test:

o Aims: To check whether the acid & gas positive screening test is due to coliform (*E coli*) or by other bacteria.

o Requirements:

1. 3 ml lactose-broth or brilliant green lactose fermentation broth in tube for lactose-broth test or
2. Agar plate (slant) for agar plate test or
3. 3 ml tryptone water for indole test
4. Medium for citrate test.

o Steps:

1. **Lactose-broth test:**

Numbers of tube giving appositive reaction out of			
1 bottle of 50 ml water	5 tube of 10 ml water	5 tube of 1 ml water	Bacterial count
0	0	0	0
0	0	1	1
0	0	2	2
0	1	0	1
0	1	1	2
0	1	1	2
0	1	2	3
0	2	0	2
0	2	1	3
0	2	2	4
0	3	0	3
0	3	1	5
0	4	0	5
1	0	0	1
1	0	1	3
1	0	2	4
1	0	3	6
1	1	0	3
1	1	1	5
1	1	2	7
1	1	3	9
1	2	0	5
1	2	1	7
1	2	2	10
1	2	3	12
1	3	0	8
1	3	1	11
1	3	2	14
1	3	3	18
1	3	4	20
1	4	0	13
1	4	1	17
1	4	2	20
1	4	3	30
1	4	4	35
1	4	5	40
1	5	0	25
1	5	1	35
1	5	2	50
1	5	3	90
1	5	4	160
1	5	5	180+

Table-3: McCrady's probability table

Quality of drinking water	MPN/ 100 ml of water	
	Coliform / 100 ml	E coli / 100 ml
Excellent	0	0
Satisfactory	1-3	0
Intermediate	4-9	0
Unsatisfactory	≥10	≥1

Table-4: Quality of drinking water according to MPN

- From all positive tubes (showing acid & gas) of screening test, transfer one loopful of medium to lactose-broth.
- Incubate the inoculated lactose-broth at 44°C (performed in thermostatically controlled water bath that do not deviate > 0.5°C from 44°C) & examined after 24 ± 2 hours.
- If no gas production is seen, further incubate up to maximum of 48 ±3 hours to check gas production.

2. **Agar plate/slant test:**
- From all positive tubes (showing acid & gas) of screening test, transfer one loopful of medium to agar plate or slant.
- The agar slants should be incubated at 37°C for 24± 2 hours.

3. **Tryptone water (indole) test**
- From all positive tubes (showing acid & gas) of screening test, transfer one loopful of medium to tryptone water.
- Incubate the tryptone water at (44.5 ±0.2°C) for 18-24 hours.
- Following incubation, add approximately 0.1ml of Kovacs reagent and mix gently.

- Results:

1. **Lactose-broth test:**
- Gas production within the Durham tube confirmed the *E coli.*
- The absence of gas formation in lactose broth confirmed no *E coli.*

2. **Agar plate/slant test:**
- Prepare the gram stained smear from the slants should be examined microscopically for GNB (coliform like *E coli*).
- The absence of GNB Gram stain constitutes a negative test (absence of coliforms in the tested sample).

3. **Tryptone water (indole) test:** Positive indole is indicated by a red colour ring over the aqueous phase of the medium which confirmed the *E coli.*

- **Advantages of MPN test:**
- Ease of interpretation, either by observation or gas emission.
- Sample toxins are diluted.
- Effective method to analyse highly turbid samples such as sediments, sludge, mud, etc. that cannot be analysed by membrane filtration.
- **Disadvantages of MPN test:**
- Results are not very accurate.
- Requires more hardware (glassware) and media.
- Probability of false positives.

ii. **Membrane filtration method:**

- **Principle:** A measured volume of water is filtered through a membrane filter with a pore size of 22μm. If bacteria present they are retained on the surface of the filter & later can grow over media on subsequent placing of membrane.
- **Steps of test:**
- Filter the water through membrane filter, which retain the water bacteria if present.
- Place the membrane filter on media facing upwards.
- Incubate at appropriate temperature for 18 hrs.
- Colonies that develop on the surface of the membrane are counted.

- After 18 hrs incubation presumptive coliform counts & *E coli* count can be done.

iii. Enzyme method:

- **Principle:** It based on detection of different enzymes of coliform & *E coli* like
  - **β- galucuronidase:** Specific for faecal *E coli.*
  - **β- galactosidase:** Specific for faecal coliform.

C. Detection of faecal *Streptococci*:

- **Principle:** Faecal *Streptococci* like *Enterococcus faecalis* etc. are present in water for a very short time, hence their detection in water suggest recent faecal contamination of water.
- **Methods:**

1. **Glucose azide broth test**
   - **Steps:**
     - All positive tubes presumptive coliform test, are subcultured on tubes containing 5 ml of glucose azide broth.
     - Incubate at 45°C for 18-24 hours.
   - **Result:** Presence of *Enterococcus faecalis* is indicated by gas production within 18 hours.
   - **Confirmation:** It is done by plating the positive tubes on Mac Conkey's agar or bile esculin agar.
   - **Specification:** It can be done to know the exact source of contamination like *E. faecalis* (human), *E. avium* (bird), *Strept bovis* (cow) & *Strept. equinus* (horse).
2. **Membrane filtration method:** Also useful for faecal *Streptococci.*

D. Detection of *Clostridium perfrigens*:

- **Principle:** *Cl perfrigens* are present in water for a very long time; hence their detection in water does not suggest recent faecal contamination of water.
- **Methods:**

1. **Litmus milk medium test**
   - **Steps:**
     - Inoculate the varying quantities of water in litmus milk medium.
     - Incubate anaerobically at 37°C for 5 days.
   - **Result:** Stormy clot (stormy fermentation) indicate the presence of *Cl perfrigens.*

E. Detection of other pathogens like *S typhi* & *V cholerae*: Such bacteria are detected by Membrane filtration method in addition to below mentioned methods.

- ***S typhi*:** Equal volume of water is added to the double strength selenite broth followed by subculturing on selective media. Growth is identified by biochemical tests & antisera.
- ***V cholerae:*** Water sample is mixed with alkaline peptone water in 1:9 ratios, followed by subculturing on selective media. Growth is identified by biochemical tests & serotyping.

II. Viruses

- Entero viruses are able to contaminate the water.
- There is no specific test to detect the viruses as indicator organisms.
- They are destroyed by chlorination with free residual chlorine at least 0.5mg/litre, for 30 minute (contact period) at pH < 8 & turbidity is ≤1 nephelometric.

III. Parasites

- Different parasites as mentioned in **table-2** are contaminating the water.
- There is no specific test to detect the parasites as indicator organisms.
- They are resistant chlorination.

Microbiology of milk

Common sources of milk contamination:

- **Animals:** Faeces, urine, infected udder, teat canal & skin.
- **Human:** Hands of human handlers.
- **Environment:** Water mixed with milk, air (dust) & utensils.

Microbes in milk:

- **According to changes done by microbes in milk:** Following are different types.

1. **Acid forming bacteria:**
   - It includes bacteria which ferments the lactose to produce acids, especially lactic acid, which leads the formation of a smooth gelatinous curd.
   - Examples: *Strept lactis, E faecalis* etc.
2. **Acid & gas forming bacteria:**
   - They produce acid & gas, which lead the formation of a smooth gelatinous curd riddled with gas bubbles.
   - Examples: Coliform bacilli (responsible for ropiness in milk after formation of acid & gas), *Cl perfrigens, Cl butyricum* etc.
3. **Alkali forming bacteria:**
   - They render the milk alkaline.
   - Examples: Aerobic spore bearers, *Alkaligenes* spp., *Achromobacter* etc.
4. **Proteolytic bacteria:**
   - It includes bacteria which breaks the protein present in milk.
   - Examples: *B subtilis, B cereus. P vulgaris* etc.
5. **Inert bacteria:**
   - These bacteria are not doing any changes in milk
   - Examples: Cocci of udder, *Achromobacter* spp. & few species of pathogenic bacteria etc.
6. **Human milk:** Human milk includes *Staph aureus, Staph epidermidis, Strept. mitis, Gaffkya tetragena* etc.

- **According to source:** → **Table-5**

Organism	Disease
Animal source	
M tuberculosis	Tuberculosis
Brucella spp.	Brucellosis
Salmonella spp.	Enteric fever & food poisoning
C burnetii	Q fever
Staph aureus	Staphylococcal food poisoning
Streptococcus spp.	Streptococcal infections
Bacillus anthracis	Anthrax
Leptospira spp.	Leptospirosis
C diphtheriae	Diphtheria
C. ulcerans	Throat ulcer
Campylobacter jejuni	Diarrhoea/dysentery
Yersinia enterocolitica	Gastroenteritis
Streptobacillus moniliformis	Haver hill fever
Cow pox virus	Cow pox
Paravaccinia (pseudocowpox) virus	Milker's nodule (node)
Coxcackie virus	Hand foot mouth disease
Tick borne encephalitis	Encephalitis
Human source	
Vibrio cholerae	Cholera
EHEC	Dysentery
Salmonella typhi & S paratyphi	Enteric fever
Shigella spp.	Dysentery
Staph aureus	Staphylococcal food poisoning
Streptococcus spp.	Streptococcal infections
Entero viruses	Enteritis
Hepatitis viruses	hepatitis

Table-5: Different sources of milk borne organisms

❖ **Mode of transmission:**

- All the organisms mentioned **table-5** are transmitted by ingestion of infected milk except like cow pox & milker's node which are transmitted by direct contact with udder during milking.
- *Streptobacillu moniliformis:* Milk contamination from nasal secretion rat.

❖ **Sterilisation/disinfection & sterility testing Of milk:** Following are the different methods of sterilisation / disinfection with sterility testing.

A. Thermised milk (equal to raw milk):

➢ **Method:** Raw milk that is heated for 15 seconds at 57-68^{0}C.

➢ **Sterility testing:**

1. By methylene blue reduction test

- **Principle:** Viable bacteria reduce the methylene blue in milk when kept in a dark place.
- **Steps:** Mix 1 ml methylene blue with 10 ml of milk in a sterile test tube & incubate at 37^{0}C in a dark place.
- **Result:** Milk is satisfactory if no change in colour in 30 minutes.
- **Advantages:**
  - Economical method.
  - It is simple & quick test useful to check the quality of milk after its arrival from the producer.

2. Resurazin test: Not significant.

B. Pasteurisation: Follow chapter → Sterilisation and disinfection

C. UHT –Ultra High Temperature method:

➢ **Method:** Milk is heated very rapidly in two stages (2nd stage is under pressure) at 125°C for a few seconds followed by rapid cooling & bottles as quickly as possible.

➢ **Sterility testing: Viable count test**

- **Steps:** Inoculate the serially diluted milk in yeast extract milk agar & then incubate at 30^{0}C or 21^{0}C (for unopened containers) for 72 hours.
- **Result:** Viable colony count in fixed amount of milk is done by multiplying the numbers of colonies with dilution factors. Viable colony count of UHT treated milk should be < 1000/ml.

D. Boiling:

➢ **Method:** Milk is heated at 100°C for a long time (up to 5 minutes).

➢ **Sterility testing: Turbidity test**

- **Principle:** In boiled milk all heat coagulable proteins are precipitated, so that it does not become turbid when ammonium sulphate is added.
- **Steps:** Add the ammonium sulphate to boiled milk.
- **Result:** Absence of turbidity is indicates adequate boiling.

E. Detection of specific pathogens:

➢ **Tubercle bacilli:** Following centrifugation of milk at 3000rpm, the deposit is inoculated over LJ medium or injected in guinea pig for isolation of bacilli.

➢ ***Brucella*:** Follow chapter → *Brucella* **(section laboratory diagnosis → animal brucellosis)**

Microbiology of air

❖ **Introduction:** Air is an important vehicle for transmission of many pathogenic organisms. A person inhale about 15 cubic metres of air per day, hence its must to know the microbial contents of air & its sterility.

❖ **Microbes in air:** Microbial contents of air are depends on place, whether indoor air or outdoor air,

➢ **Microbes in outdoor air:**

✪ **Effective factors:**

- Density of human & animal population.
- Nature of the soil.

- Density of vegetation.
- Atmospheric conditions: Humidity, temperature, wind conditions, rain fall, sunlight etc.

✪ **Microbes:** Mostly saprophytic organisms like
- Bacterial spores or spore bearing bacilli.
- *Achromobacter.*
- *Sarcina.*
- *Micrococcus.*
- Fungal spores & fungal hyphae.

➢ **Microbes in indoor air:** Indoor areas include hospital ward, operation theatre, laboratory, offices etc.

✪ **Effective factors:**
- Density of human population.
- Disturbances of clothes.
- Atmospheric conditions: Air conditioners, cleaning etc.

✪ **Microbes:** Mostly all pathogenic microorganisms causing respiratory tract infection & transmitted either via droplet nuclei or air borne route are indoor pathogens.

❖ Modes of transmission: Two modes.

- **Droplet nuclei:**
- **Air borne:**

} Follow chapter → Infections and infectious diseases

❖ Bacteriological examinations of air:

➢ **Methods:** Two methods as mentioned below.

A. Settle plate method:

- **Media required:**
  - **Blood agar:** It is preferred medium for overall fastidious, pathogenic, saprophytes & commensals.
  - **Nutrient agar:** Also a useful medium.
  - **Malt extract agar:** Useful for molds.
- **Method:**
  - Open & put the petri dish containing agar medium on surface for 30 minutes to 1 hour.
  - Bacteria carrying large dust particles present in air are settle down by gravity on the agar.
  - Incubate the plate at 37^0C for 24 hours.
- **Result:**

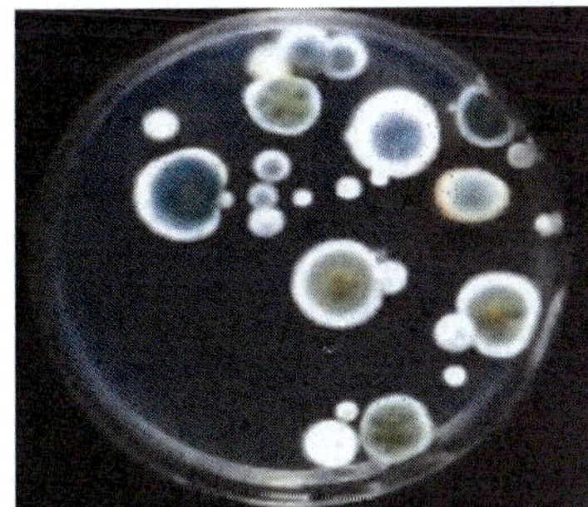

Figure-2: Colonies on settle plate

  - Colonies are developed after incubation **(fig.-2)**.
  - The numbers of the colonies formed indicate the numbers of settled particles containing bacteria.

B. Slit sampler technique:

- **Required materials:** A special equipment **called slit sampler**, as shown in **fig.-3** is required which has three parts.
  - An area to hold the petri dish.
  - Suction pump & slit.
  - Outer surface with slit.

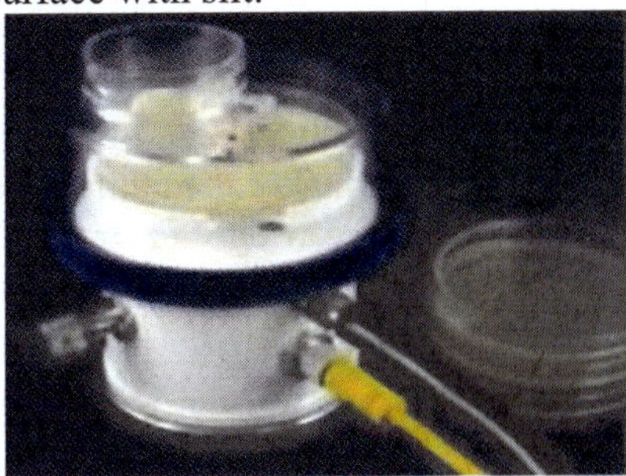

Figure-3: Slit sampler technique

- **Method:**
  - Air is sucked through the equipment at a rate of 1 cubic foot (28.3liter) per minute for 10 minutes & directed to a plate containing culture medium through the slit.
  - The plate is rotated mechanically to even spread of organisms.
  - Incubate the plate at 37^0C for 24 hours.
- **Result:**
  - Colonies are developed after incubation.
  - The numbers of the colonies formed indicate the numbers of settled particles containing bacteria.
- **Advantages:** Most efficient and convenient method for counting the number of bacteria carrying dust particles suspended in a unit volume of air.

➢ **Accepted limit of air pollution:** The upper limits of the bacterial count in air in various areas as follows.
- 50 per cubic feet in factories, offices & homes.
- 10 per cubic feet in general operation theatre.
- 1 per cubic feet in operation theatre for neurosurgery.

❖ Fumigation of indoor air & sterility testing:

➢ **Methods:**

i. Formaldehyde gas fumigation:

- **Legal aspect:** Formaldehyde is a schedule 1 chemical under the COSHH (Control of Substances Hazardous to Health) Regulations and has a Maximum Exposure Limit (MEL) of 2 ppm.
- **Target areas:** Hospital ward, operation theatre, laboratory, offices, other rooms, books, furniture, cloths, bed, pillows, bed sheet etc.
- **Biological (mechanism) actions of formaldehyde:** Formaldehyde is an alkylating agent, having bactericidal, virucidal, fungicidal & sporicidal properties & it inactivates the microorganisms by reacting with carboxyl, amino, hydroxyl and

sulphydral groups of proteins as well as amino groups of nucleic acid bases.

- **Precautions:**
- Fumigation is effective at above the temperature of 20ºC & relative humidity of 65%.
- Formalin is commercially available as 40% solution of formaldehyde in water. When formalin is heated formaldehyde vapour is generated. But, concentrations encountered during fumigation is many hundred times higher than this, so fumigation procedure must be carried out only by trained personnel under strictly defined conditions. All workers using formaldehyde must be aware of safe handling procedures.
- Under certain conditions formaldehyde can react with hydrochloric acid & chlorine containing disinfectants like hypochlorites to form chlormethyl ether, a potent lung carcinogen. So hydrochloric acid & chlorine containing disinfectants must be removed from the room before fumigation.
- **Fumigation procedure:**
- Step 1: It includes all the **preparation** as follows
- Entire block should be thoroughly cleaned before fumigation. All apparatus such as windows, doors, floor, walls, surgery table, all washable equipments, bulb, air conditioner, etc., should be cleaned according to manufacturer instructions.
- Close windows and ventilators tightly. If any openings found seal it with cellophane tape or other material to avoid the leak of fume.
- Switch off all lights, and other electrical & electronical items.
- Calculate the room size in cubic feet (Length×Breadth×Height) & calculate the required amount of formaldehyde as given in step 3.
- Adequate care must be taken by wearing cap, mask, foot cover, spectacle etc.
- Formaldehyde is irritant to eye & nose; and it has also been recognized as a potential carcinogen. So the fumigating person must be provided with the personal protective equipments (PPE).
- Paste a warning notice on the front door indicating fumigation is in progress as shown in **fig.-4.**

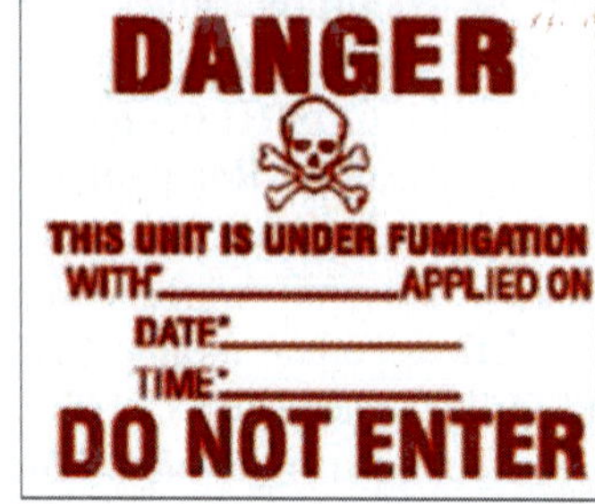

Figure-4: Fumigation symbol

- Step 2: Following are the different **fumigation procedures**.

a. Formaldehyde fumigation with electric boiler method (recommended):

- For Each 1000 cubic feet, 500 ml of formaldehyde (40% solution) added in 1000 ml of distilled water (if not available use tape water) in an electric boiler.
- Switch on the boiler, leave the room and seal the door.
- After 45 minutes (variable depending to volume present in the boils apparatus/its heating proficiency) switch off the boiler without entering in to the room (switch off the main electric supply from outside).

b. Formaldehyde fumigation with potassium permanganate ($KMnO_4$) method:

- Here the heat generation is induced by an oxidizer $KMnO_4$, which results in auto boiling and generates fume from formaldehyde.
- Take 500 ml of formaldehyde (40% solution) in 1000 ml of distilled water (if not available use tap water) for 1000 cubic feet of area, in a heat resistant bowel preferably in steel bucket and then add 450gm of $KMnO_4$ for 1000 cubic feet of area volume.
- Repeat the same in separate bucket for every another 1000 cubic feet until it reaches the complete area volume. It is important to add $KMnO_4$ to all buckets simultaneously to reduce the exposure to fume (*i.e.,* need 3 or 4 persons at different location).
- After the initiation of formaldehyde vapour, immediately leave the room and seal it for at least 12 to 24 hours.

- Step 3: Neutralization.
- Before neutralization, formaldehyde fumigation system should be taken out from the room. Then the toxicity of formaldehyde vapour should be neutralized with ammonia solution.
- Place a cotton ball and pour 300 ml of 10% ammonia (for each 500 ml of formaldehyde used) on the floor, at least 4 hours before (07 a.m.) the "sterility test".
- Formaldehyde gas reacts with ammonia gas and produce hexamine (synonym hexamethylenetetramine) which is considered a harmless substance.
- Switch on the air conditioner, at least 2 hours before the "sterility test".
- **Example:**
- Area = L×B×H = 20 × 15 × 10 = 3000 cubic feet (Note: Make it into nearest 1000, if the volume is in fraction.
- Formaldehyde required for fumigation = 500 ml for 1000 cubic feet = So, 1500 ml of formaldehyde required (to be diluted in 3000 ml of distilled water).

- Ammonia required for neutralization = 300 ml of 10% ammonia for 500 ml of formaldehyde = So 900 ml of 10% ammonia required.
- **Sterility testing:**
- It includes collection of air sample plate & swabs from different surfaces plus different equipments of room to be fumigated, before (pre fumigation sterility samples) & after (post fumigation sterility samples) the fumigation.
- Any positive culture growth from above samples indicates the repetition of fumigation.
- **Data records:** A record (log book) should be kept and properly maintained for all fumigations with following details, date & time of fumigation, date & time of neutralization, personnel involved, and the dates of "sterility test doe " & their results.
- **Advantages:**
- Low cost.
- Wide spectrum of activities like bactericidal, virucidal, fungicidal & sporicidal.
- Fumigants can reach the place where sprays, aerosols can't reach.
- Reduce residue problems in treated areas.
- Fumigants are used where standard call for **"zero microbial tolerance"** in products or living environment.
- **Disadvantages:**
- Formalin is irritant to eye & mucosa, this effect is nullified by ammonia.
- Carcinogenic for lung, nose & nasal passage.

ii. **Other methods:** Above all disadvantages of formaldehyde are overcome by using following newer methods, but these are expensive.

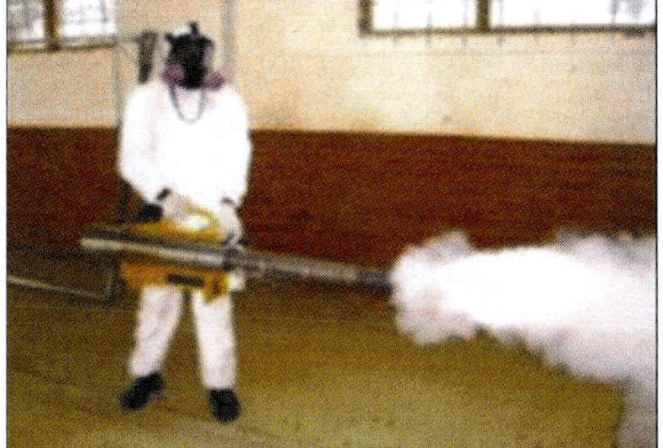

Figure-5: Fogging method

1. Specialise air flow pattern: Only purified air is circulating & contaminated air going out continuously.
2. Hydrogen peroxide (H_2O_2):
3. H_2O_2 with silver nitrate
4. Parasitic acid

(2–4: Spread by fogging machine (**fig.-5**))

5. Phosphine
6. 1,3 dichoropropane.
7. Chloropicrin.
8. Methyle isocynate.
9. Hydrogene cyanide.
10. Sulfuryl fluoride.
11. Iodoform.
12. Methyle bromide.

Question bank

Short notes

1) Bacteriological examination of water/milk/air.

Short questions

1) Define: Coliform bacteria & Most probable number (MPN) of bacteria in water.
2) Name the four milk borne pathogens.
3) How you fumigate the operation theatre?

MCQs for chapter review

MCQs

1) **All are transmitted by milk except** (AI-90)
(a) Tuberculosis (b) Brucellosis (c) Q fever (d) Leishmaniasis

Answers of MCQs & explanation

1) **(d)**
- Option a, b & c: Follow section, **Microbiology of milk & table-5**, for explanation
- Leishmaniasis : Transmitted by sand fly

Prakash

Section IX
Practical Microbiology

107 Exercises and specimens in practical examination

Learning heading & subheadings

- Exercises
- Specimens
  - Media
  - Bio-chemical tests
  - Serological tests
  - Animals
  - Slides
  - Parasite's specimens
  - Graphs or figures or pictures
  - Other specimens

Exercises

a. **Gram stain**
b. **Ziehl-Neelsen stain**
c. **Stool examination for parasites**
d. **Blood examination for parasites**
e. **Culture exercise**

1. Haemolytic colony on blood agar.
2. Pink spreading colony of *E. coli* on Mac Conkey's medium.
3. Pink mucoid colony of *K. Pneumoniae* on Mac Conkey's medium.
4. Pale/colourless colony of non-lactose fermenters on Mac Conkey's medium.
5. Pigments production by *P. aeruginosa* in nutrient agar slant.
6. Golden yellow pigment production by *Staph. aureus* in nutrient agar.
7. Lemon yellow pigment production by *Staph. citrus* in nutrient agar.
8. White pigment production by *Staph. albus* in nutrient agar.
9. Black colony by *C. diphtheriae* in potassium tellurite.
10. Black colony by *Salmonella* spp. in Wilson &Blair medium.
11. Yellow colony by *V. cholerae* in TCBS medium.
12. Semi solid agar stab for motility.
13. White colony by *Candida albicans* in SDA.
14. Brown / black / greenish-yellow colony by *Aspergillus spp.* in SDA.

Specimens

Following specimens can be ask in spotting exercise.

Media

All media described in **chapter → culture media** can be kept in practical examination as specimen for identification.

Bio-chemical tests

1. Sugar fermentation tests.
2. IMViC test.

3. Oxidase test.
4. Catalase test.
5. Urease test.
6. PPA test.
7. TSI test.
8. Slide & tube coagulase test.
9. Hanging drop preparation.

Serological tests

1. VDRL tile for VDRL test.
2. RPR card for RPR test.
3. Slide for Counter Immuno Electrophoresis (CIE) test.
4. Slide for latex particle agglutination tests like RF test & ASO test.
5. Slide Widal test.
6. Tube Widal test.
7. RPHA plate with fix microtitre well for RPHA test.
8. Coomb's test.
9. CFT.
10. ELISA plate with free microtitre well for ELISA.
11. Immuno comb test (Rapid ELISA) for HIV.
12. Immuno chromatographic test (Virucheck for HBsAg in strip form or SD HIV1/2 for HIV in biscuits form).
13. Immuno concentration test (HIV-Tridot test).

Animals

1. Nine banded armadillo (*Dasypus novemcinctus*).
2. Rabbit.
3. Guinea pig.
4. Rat.
5. Mouse.
6. Sheep.
7. Monkey.

Slides

1. GPC: Gram Positive Cocci under Gram stain.
2. GPB: Gram Positive Bacilli under Gram stain.
3. GNC: Gram Negative Cocci under Gram stain.
4. GNB: Gram Negative Bacilli under Gram stain.
5. AFB: Acid Fast Bacilli under ZN stain.
6. *Treponema pallidum* under Fontana's stain.
7. Metachromatic granules (*C. diphtheriae*) under Albert stain.
8. Bacterial spores under modified ZN stain.
9. *Candida albicans* (Pseudohyphae) under gram stain.
10. Filamentous fungi under KOH wet mount.
11. Amastigote form of *L. donovani.*
12. Fertilised eggs of *Ascaris lumbricoides.*
13. Unfertilised eggs of *Ascaris lumbricoides.*
14. Eggs of *Tinea* spp.
15. Eggs of *H. nana.*
16. Malarial parasites: Mostly
    - Ring stage of *P. vivax.*
    - Gametocytes (Crescent) of *P. falciparum.*
17. Microfilariae under Romanowsky's stain.

Parasite's specimens

1. Amoebic ulcer in intestine.
2. Amoebic abscess in liver.
3. Tape worm.
4. Hydatid cyst in liver.
5. Common round worm (*Ascaris lumbricoides*) in intestine or free form.
6. Intussusception by *Ascaris lumbricoides.*
7. Intestinal obstruction by *Ascaris lumbricoides.*
8. Hook worm.
9. Thread worm.
10. Whip worm.
11. Chylous urine.
12. Guinea worm.

Graphs or figures or pictures

1. Chart of Bacterial growth curve.
2. Figure of Biohazard symbol.
3. Figure of trophozoites/cyst of *E. histolytica.*
4. Figure of trophozoites/cyst of *G. lamblia.*
5. Figure of trophozoites of *T. vaginalis.*
6. Figure of egg of *Taenia* spp.
7. Figure of Hydatid cyst.
8. Figure of egg of *Schistosoma* spp.
9. Figure of egg of *Ancyclostoma duodenale.*
10. Figure of egg (fertilise, unfertilise & decorticated) of *A. lumbricoides.*
11. Figure of egg of *E. vermicularis.*
12. Figure of egg of *T. trichuria.*
13. Figure of microfilariae of *W. bancrofti* or *B. malayi.*

Other specimens

1. Nichrome loop.
2. Nichrome straight wire.
3. Pasteur pipette.
4. Cotton swab.
5. West's post nasal swab.
6. Candle jar.
7. McIntosh & Filde's anaerobic jar.
8. Gas Pack system.
9. Incubator.
10. Autoclave.
11. Hot air oven.
12. Water bath.
13. Inspissator.
14. Disinfections like sterillium, bacilloides, phenyl, dettol.
15. Ph strip.
16. Lovibond comparator.

17. Disposable syringe.
18. Tuberculin syringe.
19. Concavity slide & cover slip for motility testing.
20. MHA plate with antibiotic disc for antibiogram.
21. Icosahedral model of virus.

Question bank

Question of exercise

1) Stain the given smear by Gram stain & draw the labelled diagram of your findings. Report your findings to the examiner.
2) Stain the given smear by ZN stain & draw the labelled diagram of your findings. Report your findings to the examiner.
3) Study the stool sample for trophozoite, cyst or ova. Draw the labelled diagram of your findings. Report your findings to the examiner.
4) Identify the culture medium given to you. Describe the growth/cultural characteristic, identify the pathogen. Draw the labelled diagram of your findings & report your findings to the examiner.

✓ **Note:** Students have to draw the labelled diagram only in answer sheet, no need to write about steps & other details of stain performed.

Spotting questions

1) Identify the medium & write its use.
2) Identify the medium & write its method of sterilisation.
3) Identify the medium & write its type.
4) Identify the biochemical test & name the two bacteria / pathogen giving the test positive.
5) Identify the serological test & write the principle.
6) Identify the serological test & write its use.
7) Identify the animal & write its use.
8) Identify the animal & write its scientific name.
9) Identify the pathogen in smear.
10) Identify the parasite in specimens & write the name of host (hosts).
11) Identify the parasite in specimens & write its mode of transmission.
12) Identify the pathogen in graph/figure/picture.
13) Identify the parasite in specimens & answer the given question.

✓ **Note:** MCQs & the short questions given at the end of each chapter are also the part of spotting exercise.

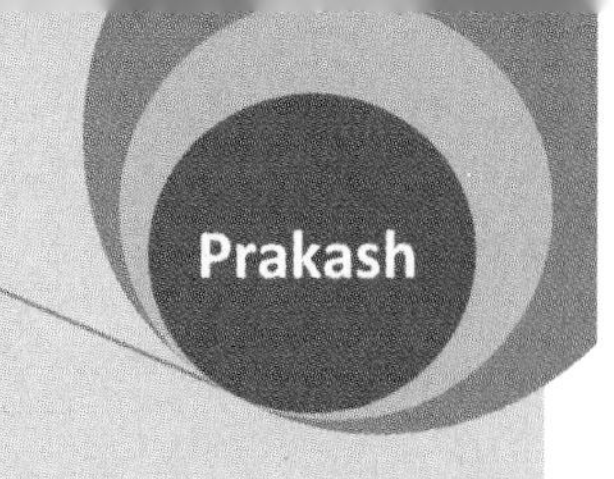

Section X

MCQs

108 MCQs for system review

✓ **Note: This chapters includes MCQs which required knowledge of many chapters of different system**

General Microbiology

1) **The term viable not cultivable is used for** (PGI, May-10, 13, Dec-00, 07)
(a) *M. leprae* (b) *M. tuberculosis* (c) *Treponema pallidum* (d) *Salmonella* (e) *Staphylococcus*
2) **Microscope used in Microbiology-** (PGI-98)
(a) Light microscope (b) Phase contrast microscope (c) Fluorescent microscope (d) All
3) **Culture media are sterilised by**
(a) Autoclave (b) Tyndallisation (c) Hot air oven (d) Radiation
4) **Electron microscopy is used for following except**
(a) To differentiate T and B lymphocytes (b) IgG deposits in kidney (c) TPI (d) Flagella
5) **Smith Noguchi medium is used for**
(a) *Salmonella* (b) *Klebsiella* (c) Spirochetes (d) *Bacillus*
6) **Lipopolysaccharide is an outer membrane seen with**
(a) Gram positive bacteria (b) Gram negative bacteria (c) a+b (d) None of above
7) **Following is mismatched**
(a) Lysozyme – Gram +Ve bacteria - Protoplast (b) Taq polymerase - *Thermus aquaticus* - PCR (c) Recombinase – Rearrangement at DNA level – Genes of Ig (d) *Listeria* – IgA protease - Loss of local immunity

Answers of MCQs & explanation

1) **(a) & (c)**
- *M. leprae* & *T. pallidum* are not cultivable in cell free media

2) **(d)**
- Microscope used in Microbiology
  - Light microscope
  - Dark- Ground (field) Illumination Microscope (DGIM)
  - Phase-Contrast Microscope (PCM)
  - Fluorescent Microscopes (FM) & staining
  - Electron Microscope (EM)

3) **(a) & (b)**
- Almost all media are sterilised by autoclave while media contains gelatin & sugars are sterilised by tyndallisation

4) **(c)**
- In TPI (*Treponema Pallidum* Immobilisation) test, *T. pallidum* are immobilized by specific antiserum in presence of complement which is examined under dark ground illumination microscope but not under electron microscope

5) **(c)**
- Smith Noguchi medium is used for anaerobic bacteria & from the given option anaerobes are spirochetes

6) **(b)**
- Lipopolysaccharide is present in gram negative bacteria

7) **(d)**
- Lysozyme acts on cell wall of Gram +Ve bacteria to form protoplast
- Taq polymerase is derived from *Thermus aquaticus* useful in PCR
- Recombinase is useful in rearrangement at DNA level for genes of Ig
- IgA protease produce by *N. meningitidis, N, gonorrhoea, H. influenzae* & *S. Pneumococcus* not by *Listeria.* It destroy the IgA resulting loss of local immunity

Immunology

1) **The following statements are true about DPT vaccine except-** (AI-04)
(a) Aluminium salt has an adjuvant effect (b) Whole killed bacteria of *Bordetella pertus* has an adjuvant effect (c) Presence of acellular pertusis components increases its immunogenicity (d) Presence of *H. influenzae* type B components increases its immunogenicity

Serological test	Use	Agent
	Precipitation	
Ascoli's thermo-precipitin test.	Anthrax	*B anthracis*
Lancefield grouping	Streptococcal disease	*Streptococci*
Elek's gel precipitation test	Toxigenicity test	*C. diphtheriae*
	Flocculation	
VDRL test	Syphilis	*T pallidum*
RPR test		
Kahn test		
	Agglutination	
Widal test	Enteric fever	*S typhi*
Weil Felix reaction.	Typhus fever	*Rickettsia*
Paul Bunnel test	Infectious mononucleosis	EBV
Cold agglutinin test	Primary atypical pneumonia	*M pneumoniae*
Streptococci MG test		
Blood grouping / cross matching	Blood transfusion	-
RA factor test	Rheumatoid Arthritis	-
ASO test	Streptolysin –O detection	*Streptococcus*
Standard Agglutination Test (SAT)	Human brucellosis	*Brucella* spp.
Coombs test	Haemolytic anaemia	-
	CFT	
Wassermann reaction	Syphilis	*T pallidum*
	Neutralisation	
Schick Test	Susceptibility & hypersensitivity to diphtheria toxin	*C. diphtheriae*
Nagler reaction	Gas gangrene	*Cl welchii*

Table-1: List of serological tests

Allergic / skin test	Use	Agent
Immediate type hypersensitivity (ITH)		
Casoni test	H cyst	*E granulosus*
Mazzotti's test	Onchocerciasis	*O. volvulus*
Delayed type hypersensitivity (DTH)		
Tuberculin test	Tuberculosis	*M tuberculosis*
Lepromin test	Leprosy	*M leprae*
Mallein test	Glanders (malleus)	*Bukholderia mallei*
Brucellin test	Human brucellosis	*Brucella* spp.
Frei's test	LGV	*C trachomatis*
Leishmanin test:	African kala azar	*L donovanii*
Frenkel's test	Toxoplasmosis	*T. gondii*
Scratch test	Ascariasis	*A. lumbricoides*

Table-2: List of allergic tests

2) **Following is/are true-**
(a) All immunogens are antigens but all antigens are not immunogens (b) All antibodies are immunoglobulins, but all immunoglobulins may not be antibodies (c) All antigens are immunogens but all immunogens are not antigens (d) All immunoglobulins are antibodies, but all antibodies may not be immunoglobulins

3) **Prozone phenomenon is a features of-** (PGI-01)
(a) Tularemia (b) Legionnaire's disease (c) Plague (d) Brucellosis

4) **All statements are correct about immunogenic technique, except-** (PGI-97)
(a) ELISA can detect both antigens and antibodies (b) Immuno fluorescence test uses fluorescein and rhodamine (c) Radio immuno assay used to quntitate antigens and haptens (d) Immunoblotting also called northern blotting

5) **Antigen-antibody complexes are detected by** (PGI-09)
(a) Western blot (b) Southern blot (c) Northern blot (d) ELISA

6) **Paul Bunnel reaction is a type of**
(a) Agglutination (b) CFT (c) Precipitation (d) Flocculation test

7) **Test based on agglutination principle is/are**
(a) Widal test (b) Weil-Felix test (c) Blood grouping (d) a+b+c

8) **Nagler reaction is type of**
(a) Neutralisation reaction (b) CFT (c) Precipitation (d) Agglutination

9) **Skin test based on neutralisation reaction is/are** (PGI, June-08)
(a) Casoni test (b) Lepromin test (c) Tuberculin test (d) Schick test

10) **Frenkel's skin test is positive i** (PGI -79, AIIMS-94)
(a) Spinal cord compression (b) Toxoplasmosis (c) Pemphigus (d) Pemphigoid

11) **Following is the helper or inducer cell**
(a) CD1 (b) CD4 (c) CD2 (d) CD8

12) **Following is the cytotoxic or suppressor cell**
(a) CD1 (b) CD4 (c) CD2 (d) CD8

13) **All of the following are glycoprotein except**
(a) Blood antigen (b) Albumin (c) Immunoglobulin (d) HCG

14) **Virus infected cells are killed by**
(a) Interferon (b) Macrophages (c) Neutrophils (d) Autolysis (e) None of above

15) **Function (s) of T lymphocytes is /are**
(a) Production of interferon (b) Lymphokine production (c) Rosette formation (d) All of above

Answers of MCQs & explanation

1) **(d)**
- DPT vaccine does not contains *H. influenzae* type B

2) **(a) & (b)**
- For explanation, follow chapters
  - Antigen (Ag)
  - Antibody (Ab) –Immunoglobulin (Ig)

3) **(d)**
- Prozone phenomenon means Ab excess while postzone phenomenon means Ag excess. Excess antibodies in serum are present in brucellosis & in secondary syphilis/ syphilis with HIV, which interfere with diagnosis. It is overcome by dilution of serum.

4) **(d)**
- ELISA can detect both antigens and antibodies
- Immuno fluorescence test uses Fluorescein Iso Thio Cyanate (FITC) (Blue-green fluorescence) or lissamine rhodamine (orange-red fluorescence)
- Radio immuno assay used in quantitation of hormones, drugs, tumour markers, IgE and viral antigens
- Immunoblotting also **called western blotting**

5) **(a) &(d)**
- Southern blot is used for DNA, Northern blot is used for RNA & Western (immuno) blot is for Ag/Ab detection.
- ELISA is also used for Ag/Ab detection

6) **(a)**
7) **(d)**
8) **(a)**

} Follow **table-1** for explanation

9) **(d)**
- Casoni test based on based on ITH while lepromin test & tuberculin test are based on DTH

10) **(b)**
- Follow **table-2** for explanation

11) **(b)** } CD4 is the helper /inducer cell while
12) **(d)** } CD8 is cytotoxic/suppressor cell

13) **(b)**
- Following are the glycoproteins
  - Ig
  - Mucin
  - Lectin
  - IFN β & γ
  - Glycophorin
  - Alkaline phosphatase
  - Collagen
  - Enzymes
  - Selectin
  - Blood group antigens
  - Transferrin
  - Ceruloplasmin
  - HLA class I & II
  - HCG (Human chorionic gonadotropin)
  - TSH
  - Plasma protein except albumin

14) **(b)**
- Virus infected cells are killed by macrophages, Tc cell & NK cells.
- Interferon has no direct action on virus but acts on other cells of same species, rendering them refractory to viral infection. It inhibits the viral transcription in infected cell.

15) **(d)**
- T lymphocytes produces lymphokines (lymphotoxin) & interferon
- T cells binds with sheep RBC (Erythrocytes = E) to form SRBC or E-rosette by CD2 receptor while B cells binds with sheep Erythrocytes (E) coated with Ab (A) & Complement (C)

to form EAC-rosette due to C3 receptors (CR2) on B cell surface.

Systemic Bacteriology

1) **False about gram positive cocci is -** (AI-08)
(a) *Staph. saprophyticus* cause UTI in female (b) Most *Enterococci* are sensitive to penicillin (c) Non pathogenic strains are coagulase negative (d) Neonatal meningitis causing streptococci hydrolyses hippurate

2) **Dental caries is caused by-** (AI-13)
(a) *Streptococcus pyogenes* (b) *Streptococcus mutans* (c) *Enterococcus* (d) *H. influenzae*

3) **In a patient of orbital cellulitis, microorganism on culture shows the greenish colonies and optochin sensitivity. The most likely organism is -** (AI-2000)
(a) *Strept viridans* (b) *Staphylococcus* (c) *Pseudomonas* (d) *Pneumococcus*

4) **Which of the following regarding bacterial drug resistance is not true** (AIIMS May-12, Nov-11, AI-12)
(a) Most bacterial drug resistance is due to production of penicillin degrading enzyme (b) Plasmid mediated resistance is always transmitted vertically (c) Complete elimination of target produce resistance to vancomycin (d) Alteration of target leads to pneumococcal resistance

5) **A man presented with 3 days H/o of lacrimation, redness & discharge from left eye. Later on he developed perforation. Discharge from his eye demonstrated gram negative cocci which were oxidase positive. Which of the following can be the probable organism?** (AIIMS May-2013)
(a) *Pseudomonas* (b) *Acinetobacter* (c) *Neisseria gonorrhoea* (d) *Moraxella catarrhalis*

6) **Gastrointestinal enteritis necriticans is caused by-** (PGI, Dec-07)
(a) *Clostridium difficile* (b) *Clostridium perfringens* (c) Botulinum (d) *C. jejuni* (e) *Pseudomonas*

7) **Swarming growth on culture is a feature of following gram positive bacterium-**
(a) *Clostridium tetani* (b) *Clostridium perfringens* (c) *Proteus mirabilis* (d) *Bacillus cereus*

8) **Heating and subsequent plating is a method used for isolating-**
(a) *Corynebacterium* (b) *Vibrio* (c) *Salmonella* (d) *Clostridium*

9) **A patient of acute lymphocytic leukemia with fever and neutropenia develops diarrhoea after administration of amoxicillin therapy. Which of the following organism is most likely to be the causative agent-** (AIIMS, Nov-05)
(a) *Salmonella typhi* (b) *Clostridium difficile* (c) *Clostridium perfringens* (d) *Shigella flexneri*

10) **Which of the following statement is true regarding pathogenicity of *Mycobacteria* species-** (AI -06)
(a) *M. tuberculosis* is more pathogenic than *M. bovis* to the human (b) *M. kansasi* can cause a disease indistinguishable from tuberculosis (c) *M. africanum* infection is acquired from the environmental sources (d) *M. marinum* is responsible for tubercular lymphadenopathy

11) **Antibodies against PGL-1 are seen in –** (AIIMS-13, AI-11)
(a) *M. leprae* (b) *M. tuberculosis* (c) *Borrelia* (d) *Brucella*

12) **Buruli ulcer is caused by**
(a) *M. tuberculosis* (b) *M. ulcerans* (c) *M. buruli* (d) *M. kansasi*

13) **Motility difference according to temperature change is shown by**
(a) *L. monocytogenes* (b) *Proteus vulgaris* (c) *Vibrio* (d) *Leptospira*

14) **Microorganism motility at 25^{0}C but not motile at 37^{0}C -** (PGI, 09, Nov-13)
(a) *Listeria monocytogenes* (b) *Campylobacter* (c) *Yersinia pestis* (d) *Streptococcus agalactiae* (d) *E. coli*

15) **A 28 year lady presented with headache, kernig sign positive. Culture showed gram positive bacilli, most probable organism is -** (AI-11)
(a) *Listeria monocytogenes* (b) *H. influenzae* (c) Meningococci (d) *Streptococcus pneumoniae*

16) **All of the following are true except -** (AI-01)
(a) *E coli* is aerobe and facultative anaerobe (b) Proteus forms uric acid stone (c) *E coli* is the motile by peritrichate flagella (d) *Proteus* causes de-amination of phenyl alanine to phenyl pyruvic acid

17) **The bacteria producing a picture resembling "pseudohaemoptysis" in a sputum sample due to prodigiosin production is**
(a) *Serratia marcesens* (b) *Erwinia herbicola* (c) *Ehrlichia seenetsu* (d) *Legionella pneumophila*

18) **Which of the following toxins acts by inhibiting the protein synthesis** (AI -04)
(a) Cholera toxin (b) Shiga toxin (c) Pertusis toxin (d) LT of enterotoxigenic *E. coli*

19) **A person returns to Delhi from Bangladesh after 2 days and has diarrhoea. Stool examination shows RBCs in stool. The likely organism causing is -** (AIIMS, Nov-99)
(a) Enteropathogenic *E. coli* (b) Enterotoxigenic *E. coli* (c) *Salmonella typhi* (d) *Shigella dysenteriae*

20) **Swarming growth on culture is characteristic of which gram negative organism** (AI -95)
(a) *Clostridium welchii.* (b) *Clostridium tetani* (c) *Bacillus cereus* (d) *Proteus mirabilis*

21) **Stalactite growth in ghee broth is due to -**
(a) *H. influenzae* (b) *C diphtheriae* (c) *Y. pestis* (d) *T pallidum*

22) **Causative agent of plague -** (AIIMS, Nov-99)
(a) *Y. pestis* (b) *Y. enterocolitica* (c) *Y. pseudotuberculosis* (d) *Pasteurella septica*

23) **Appendicitis like syndrome is caused by all except -**
(a) *Yersinia enterocolitica* (b) *Yersinia pseudotuberculosis* (c) *Pasteurella septic* (d) *Yersinia pestis*

24) **Which of the following bacteria act by increasing cAMP –** (AIIMS Nov-06, AI-07)
(a) *Vibrio cholerae* (b) *Staphylococcus aureus* (c) *E coli* heat stable toxin (d) *Salmonella*

25) **Selective medium for *Vibrios* –** (AIIMS May-08, Nov-07)
(a) TCBS (b) Stuart (c) Skirrows (d) MYPA

26) **Which organism grows in alkaline pH?**
(a) *Vibrio cholerae* (b) *E coli* (c) *Pseudomonas aeruginosa* (d) *Salmonella typhi*

27) **Swarm of gnats is a feature of**
(a) *V. cholerae* (b) *S. typhi* (c) *P. aeruginosa* (d) *E. coli*

28) **Invasive infection is caused by all except -**
(a) *Vibrio cholerae* (b) *Neisseria* (c) *Streptococci* (d) *H. influenzae*

29) **A 32 year old male, Kallu, who recently visited a sea coast presented with ulcer over the left leg. The probable causes is -**
(a) *Pasteurella multocida* (b) *Micrococcus halophilus* (c) *V. fluvialius* (d) *Neisseria gonorrhoea*

30) **Which of the following has shortest incubation period?-**
(a) Plague (b) Cholera (c) Measles (d) Typhoid

31) **Pontiac fever is caused by-** (PGI, Dec-07, Nov-01)
(a) *Legionella* (b) *Listeria* (c) Scrub typhus (d) *Leptospira* (e) *Rickettsia*

32) **Thumb print appearance in culture film smear is seen in-** (AIIMS, Nov-09, May-11)
(a) *B anthracis* (b) *Brucella* species (c) *B pertusis* (d) *Cl welchii*

33) **Whooping cough is produced by**
(a)*Y. pestis* (b) *B. pertusis* (c) *H. influenzae* (d) *P. multocida*

34) **Milk ring test is seen in-**
(a) Brucellosis (b) *Bacteroides* (c) Tuberculosis (d) Salmonellosis

35) **Positive cold agglutination test is seen in infection with-**
(a) *Mycoplasma* (b) *Chlamydiae* (c) Infectious mononucleosis (d) Varicella

36) **Which of the following is an obligate parasite-** (AI-98)
(a) *Mycoplasma* (b) *Chlamydia trachomatis* (c) Gram –ve bacilli (d) Gram +ve cocci

37) **A 23 year old male have unprotected sexual intercourse with a commercial sex worker. Two weeks later he developed a painless indurated ulcer on the glans that exuded clear serum on pressure. Inguinal lymphnode on both groin were enlarged and not tender. The most appropriate diagnostic test is-** (AIIMS, May-04)
(a) Gram stain of ulcer discharge (b) Dark field microscopy of ulcer discharge (c) Giemsa stain of lymph node aspirate (d) ELISA for HIV infection

38) **Lyme disease caused by-** (PGI, June-01)
(a) *Leptospira* (b) *Borrelia* (c) *Treponema* (d) *Bordetella* (e) Arbovirus

39) **Query fever is caused by -**
(a) *Pseudomonas* (b) *Francisella* (c) *Coxiella burnetii* (d) *R typhi*

40) **Following is grow in cell free medium except:** (PGI-99)
(a) *Rickettsiae* (b) *M. leprae* (c) *Bartonella* (d) Syphilis

41) **Granuloma with stellate abscess seen in**
(a) Tuberculosis (b) Tularemia (c) Sarcoidosis (d) *Staphylococcus*

42) **Patoc 1 strain is belong to**
(a) *L. biflexa* (b) *T pallidum* (c) *S typhi* (d) *M. bovis*

43) **Malta fever is caused by-** (PGI, Dec-07, Nov-01)
(a) *Treponema pallidum* (b) *Borrelia burgdorferi* (c) *Brucella melitensis* (d) *Pseudomonas aeruginosa*

44) **A child with fever and pharyngitis, which of the following investigation should not be done** (AIIMS-00)
(a) Widal test (b) ASO (c) Throat swab and culture (d) Chest x-ray

45) **Acute intravascular haemolysis can be caused by infection due to all of the following organisms except** (AIIMS, Nov-03, AI-03)
(a) *Clostridium tetani* (b) *Bartonella bacilliformis* (c) *Plasmodium falciparum* (d) *Babesia microti*

46) **Correct combination of incubation period is** (PGI, May-13, 11)
(a) Syphilis: 9-90 days (b) Herpes genitalis: 4-5 wk (c) LGV: 3-6 wk (d) Donovanosis: 1-4 wk (e) Chancroid: 2-3 wk

47) **Draining sinuses are seen in** (PGI-90)
(a) Mycetoma (b) Scrofula (c) Lupug vulgaris (d) Pediculosis

Answers of MCQs & explanation

1) **(b)**
- *Staph. saprophyticus* cause UTI in sexually active young female
- Most *Enterococci* are intrinsically resistant to penicillin
- Coagulase Negative Staphylococci (CoNS) are also pathogenic but less virulent than CoPS
- Neonatal meningitis causing streptococci are group B, β-haemolytic streptococci (*Strept agalactiae*) are giving hippurate hydrolyses test posiive

2) **(a)**
- *Streptococcus mutans* belong to viridans group is breaking the dietary fibres to produces the dextran which help in adhesion of bacteria, mucus, food debris & epithelial cells with teeth to produces the dental caries

3) **(d)**
- A greenish colony (on blood agar) means alpha haemolysis which is given by viridans group (*Strept mutans, Strept. sanguis, Strept. mitis, Strept. salivarius, Strept. mitior etc.*) & pneumoniae group (*Streptococcus pneumoniae*). Differences between two are given in table-1 of chapter → Pneumococcus

Organism is *Pneumococcus* has following diagnostic features
- Arranged in pair with lancet/flame in shape
- α-haemolytic colonies on blood agar
- Catalase test: Negative
- Bile solubility test: Positive

4) **(b)**
- Most bacterial drug resistance to penicillin is due to production of penicillinase (Beta-lactamase)
- Mostly plasmid transmitted horizontally
- Vancomycin resistant to *Enterococci* is due to alteration or elimination of target site like D-alanyl-D-alanine chain
- Pneumococcal resistance to Pn is due to alteration in penicillin binding protein.

5) **(c)**
- From the given options gram negative cocci which is oxidase positive is *Neisseria gonorrhoea*
- Ocular manifestations of *Neisseria gonorrhoea* are explained in chapter → Neisseriae, Moraxellaceae and Mimeae in section complications (autoinoculation)

6) **(b)**
- Necrotising enteritis or enteritis necroticans or pigbel is caused by *Clostridium perfringens* due to ingestion of pig meat with trypsin inhibitor like sweet potatoes

7) **(a)**
- *Clostridium tetani* is gram positive bacilli & it produce swarming growth on opposite half of plate after 1-2 dys anaerobic incubation
- *Clostridium perfringens* is nonmotile & not able to produce the swarming growth.
- *Proteus mirabilis* can produce swarming growth but it is gram negative bacilli
- From the genus *Bacillus, Bacillus subtilis* can produce the swarming growth but not the *Bacillus cereus*

8) **(d)**
- In *Clostridium tetani* samples are collected in three bottles of RCMM
- 1st bottle: Heated at 80 °c for 15 min
- 2nd bottle: Heated at 80 °c for 5 min and
- 3rd bottle: Left unheated.
- Purpose of heating is to kill vegetative forms & leaving spore undamage.
- Incubated at 37°c for 24-48 hr followed by subculture on blood agar daily upto 4 days and observed for growth.

9) **(b)**
- Given case is of antibiotic associated diarrhoea caused by *Clostridium difficile* where acute lymphocytic leukemia & amoxicillin therapy are the precipitating factors

10) **(b)**
- *M. tuberculosis* & *M. bovis* are equal pathogenic for human
- *M. kansasi* can cause chronic pulmonary disease resembling tuberculosis
- *M. africanum* is listed in the category of Mycobacterium tuberculosis complex (MTC) causing tuberculosis in West Africans by air borne route but pathogenicity is lower than *M. tuberculosis*. Environment is act as a source for atypical group not for MTC.
- *M. marinum* is responsible for swimming pool (fish tank) granuloma

11) **(a)**
- PGL (Phenolic Glyco Lipid Antigen)-1 is secreted by *M. leprae*, so antibodies are against the *M. leprae*. Sensitivity is 95% in untreated LL & 60% in TT cases. Titre decrease with effective therapy. It also present in non leprosy cases, so rarely useful

12) **(b) & (c)**
- *M. ulcerans* & *M. buruli* are synonym for each other, causing buruli ulcer

13) **(a)**

- Tumbling motility is the feature of *L. monocytogenes* which occurs at 25^0C but not at 37^0C
- Other bacteria given in other options are motile but it is different types & also not changed by temperature effect

14) (a)
- Tumbling motility is the feature of *L. monocytogenes* which occurs at 25^0C but not at 37^0C

15) (a)
- All options are known to cause the meningitis, but gram positive bacilli is *L. monocytogenes*

16) (b)
- *Proteus* forms the enzyme urease which cleaves the urea to ammonia and contribute to the alkalinity. Alkalinity cause the necrosis of renal tubular epithelium & precipitate the phosphate stone
- Uric acid stone forms in acidic urine, mostly in gout or Lesch-Nyhan syndrome

17) (a)
- *Serratia marcesens* produces the red pigment **called prodigiosin** & it's presence in sputum simulating the presence of blood in sputum **called pseudohaemoptysis** (Haemoptysis = Blood in sputum)

18) (b)
- Toxins act by inhibiting the protein synthesis are
- Diphtheria toxin: } By inactivation of EF-2
- *Pseudomonas* toxin:
- Shiga like toxin (SLT): } By inactivation of 60S ribosome
- Shiga toxin:
- Cholera toxin & LT of enterotoxigenic *E. coli* act through activation of c AMP
- Action of pertusis toxin: Follow chapter → *Bordetella*

19) (d)
- Given case is of traveler's diarrhoea. Enterotoxigenic *E. coli* (ETEC) is also known to cause traveller's diarrhoea from the given option. Stool contains blood (RBCs) in given case which is not the feature of ETEC, so ETEC is not the right answer
- EPEC causing watery diarrhoea without blood (RBCs), so EPEC is not the right answer
- Some author claimed that *Salmonella typhi* causing diarrhoea contains blood (RBCs) with 7- 14 days incubation period, but incubation period in given case is 2 days, so *Salmonella typhi* is not the right answer
- *Shigella dysenteriae* causing diarrhoea contains blood (RBCs) & mucus with 1-7 days incubation period, which fulfil all features of given case, so *Shigella dysenteriae* is the right answer

20) (d)
- Gram positive bacteria showing swaming are: *Clostridium tetani* & *Bacillus subtilis*
- Gram positive bacteria showing swaming are: *Proteus vulgaris, Proteus mirabilis* & *Pseudomonas aeruginosa*

21) (c)
- A characteristic growth occurs by *Y. pestis* in oil/ghee broth in flask (contains oil/ghee at top), which hangs down into broth from the surface **called 'stalactite growth'** or **called 'stalactites'**

22) (a)
- *Y pestis* causing plague
- *Y. enterocolitica* & *Y. pseudotuberculosis* causes yersiniosis characterised by acute/subacute appendicitis (**called pseudoappedicular syndrome**)
- *Pasteurella septic* causes lesions like appendicitis, meningitis, abscess, pneumonia etc.

23) (a), (b) & (c) → Follow above MCQ for explanation

24) (a)
- Cholera toxin or heat labile toxin (LT) of *Vibrio cholerae* act by c AMP
- *Staphylococcus aureus:* Produces many toxin but non of them are act through AMP
- *E coli:* Heat labile toxin (LT) act by c AMP while heat stable toxin act by c GMP
- *Salmonella:* No specific toxin production

25) (a)
- TCBS is selective medium for *Vibrio cholerae*
- Stuart is not selective but transport (holding) medium
- Skirrows is selective medium for *C. jejuni*
- MYPA (Baker's MYPA medium) is selective medium for *Bacillus cereus*

26) (a)
- *Vibrio cholerae* can grow at high (alkaline) pH about 6.4 -9.6 & high salt concentration about 0.5-1%

27) (a)
- Microscopy from young culture or from acute cholera stool reveals actively motile *Vibrio cholerae* suggests **'swarm of gnats'**

28) (a)
- *Vibrio cholerae* can cause non invasive infection like watery/secretory diarrhoea **called cholera**
- *Neisseria, Streptococci* & *H. influenzae* are causes invasive infection like meningitis

29) (c)
- *Pasteurella multocida:* It is transmitted by dog bite or contact with infected animals. Also present in human respiratory tract and in nasal sinus as commensals, which are carry to traumatic site by blood
- *Micrococcus halophilus:* It is non pathogenic, related to *Staphylococci* & no relation with sea coast
- *V. fluvialius:* Can cause wound infection on exposure to sea water
- *Neisseria gonorrhea:* Sexually transmitted & no relation with sea coast

30) (b)
- Incubation period for
- Cholera: < 24 hrs to 5 days
- Plague: Bubonic plague →2-7 days, pneumonic plague → 1-3 days & septicemic plague →2-7 days
- Measles: 10-14 days. Fever occurs after 10 day & rash occur after 14 day
- Typhoid: 7-14 days

31) (a)
- *Legionella pneumophila* causing a disease **called legionellosis** having two forms like mild influenza like symptoms **called pontiac fever** while pneumonia **called legionnair's disease**.
- *Listeria* causing a disease **called listeriosis**
- Scrub typhus is caused by *Orientia tsutsugamushi*
- *Leptospira* causing a disease **called leptospirosis** with different clinical form
- *Rickettsia* causing a disease classified in two group like typhus fever group & spotted fever group

32) (c)
- Culture smear of *B pertusis* shows loose clumps with space in between known as **'thumb print appearance'**

33) (b)
- *Y. pestis* causing plague, *B. pertusis* causing whooping cough, *H. influenzae* causing meningitis, respiratory infection etc. & *P. multocida* causing local (abscess,cellulitis etc.) & systemic lesions (like meningitis, respiratory infection, appendicitis etc.)

34) (a)
- Milk ring test is performed to diagnose the animal brucellosis from milk

Strain	Agent	Application
		Bacterial strain
Cowan I strain	*Staph. aureus*	Co-agglutination test
Strene strain	*B. anthrcis*	Used for prepare the Sterne vaccine
Carbazzo strain	*B. anthrcis*	Used for prepare the Mazzucchi vaccine
Park Williams 8 Strain	*C. diphtheriae*	Widely used for toxin production
Danish 1331	*M. bovis*	In India, WHO recommended strain of BCG for preparation of vaccine. It is prepared in BCG laboratory, Guindy, Chennai
Onco TICE	*M. bovis* (BCG)	Multiple injection of BCG vaccine has been tried in bladder cancer & in other diseases as an adjuvant therapy
O157:H7	*E coli*	All strains of *E coli* are sorbitol fermenters while O157:H7 is sorbitol non-fermenter. It diagnosed by using Sorbitol Mac Conkey's medium (also **called modified Mac Conkey's medium**
K 12 strain	*E coli*	Conjugation was 1st discovered by Joshua Lederberg & Tatum in 1946 in *E. coli* K 12 strain
Bhatanagar strain	*Citrobacter freundii*	It share common Ag **(like Vi Ag)** with *S. typhi* & *S. paratyphi C* & confusing the diagnosis
***S typhi* 901 H & O strain**	*S typhi*	For preparation of H & O antigen of widal test respectively
Ty21a	*S typhi*	Preparation of Typhoral (Live Typhoid oral) vaccine of *S typhi*
Ty2	*S typhi*	Preparation of Vi vaccine (typhim-Vi) of *S typhi*
DT 104	*S typhimurium*	Multidrug resistant strain emerged in early 1990s & associated with an increased risk of blood stream infection & hospitalization. Acquired by raw or partially cooked meat products
Bengal strain (O139)	*V cholerae*	Occurred in October 1992 in Madras (Chennai), India & later similar outbreak occurred in other part of India
American strain (H_2S +Ve) & Danish strain (H_2S -Ve)	*Brucella suis*	Biotypes of *Brucella suis* on the basis of H_2S production
Nichol's strain	*T pallidum*	- Do not grow in artificial culture media. It maintained for many decades by serial testicular passage in rabbits - Nichol's strain is useful to prepare the antigen for species specific treponemal tests
Reiter's strain, Kazan's strain	*T. phagedenis*	- Grow in artificial culture medium like **thioglycollate medium containing serum** - Reiter's strain is useful to prepare the antigen for group specific treponemal tests
Noguchi's strain	*T. refringens*	Grow in artificial culture medium like **thioglycollate medium containing serum**
Patoc 1 strain	*L. biflexa*	Antigen for genus specific (screening) tests of *Leptospira* is prepared from *L. biflexa* (non pathogenic)
TWAR strain	*Chlamydia pneumoniae*	It was 1st reported by Grayston et al. in 1986 from the adult patient with acute respiratory disease in Taiwan
		Viral strain
Oka strain.	HHV-3 (VZV)	To prepare the live attenuated vaccine of VZV
Towne 125 & AD 169 strain	HHV-5 (CMV)	To prepare the live attenuated vaccine
Brunhilde & Mahoney	Polio virus 1	For preparation of live & killed polio vaccine
Lencing & Mefi	Polio virus 2	
Leon & Sauket	Polio virus 3	
H1N1	Influenza virus A	Causing swine flu (pandemic 2009)
H5N1		Causing bird (avian) flu
Jeryl-Lynn strain	Mumps virus	To prepare the live attenuated vaccine of mumps
Edmonston strain	Measles virus	To prepare the live attenuated (injectable) vaccine of measles
Schwartz & Moraten strain		
Edmonston & Zagreb strain		
Schwartz strain	Live measles vaccine virus	It is used as a vector, in to the genome of which five structural genes from chikungunya virus have been incorporated to prepare the chikungunya vaccine.
Nakayama strain	Japanese Encephalitis virus	To prepare the killed vaccine of Japanese Encephalitis virus
Beijing strain		
Beijing P3 strain		
SA 14-14-2 strain		To prepare the live vaccine of Japanese Encephalitis virus
Asibi strain	Yellow fever virus	To prepare the live attenuated/non- neurotropic vaccine/17D vaccine of yellow fever
Flury strain	Rabies virus	To prepare the live attenuated chick embryo vaccine of rabies
Pitman Moore strain		To prepare the Human Diploid Cell culture Vaccine (HDCV) of rabies
RA 27/3 strain	Rubella virus	To prepare the live attenuated vaccine of rubella
HEV 239	HEV	China prepared the recombinant HEV vaccine by using this strain but not available globally
		Parasitic strain

Leishmania strain	*Leishmania* spp.	To prepare the vaccine cutaneous leishmaniasis

Table-3: Common strain, related agent & its application

Fever	Agent
Scarlet fever	*Strept pyogenes*
Enteric fever	*Salmonella typhi* & *Salmonella paratyphi*
Typhoid fever (step-ladder pyrexia)	*Salmonella typhi*
Paratyphoid fever	*Salmonella paratyphi*
Shanghai fever	*Pseudomonas aeruginosa*
Pontiac fever	*Legionella pneumophilla*
Mediterranean fever / Malta fever / Undulant fever	*Brucella melitensis*
Lemming fever (in Norway)	*Francisella tularensis*
Rat bite fever (RBF)	- *Streptobacillus moniliformis*: **Called haverhill fever or erythema arthriticum epidemicum or streptobacillary RBF** - *Spirillum minus*: **Called sodoku or spirillary RBF**
Relapsing fever	In USA: *B. bergdorferi* & *B. mayonii* In Europe & Asia: *B. afzelii* & *B. garinii*
Break bone fever	Dengue virus

Table-4: Common fever & etiological agents

35) (a)
- Antigens from *Mycoplasma* are producing the antibodies that agglutinate human O cell at 4°C **called cold agglutination**

36) (b)
- *Mycoplasma* , Gram –ve bacilli & Gram +ve cocci are living free in the environment or present as commensals in human or animal bodies, while *Chlamydia trachomatis* is an obligate intracellular organism in human, animal or bird's cells with tropism for squamous epithelial cells & macrophages of GIT & respiratory system

37) (b)
- Painless indurated ulcer on the glans with not tender bilateral inguinal lymphadenopathy suggestive of Syphilis caused by *T pallidum,* which is best diagnosed by DGI microscopy from the given options.

38) (b)
- Causative agent of Lyme disease was identified in1985 by Bergdorfer in USA hence **called *B. bergdorferi***. *B. mayonii* is also a causative agent of Lyme disease in USA. In Europe & Asia, *B. afzelii* & *B. garinii* are the causative agents of Lyme disease

39) (c)
- Query fever is caused by *Coxiella burnetii*
- *Pseudomonas* causing sanghai fever
- *Francisella tularensis* causing tularemia
- *R typhi* causing endemic typhus

40) (a), (b) & (d)
- *Rickettsiae, M. leprae* & Syphilis (*T pallidum*) can't grow in cell free media while *Bartonella* can grow

41) (a), (b) & (c)
- Lymph node contains granulomatous lesion with central star shaped necrosis surrounded by histiocytes, B cells & giant cells **called stellate abscess.** It present in chronic granulomatous disease (tuberculosis & sarcoidosis), tularemia, actinomycosis, nocardiosis, cat scratch disease, candidiasis & in leishmaniasis.

42) (a)
- Follow **table-3** for explanation

43) (c)
- *Treponema pallidum:* Causing syphilis
- *Borrelia burgdorferi*: Causing lyme disease
- *Pseudomonas aeruginosa:* Causing sanghai fever
- Follow **table-4** for other common fever & etiological agents

44) (a)
- Given case is of respiratory infection, by organism belong to family Streptococcaceae. Widal test is used for intestinal disease caused by *S typhi.*

45) (a)
46) (a), (c) & (d)
47) (a) & (b)
} Follow **respective chapters** for explanation

Virology

1) **Paul Bunnell test is for**
(a) Malta fever (b) Typhus fever (c) Enteric fever (d) Infectious mononucleosis

2) **Parvovirus causes** (PGI, Dec-07)
(a) Aplastic anaemia (b) Erythematosum infectiosum (c) Roseola infantum (d) Arthritis

3) **Parvovirus B19 does not causes** (AIIMS, May-08)
(a) Roseola infantum (b) Aplastic anaemia (c) Foetal hydrops

4) **Parvovirus causes**
(a) Erythematosum infectiosum (b) Exanthema subitum (c) Roseola infantum (d) Sixth disease

5) **Genital herpes simplex is diagnosed by**
(a) Gram stain (b) KOH preparation (c) Tzanck smear (d) Acid fast stain

6) **Genital infection by HPV is diagnosed by**
(a) Gram stain (b) KOH preparation (c) Tzanck smear (d) Pap smear

7) **Property of elution is found in**
(a) Myxovirus (b) Togavirus (c) Parvovirus (d) Adenovirus

8) **Which of the following pair is correct?** (PGI-05)
(a) RSV-Bronchiolitis (b) HHV5- Infectious mononucleosis (c) Parvovirus-exanthma subitum (d) HHV6-Kaposi sarcoma (e) VZV-Chickenpox

9) **Conjunctivitis is caused by all except** (AIIMS, Dec-98)
(a) CMV (b) Enterovirus 70 (c) Coxsackie virus A24 (d) Adenovirus

10) **Most common viral disease affecting parotid gland**
(a) Mumps (b) Measles (c) Rubella (d) Varicella

11) **Most common agent responsible for bronchiolitis**
(a) RSV (b) Adeno virus (c) Herpes virus (d) Influenza virus

12) **Most common cause of viral pneumonia in infant**
(a) *Rhinovirus* (b) RSV (c) Reo virus (d) CMV

13) **Which of the following pair is true** (AIIMS, May-08)
(a) Hantavirus pulmonary syndrome is caused by inhalation of rodent urine and faeces (b) KFD is caused by bite of wild animal (c) *Lyssavirus* is transmitted by tick (d) Chikungunya is caused by *Anopheles*

14) **Active immunisation following exposure is given most commonly for** (AI -99)
(a) Rabies (b) Polio (c) Plague (d) Measles

15) **Croup is most commonly due to**

(a) Respiratory syncytial virus (b) *Parainfluenzavirus* (c) Adeno virus (d) Corona virus

16) T4/T8 ratio reversal is seen in

(a) T cell lymphoma (b) Hairy cell leukemia (c) AIDS (d) Infectious mononucleosis

17) Choose the correct matches (PGI, June-02)

(a) Mumps - RA 27/3 strain (b) Rubella – Jeryl-Lynn strain (c) Measles – Edmonston-Zagreb strain (d) BCG – Danish 1331 strain

18) Nakayama strain is used to prepare which vaccine

(a) Typhoid (b) Chicken pox (c) Japanese encephalitis (d) Yellow fever

19) Latency seen viral infections (PGI, June-05, Dec-08)

(a) HSV-II (b) CMV (c) *Rotavirus* (d) HIV (e) EBV

20) Human to human transmission not seen in (PGI, June-05)

(a) SARS (b) Japanese B encephalitis (c) Bird's flu (d) Chickenpox (e) Rabies

21) Which of the following pair is correct (PGI, Dec-05)

(a) RSV - Bronchiolitis (b) Orf – Viral infection is transmitted from sheep (c) Parvo virus Bb 19 – Exanthema subitum (d) HHV6 – Kaposi sarcoma

22) Which pathogen adhere to respiratory epithelium (PGI, Dec-06)

(a) RSV (b) Influenza (c) Parainfluenza (d) HBV (e) Picorna virus

23) Which of the following contains(s) a RNA dependent DNA polymerase as a structural component of the virion

(a) Adeno viruses (b) Orthomyxo viruses (c) Rhabod viruses (d) Retro viruses

24) Break bone fever is caused by

(a) Variola (b) Coxsackie (c) Dengue (d) Adeno virus

25) Man is the only reservoir of

(a) Rabies (b) Influenzae (c) Typhoid (d) Japanese B encephalitis

26) Post exposure immunisation is done for

(a) Measles (b) Polio (c) Rabies (d) Chicken pox

Answers of MCQs & explanation

1) (d)

- Malta fever is caused by *Brucella* spp. & detected by Standard Agglutination Test (SAT) & few other serological tests
- Typhus fever is caused by *Rickettsia* spp. & detected by Weil-Felix reaction
- Enteric fever is caused by *Rickettsia* spp. & detected by Widal test
- Infectious mononucleosis is caused by EBV & detected by Paul Bunnell test
- there is reversal of T4/T8 ratio

2) (a)
3) (a) } Explained below
4) (a)

- Parvovirus B19 causes aplastic anaemia, erythematosum infectiosum (5th disease or slapped cheek disease), foetal hydrops & arthritis
- HHV-6B causes sixth disease or roseola infantum or exanthema subitum

5) (c)

- Gram stain is useful for bacteria
- KOH preparation is for fungi
- Tzanck smear is for Herpesviridae
- Acid fast stain is for acid fast organisms

6) (d)

- Gram stain is useful for bacteria
- KOH preparation is for fungi
- Tzanck smear is for Herpesviridae
- Pap smear is for cervical cancer caused by HPV

7) (a)

- Myxovirus like influenza virus has H & N peplomeres
- H is responsible to make complex with haemagglutinin (H) receptors on host cells (RBCs) & causing haemagglutination.
- N is **called neuraminidase**. It destroy the haemagglutinin (H) receptors on host cells hence **called Receptor Destroying Enzyme (RDE)** & causes reversal of haemagglutination & release the bounded virus to infect the other cells **called elution**
- This property present only in myxovirus not in other virus

8) (a) & (e)

- HHV4 (EBV)- infectious mononucleosis
- Parvovirus B19 - aplastic anaemia, erythematosum infectiosum (5th disease or slapped cheek disease), foetal hydrops & arthritis
- HHV6B-exanthea subitum (d) HHV6-Kaposi sarcoma

9) (a)

- Enterovirus 70: Causing acute hemorrhagic conjunctivitis
- Coxsackie virus A24: Rarely causing conjunctivitis
- Adenovirus: Two types eye disease
  - Epidemic kerato-conjunctivitis (Shipyard eye): By serotype 8,19 &37
  - Acute follicular (swimming pool) conjunctivitis: By serotype 3,4,7 &11

10) (a)

- Measles, rubella & varicella are the exanthematous diseases of skin

11) (a) } Explained below
12) (a)

- Adeno virus, herpes virus, influenza virus, *Rhinovirus* & reo virus are also a respiratory pathogens but RSV out rank the other pathogens & most common cause of lower respiratory tract infections like bronchitis, bronchiolitis & pneumonia in infant (< 1 year child) & young children.
- CMV is not the respiratory pathogen.

13) (a)

- Hantavirus pulmonary syndrome is caused by inhalation of aerosols arise from excreta of deer mouse & other rodents of *Sigmoidontine* family
- KFD is caused by ticks bite (Ixodid or hard tick) like *Haemaphysalis spinigera, H. turtura* etc.
- *Lyssavirus* is a genus belongs to *Rhabdoviridae* family. It has 7 species or serotypes like lyssa virus-1 as rabies virus, which is transmitted by dog bite. *Lyssavirus* is not transmitted by vector.
- Chikungunya is caused by *Aedes*

14) (a)

- For polio & plague pre-exposure prophylaxis is useful
- For measles & rabies post-exposure prophylaxis is available, but question is for most common, so answer is rabies.

15) (b)

- Parainfluenza virus-2 causes croup (acute laryngotracheobronchitis)
- Follow respective chapters for lesions produced by respiratory syncytial virus, adeno virus & corona virus.

Bacteria	
T pallidum	*R. prowazekii*
B. bergdorferi	*B. bacilliformis*
	B. (Rochalimaea) quintana
Viruses	
DNA viruses	**RNA viruses**
Some pox viruses	Measles virus
HHV 1 to 8	Rabies virus
HPV	HIV
Parasites	
T. brucei (non-flagellate latent form & flagellate latent form)	*T gondii* (tissue cyst)

Table-5: Agents causing latent infection

16) (c)
- In AIDS, HIV attack over CD4 cells, resulting decrease CD4 & there is reversal of T4/T8 ratio

17) (c) & (d) } Follow **table-3** for explanation
18) (c)

19) (a), (b), (d) & (e)
- Follow **table-5** for explanation

20) (b) & (c)
- Follow respective chapters for explanation of options.

21) (a) & (b)
- Parvo virus Bb 19: Erythema infectiosum or slapped cheek disease or 5th disease
- HHV-6: Sixth disease or roseola infantum or exanthema subitum
- HHV 8: Kaposi sarcoma

22) (a), (b) (c) & (e)
- Follow respective chapters for explanation of options.

23) (d)
- RNA dependent DNA polymerase is the reverse transcriptase, which present in viruses of family Retroviridae & Hepadnaviridae

24) (c)
- Follow **table-4** for explanation

25) (b) & (c)
- Reservoir in rabies: Two types of animal reservoirs like
  - **Domestic animals:** Dogs, cats & cattle
  - **Wild animals:** Jackals, wolves, foxes, bats, mongooses & skunks
- Reservoir in influenzae: Human, birds, animals etc.
- Reservoir in typhoid: *Salmonella typhi* is the obligate pathogen for human. Cases or carriers of *Salmonella* are the reservoir hosts.
  Reservoir in Japanese B encephalitis: *Ardeid* birds (herons & egrets) are the reservoir host while pigs are the amplifier hosts.

26) (a) & (c)
- Post exposure immunisation is done for measles, , rabies & tetanus

Mycology

1) **Fungal culture is diagnosed with**
(a) Giemsa stain (b) KOH (c) Foot pad culture (d) Albert stain

2) **Germ tube test is-**
(a) Reynold Braude phenomenon (b) Pfirffer's phenomenon (c) Theobald smith phenomenon (d) Splendore-Hoeppli phenomenon

3) **Which of the following organism cannot be cultured** (PGI, Nov-13, June-07)
(a) *Klebsiella rhinoscleromatis* (b) *Klebsiella ozaenae* (c) *Klebsiella granulomatis* (d) *Pneumocystis jiroveci* (e) *Rhinosporidium seeberi*

4) **Fungus not cultivable usually**
(a) *Rhinosporidium* (b) *Cryptococcus* (c) Dermatophytes (d) *Histoplasma*

5) **The most common organism amongst the following that causes acute meningitis in an AIDS patient is** (AI-05)
(a) *Streptococcus pneumoniae* (b) *Streptococcus agalactiae* (c) *Cryptococcus neoformans* (d) *Listeria monocytogenes*

6) **Which of the following is the most common fungal infection in immunocompetent patient** (AI-11)
(a) *Candia* (b) *Aspergillus* (c) *Cryptococcus* (d) *Penicillium*

7) **Neurotropic fungus is/are** (PGI, Dec-02)
(a) *Cryptococcus neoformans* (b) Histoplasmosis (c) *Trichophyton* (d) *Candia* (e) Aspergillosis

8) **Most fulminant fungal meningitis is caused by**
(a) *Coccidioides* (b) *Histoplasma* (c) *Cryptococcus* (d) Mucormycosis

9) **Maltese cross seen on polarizing microscopy is seen in** (AIIMS-10)
(a) *Cryptococcus* neoformans (b) *Penicillium marneffi* (c) *Blastomyces* (d) *Candida albicans*

Answers of MCQs & explanation

1) (a) & (b)
- Giemsa stain is useful for histo pathological study of fungi
- KOH is useful for wet mount preparation from samples
- Foot pad culture is useful in *M leprae*
- Albert stain is useful for *C diphtheriae*

2) (a)
- Pfirffer's phenomenon is associated with complement system
- Theobald smith phenomenon is related with anaphylaxis
- Deposition of eosinophilic material around yeast cells is due to immune phenomenon of body called Splendore-Hoeppli phenomenon

3) (d) & (e)
4) (a)
} Several attempts has been made for cultivation of *Rhinosporidium seeberi* in cell free media, cell containing media & animal culture, but successful reports are not achieved.

5) (c)
- All the microbes given in options are able to produce the meningitis, but in AIDS patient meningitis is caused by *C. neofromans* while other causes meningitis in immunocompetent individual.

6) (c)
- *Candida* causes infection in immunocompetent & also in individual with immunosuppressive disease or conditions while *Aspergillus, Cryptococcus* & *Penicillium* causes infection in person with IDDs

7) (a), (b), (d) & (e)
- Neurotropic fungus are
  - *Candida* spp.
  - *Aspergillus* spp.
  - *Cryptococcus neoformans*
  - *Histoplasma capsulatum*
  - *Blastomyces dermatitids*
  - *Sporothrix schenckii*

8) (c)
- Among the given options *Cryptococcus* is the most common fungus to cause meningitis, especially in AIDS patient when CD4 count fall below 100/cmm

9) (a)
- Maltese cross form seen in
  - Infectious diseases: Like *Babesia* spp., *Cryptococcus neoformans, P braziliensis* & *M furfur*
  - Non infectious diseases: Maltese cross form casts are present in urine in nephritic syndrome, eclampsia, renal toxicity, fat embolism, crush injury & Fabry's disease (due to aggregates of glycophospholipids)
  - Arthroscopic fluid after local trauma

Parasitology

1) **PAM (Primary Amoebic Meningoencephalitis) is caused by**
(a) *E. histolytica* (b) *N. fowleri* (c) *B. coli* (d) *G. lamblia*

2) **Cyst form is found in** (AIIMS-89)
(a) *Entamoeba fragilis* (b) *B coli* (c) *T. vaginalis* (d) *T. intestinalis*

3) **The cystic form of all are seen in man except** (AIIMS-92)
(a) *E. histolytica* (b) *Giardia* (c) *Trichomonas* (d) *Toxoplasma*

4) **Cyst phase does not exist in**
(a) *Gardnerella vaginalis* (b) *Trichomonas vaginalis* (c) *Entamoeba histolytica* (d) *Entamoeba coli*

5) **Falling leaf like motility is the characteristic of**
(a) *E. histolytica* (b) *T. vaginalis* (c) *G. lamblia* (d) All of above

6) **Which of the following infestation leads to malabsorption**

(AI-05, AIIMS -04)
(a) *Giradia lamblia* (b) *Ascaris lumbricoides* (c) *Necator americanus* (d) *Ancyclostoma duodenale*

7) **A patient present with diarrhoea. Analysis of stool on wet mount shows mobile protozoa without RBCs & pus cells. The diagnosis is** (AI-00)
(a) *Balanidium coli* (b) Giradiasis (c) *Trichomonas hominis* (d) *Entamoeba histolytica*

8) **Protozoa associated with megaoesophagus**
(a) Trypanosome (b) Amoeba (c) *Giardia* (d) *Gnathostoma*

9) **Parasitic disease affecting intestine is**
(a) Chaga's disease (b) Malaria (c) Kala azar (d) *Fasciola*

10) **Leishmania is cultured in........ medium**
(a) Chocolate agar (b) NNN (c) Tellurite (d) Sabourauds

11) **A 40 year old male from Bihar complains of pain in abdomen, having hepatosplenomegaly, peripheral smear on stain shows** (PGI, May-13, Dec-02)
(a) *Plasmodium vivax* (b) *Leishmania* (c) Microfilaria (d) None

12) **Cysticercosis is caused by** (PGI, June-05)
(a) *T solium* (b) *T saginata* (c) *A duodenale* (d) *E granulosus* (e) *E multilocularis*

13) **24 year old AIDS patient develops chronic abdominal pain, low grade fever, diarrhoea, malabsorption, Oocysts demonstrated in stool. Likely cause of his diarrhoea is**
(a) *E. histolytica* (b) *G lamblia* (c) Microsporidia (d) *Isospora belli*

14) **HIV patient with malabsorption, fever, chronic diarrhoea with acid fast positive organism. What is the causative agent?** (AIIMS, May-10)
(a) *Giardia* (b) Microsporidia (c) *Isospora* (d) *E. histolytica*

15) **Larva found in muscle is** (AIIMS, Dec-08)
(a) *Trichinella spialis* (b) *Ancyclostoma duodenale* (c) *Trichuris trichuria* (d) *Enterobius vermicularis*

16) **Larval form of which parasite resides in muscle** (AIIMS, Sept-96)
(a) *Taenia saginata* (b) *Echinococcus* (c) *Trichinella* (d) All of above

17) **Dogs are responsible for transmission of all the following except** (JIPMER-93)
(a) Hydatid disease (b) Toxoplasmosis (c) Kala azar (d) *Toxocara canis*

18) **Abdominal pain, fat malabsorption & frothy stool suggest**
(a) Amoebiasis (b) Bacillary dysentery (c) Giardiasis (d) Pancreatic enzyme deficiency

19) **Pigs are reservoir for** (AI-00)
(a) *T solium* (b) *T saginata* (c) *Trichinella spiralis* (d) *Ancyclostoma*

20) **All of the following disease may be acquired by ingestion except** (AI-94)
(a) Taeniasis (b) Guinea worm (c) Toxoplasmosis (d) Leishmaniasis

21) **Which of the following disease is transmitted by egg ingestion** (AI-95)
(a) Taeniasis (b) Trichinosis (c) Hydatidosis (d) Strongyloidosis

22) **Cercaria are infective form of**
(a) *S haematobium* (b) *P westermanii* (c) *F hepatica* (d) *T solium*

23) **All causes brain lesion except**
(a) Giardiasis (b) Tuberculosis (c) Cysticercosis (d) Bacteroides

24) **Enteropathogenic organisms are** (PGI-02)
(a) *Cryptococcus* (b) *B coli* (c) Microsporidium species (d) *E dispar* (e) *G intestinalis*

25) **Respiratory symptoms are associated with**
(a) Rocky mounted spotted fever (b) *Strongyloides* (c) *T solium* (d) *Onchocerca*

26) **Which of the following congenital infection leads to maximum CNS damage in the foetus** (AI-08)
(a) Rubella and CMV (b) Rubella and toxoplasmosis (c) CMV and toxoplasmosis (d) HIV and CMV

Answers of MCQs & explanation

1) **(b)**
- *E. histolytica* causes intestinal & extraintestinal amoebiasis. It causes cerebral amoebiasis but it is secondary due to intestinal lesion, not primary.
- *B. coli* & *G. lamblia* causes intestinal lesions.
- Follow **respective chapter** for more explanation

Entamoeba gingvalis
Dientamoeba fragilis
Trichomonas vaginalis, Trichomonas hominis (T intestialis) *Trichomonas tenax (T buccalis)*

Table-6: Parasites without cyst stage

2) **(b)** } **Explained below**
3) **(c)**
- Parasites without cystic stage are mentioned in **table-6**
- Follow section, **morphology in respective chapter** for more explanation

4) **(a) & (b)**
- *Gardnerella vaginalis* is bacterium & having no cystic stage
- Parasites without cystic stage are mentioned in **table-6**
- Follow section, **morphology in respective chapter** for more explanation

5) **(c)**
- *E. histolytica* showing crawling or gliding motility due to pseudopodium. Movement is jerky & unidirectional.
- *T. vaginalis* showing wobbling (side to side) / rotator or jerky movement
- Follow **respective chapter** for explanation

6) **(a) & (b)**
- *Giradia lamblia:* Contains sucking disc
  - It is the organ of adhesion
  - Parasite attaches to the convex surface of epithelium & cause the intestinal disturbances leading to malabsorption of fat (**called steatorrhoea**) in children & in adults.
- *Ascaris lumbrocoides:* It has antienzymatic actions like anti peptic & anti tryptic which has following two effects
  - It protect the worm from digestion by enzymes
  - Reduces the absorption of nutritional materials (malabsorption) & develop the malnutrition.

7) **(a) & (b)**
- *Balanidium coli* & *Entamoeba histolytica* causes dysentery, so RBCs & pus cells are present in stool
- Giradiasis is a case of diarrhoea, so RBCs & pus cells are not present in stool
- *Trichomonas hominis* is non pathogenic

8) **(c)**
- *T. cruzi* causing chaga's disease which causing complication in GIT (megaoesophagus & megacolon), heart (cardic myopathy & herniation of endocardium at apex of left ventricle) & lungs (dilatation of pulmonary conus)
- Amoeba causing dysentery & *Giardia* causing diarrhoea but no megaoesophagus or megacolon.
- *Gnathostoma* is known to produce larva migrans

9) **(c)**
- *T. cruzi* causing chaga's disease which causing complication in GIT like megaoesophagus & megacolon.
- Malaria affecting RBCs & spleen
- Kala azar affecting skin & lymph nodes
- *Fasciola hepatica* affecting liver

10) **(b)**
- Chocolate agar & tellurite are bacterial media
- Sabouraud's is fungal medium

11) **(b)**

- All features & location (Bihar) of patient suggesting the *Leishmania*

12) (a)
- Follow **respective chapter** for more explanation & disease produced by all given options.

13) (d)
- From the given options agents causing diarrhoea in AIDS patient are Microsporidia & *Isospora belli*. Oocyst present only in *Isospora belli.*

14) (c)
- From the given options agents causing diarrhoea in AIDS patient with acid fast natures are Microsporidia & *Isospora belli,* but malabsorption is a feature of Isospora belli
- Acid fast parasites: **Follow chapter → Microscopy and staining**

15) (a) } Parasites in which larvae are present human: → **table-7**
16) (d)

Cestodes
Spirometra spp. (In human, in muscles)
Taenia saginata (Not in human but in animal, in muscles, *C bovis*)
Taenia solium (In human & animal, in muscles & tissues, *C cellulosae*)
Echinococcus granulosus (In human & animal, in muscles & tissues, H cyst)
Nematodes
Trichinella spiralis (In human & animal in muscles)
Gnathostoma spinigerum (In human & animal in tissues)

Table-7: Parasites with larval stage in human

17) (b)
- Hydatid disease: Dog is the definitive host
- Kala azar: Canine reservoir are present in Mediterranean or infantile or Chinese or South American kala azar
- *Toxocara canis* is a parasite of dog, causing visceral larva migrans in human **called toxocariasis**
- Toxoplasmosis is transmitted by cat
- Follow **respective chapter** for explanation

18) (c) & (d)
- Abdominal pain, fat malabsorption & frothy stool are not the features of amoebiasis & bacillary dysentery but features of giardiasis & pancreatic enzyme deficiency.
- Follow **respective chapter** for more explanation

19) (a) & (c)
20) (d)
21) (a) & (c)
22) (a)
23) (a)
24) (b), (c), (d) & (e)
} Follow **respective chapter** for more explanation.

25) (a) & (b)
- Rocky mounted spotted fever: Caused by *R rickettsia*. Lung is infected in 7-16% cases
- *Strongyloides:* Larvae are infecting lungs
- Follow **respective chapter** for option 'c' & 'd'

26) (c)
- Among the all options, rubella associated with cardiac anomalies, while CMV & *Toxoplasma* are associated with brain damage.
- Follow **respective chapter** for more explanation.

Entomology

1) ***Aedes aegypticus* transmits -** (PGI, June-04)
(a) JE (b) KFD (c) Yellow fever (d) Filaria (e) Dengue

2) ***Culex* mosquito is associated with the transmission of -** (PGI, Dec-01)
(a) Malaria (b) Filariasis (c) Dengue (d) Japanese encephalitis (e) Typhus

Answers of MCQs & explanation

1) (c) & (e)
- JE: *Culex tritaeniorhynchus* is the worldwide vector including India while in India it also transmitted by *Culex vishnui complex*
- KFD: Transmitted by ticks bite (*Ixodid* or hard tick) like *Haemaphysalis spinigera, H. turtura*
- Filaria: Different types of filaria have different vectors. Not transmitted by *Aedes*

2) (b) & (d)
- Malaria: It is transmitted by *Anopheles* spp.
- Dengue: It is transmitted by *Aedes aegypticus*
- Typhus: Different type of typhus are caused by different species of *Rickettsia* which are transmitted by louse, flea, tick, or by mite

109 Image based MCQs

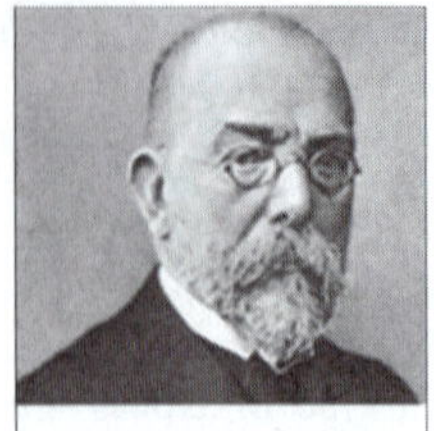

1) **Identify the scientist given in above image who was belonged to Germany**
(a) Louis Pasteur (b) Robert Koch (c) Edward Jener (d) Landsteiner

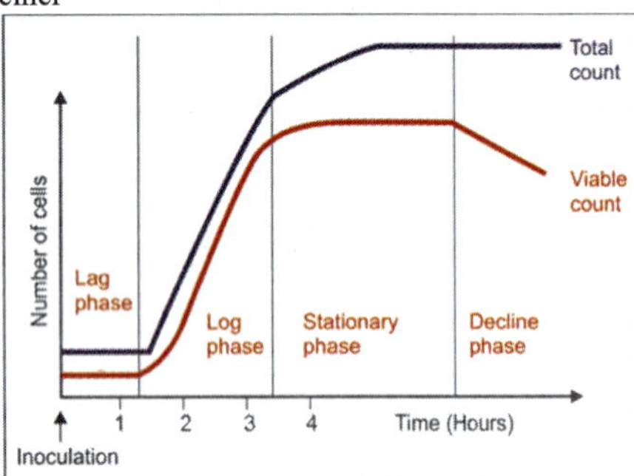

2) **Name the phase in bacterial growth curve marked by question mark (?) in above image**
(a) Lag (b) Log (c) Decline (d) Stationary

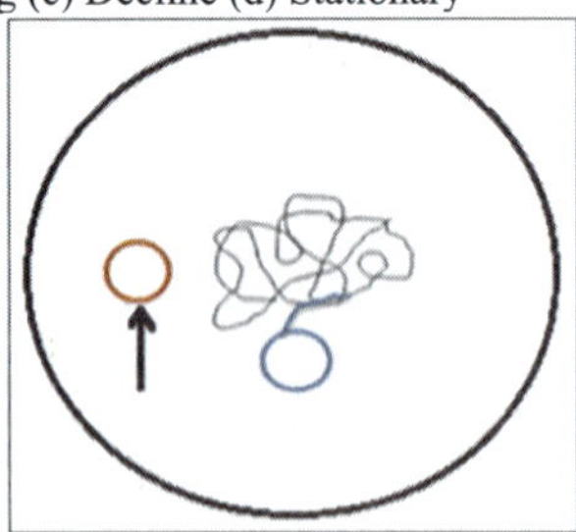

3) **Name the site marked by arrow in above image**
(a) Chromosome (b) Episome (c) Transposon (d) Plasmid

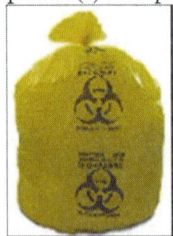

4) **Waste collected in above colour coded bag is**
(a) Body organs (b) Needle (c) Glass items (d) Food & papers

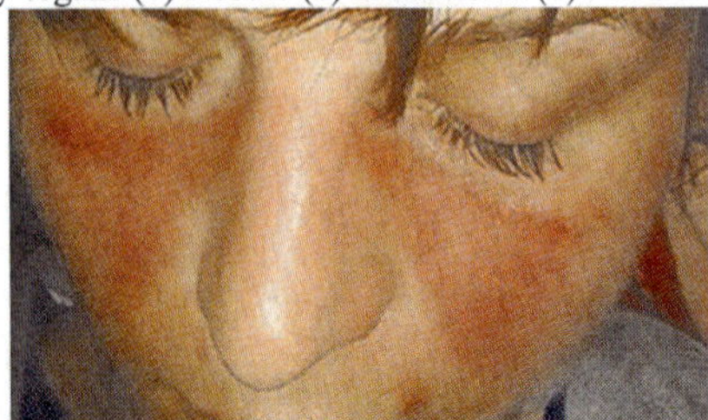

5) **Identify the disease having "butter fly rash" appearance in above image**
(a) SLE (b) Anthrax (c) Impetigo (d) Psoriasis

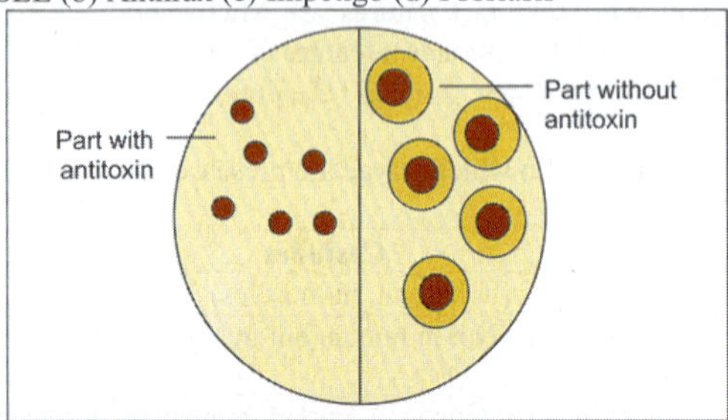

6) **Name the serological test in above image**
(a) Nagler reaction (b) CAMP test (c) Elek's gel precipitation test (d) Neutralisation based test

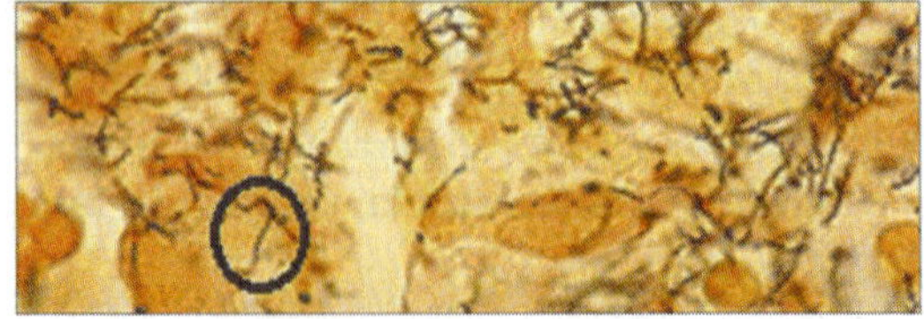

7) **The microorganism circled in the given image is the causative agent of disease that is transmitted sexually. Identify the organism.**
(a) Gonococci (b) *Treponema pallidum* (c) *Haemophilus ducreyi* (d) *Calymatobacter granulomatis*

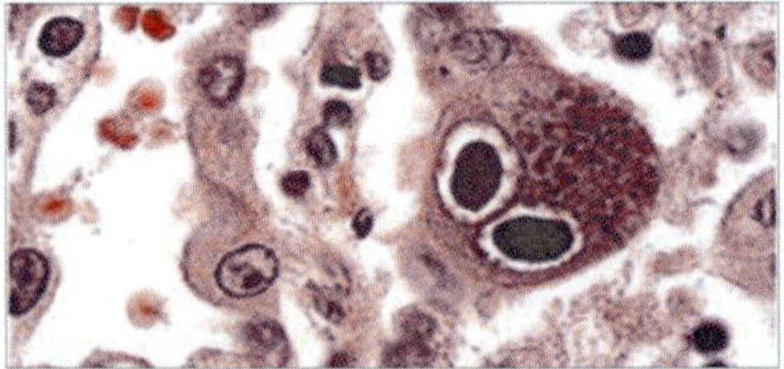

8) **Identify the organism causing inclusion body shown in above image**
(a) HSV (b) VZV (c) CMV (d) EBV

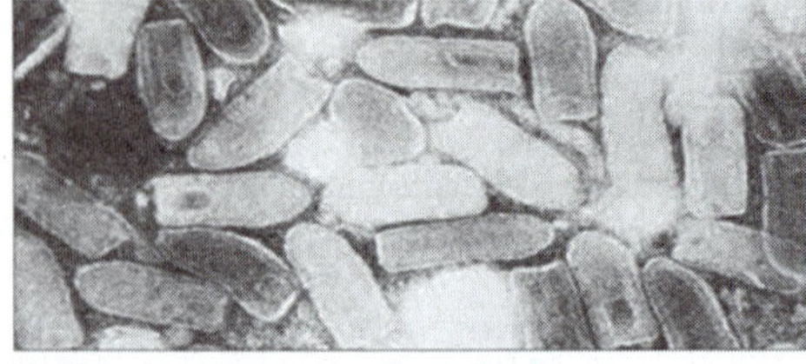

9) **Identify the virus shown in above image**
(a) Adeno virus (b) *Rotavirus* (c) Rabies virus (d) EBV

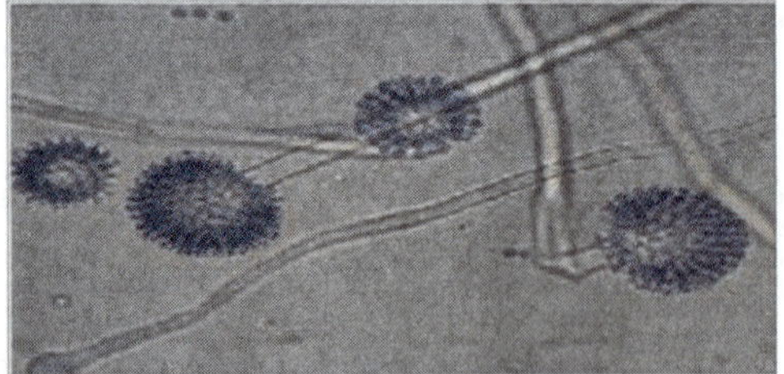

10) **A patient is having TB like clinical picture, and peripheral smear with lacto phenol cotton blue stain is showing above image. Diagnosis is**
(a) Mycoplasma (b) *Aspergillus* (c) *Cryptococcus* (d) *Candida*

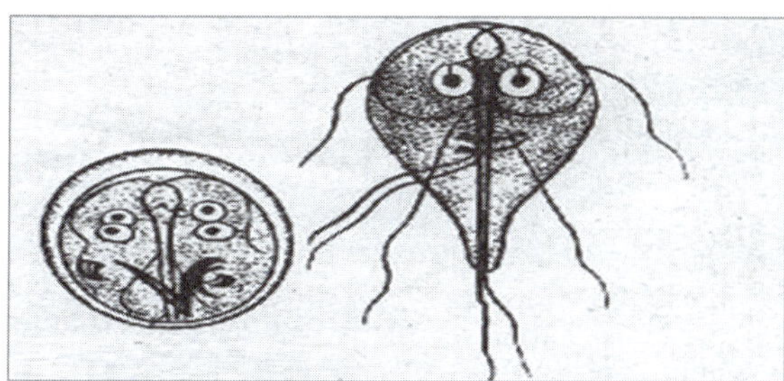

11) **An anxious mother brought her 4 year old daughter to the paediatrician. The girl was passing loose bulky stools for the past 20 days. This was often associated with pain in abdomen. The paediatrician ordered the stool examination, which showed the following organisms. Identify the organisms** (AI-03)
(a) *Entamoeba histolytica* (b) *Giardia lamblia* (c) *Cryptospiridium* (d) *E. coli*

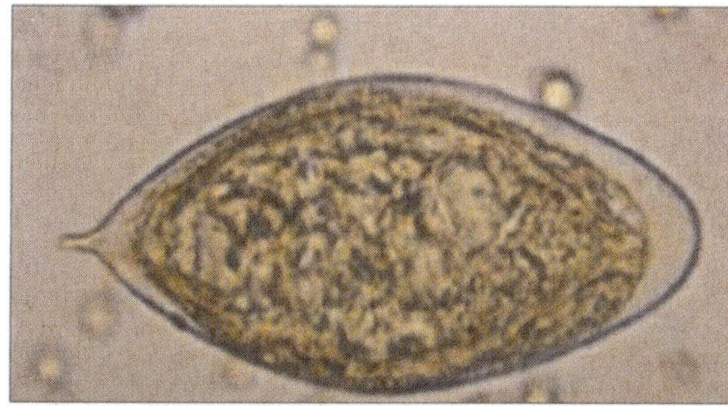

12) **The egg in above image belongs to**
(a) *Schistosoma japonicum* (b) *Schistosoma mansoni* (c) *Clonorchis sinensis* (d) *Schistosoma haematobium*

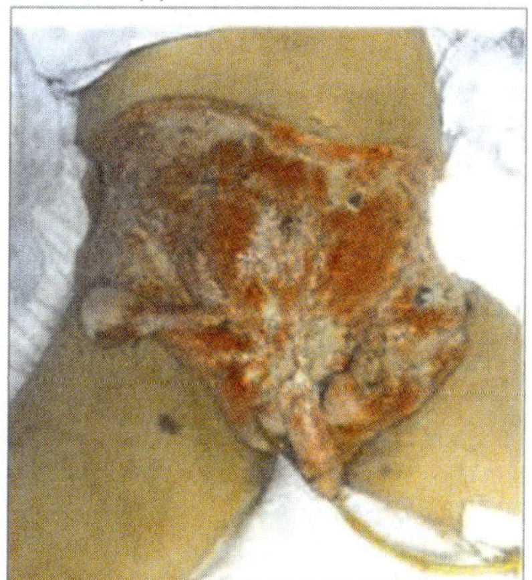

13) **Image shows the debridement of necrosed tissues in & around the external genitals. Most common clinical entity is**
(a) Fournier gangrene (b) Gas gangrene (c) Pyoderma (d) Mycetoma

Answers of MCQs & explanation

1) **(b)**
- Follow chapter, **introduction and history of Microbiology** for images of important scientists

2) **(d)**
- Follow chapter, **Physiology of bacteria** for explanation

3) **(d)**
- Follow chapter, **genetics of bacteria** for explanation

4) **(a)**
- Follow chapter, **Bio-Medical Waste (BMW) management** for explanation

5) **(a)**
- Follow chapter, **autoimmunity** for explanation

6) **(a) & (d)**
- Follow chapter, ***Clostridium* (sporing anaerobe)** for explanation

7) **(b)**
- Follow chapter, **Spirochetales** for explanation

8) **(c)**
- Given image showing bullet shape of virus indicating rabies virus
- Follow chapter, **Rhabdoviridae** for more explanation

9) **(c)**
- Given image is the owl's eye inclusion body produced by CMV
- Follow chapter, **Herpesviridae** for more explanation

10) **(b)**
- Image showing fungus with hyaline septate hyphae with exogenous conidia arranged in chain, suggestive of *Aspergillus*
- Follow chapter, **Deep mycoses** for explanation

11) **(b)**
- Follow chapter, **Intestinal, oral and genital flagellates** for explanation

12) **(d)**
- Egg in given image have terminal spine, so it is the egg of *Schistosoma haematobium*
- For morphology of egg of other option given in question: Follow chapters,
  - **Trematodes: Diecious trematodes**
  - **Trematodes: Monnoecious trematodes**

13) **(a)**
- Follow chapter, **systemic infections** for explanation

Abbreviations

+Ve: Positive
2ME: 2-mercaptoethanol
5-HT: 5-Hydroxy Tryptamine
A/t: According to
AAV: Adeno Associated Virus
Ab(s): Antibody (s)
ADCC: Antibody Dependent Cytotoxic Cells
ADS: Anti Diphtheria Serum
AFB: Acid Fast Bacilli
Ag(s): Antigen (s)
Ag-Ab reaction: Antigen-antibody reactions
AGN: Acute Glomerulo Nephritis
AGS: Anti Gas gangrene Serum
AIDS: Acquired Immuno Deficiency Disease
ALG: Anti-Lymphocyte Globulin
ALS: Anti Lymphocyte Serum
ALT: Alanine aminotransferase
AMA(s): Anti Microbial Agent(s)
AMB: Amphotericin B
AMC: Acetyl Methyl Carbinol
AMI: Antibody Mediated Immunity
APCs: Antigen-Presenting Cells
APSGN: Acute Post-Streptococcal Glomerulo Nephritis
APW: Alkaline Peptone Water
ARC: AIDS Related Complex
ARF: Acute rheumatic fever
ARF: Acute Rheumatic Fever
ART: Anti Retroviral Therapy
ASO test: Anti Streptolysin O test
ASV: Anti Snake Venom
ATG: Anti- Thymocyte Globulin
ATS: Anti Tetanus Serum
ATS: Anti-Thymocyte Serum
B/R(s): Biochemical Reaction (s)
b/w (B/W): Between
BAL: Broncho Alveolar Lavage
BB: Borderline
BCDF: B Cell Differentiation Factor
BCG: Bacillus Calmette Guerin
BCGF: B Cell Growth Factor
BCR(s): B-Cell Receptor(s)
BCYE agar: Buffered Charcoal Yeast Extract agar
BDBV: Bundibugyo virus
BEBOV: Bundibugyo ebolavirus
BFP: Biological False Positive
BFP: Biological False Positive
BHIA: Brain Heart Infusion Agar
BHIB: Brain Heart Infusion Broth
BL: Borderline Lepromatous
BMW: Bio Medical Waste
BP: Blood Pressure
BPL: Beta Propio Lactone
BSE: Bovine spongiform encephalopathy

BSL: Bio Safety Level
BT: Blood Transfusion
BT: Borderline tuberculoid
BUN: Blood Urea Nitogen
C/Cs: Cultural characteristics
C/Fs: Clinical features
C: Complement
CA MRSA: Community Acquired MRSA
C-activation: Complement activation
CAM: Chorio Allantoic Membrane
CAMP test: Christie Atkins Munch Peterson test
CBC: Complete Blood Count
CCHF: Crimean Congo Haemorrhagic Fever
CD: Cluster of Differentiation
CD: Cluster of Differention
CDC: Centres for Disease Control and Prevention
CFP-10: Culture Filtrate Protein -10
CFT: Complement Fixation Test
CFW stain: Calco Flour White stain
CGD: Chronic Granulomatous Disease
CIE: Counter Immuno Electrophoresis
CIEBOV" Côte d' Ivoire ebolavirus
CJD: Creutzfeldt Jacob Disease
CL crystals: Chacot-Leyden crystals
CLED medium: Cysteine Lactose Electrolyte Deficient medium
CMI: Cell Mediated Immunity
CMN group: *Corynebacteria Mycobacteria Nocardia* group
CMV: Cyto Megalo Virus
CNS: Central Nervous System
CoNS: Coagulase Negative *Staphylococcus*
CoPS: Coagulase Positive *Staphylococcus*
CR(s): Complement Receptor(s)
CRF: Coagulase Reacting Factor
CRP: C-Reactive Protein
CVS: Cardio Vascular System
D/D: Differential Diagnosis
DCA: Deoxy Cholate Citrate agar
DEC: Di Ethyl Carbamazine
DEET: N,N-diethyl-meta- toluamide
DGIM: Dark- Ground (field) Illumination Microscope
DHF: Dengue haemorrhagic fever
DIC: Disseminated Intravascular Coagulation
DM: Diabetes Mellitus
DP vaccine: Diphtheria & Pertusis vaccine
DPT vaccine: Diphtheria, Pertusis & Tetanus vaccine
ds: double stranded
DSS: Dengue shock syndrome
DT vaccine: Diphtheria & Tetanus vaccine
DTH: Delayed Type Hypersensitivity
e.g.: example gratia (for example)
EB: Elementary Body
EBV: Epstein-Barr Virus
EC: Exposure Code
EIA: Enzyme Immuno Assay
ELISA: Enzyme Linked Immuno Sorbent Assay
EM pathway: Embden –Mayerhof pathway
EM: Electron Microscope
ESAT-6: Early Secretory Antigen Target-6
ESBL: Extended Spectrum β-Lactamase
ET tube: Endo Tracheal tube

FITC: Fluorescein Iso Thio Cyanate
FM: Fluorescent Microscopes
FTA-ABS test: Fluorescent Treponema Antibody-ABSorption test
FTLV: Feline T-cell Lymphotropic Virus
G S L M: Glucose Sucrose Lactose Mannitol
GBS: Guillain Barre Syndrome
GC: Genital Chlamydiasis
G-CSF: Granulocyte-colony stimulating factor
GGMS stain: Grocott Gomori's Methenamine Silver stain
GI: Genital Infection
GIT: Gastro Intestinal Tract
GLC: Gas Liquid Chromatography
GM-CSF: Granulocyte macrophage -colony stimulating factor
GNB: Gram Negative Bacilli
GNC: Gram Negative Cocci
GPB: Gram Positive Bacilli
GPC: Gram Positive Cocci
GU: Gonococcal Urethritis
H & E stain: Haematoxylin & Eosin stain
H & E stain: Haematoxylin & Eosin stain
H/o: History of
HA MRSA: Hospital Acquired MRSA
HAI test: Haem Agglutination Inhibition test
HAV: Hepatitis A Virus
Hb: Haemoglobin
HBLV: Human B-cell Lymphotropic Virus
HBV: Hepatitis B Virus
HCAI(s): Health care associated infection(s)
HCC: Hepato Cellular Carcinoma
HCF(s): Health Care Facility/Facilities
HCG: Human Chorionic Gonadotropin
HCoV-EMC: Human Corona Virus-Erasmus Medical Centre
HCV: Hepatitis C Virus
HDN: Haemolytic Disease of New born
HDP: Hanging drop preparation
HDV: Hepatitis D Virus
HEV: Hepatitis E Virus
HFMD: Hand foot and mouth disease
HFV: Hepatitis F Virus
HGE: Human Granulocytic Ehrlichiosis
HGV: Hepatitis G Virus
HHV (1-8): Human Herpes Virus (1-8)
HI: Humoral Immunity
Hib: Haemophilus influenza type b
Hib: Haemophilus influenza type b
HIV: Human Immuno deficiency Virus
HLA: Human Leucocyte Antigen
HME: Human Monocytic Ehrlichiosis
HMW: High Molecules Weights
HPLC: High Performance Liquid Chromatography
HPV: Human Papilloma Virus
HPV: Human Papilloma Virus
hr: Hour
HSV-1: Herpes Simplex Virus-1
HSV-2: Herpes Simplex Virus -2
HTLV: Human T-cell Lymphotropic Virus
HTLV-I, II &III: Human T-cell Lymphotropic Virus-I, II &III
IARC: International Agency for Research on Cancer
IC: Inclusion Conjunctivitis
IC: Intracutaneous
ICC: Immuno Competent Cell
ICRC: Indian Cancer Research Centre
ICSOL: Intra Cranial Space Occupying Lesion
ICT: Immuno Chromatographic Test
ICT: Immuno Chromatographic Tests
ICTC: Integrated Counseling and Testing Centre
ID: Infecting Dose
ID: Intradermal
IDD: Immuno Deficiency Diseases
IET: Immuno Enzyme Test
IF: Immuno Fluorescent
IFA: Immuno Fluorescent Assay
IFN: Interferon
IFT: Immuno Ferritin Test
Ig (s): Immunoglobulin (s)
IGRA: Interferon Gamma Release Assay
IHA test: Indirect Haem Agglutination test
IM: Intra Muscular
IMN: Infectious mononucleosis
IN test: Indole Nitrate/Indoso Nitrate) test
IP: Incubation period
IPV: Injectable Polio Vaccine
Ir: Immune response
ITH: Immediate Type Hypersensitivity
IV catheters: Intra Venous catheter
IV: Intra Venous
JC virus: John Cunningham virus
JE: Japanese Encephalitis
JEV: Japanese encephalitis virus
KB method: Kopeloff's & Beerman's method
KFD: Kyasnur Forest Disease
KLB: Klebs- Loeffler Bacillus
KSHV: Kaposi's Sarcoma associated Herpes Virus
LAK: Lymphokine Activated Killer cells
LATS: Long Acting Thyroid Stimulator
LCB stain: Lacto Phenol cotton Blue stain
LCM virus: Lymphocytic Chorio Meninigitis virus
LCR: Ligase Chain Reaction
LD: Lethal Dose
LF: Lactose Fermenters
LGL: Large granular lymphocyte
LGV: Lympho Granuloma Venereum
LJ medium: Lowenstein Jensen medium
LL: Lepromatous Leprosy
LLF: Late Lactose Fermenters
LMW: Low Molecular Weight
LPA: Line Probe Assay
LPS: Lipopolysaccharide
LTRs: Long terminal repeat sequences
MAC: Mycobacterium Avium Complex
MAC-ELISA: IgM Antibody Capture Enzyme Linked Immuno Sorbent Assay
MAT: Microscopic Agglutination tests
MCH: Mean Corpuscular Haemoglobin
MCHC: Mean Corpuscular Haemoglobin Concentration
MCV: Mean Corpuscular Volume

MCV: Molluscum contagiosum virus
MDR: Multi Drug Resistance
MDR-TB: Multi Drug Resistance Tuberculosis
MERS-CoV: Middle-East Respiratory Syndrome-related coronavirus
MFS stain: Masson Fontana Silver stain
MHC: Major Histocompatibility Complex
MHC: Major Histocompatibility Complex
MID: Minimum Infecting Dose
MIO test: Motile Indole Ornithine test
MLD: Minimum Lethal Dose
MMR vaccine: Measles Mumps Rubella vaccine
MOHFW: Ministry of Health and Family Welfare
MOI: Multiplicity Of Infection
MRSA: Methicillin Resistance Staph Aureus
MTC: *Mycobacterium tuberculosis* complex
MW: Molecular Weight
NA: Nucleic Acid
NACO: National Aids Control Organisation (New Delhi)
NANB hepatitis: Non-A non-B hepatitis
NASBA: Nucleic Acid Sequence Base Amplification
NB: Nutrient Broth
NGOs: Non Government Organisation(s)
NGU: Non Gonococcal Urethritis
NIH: National Institute of Health
NIV: National Institute of Virology (Pune)
NK cells: Natural Killer cells
NLF: Non-Lactose Fermenters
ns: normal saline
OF test: Oxidation –Fermentation test
OMP: Outer Membrane Protein
OMP: Outer Membrane Protein
ONPG test: O-Nitro Phenyl- β-D-Galactosidase test
OPV: Oral Polio Vaccine
PAGE: Poly Acramide Gel Electrophoresis
PAIR: Puncture, Aspiration, Injection & Re aspiration
PAMPs: Pathogen Associated Molecular Patterns
PAMs: Pulmonary Alveolar Macrophages,
PAS stain: Periodic Acid Schiff stain
PCA: Passive cutaneous anaphylaxis
PCM: Phase-Contrast Microscope
PCP: Pnemo Cystis Pneumonia
PCR: Polymerase Chain Reaction
PCV: Packed Cell Volume
PDAB: Para Dimethyl Amino Bezadehyde
PEM: Protein Energy Malnutrition
PEP: Post-exposure prophylaxis
PFGE: Pulsed Field Gel Electrophoresis
PHC: Primary Health Centre
PHOL stain: Pal, Hasegawa, Ono & Lee stain
PIA: Pseudomonas Isolation Agar
PIMs: Potentially infectious materials
PJP: *P. jirovecii* pneumonia
PK reaction: Praunitz-Kustner reaction
PMNs: Poly Morphonuclear cells
Pn G: Penicillin G
Pn: Penicillin
PPA test: Phenyl Pyruvic Acid test
PPD: Purified Protein Derivative
PPE (s): Personal Protective Equipment (s)
PPI: Pulse Polio Immunisation
PPLO: Pleuro Pneumonia Like Organism
ppm = parts per million
PPNG: Penicillinase Producing *N. gonorrhoea*
PPTCT: Prevention of Parent To Child Transmission
PRAS: Pre Reduced Anaerobic System
PRNT: Plaque reduction neutralisation test
PRP: Polyribosyl Ribitol Phosphate
PRRs: Pattern Recognition Receptors
PT medium: Potassium Tellurite medium
PVC: Poly Vinyl Chloride
PW: Peptone Water
PYG agar: Peptone Yeast extract Glucose agar
PYR: L- pyrrolidonyl β-naphthylamide
RA: Rheumatoid Arthritis
RB: Reticulate Body
RBF: Rat bite fever
RCMM: Robertson's Cooked Meat Medium
RCMM: Robertson's Cooked Meat Medium
RE system: Reticulo-Endothelial system
REA: Restriction Endonuclease Analysis
RF: Rheumatoid Factor
RFLP: Restriction Fragment Length Polymorphism
RIA: Radio Immuno Assay
RNTCP: Revised National Tuberculosis Control Programme
RPR test: Rapid Plasma Reagin test
RSV: Respiratory Syncitial Virus
RSV: Respiratory Syncytial Virus
RTF: Resistance Transfer Factor
S/C: Sub Culture
SABE: Sub Acute Bacterial Endocarditis
SARS CoV: Severe Acute Respiratory Syndrome Coronoa Virus
SARS: Severe Acute Respiratory Syndrome
SARS-CoV: Severe Acute Respiratory Syndrome related coronavirus
SC: Status Code
SC: Sub Cutaneous
SCC: Squamous Cell Carcinoma
SDA: Sabouraud Dextrose Agar
SDA: Strand Displacement Amplification
SDS-PAGE: Sodium Dodycile Sulphate-Poly Acramide Gel Electrophoresis
SIM test: Sulphide Indole Motility test
SIV: Simian Immunodeficiency Virus
SLE: Systemic Lupus Erythematosus
SLT: Shiga Like Toxin
SLT: Shiga Like Toxin
Sp. / spp. : Species
SPA: Surface Protein Antigen
SPE: Streptococcal Pyrogenic Exotoxin
SPS: Sodium Polyanethol Sulphonate
ss: single stranded
SSPE: Subacute Sclerosing Pan Encephalitis
SSS: Specific Soluble Substance
SSSS: Staphylococcal Scalded Skin Syndrome
STSS: Streptococcal Toxic Shock Syndrome
SUDV or SEBOV: Sudan ebolavirus
SWG: Standard Wire Gauge
TAFV: Tai forest ebolavirus
TATA: Tumour Associated Transplant Antigen

Tc cells: T cytotoxic cells (Cytotoxic T cells)
TCBS agar: Thiosulphate Citrate Bile salt Sucrose agar
TCGF: T Cell Growth Factor
TCID: Tissue Culture Infective Dose
TCR(s): T-Cell Receptor(s)
TF: Transfer Factor
TF: Transfer Factor
Th cells: T helper cells (Helper T cells)
Th: T-helper (CD4+) cell
TIG: Tetanus Immuno Globulin
TIP: Translation Inhibiting Protein
TLRs: Toll-Like Receptors
TMA: Transcription Mediated Amplification
TNF: Tumour Necrosis Factor
TNF: Tumour Necrosis Factors
TPHA test: *T. pallidum* Haem-Agglutination test
TPI test: *Treponema pallidum* immobilisation test
TPPA test: *Treponema pallidum* particle agglutination test
TRIC: Trachoma Inclusion Conjunctivitis
TSI medium: Triple Sugar Iron Medium
TSS: Toxic Shock Syndrome
TSST: Toxic Shock Syndrome Toxin
TSTA: Tumour Specific Transplant Antigen
TT: Tetanus Toxoid
TT: Tuberculoid Type
US FDA: United State Food and Drug Administration
UV light: Ultra Violet light
UV rays: Ultraviolet rays
VDRL test: Venereal Disease Research Laboratory test
-Ve: Negative
VHF: Viral Haemorrhagic Fever
VISA: Vancomycin Intermediate Staph Aureus
VPF: Vascular Permeability Factor
VRE: Vancomycin Resistant *Enterococci*
VRSA: Vancomycin Resistant Staph Aureus
VZV: Varicella Zoster Virus
WB test: Western Blot test
WB: Western blot
WHO: World Health Organisation
XDR: Extended Drug Resistance
XDR-TB: Extended Drug Resistance Tuberculosis
XLD medium: Xylose Lysine Deoxycholate medium
ZEBOV: Zaire ebolavirus
ZN stain: Ziehl-Neelsen stain

1. Betty A. Forbes, Daniel F. Sahm, Alice S, Weiss feld. Belly & Scott's Diagnostic microbiology. 11th edition. 2002.
2. Mackie & Mc Cartney. Practical medical microbiology. 14th edition.
3. Elmer W Koneman, Stephen D Allen, William M Janda, Paul C Schreckenberger. Colour atlas and textbook of Diagnostic microbiology. 5th edition.
4. R Ananthnarayan, CK paniker, Arti Kapil (Editor). Textbook of microbiology. 9th edition. 2013.
5. BS Nagoba, Asha Pichare. Medical microbiology, Premanual for undergraduate. 2nd edition. 2012.
6. Monica Cheesbrough. District Laboratory Practice in Tropical Countries. Part-1. Cambridge Low –Price edition-1999. Reprinted 2002.
7. Surinder Kumar. Textbook of microbiology. 1st edition. 2012.
8. P Chakraborty. A textbook of microbiology. 3rd edition. 2013.
9. Apurba SS, Sandhya BK. Essential of Medical Microbiology. 1st edition. 2016.
10. Jagdish Chander. Textbook of mycology. 3rd edition. 2013 (Reprint)
11. KD Chatterjee. Parasitology (Protozoology and Helminthology). 13th edition. 2011 (Reprint).
12. Rajesh Karyakarte, Ajit Ddamle. Medical parasitology. 2003.
13. RL Ichhpujani, Rajesh Bhatia. Medical parasitology. 3rd edition. 2003 (Reprint).
14. P Chakraborty. A textbook of Medical parasitology. 2nd edition. 2005.
15. Manual on quality standard for HIV testing laboratories. National AIDS Control Organisation (NACO), Ministry of health & family welfare. March 2007.
16. Harsh Mohan. Textbook of Pathology. 7th edition. 2015.
17. Paul VK, Bagga A, Sinha A. Ghai Essential Pediatrics. 8th edition. 2014.
18. KD Tripathi. Essentials of medical Pharamacology. 7th edition. 2015 (Reprint).
19. DM Vasudev, Shreekumari S, Vaidyanathan K. Textbook of biochemistry for medical students. 8th edition. 2016.
20. K Park. Park's textbook of preventive and social medicine. 23rd edition. 2015.
21. Khurana AK. Comprehensive Ophthalmology. 6th edition. 2015
22. Infection prevention and control. An implementation handbook for public health facilities in Gujarat. 01(01) February 2017.
23. Arvind Arora. Self assessment and review of Mmicrobiology. 7th edition. 2014
24. Vinay Kamal. Textbook of Pathology. 1st edition. 2017
25. www.google.com

Index